T0295143

Genetic warning icon highlights drugs with genetic contraindications

Nursing considerations provide guidance throughout the nursing process

Life-threatening side effects are emphasized

Combinations heading identifies commonly used combination drugs

548   fexofenadine

- Give without regard to meals
- Store at room temperature; protect from moisture

SIDE EFFECTS
CNS: Insomnia, headache, dizziness
CV: Chest pain, angina, QT prolongation, peripheral edema
EENT: Xerophthalmia
GI: *Nausea, vomiting,* abdominal pain, constipation, dry mouth
GU: Dysuria, urinary retention, UTI
INTEG: Rash, angioedema
MISC: Peripheral edema, insomnia
MS: Back pain
RESP: Cough, URI
SYST: Infection

PHARMACOKINETICS
Peak 5 hr, duration up to 24 hr, rapidly absorbed, protein binding 60%, excreted in urine/feces, half-life 7 hr, metabolized by the liver (CYP2D6, CYP3A4 converted to active metabolite)

INTERACTIONS
Increase: action of fesoterodine—CYP3A4 inhibitors (antiretroviral protease inhibitors, macrolide antiinfectives, azole antifungals), avoid use with doses >4 mg
Increase: anticholinergic effect—antimuscarinics, anticholinergics
Increase: urinary frequency—diuretics
Drug/Herb
Decrease: fesoterodine—caffeine, green tea, guarana
Drug/Food
Increase: fesoteradine level—grapefruit juice
Decrease: festerodine level—cola, coffee, tea
Drug/Lab
Increase: ALT, GGT

NURSING CONSIDERATIONS
Assess:
- **Urinary patterns:** distention, nocturia, frequency, urgency, incontinence
- **Allergic reactions:** angioedema; swelling of face, tongue, throat may occur anytime during treatment; have emergency equipment nearby

- **Pregnancy/breastfeeding:** no well-controlled studies; use only if benefits outweigh fetal risk
Evaluate:
- **Therapeutic response:** absence of urinary frequency, urgency, incontinence, increase in bladder capacity
Teach patient/family:
- To avoid increased temperature, may decrease sweating
- Not to drive or operate machinery until response is known
- To avoid alcohol; drowsiness may occur
- To report immediately allergic reactions including rash; swelling of mouth, face, lips; trouble breathing
- Not to drink liquids before bedtime
- About the importance of bladder maintenance
- Not to use new medications, herbs without prescriber approval

---

fexofenadine (Rx, OTC)
(fex-oh-fi′na-deen)
Allegra Allergy Childrens, Allegra Allergy, Allegra Allergy 24-HR, Allergy Relief, Allergy Relief/Indoor/Outdoor
Func. class.: Antihistamine—2nd generation
Chem. class.: Piperidine, peripherally selective

Combinations: Allegra D

ACTION: Acts on blood vessels, GI, respiratory system by competing with histamine for H_1-receptor site; decreases allergic response by blocking pharmacologic effects of histamine, less sedating

USES: Rhinitis, allergy symptoms, chronic idiopathic urticaria

CONTRAINDICATIONS
Breastfeeding, newborn or premature infants, hypersensitivity
Precautions: Pregnancy, children, geriatric patients, respiratory disease,

♦ Canada only   Genetic warning

High Alert header highlights drugs that pose the greatest risk if administered improperly

Black Box Warnings identify serious and life-threatening adverse effects

Subheads indicate specific administration for dosing and routes of administration

Controlled Substance Schedules appear in an easy-to-spot header

Easily confused drug names are located beneath the header

Common unlabeled uses and doses are clearly indicated

800 LORazepam
NURSING CONSIDERATIONS
Assess:
- **Allergy:** hives, rash, rhinitis; monitor respiratory status
- **Beers:** avoid in older men; may decrease urinary flow and cause urinary retention
- **Pregnancy/breastfeeding:** use only if clearly needed; cautious use in breastfeeding

Evaluate:
- **Therapeutic response:** absence of running or congested nose, other allergy symptoms

Teach patient/family:
- To avoid driving, other hazardous activities if drowsiness occurs
- To avoid use of other CNS depressants

⚠ **HIGH ALERT**

loratadine/
pseudoephedrine (OTC)
(lor-at'a-deen/soo-doe-e-fedrin)
Claritin-D, Claritin-D 24 hour
Func. class.: Alpha/beta agonist, decongestant, histamine H1 antagonist

USES: Temporary relief of sinus and nasal congestion, runny nose; sneezing; itching of nose or throat and itchy, watery eyes due to common cold, hay fever (allergic rhinitis), or other upper respiratory allergies or sinusitis

CONTRAINDICATIONS
Hypersensitivity to loratadine, pseudoephedrine, or any component; within 14 days of MAOI therapy; severe hypertension, coronary heart disease

DOSAGE AND ROUTES
Adult/child ≥12 yr PO: loratadine 5 mg/pseudoephedrine 120 mg per tablet: 1 tablet q12hr (max: 2 tablets/day); loratadine 10 mg/pseudoephedrine 240 mg per tablet: 1 tablet daily (max: 1 tablet/day)
Available forms: Tabs ext rel 5/120, 10/240 mg

♣ Canada only

⚠ **HIGH ALERT**

LORazepam (Rx)
(lor-a'ze-pam)
Ativan
Func. class.: Sedative/hypnotic; antianxiety
Chem. class.: Benzodiazepine, short acting

Controlled Substance
Schedule IV

Do not confuse:
LORazepam/ALPRAZolam/clonazePAM

ACTION: Potentiates the actions of GABA, especially in the limbic system and the reticular formation

USES: Anxiety, irritability with psychiatric or organic disorders, preoperatively; insomnia; adjunct for endoscopic procedures, status epilepticus, insomnia
Unlabeled uses: Antiemetic before chemotherapy, rectal use, alcohol withdrawal, seizure prophylaxis, agitation, insomnia, sedation maintenance

CONTRAINDICATIONS
Pregnancy, breastfeeding, hypersensitivity to benzodiazepines, benzyl alcohol; closed-angle glaucoma, psychosis, history of drug abuse, COPD, sleep apnea
Precautions: Children <12 yr, geriatric patients, debilitated patients, renal/hepatic disease, addiction, suicidal ideation, abrupt discontinuation

Black Box Warning: Coadministration with other CNS depressants, abrupt discontinuation, substance abuse

DOSAGE AND ROUTES
Anxiety
- **Adult/adolescent ≥12 yr: PO** 2-3 mg/day in divided doses, max 10 mg/day
- **Geriatric: PO** 1-2 mg/day in divided doses or 0.5-1 mg at bedtime
- **Child <11 yr (unlabeled): PO** 0.025-0.05 mg/kg/dose (max q4hr)

Nbw Genetic warning

Mosby's®

2025

NURSING
DRUG
REFERENCE

Mosby's®
2025
NURSING DRUG REFERENCE

38TH EDITION

LINDA SKIDMORE-ROTH, RN, MSN, NP
Consultant
Colorado and Oklahoma

ELSEVIER

Elsevier
3251 Riverport Lane
St. Louis, Missouri 63043

MOSBY'S® 2025 NURSING DRUG REFERENCE,   ISBN: 978-0-443-12200-2
THIRTY-EIGHTH EDITION   ISSN: 1044-8470

Notices

Practitioners and researchers must always rely on their own experience and knowledge in evaluating and using any information, methods, compounds or experiments described herein. Because of rapid advances in the medical sciences, in particular, independent verification of diagnoses and drug dosages should be made. To the fullest extent of the law, no responsibility is assumed by Elsevier, authors, editors or contributors for any injury and/or damage to persons or property as a matter of products liability, negligence or otherwise, or from any use or operation of any methods, products, instructions, or ideas contained in the material herein.

Previous editions copyrighted 2024, 2023, 2022, 2021, 2020, 2019.
International Standard Book Number: 978-0-443-12200-2

Executive Content Strategist: Sonya Seigafuse
Content Development Manager: Danielle Frazier
Senior Content Development Specialist: Sarah Vora
Publishing Services Manager: Julie Eddy
Senior Project Manager: Jodi M. Willard
Design Direction: Margaret Reid

Printed in Canada

Last digit is the print number: 9   8   7   6   5   4   3   2   1

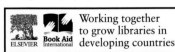

Consultants

**Sameeya Ahmed-Winston,
CPNP-PC, CPHON, BMTCN**
Nurse Practitioner—Team Lead
Children's National Hospital
Washington, DC

Meera K. Brown, PharmD, MBA
Senior Manager
CVS Health
Austin, Texas

**Janet S. Chance-Hetzler, DNP,
MSN, APRN, ACNS-BC,
AOCNS, CNE**
Assistant Professor of Nursing
Stephens College
Columbia, Missouri

Charla K. Hollin, RN, BSN
Allied Health Division Chair
University of Arkansas Rich Mountain
Mena, Arkansas

**Kathleen S. Jordan, DNP, MS,
FNP-BC, ENP-BC, ENP-C,
SANE-P, FAEN, FAANP**
Clinical Associate Professor
School of Nursing
The University of North Carolina–
Charlotte
Charlotte, North Carolina;
Nurse Practitioner
Mid-Atlantic Emergency Medical Associates
Phoenix, Arizona

**Brenda Knowles, MSN,
AGACNP-BC, FNP-C**
Nurse Practitioner
UT Erlanger Neurology
Chattanooga, Tennessee

Colleen D. Koob, DNP, RN, PNP
Dean
Beal University
Bangor, Maine

**Ludmila Kosmari, PhDc, APRN,
FNP-C**
Associate Professor
University of Texas at Arlington
Arlington, Texas

**Yvette Lowery, DNP, MSN/Ed,
FNP-c, CCRN, CEN, PCCN**
Nurse Practitioner
North Florida Regional Medical Center
Louisiana State University at Alexandria
Gainesville, Florida

**Nichole Miller, RN, MSN, DNP,
AGACNP, CCRN**
Chamberlain University
Burn Critical Care Associates
Augusta, Georgia

**Joy Susan Pendergrass, MSN,
MEd, APRN, FNP-BC**
Florida Department of Health
Nassau County, Florida
Fernandina Beach, Florida

Travis E. Sonnett, PharmD
EHRM Clinical Investigative Pharmacy
Specialist, PBM EHRM Support Team
VA Northwest Health Network (VISN 20)
PBM—Clinical Pharmacy Services
Spokane, Washington

**Daryle Wane, PhD, APRN,
FNP-BC**
BSN Program Director, Professor of
Nursing
Pasco-Hernando State College
New Port Richey, Florida

Increasingly, patients are relying on nurses to know every detail of health care. More important, nurses are expected to have these answers, especially when it comes to medication. Let *Mosby's 2025 Nursing Drug Reference* be your answer. Our indispensable, yet compact, resource contains hundreds of monographs with several easy-to-use features.

NEW FEATURES

This edition features:
- Over 50 new drugs . . . .included are monographs for:
  exagamglogene (Casgevy) for stem cell gene replacement therapy
  lovotibeglogene autotemcel (Lyfgenia) for stem cell gene replacement therapy
  momelotinib (Ojjaara) for intermediate or high-risk myelofibrosis
- An ebook with easy-to-use navigation for quick access to monographs of your choice

NEW FACTS

This edition features more than 2000 new drug facts, including:
- New drugs and dosage information
- Newly researched side effects and adverse reactions
- New and revised Black Box Warnings
- The latest precautions, interactions, and contraindications
- IV therapy updates
- Revised nursing considerations
- Updated patient/family teaching guidelines
- Updated BEERS information
- Additional combination products
- Content previously included in appendices has been moved to the monograph section for easier accessibility

ORGANIZATION

This reference is organized into two main sections:
- Individual drug monographs (in alphabetical order by generic name)
- Appendices (identified by the wide thumb tabs on the edge)
  The guiding principle behind this book is to provide fast, easy access to drug information and nursing considerations. Every detail—the paper, typeface, cover, binding, use of color, and appendices—has been carefully chosen with the user in mind.

INDIVIDUAL DRUG MONOGRAPHS

This book contains monographs for more than 1300 generic and 4500 trade medications. Common trade names are given for all drugs regularly used in the United States and Canada, with drugs available only in Canada identified by a maple leaf ♣.

The following information is provided, whenever possible, for safe, effective administration of each drug:

High-alert status: Identifies high-alert drugs with a label and icon. Visit the Institute for Safe Medication Practices (ISMP) at http://www.ismp.org for a list of medications and drug classes with the greatest potential for patient harm if they are used in error.

Tall man lettering: Uses the capitalization of distinguishing letters to avoid medication errors and is required by the FDA for drug manufacturers.

Pronunciation: Helps the nurse master complex generic names.

Rx/OTC: Identifies prescription or over-the-counter drugs.

Functional and chemical classifications: Allow the nurse to see similarities and dissimilarities among drugs in the same functional but different chemical classes.

Do not confuse: Presents drug names that might easily be confused within each appropriate monograph.

Action: Describes pharmacologic properties concisely.

Uses: List the conditions the drug is used to treat.

Unlabeled uses: Describe drug uses that may be encountered in practice but are not yet FDA approved.

Dosages and routes: List all available and approved dosages and routes for adult, pediatric, and geriatric patients.

Available forms: Include tablets, capsules, extended-release, injectables (IV, IM, SUBCUT), solutions, creams, ointments, lotions, gels, shampoos, elixirs, suspensions, suppositories, sprays, aerosols, and lozenges.

Side effects: Group these reactions by body system, with common side effects *italicized* and life-threatening reactions (those that are potentially fatal and/or permanently disabling) in red type for emphasis. *It is important to note that in some electronic versions of* Mosby's 2024 Nursing Drug Reference, *the red type may appear as* black, bold *print.*

Contraindications: List conditions under which the drug absolutely should not be given.

Precautions: List conditions that require special consideration when the drug is prescribed.

Black Box Warnings: Identify FDA warnings that highlight serious and life-threatening adverse effects.

Pharmacokinetics: Outline metabolism, distribution, and elimination.

Interactions: Include confirmed drug interactions, followed by the drug or nutrient causing that interaction, when applicable.

Drug/herb: Highlights potential interactions between herbal products and prescription or OTC drugs.

Drug/food: Identifies many common drug interactions with foods.

Drug/lab test: Identifies how the drug may affect lab test results.

Nursing considerations: Identify key nursing considerations for each step of the nursing process: Assess, Administer, Evaluate, and Teach Patient/Family. Instructions for giving drugs by various routes (e.g., PO, IM, IV) are included, with route subheadings in bold.

Compatibilities: List syringe, Y-site, additive compatibilities, and solution compatibilities if applicable and incompatibilities. If no compatibilities are listed for a drug, the necessary compatibility testing has not been done and that compatibility information is unknown. To ensure safety, assume that the drug may not be mixed with other drugs unless specifically stated.

Genetic icon ⚕: Highlights drugs with genetic contraindications.

Treatment of overdose: Provides drugs and treatment for overdoses where appropriate.

Combinations: Commonly used drug combinations are included in selected monographs.

APPENDICES

Selected New Drugs: Includes comprehensive information on over 40 key drugs approved by the FDA during the past 12 months.

Ophthalmic, Otic, Nasal, and Topical Products: Provides essential information for more than 80 ophthalmic, otic, nasal, and topical products commonly used today, grouped by chemical drug class.

Vaccines and Toxoids: Features an easy-to-use table with generic and trade names, uses, dosages and routes, and contraindications for over 40 key vaccines and toxoids.

Recently Approved Drugs: Highlights the most recently approved drugs for the market.

I am indebted to the nursing and pharmacology consultants who reviewed the manuscript and thank them for their criticism and encouragement. I would also like to thank Danielle Frazier and Sarah Vora, my editors, whose active encouragement and enthusiasm have made this book better than it might otherwise have been. I am likewise grateful to Jessica Meyer and Jodi Willard for the coordination of the production process and assistance with the development of the new edition. A special "thank you" to my son, Craig Roth, for completing the electronic files.

Linda Skidmore-Roth

Contents

INDIVIDUAL DRUG MONOGRAPHS, 1

APPENDICES, 1388

EVOLVE WEBSITE

- Additional Monographs
- Drug Categories

abacavir 1

⚠ HIGH ALERT

abacavir (Rx)

(ah-bak′ah-veer)

Ziagen

Func. class.: Antiretroviral
Chem. class.: Nucleoside reverse transcriptase inhibitor (NRTI)

Do not confuse:
abacavir/amprenavir

ACTION: Inhibitory action against HIV-1; inhibits replication of the virus by incorporating into cellular DNA by viral reverse transcriptase, thereby terminating the cellular DNA chain

USES: In combination with other antiretroviral agents for HIV-1 infection
Unlabeled uses: HIV prophylaxis following occupational exposure

CONTRAINDICATIONS

Black Box Warning: Hypersensitivity, moderate/severe hepatic disease, lactic acidosis

Precautions: Pregnancy, breastfeeding, children <3 mo, granulocyte count <1000/mm³ or HB <9.5 g/dL, severe renal disease, impaired hepatic function, HLA B5701+ (Black, White, Asian patients), abrupt discontinuation; Guillain-Barré syndrome, immune reconstitution syndrome, MI, obesity, polymyositis

DOSAGE AND ROUTES
• **Adult and adolescent ≥16 yr: PO** 300 mg bid or 600 mg/day with other antiretrovirals
• **Adolescent <16 yr and child ≥3 mo: PO** (oral solution) 8 mg/kg bid or 16 mg/kg daily, max 300 mg bid with other antiretrovirals; tablets 14-19 kg 150 mg bid or 300 mg daily; 20-24 kg 150 mg AM and 300 mg PM or 450 mg daily; ≥25 kg 300 mg bid or 600 mg daily
Hepatic dose
• **Adult: PO** (Child-Pugh A [5-6 points]) (oral solution) 200 mg bid; moderate to severe hepatic disease, do not use

HIV prophylaxis (unlabeled)
• **Adult: PO** 600 mg daily as an alternative
Available forms: Tablets 300 mg; oral solution 20 mg/mL
Administer:
• Give in combination with other antiretrovirals
• May give without regard to food q12hr around the clock
• Reduce dose in hepatic disease, use oral sol
• Storage at room temperature; protect from light; oral solution stored at room temperature; do not freeze

SIDE EFFECTS
CNS: *Fever, headache, malaise, insomnia, lethargy*
GI: *Nausea, vomiting, diarrhea, anorexia,* increase AST/ALT, hepatotoxicity, hepatomegaly with steatosis
INTEG: *Rash,* urticaria, hypersensitivity reactions
META: Lactic acidosis
OTHER: Fatal hypersensitivity reactions, MI, fat redistribution, immune reconstitution

PHARMACOKINETICS
Rapid/extensive absorption, distributed to extravascular space, then erythrocytes; 50% protein binding; extensively metabolized to inactive metabolites by the liver; half-life 1½ hr; excreted in urine, feces (unchanged); onset, peak, 1-1.5 hr, duration unknown

INTERACTIONS
• Do not coadminister with abacavir-containing products, ribavirin, interferon
Increase: possible lactic acidosis—ribavirin
Increase: abacavir levels—alcohol
Decrease: levels of methadone, may require higher dose of methadone
Drug/Lab Test
Increase: serum glucose, triglycerides, ALT, AST, amylase, CK

NURSING CONSIDERATIONS
Assess:
• Symptoms of HIV and possible infections; increased temperature baseline and throughout treatment

Side effects: *italics* = common; red = life-threatening

Black Box Warning: Lactic acidosis (elevated lactate levels, increased LFTs), severe hepatomegaly with steatosis, discontinue and do not restart; may have enlarged liver, elevated AST, ALT, lactate levels; women and the obese may be at greater risk; monitor serum lactate levels, LFTs, palpate liver for enlargement

Black Box Warning: Fatal hypersensitivity reactions: fever, rash, nausea, vomiting, fatigue, cough, dyspnea, diarrhea, abdominal discomfort; treatment should be discontinued and not restarted; those with ✹ HLA-B5701 are at great risk for hypersensitivity; obtain testing for HLA-B 5701 prior to starting treatment, register at the Abacavir Hypersensitivity Registry (800-270-0425)

• Renal studies: BUN; serum uric acid; CCr prior to, during therapy; these may be elevated

Black Box Warning: Hepatotoxicity: monitor hepatic studies prior to and monthly during therapy: bilirubin, AST, ALT, amylase, alkaline phosphatase, creatine phosphokinase, creatinine

• **Blood counts:** monitor viral load and CD4 counts during treatment; watch for decreasing granulocytes, HB; if low, therapy may have to be discontinued and restarted after recovery; blood transfusions may be required; perform hepatitis B virus (HBr) screening to confirm correct treatment
• **Resistance:** do not use triple antiretrovirals (abacavir, lamivudine, tenofovir) in treatment-naive persons
• **Immune reconstitution syndrome:** may occur anytime during treatment and is a response to CMV, *Mycobacterium avium* infection
• **Fat redistribution:** may occur anytime during treatment; buffalo hump, breast growth, moon face, facial wasting, trunk obesity

Evaluate:
• Therapeutic response: increased CD4 count, decreased viral load, decreased disease progression

Teach patient/family:
• That product is not a cure but will control symptoms; that patient is still infective, may pass HIV virus on to others, not to have sexual contact without condom, needles should not be shared, blood from infected individual should not come in contact with another's mucous membranes
• To carry emergency ID with condition, products taken; not to take other products that contain abacavir
• That body fat redistribution may occur; not to share product
• **Hypersensitivity:** to notify prescriber of sore throat, swollen lymph nodes, malaise, fever; other infections may occur; stop product and to notify prescriber immediately if skin rash, fever, cough, shortness of breath, GI symptoms occur; to advise all health care providers that allergic reaction has occurred with abacavir
• That follow-up visits must be continued because serious toxicity may occur; blood counts must be done
• To review and discuss points outlined on Medication Guide and Warning Card
• That other products may be necessary to prevent other infections and that drug is taken with other antiretrovirals
• Not to drink alcohol while taking this product
• To use exactly as prescribed, not to stop product or change dose, not to use with other products unless approved by prescriber
• **Pregnancy/breastfeeding:** to consider the use of contraception during treatment; identify if pregnancy is planned or suspected; use only if benefits outweigh risk; pregnant patients should enroll in Antiretroviral Pregnancy Registry at 800-258-4263; avoid breastfeeding

abatacept (Rx)

(ab-a-ta′sept)

Orencia, Orencia ClickJect

Func. class.: Antirheumatic agent (disease modifying)

Chem. class.: Immunomodulator

Do not confuse:
Orencia/Oracea

ACTION: A selective costimulation modulator; inhibits T lymphocytes, inhibits production of tumor necrosis factor (TNF-α), interferon-γ, interleukin-2, which are involved in immune and inflammatory reactions

USES: Polyarticular juvenile rheumatoid arthritis; moderate to severe rheumatoid arthritis; acute, chronic rheumatoid arthritis that has not responded to other disease-modifying agents; may use in combination with DMARDs; do not use with TNF antagonists (adalimumab, etanercept, inFLIXimab), anakinra

CONTRAINDICATIONS

Hypersensitivity

Precautions: Pregnancy, breastfeeding, children, geriatric patients, recurrent infections, COPD, TB, viral hepatitis, immunosuppression, neoplastic disease, respiratory infection

DOSAGE AND ROUTES

Rheumatoid arthritis/psoriatic arthritis

• **Adult:** SUBCUT 125 mg within 1 day after single IV loading dose, then 125 mg weekly; weekly SUBCUT dose may be initiated without an IV loading dose for those unable to receive an infusion

• **Adult >100 kg (220 lb):** IV INFUSION 1 g over 30 min, give at 2, 4 wk after first infusion, then q4wk

• **Adult 60-100 kg (132-220 lb):** IV INFUSION 750 mg over 30 min, give at 2, 4 wk after first infusion, then q4wk

• **Adult <60 kg (132 lb):** IV INFUSION 500 mg over 30 min, give at 2, 4 wk after first infusion, then q4wk

Juvenile rheumatoid arthritis (JRA)/ juvenile idiopathic arthritis (JIA)

• **Adolescent and child ≥6 yr and >100 kg:** IV INFUSION 1 g given over 30 min q2wk × 3 doses, then 1 g given over 30 min q4wk starting at wk 8

• **Adolescent and child ≥6 yr and 75-100 kg:** IV INFUSION 750 mg over 30 min q2wk × 2 doses, then 750 mg given over 30 min q4wk starting at wk 8

• **Adolescent and child ≥6 yr and <75 kg:** IV INFUSION 10 mg/kg given over 30 min q2wk × 3 doses, then 10 mg/kg q4wk starting at wk 8

Moderate/severe polyarticular juvenile idiopathic arthritis as monotherapy with or without methotrexate

• **Child/adolescent ≥2 yr and ≥50 kg:** SUBCUT 125 mg q1wk

• **Child/adolescent ≥2 yr and 25-50 kg:** SUBCUT 87.5 mg q1wk

• **Child/adolescent ≥2 yr and 10-25 kg:** SUBCUT 50 mg q1wk

Available forms: Lyophilized powder, single-use vials 250 mg; sol for SUBCUT injection 125 mg/mL

Administer:

• Storage in refrigerator; do not use expired vials, protect from light, do not freeze

Intermittent IV INFUSION route

• **To reconstitute,** use 10 mL sterile water for injection; insert syringe needle into vial and direct stream of sterile water for injection on the wall of vial; rotate vial until mixed; vent with needle (25 mg/mL); **further dilute** in 100 mL NS from a 100-mL infusion bag/bottle; withdraw the needed volume (2 vials remove 20 mL, 3 vials remove 30 mL, 4 vials remove 40 mL); slowly add the reconstituted solution from each vial into the infusion bag/bottle using the same disposable syringe supplied; mix gently; discard unused portions of vials; do not use if particulate is present or discolored; **give** over 30 min; use non–protein-binding filter (0.2-1.2 microns); protect from light

• Do not admix with other solutions or medications

SUBCUT route
- Use prefilled syringe for SUBCUT only (do not use for IV); allow to warm to room temperature (30-60 min); inject into fronts of thighs, outer area of upper arm, or abdomen except for 2-inch area around the navel; do not inject into tender, bruised area
- Rotate injection sites
- Use ClickJet for SUBCUT only; let warm for 30 min after removal from refrigerator, do not use if damaged or past expiration date

SIDE EFFECTS
CNS: Headache, asthenia, dizziness
CV: *Hypo/hypertension*
GI: Abdominal pain, dyspepsia, nausea, diarrhea, diverticulitis
GU: UTI, pyelonephritis
MS: Back pain
INTEG: Rash, *injection site reaction,* flushing, urticaria, pruritus
RESP: *Pharyngitis, cough, URI,* non-URI, *rhinitis,* wheezing
SYST: Anaphylaxis, malignancies, serious infections, antibody development

PHARMACOKINETICS
Half-life IV 13 days, SUBCUT 14.3 days, steady state 60 days; clearance increases with increased body weight

INTERACTIONS
- Do not give concurrently with live virus vaccines; immunizations should be brought up to date prior to treatment
- Do not use with TNF antagonists: adalimumab, etanercept, inFLIXimab; anakinra; infection may occur
- Avoid use with corticosteroids, immunosuppressives, atropine, scopolamine, halothane, nitrous oxide

NURSING CONSIDERATIONS
Assess:
- **RA:** pain, stiffness, ROM, swelling of joints during treatment baseline and periodically
- **HBV reactivation:** Screen patient at risk prior to starting treatment
- **TB:** for latent/active TB, viral hepatitis prior to beginning treatment

- For injection site pain, swelling
- Patient's overall health at each visit; product should not be given with active infections; parenteral product contains maltose, glucose monitoring must be done with glucose-specific testing
- **Infection:** sinusitis, UTI, influenza, bronchitis; serious infections have occurred; notify prescriber, therapy may need to be changed
- **Pregnancy/breastfeeding:** assess whether pregnancy is planned or suspected; if pregnant, register by calling 877-311-8972; use only if benefits outweigh fetal risk; do not breastfeed
Evaluate:
- Therapeutic response: decreased inflammation, pain in joints
Teach patient/family:
- That product must be continued for prescribed time to be effective, not to use with alcohol
- To use caution when driving; dizziness may occur
- Not to have live virus vaccinations while taking this product or use alcohol, TNF antagonists, other immunosuppressants; bring vaccinations up to date prior to use of this product
- About patient information included in packaging, including "do not shake"
- How to inject and rotate injection sites
- To immediately report signs of infection: temperature, flu like symptoms, urinary burning/stinging, sinusitis
- To avoid those with known infections
- That product contains maltrose and may lead to elevated glucose levels in some glucose testing methods
- To inform all prescribers that this product is being used

---

abemaciclib (Rx)
(a-beh′-muh-sy′-klib)
Verzenio
Func. class.: Antineoplastic
Chem. class.: Kinase inhibitors

Do not confuse:
abemaciclib/palbociclib/ribociclib

ACTION: It is an inhibitor of the cyclin-dependent kinases 4 and 6, a protein kinase inhibitor

USES: For the treatment of HR-positive, HER2-negative advanced or metastatic breast cancer with disease progression following endocrine therapy and prior chemotherapy, as monotherapy, or in combination with fulvestrant

CONTRAINDICATIONS
Hypersensitivity

Precautions: Breastfeeding, contraception requirements, hepatic disease, hepatotoxicity, infertility, neutropenia, pregnancy, pregnancy testing, reproductive risk, thromboembolic disease

DOSAGE AND ROUTES
HR-positive, HER2-negative advanced or metastatic breast cancer disease progression following endocrine therapy and prior chemotherapy, as monotherapy
• **Adult: PO** 200 mg bid until disease progression or unacceptable toxicity
HR-positive, HER2-negative advanced or metastatic breast cancer with disease progression following endocrine therapy, in combination with fulvestrant
• **Adult: PO** 150 mg bid with fulvestrant (500 mg **IM** as two 250-mg [5 mL] injections, 1 injection in each buttock, on days 1, 15, 29, and monthly thereafter) until disease progression or unacceptable toxicity. Pre- and perimenopausal women should also be treated with a gonadotropin-releasing hormone agonist
Therapeutic drug monitoring: dosage adjustments for treatment-related toxicities
Interrupt therapy per specific instructions. Restart as appropriate at the following reduced doses:
• **Starting dose:** Monotherapy, 200 mg bid; combination with fulvestrant, 150 mg bid
• **First occurrence:** Monotherapy, 150 mg bid; combination with fulvestrant, 100 mg bid

• **Second occurrence:** Monotherapy, 100 mg bid; combination with fulvestrant, 50 mg bid
• **Third occurrence:** Monotherapy, 50 mg bid; combination with fulvestrant, not applicable
Diarrhea
• **Grade 1:** Begin antidiarrheals, increase oral fluid intake. No change needed
• **Grade 2, first occurrence:** Begin antidiarrheals, increase oral fluid intake. If diarrhea does not resolve to grade ≤1 within 24 hr, hold until resolution. No change needed unless grade 2 diarrhea persists; upon resolution to grade ≤1, resume at next lower dose level
• **Grade 2, recurrent despite maximal supportive measures:** Begin antidiarrheals, increase oral fluid intake. When diarrhea resolves to grade ≤1, resume at next lower dose level
• **Grade 3 or 4, or requires hospitalization:** Begin antidiarrheals, increase oral fluid intake. When diarrhea resolves to grade ≤1, resume at next lower dose level
Hepatic dose
• **Adult: PO**
Child-Pugh A or B: no change; Child-Pugh C: reduce dosing to once per day; grade 1 (AST/ALT 1.1-3× the upper limit of normal [ULN]), without an increase in total bilirubin above 2× ULN: no change; grade 2, first occurrence (AST/ALT 3.1-5× ULN), without an increase in total bilirubin above 2× ULN: no change; if grade 2 persists, hold; after resolution to baseline or grade 1, resume at the next lower dose level; grade 2, recurrent (AST/ALT 3.1-5× ULN), without an increase in total bilirubin above 2× ULN: hold; after resolution to baseline or grade 1, resume at the next lower dose level; grade 2 or 3 (AST/ALT 3.1-20× ULN) with total bilirubin greater than 2× ULN, in the absence of cholestasis: discontinue; grade 4 (AST/ALT >20× ULN): discontinue
Available forms
Tablets 50, 100, 150, 200 mg
Administer
• With food at the same time every day
• Swallow tablets whole; do not chew, crush, or split. Do not take if broken, cracked

• If a dose is missed, do not replace missed dose; resume with the next scheduled daily dose

SIDE EFFECTS

GI: *Diarrhea, abdominal pain, anorexia, nausea, vomiting,* constipation, stomatitis, weight loss
CNS: Dizziness, drowsiness, *fatigue,* fever, headache
MS: Arthralgia
INTEG: Rash, alopecia
GU: Renal failure (rare)
HEMA: Anemia, leukemia, neutropenia, thrombocytopenia
MISC: Infection, dehydration, lung inflammation

PHARMACOKINETICS

Protein binding 96.3%; half-life 18.3 hr; fecal excretion 97.1%; metabolized in liver by CYP3A4

INTERACTIONS

Increase: abemaciclib effect—strong or moderate CYP3A4 inhibitors (itraconazole, ketoconazole); avoid concomitant use
Decrease: may decrease effect of vaccines: BCG (intravesical, live vaccines)
Decrease: abemaciclib effect—strong or moderate CYP3A4 inducers (rifampin); avoid concomitant use

NURSING CONSIDERATIONS

Assess:
• **Labs:** ANC, BMP, CBC with diff, LFTs, pregnancy testing (in those of child-bearing potential); HR+, HER2 negative status
• **Diarrhea:** at the first sign of loose stools, start antidiarrheal therapy, increase oral fluids
• **Neutropenia:** CBC baseline then q2wk for the first 2 mo, then monthly for the next 2 mo, and as needed
• **Venous thromboembolism:** monitor for signs, symptoms of thrombosis, pulmonary embolism; treat as needed
• **PE:** chest pain worse when breathing deeply or coughing, coughing up blood, dizziness, fainting, tachypnea, rapid heartbeat, irregular heartbeat, shortness of breath

• **Infection:** assess for UTI, lung infection, pharyngitis, conjunctivitis, sinusitis, vaginal infection, sepsis
• **Hepatotoxicity:** monitor LFTs baseline, then q2wk × 2 mo, monthly × next 2 mo, and then as needed; interruption in therapy or delay in treatment may be needed
• **Pregnancy/breastfeeding:** Avoid in females of reproductive potential during treatment and for at least 3 wk after last dose; can cause fetal harm or death; discontinue breastfeeding during treatment and for 3 wk after final dose. Presence in breast milk unknown. Obtain pregnancy test prior to treatment
Evaluate:
• Therapeutic outcome: decrease in size of cancerous tumor
Teach patient/family:
• **Infection:** to report the following to health care provider: increased temperature, fever, shaking, chills, cough, sore throat
• **Diarrhea:** to start antidiarrheal therapy at the first sign of loose stools, increase fluids, and notify health care provider
• **Bone marrow suppression:** Advise patient to report fatigue, fever, bruising, bleeding, blood in urine/feces
• **Thromboembolism:** to report immediately chest pain, worse when breathing deeply or coughing, coughing up blood, dizziness, fainting, tachypnea, rapid heartbeat, irregular heartbeat, shortness of breath, pain, swelling of the extremity with redness and warmth, discoloration including a bluish color
• **Pregnancy/breastfeeding:** not to use in pregnancy, breastfeeding; to use contraception during treatment and for at least 3 wk after last dose

---

⚠ HIGH ALERT

abiraterone (Rx)

(a'bir-a'ter-one)
Yonsa, Zytiga
Func. class.: Antineoplastic
Chem. class.: Androgen biosynthesis inhibitor

Do not confuse:
Zytige/Zyrtec

ACTION: Converted to abiraterone, which inhibits CYP17, the enzyme required for androgen biosynthesis; androgen-sensitive prostate cancer responds to treatment that decreases androgens

USES: Metastatic, castration-resistant prostate cancer in combination with predniSONE

CONTRAINDICATIONS

Pregnancy, women, children, breastfeeding, hypersensitivity

Precautions: Adrenal insufficiency, cardiac disease, MI, heart failure, hepatic disease, hypertension, hypokalemia, infection, surgery, ventricular dysrhythmia, stress, trauma, CYP3A4 inducers

DOSAGE AND ROUTES

• **Adult males: PO** (Zytiga) 1000 mg/day with predniSONE 5 mg bid and with GnRH (gonadotropin-releasing hormone analog) or bilateral orchiectomy; with strong CYP3A4 inducers 1000 mg bid; (Yonsa) 500 mg q day with methylprednisone 4 mg bid

Hepatic dose

• Adult males (Child-Pugh B, 7-9): PO 250 mg/day with predniSONE; permanently discontinue if AST/ALT >5 × the upper limit of normal (ULN) or total bilirubin >3 × ULN; Child-Pugh C >10, do not use

Available forms: (Zytiga) Tablets 250 mg; tabs (Yonsa) 125 mg

Administer:

PO route

• Yonsa: Give without regard to food
• Zytiga: Give whole on empty stomach 2 hr prior to or 1 hr after meals with full glass of water; do not crush, break, chew
• **Pregnancy:** women who are pregnant or who may become pregnant should not touch tablets without gloves
• Store tablets at room temperature

SIDE EFFECTS

CV: Angina, dysrhythmia exacerbation, atrial flutter/fibrillation/tachycardia, AV block, chest pain, edema, heart failure, MI, hypertension, QT prolongation, sinus tachycardia, supraventricular tachycardia, ventricular tachycardia

ENDO: Hot flashes, adrenocortical insufficiency

GI: Diarrhea, dyspepsia, hepatotoxicity

GU: Increased urinary frequency, nocturia, UTI

META: Adrenocortical insufficiency, hyperbilirubinemia, hypertriglyceridemia, hypokalemia, hypophosphatemia, *hypocalcemia*

MS: Arthralgia, myalgia, fracture

RESP: Cough, upper respiratory infection

SYST: Infection

PHARMACOKINETICS

Onset rapid, peak 2 hr, duration unknown; 99% protein binding, converted to abiraterone (active metabolite), half-life 7%-17% hr; excreted 88% (feces), 5% (urine); high-fat food increases effect, give on empty stomach; increased effect in hepatic disease

INTERACTIONS

Decrease: abiraterone effect—CYP3A4 inducers (carBAMazepine, phenytoin, rifAMPin, rifabutin, rifapentine, PHENobarbital); dose may need to be increased

Increase: action of CYP2D6/CYP2C8 substrates—dextromethorphan, thioridazine, pioglitazone; doses of these products should be reduced; avoid concurrent use if possible

Drug/Food

Increase: abiraterone action—must be taken on an empty stomach

Drug/Lab

Increase: ALT, AST, bilirubin, triglycerides, cholesterol, alkaline phosphatase

Decrease: potassium, phosphate, testosterone, lymphocytes

NURSING CONSIDERATIONS

Assess:

• **Prostate cancer:** monitor prostate-specific antigen (PSA), serum potassium, serum bilirubin baseline and periodically
• **Labs:** LFTs, BMP, serum potassium
• **Hepatotoxicity:** monitor liver function tests (AST/ALT) at baseline, every 2 wk for 3 mo, monthly thereafter in no known hepatic disease; interrupt treatment in patients without known hepatic disease at baseline who develop ALT/AST >5 × ULN

or total bilirubin >3 × ULN; patients with moderate hepatic disease at baseline, measure ALT, AST, bilirubin prior to the start of treatment, every week for 1 mo, every 2 wk for the following 2 mo, monthly thereafter; if elevations in ALT and/or AST >5 × ULN or total bilirubin >3 × ULN occur in patients with moderate hepatic impairment at baseline, discontinue and do NOT restart; obtain serum total bilirubin, AST/ALT if hepatotoxicity is suspected; elevations of AST, ALT, bilirubin from baseline provide more frequent monitoring

• Monitor B/P, pulse, edema, if hypertensive, control symptoms

• **Musculoskeletal pain, joint swelling, discomfort:** arthritis, arthralgia, joint swelling, and joint stiffness, some severe; muscle discomfort that includes muscle spasms, musculoskeletal pain, myalgia, musculoskeletal discomfort, and musculoskeletal stiffness may be relieved with analgesics

• Signs, symptoms of adrenocorticoid insufficiency (anorexia, nausea, vomiting, fatigue, weight loss); corticosteroids may need to be prescribed during stress, trauma, surgery; assess monthly for hypertension, hypokalemia, fluid retention

• **QT prolongation:** monitor ECG for QT prolongation, ejection fraction in patients with cardiac disease; small increases in the QTc interval such as <10 ms have occurred; monitor for arrhythmia exacerbation

Evaluate:

• Therapeutic response: Decreasing spread, progression of prostate cancer

Teach patient/family:

• **Pregnancy:** that women must not come into contact with tablets; to wear gloves if product needs to be handled; that males should wear condoms and use another form of contraception if partner is pregnant during use of product and for 1 wk after discontinuing treatment

• To report chest pain, swelling of joints, burning/pain when urinating, palpitations, yellow skin/eyes, light-colored stools, right upper quadrant pain

• Not to use with other medications, herbs without prescriber approval

• To take 2 hr prior to or 1 hr after meals; to swallow tablet whole, take with water (Zytiga); without regard to food (Yonsa)

• That this product, predniSONE, and a GnRH need to be used together

• Not to stop abruptly without prescriber consent

• That B/P, potassium, and possible fluid retention will be monitored at least monthly

• To immediately report jaundice of skin, eyes, clay-colored stools, dark urine; that lab work will be needed during at least first 3 mo

• To discuss all other products taken with all prescribers

• If dose is missed, skip and take next regularly scheduled dose

• Advise patient continuing labs, follow-up appointments will be needed

---

abrocitinib (Rx)

(a-broe-SYE-ti-nib)

Cibinqo

Func. class.: Antineoplastic/immunomodulating agent

Chem. class.: Janus-associated kinase (JAK) inhibitor

ACTION: Janus kinases are intracellular enzymes that transmit signals arising from cytokine interactions on the cellular membrane to influence cellular processes of immune cell function

USES: Refractory, moderate to severe atopic dermatitis in those not controlled with other therapies

CONTRAINDICATIONS

Hypersensitivity, antiplatelets (excluding low-dose aspirin)

Precautions: HIV/AIDS, breastfeeding, pregnancy, hepatitis, hepatitis exacerbation, cardiac/renal/pulmonary disease, infertility, immunosuppression, thrombocytopenia

---

Black Box Warning: Infection, stroke, thrombosis, MI, new primary malignancy

DOSAGES AND ROUTES
Adults: PO 100 mg once daily, if an adequate response is not achieved after 12 wk, may increase to 200 mg once daily
Adults who are poor CYP2C19 metabolizers: PO 50 mg once daily. If an adequate response is not achieved after 12 wk, may increase dose to 100 mg once daily
Available forms: Tablets 50, 100, 200 mg

SIDE EFFECTS
CNS: Headache, dizziness, fatigue
GI: Nausea, vomiting, upper abdominal pain, gastroenteritis
INTEG: Acne, impetigo, contact dermatitis, acne
EENT: Nasopharyngitis, herpes simplex
HEMA: Thrombocytopenia
GU: UTI
CV: Hypertension, MI
MISC: Increased CK, oropharyngeal pain, herpes zoster, influenzae

PHARMACOKINETICS
Half-life 3-5 hr, affected cytochrome P450 (CYP450) isoenzymes and drug transporters: CYP2C19, CYP2C9, CYP3A4, CYP2B6, P-glycoprotein (P-gp), organic anion transporter (OAT3), organic cation transporter (OCT1)

INTERACTIONS
Decreased abrocitinib effect: Strong inhibitors of CYP2C19: give 50 mg daily or 100 mg once daily for those patients who are not responding to 50 mg once daily
Increased bleeding: Moderate-strong inhibitors of both CYP2C19 and CYP2C9 or strong CYP2C19 or CYP2C9 inducers: Avoid concomitant use
Increased serious toxicity: P-gp substrates, monitor dosage of P-gp substrate

NURSING CONSIDERATIONS
Assess:
• **TB:** Obtain a TB before starting product, latent TB should be treated before starting this product

• Monitor CBC with differential, hemoglobin/hematocrit
• **Hepatitis:** Monitor hepatitis B serology, LFTs, plasma hepatitis C RNA baseline and periodically
• Monitor serum cholesterol profile, serum creatinine/BUN, skin cancer screening exam baseline and periodically
Evaluate:
• Therapeutic response: resolution of moderate-severe atopic dermatitis
Teach patient/family:
• Advise the patient to read the medication guide
• **Herpes zoster:** advise patients that is increased and may be serious
• **New primary cancer:** inform patients to check the skin often, as the risk of certain cancers, including skin cancers, may occur; to stay out of the sun or use protective clothing and sunscreen
• To report immediately and seek medical attention for signs/symptoms of MI, stroke, DVT, PE, retinal changes
• That vaccinations with live vaccines is not recommended during treatment, to bring vaccinations up to date before treatment
• Not to chew, crush, or split tablets
• To notify clinicians of treatment and all prescription, OTC drugs, and herbals
• **Infections:** inform patients that they may develop infections when taking abrocitinib. Instruct patients to tell their health care provider if they develop any signs or symptoms of an infection
• **Pregnancy/breastfeeding:** identify if pregnancy is planned or suspected, or if breastfeeding; advise patients to report pregnancy to 877-311-3770 and not to breastfeed; that this product may impair fertility

---

⚠ HIGH ALERT

acalabrutinib (Rx)
(a-Kal'a-broo-tin-ib)
Calquence
Func. class.: Antineoplastic
Chem. class.: Kinase inhibitor

Side effects: *italics* = common; red = life-threatening

ACTION: Second-generation kinase inhibitor, decreases proliferation of cancer cells

USES: For the treatment of mantle cell lymphoma (MCL) in patients who have received at least 1 prior therapy

CONTRAINDICATIONS
Hypersensitivity
Precautions: Serious infections, secondary malignancies, children, pregnancy, breastfeeding
Toxicity-related dosage changes
Refer to manufacturer's information
Available forms: Capsules 100 mg
Administer:
PO route
• Give whole; do not crush, chew, or break tablets
• Give without regard to food
• If dose is missed by >3 hr, skip and continue with regular schedule, do not take a double dose
• Store at room temperature

DOSAGE AND ROUTES
• **Adult: PO** 100 mg bid (approximately 12 hr apart) until disease progression
• **Hepatic dose:** Avoid use

SIDE EFFECTS
CNS: Headache, fatigue
EENT: Epistaxis
CV: Atrial fibrillation/flutter
GI: Anorexia, constipation, diarrhea, nausea, vomiting
HEMA: Thrombocytopenia, neutropenia, anemia
MS: Myalgia
RESP: Dyspnea, cough
INTEG: Rash
MISC: Infections, secondary malignancies

PHARMACOKINETICS
Onset rapid, peak 45 min, duration unknown, half-life 0.9 hr, active metabolite 6 hr, 97.5% protein binding

INTERACTIONS
Increase: Risk of bleeding: anticoagulants, antiplatelet, monitor for bleeding

Increase: Acalabrutinib level: CYP3A4 inhibitors (dilTIAZem, erythromycin, verapamil), avoid using together
Decrease: Acalabrutinib level: H2-receptor antagonists (raNITIdine), separate by 2 hr
Decrease: Acalabrutinib level: PPIs, avoid concurrent use
Decrease: Acalabrutinib level: Calcium antacids, separate by 2 hr
Decrease: Acalabrutinib level: CYP3A4 inducers, reduce dose, or avoid use

NURSING CONSIDERATIONS
Assess:
• For secondary malignancies (skin cancers)
• For atrial fibrillation/flutter
• For myelosuppression, obtain CBC monthly or more often
• For severe bleeding/hemorrhage, interruption for major surgeries may be needed
• For serious infection, fever, chills, flu-like symptoms, antibiotics may be needed
Teach patient/family:
• If dose is missed, give when remembered if less than 3 hr, if more than 3 hr, skip and take the next dose at the regularly scheduled time, do not double, to swallow whole with a whole glass of water
• To notify prescriber of severe bleeding (blood in stool or urine; prolonged or uncontrolled), that product may be interrupted for surgery (fever, chills, flulike symptoms), antibiotics may be needed
• That lab tests and follow-up exams will be needed
• Teach patient to notify prescriber of secondary malignancy (skin cancer), to use sunscreen, protective clothing. Avoid prolonged exposure to sunlight
• To report palpitations, lightheadedness, dizziness, fainting, shortness of breath, or chest discomfort
• Take at least 2 hours prior to taking cimetidine (Tagamet), famotidine (Pepcid, in Duexis), nizatidine (Axid), or ranitidine (Zantac)
• To report if pregnancy is planned or suspected, not to breastfeed during or for 2 wk following last dose

• To notify other clinicians of prescription OTC drugs and dietary or herbal supplements

acamprosate (Rx)

(a-kam-pro´sate)

Func. class.: Alcohol deterrent

Chem. class.: Synthetic amino acid neurotransmitter analog

ACTION: Not completely understood; in vitro data suggest it has affinity for type A and type B GABA receptors, lowers neuronal excitability, centrally mediated

USES: Alcohol abstinence management

CONTRAINDICATIONS

Hypersensitivity to this product or sulfites, CCr ≤30 mL/min

Precautions: Pregnancy, breastfeeding, infants, children, ethanol intoxication, renal impairment, depression, suicidal ideation, driving or operating machinery, geriatric patients

DOSAGE AND ROUTES

• **Adult: PO** 666 mg tid

Renal dosage

• **Adult: PO** CCr 30-50 mL/min 333 mg tid; CCr <30 mL/min do not use

Available forms: Delayed-release tablets 333 mg

Administer:

• Without regard to food; do not crush, chew, break delayed-release tablets

• Use only after alcohol is stopped

• Store at room temperature

SIDE EFFECTS

CNS: Anxiety, depression, dizziness, headache, insomnia, paresthesias, suicidal ideation, tremors, abnormal dreams, chills, drowsiness

CV: Palpitations, hypertension, peripheral edema

EENT: Rhinitis, pharyngitis, abnormal vision

GI: Anorexia, constipation, diarrhea, dry mouth, abdominal pain, flatulence, nausea, vomiting, taste change, weight gain

GU: Impotence

INTEG: Rash, pruritus, increased sweating

MISC: Infection, flulike symptoms

MS: Back pain, myalgias, arthralgia

RESP: Dyspnea, bronchitis

PHARMACOKINETICS

Onset unknown, peak 3-8 hr, duration unknown, half-life 20-33 hr

INTERACTIONS

Drug/Lab

Increase: LFTs, blood glucose, bilirubin, uric acid

Decrease: HB/Hct, platelets

NURSING CONSIDERATIONS

Assess:

• **Mental status:** depression, abnormal dreams, suicidal thoughts/behaviors, length of alcohol use, date of discontinuing alcohol use

• B/P baseline and periodically

• **Pregnancy/breastfeeding:** use only if benefits outweigh fetal risk; cautious use in breastfeeding, excretion unknown

Evaluate:

• Therapeutic response: continued alcohol abstinence

Teach patient/family:

• To notify prescriber of depression, abnormal thoughts, suicidal thoughts/behaviors

• To take without regard to food; not to break, crush, chew delayed-release tablets

• Not to engage in hazardous activities until effect is known; may impair thinking; monitor skills

• Not to use alcohol, to continue treatment for alcohol addiction

• **Pregnancy/breastfeeding:** to notify prescriber if pregnancy is planned or suspected; to use effective contraception; breastfeeding effects are unknown

---

⚠ HIGH ALERT

acarbose (Rx)

(ay-car´bose)

Glucobay ✦, Prandase ✦, Precose

Func. class.: Oral antidiabetic

USES: Type 2 diabetes mellitus, alone or in combination with a sulfonylurea, metformin, insulin

CONTRAINDICATIONS
Breastfeeding, hypersensitivity, diabetic ketoacidosis, cirrhosis, inflammatory bowel disease, ileus, colonic ulceration, partial intestinal obstruction, chronic intestinal disease, serum creatinine >2 mg/dL, CCr <25 mL/min

DOSAGE AND ROUTES
• **Adult:** PO 25 mg tid initially, with 1st bite of meal; maintenance dose may be increased to 50-100 mg tid; dosage adjustment at 4- to 8-wk intervals, individualized

---

acetaminophen (Rx, OTC) (Paracetamol)
(a-seat-a-mee′noe-fen)
222AF ✤, Abenol ✤, Acephen, Acephen Infant Feverall, ACET ✤, Acetab ✤, Apacet, APAP, Apra, Atasol ✤, Children's FeverAll, Fortolin ✤, Genapap, Infantaire, Mapap, NeoPAP, Novo-Gesic ✤, Pediaphen ✤, Pediatrix ✤, Q-Pap, Q-Pap Children's, Rapid Action Relief ✤, Redutemp, Ridenol, Robigesic ✤, Rounox ✤, Silapap, Taminol ✤, Tempra ✤, T-Painol, Tylenol, ✤ XS pain reliever

acetaminophen (IV) (Rx) Ofirmive
Func. class.: Nonopioid analgesic, antipyretic
Chem. class.: Nonsalicylate, paraaminophenol derivative

Combinations: With Codeine: Tablet 300 mg/15 mg, 300 mg/30 mg, 300 mg/60 mg; **With hydrocodone: Tablet:** 300 mg/5 mg, 300 mg/7.5 mg, 300 mg/10 mg; **Elixir:** 300 mg/10 mg/15 mL

Do not confuse:
acetaminophen/acetazolamide/Anacin
Aspirin Free/Anacin 3/Tylenol/Tylenol PM

ACTION: Activates descending serotonergic inhibitory pathway in CNS; antipyretic action results from (hypothalamic heat-regulating center)

USES: Mild to moderate pain or fever, arthralgia, dental pain, dysmenorrhea, headache, myalgia, osteoarthritis
Unlabeled uses: Migraine

CONTRAINDICATIONS
Hypersensitivity to this product, phenacetin aspartame, saccharin, tartrazine
Precautions: Pregnancy, breastfeeding, geriatric patients, anemia, renal/hepatic disease, chronic alcoholism, chronic malnutrition, hypovolemia (IV), G6PD deficiency

> **Black Box Warning:** Hepatotoxicity; IV (acute liver failure)

DOSAGE AND ROUTES
• **Adult/child >12 yr: PO/RECT** 325-650 mg q4-6hr prn, max 4 g/day; **weight ≥50 kg IV** 1000 mg q6hr or 650 mg q4hr prn, max single dose 1000 mg, min dosing interval 4 hr; **weight <50 kg IV** 15 mg/kg/dose q6hr or 12.5 mg/kg/dose q4hr, max single dose 15 mg/kg, min dosing interval 4 hr, max 75 mg/kg/day from all sources; **EXTENDED RELEASE** 650-1300 mg q8hr as needed, max 4 g/day
• **Child ≥2 yr and <50 kg: IV** 15 mg/kg/dose q6hr or 12.5 mg/kg/dose q4hr, max single dose 15 mg/kg, min dosing interval 4 hr, max 75 mg/kg/day from all sources
Renal dose
• **Adult: IV** CCr <30 mL/min reduce dose and prolong interval, CCr <10 mL/min **PO/RECT/IV** minimum interval of q8hr
Hepatic dose
• Adult: Mild to moderate: max 2000 mg/day; severe liver damage: contraindicated
Migraine (unlabeled)
• **Adult and adolescent: PO/RECT** 500-1000 mg, max 1 g/dose or max 4 g/day

---

Available forms: Rectal suppository 120, 325, 650 mg; soft chew tablets 80, 160 mg; capsules 500 mg; elixir 120, 160, 325 mg/5 mL; oral disintegrating tablets 80, 160 mg; oral drops 80 mg/0.8 mL, liquid 500 mg/5 mL, 160/5 mL, 1000/30 mL; extended release 650 mg, 80 mg/mL; tablets 325, 500, 650 mg; solution for injection 1000 mg/100 mL

Administer:

PO route

• Do not confuse 2 × 325 (650 mg) with 650-mg extended-release tablets

• Crushed or whole, do not crush extended-release product; chewable tablets may be chewed; give with full glass of water

• With food or milk to decrease gastric symptoms if needed

• Suspension after shaken well; check elixir, liquid, suspension concentration carefully; suspension and capsules are bioequivalent

Rectal route

• Store suppositories <80° F (27° C)

Intermittent IV INFUSION route

• No further dilution needed; do not add other medications to vial or infusion device

• For doses equal to single vial, a vented IV set may be used to deliver directly from vial; for doses less than a single vial, withdraw dose and place in an empty sterile syringe, plastic IV container, or glass bottle; infuse over 15 min

• Discard unused portion; if seal is broken, vial penetrated, or drug transferred to another container, give within 6 hr

Y-site compatibilities: Do not admix

SIDE EFFECTS

CNS: Agitation (child) (IV); headache, fatigue, anxiety (IV)

RESP: Dyspnea (IV), atelectasis (child) (IV)

CV: Hyper- and hypotension (IV)

GI: Nausea, vomiting, abdominal pain; hepatotoxicity, hepatic seizure (overdose), GI bleeding

GU: Renal failure (high, prolonged doses)

HEMA: Leukopenia, neutropenia, hemolytic anemia (long-term use), thrombocytopenia, pancytopenia

INTEG: Rash, urticaria, injection site pain

SYST: Stevens-Johnson syndrome, toxic epidermal necrolysis

TOXICITY: Cyanosis, anemia, neutropenia, jaundice, pancytopenia, CNS stimulation, delirium followed by vascular collapse, seizures, coma, death

PHARMACOKINETICS

85%-90% metabolized by liver, excreted by kidneys; metabolites may be toxic if overdose occurs; widely distributed; crosses placenta in low concentrations; excreted in breast milk; half-life 1-4 hr, protein binding 20%-50%

PO: Onset 10-30 min, peak ½-2 hr, duration 4-6 hr, well absorbed

IV: Onset rapid, peak 30-120 min, duration 3-4 hr

RECT: Onset slow, peak 1-2 hr, duration 4-6 hr, absorption varies

INTERACTIONS

Increase: renal adverse reactions—NSAIDs, salicylates; consider lower dose

Increase: methemoglobinemia—nitric oxide, prilocaine; avoid concurrent use

Increase: hypoprothrombinemia—warfarin, long-term use, high doses of acetaminophen

Increase: hepatotoxicity—barbiturates, alcohol, carBAMazepine, hydantoins, rifAMPin, rifabutin, isoniazid, diflunisal, zidovudine, lamoTRIgine, imatinib, dasatinib, mipomersen; monitor for hepatotoxicity

Decrease: absorption—colestipol, cholestyramine

Decrease: zidovudine, lamoTRIgine effect

Drug/Food

Food: decreased absorption

Drug/Herb

Increase: hepatotoxicity—St. John's wort, due to acetaminophen metabolism

Drug/Lab Test

Increase: LFTs, potassium, bilirubin, LDH, prothrombin time

Decrease: HB/Hct, WBC, RBC, platelets; albumin, magnesium, phosphate (pediatrics)

NURSING CONSIDERATIONS

Assess:

• **For fever and pain:** Type of pain, location, intensity, duration, aggravating/alleviating factors; assess for diaphoresis, fever baseline and periodically

• **Hepatic studies:** AST, ALT, bilirubin, creatinine before therapy if long-term therapy is anticipated; may cause hepatic toxicity at doses >4 g/day with chronic use

• **Renal studies:** BUN, urine creatinine, occult blood, albumin, if patient is on long-term therapy; presence of blood or albumin indicates nephritis, I&O ratio; decreasing output may indicate renal failure (long-term therapy)

• **Blood studies:** CBC, PT if patient is on long-term therapy

• **Chronic poisoning:** rapid, weak pulse; dyspnea; cold, clammy extremities; report immediately to prescriber

Black Box Warning: **Hepatotoxicity:** occurs with high doses (>4 g/day); dark urine; clay-colored stools; yellowing of skin, sclera; itching; abdominal pain; fever; diarrhea if patient is on long-term therapy; may require liver transplant, those malnourished or using alcohol chronically are at higher chance of hepatotoxicity; consult poison control with suspected acute toxicity, draw 4-hr serum level and administration of acetylcysteine based on the 4-hr level on the Rumack-Matthew nomogram

• **Potentially fatal hypersensitivity, allergic reactions:** rash, urticaria; if these occur, product may have to be discontinued
• Stevens-Johnson syndrome, toxic epidermal necrolysis may occur when beginning treatment or any other dose
• **Pregnancy/breastfeeding:** cautious use in pregnancy, breastfeeding (PO), use only if clearly needed (IV)
Evaluate:
• Therapeutic response: absence of pain using pain scoring; absence of fever
Teach patient/family:

Black Box Warning: **Hepatotoxicity:** not to exceed recommended dosage; the elixir, liquid, suspension come in sev-

eral concentrations, read label carefully; acute poisoning with liver damage may result; tell parents of children to check products carefully; that acute toxicity includes nausea, vomiting, abdominal pain; prescriber should be notified immediately; that toxicity may occur with other combination products

• Not to use with excessive alcohol, herbals, OTC products without approval of prescriber
• **To recognize signs of chronic overdose:** bleeding, bruising, malaise, fever, sore throat
• That those with diabetes may notice blood glucose monitoring changes
• To notify prescriber of pain or fever lasting more than 3 days
• Not to be used in patients <2 yr unless approved by prescriber
• **Hypersensitivity:** to stop product, call prescriber if rash occurs
• **Pregnancy/breastfeeding:** May be used when breastfeeding, short-term

TREATMENT OF OVERDOSE: Product level, gastric lavage; administer oral acetylcysteine to prevent hepatic damage *(see acetylcysteine monograph)*; monitor for bleeding

---

acetaZOLAMIDE (Rx)

(a-set-a-zole´a-mide)
Diamox ✦
Func. class.: Diuretic, carbonic anhydrase inhibitor, antiglaucoma agent, antiepileptic
Chem. class.: Sulfonamide derivative

USES: Open-angle glaucoma, angle-closure glaucoma (preoperatively, if surgery delayed), mixed, tonic-clonic, myoclonic, refractory seizures, epilepsy (petit mal, grand mal, absence), edema in HF, product-induced edema, acute altitude sickness

CONTRAINDICATIONS

Hypersensitivity to sulfonamides, severe renal/hepatic disease, electrolyte imbalances (hyponatremia, hypokalemia), hyperchloremic acidosis, Addison's disease, long-term use for closed-angle glaucoma, adrenocortical insufficiency, metabolic acidosis, acidemia, anuria

DOSAGE AND ROUTES

Angle-closure glaucoma
• **Adult: PO/IV** 250 mg q4hr or 250 mg bid for short-term therapy

Chronic open-angle glaucoma
• **Adult: PO/IV** 250 mg 1-4 times per day or 500 mg EXTENDED RELEASE bid, max 1 g/day
• **Child (unlabeled): PO** 8-30 mg/kg/day in divided doses tid or qid, or 300-900 mg/m^2/day, max 1 g/day; **IV** 5-10 mg q6hr, max 1 g/day

Edema in heart failure, drug-induced edema
• **Adult: PO/IV** 250-375 mg/day
• **Child (unlabeled): PO/IV** 5 mg/kg/day or 150 mg/m^2 in AM

Adjunct for epilepsy and myoclonic, refractory, generalized tonic-clonic, absence or mixed seizures
• **Adult: PO/IV** 8-30 mg/kg/day in 1-4 divided doses, usual range 375-1000 mg/day; **EXTENDED RELEASE** not recommended with seizures

Altitude sickness
• **Adult: PO** 250 mg twice daily starting the day before ascent and continuing for 2 to 3 days after reaching the target altitude or until descent is initiated

Renal dose
• **Adult: PO/IV** CCr 50-80 mL/min give dose ≥q6hr regular release or IV; CCr 10-50 mL/min give dose q12hr; CCr <10 mL/min, avoid use

acetylcholine ophthalmic
See Appendix B

acetylcysteine (Rx)
(a-se-teel-sis'tay-een)

Acetadote, Mucomyst ✤, Parvolex ✤

Func. class.: Mucolytic; antidote—acetaminophen

Chem. class.: Amino acid L-cysteine

Do not confuse:
acetylcysteine/acetylcholine

ACTION: Decreases viscosity of secretions by breaking disulfide links of mucoproteins; serves as a substrate in place of glutathione, which is necessary to inactivate toxic metabolites with acetaminophen overdose

USES: Acetaminophen toxicity; bronchitis; cystic fibrosis; COPD; atelectasis

CONTRAINDICATIONS
Hypersensitivity

Precautions: Pregnancy, breastfeeding, hypothyroidism, Addison's disease, CNS depression, brain tumor, asthma, renal/hepatic disease, COPD, psychosis, alcoholism, seizure disorders, bronchospasms, anaphylactoid reactions, fluid restriction, weight <40 kg, increased intracranial pressure, status asthmaticus

DOSAGE AND ROUTES
Acetaminophen toxicity
• **Adult and child: ≥41-100 kg IV** loading dose 150 mg/kg over 60 min (dilution 150 mg/kg in 200 mL of D$_5$W); then 50 mg/kg over 4 hr (dilution 50 mg/kg in 500 mL D$_5$W); then 100 mg/kg over 16 hr (dilution 100 mg/kg in 1000 D$_5$W)
• **Adult/child 21-40 kg: IV** 150 mg/kg in 100 mL diluent over 1 hr, then 50 mg/kg in 250 mL over 4 hr, then 100 mg/kg in 500 mg over 16 hr
• **Infant/child 5-20 kg: IV** 150 mg/kg in 3 mL/kg diluent over 1 hr, then 50 mg/kg in 7 mL/kg diluent over 4 hr, then 100 mg/kg in 14 mL/kg diluent over 16 hr

Bronchopulmonary disease (mucolytic)

• Give bronchodialators 15 min before acetylsteine

• **Adult and child 1-12 yr: INSTILL** 1-2 mL (10%-20% solution) q6-8hr prn or 3-5 mL (20% solution) or 6-10 mL (10% sol) tid or qid; **NEBULIZER** (face mask, mouthpiece, tracheostomy) 1-10 mL of a 20% sol, or 2-20 mL of a 10% sol, q2-8hr; **NEBULIZER** (tent, croupette) may require large dose, up to 300 mL/treatment

Tracheostomy care

• **Adult/child: INSTILL** 1-2 mL (10%-20% sol) q1-4hr directly into tracheostomy

Diagnostic bronchial lab studies

• **Adult/child: NEBULIZER** 2-3 uses of 1-2 mL of 20% sol or 2-4 mL of 10% sol

Available forms: Inhalation solution 10%, 20%; inj 20% (200 mg/mL)

Administer:
Direct intratracheal instill route

• By syringe: 1-2 mL of 10%-20% solution up to q1hr

• Decreased dose to geriatric patients; metabolism may be slowed

• Only if suction machine is available

• Only after patient clears airway by deep breathing, coughing

• Assistance with inhaled dose: bronchodilator if bronchospasm occurs; mechanical suction if cough insufficient to remove excess bronchial secretions

IV route

• **21-hr regimen:** loading dose: dilute 150 mg/kg in 200 mL D_5W; maintenance dose 1: dilute 50 mg/kg in 500 mL D_5W; maintenance dose 2: dilute 100 mg/kg in 1000 mL D_5W; give loading dose over 15 min; give maintenance dose 1 over 4 hr; give maintenance dose 2 over 16 hr, administer sequentially without time between doses

• Store in refrigerator; use within 96 hr of opening

SIDE EFFECTS

CNS: *Dizziness, drowsiness,* fever, chills
CV: Edema, flushing tachycardia
EENT: *Rhinorrhea,* pharyngitis
GI: *Nausea,* stomatitis, vomiting, anorexia
INTEG: Urticaria, rash, clamminess, pruritus
RESP: Bronchospasm, chest tightness, cough, dyspnea
MISC: Anaphylaxis, angioedema, unpleasant odor

PHARMACOKINETICS

IV: Excreted in urine, half-life 5.6 hr (adult), 11 hr (newborn), protein binding 83%, peak 5-10 min (INH)

Interactions

• Do not use with activated charcoal

NURSING CONSIDERATIONS
Assess:

• **Mucolytic use:** cough—type, frequency, character, including sputum; bronchospasm

• Rate, rhythm of respirations, increased dyspnea; sputum

• VS, cardiac status including checking for dysrhythmias, increased rate, palpitations

• ABGs for increased CO_2 retention in asthma patients

• **Antidotal use:** use within 24 hr of acetaminophen toxicity, give within 10 hr of acetaminophen to minimize hepatotoxicity; monitor LFTs, PT, BUN, creatinine, glucose, electrolytes, acetaminophen levels; inform prescriber if dose is vomited or if vomiting is persistent; 150 mg/kg may be toxic, check acetaminophen level q4hr

• **Bronchospasm:** discontinue, notify health care provider if bronchospasm occurs

• **Hypersensitivity:** anaphylaxis may occur with IV dose; if present, stop infusion, treat, restart; assess for dyspnea, swelling of face, lips, tongue; rash, itching

• Nausea, vomiting, rash; notify prescriber if these occur

• **Pregnancy/breastfeeding:** use only if clearly needed; cautious use in breastfeeding, excretion unknown

Evaluate:

• Therapeutic response: absence of purulent secretions when coughing, clear lung

sounds (mucolytic use); absence of hepatic damage with acetaminophen toxicity
Teach patient/family:
• That foul odor and smell may be unpleasant
• To clear airway for inhalation
• To report vomiting because dose may need to be repeated
• Provide adequate hydration
• Teach coughing and deep breathing
• **Acetaminophen toxicity:** Explain reason for product, expected result

---

aclidinium (Rx)

(a′kli-din′ee-um)

Tudorza Pressair, Tudorza Genuair

Func. class.: Anticholinergic, bronchodilator

Chem. class.: Synthetic quaternary ammonium compound

USES: Long-term maintenance treatment of bronchospasm in COPD, emphysema, chronic bronchitis, not indicated for initial treatment of acute episodes

CONTRAINDICATIONS
Hypersensitivity

DOSAGE AND ROUTES
• **Adults, including geriatric patients:**
ORAL INHALATION 400 mcg (1 actuation) bid; doses should be 12 hr apart

---

aclidinium/
formoterol (Rx)

Duaklir Genuair ✤, Duaklir Pressair

Func. class.: Respiratory agent

Chem. class.: Respiratory corticosteroid; long-acting β_2-agonist; respiratory long-acting muscarinic antagonist

USES: Maintenance treatment of chronic obstructive pulmonary disease (COPD)

CONTRAINDICATIONS
Hypersensitivity

DOSAGE AND ROUTES
• **Adult: INH** 1 inhalation (400 mcg aclidinium and 12 mcg formoterol per actuation) inhaled bid (morning and evening). Max: 1 INH bid

---

acyclovir (Rx)

(ay-sye′kloe-veer)

Sitavig, Zovirax

Func. class.: Antiviral

Chem. class.: Purine nucleoside analog

Combinations: Xerese: Topical cream acyclovir 5%/hydrocortisone 1%
Do not confuse:
Zovirax/Zyvox/Valtrex/Zostrix/Doribex/Valtrex/Zithromax
acyclovir/ganciclovir/Retorovir/Valcyclovir

ACTION: Converted to acyclovir monophosphate by virus-specific thymidine kinase then further converted to acyclovir triphosphate by other cellular enzymes, inhibits viral DNA synthesis

USES: Mucocutaneous herpes simplex virus, herpes genitalis (HSV-1, HSV-2), varicella infections, herpes zoster, herpes simplex encephalitis
Unlabeled uses: Bell's palsy, prevention of CMV, Epstein-Barr virus, esophagitis, hairy leukoplakia, prevention of herpes labialis, herpes simplex, herpes simplex ocular prophylaxis, keratoconjunctivitis, pharyngitis, pneumonitis, prevention of postherpetic neuralgia, proctitis, stomatitis, tracheobronchitis, varicella prophylaxis

CONTRAINDICATIONS
Hypersensitivity to this product, valACYclovir; milk protein (buccal), neonates (benzyl/alcohol)
Precautions: Pregnancy, breastfeeding, renal/hepatic/neurologic disease, electrolyte imbalance, dehydration, hypersensitivity to famciclovir, ganciclovir,

---

penciclovir, valGANciclovir, obesity, immunocompromised, geriatrics

DOSAGE AND ROUTES

Base dose in obese patients on ideal body weight, not actual body weight

Herpes simplex (recurrent)
- **Adult: PO** 400 mg 3×/day for 5 days or 200 mg 5×/day × 5 days
- **Adult and child >12 yr: IV INFUSION** 5 mg/kg over 1 hr q8hr × 7 days
- **Infant >3 mo/child <12 yr: IV INFUSION** 10 mg/kg q8hr × 7 days; if HIV infected, 5-10 mg/kg q8hr (moderate to severe)
- **Neonate: IV INFUSION** 10 mg/kg q8hr × 10 days, may use higher dose

Genital herpes, initial episodes
- **Adult: PO** 400 mg tid or 200 mg 5×/day × 7-10 days, may extend treatment if healing is not complete after 10 days; **TOP** × 5 days; **IV** 5 mg/kg q8hr or 750 mg/m²/day divided q8hr × 5-7 days

Genital herpes, episodic treatment
- **Adult: PO** 400 mg tid or 800 mg bid × 5 days or 800 mg tid × 2 days; initiate within 1 day of lesion onset

Genital herpes, suppression therapy
- **Adult: PO** 400 mg bid for up to 12 mo or 200 mg 3-5 times daily for up to 12 mo
Child<12 yr: PO 20 mg/kg bid, max 400 mg/dose

Genital herpes, initial limited, mucocutaneous HSV in immunocompromised patients, non–life-threatening
- **Adult/child ≥12 yr: TOP** cover lesions q3hr 6×/day

Herpes simplex encephalitis
- **Adult: IV** 10 mg/kg over 1 hr q8hr × 14-21 days
- **Child 3 mo-12 yr: IV** 10-15 mg/kg q8hr × 14-21 days
- **Child birth-3 mo: IV** 20 mg/kg q8hr × 21 days
- **Neonates/premature infants: IV** 10 mg/kg q12hr × 14-21 days

Herpes labialis, recurrent
- **Adult/child ≥12 yr: TOP** apply cream 5×/day for 4 days; start as soon as symptoms appear

Herpes labialis, recurrent in immunocompetent patients
- **Adult: Buccal** 50 mg as a single dose in upper gum region within 1 hr after prodromal symptoms and before cold sore formation

Herpes zoster (immunocompetent)
- **Adult: PO** 800 mg q4hr 5×/day while awake × 7-10 days; **IV** 10 mg/kg q8hr × 7 days

Herpes zoster (shingles) immunocompromised patients
- **Adult/adolescent: PO** 800 mg q4hr 5×/day for 7-10 days; **IV** 10-15 mg/kg q8hr × 10-14 days
- **Infant/child <12 yr: IV** 10 mg/kg/dose q8hr × 7-10 days

Herpes zoster (shingles) immunocompetent
- **Adult: PO** 800 mg q4hr 5×/day × 7-10 days; start within 48-72 hr of rash onset

Varicella (chickenpox)
- **Adult/child ≥2 yr: PO** 10 mg/kg/dose (max 800 mg) 4×/day × 5 days

Mucosal/cutaneous herpes simplex infections in immunosuppressed patients
- **Adult and child >12 yr: IV** 5 mg/kg q8hr × 7 days
- **Infant >3 mo/child <12: IV** 10 mg/kg q8hr × 7 days

Renal dose
- **Adult and child: PO/IV** CCr >50 mL/min 100% dose q8hr, CCr 25-50 mL/min 100% dose q12hr, CCr 10-25 mL/min 100% dose q24hr, CCr 0-10 mL/min 50% dose q24hr

Recurrent ocular herpes, prevention (unlabeled)
- **Adult/child ≥12 yr: PO** 600-800 mg every day × 8-12 mo

CMV prophylaxis (unlabeled)
- **Adult: IV** 500 mg/m² q8hr

Herpes simplex in pneumonitis/esophagitis/tracheobronchitis/proctitis/stomatitis/pharyngitis (unlabeled)
- **Adult and adolescent: IV** 5-10 mg/kg q8hr × 2-7 days or **PO** 200 mg q4hr 5×/day × 7-10 days or 400 mg 3-5×/day × ≥10 days
- **Child 6 mo-12 yr: IV** 1000 mg/day in 3-5 divided doses × 7-14 days

Herpes simplex prophylaxis for chronic suppression therapy (unlabeled)
• **Adult and adolescent: PO** 400 mg bid up to 12 mo

Available forms: Capsules 200 mg; tablets 400, 800 mg; powder for injection 500, 1000 mg; solution for injection 50 mg/mL; oral suspension 200 mg/5 mL; ointment/cream 5%; buccal tablet 50 mg

Administer:

PO route
• Do not break, crush, or chew capsules
• May give without regard to meals, with 8 oz of water
• Shake suspension before use

Buccal
• Use on the same side as the herpes labialis lesion; after removing tablet from blister, place rounded side of tablet to the upper gum above incisor tooth; hold in place for 30 sec; once adhered, the tablet will dissolve; if tablet falls off within 6 hr, reposition the same tablet, do not crush, suck, or chew tablet

Topical route
• Use finger cot or glove to cover all lesions completely; do not get in eye; wash hands after use

Intermittent IV INFUSION route
• Increase fluids to 3 L/day to decrease crystalluria; most critical during first 2 hr after IV
• **Reconstitute** 10 mL compatible solution/500 mg or 20 mL/1 g of product, 50 mg/mL, **shake, further dilute** in 100-125 mL D5W or 0.9% NaCl; use within 12 hr; **give** over at least 1 hr by infusion pump to prevent nephrotoxicity; do not reconstitute with solution containing benzyl alcohol in neonates
• **Store** at room temperature for up to 24 hr after reconstitution; if refrigerated, solution may show a precipitate that clears at room temperature; yellow discoloration does not affect potency, store vials at room temperature

Y-site compatibilities: Alemtuzumab, alfentanil, allopurinol, amikacin, aminophylline, amphotericin B cholesteryl, amphotericin B liposome, ampicillin, anidulafungin, argatroban, atracurium, bivalirudin, buprenorphine, busulfan, butorphanol, calcium chloride/gluconate, CARBOplatin, cefazolin, cefonicid, cefotaxime, cefoxitin, ceftazidime, ceftizoxime, cefTRIAXone, cefuroxime, chloramphenicol, cholesteryl sulfate complex, cimetidine, clindamycin, dexamethasone sodium phosphate, dimenhyDRINATE, DOXOrubicin, doxycycline, erythromycin, famotidine, filgrastim, fluconazole, gallium, gentamicin, granisetron, heparin, hydrocortisone sodium succinate, HYDROmorphone, imipenem/cilastatin, LORazepam, magnesium sulfate, melphalan, methylPREDNISolone sodium succinate, metoclopramide, metroNIDAZOLE, multivitamin, nafcillin, oxacillin, PACLitaxel, penicillin G potassium, PENTobarbital, perphenazine, piperacillin, potassium chloride, propofol, raNITIdine, remifentanil, sodium bicarbonate, tacrolimus, teniposide, theophylline, thiotepa, ticarcillin, tobramycin, trimethoprim-sulfamethoxazole, vancomycin, vasopressin, voriconazole, zidovudine

SIDE EFFECTS

CNS: Tremors, confusion, lethargy, hallucinations, seizures, dizziness, headache, encephalopathic changes
EENT: Gingival hyperplasia
GI: Nausea, vomiting, diarrhea, increased ALT/AST, abdominal pain, colitis
GU: Hematuria, acute renal failure, changes in menses
HEMA: Thrombotic thrombocytopenia purpura, hemolytic uremic syndrome, leukopenia (immunocompromised patients)
INTEG: Rash, urticaria, pruritus, pain or phlebitis at IV site, unusual sweating, alopecia, Stevens-Johnson syndrome
MS: Joint pain
SYST: Angioedema, anaphylaxis

PHARMACOKINETICS

Distributed widely; crosses placenta; CSF concentrations are 50% of plasma; protein binding 9%-33%
PO: Absorbed minimally, onset unknown, peak 1.5-2 hr, half-life 2.5-3.3 hr (adult); 2-3 hr (child); up to 4 hr (neonates)
Buccal: Peak 8 hr
IV: Onset immediate, peak immediate, duration unknown, half-life 20 min-3 hr (terminal); Metabolized by liver, excreted by

kidneys as unchanged product (95%), removed by hemodialysis

INTERACTIONS

Increase: CNS side effects—zidovudine

Increase: levels, toxicity—probenecid, monitor for toxicity

Increase: nephrotoxicity—aminoglycosides, foscarnet

Increase: concentrations of—entecavir, PEMEtrexed, tenofovir, theophylline

Decrease: action of hydantoins, valproic acid, monitor drug levels

Drug/Lab Test

Increase: BUN, creatinine

Decrease: WBC

NURSING CONSIDERATIONS

Assess:

• **Infection:** type of lesions, area of body covered, purulent drainage, frequency of lesions

• **Hepatic, renal studies:** AST, ALT; urinalysis, protein, BUN, creatinine, CCr, watch for increasing BUN and serum creatinine or decreased CCr; I&O ratio; report hematuria, oliguria, fatigue, weakness; may indicate nephrotoxicity; check for protein in urine during treatment

• Skin eruptions: rash, urticaria, itching

• Allergies before treatment, reaction to each medication; place allergies on chart in bright red letters

• Neurologic status with herpes encephalitis

• Provide isolation for varicella zoster and herpes zoster (disseminated)

• Provide adequate intake of fluids (2 L) to prevent deposits in kidneys, more likely to occur with rapid administration or in dehydration

Evaluate:

• Therapeutic response: absence of itching, painful lesions; crusting and healed lesions; decreased symptoms of chickenpox; healing, decreased pain with herpes zoster

Teach patient/family:

• To take as prescribed; if dose is missed, take as soon as remembered up to 1 hr before next dose; do not double dose

• That product may be taken orally before infection occurs; product should be taken when itching or pain occurs, usually before eruptions

• That sexual partners need to be told that patient has herpes because they can become infected; condoms must be worn to prevent reinfections

• Not to touch lesions to avoid spreading infection to new sites, not to use topical products on lesions, spreading may occur

• That product does not cure infection, just controls symptoms and does not prevent infecting others

• That product must be taken in equal intervals around the clock to maintain blood levels for duration of therapy

• That women with genital herpes are more likely to develop cervical cancer; to keep all gynecologic appointments

• **Topical:** Not to use around eyes, to use enough ointment to cover lesions q3hr/6× per day, use finger cot or glove to apply

• **Pregnancy/breastfeeding:** to identify if pregnancy is planned or suspected or if breastfeeding

TREATMENT OF OVERDOSE:

Discontinue product; hemodialysis

---

adalimumab (Rx)

(add-a-lim′yu-mab)

Humira, Humira Pen; Hyrimoz, (biosimilar); Abrilada (biosimilar); Hulio (biosimilar); Yusimry (biosimilar)

Func. class.: Antirheumatic agent (disease modifying), immunomodulator, anti-TNF

Chem. class.: Recombinant human IgG1 monoclonal antibody, DMARD

Do not confuse:

Humira/HumuLIN/HumaLOG

Humira Pen/Humapen Memoir

ACTION: A form of human IgG1 monoclonal antibody specific for human tumor necrosis factor (TNF-α); elevated levels of TNF-α are found in patients with rheumatoid arthritis

USES: Moderate to severe active rheumatoid arthritis who are ≥18 yr of age and who have not responded to other disease-modifying agents, juvenile rheumatoid arthritis (JRA), psoriatic arthritis, Crohn's disease, moderate to severe plaque psoriasis, ankylosing spondylitis, ulcerative colitis, noninfectious uveitis, moderate-severe hidradenitis suppurativa

CONTRAINDICATIONS

Hypersensitivity, breastfeeding, use of anakinra, abatacept

Precautions: Pregnancy, children, geriatric patients, CNS demyelinating disease, lymphoma, HF, hepatitis B carriers, mannitol hypersensitivity, latex allergy, neoplastic disease, TB

Black Box Warning: Active infections, risk of lymphomas/leukemias

DOSAGE AND ROUTES
Rheumatoid arthritis/ankylosing spondylitis/psoriatic arthritis
• **Adult:** SUBCUT 40 mg every other week or every week if not combined with methotrexate
Juvenile rheumatoid arthritis
• **Child ≥2 yr/adolescent ≥30 kg:** SUBCUT 40 mg every other week
• **Child ≥2 yr/adolescent ≥15 kg to <30 kg:** SUBCUT 20 mg every other week
• **Child ≥2 yr/adolescent 10-<15 kg:** SUBCUT 10 mg every other week
Crohn's disease/ulcerative colitis
• **Adult:** SUBCUT 160 mg given as 4 injections on day 1 or 2 injections each on days 1 and 2, then 80 mg at wk 2 and 40 mg every other week starting at wk 4
Pediatric Crohn's disease
• **Child >6 yr and ≥40 kg (88 lb):** SUBCUT 160 mg on day 1 (as 4 [40-mg] injections) or 40 mg (as 2 injections) (80 mg) × 2 days, then 80 mg after 2 wk (day 15), then 40 mg every other week (day 29)
• **Child >6 yr and 17-40 kg (37-88 lb):** SUBCUT 80 mg day 1 (as 2 [40-mg]

injections), then 40 mg after 2 wk (day 15), then 20 mg every other week (day 29)
Plaque psoriasis/noninfectious uveitis
Adult: SUBCUT 80 mg baseline as 2 injections, then 40 mg every other week starting 1 wk after initial dose (plaque psoriasis)
Child >2 yr and ≥30 kg: SUBCUT 20 mg every other week
Child ≤2 yr and ≤15 kg: SUBCUT 10 mg every other week
Moderate hidradenitis suppurativa
Adult/adolescent and ≥60 kg: SUBCUT 160 mg 1 day or split over 2 days, then 80 mg on day 15, then on day 29 give 40 mg weekly
Adolescent and 30-60 kg: SUBCUT 80 mg on day 1 then 40 mg on day 8, then 40 mg every other week
Available form: Injection prefilled pens/syringes 10 mg/0.1 mL, 10 mg/0.2 mL, 20 mg/0.2 mL, 20 mg/0.4 mL, 40 mg/0.4 mL, 40 mg/0.8 mL, 80 mg/0.8 mL; single-use vial 40 mg/0.8 mL
Administer:
SUBCUT route
• Do not admix with other solutions or medications; do not use filter; protect from light; give at 45-degree angle using abdomen, thighs; rotate injection sites; discard unused portions
• Don't inject in bruised, red, tender, abraded areas; use in SUBCUT only
Prefilled pen use:
• Using alcohol swab, clean area (do not use if solution is discolored or contains particulate), the pen is activated by removing the gray cap, pinch skin and place at 90-degree angle and press button, hold until solution is inserted, remove, use cotton ball for a few seconds, dispose of properly

SIDE EFFECTS
CNS: *Headache,* Guillain-Barré syndrome, MS
CV: *Hypertension,* HF
EENT: *Sinusitis,* optic neuritis
GI: Abdominal pain, nausea

HEMA: Leukopenia, thrombocytopenia
INTEG: *Rash, injection site reaction*
MISC: Flulike symptoms, increased cancer risk, risk of infection (TB, invasive fungal infections, other opportunistic infections), infections may be fatal; Stevens-Johnson syndrome, anaphylaxis, hyperlipidemia
RESP: *URI,* pulmonary fibrosis, bronchitis

PHARMACOKINETICS

Absorption 65%, distributed to synovial fluid, half-life 2 wk, lower clearance with advancing age (40-75 yr), onset up to 24 wk (inflammation)

INTERACTIONS

Black Box Warning: Increase: serious infections—other TNF blockers, rilonacept

Increase: infection-azathioprine
• Do not use with abatacept, anakinra, belimumab, canakinumab, natalizumab, rilonacept, tofacitinib, vedolizumab; serious infections may occur
• Do not give concurrently with live virus vaccines; immunizations should be brought up to date before treatment
Drug/Herb
Echinacea: Decreased product effect
Drug/Lab Test
Increase: ALT, cholesterol, lipids

NURSING CONSIDERATIONS
Assess:
• **RA:** pain; stiffness; ROM; swelling of joints prior to, during treatment
• **Crohn's disease/ulcerative colitis:** bowel pattern, cramping, abdominal pain, bleeding
• For injection site pain, swelling, redness—usually occurs after 2 injections (4-5 days); use cold compress to relieve pain/swelling

Black Box Warning: Infections (fever, flulike symptoms, dyspnea, change in urination, redness/swelling around any wounds), stop treatment if some serious infections including sepsis occur, may be fatal; patients with active infections should not be started on this product

• May reactivate hepatitis B in chronic carriers, may be fatal

Black Box Warning: Latent TB before therapy; treat before starting this product

• **Anaphylaxis, latex allergy:** stop therapy if lupus-like syndrome develops
• **Blood dyscrasias:** CBC, differential periodically

Black Box Warning: Neoplastic disease (lymphomas/leukemia) in children, adolescents; hepatosplenic T-cell lymphoma is more likely in adolescent males with Crohn's disease or ulcerative colitis

Evaluate:
• Therapeutic response: decreased inflammation, pain in joints, decreased joint destruction
Teach patient/family:
• About self-administration if appropriate: injection should be made in thigh, abdomen, upper arm; rotate sites at least 1 inch from old site; do not inject in areas that are bruised, red, hard; review provided medication guide with patient
• To refrigerate in container that product was received in; to dispose of needles and equipment as instructed
• That if medication is not taken when due, inject dose as soon as remembered and inject next dose as scheduled
• Not to take any live virus vaccines during treatment
• To report signs of infection, allergic reaction, TB immediately
• To advise all health care professionals of Rx, OTC, herbals, supplements taken
• **Pregnancy/breastfeeding:** To advise health care professional if pregnancy is planned or suspected or if breastfeeding; to register if pregnant at 877-311-8972
• To do regular skin assessments and report changes to provider

adefovir (Rx)

(add-ee-foh´veer)

Hepsera
Func. class.: Antiviral
Chem. class.: Nucleoside

ACTION: Inhibits hepatitis B virus DNA polymerase by competing with natural substrates and by causing DNA termination after its incorporation into viral DNA; causes viral DNA death

USES: Chronic hepatitis B

CONTRAINDICATIONS
Hypersensitivity

Precautions: Pregnancy, labor, breastfeeding, children, geriatric patients, dialysis, females, obesity, organ transplant

Black Box Warning: Severe renal disease, impaired hepatic function, lactic acidosis, HIV, hepatitis B exacerbation

DOSAGE AND ROUTES
Chronic hepatitis B
• **Adult/adolescent: PO** 10 mg/day, optimal duration unknown
Renal dose
• **Adult: PO** CCr ≥50 mL/min 10 mg q24hr; CCr 30-49 mL/min 10 mg q48hr; CCr 10-29 mL/min 10 mg q72hr; hemodialysis 10 mg q7days after dialysis
Available forms: Tablets 10 mg
Administer:
• By mouth without regard for food
• Take with full glass of water
• Store in cool environment; protect from light

SIDE EFFECTS
CNS: *Headache*
GI: *Dyspepsia,* abdominal pain, nausea, vomiting, diarrhea, hepatomegaly, flatulence, pancreatitis
GU: Hematuria, glycosuria, nephrotoxicity, Fanconi syndrome, renal failure
MISC: Fever, rash, weight loss, cough

PHARMACOKINETICS
PO: Rapidly absorbed from GI tract, peak 1¾ hr, excreted by kidneys 45%, terminal half-life 7.48 hr

INTERACTIONS
• Do not use in combination with emtricitabine/tenofovir, emtricitabine/rilpivirine, emtricitabine/efavirenz/tenofovir

Increase: serum concentrations and possible nephrotoxicity—aminoglycosides, memantine, emtricitabine, efavirenz, dofetilide, digoxin, cycloSPORINE, aMILoride, quiNINE, quiNIDine, procainamide, PEMEtrexed, midodrine, metFORMIN, NSAIDs, vancomycin, trospium, triamterene, tenofovir, tacrolimus, ranitidine, cimetidine, morphine

Black Box Warning: Increase: lactic acidosis, severe hepatomegaly, NNRTIs, NRTIs, antiretroviral protease inhibitors

Drug/Lab Test
Increase: ALT, AST, amylase, creatine kinase

NURSING CONSIDERATIONS
Assess

Black Box Warning: Nephrotoxicity: increasing CCr, BUN

Black Box Warning: HIV antibody testing before beginning treatment, HIV resistance may occur in chronic hepatitis B patients

Black Box Warning: For lactic acidosis, severe hepatomegaly with stenosis; for use of NNRTIs, NRTIs, antiretroviral protease inhibitors (PIs), lactic acidosis with severe hepatomegaly is more common in females, obese patients, and with prolonged nucleoside use

• Geriatric patients more carefully; may develop renal, cardiac symptoms more rapidly

Black Box Warning: For exacerbations of hepatitis after discontinuing treatment, monitor LFTs, hepatitis B serology

• Pregnancy: if planned or suspected; if pregnant call the Pregnancy Registry: 800-258-4263
Evaluate:
• Therapeutic response: decreased symptoms of chronic hepatitis B, improving LFTs

---

Side effects: *italics* = common; red = life-threatening

Teach patient/family:
- That optimal duration of treatment is unknown; that product is not a cure; that transmission may still occur
- To avoid use with other medications unless approved by prescriber
- To notify prescriber of decreased urinary output
- Not to stop abruptly unless directed; worsening of hepatitis may occur
- To report immediately dyspnea, nausea, vomiting, abdominal pain, weakness, dizziness, cold extremities
- To notify prescriber if pregnancy is planned or suspected; avoid breastfeeding

---

⚠ HIGH ALERT

adenosine (Rx)
(a-den'oh-seen)
Adenocard
Func. class.: Antidysrhythmic
Chem. class.: Endogenous nucleoside

ACTION: Slows conduction through AV node, can interrupt reentry pathways through AV node, and can restore normal sinus rhythm in patients with paroxysmal supraventricular tachycardia (PSVT)

USES: PSVT, as a diagnostic aid to assess myocardial perfusion defects in CAD, Wolff-Parkinson-White syndrome
Unlabeled uses: Wide-complex tachycardia diagnosis

CONTRAINDICATIONS
Hypersensitivity, second- or third-degree AV block, sick sinus syndrome, bradycardia, asystole, COPD, asthma, severe respiratory conditions
Precautions: Pregnancy, breastfeeding, children, geriatric patients

DOSAGE AND ROUTES
Converting paroxysmal supraventricular tachycardia to sinus rhythm
- **Adult and child >50 kg (110 lb): IV BOL** 6 mg; if conversion to normal sinus rhythm does not occur within 1-2 min, give 12 mg by rapid **IV BOL**; may repeat 12-mg dose again in 1-2 min
- **Infant and child <50 kg (110 lb): IV BOL** 0.1 mg/kg; if not effective, increase dose by 0.05-0.1 mg/kg q2min to a max of 0.3 mg/kg/dose
- **Neonate: IV BOL** 0.05 mg/kg by rapid **IV BOL,** may increase by 0.05 mg/kg q2min, max 0.3 mg/kg/dose

Diagnostic use
- **Adult/child >50 kg:** IV 140 mcg/kg/min × 6 min (0.84 mg/kg total)
Available forms: 3 mg/mL sol for injection
Administer:

IV, direct route
- Warm to room temperature; crystals will dissolve
- Undiluted; give 6 mg or less by rapid injection over 1-2 sec; if using an IV line, use port near insertion site, flush with NS (20 mL), then elevate arm, dose reduction recommended if given by central line
- Store at room temperature; solution should be clear; discard unused product

IV intermittent infusion
Diagnostic
- Use 30-mL vial undiluted (3 mg/mL), give at 140 mcg/kg/min over 6 min (total 0.84 mg/kg)
- Thallium-201 should never be given after 3 min of infusion

SIDE EFFECTS
CNS: Light headedness, dizziness, arm tingling, numbness, headache; seizures
CV: Chest pain, pressure, atrial tachydysrhythmias, sweating, palpitations, hypotension, *facial flushing,* AV block, cardiac arrest, ventricular dysrhythmias, atrial fibrillation
GI: *Nausea,* metallic taste
RESP: *Dyspnea, chest pressure,* hyperventilation, bronchospasm (asthmatics)
MS: Back pain

PHARMACOKINETICS
Cleared from plasma in <30 sec, half-life 10 sec, converted to inosine/adenosine monophosphate

---

INTERACTIONS

Increase: risk for higher degree of heart block—carBAMazepine

Increase: risk for ventricular fibrillation—digoxin, verapamil; monitor ECG

Increase: effects of adenosine—dipyridamole; adenosine dose may need to be reduced

Decrease: activity of adenosine—theophylline or other methylxanthines (caffeine); adenosine dose may need to be increased

Drug/Lifestyle

Increase: tachycardia, hypertension (smoking)

Drug/Herb

Increase: adenosine effect—ginger

Decrease: adenosine effect—guarana, green tea

NURSING CONSIDERATIONS

Assess:

• **Cardiopulmonary status:** B/P, pulse, respiration, rhythm, ECG intervals (PR, QRS, QT); check for transient dysrhythmias (PVCs, PACs, sinus tachycardia, AV block)

• **Respiratory status:** rate, rhythm, lung fields for crackles; watch for respiratory depression; bilateral crackles may occur in HF patient; increased respiration, increased pulse, product should be discontinued

• CNS effects: dizziness, confusion, psychosis, paresthesias, seizures; product should be discontinued

• **Pregnancy/breastfeeding: identify if pregnancy is planned or suspected, or if breastfeeding; use only if benefits outweigh fetal risk; do not breastfeed**

Evaluate:

• Therapeutic response: normal sinus rhythm or diagnosis of perfusion defect

Teach patient/family:

• To report facial flushing, dizziness, sweating, palpitations, chest pain; usually transient; chest pressure may occur immediately after administration

• To report IV discomfort

• **Pregnancy/breastfeeding:** to advise prescriber if pregnancy is planned or suspected or if breastfeeding; do not breastfeed

TREATMENT OF OVERDOSE:

Defibrillation, vasopressor for hypotension, aminophylline

> **⚠ HIGH ALERT**

ado-trastuzumab (Rx)

(a'doe-tras-tooz'ue-mab)

Kadcyla

Func. class.: Antineoplastic-biologic response modifier

Chem. class.: Signal transduction inhibitors (STIs), humanized anti-HER2 antibody

Do not confuse:

ado-trastuzumab/trastuzumab

ACTION: Humanized ⟨⟩ anti-HER2 monoclonal antibody that is linked to DM1, a small molecule microtubular inhibitor; once the antibody is bound to the HER2 receptor, the complex is internalized and the DM1 is released to bind with tubulin to lead to apoptosis

USES: Breast cancer; metastatic with overexpression of HER2, who previously received trastuzumab and a taxane, separately or in combination

CONTRAINDICATIONS

Hypersensitivity to this product, Chinese hamster ovary cell protein

Black Box Warning: Pregnancy

Precautions: Breastfeeding, children, pulmonary disease, acute bronchospasm, anticoagulant, ⟨⟩ Asian patients, asthma, COPD, extravasation, fever, hepatitis, human antihuman antibody, hypotension, neuropathy, interstitial lung disease/pneumonitis; extravasation; thrombocytopenia

Black Box Warning: Heart failure, hepatotoxicity

DOSAGE AND ROUTES

• **Adult: IV** 3.6 mg/kg over 30-90 min q3wk ×14 wk; give first infusion over 90 min; if tolerated, give over 30 min, max 3.6 mg/kg

Dosage adjustments for toxicities

Hepatotoxicity:

• **AST/ALT >5 to ≤20 × ULN:** withhold, resume at a reduced dose when AST/ALT is ≤5 × ULN; first dose reduction: reduce the dose to 3 mg/kg; second dose reduction: reduce the dose to 2.4 mg/kg; requirement for further dose reduction: discontinue **AST/ ALT >20× ULN:** discontinue

• **Total bilirubin >3 to ≤10× ULN:** withhold, resume treatment at a reduced dose when total bilirubin recovers to ≤1.5; first dose reduction: reduce the dose to 3 mg/kg; second dose reduction: reduce the dose to 2.4 mg/kg; requirement for further dose reduction: discontinue treatment

• **Total bilirubin >10× ULN:** permanently discontinue; permanently discontinue treatment in patients with AST/ALT >3× ULN and total bilirubin >2× ULN; permanently discontinue treatment in patients diagnosed with nodular regenerative hyperplasia (NRH)

• **Left ventricular ejection fraction (LVEF):** *LVEF 40%-45% and decrease is <10% from baseline:* continue; repeat LVEF assessment within 3 wk; *LVEF 40%-45% and decrease is ≥10% from baseline:* withhold; repeat LVEF assessment within 3 wk; if LVEF remains ≥10% from baseline, discontinue; *LVEF <40%:* withhold; repeat LVEF assessment within 3 wk; if LVEF remains <40%, discontinue; *symptomatic heart failure (HF):* discontinue

Thrombocytopenia:

• **Platelet count 25,000/mm³ to <50,000/mm³:** withhold; resume at same dose when platelet count recovers to ≥75,000/mm³

• **Platelet count <25,000/mm³:** withhold; resume at a reduced dose when platelet count recovers to ≥75,000/mm³: first reduction: reduce the dose to 3 mg/kg; second reduction: reduce the dose to 2.4 mg/kg; requirement for further reduction: discontinue

Pulmonary toxicity:

• Permanently discontinue in interstitial lung disease or pneumonitis

Peripheral neuropathy:

• Withhold in grade 3 or 4 peripheral neuropathy; resume upon resolution to ≤grade 2

Available forms: lyophilized powder 100, 160 mg/vial

Administer:

IV route

• Visually inspect for particulate matter and discoloration before use

• Give as infusion with a 0.2- or 0.22-micron in-line filter; do not administer as an IV push or bolus

• Use cytotoxic handling procedures; do not mix with, or administer as an infusion with, other IV products

Reconstitution:

• Slowly inject 5 mL of sterile water for injection into each 100-mg vial or 8 mL of sterile water for injection into each 160-mg vial to yield a single-use solution of 20 mg/mL

• Direct the stream of sterile water toward the wall of the vial

• Gently swirl the vial; do not shake

• After reconstitution, withdraw amount and dilute immediately in 250 mL of 0.9% sodium chloride; gently invert the bag to mix

• The reconstituted single-use product does not contain a preservative; use the diluted solution immediately or store at 36° F-46° F (2° C-8° C) for up to 24 hr after reconstitution; discard any unused drug after 24 hr; do not freeze

IV infusion

• Closely monitor for possible subcutaneous infiltration during administration

• **First infusion:** give over 90 min; the infusion rate should be slowed or interrupted if the patient develops an infusion-related reaction; observe for at least 90 min following the initial dose for fever, chills, or other infusion-related reactions; permanently discontinue for life-threatening infusion-related reactions

• **Subsequent infusions:** administer over 30 min if prior infusions were well tolerated; the infusion rate should be slowed or interrupted if the patient develops an infusion-related reaction; observe for at least 30 min after the infusion; permanently discontinue for life-threatening infusion-related reactions

SIDE EFFECTS

CNS: Dizziness, insomnia, neuropathy, chills, fatigue, fever, flushing, headache
CV: Hypertension, peripheral edema, left ventricular dysfunction
EENT: Blurred vision, conjunctivitis, stomatitis
GI: Diarrhea, nausea, vomiting, constipation, dyspepsia, hepatotoxicity
HEMA: Anemia, bleeding, thrombocytopenia
INTEG: Rash, infusion-related reactions
MS: Arthralgia, pain
RESP: Cough, dyspnea, pneumonitis, interstitial lung disease
SYST: Anaphylaxis
OTHER: Elevated LFTs, hand-foot syndrome

PHARMACOKINETICS

93% protein binding, metabolized in the liver by CYP3A4, half-life 4 days

INTERACTIONS

Belimumab, natalizumab, live virus vaccines: Increased adverse reactions
Increase: bleeding risk—warfarin, platelet inhibitors, anticoagulants
Increase: ado-trastuzumab toxicity—CYP3A4 inhibitors (clarithromycin, ketoconazole, ritonavir, saquinavir, atazanavir); avoid concurrent use
Drug/Herb
Echinacea: Decreased product effect
Drug/Lab
Increase: ALT/AST, bilirubin
Decrease: potassium, platelets

NURSING CONSIDERATIONS
Assess:
• HER-2-positive breast cancer: confirm status
• Labs: CBC, LFTs, ECG baseline; potassium, LFTs before each treatment
• Hypersensitivity: monitor during each infusion
• Pregnancy test, CBC, differential, LFTs

Black Box Warning: HF, other cardiac symptoms: dyspnea, coughing; gallop

• **Cardiotoxicity:** monitor LVEF, if >45% continue dose; if 40%-45% and <10% from baseline, continue or reduce, repeat LVEF in 3 wk; if LVEF 40%-45% with decrease >10% from baseline, hold and repeat testing in 3 wk, discontinue if no improvement within 10% of baseline, LVEF <40%, or symptomatic HF
• Symptoms of infection; may be masked by product
• CNS reaction: LOC, mental status, dizziness, confusion

Black Box Warning: Hypersensitivity reactions, anaphylaxis

Black Box Warning: Hepatotoxicity: monitor LFTs baseline and prior to each dose; fatal liver damage may occur; reduced dose or discontinuing treatment may be required; monitor for infusion reactions during and for 1.5 hr after infusion; slowing infusion may be needed; monitor LFTs, bilirubin baseline and prior to each dose

• **Infusion reactions that may be fatal:** fever, chills, nausea, vomiting, pain, headache, dizziness, hypotension; discontinue product
• **Pulmonary toxicity:** dyspnea, interstitial pneumonitis, pulmonary hypertension, ARDS; can occur after infusion reaction; those with lung disease may have more severe toxicity, discontinue in those with pneumonitis, interstitial lung disease
• **Bleeding:** monitor for bleeding; grade 3 or 4 bleeding with fatalities has occurred; check platelets baseline and prior to each dose

Black Box Warning: Hepatic disease: may be fatal; monitor LFTs, bilirubin baseline and before each dose

Evaluate:
• Therapeutic response: decrease in size, spread of breast cancer
Teach patient/family:
• Reason for product, expected result
• To take acetaminophen for fever
• To avoid hazardous tasks because confusion, dizziness may occur
• To report signs of infection: sore throat, fever, diarrhea, vomiting; bleeding; decreased heart function/SOB with exertion
• To report weight gain; swelling of the ankles, feet; fatigue; cough; bleeding

Side effects: *italics* = common; red = life-threatening

• **Infusion reactions:** to report pain at infusion site

aducanumab-avwa (Rx)
(a-due-KAN-ue-mab-avwa)
Aduhelm
Func. class.: Alzheimer agent
Chem. class.: Amyloid beta–directed antibody

ACTION:
A human immunoglobulin gamma 1 (IgG1) monoclonal antibody directed against amyloid beta, reduces amyloid beta plaques

USES:
Alzheimer disease

CONTRAINDICATIONS
None
Precautions: Amyloid-related imaging abnormalities (ARIAs), hypersensitivity, angioedema

DOSAGE AND ROUTES
• **Adult:** IV Titration, 1 mg/kg IV over 1 hour every 4 wk and at least 21 days apart for infusions 1 and 2; then 3 mg/kg IV over 1 hr every 4 wk and at least 21 days apart for infusions 3 and 4; and then 6 mg/kg IV over 1 hr every 4 wk and at least 21 days apart for infusions 5 and 6
Available forms: Injection 170 mg/1.7 mL (100 mg/mL), 300 mg/3 mL (100 mg/mL) solution single-dose vials
Administer:
• Titrate
• Obtain a recent (within 1 yr) brain MRI before use and before the 7th and 12th infusions. If severe ARIA-H is observed, may continue with caution only after a clinical evaluation and a follow-up MRI demonstrate radiographic stabilization

• Dilution in 100 mL of 0.9% Sodium Chloride Injection, USP, is required before administration. Give over 1 hr, use a 0.2- or 0.22-micron in-line filter
• Storage: Store in original carton until use, protect from light, refrigerated, do not freeze or shake; combined time out of refrigeration with protection from light max 24 hr at room temperature

SIDE EFFECTS
CNS: Headache
CV: Edema
HEMA: Microhemorrhage
MS: Falls
Syst: ARIA

INTERACTIONS
None known

PHARMACOKINETICS
Onset, peak, duration unknown

NURSING CONSIDERATIONS
Assess:
• **ARIA:** Assess for headache, confusion, dizziness, vision changes, nausea; notify prescriber
• **Hypersensitivity:** Assess for itching, rash, angioedema
Evaluate:
• Therapeutic response: Decreasing symptoms of Alzheimer disease (confusion)
Teach patient/family:
• **ARIA:** Teach patient that ARIA may occur with temporary swelling in areas of the brain, small spots of bleeding on the brain; to report headache, confusion, dizziness, vision changes, nausea. That MRIs will be needed
• **Hypersensitivity:** Inform patient that hypersensitivity, including angioedema, urticaria, may occur, to contact health care provider

afamelanotide (Rx)
(aˊfa-me-lanˊoh-tide)
Scenesse
Func. class.: Dermatologic agent
Chem. class.: Melanocortin receptor agonist

ACTION:
Increases production of eumelanin in the skin without exposure to sunlight or artificial UV light

USES:
To increase light exposure in those with phototoxic reactions from erythropoietic protoporphyria

CONTRAINDICATIONS
None
Precautions: Not approved in children

DOSAGE AND ROUTES
• **Adult:** SUBCUT 16 mg implanted above the anterior suprailiac crest q2mo
Available forms: Implant, SUBCUT 16 mg
Administer:
• This product should be implanted by a health care professional proficient in the SUBCUT implantation procedure
• Patients should maintain sun and light protection measures during treatment to prevent phototoxic reactions
• Monitor patient for 30 min after implant
• Leave dressing in place for 24 hr
• Store in refrigerator, protect from light

SIDE EFFECTS
CNS: Dizziness, fatigue, drowsiness
GI: Nausea
INTEG: Site reaction, melanocytic nevus, hyperpigmentation, skin irritation/discoloration
ENDO: Porphyria
RESP: Oropharyngeal pain, cough, respiratory tract infection

PHARMACOKINETICS
Onset unknown, peak 36 hr, duration 96 hr, half-life 15 hr

INTERACTIONS
None known

NURSING CONSIDERATIONS
Assess:
• **Skin pigmentation:** Increased skin pigmentation and darkening of preexisting nevi and ephelides may occur; obtain a full-body skin examination (twice yearly)

• **Phototoxic reactions:** Maintain sun and light protection measures during treatment to prevent phototoxic reactions
• **Pregnancy/breastfeeding:** Not known if safe in pregnancy or breastfeeding
Evaluate:
• Therapeutic response: Prevention of phototoxic reactions
Teach patient/family:
• To contact their health care provider if implant is expelled
• To remove dressing 24 hr after implant
• To monitor site and report reactions to their health care provider
• To maintain sun and light protection measures during treatment
• That darkening of preexisting nevi or other skin abnormalities may occur
• To schedule twice-yearly full-body skin exams

⚠ HIGH ALERT

afatinib (Rx)
(a-fat′i-nib)
Gilotrif
Func. class.: Antineoplastic biologic response modifiers

USES: Treatment of non–small-cell lung cancer whose tumors have epidermal growth factor receptor exon 19 deletions or 21 substitution mutations

CONTRAINDICATIONS
Pregnancy, hypersensitivity

DOSAGE AND ROUTES
• **Adult:** PO 40 mg daily until disease progression or unacceptable toxicity
Dose adjustments for toxicities:
• **Hepatotoxicity:** Hold in worsening liver function; when toxicity resolves to grade 1 or less, resume at a reduced dose (10 mg/day less than the dose causing hepatotoxicity); permanently discontinue for severe drug-induced hepatic impairment or if hepatotoxicity persists at a dose of 20 mg/day
• **Grade 2 or higher renal toxicity (CCr >1.5 × ULN):** Hold until the toxicity resolves to grade 1 or less (CCr <1.5 × ULN),

then resume at a reduced dose (10 mg/day less than the dose causing nephrotoxicity); permanently discontinue if nephrotoxicity persists at a dose of 20 mg/day

aflibercept (Rx)
(a-fli-ber'sept)
Eylea
Func. class.: Vascular endothelial growth factor inhibitor signal transduction inhibitor (STI) (ophthalmic)

USES: For treatment of neovascular (wet) age-related macular degeneration (AMD), macular edema after central retinal vein occlusion, diabetic retinopathy with diabetic macular edema

DOSAGE AND ROUTES
Neovascular age-related macular degeneration (wet)
Adult: Intravitreal injection 2 mg (0.05 mL) into affected eye q4wk × 12 wk, then 2mg q8wk
Diabetic macular edema/retinopathy
Adult: Intravitreal injection 2 mg (0.05 mL) q4wk × 5 injections, then 2 mg (0.05 mL) q8wk
Macular edema
Adult: Intravitreal injection: 2 mg (0.05 mL) q4wk
Available forms: Intravitreal injection 2 mg (0.05 mL) single-use vial
• **Adult: Intravitreal injection** 2 mg (0.05 mL) into affected eye(s) q4wk × 12 wk, then 2 mg (0.05 mL) q8wk

albuterol (Rx)
(al-byoo'ter-ole)
Airomir ♣, ProAir HFA, ProAir RespiClick, Proventil HFA, Ventolin Diskus ♣, Ventolin Nebules ♣, Ventolin HFA
Func. class.: Bronchodilator
Chem. class.: Adrenergic β$_2$-agonist, sympathomimetic, bronchodilator

Combinations: Combivent Respimat: albuterol/ipratropium 100 mcg/20 mcg/actuation; **DuoNEB:** 3 mg/0.5 mg/3 mL

Do not confuse:
albuterol/atenolol/Albutein
Proventil/Prinivil

ACTION: Causes bronchodilation by action on β$_2$ (pulmonary) receptors by increasing levels of cAMP

USES: Prevention of exercise-induced asthma, acute bronchospasm, bronchitis, emphysema, bronchiectasis, or other reversible airway obstruction
Unlabeled uses: Hyperkalemia in dialysis patients, COPD, emphysema

CONTRAINDICATIONS
Hypersensitivity to sympathomimetics
Precautions: Pregnancy, breastfeeding, cardiac/renal disease, hyperthyroidism, diabetes mellitus, hypertension, prostatic hypertrophy, angle-closure glaucoma, seizures, exercise-induced bronchospasm (aerosol) in children <12 yr, hypoglycemia, tachydysrhythmias, severe cardiac disease, heart block

DOSAGE AND ROUTES
Bronchospasm prophylaxis
• **Adult and child ≥4 yr: INH** (metered-dose inhaler) 2 puffs (180 mcg) q4-6hr as needed; **>12 yr INH** (powdered inhaler) (ProAir RespiClick) 180 mcg (2 INH) q4-6hr as needed
• **Adult and child ≥13 yr: PO** (ext rel) 4-8 mg q12hr, max 32 mg/day; **PO** (regular release) 2-4 mg tid, max 32 mg/day
• **Child 6-12 yr: PO** (extended release) 4 mg q12hr, max 24 mg/day; **PO** (regular release) 6-13 yr 2 mg tid-qid, max 24 mg/day
• **Child 2-5 yr: PO** 0.1 mg/kg tid, max 12 mg/day
• **Adult and child ≥15 yr: PO** (syrup) 2-4 mg tid-qid, max 32 mg/day
• **Child 6-14 yr: PO** (syrup) 2 mg tid-qid, max 24 mg/day
• **Child 2-5 yr: PO** (syrup) 0.1 mg/kg tid, max 12 mg/day

Acute bronchospasm
Adult/child >12 yr: INH 4-8 puffs q20min × 3 doses then taper; NEB 2.5 mg q20min × 3 doses then 2.5-10 mg q1-4hr or 10-15 mg continuously
Child <12 yr: INH 4-8 puffs q20min × 3 doses, then q1-4hr as needed; NEB: 0.15 mg/kg q20min × 3 doses, then 0.15-0.3 mg/kg q1-4hr as needed, max 10 mg q1-4hr as needed or 0.5 mg/kg/hr continuously

Asthma (unlabeled)
• **Child <4 yr:** INH (metered-dose inhaler) 180-600 mcg q2 min, max 6 doses; persistent asthma 2 puffs (HFA) q4-6hr

To prevent exercise-induced bronchospasm (not ProAir RespiClick)
• **Adult/child ≥4 yr:** INH 2 puffs before exercise, max 12 puffs/24 hr
• **Adult/child ≥12 yr:** INH (ProAir RespiClick) 2 puffs 15-30 min prior to exercise

Hyperkalemia (unlabeled)
• **Adult:** ORAL INH (albuterol nebulizer solution) 10-20 mg over 15 min
Available forms: INH aerosol 100 mcg/actuation ✦, INH powder 108 mcg/actuation; syrup 2 mg/5 mL; tablets 2, 4 mg; ext rel 4, 8 mg; INH sol 0.63 mg/3 mL, 1.25 mg/3 mL, 2.5 mg/3 mL, 0.5 mg/mL ✦, 1 mg/mL ✦, 2 mg/mL ✦, 5 mg/1 mL ✦
Administer:
• Store in light-resistant container; do not expose to temperatures of more than 86° F (30° C)
PO route
• Do not break, crush, or chew extended-release tablets; give with meals to decrease gastric irritation
• **Oral solution** to children (no alcohol, sugar)
Inhalation route
• For geriatric patients and children, a spacing device is advised
• After shaking metered-dose inhaler, prime before first use, a spacer may be needed, exhale, place mouthpiece in mouth, inhale slowly while depressing inhaler, hold breath, remove, exhale slowly; give INH at least 1 min apart
• Rinse mouth with water after use

• **NEB/IPPB** dilute 5 mg/mL solution/2.5 mL 0.9% NaCl for INH; other solutions do not require dilution; for NEB O_2 flow or compressed air 6-10 L/min, 1 treatment lasts 10 min; IPPB 5-20 min
ProAir Respistick:
• Prior to using for the first time, check that the number "200" is showing. Do not wash or put any part of the inhaler in water; if the mouthpiece needs cleaning, wipe with a dry cloth or tissue; when there are "20" doses left, the counter will change to red; refill

SIDE EFFECTS
CNS: *Tremors, anxiety,* insomnia, headache, stimulation, *restlessness*
CV: Angina, hypo/hypertension, dysrhythmias, chest pain
EENT: Dry nose, irritation of nose and throat
GI: Nausea, vomiting
MISC: Hyperglycemia
RESP: Paradoxical bronchospasm

PHARMACOKINETICS
Extensively metabolized in the liver and tissues, crosses placenta, breast milk, blood-brain barrier, half-life 2.7-6 hr, well absorbed
PO: Onset ½ hr, peak 2-3 hr, duration 4-6 hr
PO-ER: Onset ½ hr, peak 2-3 hr, duration 8-12 hr
INH: Onset 5-15 min, peak 1.5-2 hr, duration 2-6 hr, half-life 4 hr

INTERACTIONS
Decrease: digoxin level—digoxin
Increase: CNS stimulation—CNS stimulants
Increase: ECG changes/hypokalemia—potassium-losing diuretics
Increase: action of aerosol bronchodilators
Increase: action of albuterol—tricyclics, MAOIs, other adrenergics; avoid use
Increase: CV effects—atomoxetine, selegiline
Decrease: albuterol—other β-blockers (caredilol, labetalol, metoprolol)

Side effects: *italics* = common; red = life-threatening

Drug/Herb
Increase: stimulation—caffeine (cola nut, green/black tea, guarana, yerba maté, coffee, chocolate)
Drug/Lab Test
Decrease: potassium

NURSING CONSIDERATIONS
Assess:
• **Respiratory function:** vital capacity, pulse oximetry, forced expiratory volume, ABGs, VBGs; lung sounds, heart rate and rhythm, B/P, sputum (baseline and peak); whether patient has received theophylline therapy before giving dose
• **Labs:** Blood glucose, potassium
• Patient's ability to self-medicate
• Trouble breathing with wheezing, hold medication, notify prescriber if bronchospasm occurs
• **Pregnancy/breastfeeding:** identify if pregnancy is planned or suspected; use only if necessary; avoid breastfeeding
Evaluate:
• Therapeutic response: absence of dyspnea, wheezing; improved airway exchange; improved ABGs, VBGs
Teach patient/family:
• To use exactly as prescribed; to take missed dose when remembered, alter dosing schedule; not to use OTC medications; that excess stimulation may occur, to use this product before other medications, allow 5 min between each
• About use of inhaler: review package insert with patient; use demonstration, return demonstration; shake, prime before first use and when not used for >2 wk; release 4 test sprays into air, away from the face; about when empty and when to renew, a bad taste may occur
• To avoid getting aerosol in eyes (blurring of vision may result) or use near flames or sources of heat
• Do not wash inhaler, wipe with dry cloth, to discard product when counter changes to red
• To avoid smoking, smoke-filled rooms, persons with respiratory infections
• That paradoxical bronchospasm may occur; to stop product immediately, call prescriber, usually from first dose of new inhaler
• To limit caffeine products such as chocolate, coffee, tea, colas
• **Pregnancy/breastfeeding:** to advise prescriber if pregnancy is planned or suspected, or if breastfeeding
• To notify health care professional immediately if product does not relieve symptoms, corticosteroids may be needed

TREATMENT OF OVERDOSE: Administer β_1-adrenergic blocker, IV fluids

---

albumin, human 5% (Rx)
(al-byoo′min)
AlbuKed 5%, Albuminex 5%, AlbuRx 5%, Flexbumin 5%, Albutein 5%, Plasbumin-5
albumin, human 25%
Albutein 25%, Plasbumin-25
Func. class.: Plasma volume expander

USES: Restores plasma volume after burns, hyperbilirubinemia, shock, hypoproteinemia, prevention of cerebral edema, cardiopulmonary bypass procedures, ARDS, nephrotic syndrome

CONTRAINDICATIONS
Hypersensitivity, HF, severe anemia, renal insufficiency, pulmonary edema

DOSAGE AND ROUTES
Burns
• **Adult: IV** dose to maintain plasma albumin at 3-4 mg/dL
Hypovolemic shock
• **Adult: IV** rapidly give 5% solution, when close to normal, infuse at ≤2-4 mL/min (25% sol ≤1 mL/min)
• **Child: IV** 0.5-1 g/kg/dose 5% solution, may repeat as needed, max 6 g/kg/day
Nephrotic syndrome
• **Adult: IV** 100-200 mL of 25% and loop diuretic × 7-10 days

Hypoproteinemia
• **Adult:** IV 25 g, may repeat in 15-30 min, or 50-75 g of 25% albumin infused at ≤2 mL/min
• **Child and infant:** IV 0.5-1 g/kg/dose over 2-4 hr, may repeat q1-2days
Hyperbilirubinemia/erythroblastosis fetalis
• **Child:** IV 1 g/kg 1-2 hr before transfusion

▲ HIGH ALERT

alectinib (Rx)
[al-ek'ti-nib]
Alecensa, Alecensaro ✦
Func. class.: Antineoplastics
Chem. class.: Tyrosine kinase inhibitor

alendronate/risedronate

Combinations: Fosamax D:
alendronate 70 mg/vitamin D analogue 2800 IU; 70 mg/5600 IU

ACTION: Targets ALK, RET genes, decreasing proliferation of cancer cells

USES: For the treatment of metastatic, ALK-positive, non–small-cell lung cancer (NSCLC), pregnancy, breastfeeding

CONTRAINDICATIONS
Hypersensitivity, pregnancy, breastfeeding

PRECAUTIONS: Child: Liver disease, pulmonary disease

DOSAGE AND ROUTES
• **Adult: PO** 600 mg bid, with food, until disease progression or unacceptable toxicity
Hepatic Dose
Adult: Child-Pugh Class C 450 mg bid
Available forms: Capsules 150 mg
Administer
• Use cytotoxic handling procedures
• Give capsule whole; do not open, cut, or break
• Use with food
• Do not double doses; if dose is missed, give at next regularly scheduled time

• Storage: Protect from light, store at room temperature below 86° F (30° C)

SIDE EFFECTS
CV: Bradycardia, edema
CNS: Headache, fatigue
HEMA: Anemia, neutropenia, lymphopenia
GI: Vomiting, nausea, anorexia, constipation, diarrhea, hepatotoxicity, increased weight
META: Hypocalcemia, hyperglycemia, hypokalemia, hyponatremia
MS: Myalgia
RESP: Dyspnea, cough
INTEG: Rash, photosensitivity

PHARMACOKINETICS
Onset unknown, peak 4 hr, duration unknown, 99% protein binding, metabolized by the liver, excreted by the kidney

INTERACTIONS
Increased: bradycardia, other products causing bradycardia, monitor carefully

NURSING CONSIDERATIONS
Assess:
• **Bradycardia:** Heart rate <50 beats per min. Monitor heart rate and B/P regularly. If symptomatic bradycardia (non-life-threatening) occurs, withhold treatment until recovery to asymptomatic bradycardia or to a heart rate of ≥60 beats per min
• **Hepatotoxicity:** Monitor liver function tests (ALT, AST, and total bilirubin) every 2 wk during the first 3 mo and then once a mo and as needed; monitor more frequently in patients who develop transaminase and bilirubin elevations. May require therapy interruption, dose reduction, or permanent discontinuation
• **Myalgia:** Monitor for muscle pain, tenderness, or weakness. Assess CPK every 2 wk for the first mo of therapy and then as needed
• **Photosensitivity:** Patients should avoid sun exposure (during treatment and for 7 days after the final dose) and use a sunscreen

• **Pulmonary toxicity:** Monitor for ILD/pneumonitis; evaluate worsening of respiratory symptoms or signs/symptoms of ILD/pneumonitis (cough, dyspnea, fever). Immediately interrupt for confirmed ILD/pneumonitis; permanently discontinue if these occur

• **Renal toxicity:** Monitor for renal toxicity, may require discontinuation

• **Pregnancy/breastfeeding:** Do not use during pregnancy or breastfeeding, use contraception during and for 1 wk after last dose if of childbearing potential; males should use contraception during and for 3 mo after last dose if female partner is of childbearing potential

Patient/family teaching

• To report constipation, vomiting, nausea, diarrhea, weight gain, headache if these are severe or do not go away

• To report liver problems like dark urine, fatigue, lack of appetite, nausea, abdominal pain, light-colored stools, vomiting, or yellow skin

• To report symptoms of infection

• To report lung problems like shortness of breath or other trouble breathing, cough that is new or worse

• To report kidney problems like unable to pass urine, blood in the urine, change in amount of urine passed, or weight gain

• To report high blood sugar like confusion, fatigue, increased thirst, increased hunger, passing a lot of urine, flushing, fast breathing, or breath that smells like fruit

• To report electrolyte problems like mood changes, confusion, muscle pain or weakness, abnormal heartbeat, seizures, lack of appetite, or severe nausea or vomiting

• To report severe loss of strength and energy

• To report slow heartbeat, dizziness, passing out

• To report muscle pain, back pain, muscle weakness

• To report swelling in arms, legs, or vision changes

• To report allergic reactions, like rash; hives; itching; red, swollen, blistered; wheezing; tightness in the chest or throat; trouble breathing, swallowing, or talking; unusual hoarseness; or swelling of the mouth, face, lips, tongue, or throat

• To notify your prescriber if pregnancy is planned or suspected, or if breastfeeding

---

alendronate (Rx)

(al-en-drone′ate)

Binosto, Fosamax, Fosamax plus D, Fosavance ✦

Func. class.: Bone-resorption inhibitor
Chem. class.: Bisphosphonate

Do not confuse:
Fosamax/Flomax
alendronate/risedronate

Combinations: Fosamax D:
alendronate 70 mg/vitamin D analogue 2800 IU; 70 mg/5600 IU

ACTION: Decreases rate of bone resorption and may directly block dissolution of hydroxyapatite crystals of bone; inhibits osteoclast activity

USES: Treatment and prevention of osteoporosis in postmenopausal women, treatment of osteoporosis in men, Paget's disease, treatment of corticosteroid-induced osteoporosis in postmenopausal women not receiving estrogen and in men who are on continuing corticosteroid treatment with low bone mass

CONTRAINDICATIONS

Hypersensitivity to bisphosphonates, delayed esophageal emptying, inability to sit or stand for 30 min, hypocalcemia, pregnancy, breastfeeding, children, CCr <35 mL/min

Precautions: Esophageal disease, ulcers, gastritis, poor dental health, increased esophageal cancer risk

DOSAGE AND ROUTES

Osteoporosis in postmenopausal women

• **Adult and geriatric:** PO 10 mg/day or 70 mg/wk

Paget's disease
• **Adult and geriatric: PO** 40 mg/day × 6 mo; consider retreatment for relapse
Prevention of osteoporosis in postmenopausal women (excluding Binosto and oral solution)
Adult/postmenopausal female: PO 5 mg/day or 35 mg/wk
Glucocorticoid-induced osteoporosis in those receiving glucocorticosteroids
• **Adult: PO** 5 mg/day; those not receiving estrogen 10 mg/day
Androgen deprivation therapy/osteoporosis prevention
Adult: PO 70 mg weekly
Renal dose
• **Adult: PO** CCr ≤35 mL/min, not recommended
Available forms: Tablets 5, 10, 35, 40, 70 mg; tablets 70 mg with 2800 IU vitamin D_3, 70 mg with 5600 IU vitamin D_3; oral sol 70 mg/75 mL; effervescent tablet 70 mg
Administer:
• For 6 mo to be effective for Paget's disease
• Store in cool environment, out of direct sunlight
• **Tablet:** take with 8 oz of water 30 min before first food, beverage, or medication of the day
• Do not lie down for ≥30 min after dose; do not take at bedtime or before rising
• **Oral solution:** use oral syringe or calibrated device; give in AM with ≥2 oz of water ≥30 min before food, beverage, or medication
• **Effervescent tablet:** Dissolve in 4 oz of water, after 5 min, stir and drink

SIDE EFFECTS
RESP: Asthma exacerbation
CV: Atrial fibrillation
INTEG: Rash, photosensitivity
CNS: Headache
GI: *Abdominal pain, constipation, nausea, vomiting, esophageal ulceration,* acid reflux, dyspepsia, esophageal perforation, diarrhea, esophageal cancer

META: Hypophosphatemia, hypocalcemia
MS: Bone pain, osteonecrosis of the jaw, bone fractures

PHARMACOKINETICS
Protein binding 78%, rapidly cleared from circulation, taken up mainly by bones, eliminated primarily through kidneys, bound to bone, half-life >10 yr

INTERACTIONS
Increase: GI adverse reactions—NSAIDs, salicylates, H_2 blockers, proton pump inhibitors, gastric mucosal agents; monitor for GI reactions
Decrease: absorption—antacids, calcium supplements; give alendronate at least 30-60 min before other products
Drug/Food
Decrease: absorption when used with caffeine, orange juice, food; take food at least 30 min after alendronate
Drug/Lab Test
Decrease: calcium, phosphate, alkaline phosphatase

NURSING CONSIDERATIONS
Assess:
• Hormonal status of women before treatment, history of fractures
• **For osteoporosis:** bone density test before and during treatment
• **For Paget's disease:** increased skull size, bone pain, headache; decreased vision, hearing; alkaline phosphatase levels, baseline and periodically, 2× upper limit of normal is indicative of Paget's disease
• **Labs:** Alkaline phosphatase, serum calcium, phosphate; serum creatinine/BUN, serum vitamin D baseline and periodically
• **For hypercalcemia:** paresthesia, twitching, laryngospasm; Chvostek's, Trousseau's signs
• Dental status: regular dental exams should be performed; dental extractions (cover with antiinfectives before procedure)
• **MS pain:** may occur in a few days or years later, symptoms usually resolve after discontinuing

Side effects: *italics* = common; red = life-threatening

Evaluate:
• Therapeutic response: increased bone mass, absence of fractures
Teach patient/family:
• To remain upright for 30 min after dose to prevent esophageal irritation; if dose is missed, skip dose, do not double doses or take later in day; to take in AM before food, other meds; to take with 6-8 oz of water only (no mineral water)
• To take calcium, vitamin D if instructed by health care provider
• To use sunscreen, protective clothing to prevent photosensitivity
• To avoid smoking, alcohol intake, which increase osteoporosis
• To perform weight-bearing exercise to increase bone density
• To maintain good oral hygiene, to use antiinfectives before dental procedures as directed by prescriber
• **Pregnancy/breastfeeding:** to inform prescriber if pregnancy is planned or suspected; that cautious use is advised in breastfeeding

alfuzosin (Rx)
(al-fyoo'zoe-sin)
Uroxatral, Xatral ♣
Func. class.: Urinary tract, antispasmodic, α₁-agonist

USES: Symptoms of benign prostatic hyperplasia

DOSAGE AND ROUTES
• **Adult:** PO EXTENDED RELEASE 10 mg/day

Available forms: Tablets, extended release 10 mg

alirocumab (Rx)
(al'-i-rok'-ue-mab)
Praluent
Func. class.: Antilipemic

USES: Heterozygous, familial hypercholesterolemia, atherosclerotic disease

DOSAGE AND ROUTES
• **Adult: SUBCUT** 75 mg q2wk, may increase to 150 mg q2wk if needed after 4-8 wk or 300 mg q4wk
Available forms: Injection: 75 mg/mL, 150 mg/mL (single-dose pens/syringes)

aliskiren (Rx)
(a-lis'kir-en)
Rasilez ♣, Tekturna
Func. class.: Antihypertensive
Chem. class.: Direct renin inhibitor

ACTION: Renin inhibitor that acts on the renin-angiotensin system (RAS)

USES: Hypertension, alone or in combination with other antihypertensives

Black Box Warning: Pregnancy

Precautions: Breastfeeding, children, geriatric patients, angioedema, aortic/renal artery stenosis, cirrhosis, CAD, dialysis, hyper/hypokalemia, hyponatremia, hypotension, hypovolemia, renal/hepatic disease, surgery, diabetes

DOSAGE AND ROUTES
• **Adult/child ≥6 yr and >50 kg: PO** 150 mg/day, may increase to 300 mg/day if needed, max 300 mg/day
Child ≥6 yr and 20-50 kg: PO 75 mg daily, max 150 mg/day
Available forms: Tablets 150, 300 mg
Administer:
• May use with other antihypertensives
• Do not use with a high-fat meal
• Daily with a full glass of water; titrate up to achieve correct dose
• Do not discontinue abruptly; correct electrolyte/volume depletion before treatment
• Store in tight container at room temperature

SIDE EFFECTS
CV: Orthostatic hypotension, hypotension
CNS: Headache, dizziness, seizures
GI: *Diarrhea*
GU: Renal stones, increased uric acid

INTEG: Rash
META: Hyperkalemia
MISC: Angioedema, cough

PHARMACOKINETICS
Poorly absorbed, bioavailability 2.5%, peak 1-3 hr, steady state 7-8 days, 91% excreted unchanged in the feces, half-life 24 hr

INTERACTIONS
• Do not use with ACE inhibitors, angiotensin II receptor antagonists in diabetes mellitus
Increase: potassium levels—ACE inhibitors, angiotensin II receptor antagonists, potassium supplements, potassium-sparing diuretics
Increase: hypotension—other antihypertensives, diuretics
Increase: aliskiren levels—atorvastatin, itraconazole, ketoconazole, cycloSPORINE; concurrent use is not recommended
Decrease: levels of warfarin
Drug/Food
Decrease: aliskiren effect—high-fat meal, grapefruit
Drug/Lab Test
Increase: uric acid, BUN, serum creatinine, potassium

NURSING CONSIDERATIONS
Assess:
• Renal studies: uric acid, serum creatinine, BUN may be increased; hyperkalemia may occur; correct salt depletion, hyperkalemia, volume before starting therapy
• **Allergic reactions:** angioedema may occur (swelling of face; trouble breathing, swallowing)
• Daily dependent edema in feet, legs; weight, B/P, orthostatic hypotension
• **Diabetes:** identify the use of ACE inhibitors, angiotensin II receptor antagonists; if in use, do not use aliskiren
Evaluate:
• Therapeutic response: decrease in B/P
Teach patient/family:
• About the importance of complying with dosage schedule even if feeling better; that if dose is missed, take as soon as possible; that if it is almost time for the next dose, take only that dose; do not double dose; do not take with high-fat meal or grapefruit
• How to take B/P and normal reading for age group
• Not to use OTC products including herbs, supplements unless approved by prescriber
• **To report to prescriber immediately:** dizziness, faintness, chest pain, palpitations, uneven or rapid heartbeat, headache, severe diarrhea, swelling of tongue or lips, trouble breathing, difficulty swallowing, tightening of the throat
• Not to operate machinery or perform hazardous tasks if dizziness occurs
• To rise slowly to avoid faintness

Black Box Warning: Pregnancy: To notify if pregnancy is planned or suspected; if pregnant, product will need to be discontinued

allopurinol (Rx)
(al-oh-pure′i-nole)
Aloprim, Zyloprim
Func. class.: Antigout drug, antihyperuricemic
Chem. class.: Xanthine oxidase inhibitor

Do not confuse:
Zyloprim/Zovirax/zolpidem
alendronate/risedronate

Combinations: Fosamax D:
alendronate 70 mg/vitamin D analogue 2800 IU; 70 mg/5600 IU

ACTION: Inhibits the enzyme xanthine oxidase, reducing uric acid synthesis

USES: Chronic gout, hyperuricemia associated with malignancies, recurrent calcium oxalate calculi, uric acid calculi

CONTRAINDICATIONS
Hypersensitivity

Precautions: Pregnancy, breastfeeding, children, renal/hepatic disease

DOSAGE AND ROUTES
Increased uric acid levels in malignancies
- **Adult/child >10 yr: PO** 600-800 mg/day in divided doses for 2-3 days; start up to 1-2 days before chemotherapy; **IV INFUSION** 200-400 mg/m^2/day, 24-48 hr before chemotherapy, may be divided at 6-, 8-, 12-hr intervals; max 600 mg/day
- **Child 6-10 yr: PO** 300 mg/day, adjust dose after 48 hr; max 400 mg/day
- **Child <6 yr: PO** 150 mg/day, adjust dose after 48 hr
- **Child ≤10 yr: IV INFUSION** 200 mg/m^2/day, initially as a single dose or divided q6-12hr

Recurrent calculi
- **Adult: PO** 200-300 mg/day in a single dose or divided bid-tid

Uric acid nephropathy prevention
- **Adult and child >10 yr: PO** 600-800 mg/day × 2-3 days

Gout (mild)
- **Adult: PO** 100 mg/day, titrating upward, max 800 mg/day

Recurrent uric acid calcium exalate calculi
Adult: PO 300 mg/day in 1 or 2-3 divided doses; titrate dose to 24-hr urinary urate level

Renal dose
- **Adult: PO/IV** CCr 81-100 mL/min 300 mg/day; CCr 61-80 mL/min 250 mg/day; CCr 41-60 mL/min 200 mg/day; CCr 21-40 mL/min 150 mg/day; CCr 10-20 mL/min 100-200 mg/day; CCr 3-9 mL/min 100 mg/day or 100 mg every other day; CCr <3 mL/min 100 mg q24hr or longer or 100 mg every 3rd day

Available forms: Tablets, scored 100, 300 mg; powder for injection 500 mg/vial

Administer:
PO route
- With meals to prevent GI symptoms; may crush, add to foods or fluids
- Begin 1-2 days before antineoplastic therapy

Intermittent IV INFUSION route
- Use in tumor lysis prior to start of chemotherapy (24-48 hr)
- Reconstitute 30-mL vial with 25 mL of sterile water for inj; dilute to desired concentrations (≤6 mg/mL) with 0.9% NaCl for inj or D$_5$W for inj; begin infusion within 10 hr

Y-site compatibilities: Acyclovir, aminophylline, amphotericin B lipid complex, anidulafungin, argatroban, atenolol, aztreonam, bivalirudin, bleomycin, bumetanide, buprenorphine, butorphanol, calcium gluconate, CARBOplatin, caspofungin, ceFAZolin, cefoTEtan, cefTAZidime, ceftizoxime, cefTRIAXone, cefuroxime, CISplatin, cyclophosphamide, DACTINomycin, DAUNOrubicin citrate liposome, dexamethasone, dexmedetomidine, DOCEtaxel, DOXOrubicin liposomal, enalaprilat, etoposide, famotidine, fenoldopam, filgrastim, fluconazole, fludarabine, fluorouracil, furosemide, gallium, ganciclovir, gatifloxacin, gemcitabine, gemtuzumab, granisetron hydrochloride, heparin, hydrocortisone phosphate, hydrocortisone succinate, HYDROmorphone, ifosfamide, linezolid injection, LORazepam, mannitol, mesna, methotrexate, metroNIDAZOLE, milrinone, mitoXANtrone, morphine, nesiritide, octreotide, oxytocin, PACLitaxel, pamidronate, pantoprazole, PEMEtrexed, piperacillin, piperacillin-tazobactam, plicamycin, potassium chloride, raNITIdine, sodium acetate, sulfamethoxazole-trimethoprim, teniposide, thiotepa, ticarcillin, ticarcillin-clavulanate, tigecycline, tirofiban, vancomycin, vasopressin, vinBLAStine, vinCRIStine, voriconazole, zidovudine, zoledronic acid

SIDE EFFECTS
GI: *Nausea, vomiting, malaise,* diarrhea, hepatitis
INTEG: Rash
CV: Hypo- and hypertension, HF (IV use)
CNS: Drowsiness
GU: Renal failure
MISC: Hypersensitivity, bone marrow depression
MS: Acute gouty attack

PHARMACOKINETICS
Protein binding <1%, half-life 1-2 hr
PO: Peak 1.5 hr; excreted in feces, urine
IV: Peak up to 30 min

INTERACTIONS
Alcohol, diazoxide: increased urate risk, may need dosage increased
Increase: rash—ampicillin, amoxicillin; avoid concurrent use
Increase: action of oral anticoagulants
Increase: hypersensitivity, toxicity—ACE inhibitors, thiazides
Increase: bone marrow depression—(mercaptopurine, azaTHIOprine)

NURSING CONSIDERATIONS
Assess:
• **For gout:** joint pain, swelling; may use with NSAIDs for acute gouty attacks; effect may take several weeks
• **Labs:** CBC, AST, ALT, BUN, creatinine, uric acid levels, BMP; LFTs (hepatic disease) before starting treatment, periodically
• I&O ratio; increase fluids to 2 L/day to prevent stone formation and toxicity
• For rash, hypersensitivity reactions, discontinue allopurinol immediately, after rash is resolved, treatment may continue at a lower dose
Evaluate:
• Therapeutic response: decreased pain in joints, decreased stone formation in kidneys, decreased uric acid levels
Teach patient/family:
• To take as prescribed; if dose is missed, take as soon as remembered; do not double dose; tablets may be crushed
• To increase fluid intake to 2 L/day
• To report skin rash, stomatitis, malaise, fever, aching; product should be discontinued
• To avoid hazardous activities if drowsiness or dizziness occurs
• To avoid alcohol, caffeine; will increase uric acid levels
• An alkaline diet may be required
• That follow-up examinations and blood work will be needed
• To identify triggers and avoid

• To avoid large doses of vitamin C; kidney stone formation may occur
• To reduce dairy products, refined sugars, sodium, meat if taking for calcium oxalate stones; to identify triggers and avoid

almotriptan (Rx)
(al-moh-trip′tan)
Func. class.: Antimigraine agent, abortive
Chem. class.: 5-HT₁-receptor agonist, triptan

Do not confuse:
almotriptan/alvinopan

ACTION: Binds selectively to the vascular 5-HT$_{1B/1D/1F}$-receptors, exerts antimigraine effect

USES: Acute treatment of migraine with or without aura (adult/adolescent/child ≥12 yr)

CONTRAINDICATIONS
Hypersensitivity, acute MI, angina, CV disease, CAD, stroke, vasospastic angina, ischemic heart disease or risk for, peripheral vascular syndrome, uncontrolled hypertension, basilar or hemiplegic migraine
Precautions: Pregnancy, postmenopausal women, men >40 yr, breastfeeding, children <18 yr, geriatric patients, risk factors for CAD, MI; hypercholesterolemia, obesity, diabetes, impaired renal/hepatic function, sulfonamide hypersensitivity, cardiac dysrhythmias, Raynaud's disease, tobacco smoking, Wolff-Parkinson-White syndrome

DOSAGE AND ROUTES
Migraine headache
• **Adult, adolescent, and child ≥12 yr:** **PO** 6.25 or 12.5 mg; may repeat dose after 2 hr; max 2 doses/24 hr or 4 treatment cycles within any 30-day period; max of 25 mg/day
Use with CYP3A4 inhibitors
Adult: PO 6.25 mg, max 12.5 mg/day
Hepatic/renal dose
• **Adult: PO** (CCr 10-30 mL/min) 6.25 mg initially, max 12.5 mg

Available forms: Tablets 6.25, 12.5 mg
Administer:
- Avoid using more than 2×/24 hr; rebound headache may occur
- Swallow tablets whole; do not break, crush, chew tablets, without regard to food

SIDE EFFECTS

CNS: *Dizziness,* headache, seizures, paresthesias
CV: Coronary artery vasospasm, MI, ventricular fibrillation, ventricular tachycardia
GI: Nausea, xerostomia
INTEG: Sweating, rash

PHARMACOKINETICS

Onset of pain relief 2 hr; peak 1-3 hr; duration 3-4 hr; bioavailability 70%; protein binding 35%; metabolized in the liver (metabolite), metabolized by MAO-A, CYP2D6, CYP3A4; excreted in urine (40%), feces (13%); half-life 3-4 hr

INTERACTIONS

Increase: serotonin syndrome—SSRIs, SNRIs, serotonin-receptor agonists, sibutramine
Increase: vasospastic effects—ergot, ergot derivatives, other 5-HT1 agonists; avoid concurrent use
Increase: almotriptan effect—MAOIs; do not use together
Increase: plasma concentration of almotriptan—(CYP3A4 inhibitors) itraconazole, ritonavir, erythromycin, ketoconazole; avoid concurrent use in renal/hepatic disease, use 6.25 mg/day max 12.5 mg/day
Drug/Herb
Avoid use with feverfew
Increase: serotonin syndrome—St. John's wort

NURSING CONSIDERATIONS
Assess:
- **Migraine:** pain location, aura, duration, intensity, nausea, vomiting; quiet, calm environment with decreased stimulation from noise, bright light, excessive talking
- **Serotonin syndrome:** in those taking SSRIs, SNRIs; agitation, confusion, hallucinations, diaphoresis, hypertension, diarrhea, fever, tremors; usually occurs when dose is increased
- B/P; signs/symptoms of coronary vasospasms
- For stress level, activity, recreation, coping mechanisms
- **Neurologic status:** LOC, blurring vision, nausea, vomiting, tingling, hot sensation, burning, feeling of pressure, numbness, flushing preceding headache
- **Tyramine foods** (pickled products, beer, wine, aged cheese), food additives, preservatives, colorings, artificial sweeteners, chocolate, caffeine, which may precipitate these types of headaches
Evaluate:
- Therapeutic response: decrease in severity of migraine
Teach patient/family:
- To report chest pain, drowsiness, dizziness, tingling, flushing
- To notify prescriber if pregnancy is planned or suspected; to avoid breastfeeding
- That if 1 dose does not relieve migraine, to take another after 2 hr, max 4 treatment cycles in 30 days; do not take MAOIs for ≥24 hr
- That product does not prevent or reduce number of migraine attacks; use to relieve attack only
- **Serotonin syndrome:** To report immediately signs of serotonin syndrome
- To report immediately chest tightness or pain
- Not to drive or operate machinery until reaction is known, drowsiness, dizziness may occur
- To inform all health care professionals of all OTC, Rx, herbals, supplements taken

---

⚠ HIGH ALERT

alogliptin (Rx)
(al'oh-glip'tin)
Nesina
Func. class.: Antidiabetic
Chem. class.: Dipeptidyl peptidase-4 (DPP-4) inhibitor

ACTION: A dipeptidyl-peptidase-IV (DDP-IV) inhibitor potentiates the effects of the incretin hormones by inhibiting their breakdown by DDP-IV

USES: Type 2 diabetes mellitus (T2DM)

CONTRAINDICATIONS
Hypersensitivity, ketoacidosis, type 1 diabetes

Precautions: Pregnancy, breastfeeding, hepatic disease, burns, diarrhea, fever, GI obstruction, hyper/hypoglycemia, hyper/hypothyroidism, hypercortisolism, children, ileus, malnutrition, pancreatitis, surgery, trauma, vomiting, kidney disease, adrenal insufficiency, angioedema

DOSAGE AND ROUTES
• **Adult:** PO 25 mg/day
Renal dose
• **Adult:** PO CCr 30-59 mL/min: 12.5 mg every day; CCr <30 mL/min: 6.25 mg every day; intermittent hemodialysis: 6.25 mg every day; give without regard to the timing of hemodialysis
Available forms: Tablets 6.25, 12.5, 25 mg
Administer:
• Without regard to food

SIDE EFFECTS
CNS: Headache
GI: Pancreatitis, hepatotoxicity
CV: Heart failure
SYST: Rash, hypersensitivity, angioedema, Stevens-Johnson syndrome, anaphylaxis

PHARMACOKINETICS
20% protein binding, excreted unchanged (urine), peak 1-2 hr, duration up to 24 hr, effect decreased in liver disease and increased in kidney disease, half-life 21 hr

INTERACTIONS
Increase: hypoglycemia—insulin, androgens, pegvisomant, sulfonylureas; dosage adjustment may be needed
Decrease: hypoglycemia—danazol, thiazides; adjust dose
Drug/Lab Test
Increase: LFTs
Decrease: glucose

NURSING CONSIDERATIONS
Assess:
• **Diabetes:** monitor blood glucose, glycosylated hemoglobin A1c (A1c), LFTs, serum creatinine/BUN baseline and throughout treatment
• **Pancreatitis:** can occur during use; monitor for severe abdominal pain, with or without vomiting
• **Hypersensitivity reactions:** angioedema, Stevens-Johnson syndrome; product should be discontinued
• **HF:** Assess for risk of HF in those with known HF or kidney disease
Evaluate:
• Positive therapeutic response: decrease in polyuria, polydipsia, polyphagia, clear sensorium, absence of dizziness, improvement in A1c
Teach patient/family:
• **Hepatotoxicity:** To report yellowing of skin, eyes, dark urine, clay-colored stools, nausea, vomiting
• That diabetes is a lifelong condition, product does not cure disease
• That all food in diet plan must be eaten to prevent hypoglycemia; to continue with weight control, dietary medical nutrition therapy, physical activity, hygiene
• To carry emergency ID with prescriber, medications, and condition listed
• To test blood glucose using a blood glucose meter, and urine ketones
• To report allergic reactions, nausea, vomiting, abdominal pain, dark urine
• **Hypersensitivity:** To notify health care professional and stop taking product if rash; trouble breathing; swelling of face, lips, tongue occur
• To notify all health care professionals of OTC, Rx, herbs, supplements used
• **Pregnancy/breastfeeding:** To report if pregnancy is planned or suspected, or if breastfeeding

alosetron (Rx)
(ah-loss′a-tron)
Lotronex
Func. class.: Anti-IBS agent

Side effects: *italics* = common; red = life-threatening

USES: Severe, chronic, diarrhea-predominant irritable bowel syndrome (IBS) in women who have failed conventional therapy

CONTRAINDICATIONS
Crohn's disease, severe hepatic disease, diverticulitis, toxic megacolon, GI adhesions/strictures/obstruction/perforation, thrombophlebitis, ulcerative colitis

Black Box Warning: Ischemic colitis, severe constipation

DOSAGE AND ROUTES
• **Adult woman: PO** 0.5 mg bid, may increase to 1 mg bid after 4 wk if well tolerated; if symptoms are not controlled after 4 wk of treatment with 1 mg bid, discontinue
Available forms: Tablets 0.5 mg, 1 mg

⚠ HIGH ALERT

alpelisib (Rx)
(al-peh-lih'-sib)
Piqray, Vijoice
Func. class.: Antineoplastic
Chem. class.: Small molecule antineoplastic phosphatidylinositol-3-kinase (PI3K) inhibitors

---

Do not confuse:
alpebelisib/duvelisib/copanlisib/idelalisib

ACTION: In breast cancer cell lines, inhibits the phosphorylation of PI3K downstream targets, including Akt, and showed activity in cell lines harboring a ⁄⊙⍺ *PI3KCA* mutation

USES: Hormone receptor (HR)–positive, *HER2*–negative, ⁄⊙⍺ *PIK3CA*-mutated, advanced or metastatic breast cancer in men and postmenopausal women after progression on or after an endocrine-based regimen, in combination with fulvestrant

CONTRAINDICATIONS
Hypersensitivity, pregnancy
Precautions:
Breastfeeding, chronic lung disorders, contraceptive requirement, diabetes mellitus, diarrhea, hyperglycemia, infertility, interstitial lung disease, male- mediated teratogenicity

DOSAGE AND ROUTES
Breast Cancer
Adult: PO 300 mg PO daily with food, in combination with fulvestrant (500 mg IM on days 1, 15, and 29 and monthly thereafter) until disease progression or unacceptable toxicity

PIK3CA PROS
Adult: PO 250 mg q day
Child 2-17 yr: PO 50 mg q day; may increase to 125 mg q day after 24 wk in those ≥6 yr
Available forms: Piqray: Tablets 50, 100, 200 mg; Vijoice: 50, 125, 200 mg
Administer:
Piqray:
• Give with food at approximately the same time each day
• Do not crush, chew, or split; do not use any tablet that is broken, cracked, or otherwise not intact
• If a dose is missed, it can be taken with food within 9 hr after the time it is usually taken. After more than 9 hr, skip the dose for that day and resume dosing on the following day at the usual time
• If vomiting occurs, do not administer an additional dose on that day. Resume dosing the following day at the usual time
Vijoice
• Give with food
• Do not cut, break, chew; do not use if broken
• If unable to swallow, place tablets in glass of 2-4 ounces of water, let stand 5 min, crush tablets with a spoon, give immediately, add more water and stir to remove other product and administer

SIDE EFFECTS
CNS: *Fever, headache*
ENDO: Hypoglycemia, hyperglycemia
INTEG: *Rash, pruritus*
GU: Renal dysfunction

RESP: Pneumonitis
GI: *Nausea, vomiting, diarrhea, abdominal pain, anorexia, weight loss*
SYST: Infection, anaphylaxis, Stevens-Johnson syndrome

PHARMACOKINETICS
89% protein binding, half-life 8-9 hr; 81% excreted in feces (36% unchanged, 32% as metabolite), 14% excreted in urine (2% unchanged, 7.1% metabolite); affected by CYP2C9, CYP3A4, BCRP; peak 2-4 hr

INTERACTIONS
Avoid use with CYP3A4 inhibitors, inducers, substrates

Drug/Lab Test
Increase: LFTs, GGT, lipase, creatinine, ALT, aPTT
Decrease: hgb, platelets, calcium, magnesium, serum albumin, potassium

NURSING CONSIDERATIONS
Assess:
• **Diabetes mellitus:** Fasting blood glucose and hemoglobin A1c (HbA1c) should be monitored before starting treatment and any antidiabetic treatment change; continue to monitor blood glucose weekly for the first 2 wk, then q4wk; monitor HbA1c q3mo
• **Severe diarrhea:** May use with antidiarrheal medication (loperamide). An interruption of therapy, dose reduction, or discontinuation of therapy may be necessary
• **Pancreatitis:** Monitor for nausea, vomiting, abdominal pain, discontinue product if symptoms occur; amylase (urine/serum), amylase/CCr ratio, lipase glucose, electrolytes
• **HF:** monitor for edema in feet/legs, SOB, increased weight >5 lb, during treatment
• Monitor baselines in renal function periodically
• **Severe hypersensitivity reactions (anaphylaxis and anaphylactic shock):** Monitor for severe hypersensitivity reactions (dyspnea, flushing, rash, fever, or tachycardia); permanently discontinue if this occurs

• **Pregnancy/breastfeeding:** Do not use in pregnancy/breastfeeding. Obtain pregnancy testing before use
Evaluate:
• Therapeutic response: Decreased disease progression in breast cancer
Teach patient/family:
• **Pregnancy/breastfeeding:** To report planned or suspected pregnancy; to use effective contraception during treatment and for at least 1 mo after the last dose; to avoid breastfeeding
• To report new or worsening side effects
• To take tablets whole, not to crush or chew; to take with food
• Preexisting chronic lung disease (CLD); severe pneumonitis/interstitial lung disease: Advise patients to immediately report any new or worsening respiratory symptoms (hypoxia, cough, dyspnea)
• Diarrhea: Teach patients to begin antidiarrheal treatment, increase oral fluids, and notify their health care provider if diarrhea occurs

---

> **⚠ HIGH ALERT**

ALPRAZolam (Rx)
(al-pray'zoe-lam)
Apo-Alpraz ✦, Xanax, Xanax XR
Func. class.: Antianxiety
Chem. class.: Benzodiazepine (short/intermediate acting)

Controlled Substance Schedule IV

Do not confuse:
ALPRAZolam/LORazepam
Xanax/Zantac/Zyrtec/Fanapt/Tenex

ACTION: Depresses subcortical levels of CNS, including limbic system, reticular formation, may be mediated by GABA

USES: Anxiety, panic disorders with or without agoraphobia, anxiety with depressive symptoms

CONTRAINDICATIONS
Pregnancy, breastfeeding, hypersensitivity to benzodiazepines, closed-angle glaucoma, psychosis, addiction

---

Side effects: *italics* = common; red = life-threatening

Precautions: Geriatric patients, debilitated patients, hepatic disease, obesity, severe pulmonary disease

DOSAGE AND ROUTES
Anxiety disorder
• **Adult: PO** 0.25-0.5 mg tid, may increase q3-4days if needed, max 4 mg/day in divided doses
• **Geriatric: PO** 0.25 mg bid; increase by 0.125 mg as needed
Panic disorder
• **Adult: PO** 0.5 mg tid, may increase up to 1 mg/day q3-4days, max 10 mg/day; **EXTENDED RELEASE** (Xanax XR) give daily in AM, 0.5-1 mg initially, maintenance 3-6 mg/day, max 10 mg/day
Hepatic dose
• Reduce dose by 50%-60%
Available forms: Tablets 0.25, 0.5, 1, 2 mg; extended-release tablets (Xanax XR) 0.5, 1, 2, 3 mg; orally disintegrating tablets 0.25, 0.5, 1, 2 mg; oral solution 1 mg/mL
Administer:
• Tablets may be crushed, mixed with food, fluids if patient is unable to swallow medication whole; do not break, crush, chew extended release (XR), give extended-release tablets in AM; conversion from regular-release tablets to extended release is at same dose
• With food or milk for GI symptoms; high-fat meal will decrease absorption
• To discontinue, decrease by 0.5 mg q3days
• May divide total daily doses into more times/day if anxiety occurs between doses
• **Orally disintegrating tablets:** place on tongue to dissolve and swallow; protect from moisture, discard unused portion of tablet if split
• **Oral solution:** mix with water, juice, applesauce, or other soft foods; use calibrated dropper supplied

SIDE EFFECTS
CNS: *Dizziness, drowsiness,* confusion, headache, stimulation, poor coordination, suicide
EENT: *Blurred vision*
GI: Constipation, dry mouth, nausea, vomiting, anorexia, diarrhea, weight gain/loss
GU: Decreased libido
INTEG: Rash, dermatitis

PHARMACOKINETICS
PO: Well absorbed; widely distributed; onset 30 min; peak 1-2 hr; duration 4-6 hr; *oral disintegrating tablet* peak 1.5-2 hr; therapeutic response 2-3 days; metabolized by liver (CYP3A4), excreted by kidneys; crosses placenta, breast milk; half-life 12-15 hr, protein binding 80%

INTERACTIONS
Increase: ALPRAZolam action—CYP3A4 inhibitors (cimetidine, disulfiram, erythromycin, FLUoxetine, isoniazid, itraconazole, ketoconazole, metoprolol, propranolol, valproic acid); do not use together

Black Box Warning: **Increase:** CNS depression—anticonvulsants, alcohol, antihistamines, sedative/hypnotics, opioids; avoid concurrent use

Decrease: sedation—xanthines
Decrease: ALPRAZolam action—CYP3A4 inducers (barbiturates, carBAMazepine rifAMPin), adjust dose as needed
Decrease: action of levodopa
Drug/Herb
Increase: CNS depression—kava, melatonin, St. John's wort, valerian
Drug/Food
Increase: product level—grapefruit juice; avoid concurrent use
Drug/Lab Test
Increase: AST/ALT, alkaline phosphatase

NURSING CONSIDERATIONS
Assess:
• Mental status: anxiety, mood, sensorium, orientation, affect, sleeping pattern, drowsiness, dizziness, especially in geriatric patients both before and during treatment, suicidal thoughts, behaviors
• **Labs:** AST, ALT, bilirubin, creatinine, LDH, alkaline phosphatase, CBC; may cause neutropenia, decreased Hct, increased LFTs

Black Box Warning: For use with other CNS depressants or opioids, monitor for respiratory depression

• **Physical dependency, withdrawal symptoms:** anxiety, panic attacks, agitation, seizures, headache, nausea, vomiting, muscle pain, weakness; withdrawal seizures may occur after rapid decrease in dose or abrupt discontinuation

• **Beers:** avoid in older adults; increased risk of cognitive impairment

Evaluate:

• Therapeutic response: decreased anxiety, restlessness, sleeplessness, panic attacks

Teach patient/family:

• Not to double doses; to take exactly as prescribed; if dose is missed, take within 1 hr as scheduled; that product may be taken with food

• Not to use for everyday stress or for more than 4 mo unless directed by prescriber; not to take more than prescribed amount; that product may be habit forming; that memory impairment is a result of long-term use

• To avoid OTC preparations unless approved by prescriber, not to use with grapefruit juice

• Not to discontinue medication abruptly after long-term use

• To avoid driving, activities that require alertness because drowsiness may occur

• To avoid alcohol, other psychotropic medications unless directed by prescriber

• To rise slowly or fainting may occur, especially among geriatric patients

• That drowsiness may worsen at beginning of treatment

• **Oral disintegrating tablet:** to place on tongue and allow to dissolve; swallow; if only half tablet required, discard other half

• **Oral solution:** to mix with water, juice, or other soft foods; to use measuring device supplied

• **Pregnancy/breastfeeding:** If planned or suspected; not to use in pregnancy, to avoid breastfeeding

TREATMENT OF OVERDOSE:
VS, supportive care, flumazenil

alprostadil (Rx)

(al-pros′ta-dil)

Caverject, Caverject Impulse, Edex, Muse, Prostin VR Pediatric

Func. class.: Hormone

USES: To maintain patent ductus arteriosus (temporary treatment), erectile dysfunction

CONTRAINDICATIONS
Hypersensitivity, respiratory distress syndrome, those at risk for priapism

Black Box Warning: Apnea

DOSAGE AND ROUTES
Patent ductus arteriosus (Prostin VR Pediatric)

• **Infant: IV INFUSION** 0.05-0.1 mcg/kg/min until desired response, then reduce to lowest effective amount, max 0.4 mcg/kg/min

Erectile dysfunction of vasculogenic or mixed etiology, psychogenic

• **Men: INTRACAVERNOSAL** 2.5 mcg, may increase by 2.5 mcg, may then increase by 5-10 mcg until adequate response occurs (max 60 mcg/dose); **INTRAURETHRAL** 125-250 mcg, max 2 doses/24 hr, max dose 1000 mcg; administer as needed to achieve erection

Available forms: injection 500 mcg/mL; intracavernosal injection 10 mcg/vial, 20 mcg/vial, 40 mcg/vial; urethral suppository 125, 250, 500, 1000 mcg

⚠ HIGH ALERT

alteplase (Rx)

(al-ti-plaze′)

Activase, Activase rt-PA ✚, Cathflo Activase

Func. class.: Thrombolytic enzyme
Chem. class.: Tissue plasminogen activator (TPA)

Do not confuse:
alteplase/Altace
Activase/Cathflo Activase/TNKase

ACTION: Produces fibrin conversion of plasminogen to plasmin; able to bind to fibrin, convert plasminogen in thrombus to plasmin, which leads to local fibrinolysis, limited systemic proteolysis

USES: Lysis of obstructing thrombi associated with acute MI, ischemic conditions that require thrombolysis (i.e., PE, unclotting arteriovenous shunts, acute ischemic CVA), central venous catheter occlusion (Cathflo)
Unlabeled uses: Acute ischemic stroke 3-4.5 hr after symptoms begin

CONTRAINDICATIONS

Active internal bleeding, history of CVA, severe uncontrolled hypertension, intracranial/intraspinal surgery/trauma (within 3 mo), aneurysm, brain tumor, platelets <100,000 mm³, bleeding diathesis including INR >1.7 or PR >15 sec, arteriovenous malformation, subarachnoid hemorrhage, intracranial hemorrhage, uncontrolled hypertension, seizure at onset of stroke
Precautions: Pregnancy, breastfeeding, children, geriatric patients, neurologic deficits, mitral stenosis, recent GI/GU bleeding, diabetic retinopathy, subacute bacterial endocarditis, arrhythmias, diabetic hemorrhage retinopathy, CVA, recent major surgery, hypertension, acute pericarditis, hemostatic defects, significant hepatic disease, septic thrombophlebitis, occluded AV cannula at seriously infected site

DOSAGE AND ROUTES
MI (standard infusion) (Activase)
• **Adult >65 kg:** 100 mg total given over 3 hr as follows: 60 mg given over first hour (6- to 10-mg bolus over 1-2 min), then 20 mg given over second hour, then 20 mg over third hour
• **Adult <65 kg:** 1.25 mg/kg over 3 hr: 0.75 mg/kg over first hour (0.075-0.125 mg/kg given as a bolus over first 1-2 min), then 0.25 mg/kg over second hour, then 0.25 mg/kg over third hour, max 100 mg
MI (accelerated infusion) (Activase)
• **Adult ≥67 kg:** 100 mg total dose: give 15-mg **IV BOL**, then 50 mg over 30 min, then 35 mg over 60 min

• **Adult <67 kg:** 15-mg **IV BOL**, then 0.75 mg/kg (max 50 mg) over 30 min, then 0.5 mg/kg (max 35 mg) over next 60 min
Acute pulmonary embolism (Activase)
• **Adult: IV** 100 mg over 2 hr, then heparin
Acute ischemic stroke (Activase)
• **Adult/child IV** 0.9 mg/kg, max 90 mg; give as **INFUSION** over 1 hr, give 10% of dose **IV BOL** over first minute
Occluded venous access devices (Cathflo Activase)
• **Adult/child ≥30 kg: IV** 2 mg/2 mL instilled in occluded catheter, may repeat if needed after 2 hr
• **Child 10-29 kg: IV** 110% of lumen volume, max 2 mg/2 mL instilled in occluded catheter, may repeat if needed after 2 hr
Available forms: Powder for injection 50 mg (29 million international units/vial), 100 mg (58 million international units/vial); Cathflo Activase: lyophilized powder for injection 2 mg
Administer: (Activase)
Intermittent IV INFUSION route
• After reconstituting with provided diluent, add amount of sterile water for injection (no preservatives) 20-mg vial/20 mL or 50-mg vial/50 mL to make 1 mg/mL, mix by slow inversion or dilute with NaCl, D₅W to a concentration of 0.5 mg/mL; 1.5 to <0.5 mg/mL may result in precipitation of product; use 18G needle; flush line with NaCl after administration, give over 3 hr for MI, 2 hr for PE
• Pressure for 30 sec to minor bleeding sites; 30 min to sites of arterial puncture followed by pressure dressing; inform prescriber if this does not attain hemostasis; apply pressure dressing
• Store powder at room temperature or refrigerate; protect from excessive light
• Heparin therapy after thrombolytic therapy is discontinued, TT, ACT, or APTT less than 2× control (about 3-4 hr); treatment can be initiated before coagulation study results obtained, infusion should be discontinued if pretreatment INR >1.7, PT >15 sec, or elevated APTT is identified
• Use reconstituted IV solution within 8 hr or discard
• Avoid invasive procedures, injections, rectal temperature

- **Cathflo Activase:** Use product after other options used for declotting a line; reconstitute by using 2.2 mL of sterile water provided and injecting in vial, direct flow into powder (1 mg/mL), foam will disappear after standing; swirl, do not shake, solution will be pale yellow or clear, use within 8 hr, instill 2 mL of reconstituted solution into occluded catheter, try to aspirate after ½ hr; if unable to remove, allow 2 hr, a second dose may be used; aspirate 5 mL of blood to remove clot and product, irrigate with normal saline

SIDE EFFECTS
INTEG: Urticaria, rash
SYST: GI, GU, intracranial, retroperitoneal bleeding, anaphylaxis, fever

PHARMACOKINETICS
Cleared by liver, 80% cleared within 10 min of product termination, onset immediate, half-life 35 min, peak 1 hr

INTERACTIONS
Increase: bleeding—anticoagulants, salicylates, dipyridamole, other NSAIDs, abciximab, eptifibatide, tirofiban, clopidogrel, ticlopidine, some cephalosporins, low-molecular-weight heparins, thrombolytics, plicamycin, valproic acid; monitor for bleeding
Drug/Herb
Increase: risk for bleeding—feverfew, garlic, ginger, ginkgo, ginseng, green tea
Drug/Lab Test
Increase: PT, APTT, TT, plasminogen, fibrinogen levels

NURSING CONSIDERATIONS
Assess:
- Perform noncontrast CT of brain or MRI to rule out intracranial hemorrhage prior to systemic administration
- Treatment is not recommended in patients with acute ischemic stroke >4.5 hr after symptom onset, with minor neurologic deficit, or with rapidly improving symptoms
- VS, B/P, pulse, respirations, neurologic signs, temperature at least q4hr; temperature >104° F (40° C) indicates internal bleeding; monitor rhythm; ventricular dysrhythmias may occur with hyperperfusion; monitor heart, breath sounds, neurologic status, peripheral pulses; assess neurologic status, neurologic change may indicate intracranial bleeding
- **For bleeding:** during first hour of treatment and 24 hr after procedure: hematuria, hematemesis, bleeding from mucous membranes, epistaxis, ecchymosis; guaiac all body fluids, stools; do not use 150 mg or more total dose; intracranial bleeding may occur; do not use in severe uncontrolled hypertension, aneurysm, head trauma, for MI, pulmonary embolism; obtain noncontrast CT of brain or MRI to take out intracranial hemorrhage prior to systemic use
- **Hypersensitivity:** fever, rash, itching, chills, facial swelling, dyspnea, notify prescriber immediately; stop product, keep resuscitative equipment nearby; mild reaction may be treated with antihistamines
- Previous allergic reactions or streptococcal infection; alteplase may be less effective
- Blood studies (Hct, platelets, PTT, PT, TT, APTT) before starting therapy; PT or APTT must be less than 2× control before starting therapy; TT or PT q3-4hr during treatment
- **MI:** ECG continuously, cardiac enzymes, radionuclide myocardial scanning/coronary angiography; chest pain intensity, character; monitor those with major early infarct signs on CT scan with substantial edema, mass effect, midline shift
- **PE:** pulse, B/P, ABGs, rate/rhythm of respirations
- **Occlusion:** have patient exhale then hold breath when connecting/disconnecting syringe to prevent air embolism
- **Acute ischemic stroke:** assess neurologic symptoms of stroke, speech, weakness, on one side of body, must be used within 3-4.5 hr of onset of symptoms
- **DVT/arterial thrombosis:** check pulses in affected extremities often; obtain angiography/venography, complete duplex ultrasound, D-dimer blood test
- **Pregnancy/breastfeeding:** usually considered contraindicated in pregnancy

except in serious conditions; use cautiously in breastfeeding

Evaluate:

• Therapeutic response: lysis of thrombi, adequate hemodynamic state, absence of HF, cannula/catheter lack of occlusion

Teach patient/family:

• The purpose and expected results of the treatment; to report adverse reactions, bleeding

---

aluminum hydroxide (OTC)

AlternaGel, Alu-Cap, Almagel Plus ✤, Alu-Tab, Amphojel, Basaljel, Diovol Plus ✤, Gelusil ✤, Mucaine ✤

Func. class.: Antacid, hypophosphatemic

Chem. class.: Aluminum product, phosphate binder

ACTION: Neutralizes gastric acidity; binds phosphates in GI tract; these phosphates are then excreted

USES: Antacid, hyperphosphatemia in chronic renal failure; adjunct in gastric, peptic, duodenal ulcers; hyperacidity, reflux esophagitis; heartburn, stress ulcer prevention in critically ill, GERD

CONTRAINDICATIONS

Hypersensitivity to product or aluminum products

Precautions: Pregnancy, breastfeeding, geriatric patients, fluid restriction, decreased GI motility, GI obstruction, dehydration, renal disease, sodium-restricted diets, GI bleeding, hypokalemia

DOSAGE AND ROUTES
Antacid

• **Adult: PO** 500-1500 mg 3-6× daily, max 6 doses/day

Hyperphosphatemia

• **Adult: PO** Suspension 30-40 mL (regular) or 15-20 mL (concentrated) tid-qid

• **Child: PO** 50-150 mg/kg/day in 4-6 divided doses

Available forms: Suspension 320 mg/5 mL, 450 mg/5 mL, 600 mg/5 mL, 675 mg/5 mL; capsules 475, 500 mg; tablets 300, 500, 600 mg

Administer: 2 tsp (10 mL) will neutralize 20 mEq of acid

PO route

• Give 2 hr before or 6 hr after fluoroquinolones

• **Hyperphosphatemia:** Give with 8 oz water, meals unless contraindicated

• Laxatives or stool softeners if constipation occurs, especially for geriatric patients

• After shaking suspension

NG route

• By nasogastric tube if patient unable to swallow

SIDE EFFECTS

GI: *Constipation,* anorexia, fecal impaction, nausea, vomiting, cramps

META: *Hypophosphatemia*

PHARMACOKINETICS

PO: Onset 20-40 min, duration 1-3 hr, excreted in feces, onset 20-40 min, peak 30 min, duration 1-3 hr

INTERACTIONS

Decrease: effectiveness of—allopurinol, amprenavir, cephalosporins, corticosteroids, delavirdine, digoxin, fluoroquinolones, gabapentin, gatifloxacin, H_2 antagonists, iron salts, isoniazid, ketoconazole, penicillAMINE, phenothiazines, phenytoin, quiNIDine, quinolones, tetracyclines, thyroid hormones, ticlopidine, anticholinergics; separate by at least 4-6 hr

Drug/Food

Decrease: product effect—high-protein meal

NURSING CONSIDERATIONS
Assess:

• **GI pain:** location, intensity, duration, character, aggravating, alleviating factors; monitor for blood in stools, emesis, sputum in ulcer disease

• Phosphate, magnesium, calcium levels, product is bound in GI system

---

• **Hypophosphatemia:** anorexia, weakness, fatigue, bone pain, hyporeflexia
• Constipation; increase fiber in diet if needed, may use stool softeners or laxatives; record amount and consistency of stools
• **Pregnancy/breastfeeding:** may use occasionally at recommended dose in pregnancy, breastfeeding

Evaluate:
• Therapeutic response: absence of GI pain, decreased acidity, healed ulcers, decreased phosphate levels

Teach patient/family:
• Not to use for prolonged periods for patients with low serum phosphate or patients on low-sodium diets; to shake liquid well
• That stools may appear white or speckled
• To check with prescriber after 2 wk of self-prescribed antacid use
• To separate from other medications by 2 hr
• **Hyperphosphatemia:** to avoid phosphate foods (most dairy products, eggs, fruits, carbonated beverages) during product therapy
• To notify prescriber of black tarry stools, which may indicate bleeding

alvimopan (Rx)
(al-vim′oh-pan)
Entereg
Func. class.: Functional GI disorder agent

USES: Prevention of postoperative ileus

CONTRAINDICATIONS
Those who have taken therapeutic doses of opioids for more than 7 consecutive days immediately before starting alvimopan, end-stage renal disease, Child-Pugh C

DOSAGE AND ROUTES
• **Adult/geriatric patient: PO** 12 mg 30 min-5 hr before surgery, then 12 mg bid beginning the day after surgery; max 7 days or hospital discharge; max 15 doses

Opiate agonist–induced constipation (unlabeled)
• **Adult: PO** 0.5 mg or 1 mg every day
Renal/hepatic dosage
• **Adult: PO** do not use in end-stage renal disease or Child-Pugh Class C
Available forms: Capsules 12 mg

amantadine (Rx)
(a-man′ta-deen)
Gocovri, Osmolex ER
Func. class.: Antiviral, antiparkinsonian agent
Chem. class.: Tricyclic amine

Do not confuse:
amantadine/raNITIdine/rimantidine/ amiodarone

ACTION: Prevents uncoating of nucleic acid in viral cell, thereby preventing penetration of virus to host; causes release of DOPamine from neurons

USES: Prophylaxis or treatment of influenza type A, EPS, parkinsonism, Parkinson's disease

CONTRAINDICATIONS
Hypersensitivity, breastfeeding, children <1 yr, eczematic rash
Precautions: Pregnancy, geriatric patients, epilepsy, HF, orthostatic hypotension, psychiatric disorders, renal/hepatic disease, peripheral edema, CV disease

DOSAGE AND ROUTES
Parkinson's disease
• **Adult: PO** 100 mg bid (monotherapy); after 7 days may increase to 400 mg in divided doses; Osmolex SR: initial dosage 129 mg daily in the AM; may increase weekly, max 322 mg daily in the AM
Influenza type A
• **Adult and child ≥13 yr: PO** 200 mg/day in single dose or divided bid
• **Geriatric: PO** No more than 100 mg/day
• **Child 1-8 yr: PO** 4.4-8.8 mg/kg/day divided bid-tid, max 150 mg/day

Drug-induced EPS

• **Adult: PO** 100 mg bid, up to 300 mg/day in divided doses; **EXTENDED RELEASE** Osmolex ER: 129 mg once daily in the morning, initially. May increase at weekly intervals as needed. Max: 322 mg/day

Amantadine: Drug-induced EPS extended release dosing should remove Gocovri and add Osmolex ER: 129 mg PO once daily in the morning, initially. May increase at weekly intervals as needed. Max: 322 mg/day. Gocovri is indicated/dosed for Parkinson's disease with drug induced dyskinesia in patients receiving levodopa, or adjunct therapy for "off" episodes for patients on carbidopa/levodopa

Renal dose

• **Adult: PO** CCr 30-50 mL/min 200 mg first day then 100 mg/day; CCr 15-29 mL/min 100 mg first day, then 100 mg on alternate days; CCr 15 mL/min reduce dose and interval to 200 mg q7days

Available forms: Capsules 100 mg; oral solution 50 mg/5 mL; tablets 100 mg; extended release (Osmolex ER) 129, 193, 258 mg; extended release (Gocovri) 68.5, 137 mg

Administer:

• **Prophylaxis:** before exposure to influenza; continue for 10 days after contact; **treatment:** initiate within 24-48 hr of onset of symptoms, continue for 24-48 hr after symptoms disappear

• After meals for better absorption to decrease GI symptoms; at least 4 hr before bedtime to prevent insomnia

• In divided doses to prevent CNS disturbances: headache, dizziness, fatigue, drowsiness

• Store in tight, dry container

SIDE EFFECTS

CNS: *Headache, dizziness,* drowsiness, fatigue, *anxiety,* psychosis, *depression, hallucinations,* tremors, seizures, confusion, *insomnia*

CV: *Orthostatic hypotension,* HF

EENT: Blurred vision

GI: *Nausea, vomiting,* constipation, dry mouth, anorexia

GU: *Frequency, retention*

HEMA: Leukopenia, agranulocytosis

INTEG: Photosensitivity, dermatitis, livedo reticularis

PHARMACOKINETICS

PO: Onset 48 hr, peak 1-4 hr, half-life 24 hr, not metabolized, excreted in urine (90%) unchanged, crosses placenta, excreted in breast milk

INTERACTIONS

Increase: anticholinergic response—atropine, other anticholinergics; reduce dose of anticholinergics

Increase: CNS stimulation—CNS stimulants

Decrease: amantadine effect—metoclopramide, phenothiazines

Decrease: renal excretion of amantadine—triamterene, hydroCHLOROthiazide

Decrease: effect—S/B H1N1 influenza A virus vaccine; avoid use 2 wk before or 48 hr after amantadine

Drug/Lab Test

Increase: BUN, creatinine, alkaline phosphatase, CK, LDH, bilirubin, AST, ALT, GGT

NURSING CONSIDERATIONS

Assess:

• Mental status: may cause increased psychiatric disorders especially in the elderly

• **HF:** weight gain, jugular venous distention, dyspnea, crackles

• Skin eruptions, photosensitivity after administration of product

• Serum creatinine, BUN in renal impairment

• Reaction to each medication

• Signs of infection

• **Livedo reticularis:** mottling of the skin, usually red; edema; itching in lower extremities, usually in Parkinson's disease

• **Parkinson's disease:** gait, tremors, akinesia, rigidity, may be effective if anticholinergics have not been effective

• **Toxicity:** confusion, behavioral changes, hypotension, seizures

Evaluate:

• Therapeutic response: absence of fever, malaise, cough, dyspnea with infection; tremors, shuffling gait with Parkinson's disease

Teach patient/family:
• To change body position slowly to prevent orthostatic hypotension
• About aspects of product therapy: to report dyspnea, weight gain, dizziness, poor concentration, dysuria, complex sleep behaviors
• To avoid hazardous activities if dizziness, blurred vision occurs
• **Parkinson's disease:** to take product exactly as prescribed; parkinsonian crisis may occur if product is discontinued abruptly; not to double dose; if a dose is missed, not to take within 4 hr of next dose; capsules may be opened and mixed with food
• To avoid alcohol
• **Pregnancy/breastfeeding:** Avoid use in pregnancy; identify if pregnancy is suspected; avoid breastfeeding

TREATMENT OF OVERDOSE:
Maintain airway, administer EPINEPHrine, aminophylline, O₂, IV corticosteroids, physostigmine

---

ambrisentan (Rx)
(am-bri-sen′tan)
Letairis, Volibris ✦
Func. class.: Antihypertensive

ACTION: Endothelin-A receptor antagonist; endothelin-A is a vasoconstrictor

USES: Pulmonary arterial hypertension, alone or in combination with other antihypertensives in WHO class II (significant exertion), III (mild exertion)

CONTRAINDICATIONS
Breastfeeding, hypersensitivity, idiopathic pulmonary fibrosis (IPF)

Black Box Warning: Pregnancy

Precautions: Children, females, geriatric patients, hepatitis, anemia, heart failure, jaundice, peripheral edema, hepatic disease, pulmonary disease

DOSAGE AND ROUTES
• **Adult:** PO 5 mg/day; may increase q4wk to max 10 mg/day if needed

Hepatic dose
• **Adult: PO** Discontinue if AST/ALT >5× ULN, or if elevations are accompanied by bilirubin >2× ULN, or other signs of liver dysfunction
Available forms: Tablets 5, 10 mg
Administer:
• Do not break, crush, chew tablets
• Daily with a full glass of water without regard to food
• Do not discontinue abruptly

Black Box Warning: Only those facilities enrolled in the LEAP program (866-664-5327) may administer this product

• Store in tight container at room temperature

SIDE EFFECTS
CNS: *Headache,* fever, flushing, fatigue
CV: Orthostatic hypotension, hypotension, *peripheral edema,* palpitations
EENT: Sinusitis, rhinitis
GI: Abdominal pain, constipation, anorexia, hepatotoxicity
GU: Decreased sperm counts
HEMA: *Anemia*
INTEG: Rash, angioedema
RESP: Pharyngitis, dyspnea, pulmonary edema, veno-occlusive disease (VOD)

PHARMACOKINETICS
Rapidly absorbed, peak 2 hr, protein binding 99%, metabolized by CYP3A4, CYP2C19, UGTa, terminal half-life 15 hr, effective half-life 9 hr

INTERACTIONS
• Possibly increase ambrisentan: cimetidine, clopidogrel, efavirenz, felbamate, FLUoxetine, modafinil, OXcarbazepine, ticlopidine
Increase: hypotension—other antihypertensives, diuretics, MAOIs
Increase: ambrisentan—CYP3A4 inhibitors (amprenavir, aprepitant, atazanavir, clarithromycin, conivaptan, cycloSPORINE, dalfopristin, danazol, darunavir, erythromycin, estradiol, imatinib, itraconazole, ketoconazole, nefazodone, nelfinavir, quinupristin, ritonavir, RU-486, saquinavir, tamoxifen, telithromycin, troleandomycin, zafirlukast); CYP2C19/CYP3A4 (chloramphenicol, delavirdine,

fluconazole,   fluvoxaMINE,   isoniazid,
voriconazole)
Decrease: ambrisentan—CYP3A4 induc-
ers (carBAMazepine, PHENobarbital, phe-
nytoin, rifAMPin)
Decrease: ambrisentan absorption—meflo-
quine, niCARDipine, propafenone, quiNI-
Dine, ranolazine, tacrolimus, testosterone
Drug/Herb
Need for ambrisentan dosage change:
St. John's wort, ephedra (ma huang)
Drug/Food
Avoid use with grapefruit products
Drug/Lab Test
Increase: LFTs, bilirubin
Decrease: Hct, HB

NURSING CONSIDERATIONS
Assess:
• **Pulmonary status:** improvement in
breathing, ability to exercise; pulmonary
edema that may indicate veno-occlusive
disease
• Blood studies: CBC with differential;
Hct, HB may be decreased
• Liver function tests: AST, ALT, bilirubin

Black Box Warning: Assess pregnancy
status before giving this product and
monthly and 1 mo after concluding therapy; pregnancy

• **Hepatotoxicity:** nausea, vomiting, ab-
dominal pain/cramping, jaundice, an-
orexia, itching
• **Beers:** use in older adults cautiously;
may exacerbate syncope
Evaluate:
• Therapeutic response: decrease in
B/P; decreased shortness of breath
Teach patient/family:
• The importance of complying with
dosage schedule even if feeling better
• The importance of follow-up with labs
• That sperm count may be decreased

Black Box Warning: To notify if pregnancy
is planned or suspected (if pregnant,
product will need to be discontinued, pregnancy test done monthly); to use 2 contraception methods while taking this product
and for 1 mo after concluding therapy

• Not to use OTC products, including
herbs, supplements, unless approved by
prescriber
• To take tablet whole; not to crush, chew
• **To report to prescriber immediately:**
dizziness, faintness, chest pain, palpitations, uneven or rapid heart rate, headache, edema, weight gain
• **To report hepatic dysfunction:** nau-
sea/vomiting, anorexia, fatigue, jaundice,
right upper quadrant abdominal pain,
itching, fever, malaise

amikacin (Rx)
(am-i-kay'sin)
Func. class.: Antiinfective
Chem. class.: Aminoglycoside

Do not confuse:
amikacin/amicar/anakinra

ACTION: Interferes with protein
synthesis in bacterial cells by binding
to ribosomal subunits, which causes
misreading of genetic code; inaccurate peptide sequence forms in protein chain, thereby causing bacterial
death

USES: Severe systemic infections of
CNS, respiratory tract, GI tract, urinary
tract, bone, skin, soft tissues caused by
Staphylococcus aureus (MSSA), *Pseudomonas aeruginosa, Escherichia
coli, Enterobacter, Acinetobacter,
Providencia, Citrobacter, Serratia,
Proteus, Klebsiella pneumoniae*
Unlabeled   uses: *Mycobacterium
avium* complex (MAC) (intrathecal or
intraventricular) in combination

CONTRAINDICATIONS
Pregnancy, hypersensitivity to aminoglycosides, sulfites
Precautions: Breastfeeding, neonates,
geriatric patients, myasthenia gravis, Parkinson's disease, mild to moderate infections, dehydration

Black Box Warning: Hearing impairment, renal/neuromuscular disease

DOSAGE AND ROUTES
• **Adult/child: IV INFUSION** 15 mg/kg/day in 2-3 divided doses q8-12hr in 100-200 mL D$_5$W over 30-60 min, max 1.5 g/day; **pulse dosing** (once-daily dosing) may be used with some infections; **IM** 10-15 mg/kg/day in divided doses q8-12hr; or extended-interval dosing as an alternative dosing regimen
• **Neonate: IV/IM** 10 mg/kg initially, then 7.5 mg/kg q8-12hr
Renal dose (extended-interval dosing)
• **Adult: IV** CCr 40-59 mL/min 15 mg/kg q36hr; CCr 20-39 mL/min 15 mg/kg q48hr; <20 mL/min adjust based on serum concentrations and MIC (use traditional dosing)
***Mycobacterium avium* complex (MAC)**
• **Adult: IM/IV** 15-20 mg/kg/day or 5× per week
Adolescent: IV 10-15 mg/kg/dose q day, max 1.5 g/day plus clarithromycin or azithromycin and ethambutol for HIV
• **Child: IV** 15-30 mg/kg/day divided q12-24hr as part of multiple-drug regimen, max 1.5 g/day
Available forms: Injection 50, 250 mg/mL; suspension for oral inhalation 590 mg/8.4 mL
Administer:
• Obtain C&S before administration; begin treatment before results are received
IM route
• Inject in large muscle mass; rotate injection sites
• Obtain peak 1 hr after IM, trough before next dose
Intermittent IV INFUSION route
• Dilute 500 mg of product/100-200 mL of D$_5$W, 0.9% NaCl (10 mg/mL) and give over ½-1 hr; dilute in sufficient volume to allow for infusion over 1-2 hr (infants); flush after administration with D$_5$W or 0.9% NaCl; solution clear or pale yellow; discard if precipitate or dark color develops
• In children, amount of fluid will depend on ordered dose; in infants, infuse over 1-2 hr
• In evenly spaced doses to maintain blood level, separate from penicillins by at least 1 hr

Y-site compatibilities: Acyclovir, alatrofloxacin, aldesleukin, alemtuzumab, alfentanil, amifostine, aminophylline, amiodarone, amsacrine, anidulafungin, argatroban, ascorbic acid, atracurium, atropine, aztreonam, benztropine, bivalirudin, bumetanide, buprenorphine, butorphanol, calcium chloride/gluconate, CARBOplatin, caspofungin, ceFAZolin, cefepime, cefonicid, cefotaxime, cefoTEtan, cefOXitin, cefTAZidime, ceftizoxime, cefTRIAXone, cefuroxime, chloramphenicol, chlorproMAZINE, cimetidine, cisatracurium, CISplatin, clindamycin, codeine, cyanocobalamin, cyclophosphamide, cycloSPORINE, cytarabine, DACTINomycin, DAPTOmycin, dexamethasone, dexmedetomidine, digoxin, diltiazem, diphenhydrAMINE, DOBUTamine, DOCEtaxel, DOPamine, doripenem, doxacurium, DOXOrubicin, doxycycline, enalaprilat, ePHEDrine, EPINEPHrine, epirubicin, epoetin alfa, eptifibatide, ertapenem, erythromycin, esmolol, etoposide, famotidine, fentaNYL, filgrastim, fluconazole, fludarabine, fluorouracil, foscarnet, furosemide, gemcitabine, gentamicin, glycopyrrolate, granisetron, hydrocortisone, HYDROmorphone, IDArubicin, ifosfamide, IL-2, imipenem/cilastin, isoproterenol, ketorolac, labetalol, levofloxacin, lidocaine, linezolid, LORazepam, magnesium sulfate, mannitol, mechlorethamine, melphalan, meperidine, metaraminol, methotrexate, methoxamine, methyldopate, methylPREDNISolone, metoclopramide, metoprolol, metroNIDAZOLE, midazolam, milrinone, mitoXANtrone, morphine, multivitamins, nafcillin, nalbuphine, naloxone, niCARdipine, nitroglycerin, nitroprusside, norepinephrine, octreotide, ondansetron, oxaliplatin, oxytocin, PACLitaxel, palonosetron, pantoprazole, papaverine, PEMEtrexed, penicillin G, pentazocine, perphenazine, PHENobarbital, phenylephrine, phytonadione, piperacillin/tazobactam, potassium chloride, procainamide, prochlorperazine, promethazine, propranolol, protamine, pyridoxine, quinupristin/dalfopristin, ranitidine, remifentanil, riTUXimab, rocuronium, sargramostim, sodium acetate, sodium bicarbonate, succinylcholine, SUFentanil, tacrolimus, teniposide, theophylline, thiamine, thiotepa, ticarcillin/clavulanate, tigecycline, tirofiban, tobramycin, tolazoline, trimethaphan, urokinase, vancomycin, vasopressin, vecuronium, verapamil, vinCRIStine, vinorelbine, voriconazole, warfarin, zidovudine, zoledronic acid

SIDE EFFECTS

CNS: Dizziness, vertigo
EENT: *Ototoxicity,* deafness
GU: Nephrotoxicity
HEMA: Eosinophilia, anemia
INTEG: *Rash,* burning, urticaria, dermatitis, alopecia
RESP: Apnea
SYST: Hypersensitivity

PHARMACOKINETICS

IM: Onset rapid, peak 1 hr, leads to unpredictable concentrations, IV preferred
IV: Onset immediate, peak 15-30 min, half-life 2 hr, prolonged up to 7 hr in infants; not metabolized; excreted unchanged in urine; crosses placenta; removed by hemodialysis

INTERACTIONS

Increase: masking ototoxicity: dimenhyDRINATE, ethacrynic acid
Increase: neurotoxicity—NSAIDs

Black Box Warning: Increase: nephrotoxicity—cephalosporins, acyclovir, vancomycin, amphotericin B, cycloSPORINE, loop diuretics, cidofovir

Black Box Warning: Increase: ototoxicity—IV loop diuretics

Black Box Warning: Increase: neuromuscular blockade, respiratory depression—anesthetics, nondepolarizing neuromuscular blockers

Decrease: amikacin effect in renal disease—parenteral penicillins, cephalosporins do not combine
Drug/Lab Test
Increase: BUN, creatinine, AST/ALT, alkaline phosphatase, bilirubin, LDH
Decrease: serum potassium, sodium, calcium, magnesium

NURSING CONSIDERATIONS
Assess:
• Weight before treatment; calculation of dosage is usually based on ideal body weight but may be calculated on actual body weight; in those underweight and not obese, use total body weight (TBW) instead of ideal body weight
• IV site for thrombophlebitis including pain, redness, swelling q30min; change site if needed; apply warm compresses to discontinued site

Black Box Warning: Nephrotoxicity: renal impairment; obtain urine for CCr, BUN, serum creatinine; in renal impairment; nephrotoxicity may be reversible if product is stopped at first sign; I&O ratio; urinalysis daily for proteinuria, cells, casts; report sudden change in urine output

Black Box Warning: Ototoxicity: deafness: audiometric testing, ringing, roaring in ears, vertigo; assess hearing before, during, after treatment

• **Dehydration:** high specific gravity, decrease in skin turgor, dry mucous membranes, dark urine, keep well hydrated 2000 mL/day
• **Overgrowth of infection:** increased temperature, malaise, redness, pain, swelling, perineal itching, diarrhea, stomatitis, change in cough, sputum
• **Vestibular dysfunction:** nausea, vomiting, dizziness, headache; product should be discontinued if severe

Black Box Warning: Neuromuscular blockade; respiratory paralysis may occur; more common in those receiving anesthetics, neuromuscular blockers; use of calcium salts may be used to reverse effect

Evaluate:
• Therapeutic response: absence of fever, draining wounds; negative C&S after treatment

Teach patient/family:
- To report headache, dizziness, symptoms of overgrowth of infection, renal impairment, symptoms of nephrotoxicity, hepatotoxicity
- Teach patient to report trouble breathing, weakness, pain at infusion site
- Advise patient not to use other medications, herbals, supplements without discussing with prescriber
- Inform the patient to keep well hydrated
- **Ototoxicity:** To report loss of hearing; ringing, roaring in ears; feeling of fullness in head
- **To report hypersensitivity:** rash, itching, trouble breathing, facial edema; notify health care provider
- **Pregnancy/breastfeeding:** tell prescriber if pregnancy is planned or suspected or if breastfeeding; do not use in pregnancy, breastfeeding

TREATMENT OF HYPERSENSITIVITY: Hemodialysis, exchange transfusion in the newborn, monitor serum levels of product, may give ticarcillin or carbenicillin

---

aMILoride (Rx)
(a-mill'oh-ride)
Midamor ✤
Func. class.: Potassium-sparing diuretic
Chem. class.: Pyrazine

Do not confuse:
aMILoride/amLODIPine/amiodarone

ACTION: Inhibits sodium, potassium ion exchange in the distal tubule, cortical collecting duct, resulting in inhibition of sodium reabsorption and decreasing potassium secretion

USES: Edema in HF in combination with other diuretics, for hypertension, adjunct with other diuretics to maintain potassium

CONTRAINDICATIONS
Anuria, hypersensitivity, diabetic nephropathy, renal failure

Black Box Warning: Hyperkalemia

Precautions Pregnancy, breastfeeding, children, geriatric patients, dehydration, diabetes, respiratory acidosis, hyponatremia, impaired renal function

DOSAGE AND ROUTES
Hypertension
- **Adult: PO** 5-10 mg/day in 1-2 divided doses; may be increased to 10-20 mg/day if needed
- **Infant/child (6-20 kg): PO** 0.4-0.625 mg/kg daily, max 20 mg/day, dose daily max 20 mg/day
Renal dose
- **Adult: PO** CCr 10-50 mL/min reduce dose by 50%; CCr <10 mL/min contraindicated

Available forms: Tablets 5 mg
Administer:
- In AM to avoid interference with sleep if using as diuretic; if second daily dose is needed, give in late afternoon
- With food; if nausea occurs, absorption may be decreased slightly

SIDE EFFECTS
CNS: *Headache,* dizziness, weakness, paresthesias, tremors, depression, anxiety, encephalopathy
CV: *Orthostatic hypotension,* dysrhythmias, chest pain
ELECT: Hyperkalemia, dehydration, hyponatremia
GI: *Nausea, diarrhea,* dry mouth, *vomiting, anorexia,* cramps, constipation, abdominal pain, jaundice
INTEG: *Rash, pruritus,* Stevens-Johnson syndrome, toxic epidermal necrolysis
MS: Cramps

PHARMACOKINETICS
Absorption variable 20%-90%; widely distributed; onset 2 hr; peak 6-10 hr; duration 24 hr; excreted in urine, feces; half-life 6-9 hr, crosses placenta

INTERACTIONS

Black Box Warning: **Hyperkalemia:** avoid concurrent use with other potassium-sparing diuretics, potassium products, ACE inhibitors, salt substitutes,

---

Side effects: *italics* = common; red = life-threatening

cycloSPORINE, tacrolimus; if together, monitor potassium level

Increase: lithium toxicity: lithium; moni-
tor lithium levels
Increase: action of antihypertensives
Decrease: effect of aMILoride—NSAIDs;
avoid concurrent use
Drug/Herb
Increase: effect—hawthorn, horse
chestnut
Drug/Food
• Possible hyperkalemia: foods high in
potassium, potassium-based salt substitutes
Drug/Lab Test
Increase: LFTs, BUN, potassium, sodium,
bilirubin, calcium, cholesterol
Decrease: Potassium, magnesium, sodium
Interference: GTT

NURSING CONSIDERATIONS
Assess:
• Heart rate; B/P lying, standing; postural hypotension may occur
• Electrolytes: potassium, sodium, chloride; glucose (serum), BUN, CBC, serum
creatinine, blood pH, ABGs, periodic ECG

> **Black Box Warning: Hyperkalemia:** fa-
> tigue, weakness, paresthesia, confusion,
> dyspnea, dysrhythmias, ECG changes;
> including hyperacute T waves; monitor
> potassium level at baseline and dosage
> changes, hyperkalemia is more com-
> mon in renal disease, geriatric patients,
> diabetes; if potassium ≥5.5 mEq/L, im-
> mediately notify prescriber; discontinue
> aMILoride 3 days before GTT

• **Fluid volume status:** distended neck
veins; crackles in lungs; color, quality,
and specific gravity of urine; skin turgor;
adequacy of pulse; moist mucous membranes; bilateral lung sounds; peripheral
pitting edema; dehydration; symptoms of
decreasing output; thirst; hypotension;
dry mouth should be reported
• **Hypokalemia:** weakness, polyuria,
polydipsia, fatigue, ECG U wave

• **Pregnancy/breastfeeding:** identify if
pregnancy is planned or suspected or if
breastfeeding; use only if clearly needed
• **Beers:** avoid in older adults; may
decrease sodium, increase potassium,
decrease Ccr; use with caution; may
exacerbate or cause inappropriate antidiuretic hormone secretion/hyponatremia;
monitor sodium level carefully
Evaluate:
• Therapeutic response: improvement
in edema of feet, legs, sacral area daily if
medication is being used for HF; decreased B/P; prevention of hypokalemia
(diuretics)
Teach patient/family:
• To take as prescribed; if dose is
missed, to take when remembered within
1 hr of next dose; to take with food or
milk for GI symptoms; to take early in day
to prevent nocturia; to avoid alcohol; not
to use other products unless approved by
prescriber
• To maintain a weekly record of weight,
notify health care professional of weight
loss >5 lb
• About adverse reactions: to report
muscle cramps, weakness, nausea, dizziness, blurred vision
• **Hyperkalemia:** to avoid potassium-
rich foods: oranges, bananas, salt substitutes, dried fruits, potassium supplements; refer to dietician for assistance,
planning
• To rise slowly from sitting to standing
to avoid orthostatic hypotension
• To avoid hazardous activities if dizziness occurs
• To continue other medical treatments
(exercise, weight loss, relaxation techniques, cessation of smoking)
• To continue taking medication even if
feeling better, this product controls
symptoms but does not cure condition,
to use as directed, not to double or skip
doses
• Not to exercise in hot weather or stand
for prolonged periods since orthostatic
hypotension is enhanced

• How to take own B/P, pulse, and record

TREATMENT OF OVERDOSE:
Lavage if taken orally, monitor electrolytes, administer sodium bicarbonate for potassium >6.5 mEq/L, IV glucose, Kayexalate as needed; monitor hydration, CV, renal status

amino acids (Rx)
(a-mee′noe)
amino acid infusions (crystalline) (Rx)
Aminosyn, Aminosyn II, Aminosyn-PF, Clinisol, FreAmine III, Premasol, Travasol, TrophAmine
amino acid infusions/ dextrose (Rx)
Aminosyn II with dextrose, Clinimix, Amino Acid Infusions/ electrolytes
aminosyn with electrolytes (Rx)
Aminosyn II with electrolytes, FreAmine III with electrolytes, ProcalAmine with electrolytes, Travasol with electrolytes
amino acid infusions/ electrolytes/dextrose (Rx)
Aminosyn II with electrolytes in dextrose
amino acid infusions (hepatic failure) (Rx)
HepatAmine, Hepatasol
amino acid infusions (high metabolic stress) (Rx)
Aminosyn-HBC, FreAmine HBC
amino acid infusions (renal failure) (Rx)
Aminosyn-RF, NephrAmine
Func. class.: Nutritional supplement/ protein

ACTION: Needed for anabolism to maintain structure, decrease catabolism, promote healing

> **Black Box Warning: Central infusions:** administration by central venous catheter should be used only by those familiar with technique and complications

USES: Hepatic encephalopathy, cirrhosis, hepatitis, nutritional support in cancer; burn or solid organ transplant patients; to prevent nitrogen loss when adequate nutrition by mouth, gastric, or duodenal tube cannot be obtained

CONTRAINDICATIONS
Hypersensitivity, severe electrolyte imbalances, anuria, severe liver damage, maple syrup urine disease, PKU, azotemia, ❦ genetic disease of amino acid metabolism
Precautions: Pregnancy, breastfeeding, children, renal disease, diabetes mellitus, HF, sulfite sensitivity

DOSAGE AND ROUTES
Nutritional support (cirrhosis, hepatic encephalopathy, hepatitis)
• **Adult:** IV 80-120 g/day amino acids/ 12-18 g nitrogen of hepatic failure formula
TPN
• **Adult:** IV 1-1.5 g/kg/day
Metabolic stress (severe)
• **Adult:** IV 1.5 g/kg; use formula for high metabolic stress
Renal failure (nutritional support)
• **Adult:** IV Aminosyn-RF 300-600 mL/70% dextrose/day; NephrAmine 250-500 mL/70% dextrose/day; the total daily dosage is calculated based on the daily protein requirements, as well as the patient's metabolic and clinical response. Check product instructions for specific directions
• **Child:** IV 2-3 g/kg/day
Available forms:
Injection: 250, 500, 1000, 2000 mL, containing amino acids in various concentrations; amino acid infusions, crystalline: Aminosyn: 3.5%, 5%, 7%, 8.5%,

10%; Aminosyn II: 3.5%, 5%, 7%, 8.5%, 10%, 15%; Aminosyn-PF: 7%, 10%; Clinisol: 15%; FreAmine III: 8.5%, 10%; Premasol: 6%, 10%; Travasol: 10%; TrophAmine: 6%, 10%

Amino acid infusion/dextrose: Aminosyn II: 3.5% in 5% dextrose, 4.25% in 20% dextrose, 4.25% in 10% dextrose, 4.25% in 25% dextrose; Clinimix: 2.75% in 5% dextrose, 4.25% in 5% dextrose, 4.25% in 10% dextrose, 4.25% in 20% dextrose, 4.25% in 25% dextrose, 5% in 10% dextrose, 5% in 15% dextrose, 5% in 20% dextrose, 5% in 25% dextrose

Amino acid infusions/electrolytes: Aminosyn: 3.5%, 7%, 8.5%; Aminosyn II: 3.5%, 7%, 8.5%; FreAmine III: 3%, 8.5%; ProcalAmine: 3%; Travasol: 3.5%, 5.5%, 8.5%

Amino acid infusions/electrolytes/dextrose: Aminosyn II: 3.5% with electrolytes in 5% dextrose, 3.5% with electrolytes in 25% dextrose, 4.25% with electrolytes in 10% dextrose, 4.25% with electrolytes in 20% dextrose, 4.25% with electrolytes in 25% dextrose; amino acid infusions (hepatic failure): HepatAmine: 8%; Hepatasol: 8%

Amino acid infusions (high metabolic stress): Aminosyn-HBC 7%; Freamine HBC: 6.9%; amino acid infusions (renal failure): Aminosyn-RF: 5.2%; NephrAmine: 5.4%

Administer:
Continuous IV INFUSION route
• Up to 40% protein and dextrose (up to 12.5%) via peripheral vein; stronger solution requires central IV administration
• TPN only mixed with dextrose to promote protein synthesis
• Immediately after mixing under strict aseptic technique, use infusion pump, in-line filter (0.22 μm) unless mixed with fat emulsion and dextrose (3 in 1); use careful monitoring technique; do not speed up infusion; pulmonary edema, glucose overload will result

SIDE EFFECTS
CNS: Dizziness, headache, confusion, loss of concentration, fever

CV: Hypertension, HF/pulmonary edema, flushing, thrombosis
ENDO: Hyperglycemia, rebound hypoglycemia, electrolyte imbalances, hyperosmolar hyperglycemic nonketotic syndrome, alkalosis, hypophosphatemia, hyperammonemia, dehydration, hypocalcemia
GI: Nausea, abdominal pain, cholestasis
GU: Glycosuria osmotic diuresis
INTEG: Extravasation necrosis, phlebitis at injection site

INTERACTIONS
Individual Drugs
Decrease: Protein-sparing effects—tetracycline
Drug/Lab Test
Increase: LFTs, ammonia, glucose
Decrease: Potassium, phosphate, glucose

NURSING CONSIDERATIONS
Assess:
• Electrolytes (potassium, sodium, phosphate, chloride, magnesium, bicarbonate, blood glucose, ammonia, ketones)
• Renal/hepatic studies: BUN, creatinine, ALT, AST, bilirubin
• Weight changes, triglycerides before and after infusion; vitamin A level with renal disease
• **Injection site for extravasation:** redness along vein, edema at site, necrosis, pain, hard tender area; site should be changed immediately; discontinue infusion, culture tubing and solution
• **Sepsis:** chills, fever, increased temperature, if sepsis is suspected
• **For impending hepatic coma:** asterixis, confusion, uremic fetor, lethargy
• **Hyperammonemia:** nausea, vomiting, malaise, tremors, anorexia, seizures
• Change of dressing and IV tubing every 24-48 hr to prevent infection if chills, fever, other signs of infection occur
Evaluate:
• Therapeutic response: weight gain, decrease in jaundice with liver disorders, increased LOC
Teach patient/family:
• Reason for use of TPN
• To report chills, sweating at once; risk for infection is higher

- About infusion pump, how to care for tubing/site; and blood glucose

⚠ HIGH ALERT

amiodarone (Rx)

(a-mee-oh′da-rone)

Cordarone ✤, Nexterone, Pacerone

Func. class.: Antidysrhythmic (class III)
Chem. class.: Iodinated benzofuran derivative

Do not confuse:
amiodarone/amantadine

ACTION: Prolongs duration of action potential and effective refractory period, noncompetitive α- and β-adrenergic inhibition; increases PR and QT intervals, decreases sinus rate, decreases peripheral vascular resistance

USES: Hemodynamically unstable ventricular tachycardia, supraventricular tachycardia, ventricular fibrillation not controlled by first-line agents

CONTRAINDICATIONS

Pregnancy, breastfeeding, neonates, infants, severe sinus node dysfunction, hypersensitivity to this product/iodine/benzyl alcohol, cardiogenic shock, second-to third-degree AV block, bradycardia
Precautions: Children, goiter, Hashimoto's thyroiditis, electrolyte imbalances, HF, respiratory disease, torsades de pointes

Black Box Warning: Hepatotoxicity, cardiac arrhythmias, pneumonitis, pulmonary fibrosis; requires an experienced clinician

DOSAGE AND ROUTES
Ventricular dysrhythmias
Adult: PO Loading dose 800-1600 mg/day for 1-3 wk, then 600-800 mg/day for 1 mo, maintenance 400 mg/day; **IV** loading dose **(first rapid)** 150 mg over the first 10 min, then slow 360 mg over the next 6 hr, **maintenance** 540 mg given

over the remaining 18 hr, decrease rate of the slow infusion to 0.5 mg/min
Supraventricular tachycardia
- **Adult:** PO 600-800 mg/day × 1 wk until desired response, then decrease to 400 mg/day × 3 wk, then 200-400 mg/day (maintenance)
- **Child:** PO 10 mg/kg/day × 10 days or until desired response, then decrease to 5 mg/kg/day for several weeks, then decrease to 2.5 mg/kg/day or lower (maintenance)
Conversion of atrial fibrillation to sinus rhythm (unlabeled)
- **Adult: IV** 5-7 mg/kg over 30-60 min, then 1.2-1.8 mg/kg **CONTINUOUS IV INFUSION** or PO divided doses
Available forms: Tablets 100, 200, 400 mg; injection 50 mg/mL
Administer:
PO route
- May be used with/without food but be consistent

IV, direct route
- **Peripheral:** max 2 mg/mL for more than 1 hr; preferred through central venous line with in-line filter; concentrations of more than 2 mg/mL should be given by central line
- **Cardiac arrest:** give 300 mg IV bolus; diluted to a total volume of 20 mL D₅W; may repeat 150 mg after 3-5 min

Intermittent IV INFUSION route
- **Rapid loading:** add 3 mL (150 mg), 100 mL D₅W (1.5 mg/mL), give over 10 min
- **Slow loading:** add 18 mL (900 mg), 500 mL D₅W (1.8 mg/mL), give over next 6 hr

Continuous IV INFUSION route
- After 24 hr, dilute 50 mL to 1-6 mg/mL; give 1-6 mg/mL at 1 mg/min for the first 6 hr, then 0.5 mg/min

Y-site compatibilities: Amikacin, clindamycin, DOBUTamine, DOPamine, doxycycline, erythromycin, esmolol, gentamicin, insulin, isoproterenol, labetalol, lidocaine, metaraminol, metroNIDAZOLE, midazolam, morphine, nitroglycerin, norepinephrine, penicillin G potassium, phenylephrine, potassium chloride, procainamide, tobramycin, vancomycin

SIDE EFFECTS

CNS: *Headache, dizziness,* involuntary movement, *tremors, peripheral neuropathy,* malaise, *fatigue,* ataxia, *paresthesias,* insomnia, confusion, hallucinations

CV: *Hypotension, bradycardia,* HF, dysrhythmias

EENT: *Corneal microdeposits,* dry eyes

ENDO: *Hypo*/hyperthyroidism

GI: *Nausea, vomiting,* diarrhea, abdominal pain, *anorexia, constipation,* hepatotoxicity, pancreatitis

GU: Epididymitis, ED

INTEG: Rash, photosensitivity, blue-gray skin discoloration, alopecia, spontaneous ecchymosis, toxic epidermal necrolysis, urticaria, pancreatitis, phlebitis (IV)

MISC: Flushing, abnormal taste or smell, edema, abnormal salivation

RESP: Pulmonary fibrosis/toxicity, ARDS

PHARMACOKINETICS

PO: Onset 1-3 wk, peak 3-7 hr; **IV:** Onset 2 hr, peak 3-7 hr; half-life 26-107 days, increased in geriatric patients, metabolized by liver (an inhibitor of CYP1A2, CYP3A4, CYP2C8, CYP2C9, CYP2C19, CYP2A6, CYP2B6, CYP2D6, P-glycoprotein), excreted by kidneys, 99% protein binding

INTERACTIONS

Increase: QT prolongation—azoles, fluoroquinolones, macrolides, loratadine, traZODone

Increase: amiodarone concentrations, possible serious dysrhythmias—protease inhibitors; reduce dose

Increase: myopathy—HMG-CoA reductase inhibitors; monitor for myopathy

Increase: bradycardia, sinus arrest, AV block—β-blockers, calcium channel blockers; use cautiously

Increase: levels of cycloSPORINE, dextromethorphan, digoxin, disopyramide, flecainide, methotrexate, phenytoin, procainamide, quiNIDine, theophylline, class I antidysrhythmics

Increase: anticoagulant effects—dabigatran, warfarin, dose may need to be decreased (warfarin)

Drug/Herb
St. John's wort may decrease amiodarone level

Drug/Food
Toxicity: grapefruit juice

Drug/Lab Test
Increase: T$_4$, ALT, AST, GGT alkaline phosphatase, cholesterol, lipids, PT, INR
Decrease: T$_3$

NURSING CONSIDERATIONS
Assess:

Black Box Warning: Cardiac dysrhythmias: ECG continuously to determine effectiveness; measure PR, QRS, QT intervals; check for PVCs, other dysrhythmias, B/P continuously for hypo/hypertension; report dysrhythmias, slowing heart rate; monitor amiodarone level: therapeutic 1-2.5 mcg/mL; toxic >2.5 mcg/mL

Black Box Warning: Pulmonary toxicity: dyspnea, fatigue, cough, fever, chest pain; product should be discontinued; for ARDS, pulmonary fibrosis, crackles, tachypnea, increased at higher doses (>400 mg/day), toxicity is common, monitor chest x-ray, PFTs with diffusion capacity

• **Stevens-Johnson syndrome:** monitor for rash, blistering; discontinue immediately, notify prescriber

Black Box Warning: Hepatotoxicity: monitor hepatic enzymes; rarely fatal hepatotoxicity has occurred

• Electrolytes (sodium, potassium, chloride); hepatic studies: AST, ALT, bilirubin, alkaline phosphatase; for dehydration, hypovolemia; monitor PT, INR if using warfarin

• CNS symptoms: confusion, psychosis, numbness, depression, involuntary movements; product should be discontinued

• **Hypothyroidism:** lethargy; dizziness; constipation; enlarged thyroid gland; edema of extremities; cool, pale skin

• **Hyperthyroidism:** restlessness; tachycardia; eyelid puffiness; weight loss; frequent urination; menstrual irregularities; dyspnea; warm, moist skin; may cause fatal thyrotoxicosis, cardiac dysrhythmias; may need to discontinue product

• Ophthalmic exams at baseline and periodically (PO); to prevent corneal deposits, use methylcellulose

• Cardiac rate, respirations: rate, rhythm, character, chest pain; start with patient hospitalized and monitored up to 1 wk; for rebound hypertension after 1-2 hr

• **Beers:** Avoid as first-line therapy for atrial fibrillation in older adults unless heart failure or substantial left ventricular hypertrophy is present

Evaluate:

• Therapeutic response: decrease in ventricular tachycardia, supraventricular tachycardia, fibrillation

Teach patient/family:

• To take this product as directed; to avoid missed doses; not to use with grapefruit juice; not to discontinue abruptly, not to use other drugs, herbs without prescriber approval, many interactions

• To use sunscreen or stay out of sun to prevent burns; that dark glasses may be needed for photophobia

• To report side effects immediately; more common at high dose and longer duration

• That skin discoloration is usually reversible

• To report vision changes, weight change, rash, blistering, numbness, temperature intolerance

• **Pregnancy/breastfeeding:** Identify if pregnancy is planned or suspected or if breastfeeding; not to be used in pregnancy, breastfeeding

TREATMENT OF OVERDOSE:

O_2, artificial ventilation, ECG, administer DOPamine for circulatory depression, administer diazePAM, thiopental for seizures, isoproterenol

---

amisulpride (Rx)

(a′mi-sul′pride)

Barhemsys

Func. class.: Antiemetic

ACTION:

Blocks dopamine receptors (dopamine-2 and dopamine-3). Decrease chemoreceptor trigger zone (CTZ) responsible for vomiting

USES:

Prevention/treatment of postoperative nausea/vomiting

CONTRAINDICATIONS

Hypersensitivity

Precautions: QT prolongation, pregnancy, child, renal disease, infertility, pre-existing arrhythmias/cardiac conduction disorders, hypokalemia, hypomagnesemia, congestive heart failure

DOSAGE AND ROUTES

Prevention of postoperative nausea/vomiting

Adult: IV 5 mg as a single dose given over 1-2 min at the time of induction of anesthesia

Treatment of postoperative nausea/vomiting

Adult: IV 10 mg as a single dose given over 1-2 min for nausea/vomiting after surgery

Renal dose

Adult: IV CCr <30 mL/min: Avoid use

Available forms: Injection 5 mg/2 mL (2.5 mg/mL), 10 mg/4 mL (2.5 mg/mL) single-dose vial

Administer:

• Visually inspect for particulate matter and discoloration, discard if present

• Dilution is not needed

• Protect from light, give within 12 hr of removing from carton

Solution compatibilities. Water for injection, D_5W, 0.9% NaCl

---

Side effects: *italics* = common; red = life-threatening

SIDE EFFECTS
CNS: Chills, agitation, seizures, confusion, insomnia, somnolence, EPS, confusion, psychiatric symptoms
CV: Postural hypotension bradycardia, torsades de pointes, ventricular tachycardia, prolonged QT
META: Hypokalemia, hypomagnesemia
GI: Abdominal distention, increased LFTs
HEMA: Agranulocytosis
SYST: Neuroleptic malignant syndrome, angioedema, hypersensitivity

PHARMACOKINETICS
Onset rapid, peak end of dose, duration unknown, half-life 4-5 hr, protein binding 25%-30%

INTERACTIONS
Increase: antagonism—DOPamine agonists (levodopa), avoid using together
Increase: QT prolongation—drugs that increase QT prolongation (ondansetron), monitor ECG

NURSING CONSIDERATIONS
Assess:
• Monitor B/P baseline and periodically, monitor for postural hypotension
• Monitor for abdominal pain, caused from abdominal distension
• **QT prolongation:** Monitor ECG if other QT prolongation medications are used or history of QT prolongation
• **Pregnancy/breastfeeding:** Identify if pregnant or breastfeeding
Evaluate:
• Therapeutic response: Absence of nausea/vomiting
Teach patient/family:
• **QT prolongation:** Instruct patients to contact their health care provider immediately about change in their heart rate, lightheadedness, syncope
• Teach patients to report to their health care provider if they are taking drugs that prolong the QT interval
• **Pregnancy/breastfeeding:** Suggest pumping and discarding breast milk for 48 hr after product use

amitriptyline (Rx)
(a-mee-trip'ti-leen)
Elavil ✦, Levate ✦
Func. class.: Antidepressant—tricyclic
Chem. class.: Tertiary amine

Combinations: amitriptyline/chlordiazepoxide 12.5 mg/5 mg, 25 mg/10 mg
Do not confuse:
amitriptyline/nortriptyline/aminophylline

ACTION: Blocks reuptake of norepinephrine, serotonin into nerve endings, thereby increasing action of norepinephrine, serotonin in nerve cells

USES: Major depressive disorder

CONTRAINDICATIONS
Hypersensitivity to tricyclics; recovery phase of myocardial infarction
Precautions: Pregnancy, breastfeeding, geriatric patients, seizure disorders, prostatic hypertrophy, schizophrenia, psychosis, severe depression, increased intraocular pressure, closed-angle glaucoma, urinary retention, renal/hepatic/cardiac disease, hyperthyroidism, electroshock therapy, elective surgery

Black Box Warning: Children <12 yr, suicidal patients

DOSAGE AND ROUTES
Depression
• **Adult: PO** Initially, 75 mg/day divided, or 50-100 mg daily at bedtime, max outpatient 150 mg/day, max inpatient 300 mg/day
• **Adolescents: PO** 10 mg tid and 20 mg at bedtime, then titrate
• **Geriatric: PO** Initially, 10-25 mg at bedtime; may increase by 10-25 mg weekly, max 150 mg/day
Available forms: Tablets 10, 25, 50, 75, 100, 150 mg
Administer:
• Increase fluids, bulk in diet if constipation, urinary retention occur, especially in geriatric patients
• With food, milk for GI symptoms

- Crushed if patient unable to swallow medication whole, give with food, fluids
- Dosage at bedtime if oversedation occurs during day; may take entire dose at bedtime; geriatric patients may not tolerate once-daily dosing; use tapering when withdrawing product
- Store at room temperature; do not freeze

SIDE EFFECTS
CNS: *Dizziness, drowsiness,* confusion, headache, anxiety, tremors, weakness, *insomnia,* EPS (geriatric patients), seizures, suicidal thoughts, anxiety
CV: *Orthostatic hypotension,* ECG changes, tachycardia, hypertension, palpitations, dysrhythmias, QT prolongation
EENT: *Blurred vision,* tinnitus, mydriasis
GI: *Constipation, dry mouth,* weight gain, nausea, vomiting, paralytic ileus, epigastric distress, hepatitis, diarrhea, constipation
GU: *Urinary retention,* sexual dysfunction
HEMA: Agranulocytosis, thrombocytopenia, eosinophilia, leukopenia, aplastic anemia
INTEG: Rash, urticaria, sweating, photosensitivity
SYST: Hypersensitivity

PHARMACOKINETICS
Onset 45 min; peak 2-12 hr, protein binding >95%; metabolized by liver to nortriptyline; excreted in urine, feces; crosses placenta; excreted in breast milk; half-life 30-46 hr; antidepressant action up to 30 days, peak 2-6 wk, duration up to several weeks

INTERACTIONS
Increase: Hyperpyretic crisis, seizures, hypertensive episode—MAOIs; do not use within 14 days of MAOIs
Increase: risk for agranulocytosis—antithyroid agents
Increase: QT prolongation—procainamide, quiNIDine, amiodarone, tricyclics, class IA, III antidysrhythmics; may need dosage change

Increase: amitriptyline levels, toxicity—cimetidine, FLUoxetine, phenothiazines, oral contraceptives, antidepressants, carBAMazepine, class IC antidysrhythmics, ritonavir
Increase: effects of direct-acting sympathomimetics (EPINEPHrine), alcohol, barbiturates, benzodiazepines, CNS depressants, opioids, sedative/hypnotics
Increase: serotonin syndrome—linezolid, methylene blue; use cautiously
Increase: hypertensive crisis—cloNIDine
Drug/Herb
Increase: serotonin syndrome—SAM-e, St. John's wort, yohimbe; avoid concurrent use
Increase: CNS depression—kava, hops, chamomile, lavender, valerian
Drug/Lab Test
Increase: blood glucose, LFTs
Decrease: WBCs, platelets, granulocytes, blood glucose

NURSING CONSIDERATIONS
Assess:
- B/P lying, standing; pulse if systolic B/P drops 20 mm Hg, hold product, notify prescriber; take vital signs more frequently with CV disease; ECG baseline and frequently in cardiac patients; avoid use immediately after MI
- **Labs:** CBC, leukocytes, differential, cardiac enzymes if patient is receiving long-term therapy; thyroid function tests; AST, ALT, bilirubin
- Weight weekly; appetite may increase with product
- EPS primarily in geriatric patients: rigidity, dystonia, akathisia
- Paralytic ileus, glaucoma exacerbation

Black Box Warning: Suicidal thinking, behavior: mood, sensorium, affect, suicidal tendencies; increase in psychiatric symptoms: depression, panic; suicidal tendencies are higher in those ≤24 yr, restrict amount of product available, avoid use in child <12 yr

- Urinary retention, constipation: constipation is most likely to occur in children and geriatric patients

• **Withdrawal symptoms:** headache, nausea, vomiting, muscle pain, weakness; do not usually occur unless product was discontinued abruptly
• **Alcohol consumption:** if alcohol is consumed, hold dose until morning
• **Pain syndromes (unlabeled):** intensity, location, severity; use pain scale; product may be taken for 1-2 mo before effective
• **Sexual dysfunction:** erectile dysfunction, decreased libido
• **Beers** Avoid in older adults; highly anticholinergic, sedating, orthostatic hypotension

Evaluate:
• Therapeutic response: decrease in depression, absence of suicidal thoughts

Teach patient/family:
• To take medication as directed (usually at bedtime); not to double dose; that therapeutic effects may take 2-3 wk; not to discontinue medication quickly after long-term use, usually used for at least 3-4 mo: may cause nausea, headache, malaise
• To use caution when driving, performing other activities that require alertness because of drowsiness, dizziness, blurred vision; to avoid rising quickly from sitting to standing (especially geriatric patients); how to manage anticholinergic effects
• To avoid alcohol, other CNS depressants
• To wear sunscreen or large hat when outdoors; photosensitivity occurs
• **Pregnancy/breastfeeding:** Identify if pregnancy is planned or suspected or if breastfeeding

Black Box Warning: To watch for suicide; advise to watch closely for suicidal thinking, behavior, making a plan or attempts, panic attacks, change in mood

• That follow-up examinations will be needed
• That all health care professionals should be notified the product is being used

TREATMENT OF OVERDOSE: ECG monitoring, administer anticonvulsant, sodium bicarbonate

amLODIPine (Rx)
(am-loe′di-peen)
Katerzia, Norvasc
Func. class.: Antianginal, antihypertensive, calcium channel blocker
Chem. class.: Dihydropyridine

Combinations: Azor: 5 mg/20 mg, 10 mg/20 mg, 5 mg/40 mg, 10 mg/40 mg amlodipine/olmesartan; **Cadut:** 2.5 mg/10 mg, 2.5 mg/20 mg, 2.5 mg/40 mg, 5 mg/10 mg, 10 mg/10 mg, 5 mg/20 mg, 5 mg/40 mg, 10 mg/40 mg, 5 mg/80 mg, 10 mg/80 mg amlodipine/atorvastatin; **Lotrel:** 2.5 mg/10 mg, 5 mg/10 mg, 5 mg/20 mg, 5 mg/40 mg, 10 mg/20 mg, 10 mg/40 mg amlodipine/benazepril; **Exforge:** 5 mg/160 mg/12.5 mg, 5 mg/160 mg/25 mg, 10 mg/160 mg/25 mg, 10 mg/320 mg/25 mg, amlodipine/valsartan/hydrochlorothiazide; **Prestalia:** 2.5 mg/3.5 mg, 5 mg/7 mg, 10 mg/14 mg amlodipine/peridopril; **Tribenzor:** 5 mg/20 mg/12.5 mg, 5 mg/40 mg/12.5 mg; 10 mg/40 mg/25 mg amlopidine/olmesartan/hydrochlorothiazide; **Twynsta:** 5 mg/40 mg, 5 mg/80 mg, 10 mg/40 mg, 10 mg/80 mg amlodipine/telmisartan

Do not confuse:
amLODIPine/aMILoride

ACTION: Inhibits calcium ion influx across cell membrane during cardiac depolarization; produces relaxation of coronary vascular smooth muscle, peripheral vascular smooth muscle; dilates coronary vascular arteries; increases myocardial O_2 delivery in patients with vasospastic angina

USES: Chronic stable angina pectoris, hypertension, variant angina (Prinzmetal's angina)

CONTRAINDICATIONS

Hypersensitivity to this product or dihydropyridine, severe aortic stenosis, severe obstructive CAD, B/P systolic <90 mm Hg

Precautions: Pregnancy, breastfeeding, children <6 yr, geriatric patients, HF, hypotension, hepatic injury, GERD

DOSAGE AND ROUTES
Coronary artery disease
• **Adult: PO** 5-10 mg/day
• **Geriatric: PO** 5 mg/day, max 10 mg/day
Hypertension
• **Adult: PO** 2.5-5 mg/day initially, max 10 mg/day
• **Geriatric: PO** 2.5 mg/day, may increase to 5 mg/day, max 10 mg/day
• **Child 6-17 yr (unlabeled): PO** 2.5-5 mg/day
• **Child 1-5 yr (unlabeled): PO** 0.1 mg/kg/dose daily initially, max 0.6 mg/kg/dose
Hepatic dose
• **Adult: PO** 2.5 mg/day; may increase to 10 mg/day (antihypertensive); 5 mg/day, may increase to 10 mg/day (antianginal)

Available forms: Tablets 2.5, 5, 10 mg; suspension 1 mg/mL

Administer:
• Once a day without regard to meals
• Shake suspension before using

SIDE EFFECTS

CNS: *Headache,* fatigue, dizziness, somnolence
CV: *Peripheral edema,* bradycardia, hypotension, angina, edema, palpitations
GI: Nausea, abdominal pain, anorexia, gingival hyperplasia, dyspepsia
INTEG: Rash, pruritus
OTHER: Flushing

PHARMACOKINETICS

Peak 6-12 hr; half-life 30-50 hr; increased in geriatric patients, hepatic disease; metabolized by liver (CYP3A4); excreted in urine (90% as metabolites); protein binding >93%

INTERACTIONS

Antihypertensives, nitrates, fentaNYL, quiNIDine, alcohol: increased hypotension

Lithium: increased lithium toxicity
NSAIDs: decreased effect of NSAIDs
Increase: amLODIPine level—strong CPY3A4 inhibitors (clarithromycin, ketoconazole, ritonavir)
Increase: level of cycloSPORINE
Increase: myopathy—simvastatin

NURSING CONSIDERATIONS
Assess:
• **Vitals:** B/P, pulse, respirations, ECG; some patients have developed severe angina, acute MI after calcium channel blockers if obstructive CAD is severe
• Monitor compliance with number of prescription refills
• Fluid volume status, peripheral edema, dyspnea, jugular vein distention, crackles
• **Angina:** intensity, location, duration of pain
• **Pregnancy/breastfeeding:** identify if pregnancy is planned or suspected, or if breastfeeding
Evaluate:
• Therapeutic response: decreased anginal pain, decreased B/P, increased exercise tolerance
Teach patient/family:
• To take product as prescribed, not to double or skip dose, to take even if feeling better
• To avoid hazardous activities until stabilized on product, dizziness is no longer a problem
• To comply in all areas of medical regimen: diet, exercise, stress reduction, product therapy, smoking cessation
• To notify prescriber of irregular heartbeat; shortness of breath; swelling of feet, face, hands; severe dizziness; constipation; nausea; hypotension; if chest pain does not improve, use nitroglycerin when angina is severe
• To use correct technique when monitoring pulse; to contact prescriber if pulse <50 bpm
• To change positions slowly to prevent orthostatic hypotension
• To continue with good oral hygiene to prevent gingival disease

---

Side effects: *italics* = common; red = life-threatening

• To use sunscreen, protective clothing to prevent photosensitivity
• To notify all health care providers of use of this product
• **Angina:** advise patient to continue with nitrates or beta blockers, not to discontinue
• Advise patient to discuss with health care provider all Rx, OTC, herbals, and supplements used
• Advise patient to notify health care provider of upcoming surgeries or procedures
• **Pregnancy/breastfeeding:** Advise patient to report if pregnancy is planned or suspected or if breastfeeding

TREATMENT OF OVERDOSE:
Defibrillation, β-agonists, IV calcium inotropic agents, diuretics, atropine for AV block, vasopressor for hypotension

---

amoxicillin (Rx)
(a-mox-i-sill′in)
Amoxil ✿, Moxatag
Func. class.: Antiinfective, antiulcer
Chem. class.: Aminopenicillin

Do not confuse:
amoxacillin/amoxapine

ACTION: Interferes with cell wall replication of susceptible organisms; bactericidal: lysis mediated by bacterial cell wall autolysins

USES: Treatment of skin, respiratory, GI, GU infections, otitis media, gonorrhea; for gram-positive cocci *(Staphylococcus aureus, Streptococcus pyogenes, Streptococcus faecalis, Streptococcus pneumoniae)*, gram-negative cocci *(Neisseria gonorrhoeae, Neisseria meningitidis)*, gram-positive bacilli *(Corynebacterium diphtheriae, Listeria monocytogenes)*, gram-negative bacilli *(Haemophilus influenzae, Escherichia coli, Proteus mirabilis, Salmonella)*; gastric ulcer, β-lactase–negative organisms, prophylaxis of bacterial endocarditis; for treatment of ulcers due to *Helicobacter pylori*
Unlabeled uses: Lyme disease in child <8 yr, anthrax treatment and prophylaxis, cervicitis, *Chlamydia trachomatis,* dental abscess/infection, dyspepsia, nongonococcal urethritis, periodontitis, typhoid fever

CONTRAINDICATIONS
Hypersensitivity to this product or beta-lactams
Precautions: Pregnancy, breastfeeding, neonates, hypersensitivity to cephalosporins, carbapenems; severe renal disease, mononucleosis, phenylketonuria, diabetes, geriatric patients, asthma, child, colitis, dialysis, eczema, pseudomembranous colitis, syphilis

DOSAGE AND ROUTES
Tonsillitis and/or pharyngitis (rheumatic fever prophylaxis) secondary to *Streptococcus pyogenes*
• **Adult/adolescent/child ≥12 yr:** PO (Moxatag 775-mg extended-release tablets) 775 mg/day, given within 1 hr of completing a meal, for 10 days
• **Adult:** PO (immediate-release) 1 g/day or 500 mg bid for 10 days
• **Infant/child/adolescent:** PO (immediate-release) 25 mg/kg/dose (max 500 mg/dose) bid for 10 days
Sinusitis
• **Child ≥2 yr/adolescent:** PO (immediate-release) **standard-dose therapy,** 45 mg/kg/day divided q12h; **high-dose therapy,** 80-90 mg/kg/day divided q12h (max 2 g/dose)
• **Child <2 yr:** PO Treat with amoxicillin/clavulanate, not amoxicillin alone
Acute otitis media
• **Adult:** PO (immediate-release) 500 mg q12h or 250 mg q8h for mild/moderate infections; 875 mg q12h or 500 mg q8h for severe infections
• **Infant ≥6 mo/child/adolescent:** PO (immediate-release) 80-90 mg/kg/day divided q12h

---

• **Infant 4-5 mo: PO** (immediate-release) 80-90 mg/kg/day divided q12h for 10 days
• **Infant ≤3 mo: PO** (immediate-release) 30 mg/kg/day divided q12h

Most respiratory Infections
• **Adult: PO** (immediate-release) 500 mg q12h or 250 mg q8h (mild-moderate infections); 875 mg 12 hr or 500 mg q8hr (severe infections)
• **Infant >3 mo/child/adolescent: PO** (immediate-release) 20 mg/kg/day divided q8h (max 250 mg/dose) or 25 mg/ kg/day divided q12h (max 500 mg/day)
• **Neonate/infant ≤3 mo: PO** (immediate-release) 30 mg/kg/day divided q12h

H. pylori
• **Adult: PO** 1000 mg bid with lansoprazole 30 mg bid with clarithromycin 500 mg bid × 14 days or 1000 mg bid with omeprazole 20 mg bid, with clarithromycin 500 mg bid × 14 days or 1000 mg bid with esomeprazole 40 mg daily with clarithromycin 500 mg bid × 10 days; or 1000 mg tid with lansoprazole 30 mg tid × 14 days

Gonorrhea
• **Adult/child ≥40 kg: PO** × 3 g single dose
• **Child >2 yr and <40 kg: PO** 50 mg/kg with probenecid 25 mg/kg single dose

Endocarditis prevention
• **Adult: PO** 2 g 60 min prior to procedure
• **Child: PO** 50 mg/kg 60 min prior to procedure, max adult dose

UTI, including cystitis
Mild to moderate infections caused by highly susceptible organisms
• **Adult: PO** (immediate-release) 500 mg q12h or 250 mg q8h
• **Infant >3 mo/child/adolescent: PO** (immediate-release) 20 mg/kg/day divided q8h (max 250 mg/dose) or 25 mg/ kg/day divided q12h (max 500 mg/dose)
• **Neonate/infant ≤3 mo: PO** (immediate-release) 30 mg/kg/day divided q12h

Renal disease
• **Adult: PO** CCr 10-30 mL/min 250-500 mg q12hr; CCr <10 mL/min 250-500 mg q24hr; do not use 775-, 875-mg strength if CCr <30 mL/min

Available forms: Capsules 250, 500 mg; chewable tablets 125, 200, 250, 400 mg; tablets, 500, 875 mg; extended-release tablets (Moxatag) 775 mg; powder for suspension 125, 200, 250, 400 mg/5 mL; suspension 50 mg/mL

Administer:
PO route
• Identify allergies before use
• **Suspension:** shake well before each dose; use calibrated spoon, oral syringe, or measuring cup; may be used alone, mixed in drinks; use immediately; discard unused portion after 14 days, store in refrigerator
• Give around the clock; capsules may be emptied, mixed with liquids if needed without regard to food
• **Extended release:** do not crush, chew, break; take with food within 1 hr of finishing a meal

SIDE EFFECTS
CNS: Seizures, agitation, confusion, dizziness, insomnia
GI: *Nausea, vomiting, diarrhea,* pseudomembranous colitis
HEMA: Anemia, bone marrow depression, granulocytopenia, hemolytic anemia, eosinophilia, thrombocytopenia, agranulocytosis
INTEG: *Urticaria, rash*
SYST: Anaphylaxis, serum sickness, overgrowth of infection, anaphylaxis, hypersensitivity

PHARMACOKINETICS
PO: Peak 1-2 hr, duration 6-8 hr, half-life 1-1⅓ hr extended in renal disease, metabolized in liver, excreted in urine, crosses placenta, enters breast milk

INTERACTIONS
Increase: rash—allopurinol
Increase: amoxicillin level—probenecid; used for this reason
Increase: anticoagulant action—warfarin
Increase: methotrexate levels—methotrexate; monitor for toxicity
Decrease: contraceptive effect possible—hormonal contraceptives
Drug/Lab Test

Side effects: *italics* = common; red = life-threatening

Increase: AST/ALT, alkaline phosphatase, LDH, eosinophils
Decrease: HB, WBC, platelets
Interference: urine glucose test (Clinitest, Benedict's reagent)

NURSING CONSIDERATIONS
Assess:
• C&S may be drawn before product therapy; product may be given as soon as culture is taken
• **CDAD:** bowel pattern before, during treatment; diarrhea, cramping, blood in stool; report to prescriber immediately, product should be discontinued, may occur even weeks after discontinuing product; do not use antidiarrheals or other product
• Skin eruptions after administration of penicillin to 1 wk after discontinuing product; rash is more common if allopurinol is taken concurrently
• **Pregnancy/breastfeeding:** identify if pregnancy is planned or suspected or if breastfeeding; use only if clearly needed; appears in breast milk, use cautiously in breastfeeding; advise those taking oral contraceptives to use alternative contraceptive, contraceptive may be decreased
• **Anaphylaxis:** rash, itching, dyspnea, facial/laryngeal edema
Evaluate:
• Therapeutic response: absence of infection; prevention of endocarditis, resolution of ulcer symptoms
Teach patient/family:
• That capsules may be opened, contents taken with fluids; that chewable form is available; to take as prescribed, not to double dose
• All aspects of product therapy: to complete entire course of medication to ensure organism death; that culture may be taken after completed course of medication
• To report sore throat, fever, fatigue, diarrhea (superinfection or agranulocytopenia), blood in stool, abdominal pain (pseudomembranous colitis)
• That product must be taken in equal intervals around the clock to maintain blood levels; to take without regard to food, that

capsules may be opened, contents taken with fluids; that chewable form is available; to take as prescribed, not to double dose
• To wear or carry emergency ID if allergic to penicillins
• Advise patient with rheumatic heart disease to use antibiotics before significant dental or medical/surgical procedures

TREATMENT OF ANAPHYLAXIS: Withdraw product, maintain airway; administer EPINEPHrine, aminophylline, O_2, IV corticosteroids

amoxicillin/clavulanate (Rx)
(a-mox-i-sill'in)

Augmentin, Augmentin ES, Augmentin XR, Clavulin ✦
Func. class.: Broad-spectrum antiinfective
Chem. class.: Aminopenicillin β-lactamase inhibitor

ACTION: Bacteriocidal, interferes with cell wall replication of susceptible organisms; lysis mediated by bacterial cell wall autolytic enzymes, combination increases spectrum of activity against β-lactamase–resistant organisms

USES: Lower respiratory tract infections, sinus infections, pneumonia, otitis media, impetigo, skin infection, UTI; effective for *Actinomyces* sp., *Bacillus anthracis*, *Bacteroides* sp., *Bordetella pertussis*, *Borrelia burgdorferi*; *Brucella* sp., *Burkholderia pseudomallei*, *Clostridium perfringens/tetani*, *Corynebacterium diphtheriae*, *Eikenella corrodens*, *Enterobacter* sp., *Enterococcus faecalis*, *Erysipelothrix rhusiopathiae*, *Escherichia coli*, *Eubacterium* sp., *Fusobacterium* sp., *Haemophilus ducreyi/parainfluenzae* (positive/negative beta-lactamase), *Helicobacter pylori*, *Klebsiella* sp., *Lactobacillus* sp., *Listeria monocytogenes*, *Moraxella catarrhalis*, *Neisseria gonorrhoeae/meningitidis*, *Nocardia brasiliensis*, *Peptococcus* sp.,

Peptostreptococcus sp., *Prevotella mela-ninogenica, Propionibacterium* sp., *Shigella* sp., *Staphylococcus aureus (MSSA)/epidermidis/saprophyticus, Streptococcus agalactiae (group B streptococci)/dysgalactiae/pneumoniae/pyogenes (group A streptococci), Treponema pallidum, Vibrio cholerae, Viridans streptococci*

CONTRAINDICATIONS
Hypersensitivity to penicillins, severe renal disease, dialysis
Precautions: Pregnancy, breastfeeding, neonates, children, hypersensitivity to cephalosporins; renal/GI disease, asthma, colitis, diabetes, eczema, leukemia, mononucleosis, viral infections, phenylketonuria

DOSAGE AND ROUTES
Most infections
• **Adult/child >40 kg:** 250 mg q8hr or 500 mg q12hr
Recurrent/persistent otitis media *(Streptococcus pneumoniae, Haemophilus, Moraxella catarrhalis)*
• **Child ≥3 mo to <2 yr: PO** 90 mg/kg/day (600 mg amoxicillin/42.9 mg clavulanate/5 mL) q12hr × 10 days
Lower respiratory infections, otitis media, sinusitis, skin/skin structure infections, UTIs
• **Adult: PO** 250-500 mg q8hr or 500-875 mg q12hr, depending on severity of infection
• **Child ≤40 kg: PO** 20-90 mg/kg/day in divided doses q8-12hr
Community-acquired pneumonia or acute bacterial sinusitis
• **Adult: PO** 2000 mg/125 mg (Augmentin XR) q12hr × 7-10 days (pneumonia), 10 days (sinusitis)
Renal disease
• **Adult: PO** CCr 10-30 mL/min dose q12hr; CCr <10 mL/min dose q24hr; do not use 875-mg strength or ext rel if CCr <30 mL/min; Augmentin XR is contraindicated with renal disease
Available forms: Tablets 250, 500, 875 mg amoxicillin/125 mg clavulanate; chewable tablets 200 mg amoxacillin/28.5 clavulanate, 400 mg amoxicillin/57 mg clavulanate; powder for oral suspension 250 mg amoxicillin/28.5 mg clavulanate, 200 amoxicillin mg/28.5 clavulanate mg, 400 amoxicillin mg/57 clavulanate mg, 600/42.9 mg/5 mL clavulanate extended-release tablets (XR) 1000 mg amoxicillin/62.5 mg clavulanate; powder for oral suspension (ES) 600 mg amoxicillin/42.9 mg clavulanate

Administer:
PO route
• Do not break, crush, chew extended-release product
• Only as directed; two 250-mg tablets not equivalent to one 500-mg tablet due to strength of clavulanate
• Shake suspension well before each dose; may be used alone, mixed in drinks; use immediately, discard unused portion of suspension after 14 days, store in refrigerator
• Give around the clock
• Give with light meal for increased absorption, fewer GI effects, confusion, behavioral changes

SIDE EFFECTS
CNS: Headache, fever, seizures, agitation, insomnia
GI: *Nausea, diarrhea, vomiting,* increased AST/ALT, CDAD
GU: *Vaginitis*
HEMA: Anemia, bone marrow depression, granulocytopenia, leukopenia, eosinophilia, thrombocytopenic purpura
INTEG: *Rash,* urticaria
SYST: Anaphylaxis, respiratory distress, serum sickness

PHARMACOKINETICS
PO: Peak 1-2.5 hr, duration 8-12 hr, half-life 1-1⅓ hr, metabolized in liver, excreted in urine, crosses placenta, excreted in breast milk, removed by hemodialysis

INTERACTIONS
Increase: amoxicillin levels—probenecid, used for this reason
Increase: anticoagulant effect—warfarin; monitor closely, dose adjustment may be needed
Increase: skin rash—allopurinol

Decrease: contraceptive effect—oral contraceptives
Drug/Food
Decrease: absorption by a high-fat meal
Drug/Lab Test
Increase: AST/ALT, alkaline phosphatase, LDH
Interference: urine glucose tests (Clinitest, Benedict's reagent, cupric SO$_4$)

NURSING CONSIDERATIONS
Assess:
• **Infection:** For signs/symptoms of infection (characteristics of wounds, sputum, urine, stool, WBC >10,000/mm^3, earache, fever, obtain baseline and during treatment
• **Superinfection:** Perineal itching, fever, malaise, redness, pain, swelling, rash, diarrhea, change in cough sputum; if large doses are given or geriatrics
• Hepatic studies: AST, ALT baseline, periodically in hepatic disease, discontinue if hepatitis occurs
• Blood studies: WBC
• C&S may be drawn before product therapy; product may be given as soon as culture is taken
• **CDAD:** bowel pattern before, during treatment; diarrhea, cramping, blood in stools; report to prescriber
• **Anaphylaxis:** rash, itching, dyspnea, facial/laryngeal edema; skin eruptions after administration of penicillin to 1 wk after discontinuing product, adrenaline, suction, tracheostomy set, endotracheal intubation equipment on unit
Evaluate:
• Therapeutic response: absence of infection
Teach patient/family:
• To take as prescribed, not to double or skip doses
• All aspects of product therapy: to complete entire course of medication to ensure organism death, that culture may be taken after completed course of medication
• That product must be taken in equal intervals around the clock to maintain blood levels

• To report sore throat, fever, fatigue (superinfection or agranulocytosis); diarrhea, cramping, blood in stools (pseudomembranous colitis)
• To wear or carry emergency ID if allergic to penicillins
• **Pregnancy/breastfeeding:** To notify health care professional if pregnancy is planned or suspected or if breastfeeding; to use another form of contraception if taking oral contraceptives, effect may be decreased

TREATMENT OF HYPERSENSITIVITY: Withdraw product, maintain airway, administer EPINEPHrine, O$_2$, IV corticosteroids for anaphylaxis

---

⚠ HIGH ALERT

amphotericin B lipid complex (ABLC) (Rx)
(am-foe-ter′i-sin)
Abelcet
Func. class.: Antifungal
Chem. class.: Amphoteric polyene

Do not confuse:
Abelcet/amphotericin B

ACTION: Increases cell membrane permeability in susceptible fungi by binding sterols; alters cell membrane, thereby causing leakage of cell components, cell death

USES: Indicated for the treatment of invasive fungal infections in patients who cannot tolerate or have failed conventional amphotericin B therapy; broad-spectrum activity against many fungal, yeast and mold pathogen infections, including *Aspergillus, Zygomycetes, Fusarium, Cryptococcus,* and many hard-to-treat *Candida* species; *Aspergillus fumigatus, Aspergillus* sp., *Blastomyces dermatitidis, Candida albicans, Candida guilliermondii, Candida* sp., *Candida stellatoidea, Candida tropicalis, Coccidioides*

---

immitis, Cryptococcus sp., *Histoplasma* sp., sporotrichosis

CONTRAINDICATIONS

Hypersensitivity

Precautions: Anemia, breastfeeding, cardiac disease, children, electrolyte imbalance, geriatric patients, hematologic/hepatic/renal disease, hypotension, pregnancy

DOSAGE AND ROUTES

• **Adult: IV** 3-5 mg/kg/day
Renal dose
• **Adult: IV** CCr <10 mL/min give 5 mg/kg q24-36hr
Available forms: Suspension for injection 5 mg/mL
Administer:
• **Do not confuse the 4 different types; these are not interchangeable:** conventional amphotericin B, amphotericin B cholesteryl, amphotericin B lipid complex, amphotericin B liposome
• May premedicate with acetaminophen, diphenhydrAMINE
• Use only after C&S confirms organism
IV route
• Give product only after C&S confirms organism, product needed to treat condition; make sure product is used for life-threatening infections
• Handle with aseptic technique, amphotericin B lipid complex (ABLC) has no preservatives; visually inspect parenteral products for particulate matter and discoloration before use
Filtration and dilution:
• Before dilution, store at 36° F-46° F (2° C-8° C), protected from moisture and light; do not freeze; the diluted, ready-for-use admixture is stable for up to 48 hours at 36° F-46° F (2° C-8° C) and an additional 6 hr at room temperature; do not freeze
• Prepare by shaking the vial until no yellow sediment remains
• Transfer the amount of drug from the required number of vials into one or more sterile syringes using an 18-gauge needle

• Attach the provided 5-micron filter needle to the syringe; inject the syringe contents through the filter needle into an IV bag containing the D₅W injection; each filter needle may be used on the contents of no more than four 100-mg vials
• The suspension must be diluted with D₅W injection (1 mg/mL); for pediatric patients and patients with cardiovascular disease, the final concentration may be 2 mg/mL; DO NOT USE SALINE SOLUTIONS OR MIX WITH OTHER DRUGS OR ELECTROLYTES
• The diluted ready-for-use admixture is stable for up to 48 hr at 36° F-46° F (2° C-8° C) and an additional 6 hr at room temperature; do not freeze
IV INFUSION
• Flush IV line with D₅W injection before use or use a separate IV line; DO NOT USE AN IN-LINE FILTER
• Before infusion, shake the bag until thoroughly mixed; max rate 2.5 mg/kg/hr; if the infusion time exceeds 2 hr, mix by shaking the infusion bag every 2 hr

Y-site compatibilities: acyclovir, allopurinol, aminocaproic acid, aminophylline, amiodarone, anidulafungin, argatroban, arsenic trioxide, atracurium, azithromycin, aztreonam, bumetanide, buprenorphine, busulfan, butorphanol, CARBOplatin, carmustine, ceFAZolin, cefepime, cefotaxime, cefoTEtan, cefOXitin, cefTAZidime, ceftizoxime, cefTRIAXone, cefuroxime, chloramphenicol, chlorproMAZINE, cimetidine, cisatracurium, clindamycin, cyclophosphamide, cycloSPORINE, cytarabine, DACTINomycin, dexamethasone, digoxin, diphenhydrAMINE, DOCEtaxel, doxacurium, DOXOrubicin liposomal, enalaprilat, EPINEPHrine eptifibatide, ertapenem, etoposide, famotidine, fentaNYL, fludarabine, fluorouracil, fosphenytoin, furosemide, ganciclovir, granisetron, heparin, hydrocortisone, HYDROmorphone, ifosfamide, insulin, regular ketorolac, lepirudin, lidocaine, linezolid, LORazepam, mannitol, melphalan, meperidine, methotrexate, methylPREDNISolone, metoclopramide, mitoMYcin, mivacurium, nafcillin, nesiritide, nitroglycerin, nitroprusside, octreotide, oxaliplatin, PACLitaxel, pamidronate, pantoprazole, PEMEtrexed, pentazocine, PENTobarbital, PHENobarbital, phentolamine, piperacillin-tazobactam, procainamide, raNITIdine, succinylcholine, SUFentanil, tacrolimus, telavancin, teniposide, theophylline, thiopental, thiotepa, ticarcillin, ticarcillin-clavulanate, trimethobenzamide, verapamil, vinBLAStine, vinCRIStine, zidovudine, zoledronic acid

SIDE EFFECTS

CNS: *Headache, fever, chills,* confusion, anxiety, insomnia
CV: Hypotension, cardiac arrest, chest pain, hypertension, tachycardia, edema
GI: *Nausea, vomiting, anorexia,* diarrhea, cramps, bilirubinemia
GU: Nephrotoxicity
HEMA: Anemia, thrombocytopenia, agranulocytosis, leukopenia
INTEG: *Burning, irritation,* pain, necrosis at injection site with extravasation, rash, pruritus, dermatitis
META: Hyponatremia, hypomagnesemia, hypokalemia
MS: Arthralgia, myalgia, generalized pain, weakness, weight loss
RESP: Dyspnea, wheezing, respiratory failure
SYST: Toxic epidermal necrolysis, exfoliative dermatitis, anaphylaxis, sepsis, infection

PHARMACOKINETICS

IV: half-life 7 days

INTERACTIONS

• Do not use with cidofovir
Increase: nephrotoxicity—other nephrotoxic antibiotics (aminoglycosides, CISplatin, vancomycin, cycloSPORINE, polymyxin B), antineoplastics, pentamidine, salicylates, tacrolimus, tenofovir; use cautiously
Increase: hypokalemia—corticosteroids, digoxin, skeletal muscle relaxants, thiazides, loop diuretics; monitor electrolytes
Decrease: amphotericin B lipid complex—azole antifungals; may still be used concurrently in serious resistant infections

Drug/Lab Test
Increase: AST/ALT, alkaline phosphatase, BUN, creatinine, LDH, bilirubin
Decrease: magnesium, potassium, HB, WBC, platelets

NURSING CONSIDERATIONS

Assess:
• VS every 15-30 min during first infusion; note changes in pulse, B/P
• Blood studies: CBC, potassium, sodium, calcium, magnesium every 2 wk; BUN, creatinine 2-3 ×/wk
• Weight weekly; if weight increases by more than 2 lb/wk, edema is present; renal damage should be considered
• **For renal toxicity:** increasing BUN, serum creatinine; if BUN is >40 mg/dL or if serum creatinine is >3 mg/dL, product may be discontinued, dosage reduced, I&O ratio; watch for decreasing urinary output, change in specific gravity; discontinue product to prevent permanent damage to renal tubules
• **For hepatotoxicity:** increasing AST, ALT, alkaline phosphatase, bilirubin
• **For allergic reaction:** dermatitis, rash; product should be discontinued, antihistamines (mild reaction) or EPINEPHrine (severe reaction) should be administered
• **For hypokalemia:** anorexia, drowsiness, weakness, decreased reflexes, dizziness, increased urinary output, increased thirst, paresthesias
• **Infusion reactions:** fever, chills, pain, swelling at site
Evaluate:
• Therapeutic response: resolution of infection, negative C&S for infecting organism
Teach patient/family:
• That long-term therapy may be needed to clear infection (2 wk-3 mo, depending on type of infection), frequent blood draws will be needed
• To notify prescriber of bleeding, bruising, or soft tissue swelling, neurologic, renal symptoms
• **Pregnancy/breastfeeding:** to advise prescriber if pregnancy is planned or suspected; not to breastfeed

amphotericin
B liposomal (LAmB) (Rx)
(am-foe-ter′i-sin)
AmBisome
Func. class.: Antifungal
Chem. class.: Amphoteric polyene

Do not confuse:
AmBisome/amphotericin B

ACTION: Increases cell membrane permeability in susceptible fungi by binding to membrane sterols; alters cell membrane, thereby causing leakage of cell components, cell death

THERAPEUTIC OUTCOME
Resolution of infection

USES: Empiric therapy for presumed fungal infection in febrile neutropenic patients; treatment of cryptococcal meningitis in HIV-infected patients; treatment of *Aspergillus* sp., *Candida* sp., and/or *Cryptococcus* sp. infections refractory to amphotericin B deoxycholate, or in patients where renal impairment or unacceptable toxicity precludes the use of amphotericin B deoxycholate *(Aspergillus flavus, Aspergillus fumigatus, Blastomyces dermatitidis, Candida albicans, Candida krusei, Candida lusitaniae, Candida parapsilosis, Candida tropicalis, Cryptococcus neoformans);* treatment of visceral leishmaniasis
Unlabeled uses: Coccidioidomycosis, histoplasmosis

CONTRAINDICATIONS
Hypersensitivity
Precautions: Anemia, breastfeeding, cardiac disease, children, electrolyte imbalance, geriatric patients, hematologic/hepatic/renal disease, hypotension, pregnancy, severe bone marrow depression

DOSAGE AND ROUTES
Systemic fungal infections
• **Adults and children:** IV 3-6 mg/kg/dose q24hr

Esophageal candidiasis (unlabeled) in HIV-infected patients
• **Adults/adolescents:** IV 3-4 mg/kg/dose q24hr for 14 to 21 days
Cryptococcal meningitis in HIV patients
• **Adults/adolescents/children/infants:** IV 6 mg/kg/dose q24hr
Visceral leishmaniasis
• **Adult:** IV 3 mg/kg q24hr on days 1-5, then 3 mg/kg q24hr on days 14, 21 (immunocompetent); 4 mg/kg q24hr on days 1-5, then 4 mg/kg q24hr on days 10, 17, 24, 31, 38 (immunosuppressed)
Severe disseminated (nonmeningeal) or diffuse pulmonary coccidioidomycosis (unlabeled) in HIV-infected patients
• **Adults:** IV 3-5 mg/kg/dose q24hr
Histoplasmosis (unlabeled)
Adults: IV 3 mg/kg/dose daily depending on the type of histoplasmosis and concomitant conditions
Infant/child/adolescent: IV 3-5 mg/kg/dose daily
Renal dose
• **Adult:** IV CCr <10 mL/min use 3 mg/kg q24hr
Available forms: Powder for injection 50-mg vial
Administer:
• **Do not confuse the 4 different types; these are not interchangeable:** conventional amphotericin B, amphotericin B cholesteryl, amphotericin B lipid complex, amphotericin B liposome
• May premedicate with acetaminophen, diphenhydrAMINE
IV route
• Give after C&S confirms organism and product needed to treat condition
• Use for life-threatening infections
• Administer by IV infusion only; use aseptic technique, as LAmB does not contain any preservatives
• Visually inspect for particulate and discoloration
Reconstitution
• LAmB *must* be reconstituted using sterile water for injection (without a bacteriostatic agent); DO NOT RECONSTITUTE WITH SALINE OR ADD SALINE TO THE

RECONSTITUTED SUSPENSION, DO NOT MIX WITH OTHER DRUGS; doing so can cause a precipitate to form
• Reconstitute vials containing 50 mg of LAmB/12 mL of sterile water (4 mg/mL)
• Immediately after the addition of water, SHAKE VIGOROUSLY; the suspension should be yellow and translucent; visually inspect vial for particulate matter and continue shaking until completely dispersed
• Store suspension for up to 24 hr refrigerated if using sterile water for injection; do not freeze

Filtration and dilution
• Calculate the amount of reconstituted (4 mg/mL) suspension to be further diluted and withdraw this amount into a sterile syringe
• Attach the provided 5-micron filter to the syringe; inject the syringe contents through the filter into the appropriate amount of D_5W injection; use only one filter per vial
• The suspension must be diluted with D_5W injection (1-2 mg/mL) before administration; for infants and small children, lower concentrations (0.2-0.5 mg/mL) may be appropriate to provide sufficient volume for infusion
• Use injection of LAmB within 6 hr of dilution with D_5W

IV INFUSION
• Flush line with D_5W injection before infusion; if this cannot be done, then a separate IV line must be used
• An in-line membrane filter may be used with pore diameter if the filter is not less than 1 micron
• Administer using a controlled infusion device over a period of 120 min; infusion time may be reduced to 60 min in patients who tolerate the infusion; if discomfort occurs, the duration of infusion may be increased
• Store protected from moisture and light; diluted solution is stable for 24 hr at room temperature

Acetaminophen and diphenhydrAMINE
• 30 min before infusion to reduce fever, chills, headache

Y-site compatibilities: Acyclovir, amifostine, aminophylline, anidulafungin, atropine, azithromycin, bivalirudin, bumetanide, buprenorphine, busulfan, butorphanol, CARBOplatin, carmustine, ceFAZolin, ceFOXitin, ceftizoxime, cefTRIAXone, cefuroxime, cimetidine, clindamycin, cyclophosphamide, cytarabine, DACTINomycin, DAPTOmycin, dexamethasone, dexmedetomidine, diphenhydrAMINE, doxacurium, enalaprilat, ePHEDrine, EPINEPHrine, eptifibatide, ertapenem, esmolol, etoposide, famotidine, fenoldopam, fentaNYL, fludarabine, fluorouracil, fosphenytoin, furosemide, granisetron, haloperidol, heparin, hydrocortisone, HYDROmorphone, ifosfamide, isoproterenol, ketorolac, levorphanol, lidocaine, linezolid, mesna, methotrexate, methylPREDNISolone, metoprolol, milrinone, mitoMYcin, nesiritide, nitroglycerin, nitroprusside, octreotide, oxaliplatin, oxytocin, palonosetron, pancuronium, pantoprazole, PEMEtrexed, PENTobarbital, PHENObarbital, phenylephrine, piperacillin/tazobactam, potassium chloride, procainamide, raNITIdine, SUFentanil, tacrolimus, theophylline, thiopental, thiotepa, ticarcillin/clavulanate, tigecycline, trimethoprim-sulfamethoxazole, vasopressin, vinCRIStine, voriconazole, zidovudine

SIDE EFFECTS
CNS: *Headache, fever, chills,* peripheral nerve pain, insomnia
CV: Hypotension, cardiac arrest, tachycardia, edema, flushing
GI: *Nausea, vomiting, anorexia,* diarrhea, cramps, GI hemmorrhage, hyperbilirubinemia
GU: Nephrotoxicity
HEMA: Anemia, thrombocytopenia, agranulocytosis, leukopenia
INTEG: *Burning, irritation,* pain, necrosis at injection site with extravasation, flushing, dermatitis, skin rash (topical route)
MS: Arthralgia, myalgia
RESP: Dyspnea, cough
SYST: Stevens-Johnson syndrome, toxic epidermal necrolysis, exfoliative dermatitis, anaphylaxis

PHARMACOKINETICS
IV: Metabolized in liver; excreted in urine (metabolites), breast milk; protein

binding 90%; poorly penetrates CSF, bronchial secretions, aqueous humor, muscle, bone; half-life 4-6 days

INTERACTIONS

Increase: nephrotoxicity—other nephrotoxic antibiotics (aminoglycosides, antineoplastics, CISplatin, vancomycin, cycloSPORINE, polymyxin B)

Increase: hypokalemia—corticosteroids, digoxin, skeletal muscle relaxants, thiazides, loop diuretics

Decrease: amphotericin B liposomal—azole antifungals, may be used concurrently in serious resistant infections

NURSING CONSIDERATIONS
Assess:

• VS every 15-30 min during first infusion; note changes in B/P

• Blood studies: CBC, potassium, sodium, calcium, magnesium every 2 wk, BUN, creatinine 2-3×/wk

• Weight weekly; if weight increases by more than 2 lb/wk, edema is present; renal damage should be considered

• **For renal toxicity:** increasing BUN, serum creatinine; if BUN is >40 mg/dL or if serum creatinine is >3 mg/dL, product may be discontinued, dosage reduced; I&O ratio; watch for decreasing urinary output, change in specific gravity; discontinue product to prevent permanent damage to renal tubules

• **For hepatotoxicity:** increasing AST, ALT, alkaline phosphatase, bilirubin, monitor LFTs

• **For allergic reaction:** dermatitis, rash; product should be discontinued, antihistamines (mild reaction) or EPINEPHrine (severe reaction) administered

• **For hypokalemia:** anorexia, drowsiness, weakness, decreased reflexes, dizziness, increased urinary output, increased thirst, paresthesias

• **Infusion reaction:** chills, fever, pain, swelling at site

Evaluate:

• Therapeutic response: resolution of infection, negative C&S for infecting organism

Teach patient/family:

• That long-term therapy may be needed to clear infection (2 wk-3 mo, depending on type of infection), that frequent blood draws will be needed

• To notify prescriber of bleeding, bruising, or soft tissue swelling, renal, neurologic side effects

• **Pregnancy/breastfeeding:** To notify health care professional if pregnancy is planned or suspected, not to breastfeed

---

ampicillin (Rx)

(am-pi-sill'in)

Func. class.: Antiinfective—broad-spectrum

Chem. class.: Aminopenicillin

Do not confuse:

ampicillin/aminophylline/amoxicillin

ACTION: Interferes with cell wall replication of susceptible organisms; the cell wall, rendered osmotically unstable, swells, bursts from osmotic pressure; lysis mediated by cell wall autolysins

USES: Effective for gram-positive cocci *(Staphylococcus aureus, Streptococcus pyogenes, Streptococcus faecalis, Streptococcus pneumoniae),* gram-negative cocci *(Neisseria meningitidis),* gram-negative bacilli *(Haemophilus influenzae, Proteus mirabilis, Salmonella, Shigella, Listeria monocytogenes),* gram-positive bacilli; meningitis, GI/GU/respiratory infections, endocarditis, septicemia, otitis media, skin infection, bacterial endocarditis

CONTRAINDICATIONS

Hypersensitivity to penicillins, antimicrobial resistance

Precautions: Pregnancy, breastfeeding, neonates, hypersensitivity to cephalosporins, renal disease, mononucleosis

DOSAGE AND ROUTES
Systemic infections

• **Adult and child ≥40 kg: PO** 250-500 mg q6hr; **IV/IM** 2-8 g/day in divided doses q4-6hr

• **Child <40 kg: PO** 50-100 mg/kg/day in divided doses q6-8hr; **IV/IM** 100-150 mg/kg/day in divided doses q6hr

Bacterial meningitis

• **Adult and adolescent: IM/IV** 150-200 mg/kg/day in divided doses q3-4 hr; IDSA dose **IV** 2 g q4hr

• **Infant and child: IM/IV** 150-200 mg/kg/day in divided doses q3-4hr; IDSA dose IV 200-400 mg/kg/day in divided doses q6hr

• **Neonate >7 days and >2000 g: IM/IV** 200 mg/kg/day in divided doses q6hr; IDSA dose; **IV** 200 mg/kg/day in divided doses q6-8hr

Prevention of bacterial endocarditis

• **Adult: IM/IV** 2 g 30 min prior to procedure

• **Child: IM/IV** 50 mg/kg 30 min prior to procedure, max 2 g

GI/GU infections other than N. gonorrhoeae

• **Adult and child >20 kg: PO** 500 mg q6hr, may use larger dose for more serious infections

• **Child <40 kg: PO** 50 mg/kg/day in divided doses q6-8hr

Renal disease

• **Adult and child:** CCr 10-50 mL/min extend to q6-12hr; CCr <10 mL/min extend to q12-16hr

Available forms: Powder for injection 125, 250, 500 mg, 1, 2, 10 g/vial; capsules 250, 500 mg; powder for oral suspension 125, 250 mg/5 mL

Administer:

• Check allergies before using; obtain C&S before using; begin before results are received

PO route

• Give in even doses around the clock, store caps in tight container, store after reconstituting in refrigerator up to 2 wk, 1 wk room temperature

• Tablets may be crushed or capsules opened and mixed with water

• On empty stomach with plenty of water for best absorption (1-2 hr before meals or 2-3 hr after meals)

• Shake suspension well before each dose; store after reconstituting in refrigerator up to 2 wk, 1 wk room temperature

IM route

• **Reconstitute** by adding 0.9-1.2 mL/125-mg vial; 0.9-1.9 mL/250-mg vial; 1.2-1.8 mL/500-mg vial; 2.4-7.4 mL/1-g vial; 6.8 mL/2-g vial

IV route

IV direct

• After diluting with sterile water 0.9-1.2 mL/125-mg product, administer over 3-5 min (up to 500 mg), 10-15 min (>500 mg)

Intermittent IV INFUSION route

• May be diluted in 50 mL or more of D_5W, D_5 0.45% NaCl to a concentration of 30 mg/mL or less; IV solution is stable for 1 hr; give at prescribed rate, do not give in same tubing as aminoglycosides, separate by ≥1 hr

Y-site compatibilities: Acyclovir, alemtuzumab, alprostadil, amifostine, aminocaproic acid, anidulafungin, argatroban, atenolol, azithromycin, bivalirudin, bleomycin, CARBOplatin, carmustine, CISplatin, clarithromycin, cyclophosphamide, cytarabine, DACTINomycin, DAPTOmycin, DAUNOrubicin liposome, dexmedetomidine, dexrazoxane, DOCEtaxel, doxacurium, doxapram, DOXOrubicin liposome, eptifibatide, etoposide, etoposide phosphate, filgrastim, fludarabine, fluorouracil, foscarnet, gallium, gatifloxacin, gemcitabine, gemtuzumab, granisetron, hetastarch, ifosfamide, irinotecan, lepirudin, leucovorin, levoFLOXacin, linezolid, mannitol, mechlorethamine, melphalan, methotrexate, metroNIDAZOLE, milrinone, octreotide, ofloxacin, oxaliplatin, PACLitaxel, palonosetron, pamidronate, pancuronium, pantoprazole, PEMEtrexed, penicillin G potassium, perphenazine, potassium acetate, propofol, remifentanil, riTUXimab, rocuronium, sodium acetate, teniposide, thiotepa, tigecycline, tirofiban, TNA, trastuzumab, vecuronium, vinBLAStine, vinCRIStine, vitamin B/C, voriconazole, zoledronic acid

SIDE EFFECTS

CNS: Seizures (high doses)

GI: *Nausea, vomiting, diarrhea,* CDAD, stomatitis
HEMA: Anemia, bone marrow depression, granulocytopenia, leukopenia, eosinophilia
INTEG: *Rash, urticaria*
MISC: Anaphylaxis, serum sickness

PHARMACOKINETICS

Half-life 50-110 min; excreted in urine, bile, breast milk; crosses placenta; removed by dialysis
PO: Peak 2 hr, duration 6-8 hr
IM: Peak 1 hr, duration 6-8 hr
IV: Peak rapid, duration 6-8 hr

INTERACTIONS

Increase: bleeding—oral anticoagulants, monitor INR/PT
Increase: ampicillin concentrations—probenecid, used for this action
Increase: ampicillin-induced skin rash—allopurinol, monitor for rash
Decrease: ampicillin level—H_2 antagonists, proton pump inhibitors, separate by 2 hr

Drug/Lab Test

Increase: eosinophils, ALT, AST
Decrease: conjugated estrogens during pregnancy, HB, WBC, platelets
False positive: urine glucose, direct Coomb's test
Interference: urine glucose (Clinitest, Benedict's reagent, cupric SO_4)

NURSING CONSIDERATIONS

Assess:

• **Infection:** characteristics of wound, sputum; urine, stool, earache, fever WBC baseline, periodically; C&S before product therapy, product may be taken as soon as culture is taken
• Hepatic studies: AST, ALT
• Blood studies: WBC, RBC, HB, Hct, bleeding time
• **CDAD:** bowel pattern before/during treatment
• Skin eruptions after administration of penicillin to 1 wk after discontinuing product; identify allergies before using

• Respiratory status: rate, character, wheezing, tightness in chest
• **Anaphylaxis:** rash, itching, dyspnea, facial swelling; stop product, notify prescriber, have emergency equipment available

Evaluate:

• Therapeutic response: absence of fever, draining wounds, resolution of infection

Teach patient/family:

• To take oral ampicillin on empty stomach with full glass of water; to use alternative contraception
• All aspects of product therapy: to complete entire course of medication to ensure organism death (10-14 days); that culture may be taken after completed course of medication
• To report sore throat, fever, fatigue, diarrhea (may indicate superinfection); to report rash, other signs of allergy
• That product must be taken in equal intervals around the clock to maintain blood levels
• To wear or carry emergency ID if allergic to penicillins
• **CDAD:** diarrhea with blood or pus; notify prescriber
• **Pregnancy/breastfeeding:** Identify if pregnancy is planned or suspected or if breastfeeding; to use additional contraception if using oral contraception, effect may be decreased

TREATMENT OF ANAPHYLAXIS: Withdraw product, maintain airway; administer EPINEPHrine, aminophylline, O_2, IV corticosteroids

---

ampicillin, sulbactam (Rx)

Unasyn
Func. class.: Antiinfective—broad-spectrum
Chem. class.: Aminopenicillin with β-lactamase inhibitor

ACTION: Interferes with cell wall replication of susceptible organisms; the cell wall, rendered osmotically unstable, swells, bursts from osmotic pressure; lysis due to cell wall autolytic enzymes; combination extends spectrum of activity by β-lactamase inhibition

USES: Skin infections, intraabdominal infections, cellulitis, diabetic foot ulcer, nosocomial pneumonia, gynecologic infections; *Acinetobacter* sp., *Actinomyces* sp., *Bacillus anthracis, Bacteroides* sp., *Bifidobacterium* sp., *Bordetella pertussis, Borrelia burgdorferi, Brucella* sp., *Clostridium* sp., *Corynebacterium diphtheriae/xerosis, Eikenella corrodens, Enterococcus faecalis, Erysipelothrix rhusiopathiae, Escherichia coli, Eubacterium* sp., *Fusobacterium* sp., *Gardnerella vaginalis, Haemophilus influenzae* (β-lactamase negative/positive), *Helicobacter pylori, Klebsiella* sp., *Lactobacillus* sp., *Leptospira* sp., *Listeria monocytogenes, Moraxella catarrhalis, Morganella morganii, Neisseria gonorrhoeae, Pasteurella multocida, Peptococcus* sp., *Peptostreptococcus* sp., *Porphyromonas* sp., *Prevotella* sp., *Propionibacterium* sp., *Proteus mirabilis, Proteus vulgaris, Providencia rettgeri, Providencia stuartii, Salmonella* sp., *Shigella* sp., *Staphylococcus aureus (MSSA)/epidermidis/saprophyticus, Streptococcus agalactiae/dysgalactiae/pneumoniae/pyogenes, Treponema pallidum,* viridans streptococci

CONTRAINDICATIONS

Hypersensitivity to penicillins, sulbactam
Precautions: Pregnancy, breastfeeding, neonates, hypersensitivity to cephalosporins/carbapenems, renal disease, mononucleosis, viral infections, syphilis

DOSAGE AND ROUTES

• **Adult/adolescent/child ≥40 kg: IM/IV** 1.5-3 g q6hr, max 4 g/day sulbactam
• **Child >1 yr: IV** 150-300 mg/kg/day divided q6hr
Infant: IM/IV ≥1 mo: 100-150 mg ampicillin/kg/day divided q6hr

Renal disease
• **Adult ≥40 kg: IM/IV** CCr 15-30 mL/min dose q12hr; CCr 5-15 mL/min dose q24hr
Available forms: Powder for injection 1.5 g (1 g ampicillin, 0.5 g sulbactam), 3 g (2 g ampicillin, 1 g sulbactam), 15 g (10 g ampicillin, 5 g sulbactam)
Administer:
IM route
• Reconstitute by adding 3.2 mL sterile water/1.5-g vial; 6.4 mL/3-g vial, give deep in large muscle, aspirate
• Do not use IM in child
Direct IV route
• After reconstituting 1.5 g/3.2 mL sterile water for injection or 3 g/6.4 mL (250 mg ampicillin/125 mg sulbactam), allow to stand until foaming stops; may give over 15 min, inject slowly, use within 1 hr of reconstitution
Intermittent IV INFUSION route
• Reconstitute as IV direct, then dilute further in 50 mL or more of D₅W, NaCl; administer within 1 hr after reconstitution; give over 15-30 min, separate doses from aminoglycosides by ≥1 hr

Y-site compatibilities: Alemtuzumab, amifostine, aminocaproic acid, anidulafungin, argatroban, atenolol, bivalirudin, bleomycin, CARBOplatin, carmustine, cefepime, CISplatin, codeine, cyclophosphamide, cytarabine, DAPTOmycin, DAUNOrubicin liposome, dexmedetomidine, DOCEtaxel, doxacurium, DOXOrubicin liposomal, eptifibatide, etoposide, fenoldopam, filgrastim, fludarabine, fluorouracil, foscarnet, gallium, gatifloxacin, gemcitabine, granisetron, hetastarch, irinotecan, levoFLOXacin, linezolid, methotrexate, metroNIDAZOLE, octreotide, oxaliplatin, PACLitaxel, palonosetron, pamidronate, pancuronium, pantoprazole, PEMEtrexed, remifentanil, riTUXimab, rocuronium, tacrolimus, teniposide, thiotepa, tigecycline, tirofiban, TNA, TPN, trastuzumab, vecuronium, vinCRIStine, voriconazole, zoledronic acid

SIDE EFFECTS

CNS: Coma, seizures (high dose)
GI: *Nausea, vomiting, diarrhea,* abdominal pain, CDAD, hepatotoxicity

HEMA: Anemia, bone marrow depression, granulocytopenia, leukopenia, eosinophilia
INTEG: Injection site reactions, rash, urticaria
MISC: Anaphylaxis, serum sickness, Stevens-Johnson syndrome

PHARMACOKINETICS
IV: Peak 5 min, IM 1 hr; half-life 50-110 min (ampicillin) 1-1.4 hr (sulbactam), 10%-50% metabolized in liver, 75%-85% of both products excreted in urine, excreted in breast milk, crosses placenta

INTERACTIONS
Increase: bleeding risk—oral anticoagulants; check INR, PT
Increase: ampicillin-induced skin rash—allopurinol, check for rash
Increase: ampicillin level—probenecid
Increase: methotrexate level—methotrexate
Decrease: contraception effect—oral contraceptives, use additional contraception
Drug/Lab Test
Decrease: hct/HB, RBC, WBC, neutrophils, lymphocytes
False positive: urine glucose, urine protein

NURSING CONSIDERATIONS
Assess:
• For previous sensitivity to penicillin or cephalosporins, cross-sensitivity is common
• **Infection:** characteristics of wound, sputum; take temperature, WBC count, check allergies before using; C&S before product therapy, product may be given as soon as culture is taken
• **CDAD:** bowel pattern before, during treatment
• Hepatic studies: AST, ALT if on long-term therapy or impaired liver function
• **Anaphylaxis:** skin eruptions after administration of ampicillin to 1 wk after discontinuing product
Evaluate:
• Therapeutic response: absence of fever, draining wounds; negative C&S
Teach patient/family:
• To report superinfection: vaginal itching; loose, foul-smelling stools; black furry tongue

• **CDAD:** to report immediately to health care provider symptoms of fever, diarrhea with pus, blood, mucus; may occur up to 4 wk after treatment
• To wear or carry emergency ID if allergic to penicillin products
• **Pregnancy/breastfeeding:** If pregnancy is planned or suspected; use additional contraception if using oral contraceptives

TREATMENT OF ANAPHYLAXIS: Withdraw product, maintain airway; administer EPINEPHrine, aminophylline, O_2, IV corticosteroids

---

anakinra (Rx)
(an-ah-kin'rah)
Kineret
Func. class.: Antirheumatic (DMARD), immunomodulator

USES: Reduction in signs and symptoms of moderate to severe active rheumatoid arthritis in patients ≥18 yr who have not responded to other disease-modifying agents, neonatal-onset multisystem inflammatory disease

CONTRAINDICATIONS
Hypersensitivity to *Escherichia coli*–derived proteins, latex; sepsis

DOSAGE AND ROUTES
Rheumatoid arthritis
• **Adult:** SUBCUT 100 mg/day at same time of the day
Neonatal-onset multisystem inflammatory disease
• **Adult/child:** SUBCUT 1-2 mg/kg/day, may increase by 0.5-1 mg to max 8 mg/kg/day
Renal dose
• **Adult:** SUBCUT CCr <30 mL/min 100 mg every other day

Available forms: Injection 100-mg/0.67-mL prefilled syringe

⚠ HIGH ALERT

anastrozole (Rx)

(an-a-stroh'zole)

Arimidex

Func. class.: Antineoplastic

Chem. class.: Aromatase inhibitor

ACTION: Highly selective nonsteroidal aromatase inhibitor that lowers serum estradiol concentrations; many breast cancers have strong estrogen receptors

USES: Advanced breast carcinoma in estrogen receptor–positive patients (postmenopausal); patients with advanced disease taking tamoxifen, adjunct therapy

Unlabeled uses: Breast cancer risk reduction (postmenopausal women)

CONTRAINDICATIONS

Pregnancy, breastfeeding, hypersensitivity

Precautions: Children, geriatric patients, premenopausal women, osteoporosis, hepatic/cardiac disease

DOSAGE AND ROUTES

• **Adult:** PO 1 mg/day

Breast cancer risk reduction (postmenopausal women) (unlabeled)

Adult: PO 1 mg/day × 5 yr

Available forms: Tablets 1 mg

Administer:

• Use cytotoxic handling procedures

• Give without regard to meals at same time of day

• Store in light-resistant container at room temperature

SIDE EFFECTS

CNS: *Hot flashes, headache, lightheadedness,* depression, dizziness, confusion, insomnia, anxiety, fatigue, mood changes

CV: Chest pain, *hypertension,* thrombophlebitis, *edema,* angina

GI: *Nausea, vomiting,* altered taste leading to anorexia, diarrhea, constipation, abdominal pain, dry mouth

GU: Vaginal bleeding, vaginal dryness, pelvic pain

INTEG: *Rash,* Stevens-Johnson syndrome, anaphylaxis, angioedema

MISC: Hypercholesterolemia

MS: Bone pain, myalgia, back pain, arthralgia, fractures

RESP: Cough, sinusitis, dyspnea

EENT: Pharyngitis

PHARMACOKINETICS

Peak 4-7 hr; half-life 50 hr; metabolized in liver 85%, excreted in feces, urine, terminal half-life 50 hr

INTERACTIONS

• Do not use with oral contraceptives, estrogen, tamoxifen, androstenedione, DHEA, may decrease the action of anastrozole

Drug/Lab Test

Increase: AST, ALT, cholesterol

NURSING CONSIDERATIONS

Assess:

• Bone mineral density, cholesterol, lipid panel, periodically

• **Serious skin reactions:** Stevens-Johnson syndrome

• **Pregnancy:** Identify that patient is not pregnant before starting

Evaluate:

• Therapeutic response: decreased tumor size, spread of malignancy

Teach patient/family:

• To report any complaints, side effects to prescriber

• That vaginal bleeding, pruritus, hot flashes are reversible after discontinuing treatment

• To report continued vaginal bleeding immediately

• That tumor flare—increase in size of tumor, increased bone pain—may occur and will subside rapidly; may take analgesics for pain

• **Pregnancy/breastfeeding:** to tell prescriber if pregnancy is planned or suspected; do not use in pregnancy and for 3 wk after last dose or breastfeeding during or for 15 days after product is stopped

• To take adequate calcium and vitamin D due to risk for bone loss/fractures

• That follow-up exams will be needed

• Advise patient to report side effects to health care provider: hepatic: yellowing of skin, eyes, right abdominal pain; skin: rash, blisters, ulcerations; allergy: allergy: swelling of face, lips, tongue, breathing difficulties

antithymocyte

See lymphocyte immune globulin

anidulafungin (Rx)

(a-nid-yoo-luh-fun′jin)

Eraxis

Func. class.: Antifungal, systemic
Chem. class.: Echinocandin

ACTION: Inhibits fungal enzyme synthesis; causes direct damage to fungal cell wall

USES: Esophageal candidiasis, *Candida albicans, C. glabrata, C. parapsilosis, C. tropicalis*

CONTRAINDICATIONS

Hypersensitivity to product, other echinocandins

Precautions: Pregnancy, breastfeeding, children, severe hepatic disease

DOSAGE AND ROUTES

Candidemia and other *Candida* infections

• **Adult: IV** 200-mg loading dose on day 1, then 100 mg/day, continue treatment for 2 weeks after documented clearance of Candida from bloodstream and resolution of symptoms

Child ≥1 mo: IV 3 mg/kg loading dose on day 1 (max 200 mg), then 1.5 mg/kg q day (max 100 mg) × 14 days after last positive culture

Esophageal candidiasis

• **Adult: IV** 200 mg/day × 14-21 days or 200 mg q day × 14-21 days

Available forms: Powder for injection, lyophilized 50 mg/vial, 100 mg/vial for IV use

Administer:

IV route

• Obtain C&S tests before starting treatment
• Visually inspect prepared infusions for particulate matter and discoloration, do not use if present; give by IV infusion only, after dilution
• **Reconstitution:** Reconstitute each 50-mg or 100-mg vial/15 mL or 30 mL of sterile water for injection, respectively (3.33 mg/mL)
• **Storage:** Reconstituted solutions are stable for up to 24 hr at room temperature

• **Dilution:** Do not use any other diluents besides D₅W or sodium chloride 0.9% (NS)
• **Preparation of the 100-mg daily infusion:** Withdraw the contents of one 100-mg reconstituted vial OR two 50-mg reconstituted vials and add to an IV infusion bag or bottle containing 100 mL of D₅W or NS to give a total infusion volume of 130 mL
• **Preparation of a 50-mg daily infusion:** Withdraw the contents of one 50-mg reconstituted vial and add to an IV infusion bag or bottle containing 50 mL of D₅W or NS to give a total infusion volume of 65 mL
• **Storage:** Diluted solutions are stable for up to 48 hr at temperatures up to 77° F (25° C) or for 72 hr if stored frozen

Intermittent IV Infusion

• Do not mix or co-infuse with other medications
• Administer as a slow IV infusion at a rate of 1.4 mL/min or 84 mL/hr; the minimum duration of infusion is 180 min for the 200-mg dose, 90 min for the 100-mg dose, and 45 min for the 50-mg dose
• Store reconstituted vials at 59° F-86° F (15° C-30° C) for up to 24 hr, do not freeze (dehydrated alcohol); store reconstituted vials at 36° F-46° F (2.2° C-7.7° C) (sterile water) for up to 24 hr, do not freeze

Y-site compatibilities: Acyclovir, alemtuzumab, alfentanil, allopurinol, amifostine, amikacin, aminocaproic acid, aminophylline, amiodarone, amphotericin B lipid complex, amphotericin B liposome, ampicillin, ampicillin sulbactam, argatroban, arsenic trioxide, atenolol, atracurium, azithromycin, aztreonam, bivalirudin, bleomycin, bumetanide, buprenorphine, busulfan, butorphanol, calcium chloride/gluconate, CARBOplatin, carmustine, caspofungin, ceFAZolin, cefepime, cefotaxime, cefoTEtan, cefOXitin, cefTAZidime, ceftizoxime, cefTRIAXone, cefuroxime, chloramphenicol, chlorproMAZINE, cimetidine, ciprofloxacin, cisatracurium, CISplatin, clindamycin, cyclophosphamide, cycloSPORINE, cytarabine, dacarbazine, DACTINomycin, DAUNOrubicin liposome, DAUNOrubicin hydrochloride, dexamethasone, dexmedetomidine, dexrazoxane, digoxin, diltiazem, diphenhydrAMINE, DOBUtamine, DOCEtaxel, dolasetron, DOPamine, doripenem, doxacurium, DOXOrubicin, DOXOrubicin liposomal, doxycycline, droperidol, enalaprilat, ePHEDrine, EPINEPHrine, epiRUBicin, eptifibatide, erythromycin, esmolol, etoposide, etoposide phosphate, famotidine, fenoldopam, fentaNYL, fluconazole, fludarabine, fluorouracil, foscarnet, fosphenytoin, furosemide, gallium nitrate, ganciclovir, gatifloxacin, gemcitabine, gentamicin, glycopyrrolate, granisetron, haloperidol, heparin, hydrALAZINE, hydrocortisone, HYDROmorphone, hydrOXYzine, IDArubicin, ifosfamide, imipenem-cilastatin, inamrinone, insulin (regular), irinotecan, isoproterenol, ketorolac, labetalol, leucovorin, levoFLOXacin, lidocaine, linezolid injection, LORazepam, mannitol, mechlorethamine, melphalan, meperidine, meropenem, mesna, metaraminol, methotrexate, methyldopate, methylPREDNISolone, metoclopramide, metoprolol, metroNIDAZOLE, midazolam, milrinone, mitoMYcin, mitoXANTRONE, mivacurium, morphine, moxifloxacin, mycophenolate mofetil, nafcillin, naloxone, nesiritide, niCARdipine, nitroglycerin, nitroprusside, norepinephrine, octreotide, ondansetron, oxaliplatin, oxytocin, PACLitaxel, palonosetron, pamidronate, pancuronium, pantoprazole, PEMEtrexed, pentamidine, pentazocine, PENTobarbital, PHENobarbital, phentolamine, phenylephrine, piperacillin/tazobactam, polymyxin B, potassium acetate/chloride, procainamide, prochlorperazine, promethazine, propranolol, quiNIDine, quinupristin-dalfopristin, raNITIdine, remifentanil, rocuronium, sodium acetate, streptozocin, succinylcholine, SUFentanil, sulfamethoxazoletrimethoprim, tacrolimus, teniposide, theophylline, thiopental, thiotepa, ticarcillin, ticarcillin/clavulanate, tirofiban, tobramycin, topotecan, trimethobenzamide, vancomycin, vasopressin, vecuronium, verapamil, vinBLAStine, vinCRIStine, vinorelbine, voriconazole, zidovudine, zoledronic acid

SIDE EFFECTS

CNS: Dizziness, *headache*, fever, depression
CV: DVT, hypotension, chest pain, edema
GI: *Nausea, anorexia, vomiting, diarrhea*
META: Hypokalemia
RESP: Dyspnea, cough
HEMA: Anemia, thrombocytopenia
INTEG: *Rash*, urticaria, itching, flushing
META: Hyperkalemia
GU: UTI
EENT: Oral candidiasis
MS: *Back pain*

PHARMACOKINETICS

Steady state after loading dose, half-life 40-50 hr, protein binding 99%, crosses placenta, no metabolism, onset up to 24 hr

INTERACTIONS

None known

Drug/Lab Test
Increase: amylase, bilirubin, creatinine, lipase, PT, alkaline phosphatase, AST, ALT
Decrease: Magnesium, potassium, glucose

NURSING CONSIDERATIONS

Assess:
• **Infection:** clearing of cultures during treatment; obtain culture at baseline and throughout treatment; product may be started as soon as culture is taken, those with HIV pharyngeal candidiasis may need additional antifungals
• Hepatic studies before, during treatment: bilirubin, AST, ALT, alkaline phosphatase, as needed; also uric acid
• **GI symptoms:** frequency of stools, cramping; if severe diarrhea occurs, electrolytes may need to be given

Evaluate:
• Therapeutic response: decreased symptoms of *Candida* infection, negative culture

Teach patient/family:
• The reason for product, expected result

- **Anaphylaxis:** To report anaphylaxis symptoms immediately
- **Pregnancy/breastfeeding:** to notify prescriber if pregnancy is suspected, planned; to avoid breastfeeding

anifrolumab (Rx)

(an-i-FROL-ue-mab)

Saphnelo

Func. class.: Monoclonal antibody
Chem. class.: Type 1 interferon receptor antagonist

ACTION:
Binds to subunit 1 of the type I interferon, inhibition of type I IFN, blocks plasma cell differentiation and normalizes peripheral T-cells

USES:
Systemic lupus erythematosus

CONTRAINDICATIONS
Anaphylaxis

Precautions: Serious infections, hypersensitivity, malignancy, pregnancy, breastfeeding

DOSAGE AND ROUTES
- **Adult: IV INF** 300 mg over 30 min q4wk
Available forms: Injection: 300 mg/2 mL (150 mg/mL) in a single-dose vial
Administer:
IV INF route
- Visually inspect for particulates and discoloration, product should be clear to opalescent, colorless to slightly yellow; discard if cloudy, discolored or visible particles are present
- Do not shake
- Withdraw and discard 2 mL of solution from a 100 mL 0.9% NaCl injection, USP infusion bag
- Withdraw 2 mL of solution from the vial and add to the infusion bag, mix the solution by gentle inversion, do not shake
- Discard any unused portion
- Use immediately after preparation; if not used immediately, store diluted solution at room temperature (59° F-77° F, 15° C-25°

C) for ≤4 hr, or refrigerated (36° F-46° F, 2° C-8° C) for ≤24 hr; do not freeze, protect from light; if refrigerated, allow to come to room temperature before use
- Give over 30 min; use an infusion line containing a sterile, low-protein-binding 0.2 or 0.22 micron in-line filter
- Flush with 25 mL normal saline after completion, do not admix or administer through same line
- Dispose of any equipment as per agency policy

SIDE EFFECTS
- **RESP:** Nasopharyngitis, URI, bronchitis, cough
- **INTEG:** Infusion-related reactions
- **SYST:** Herpes zoster

INTERACTIONS
Avoid use with other biologic therapies, live, live-attenuated vaccines

PHARMACOKINETICS
Onset, peak, duration unknown

NURSING CONSIDERATIONS
Assess:
- **Serious infections:** Assess for active and chronic infections, avoid starting treatment in those with active infections
- **Hypersensitivity:** Serious hypersensitivity reactions, including anaphylaxis and angioedema have been reported
- **Malignancy:** Assess history of past or present malignancies, assess risk factors for malignancy before use
- **Immunizations:** Avoid use of live or live-attenuated vaccines in patients receiving, bring immunizations up to date before use
Evaluate:
- Therapeutic response: Decreasing effects of SLE
Teach patient/family:
- **Serious, chronic infections:** Teach patient to report signs, symptoms of infection (flulike symptoms, URI, bronchitis, or worsening of chronic infections)
- **Hypersensitivity:** Inform patient to report any allergic reactions, including itching, rash, trouble breathing, immediately to health care provider

Side effects: *italics* = common; red = life-threatening

• **Malignancy:** Consider the individual benefit and risk in patients with known risk factors for malignancy before prescribing
• **Immunization:** Bring immunizations up to date before use
• **Pregnancy/breastfeeding:** Notify health care provider if pregnancy is planned or suspected or if breastfeeding

---

antihemophilic factor Fc fusion protein (Rx)
(an-tee-hee-moe-fil'ik fak'tor)

Eloctate
Func. class.: Hemostatic

USES: Hemophilia A (congenital factor VIII deficiency), control/prevention of bleeding, perioperative management of surgical bleeding

DOSAGE AND ROUTES
Hemophilia A (congenital factor VIII deficiency)
• **Adults, adolescents, children, infants, and neonates:** IV INFUSION Infuse dose ≤10 mL/min; dose (IU) = body weight (kg) × desired factor VIII increase (IU/dL or % of normal) × 0.5 (IU/kg per IU/dL) *OR* estimated increment of factor VIII (IU/dL or % of normal) = [total dose (IU)/body weight (kg)] × 2 (IU/dL per IU/kg)

Control/prevention of bleeding
• **Adults, adolescents, children, infants, and neonates:** Dose and duration of treatment depend on the severity of the factor VIII deficiency, the location and extent of bleeding, and the patient's clinical condition

Perioperative management of surgical bleeding
• **Adults, adolescents, children, infants, and neonates:** Dose and duration of treatment depend on the severity of the factor VIII deficiency, the location and extent of bleeding, and the patient's clinical condition

Routine bleeding prophylaxis to prevent/reduce the frequency of bleeding episodes
• **IV** Initially, 50 IU/kg q4days; adjust dose based on response

---

⚠ HIGH ALERT

apalutamide (Rx)
(a'puh-loo'tuh-mide)

Erleada
Func. class.: Antineoplastic
Chem. class.: Anti-androgen receptor inhibitor

ACTION: An androgen receptor inhibitor that binds directly to the ligand-binding domain of the androgen receptor. It inhibits androgen receptor translocation and DNA binding and impedes androgen receptor–mediated transcription

USES: For the treatment of non-metastatic castration-resistant prostate cancer

CONTRAINDICATIONS
Pregnancy
Precautions: Bone fractures, breastfeeding, contraception requirements, driving or operating machinery, geriatric patients, infertility, male-mediated teratogenicity, reproductive risk, seizure disorder, seizures

DOSAGE AND ROUTES
Nonmetastatic, castration-resistant prostate cancer
• **Adults:** PO 240 mg daily until disease progression or toxicity; a gonadotropin-releasing hormone (GnRH) analog should be given concurrently or a bilateral orchiectomy should have been performed
Available forms: Tablet 60 mg

SIDE EFFECTS
CNS: Fatigue
CV: Hypertension, peripheral edema, heart failure, MI
GI: Diarrhea, anorexia, nausea, weight loss

GU: Hot flashes
HEMA: Anemia, leukopenia, lymphopenia
INTEG: Rash
META: Hypercholesterolemia, hypertriglyceridemia, hyperkalemia
MS: Arthralgia, bone fractures

PHARMACOKINETICS
96% plasma protein binding, primarily metabolized by CYP2C8 and CYP3A4 to its active metabolite, half-life 3 days, excreted 65% urine (unchanged), 24% feces (unchanged)

INTERACTIONS
Decrease: effects of CYP3A4 substrates—abemaciclib, cycloSPORINE, tacrolimus, sirolimus, DOCEtaxel, tamoxifen, PACLitaxel, cyclophosphamide, DOXOrubicin, erlotinib, etoposide, ifosfamide, teniposide, vinBLAStine, vinCRIStine, vindesine, imatinib, irinotecan, sorafenib, sunitinib, vemurafenib, temsirolimus, anastrozole, gefitinib, azole antifungals, macrolides, clarithromycin, erythromycin, telithromycin, dapsone, tricyclic antidepressants, SSRIs, some miscellaneous antidepressants, antipsychotics, opioids, benzodiazepines, some hypnotics, busPIRone, statins, calcium channel blockers, class I/III antidysrhythmics, PDE5 inhibitors, sex hormone agonists/antagonists, H1-receptor antagonists, protease inhibitors, non-nucleoside reverse transcriptase inhibitors; avoid concurrent use

NURSING CONSIDERATIONS
Assess
• **Possible bone fractures:** monitor and manage patients at risk for bone fractures; consider the use of bone-targeted agents. Falls and fractures are possible
• **Seizures:** use with caution in those with pre-existing seizure disorders; permanently discontinue if seizure occurs
• **Geriatric patients:** may be at increased risk for related adverse reactions; monitor closely for adverse reactions
• **Pregnancy/breastfeeding:** contraindicated in pregnancy, male infertility is a possibility

Evaluate:
• Therapeutic response: decrease in prostatic size, decrease in spread of cancer
Teach patient/family
• **Male-mediated teratogenicity:** that product is not indicated for use in females; that males with female partners of reproductive potential should avoid pregnancy and use effective contraception during and for at least 3 mo after treatment; that product may impair male fertility
• **Seizures:** about an increase in the risk of seizure and the risk of engaging in any activity where sudden loss of consciousness could cause harm to themselves or others (driving or operating machinery). It is unknown whether antiepileptic medications will prevent seizures

⚠ **HIGH ALERT**

apixaban (Rx)
(a-pix´-a-ban)
Eliquis
Func. class.: Anticoagulant
Chem. class.: Factor Xa inhibitor

ACTION: Inhibits factor Xa and thereby decreases thrombin and clot formation

USES: Deep venous thrombosis (DVT) after hip or knee replacement, to prevent stroke and embolism in atrial fibrillation (nonvalvular)

CONTRAINDICATIONS
Hypersensitivity, active bleeding, severe hepatic disease
Precautions: Breastfeeding, dialysis, hepatic/renal disease, labor, pregnancy, surgery, prosthetic heart valves, antiphospholipid syndrome, dysfunctional uterine bleeding, geriatrics, mitral stenosis

Black Box Warning: Abrupt discontinuation, epidural, spinal anesthesia, lumbar puncture

Side effects: *italics* = common; red = life-threatening

DOSAGE AND ROUTES

DVT or pulmonary embolism (PE)
• **Adult: PO** 10 mg bid × 7 days, then 5 mg bid ≥6 mo, to reduce recurrence >6 mo 2.5 mg bid; use with strong CYP3A4 and P-gb inhibitors: 2.5 mg

Stroke prophylaxis and systemic embolism prophylaxis
• **Adult: PO** 5 mg bid; in those with any 2 of the following—age ≥80 yr, body weight ≤60 kg, or serum creatinine ≥1.5 mg/dL—reduce the dose to 2.5 mg bid. Also decrease the dose to 2.5 mg bid (strong inhibitor of both CYP3A4 and P-glycoprotein)

Reduction in risk of recurrent DVT and/or PE after completion of treatment for acute DVT or PE
• **Adult:** 2.5 mg bid daily after at least 6 mo of treatment for DVT or PE

DVT prophylaxis and PE prophylaxis in patients undergoing knee or hip replacement surgery; avoid use in CYP3A4 and P-gb inhibitors
• **Adult:** 2.5 mg bid × 12 days after knee replacement surgery or for 35 days after hip replacement surgery. Give initial dose 12-24 hr after surgery

Renal dose:
• No dosage adjustment needed when used for treatment/prevention of venous thromboembolism
• **Adult: PO** serum CCr ≥1.5 mg/dL, ≤60 kg, and/or ≥80 yr; if 2 of these 3 characteristics are present, then decrease dose to 2.5 mg bid

Hemodialysis end-stage renal disease maintained on hemodialysis
• **Adult: PO** 5 mg bid; reduce to 2.5 mg bid if patient is ≥80 yr or ≤60 kg

Available forms: Tablets 2.5, 5 mg

Administer:
• May be taken without regard to food
• If unable to swallow whole, may crush and suspend the tablet in 60 mL 5% dextrose solution; give immediately via NG
• If a dose is missed, it should be taken as soon as possible on the same day. Twice-daily dosing should be resumed.

Do not double the dose to make up for a missed dose
• Converting from warfarin: obtain INR when <2.0, start apixaban; from other anticoagulants, stop one and start the other at next dosing time

SIDE EFFECTS
CNS: Syncope, intracranial bleeding
CV: Hypotension
HEMA: Severe bleeding
INTEG: Rash
MISC: Hypersensitivity

PHARMACOKINETICS
Peak 3-4 hr, half-life 12 hr

INTERACTIONS
Increase: bleeding risk—antiplatelets, other anticoagulants, salicylates, NSAIDs, SNRIs, SSRIs, thrombolytics; avoid concurrent use
Increase: apixaban effect—CYP3A4 inhibitors, P-gp; give 2.5 mg apixaban
Decrease: apixaban effect—strong inducers of CYP3A4 and also P-glycoprotein (carBAMazepine, ketoconazole, itraconazole, phenytoin, rifAMPin); use lower dose

Drug/Herb
Decrease: apixaban effect—St. John's wort; avoid concurrent use

Drug/Lab Test
Increase: PT, PTT, INR, coagulation studies

NURSING CONSIDERATIONS
Assess:
• **Bleeding:** bleeding may occur from any body system; may be fatal if severe

Black Box Warning: Neurologic status: monitor for impairment, including numbness, paresthesia, weakness, confusion, back pain, bowel/bladder impairment; notify prescriber immediately

Black Box Warning: Abrupt discontinuation: do not discontinue abruptly; if bleeding occurs, consider using another anticoagulant to prevent thromboembolic events

Black Box Warning: Epidural, spinal anesthesia, lumbar puncture: avoid use in these conditions, risk of hematoma and permanent paralysis, may be increased with use of other anticoagulants, thrombolytics, antiplatelets

• **Hypersensitivity:** rash, itching, chills, fever; report to prescriber
• **Beers:** avoid in older adults; may cause increased risk of bleeding, decreased creatinine clearance
Evaluate:
Therapeutic response: prevention/treatment of DVT, adequate anticoagulation
Teach patient/family:

Black Box Warning: Not to discontinue without prescriber approval; stroke, clots may occur

• **Bleeding:** to report bleeding, bruising, confusion, weakness, numbness of limbs
• To avoid OTC products, supplements, herbs unless approved by prescriber; serious product interactions may occur
• To carry emergency ID with product taken; to inform all health providers of product use
• To report hypersensitivity reactions: rash, chills, fever, itching
• **Pregnancy/breastfeeding:** To avoid breastfeeding; it is not known if the product appears in breast milk; to notify prescriber if pregnancy is planned or suspected
• **Overdose:** give andexanet alfa

apomorphine (Rx)
(ah-poe-more'feen)
Apokyn, Kynmobi, Movapo ✿
Func. class.: Antiparkinson agent
Chem. class.: DOPamine agonist, non-ergot

USES: For use as rescue of "off" episodes associated with advanced Parkinson's disease
CONTRAINDICATIONS
Hypersensitivity to this product, sulfites, or benzyl alcohol, IV use, major

psychotic disorder; concurrent treatment with drugs of the 5-HT$_3$ antagonist class (e.g., ondansetron, granisetron, alosetron)

DOSAGE AND ROUTES
• **Adult: Test dose: SUBCUT** 0.2 mL (2 mg) (test dose) where B/P can be closely monitored (before dose and 20, 40, 60 min after); if tolerated and patient responds, then begin with 0.2 mL (2 mg); may increase by 1 mg every few days, max 0.6 mL (6 mg)
• **Usual dosage: SUBCUT** 0.3-0.6 mL (3-6 mg), average frequency tid
• **SL:** 10 mg as needed at ≥2 hr for "off" episodes" up to a max 5 doses daily

Available forms: Solution for injection 10 mg/mL with benzyl alcohol

apraclonidine ophthalmic
See Appendix B

apremilast (Rx)
(a-pre'mi-last)
Otezla
Func. class.: Musculoskeletal agents: disease-modifying antirheumatic drugs (DMARDs)
Chem. class.: Phosphodiesterase-4 inhibitors

ACTION: A phosphodiesterase-4 (PDE4) inhibitor specific for cyclic adenosine monophosphate (cAMP). Inhibition of PDE4 results in an increase in intracellular concentration of cAMP, with a partial inhibition of proinflammatory mediators and an increase in the production of some antiinflammatory mediators

USES: Treatment of active psoriatic arthritis; severe plaque psoriasis (in those not a candidate for phototherapy)/ oral ulcers in Behcet disease

Side effects: *italics* = common; red = life-threatening

CONTRAINDICATIONS
Hypersensitivity

Precautions: Pregnancy, breastfeeding, depression/suicidal, renal disease (CCr <30 mL/min)

DOSAGES AND ROUTES
Active psoriatic arthritis/severe plaque psoriasis/oral ulcers in Behcet's disease
• **Adult:** PO day 1: 10 mg **PO** AM; day 2: 10 mg AM and PM; day 3: 10 mg AM and 20 mg PM; day 4: 20 mg AM and PM; day 5: 20 mg AM and 30 mg PM; day 6 and thereafter: 30 mg bid

Renal dose
• **Adult:** PO CCr ≥30 mL/min: no change; CCr <30 mL/min: 30 mg every day. Initially, 10 mg AM days 1-3; 20 mg AM days 4 and 5; 30 mg every day for day 6 and thereafter

Available forms: Tablets 10, 20, 30 mg; starter pack

Administer:
• Give whole; do not crush, break, or chew; give without regard to meals

SIDE EFFECTS
CNS: *Headache,* depression, suicidal ideation, fatigue, insomnia

GI: Diarrhea, nausea, vomiting, abdominal pain, frequent bowel movements, dyspepsia, weight loss

RESP: URI, pharyngitis, bronchitis

SYST: Hypersensitivity reactions

MS: Back pain

PHARMACOKINETICS
68% protein binding; metabolized by CYP3A4; half-life 6-9 hr; excreted urine 58%, feces 39%; peak 2.5 hr

INTERACTIONS
Decrease: apremilast—CYP3A4 inducers (rifAMPin, isoniazid, pyrazinamide, barbiturates, phenytoin, carBAMazepine, enzalutamide); avoid concurrent use

Drug/Herb
Decrease: apremilast—CYP3A4 inducers (St. John's wort); avoid concurrent use

NURSING CONSIDERATIONS
Assess:
• **Psoriatic arthritis/severe plaque psoriasis:** assess for hypersensitivity reactions

• For depression and suicidal ideation, mood changes

• For renal failure or severe renal impairment (CrCl <30 mL/min), dosage reduction is required

• For significant or unexplained weight loss; report weight loss, as therapy may need to be discontinued

• **Pregnancy and breastfeeding:** if pregnancy is planned or suspected; use only if benefits outweigh fetal risk; if used during pregnancy, call 877-311-8972; cautious use in breastfeeding

Evaluate:
• Therapeutic response: resolution of symptoms of psoriatic arthritis or plaque psoriasis

Teach patient/family:
• To report new rash, hypersensitivity reactions; report change in urine output, renal disease history

• To be alert for depression and suicidal ideation, mood changes; if these occur, notify prescriber immediately

---

aprepitant (PO) (Rx)
(ap-re′pi-tant)
Cinvanti, Emend
Aponvie, fosaprepitant (IV) (Rx)
Emend
Func. class.: Antiemetic
Chem. class.: Substance P/neurokinin antagonist

Do not confuse:
aprepitant/fosaprepitant

ACTION: Selective antagonist of human substance P/neurokinin 1 (NK$_1$) receptors that decreases emetic reflex

USES: Prevention of nausea/vomiting associated with cancer chemotherapy (highly emetogenic/moderately emetogenic), including high-dose CISplatin; used in combination with other antiemetics; postoperative nausea/vomiting

CONTRAINDICATIONS
Hypersensitivity to this product, polysorbate 80, pimozide

Precautions: Pregnancy, breastfeeding, children, geriatric patients, hepatic disease

DOSAGE AND ROUTES
Prevention of nausea/vomiting after chemotherapy
• **Adult: PO** Day 1 (1 hr before chemotherapy) aprepitant 125 mg with 12 mg dexamethasone **PO,** with 32 mg ondansetron **IV;** day 2 aprepitant 80 mg with 8 mg dexamethasone **PO;** day 3 aprepitant 80 mg with 8 mg dexamethasone **PO;** day 4 only dexamethasone 8 mg **PO; Adult: IV** (Cinvanti): (HEC) On day 1 130 mg over 30 min before chemotherapy; 3-day regimen (MEC) on day 1 100 mg over 30 min, given 30 min before chemotherapy, on day 2 and 3 80 mg PO 1 hr before chemotherapy, given in AM if no chemotherapy is given
Child ≥12 yr: PO capsules 125 mg 1 hr prior to chemotherapy; suspension 3 mg/kg 1 hr prior to chemotherapy, max 125 mg
IV INFUSION
150 mg fosaprepitant over 15 min, 30 min prior to chemotherapy
Prevention of postoperative nausea/vomiting
• **Adult: PO** 40 mg within 3 hr of induction of anesthesia
Available forms: Capsules 40, 80, 125 mg; combo pack capsules 80-125 mg; powder for oral suspension 125 mg/pouch; emulsion for injection: 32 mg/4.4 mL, 130 mg/18 mL
Administer:
• Give with dexamethasone and a 5-HT3 antagonist
PO route
• Do not break, crush, or chew
• PO on 3-day schedule, give with full glass of water 1 hr before chemotherapy, with or without food, given with other antiemetics
• Do not open or break capsules
• **Suspension:** Use for children unable to swallow capsules, administer slowly, store at room temperature
• Store at room temperature; keep in original bottles, blisters
Intermittent IV INFUSION route (Fosaprepitant-Emend)
• Use IV on day 1 of 3-day regimen
• **Reconstitution:** use aseptic technique; inject 5 mL 0.9% NaCl into the vial,

directing stream to wall of vial to prevent foam; swirl (do not shake)
• Prepare infusion bag 145 mL/150 mg; do not dilute, reconstitute with calcium, magnesium, including LR, Hartmann's solution
• Withdraw entire volume from vial, transfer to infusion bag; total volume 115 mL (1 mg/1 mL)
• Gently invert bag; reconstituted solution stable for 24 hr at lower room temperature or (<77° F/<25° C)
• Visually inspect for particulates, discoloration
• Infuse over 30 min, stable for 24 hr at room temperature, 30 min prior to chemotherapy, pediatrics use CVAD
• Monitor for IV site reactions
Aprepitant (Cinvanti)
• Withdraw 18 mL for the 130-mg dose or 14 mL for the 100-mg dose from the vial and transfer it into an infusion bag filled with 100 mL of 0.9% NaCl or D₅W
• Gently invert the bag 4 to 5 times. Avoid shaking
• Before using, inspect the bag for particulate matter and discoloration. Discard if present

SIDE EFFECTS
CNS: *Headache, dizziness,* insomnia, weakness, headache, fever
CV: Bradycardia, hypo/hypertension
GI: *Diarrhea, constipation,* abdominal pain, *nausea,* vomiting, heartburn
HEMA: Anemia
INTEG: Pruritus, rash, urticaria, injection reaction
MISC: Fatigue, dehydration, fever, alopecia

PHARMACOKINETICS
Absorption 60%-65%, peak 4 hr (PO) infusion's end (IV), metabolized in liver by CYP3A4 enzymes to active metabolite, half-life 9-12 hr, 95% protein bound, not excreted in kidneys, crosses blood-brain barrier

INTERACTIONS
Increase: levels of each product—ALPRAZolam, midazolam, triazolam; decrease benzodiazepine dose
Increase: aprepitant action—CYP3A4 inhibitors (ketoconazole, itraconazole,

nefazodone, troleandomycin, clarithromycin, ritonavir, nelfinavir, diltiaZEM)

Pimozide: increase levels, torsade de pointes risk, do not use together

Dexamethasone, methylprednisone: increased effect of each

Increase: action of CYP3A4 substrates (pimozide, dexamethasone, methylPREDNISolone, midazolam, ALPRAZolam, triazolam, DOCEtaxel, PACLitaxel, etoposide, irinotecan, imatinib, ifosfamide, vinorelbine, vinBLAStine, vinCRIStine), avoid concurrent use

Decrease: aprepitant action—CYP3A4 inducers (rifAMPin, carBAMazepine, phenytoin)

Decrease: action of CYP2C9 substrates (warfarin, phenytoin), hormonal contraceptives

Decrease: action of both products—PARoxetine

Hormonal contraceptives: decreased action by contraceptives, use a nonhormonal option

Drug/Food

Decrease: effect—grapefruit juice

Drug/Lab

Increase: AST/ALT, alkaline phosphatase

Decrease: HB,WBC

NURSING CONSIDERATIONS
Assess:
• **For hypersensitivity reactions:** pruritus, rash, urticaria, anaphylaxis
• CV status: hypo/hypertension, bradycardia, tachycardia, DVT
• For absence of nausea, vomiting during chemotherapy
• For drug/herb/supplement interactions, as there are many
• CBC, LFTs, creatinine baseline and periodically

Evaluate:
• Therapeutic response: absence of nausea, vomiting during cancer chemotherapy, or post-op

Teach patient/family:
• To take only as prescribed; to take first dose 1 hr prior to chemotherapy or within 3 hr of surgery to prevent nausea, vomiting
• To report all medications and herbals to prescriber before taking this medication
• That those patients also taking warfarin should have clotting monitored

closely during 2-wk period after administration of aprepitant

• **Pregnancy/breastfeeding:** to use nonhormonal form of contraception while taking this agent and for 1 mo thereafter; oral contraceptive effect may be decreased; to avoid breastfeeding

---

arformoterol (Rx)
(ar-for-moe′ter-ole)
Brovana
Func. class.: Long-acting adrenergic β_2-agonist, sympathomimetic, bronchodilator

---

USES: Maintenance bronchospasm prevention in COPD, including chronic bronchitis, emphysema

CONTRAINDICATIONS
Hypersensitivity to sympathomimetics, product, racemic formoterol; tachydysrhyhmias, severe cardiac disease, heart block, children, monotherapy in asthma

DOSAGE AND ROUTES
COPD
• **Adult: NEB** 15 mcg, bid, AM, PM, max 30 mcg/day

Available forms: solution for inhalation 15-mcg/2-mL vials

⚠ HIGH ALERT

argatroban (Rx)
(are-ga-troe′ban)
Func. class.: Anticoagulant
Chem. class.: Direct thrombin inhibitor

Do not confuse:
argatroban/Aggrastat

ACTION: Direct inhibitor of thrombin; it reversibly binds to thrombin active site

USES: Anticoagulation prevention/treatment of thrombosis in heparin-induced thrombocytopenia; adjunct to percutaneous coronary intervention

(PCI) in those with history of HIT, deep vein thrombosis, pulmonary embolism

CONTRAINDICATIONS
Hypersensitivity, overt major bleeding
Precautions: Pregnancy, breastfeeding, children, intracranial bleeding, renal function impairment, hepatic disease, severe hypertension, after lumbar puncture, spinal anesthesia, major surgery/trauma, congenital/acquired bleeding, GI ulcers, abrupt discontinuation

DOSAGE AND ROUTES
Prevention/treatment of thrombosis (heparin-induced thrombocytopenia)
• **Adult: CONT IV INFUSION** 2 mcg/kg/min; adjust dose until steady-state aPTT is 1.5-3 × initial baseline, max 100 sec, max dose 10 mcg/kg/min
Hepatic dose
• **Adult: CONT INFUSION** 0.5 mcg/kg/min; adjust rate based on aPTT
Percutaneous coronary intervention (PCI) in HIT
• **Adult: IV INFUSION** 25 mcg/kg/min and bolus of 350 mcg/kg given over 3-5 min, check ACT 5-10 min after bolus completed, proceed if ACT >300 sec; if ACT <300 sec, give another 150 mcg/kg bolus, increase infusion rate to 30 mcg/kg/min, recheck ACT in 5-10 min; if ACT >450 sec, decrease infusion rate to 15 mcg/kg/min, recheck ACT in 5-10 min; when ACT is therapeutic, continue for duration of procedure
Available forms: Injection 100 mg/mL (2.5 mL; must dilute 100-fold), 50 mg/50 mL, 125 mg/125 mL
Administer:
• Avoid all IM injections that may cause bleeding
• Discontinue all other anticoagulants before use of argotroban
IV, direct route
• **For PCI:** 350 mg/kg bolus, over 3-5 min and continuous infusion of 25 mcg/kg/min; check ACT 5-10 min after bolus
Continuous IV INFUSION route
• **Dilute** in 0.9% NaCl, D₅W, LR to a final concentration of 1 mg/mL; mix by repeated inversion of the diluent bag for 1 min; may briefly be slightly hazy use after clearing

• Protect from sunlight
• Dosage adjustment may be made after review of aPTT, max 10 mcg/kg/min
• Stable at room temperature for 24 hr, 96 hr refrigerated, do not place in direct sunlight

SIDE EFFECTS
CNS: *Fever,* intracranial bleeding, headache
CV: Atrial fibrillation, coronary thrombosis, MI, myocardial ischemia, coronary occlusion, ventricular tachycardia, bradycardia, *chest pain, hypotension*
GI: *Nausea, vomiting, abdominal pain, diarrhea,* GI bleeding
HEMA: Bleeding
SYST: Anaphylaxis

PHARMACOKINETICS
Metabolized in liver, distributed to extracellular fluid, 54% plasma protein binding, half-life 39-51 min, excreted in feces, peak 1-2 hr (anticoagulant action)

INTERACTIONS
Increase: bleeding risk—antiplatelets, NSAIDs, salicylates, dipyridamole, clopidogrel, ticlopidine, heparin, warfarin, glycoprotein IIb/IIIa antagonists (abciximab, tirofiban, eptifibatide); thrombolytics (alteplase, reteplase, urokinase, tenecteplase), other anticoagulants; avoid using concurrently
Drug/Herb
Increase: bleeding risk—ginger, garlic, ginkgo, horse chestnut
Drug/Lab
Decrease: HB/Hct

NURSING CONSIDERATIONS
Assess:
• Obtain baseline aPTT prior to treatment, do not start if aPTT ratio ≥2.5, then aPTT 4 hr after initiation of treatment and at least daily thereafter; if aPTT is above target, stop infusion for 2 hr, then restart at 50%, take aPTT in 4 hr; if below target, increase infusion rate of 0.21 mg/kg/hr without checking for coagulation abnormalities, do not use with other parenteral anticoagulants; monitor Hct/Hb and platelets baseline and periodically

- **Bleeding:** gums; petechiae; ecchymosis; black, tarry stools; hematuria/epistaxis; decreased B/P, Hct; vaginal bleeding, possible hemorrhage
- **Anaphylaxis:** dyspnea, rash during treatment
- Fever, skin rash, urticaria
- **Pregnancy/breastfeeding:** if pregnancy is planned or suspected; if pregnant, use only if benefits outweigh fetal risk; do not breastfeed, excretion unknown

Evaluate:
- Therapeutic response: prevention of thrombosis

Teach patient/family:
- Reason for product, expected results
- To use a soft-bristle toothbrush to avoid bleeding gums; avoid contact sports; use electric razor; avoid IM injection
- To report any signs of bleeding: gums, under skin, urine, stool; trouble breathing, wheezing, skin rash
- **Pregnancy/breastfeeding:** to notify prescriber if planning to become pregnant, breastfeeding
- Not to use OTC meds, herbal products unless approved by prescriber
- To notify prescriber of hepatic/GI disease, recent surgery, injury
- **Overdose:** discontinue, monitor coagulation studies

ARIPiprazole (Rx)

(a-rip-ip-pra'zol)

Abilify, Abilify Discmelt, Abilify Maintena, Abilify MyCite

Aripiprazole lauroxil

Aristada, Aristada Initio

Func. class.: Antipsychotic
Chem. class.: Quinolinone

Do not confuse:
ARIPiprazole/RABEprazole

ACTION: Exact mechanism unknown; may be mediated through both DOPamine type 2 (D_2, D_3) and serotonin type 2 ($5\text{-}HT_{1A}$, $5\text{-}HT_{2A}$) antagonism, DOPamine system stabilizer

USES: Schizophrenia and bipolar disorder (adults and adolescents), mania, major depressive disorder, short-term mania or mixed episodes of bipolar disorder; irritability in patients with autism

CONTRAINDICATIONS

Breastfeeding, hypersensitivity, seizure disorders

Precautions: Pregnancy, geriatric patients, renal/hepatic/cardiac disease, neutropenia

Black Box Warning: Children with depression; suicidal ideation; dementia

DOSAGE AND ROUTES
Major depressive disorder
- **Adult:** PO 2-5 mg/day as an adjunct to other antidepressant treatment; adjust by 5 mg at ≥1 wk (range, 2-15 mg/day)

Schizophrenia
- **Adult:** PO 10-15 mg/day; if needed, dosage may be increased to 30 mg/day after 2 wk; maintenance 15 mg/day; periodically reassess; **(Aristada Maintena) IM/extended release** (monthly injection suspension) 400 mg monthly; IM (Aristada Initio) 675 mg once with 30 mg aripiprazole with first dose IM
- **Adolescent 13-17 yr:** PO 2 mg/day, may increase to 5 mg after 2 days, then 10 mg after 2 more days, max 30 mg/day

Bipolar disorder
- **Adult:** PO 15 mg/day, may increase to 30 mg if needed (monotherapy); adjunctive to lithium or valproate **PO** 10-15 mg daily, may increase to 30 mg if needed; **IM** (Abilify Maintena) 400 mg monthly, start with oral product to determine tolerability, use PO product for 14 days during beginning therapy with IM
- **Child >10 yr, adolescent:** PO 2 mg, titrate to 5 mg/day after 2 days to target of 10 mg/day after another 2 days

Agitation with bipolar disorder/ schizophrenia
- **Adult:** IM 9.75 mg as a single dose, may start with a lower dose, max 30 mg/day

Irritability associated with autism
- **Child ≥6 yr, adolescent:** PO 2 mg/day, increase to 5 mg/day after 1 wk, may in-

---

crease to 10-15 mg/day if needed; dose changes should not occur more frequently than q1wk

Tourette's syndrome

- **Child 6-18 yr ≥50 kg: PO** 2 mg/day × 2 days, then increase to 5 mg/day, target 10 mg/day on day 8
- **Child 6-18 yr <50 kg: PO** 2 mg/day, increase to 5 mg/day after 2 days; may increase to 10 mg/day; adjust dose ≥1 wk

Potential CYP2D6 inhibitor, strong CYP3A4 inhibitors

- **Adult: PO** reduce to 50% of usual dose; increase dose when CYP2D6, CYP3A4 inhibitors withdrawn

Combination of strong CYP3A4/CYP2D6 inhibitors

- **Adult: PO** reduce to 25% of usual dose

Available forms: Tablets 2, 5, 10, 15, 20, 30 mg; injection 9.75 mg/1.3 mL; orally disintegrating tablet 10, 15 mg; oral solution 1 mg/mL; suspension for injection 441 mg/1.6 mL, 662 mg/2.4 mL, 882 mg/3.2 mL in prefilled syringes (Aristada); 675 mg/2.4 mL (Arisada Initio); Tablet 2, 5, 10, 15, 20, 30 mg (Abilify MyCite with sensor)

Administer:

PO route

- Store in tight, light-resistant container
- May be given without regard to meals
- **Orally disintegrating tablets:** do not open blister until ready to use, do not push tablet through foil; place on tongue, allow to dissolve, swallow, do not divide
- **Oral liquid:** use calibrated measuring device
- **Oral solution:** can be substituted for tablet mg per mg, up to 25-mg dose. Patients receiving 30-mg tablets should receive 25 mg, immediate release of solution

IM (extended release) route

- **Mycite tablets:** May give without regard to meals
- Swallow tablets whole; do not divide, crush, or chew
- The tablets are embedded with an ingestible event marker (IEM) intended to track drug ingestion with a wearable sensor (Mycite patch) and smartphone app

- Although most ingestions will be detected within 30 min, it may take up to 2 hr for the app and web portal to detect ingestion of the tablet. If the tablet is not detected after ingestion, do not repeat the dose
- It is not recommended to use the tablets to track drug ingestion in "real time" or during an emergency because detection may be delayed or not occur

Schizophrenia (Aristada/Aristada INITIO)

- Use PO first before using these products to raise tolerability to product
- May give IM 1 dose of Aristada INITIO 675 mg (in either deltoid or gluteal muscle) and 1 dose of PO ARIPiprazole 30 mg with the first Aristada injection
- The first Aristada injection may be given on the same day as Aristada INITIO or up to 10 days after
- Avoid injecting both Aristada INITIO and Aristada concomitantly into the same site OR
- Give 21 consecutive days of PO ARIPiprazole with the first Aristada injection
- Depending on individual patient's needs, treatment with Aristada can be initiated at a dose of 441 mg (monthly in deltoid or gluteal), 662 mg (monthly in gluteal), or 882 mg (monthly or every 6 wk in gluteal) or 1064 mg (every 2 mo in gluteal). The 441-mg, 662-mg, 882-mg, and 1064-mg doses correspond to 300 mg, 450 mg, 600 mg, and 724 mg of ARIPiprazole, respectively
- **Mycite patch:** The patch detects the signal from the IEM sensor embedded in the tablet after ingestion and transmits data to a smartphone
- Apply only when instructed by the Mycite app to the left side of the body just above the lower edge of the rib cage
- Ensure that the app is paired with the patch before use. The status of the patch is indicated by a status icon in the app to inform the user that the patch is properly adhered and fully functioning
- Do not place the patch where the skin is scraped, cracked, inflamed, or irritated or in an area that overlaps the most recently removed patch

• Do not remove the patch when showering, swimming, or exercising
• Change the patch weekly or sooner if needed. The app will prompt you to change the patch and will direct you to apply and remove the patch correctly
• Remove the patch when having an MRI and replace it with a new one as soon as possible. If there is skin irritation, remove the patch
• Give IM only; inject slowly, deeply into muscle mass; discard unused portion; do not give IV or SUBCUT
• Available as ready to use
• Extended release monthly (Abilify Maintena)

SIDE EFFECTS

CNS: *Drowsiness, insomnia, agitation, anxiety, headache,* seizures, neuroleptic malignant syndrome, *lightheadedness, akathisia, tremor,* suicidal ideation, tardive dyskinesia, EPS
CV: Orthostatic hypotension, tachycardia, chest pain, hypertension, peripheral edema
EENT: *Blurred vision, rhinitis*
GI: *Constipation, nausea, vomiting, weight gain*
INTEG: *Rash, dry skin, sweating*
META: Hyperglycemia
MS: Myalgia
RESP: *Cough,* dyspnea, hypercholesterolemia
HEMA: Agranulocytosis, anemia, leukemia
SYST: Death among geriatric patients with dementia, hypersensitivity

PHARMACOKINETICS

PO: Absorption 87%; extensively metabolized by liver to a major active metabolite by CYP3A4/CYP2D6; plasma protein binding >99%; half-life 75 hr; excretion via urine 25%, feces 55%; clearance decreased in geriatric patients

INTERACTIONS

Increase: effects of ARIPiprazole—CYP3A4 inhibitors (ketoconazole, erythromycin), CYP2D6 inhibitors (quiNIDine, FLUoxetine, PARoxetine); reduce dose of ARIPiprazole
Increase: sedation—other CNS depressants, alcohol

Increase: EPS—other antipsychotics, lithium
Decrease: ARIPiprazole level—famotidine, valproate
Decrease: effects of ARIPiprazole—CYP3A4 inducers (carBAMazepine); dose of ARIPiprazole may need to be increased
Increase: antihypertensive effect—antihypertensives; monitor B/P
Drug/Herb
Decrease: ARIPiprazole effect—St. John's wort
Drug/Lab
False positive: amphetamine drug screen

NURSING CONSIDERATIONS
Assess:

Black Box Warning: Mental status before initial use; children/young adults may exhibit suicidal thoughts/behaviors; smallest amount of product should be given; elderly with dementia-related psychosis are at increased risk of death

• AIMS assessment, neurologic function, LFTs, weight, lipid profile, blood glucose monthly
• Affect, orientation, LOC, reflexes, gait, coordination, sleep pattern disturbances
• B/P standing and lying; also pulse, respirations; take q4hr during initial treatment; establish baseline before starting treatment; report drops of 30 mm Hg; watch for ECG changes
• Dizziness, faintness, palpitations, tachycardia on rising
• EPS, including akathisia (inability to sit still, no pattern to movements), tardive dyskinesia (bizarre movements of the jaw, mouth, tongue, extremities), pseudoparkinsonism (rigidity, tremors, pill rolling, shuffling gait)
• **Neuroleptic malignant syndrome:** hyperthermia, increased CPK, altered mental status, muscle rigidity; notify prescriber immediately
• **Beers:** avoid in older adults, high risk of delirium, CVA; may use in schizophrenia, bipolar disorder, or short-term as antiemetic in chemotherapy
Evaluate:
• Therapeutic response: decrease in emotional excitement, hallucinations, de-

lusions, paranoia; reorganization of patterns of thought, speech

Teach patient/family:
• That orthostatic hypotension may occur; to rise from sitting or lying position gradually
• To avoid hot tubs, hot showers, tub baths; hypotension may occur
• To avoid abrupt withdrawal of this product; EPS may result; product should be withdrawn slowly
• To avoid OTC preparations (cough, hay fever, cold) unless approved by prescriber because serious product interactions may occur; to avoid use with alcohol, CNS depressants because increased drowsiness may occur
• To avoid hazardous activities if drowsy, dizzy
• About compliance with product regimen
• To report impaired vision, tremors, muscle twitching
• That examinations and blood work will be needed during treatment
• That weight gain may occur, to notify health care professional of large weight gain
• That heat stroke may occur in hot weather; to take extra precautions to stay cool

Black Box Warning: To report suicidal thoughts/behaviors, dementia immediately

• **Pregnancy/breastfeeding:** Identify if pregnancy is planned or suspected; pregnant patient should be enrolled in the National Pregnancy Registry for Atypical Antipsychotics 866-961-2388; avoid breastfeeding; use only if benefits outweigh fetal risk

TREATMENT OF OVERDOSE: Lavage if orally ingested; provide airway; *do not induce vomiting*

armodafinil (Rx)
(ar-moe-daf′in-il)
Nuvigil
Func. class.: CNS stimulant

Controlled Substance Schedule IV

ACTION: May inhibit dopamine reuptake, unknown

USES: Narcolepsy, obstructive sleep apnea/hypoapnea syndrome, circadian rhythm disruption (shift-work sleep problems)

CONTRAINDICATIONS
Hypersensitivity to this product or modafinil

DOSAGE AND ROUTES
Narcolepsy, obstructive sleep apnea/hypoapnea syndrome
• Adult and adolescent ≥17 yr: PO 150-250 mg in AM
Circadian rhythm disruption (shift-work sleep problems)
• Adult and adolescent ≥17 yr: PO 150 mg at start of shift
Available forms:
Tablets 50, 150, 200, 250 mg
Administer
• Give with or without food consistently at same time of the day

SIDE EFFECTS
CV: Increased B/P, pulse, palpitations
CNS: Anxiety, dizziness, depression, fatigue, headache, insomnia, migraine, paresthesia, tremor, suicidal thoughts/behaviors, mania, hallucinations, delusions
GI: Anorexia, nausea, vomiting, constipation, diarrhea, dry mouth
GU: Polyuria
RESP: Dyspnea
INTEG: Dermatitis, allergic reactions, Stevens-Johnson syndrome
MISC: Flulike symptoms

PHARMACOKINETICS
Onset unknown, peak 2 fasting hr, duration unknown, half-life 15 hr, 60% protein binding

INTERACTIONS
Increased: Levels of drugs metabolized by CYP2C19 (diazepam, phenytoin, propranolol), monitor carefully, dosage reduction may be needed
Increased: Level of armodafinil—CYP3A4 inhibitors (erythromycin)
Decrease: Levels of drugs metabolized by CYP3A4 (midazolam, cyclosporine)
Decrease: Level of armodafinil—CYP3A4 inducers (carbamazepine, rifampin)
Decrease: Effect of hormonal contraceptives, use alternative contraception

Side effects: *italics* = common; red = life-threatening

Drug/Food
Decrease: Onset of medication: food
Drug/Lab
Increase: Alkaline phosphatase, GGT

NURSING CONSIDERATIONS
Assess:
• Cardiac status: Monitor for changes in B/P, pulse, ECG, chest pain
• Monitor for Stevens-Johnson syndrome/toxic epidermal necrolysis (red, swollen, blistered, or peeling skin [with or without fever]; red or irritated eyes; or sores in mouth, throat, nose, or eyes), to stop product immediately and notify prescriber
• Monitor for suicidal thoughts/behaviors, mania, hallucinations, delusions
• Monitor for continued sleepiness or inability to stay awake
• Identify all products taken, OTC, Rx, supplements, herbal products, to avoid drug interactions
• DRESS: Monitor for rash, fever, facial swelling, lymphadenopathy; although rare, occurs with other system involvement
Teach patient/family:
• To report trouble sleeping, nausea, dry mouth, depression, swollen glands, behavioral changes, chest pain, dark urine, change in vision, yellow skin, trouble breathing, bruising, bleeding
• To report Stevens-Johnson syndrome/toxic epidermal necrolysis (red, swollen, blistered, or peeling skin [with or without fever]); red or irritated eyes; or sores in mouth, throat, nose, or eyes; to stop product immediately and notify prescriber
• To report immediately suicidal thoughts/behaviors, mania, hallucinations, delusions
• To use alternative contraception if taking hormonal contraceptives during and for 1 mo after last dose
• To notify prescriber if pregnancy is planned or suspected, or if breastfeeding
• To use product at the same time of the day, with or without food consistently
• To avoid driving or other hazardous activities until response is known, dizziness may occur

• To report all products taken to other health care providers
Evaluate:
• Therapeutic response: Ability to stay awake

---

ascimimib (Rx)
(as-KIM-i-nib)
Scemblix
Func. class.: Antineoplastic
Chem. class.: Kinase inhibitor

ACTION:
Inhibits the ABL1 kinase activity of a fusion protein by binding to the ABL pocket, showed activity against wild-type BCR-ABL1 and several mutant forms of the kinase, including the T315I mutation

USES:
Philadelphia chromosome–positive myeloid leukemia

CONTRAINDICATIONS
Hypersensitivity, pregnancy, breastfeeding
Precautions: Myelosuppression, pancreatic/CV toxicity, hypertension, pregnancy

DOSAGE AND ROUTES
PH+ CML in CP
• **Adult: PO** 80 mg daily or 40 mg bid
Ph+ CML in CP with T315I Mutation
• **Adult: PO** 200 mg bid
Available forms: Film-coated tablets 20, 40 mg
Administer:
• Avoid food for at least 2 hr before and 1 hr after use
• Swallow tablets whole; do not break, crush, or chew
• Skip any missed dose and take the next dose at the regular time if missed by >12 hr for daily dosing or >6 hr with bid dosing

SIDE EFFECTS
RESP: URI
GI: Nausea, vomiting, diarrhea, abdominal pain, anorexia, constipation
MS: MS pain
CNS: Fatigue, dizziness, fever
INTEG: Rash

INTERACTIONS

Increase: adverse reactions—strong CYP3A4 inhibitors, certain substrates of CYP3A4, certain P-gp substrates
Avoid use with itraconazole oral solution, with substrates of CYP2C9

Drug/Lab Test:
Increase: Triglycerides, creatine kinase, alanine aminotransferase, lipase, amylase
Decrease: Platelets, neutrophils, HCT

PHARMACOKINETICS

97% protein binding, half-life 5.5-9 hr, peak 2.5 hr, onset, duration unknown

NURSING CONSIDERATIONS
Assess:

• **Hypersensitivity:** Monitor patients for signs and symptoms of hypertension, B/P often and provide treatment as needed
• **CV toxicity:** Monitor those with history of CV risk factors for adverse reactions, QTc prolongation
• **Myelosuppression:** Monitor CBC baseline and q2mo during first 3 mo and monthly thereafter during therapy and interrupt treatment or reduce dose if needed, severe thrombocytopenia and neutropenia may occur
• **Toxicity and pancreatitis:** Monitor serum lipase and amylase baseline and during treatment. Interrupt, then resume at reduced dose or discontinue based on severity. Evaluate for pancreatitis when lipase elevation is accompanied by abdominal pain, nausea, vomiting
• **Hypertension:** Monitor B/P baseline and often, manage hypertension with antihypertensives as prescribed, interrupt, reduce dose, or stop if not medically controlled
• **Pregnancy/breastfeeding:** Obtain pregnancy test in females of reproductive potential, can cause fetal harm. Advise females of reproductive potential of the potential risk and to use effective contraception during and for 1 wk after last dose; to discontinue breastfeeding during and for 1 wk after last dose, may cause infertility

Evaluate:
• Therapeutic response: Prevention of increase in CML

Teach patient/family:
• **Hypersensitivity:** Advise patient to report immediately itching, rash, trouble breathing
• **CV toxicity:** Teach patient to report
• **Myelosuppression:** Advise patient to report excessive fatigue
• **Pancreatitis and toxicity:** Teach patient to report severe abdominal pain, nausea, vomiting
• **Pregnancy/breastfeeding:** Teach patient product can cause fetal harm, that females of reproductive potential should use effective contraception during and for 1 wk after last dose; to discontinue breastfeeding during and for 1 wk after last dose

---

asenapine (Rx)
(a-sen′a-peen)
Saphris, Secuado
Func. class.: Antipsychotic, atypical; DOPamine-serotonin antagonist
Chem. class.: Dibenzapine

ACTION: Unknown; may be mediated through both DOPamine type 2 (D2) and serotonin type 2 (5-HT2A) antagonism

USES: Bipolar 1 disorder, schizophrenia

CONTRAINDICATIONS
Breastfeeding, hypersensitivity
Precautions: Pregnancy, children, geriatric patients, cardiac/renal/hepatic disease, breast cancer, Parkinson's disease, dementia, seizure disorder, CNS depression, agranulocytosis, QT prolongation, torsades de pointes, suicidal ideation, substance abuse, diabetes mellitus

> **Black Box Warning:** Increased mortality in elderly patients with dementia-related psychosis

DOSAGE AND ROUTES
Schizophrenia
• **Adult: SL** 5 mg bid, may increase to 10 mg bid after 1 wk, max 20 mg/day; TD 3.8 mg/24 hr patch q day, may increase to 5.7 mg/24 hr or 7.6 mg/24 hr after 1 wk

---

Side effects: *italics* = common; red = life-threatening

Acute mania/mixed episodes (bipolar 1 disorder, monotherapy)

- **Adult:** SL 10 mg bid, may decrease to 5 mg bid as needed, max 20 mg/day; with lithium or valproate 5 mg bid, may increase to 10 mg bid
- **Child 10-17 yr:** SL 2.5 mg bid, may increase after 3 days to 5 mg bid, then after 3 more days 10 mg bid can be tolerated

Available forms: SL tablet 2.5, 5, 10 mg; transdermal 3.8 mg/24 hr, 5.7 mg/24 hr, 7.6 mg/24 hr

Administer:

- Anticholinergic agent to be used for EPS
- Store in tight, light-resistant container
- **SL tablet:** remove tablet; place tablet under tongue; after it dissolves, swallow; advise patient not to chew, crush, swallow tablets; not to eat, drink for 10 min

Transdermal

- Open when ready to use, apply patch to clean, dry skin on hip, upper arm, upper back, abdomen; use for 24 hr
- Rotate sites each time
- Do not use if open
- Lifting may occur and should be pressed firmly, if unable to attach, use a new one
- May be worn during shower

SIDE EFFECTS

CNS: *EPS, pseudoparkinsonism, akathisia, dystonia, tardive dyskinesia; drowsiness, insomnia, agitation, anxiety, headache,* seizures, neuroleptic malignant syndrome, dizziness, suicidal ideation
CV: Orthostatic hypotension, tachycardia; QT prolongation
ENDO: Hyperglycemia
GI: *Nausea,* vomiting, oral hypoesthesia/paresthesia (SL)
HEMA: Agranulocytosis, anemia, leukopenia
INTEG: Serious allergic reactions (anaphylaxis, angioedema)

PHARMACOKINETICS

Extensively metabolized by the liver by CYP3A4/UGTA14, protein binding 95%, peak 0.5-1.5 hr, half-life 24 hr, excreted urine 50%, feces 40% (metabolites)

INTERACTIONS

Increase: sedation—other CNS depressants, alcohol
Increase: EPS—CYP2D6 inhibitors/substrates (SSRIs)
Increase: serotonin syndrome—SSRIs
Increase: Seizure risk—buPROPion
Increase: EPS—other antipsychotics
Increase: asenapine excretion—carBAMazepine
Increase: QT prolongation—class IA/III antidysrhythmics, some phenothiazines, β-agonists, local anesthetics, tricyclics, haloperidol, methadone, chloroquine, clarithromycin, droperidol, erythromycin, pentamidine; avoid concurrent use
Decrease: asenapine action—CYP2D6 inducers (carBAMazepine, barbiturates, phenytoins, rifAMPin)

Drug/Herb
Increase: CNS depression—kava
Increase: EPS—betel palm, kava

Drug/Lab Test
Increase: prolactin levels, glucose, cholesterol, LFTs, lipids, triglycerides
Decrease: sodium

NURSING CONSIDERATIONS
Assess:

> **Black Box Warning:** Mental status before initial administration; watch for suicidal thoughts and behaviors; dementia and death may occur among elderly patients

- Affect, orientation, LOC, reflexes, gait, coordination, sleep pattern disturbances
- B/P standing and lying; also pulse, respirations; take these during initial treatment; establish baseline before starting treatment; report drops of 30 mm Hg; watch for ECG changes; QT prolongation may occur
- Dizziness, faintness, palpitations, tachycardia on rising
- **EPS,** including akathisia, tardive dyskinesia (bizarre movements of the jaw, mouth, tongue, extremities), pseudoparkinsonism (rigidity, tremors, pill rolling, shuffling gait)
- **Neuroleptic malignant syndrome:** hyperthermia, increased CPK, altered mental status, muscle rigidity

• Weight, thyroid function studies, serum prolactin, lipid profile, serum electrolytes, creatinine, pregnancy test, neurologic function, LFTs, glycosylated hemoglobin A1c, CBC, blood glucose, AIMS assessment baseline and periodically

• Supervised ambulation until patient stabilized on medication; do not involve patient in strenuous exercise program because fainting is possible; patient should not stand still for a long time

• **Beers:** avoid use in older adults; high risk of delirium, CVA, worsening parkinsonian symptoms, increased CNS effects; may use in schizophrenia, bipolar disorder, or as antiemetic in chemotherapy

Evaluate:

• Therapeutic response: decrease in emotional excitement, hallucinations, delusions, paranoia; reorganization of patterns of thought, speech

Teach patient/family:

• That orthostatic hypotension may occur; to rise from sitting or lying position gradually

• To avoid hot tubs, hot showers, tub baths; hypotension may occur

• To avoid abrupt withdrawal of this product; EPS may result; product should be withdrawn slowly

• To avoid OTC preparations (cough, hay fever, cold) unless approved by prescriber; serious product interactions may occur; to avoid use of alcohol, opioids, increased drowsiness may occur

• That weight gain is common

• How to take prescribed product

• To avoid hazardous activities if drowsy, dizzy

• About compliance with product regimen

• That heat stroke may occur in hot weather; to take extra precautions to stay cool

• To notify provider if history of diabetes in patient or family; if so, blood sugar should be checked before starting this product

Black Box Warning: To report suicidal thoughts/behaviors, dementia immediately

• **Pregnancy/breastfeeding:** use only if benefits outweigh fetal risk; identify if pregnancy is planned or suspected; if pregnant, register at National Pregnancy Registry for Atypical Antipsychotics (866-961-2388)

TD route

• Teach patient how to apply patch

• Advise patient to report irritation, rash, itching at site; may be more frequent in African Americans or if worn for an extended period

SL route

• Teach patient to let dissolve under tongue, not to chew or swallow whole

• Advise patient not to eat or drink anything for 10 min

TREATMENT OF OVERDOSE:

Lavage if orally ingested; provide airway; *do not induce vomiting*

---

aspirin (acetylsalicylic acid, ASA) (OTC)

(as′pir-in)

Acuprin, Asaphen ♣, Asatab ♣, A.S.A. Ascriptin Enteric, Aspergum, Aspir-Low, Aspir-trin, Bayer Aspirin, Easprin, Ecotrin, Entrophen ♣, Halfprin, Lowprin ♣, Novasen ♣, Rivasa ♣, Sloprin, St. Joseph Adult, Zorprin

Func. class.: Nonopioid analgesic, nonsteroidal antiinflammatory, antipyretic, antiplatelet

Chem. class.: Salicylate

Combinations: 25 mg/200 mg aspirin/dipyridamole; **Fiorinal:** 325 mg/50 mg/40 mg aspirin/butalbital/caffeine: **Loratab/ASA:** 325 mg/5 mg, aspirin/hydrocodone; **Percodan:** 325 mg/2.25 mg; 325 mg/4.5 mg aspirin/oxyCODONE; **Yosprala:** 325 mg/40 mg, 81 mg/40 mg aspirin/omeprazole

Do not confuse:

Aspirin/Anacin Adult Low/Anacin-3

ACTION:

Blocks pain impulses by blocking COX-1 in CNS, reduces

inflammation by inhibition of prostaglandin synthesis; antipyretic action results from vasodilation of peripheral vessels; decreases platelet aggregation

USES: Mild to moderate pain or fever, including rheumatoid arthritis (RA), osteoarthritis, thromboembolic disorders; TIAs, rheumatic fever, post-MI, prophylaxis of MI, ischemic stroke, angina, acute MI
Unlabeled uses: Colorectal cancer prophylaxis, venous thromboembolism, extended treatment to prevent recurrence, Kawasaki disease

CONTRAINDICATIONS
Pregnancy, breastfeeding, children <12 yr, children with flulike symptoms, hypersensitivity to salicylates, tartrazine (FD&C yellow dye #5), GI bleeding, bleeding disorders, vitamin K deficiency, peptic ulcer, acute bronchospasm, agranulocytosis, increased intracranial pressure, intracranial bleeding, nasal polyps, urticaria
Precautions: Abrupt discontinuation, acetaminophen/NSAIDs hypersensitivity, acid/base imbalance, alcoholism, ascites, asthma, bone marrow suppression in elderly patients, dehydration, G6PD deficiency, gout, heart failure, anemia, renal/hepatic disease, pre/postoperatively, gastritis

DOSAGE AND ROUTES
Pain/fever
• **Adult:** PO/RECT 325-1000 mg q4hr prn, max 4 g/day; extended-release tablets 650 mg q8hr or 800 mg q12hr
• **Child 2-11 yr:** PO 10-15 mg/kg/dose q4hr, max 4 g/day
RA, osteoarthritis, other inflammatory conditions
• **Adult:** PO 2.4 g/day in divided doses q4-6hr, maintenance 3.6-5.4 g/day; **EXTENDED RELEASE** 650 mg q8hr or 800 mg q12hr; target salicylate level 150-300 mcg/mL
Juvenile RA
• **Child:** PO/RECT 90-130 mg/kg/day in divided doses, target salicylate level 150-300 mcg/mL

Thromboembolic disorders
• **Adult:** PO 325-650 mg/day or bid
Transient ischemic attacks
• **Adult:** PO 50-325 mg/day (grade 1A)
Evolving MI with ST segment elevation (STEMI)
• **Adult:** PO 160-325 mg nonenteric, chewed and swallowed immediately, maintenance 75-162 mg daily
MI, stroke prophylaxis
• **Adult:** PO 75-325 mg/day
Prevention of recurrent MI/antiplatelet
• **Adult:** PO 75-325 mg/day
CABG
• **Adult:** PO 325 mg/day starting 6 hr postprocedure, continue for 1 yr
PTCA
• **Adult:** PO 325 mg 2 hr before surgery, then 160-325 mg daily
Prevention of colorectal cancer in those who are carriers of hereditary nonpolyposis colon cancer Lynch syndrome (unlabeled)
Adult: PO 600 mg daily × 2 yr
Venous thromboembolism to prevent recurrence (unlabeled)
Adult: PO 100 mg/day
Available forms: capsules 325 ♣; capsules extended release 162.5; tablets 81, 162.5, 325, 500, 650, 975 mg; chewable tablets 81 mg; suppository 60, 120, 150 ♣, 160 ♣, 200, 300, 600, 650 ♣ mg; enteric-coated tablets 81, 162 ♣, 325, 500 mg; delayed-release tablets 81, 325, 500 mg ♣
Administer:
PO route
• Do not break, crush, or chew enteric product
• Crushed or whole (regular PO product), chewable tablets may be chewed
• With food or milk to decrease gastric symptoms; separate by 2 hr from enteric products
• With 8 oz of water; sit upright for ½ hr after dose to facilitate product passing into stomach
Rectal route
• Place suppository in refrigerator for at least 30 min before removing wrapper

SIDE EFFECTS

CNS: Confusion, seizures, headache, intracranial hemorrhage

CV: Tachycardia, hypotension, dysrhythmias

EENT: Tinnitus, hearing loss

ENDO: Hypoglycemia, hypokalemia

GI: *Nausea, vomiting,* GI bleeding, pancreatitis, hepatotoxicity

GU: Increased BUN, creatinine, interstitial nephritis, renal failure syndrome

HEMA: Thrombocytopenia, leukopenia, DIC, increased PT, aPTT, bleeding time

INTEG: *Rash,* urticaria, bruising

SYST: Reye's syndrome (children), anaphylaxis, laryngeal edema, angioedema

PHARMACOKINETICS

Enteric metabolized by liver; inactive metabolites excreted by kidneys; crosses placenta; excreted in breast milk; half-life 15-20 min, up to 30 hr in large dose; rectal products may be erratic; protein binding 90%

PO: Onset 15-30 min, peak 1-2 hr, duration 4-6 hr, well absorbed

PO: Enteric coated: onset 10-30 min, duration 2-4 hr

RECT: Onset slow, duration 4-6 hr

INTERACTIONS

Increase: gastric ulcer risk—corticosteroids, antiinflammatories, NSAIDs, alcohol

Increase: bleeding—alcohol, plicamycin, cefamandole, thrombolytics, ticlopidine, clopidogrel, tirofiban, eptifibatide, anticoagulants; monitor for bleeding

Increase: effects of insulin, methotrexate, thrombolytic agents, penicillins, phenytoin, valproic acid, oral hypoglycemics, sulfonamides; monitor for increased effects of each product

Increase: salicylate levels—urinary acidifiers, ammonium chloride, nizatidine

Increase: hypotension—nitroglycerin

Decrease: effects of aspirin—antacids (high doses), urinary alkalizers, corticosteroids; monitor for decreased effects

Decrease: antihypertensive effect—ACE inhibitors, monitor B/P

Decrease: effects of probenecid, spironolactone, sulfinpyrazone, sulfonylamides, NSAIDs, β-blockers, loop diuretics

Drug/Herb

Increase: risk of bleeding—feverfew, garlic, ginger, ginkgo, ginseng *(Panax),* horse chestnut

Drug/Food

Increase: risk of bleeding—fish oil (omega-3 fatty acids)

• Foods that acidify urine may increase aspirin level

Drug/Lab Test

Increase: coagulation studies, LFTs, serum uric acid, amylase, CO_2, urinary protein

Decrease: serum potassium, cholesterol

Interference: VMA, 5-HIAA, xylose tolerance test, TSH, pregnancy test

NURSING CONSIDERATIONS

Assess:

• **Pain:** character, location, intensity; ROM before and 1 hr after administration

• **Fever:** temperature before and 1 hr after administration

• Hepatic studies: AST, ALT, bilirubin, creatinine if patient is receiving long-term therapy

• Renal studies: BUN, urine creatinine; I&O ratio; decreasing output may indicate renal failure (long-term therapy)

• Blood studies: CBC, Hct, HB, PT if patient is receiving long-term therapy

• **Hepatotoxicity:** dark urine, clay-colored stools, yellowing of skin, sclera, itching, abdominal pain, fever, diarrhea if patient is receiving long-term therapy

• **DRESS:** Monitor for rash, facial swelling, fever, lymphadenopathy, blood count abnormalities; discontinue

• **Allergic reactions:** rash, urticaria; if these occur, product may have to be discontinued; patients with asthma, nasal polyps, allergies: severe allergic reaction may occur

• **Ototoxicity:** tinnitus, ringing, roaring in ears; audiometric testing needed before, after long-term therapy

• **Salicylate level:** therapeutic level 150-300 mcg/mL for chronic inflammation
• **Beers:** avoid chronic use in older adults; GI bleeding may occur
• **Pregnancy/breastfeeding:** do not use in first trimester; may cause fetal harm; use only if benefits outweigh fetal risks (second/third trimester); avoid breastfeeding

Evaluate:
• Therapeutic response: decreased pain, inflammation, fever

Teach patient/family:
• To report any symptoms of hepatotoxicity, renal toxicity, visual changes, ototoxicity, allergic reactions, bleeding (long-term therapy)
• To avoid if allergic to tartrazine
• Not to exceed recommended dosage; acute poisoning may result
• To read labels on other OTC products because many contain aspirin, salicylates
• That the therapeutic response takes 2 wk (arthritis)
• To report tinnitus, confusion, diarrhea, sweating, hyperventilation
• To avoid alcohol ingestion; GI bleeding may occur
• That patients who have allergies, nasal polyps, asthma may develop allergic reactions
• To discard tablets if vinegar-like smell is detected
• That medication is not to be given to children or teens with flulike symptoms or chickenpox, because Reye's syndrome may develop
• To take with a full glass of water
• **Pregnancy/breastfeeding:** to inform prescriber if pregnancy is planned or suspected; avoid breastfeeding

TREATMENT OF OVERDOSE: Lavage, monitor electrolytes, VS

---

atazanavir (Rx)

(at-a-za-na′veer)

Reyataz

Func. class.: Antiretroviral
Chem. class.: Protease inhibitor

ACTION: Inhibits human immunodeficiency virus (HIV-1) protease, which prevents maturation of the infectious virus

USES: HIV-1 infection in combination with other antiretroviral agents

CONTRAINDICATIONS
Hypersensitivity, Child-Pugh Class C
Precautions: Pregnancy, breastfeeding, children, geriatric patients, hepatic disease, alcoholism, drug resistance, AV block, diabetes, dialysis, females, hemophilia, hypercholesterolemia, immune reconstitution syndrome, lactic acidosis, pancreatitis, cholelithiasis, serious rash

DOSAGE AND ROUTES
Antiretroviral-naive patients
• **Adult:** PO 400 mg/day (unable to take ritonavir); 300 mg with ritonavir 100 mg/day
• **Child ≥6 yr/adolescent ≥40 kg:** PO 300 mg with ritonavir 100 mg daily, or 400 mg/day (unable to take ritonavir)
• **Child ≥6 yr/adolescent Capsules, ≥6 years, ≥35-39 kg:** atazanavir 300 mg with ritonavir 100 mg orally once daily with food
• **Child ≥6 yr/adolescent Capsules, ≥6 years, 15 kg to less than 35 kg:** atazanavir 200 mg with ritonavir 100 mg orally once daily with food
Antiretroviral-experienced patients
• **Adult:** PO 300 mg with ritonavir 100 mg daily
• **Pregnant adults/adolescents (second/third trimester) with H_2 blocker or tenofovir:** PO 400 mg with ritonavir 100 mg daily
• **Child ≥6 yr/adolescent ≥40 kg:** PO 300 mg with ritonavir 100 mg daily
• **Child ≥6 yr/adolescent 20 to <40 kg:** PO 200 mg with ritonavir 100 mg daily
• **Children and adolescents ≥25 kg:** PO (oral powder) 300 mg q24hr with ritonavir 100 mg q24hr
• **Children 15 to 24 kg:** PO (oral powder) 250 mg q24hr with ritonavir 80 mg q24hr
• **Infants and children ≥3 mo and 5 to 14 kg:** PO (oral powder) 200 mg q24hr with ritonavir 80 mg q24hr

Hepatic dose
• **Adult:** PO Child-Pugh B: 300 mg/day; Child-Pugh C: do not use
Renal dose
• **Adult**: PO Therapy-naive and HD: 300 mg daily; with ritonavir: 100 mg daily; therapy experienced and HD: do not use
Available forms: Capsules 100, 150, 200, 300 mg; oral powder 50 mg/packet
Administer:
• **Capsules:** With food; 2 hr before or 1 hr after antacid or didanosine; swallow capsule whole, do not open
• **Oral powder:** Use with food or beverage; mix 1 tablespoon of food with powder, feed, then add another tablespoon of food to container, mix, and feed; or mix with 30 mL of liquid, give, then add another 15 mL of liquid to cup to remove residual, give; use within 1 hr of mixing

SIDE EFFECTS
CNS: Headache, depression, dizziness, insomnia, peripheral neuropathy
CV: Increased PR interval
GI: Vomiting, *diarrhea, abdominal pain, nausea,* hepatotoxicity, cholelithiasis
INTEG: *Rash,* Stevens-Johnson syndrome, *photosensitivity,* DRESS
MISC: Fatigue, fever, arthralgia, back pain, cough, lipodystrophy, pain, gynecomastia, nephrolithiasis; lactic acidosis, hyperbilirubinemia (pregnancy, females, obesity), immune reconstitution syndrome

PHARMACOKINETICS
Rapidly absorbed, absorption increased with food, peak 2½ hr, 86% protein bound, extensively metabolized in liver by CYP3A4, 27% excreted unchanged in urine/feces (minimal), half-life 7 hr

INTERACTIONS
Increase: levels, toxicity of immunosuppressants (cycloSPORINE, sirolimus, tacrolimus), sildenafil, antifungals (itraconazole, ketoconazole, voriconazole), tricyclic antidepressants, warfarin, calcium channel blockers, clarithromycin, clorazepate, diazePAM, irinotecan, HMG-CoA reductase inhibitors, antidysrhythmics, midazolam, triazolam, ergots, pimozide, other protease inhibitors; monitor for toxicity (amprenavir, darunavir, fosamprenavir, indinavir, nelfinavir, ritonavir, saquinavir)
Increase: effects of estrogens, oral contraceptives (unboosted), decreased (boosted with ritonavir)
Increase: atazanavir levels—CYP3A4 substrates, CYP3A4 inhibitors
Increase: hyperbilirubinemia—indinavir
Decrease: telaprevir level when used with atazanavir and ritonavir
Increase: QT prolongation—salmeterol, clarithromycin, romiDEPsin, ranolazine; dose reduction of each of these products may be needed
Increase: effect of alfuzosin, ARIPiprazole, benzodiazepine, brentuximab, cabazitaxel, carBAMazepine, cilostazol, colchicine, corticosteroids, eletriptan, eplerenone, crizotinib, DOCEtaxel, ixabepilone, iloperidone, lurasidone, maraviroc, muscarinic receptor antagonists, nilotinib, opioids, vinca alkaloids (vinCRIStine, vinBLAStine), vilazodone, vasopressin antagonists, dasatinib, lapatinib, SORAfenib, traZODone, risperIDONE, raltegravir, QUEtiapine
Decrease: atazanavir levels—CYP3A4 inducers, rifAMPin, antacids, didanosine, efavirenz, proton pump inhibitors, H$_2$-receptor antagonists; give atazanavir 2 hr before or 1 hr after these products
Drug/Herb
Decrease: atazanavir levels—St. John's wort; avoid concurrent use
Increase: myopathy, rhabdomyolysis—red yeast rice
Drug/Lab Test
Increase: AST, ALT, total bilirubin, amylase, lipase, CK
Decrease: HB, neutrophils, platelets
Drug/Food
Increased drug bioavailability (to be taken with food)

NURSING CONSIDERATIONS
Assess:
• **For hepatic failure; hepatic studies:** ALT, AST, bilirubin; do not use in Child-Pugh C
• For lactic acidosis, hyperbilirubinemia (females, pregnancy, obesity); if pregnant, call Antiretroviral Pregnancy Registry 800-

258-4263; do not breastfeed; use additional contraception when boosted with ritonavir

• PR interval in those taking calcium channel blockers, digoxin, monitor ECG

• For signs of infection, anemia, neph-rolithiasis

• Bowel pattern before, during treatment; if severe abdominal pain with bleeding occurs, product should be discontinued; monitor hydration

• Viral load, CD4 count throughout treatment

• Monitor blood glucose in those with diabetes

• Monitor for opportunistic infections/autoimmune disorder during treatment

• **Serious rash (Stevens-Johnson syndrome, DRESS):** most rashes last 1-4 wk; if serious, discontinue product

• **Immune reconstitution syndrome:** time of onset is variable when given with combination antiretroviral therapy

Evaluate:

• Therapeutic response: increasing CD4 counts; decreased viral load, resolution of symptoms of HIV-1 infection

Teach patient/family:

• To take as prescribed with other anti-retrovirals as prescribed; if dose is missed, to take as soon as remembered up to 1 hr before next dose; not to double dose or share with others

• That product must be taken daily to maintain blood levels for duration of therapy

• To report yellowing of skin, sclera

• To notify prescriber if diarrhea, nausea, vomiting, rash occurs; dizziness, light-headedness may occur; ECG may be altered

• That product interacts with many products, including St. John's wort; to advise prescriber of all products, herbal products used

• That redistribution of body fat may occur, the effect is not known

• That product does not cure HIV-1 infection, prevent transmission to others; only controls symptoms

• That if taking phosphodiesterase type 5 inhibitor with atazanavir, there may be increased risk of phosphodiesterase type 5 inhibitor–associated adverse events (hypotension, prolonged penile erection); to notify physician promptly of these symptoms

• **Pregnancy/breastfeeding:** that registration with Antiretroviral Pregnancy Registry is strongly encouraged for pregnant patients; to notify prescriber if pregnancy is planned or suspected; to use additional contraception when boosted with ritonavir

---

⚠ HIGH ALERT

atenolol (Rx)

(a-ten′oh-lole)

Tenormin, Tenoretic ✦

Func. class.: Antihypertensive, antianginal

Chem. class.: β-Blocker, β_1-, β_2-blocker (high doses)

Combination: atenolol 100 mg/chlorthalidone 25 mg, atenolol 50 mg/chlorthalidone 25 mg

Do not confuse:

atenolol/albuterol

Tenormin/thiamine/Imuran

ACTION: Competitively blocks stimulation of β-adrenergic receptor within vascular smooth muscle; produces negative chronotropic activity (decreases rate of SA node discharge, increases recovery time), slows conduction of AV node, decreases heart rate, negative inotropic activity decreases O_2 consumption in myocardium; decreases action of renin-aldosterone-angiotensin system at high doses, inhibits β_2 receptors in bronchial system at higher doses

USES: Hypertension, angina pectoris; suspected or known MI (IV use); MI prophylaxis

CONTRAINDICATIONS

Pregnancy, hypersensitivity to β-blockers, cardiogenic shock, second- or third-degree heart block, sinus bradycardia, cardiac failure

---

Precautions: Breastfeeding, major surgery, diabetes mellitus, thyroid/renal disease, HF, COPD, asthma, well-compensated heart failure, dialysis, myasthenia gravis, Raynaud's disease, pulmonary edema

Black Box Warning: Abrupt discontinuation

DOSAGE AND ROUTES
Hypertension
• **Adult: PO** 25-50 mg/day, increasing q1-2wk to 100 mg/day; may increase to 200 mg/day for **angina**, up to 100 mg/day for hypertension
• **Child: PO** 0.8-1 mg/kg/dose initially; range, 0.8-1.5 mg/kg/day; max 2 mg/kg/day; max 2 mg/kg/day up to 100 mg/day
• **Geriatric: PO** 25 mg/day initially
Post-MI
• **Adult: PO** 50 mg bid, max 100 mg/day in 1-2 divided doses for 6-9 days or until discharge
Renal disease
• **Adult: PO** CCr 15-35 mL/min, max 50 mg/day; CCr <15 mL/min, max 25 mg/day; hemodialysis 25-50 mg after dialysis
Available forms: Tablets 25, 50, 100 mg
Administer:
PO route
• Before meals, at bedtime; tablet may be crushed, swallowed whole, same time of day
• Reduced dosage with renal dysfunction
• Store protected from light, moisture; place in cool environment

SIDE EFFECTS
CNS: *Insomnia, fatigue, dizziness, mental changes,* memory loss, depression, lethargy, drowsiness, strange dreams
CV: Profound hypotension, bradycardia, HF
ENDO: Hypo- and hyperglycemia
GI: *Nausea, diarrhea,* vomiting, constipation
GU: Impotence, decreased libido, urinary frequency
MS: Back, joint pain
MISC: Lupus syndrome
INTEG: Rash
RESP: Bronchospasm, dyspnea, wheezing, pulmonary edema

PHARMACOKINETICS
PO: Peak 2-4 hr; onset 1 hr; duration 24 hr; half-life 6-7 hr; excreted unchanged in urine, feces (50%); protein binding 5%-15%

INTERACTIONS
• Mutual inhibition: sympathomimetics (cough, cold preparations)
Increase: hypotension, bradycardia—reserpine, hydrALAZINE, methyldopa, prazosin, anticholinergics, digoxin, diltiaZEM, verapamil, cardiac glycosides, calcium channel blockers, antihypertensives; monitor and adjust dose if needed
Increase: hypoglycemia—insulins, oral antidiabetics
Increase: hypertension—amphetamines, ePHEDrine, pseudoephedrine
Increase: toxicity risk—dolasetron; lidocaine (IV)
Decrease: atenolol effect—salicylates, rifamycins, penicillins, NSAIDs, calcium carbonate, aluminum antacids
Drug/Herb
Increase: atenolol effect—hawthorn
Decrease: atenolol effect—ephedra (ma huang)
Drug/Lab Test
Increase: BUN, potassium, triglycerides, uric acid, ANA titer, platelets, alkaline phosphatase, creatinine, LDH, AST/ALT
Decrease: glucose

NURSING CONSIDERATIONS
Assess:
• I&O, weight daily; watch for HF (rales/crackles, jugular vein distention, weight gain, edema)
• **Hypertension:** B/P, pulse q4hr; note rate, rhythm, quality; apical/radial pulse before administration; notify prescriber of any significant changes (<50 bpm); ECG
• **Hypoglycemia:** may be masked in diabetes mellitus (tachycardia, sweating)
• **Angina:** monitor number and character of anginal attacks

Black Box Warning: Taper gradually, do not discontinue abruptly, may precipitate angina, MI

Side effects: *italics* = common; red = life-threatening

• If pregnancy is planned or suspected; do not use in pregnancy, breastfeeding

Evaluate:

• Therapeutic response: decreased B/P after 1-2 wk, increased activity tolerance, decreased anginal pain

Teach patient/family:

Black Box Warning: Not to discontinue product abruptly, taper over 2 wk (angina); to take at same time each day as directed

• Not to use OTC products unless directed by prescriber
• To report bradycardia, dizziness, confusion, depression, fever
• To take pulse at home; advise when to notify prescriber (heart rate <50 bpm)
• To limit alcohol, smoking, sodium intake
• To comply with weight control, dietary adjustments, modified exercise program
• To carry emergency ID to identify product, allergies, conditions being treated
• To avoid hazardous activities if dizziness is present
• To change position slowly to limit orthostatic hypotension
• That product may mask symptoms of hypoglycemia in diabetic patients
• **Pregnancy/breastfeeding:** if pregnancy is planned or suspected; do not use in pregnancy, breastfeeding; to use contraception while taking this product; to avoid breastfeeding

TREATMENT OF OVERDOSE:
Lavage, IV atropine for bradycardia, IV theophylline for bronchospasm, dextrose for hypoglycemia, digoxin, O$_2$, diuretic for cardiac failure, hemodialysis

---

⚠ HIGH ALERT

atezolizumab (Rx)
(a-te-zoe-liz'ue-mab)

Tecentriq

Func. class.: Antineoplastic
Chem. class.: Monoclonal antibody

ACTION: Binds to PD-1, resulting in an antitumor response

USES: Treatment of locally advanced or metastatic urothelial carcinoma, including bladder cancer and other urinary system cancers, in patients who progress during or following platinum-containing chemotherapy for advanced disease, or within 12 months of neoadjuvant or adjuvant platinum-containing chemotherapy; triple-negative breast cancers (PD-1 expression) in combination; nonsquamous NSCLC with no EGFR or ALK gene aberrations

CONTRAINDICATIONS
Hypersensitivity

DOSAGE AND ROUTES
Breast cancer (triple negative), locally advanced or metastatic 🔬⚕
• **Adult:** IV: 840 mg on days 1 and 15 q4wk with protein-bound paclitaxel until disease progression or unacceptable toxicity

Hepatocellular carcinoma, unresectable or metastatic
• **Adult:** IV: 1200 mg q3wk with bevacizumab on the same day until disease progression or unacceptable toxicity; if bevacizumab is discontinued due to unacceptable toxicity, may continue atezolizumab monotherapy at 840 mg q2wk or 1200 mg q3wk or 1680 mg q4wk until disease progression or unacceptable toxicity

Melanoma, unresectable or metastatic (BRAF V600 mutation-positive) 🔬⚕
• **Adult:** IV: 840 mg q2wk with cobimetinib and vemurafenib until disease progression or unacceptable toxicity; before starting atezolizumab, patients should receive 28 days of cobimetinib and vemurafenib

Non–small-cell lung cancer (NSCLC), metastatic 🔬⚕
• **Adult:** IV: First-line treatment NSCLC (single agent): 840 mg q2wk or 1200 mg q3wk or 1680 mg q4wk; continue

until disease progression or unacceptable toxicity; first-line treatment, nonsquamous NSCLC: 1200 mg on day 1 q3wk with bevacizumab, paclitaxel, and carboplatin × 4 to 6 cycles, then atezolizumab 1200 mg on day 1, followed by bevacizumab q3wk until disease progression or unacceptable toxicity; previously treated NSCLC: 840 mg q2wk or 1200 mg q3wk or 1680 mg q4wk; continue until disease progression or unacceptable toxicity

Small cell lung cancer (extensive stage), first-line treatment
• **Adult: IV:** Induction: 1200 mg on day 1 q3wk with carboplatin and etoposide × 4 cycles, then maintenance therapy of monotherapy of atezolizumab at 840 mg q2wk or 1200 mg q3wk or 1680 mg q4wk; continue until disease progression or unacceptable toxicity

Urothelial carcinoma, locally advanced or metastatic 🕊⊘
• **Adult: IV:** 840 mg q2wk or 1200 mg q3wk or 1680 mg q4wk; continue until disease progression or unacceptable toxicity

AVAILABLE FORMS:
Injection 840 mg/14 mL, 1200 mg/20 mL single-dose vials

ADMINISTER
IV Route
• Visually inspect parenteral products for particulate matter and discoloration prior to use, discard if present
• Withdraw 20 mL of product and dilute with 250 mL in a polyvinyl chloride (PVC), polyethylene (PE), or polyolefin (PO) infusion bag containing 0.9% sodium chloride injection
• Mix by gentle inversion; do not shake
• *Storage after dilution:* Store diluted solution at room temperature for no more than 6 hr (including infusion time) or under refrigeration 36° F to 46° F (2° C to 8° C) for no more than 24 hr from the time of preparation
• Give atezolizumab prior to chemotherapy or other antineoplastic agents when given on the same day

• Do not infuse through the same IV line with other drugs
• Give first dose with or without a sterile, nonpyrogenic, low protein-binding in-line filter (0.2 to 0.22 micron) over 60 min; do not administer atezolizumab as an IV push or bolus. If tolerated, all subsequent infusions may be infused over 30 min
• Interrupt or slow administration for grade 2 infusion–related reactions; the infusion may resume when symptoms have resolved to grade 0 or 1, permanently discontinue atezolizumab for grade 3 or 4 infusion–related reactions

SIDE EFFECTS
CV: Peripheral edema, venous thromboembolism
CNS: Confusion, fatigue, fever
GI: Nausea, vomiting, abdominal pain, constipation, anorexia, diarrhea, obstruction, immunomediated colitis, immunomediated hepatitis, increased LFTs
GU: Hematuria, UTI, obstruction
HEMA: Anemia, lymphopenia
MS: Back/neck pain, arthralgia, myalgia
RESP: Dyspnea, cough, immunomediated pneumonitis, ILD
INTEG: Rash, pruritus, Stevens-Johnson syndrome
MISC: Infection, infusion-related reactions, hypo/hyperthyroidism

PHARMACOKINETICS
Onset unknown, peak unknown, duration unknown, half-life 27 days
Interactions
None known

NURSING CONSIDERATIONS
Assess:
• **Adrenal insufficiency:** Monitor for adrenal insufficiency (fatigue, joint/muscle pain, dizziness, nausea) usually within 5.7 mo. Withhold for grade 2 or higher and give systemic corticosteroids (1 to 2 mg/kg/day prednisone or equivalent) followed by a taper and administer hormone replacement as indicated
• **Cardiovascular toxicity:** Monitor for myocarditis. May require treatment interruption, discontinuation, systemic corti-

costeroids, and/or other immunosuppressive therapy (ASCO)

• **Diabetes mellitus:** For type 1 diabetes, initiate insulin treatment as indicated. Monitor for hyperglycemia and other signs/symptoms of diabetes; withhold therapy for grade 2 or higher hyperglycemia

• **Gastrointestinal toxicity:** Immune-mediated colitis or diarrhea (defined as requiring systemic corticosteroids) has occurred. Monitor for signs/symptoms of colitis and diarrhea. Withhold treatment for grade 2 or 3 diarrhea or colitis. For grade 2 or higher diarrhea or colitis, if symptoms persist for >5 days or recur, administer systemic corticosteroids (1 to 2 mg/kg/day prednisone equivalent). Discontinue permanently for grade 4 diarrhea or colitis

• **Hepatotoxicity:** Immune-mediated hepatitis and liver test abnormalities, including grades 3 and 4 and fatal cases, have occurred. Monitor for signs/symptoms of hepatitis (during and after treatment), including liver function tests (AST, ALT, and bilirubin). Give systemic corticosteroids (1 to 2 mg/kg/day prednisone or equivalent) followed by a taper for grade 2 or higher transaminase and/or bilirubin elevations. For grade 2 toxicity, withhold treatment until grade 1 or resolved or corticosteroid dose is ≤10 mg/day prednisone (or equivalent); permanently discontinue for grade 3 or 4 immune-mediated hepatitis

• **Infection:** Monitor for signs/symptoms of infection. Withhold treatment for grade 3 or higher infections; may resume once clinically stable

• **Infusion-related reactions:** Monitor for signs/symptoms of infusion reactions. Interrupt or slow the infusion in those with grade 1 or 2 infusion reactions; may premedicate with subsequent doses. Permanently discontinue for grade 3 or 4 infusion reactions

• **Ocular toxicity:** Uveitis and iritis have been reported. May require systemic corticosteroids to reduce the risk of permanent vision loss

• **Pulmonary toxicity:** Immune-mediated pneumonitis and interstitial lung disease may occur. Monitor for signs (with radiographic imaging) and symptoms of pneumonitis. Give systemic corticosteroids (1 to 2 mg/kg/day prednisone or equivalent) followed by a taper for grade 2 or higher pneumonitis. For grade 2 toxicity, withhold treatment until grade 1 or resolved or corticosteroid dose is ≤10 mg/day prednisone (or equivalent); permanently discontinue for grade 3 or 4 pneumonitis

• **Thyroid disorders:** Hypothyroidism, hyperthyroidism, and acute thyroiditis (rare) have occurred. Monitor thyroid function prior to and periodically during treatment. For hypothyroidism, initiate thyroid replacement. For grade 2 or higher hyperthyroidism, withhold

Teach patient/family:

• To report all severe reactions, as these may require corticosteroids or discontinuation (infection, immune-mediated reactions, allergic reactions)

• To report of infusion reaction (back pain, neck pain, chills, tremors, dizziness, passing out, fever, flushing, itching, rash, shortness of breath, swelling of the face, or wheezing)

• To report bowel problems (black, tarry, or bloody stools; fever; mucus in stools; vomiting; vomiting blood; severe abdominal pain; constipation; or diarrhea)

• To report liver problems (dark urine, fatigue, lack of appetite, nausea, abdominal pain, light-colored stools, vomiting, or yellow skin)

• To report UTI (blood in the urine, burning or painful urination, passing a lot of urine, fever, lower abdominal pain, or pelvic pain)

• To report lung problems (like shortness of breath or other trouble breathing, cough that is new or worse)

• To report kidney problems (unable to pass urine, blood in the urine, change in amount of urine passed, or weight gain)

• To report Stevens-Johnson syndrome/toxic epidermal necrolysis (red, swollen, blistered, or peeling skin [with or without fever]; red or irritated eyes; or sores in mouth, throat, nose, or eyes)

- To report mood changes, behavioral changes, weight changes, constipation, deeper voice, dizziness, passing out, cold sensation, severe fatigue, hair loss, persistent headache, or decreased sex drive
- To report pancreatitis (severe abdominal pain, severe back pain, severe nausea, or vomiting)
- To report signs of an allergic reaction (rash; hives; itching; red, swollen, blistered, or peeling skin with or without fever; wheezing; tightness in the chest or throat; trouble breathing, swallowing, or talking; unusual hoarseness; or swelling of the mouth, face, lips, tongue, or throat)

Evaluate

- Therapeutic response: Decreasing progression of cancer

---

atogepant (Rx)

(a-TOE-je-pant)

Qulipta

Func. class.: Migraine agent
Chem. class.: Calcitonin gene-related peptide

ACTION:
Centrally, CGRP is involved in transmission through neurons and pain modulation in the brainstem

USES:
Migraine prevention

CONTRAINDICATIONS
None
Precautions: Breastfeeding, pregnancy, hepatic disease, CYP3A4 inhibitors, OATP inhibitors

DOSAGE AND ROUTES
- **Adult: PO** 10, 30, or 60 mg daily; if used with strong CYP3A4 inhibitor: 10 mg daily; strong and moderate CYP3A4 inducers: 30 mg or 60 mg daily; OATP inhibitors: 10 mg or 30 mg daily
Available forms: Tablets 10, 30, 60 mg
Administer:
- Take without regard to food

SIDE EFFECTS
- **CNS:** Fatigue
- **GI:** Nausea, constipation

INTERACTIONS
Dose modifications may be needed with CYP3A4 inhibitors or OATP inhibitors

PHARMACOKINETICS
Onset, duration unknown, peak 1-2 hr; half-life 11 hr

NURSING CONSIDERATIONS
Assess:
- **Migraines:** Identify severity, triggers, nausea, auras, and if this product lessens the number of migraines
- **Pregnancy/breastfeeding:** May cause fetal harm, discontinue breastfeeding
- **Severe hepatic disease:** Avoid use in patients with severe hepatic impairment

Evaluate:
- Therapeutic response: Prevention of migraine

Teach patient/family:
- **Migraines:** Teach patient to keep a record of number of migraines, triggers, character
- **Pregnancy/breastfeeding:** Teach patient to report if pregnancy is planned or suspected or if breastfeeding
- **Interactions:** Inform patients that this product may interact with some other drugs and that dosage modifications may be recommended when used with some other drugs. Advise patients to report to their health care provider the use of other Rx, OTC, herbals, grapefruit juice

---

atomoxetine (Rx)

(at-o-mox'eh-teen)

Strattera

Func. class.: Psychotherapeutic—miscellaneous (ADHD)
Chem. class.: Selective norepinephrine reuptake inhibitor

Do not confuse:
atomoxetine/atorvastatin

ACTION: Selective norepinephrine reuptake inhibitor; may inhibit the presynaptic norepinephrine transporter

USES:
Attention-deficit/hyperactivity disorder

CONTRAINDICATIONS
Hypersensitivity, closed-angle glaucoma, MAOI therapy, history of pheochromocytoma

Precautions: Pregnancy, breastfeeding, hepatic disease, angioedema, bipolar disorder, dysrhythmias, CAD, hypo/hypertension, arteriosclerosis, cardiac disease, cardiomyopathy, heart failure, jaundice

> **Black Box Warning:** Children <6 yr, suicidal ideation

DOSAGE AND ROUTES
ADHD
• **Adult and child >6 yr and >70 kg: PO** 40 mg/day, increase after 3 days to target daily dose of 80 mg in AM or evenly divided doses AM, late afternoon; max 100 mg/day
• **Child >6 yr and ≤70 kg: PO** 0.5 mg/kg/day, increase after 3 days to target daily dose of 1.2 mg/kg in AM or evenly divided doses AM, late afternoon; max 1.4 mg/kg/day or 100 mg/day, whichever is less
Hepatic dose
• **Adult/Child PO Child-Pugh B:** reduce dose by 50%; Child-Pugh C: reduce dose by 75%
Strong CYP2D6 inhibitors
Adult/child: PO, reduce dose if needed
Available forms: Capsules 10, 18, 25, 40, 60, 80, 100 mg
Administer:
• Whole; do not break, crush, chew
• Gum, hard candy, frequent sips of water for dry mouth
• Without regard to food

SIDE EFFECTS
CNS: *Insomnia,* dizziness, irritability, crying, mood swings, fatigue, lethargy, paresthesia, suicidal ideation
CV: *Palpitations,* hot flushes, tachycardia, increased B/P, palpitations, orthostatic hypotension, QT prolongation

GI: Dyspepsia, nausea, anorexia, dry mouth, weight loss, vomiting, diarrhea, constipation, hepatotoxicity
GU: Urinary hesitancy, retention, dysmenorrhea, erectile disturbance, ejaculation failure, impotence, prostatitis
INTEG: Sweating, rash
MISC: Rhabdomyolysis, angioneurotic edema, anaphylaxis

PHARMACOKINETICS
Peak 1-2 hr duration up to 24 hr, metabolized by liver, some are poor metabolizers ᴿ⁰ᵪ, excreted by kidneys, 98% protein binding, half-life 5 hr

INTERACTIONS
Increase: hypertensive crisis—MAOIs or within 14 days of MAOIs, vasopressors
Increase: cardiovascular effects of albuterol, pressor agents
Increase: effects of atomoxetine—CYP2D6 inhibitors (amiodarone, cimetidine [weak], clomiPRAMINE, delavirdine, gefitinib, imatinib, propafenone, quiNIDine [potent], ritonavir, citalopram, escitalopram, FLUoxetine, sertraline, PARoxetine, thioridazine, venlafaxine)

NURSING CONSIDERATIONS
Assess:

> **Black Box Warning: Mental status:** mood, sensorium, affect, stimulation, memory loss, confusion, insomnia, aggressiveness, suicidal ideation in children/young adults, to notify prescriber immediately

• VS, B/P; check patients with cardiac disease more often for increased B/P
• **Hepatic injury:** may cause liver failure: monitor LFT; assess for jaundice, pruritus, flulike symptoms, upper right quadrant pain
• **Priapism:** monitor for urinary function (hesitancy, retention), sexual changes
• Appetite, sleep, speech patterns
• **ADHD:** For increased attention span, decreased hyperactivity with ADHD, growth rate, weight; therapy may need to be discontinued
Evaluate:
• Therapeutic response: decreased hyperactivity (ADHD), improved attention

Teach patient/family:
• To avoid OTC preparations, other medications, herbs, supplements unless approved by prescriber; no tapering needed when discontinuing product
• To avoid alcohol ingestion
• To avoid hazardous activities until stabilized on medication
• To get needed rest; patients will feel more tired at end of day; not to take dose late in day, insomnia may occur

Black Box Warning: To report suicidal ideation immediately

• To notify prescriber immediately if erection >4 hr
• To report immediately fainting, chest pain, difficulty breathing
• **Pregnancy/breastfeeding:** to notify prescriber if pregnancy is planned or suspected, or if breastfeeding; avoid in pregnancy or breastfeeding, those who took this product during pregnancy should register with the National Pregnancy Registry for ADHD medication: 866-961-2388

atorvastatin (Rx)

(a-tore′va-stat-in)

Lipitor

Func. class.: Antilipidemic

Chem. class.: HMG-CoA reductase inhibitor (statin)

Combinations: Cadut: 2.5 mg/10 mg, 2.5 mg/20 mg, 2.5 mg/40 mg, 5 mg/10 mg, 10 mg/10 mg, 5 mg/20 mg, 5 mg/40 mg, 10 mg/40 mg, 5 mg/80 mg, 10 mg/80 mg amlodipine/atorvastatin

Do not confuse:
atorvastatin/atomoxetine
Lipitor/Loniten/ZyrTEC

ACTION: Inhibits HMG-CoA reductase enzyme, which reduces cholesterol synthesis; high doses lead to plaque regression

USES: As adjunct for primary hypercholesterolemia (types Ia, Ib), elevated triglyceride levels, prevention of CV disease by reduction of heart risk in those with mildly elevated cholesterol, heterozygous familial hypercholesterolemia in pediatric patients ✧⊗, intensive lipid-lowering after an ACS event, noncardioembolic stroke/TIA, to reduce total/LDL cholesterol in homozygous familial hypercholesterolemia ✧⊗

CONTRAINDICATIONS

Pregnancy, breastfeeding, hypersensitivity, active hepatic disease, use with strong CYP3A4 inhibitors

Precautions: Previous hepatic disease, alcoholism, severe acute infections, trauma, severe metabolic disorders, electrolyte imbalance, use with azole antifungals

DOSAGE AND ROUTES

• **Adult: PO** 10-20 mg/day, usual range 10-80 mg/day, dosage adjustments may be made in 2- to 4-wk intervals, max 80 mg/day; patients who require >45% reduction in LDL may be started at 40 mg/day; concurrent use with clarithromycin, itraconazole, saquinavir/ritonavir, derunavir, fosamprenivir, fosamprenavir/ritonavir max 20 mg/day
• **Child 10-17 yr: PO** 10 mg daily, adjust q4wk, max 40 mg/day

Available forms: Tablets 10, 20, 40, 80 mg

Administer:
• Total daily dose at any time of day without regard to meals
• Store in cool environment in tight container protected from light

SIDE EFFECTS

CNS: Headache, asthenia, insomnia
EENT: Lens opacities
GI: *Abdominal cramps, constipation, diarrhea, flatus, heartburn,* dyspepsia, liver dysfunction, pancreatitis, nausea, increased serum transaminase
GU: Impotence, UTI
INTEG: Rash
MISC: Hypersensitivity; gynecomastia (child)
MS: Arthralgia, myalgia, rhabdomyolysis, myositis
RESP: Pharyngitis, sinusitis

Side effects: *italics* = common; red = life-threatening

PHARMACOKINETICS
Peak 1-2 hr, metabolized in liver, highly protein-bound, excreted primarily in urine, half-life 14 hr, protein binding 98%

INTERACTIONS
Increase: rhabdomyolysis—azole antifungals, cycloSPORINE, erythromycin, niacin, gemfibrozil, clofibrate, amiodarone, boceprevir, nelfinavir, lopinavir/ritonavir, macrolides, tacrolimus, telaprevim; do not use together
Increase: serum level of digoxin
Increase: toxicity, decreased metabolism of HMG-CoA: colchicine, diltiazem, fibric acid derivatives, protease inhibitors
Increase: levels of oral contraceptives
Increase: levels of atorvastatin, myopathy—CYP3A4 inhibitors
Increase: effects of warfarin
Decrease: atorvastatin levels—colestipol, antacids, cholestyramine
Drug/Herb
Decrease: effect—St. John's wort
Drug/Food
• Possible toxicity when used with grapefruit juice (large amounts); oat bran may reduce effectiveness
Drug/Lab Test
Increase: ALT, AST, CK

NURSING CONSIDERATIONS
Assess:
• **Hypercholesterolemia:** diet, obtain diet history including fat, cholesterol in diet; cholesterol triglyceride levels periodically during treatment; check lipid panel 6-12 wk after changing dose
• Hepatic studies q1-2mo, at initiation, 6, 12 wk after initiation or change in dose, periodically thereafter; AST, ALT, LFTs may be increased
• Bowel status: constipation, stool softeners may be needed; if severe, add fiber, water to diet
• **Rhabdomyolysis:** for muscle pain, tenderness, obtain CPK baseline; if markedly increased, product may need to be discontinued; many drug interactions may increase possibility for rhabdomyolysis
• **Pregnancy/breastfeeding:** do not breastfeed or use in pregnancy

Evaluate:
• Therapeutic response: decrease in LDL, total cholesterol, triglycerides, CAD; increase in HDL:LDL ratio
Teach patient/family:
• That compliance is needed for positive results to occur, not to skip or double doses
• That blood work and eye exam will be necessary during treatment
• To report blurred vision, severe GI symptoms, headache, muscle pain, and weakness; to avoid alcohol
• That previously prescribed regimen will continue: low-cholesterol diet, exercise program, smoking cessation
• **Pregnancy/breastfeeding:** identify if pregnancy is planned or suspected, or if breastfeeding

---

atovaquone (Rx)
(a-toe′va-kwon)
Mepron
Func. class.: Antiinfective
Chem. class.: Analog of ubiquinone

ACTION: Interferes with DNA/RNA synthesis in protozoa

USES: *Pneumocystis jiroveci* infections in patients intolerant of trimethoprim-sulfamethoxazole; prophylaxis

CONTRAINDICATIONS
Hypersensitivity or history of developing life-threatening allergic reactions to any component of the formulation, benzyl alcohol sensitivity
Precautions: Pregnancy, breastfeeding, neonates, hepatic disease, GI disease, respiratory insufficiency

DOSAGE AND ROUTES
Acute, mild, moderate
Pneumocystis jiroveci **pneumonia**
• **Adult and adolescent 13-16 yr: PO** 750 mg with food bid for 21 days
Pneumocystis jiroveci **pneumonia, prophylaxis**
• **Adult and adolescent >13 yr: PO** 1500 mg/day with meal
Available forms: Suspension 750 mg/5 mL

Administer:
• If vomiting occurs after ingestion, notify prescriber
• With high-fat food to increase absorption of product and higher plasma concentrations
• Oral suspension; shake gently before using
• All contents of foil pouch, pour in spoon or directly into mouth

SIDE EFFECTS

CNS: *Dizziness, headache, anxiety, insomnia,* asthenia, fever
CV: Hypotension
GI: *Nausea, vomiting, diarrhea,* anorexia, increased AST/ALT, acute pancreatitis, constipation, abdominal pain
HEMA: Anemia, neutropenia
INTEG: Pruritus, urticaria, *rash*
META: Hypoglycemia, hyponatremia
OTHER: Cough, dyspnea

PHARMACOKINETICS

Excreted unchanged in feces (94%), protein binding (99%), half-life 2-3 days, peak 1-8 hr

INTERACTIONS

Increase: level of—zidovudine; monitor for toxicity
Decrease: effect of atovaquone—metoclopramide, rifAMPin, rifabutin, tetracycline; avoid concurrent use
Drug/Food
Increased absorption with food
Drug/Lab Test
Increase: AST, ALT, alk phos
Decrease: glucose, neutrophils, HB, sodium

NURSING CONSIDERATIONS

Assess:
• **Infection:** WBC, vital signs; sputum baseline, periodically; obtain specimens needed before giving first dose
• Bowel pattern before, during treatment
• Respiratory status: rate, character, wheezing, dyspnea; risk for respiratory infection
• Allergies before treatment, reaction to each medication
Evaluate:
• Therapeutic response: C&S negative
• Decreased infection signs/symptoms

Teach patient/family:
• To take with food to increase plasma concentrations
• **Pregnancy/breastfeeding:** identify if pregnancy is planned or suspected; use cautiously in breastfeeding
• To take product as prescribed, not to skip or double dose

---

atovaquone/proguanil (Rx)

(a-toe'va-kwon)

Malarone, Malarone Pediatric
Func. class.: Antimalarial
Chem. class.: Aromatic diamide derivative

ACTION: The constituents of Malarone, atovaquone, and proguanil hydrochloride interfere with 2 different pathways involved in DNA/RNA synthesis in protozoa

USES: Malaria, malaria prophylaxis

CONTRAINDICATIONS

Hypersensitivity to this product, malaria prophylaxis in patients with severe renal impairment
Precautions: Pregnancy, breastfeeding, children, hepatic/GI/renal disease

DOSAGE AND ROUTES

Treatment of acute, uncomplicated *Plasmodium falciparum* malaria
Malarone adult-strength tablets
• **Adult/adolescent/child >40 kg:** PO 4 adult-strength tablets every day as a single dose × 3 consecutive days
• **Child 31-40 kg:** PO 3 adult-strength tablets every day as a single dose × 3 consecutive days
• **Child 21-30 kg:** PO 2 adult-strength tablets every day as a single dose × 3 consecutive days
• **Infant/child 11-20 kg:** PO 1 adult-strength tablet every day × 3 consecutive days
Malarone pediatric tablets
• **Infant/child 11-20 kg:** PO 4 pediatric tablets every day × 3 consecutive days
• **Infant/child 9-10 kg:** PO 3 pediatric tablets every day × 3 consecutive days

• **Infant/child 5-8 kg: PO** 2 pediatric tablets every day × 3 consecutive days
***P. falciparum* malaria prophylaxis, including chloroquine resistance areas**
Malarone adult-strength tablets
• **Adult/adolescent/child >40 kg: PO** 1 adult-strength tablet every day; begin prophylaxis 1-2 days before entering the endemic area; continue daily during the stay and for 7 days after leaving the area
Malarone pediatric tablets
• **Child 31-40 kg: PO** 3 pediatric tablets every day; begin prophylaxis 1-2 days before entering the endemic area; continue daily during the stay and for 7 days after leaving the area
• **Child 21-30 kg: PO** 2 pediatric tablets every day; begin prophylaxis 1-2 days before entering the endemic area; continue daily during the stay and for 7 days after leaving the area
• **Infant/child 11-20 kg: PO** 1 pediatric tablet every day; begin prophylaxis 1-2 days before entering the endemic area; continue daily during the stay and for 7 days after leaving the area
Renal dose
• **Adult: PO** CCr <30 mL/min, do not use for prophylaxis
Available forms: Tablets (adult) 250 mg atovaquone/proguanil 100 mg; tablets (pediatric) 62.5 atovaquone/proguanil 25 mg
Administer:
• Give with food or with milk or milk-based drink (nutritional supplement shake) to enhance oral absorption of atovaquone; food with high fat content is desired
• Give dose at the same time each day; administer a repeat dose if vomiting occurs within 1 hr after dosing
• Tablets may be crushed and mixed with condensed milk for children unable to swallow whole tablets

SIDE EFFECTS
CNS: *Dizziness, headache, anxiety, insomnia,* asthenia, fever
CV: Hypotension
GI: *Nausea, vomiting, diarrhea,* anorexia, increased AST/ALT, acute pancreatitis, constipation, abdominal pain

INTEG: Pruritus
OTHER: Cough, dyspnea

PHARMACOKINETICS
Atovaquone excreted unchanged in feces (94%), highly protein-bound (99%), proguanil 75% protein-bound, 40%-60% excreted in urine, hepatic metabolism; half-life 2-3 days

INTERACTIONS
Increase: level of warfarin; monitor INR
Decrease: effect of atovaquone—rifAMPin, rifabutin, tetracycline, metoclopramide; avoid using concurrently
Drug/Lab
Increase: AST, ALT, alkaline phosphatase
Decrease: glucose, neutrophils, HB

NURSING CONSIDERATIONS
Assess:
• **Malaria:** identify when the patient will be entering an area with malaria
• Bowel pattern before, during treatment
• Respiratory status: rate, character, wheezing, dyspnea; risk for respiratory infection
• Allergies before treatment, reaction to each medication
• CBC, LFTs, serum amylase, creatinine/BUN, sodium; increases in LFTs can persist for 4 wk after discontinuation of treatment
• **Pregnancy/breastfeeding:** identify if pregnancy is planned or suspected; avoid in breastfeeding if possible
Evaluate:
• Therapeutic response: resolution/prevention of malaria
Teach patient/family:
• To take with food to increase plasma concentrations, at same time of day
• To take whole course of treatment
• That product may be crushed and mixed with fluid if unable to swallow

---

⚠ HIGH ALERT

atracurium (Rx)
(a-tra-kyoor'ee-um)
Func. class.: Neuromuscular blocker (nondepolarizing)

USES: Facilitation of endotracheal intubation, skeletal muscle relaxation during mechanical ventilation, surgery, or general anesthesia

CONTRAINDICATIONS
Hypersensitivity

Black Box Warning: Respiratory insufficiency

DOSAGE AND ROUTES
• **Adult and child >2 yr: IV BOLUS** 0.4-0.5 mg/kg, then 0.08-0.1 mg/kg 20-45 min after first dose if needed for prolonged procedures; give smaller doses with halothane
• **Child 1 mo-2 yr: IV BOLUS** 0.3-0.4 mg/kg
Available forms: Injection 10 mg/mL

⚠ HIGH ALERT

atropine (Rx)
(a′troe-peen)
Atropen
Func. class.: Antidysrhythmic, anticholinergic parasympatholytic, antimuscarinic
Chem. class.: Belladonna alkaloid

ACTION: Blocks acetylcholine at parasympathetic neuroeffector sites; increases cardiac output, heart rate by blocking vagal stimulation in heart; dries secretions by blocking vagus

USES: Bradycardia <40-50 bpm, bradydysrhythmia, reversal of anticholinesterase agents, insecticide poisoning, blocking cardiac vagal reflexes, decreasing secretions before surgery, antispasmodic with GU, biliary surgery, bronchodilator, AV heart block
Unlabeled uses: Stress endocardiopathy

CONTRAINDICATIONS
Hypersensitivity to belladonna alkaloids, closed-angle glaucoma, GI obstructions, myasthenia gravis, thyrotoxicosis, ulcerative colitis, prostatic hypertrophy, tachycardia/tachydysrhythmias, asthma, acute hemorrhage, severe hepatic disease, myocardial ischemia, paralytic ileus

Precautions: Pregnancy, breastfeeding, children <6 yr, geriatric patients, renal disease, HF, hyperthyroidism, COPD, hypertension, intraabdominal infection, Down syndrome, spastic paralysis, gastric ulcer

DOSAGE AND ROUTES
Symptomatic bradycardia
• **Adult: IV BOLUS** 0.5-1 mg given q3-5min, max 3 mg
• **Child: IV BOLUS** 0.02 mg/kg, may repeat ×1; max single dose 0.5 mg, max total dose 1 mg
Bradysystolic arrest
Adult: IV 1 mg q3-5min, max total dose 3 mg
Organophosphate/carbamate/nerve agent poisoning
• **Adult and child: IM/IV** 1-2 mg q20-30min until muscarinic symptoms disappear; may need 6 mg every hr
• **Adult and child >90 lb, usually >10 yr: AtroPen** 2 mg
• **Child 40-90 lb, usually 4-10 yr: AtroPen** 1 mg
• **Child 15-40 lb: AtroPen** 0.5 mg
• **Infant <15 lb: IM/IV** 0.05 mg/kg q5-20min as needed
Presurgery (decreasing secretions)
• **Adult and child >20 kg: SUBCUT/IM/IV** 0.4-0.6 mg 30-60 min before anesthesia
• **Child <20 kg: IM/SUBCUT** 0.01 mg/kg up to 0.4 mg, ½-1 hr preop, max 0.6 mg/dose
Bronchospasm
Adult: INH 0.025-0.05 mg/kg/dose q4-6 hr as needed, max 2.5 mg/dose
Child: INH 0.03-0.05 mg/kg/dose 3-4 times per day, max 2.5 mg/dose
Stress endocardiography (unlabeled)
Adult: IV 0.25-0.5 up to a total dose of 1-2 mg until 85% of target HR is achieved
Available forms: Injection 0.05, 0.1, 0.4, 0.8, 1 mg/mL; AtroPen 0.25, 0.5, 1, 2 mg/0.7 mL Injection prefilled autoinjectors
Administer:
IM route
• Atropine flush may occur in children and is not harmful, usually 15-20 min after use
AtroPen
• Use no more than 3 AtroPen injections unless under the supervision of trained medical provider

• Use as soon as symptoms appear (tearing, wheezing, muscle fasciculations, excessive oral secretions), may use through clothing

IV route

• Undiluted or diluted with 10 mL sterile water; give at 0.6 mg/min through **Y**-tube or 3-way stopcock; do not add to IV solution; may cause paradoxical bradycardia for 2 min

Y-site compatibilities: Amrinone, etomidate, famotidine, heparin, hydrocortisone, meropenem, nafcillin, potassium chloride, SUFentanil, vitamin B/C

Endotracheal route

• Dilute with 5-10 mL of 0.9% NaCl, inject into endotracheal tube, then positive pressure ventilation

SIDE EFFECTS

CNS: Headache, dizziness, involuntary movement, confusion, flushing, drowsiness
CV: Tachycardia, bradycardia
EENT: Blurred vision, photophobia, dry eyes
GI: Dry mouth, constipation
RESP: Tachypnea, pulmonary edema
GU: Retention, hesitancy, impotence
INTEG: Flushing, decreased sweating

PHARMACOKINETICS

Half-life 4-5 hr, excreted by kidneys unchanged (50%), metabolized in liver, crosses placenta, excreted in breast milk
IM/SUBCUT: Onset 15-50 min, peak 30 min, duration 4-6 hr, well absorbed
IV: Peak 2-4 min, duration 4-6 hr

INTERACTIONS

Increase: mucosal lesions—potassium chloride tablet; avoid concurrent use
Increase: anticholinergic effects—tricyclics, amantadine, antiparkinson agents, phenothiazines, antidysrhythmics
Increase: altered response—β-blockers
Decrease: absorption—ketoconazole, levodopa
Decrease: effect of atropine—antacids

NURSING CONSIDERATIONS

Assess:

• I&O ratio; check for urinary retention, daily output

• VS during treatment, ECG for ectopic ventricular beats, PVC, tachycardia in cardiac patients
• For bowel sounds, constipation, abdominal distention, if constipation occurs add fluids, bulk in diet
• **Beers:** avoid in older adults; highly anticholinergic, high risk of delirium, in men decreased urinary flow

Evaluate:

• Therapeutic response: decreased dysrhythmias, increased heart rate, secretions; GI, GU spasms; bronchodilation

Teach patient/family:

• To report blurred vision, chest pain, allergic reactions, constipation, urinary retention; to use sunglasses to protect the eyes
• Not to perform strenuous activity in high temperatures; heat stroke may result
• To take as prescribed; not to skip or double doses
• Not to operate machinery if drowsiness occurs
• Not to take OTC products, herbals, supplements without approval of prescriber
• Not to freeze or expose to light (Atro-Pen)
• To use sunglasses for photophobia
• **Pregnancy/breastfeeding:** identify if pregnant or if breastfeeding; use only if benefits outweigh fetal risk

TREATMENT OF OVERDOSE:

O_2, artificial ventilation, ECG; administer DOPamine for circulatory depression; administer diazePAM or thiopental for seizures; assess need for antidysrhythmics

---

atropine ophthalmic
See Appendix B

---

avacopan (Rx)
(a-va-KOE-pan)
Tavneos
Func. class.: Immunomodulating agent
Chem. class.: Complement 5a receptor (C5aR) antagonist

ACTION:
Blocks C5a-mediated neutrophil activation and migration. The precise mechanism is unknown

USES:
Antineutrophil cytoplasmic autoantibody (ANCA)–associated vasculitis in combination

CONTRAINDICATIONS
Hypersensitivity
Precautions: Hepatotoxicity, angioedema, hepatitis B virus reactivation, serious infections

DOSAGE AND ROUTES
• **Adult: PO** 30 mg (three 100 mg capsules bid with food; reduce to 30 mg daily when used with strong CYP3A4 inhibitors
Available forms: Capsule 10 mg
Administer:
• Capsules should not be crushed, chewed, or opened
• If a dose is missed, wait until the usual scheduled time to take the regular dose, do not double

SIDE EFFECTS
CNS: Headache, paresthesia, fatigue, dizziness
GI: Nausea, diarrhea, vomiting, abdominal pain
CV: Hypotension
INTEG: Rash

INTERACTIONS
Avoid use with strong and moderate CYP3A4 enzyme inducers, strong CYP3A4 enzyme inhibitors: Reduce avacopan dose to 30 mg daily
Sensitive CYP3A4 substrates: Monitor for adverse reactions and reduce dose of sensitive CYP3A4 substrates

PHARMACOKINETICS
Protein binding: 99.99%

NURSING CONSIDERATIONS
Assess:
• Monitor LFTs, alkaline phosphatase, total bilirubin baseline

• Monitor hepatitis B virus (HBV) serology: Screen patients for HBV infection by measuring HBsAg and anti-HBc baseline
Evaluate:
• Therapeutic response: Decreasing vasculitis
Teach patient/family:
• Instruct the patient to swallow whole, not to chew or crush. If a dose is missed, take at next regular dose time, to discuss all OTC, Rx, and herbals taken
• **Hypersensitivity:** Advise patients to seek immediate medical attention for angioedema (swelling of face, extremities, eyes, lips, tongue; and difficulty in swallowing or breathing) and to stop the drug immediately
• **Hepatotoxicity:** Advise patients to contact their health care provider immediately for signs or symptoms of liver problems; yellowing of the skin or the white part of the eyes, dark or brown urine, pain on the upper right side of the abdomen, bleeding or bruising anywhere
• **Infections:** Inform patients that serious infections have been reported, including reactivation of hepatitis B infection. Instruct patients to contact their health care provider immediately if they develop any signs or symptoms of an infection
• **Breastfeeding:** Teach patient to consider benefits/risk during breastfeeding

avanafil (Rx)
(a-van′a-fil)
Stendra
Func. class.: Impotence agent

USES: Treatment of erectile dysfunction

CONTRAINDICATIONS
Hypersensitivity, severe renal/hepatic disease, current nitrates/nitrites, patients <18 yr

DOSAGE AND ROUTES
Erectile dysfunction
• **Adult: PO** 100 mg 30 min before sexual activity, dose may be reduced to

50 mg or increased to 200 mg; usual max dose frequency is 1 time/day

Dosage adjustments

Potent CYP3A4 inhibitors/nitrates

• Do not use

Moderate CYP3A4 inhibitors/ α-blockers

• Max 50 mg/day

Hepatic dosage/severe renal disease

Child-Pugh C: Not recommended

Available forms: Tablets 50,100, 200 mg

⚠ HIGH ALERT

avapritinib (Rx)

(a'va-pri'ti-nib)

Ayvakit

Func. class.: Antineoplastic

Chem. class.: Tyrosine kinase inhibitor

ACTION: Blocks PDGFRA and KIT exon 11, 11/17, 17 mutations

USES: Unresectable/metastatic GI stromal tumor (GIST) with these mutations

CONTRAINDICATIONS

Hypersensitivity, pregnancy, breastfeeding

Precautions: Intracranial hemorrhage

DOSAGE AND ROUTES

• **Adult:** PO 300 mg daily on an empty stomach, continue until disease progression or unacceptable toxicity

Systemic mast cell disease

• **Adult:** PO 200 mg daily on empty stomach, continue until disease progression or unacceptable toxicity

Available forms: Tablet 100 mg, 200 mg, 300 mg

Administer:

• Give on an empty stomach, at least 1 hr before or 2 hr after a meal

• If a dose is missed, do not take if next dose is due within 8 hr

• Give antiemetics to prevent nausea and vomiting

• Store at room temperature

SIDE EFFECTS

CV: Edema

INTEG: Alopecia, hair discoloration, rash

GI: Abdominal pain, constipation, anorexia, diarrhea, dysgeusia, dyspepsia, nausea/vomiting

CNS: CNS toxicity, cognitive dysfunction, dizziness, fatigue, headache, memory impairment, mood/sleep disorder, fever

MS: Asthenia

EENT: Tearing, periorbital edema

RESP: Dyspnea, pleural effusion

PHARMACOKINETICS

Onset unknown, peak 2-4 hr, duration unknown, half-life 32-57 hr, protein binding 98.8%

INTERACTIONS

Increase avapritinib effect: Moderate/ strong CYP3A4 inhibitors, avoid using together

Decrease avapritinib effect: Moderate/ strong CYP3A4 inducers, avoid using together

Drug/Lab: Increase: LFTs, bilirubin, serum creatinine, INR, PTT, thrombocytopenia

Decrease: Serum albumin, serum magnesium, serum phosphate, serum potassium/sodium, neutrophils, leukocytes

NURSING CONSIDERATIONS

Assess:

• Assess for PDGFRA exon 18 mutations before use

• Assess for pregnancy before use in females of reproductive potential, males with female partners of reproductive potential should use contraception during and for 6 wk after last dose

• Monitor CNS effects (cognitive impairment, dizziness, sleep/mood/speech disorders), intracranial hemorrhage

---

Evaluate:
• Therapeutic response: Decrease in spread of GI stromal tumor
Teach patient/family:
• To report adverse reactions immediately: Severe headache, cognitive changes, shortness of breath, change in vision
• About reason for treatment, expected results
• That effect on male infertility is unknown
• Not to stop or change dose
• To avoid hazardous activities until response is known, dizziness may occur
• To take on empty stomach
• To avoid OTC products unless approved by prescriber
• To notify prescriber if pregnancy is planned or suspected; not to breastfeed; to use effective contraception during and for 6 wk after last dose, females of reproductive potential and males with female partners of reproductive potential

axicabtagene ciloleucel (Rx)

(ax-i-cab′tay-jeen sye-lo′loo-sel)
Yescarta
Func. class.: Antineoplastic, cellular immunotherapies

USES: For the treatment of non-Hodgkin's lymphoma
CONTRAINDICATIONS
Hypersensitivity

Black Box Warning: Cytokine release syndrome

DOSAGE AND ROUTES
Large B-cell lymphoma
• **Adult: IV** 2×10^6 CAR-positive viable T cells per kg of body weight (max dose of 2×10^8 CAR-positive viable T cells) as a single IV dose
Therapeutic drug monitoring: management of treatment-related toxicity; refer to package insert

Available forms: Infusion bag: 2×10^6 chimeric antigen receptor–positive T cells/kg

⚠ HIGH ALERT

A

axitinib (Rx)

Inlyta
Func. class.: Antineoplastics, biologic response modifiers, signal transduction inhibitors (STIs)
Chem. class.: Tyrosine kinase inhibitor

ACTION: Inhibits receptor tyrosine kinases including vascular endothelial growth factor receptor 1 (VEGFR-1), VEGFR-2, and VEGFR-3; inhibits tumor growth and phosphorylation of VEGFR-2 and VEGF-mediated endothelial cell proliferation

USES: Treatment of advanced renal cell cancer after failure of 1 prior systemic therapy

CONTRAINDICATIONS
Pregnancy, breastfeeding
Precautions: Risk for or history of thromboembolic disease, recent bleeding, untreated brain metastasis, recent GI bleeding, GI perforation, fistula, surgery, moderate hepatic disease, uncontrolled hypertension, hyper/hypothyroidism, proteinuria, infertility, end-stage renal disease (CrCl <15 mL/min); not intended for use in adolescents, children, infants, neonates

DOSAGE AND ROUTES
Advanced renal cell carcinoma after failure of 1 systemic therapy
• **Adult: PO** 5 mg bid (at 12-hr intervals), may increase to 7 mg bid and then to 10 mg bid in intervals of 6 wk
First-line treatment of advanced renal cell cancer, with pembrolizumab
• **Adults: PO** 5 mg bid with pembrolizumab 200 mg IV on day 1 q3wk or 400 mg IV on day 1 q6wk. The axitinib dosage may be increased to 7 mg bid and then to 10 mg bid q6wk or longer in normotensive patients
First-line treatment of advanced renal cell cancer, with avelumab
• **Adults: PO** 5 mg bid with avelumab 800 mg IV over 1 hr q2wk until disease progression or unacceptable toxicity.

Side effects: *italics* = common; red = life-threatening

The axitinib dosage may be increased to 7 mg bid and then to 10 mg bid in normotensive patients

• **Adult receiving a strong CYP3A4/5 inhibitor:** Reduce dose by ½, adjust as needed
Available forms: Tablets 1, 5 mg
Administer:

• Premedicate with antihistamine and acetaminophen 30-60 min prior to each dose
• Use safe handling precautions
• Give with or without food; swallow tablet whole with a glass of water
• If patient vomits or misses a dose, an additional dose should not be taken; the next dose should be taken at the usual time
• Store at room temperature

SIDE EFFECTS

CNS: Dizziness, headache, reversible posterior leukoencephalopathy syndrome (RPLS), fatigue
CV: Hypertension, arterial thromboembolic events (ATE), venous thromboembolic events (VTE)
ENDO: Hypothyroidism, hyperthyroidism
GI: Lower GI bleeding/perforation/fistula, abdominal pain, constipation, diarrhea, dysgeusia, dyspepsia, dysphonia, hemorrhoids, nausea, mucosal inflammation, stomatitis, vomiting, increased ALT/AST
GU: Proteinuria
HEMA: Bleeding, intracranial bleeding, anemia, polycythemia, decreased/increased hemoglobin, lymphopenia, thrombocytopenia, neutropenia
INTEG: Palmar-plantar erythrodysesthesia (hand and foot syndrome), rash, dry skin, pruritus, alopecia, erythema
MISC: Weight loss, dehydration, metabolic and electrolyte laboratory abnormalities
MS: Asthenia, arthralgia, musculoskeletal pain, myalgia
RESP: Cough, dyspnea

PHARMACOKINETICS

Absorption: bioavailability 58%; distribution: protein binding >99%; metabolized in liver by CYP3A4/5, CYP1A2, CYP2C19, and UGT1A1; metabolites are carboxylic acid, sulfoxide, and *N*-glucuronide; excretion 41% in feces and 23% in urine, 12% unchanged; half-life: 2.5-6.1 hr; steady state 2-3 days; onset unknown, peak 2.5-4.1 hr, increased in moderate hepatic disease; duration unknown

INTERACTIONS

Increase: effect of axitinib—CYP3A4/5 inhibitors, strong/moderate (ketoconazole, boceprevir, chloramphenicol, conivaptan, delavirdine, fosamprenavir, imatinib, indinavir, isoniazid, itraconazole, dalfopristin, quinupristin, posaconazole, ritonavir, telithromycin, tipranavir [boosted with ritonavir], darunavir [boosted with ritonavir], aldesleukin [IL-2], amiodarone, aprepitant, fosaprepitant, atazanavir, bromocriptine, clarithromycin, crizotinib, danazol, diltiaZEM, dronedarone, erythromycin, fluvoxaMINE, lanreotide, lapatinib, miconazole, miFEPRIStone, nefazodone, nelfinavir, niCARdipine, octreotide, pantoprazole, saquinavir, tamoxifen, verapamil, voriconazole, grapefruit juice); avoid using together, or reduce axitinib
Decrease: effect of axitinib—CYP3A4/5 inducers, strong/moderate (rifAMPin, carBAMazepine, dexamethasone, phenytoin, PHENobarbital, rifabutin, rifapentine, St. John's wort, ethanol, bexarotene, bosentan, efavirenz, etravirine, griseofulvin, metyraPONE, modafinil, nafcillin, nevirapine, OXcarbazepine, vemurafenib, pioglitazone, topiramate); avoid using together
Increase or decrease: effect of axitinib—CYP3A4/5 inhibitors and inducers (quiNINE)
Drug/Lab Test
Increase: creatinine, lipase, amylase, potassium
Decrease: bicarbonate, calcium, albumin, glucose, phosphate, sodium
Increase or decrease: sodium, glucose
Drug/Food
Increase: drug effect—grapefruit or grapefruit juice
Drug/Herb
Decrease: effect of axitinib—St. John's wort

NURSING CONSIDERATIONS
Assess:
• **Bleeding:** monitor for GI bleeding or perforation; temporarily discontinue therapy if any bleeding that requires treatment

- **Surgery:** discontinue ≥24 hr before surgery; may be resumed after adequate wound healing
- **Hepatic/renal disease:** dosage should be reduced in patients with moderate (Child-Pugh Class B) hepatic disease; monitor liver function tests (ALT, AST, bilirubin) before and periodically during therapy; monitor CCr before and during treatment
- **Hypertension:** B/P should be well controlled before starting treatment; monitor for hypertension and administer antihypertensive therapy as needed before and during therapy; dose should be reduced for persistent hypertension; therapy should be discontinued if B/P remains elevated after a dosage reduction or if there is evidence of hypertensive crisis; after discontinuation, monitor B/P for hypotension in those receiving antihypertensives
- **Hyper/hypothyroidism:** monitor thyroid function tests before and periodically during therapy; thyroid disease should be treated with thyroid medications
- Monitor for proteinuria before and periodically during therapy; product may need to be decreased or discontinued if moderate to severe proteinuria occurs
- **RPLS:** monitor for headache, seizures, visual changes, confusion, drowsiness, hemiplegia, discontinue product if these occur
- **Pregnancy/breastfeeding:** determine if the patient is pregnant or breastfeeding before using this product; may also cause infertility; do not use in pregnancy and for 1 wk after last dose or breastfeeding; obtain pregnancy test in women of child-bearing potential before starting therapy

Evaluate:
- Therapeutic response: decreased spread of malignancy

Teach patient/family:
- That product will be discontinued ≥24 hr before surgery; may be resumed after adequate wound healing
- To notify prescriber of bleeding that is severe or that requires treatment

- That laboratory testing will be required before and periodically during product use
- How to monitor B/P and that B/P products should be continued as directed by prescriber
- That product may be taken without regard to meals
- To report all adverse reactions, including neurologic, GI bleeding
- To avoid use with grapefruit/grapefruit juice, St. John's wort
- Pregnancy/breastfeeding: to use contraception during treatment, and for 1 wk after last dose or to avoid use of this product; to notify prescriber if pregnancy is planned or suspected; not to breastfeed

⚠ HIGH ALERT

azaCITIDine (Rx)
(a-za-sie-ti'deen)
Onureg, Vidaza
Func. class.: Antineoplastic
Chem. class.: Pyrimidine nucleoside analogue

Do not confuse:
azaCITIDine/azaTHIOprine

ACTION: Cytotoxic by producing damage to double-strand DNA during DNA synthesis

USES: Myelodysplastic syndrome (MDS), acute myelogenous leukemia (AML)

CONTRAINDICATIONS
Pregnancy, hypersensitivity to product or mannitol, advanced malignant hepatic tumors
Precautions: Breastfeeding, children, geriatric patients, renal/hepatic disease, baseline albumin <30 g/L; a man should not father a child while taking product

DOSAGE AND ROUTES
Myelodysplastic syndrome/AML
- **Adult:** PO 300 mg daily on days 1-14 (28-day cycle); **SUBCUT/IV** 75 mg/m^2/day × 7

days q4wk, dose may be increased to 100 mg/m^2 if no response seen after 2 treatment cycles; minimum treatment, 4 cycles

Available forms: Powder for injection 100 mg; tablets 200, 300 mg

Administer:

• Use cytotoxic handling procedures

SUBCUT route

• **Reconstitute** with 4 mL sterile water for injection (25 mg/mL), inject diluents slowly into vial, invert vial 2-3 times, gently rotate; solution will be cloudy, use immediately; divide doses >4 mL into 2 syringes; invert contents 2-3 times, gently roll syringe between the palms for 30 sec immediately before administration, rotate injection site

Intermittent IV INFUSION route

• **Reconstitute** each vial with 10 mL sterile water for injection, shake well until all solids are dissolved, withdraw solution (10 mg/mL), inject in 50-100 NS or LR infusion, run over 10-40 min

SIDE EFFECTS

CNS: *Anxiety, depression, dizziness, fatigue, headache, fever, insomnia*

CV: Cardiac murmur, hypotension, tachycardia, peripheral edema, *chest pain*

GI: *Diarrhea, nausea, vomiting,* anorexia, *constipation,* abdominal pain, distention, tenderness, hemorrhoids, mouth hemorrhage, tongue ulceration, stomatitis, dyspepsia, hepatotoxicity, hepatic coma

GU: Renal failure, renal tubular acidosis, dysuria, UTI

HEMA: Leukopenia, anemia, thrombocytopenia, neutropenia, febrile neutropenia, ecchymosis, petechiae

INTEG: *Irritation at site, rash,* sweating, pyrexia, pruritus

META: Hypokalemia

MS: Weakness, arthralgia, muscle cramps, myalgia, back pain

RESP: Cough, *dyspnea, pharyngitis,* pleural effusion

PHARMACOKINETICS

Rapidly absorbed, peak ½ hr, metabolized in the liver, half-life 4 hr, excreted in urine

INTERACTIONS

Increase: bone marrow suppression—other antineoplastics

Increase: bleeding—anticoagulants

Drug/Lab

Increase: BUN, creatinine

Decrease: WBC, platelets, neutrophils, potassium

NURSING CONSIDERATIONS

Assess:

• For CNS symptoms: fever, headache, chills, dizziness

• **Bone marrow suppression/hematologic response:** CBC with differential, baseline WBC ≥3000/mm^3, absolute neutrophil count (ANC) ≥1500/mm^3, platelets >75,000/mm^3, adjust dose based on nadir; ANC <500/mm^3, platelets <25,000/mm^3, give 50% dose next course; ANC 500-1500/mm^3, platelets 25,000-50,000/mm^3, give 67% next course; bruising, bleeding, blood in stools, urine, sputum, emesis; myelodysplastic syndrome (MDS), splenomegaly

• Buccal cavity for dryness, sores or ulceration, white patches, oral pain, bleeding, dysphagia

• **Myelodysplastic syndrome:** severe anemia, cytopenias, splenomegaly

• **TLS:** Monitor for TLS even with allopurinol, monitor electrolytes, uric acid, serum creatinine baseline and periodically

• Blood studies: BUN, bicarbonate, creatine, LFTs

• Increased fluid intake to 2-3 L/day to prevent dehydration unless contraindicated

• Rinsing of mouth tid-qid with water, club soda; brushing of teeth bid-tid with soft brush or cotton-tipped applicator for stomatitis; use unwaxed dental floss

Evaluate:

• Therapeutic response: improvement in blood counts with refractory anemia, or refractory anemia with excess blasts

Teach patient/family:

• To avoid crowds, persons with known infections; not to receive immunizations

• To avoid foods with citric acid or hot or rough texture if stomatitis is present; to drink adequate fluids

• To report stomatitis; any bleeding, white spots, ulcerations in mouth; to examine mouth daily, report symptoms, infection site reactions, pruritus, fever

• **Pregnancy/breastfeeding:** to use contraception during and for 6 mo after therapy; not to breastfeed; not to father a child while receiving product

---

azaTHIOprine (Rx)

(ay-za-thye′oh-preen)

Azasan, Imuran

Func. class.: Immunosuppressant

Chem. class.: Purine antagonist

Do not confuse:

azaTHIOprine/azaCITIDine

ACTION: Produces immunosuppression by inhibiting purine synthesis in cells

USES: Renal transplants to prevent graft rejection, refractory rheumatoid arthritis

Unlabeled uses: Chronic ulcerative colitis, Crohn's disease, autoimmune hepatitis, dermatomyositis, thrombocytopenic purpura, lupus nephritis, polymyositis, pulmonary fibrosis, systemic lupus erythematosus (SLE), Wegener's granulomatosis, vasculitis, atopic dermatitis

CONTRAINDICATIONS

Pregnancy, hypersensitivity, breastfeeding

Precautions: Severe renal/hepatic disease, geriatric patients, ♦ thiopurine methyltransferase deficiency, infection, bone marrow suppression; must be used by an experienced clinician

Black Box Warning: Neoplastic disease

DOSAGE AND ROUTES

Immunosuppression in kidney transplantation

• **Adult and child: PO/IV** 3-5 mg/kg/day, then maintenance **(PO)** of ≥1-3 mg/kg/day

Child/adolescent (unlabeled): PO 1-2 mg/kg/day with tacrolimus and corticosteroids

Renal dose

• **Adult: PO** Give lower dose in tubular necrosis in immediate postcadaveric transplant period

Refractory rheumatoid arthritis

• **Adult: PO** 1 mg/kg/day, may increase dose after 2 mo by 0.5 mg/kg/day and then q4wk, max 2.5 mg/kg/day

Lupus nephritis/SLE/Wegener's granulomatosis/idiopathic pulmonary fibrosis/multiple sclerosis (unlabeled)

• **Adult: PO** 2-3 mg/kg/day

Atopic dermatitis (unlabeled)

• **Adult/adolescent ≥16 yr: PO** 2.5 mg/kg/day

Crohn's disease, ulcerative colitis (unlabeled)

• **Adult/child: PO** 50 mg/day; may increase by 25 mg/day q1-2wk up to 2-3 mg/kg/day, if tolerated

Available forms: Tablets 50, 75, 100 mg; powder for injection 50 mg ♦, 100 mg/vial

Administer:

• For several days before transplant surgery

• All medications PO if possible; avoid IM injection because bleeding may occur

PO route

• With meals to reduce GI upset

IV route

• Prepare in biologic cabinet with gown, gloves, mask

Direct IV

• **Dilute** to 10 mg/mL with 0.9% NaCl, 0.45% NaCl, D₅W, **give** over 5 min

Intermittent IV INFUSION route

• **Reconstitute** 100 mg/10 mL of sterile water for injection; rotate to dissolve; **further dilute** with 50 mL or more saline or glucose in saline, **give** over ½-1 hr

Y-site compatibilities: Alfentanil, atracurium, atropine, benztropine, calcium gluconate, cycloSPORINE, enalaprilat, epoetin alfa, erythromycin, fentaNYL, fluconazole, folic acid, furosemide, glycopyrrolate, heparin, insulin, mannitol, mechlorethamine, metoprolol, naloxone,

---

nitroglycerin, oxytocin, penicillin G, potassium chloride, propranolol, protamine, SUFentanil, trimethaphan, vasopressin

SIDE EFFECTS
CNS: Progressive multifocal leukoencephalopathy
EENT: Retinopathy
Resp: Pulmonary edema
GI: *Nausea, vomiting,* stomatitis, esophagitis, pancreatitis, hepatotoxicity, jaundice, hepatic veno-occlusive disease
HEMA: Leukopenia, thrombocytopenia, anemia, pancytopenia, bleeding
INTEG: Rash, alopecia
MISC: Serum sickness, Raynaud's symptoms, secondary malignancy, infection, chills, fever
MS: Arthralgia, muscle wasting

PHARMACOKINETICS
Metabolized in liver, excreted in urine (active metabolite), crosses placenta, half-life 3 hr

INTERACTIONS
Increase: leukopenia—ACE inhibitors, sulfamethoxazole-trimethoprim; monitor for increased leukopenia
Increase: myelosuppression—cycloSPORINE, antineoplastics; monitor for increased myelosuppression
Increase: action of azaTHIOprine—allopurinol; decrease dose of allopurinol, or avoid using
Decrease: immune response—vaccines, toxoids
Drug/herb
Decrease: product's effect—cat's-claw, echinacea; avoid concurrent use
Drug/Lab Test
Increase: LFTs
Decrease: uric acid
Interference: CBC, differential count

NURSING CONSIDERATIONS
Assess:
• **For infection:** increased temperature, WBC; sputum, urine, vital signs baseline and during treatment
• I&O, weight daily; report decreasing urine output; toxicity may occur

• **Bone marrow suppression:** severe leukopenia, pancytopenia, thrombocytopenia; HB, WBC, platelets during treatment monthly; if leukocytes are <3000/mm³ or platelets <100,000/mm³, product should be discontinued; CBC
• **Hepatotoxicity:** if dark urine, jaundice, itching, light-colored stools, increased LFTs, product should be discontinued; hepatic studies: alkaline phosphatase, AST, ALT, bilirubin
• **Arthritis:** pain; ROM; swelling; mobility before, during treatment
Evaluate:
• Therapeutic response: absence of graft rejection, immunosuppression in autoimmune disorders
Teach patient/family:
• To take as prescribed; not to miss doses; if dose is missed on daily regimen, to skip dose; if taking multiple doses/day, to take as soon as remembered
• That therapeutic response may take 3-4 mo with RA; to continue with prescribed exercise, rest, other medications
• To report fever, rash, severe diarrhea, chills, sore throat, fatigue because serious infections may occur; report unusual bleeding, bruising; signs/symptoms of renal/hepatic toxicity
• To avoid vaccinations, bring up to date before use
• To avoid crowds to reduce risk for infection
• That treatment is ongoing to prevent transplant rejection
• To avoid use with OTC, herbals, supplements unless approved by prescriber
• **RA:** Advise patient to continue with other prescribed treatment, other medications, physical therapy

azelaic acid (Rx)
(aze-eh-lay'ik)
Azelex, Finacea
Func. class.: Antiacne agent
Chem. class.: Dicarboxylic acid

USES: Mild to moderate inflammatory acne vulgaris, rosacea

CONTRAINDICATIONS
Hyper-sensitivity

DOSAGE AND ROUTES
Adult/child ≥12 yr: Apply a thin film and massage into affected areas bid AM and PM
Available forms: Cream 20%, gel 15%

---

azelastine (ophthalmic) (Rx)
(ah-zell'ah-steen)
Optivar
Func. class.: Antihistamine (ophthalmic)
Chem. class.: H$_1$ receptor antagonist

ACTION: Decreases the allergic response by inhibiting histamine release

USES: Pruritus from allergic conjunctivitis

CONTRAINDICATIONS
Hyper-sensitivity
Precautions: Pregnancy, breastfeeding, child <3 yr

DOSAGE AND ROUTES
• **Adult/child ≥3 yr: OPHTH** 1 drop into each affected eye bid
Available forms: Ophthalmic solution: 0.05%
Administer:
• Tip of dropper should not touch the eye
• Store upright and tightly closed at room temperature

SIDE EFFECTS
CNS: Headache
EENT: Eye burning/stinging/irritation, blurred vision, rhinitis, bitter taste
INTEG: Pruritus
RESP: Asthma, dyspnea, wheezing

PHARMACOKINETICS
Onset 3 min, duration 8 hr, half-life 22 hr, protein binding 88%

NURSING CONSIDERATIONS
Assess:
• Eyes: for itching, redness, use of soft or hard contact lenses
Evaluate:
• Therapeutic response: absence of redness, itching in the eyes
Teach patient/family:
• To use in the eyes only; not to touch dropper to eye/eyelid
• Not to wear contact lenses if eyes are red and itching
• To wait at least 10 min before inserting contact lenses; soft contact lenses can absorb preservative

---

azelastine nasal agent
See Appendix B

---

azilsartan (Rx)
(a-zill-sar'tain)
Edarbi
Func. class.: Antihypertensive-ARB

USES: Hypertension, alone or in combination with other antihypertensives

CONTRAINDICATIONS

Black Box Warning: Pregnancy

DOSAGE AND ROUTES
• **Adult: PO** 80 mg/day, may give an initial dose of 40 mg/day in patients receiving high-dose diuretic therapy
Available forms: Tablets 40, 80 mg

---

azithromycin (Rx)
(ay-zi-thro-my'sin)
AzaSite, Zithromax, Zmax
Func. class.: Antiinfective
Chem. class.: Macrolide

Do not confuse:
azithromycin/erythromycin
Zithromax/Zinacef

ACTION: Binds to 50S ribosomal subunits of susceptible bacteria and suppresses protein synthesis; much greater spectrum of activity than erythromycin; more effective against gram-negative organisms

USES: Mild to moderate infections of the upper respiratory tract, lower respiratory tract; uncomplicated skin and skin structure infections caused by *Bacillus anthracis, Bacteroides bivius, Bordetella pertussis, Borrelia burgdorferi, Campylobacter jejuni, CDC coryneform group G, Chlamydia trachomatis, Chlamydophila pneumoniae, Clostridium perfringens, Gardnerella vaginalis, Haemophilus ducreyi, influenzae* (beta-lactamase negative/positive), *Helicobacter pylori, Klebsiella granulomatis, Legionella pneumophila, Moraxella catarrhalis, Mycobacterium avium-intracellulare, Mycoplasma genitalium/hominis/pneumoniae, Neisseria gonorrhoeae, Peptostreptococcus* sp., *Prevotella bivia, Rickettsia tsutsugamushi, Salmonella typhi, Staphylococcus aureus (MSSA)/epidermidis, Streptococcus* sp., *Toxoplasma gondii, Treponema pallidum, Ureaplasma urealyticum, Vibrio cholerae, Viridans streptococci;* **PO:** acute pharyngitis/tonsillitis (group A streptococcal); acute skin/soft tissue infections; community-acquired pneumonia; **Ophthalmic:** bacterial conjunctivitis

Unlabeled uses: Babesiosis, cholera, COPD, cystic fibrosis, dental abscess/infection, granuloma inguinale, Lyme disease, lymphogranuloma venereum, MAC, periodontitis, pertussis, prostatitis, shigellosis, syphilis, typhoid fever

CONTRAINDICATIONS

Hypersensitivity to azithromycin, erythromycin, any macrolide, hepatitis, jaundice
Precautions: Pregnancy, breastfeeding; geriatric patients; renal/hepatic/cardiac disease; <6 mo for otitis media; <2 yr for

pharyngitis, tonsillitis, QT prolongation, ulcerative colitis, torsades de pointes, sunlight exposure, sodium restriction, myasthenia gravis, CDAD, contact lenses, hypokalemia, hypomagnesemia

DOSAGE AND ROUTES
Most infections
• **Adult: PO** 500 mg on day 1, then 250 mg/day on days 2-5 for a total dose of 1.5 g or 500 mg a day × 3 days
• **Child 2-15 yr: PO** 10 mg/kg on day 1, then 5 mg/kg × 4 days
MAC in HIV:
Adult: PO 500-600 mg daily
Cervicitis, chlamydia, chancroid, nongonococcal urethritis, syphilis
• **Adult: PO** 1 g single dose
Gonorrhea
• **Adult: PO** 1 g single dose with ceftriaxine 250 mg IM
Lower respiratory tract infections
• **Adult: PO** 500 mg day 1, then 250 mg × 4 days
• **Child: PO** 5-12 mg/kg/day × 5 days
Bacterial conjunctivitis
• **Adult/child ≥1 yr: Ophthalmic** Instill 1 drop in affected eye bid × 2 days, then 1 drop in eye daily × 5 days
Lyme disease (unlabeled)
• **Adult: PO** 500 mg/day × 7 days
Traveler's diarrhea
• **Adult: PO** 1000 mg as a single dose
Pertussis (unlabeled)
• **Adult: PO** 500 mg on day 1, then 250 mg/day for 2-5 days
• **Infant ≥6 mo and child: PO** 10 mg/kg/day (max 500 mg) on day 1, then 5 mg/kg/day (max 250 mg) on days 2-5
• **Infant <6 mo: PO** 10 mg/kg/day × 5 days
Cystic fibrosis (unlabeled)
Adult: PO 500 mg (≥40 kg); 250 mg (<40 kg) 3×/wk or 250 mg daily
COPD (unlabeled)
Adult: PO 250-500 mg 3×/wk or 250 mg daily

Available forms: Tablets 250, 500, 600 mg; powder for injection 500 mg; suspension 100, 200 mg/5 mL, 1 g single-dose powder for suspension; extended-release powder for suspension 2 (ZMAX); ophthalmic drops 1% solution

Administer:

Ophthalmic route

• Store in refrigerator
• Do not touch dropper to eye

PO route

• **Suspension** 1 hr before meal or 2 hr after meal; reconstitute 1 g packet for suspension with 60 mL water, mix, rinse glass with more water and have patient drink to consume all medication; packets not for pediatric use
• Store at room temperature

Intermittent IV INFUSION route

• **Reconstitute** 500 mg of product with 4.8 mL sterile water for injection (100 mg/mL); shake, **dilute** with 250 or 500 mL 0.9% NaCl, 0.45% NaCl, or LR to 1-2 mg/mL; diluted solution stable for 24 hr or 7 days if refrigerated
• **Give** 1 mg/mL solution over 3 hr or 2 mg/mL solution over 1 hr; never give IM or as bolus
• Reconstituted product is stable for 24 hr at room temperature or 7 days refrigerated

Y-site compatibilities: Acyclovir, alatrofloxacin, alemtuzumab, alfentanil, aminocaproic acid, aminophylline, amphotericin B liposome/lipid complex, ampicillin, ampicillin-sulbactam, anidulafungin, atenolol, bivalirudin, bleomycin, bumetanide, buprenorphine, butorphanol, calcium chloride/gluconate, CARBOplatin, carmustine, ceFAZolin, cefepime, cefoTEtan, cefOXitin, ceftaroline, cefTAZidime, ceftizoxime, cimetidine, cisatracurium, CISplatin, cyclophosphamide, cycloSPORINE, cytarabine, DAPTOmycin, DAUNOrubicin liposome, dexamethasone, dexmedetomidine, dexrazoxane, digoxin, diltiaZEM, diphenhydrAMINE, DOBUTamine, DOCEtaxel, dolasetron, doripenem, doxacurium, DOXOrubicin liposomal, doxycycline, droperidol, enalaprilat, EPINEPHrine, epiRUBicin, eptifibatide, ertapenem, esmolol, etoposide, etoposide phosphate, fenoldopam, fluconazole, fluorouracil, foscarnet, fosphenytoin, gallium, ganciclovir, gatifloxacin, gemcitabine, granisetron, haloperidol, heparin, hydrocortisone phosphate/

succinate, HYDROmorphone, hydrOXYzine, IDArubicin, ifosfamide, inamrinone, irinotecan, isoproterenol, labetalol, lepirudin, magnesium sulfate, mannitol, meperidine, meropenem, mesna, mechlorethamine, methohexital, methotrexate, methylPREDNISolone, metoclopramide, metroNIDAZOLE, milrinone, minocycline, mivacurium, nalbuphine, naloxone, nesiritide, nitroglycerin, nitroprusside, octreotide, ofloxacin, ondansetron, oxaliplatin, oxytocin, PACLitaxel, palonosetron, pamidronate, pantoprazole, PEMEtrexed, PENTobarbital, phenylephrine, piperacillin, potassium acetate/phosphates, procainamide, prochlorperazine, promethazine, propranolol, raNITidine, remifentanil, rocuronium, sodium acetate, succinylcholine, SUFentanil, sulfamethoxazole-trimethoprim, tacrolimus, telavancin, teniposide, thiotepa, ticarcillin, tigecycline, tirofiban, TPN, trimethobenzamide, vancomycin, vasopressin, vecuronium, verapamil, vinCRIStine, voriconazole, zidovudine, zoledronic acid

SIDE EFFECTS

CNS: Dizziness, headache, seizures, fatigue
CV: Palpitations, chest pain, QT prolongation, torsades de pointes (rare)
EENT: Hearing loss, tinnitus
GI: *Nausea, diarrhea,* hepatotoxicity, abdominal pain, stomatitis, heartburn, dyspepsia, flatulence, melena, cholestatic jaundice, CDAD
GU: Vaginitis, nephritis
HEMA: Anemia, leukopenia, thrombocytopenia
INTEG: Rash, urticaria, pruritus, photosensitivity, pain at injection site
SYST: Angioedema, Stevens-Johnson syndrome, toxic epidermal necrolysis

PHARMACOKINETICS

PO: Peak 2-4 hr, duration 24 hr
IV: Peak end of infusion; duration 24 hr; half-life 11-57 hr; excreted in bile, feces, urine primarily as unchanged product; may be inhibitor of P-glycoprotein

INTERACTIONS

Increase: ergot toxicity—ergotamine

Side effects: *italics* = common; red = life-threatening

Increase: dysrhythmias—pimozide; fatal reaction, do not use concurrently

Increase: QT prolongation—amiodarone, quiNIDine, nilotinib, droperidol, methadone, propafenone, fluoroquinolones, lithium, paliperidone

Increase: effects of oral anticoagulants, digoxin, theophylline, methylPREDNISolone, cycloSPORINE, bromocriptine, disopyramide, triazolam, carBAMazepine, phenytoin, tacrolimus, nelfinavir

Decrease: clearance of triazolam

Decrease: absorption of azithromycin—aluminum, magnesium antacids, separate by ≥2 hr

Drug/Lab Test

Increase: CPK, ALT, AST, bilirubin, BUN, creatinine, alkaline phosphatase, potassium, blood glucose

Drug/Food

Decrease: absorption—food (suspension)

Decrease: blood glucose, potassium, sodium

NURSING CONSIDERATIONS

Assess:

• I&O ratio; report hematuria, oliguria with renal disease

• Hepatic studies: AST, ALT, CBC with differential

• Renal studies: urinalysis, protein, blood

• C&S before product therapy; product may be taken as soon as culture is taken; C&S may be repeated after treatment

• **QT prolongation, torsades de pointes:** assess for patients with serious bradycardia, ongoing proarrhythmic conditions, or elderly; more common in these patients

• **Serious skin reactions:** Stevens-Johnson syndrome, toxic epidermal necrolysis, angioedema; discontinue if rash develops, treat symptomatically

• **Superinfection:** sore throat, mouth, tongue; fever, fatigue, diarrhea, anogenital pruritus

• **CDAD:** diarrhea, abdominal pain, fever, fatigue, anorexia; obtain CBC, serum albumin

• Bowel pattern before, during treatment

• Respiratory status: rate, character; wheezing, tightness in chest: discontinue product

• Cardiovascular death has occurred in those with serious bradycardia or ongoing hypokalemia, hypomagnesemia; avoid use

• **Pregnancy/breastfeeding:** use only if clearly needed; cautious use in breastfeeding, excreted in breast milk

Evaluate:

• Therapeutic response: C&S negative for infection; decreased signs of infection

Teach patient/family:

• To report sore throat, fever, fatigue, severe diarrhea, anal/genital itching (may indicate superinfection)

• Not to take aluminum-magnesium–containing antacids simultaneously with this product (PO)

• To notify nurse of diarrhea, dark urine, pale stools; yellow discoloration of eyes, skin; severe abdominal pain

• To complete dosage regimen

• To take ZMAX 1 hr before or 2 hr after a meal; shake well before use

• To use protective clothing or stay out of the sun, photosensitivity may occur

TREATMENT OF HYPERSENSITIVITY: Withdraw product, maintain airway; administer EPINEPHrine, aminophylline, O_2, IV corticosteroids

azithromycin ophthalmic
See Appendix B

aztreonam (Rx)
(az-tree′oh-nam)

Azactam, Cayston

Func. class.: Antibiotic—miscellaneous

Chem. class.: Monobactam

ACTION: Bactericidal, inhibits cell wall synthesis

USES: UTI; septicemia; skin, muscle, bone infection; lower respiratory tract, intraabdominal infections; other infections caused by gram-negative organisms

CONTRAINDICATIONS
Hypersensitivity to product, severe renal disease

DOSAGE AND ROUTES
Urinary tract infections
• **Adult: IM/IV** 500 mg-1 g q8-12hr
Systemic infections
• **Adult: IM/IV** 1-2 g q8-12hr
• **Child: IM/IV** 90-120 mg/kg/day in divided doses q6-8hr; max 8 g/day **IV**
Severe systemic infections
• **Adult: IM/IV** 2 g q6-8hr; max 8 g/day; continue treatment for 48 hr after negative culture or until patient is asymptomatic
Cystic fibrosis with *Pseudomonas aeruginosa*
• **Adult, adolescent, child ≥7 yr: NEB** 75 mg tid × 28 days, then 28 days off; give q4hr or more; give bronchodilator before aztreonam
Available forms:
Inhalation 75-mg ampule (Cayston); injection 500 mg, 1-g, 2-g vials; injection premixed 1 g/50 mL, 2 g/50 mL
Administer:
IV Route
• Visually inspect parenteral products for particulate matter and discoloration prior to administration whenever solution and container permit
• For IV push, reconstitute each vial with 6 to 10 mL of sterile water for injection
• For intermittent IV infusion, reconstitute with at least 3 mL of sterile water for injection per g of aztreonam. FURTHER DILUTION IS NECESSARY FOR IV INFUSION
• Shake immediately and vigorously
• Storage: Use within 48 hr if kept at room temperature 59° F-98° F (15° C-30°

C) or within 7 days if kept under refrigeration 38° F-48° F (2° C-8° C)
Intermittent IV Infusion
• Further dilute the appropriate dose in a compatible IV solution
• If using a volume control administration set, the final dilution of aztreonam max 20 mg/mL
• Shake immediately and vigorously
Premixed Galaxy IV Solution
• Thaw frozen containers at room temperature 77° F (25° C) or under refrigeration 36° F-46° F (2° C-8° C).
• Contents of the solution may precipitate in the frozen state and should dissolve with little or no agitation once the solution has reached room temperature
• Storage: The thawed solution is stable for 48 hr at room temperature or 14 days under refrigeration
Intermittent IV Injection Route
• Slowly inject directly into a vein or the tubing of a suitable administration set over 3 to 5 min
Intermittent IV Infusion Route
• Infuse appropriate dose IV over 20 to 60 min
• For neonates, an infusion time of 15 min has been recommended
• For premixed bags, do not use plastic containers in series connections, as this could result in an embolism
IM Route
• Reconstitute vials with at least 3 mL of an appropriate diluent per g of aztreonam
• Shake immediately and vigorously
• In adults, inject doses of 1 g or less deeply into a large muscle upper outer quadrant of the gluteus maximus or lateral part of the thigh
• Do not admix with any local anesthetic agent
Inhalation Route
• Do not reconstitute aztreonam for inhalation until ready to use
• Twist the tip off of the provided 1 mL sterile diluent (0.17% sodium chloride) ampule and squeeze contents into the aztreonam vial

• Gently swirl until the contents have completely dissolved

• Have patient use a bronchodilator before nebulized solution. A short-acting bronchodilator can be administered 15 min to 4 hr before aztreonam. A long-acting bronchodilator can be administered 30 min to 12 hr before aztreonam.

• Administer aztreonam immediately after reconstitution using an Altera Nebulizer System only. Do not administer via any other nebulizer

• Do not mix with any other drugs

• Administration typically takes 2-3 min via the nebulizer mouthpiece

SIDE EFFECTS

CV: Hypotension, chest pain, thrombophlebitis

CNS: Confusion, headache, insomnia, fever, seizures

EENT: Nasal congestion, sore throat

GI: Pseudomembranous colitis, diarrhea, abdominal pain, nausea, vomiting

RESP: Cough dyspnea, bronchospasm

HEMA: Anemia, thrombocytopenia, neutropenia, pancytopenia

INTEG: Rash, injection site reactions, allergic reactions

PHARMACOKINETICS

IV: onset unknown, peak immediate, duration unknown; **IM:** onset unknown, peak <1 hr, duration unknown; inhalation: onset unknown, 1 hr, duration unknown; half-life 1½-2 hr

INTERACTIONS

Increase: Synergism: aminoglycosides, monitor renal studies

Increase: Antagonism: cefoxitin, imipenem, avoid concurrent use

NURSING CONSIDERATIONS

Assess:

• Monitor LFTs and renal function studies

• Monitor for overgrowth of infection and superinfection

• Monitor for allergic reactions, also those allergic to penicillin and cephalosporins

• May use with other antiinfectives for coverage of gram-positive and anaerobic infections

• Monitor for CDAD that can occur up to 2 mo after using

Teach patient/family:

• That IM injection is painful

• To report continuing signs/symptoms of infection

• To use bronchodilator, then inhalation product

• To report if pregnancy is planned or suspected or if breastfeeding

Evaluate:

• Therapeutic response: Decreased signs/symptoms of UTI or cystic fibrosis

---

bacitracin topical
See Appendix B

---

baclofen (Rx)
(bak'loe-fen)
Gablofen, Lioresal Intrathecal,
Lyvispah
Func. class.: Skeletal muscle
relaxant, central acting
Chem. class.: GABA chlorophenyl
derivative

Do not confuse:
baclofen/Bactroban/bacitracin

ACTION: Inhibits synaptic responses
in CNS by stimulating GABAb receptor
subtype, which decreases neurotransmitter function; decreases frequency, severity of muscle spasms

USES: Spasticity with spinal cord
injury, multiple sclerosis
Unlabeled uses: Neuropathic pain, trigeminal neuralgia

CONTRAINDICATIONS
Hypersensitivity, epidural, IM, IV, SUB-
CUT administration
Precautions: Pregnancy, breastfeeding,
geriatric patients, peptic ulcer disease,
renal/hepatic disease, stroke, seizure disorder, diabetes mellitus, psychosis,
abrupt discontinuation (intrathecal), CNS
depressants, especially opiates

DOSAGE AND ROUTES
**Spasticity in multiple sclerosis/
spinal cord injury**
• **Adult/child ≥12 yr: PO** 5 mg tid × 3
days, then 10 mg tid × 3 days, then 15
mg tid × 3 days, then 20 mg tid × 3 days,
then titrated to response, max 80 mg/day
(20 mg qid); **INTRATHECAL** use
implantable intrathecal infusion pump;
use screening trial of 3 separate bolus
doses if needed 24 hr apart (50 mcg,
75 mcg, 100 mcg)
• **Child 8-11 yr:** As above; max 60 mg/day

• **Child >2-7 yr: PO** 10-15 mg/day
divided q8hr; titrate q3days by 5-15 mg/
day to max 40 mg/day
• **Child: INTRATHECAL** initial test dose
same as adult; for small children, initial
dose of 25 mcg/dose may be used;
25-1200 mcg/day infusion titrated to
response in screening phase
**Neuropathic pain including
trigeminal neuralgia (unlabeled)**
• **Adult: PO** 10 mg tid, may increase by
10 mg every other day; max 80 mg/day
Renal dose
• **Adult:** PO/IT CCr 50-80 mL/min: reduce
dose by 33%; CCr 30-50 mL/min: reduce
dose by 50%
Available forms: Tablets 5, 10, 20 mg;
IT injection 50 mcg/mL, 500 mcg/mL,
1000 mcg/mL, 2000 mcg/mL; oral granules 5-, 10-, 20-mg packets; oral solution
5 mg/5 mL (1 mg/mL)
Administer:
PO route
• With meals for GI symptoms
• When discontinuing taper over 2 wk
• Store in a tight container at room temperature
IT route
For screening, dilute to 50 mcg/mL with
NaCl for injection (preservative free); give
test dose over 1 min; watch for decreasing
muscle tone, frequency of spasm; if inadequate, use 2 more test doses q24hr, those
with inadequate response should not
receive chronic IT therapy; **maintenance
infusion** via implantable pump of 500-
2000 mcg/mL because individual titration
is required, may cause tolerance and need
to taper over 2-4 wk and then restart
• Do not give IT dose by injection, IV,
IM, SUBCUT, epidural

Black Box Warning: Do not discontinue
IT abruptly; may be fatal

SIDE EFFECTS
CNS: *Dizziness, weakness, fatigue, drowsiness,* headache, *disorientation,* insomnia,
paresthesias, tremors; seizures (IT)
CV: Hypotension, bradycardia, flushing,
edema

Side effects: *italics* = common; red = life-threatening

EENT: Nasal congestion, blurred vision, tinnitus
GI: *Nausea,* constipation, dry mouth, anorexia, weight gain
GU: Urinary frequency, hematuria
INTEG: Rash, pruritus
RESP: Dyspnea
MISC: Hypersensitivity, sweating, hyperglycemia

PHARMACOKINETICS

IT: Peak 4 hr, duration 4-8 hr, half-life 2½-4 hr, PO; 1.5-4 hr IT partially metabolized in liver, excreted in urine (unchanged), protein binding 30%; CSF levels with plasma levels 100× that of the oral route

INTERACTIONS

Increase: CNS depression—alcohol, tricyclics, opiates, barbiturates, sedatives, hypnotics, MAOIs, antihistamines; increases CNS depression; avoid concurrent use

> **Black Box Warning:** Increased respiratory depression, death—opiates; avoid concurrent use; limit quantity provided

Increase: hypotension—antihypertensives
Drug/Herb
Increase: CNS depression—kava, valerian, chamomile
Drug/Lab Test
Increase: AST, ALT, alkaline phosphatase, blood glucose, CK

NURSING CONSIDERATIONS
Assess:

• **MS:** Assess for spasms, spasticity, improvement should occur

> • **Black Box Warning: Abrupt discontinuation;** serious adverse reactions may occur (intrathecal), may cause spasticity/rigidity, fever, change in mental status, death

> • **Black Box Warning: Intrathecal:** Have emergency equipment nearby; assess test dose and titration; if no response, check pump, catheter for proper functioning, when switching to IT, avoid overdose by discontinuing other PO antispasmodic by tapering

• B/P, weight, blood glucose, hepatic function periodically

• **Seizures (IT):** for increased seizure activity with seizure disorders; product decreases seizure threshold; EEG in epileptic patients
• **Withdrawal symptoms:** agitation, tachycardia, insomnia, hyperpyrexia
• **Allergic reactions:** rash, fever, respiratory distress
• Severe weakness, numbness in extremities
• **CNS depression:** dizziness, drowsiness
Evaluate:
• Therapeutic response: decreased pain, spasticity, ability to perform ADLs
Teach patient/family:

> • **Black Box Warning: IT:** Not to discontinue medication quickly; hallucinations, spasticity, tachycardia will occur; product should be tapered off over 1-2 wk, especially intrathecal form; teach proper care of IT site

> • **Black Box Warning:** Not to take with alcohol, other CNS depressants, opioids

• To avoid hazardous activities if drowsiness, dizziness occurs; to rise slowly to prevent orthostatic hypotension; if taken with opioids and suppressed breathing, dizziness occurs, request emergency services
• To avoid using OTC medications; not to take cough preparations, antihistamines unless directed by prescriber; to take PO with food or milk
• To take as prescribed, not to skip or double doses, take missed dose within 1 hr, if doses are missed withdrawal symptoms may occur
• **Hypersensitivity:** advise patient to report itching, hives, rash
• **Orthostatic hypotension:** advise patient to change positions slowly
• To notify prescriber if nausea, headache, tinnitus, insomnia, confusion, constipation, inadequate or painful urination continues
• **MS:** may require 1-2 mo for full response
• **Pregnancy/breastfeeding:** to notify prescriber if pregnancy is planned or suspected; avoid breastfeeding, pregnancy; may cause neonatal withdrawal symptoms in the infant (seizures, tremors) shortly after birth

TREATMENT OF OVERDOSE:
Induce emesis in conscious patient, dialysis, physostigmine to reduce life-threatening CNS side effects

---

baloxavir marboxil (Rx)
(ba-lox′a′veer mar-box′el)
Xofluza
Func. class.: Antiviral—influenza
Chem. class.: Endonuclease inhibitor

ACTION: Baloxavir, the active metabolite of baloxavir marboxil, is responsible for the drug's antiviral activity; inhibits the activity of polymerase acidic (PA) protein, an influenza virus–specific enzyme

USES: Treatment of acute uncomplicated influenza A virus or influenza B virus infection

CONTRAINDICATIONS
Hypersensitivity
Precautions: Bacterial infections, child <12 yr

DOSAGE AND ROUTES
• **Adult/adolescent/child >5 yr ≥80 kg:**
PO 80 mg single dose; **20-79 kg:** 40 mg single dose
Available forms: Tablets 20 mg, 40 mg
Administer:
• Begin treatment within 48 hr of symptom onset
• Administer with or without food
• Avoid with dairy products, calcium-fortified beverages, laxatives, antacids, or oral supplements (calcium, iron, magnesium, selenium, zincs), other calcium-containing agents

SIDE EFFECTS
CNS: Headache
GI: Diarrhea, nausea, vomiting
RESP: Bronchitis, nasopharyngitis

PHARMACOKINETICS
Protein binding >92%, metabolized by metabolic pathway by UGT1A3, CYP3A4, excretion urine 14.7%, feces 80%, onset unknown, peak 4 hr, duration unknown, half-life 79 hr

INTERACTIONS
• Avoid use with laxatives, antacids, oral supplements (calcium, iron, magnesium, selenium, zinc), dairy products, may decrease baloxavir level
• Avoid use with live attenuated influenza vaccines

NURSING CONSIDERATIONS
Assess:
• **Flulike symptoms:** duration, onset, specific symptoms (fever, cough, muscle aches and pains)
• **Pregnancy/breastfeeding:** no adverse effects in animals regarding pregnancy and breastfeeding; influenza may pose health hazard to mother and fetus

Evaluate:
• **Therapeutic response:** relief of symptoms of influenza A or B

Teach patient/family:
• **Pregnancy/lactation:** to notify health care provider if pregnancy is planned or suspected, or if breastfeeding
• To take within 48 hr of flu symptoms
• To avoid use with laxatives, antacids, oral supplements (calcium, iron, magnesium, selenium, zinc), dairy products
• To avoid use with live attenuated influenza vaccines

---

baricitinib (Rx)
(bar i sye′ti nib)
Olumiant
Func. class.: Antirheumatic, antiinflammatory
Chem. class.: JAK inhibitor

ACTION: An oral Janus kinase (JAK) inhibitor. Janus kinases are enzymes that transmit signals arising from cytokine or growth factor receptor interactions

USES: Treatment of moderately to severely active rheumatoid arthritis in patients who have had an inadequate response to 1 or more tumor necrosis factor (TNF) antagonists

CONTRAINDICATIONS
Hypersensitivity

Side effects: *italics* = common; red = life-threatening

Precautions: Vaccinations, lipid elevations, anemia, lymphopenia, neutropenia, GI perforation, viral reactivation, TB

Black Box Warning: Hepatitis exacerbation, hepatotoxicity, lactic acidosis, HIV

DOSAGE AND ROUTES
• **Adult: PO** 2 mg daily; may give with or without methotrexate or other nonbiologic disease-modifying antirheumatic drugs (DMARDs)
Available forms: Tablets 2 mg
Administer:
• Without regard to food

SIDE EFFECTS
EENT: Rhinitis, sinusitis
GI: Nausea, GI perforation, hepatotoxicity
INTEG: Skin cancer
RESP: Pulmonary embolism
SYST: Infection, new primary malignancy

PHARMACOKINETICS
Protein binding 45%-50%, metabolized by CYP3A4, excreted 75% urine, 20% feces, half-life 24 hr

INTERACTIONS
Increase: effect of product—strong OAT3 inhibitors (probenecid)

NURSING CONSIDERATIONS
Assess:
• For pain, swelling in joints, ADLs, aggravating factors
• CBC with differential, hemoglobin/hematocrit, LFTs, serum cholesterol profile, serum creatinine/BUN, tuberculin skin test baseline and periodically
• For new primary malignancies, skin cancer screening exam
• **Pregnancy/breastfeeding:** do not use in pregnancy, breastfeeding
Evaluate:
• Therapeutic response: decreased pain, swelling of joints; slowing of destruction of joints; increased physical function
Teach patient/family:
• About the potential benefits and risk of this product

• **Infections:** that infections are more common; to report any symptoms of infection to health care provider
• **New malignancies:** that product may increase the risk of new cancers, including lymphoma; to notify health care provider
• **Thrombosis:** that DVT and PE may occur; to report any symptoms to health care provider
• That lab work will be needed on a continuing basis
• **Pregnancy/breastfeeding:** not to breastfeed during therapy

---

basiliximab (Rx)
(bas-ih-liks′ih-mab)
Simulect
Func. class.: Immunosuppressant

USES: Acute allograft rejection in renal transplant patients when used with cycloSPORINE and corticosteroids

CONTRAINDICATIONS
Mannitol, murine protein hypersensitivity, pregnancy, breastfeeding
Precautions: Children, geriatric patients, human antimurine antibody, infections, neoplastic disease, vaccination

Black Box Warning: Requires a specialized care setting and experienced clinician

DOSAGE AND ROUTES
Acute kidney transplant rejection prophylaxis
• **Adults, adolescents, and children ≥35 kg: IV** 20 mg within 2 hr before transplantation, then 20 mg IV 4 days after surgery
• **Children and adolescents <35 kg: IV** 10 mg within 2 hr before transplantation, then 10 mg IV 4 days after transplantation

For acute liver transplant rejection prophylaxis (unlabeled)

• **Adults: IV** 20 mg within 2 hr of graft reperfusion, then 20 mg IV 4 days after transplantation
Available forms: injection 10, 20 mg vials

beclomethasone, inhalation (Rx)
(be-kloe-meth′a-sone)
QVAR RediHaler
beclamethasone nasal (Rx)
Beconase AQ, Beclovent ♣, Vanceril ♣
Func. class.: Antiasthmatic
Chem. class.: Corticosteroid

Do not confuse:
beclomethasone/betamethasone

ACTION: Prevents inflammation by suppression of the migration of polymorphonuclear leukocytes, fibroblasts, and the reversal of increased capillary permeability and lysosomal stabilization; does not suppress hypothalamus and pituitary function

USES: Chronic asthma, allergic/vasomotor rhinitis, nasal polyps

CONTRAINDICATIONS
Hypersensitivity, status asthmaticus (primary treatment)
Precautions: Pregnancy, breastfeeding, children <12 yr, nasal disease/surgery, nonasthmatic bronchial disease; bacterial, fungal, viral infections of mouth, throat, lungs; HPA suppression, osteoporosis, Cushing's syndrome, diabetes mellitus, measles, cataracts, corticosteroid hypersensitivity, glaucoma, herpes infection

DOSAGE AND ROUTES
Chronic asthma
• **Adult and child ≥12 yr: INH** 40-80 mcg bid (alone) or 40-160 mcg bid (previous inhaled corticosteroids); max

320 mcg bid; **Nasal:** 1-2 sprays in each nostril bid
• **Child 4-11 yr: INH** 40 mcg bid; max 80 mcg bid; **Nasal** 1-2 sprays in each nostril bid

Seasonal, perennial rhinitis; nasal polyp recurrence
• **Adult/child ≥12 yr: Nasal** 1-2 sprays in each nostril bid
• **Child 6-11 yr: Nasal** 1 spray in each nostril bid, may increase to 2 sprays bid as needed, decrease to 1 spray each nostril bid after symptoms are controlled
Available forms: Oral inhalation 40, 80/actuation; nasal suspension 42 mcg/spray
Administer:
• **Oral inhalation:** No shaking, spacer, or priming needed
• **Nasal:** Shake, invert, tilt head backward, insert nozzle into nostril, compress activator, inhale through nose, exhale through mouth

SIDE EFFECTS
CNS: *Headache,* psychiatric/behavioral changes (child)
EENT: *Hoarseness, candidal infection of oral cavity, sore throat,* loss of taste/smell, dysgeusia, pharyngitis, rhinitis, sinusitis, cataracts, fungal infections, epistaxis
ENDO: HPA suppression
GI: Dry mouth, dyspepsia
MISC: Angioedema, adrenal insufficiency, facial edema, Churg-Strauss syndrome (rare)
RESP: Bronchospasm, wheezing, cough
Nasal
CNS: Headache, dizziness
EENT: Nasal burning/irritation, sneezing
GI: Dry mouth, esophageal candidiasis
RESP: Cough

PHARMACOKINETICS
INH: Onset 1-4 wk, peak ½ hr; duration unknown; excreted in feces, urine (metabolites); half-life 2.8 hr; crosses placenta; metabolized in lungs, liver (by CYP3A)

Side effects: *italics* = common; red = life-threatening

NURSING CONSIDERATIONS
Assess:

- **Bronchospasm:** use short-acting bronchodilator
- **Fungal infections:** assess mucous membranes often for infection
- Adrenal function periodically for HPA axis suppression during prolonged therapy; monitor growth/development, taper corticosteroids
- **Vision changes:** monitor for vision changes, cataracts may occur
- Decreased bone density; monitor with bone density test
- **Bronchospasm:** discontinue immediately and treat with short-acting bronchodilator
- Provide gum, rinsing of mouth for dry mouth
- **Beers:** avoid in older adults; high risk of delirium

Evaluate:

- Therapeutic response: decreased dyspnea, wheezing, dry crackles; nasal polyps are reduced

Teach patient/family:

- To take as prescribed, not to double or skip doses, not to use for acute asthma
- To gargle/rinse mouth after each use to prevent oral fungal infections
- To notify prescriber if therapeutic response decreases; dosage adjustment may be needed
- Proper administration technique and cleaning technique, no need to prime
- About all aspects of product usage, including cushingoid symptoms
- About **adrenal insufficiency symptoms:** nausea, anorexia, fatigue, dizziness, dyspnea, weakness, joint pain, depression
- To check growth in child on long-term therapy
- To taper PO products before starting inhalation products
- That peak response may take up to 1 mo
- To carry medical alert ID with corticosteroid user listed
- Not be used to treat acute bronchospasm

- **Allergic reaction:** To inform health care professional of rash; itching; swelling of face, lips; trouble breathing
- **Pregnancy/breastfeeding:** To notify prescriber if pregnancy is planned or suspected; may breastfeed

bedaquiline (Rx)
(bed-ak′-wi-leen)

Sirturo

Func. class.: Antiinfective/antituberculotic

USES: For use as part of a combination regimen to treat pulmonary multidrug-resistant tuberculosis infection (MDR-TB) in adults/children when other effective treatment regimens are not available

CONTRAINDICATIONS
Hypersensitivity

Precautions: Alcoholism, bradycardia, breastfeeding, arrhythmias, cardiac disease, children, coronary artery disease, diabetes mellitus, females, geriatric patients, heart failure, hepatic disease, hypertension, hypocalcemia, hypokalemia, hypomagnesemia, malnutrition, MI, pregnancy, syncope, thyroid disease

Black Box Warning: QT prolongation, increased mortality risk

DOSAGE AND ROUTES
- **Adults/child ≥5 yr and ≥30 kg: PO** 400 mg daily × 2 wk, then reduce dose to 200 mg 3×/wk with food (≥48 hr between doses). Total duration is 24 wk
- **Child ≥5 yr and 15-29 kg: PO** 200 mg daily for 2 wk, then 100 mg 3 times a week spaced 48 hr apart for 22 wk, total duration 24 wk

Available forms: Tablets 20, 100 mg

belantamab mafodotin-blmf (Rx)

(bel-an'ta-mab ma-foe-doe'tin)

Blenrep

Func. class.: Antineoplastic agent
Chem. class.: Anti-BCMA

ACTION: A humanized antibody targeted against B-cell maturation antigen (BCMA) that is expressed on multiple myeloma cells

USES: Treatment of relapsed/refractory multiple myeloma in those who have received ≥4 prior therapies

CONTRAINDICATIONS

Hypersensitivity

Black Box Warning: Ocular toxicity, restricted access

Precautions: Bleeding, breastfeeding, driving/operating machinery, geriatric, pregnancy, infusion-related reactions, requires a specialized care setting, requires an experienced clinician, thrombocytopenia, visual impairment

DOSAGE AND ROUTES
Multiple myeloma
Adult IV: 2.5 mg/kg q3wk until disease progression/unacceptable toxicity
Available forms: IV solution preservative-free 100-mg/vial
Administer:
• Allow to warm to room temperature for 10 min
• Reconstitute 100 mg/2 mL SWFI (50 mg/mL); gently swirl
• Solution should be clear to opalescent, colorless-yellow-brown liquid; discard if particulates are observed
• Withdraw needed amount and dilute in a 250-mL NS infusion bag (0.2-2 mg/mL), use only infusion bag of PVC or polyolefin
• Mix by gentle inversion; do not shake
• Solutions diluted for infusion should be clear and colorless; discard if particulate matter is observed

• Do not admix
• Give over ≥30 min using PVC or polyolefin infusion set, may use a polyethersulfone-based filter (0.2 micron)
• Do not give with other medications
• If refrigerated, allow to warm to room temperature prior to use; use within 6 hr including time to warm and infusion time
• Assess for infusion-related reactions
• Store vials refrigerated; reconstituted solution may be stored refrigerated or room temperature for ≤4 hr; discard if not diluted within 4 hr; solutions diluted for infusion may be stored refrigerated ≤24 hr

SIDE EFFECTS
CNS: Fatigue, fever, asthenia
GI: Constipation, anorexia, diarrhea, nausea, vomiting, increased LFTs
GU: Increased serum creatinine, renal insufficiency, albuminuria
META: Decreased serum albumin, hypokalemia, hyponatremia, increased gamma-glutamyl transferase, hyperglycemia, hypercalcemia
HEMA: Decreased hgb, decreased neutrophils, lymphocytopenia, thrombocytopenia
MS: Arthralgia, back pain, increased CPK
EENT: Blurred vision, decreased visual acuity, dry eye syndrome, epithelial keratopathy, eye irritation, photophobia
RESP: URI, pneumonia
MISC: Infusion-related reaction, sepsis

PHARMACOKINETICS
Onset of response 1.4 mo, peak end of infusion, duration of response ≥6 mo, half-life 14 days

INTERACTIONS
Increased: myelosuppression—BCG (intravesical), chloramphenicol (ophthalmic), cladribine, clozapine, deferiprone, promazine, salicylates

NURSING CONSIDERATIONS
Assess:
• Monitor CBC at baseline and as needed
• Obtain hepatitis B virus screening with hepatitis B surface antigen (HBsAg), hepatitis B core antibody (anti-HBc), total Ig or

IgG, and antibody to hepatitis B surface antigen (anti-HBs) prior to use, may start treatment before results are received
• Monitor for bleeding, infusion site reactions

Black Box Warning: REMS: Ocular toxicity: is available only through a restricted program under a Risk Evaluation and Mitigation Strategy (REMS) called the BLENREP REMS; obtain ophthalmic exams (visual acuity/slit lamp) baseline within 3 wk of first dose, prior to each dose, and for worsening ocular symptoms

• **Pregnancy/breastfeeding:**   Obtain pregnancy testing prior to use in females of reproductive potential; contraception is needed during and for 4 mo after the last dose; males with female partners of reproductive potential should use contraception during and for 6 mo after the last dose
Evaluate:
• Therapeutic response: Decreasing spread of multiple myeloma
Teach patient/family:
• To use preservative-free lubricant eye drops and avoid contact lenses, that ophthalmic testing will be needed during treatment
• Identify if pregnancy is planned or suspected, or if breastfeeding; discuss contraception

---

belatacept (Rx) REMS
(bel-a-ta'sept)
Nulojix
Func. class.: Immunosuppressant
Chem. class.: Fusion protein

ACTION: Activated T-lymphocytes are the mediators of immunologic rejection. This product is a selective T-cell costimulation blocker; blocks the CD28 mediated costimulation of T lymphocytes by binding to CD80 and CD86 on antigen-presenting cells; inhibits T-lymphocyte proliferation and the production of the cytokines

USES: Kidney transplant rejection prophylaxis given with basiliximab induction, mycophenolate mofetil, corticosteroids

CONTRAINDICATIONS
Hypersensitivity, Epstein-Barr virus (EBV) seronegative, EBV status unknown
Precautions: Breastfeeding, child/infant/neonate, pregnancy, diabetes mellitus, progressive multifocal leukoencephalopathy, immunosuppression, sunlight exposure, TB

Black Box Warning: Infection, organ transplant, requires an experienced clinician and specialized care setting, secondary malignancy, posttransplant lymphoproliferation disorder (PLD), immunosuppression

DOSAGE AND ROUTES
• **Adult: IV** 10 mg/kg give over 30 min the day of transplantation (day 1) but before transplantation, on day 5 96 hr after the day 1 dose, at the end of wk 2, at the end of wk 4, at the end of wk 8, and at the end of wk 12; *maintenance* 5 mg/kg rounded to the nearest 12.5-mg increment; give over 30 min at the end of wk 16 and q4wk ± 3 days thereafter
Available forms: Powder for injection 250 mg
Administer:

Black Box Warning: Only providers skilled in the use of immunosuppressants and the management of transplants should use these products

IV route
• Visually inspect for particulate matter, discoloration; discard if present
• Calculate the number of vials required
• Reconstitute each vial/10.5 mL of either sterile water for injection, 0.9% sodium chloride, D_5W, using the silicone-free disposable syringe provided and an 18-21G needle; for additional silicone-free disposable syringes, call 888-685-6549;

discard any solution prepared using siliconized syringes

• Inject diluent into the vial and direct the stream to the glass wall; rotate and invert with gentle swirling; do not shake, when reconstituted (25 mg/mL), product should be clear to slightly opalescent and colorless to pale yellow; do not use if opaque particles, discoloration, or other foreign particles are present

• Calculate the total volume of the reconstituted 25 mg/mL solution required; further dilute with a volume of infusion fluid equal to the volume of the reconstituted drug solution required; use either NS or D_5W if drug was reconstituted with SWFI; use NS if drug was reconstituted with NS; use D_5W if drug was reconstituted with D_5W; with the same silicone-free disposable syringe; final concentrations 2-10 mg/mL; but total infusion volumes ranging from 50 to 250 mL may be used; discard any unused solution; after reconstitution, immediately transfer the reconstituted solution to the infusion bag or bottle; complete within 24 hr

• Give over 30 min; use an infusion set and a sterile, nonpyrogenic, low–protein-binding filter (0.2-1.2 mm); use a separate line

• Store refrigerated, protected from light ≤24 hr; max 4 hr of the total 24 hr can be at room temperature and room light

SIDE EFFECTS

CV: Hypo/hypertension
CNS: Progressive multifocal leukoencephalopathy (PML), headache, fever
GI: Abdominal pain, constipation, diarrhea, nausea, vomiting
GU: Proteinuria
HEMA: Anemia, neutropenia, leukopenia
INTEG: Infusion reaction
META: Hyperglycemia, hyper/hypokalemia
SYST: Secondary malignancy, posttransplant lymphoproliferation disorder, wound dehiscence

PHARMACOKINETICS

Half-life, 6.1-15.1 days steady state by wk 8 after transplantation and by mo 6 during maintenance phase, peak infusion end

INTERACTIONS

Increase: effect, toxicity—mycophenolic acid

• Do not use 30 days before or with this product: live virus vaccines

NURSING CONSIDERATIONS
Assess:

Black Box Warning: Transplant rejection: flulike symptoms, decreasing urinary output, malaise; some may experience pain in area (rare; monitor BUN/creatinine)

Black Box Warning: Infection: monitor for fever, chills, increased WBC, wound dehiscences; immunosuppression occurs

Black Box Warning: Posttransplant lymphoproliferation disorder: may lead to secondary malignancy (lymphoma) or infectious mononucleosis–like lesions (mood change, confusion, memory loss, change in gait, talking); treat with antivirals or immunosuppressant; product may need to be discontinued

• Monitor for IV infusion reactions (redness, swelling at site)
• **PML:** apathy, confusion, ataxia
• **Pregnancy/breastfeeding:** use only if benefits outweigh risk to the fetus; pregnant females should enroll in the National Transplant Pregnancy Registry by calling 877-955-6877; use adequate contraception during treatment and for 4 mo after last dose; discontinue breastfeeding or product; excretion in breast milk is unknown
Evaluate:
• Therapeutic response: absence of renal transplant rejection
Teach patient/family:
• Reason for product and expected result; use REMS guidelines
• To avoid exposure to sunlight, tanning beds; risk of secondary malignancy, including skin cancer
• To avoid crowds, persons with known infections
• That repeated lab test will be needed
• To avoid with vaccines; to inform providers of all OTC, prescription medications, herbs, supplements
• That immunosuppressants will be needed for life to prevent rejection; to

call provider immediately if symptoms of rejection/infection arise

belimumab (Rx)

(be-lim'ue-mab)

Benlysta

Func. class.: Immunosuppressant, monoclonal antibody

Chem. class.: Disease-modifying antirheumatic drugs (DMARDs)

ACTION: Inhibits B-lymphocyte stimulator (BLyS), needed for B-cell survival

USES: Active, autoantibody-positive, systemic lupus erythematosus (SLE) in combination with standard therapy

CONTRAINDICATIONS

Hypersensitivity

Precautions: Pregnancy, breastfeeding, children/infants, geriatric patients, ✱☜✍ patients of African descent, depression, immunosuppression, infection, suicidal ideation, vaccination, secondary malignancy, cardiac disease; requires experienced clinician

DOSAGE AND ROUTES

• **Adult: IV** 10 mg/kg over 1 hr q2wk for the first 3 doses, then q4wk; **SUBCUT** 200 mg weekly

• **Child/adolescent 5-17 yr:** IV 10 mg/kg/dose over 1 hr q2wk × 3 doses, then q4wk

Available forms: Powder for IV injection 120, 400 mg; SUBCUT autoinjector 200 mg/mL, prefilled syringe

Administer:

• Only health care providers prepared to manage anaphylaxis should administer this product; may give premedication for prophylaxis against infusion and hypersensitivity reactions (antihistamine, antipyretic)

Intermittent IV INFUSION route ○—

• Visually inspect for particulate matter and discoloration whenever solution and container permit

• **Give** as IV infusion only; do not give IV bolus or push; give over 1 hr and slow or stop if infusion reactions occur

• Do not give with any other agents in the same IV line

• Allow to stand at room temperature for 10-15 min before using

• **Reconstitute** with the appropriate amount of sterile water for injection (80 mg/mL); add 1.5 mL of sterile water (120 mg/vial) or 4.8 mL of sterile water (400 mg/vial)

• Direct the stream of sterile water toward the side of the vial; gently swirl for 60 sec, allow to sit during reconstitution, gently swirl for 60 sec until powder is dissolved; do not shake

• Solution should be opalescent and colorless to pale yellow and without particles; small air bubbles are expected; protect from sunlight

• **Dilution:** dilute only in normal saline for injection, 0.45% NaCl, lactated Ringer's; dilute reconstituted solution with enough compatible solution to 250 mL; from a 250-mL infusion bag or bottle of compatible solution, withdraw and discard a volume equal to the volume of the reconstituted solution required for dose; add the required volume of the reconstituted solution to the infusion bag/bottle; gently invert to mix

• Discard any unused solution

• Store in refrigerator or at room temperature; total time from reconstitution to completion of infusion max 8 hr

SUBCUT route

• Allow 30 min to reach room temperature

• Inspect for particulate matter and discoloration; product should be clear to opalescent and colorless to pale yellow. It is normal to see air bubbles

• Do not use the autoinjector or prefilled syringe if dropped on a hard surface

• Protect from light and store refrigerated at 36° F-46° F (2° C-8° C) until time of use. Do not freeze. Do not shake. Avoid exposure to heat

• Do not administer where skin is tender, bruised, erythematous, or hard

• Rotate injection site with each dose

• **Missed dose:** if a dose is missed, administer as soon as possible. Do not give 2 doses on same day

SIDE EFFECTS

CNS: Headache, dizziness, *depression,* fever, *insomnia, migraine,* suicidal ideation, progressive multifocal leukoencephalopathy
GU: UTI
CV: Bradycardia
GI: *Nausea, diarrhea*
MISC: Rash, allergic reactions, myalgia
SYST: Anaphylaxis, angioedema, antibody formation, secondary malignancy, infection, influenza, infusion reactions

INTERACTIONS

• Don't use with cyclophosphamide (IV)
• Don't use with live virus vaccines within 30 days of belimumab; response to vaccine will be decreased

Drug/Herb
Decrease belimumab effect—echinacea

Drug/Lab Test
Decrease: leukocytes

PHARMACOKINETICS

Half-life 19.4 days, SUBCUT 18.3 days. Onset, peak duration unknown

NURSING CONSIDERATIONS
Assess:

• **SLE improvement:** monitor for decreasing fever, malaise, fatigue, joint pain, myalgias
• **Progressive multifocal leukoencephalopathy:** apathy, confusion, ataxia, cognitive problems; if diagnosed, discontinue
• **Suicidal ideation:** more common in those with preexisting depression
• **Infection:** determine if a chronic or acute infection is present, may be fatal; do not begin therapy if any products are being used for a chronic infection; leukopenia may occur and susceptibility to infections is increased
• **Anaphylaxis** (angioedema, rash, pruritus, wheezing), infusion site reactions: if these occur, stop infusion, provide antihistamines, corticosteroids, have emergency equipment nearby
• ⏣ **African descent patients:** use cautiously in these patients; may not respond to this product
• **Pregnancy/breastfeeding:** determine if pregnant or if pregnancy is planned or suspected; if pregnant, enroll in registry

(877-681-6296); do not breastfeed; contraception is required during and for 4 mo after conclusion of therapy

Evaluate:
• Positive response: decreasing symptoms of SLE; decreasing fatigue, fever, malaise

Teach patient/family:
• To seek treatment immediately for serious hypersensitive reactions
• Not to receive live vaccinations during treatment; bring up to date before treatment
• That compliance is required
• **Infection:** To report fever, shortness of breath, diarrhea, urinary frequency/burning, sweating, chills; to avoid others with known infections
• To report history of cancer in patient or family
• SUBCUT injection technique, must give at same time of day every week
• To take as prescribed, not to double or skip doses; if dose is missed, then take as soon as remembered, then resume correct schedule, provide "Medication Guide" and go over with patient

---

⚠ HIGH ALERT

belinostat (Rx)
(beh-lih'noh-stat')
Beleodaq
Func. class.: Antineoplastic-biologic response modifier
Chem. class.: Histone deacetylase inhibitor

Do not confuse:
belinostat/beractant

ACTION: A class I and II inhibitor of the histone deacetylase (HDAC) enzymes. Overexpression of ⏣ HDACs is present in some cancer cells. HDAC inhibitors have been shown to activate differentiation, inhibit the cell cycle, and induce apoptosis

USES: For the treatment of relapsed or refractory peripheral T-cell lymphoma (PTCL)

CONTRAINDICATIONS

Hypersensitivity, pregnancy

Precautions: Hematologic toxicity (thrombocytopenia, leukopenia, neutropenia, lymphopenia, anemia), serious infections (pneumonia, sepsis), fatal hepatic toxicity, tumor lysis syndrome (TLS), breastfeeding

DOSAGE AND ROUTES

• **Adult:** IV 1000 mg/m^2 over 30 min on days 1-5 q21days. Reduce the dose to 750 mg/m^2 in those who are ✷☞ homozygous for the UGT1A1∗28 allele. Cycles should be repeated until disease progression or unacceptable toxicity

Available forms: Powder for injection 500 mg (single-use vial)

Administer:

Intermittent IV route

• Reconstitution: Add 9 mL of sterile water for injection/500 mg, swirl until there are no visible particles (50 mg/mL); stable at room temperature for up to 12 hr

• Withdraw amount from the reconstituted vial and further dilute in 250 mL 0.9% sodium chloride for injection, the final solution is stable at room temperature for up to 36 hr, including infusion time; use a 0.22-micron in-line filter; give over 30 min; if pain occurs at infusion site, run over 45 min

Dose adjustments due to treatment-related toxicity

Hematologic toxicities:

• Do not begin the next cycle until the neutrophil count (ANC) is ≥1000/mm^3 and platelet count ≥50,000/mm^3

• ANC nadir ≥500/mm^3 *and* platelet count nadir ≥25,000/mm^3: no dose adjustment

• ANC nadir <500/mm^3 (any platelet count): begin next cycle of treatment at a reduced dose of 750 mg/m^2

• Platelet nadir <25,000/mm^3 (any ANC): begin next cycle of treatment at a reduced dose of 750 mg/m^2

SIDE EFFECTS

CNS: Fatigue, headache, dizziness, fever, chills

CV: Hypotension, QT prolongation

GI: *Constipation, anorexia, abdominal pain, nausea, vomiting, diarrhea,* hepatotoxicity

HEMA: Anemia, thrombocytopenia, neutropenia

RESP: Dyspnea, cough

INTEG: Injection site reactions, rash, phlebitis

MISC: Hypokalemia

SYST: Multiorgan failure, tumor lysis syndrome (TLS), serious infections

PHARMACOKINETICS

Half-life of 1.1 hr; 92.9%-95.8% protein bound, 80%-90% metabolized by hepatic UGT1A1; metabolized in the liver, 40% excreted renally, primarily as metabolites; onset, peak, duration unknown

INTERACTIONS

Increase: belinostat—strong UGT1A1 inhibitors (atazanavir, indinavir); avoid concurrent use if possible

Increase: QT prolongation—drugs that prolong QT, assess often

Drug/Lab

Increase: creatinine, LDH

Decrease: platelets, neutrophils, RBC, potassium

NURSING CONSIDERATIONS

Assess:

• **Hematologic toxicity (thrombocytopenia, leukopenia, neutropenia, lymphopenia, anemia):** monitor CBC before starting and every week. Dose modifications may be necessary in patients with bone marrow suppression and should be determined by the ANC and platelet count nadirs of the previous cycle. Platelet counts should be ≥50,000/mm^3 and ANC >1000/mm^3 before starting each cycle

• **Serious infections (pneumonia, sepsis):** may be fatal. Do not use in those with an active infection. Use caution in patients with a history of extensive or intensive chemotherapy, as they may be at higher risk of life-threatening infections; monitor for dyspnea, cough, characteristics of sputum

• **Fatal hepatic toxicity:** monitor LFTs before the start of each cycle. Those with signs of hepatic disease may require dose modification or discontinuation

• **Tumor lysis syndrome (TLS):** those with high tumor burden or advanced-stage disease are at greater risk for development of TLS; consider tumor lysis prophylaxis with antihyperuricemic agents and hydration beginning 12-24 hr before treatment; for TLS treatment, administer aggressive IV hydration, antihyperuricemic agents, correct electrolyte abnormalities, and monitor renal function
• **Renal studies:** monitor BUN/creatinine periodically; if renal disease is present, use cautiously
• **Pregnancy/breastfeeding:** consider discontinuing breastfeeding; identify whether the patient is pregnant before using; do not use if pregnant

Evaluate:
• Therapeutic response: prevention of spread of disease

Teach patient/family:
• To avoid use in breastfeeding; not to use in pregnancy; that fertility may be impaired
• To report infusion site reactions, rash, severe constipation or diarrhea, abdominal pain, nausea, vomiting
• **Bleeding:** to report increased bruising, bleeding, melanotic or dark tarry stools
• **Tumor lysis syndrome:** to report immediately fatigue, dark urine, nausea, weakness, confusion, change in heart rate
• **Infection:** to report sore throat, cough, trouble breathing, flulike symptoms
• **Hepatic toxicity:** to report dark urine, anorexia, yellow skin/eyes, itching, abdominal pain
• That compliance is needed with product and lab testing

belumosudil (Rx)
(bel-ue-moe-soo-dil)
Rezurock
Func. class.: Immunosupressant

USES: Graft versus host disease when other treatments have not worked

DOSAGE AND ROUTES
• **Adult/child** ≥12 yr 200 mg daily
Available forms: Tablet 200 mg

belzutifan (Rx)
(bel-ZOO-ti-fan)
Welireg
Func. class.: Misc. antineoplastic
Chem. class.: Kinase inhibitor

ACTION: Inhibits hypoxia-inducible factor that plays a role in oxygen sensing by regulating genes that promote adaptation to hypoxia

USES: von Hippel-Lindau disease who require therapy for renal cell carcinoma, NS hemangioblastomas/pancreatic neuroendocrine tumors not requiring immediate surgery

CONTRAINDICATIONS
Hypersensitivity

Black Box Warning: Pregnancy

Precautions: Anemia, hypoxia, breastfeeding

DOSAGE AND ROUTES
• **Adult: PO** 120 mg daily until disease progression or unacceptable toxicity
Available forms: Tabs 40 mg
Administer:
• Take at the same time each day, use without regard to food
• Swallow tablets whole. Do not chew, crush, split
• If a dose is missed, take as soon as possible on the same day. Resume the regular daily dose schedule the next day. Do not take dose to make up for a missed dose
• If vomiting occurs after taking, do not retake the dose. Take the next dose on the next day

SIDE EFFECTS
CNS: Fatigue, headache, dizziness
GI: Nausea
RESP: Hypoxia
HEMA: Anemia

INTERACTIONS
Increased: belzutifan effect—UGT2B17 or CYP2C19 inhibitors, monitor for anemia and hypoxia

Increased: contraceptive failure—hormonal contraceptives, use alternative contraceptive measures

Avoid use with sensitive CYP3A4 substrates

PHARMACOKINETICS
Peak 1-2 hr

NURSING CONSIDERATIONS
Assess:
• **Hypoxia:** Monitor O_2 saturation baseline and periodically; for decreased O_2 saturation with exercise (pulse oximeter <88% or PaO_2 ≤55 mm Hg), consider withholding until pulse oximetry with exercise is greater than 88%, then resume at the same dose or at a reduced dose. For decreased oxygen saturation at rest (pulse oximeter <88% or PaO_2 ≤55 mm Hg) or urgent intervention indicated, withhold until resolved and resume at a reduced dose or discontinue. For life-threatening hypoxia or for recurrent symptomatic hypoxia, permanently discontinue

• **Anemia:** Monitor for anemia baseline and periodically. Closely monitor patients who are dual UGT2B17/CYP2C19 poor metabolizers, transfusions may be needed, HB <9 g/dL, withhold until ≥9 g/dL, then resume at reduced dose or permanently discontinue depending on the severity of anemia. For life-threatening anemia or when urgent intervention is indicated, withhold until HB ≥9 g/dL, then resume at a reduced dose or permanently discontinue

Black Box Warning: **Pregnancy/lactation:** Obtain a pregnancy test before starting treatment. A nonhormonal contraceptive should be used during and for 1 wk after last dose. Both males and females should use contraceptives; infertility may occur, and it is not known if it is reversible

Evaluate:
• Therapeutic response: Prevention of spread of cancer

Teach patient/family:
• Teach the patient to take without regard to food, if vomiting occurs do not retake dose

• Laboratory testing will be needed, if blood counts are low, a transfusion may be needed

• Advise health care provider if tired, short of breath, chest pain or rapid heartbeat occurs

Black Box Warning: **Pregnancy/lactation:** Do not use in pregnancy, use a nonhormonal contraceptive during and for 1 wk after last dose. Because hormonal contraceptives may not work, both males and females should use effective contraception; infertility may occur and it isn't known if reversible

---

bempedoic acid (Rx)
(bem′pe-doe′ik as′id)

Nexletol

Func. class.: Antilipemic

Chem. class.: Adenosine triphosphate–citrate lyase inhibitor

ACTION: Lowers low-density lipoprotein cholesterol (LDL-C) by inhibiting cholesterol synthesis in the liver

USES: Atherosclerotic CV disease, heterozygous familial hypercholesterolemia, as an adjunct to diet and statin therapy

CONTRAINDICATIONS
Hypersensitivity

Precautions: Severe renal/hepatic disease, myopathy, tendon rupture, children, hyperuricemia

DOSAGE AND ROUTES
• **Adult: PO** 180 mg daily

Available forms: Tabs 180 mg

Administer:
• Give without regard to food

- Store in original package (with desiccant) at room temperature

SIDE EFFECTS
ENDO: Hyperuricemia
CV: Atrial fibrillation
GI: Abdominal distress
GU: BPH
HEMA: Anemia, leukopenia
MS: Back/limb pain, muscle spasm, gout
RESP: URI

PHARMACOKINETICS
Onset/duration unknown, peak 3.5 hr, half-life 21 hr

INTERACTIONS
Increase: effect of—OATP1B1/1B3 (SLCO1B1/1B3) inhibitors, avoid combination
Increase: myopathy risk—pravastatin, simvastatin, avoid pravastatin doses of >40 mg/day, simvastatin doses >30 mg/day
Drug/Lab Test:
Increase: LFTs, BUN, serum creatinine, CK

NURSING CONSIDERATIONS
Assess:
- Monitor lipid panel 3-4 mo after starting treatment
- **Myopathy/tendon rupture:** Assess for muscle tenderness, spasms, weakness; monitor doses of statins; notify provider immediately of tendon rupture, discontinue product
- **Hyperuricemia:** Monitor uric acid levels if needed and assess for signs/symptoms of gout, if indicated use urate-lowering products
- **Pregnancy/breastfeeding:** Do not use in pregnancy, avoid breastfeeding
Evaluate:
- Therapeutic response: Decrease in LDL-C levels
Teach patient/family:
- **Hyperuricemia:** Teach patients about the risk of elevated serum uric acid levels, with possibility of gout, that lab exams will be needed, to contact prescriber if signs/symptoms of gout develop
- **Tendon rupture risk:** Advise patients of tendon rupture, to rest at the first sign

of tendinitis or tendon rupture, immediately contact provider
- Myopathy risk (simvastatin or pravastatin): Teach patients to notify providers if they are taking simvastatin or pravastatin, myopathy risk is increased with use of these products
- Pregnancy/breastfeeding: Teach patient to notify prescriber if pregnancy is planned or suspected or if breastfeeding

benazepril (Rx)
(ben-aze'uh-pril)
Lotensin
Func. class.: Antihypertensive
Chem. class.: Angiotensin-converting enzyme (ACE) inhibitor

Do not confuse:
benazepril/Benadryl
Lotensin/lovastatin

ACTION: Selectively suppresses renin-angiotensin-aldosterone system; inhibits ACE, thus preventing conversion of angiotensin I to angiotensin II

USES: Hypertension, alone or in combination with thiazide diuretics

CONTRAINDICATIONS
Breastfeeding, children, hypersensitivity to ACE inhibitors, hereditary angioedema

Black Box Warning: Pregnancy

Precautions: Geriatric patients, impaired renal/hepatic function, dialysis patients, hypovolemia, blood dyscrasias, HF, asthma, bilateral renal artery stenosis, Black patients

DOSAGE AND ROUTES
Hypertension
- **Adult: PO** 10 mg/day initially, then 20-40 mg/day divided bid or daily (without a diuretic); reduce initial dose to 5 mg **PO** daily (with a diuretic); increase as needed, max 80 mg/day
- **Child ≥6 yr: PO** 0.2 mg/kg/day, increase as needed; max 0.6 mg/kg/day or 40 mg/day, whichever is lower.

Renal dose
• **Adult:** PO CCr <30 mL/min or CCr >3 mg/dL, use 5 mg daily, max 40 mg/day
• **Child ≥6 yr:** PO CCr <30 mL/min, do not use

Available forms: Tablets 5, 10, 20, 40 mg

Administer:
• May give without regard to food
• Do not discontinue product abruptly
• ⬥ Black patients' response to this drug is less, may need to be combined with other products
• Store in a tight container at 86° F (30° C) or less

SIDE EFFECTS

CNS: Insomnia, headache, dizziness, fatigue
CV: Hypotension, postural hypotension
GI: Nausea, constipation, vomiting, diarrhea
GU: Increased BUN, creatinine, decreased libido, impotence, renal insufficiency
INTEG: Rash, flushing, sweating
MISC: Angioedema, Stevens-Johnson syndrome, hypersensitivity, dry cough

PHARMACOKINETICS

Onset 1 hr, peak 1-2 hr fasting, 2-4 hr after food, duration 24 hr; protein binding 89%-95%; half-life 10-11 hr; metabolized by liver (metabolites); excreted in urine 33%

INTERACTIONS

Increase: hypotension—phenothiazines, nitrates, acute alcohol ingestion, diuretics, other antihypertensives; may need to reduce dose, monitor B/P
Increase: hyperkalemia—potassium-sparing diuretics, potassium supplements; monitor potassium, BUN, creatinine
Increase: hypotension, hyperkalemia in diabetes, renal disease—aliskiren; do not use in diabetes, avoid use in GFR <60 mL/min
Increase: myelosuppression—azaTHIOprine
Increase: serum levels of lithium, digoxin; may cause toxicity; monitor lithium or digoxin levels
Decrease: hypotensive effects—NSAIDs, COX-2 inhibitors; monitor B/P

Drug/Herb
Increase: antihypertensive effect—hawthorn
Decrease: antihypertensive effect—ephedra (ma huang); avoid concurrent use

Drug/Lab Test
Increase: AST, ALT, alkaline phosphatase, bilirubin, uric acid, blood glucose, potassium, BUN, creatinine

NURSING CONSIDERATIONS

Assess:
• **Hypertension:** B/P, pulse at baseline, periodically; orthostatic hypotension, syncope when used with diuretic; notify prescriber of changes; monitor compliance
• **Renal studies:** protein, BUN, creatinine; increased levels may indicate nephrotic syndrome; monitor urine for protein; LFTs, uric acid, glucose may be increased; diuretic should be discontinued 3 days before use; if hypertension is not controlled, a diuretic can be added; measure B/P at peak 2-4 hr and trough (before next dose); ⬥ this product is less effective in patients of African descent; CBC, ALT/AST, alkaline phosphatase
• Potassium levels, although hyperkalemia rarely occurs
• **Allergic reactions:** rash, fever, pruritus, urticaria; product should be discontinued if antihistamines fail to help; **Stevens-Johnson syndrome; angioedema** is more common in patients of African descent
• **Renal symptoms:** polyuria, oliguria, frequency, dysuria

Evaluate:
• Therapeutic response: decrease in B/P; decreased HF (unlabeled)

Teach patient/family:
• Not to use OTC products (cough, cold, allergy) unless directed by prescriber; not to use salt substitutes that contain potassium without consulting prescriber
• The importance of complying with dosage schedule, even if feeling better

Black Box Warning: To notify prescriber of pregnancy; product will need to be discontinued immediately; do not breastfeed

---

🍁 Canada only   ⬥ Genetic warning

- To rise slowly to sitting or standing position to minimize orthostatic hypotension
- To notify prescriber of mouth sores; sore throat; fever; swelling of hands or feet; irregular heartbeat; chest pain; bruising; bleeding; swelling of face, tongue, lips; difficulty breathing; signs of infection; cough
- To report excessive perspiration, dehydration, vomiting, diarrhea; may lead to fall in B/P; to use caution in hot weather, strenuous exercise; to consume adequate fluids
- That product may cause dizziness, fainting, light headedness; that this may occur during first few days of therapy
- That product may cause skin rash or impaired perspiration
- **Diabetes:** blood glucose, glucose may be decreased, especially during early treatment
- **Hypertension:** how to take B/P and normal readings for age group
- **Pregnancy/breastfeeding:** to notify prescriber if pregnancy is planned or suspected or if breastfeeding, not to use in pregnancy, breastfeeding

TREATMENT OF OVERDOSE: 0.9% NaCl IV infusion, hemodialysis

⚠ HIGH ALERT

bendamustine (Rx)
(ben-da-muss′teen)

Bendeka, Treanda
Func. class.: Antineoplastic alkylating agent

USES: Chronic lymphocytic leukemia, indolent B-cell non-Hodgkin's lymphoma that has progressed or within 6 mo use of rituximab regimen

CONTRAINDICATIONS
Pregnancy, fetal harm may occur; breastfeeding, children, hepatic disease, renal impairment, hypersensitivity to product or mannitol
Precautions: Hyperuricemia, infusion-related reactions, myelosuppression, infection, skin reactions

DOSAGE AND ROUTES
Chronic lymphocytic leukemia
- **Adult: IV INFUSION** 100 mg/m^2 over 30 min (Treanda) or 10 min (Bendeka) on days 1, 2 q28days up to 6 cycles
Non-Hodgkin's lymphoma
- **Adult: IV INFUSION** 120 mg/m^2 over 60 min (Treanda) or 10 min (Bendeka) on days 1, 2 q21days up to 8 cycles
Mantle cell lymphoma (unlabeled)
- **Adult: IV INFUSION** 90 mg/m^2 on days 1, 2 with rituximab on day 1 q28days for 6 cycles

Renal/hepatic dose
- **Adult: IV INFUSION** CCr <30 mL/min, do not use; AST or ALT 2.5-10 × ULN or bilirubin 1.5-3 × ULN, do not use
Available forms: Solution for injection 100-mg/4-mL vials; lyophilized powder for injection: 25-, 100-mg single-use vials

benzocaine topical
See Appendix B

benzonatate (Rx)
(ben-zoe′na-tate)

Tessalon Perles, Zonatuss
Func. class.: Antitussive, nonopioid

USES: Nonproductive cough

CONTRAINDICATIONS
Hypersensitivity

DOSAGE AND ROUTES
- **Adult and child ≥10 yr: PO** 100-200 mg up to tid; max 600 mg/day
Available forms: Capsules 100, 150, 200 mg

benztropine (Rx)
(benz′troe-peen)

Cogentin
Func. class.: Anticholinergic, antiparkinson agent
Chem. class.: Tertiary amine

Side effects: *italics* = common; red = life-threatening

Do not confuse:
benztropine/bromocriptine

ACTION: Blockade of central acetylcholine receptors, balances cholinergic activity

USES: Parkinson's symptoms, EPS associated with neuroleptic products, acute dystonic reactions

CONTRAINDICATIONS
Children <3 yr, hypersensitivity, closed-angle glaucoma, dementia, tardive dyskinesia
Precautions: Pregnancy, breastfeeding, geriatric patients, tachycardia, renal/hepatic disease, substance abuse history, dysrhythmias, hypo/hypertension, myasthenia gravis, GI/GU obstruction, peptic ulcer, megacolon, prostate hypertrophy, psychosis

DOSAGE AND ROUTES
Drug-induced EPS (not tardive dyskinesia)
• Adult: **IM/IV/PO** 1-4 mg daily/bid; give **PO** dose as soon as possible
• Child >3 yr: **IM/IV/PO** 0.02-0.05 mg/kg/dose 1-2×/day
Transient EPS
• Adult: **PO/IM/IV** 1-2 mg bid or tid, after ≤2 wk discontinue and see if still required
Parkinson's symptoms
• Adult: **PO/IM** 0.5-1 mg at bedtime; increase to 0.5 mg q5-6days titrated to patient response, max 6 mg/day
Acute dystonic reactions
• Adult: **IM/IV** 1-2 mg, may increase to 1-2 mg bid **(PO)**
Postencephalitic parkinsonism
• Adult: **PO/IM/IV** 2 mg/day in 1 dose or divided, max 6 mg/day
Available forms: Tablets 0.5, 1, 2 mg; injection 1 mg/mL in 2-mL ampule
Administer:
PO route
• With or after meals to prevent GI upset; may give with fluids other than water
• At bedtime to avoid daytime drowsiness with parkinsonism
• Store at room temperature
IM route
• Inject deeply in muscle; use filtered needle to remove solution from ampule

IV, direct route
• Use in emergencies, not used often; rate 1 mg/min

Y-site compatibilities: Alfentanil, amikacin, aminophylline, ascorbic acid injection, atracurium, atropine, azaTHIOprine, aztreonam, bumetanide, buprenorphine, butorphanol, calcium chloride, gluconate, ceFAZolin, cefotaxime, cefoTEtan, cefOXitin, cefTAZidime, ceftizoxime, cefTRIAXone, cefuroxime, chlorproMAZINE, cimetidine, clindamycin, cyanocobalamin, cycloSPORINE, dexamethasone, digoxin, diphenhydrAMINE, DOBUTamine, DOPamine, doxycycline, enalaprilat, ePHEDrine, epinephrine, epoetin alfa, erythromycin lactobionate, esmolol, famotidine, fentaNYL, fluconazole, folic acid (as sodium salt), gentamicin, glycopyrrolate, heparin, hydrocortisone sodium succinate, hydrOXYzine, imipenem-cilastatin, inamrinone, insulin (regular), isoproterenol, ketorolac, labetalol, lactated Ringer's, lidocaine, magnesium sulfate, mannitol, meperidine, metaraminol, methyldopate, methylPREDNISolone, metoclopramide, metoprolol, midazolam, minocycline, morphine, multiple vitamins injection, nafcillin, nalbuphine, naloxone, netilmicin, nitroglycerin, nitroprusside, norepinephrine, ondansetron, oxacillin, oxytocin, papaverine, penicillin G potassium/sodium, pentamidine, pentazocine, PHENobarbital, phentolamine, phenylephrine, phytonadione, piperacillin, polymyxin B, potassium chloride, procainamide, prochlorperazine, promethazine, propranolol, protamine, pyridoxine, quiNIDine, ranitidine, Ringer's injection, sodium bicarbonate, succinylcholine, SUFentanil, tacrolimus, theophylline, thiamine, ticarcillin, ticarcillin-clavulanate, tobramycin, tolazoline, urokinase, vancomycin, vasopressin, verapamil

SIDE EFFECTS

CNS: Hallucinations, depression, dizziness, memory loss; *confusion;* delirium (geriatric headache, sedation)
CV: Palpitations, tachycardia, hypotension, bradycardia
EENT: Blurred vision, photophobia

GI: *Dry mouth, constipation,* nausea
GU: Urinary hesitancy/retention
INTEG: Rash
MISC: Decreased sweating

PHARMACOKINETICS

PO: Onset 1 hr, peak 7 hr, duration 24 hr
IM/IV: Onset 15 min, duration 6-10 hr

INTERACTIONS

Increase: anticholinergic effect—antihistamines, phenothiazines, tricyclics, disopyramide, quiNIDine; reduce dose

Decrease: absorption—antidiarrheals, antacids

Decrease: anticholinergic effect of—cholinergics; monitor response

Drug/Herb

Increase: anticholinergic action—jimsonweed, *Scopola*

NURSING CONSIDERATIONS

Assess:

• **Parkinsonism:** EPS, shuffling gait, muscle rigidity, involuntary movements, loss of balance, tardive dyskinesia; may exacerbate symptoms

• Monitor vital signs B/P, pulse in IM/IV dosing, patient should remain recumbent for 1 hr after use

• I&O ratio; commonly causes decreased urinary output; urinary hesitancy, retention; palpate bladder if retention occurs

• Constipation: increase fluids, bulk, exercise if this occurs, paralytic ileus may occur

• Mental status: affect, mood, CNS depression, worsening of mental symptoms during early therapy

• Use caution during hot weather; product may increase susceptibility to heat stroke by decreasing sweating

• With benztropine "buzz" or "high," patients may imitate EPS

• Hard candy, gum, frequent drinks to relieve dry mouth

• **Withdrawal symptoms:** do not discontinue abruptly; taper

• **Beers:** avoid in older adults; high risk of delirium, CNS effects, decreased urinary flow

• **Pregnancy/breastfeeding:** Unknown

Evaluate:

• Therapeutic response: absence of involuntary movements after 2 days of treatment

Teach patient/family:

• To report urinary hesitancy/retention, dysuria

• That tablets may be crushed, mixed with food; may take whole dose at bedtime if approved by prescriber

• Not to discontinue product abruptly; to taper off over 1 wk or withdrawal symptoms may occur (EPS, tremors, insomnia, tachycardia, restlessness); to take as directed; not to double dose

• To avoid driving, other hazardous activities; drowsiness/dizziness may occur

• To avoid OTC medications: cough, cold preparations with alcohol, antihistamines, antacids, antidiarrheals within 2 hr unless directed by prescriber

• To change positions slowly to prevent orthostatic hypotension

• To use good oral hygiene, frequent sips of water, sugarless gum for dry mouth

• To avoid strenuous exercise or activities in hot weather; overheating may occur

• That routine exams will be needed

• To separate antacids by 2 hr of this product

---

bepotastine (Rx)

(beh-pot'uh-steen)
Bepreve
Func. class.: Antihistamine (ophthalmic)
Chem. class.: Histamine-1 receptor antagonist

USES: Ocular pruritus associated with signs/symptoms of allergic conjunctivitis

CONTRAINDICATIONS

Hypersensitivity
Precautions: Pregnancy, breastfeeding, children, contact lenses

DOSAGE AND ROUTES

• **Adult/child ≥2 yr: OPHTH** Instill 1 drop in affected eye bid, max 2 drops/day in each eye

Available forms: Opthalmic solution 1.5%

betamethasone (augmented) topical
See Appendix B

betamethasone dipropionate (Rx)
(bay-ta-meth´a-sone)
Betaderm ✦, Betagel ✦, Betaprolene Cream ✦, Betaflam ✦, Betnesol ✦, Celestoderm V ✦, Diprolene, Diprolene AF, Servivo
betamethasone valerate
Luxiq
Func. class.: Corticosteroid, topical

ACTION: Crosses cell membrane to attach to receptors to decrease inflammation, itching; inhibits multiple inflammatory cytokines

USES: Inflammation/itching corticosteroid-responsive dermatoses on the skin/scalp

CONTRAINDICATIONS
Hypersensitivity, use of some preparations on face, axilla, groin
Precautions: Pregnancy, skin infections

DOSAGE AND ROUTES
• **Adult:** TOP 1-2 times/day (dipropionate) or 1-3 times/day (valerate); or apply spray 0.05% bid up to 4 wk (plaque psoriasis, mild to moderate)
Available forms: dipropionate: gel, lotion, ointment, cream, spray 0.05%; **valerate:** cream, lotion, ointment 0.1%, foam 0.12%

SIDE EFFECTS
INTEG: Burning, folliculitis, pruritus, dermatitis, maceration, erythema
MISC: Hyperglycemia, glycosuria, Cushing's syndrome, HPA axis suppression

PHARMACOKINETICS
Unknown

NURSING CONSIDERATIONS
Assess:
• **Skin reactions:** burning, pruritus, folliculitis, dermatitis
• **HPA axis suppression:** usually rare with topical products
Evaluate:
• Decreased itching; inflammation on the skin, scalp
Teach patient/family:
Topical route:
• That betamethasone valerate may be used with occlusive dressings for psoriasis or recalcitrant conditions; not to use dipropionate with occlusive dressings
• Avoid use of topical corticosteroids on face
Cream/ointment/lotion:
• To apply sparingly in a thin film, using gloves, and to rub gently into the cleansed, slightly moist affected area
• Not to use on broken, wet skin; area of infection; face or groin; axilla
Gel:
• To apply sparingly in a thin film, using gloves, and to rub gently into the cleansed, slightly moist affected area
Scalp foam:
• Gently massage into affected area until foam disappears; repeat until entire affected scalp area is treated
• That treatment should be limited to 2 wk

⚠ HIGH ALERT

betaxolol (Rx)
(beh-tax´oh-lol)
Betoptic-S, Kerlone
Func. class.: Antiglaucoma
Chem. class.: Beta-blocker

USES: Treatment of chronic open-angle glaucoma and ocular hypertension; **PO** for hypertension

CONTRAINDICATIONS
Hypersensitivity, AV block, heart failure, bradycardia, sick sinus syndrome
Precautions: Abrupt discontinuation, children, pregnancy, breastfeeding, asthma,

---

COPD, depression, diabetes mellitus, myasthenia gravis, hyperthyroidism, pulmonary disease, angle-closure glaucoma

DOSAGE AND ROUTES
Chronic open-angle glaucoma
• **Adult:** Instill 1-2 drops in the affected eye(s) bid
Hypertension
• **Adult: PO** 10 mg/day, may increase to 20 mg after 1-2 wk; may be used with or without diuretics
Geriatric
• **PO** Initially, 5 mg/day, may increase 5 mg/day q2wk, max 20 mg/day

Available forms: Opthalmic solution 0.5%; tablets 10, 20 mg; opthalmic suspension 0.25%

---

bethanechol (Rx)
(be-than′e-kole)
Duvoid ✤
Func. class.: Urinary tract stimulant, cholinergic
Chem. class.: Synthetic choline ester

ACTION: Stimulates muscarinic ACH receptors directly; mimics effects of parasympathetic nervous system stimulation; stimulates gastric motility, micturition; increases lower esophageal sphincter pressure

USES: Urinary retention (postoperative, postpartum), neurogenic atony of bladder with retention
Unlabeled uses: Ileus, GERD, anticholinergic syndrome

CONTRAINDICATIONS
Hypersensitivity, severe bradycardia, asthma, severe hypotension, hyperthyroidism, peptic ulcer, parkinsonism, seizure disorders, CAD, COPD, coronary occlusion, mechanical obstruction, peritonitis, recent urinary/GI surgery, GI/GU obstruction
Precautions: Pregnancy, breastfeeding, children <8 yr, hypertension

DOSAGE AND ROUTES
• **Adult: PO/SUBCUT** 10-50 mg bid-qid

• **Child (unlabeled): PO** 0.5 mg/kg/day in 3-4 divided doses
Ileus (unlabeled)
• **Adult: PO** 10-20 mg tid-qid
Available forms: Tablets 5, 10, 25, 50 mg
Administer:
• To avoid nausea, vomiting, take on an empty stomach
• Only after all other cholinergics have been discontinued; cholinergic effects at higher doses may be cumulative
• Store at room temperature

SIDE EFFECTS
CNS: Dizziness, headache, malaise
CV: Hypotension, bradycardia, reflex tachycardia, cardiac arrest, circulatory collapse
EENT: Miosis, increased salivation, lacrimation, blurred vision
GI: *Nausea, bloody diarrhea, belching, vomiting, cramps, fecal incontinence*
GU: Urgency
INTEG: Rash, urticaria, flushing, increased sweating
RESP: Acute asthma, dyspnea, bronchoconstriction

PHARMACOKINETICS
PO: Onset 30-90 min, peak 60-90 min, duration 6 hr

INTERACTIONS
Increase: severe hypotension—ganglionic blockers; avoid concurrent use
Increase: action or toxicity—cholinergic agonists, anticholinesterase agents; avoid concurrent use
Decrease: action of anticholinergics, procainamide, quiNIDine, belladonna; monitor for adequate effect
Drug/Lab Test
Increase: AST, lipase/amylase, bilirubin

NURSING CONSIDERATIONS
Assess:
• **Urinary patterns:** retention, urgency
• B/P, pulse: observe after parenteral dose for 1 hr; may need to use atropine SUBCUT 0.6 mg or IV push slowly for bronchoconstriction
• I&O ratio: check for urinary retention, urge incontinence

- **Toxicity:** bradycardia, hypotension, bronchospasm, headache, dizziness, seizures, respiratory depression; product should be discontinued if toxicity occurs
- **Orthostatic hypotension:** monitor frequently, monitor ambulation to prevent falling
- **Pregnancy/breastfeeding:** use only if clearly needed; discontinue breastfeeding or product

Evaluate:

- Therapeutic response: absence of urinary retention, abdominal distention

Teach patient/family:

- To take product exactly as prescribed; 1 hr before meals or 2 hr after meals to avoid nausea
- To make position changes slowly; orthostatic hypotension may occur
- To avoid driving, hazardous activities until effects are known

TREATMENT OF OVERDOSE: Administer atropine 0.6-1.2 mg IV or IM (adult)

⚠ HIGH ALERT

betrixaban (Rx)

(be-trix′-a-ban)

Bevyxxa

Func. class.: Anticoagulant
Chem. class.: Selective factor Xa inhibitor

ACTION: Inhibits factor Xa; neutralization of factor Xa interrupts blood coagulation and thrombin formation

USES: Prevention/treatment of deep venous thrombosis' PE in at-risk, acutely ill, hospitalized medical patients

CONTRAINDICATIONS

Hypersensitivity, active major bleeding

Precautions: Pregnancy, breastfeeding, children, geriatric patients, hepatic disease, renal disease

Black Box Warning: Spinal/epidural anesthesia, lumbar puncture

DOSAGE AND ROUTES

DVT prophylaxis, pulmonary embolism prophylaxis in at-risk, acutely ill, hospitalized medical patients

- **Adult: PO** 160 mg once, followed by 80 mg/day for 35-42 days

Renal dose

Adult: PO CCr 15-<30 mL/min 80 mg, then 40 mg daily × 35-42 days

Concomitant use of P-gp inhibitors: Reduce initial dose to 80 mg as a single dose, then 40 mg once daily for 35-42 days

Available forms: Capsules 40, 80 mg

Administer:

- Give with food at same time of day
- If a dose is missed, take as soon as remembered on the same day; do not double
- Store at room temperature

PHARMACOKINETICS

Onset unknown, peak 3-4 hr, duration >72 hr, protein binding 60%, half-life 19-27 hr; excreted in urine 11%, feces 85%

INTERACTIONS

Increase: bleeding risk—salicylates, NSAIDs, abciximab, eptifibatide, tirofiban, clopidogrel, dipyridamole, quiNIDine, valproic acid, P-gp inhibitors

Drug/Herb

Increase: bleeding risk—feverfew, garlic, ginger, ginkgo, ginseng, green tea, horse chestnut, kava

Drug/Lab

Decrease: potassium

NURSING CONSIDERATIONS

Assess:

Black Box Warning: Monitor patients who have received epidural/spinal anesthesia or lumbar puncture for neurologic impairment, including spinal hematoma; may lead to permanent disability or paralysis

- **Hepatic impairment:** avoid use
- **Renal impairment:** dose reduction is required

- For bleeding: gums, petechiae, ecchymosis, black tarry stools, hematuria; decreased Hct; notify prescriber
- For risk of hemorrhage if coadministering with other products that may cause bleeding
- For hypersensitivity: rash, fever, chills; notify prescriber
- Monitor QTc interval if needed in cardiac patients
- **Pregnancy/breastfeeding:** consider risks of bleeding and stroke; use only if benefits outweigh risks; consider potential adverse effects before breastfeeding
- **Beers:** avoid in older adults; increased risk of bleeding, lower CCr

Evaluate:
- Therapeutic response: prevention of DVT

Teach patient/family:
- To use soft-bristle toothbrush to avoid bleeding gums; to use electric razor
- To report any signs of bleeding: gums, under skin, urine, stools; bleeding risk may continue up to 72 hr after stopping therapy
- To avoid OTC products containing aspirin, NSAIDs
- To take with food

Black Box Warning: Spinal/epidural hematoma: in those that received spinal/epidural anesthesia; weakness in lower extremities, bowel bladder involvement

⚠ HIGH ALERT

bevacizumab (Rx)
(beh-va-kiz'you-mab)
Avastin; MVASi (biosimilar) ♣, Zirabev (biosimilar)
Func. class.: Antineoplastic—miscellaneous
Chem. class.: Monoclonal antibody

Do not confuse:
Avastin/Astelin

ACTION: Monoclonal antibody selectively binds to and inhibits activity of human vascular endothelial growth factor (VEGF) to reduce microvascular growth and metastatic disease progression

USES:

Avastin: Heptocelluler carcinoma (unresectable/metastatic)
Avatin or Zirbev: Epithelial ovarian, fallopian, peritoneal carcinoma in those who have received ≤2 other systemic treatments
Avastin, Mvasi, Zirabev: Metastatic carcinoma of the colon or rectum in combination with glioblastoma, non–small cell lung cancer
Unlabeled uses: Adjunctive for ovarian cancer, (wet) macular degeneration, unresectable malignant pleural mesothelioma, diabetic macular edema

CONTRAINDICATIONS
Hypersensitivity, serious bleeding, hypertensive crisis, recent surgery
Precautions: Pregnancy, breastfeeding, children, geriatric patients, HF, blood dyscrasias, CV disease, hypertension, surgery, thromboembolic disease, hamster protein/murine hypersensitivity

Black Box Warning: GI perforation, wound dehiscence, bleeding

DOSAGE AND ROUTES
Non–small-cell lung cancer
- **Adult:** IV 15 mg/kg over 60-90 min with CARBOplatin and PACLitaxel q3wk
Platinum-resistant recurrent epithelial ovarian, fallopian tube, or primary peritoneal cancer (Avastin only)
- **Adult:** IV 10 mg/kg q2wk with PACLitaxel and pegylated liposomal DOXOrubicin or topotecan weekly; or 15 mg/kg q3wk with topotecan
Platinum-sensitive recurrent epithelial ovarian, fallopian tube, or primary peritoneal cancer (Avastin only)
- **Adult:** IV 15 mg/kg q3wk with CARBOplatin and PACLitaxel for ≤6 cycles 8 cycles, then continue bevacizumab (single agent): 15 mg/kg q3wk until progression
Stage III/IV epithelial ovarian, fallopian tube, or primary peritoneal cancer after resection (Avastin only)
- **Adult:** IV 15 mg/kg q3wk with CARBOplatin and PACLitaxel for ≤6 cy-

cles, then 15 mg/kg q3wk (single agent) for 22 cycles

Metastatic colorectal cancer with fluoropyrimidine-irinotecan–based or fluoropyrimidine-oxaliplatin–based or fluoropyrimidine-oxaliplatin–based treatment for second-line after progression
• **Adult: IV** 5 mg/kg q2wk or 7.5 mg/kg q3wk

Persistent, recurrent, or metastatic cervical cancer with PACLitaxel and CISplatin or PACLitaxel and topotecan
• **Adult: IV** infusion 15 mg/kg q3wk

First- or second-line treatment of metastatic colon or rectal cancer with 5-FU
• **Adult: IV** infusion 5 mg/kg q14days if used with bolus irinotecan, 5-FU, and leucovorin; or 10 mg/kg q14days if used with oxaliplatin, F-FU, and leucovorin (FOLOX 4); rates vary

With CARBOplatin and PACLitaxel as first-line in treatment of unresectable, recurrent, locally advanced, or metastatic nonsquamous NSCLC
• **Adult: IV** infusion 15 mg q3wk

Unresectable or metastatic hepatocellular cancer (HCC) in patients who have not received prior systemic therapy, with atezolizumab
• **Adult: IV** 15 mg/kg q3wk give with atezolizumab (840 mg IV q2wk or 1200 mg IV q3wk or 1680 mg IV q4wk) until disease progression or unacceptable toxicity

Unresectable malignant pleural mesothelioma (unlabeled)
• **Adult: IV** 15mg/kg q3wk with CISplatin and pemetrexed for up to 6 cycles, then bevacizumab 15 mg/kg q3wk maintenance until disease progression or toxicity

Diabetic macular edema (unlabeled)
• **Adult: Intravitreal** 1.25 mg (0.05 mL), repeat q4wk depending on response

Neovascular (wet) age-related macular degeneration (AMD) (unlabeled)
• **Adult/geriatric patients: INTRAVITREAL INJECTION** 1.25 mg (0.05 mL) monthly into affected eye × 3 mo
Available forms: Solution for injection 25 mg/mL
Administer:

Intermittent IV INFUSION route
• Do not give by IV bolus, IV push; do not shake vial, do not admix, do not freeze
• Withdraw amount of product to be given, dilute in 100 mL 0.9% NaCl, discard any unused portion

Black Box Warning: **Wound dehiscence:** discontinue 28 days prior to elective surgery, do not give for ≥28 days after surgery; make sure wound is healed before giving product

• Give as IV infusion over 90 min for first dose and 60 min thereafter if well tolerated; subsequent infusion may be given over 30 min; do not admix with dextrose
• Store refrigerated up to 8 hr (diluted)

SIDE EFFECTS
CNS: *Asthenia, dizziness,* abnormal gait, syncope, headache, confusion
CV: Deep vein thrombosis, arterial thrombosis, hypo/hypertension, heart failure
GI: Nausea, vomiting, *anorexia, diarrhea,* constipation, *abdominal pain,* colitis, taste change, dyspepsia, stomatitis, GI hemorrhage/perforation
GU: Proteinuria, vaginal hemorrhage
HEMA: Leukopenia, neutropenia, thrombocytopenia
META: Bilirubinemia, hypokalemia
MISC: Exfoliative dermatitis, *alopecia*
RESP: Dyspnea, upper respiratory tract infection, hemoptysis
INTEG: Skin discoloration, infusion reactions, dry skin, skin ulcer, palmar-plantar erythrodysesthesia

PHARMACOKINETICS
Half-life 20 days, steady-state 100 days

INTERACTIONS
• Avoid concurrent use with SUNItinib; microangiopathic hemolytic anemia may occur

Increase: CV toxicity antineoplastics

Increase: osteonecrosis of the jaw—biophosphates

Decrease: immune response to live virus vaccines

Drug/Lab

Increase: bilirubin

Decrease: neutrophil, platelets, WBC, potassium

NURSING CONSIDERATIONS
Assess:
• B/P; take frequently if hypertension develops, discontinue if hypertensive crisis occurs
• For symptoms of infection; may be masked by product
• **CNS reaction:** dizziness, confusion
• **HF:** crackles, jugular venous distention, dyspnea during treatment
• **GU status (proteinuria):** nephrotic syndrome may occur; monitor urinalysis for increasing protein level; product should be held if protein ≥2 g/24 hr; resume when <2 g/24 hr

Black Box Warning: **Wound dehiscence:** hold for ≥28 days until incision is healed, discontinue 28 days prior to elective surgery; if wound dehicence occurs discontinue

Black Box Warning: **GI perforation** (constipation, fever, abdominal pain, nausea, vomiting), **serious bleeding** (bleeding from any orifice, stroke, deep vein thrombosis), **nephrotic syndrome, hypertensive crisis;** product should be discontinued permanently; surgery should be postponed

• **Thromboembolic events:** monitor for stroke, TIA, MI; usually occurs in geriatric patients who used this product previously
• **Fistulas:** may occur within 6 mo of beginning treatment, may be fatal

• **Reversible posterior leukoencephalopathy syndrome (RPLS):** discontinue if this disorder develops (headache, vision changes, seizures, altered mental status); MRI may be ordered, occurs 16 hr-1 yr after beginning treatment
• **Infusion reactions:** Monitor for headache, increased B/P, chest pain, sweating, wheezing or trouble breathing; provide antihistamine, corticosteroids, if severe epinephrine
• **Pregnancy/breastfeeding:** drug may lead to fetal harm; do not use in pregnancy, do not breastfeed during and for 6 mo after last dose; use contraception during and for 6 mo after last dose

Evaluate:
• Therapeutic response: decrease in size of tumors

Teach patient/family:
• To avoid hazardous tasks because confusion, dizziness may occur
• To report signs of infection: sore throat, fever, diarrhea, vomiting

Black Box Warning: **Hemorrhage/ bleeding:** to report bleeding, changes in urinary patterns, edema, abdominal pain

• To avoid live virus vaccines
• About the need to discontinue product 1 mo before surgery and not to restart until wound is healed
• **Pregnancy/breastfeeding:** that fetal harm may occur, not to breastfeed, not to become pregnant while taking this product or for 6 mo after discontinuing treatment; discuss possible infertility with patient

---

bezlotoxumab (Rx)
(bez'loe-tox'ue-mab)
Zinplava
Func. class.: Antidiarrheal

USES: For *Clostridium difficile* infection (CDI) in patients who are receiving antibacterial treatment of CDI and are at a high risk for CDI recurrence

---

CONTRAINDICATIONS
Hypersensitivity

Precautions: Breastfeeding, pregnancy, heart failure

DOSAGE AND ROUTES
• **Adult:** IV 10 mg/kg as a single dose
Available forms: Solution for injection 25 mg/mL

---

bictegravir/emtricitabine/tenofovir alafenamide (Rx)
(bik-teg´-ra-veer/em-try-sye´tah-been/ten-of´oh-veer al´e´fen´a-mide)

Biktarvy
Func. class.: HIV antivirals
Chem. class.: Integrase strand transfer inhibitor (INSTI); nucleoside and nucleotide reverse transcriptase inhibitor (NRTI) combinations

---

ACTION: A 3-drug combination of bictegravir (BIC), an HIV-1 integrase strand transfer inhibitor (INSTI), and emtricitabine (FTC) and tenofovir alafenamide (TAF), both HIV-1 nucleoside analog reverse transcriptase inhibitors (NRTIs)

USES: Complete regimen for the treatment of HIV-1 infection in adults who have no antiretroviral treatment history or to replace the current antiretroviral regimen in those who are virologically suppressed (HIV-1 RNA <50 copies per mL)

CONTRAINDICATIONS
Do not use with dofetilide, rifAMPin; hypersensitivity
Precautions: Alcoholism, breastfeeding, Graves' disease, pregnancy, hepatic impairment, HIV resistance, immune reconstitution syndrome, infection resistance, osteoporosis, renal impairment, lactic acidosis/severe hepatomegaly with steatosis, suicidal ideation

Black Box Warning: Hepatitis B and HIV coinfection, hepatitis B exacerbation

DOSAGE AND ROUTES
• **Adult:** 1 tablet daily
Available forms: Tablets 50 mg bictegravir, 200 mg emtricitabine, 25 mg tenofovir alafenamide

Administer:
• With or without food
• Do not use 2 hr before or after dairy products or antacids that contain aluminum, magnesium, or calcium

SIDE EFFECTS
CNS: Fatigue, abnormal dreams, headache, depression, suicidal ideation
GI: Nausea, vomiting, diarrhea, steatosis, hepatomegaly, exacerbation of HBV infection
HEMA: Immune reconstitution syndrome
MISC: Lactic acidosis, rash

PHARMACOKINETICS
Bictegravir: Protein binding >99%, elimination via metabolism, mediated by CYP3A and UGT1A1 enzymes; excreted in feces (60.3%), urine (35%), half-life 17.3 hr
Emtricitabine: Protein binding <4%, excreted in urine (70%), feces (13.7%), half-life 10 hr
Tenofovir AF: Protein binding 80%, elimination via metabolism (more than 80% of dose), excreted in feces (31.7%), elimination of metabolite via kidneys (70%-80%) by a combination of glomerular filtration and active tubular secretion, half-life 0.51 hr; metabolite half-life of 150-180 hr

INTERACTIONS
• Do not use with other antiretrovirals for HIV, rifAMPin
Increase: effect of metFORMIN
Increase: effect of this HIV combination product—OCT2 and MATE1 (dofetilide); CYP3A4 inhibitors, UGT1A1 inhibitors
Decrease: concentration of this HIV combination product—carBAMazepine, OXcarbazepine, phenobarbital, phenytoin; use alternative anticonvulsants

---

Decrease: concentration of this HIV combination product—products that inhibit P-gp and BCRP

Drug/Herb
Avoid use with St. John's wort

NURSING CONSIDERATIONS
Assess:
• **HIV:** symptoms and change in severity; opportunistic infections may occur with HIV; assess for these infections throughout therapy
• **Osteoporosis and bone mineral loss:** assess those who have had prior fractures, osteoporosis, or mineral bone loss
• **Hepatitis B infection:** before use, test for hepatitis B virus infection; monitor hepatitis B serology, plasma hepatitis C RNA
• **Lab testing:** before use and periodically during treatment, assess serum creatinine, estimated CCr, urine glucose, urine protein, serum phosphorus in those with chronic kidney disease
• Monitor blood glucose, CBC with differential, CD4+ T-cell count, LFTs, plasma HIV RNA, pregnancy testing (if applicable), serum bilirubin (total and direct), serum cholesterol, BUN, serum lipid profile, urinalysis

Black Box Warning: Exacerbations of HBV in coinfection with HBV: monitor for several months after treatment especially in hepatotoxicity

• **Pregnancy/breastfeeding:** for pregnant women, therapy should begin immediately after HIV diagnosis. Therapy may be initiated before drug resistance testing results are available; modify based on the assay
• **Depression and suicidal ideation:** although rare, has occurred in those with depression before treatment
• **Immune reconstitution syndrome:** that patients may develop an inflammatory response to opportunistic infections (such as *Mycobacterium avium* infection, cytomegalovirus, *Pneumocystis jirovecii*

pneumonia [PCP], or TB), autoimmune disorders (Graves' disease, polymyositis, and Guillain-Barré syndrome); response may occur during or many months after starting treatment
Evaluate:
• Therapeutic response: improving signs and symptoms of HIV, improving CD4+ counts, plasma HIV RNA with only moderate side effects

TEACH PATIENT/FAMILY
• To take as directed, not to skip or double doses; if missed, to take when remembered; not to share with others
• That product is not a cure; that patient is still infective and may transmit infection to others via sexual contact, blood transfusions, or sharing needles; to practice safe sex, as using a condom will prevent transmission from person to person; not to donate blood
• That lab testing will be required periodically during treatment
• **Lactic acidosis/hepatomegaly with stenosis:** to report immediately nausea, vomiting, abdominal pain, severe weakness
• To inform all health care providers of OTC, Rx, herbal products, supplements taken; not to start or stop without consent of prescriber; to avoid St. John's wort
• Not to use antacids, dairy products 2 hr before or after this product
• **Pregnancy/breastfeeding:** to notify health care provider if pregnancy is planned or suspected; if pregnant, to enroll in the Antiretroviral Pregnancy Registry (800-258-4263); to avoid breastfeeding

bimatoprost (ophthalmic/topical) (Rx)
(by-mat'oh-prost)
Durysta, Latisse, Lumigan
Func. class.: Antiglaucoma agent

Do not confuse:
bimatoprost/travoprost

USES: Increased intraocular pressure in those with open-angle glaucoma/ocular hypertension (Lumigan); eyelash hypotrichosis (Latisse)

CONTRAINDICATIONS
Hypersensitivity to this product, benzalkonium chloride
Precautions: Children, intraocular inflammation, closed-angle glaucoma, macular edema, contact lenses, ocular infection, surgery, trauma; corneal abrasion, iritis, urethritis

DOSAGE AND ROUTES
Increased intraocular pressure/ ocular hypertension (Lumigan)
• **Adult: OPHTH Instill** 1 drop in each affected eye (conjunctival sac) every night
Eyelash hypotrichosis (Latisse)
• **Adult: Apply** 1 drop to skin of upper eyelid margin at base of eyelashes every night using a new supplied disposable sterile applicator
Available forms: Ophthalmic solution 0.01%; topical solution 0.03%; implant

---

binimetinib (Rx)
(bih´-nee-meh´-tih-nib)
Mektovi
Func. class.: Antineoplastic

USES: Treatment of unresectable/metastatic melanoma (BRAF V600E or V600K mutations) with encorafenib

CONTRAINDICATIONS
Hypersensitivity

DOSAGE AND ROUTES
• **Adult: PO** 45 mg bid with encorafenib
PO 450 mg daily until disease progression
Available forms: Tablets 15 mg

bisacodyl (Rx, OTC)
(bis-a-koe´dill)
Peglyte ✦, Bisacolax, Bisacolax, Correctol, Carter's Little Pills ✦, Codulax ✦, Ducodyl, Doxidan, Dulcolax, Ex-Lax Ultra, Femilax, Fleet, Laxative for Women ✦, Silver Bullet Suppository ✦, The Magic Bullet ✦ Soflax-Ex ✦
Func. class.: Laxative, stimulant
Chem. class.: Diphenylmethane

Do not confuse:
Dulcolax (bisacodyl)/Dulcolax (docusate)

ACTION: Acts directly on intestine by increasing peristalsis; thought to irritate colonic intramural plexus

USES: Short-term treatment of constipation; bowel or rectal preparation for surgery, examination

CONTRAINDICATIONS
Hypersensitivity, abdominal pain, nausea, vomiting, appendicitis, acute surgical abdomen, ulcerated hemorrhoids, acute hepatitis, fecal impaction, intestinal/ biliary tract obstruction
Precautions: Pregnancy, breastfeeding, rectal fissures, severe CV disease

DOSAGE AND ROUTES
• **Adult and child ≥12 yr: PO** 5-15 mg in PM or AM; may use up to 30 mg for bowel or rectal preparation; **RECT** 10 mg as a single dose; 30-mL enema
• **Child 6-11 yr: PO** 5 mg as a single dose; **RECT** 5 mg as a single dose
Available forms: Tablets delayed release 5, 10 mg; enteric-coated tablets 5 mg; suppository 5, 10 mg; rectal solution 10 mg/30 mL
Administer:
PO route
• Use lowest dose
• Swallow tablets whole with full glass of water; do not break, crush, chew tablets

---

• Take alone only with water for better absorption; do not take within 1 hr of other products or within 1 hr of antacids, milk, H$_2$ antagonists; do not take enteric product with proton-pump inhibitors

• In AM or PM

Rectal route

• Insert high in rectum end first, effect in 15 min-1 hr

SIDE EFFECTS

CNS: Muscle weakness
GI: *Nausea, anorexia, cramps,* diarrhea, rectal burning (suppositories)
META: Protein-losing   enteropathy (extended use), hypokalemia (extended use), tetany

PHARMACOKINETICS

Small amounts absorbed/metabolized by liver; excreted in urine, bile, feces, breast milk
PO: Onset 6-10 hr
RECT: Onset 15-60 min

INTERACTIONS

Increase: gastric irritation—antacids, milk, H$_2$ blockers, gastric acid pump inhibitors
Decrease: absorption with antacids, H$_2$ blockers, gastric acid pump inhibitors
Drug/Food
Increase   irritation—dairy   products, separate by 2 hr
Drug/Lab
Increase: sodium phosphate
Decrease: calcium, magnesium
Drug/Herb
Increase: laxative action—flexibility of the valley, pheasant's eye, senna, squill

NURSING CONSIDERATIONS
Assess:

• Blood, urine electrolytes if product is used often by patient

• I&O ratio to identify fluid loss

• Cause of constipation; identify whether fluids, bulk, exercise missing from lifestyle; determine use of constipating products

• **GI symptoms:** cramping, rectal bleeding, nausea, if these symptoms occur, product should be discontinued

• Multiple products/routes may be used for bowel prep

Evaluate:

• Therapeutic response: decrease in constipation, removal of stool from colon

Teach patient/family:

• Not to use laxatives for long-term therapy because bowel tone will be lost; 1-wk use is usually sufficient

• That normal bowel movements do not always occur daily

• Not to use in presence of abdominal pain, nausea, vomiting

• To notify prescriber if constipation is unrelieved or if symptoms of electrolyte imbalance occur: muscle cramps, pain, weakness, dizziness

• To take with a full glass of water; if using with dairy products separate by 2 hr; to separate from other foods by 1 hr

• Identify bulk, water, constipating products, exercise in patient's life

---

bismuth subsalicylate (OTC)

(bis'muth sub-sal-iss'uh-late)

Bismatrol, Kaopectate, Kao-Tin, Peptic Relief, Pepto-Bismol, Pink Bismuth, Kaopectolin, K-Pek, Maalox Total Stomach Relief, Stomach Relief

Func. class.: Antidiarrheal, weak antacid
Chem. class.: Salicylate

Do not confuse:
Kaopectate/Kayexalate

ACTION: Inhibits the prostaglandin synthesis responsible for GI hypermotility, intestinal   inflammation;   stimulates absorption of fluid and electrolytes; binds toxins produced by *Escherichia coli*

USES: Relief of diarrhea, heartburn, indigestion, nausea, upset stomach

CONTRAINDICATIONS

Children <3 yr, children with chickenpox, history of GI bleeding, flulike symptoms, hypersensitivity to product or salicylates, PUD

Side effects: *italics* = common; red = life-threatening

Precautions: Pregnancy, breastfeeding, geriatric patients, gout, diabetes mellitus, bleeding disorders, previous hypersensitivity to NSAIDs, *Clostridium difficile*–associated diarrhea when used with anti-infectives for *Helicobacter pylori*

DOSAGE AND ROUTES
Antidiarrheal/gastric distress
• **Adult/adolescent: PO** 524 mg (2 tablets or 30 mL) q30-60min as needed, max 8 doses/day; or 1050 mg (30 mL) hourly as needed, max 4 doses/day
H. pylori
• **Adult/adolescent: PO** 525 mg qid, max 4.2 g/24 hr; given with metroNIDAZOLE or tetracycline and acid-suppressive therapy × 14 days
Traveler's diarrhea (unlabeled)
• **Adult: PO** 30 mL q30min (8×/day regular strength, 4×/day max strength)
Available forms: Tablets 262 mg; chewable tablets 262 mg; liquid 262 mg/15 mL, 525 mg/15 mL
Administer:
• Increase fluids to rehydrate patient
• **Suspension:** shake liquid before using; use measuring cup, syringe
• Tablets can be chewed, dissolved in mouth; caplets to be swallowed whole with water

SIDE EFFECTS
CNS: Confusion, twitching, neurotoxicity (high doses)
EENT: Hearing loss, tinnitus, metallic taste, blue gums, black tongue
GI: Increased fecal impaction (high doses), dark stools, constipation, diarrhea, nausea
HEMA: Increased bleeding time
MISC: Reye's syndrome

PHARMACOKINETICS
PO: Onset 1 hr, peak 2 hr, duration 4 hr

INTERACTIONS
Increase: toxicity—salicylates, methotrexate
Increase: effect of anticoagulants (PO), antidiabetics (PO)
Decrease: absorption of tetracycline, quinolones, phenytoin; separate for ≥2 hr

Drug/Lab Test
Interference: radiographic studies of GI system

NURSING CONSIDERATIONS
Assess:
• **Diarrhea:** bowel pattern before product therapy, after treatment
• **GI status:** abdominal pain, nausea, heartburn, bowel sounds
• **Pregnancy/breastfeeding:** avoid in pregnancy; do not breastfeed
• Electrolytes K, Na, Cl if diarrhea is severe or continues long term; assess skin turgor, other signs of dehydration
Evaluate:
• Therapeutic response: decreased diarrhea, absence of diarrhea when traveling; resolution of ulcers
Teach patient/family:
• To chew, dissolve tablets in mouth; not to swallow whole; to shake liquid before using, maintain hydration
• To avoid other salicylates unless directed by prescriber; not to give to children, possibility of Reye's syndrome
• That stools may turn black; that tongue may darken; that impaction may occur in debilitated patients
• To stop use if symptoms do not improve within 2 days or become worse, or if diarrhea is accompanied by high fever
• To separate quinolones, phenytoin, tetracyclines by ≥2 hr

⚠ HIGH ALERT

bisoprolol (Rx)
(bis-oh′pro-lole)
Func. class.: Antihypertensive
Chem. class.: β_1-blocker

Do not confuse:
bisoprolol/buPROPion/busPIRone

ACTION: Blocks stimulation of β_1-adrenergic receptors within cardiac muscle (decreases rate of SA node discharge, increases recovery time), slows conduction of AV node, decreases heart rate, which decreases O_2 consumption in myocardium; decreases renin-angiotensin-aldosterone system; inhibits beta 2 receptors (bronchial/vascular smooth muscle) at high doses

USES: Mild to moderate hypertension
Unlabeled uses: Heart failure with reduced ejection fraction

CONTRAINDICATIONS

Hypersensitivity to beta-blockers, cardiogenic shock, heart block (second, third degree), sinus bradycardia, acute cardiac failure
Precautions: Pregnancy, breastfeeding, children, major surgery, diabetes mellitus, HF, thyroid/renal/hepatic disease, COPD, asthma, well-compensated heart failure, aortic or mitral valve disease, peripheral vascular disease, myasthenia gravis, abrupt discontinuation

DOSAGE AND ROUTES
Hypertension
• **Adult: PO** 5 mg/day; reduce to 2.5 mg in bronchospastic disease; may increase to 20 mg/day if necessary; max 20 mg/day
Heart failure with reduced injection fraction (unlabeled)
Adult: PO 1.25 mg daily, max 10 mg daily
Renal/hepatic dose
• **Adult: PO** CCr <40 mL/min 2.5 mg, titrate upward
Available forms: Tablets 5, 10 mg
Administer:
• Take apical pulse before each dose, if <50 bpm, withhold
• Do not crush, swallow whole; may give without regard to meals, at same time of day
• Store protected from light, moisture; at room temperature

SIDE EFFECTS
CNS: Insomnia, fatigue, dizziness, headache
CV: Bradycardia, HF, postural hypotension, peripheral edema, cold extremities
EENT: Blurred vision, dry mouth
ENDO: Hypoglycemia
GI: Nausea, diarrhea, vomiting

INTEG: Rash, sweating
RESP: Dyspnea, cough

PHARMACOKINETICS
Onset 1-2 hr, peak 2-4 hr, duration unknown, half-life 9-12 hr, 50% excreted unchanged in urine, protein binding 30%-36%, metabolized in liver to inactive metabolites

INTERACTIONS
Increase: myocardial depression—calcium channel blockers, phenytoin (IV), verapamil
Increase: antihypertensive effect—ACE inhibitors, alpha-blockers, calcium channel blockers, diuretics, nitrates
Increase: bradycardia—digoxin, amiodarone cloNIDine, dilTIAZem, verapamil, reserpine, guanethidine
Increase: antidiabetic effect—antidiabetics; may mask hypoglycemic symptoms
Increase: peripheral ischemia—ergots
Decrease: antihypertensive effect—NSAIDs, salicylates
Drug/Herb
Increase: Beta-blocking effect—hawthorn
Decrease: Beta-blocking effect—ephedra, licorice root
Drug/Lab Test
Increase: AST, ALT, blood glucose, BUN, uric acid, potassium, creatinine, phosphorus

NURSING CONSIDERATIONS
Assess:
• **Hypertension:** B/P, pulse during beginning treatment, periodically thereafter; pulse: note rate, rhythm, quality; apical/radial pulse prior to administration; notify prescriber of any significant changes (pulse <50 bpm); monitor ECG baseline and periodically
• Baselines of renal, hepatic studies prior to beginning therapy
• **Heart failure:** I&O, weight daily; increased weight, jugular venous distention, dyspnea, crackles; edema in feet, legs daily; avoid use in severe heart failure
• Skin turgor, dryness of mucous membranes for hydration status, especially for geriatric patients

• **Abrupt discontinuation:** Taper over 1 wk, abrupt discontinuation may increase angina
• **Surgery:** Do not discontinue before surgery
• **Pregnancy/breastfeeding:** Use only if clearly needed in pregnancy, use cautiously in breastfeeding

Evaluate:
• Therapeutic response: decreased B/P after 1-2 wk

Teach patient/family:
• Not to discontinue product abruptly, taper over 1 wk; may cause precipitate angina, rebound hypertension; evaluate noncompliance
• Not to use OTC products that contain alpha-adrenergic stimulants (e.g., nasal decongestants, OTC cold preparations) unless directed by prescriber
• To report slow heart rate, dizziness, confusion, depression, fever, cold extremities
• To take pulse at home; advise when to notify prescriber
• To avoid alcohol, smoking; to limit sodium intake
• To comply with weight control, dietary adjustments, modified exercise program
• To carry emergency ID to identify product, allergies
• To avoid hazardous activities if dizziness is present
• **To report symptoms of heart failure:** difficulty breathing especially on exertion or when lying down, night cough, swelling of extremities
• That if diabetic, product may mask signs of hypoglycemia or alter blood glucose levels

Pregnancy/breastfeeding: To notify health care professional if pregnancy is planned or suspected or if breastfeeding

TREATMENT OF OVERDOSE:
Lavage, IV atropine for bradycardia; IV theophylline for bronchospasm; digoxin, O_2, diuretic for cardiac failure; hemodialysis, IV glucose for hypoglycemia; IV diazePAM or phenytoin for seizures

---

⚠ HIGH ALERT

bivalirudin (Rx)
(bye-val-i-rue′din)
Angiomax
Func. class.: Anticoagulant
Chem. class.: Direct thrombin inhibitor

ACTION: Direct inhibitor of thrombin that is highly specific; able to inhibit free and clot-bound thrombin

USES: Unstable angina in patients undergoing percutaneous transluminal coronary angioplasty (PTCA), used with aspirin; heparin-induced thrombocytopenia, with/without thrombosis syndrome, PCI with IIb/IIIa
Unlabeled: ST-elevation MI (primary PCI), non-ST elevation, ACS (moderate-high risk) early invasive strategy

CONTRAINDICATIONS
Hypersensitivity, active bleeding, cerebral aneurysm, intracranial hemorrhage, recent surgery, CVA
Precautions: Pregnancy, breastfeeding, children, geriatric patients, renal function impairment, hepatic disease, asthma, blood dyscrasias, thrombocytopenia, GI ulcers, hypertension, inflammatory bowel disease, vitamin K deficiency, asthma

DOSAGE AND ROUTES

Anticoagulation in unstable angina in those undergoing PTCA or PCI with provisional use of platelet glycoprotein inhibitor
• **Adult:** IV BOLUS 0.75 mg/kg, then **IV INFUSION** 1.75 mg/kg/hr for 4 hr; another **IV INFUSION** may be used at 0.2 mg/kg/hr for ≤20 hr; this product is intended to be used with aspirin (325 mg/day) adjusted to body weight

Patients undergoing PCI at risk for HIT/HITTS or ST elevation in patients undergoing primary PCI (unlabeled)
Adult: IV BOLUS 0.75 mg/kg, then continuous infusion 1.75 mg/kg/hr for duration of procedure, may give another infu-

sion after 4 hr of 0.2 mcg/kg/hr up to 20 hr, give with aspirin 325 mg

ST-elevation MI (undergoing primary PCI) (unlabeled)
Adults: 0.75 mg/kg/IV bolus, then 1.75 mg/kg IV infusion for duration. May give additional 0.3 mg/kg bolus dose if needed. May continue bolus dose if needed. May continue infusion at 1.75 mg/kg for up to 4 hr after procedure. If infusion is continued, may continue infusion at 0.2 mg/kg for up to 20 hr

Non-ST-elevation ACS (moderate to high risk) (early invasive strategy) (unlabeled)
Adults: If initiating during PCI, give 0.75 mg/kg IV bolus, followed by 1.75 mg/kg/hr IV infusion for duration of procedure. May give additional 0.3 mg/kg bolus dose if needed. May continue infusion at 1.75 mg/kg for up to 4 hr after procedure. If infusion is continued and an additional infusion is necessary, may continue infusion at a reduced dose of 0.2 mg/kg for up to 20 hr. If unfractionated heparin was given before procedure, wait 30 min before using bivalirudin. If initiating before PCI or diagnostic angiography, give 0.1 mg/kg IV bolus, then by 0.25 mg/kg IV infusion, continue until angiogram or PCI

Renal dose
• **Adult:** IV CCr ≥30 mL/min no adjustment; CCr 10-29 mL/min consider reducing to 1 mL/kg/hr; hemodialysis 0.25 mg/kg/hr, same bolus dose

Available forms: Injection, lyophilized 250 mg/vial

Administer:
• Before PTCA; give with aspirin (325 mg)
• Store reconstituted vials in refrigerator for up to 24 hr; store diluted concentrations at room temperature for 24 hr

IV, direct route
• Dilute by adding 5 mL of sterile water for injection/250 mg bivalirudin, swirl until dissolved, further dilute in 50 mL of D₅W or 0.9% NaCl (5 mg/mL), give by bolus injection 0.75 mg/kg, then intermittent infusion

Intermittent IV INFUSION route
• To each 250-mg vial add 5 mL of sterile water for injection, swirl until dissolved, further dilute in 500 mL D₅W or 0.9% NaCl (0.5 mg/mL); give infusion after bolus dose at a rate of 1.75 mg/kg/hr; may give an additional infusion at 0.2 mg/kg/hr

Y-site compatibilities: Abciximab, acyclovir, alfentanil, allopurinol, amifostine, amikacin, aminocaproic acid, aminophylline, amphotericin B liposome, ampicillin, ampicillin-sulbactam, anidulafungin, argatroban, arsenic trioxide, atenolol, atracurium, atropine, azithromycin, aztreonam, bleomycin, bumetanide, buprenorphine, busulfan, butorphanol, calcium chloride/gluconate, capreomycin, CARBOplatin, carmustine, ceFAZolin, cefepime, cefotaxime, cefoTEtan, cefOXitin, cefTAZidime, ceftizoxime, cefTRIAXone, cefuroxime, chloramphenicol, cimetidine, ciprofloxacin, cisatracurium, CISplatin, clindamycin, cyclophosphamide, cycloSPORINE, cytarabine, dacarbazine, DACTINomycin, DAPTOmycin, DAUNOrubicin, DAUNOrubicin liposome, dexamethasone, dexmedetomidine, dexrazoxane, digoxin, diltiazem, diphenhydrAMINE, DOCEtaxel, dolasetron, DOPamine, DOXOrubicin, DOXOrubicin liposomal, doxycycline, droperidol, enalaprilat, ePHEDrine, EPINEPHrine, epirubicin, epoprostenol, eptifibatide, ertapenem, erythromycin, esmolol, etoposide, etoposide phosphate, famotidine, fenoldopam, fentaNYL, fluconazole, fludarabine, fluorouracil, foscarnet, fosphenytoin, furosemide, gallium, ganciclovir, gatifloxacin, gemcitabine, gentamicin, glycopyrrolate, granisetron, haloperidol, heparin, hydrALAZINE, hydrocortisone, HYDROmorphone, hydrOXYzine, IDArubicin, ifosfamide, imipenem-cilastatin, inamrinone, insulin (regular), irinotecan, isoproterenol, ketorolac, labetalol, leucovorin, levofloxacin, lidocaine, linezolid, LORazepam, magnesium, mannitol, mechlorethamine, melphalan, meperidine, meropenem, mesna, methohexital, methotrexate, methyldopate, methylPREDNISolone, metoclopramide, metoprolol, metroNIDAZOLE, midazolam, milrinone, mitoMYcin, mito-XANtrone, mivacurium, morphine, moxifloxacin, mycophenolate mofetil, nafcillin, nalbuphine, naloxone, nesiritide, niCARdipine, nitroglycerin, nitroprusside, norepinephrine, octreotide, ofloxacin, ondansetron, oxaliplatin, oxytocin, PACLitaxel, palonosetron, pamidronate, pancuronium, PEMEtrexed, PENTobarbital, PHENobarbital, phenylephrine, piperacillin, piperacillin-tazobactam, polymyxin B, potassium acetate/chloride/phosphates, procainamide, promethazine, propranolol, ranitidine, remifentanil, rocuronium, sodium acetate/bicarbonate/phosphates, streptozocin, succinylcholine, SUFentanil, sulfamethoxazole-trimethoprim, tacrolimus, teniposide, theophylline, thiopental, thiotepa, ticarcillin, ticarcillin-clavulanate, tigecycline, tirofiban, tobramycin, topotecan, vasopressin, vecuronium, verapamil, vinBLAStine, vinCRIStine, vinorelbine, voriconazole, warfarin, zidovudine, zoledronic acid

SIDE EFFECTS

CNS: *Headache, insomnia, anxiety, nervousness*
CV: *Hypo/hypertension, bradycardia,* ventricular fibrillation
GI: *Nausea, vomiting, abdominal pain, dyspepsia*
HEMA: Hemorrhage, thrombocytopenia
MISC: Pain at injection site, pelvic pain, urinary retention, fever, anaphylaxis, infection
MS: *Back pain*
GU: Urinary retention, renal failure, oliguria

PHARMACOKINETICS

Excreted in urine, half-life 25 min, onset rapid, peak immediate duration 1 hr, no protein binding

INTERACTIONS

Increase: bleeding risk—abciximab, anticoagulants, aspirin, thrombolytics, cephalosporins, use together cautiously
Drug/Herb
Increase: bleeding risk—angelica, chamomile, devil's claw, dong quai, garlic, ginger, ginkgo, ginseng, horse chestnut, licorice, saw palmetto; avoid concurrent use

NURSING CONSIDERATIONS

Assess:
• **Bleeding:** check arterial and venous sites, IM injection sites, catheters; all punctures should be minimized; fall in B/P or Hct may indicate hemorrhage; hematoma, hemorrhage at puncture site are more common in the elderly; monitor coagulation studies, Hct before use; baseline and periodic ACT, aPTT, PT, INR, TT, platelets, HB, Hct
• CV status: B/P; watch for hypo/hypertension, bradycardia
• Neurologic status: any focal or generalized deficits should be reported immediately
• **PCI use:** possible thrombosis, stenosis, unplanned stent, prolonged ischemia, decreased reflow
• **Renal function:** dosage reductions may be required
Pregnancy/breastfeeding: use only if clearly needed, use cautiously in breastfeeding
Evaluate:
• Therapeutic response: anticoagulation with PTCA, PCI; resolution of heparin-induced thrombocytopenia, thrombosis syndrome
Teach patient/family:
• About the reason for the product and expected results
• To report black, tarry stools; blood in urine; difficulty breathing
• Not to use any OTC, herbal products unless approved by prescriber
• Not to use hard-bristle toothbrush or regular razor to avoid any injury; hemorrhage may result
• **Pregnancy/breastfeeding:** Report if pregnancy is planned or suspected or if breastfeeding

---

⚠ HIGH ALERT

bleomycin (Rx)

(blee-oh-mye′sin)
Func. class.: Antineoplastic, antibiotic
Chem. class.: Glycopeptide

ACTION: Inhibits synthesis of DNA, RNA, protein; derived from *Streptomyces verticillus;* phase specific to the G_2 and M phases; a nonvesicant, sclerosing agent

USES: Squamous cell carcinoma of head, neck, penis, cervix, vulva; Hodgkin's/non-Hodgkin's disease; testicular carcinoma; as a sclerosing agent for malignant pleural effusion

CONTRAINDICATIONS
Pregnancy, breastfeeding, hypersensitivity

Precautions: Patients >70 yr old, renal/hepatic disease, respiratory disease, max lifetime dose 400 units, fever

> **Black Box Warning:** Pulmonary fibrosis; requires specialized care setting, experienced clinician

DOSAGE AND ROUTES
Test dose
• **Adult/child (unlabeled): IM/IV/SUBCUT** ≤2 units for first 2 doses followed by 24 hr of observation
Non-Hodgkin's lymphoma, testicular cancer, squamous cell carcinoma
• **Adult/child: SUBCUT/IV/IM** After test dose 0.25-0.5 unit/kg 1-2×/wk or 10-20 units/m², then 1 unit/day or 5 units/wk; max total dose of 400 units during lifetime
Hodgkin's lymphoma
• **Adult/adolescent ≥15 yr: SUBCUT/IV/IM** After test dose 5-20 units/m² may be given in combination
Malignant pleural effusion
• **Adult: BOLUS INTRAPLEURAL** 60 units as a single dose
Renal dose
• **Adult/child:** CCr 40-50 mL/min reduce dose by 30%; CCr 30-39 mL/min reduce dose by 40%; CCr 20-29 mL/min reduce dose by 45%; CCr 10-19 mL/min reduce dose by 55%; CCr 5-10 mL/min reduce dose by 60%

Available forms: Powder for injection, 15, 30 units/vial
Administer:
• Antiemetic 30-60 min prior to giving product to prevent vomiting
• Topical or systemic analgesics for pain of stomatitis as ordered; antihistamines and antipyretics for fever, chills
• May be given IM, SUBCUT, IV, intrapleurally, intralesionally, intraarterially
IM/SUBCUT route
• After reconstituting 15 units/1-5 mL or 30 units/2-10 mL of 0.9% NaCl or bacteriostatic water for injection, max concentration 5 units/mL, rotate injection sites; do not use products that contain benzyl alcohol when giving to neonates or that contain dextrose because of loss of potency
IV route
• Use cytotoxic handling procedures
• After reconstituting 15- or 30-unit vial with 5 or 10 mL of NS, respectively, inject slowly over 10 min or, after further dilution with 50-100 mL 0.9% NaCl, give at prescribed rate
• For patients with lymphoma, give 2 test doses of 2-5 units before initial dose; monitor for anaphylaxis
• Store for 2 wk after reconstituting if refrigerated or for 24 hr at room temperature; discard unused portions

Y-site compatibilities: Acyclovir, alfentanil, allopurinol, amifostine, amikacin, aminocaproic acid, aminophylline, amiodarone, ampicillin, ampicillin-sulbactam, anidulafungin, atenolol, atracurium, azithromycin, aztreonam, bivalirudin, bumetanide, buprenorphine, busulfan, butorphanol, calcium chloride/gluconate, CARBOplatin, carmustine, caspofungin, ceFAZolin, cefepime, cefotaxime, cefoTEtan, cefOXitin, cefTAZidime, ceftizoxime, cefTRIAXone, cefuroxime, chloramphenicol, chlorproMAZINE, cimetidine, ciprofloxacin, cisatracurium, CISplatin, clindamycin, codeine, cyclophosphamide, cycloSPORINE, cytarabine, dacarbazine, DACTINomycin, DAPTOmycin, DAUNOrubicin, dexamethasone, dexmedetomidine, dexrazoxane, digoxin, diltiazem, diphenhydrAMINE, DOBUTamine, DOCEtaxel, DOPamine, doxacurium, DOXOrubicin, DOXOrubicin liposomal, doxycycline, droperidol, enalaprilat, ePHEDrine, EPINEPHrine, epirubicin, ertapenem, erythromycin, esmolol, etoposide, famotidine, fenoldopam, fentaNYL, filgrastim, fluconazole, fludarabine, fluorouracil, foscarnet, fosphenytoin, furosemide, ganciclovir, gatifloxacin, gemcitabine, gentamicin, glycopyrrolate, granisetron, haloperidol, heparin, hydrALAZINE, hydrocortisone sodium succinate, HYDROmorphone, hydrOXYzine, IDArubicin, ifosfamide, imipenem-cilastatin, inamrinone, insulin (regular), irinotecan, isoproterenol, ketorolac, labetalol, leucovorin, levofloxacin, levorphanol, lidocaine, linezolid, LORazepam, magnesium sulfate, mannitol, mechlorethamine, melphalan, meperidine, meropenem, mesna, metaraminol, methohexital, methotrexate, methyldopate, methylPREDNISolone, metoclopramide, metoprolol, metroNIDAZOLE, midazolam, milrinone, minocycline, mitoMYcin, mitoXANtrone, mivacurium, morphine, nafcillin, nalbuphine, naloxone, nesiritide, niCARdipine, nitroglycerin, nitroprusside, norepinephrine, octreotide, ondansetron, oxaliplatin, palonosetron, pamidronate, pancuronium, pantoprazole, PEMEtrexed, pentamidine, pentazocine, PENTobarbital, PHENobarbital, phenylephrine, piperacillin, piperacillin-tazobactam, polymyxin B, potassium chloride, potassium phosphates, procainamide, prochlorperazine, promethazine, propranolol, quiNIDine, ranitidine, remifentanil, riTUXimab, rocuronium, sargramostim, sodium acetate, sodium bicarbonate, sodium phosphates, succinylcholine, SUFentanil, sulfamethoxazole-trimethoprim, tacrolimus, teniposide, theophylline, thiopental, thiotepa, ticarcillin, ticarcillin-clavulanate, tirofiban, tobramycin, tolazoline, trastuzumab, trimethobenzamide, vancomycin, vasopressin, vecuronium, verapamil, vinBLAStine, vinCRIStine, vinorelbine, voriconazole, zidovudine

SIDE EFFECTS

CNS: Pain at tumor site, headache, confusion, *fever*, chills, malaise
CV: Hypotension, peripheral vasoconstriction
GI: *Nausea, vomiting, anorexia, stomatitis, weight loss*
GU: Hemolytic-uremic syndrome
INTEG: *Rash, alopecia,* hyperpigmentation
RESP: Fibrosis, pneumonitis, wheezing, pulmonary toxicity
SYST: Anaphylaxis

PHARMACOKINETICS

Half-life 2-4 hr; when CCr is >35 mL/min, half-life is increased with lower clearance; metabolized in liver; 70% excreted in urine (unchanged) **IV, IM, SUBCUT:** Peak 30-60 min

INTERACTIONS

• Avoid live virus vaccines concurrently; adverse reactions may occur
Increase: bleomycin toxicity—cisplatin
Increase: oxygen requirements—anesthesia
Decrease: serum phenytoin levels—phenytoin, fosphenytoin; check drug level periodically
Drug/Lab Test
Increase: uric acid

NURSING CONSIDERATIONS
Assess:
• IM test dose of 1-2 units in patients with lymphoma before first 2 doses
• CBC, differential baseline and periodically, thrombocytopenia, leukopenia may occur (nadir 12 days)

Black Box Warning: Pulmonary toxicity/ fibrosis: risk increases >70 yr; pulmonary function tests; chest x-ray before, during therapy, should be obtained q2wk during treatment; pulmonary diffusion capacity for carbon monoxide (DLCO) monthly, if <40% of pretreatment value, stop treatment; treat pulmonary infection before treatment; dyspnea, crackles, unproductive cough, chest pain, tachypnea, fatigue, increased pulse, pallor, lethargy, more common in the elderly, radiation therapy, pulmonary disease; usually occurs with cumulative doses >400 units

• Temperature; fever may indicate beginning infection
• Renal status: serum creatinine/BUN; CBC
• Effects of alopecia, skin color alterations on body image; discuss feelings about body changes
• Buccal cavity q8hr for dryness, sores, ulceration, white patches, oral pain, bleeding, dysphagia
• Local irritation, pain, burning, discoloration at injection site
• **Anaphylaxis:** rash, pruritus, urticaria, purpuric skin lesions, itching, flushing, wheezing, hypotension; have emergency equipment available

Black Box Warning: **Idiosyncratic reaction:** severe reaction in those with lymphoma, hypotension, mental confusion, fever, chills, wheezing in lymphoma

Black Box Warning: Requires a specialized care setting and experienced clinician due to severe reactions

• Rinsing of mouth tid-qid with water, club soda; brushing of teeth with soft brush or cotton-tipped applicators for stomatitis; use unwaxed dental floss
• **Pregnancy/breastfeeding:** do not use in pregnancy/breastfeeding
Evaluate:
• Therapeutic response: decrease in size of tumor
Teach patient/family:
• To report any changes in breathing, coughing, fever
• That hair may be lost during treatment and that wig or hairpiece may make patient feel better; that new hair may be different in color, texture
• To report any bleeding, white spots, ulcerations in mouth; to examine mouth daily and report symptoms; to report decreased urination
• That continuing exams and lab work will be needed
• **Skin toxicity:** To report rash, color changes, sensitivity, irritation
• **Stomatitis:** Teach patient that mouth ulcerations, redness may occur, use soft toothbrush

• **Pregnancy/breastfeeding:** to use contraception during treatment; to avoid breastfeeding
• Not to receive vaccines during treatment

⚠ *HIGH ALERT*

bortezomib (Rx)
(bor-tez′oh-mib)
Velcade
Func. class.: Antineoplastic—miscellaneous
Chem. class.: Proteasome inhibitor

ACTION: Reversible inhibitor of chymotrypsin-like activity; causes delay in tumor growth by disrupting normal homeostatic mechanisms

USES: Multiple myeloma previously untreated or when at least 2 other treatments have failed; mantle cell lymphoma in patients who have received ≥1 prior therapy

CONTRAINDICATIONS
Pregnancy, breastfeeding; hypersensitivity to product, boron, mannitol
Precautions: Children, geriatric patients, peripheral neuropathy, cardiac/hepatic disease, hypotension, tumor lysis syndrome, thrombocytopenia, infection, diabetes mellitus, bone marrow suppression, intracranial bleeding, injection site irritation

DOSAGE AND ROUTES
Multiple myeloma (previously untreated)
• **Adult: IV BOL/SUBCUT** Give for nine 6-wk cycles; cycles 1-4, 1.3 mg/m²/dose given on days 1, 4, 8, 11, then a 10-day rest period (days 12-21), then give again on days 22, 25, 29, 32, then a 10-day rest period (days 33-42); given with melphalan (9 mg/m²/day on days 1-4) and predniSONE (60 mg/m²/day on days 1-4); during cycles 5-9, give bortezomib 1.3 mg/m²/dose on days 1, 8, 22, 29 with melphalan (9 mg/m²/day on days 1-4) and predniSONE (60 mg/m²/day on days 1-4); this 6-wk cycle is

---

considered 1 course; at least 72 hr should elapse between consecutive doses

Mantle cell lymphoma in combination (previously untreated)

• **Adult:** IV **BOL/SUBCUT** 1.3 mg/m²/dose on days 1, 4, 8, 11 followed by a 10-day rest period (days 12-21); ×6 (3-wk) cycles with rituximab 375 mg/m², cyclophosphamide 750 mg/m², DOXOrubicin 50 mg/m² all on day 1, and predniSONE 100 mg/m² daily on days 1-5, give bortezomib before rituximab

Relapsed multiple myeloma or mantle cell lymphoma

• **Adult:** IV **BOL/SUBCUT** 1.3 mg/m²/2 × per wk on days 1, 4, 8, 11 followed by a 10-day rest period

Hepatic dose

• **Adult:** IV bilirubin >1.5 × ULN, reduce to 0.7 mg/m² during cycle 1; consider dose escalation to 1 mg/m² or further reduction to 0.5 mg/m² during next cycles based on tolerability

Available forms: Lyophilized powder for injection 3.5 mg

Administer:

• IV and SUBCUT concentrations are different

IV bolus route

• **Reconstitute** each vial with 3.5 mL of 0.9% NaCl (1 mg/mL); solution should be clear/colorless; **inject** as bolus over 3-5 sec
• Store unopened product at room temperature, protect from light
• Wear protective clothing during handling, preparation; avoid contact with skin
• Check for extravasation at injection site

SUBCUT route

• Reconstitute with 1.4 mL of NS to a final concentration of 2.5 mg/mL; if injection site reaction occurs, reconstitute vial with 3.5 mL of NS to a final concentration of 1 mg/mL or consider IV administration; use within 8 hr
• Administer calculated dose into the thigh or abdomen; rotate sites with each injection; inject at least 1 inch from old sites
• Space apart consecutive doses by at least 72 hr. Consider SUBCUT in patients with preexisting peripheral neuropathy or at high risk for the condition

SIDE EFFECTS

CNS: Posterior reversible encephalopathy syndrome (PRES), progressive multifocal leukoencephalopathy (PML), dizziness, headache, *peripheral neuropathy,* fever, headache, *fatigue, malaise, weakness*

CV: *Hypotension,* edema

GI: Abdominal pain, *constipation, diarrhea, nausea, vomiting,* anorexia, hepatotoxicity

HEMA: *Anemia,* neutropenia, thrombocytopenia

MISC: Tumor lysis syndrome

RESP: Cough, pneumonia, dyspnea

PHARMACOKINETICS

Half-life 9-15 hr, protein binding 83%, metabolized by CYP450 enzymes (3A4, 2D6, 2C19, 2C9, 1A2), onset, peak, duration unknown

INTERACTIONS

Increase: risk for bleeding—anticoagulants, NSAIDs, platelet inhibitors, salicylates, thrombolytics

Increase: peripheral neuropathy—amiodarone, antivirals (amprenavir, atazanavir, didanosine, lamiVUDine, 3TC, ritonavir, stavudine, zidovudine), chloramphenicol, CISplatin, colchicine, cycloSPORINE, dapsone, disulfiram, DOCEtaxel, gold salts, HMG-CoA reductase inhibitors, iodoquinol, INH, metroNIDAZOLE, nitrofurantoin, oxaliplatin, PACLitaxel, penicillamine, phenytoin, sulfaSALAzine, thalidomide, vinBLAStine, vinCRIStine, zalcitabine ddc, isoniazid, statins, others

Drug/Herb

Increase: toxicity or decrease efficacy—St. John's wort

Drug/Lab

Increase: LFTs, glucose

Decrease: platelets

NURSING CONSIDERATIONS

Assess:

• VS baseline and frequently, hypotension may occur, patients who are dehydrated are at greater risk
• **GI toxicity:** nausea, vomiting, diarrhea, constipation, may require antiemetics, antidiarrheals

- **Thrombocytopenia, neutropenia:** CBC baseline and periodically, platelets before each dose, dose adjustment may be required (nadir 11 platelets)
- **Peripheral neuropathy:** discomfort, burning, stinging in extremities; may use SUBCUT in those at risk
- **Pregnancy/breastfeeding:** do not use in pregnancy, breastfeeding during or for 2 mo after last dose
- **Fatal pulmonary toxicity:** assess for risk factors or new or worsening pulmonary symptoms
- **Tumor lysis syndrome:** usually in patients with a high tumor burden (hyperkalemia, hyperuricemia, hyperphosphatemia, renal failure)
- **PRES:** headache, malaise, confusion, seizures, blindness, hypertension, usually occurs within a few hours up to 1 yr after starting treatment, most symptoms do not need treatment, MRI confirms
- **PML:** for new infections of the brain

Evaluate:
- Therapeutic response: improvement of multiple myeloma symptoms

Teach patient/family:
- To monitor blood glucose levels if diabetic
- To contact prescriber about new or worsening peripheral neuropathy, severe vomiting, diarrhea, easy bruising, bleeding, infection
- To avoid driving, operating machinery until effect is known
- To avoid using other medications unless approved by prescriber
- About bleeding risk; to report bruising, bleeding
- To immediately report headache, confusion, lethargy (PRES)
- **Pregnancy/breastfeeding:** To use contraception while taking this product and for 2 mo after last dose; not to breastfeed during and for 2 mo after last dose

bosentan (Rx) REMS
(boh´sen-tan)
Tracleer
Func. class.: Vasodilator
Chem. class.: Endothelin receptor antagonist

Do not confuse:
Tracleer/Tricor

ACTION: Peripheral vasodilation occurs via the antagonism of the effect of endothelin on endothelium and vascular smooth muscle

USES: Pulmonary arterial hypertension with WHO class III, IV symptoms
Unlabeled uses: Septic shock to improve microcirculatory blood flow, functional class II pulmonary arterial hypertension

CONTRAINDICATIONS
Hypersensitivity, CVA, CAD

Black Box Warning: Pregnancy

Precautions: Breastfeeding, children, geriatric patients, mitral stenosis, anemia, edema, jaundice, hypovolemia, hypotension

Black Box Warning: Hepatic disease, requires an experienced clinician, contraceptive requirements, pregnancy testing, only those registered with the Tracleer REMS program (866-228-3546) may use this product

DOSAGE AND ROUTES
Pulmonary hypertension (pulmonary arterial hypertension WHO Group 1)
- **Adults/adolescents >40 kg: PO** tablet 62.5 mg bid × 4 wk, then increase to 125 mg bid
- **Adults/adolescents ≤40 kg: PO** tablet 62.5 mg bid
- **Children 21-40 kg (unlabeled): PO** tablet 62.5 mg bid, initiate at half of maintenance dose and increase to target dosage after 4 wk
- **Infants/children 10-20 kg (unlabeled): PO** 31.25 mg bid, initiate at half of maintenance dose and increase to target dosage after 4 wk
- **Infants <10 kg (unlabeled): PO** 2 mg/kg/dose bid, initiate at half of maintenance dose and increase to target dosage after 4 wk
- **Children 3-12 yr and 25-40 kg: PO** tablet for suspension 64 mg bid

• **Children 3-12 yr and 17-24 kg: PO**
tablet for suspension 48 mg bid
• **Children 3-12 yr and 9-16 kg: PO**
tablet for suspension 32 mg bid
• **Children 3-12 yr and 4-8 kg: PO** tablet for suspension 16 mg bid

Hepatic dose
• **Adult: PO** baseline AST/ALT <3 × ULN no dosage change, monitor LFTs monthly, reduce or interrupt if elevated; AST/ALT >3 and ≤5 × ULN repeat test, if confirmed reduce to 62.5 mg bid or interrupt; monitor LFTs q2wk, if interrupted, restart when LFTs <3 × ULN, check LFTs within 3 days; increase in AST/ALT >5 and ≤5 × ULN; during treatment repeat test to confirm, discontinue, monitor LFTs q2wk until LFTs <3 × ULN, restart at starting dose; AST/ALT >8 × ULN discontinue permanently

Persistent pulmonary hypertension of the newborn (PPHN) (unlabeled)
• **Premature and term neonates ≥34 wk gestation: PO** 1 mg/kg/dose bid
Available forms: Tablets 62.5, 125 mg; tablet for oral suspension 32 mg
Administer:
• Give without regard to meals
• Only available through the TAP program; 866-228-3546
• Use water to disperse tablets for oral suspension
• Do not stop product abruptly; taper
• Store at room temperature

SIDE EFFECTS
CNS: Headache, flushing, fatigue, fever
CV: Hypotension, chest pain, palpitations, edema of lower limbs, fluid retention
GI: Abnormal hepatic function, diarrhea, dyspepsia, hepatotoxicity
HEMA: Anemia, leukopenia, neutropenia, lymphopenia, thrombocytopenia
INTEG: Pruritus, anaphylaxis, rash, Stevens-Johnson syndrome, toxic epidermal necrolysis
MISC: Oligospermia, tumor lysis syndrome, respiratory infection, arthralgia
SYST: Secondary malignancy

PHARMACOKINETICS
Metabolized by inducer of CYP2C9, CYP3A4, possibly CYP2C19; metabolized by the liver; terminal half-life 5 hr; steady-state 3-5 days

INTERACTIONS
• Do not coadminister cycloSPORINE with bosentan; bosentan is increased, cycloSPORINE is decreased
• Do not coadminister glyBURIDE with bosentan; glyBURIDE is decreased significantly, bosentan is also decreased, hepatic enzymes may be increased
Increase: bosentan effects—CYP2C9, CYP3A4 inhibitors, avoid using together
Increase: bosentan level—ketoconazole, assess for adverse reactions
Decrease: effects of warfarin, hormonal contraceptives, statins, use 2 forms of contraception if using with hormonal contraceptives

Drug/Lab Test

Black Box Warning: Increase: ALT, AST

Decrease: Hb, Hct

NURSING CONSIDERATIONS
Assess:
• **Serious skin toxicities:** angioedema occurring 8-21 days after initiating therapy
• B/P, pulse during treatment until stable
• Blood studies: Hct, HB after 1 mo, 3 mo, then every 3 mo; may be decreased
• **Pulmonary hypertension/HF:** fluid retention, weight gain, increased leg edema; may occur within weeks

Black Box Warning: Hepatic toxicity: vomiting, jaundice; product should be discontinued; hepatic studies: AST, ALT, bilirubin; hepatic enzymes may increase; if ALT/AST >3 × and ≤5 × ULN, decrease dose or interrupt treatment and monitor AST/ALT q2wk; if bilirubin >2 × ULN or signs of hepatitis or hepatic disease are present, stop treatment

Black Box Warning: Experienced clinician: must be enrolled in the Tracleer REMS program (866-228-3546) and comply with requirements

Black Box Warning: Pregnancy: perform pregnancy testing prior to and during treatment in all female patients of childbearing potential, do not use unless a negative serum or urine pregnancy test is confirmed during the first 5 days of a normal menstrual period and at least 11 days after the last unprotected sex then monthly; do not use hormonal contraceptive as sole method

• **Beers:** use with caution in older adults; syncope may be exacerbated
Evaluate:
• Therapeutic response: decrease in pulmonary hypertension
Teach patient/family:
• To report jaundice, dark urine, joint pain, fatigue, malaise, bruising, easy bleeding, fluid retention

Black Box Warning: Patient must use nonhormonal contraception during and ≥1 mo after conclusion of treatment and another method, discuss risk of low sperm count, obtain monthly pregnancy test, do not breastfeed

• That lab work will be required periodically
• To take without regard to food; not to take new meds/herbs without prescriber approval; to take in AM or PM

⚠ **HIGH ALERT**

bosutinib (Rx)
(boe-sue′ti-nib)
Bosulif
Func. class.: Antineoplastic biologic response modifiers
Chem. class.: Signal transduction inhibitors (STIs), tyrosine kinase inhibitor

USES: Treatment of CML (chronic accelerator phase); ⊘℞ Philadelphia chromosome–positive patients in blast-cell crisis
Contraindications: Pregnancy, hypersensitivity

DOSAGE AND ROUTES
Newly diagnosed chronic phase PHxCML
• **Adult: PO** 400 mg daily with food, may increase to 600 mg/day in those who have not developed grade 3 toxicity or who do not reach complete hematologic

response by wk 8 or complete cytogenic response (CCyR) by wk 12
Chronic accelerated or blast phase Philadelphia chromosome–positive (PH+) CML ⊘℞
Adult: PO 500 mg daily with food, may use escalation to 600 mg daily in those not reaching hematologic response by wk 8 or complete cytogenia response by wk 12
Hepatic dosage
• **Adult: PO** Any baseline hepatic impairment: start at 200 mg/day; liver transaminase >5 × ULN, hold dose until levels are ≤2.5 × ULN, then resume at 400 mg/day; liver transaminase level ≥3 × ULN and bilirubin >2 × ULN and alkaline phosphatase <2 × ULN, discontinue
Available forms: 100, 400, 500 mg tablets

bremelanotide injection (Rx)
(bre′me-lan′oh-tide)
Vyleesi
Func. class.: Sexual dysfunction agent
Chem. class.: Melanocortin receptor agonists

ACTION: Nonselectively activates several receptor subtypes. The mechanism is unknown. It may activate selected brain pathways involved in normal sexual responses

USES: Premenopausal women with acquired, generalized hypoactive sexual desire disorder

CONTRAINDICATIONS
Hypersensitivity, men, postmenopausal women, cardiac disease
Precautions: Pregnancy, breastfeeding, contraception requirement, geriatric, hepatic disease, hypertension, renal dysfunction, skin hyperpigmentation

DOSAGE AND ROUTES
• **Adult premenopausal women: SUBCUT** 1.75 mg as needed, at least 45 min prior to anticipated sexual activity; max: 1 dose/24 hr
Available forms: Autoinjector solution for injection 1.75 mg/0.3 mL

Administer:
SUBCUT route

• Visually inspect parenteral products for particulate matter and discoloration before use. Do not use injections that are unusually cloudy, discolored, or contain particulate; injection is clear and colorless
• Inject SUBCUT into the abdomen or thigh. Do not administer within 2 inches around the umbilicus or where the skin is tender, bruised, red, hard, thick, or scaly
• The dose is administered at least 45 min before anticipated sexual activity
• Not to be used more than 1 dose/24 hr. No more than 8 doses/mo
• Discard the used autoinjector in a sharps container after use

SIDE EFFECTS

CNS: *Flushing, headache*
INTEG: *Injection site reactions*
GI: *Nausea,* hepatitis
GU: Hot flashes
CV: Hypertension

PHARMACOKINETICS

21% binds to human serum protein, half-life 1.9-4 hr; metabolism involves multiple hydrolyses of the amide bond of the cyclic peptide; excreted 64.8% urine, 22.8% feces

INTERACTIONS

Decreased: effect of naltrexone; do not use together

NURSING CONSIDERATIONS
Assess:

• **Sexual arousal:** identify characteristics of lack of sexual arousal, length of time, other treatments administered in the past
• **Hypertension/cardiac disease:** monitor B/P before starting treatment and periodically ensure B/P is well controlled
• **Nausea/vomiting:** is a common side effect, may require an antiemetic; product may need to be discontinued for persistent or severe nausea or antiemetic therapy initiated for those patients who are bothered by nausea
• **Skin hyperpigmentation:** may be more common in those with darker skin and with daily dosing, more common on face, gingiva, and breast; may be permanent

• **Severe hepatic/renal disease (Child-Pugh C; score 10-15) or severe renal impairment (eGFR <30 mL/min/1.73 m²):** may have an increase in severity of adverse reactions
• **Pregnancy/breastfeeding:** contraception requirements are advised; females of child-bearing potential should be counseled regarding appropriate methods of contraception while on therapy; discontinue if pregnancy is suspected; pregnant women are encouraged to call the Bremelanotide Pregnancy Exposure Registry at (877) 411-2510; avoid breastfeeding—no data are available regarding safety

Evaluate:
• Therapeutic response
• Sexual arousal

Teach patient/family:

• **Sexual arousal:** report if product has resolved lack of sexual arousal
• **Hypertension/cardiac disease:** teach patient that B/P will be evaluated periodically
• **Nausea/vomiting:** teach patient to report nausea and vomiting, may require an antiemetic
• **Skin hyperpigmentation:** teach patient to report skin hyperpigmentation; product may need to be discontinued
Train the patient on the use of the autoinjector, to read the manufacturer-provided instructions for use
• **Pregnancy/breastfeeding:** counsel patients on need for contraception; females of childbearing potential should be counseled regarding appropriate methods of contraception while on therapy; advise patient to discontinue if pregnancy is suspected; pregnant women are encouraged to call the Bremelanotide Pregnancy Exposure Registry at (877) 411-2510; avoid breastfeeding

---

⚠ HIGH ALERT

brentuximab (Rx)
(bren-tuk'see-mab)

Adcetris
Func. class.: Antineoplastic
Chem. class.: Monoclonal antibody

Controlled Substance Schedule IV

ACTION: The anticancer activity is due to the binding of ⊗ tubulin and disrupts the microtubule network within the cell, inducing cell cycle arrest and apoptotic death of the cells

USES: Hodgkin's disease after failure of autologous stem cell transplant (ASCT) or after failure of at least 2 prior multiagent chemotherapy regimens in patients who are not ASCT candidates; non-Hodgkin's lymphoma (NHL); systemic anaplastic large cell lymphoma (sALCL) after failure of at least 1 prior multiagent chemotherapy regimen, previously untreated systemic ALCL or other CD30-expressing peripheral T-cell lymphoma (PTCL)

CONTRAINDICATIONS
Hypersensitivity, pregnancy, use with bleomycin, breastfeeding, CCr <30 mL/min, hepatic disease in neonate or child or severe (Child-Pugh class B-C)

Precautions: Breastfeeding, children, infants, neonates, neutropenia, peripheral neuropathy, tumor lysis syndrome (TLS)

Black Box Warning: Progressive multifocal leukoencephalopathy

DOSAGE AND ROUTES
• **Adult:** IV 1.8 mg/kg q3wk until disease progression or unacceptable toxicity

Renal dose
• **Adult:** IV CCr <30 mL/min, avoid use
Hepatic dose
• **Adult:** IV (Child-Pugh A) 1.2 mg/kg q3wk, max 120 mg; (Child-Pugh B or C avoid use)
Previously untreated stage III or IV cHL
Adult: IV 1.2 mg/kg (max 180 mg) q2wk until max 12 doses given or disease progression or unacceptable toxicity
Renal dose
Adult: IV CCr <30 mL/min, avoid use
Hepatic dose
Adult IV: (Child-Pugh A) 0.9 mg/kg (max 90 mg) q2wk to max 12 doses or disease progression or unacceptable toxicity; (Child-Pugh C) avoid use

Available forms: Powder for injection 50 mg/vial
Administer:
Intermittent IV INFUSION route
• Visually inspect for particulate matter and discoloration whenever solution and container permit
• Only as an IV infusion, do not give as an IV push or bolus
• Use cytotoxic handling procedures
• Do not mix, or administer as an infusion, with other IV products
• Calculate the dose (mg) and the number of vials required. For patients weighing >100 kg, use 100 kg to calculate the dose; reconstitute each 50-mg vial per 10.5 mL of sterile water for injection (5 mg/mL)
• Direct the stream of sterile water toward the wall of the vial and not directly at the cake or powder; gently swirl the vial, do not shake
• Discard any unused portion left in the vial
• After reconstitution, dilute immediately with ≥100 mL of 0.9% sodium chloride, 5% dextrose, or lactated Ringer's solution to a final concentration (0.4 mg/mL-1.8 mg/mL)
• Infuse over 30 min
• Use the diluted solution immediately or store in refrigerator for ≤24 hr after reconstitution; do not freeze

SIDE EFFECTS
CNS: Headache, dizziness, *fever*, peripheral neuropathy, anxiety, chills, *fatigue*, insomnia, night sweats, progressive multifocal leukoencephalopathy
CV: Peripheral edema
GI: *Abdominal pain, nausea, vomiting,* constipation, *diarrhea,* weight loss, GI hemorrhage/perforation/obstruction
INTEG: *Rash,* pruritus, alopecia, xerosis
RESP: Pneumothorax, pneumonitis dyspnea, *cough*
SYST: Anaphylaxis, tumor lysis syndrome, Stevens-Johnson syndrome, infusion reactions, toxic epidermal necrolysis
HEMA: Anemia, neutropenia, thrombocytopenia, lymphadenopathy

Side effects: *italics* = common; red = life-threatening

PHARMACOKINETICS

Onset rapid, peak 1-3 days, duration unknown, protein binding is 68%-82%, only a small amount is metabolized; potent inhibitors or inducers of CYP3A4 may alter action; half-life is 4-6 days

INTERACTIONS

Increase: brentuximab action—CYP3A4 inhibitors, P-gp inhibitors, ketoconazole, boceprevir, delavirdine, isoniazid, indinavir, itraconazole, dalfopristin, quinupristin, telithromycin, tipranavir, rifAMPin, ritonavir

Increase: toxicity live virus vaccines

Increase: pulmonary toxicity—bleomycin; do not use together

Decrease: brentuximab action—CYP3A4 inducers

Drug/Herb

Increase: brentuximab component action—St. John's wort

Drug/Lab

Increase: ALT/AST, bilirubin

Decrease: WBC, platelets, RBCs

NURSING CONSIDERATIONS

Assess:

• **Pulmonary toxicity:** cough, trouble breathing, report immediately

• **Infection:** report immediately, fever, chills

• **Tumor lysis syndrome (TLS):** assess for hyperkalemia, hypophosphatemia, hypocalcemia; may develop renal failure; may use allopurinol or rasburicase to prevent TLS; monitor serum BUN/creatinine

Black Box Warning: **Peripheral neuropathy, progressive multifocal leukoencephalopathy:** assess for weakness or paralysis, vision loss, impaired speech, and cognitive deterioration; often fatal

• Monitor CBC and differential, LFTs, serum bilirubin (direct and indirect), electrolytes, uric acid, neurologic function

• **Bone marrow suppression:** monitor CBC before each dose

• **GI toxicity:** monitor for changes in bowel habits, bowel obstruction, constipation, pancreatitis

• **Anaphylaxis:** monitor for symptoms; high risk during administration

• **Stevens-Johnson syndrome:** monitor and report skin reactions or rash; discontinue if toxic epidermal necrolysis or Stevens-Johnson syndrome occurs

• **Pregnancy:** determine if pregnancy is planned or suspected; do not use in pregnancy/breastfeeding; reliable contraception should be used

Evaluate:

• Decreasing symptoms of Hodgkin's disease (decreased lymph nodes, night sweats, weight loss, splenomegaly, hepatomegaly)

Teach patient/family:

• To report immediately weakness, change in vision, impaired speech, peripheral neuropathy, neutropenia if severe, rash, change in bowel habits

• **Meds:** Instruct patient to discuss all Rx, OTC, herbals, supplements with health care provider

• **Hyperglycemia:** Teach patient that product may cause hyperglycemia, to report to health care provider increased thirst, dry mouth, increased urination, blurred vision, tiredness

• **Hepatotoxicity:** AST/ALT, bilirubin baseline and periodically; if elevated, product may need to be discontinued or decreased

• **Pulmonary toxicity:** dyspnea, cough; if these occur, product may need to be discontinued

• **Infusion site reactions:** check site frequently, if reaction occurs (redness, swelling at site), stop infusion, give antihistamines

• To use reliable contraception; not to breastfeed during and for 6 mo after last dose, males with a partner of reproductive potential should also use contraceptive; fertility may be decreased in males

brexanolone (Rx)

REMS

(brek-san'oh-lone)

Zulresso

Func. class.: Antidepressant

Chem. class.: GABA modulator, corticosteroid

Controlled substance: IV

ACTION: Not fully known but thought to be related to its positive modulation of γ-aminobutyric acid A (GABA-A) receptors; GABA is a major inhibitory neurotransmitter in the brain

USES: Postpartum depression

CONTRAINDICATIONS
Hypersensitivity, CCr 15 mL/min

Precautions: Abrupt discontinuation, driving or hazardous activities, breastfeeding, coadministration with other CNS depressants, alcohol use, hypoxia, pregnancy, renal failure, suicidal ideation, child/young adult

Black Box Warning: CNS depression, loss of consciousness; requires a specialized setting

DOSAGE AND ROUTES
Adult females: continuous IV: Give over a total of 60 hr (2.5 days) as follows: 0 to 4 hr: initiate with a dose of 30 mcg/kg/hr; 4 to 24 hr: increase dose to 60 mcg/kg/hr; 24 to 52 hr: increase dose to 90 mcg/kg/hr; 52 to 56 hr: decrease dose to 60 mcg/kg/hr; 56 to 60 hr: decrease dose to 30 mcg/kg/hr

Available forms: Solution for injection 100 mg/20 mL (5 mg/mL)

Administer:
• The vials require dilution
• Visually inspect; vial should be clear, colorless without particulate matter and discoloration; do not use discolored vials or vials with particulate matter
• 5 infusion bags will be required for the 60-hr infusion; additional bags will be needed for those ≥90 kg
• Prepare and store in a polyolefin, non-DEHP, nonlatex bag only; do not use in-line filter
• Dilute in the infusion bag immediately after the initial puncture of the vial
• Withdraw 20 mL of product from the vial and place in the infusion bag; dilute with 40 mL of sterile water for injection, and further dilute with 40 mL of 0.9% sodium chloride injection (total volume of 100 mL) to achieve a target concentration of 1 mg/mL
• Immediately place the infusion bag in refrigerator until use
• Give as a continuous IV infusion over a total of 60 hr (2.5 days) via a dedicated line; do not inject other medications into the infusion bag or admix
• Use a programmable infusion pump, prime infusion sets with admixture prior to inserting into the pump and connecting to the venous catheter
• A health care provider must be available on site to continuously monitor
• Initiate treatment early enough during the day to allow for recognition of excessive sedation
• After the product is diluted, it can be stored in infusion bags under refrigerated conditions for up to 96 hr
• Each diluted product can be used for up to 12 hr of infusion time at room temperature; discard any unused product after 12 hr of infusion

SIDE EFFECTS
CNS: Sedation, drowsiness, loss of consciousness, suicidal ideation, dizziness
CV: Tachycardia
GI: Dry mouth, diarrhea, dyspepsia
RESP: Hypoxia
INTEG: Injection site reaction, flushing

PHARMACOKINETICS
Extensive distribution into tissues, protein binding >99%, extensively metabolized by non-CYP pathways including keto-reduction, glucuronidation, and sulfation; half-life 9 hr; excreted as metabolites in feces (47%) and urine (42%); less than 1% of the drug is excreted as unchanged

INTERACTIONS
None known

NURSING CONSIDERATIONS
Assess:
• Monitor for hypoxia using continuous pulse oximetry with an alarm; if hypoxia occurs, discontinue and do not reinitiate

Black Box Warning: Assess for excessive sedation q2hr during planned, non-sleep periods, and stop the infusion if excessive sedation occurs until the symptom resolves; thereafter, the infusion may be resumed at the same or lower dose

• Available only through the Zulresso Risk Evaluation and Mitigation Strategy (Zulresso REMS) program; risks of serious adverse outcomes (excessive sedation or sudden loss/alteration of consciousness)

Side effects: *italics* = common; red = life-threatening

• **Suicidal ideation:** assess for suicidal thoughts and behavior; more common in young adults
Evaluate:
• Therapeutic response: decrease in postpartum depression, improved mood
Teach patient/family:
• Reason for product and expected result, advise patient to read medication guide before treatment starts
• To discuss all Rx, OTC, herbals and supplements with health care provider
• To report pain, inflammation at injection site
• **Excessive sedation and sudden loss of consciousness:** excessive sedation or loss of consciousness can occur; checking q2hr for these symptoms will be required; if these occur, tell your health care provider
• A family member or caregiver needs to help care for you and your children during the infusion
• Not to drive or engage in hazardous tasks while sleepiness occurs
• Not to use alcohol or other CNS depressants
• **Pregnancy/breastfeeding:** to identify if pregnancy is planned or suspected or if breastfeeding; if pregnant, register with the National Pregnancy Registry for Antidepressants at 844-405-6185 or visit https://womensmentalhealth.org/clinical-and-research-programs/pregnancyregistry/antidepressants/

---

brexpiprazole (Rx)
brex-pip′-ra-zole
Rexulti
Func. class.: Antipsychotic, atypical
Chem. class.: Serotonin-dopamine activity modulator (SDAM)

ACTION: May exert its effects through a combination of partial agonist activity at dopaminergic D-2 receptors, serotonergic 5-HT1A receptors, antagonist activity at serotonergic 5-HT2A receptors

USES: Adjunctive treatment of major depressive disorder, schizophrenia

CONTRAINDICATIONS
Hypersensitivity
Precautions: Elderly patients, stroke, neuroleptic malignant syndrome, tardive dyskinesia, leukopenia, neutropenia, agranulocytosis, orthostatic hypotension, seizures, cognitive impairment, pregnancy, breastfeeding

DOSAGE AND ROUTES
Schizophrenia
• **Adult: PO** Initially, 1 mg daily on days 1-4; increase to 2 mg daily on days 5-7, then increase to 4 mg daily on day 8 based on response and tolerability. Recommended dose range 2-4 mg/day (max: 4 mg/day)
Adjunctive treatment of major depressive disorder
• **Adult: PO** Initially, 0.5 to 1 mg daily; after titration to 1 mg/day, increase to target dose of 2 mg/day; titrate dosage at weekly intervals based on response and tolerability; max 3 mg/day
Hepatic dose
• **Adult: PO** Mild hepatic impairment: no change; moderate to severe hepatic impairment (Child-Pugh score ≥7): max 2 mg/day for major depressive disorder, 3 mg/day for schizophrenia
Renal dose
• **Adult: PO** CCr ≥60 mL/min: no change; CCr <60 mL/min, including end-stage renal disease (ESRD): max 2 mg/day for major depression, 3 mg/day for schizophrenia
Available forms: Tablets 0.25, 0.50, 1, 2, 3, 4 mg
Administer:
• Initiate treatment at low end of dosage range in geriatric adults
• Periodically reassess for need of continued maintenance therapy
• Give without regard to food
• If dose is missed, give when remembered; if close to next dose, skip missed dose and give regular dose

SIDE EFFECTS
CNS: Akathisia, fatigue, drowsiness, dizziness, tremor, sedation, insomnia, EPS
EENT: Blurred vision, dry mouth, nasopharyngitis
GI: Constipation, diarrhea, nausea, flatulence, abdominal cramping/pain
GU: UTI
MISC: Weight gain, myalgia

PHARMACOKINETICS
Half-life 91 hr, onset unknown, peak 4 hr, duration unknown

INTERACTIONS
Increase: temperature—anticholinergics
Increase: CNS depression—other CNS depressants, use cautiously
Increase: brexpiprazole effect—strong CYP2D6 inhibitors, strong CYP3A4 inhibitors, may need dose reduction

Drug/Herb:
Decrease: brexpiprazole effect—St. John's wort; may need to increase product dose

Drug/Food:
Increase: brexpiprazole effect—grapefruit juice; avoid using together

NURSING CONSIDERATIONS
Assess:
• **Hypersensitivity:** rash, facial swelling, urticaria, and anaphylaxis have been observed; discontinue immediately
• **Vitals:** Monitor B/P, pulse, respirations

Black Box Warning: Suicidal ideation: provide close supervision and control; give the smallest quantity to reduce the risk of overdose. In those who exhibit changes in symptoms, worsening of depression, suicidality, or other changes in mood or behavior, a decision should be made to change or discontinue treatment. If discontinuing, taper as rapidly as possible, abrupt discontinuation of drug can cause adverse symptoms. Children and young adults <24 yr are at increased risk

• **Neuroleptic malignant syndrome:** Monitor for fever, severe muscle rigidity, seizures, hyper-/hypotension, altered LOC, diaphoresis, tachypenia; notify health care provider immediately

• Akathsia, dystonic reaction: Monitor for agitation, overwhelming sense of tremor, inability to sit still; twitching, twisting movements when muscles contract involuntarily
• **Tardive dyskinesia:** periodic evaluation for movement disorders (AIMS) is recommended. If signs and symptoms of tardive dyskinesia appear, consider discontinuation
• **Seizure disorder:** use cautiously in patients with history of seizure disorder or with conditions that may lower the seizure threshold. Conditions that lower the seizure threshold may be more prevalent in patients 65 yr or older
• **Orthostatic hypotension:** dizziness, light headedness, tachycardia, and occasionally syncope. Risks are generally greatest at beginning of treatment and during dose escalation. Patients at higher risk include those with dehydration, hypovolemia, treatment with antihypertensive medications, history of cardiac disease (HF, MI, CAD, ischemia, or conduction abnormalities), history of cerebrovascular disease, and patients who are antipsychotic-naive. Monitor orthostatic vital signs, such as pulse and B/P. Complete fall risk assessments in at-risk patients on long-term antipsychotic therapy
• **Hematologic disease:** those with a history of clinically significant low WBC count or drug-induced leukopenia/neutropenia should have frequent CBC assessments in first few months of treatment. Discontinue in patients with ANC <1000/mm^3
• **Pregnancy/breastfeeding:** use only when benefits outweigh fetal risks. Neonates exposed to antipsychotics in the third trimester of pregnancy are at risk for extrapyramidal and/or withdrawal symptoms after delivery. Enroll patient in National Pregnancy Registry for Psychiatric Medications (866-961-2388). Consider benefits/risks of breastfeeding

Teach patient/family:
• To use caution when driving or operating machinery or performing other tasks that require mental alertness until the effects are known
• To avoid ethanol ingestion during treatment. Somnolence could lead to falls with the potential for fractures and other injuries

• To watch for suicidal behaviors or thoughts by family or impulsive urges
• That dystonic reactions may occur
• To rise slowly from sitting or lying, orthostatic hypotension may occur
• To report if pregnancy is planned or suspected or if breastfeeding
• To report all products taken to prevent drug interactions

⚠ HIGH ALERT

brigatinib (Rx)

(bri-ga´-ti-nib)

Alunbrig

Func. class.: Antineoplastic

USES: Advanced ALK-positive metastatic non–small-cell lung cancer who have progressed on or are intolerant to crizotinib

DOSAGE AND ROUTES

• **Adult: PO** 90 mg/day × 7 days; if tolerated during the first 7 days, increase to 180 mg/day. Continue until disease progression or unacceptable toxicity

Available forms: Tablets 30, 90, 180 mg

---

brimonidine (ophthalmic) (Rx)

(bri-moe´ni-deen)

Alphagan P, Lumify, Mirvaso, Qoliana

Func. class.: Antiglaucoma
Chem. class.: Selective α_2 agonist

Do not confuse:
brimonidine/bimatoprost

ACTION: Select α-agonist that decreases aqueous humor and increases outflows

USES: Treatment of chronic open-angle glaucoma and ocular hypertension

CONTRAINDICATIONS
Hypersensitivity, AV block, heart failure, bradycardia, sick sinus syndrome, within 14 days of MAOI therapy
Precautions: Breastfeeding, depression, cerebrovascular disease, hepatic/renal impairment, Raynaud's phenomenon, orthostatic hypotension, thromboangiitis obliterans

DOSAGE AND ROUTES
Reduce IOP/ocular HNT or open-angle glaucoma
• **Adult/child >2 yr:** Instill 1 drop in the affected eye(s) tid
Persistent erythmea of rosacea (Mirvaso)
Adult: Gel Apply pea-size amount to several areas of the face daily

Redness in eye from irritation
Adult/child ≥5 yr: Opthalmic solution 1 drop in affected eye q6-8h, no more than qid

Available forms: Ophthalmic solution 0.1%, 0.15%, 0.2%

SIDE EFFECTS
RESP: Cough, dyspnea, bronchitis, pharyngitis
CNS: Headache, dizziness, somnolence
CV: Hyper/hypotension, hypercholesterolemia
EENT: Eye stinging/burning, tearing, photophobia, change in vision, sinus infection, blurred vision, pruritus, photophobia, eyelid erythema, ocular pain, nasal dryness

PHARMACOKINETICS
Peak ½-2 hr, half-life 2 hr

INTERACTIONS
Increase: intraocular pressure reduction—apraclonidine, dorzolamide, pilocarpine, timolol
Increase: effects of—CNS depressants
Decrease: B/P—beta-blockers, antihypertensives
Decrease: brimonidine effect—tricyclic antidepressants, may cause HTN crisis MAOIs, linezolid

---

NURSING CONSIDERATIONS
Assess:
• Glaucoma: monitor intraocular pressure
• Redness, flushing, whitening after gel, will resolve after discontinuation, do not use gel on wounds
Evaluate:
• Decreasing intraocular pressure
Teach patient/family:
• That drug is for ophthalmic use only
• Not to touch the tip of the dropper to the eye, fingertips, or other surface to prevent contamination
• Not to use alcohol
• To wait 15 min before inserting soft contact lenses
• To avoid hazardous activities until response is known
• To wash hands prior to and after use; to teach proper use
• That if more than one topical ophthalmic drug product is being used, the drugs should be administered at least 5 min apart
• To avoid contamination or the spread of infection by not using dropper for more than one person

brinzolamide ophthalmic
See Appendix B

brivaracetam (Rx)
(briv-a-ra′se-tam)
Briviact
Func. class.: Anticonvulsant
Controlled Substance V

ACTION: The exact mechanism is not known, may occur in modulation of synaptic vesicle proteins; additional anticonvulsant activity may be related to the modulation of voltage-dependent sodium channels

USES: For the adjunctive treatment of partial-onset seizures

CONTRAINDICATIONS
Hypersensitivity
Precautions: Abrupt discontinuation, breastfeeding, depression, driving or operating machinery, geriatric patients, hepatic disease, pregnancy, suicidal ideation, ⚠ poor metabolizers of CYP2C19

DOSAGE AND ROUTES
• **Adult/adolescent ≥16: PO/IV** 50 mg bid. Adjust dose to 25 mg bid or 100 mg bid based on clinical response; max 100 mg bid. Use **IV** when **PO** is temporarily not feasible
• **Child/adolescent 4-15 yr and ≥50 kg: PO** 25-50 mg bid
• **Child/adolescent 4-15 yr and 20-49 kg: PO** 0.5-1 mg/kg/dose bid; maintenance 0.5-2 mg/kg/dose twice daily
• **Child/adolescent 4-12 yr and 11-19 kg: PO** 0.5-1.25 mg/kg/dose bid; maintenance 0.5-2.5 mg/kg/dose twice daily; max 5 mg/kg/day
Infant/Child <11 kg: PO 0.75 to 1.5 mg/kg/dose BID, adjust based on clinical response and tolerability
With rifampin use: Adult/child: Increase brivaracetam by up to double dose
Available forms:
• Tablets 10, 25, 50, 75, 100; oral solution 10 mg/mL; solution for injection 50 mg/5 mL (10 mg/mL), single-dose vial
Administer:
• May be administered without regard to meals
• To discontinue, gradually reduce the dose to minimize the risk for increased seizure frequency and status epilepticus
Tablets:
• Swallow tablets whole; do not crush or chew
Oral solution:
• No dilution is necessary
• Measure and administer oral solution using a calibrated measuring device
• A nasogastric tube or gastrostomy tube may be used for administration
• **Storage:** discard any unused solution 5 mo after first opening the bottle

IV Infusion

• Visually inspect, do not use if discoloration or particulate matter is present; injection is a clear, colorless solution
• May be given IV without further dilution or may be mixed with a diluent, including 0.9% NaCl injection, LR injection, or D_5 injection
• Infuse over 2 to 15 min
• **Storage:** after dilution, the solution may be stored ≤4 hr at room temperature and may be stored in polyvinyl chloride (PVC) bags; discard any unused injection vial contents; for single dose only

SIDE EFFECTS

CNS: Dizziness, drowsiness, ataxia, euphoria, fatigue, irritability, depression, emotional lability, hallucinations, psychosis, suicidal ideation

GI: Constipation, nausea, vomiting

HEMA: Leukopenia

INTEG: Angioedema, infusion site pain

RESP: Bronchospasm

PHARMACOKINETICS

Protein binding 20%, primarily metabolized by hydrolysis to form a hydroxy metabolite, metabolized by CYP2C19, excreted in urine 95%, feces <1%, half-life 9 hr, all forms may be used interchangeably, peak 1 hr without food, high-fat meal slows absorption

INTERACTIONS

Increase: sedation—TCAs, antihistamines, benzodiazepines, other CNS depressants
Increase: possible toxicity—carBAMazepine
Decrease: brivaracetam absorption—sevelamer

Drug/Lab Test:
Increase: LFTs
Decrease: Hct/HB, WBC, RBC

NURSING CONSIDERATIONS

Assess:
• **Seizures:** type, location, duration, character; provide seizure precautions
• **Renal studies:** urinalysis, BUN, urine creatinine q3mo
• **Blood studies:** CBC, LFTs
• **Mental status:** mood, sensorium, affect, behavioral changes, suicidal

thoughts/behaviors; if mental status changes, notify prescriber
• Assistance with ambulation during early part of treatment; dizziness, drowsiness occurs, sedation
• **Hypersensitivity:** Angioedema, product should be discontinued immediately, treat
• **DRESS:** Rash, hepatitis, fever, eosinophilia, discontinue immediately, treat
• **Pregnancy/breastfeeding:** use only if benefits outweigh fetal risk; pregnant patients should be registered at the North American Antiepileptic Drug Pregnancy Registry (888-233-2334); discontinue breastfeeding or product; excretion is unknown

Evaluate:
• Therapeutic response: decreased seizure activity

Teach patient/family:
• To carry emergency ID stating patient's name, medications taken, condition, prescriber's name and phone number
• How to use oral solution, use calibrated device to measure
• Advise patient to discuss with health care provider all Rx, OTC, herbals, and supplements taken
• To notify prescriber if pregnancy is planned or suspected
• To avoid driving, other activities requiring alertness until response is known; drowsiness occurs when beginning therapy
• To obtain medical care immediately for angioedema, bronchospasm
• Not to discontinue quickly after long-term use; withdrawal seizure may occur; date bottle, throw away oral solution after 5 mo
• Not to breastfeed; to notify prescriber immediately if pregnancy is planned or suspected
• To report immediately suicidal thoughts/behaviors, psychotic symptoms (hallucination, delusions, or unusual behaviors)

---

brodalumab (Rx) REMS
(broe-dal′-ue-mab)
Siliq
Func. class.: Immunosuppressive
Chem. class.: Recombinant human IgG2 monoclonal antibody

Do not confuse:
Siliq/Actiq

ACTION: Human IgG2 monoclonal antibody that binds to interleukin-17 receptor A (IL-17RA) and prevents IL-17 cytokines from activating the receptor

USES: For the treatment of moderate to severe plaque psoriasis in adult patients who are candidates for phototherapy or systemic therapy and who have failed to respond or have lost response to other systemic therapies

CONTRAINDICATIONS
Hypersensitivity, Crohn's disease
Precautions: Pregnancy, breastfeeding, children, depression, geriatric patients, immunosuppression, infection, suicidal ideation, vaccination

Black Box Warning: Suicidal ideation

DOSAGE AND ROUTES
• **Adult: SUBCUT** 210 mg at wk 0, 1, and 2, then 210 mg q2wk; discontinue if inadequate response after 12-16 wk
• **Available forms:** Prefilled syringe 210 mg/1.5 mL

Administer:
SUBCUT route
• Remove prefilled syringe from refrigerator and allow to reach room temperature (about 30 min) without removing the needle cap; once brought to room temperature, do not return to the refrigerator
• If needed, the prefilled syringe may be stored at room temperature for up to 14 days
• Discard after 14 days
• Do not shake
• Visually inspect for particulate matter and discoloration; do not use if discolored, cloudy, or foreign particulate matter is present
• Do not use where skin is tender, bruised, red, hard, thick, scaly, or affected by psoriasis
• Each single-use prefilled syringe contains 210 mg/1.5 mL of product. Inject the entire 1.5 mL contents of the syringe.

No preservatives are present; discard unused portion
• Protect from light, do not freeze

Black Box Warning: The drug is available only through a restricted program (Siliq Risk Evaluation and Mitigation Strategy [REMS] Program). Prescribers must be certified in the program. Patients must sign a patient-prescriber agreement form. For information, visit the Siliq REMS website or call 855-511-6135

SIDE EFFECTS
CNS: Headache, fatigue, suicidal ideation
EENT: Sinusitis
GI: Nausea, diarrhea
MS: Arthralgia
INTEG: Erythema, pruritus
HEMA: Bleeding, neutropenia
MISC: Infection, injection site reactions, antibody formation, pharyngitis, TB

PHARMACOKINETICS
Onset unknown, peak 3 days, duration unknown, half-life unknown

INTERACTIONS
Increase: altered effect of each product—CYP450 enzymes (carBAMazepine, cyclosporine, ethosuximide, fosphenytoin, phenytoin, tacrolimus, theophylline, aminophylline, warfarin); monitor if products are initiated or discontinued; dose adjustments may be needed
• Do not give concurrently with live virus vaccines; bring immunizations up-to-date before treatment
Drug/Lab
Decrease: ANC

NURSING CONSIDERATIONS
Assess:
• For injection site pain, swelling, redness; use cold compress to relieve pain/swelling
• **Infection:** fever, flulike symptoms, dyspnea, change in urination, redness/swelling around any wounds; stop treatment if present; serious infections including sepsis may occur, may be fatal; patients with active infections should not be started on this product

• **TB:** test for TB before starting product; do not use in active TB; for latent TB, give antituberculosis therapy before use of product; monitor closely for signs and symptoms of active TB infection during and after treatment

• **Pregnancy/breastfeeding:** no data for use in pregnancy, breastfeeding; excretion in breast milk unknown

Black Box Warning: Suicidal ideation: assess risks and benefits of treatment when considering use in those with a history of depression or psychosis

Evaluate:
• Therapeutic response: decrease in lesions

Teach patient/family:
• About self-administration if appropriate: injection should be made in thigh, abdomen, upper arm; rotate sites at least 1 inch from old site; do not inject in areas that are bruised, red, hard; not to use if dropped on hard surface, use new syringe

• That if medication is not taken when due, to inject dose as soon as remembered and inject the next dose as scheduled

• Not to take any live virus vaccines during treatment

• To report signs of infection (fever, sweats, or chills; muscle aches; weight loss; cough; warm, red, or painful skin or sores on the body different from psoriasis; diarrhea or stomach pain; shortness of breath; blood in phlegm [mucus]; burning in urination or urinating more often than normal); allergic reactions (itching, rash)

• To tell provider of all prescription and OTC medications, herbals, and supplements currently taken

• That a patient-prescriber agreement form is required to be signed

Black Box Warning: Suicidal ideation: to seek medical attention for suicidal ideation, new-onset or worsening depression, anxiety, or other mood changes

brolucizumab-dbll (Rx)
(broe-lue-siz′-ue-mab-dbll)
Beovu
Func. class.: Ophthalmic agent
Chem. class.: VEGF inhibitor

ACTION: Binds to VEGF, suppresses endothelial cell proliferation, neovascularization, and vascular permeability

USES: Neovascular (wet) age-related macular degeneration

CONTRAINDICATIONS
Ocular/periocular infections, active intraocular inflammation, hypersensitivity
Precautions: Endophthalmitis, retinal detachment, retinal vasculitis and/or retinal vascular occlusion, increased IOP, arterial thromboembolic events

DOSAGE AND ROUTES
• **Adult: Intravitreal injection** 6 mg (0.05 mL of 120 mg/mL solution) monthly × 3 doses, then 6 mg (0.05 mL) q8-12wk
Available forms: Intravitreal injection: 6 mg/0.05 mL solution single-dose vial
Administer:
• Given by ophthalmologist
• Inspect solution for discoloration or particulate matter, do not use if present
• Vial is for single use, discard unused portion
• Refrigerate vial, do not freeze. Store the vial in the outer carton to protect from light; before use, the unopened glass vial may be kept at room temperature for ≤24 hr

SIDE EFFECTS
EENT: Blurred vision, cataract, conjunctival hemorrhage, eye pain, floaters

PHARMACOKINETICS
Onset, duration unknown, peak 24 hr, half-life 4.4 days

INTERACTIONS
None known

NURSING CONSIDERATIONS
Assess:
• Monitor IOP for 30 min after injection
• Assess for arterial thromboembolic events after injection
• **Pregnancy/breastfeeding:** Not to use in pregnancy, use contraception if woman is of childbearing potential; not to breastfeed during or for 1 mo after conclusion of treatment
Evaluate:
• Therapeutic response: Prevention of loss of sight
Teach patient/family:
• Inform patients that after injection endophthalmitis, retinal detachment, retinal vasculitis, retinal vascular occlusion may occur; if the eye becomes red, sensitive to light, painful, or change in vision occurs, immediately contact ophthalmologist
• Teach patients that temporary visual disturbances may occur after injection
• Advise patients not to drive or use machinery until reaction is known

---

bromfenac
(ophthalmic) (Rx)
(brom′fen-ak)
BromSite, Prolensa, Xibrom
Func. class.: Antiinflammatory (ophthalmic)

USES: To reduce pain and inflammation after cataract surgery

CONTRAINDICATIONS
Hypersensitivity to this product, sulfites, NSAIDs, salicylates
Precautions: Bleeding disorders, complicated ocular surgery, corneal denervation, diabetes mellitus, rheumatoid arthritis, dry eye syndrome, pregnancy, breastfeeding
Do not administer while wearing contact lenses

DOSAGE AND ROUTES
Ophthalmic dosage (Bromday 0.09% solution or Prolensa 0.07% solution)
• **Adults:** One drop (0.07 mg or 0.09 mg) instilled into affected eye(s) once daily beginning 24 hours prior to cata-

ract surgery, continued on the day of surgery, and through the first 14 days of the postoperative period.
Ophthalmic dosage (Xibrom 0.09% solution)
• **Adults:** One drop (0.09 mg) instilled into affected eye(s) twice daily beginning 24 hours after cataract surgery, continued through the first 14 days of the postoperative period.
Ophthalmic dosage (BromSite 0.075% solution)
• **Adults:** One drop (0.075 mg) instilled into affected eye(s) twice daily beginning 1 day prior to surgery, continued on the day of surgery, and through the first 14 days of the postoperative period.
Available forms: Opthalmic solution 0.07%, 0.075%, 0.09%

⚠ **HIGH ALERT**

bromocriptine (Rx)
(broe-moe-krip′teen)
Cycloset, Parlodel
Func. class.: Antiparkinson agent
Chem. class.: Dopamine receptor agonist

Do not confuse:
Parlodel/pindolol/
bromocriptine/benztropine/brimonidine

ACTION: Inhibits prolactin release by activating postsynaptic dopamine receptors; activation of striatal dopamine receptors may be reason for improvement in Parkinson's disease

USES: Parkinson's disease, amenorrhea/galactorrhea caused by hyperprolactinemia, infertility, acromegaly, pituitary adenomas, adjunct for type 2 diabetes
Unlabeled uses: Neuroleptic malignant syndrome, mastalgia

CONTRAINDICATIONS
Basilar migraine, hemiplegic migraine, breastfeeding, uncontrolled hypertension, severe peripheral vascular disease; hypersensitivity to ergot, bromocriptine; preeclampsia/eclampsia

---

Side effects: *italics* = common; red = life-threatening

Precautions: Pregnancy, breastfeeding, children, renal/hepatic disease, pituitary tumors, peptic ulcer disease, sulfite hypersensitivity, pulmonary fibrosis, dementia, GI bleeding, bipolar disorder, abrupt discontinuation, acute MI, angina, type 1 diabetes mellitus

DOSAGE AND ROUTES
Parkinson's disease (not Cycloset)
• **Adult:** PO 1.25 mg bid with meals; may increase q2-4wk by 2.5 mg/day, max 30 mg/day; levodopa should be continued while bromocriptine is being instituted

Amenorrhea/galactorrhea from hyperprolactinemia; hypogonadism, infertility (not Cycloset)
• **Adult, adolescent ≥16 yr:** PO 1.25-2.5 mg with meals; may increase by 2.5 mg q3-7days, usual range 2.5-15 mg/day, max 30 mg/day
• **Child 11-15 yr:** PO 1.25-2.5 mg daily

Acromegaly (not Cycloset)
• **Adult:** PO 1.25-2.5 mg at bedtime; may increase by 1.25-2.5 mg q3-7days; usual range 20-30 mg/day, max 100 mg/day

Pituitary adenoma (not Cycloset)
• **Adult/adolescent ≥16 yr:** PO 1.25 mg bid-tid; may increase over several weeks to 10-20 mg/day

Type 2 diabetes (Cycloset only)
• **Adult:** PO (initially) 0.8 mg daily in AM within 2 hr of waking; titrate by 0.8 mg/day no more than weekly to max 1.6-4.8 mg/day
• **CYP3A4 inhibitors:** max 1.6 mg daily if used with moderate inhibitors
Available forms: Capsules 5 mg; tablets 2.5 mg (Parodel), 0.8 mg (Cycloset)
Administer:
• With meal to prevent GI symptoms; Cycloset: give with food in AM within 2 hr of waking
• At bedtime so dizziness, orthostatic hypotension do not occur
• Store at room temperature in tight, light-resistant container

SIDE EFFECTS
CNS: *Headache,* depression, restlessness, anxiety, nervousness, confusion, seizures, *hallucinations,* dizziness, fatigue, drowsiness, abnormal involuntary movements, psychosis, weakness

CV: Orthostatic hypotension, decreased B/P, palpitations, extrasystole, shock, dysrhythmias, bradycardia, MI
EENT: Blurred vision, diplopia, burning eyes, nasal congestion
GI: *Nausea, vomiting, anorexia,* cramps, constipation, diarrhea, dry mouth, GI hemorrhage
GU: Frequency, retention, incontinence, diuresis
INTEG: *Rash on face, arms;* alopecia; coolness, pallor of fingers, toes; peripheral edema
META: Hypoglycemia

PHARMACOKINETICS
Onset 2 hr, peak 1-3 hr, duration 4-8 hr, 90%-96% protein bound, half-life 3 hr, metabolized by liver (inactive metabolites), 85%-98% excreted in feces, >90% undergoes first-pass metabolism

INTERACTIONS
• Disulfiram-like reaction: alcohol
Increase: action of antihypertensives, levodopa, chloramphenicol, probenecid, salicylates, sulfonamides; dose of both products may need to be adjusted
Decrease: action of bromocriptine—phenothiazines, oral contraceptives, progestins, estrogens, haloperidol, loxapine, methyldopa, metoclopramide, MAOIs, reserpine; dose may need to be decreased
Decrease/increase: effect of Cycloset—CYP3A4 inhibitors/inducers; use cautiously
Decrease: effect of Cycloset—butyrophenones, metoclopramide, phenothiazine, thioxanthenes; avoid concurrent use
Drug/Lab Test
Increase: growth hormone, AST, ALT, CK, BUN, uric acid, alkaline phosphatase

NURSING CONSIDERATIONS
Assess:
• B/P; establish baseline, compare with other readings; this product decreases B/P and causes orthostatic hypotension; obtain chest x-ray baseline
• Monitor for reactions that usually occur at start of treatment (nausea, dizziness, orthostatic hypotension)
• **Parkinson's symptoms:** pill rolling, shuffling gait, restlessness, tremors, pos-

tural instability before and during treatment
• **Neuroleptic malignant syndrome:** decrease in temperature and sweating, lower pulse rate, and lessening of seizures indicate resolution of symptoms
• Change in size of soft tissue volume with acromegaly
• **CNS symptoms:** CNS depression, hallucinations, vertigo; report symptoms immediately
• **Pregnancy:** fertility may occur before onset of menses after pregnancy; use pregnancy testing q4wk or if menstruation does not occur, use alternative contraceptive methods other than oral contraceptives/subdermal implants during treatment; do not use in breastfeeding
Evaluate:
• Therapeutic response (Parkinson's disease): decreased dyskinesia, drooling, spasm, rigidity
Teach patient/family:
• That tablets may be crushed, mixed with food; Cycloset to be taken within 2 hr of rising; that 8 wk are needed for full effect
• To change position slowly to prevent orthostatic hypotension
• To use contraceptives during treatment with this product; that pregnancy may occur; to use methods other than oral contraceptives/subdermal implants
• That therapeutic effect for Parkinson's disease may take 2 mo, titrate slowly
• To avoid hazardous activity if dizziness occurs
• To report symptoms of MI immediately
• To take with food, avoid alcohol

budesonide (Rx)
(byoo-des'oh-nide)
Inhalation
Pulmicort Respules, Pulmicort Flexhaler
Nasal
Rhinocort Allergy
Systemic
Entocort EC, Tarpeyo, Uceris
Func. class.: Glucocorticoid
Chem. class.: Nonhalogenated

ACTION: Prevents inflammation by depressing migration of polymorphonuclear leukocytes and fibroblasts, reversal of increased capillary permeability, and lysosomal stabilization; does not suppress hypothalamus or pituitary function

USES: Rhinitis; prophylaxis for asthma; Crohn's disease, ulcerative colitis, nasal polyps
Unlabeled uses: Microscopic colitis, laryngotracheobronchitis (croup)

CONTRAINDICATIONS
Hypersensitivity, status asthmaticus, acute bronchospasm
Precautions: Pregnancy, breastfeeding; children; TB; fungal, bacterial, systemic viral infections; ocular herpes simplex; nasal septal ulcers; hepatic disease, diabetes, GI disease, increased intraocular pressure

DOSAGE AND ROUTES
Rhinitis
• **Adult and child >12 yr: SPRAY/INH** 2 sprays in each nostril AM, PM or 4 sprays in each nostril AM
Asthma
• **Adult: INH** 360 mcg bid, max 720 mcg bid
• **Child 1-8 yr previously taking bronchodilator alone: NEB** (Respules) 0.5 mg daily or 0.25 mg bid; suspension via jet nebulizer, max 0.5 mg daily; previously using inhaled corticosteroid 0.5 mg daily or 0.25 mg bid suspension via jet nebulizer, max 0.5 mg bid
Crohn's disease/ulcerative colitis (Uceris)
• **Adult: PO** 9 mg/day AM × 8 wk
Primary nephropathy (Tarpeyo)
• **Adult: PO** 16 mg daily
Laryngotracheobronchitis (croup) (unlabeled)
• **Infant ≥3 mo-child ≤5 yr: NEB** (Pulmicort Respules INH suspension) 2 mg inhaled as a single dose
Available forms: Dry powder for INH 90, 100 ✤, 180, 200, 400 ✤; 32 mcg/actuation (Rhinocort Aqua) nasal spray; suspension for INH 0.5 mg/2 mL, 0.25 mg/2 mL; capsule 3 mg; extended-release tablet

(Uceris) 9 mg, rectal foam 2 mg/actuation; delayed-release capsule 4 mg

Administer:

PO route (Crohn's disease/ulcerative colitis)

• Swallow capsules whole; do not break, crush, chew; take in AM
• May repeat 8-wk course if needed; may taper to 6 mg/day for 2 wk before cessation
• Store at 59° F-86° F (15° C-30° C); keep away from heat, open flame

Rectal foam route

• Product is flammable, may use before bedtime, applicators are single use only

Inhalation route

• Prime inhaler before initial use only. Do not shake; do not use with spacer. After inhalation, rinse and spit with water

Nasal route

• Shake gently before use
• Prime by actuating 8 times before initial use
• Reprime if not used for 2 consecutive days. If not used for 14 days, rinse the applicator and reprime until a fine mist appears

SIDE EFFECTS

CNS: *Headache,* insomnia, hypertonia, syncope, dizziness, drowsiness

CV: Chest pain, hypertension, sinus tachycardia, palpitation

EENT: *Sinusitis, pharyngitis,* rhinitis, oral candidiasis

ENDO: Adrenal insufficiency, growth suppression in children

GI: Dry mouth, dyspepsia, nausea, vomiting, abdominal pain

MISC: Ecchymosis, fever, *hypersensitivity,* flulike symptoms, epistaxis, dysuria

MS: Back pain, myalgias, fractures

RESP: Nasal irritation, cough, nasal bleeding, *respiratory infections,* bronchospasm

PHARMACOKINETICS

Peak: Respules 4-6 wk, Rhinocort Aqua 2 wk, half-life 2-3.6 hr

Onset: Respules 2-8 days, Rhinocort Aqua 10 hr

Enters breast milk

INTERACTIONS

Increase: budesonide effect—CYP3A inhibitors; dose adjustment may be needed
• Avoid concurrent use of varicella live vaccine in pediatric patients

NURSING CONSIDERATIONS

Assess:

• Respiratory status: rate, rhythm, increase in bronchial secretions, wheezing, chest tightness; provide fluids to 2 L/day to decrease thickness of secretions; check for oral candidiasis
• **Bronchospasm:** stop treatment, give bronchodilator
• **Crohn's disease/ulcerative colitis:** assess for improvement in symptoms, decreased stools, abdominal cramps, urgency
• **HPA axis suppression:** do not stop abruptly, taper
• Viral infections: corticosteroid use can mask infections
• Increased intraocular pressure: discontinue use if this occurs
• **Beers:** avoid in older adults; high risk of delirium
• **Pregnancy/breastfeeding:** fetal harm appears remote; excreted in breast milk; consider risk factors in continuing breastfeeding

Evaluate:

• Therapeutic response: absence of asthma, rhinitis

Teach patient/family:

• To notify prescriber of pharyngitis, nasal bleeding, oral candidiasis
• Not to exceed recommended dose because adrenal suppression may occur
• To carry emergency ID that identifies steroid use
• To read and follow package directions
• To prevent exposure to infections (especially viral)
• To use good oral hygiene if using nebulizer or inhaler
• To avoid breastfeeding
• That burning or stinging may occur with first few doses of inhalation use
• That product is not a bronchodilator and not to be used for asthma; to use regularly

- How to use as described in "Administer"
- To notify prescriber if symptoms persist after weeks, that results usually take 2 wk
- To notify prescriber if exposure to measles, chickenpox occurs

bumetanide (Rx)

(byoo-met′a-nide)

Bumex, Burinex ✦

Func. class.: Loop diuretic, antihypertensive

Chem. class.: Sulfonamide derivative

ACTION: Acts on ascending loop of Henle by inhibiting reabsorption of chloride, sodium

USES: Edema in heart failure, renal disease, hepatic disease

CONTRAINDICATIONS

Hypersensitivity to sulfonamides, anuria, hepatic coma

Black Box Warning: Fluid and electrolyte depletion

Precautions: Pregnancy, breastfeeding, neonates, ascites, severe renal disease, hepatic cirrhosis, blood dyscrasias, ototoxicity, hyperuricemia, hypokalemia, hyperglycemia, oliguria, hypomagnesemia, hypovolemia

Black Box Warning: Dehydration

DOSAGE AND ROUTES

- **Adult and adolescent: PO** 0.5-2 mg/day; **IV/IM** 0.5-1 mg; may give second or third dose at 2-3 hr intervals, not to exceed 10 mg/day
- **Child and infant (unlabeled): PO/IM/IV** 0.015-0.1 mg/kg dose q6-24hr, max 10 mg/day
- **Neonates (unlabeled): PO/IM/IV** 0.01-0.05 kg/dose q12-24hr

Available forms: Tablets 0.5, 1, 2, 5 ✦ mg; injection 0.25 mg/mL

PO route

- Use in AM to prevent nocturia
- Without regard to food

IV, direct route

- Direct IV undiluted slowly over 1-2 min through Y-tube, 3-way stopcock, or hep-lock

Intermittent IV INFUSION route

- Dilute in LR, D₅W, 0.9% NaCl (rarely given by this method), give over 12 hr with renal disease; give at 4 mg/min or less, use infusion pump, protect from light

Y-site compatibilities: Acyclovir, alfentanil, allopurinol, amifostine, amikacin, aminocaproic acid, aminophylline, amiodarone, amoxicillin, amphotericin B lipid complex (Abelcet), amphotericin B liposome (AmBisome), anidulafungin, ascorbic acid injection, atenolol, atracurium, atropine, aztreonam, benztropine, bivalirudin, bleomycin, buprenorphine, butorphanol, calcium chloride/gluconate, CARBOplatin, caspofungin, cefamandole, ceFAZolin, cefepime, cefmetazole, cefonicid, cefotaxime, cefoTEtan, cefOXitin, cefTAZidime, ceftizoxime, ceftobiprole, cefTRIAXone, cefuroxime, cephapirin, chloramphenicol, cimetidine, cisatracurium, CISplatin, cladribine, clarithromycin, clindamycin, codeine, cyanocobalamin, cyclophosphamide, cycloSPORINE, cytarabine, DACTINomycin, DAPTOmycin, dexamethasone, dexmedetomidine, digoxin, diltiazem, diphenhydrAMINE, DOBUTamine, DOCEtaxel, DOPamine, doripenem, doxacurium, DOXOrubicin, doxycycline, enalaprilat, ePHEDrine, EPINEPHrine, epirubicin, epoetin alfa, eptifibatide, ertapenem, erythromycin, esmolol, etoposide, famotidine, fentaNYL, filgrastim, fluconazole, fludarabine, fluorouracil, folic acid, furosemide, gatifloxacin, gemcitabine, gentamicin, glycopyrrolate, granisetron, heparin, hydrocortisone sodium succinate, HYDROmorphone, hydrOXYzine, IDArubicin, ifosfamide, imipenem-cilastatin, indomethacin, insulin (regular), irinotecan, isoproterenol, ketorolac, labetalol, levofloxacin, lidocaine, linezolid, LORazepam, magnesium sulfate, mannitol, mechlorethamine, melphalan, meperidine, metaraminol, methotrexate, methoxamine, methyldopa, methylPREDNISolone, metoclopramide, metoprolol, metroNIDAZOLE, mezlocillin, micafungin, miconazole, milrinone, mito-XANtrone, morphine, moxalactam, multiple vitamins injection, mycophenolate, nafcillin, nalbuphine, naloxone, netilmicin, nitroglycerin, nitroprusside, norepinephrine, octreotide, ondansetron, oxacillin, oxaliplatin, oxytocin, palonosetron, pamidronate, pancuronium, pantoprazole, PEMEtrexed, penicillin G potassium/sodium, pentazocine, PENTobarbital, PHENobarbital, phenylephrine, phytonadione, piperacillin, piperacillin-tazobactam, polymyxin B, potassium chloride, procainamide, promethazine, propofol, propranolol, protamine, pyridoxine, quiNIDine, ranitidine, remifentanil, rifampin, ritodrine, riTUXimab, rocuronium, sodium acetate, sodium bicarbonate, succinylcholine, SUFentanil, tacrolimus, teniposide, theophylline, thiamine, thiotepa, ticarcillin, ticarcillin-clavulanate, tigecycline, tirofiban, TNA, tobramycin, tolazoline, TPN, traMADol, trastuzumab, trimetaphan, urokinase, vancomycin, vasopressin, vecuronium, verapamil, vinCRIStine, vinorelbine, voriconazole

SIDE EFFECTS

CNS: *Headache,* fatigue, weakness, *dizziness, encephalopathy*
CV: *Hypotension,* ECG changes, dehydration
EENT: *Loss of hearing*
ELECT: *Hypokalemia, hypochloremic alkalosis, hypomagnesemia, hyperuricemia, hypocalcemia, hyponatremia*
ENDO: *Hyperglycemia*
GI: Dry mouth, upset stomach, vomiting, diarrhea, nausea
GU: *Polyuria,* glycosuria
INTEG: *Rash, pruritus,* SJS, toxic epidermal necrolysis
MS: *Myalgia, arthralgia*

PHARMACOKINETICS

Excreted by kidneys (50% unchanged), feces (20%); crosses placenta; excreted in breast milk; protein binding >72%; half-life 1-1½ hr
PO: Onset ½-1 hr, peak 1-2 hr, duration 3-6 hr
IM: Onset 40 min, peak 1-2 hr, duration 4-6 hr

IV: Onset 5 min, peak 15-30 min, duration 3-6 hr

INTERACTIONS

Increase: ototoxicity—aminoglycosides, avoid concurrent use
Increase: hypokalemia—corticosteroids, diuretics, laxatives (stimulants); monitor closely
Increase: diuresis—other diuretics, monitor for dehydration and electrolyte imbalances
Increase: toxicity—lithium, digoxin, monitor levels of each
Increase: hypotension, antihypertensives, nitrates
Decrease: diuretic effect—NSAIDs, monitor carefully
Decrease: antidiabetic effects—antidiabetics, monitor glucose
Drug/Herb
Increase: effect—hawthorn, horse chestnut, avoid using together
Decrease: effect of bumetanide—ginseng, ephedra
Drug/Lab
Increase: glucose
Decrease: chloride, potassium, sodium, calcium, phosphorus

NURSING CONSIDERATIONS
Assess
• For tinnitus, hearing loss, ear pain; obtain audiometric testing for long-term IV treatment

Black Box Warning: Dehydration: weight, I&O daily to determine fluid loss; if urinary output decreases or azotemia occurs, product should be discontinued; safest dosage schedule is alternate days

• B/P lying, standing; postural hypotension may occur

Black Box Warning: Fluid and electrolyte depletion: potassium, sodium, calcium; include BUN, blood glucose, CBC, serum creatinine, blood pH, ABGs, uric acid, calcium, magnesium; severe electrolyte depletion should be corrected before starting treatment

• Blood glucose if patient is diabetic; blood uric acid levels in those with gout
• Improvement in edema of feet, legs, sacral area daily if medication is being used for HF
• Signs of metabolic alkalosis: drowsiness, restlessness
• **Hypokalemia:** postural hypotension, malaise, fatigue, tachycardia, leg cramps, weakness
• Rashes, temperature elevation daily
• Confusion, especially in geriatric patients; take safety precautions if needed
• **Digoxin toxicity** in patients taking digoxin products: anorexia, nausea, vomiting, confusion, paresthesia, muscle cramps; **lithium toxicity** in those taking lithium
• **Beers:** use cautiously in older adults; may cause or exacerbate syndrome of inappropriate antidiuretic hormone secretion

Evaluate:
• Therapeutic response: decreased edema, B/P

Teach patient/family:
• To increase fluid intake to 2-3 L/day unless contraindicated; to take potassium supplement; to rise slowly from lying or sitting position
• To recognize adverse reactions: muscle cramps, weakness, nausea, dizziness, edema, weight gain
• To take with food, milk for GI symptoms; to avoid alcohol
• To take early in day to prevent nocturia; if another dose is needed, take after noon, not to double or miss dose
• To take B/P, pulse, weight weekly
• That orthostatic hypotension may occur, to avoid rising rapidly
• To continue other medical regimens
• That continuing exams and blood work will be needed
• To notify other health care professionals of condition being treated, medications taken
• **Pregnancy/breastfeeding:** To report if pregnancy is planned or suspected or if breastfeeding

TREATMENT OF OVERDOSE:
Lavage if taken orally; monitor electrolytes; administer dextrose in saline; monitor hydration, CV, renal status

---

B

⚠ HIGH ALERT

buprenorphine (Rx)
REMS
(byoo-pre-nor'feen)
Belbuca, Buprenex, Butrans, Probuphine, Sublocade
Func. class.: Opioid analgesic, partial agonist
Chem. class.: Thebaine derivative

Controlled Substance Schedule III

ACTION: Depresses pain impulse transmission at the spinal cord level by interacting with opioid receptors, partial agonist at μ-opioid receptor

USES: Moderate to severe pain, opiate agonist withdrawal/dependence

CONTRAINDICATIONS
Hypersensitivity, ileus, status asthmaticus

Black Box Warning: Respiratory depression

Precautions: Pregnancy, breastfeeding, substance abuse/alcoholism, increased intracranial pressure, MI (acute), severe heart disease, respiratory depression, renal/hepatic/pulmonary disease, hypothyroidism, Addison's disease, QT prolongation, accidental exposure, neonatal opioid withdrawal syndrome

Black Box Warning: Potential for overdose/poisoning, substance abuse, IM, coadministration with other CNS depressants, implant insertion and removal

DOSAGE AND ROUTES
Moderate/severe pain
• **Adult/child ≥13 yr: IM/IV** 0.3 mg q4-6hr as needed: **TD** each patch is worn for 7 days (moderate-severe pain); **opioid-naive patients** (those taking <30 mg of oral morphine or equivalent before beginning treatment with TD buprenorphine), 5 mcg/hr q7days, overestimating dose can

---

Side effects: *italics* = common; red = life-threatening

be fatal; **conversion from other opiate agonist therapy,** titrate from other opioids for up to 7 days to no more than 30 mg oral morphine or equivalent before beginning TD therapy, begin with 5 mcg/hr q7days; for those with daily dose of 30-80 mg oral morphine or equivalent, start with 10 mcg/hr q7days; for those taking >80 mg oral morphine or equivalent, start with 20 mcg/hr q7days

• **Geriatric/debilitated patients: IM/IV** 0.15 mg slowly
• **Child 2-12 yr: IM/IV** 2-6 mcg/kg q4-8hr, give IV over ≥2 min

Opioid dependence

Adult: SL 8 mg on day 1 and 16 mg on day 2, titrate in increments of 2 or 4 mg up or down to needed, maintenance dose 4-24 mg SL daily; **Implant:** 4 implants (320 mg buprenorphine hydrochloride) subdermally in the inner side of the upper arm and leave in place for 6 mo; **Ext Rel (Brixadi) SUBCUT:** For patients taking 6 mg/day or less of SL buprenorphine, use 8 mg/wk; for 8 to 10 mg/day SL, switch to 16 mg/wk or 64 mg/mo; for 12 to 16 mg/day SL, switch to 24 mg/wk or 96 mg/mo; for 18 to 24 mg/day SL, switch to 32 mg/wk; for 128 mg/mo SUBCUT Max: 32 mg/wk or 128 mg/mo.

Hepatic dose

Adult TD (mild-moderate): 5 mcg/hr system initially
Buccal (severe hepatic disease): decrease dose by 50%, titrate upward by 75 mcg q12hr ≥q4days

Available forms: Injection 0.3 mg/mL (1-mL vials); SL tablet 2, 8 mg as base; TD system 5, 7.5, 10, 15, 20 mcg/hr (weekly); dissolving film (buccal) 75, 150, 300, 450, 600, 750, 900 mcg; solution for injection, extended release 100 mg/0.5 mL, 300 mg/1.5 mL; SD implant 74.2 mg/implant

Administer:

SL route
• Do not chew; dissolve under tongue, use 2 or more at same time

Transdermal route (REMS)
• Apply to clean, dry, intact skin; each patch should be worn for 7 days, do not exceed dose, QTC prolongation may oc-

cur; do not apply direct heat source to patch, will increase absorption of product, may use first-aid tape if edge of patch is not adhering
• Apply to upper outer arm, upper chest/back, or side of chest

Subcut route (extended-release injection—Sublocade)
• Inject only in abdominal region. DO NOT use IM/IV
• Visually inspect for particulate matter, discoloration before use; product is clear, colorless to yellow to amber solution
• Give monthly with a minimum of 26 days between doses
• Use only the syringe and safety needle included. Do not attach the needle until time of use
• Do not inject into an area where skin is irritated, reddened, bruised, infected, or scarred
• Do not rub area after injection
• To avoid irritation, rotate injection site with each injection
• Injection site should be examined for infection, evidence of tampering, or attempts to remove the depot
• **Storage:** Store unopened prefilled syringes in the refrigerator in original packaging; do not freeze. Discard injection if left at room temperature for longer than 7 days

Subdermal route (Probuphine)
• Inserted in inner side of upper arm
• Maintenance dose must be 8 mg/day or less
• Use guideline from manufacturer
• Available from REMS program (844-859-6341), health care professional must complete training program
• Inserts are removed after 6 mo, if other insert is not used, use transmucosal

IM route
• In deep muscle mass

IV, direct route
• **Give** undiluted over ≥2 min, titrate to patient response; rapid injection will increase side effects
• With antiemetic if nausea, vomiting occur
• When pain is beginning to return; determine dosage interval by patient response

Y-site compatibilities: Acyclovir, alfentanil, allopurinol, amifostine, amikacin, aminocaproic acid, amphotericin B liposome (AmBisome), anidulafungin, ascorbic acid injection, atenolol, atracurium, atropine, aztreonam, benztropine, bivalirudin, bleomycin, bumetanide, butorphanol, calcium chloride/gluconate, CARBOplatin, cefamandole, ceFAZolin, cefepime, cefotaxime, cefoTEtan, cefOXitin, cefTAZidime, ceftizoxime, cefTRIAXone, cefuroxime, chloramphenicol, chlorproMAZINE, cimetidine, cisatracurium, CISplatin, cladribine, clindamycin, cyanocobalamin, cyclophosphamide, cycloSPORINE, cytarabine, D₅W-dextrose 5%, DACTINomycin, DAPTOmycin, dexamethasone, dexmedetomidine, digoxin, diltiazem, diphenhydrAMINE, DOBUTamine, DOCEtaxel, DOPamine, doxacurium, DOXOrubicin HCl, doxycycline, enalaprilat, ePHEDrine, EPINEPHrine, epirubicin, epoetin alfa, eptifibatide, ertapenem, erythromycin, esmolol, etoposide, famotidine, fenoldopam, fentaNYL, filgrastim, fluconazole, fludarabine, gatifloxacin, gemcitabine, gentamicin, glycopyrrolate, granisetron, heparin, hydrocortisone, hydrOXYzine, IDArubicin, ifosfamide, imipenem-cilastatin, inamrinone, insulin (regular), irinotecan, isoproterenol, ketorolac, labetalol, lactated Ringer's injection, levofloxacin, lidocaine, linezolid, LORazepam, magnesium sulfate, mannitol, mechlorethamine, melphalan, meperidine, metaraminol, methicillin, methotrexate, methoxamine, methyldopate, methylPREDNISolone, metoclopramide, metoprolol, metroNIDAZOLE, mezlocillin, miconazole, midazolam, milrinone, minocycline, mitoXANtrone, morphine, moxalactam, multiple vitamins injection, mycophenolate mofetil, nafcillin, nalbuphine, naloxone, nesiritide, netilmicin, nitroglycerin, nitroprusside, norepinephrine, octreotide, ondansetron, oxacillin, oxaliplatin, oxytocin, palonosetron, pamidronate, pancuronium, papaverine, PEMEtrexed, penicillin G potassium/sodium, pentamidine, pentazocine, phenylephrine, phytonadione, piperacillin, piperacillin-tazobactam, polymyxin B, potassium chloride, procainamide, prochlorperazine, promethazine, propofol, propranolol, protamine, pyridoxine, quiNIDine, ranitidine, remifentanil, Ringer's injection, riTUXimab, rocuronium, sodium acetate, succinylcholine, SUFentanil, tacrolimus, teniposide, theophylline, thiamine, thiotepa, ticarcillin, ticarcillin-clavulanate, tigecycline, tirofiban, TNA (3-in-1), tobramycin, tolazoline, TPN, trastuzumab, trimetaphan, urokinase, vancomycin, vasopressin, vecuronium, verapamil, vinCRIStine, vinorelbine, voriconazole

SIDE EFFECTS

CNS: *Drowsiness, dizziness, confusion, headache, sedation, euphoria, hallucinations, strange dreams*
CV: Palpitations, QT prolongation, hypo/hypertension
EENT: Tinnitus, blurred vision, *miosis*, diplopia
GI: *Nausea,* vomiting, anorexia, constipation, dry mouth, hepatotoxicity
GU: Urinary retention
INTEG: *Rash,* diaphoresis, pruritus
RESP: Respiratory depression, bronchospasm
MISC: Anaphylaxis, angioedema, dependency

PHARMACOKINETICS

Metabolized in liver by CYP3A4, excreted by kidneys and in feces, crosses placenta, excreted in breast milk, half-life 2½-3½ hr, 96% bound to plasma proteins
IM: Onset 15 min, peak 1 hr, duration 6-10 hr
SL: Onset, peak, duration unknown, half-life 37 hr
IV: Onset 1 min, peak 5 min, duration 6 hr, half-life 2.2 hr
TD: Half-life 26 hr
Epidural: Duration dose dependent

INTERACTIONS

Increase: effect with other CNS depressants—alcohol, opioids, sedative/hypnotics, antipsychotics, skeletal muscle relaxants, MAOIs

Side effects: *italics* = common; red = life-threatening

Increase: buprenorphine effect—CYP3A4 inhibitors (erythromycin, indinavir, ketoconazole, ritonavir, saquinavir)

Increase: QT prolongation—class IA, III antidysrhythmics

Increase: serotonin syndrome 5-HT3 antagonists, linezolid, methylene blue, MAOIs, SSRIs, SNRIs, tricyclics

Decrease: buprenorphine effect—CYP3A4 inducers (carBAMazepine, PHENobarbital, phenytoin, rifampin)

Drug/Herb

Increase: CNS depression—chamomile, kava, St. John's wort

NURSING CONSIDERATIONS
Assess:

• **Pain:** intensity, location, type before treatment, after 5, 15, 30 min (IV); need for pain medication, tolerance

> **Black Box Warning: Accidental exposure:** keep away from children and pets; may be fatal

• I&O ratio; check for decreasing output; may indicate urinary retention
• Bowel pattern; severe constipation can occur
• CNS changes, dizziness, drowsiness, hallucinations, euphoria, LOC, pupil reaction; withdrawal in opioid-dependent persons
• Allergic reactions: rash, urticaria

> **Black Box Warning: Respiratory dysfunction:** respiratory depression, character, rate, rhythm; notify prescriber if respirations are <12/min, may be fatal

> **Black Box Warning: Potential for overdose** may occur from chewing, swallowing, snorting, or injecting extracted product from TD formulation

• **QT prolongation:** in those taking class Ia, III antidysrhythmics; patients with hypokalemia, cardiac instability (TD), max TD 20 mcg/hr q7day
• **Beers:** avoid in older adults unless safer alternatives are not available, may cause impaired psychomotor function, syncope

• **Pregnancy/breastfeeding:** avoid use in pregnancy and breastfeeding; in those using product and breastfeeding, watch infant for decreased respiration, lethargy, decreased heart rate

Evaluate:

• Therapeutic response: decrease in pain, decreased withdrawal symptoms

Teach patient/family:

• To report any symptoms of CNS changes, allergic reactions

> **Black Box Warning:** That psychologic dependence leading to substance abuse may result when used for extended periods; that long-term use is not recommended

• That product can cause serious breathing problems; call provider right away if feeling faint, dizzy, or if breathing gets much slower than normal
• To avoid hazardous activities such as driving unless reaction is known
• Do not start new meds/herbs without prescriber approval; do not double, skip doses
• Start stool softener/laxatives to lessen constipation
• **SL route:** to place under tongue and allow to dissolve
• **Transdermal route:** how to apply and dispose of patch; not to use a heating pad or other heat source; do not cut

TREATMENT OF OVERDOSE:
Naloxone 0.4 mg ampule diluted in 10 mL 0.9% NaCl given by direct IV push 0.02 mg q2min (adult)

---

buPROPion (Rx)
(byoo-proe′pee-on)
Aplenzin, Forfivo XL, Wellbutrin XL, Wellbutrin SR, Zyban
Func. class.: Antidepressant—miscellaneous smoking deterrent
Chem. class.: Aminoketone

Do not confuse:
buPROPion/busPIRone
Zyban/Diovan

ACTION: Inhibits reuptake of DOPamine, norepinephrine, serotonin

USES: Depression (Wellbutrin), smoking cessation (Zyban); seasonal affective disorder, substance abuse, glaucoma, smoking, cardiac disease, heart failure

Unlabeled uses: ADHD (adult)

CONTRAINDICATIONS
Hypersensitivity, head trauma, stroke, intracranial mass, eating disorders, seizure disorders, use with MAOIs, ritonavir, severe stroke
Precautions: Pregnancy, breastfeeding, geriatric patients, renal/hepatic disease, recent MI, cranial trauma, seizure disorder, substance abuse, glaucoma, smoking, cardiac disease, heart failure, head trauma, stroke, intracranial mass, Tourette's syndrome, tics, tobacco smoking, abrupt discontinuation

Black Box Warning: Children <18 yr, suicidal thinking/behavior (young adults)

DOSAGE AND ROUTES
Depression
• **Adult:** IR 100 mg bid initially, then increase after 3 days to 100 mg tid if needed, max 150 mg single dose; **ER/SR** initially 150 mg AM, increase to 300 mg/day if initial dose is tolerated, after no less than 4 days; after several weeks, titrate to 200 mg bid; **Aplenzin** 174 mg q AM, may increase to 348 mg q AM on day 4, may increase to 522 mg after several weeks if needed; **Forfivo XL** (not for initial treatment) 450 mg daily after titration with another product (300 mg/day × ≥2 wk)
• **Geriatric:** PO 50-100 mg/day, may increase by 50-100 mg q3-4days
Smoking cessation
• **Adult:** SR 150 mg daily × 3 days, then 150 mg bid for remainder of treatment
Seasonal affective disorder
• **Adult:** PO (Wellbutrin XL) 150 mg as a single dose in the AM, after 1 wk may be increased to 300 mg/day; (Aplenzin) 174 mg daily in AM, after 7 days may increase to 348 mg daily
Hepatic dose
Adult: PO (moderate-severe) Aplenzin max 174 mg every other day

Available forms: Tablets 75, 100 mg; extended-release tablet (XL) 100, 150, 200, 300, 450 mg; (SR-12 hr, XL-24 hr); tablet extended release (Aplenzin) 174, 348, 522 mg
Administer:
PO route
• When switching to Aplenzin from Wellbutrin, Wellbutrin SR or XL, use these equivalents: 174 mg buPROPion HBr = 150 mg buPROPion HCl; 348 mg buPROPion HBr = 300 mg buPROPion HCl; 522 mg buPROPion HBr = 450 mg buPROPion HCl
• **Wellbutrin immediate release,** separate by ≥6 hr, give in 3 divided doses; **Wellbutrin XL,** give daily in AM; **Zyban SR,** give in 2 divided doses, ≥8 hr apart; **Aplenzin ER,** give daily in AM, a larger dose of Aplenzin is needed because these products are not equivalent
• Do not break, crush, chew sustained-release, extended-release tablet
• At evenly spaced times to prevent seizures; seizure risk increases with high doses
• Increase fluids, bulk in diet if constipation occurs
• Do not use with SSRIs, linezolid, methylene blue, MAOIs
• With food, milk for GI symptoms
• Sugarless gum, hard candy, frequent sips of water for dry mouth
• Avoid giving at night to prevent insomnia

SIDE EFFECTS
CNS: *Headache, agitation, dizziness, akinesia, confusion,* seizures, delusions, *insomnia, sedation, tremors,* suicidal/homicidal ideation, flushing
CV: Dysrhythmias, hypertension, palpitations, *tachycardia,* hypotension, chest pain, chills
EENT: *Blurred vision, auditory disturbance*
GI: *Nausea, vomiting,* anorexia, diarrhea, *dry mouth,* increased appetite, *constipation,* altered taste
GU: Impotence, urinary frequency, retention
INTEG: *Rash,* pruritus, *sweating*
MISC: *Hot flashes*

Side effects: *italics* = common; red = life-threatening

PHARMACOKINETICS
Onset 1-4 wk, half-life 14 hr (immediate release), extensively metabolized by liver, some conversion to active metabolites, protein binding 84%, excreted in urine and feces

INTERACTIONS
• Do not use within 14 days of MAOIs

Increase: adverse reactions: amantadine, haloperidol seizures—levodopa, MAOIs, phenothiazines, antidepressants, benzodiazepines, alcohol, theophylline, systemic steroids

Increase: serotonin syndrome—SSRIs, methylene blue, linezolid, traMADol, traZODone, tricyclic antidepressants, cyclobenzaprine; do not use together

Increase: action of citalopram

Decrease: effect of tamoxifen

Decrease: buPROPion effect—carBAMazepine, cimetidine, PHENobarbital, phenytoin or other products (CYP2D6); CYP2B6 inducers

Drug/Herb
Increase: CNS depression—kava, valerian

Drug/Lab Test
Positive: urine drug screen for amphetamine possible

NURSING CONSIDERATIONS
Assess:
• **Smoking:** for smoking cessation after 7-12 wk; if progress has not been made, product should be discontinued, begin smoking cessation while patient is still smoking, start smoking cessation after 7 days
• For increased risk of seizures; if patient has excessively used CNS depressants and OTC stimulants, dosage of buPROPion should not be exceeded
• Monitor weight regularly, monitor VS baseline and periodically

Black Box Warning: **Mental status:** mood, sensorium, affect, suicidal/homicidal tendencies, increase in psychiatric symptoms, assess for mania in those with bipolar disorder

• **Beers:** avoid in older adults; lowers seizure threshold, may be acceptable for those with well-controlled seizures for which other treatment has been ineffective

Evaluate:
• Therapeutic response: decreased depression, ability to perform daily activities, ability to sleep throughout the night, smoking cessation

Teach patient/family:
• That therapeutic effects may take 2-4 wk; not to increase dose without prescriber's approval; that treatment for smoking cessation lasts 7-12 wk
• To use caution when driving, performing other activities that require alertness; sedation, blurred vision may occur
• To avoid alcohol, other CNS depressants; alcohol may increase risk of seizures
• Not to chew, crush tablets
• That extended-release shell may be seen in stools, tablet odor is unpleasant
• That exams and lab work will be needed
• To notify health care professionals of all Rx, herbals, supplements taken, not to start new product unless discussed prior to use
• Not to use with nicotine patches unless directed by prescriber; may increase B/P
• To notify prescriber immediately if urinary retention occurs
• That risk of seizures increases when dose is exceeded or if used with alcohol or other CNS depressants; if patient has seizure disorder

Black Box Warning: That suicidal/homicidal ideas, behaviors, hostility, depression may occur in children or young adults, to report immediately

• **Serotonin syndrome:** monitor for increased B/P, pulse, fever, agitation, tremor, sweating, diarrhea; usually caused when combined with other products on interaction list; immediately stop drug and report symptoms to prescriber
• **Pregnancy/breastfeeding:** to notify prescriber if pregnancy is suspected, planned, or if breastfeeding

TREATMENT OF OVERDOSE:
ECG monitoring; lavage; administer anticonvulsant

burosumab-twza (Rx)

(bur-oh′sue-mab)

Crysvita

Func. class.: Fibroblast growth factor blocking antibody

USES: ⚠ X-linked hypophosphatemia (XLH) in adult and pediatric patients 1 yr of age and older

CONTRAINDICATIONS

Use with oral phosphate or active vitamin D analogs; serum phosphorus is within or above the normal range for age; severe renal impairment or end-stage renal disease

DOSAGE AND ROUTES

• **Adult: SUBCUT** 1 mg/kg body weight rounded to nearest 10 mg (max 90 mg) q4wk

• **Child 1-18 yr: SUBCUT** 0.8 mg/kg body weight rounded to nearest 10 mg (max 90 mg) q2wk. Dose may be increased up to approximately 2 mg/kg (max 90 mg) q2wk to achieve normal serum phosphorus

Available forms: Solution for injection 10, 20, 30 mg/mL

⚠ HIGH ALERT

busPIRone (Rx)

(byoo-spye′rone)

Func. class.: Antianxiety, sedative

Chem. class.: Azaspirodecanedione

Do not confuse:

busPIRone/buPROPion

ACTION: Acts by inhibiting the action of serotonin (5-HT); has shown little potential for abuse; a good choice with substance abuse

USES: Generalized anxiety disorders

CONTRAINDICATIONS

Children <18 yr, hypersensitivity, MAOIs

Precautions: Pregnancy, breastfeeding, geriatric patients, impaired hepatic/renal function

DOSAGE AND ROUTES

Anxiety disorders

• **Adult: PO** 7.5 mg bid; may increase by 5 mg/day q2-3days, max 60 mg/day

Hepatic/renal dose

• **Adult: PO** Do not use in severe renal/ hepatic disease

Available forms: Tablets 5, 7.5, 10, 15, 30 mg

Administer:

• With food, milk for GI symptoms; avoid grapefruit juice; give drug at same time of day, with/without food consistently

• Crushed if patient unable to swallow medication whole

• Sugarless gum, hard candy, frequent sips of water for dry mouth

SIDE EFFECTS

CNS: *Dizziness, headache, stimulation, insomnia, nervousness, numbness, paresthesia, incoordination*

CV: *Tachycardia, palpitations,* hypo/ hypertension, chest pain

EENT: *Sore throat, tinnitus, blurred vision, nasal congestion;* change in taste, smell

GI: *Nausea, dry mouth, diarrhea, constipation,* increased appetite

GU: Frequency, hesitancy, change in libido

INTEG: *Rash,* edema, pruritus, alopecia, dry skin

MISC: *Sweating,* fatigue, fever

MS: *Pain, weakness,* muscle cramps, myalgia

RESP: Hyperventilation, chest congestion, shortness of breath

PHARMACOKINETICS

Onset, duration unknown; Peak 40-90 min, half-life 2-4 hr, rapidly absorbed, metabolized by liver (CYP3A4), excreted in feces, protein binding 86%

INTERACTIONS

Increase: busPIRone—CYP3A4 inhibitors (erythromycin, itraconazole, nefazodone, ketoconazole, ritonavir, verapamil,

---

Side effects: *italics* = common; red = life-threatening

dilTIAZem, several other protease inhibitors), dosage decrease may be needed

Increase: B/P—procarbazine, MAOIs; avoid using together

Increase: CNS depression—psychotropic products, alcohol (avoid use), monitor closely if used together

Increase: serotonin syndrome—SSRIs, SNRIs, serotonin receptor agonists

Decrease: busPIRone effects—rifAMPin

Decrease: busPIRone action—CYP3A4 inducers (rifAMPin, phenytoin, PHENobarbital, carBAMazepine, dexamethasone), dosage increase may be needed

Drug/Herb
Increase: CNS depression—chamomile, kava kava, valerian
Drug/Food
Increase: peak concentration of busPIRone—grapefruit juice

NURSING CONSIDERATIONS
Assess:
• B/P lying, standing; pulse; if systolic B/P drops 20 mm Hg, hold product, notify prescriber
• CNS reactions because some may be unpredictable
• Mental status: mood, sensorium, affect, sleeping pattern, drowsiness, dizziness; withdrawal symptoms when dose reduced, product discontinued
• Safety measures if drowsiness, dizziness occurs
• **Beers:** avoid in older adults with delirium or at high risk for delirium
Evaluate:
• Therapeutic response: decreased anxiety, restlessness, sleeplessness
Teach patient/family:
• That product may be taken consistently with/without food
• To avoid OTC products, alcohol ingestion, other psychotropic medications unless approved by prescriber; to avoid large amounts of grapefruit juice
• To avoid activities that require alertness because drowsiness may occur
• Not to discontinue medication abruptly after long-term use; if dose is missed, do not double

• To rise slowly because fainting may occur, especially among geriatric patients
• That drowsiness may worsen at beginning of treatment; that 2 wk of therapy may be required before therapeutic effects occur, max effect 3-6 wk
• **Serotonin syndrome:** to report immediately (fever, tremor, sweating, diarrhea, delirium)
• **Pregnancy/breastfeeding:** report if pregnancy is planned or suspected or if breastfeeding, use in pregnancy and breastfeeding isn't recommended

---

⚠ *HIGH ALERT*

busulfan (Rx)
(byoo-sul′fan)
Busulfex, Myleran
Func. class.: Antineoplastic alkylating agent

USES: Chronic myelocytic leukemia, bone marrow ablation, stem cell transplant preparation with CML

CONTRAINDICATIONS
Pregnancy, breastfeeding, blastic phase of chronic myelocytic leukemia, hypersensitivity

Precautions: Women of childbearing age, leukopenia, anemia, hepatotoxicity, renal toxicity, seizures, tumor lysis syndrome, hyperkalemia, hyperphosphatemia, hypocalcemia, hyperuricemia, radiation, chemotherapy, male-mediated teratogenicity, veno-occlusive disease (VOD), sinusoidal obstruction syndrome, head trauma

> **Black Box Warning:** Thrombocytopenia, neutropenia, new primary malignancy, bone marrow suppression

DOSAGE AND ROUTES
Chronic myelocytic leukemia
• **Adult:** PO Induction dosing is 60 mcg/kg or 1.8 mg/m^2 every day; usual dose is 4 to 8 mg
• **Child:** PO 0.06-0.12 mg/kg/day or 1.8-4.6 mg/m^2/day

Allogenic hematopoietic stem cell transplantation

• **Adult: IV** 0.8 mg/kg over 2 hr, q6hr × 4 days (total 16 doses); give cyclophosphamide **IV** 60 mg/kg over 1 hr daily for 2 days starting after 16th dose of busulfan; **PO** (unlabeled) 1 mg/kg q6hr × 16 doses

• **Adolescent and child >12 kg (unlabeled): IV** 0.8 mg/kg over 2 hr q6hr × 16 doses (4 days), then high-dose cyclophosphamide 50 mg/kg/day × 4 days

• **Infant/child ≤12 kg (unlabeled): IV** 1.1 mg/kg over 2 hr q6hr × 16 doses (4 days), then high-dose cyclophosphamide 50 mg/kg/day × 4 days

Available forms: Injection 6 mg/mL, tablets 2 mg

---

butoconazole vaginal antifungal
See Appendix B

⚠ HIGH ALERT

butorphanol (Rx)
(byoo-tor′fa-nole)
Func. class.: Opioid analgesic
Chem. class.: Mixed opioid antagonist, partial agonist

Controlled Substance Schedule IV

ACTION: Depresses pain impulse transmission at the spinal cord level by interacting with opioid receptors

USES: Moderate to severe pain, general anesthesia induction/maintenance, headache, migraine, preanesthesia

CONTRAINDICATIONS
Hypersensitivity to product, preservative; addiction (opioid)

Precautions: Pregnancy, breastfeeding, children <18 yr, addictive personality, increased intracranial pressure, renal/hepatic disease, ileus, COPD, potential for overdose

Black Box Warning: Coadministration with other CNS depressants, respiratory depression, accidental exposure (intranasal), neonatal opioid withdrawal syndrome, substance abuse

DOSAGE AND ROUTES
Moderate-severe pain

• **Adult: IM** 1-4 mg q3-4hr prn; **IV** 0.5-2 mg q3-4hr prn; **INTRANASAL** 1 spray in 1 nostril, may give another dose 1-1½ hr later; repeat if needed 3-4 hr after last dose

• **Geriatric: IV** ½ adult dose at 2× the interval; **INTRANASAL** if no relief after 90-120 min, may repeat with 1 spray

Anesthesia—maintenance in balanced anesthesia; anesthetic adjunct

• **Adult: IV** Initially, 2 mg shortly before anesthesia induction. Maintenance, 0.5-1 mg **IV** during anesthesia, up to 0.06 mg/kg; usual total dose, 4-12.5 mg (approximately 0.06 to 0.18 mg/kg)

Atrial cardioversion—pain

• **Adult: INTRANASAL** 1 mg 30 min before internal atrial defibrillation shock

Renal/hepatic dose

• **Adult: INTRANASAL** max 1 mg followed by 1 mg after 90-120 min; IM/IV give 50% of dose (0.5 mg IV, 1 mg IM), do not repeat within 6 hr

Available forms: Injection 1, 2 mg/mL; nasal spray 10 mg/mL

Administer:

• With antiemetic if nausea, vomiting occur

• When pain is beginning to return; determine dosage interval according to patient response

• Store in light-resistant container at room temperature

Nasal route

• Prime before first use, point sprayer away from the face, pump activator 7× until a fine, wide spray occurs; if not used for 48 hr, reprime by pumping 1-2×

• If more than 1 spray is needed, use other nostril

Side effects: *italics* = common; red = life-threatening

- Do not share with others
- Nasal congestion/irritation may occur

IM route

- Deeply in large muscle mass

IV direct route

- Undiluted at a rate of <2 mg/>3-5 min, titrate to patient response; inject directly in vein or tubing of free-flowing compatible IV infusion

Y-site compatibilities: Acyclovir, alfentanil, allopurinol, amifostine, amikacin, aminocaproic acid, aminophylline, amphotericin B liposome (AmBisome), anidulafungin, ascorbic acid injection, atenolol, atracurium, atropine, aztreonam, benztropine, bivalirudin, bleomycin, bumetanide, buprenorphine, calcium chloride/gluconate, CARBOplatin, caspofungin, cefamandole, ceFAZolin, cefepime, cefotaxime, cefoTEtan, cefOXitin, cefTAZidime, ceftizoxime, cefTRIAXone, cefuroxime, cephalothin, chlorproMAZINE, cimetidine, cisatracurium, CISplatin, cladribine, clindamycin, cyanocobalamin, cyclophosphamide, cycloSPORINE, cytarabine, DACTINomycin, DAPTOmycin, dexamethasone phosphate, dexmedetomidine, digoxin, diltiazem, diphenhydrAMINE, DOBUTamine, DOCEtaxel, DOPamine, doxacurium, DOXOrubicin, DOXOrubicin liposomal, doxycycline, enalaprilat, ePHEDrine, EPINEPHrine, epirubicin, epoetin alfa, eptifibatide, ertapenem, erythromycin, esmolol, etoposide, famotidine, fenoldopam, fentaNYL, filgrastim, fluconazole, fludarabine, fluorouracil, gatifloxacin, gemcitabine, gentamicin, glycopyrrolate, granisetron, heparin, hydrocortisone, hydrOXYzine, IDArubicin, ifosfamide, imipenem-cilastatin, irinotecan, isoproterenol, ketorolac, labetalol, lactated Ringer's injection, levofloxacin, lidocaine, linezolid injection, LORazepam, magnesium, mannitol, mechlorethamine, melphalan, meperidine, metaraminol, methicillin, methotrexate, methoxamine, methyldopate, methylPREDNISolone, metoclopramide, metoprolol, metroNIDAZOLE, mezlocillin, milrinone, minocycline, mitoXANtrone, morphine, multiple vitamins injection, mycophenolate mofetil, nafcillin, nalbuphine, naloxone, nesiritide, netilmicin, niCARdipine, nitroglycerin, nitroprusside, norepinephrine, octreotide, ondansetron, oxacillin, oxaliplatin, oxytocin, palonosetron, pamidronate, pancuronium, papaverine, PEMEtrexed, penicillin G potassium/sodium, pentazocine, PHENobarbital, phenylephrine, phytonadione, piperacillin, piperacillin-tazobactam, polymyxin B, potassium chloride, procainamide, prochlorperazine, promethazine, propofol, propranolol, protamine, pyridoxine, quiNIDine, ranitidine, remifentanil, Ringer's injection, riTUXimab, rocuronium, sargramostim, sodium acetate, succinylcholine, SUFentanil, tacrolimus, teniposide, theophylline, thiamine, thiotepa, ticarcillin, ticarcillin-clavulanate, tigecycline, tirofiban, TNA, tobramycin, tolazoline, TPN, trastuzumab, urokinase, vancomycin, vasopressin, vecuronium, verapamil, vinCRIStine, vinorelbine, voriconazole

SIDE EFFECTS

CNS: *Drowsiness, dizziness, confusion, headache, sedation, euphoria, weakness, hallucinations,* insomnia (nasal)

CV: Palpitations, bradycardia, hypotension

EENT: Tinnitus, blurred vision, miosis, diplopia, nasal congestion, unpleasant taste

GI: *Nausea, vomiting, anorexia, constipation, cramps*

GU: Urinary retention

INTEG: Rash, urticaria, bruising, flushing, diaphoresis, pruritus

RESP: Respiratory depression

PHARMACOKINETICS

Metabolized by liver, excreted by kidneys, crosses placenta, excreted in breast milk, half-life 2-9 hr, protein binding 80%

IM: Onset 5-15 min, peak 30-60 min, duration 3-4 hr

INTRANASAL: Onset within 15 min, peak 1-2 hr, duration 4-5 hr

IV: Onset 1 min, peak 4-5 min, duration 2-4 hr

INTERACTIONS

Black Box Warning: Increase: CNS effects—alcohol, benzodiazepines, opioids, sedative/hypnotics, antipsychotics, skeletal muscle relaxants, other CNS depressants, MAOIs

Increase: butorphanol effect—CYP3A4 inhibitors (azoles, macrolides, protease inhibitors), monitor for severe respiratory depression
Increase: serotonin syndrome—SSRIs and other serotonergic agents, monitor for serotonin syndrome
Decrease: butorphanol effect—CYP3A4 inducers (carBAMazepine, phenytoin, rifAMPin), dosage increase may be needed
Drug/Herb
St. John's wort: Increased serotonin syndrome risk

NURSING CONSIDERATIONS
Assess:
• For decreasing output; may indicate urinary retention
• For withdrawal symptoms in opioid-dependent patients; PE, vascular occlusion, abscesses, ulcerations
• CNS changes: dizziness, drowsiness, hallucinations, euphoria, LOC, pupil reaction
• Allergic reactions: rash, urticaria

Black Box Warning: Respiratory dysfunction: respiratory depression, character, rate, rhythm; notify prescriber if respirations are <10/min

Black Box Warning: Neonatal opioid withdrawal: if mother used this product for prolonged periods during pregnancy, monitor neonate for withdrawal

Black Box Warning: Substance abuse: identify if there has been substance abuse (including alcoholism) in the past or present; addiction is more common in these patients

Black Box Warning: Accidental exposure (intranasal): keep out of reach of children

Black Box Warning: Avoid with benzodiazepines

• Need for pain medication, physical dependence
• Safety measures: night-light, call bell within easy reach, assistance with ambulation, especially for geriatric patients
• **Pregnancy/breastfeeding:** use only if benefits outweigh risks; usually compatible with breastfeeding
Evaluate:
• Therapeutic response: decrease in pain
Teach patient/family:

Black Box Warning: To report any symptoms of CNS changes, if using with other opioids, benzodiazepines, alcohol, or other CNS depressants, to seek medical care immediately for stupor, slow breathing, severe sleepiness

Black Box Warning: Accidental overdose: May be fatal, keep out of reach of children

• To report all products taken (OTC, Rx, herbs, supplements)
• That physical dependency may result when used for extended periods
• That withdrawal symptoms may occur: nausea, vomiting, cramps, fever, faintness, anorexia
• How to use nasal product
• To avoid hazardous activities, to have help getting out of bed or walking

TREATMENT OF OVERDOSE:
Naloxone 0.4-2 mg IV, IM/SUBCUT/O_2, IV fluids, vasopressors

cabozantinib (Rx)

(ka-boe-zan'ti-nib)

Cabometyx, Cometriq

Func. class.: Antineoplastic, biologic response modifier, signal transduction inhibitor

Chem. class.: Multi-tyrosine kinase inhibitor

ACTION: Blocks abnormal tyrosine kinase proteins ✍⚕ (RET, MET, VEGFR-1, VEGFR-2, VEGFR-3, KIT, TRKB, FLT-3, AXL, TIE-2, ROS1, TYRO3, and MER); inhibits these receptor tyrosine kinases (RTKs) that are responsible for the control of cell migration, metabolism, proliferation, and differentiation

USES: In patients with progressive, metastatic medullary thyroid cancer, advanced renal cell cancer (RCC) who have received prior anti-angiogenic therapy

CONTRAINDICATIONS

Hypersensitivity, pregnancy

Black Box Warning: Bleeding, fistula, GI perforation

Precautions: Breastfeeding, contraception requirements, dental disease, dental work, diarrhea, encephalopathy, GI bleeding, hypertension, infertility, MI, proteinuria, reproductive risk, skin disease, surgery, thromboembolic disease, wound dehiscence

DOSAGE AND ROUTES

Progressive, metastatic medullary thyroid cancer (capsules only; do not substitute with tablets):
• **Adult:** PO 140 mg daily on an empty stomach until disease progression or unacceptable toxicity occurs

Advanced RCC in patients who have received prior anti-angiogenic therapy (tablets only; do not substitute with capsules):
• **Adult:** PO 60 mg daily on an empty stomach until disease progression or unacceptable toxicity

Hepatic dose
Cometriq capsules:
• Mild or moderate hepatic impairment (Child-Pugh class A or B): reduce the starting dose to 80 mg daily; severe hepatic impairment (Child-Pugh class C): do not use
Cabometyx tablets:
• Mild or moderate hepatic impairment (Child-Pugh class A or B): reduce the starting dose to 40 mg daily; severe hepatic impairment (Child-Pugh class C): do not use

Available forms: Capsules 60, 100, 140 mg; tablets 20, 40, 60 mg

Administer:
• Do not substitute tablets with capsules
• Take on an empty stomach; do not eat for at least 2 hr prior to and at least 1 hr after taking, swallow capsules and tablets whole; do not open or crush
• Do not take with grapefruit juice or nutritional supplements that are known to inhibit CYP450
• Do not take a missed dose within 12 hr of the next dose. If the next dose is in 12 hr or more, take the missed dose; if the next dose is in <12 hr, skip and take the next dose at the scheduled time
Cometriq capsules:
• **Strong CYP3A4 inhibitors:** Avoid concomitant use if possible. If a strong CYP3A4 inhibitor is required, reduce the daily dose by 40 mg; resume the prior dose after 2 to 3 days if the strong CYP3A4 inhibitor is discontinued
• **Strong CYP3A4 inducers:** If a strong CYP3A4 inducer is required, increase the daily dose by 40 mg as tolerated. Max 180 mg/day. Resume the prior dose after 2 to 3 days if the strong CYP3A4 inducer is discontinued
Cabometyx tablets:
• **Strong CYP3A4 inhibitors:** Reduce the daily dose by 20 mg; resume the prior dose after 2 to 3 days if the strong CYP3A4 inhibitor is discontinued
• **Strong CYP3A4 inducers:** Increase the daily dose by 20 mg as tolerated. Max 80 mg/day. Resume the prior dose after

2 to 3 days if the strong CYP3A4 inducer is discontinued

SIDE EFFECTS
RESP: Cough, dyspnea
CNS: Dizziness, headache, fatigue
CV: Hypertension, hypertriglyceridemia
EENT: Rash, erythema, hair discoloration, oral ulceration, stomatitis
META: Hyperbilirubinemia, hyperglycemia, hypocalcemia, hypokalemia, hypoalbuminemia, hypomagnesemia, hyponatremia, hypophosphatemia
MISC: Arthralgia, asthenia, dysgeusia, hand and foot syndrome, hypothyroidism, dysphonia
GI: Anorexia, nausea, vomiting, weight loss, abdominal pain, diarrhea, constipation, dyspepsia
HEMA: Thrombocytopenia, lymphopenia, neutropenia, anemia

PHARMACOKINETICS
Protein binding ≥99.7%, half-life 55 hr, excretion 54% feces (43% as unchanged drug), 21% urine, peak 2-5 hr
• Metabolized in the liver and is a substrate of CYP3A4

INTERACTIONS
Increase: GI bleeding—warfarin, NSAIDs
Increase: cabozantinib effects—CYP3A4 inhibitors (amprenavir, bocenavir, delavirdine, ketoconazole, indinavir, itraconazole, dalfopristin/quinupristin, ritonavir, tipranavir, fluconazole, isoniazid, miconazole)
Decrease: cabozantinib effects—CYP3A4 inducers (rifAMPin, rifapentine, rifabutin, primadone, phenytoin, phenobarbital, nevirapine, nafcillin, modafinil, griseofulvin, etravirine, efavirenz, barbiturates, bexarotene, bosentan, carBAMazepine, enzalutamide, dexamethasone)
Drug/Food
Increase: cabozantinib effects—grapefruit juice
Drug/Herb
Decrease: cabozantinib effects—St. John's wort

Drug/Smoking
Decrease: cabozantinib effects—smoking, dose may need to be increased
Drug/Lab
Increase: INR, PT, AST, ALT, bilirubin

NURSING CONSIDERATIONS
Assess:

Black Box Warning: **GI perforation/bleeding:** some cases have been fatal, usually occurs in those using NSAIDs, taxanes, or those with diverticulitis or peptic ulcer disease, discontinue if these occur

• **Serious arterial and venous thromboembolic disease:** some have been fatal, permanently discontinue if myocardial infarction or any other arterial thromboembolic complication occurs
• **Wound dehiscence:** temporary suspension of therapy is recommended at least 28 days before scheduled surgery, including dental surgery. Resume based on adequate wound healing. Hold in those who develop wound dehiscence or wound healing complications
• **Hypertension:** monitor BP prior to and regularly during treatment, hold in those not adequately controlled; resume at a reduced dose. Permanently discontinue if malignant hypertension, hypertensive crisis, or persistent uncontrolled hypertension despite optimal management
• **Dental disease:** oral examination prior to starting therapy to evaluate for dental disease; good oral hygiene practices should be encouraged. Discontinue at least 28 days before invasive dental work or surgery. Osteonecrosis of the jaw (ONJ) has been reported; permanently discontinue capsules (Cometriq) in those who develop ONJ
• **Palmar-plantar erythrodysesthesia (hand and foot syndrome):** hold in those who develop intolerable grade 2 or grade 3 or 4 hand and foot syndrome, resume at a reduced dose when toxicity has improved to grade 1

• **Proteinuria:** monitor urine protein regularly; permanently discontinue in nephrotic syndrome

• **Severe diarrhea:** those with preexisting diarrhea should be treated prior to receiving this product; hold (Cabometyx) therapy for intolerable grade 2 diarrhea, for grade 3 or higher diarrhea that cannot be managed with standard antidiarrheal treatments until improvement to grade 1 or less; a dose reduction may be necessary. Fluid and electrolyte replacement if dehydrated

• **Reversible posterior leukoencephalopathy syndrome (RPLS):** assess for seizures, headache, visual disturbances, confusion, and altered mental status. Discontinue if RPLS is suspected or diagnosed; confirm by MRI

• **Pregnancy/breastfeeding:** assess if pregnancy is planned or suspected. Females of reproductive potential should avoid becoming pregnant during treatment; women who become pregnant while receiving product should be apprised of the potential hazard to the fetus

• Counsel patients about the reproductive risk and contraception requirements. Females and men with female partners who are able to become pregnant should avoid pregnancy and use effective contraception during and for ≥4 mo after the last dose. Obtain pregnancy testing prior to initiation; do not breastfeed

Evaluate:

• **Therapeutic response:** decreased spread of cancer

Teach patient/family:

• To report adverse reactions immediately, SOB, severe abdominal pain, persistent diarrhea, severe hypertension, bleeding

• About reason for treatment, expected results

• To use reliable contraception during treatment and for ≥4 mo after treatment

---

⚠ HIGH ALERT

calcitonin (salmon) (Rx)
Miacalcin
Func. class.: Parathyroid agent (calcium regulator)
Chem. class.: Polypeptide hormone

Do not confuse:
Calcitonin/calcitriol/calcifediol/calcium

ACTION: Decreases bone resorption, blood calcium levels; increases deposits of calcium in bones; opposes parathyroid hormone

USES: Paget's disease, postmenopausal osteoporosis, hypercalcemia

CONTRAINDICATIONS
Hypersensitivity to this product, fish
Precautions: Pregnancy, breastfeeding, children, hypotension, hypocalcemia, secondary malignancy

DOSAGE AND ROUTES
Postmenopausal osteoporosis
• **Adult: SUBCUT/IM** 100 units every other day; **INTRANASAL** 200 units (1 spray) daily, alternating nostrils daily
Paget's disease
• **Adult: SUBCUT/IM** 100 units/day; maintenance 50 units daily, every other day, or 3× per wk
Hypercalcemia
• **Adult: SUBCUT/IM** 4 units/kg q12hr, increase to 8 units/kg q12hr if response is unsatisfactory, may increase to 8 units/kg q6hr if needed after 2 more days

Available forms: Injection 200 units/mL; nasal spray 200 units/actuation
Administer:
• Store at <77° F (25° C); protect from light
SUBCUT route
• Rotate injection sites; use within 2 hr of reconstitution; **give** at bedtime to minimize nausea, vomiting
IM route
• After test dose of 10 units/mL, 0.1 mL intradermally; watch for 15 min; **give**

---

only with EPINEPHrine, emergency meds available

• IM inject slowly into deep muscle mass; rotate sites; preferred route if volume is >2 mL; use within 2 hr of reconstitution

Nasal route

• Prime pump before first dose

• Use at bedtime; alternate nostrils daily, prime to get full spray before first dose, store in refrigerator

• Allow to come to room temperature before using

• Discard after 30 days

SIDE EFFECTS

CNS: Headache (nasal)
EENT: Eye pain (nasal)
GI: Nausea, *diarrhea, vomiting, anorexia,* (IM/SUBCUT)
GU: Nocturia, frequency
INTEG: Rash, flushing, reaction at injection site
MS: Backache, myalgia, arthralgia
RESP: Dyspnea, flulike symptoms, bronchospasm
SYST: Anaphylaxis, infection

PHARMACOKINETICS

IM/SUBCUT: Onset 15 min, peak 2 hr, duration 6-8 hr, metabolized by kidneys, excreted as inactive metabolites via kidneys

INTERACTIONS

Decrease: lithium effect; monitor lithium level
Decrease: effect of nasal spray— bisphosphonates (Paget's disease); monitor for adequate effect

NURSING CONSIDERATIONS
Assess:

• Anaphylaxis, hypersensitivity reaction (rash, fever, inability to breathe); emergency equipment should be nearby

• GI symptoms, polyuria, flushing, head swelling, tingling, headache; may indicate hypercalcemia

• Nutritional status; diet for sources of vitamin D (milk, some seafood), calcium (dairy products, dark green vegetables), phosphates

• **Postmenopausal osteoporosis:** vitamin D (50-135 international units/dL), alkaline phosphatase baseline, q3-6mo; monitor urine hydroxyproline with Paget's disease, biochemical markers of bone formation/absorption, radiologic evidence of fracture; bone density

• **Toxicity (can occur rapidly),** increased drug level; have parenteral calcium on hand if calcium level drops too low; check for tetany (irritability, paresthesia, nervousness, muscle twitching, seizures, tetanic spasms)

Evaluate:

• Therapeutic response: calcium levels 9-10 mg/dL, decreasing symptoms of Paget's disease

Teach patient/family:
SUBCUT route/IM route

• About the method of injection if patient will be responsible for self-medication; to rotate sites, not to inject into broken, irritated skin; provide written instructions

• To report difficulty swallowing, any changes in side effects to prescriber immediately

• To report immediately signs/symptoms of hypocalcemia: tetany, seizures

• **Pregnancy/breastfeeding:** to advise prescriber if pregnancy is planned or suspected or if breastfeeding

• **Postmenopausal osteoporosis:** to take vitamin D and calcium differential; that nausea, vomiting, and facial flushing occur often

Nasal route

• To use alternating nostrils; to use after allowing to warm to room temperature; to prime to get full spray; to discard after 30 days

---

calcitriol vitamin D$_3$ (Rx)
(kal-sih-try′ole)
Rocaltrol, Vectical
Func. class.: Parathyroid agent (calcium regulator)
Chem. class.: Vitamin D hormone

Do not confuse:
calcitriol/Calciferol/calcitonin/calcium

ACTION: Increases intestinal absorption of calcium; provides calcium for bones; increases renal tubular reabsorption of phosphate

USES: Hypocalcemia with chronic renal disease, hyperparathyroidism, pseudohypoparathyroidism, renal osteodystrophy; plaque psoriasis (TOP)

CONTRAINDICATIONS
Hypersensitivity, hyperphosphatemia, hypercalcemia, vitamin D toxicity
Precautions: Pregnancy, breastfeeding, renal calculi, CV disease

DOSAGE AND ROUTES
Hypocalcemia in long-term dialysis
• **Adult:** PO 0.25 mcg/day
• **Adult and child ≥13 yr IV** 0.5 mcg (0.01 mcg/kg) 3× per wk, may increase by 0.25-0.5 mcg/dose q2-4wk
• **Child 1-5 yr:** PO 0.25-2 mcg/day; IV 0.01-0.05 mcg/kg 3× per wk
Hypoparathyroidism
• **Adult and child ≥6 yr:** PO 0.25 mcg/day, may increase q2-4wk, maintenance 0.5-2 mcg/day
• **Child <1 yr:** PO 0.04-0.08 mcg/kg/day
Management of secondary parathyroidism with bone disease in predialysis (CCr 15-55 mL/min)
• **Adult/child ≥3 yr:** PO 0.25 mcg/day, may increase to 0.5 mcg/day
Mild-moderate plaque psoriasis
Adult/child 7-17 yr: TOP apply to affected area bid, max 200 g/wk
Child 2-6 yr: TOP apply to affected area bid, max 100 g/wk
Available forms: Capsules 0.25, 0.5 mcg; injection 1 mcg/mL; oral solution 1 mcg/mL; topical 3 mcg/g
Administer:
PO route
• Do not break, crush, chew capsules
• Give without regard to meals
• Store protected from light, heat, moisture
Topical route
• Rub into skin
IV route
• **Hypocalcemia:** Give by direct IV over 1 min through catheter at hemodialysis conclusion

SIDE EFFECTS
CNS: Drowsiness, headache, vertigo
CV: Hypertension, dysrhythmias, edema
EENT: Blurred vision, photophobia, rhinorrhea
ENDO: Hypercalcemia
GI: Nausea, vomiting, jaundice, anorexia, dry mouth, constipation, cramps, metallic taste, pancreatitis
GU: Polyuria
MS: Myalgia, arthralgia, weakness
SYST: Anaphylaxis
INTEG: Pain at injection site, rash, pruritus

PHARMACOKINETICS
IV: Onset immediate, duration 3-5 days
TOPICAL: Onset, peak, duration unknown
PO: Absorbed readily from GI tract, peak 10-12 hr, duration 3-5 days, half-life 5-8 hr, undergoes hepatic recycling, excreted in bile

INTERACTIONS
Increase: hypercalcemia—thiazide diuretics, calcium supplements
Increase: cardiac dysrhythmias—cardiac glycosides, verapamil; use cautiously
Increase: hypermagnesemia—magnesium antacids/supplements, avoid using together
Increase: toxicity—other vitamin D products, avoid using together
Increase: metabolism of vitamin D—phenytoin
Decrease: absorption of calcitriol—cholestyramine, mineral oil, fat-soluble vitamins; avoid concurrent use
Drug/Food
Large amounts of high-calcium foods may cause hypercalcemia
Drug/Lab Test
Increase: AST/ALT, BUN, creatinine
False increase: Cholesterol
Interference: Alkaline phosphatase, electrolytes

NURSING CONSIDERATIONS
Assess:
• **Vitamin D deficiency:** Baseline and periodically
• May increase calcium; should be kept at 9-10 mg/dL, vitamin D 50-135 units/dL, phosphate 70 mg/dL; toxic reactions may occur rapidly

• Serum calcium, phosphate 2× per wk during beginning treatment; serum calcium magnesium, alkaline phosphatase and intact PTH ≤ monthly

• **Hypercalcemia:** dry mouth, metallic taste, polyuria, bone pain, muscle weakness, headache, fatigue, change in level of consciousness, dysrhythmias, increased respirations, anorexia, nausea, vomiting, cramps, constipation; **hypocalcemia:** paresthesia, twitching, Chvostek's sign, Trousseau's sign

• Nutritional status, diet for sources of vitamin D (milk, some seafood); calcium (dairy products, dark green vegetables), phosphates (dairy products) must be avoided

• Restrict sodium, potassium if required; restriction of fluids if required for chronic renal failure

• Height, weight in children, baseline and periodically if on long-term high-dose therapy

Evaluate:

• Therapeutic response: calcium 9-10 mg/dL; decreasing symptoms of hypocalcemia, hypoparathyroidism

Teach patient/family:

• **About symptoms of hypercalcemia:** renal stones, nausea, vomiting, anorexia, lethargy, thirst, bone or flank pain, confusion

• To follow prescribed diet, to avoid products with sodium: cured meats, dairy products, cold cuts, olives, beets, pickles, soups, meat tenderizers with chronic renal failure; products with potassium: oranges, bananas, dried fruit, peas, dark green leafy vegetables, milk, melons, beans

• To avoid OTC products that contain calcium, potassium, sodium with chronic renal failure, to take as prescribed, not to double or skip doses

• To monitor weight weekly; to maintain fluid intake

• To continue with exams and lab work

• To avoid large doses of vitamins or supplements

• **Pregnancy/breastfeeding:** identify if pregnancy is planned or suspected or if breastfeeding; do not breastfeed

TREATMENT OF OVERDOSE: Discontinue treatment, diuretics, hemodialysis

---

calcium carbonate (OTC) C

Calcarb, Calci-Chew, Calci-Mix, Maalox Antacid, Mylanta, Oysterase, Os-Cal, Rolaids, Tums

Func. class.: Antacid, calcium supplement

Chem. class.: Calcium product

Do not confuse:
calcium/calcitriol/calcitonin

ACTION: Neutralizes gastric acidity

USES: Antacid, calcium supplement

CONTRAINDICATIONS
Hypersensitivity, hypercalcemia

Precautions: Pregnancy, breastfeeding, geriatric patients, fluid restriction, decreased GI motility, GI obstruction, dehydration, renal disease, hyperparathyroidism, bone tumors

DOSAGE AND ROUTES
Hypocalcemia prevention, osteoporosis

• **Adult: PO** 1-2 g

• **Adult 19-50 yr: PO** 1000 mg/day elemental calcium (2500 mg/day calcium carbonate)

Chronic hypocalcemia

• **Adult: PO** 2-4 g/day elemental calcium (5-10 g/day calcium carbonate) in 3-4 divided doses

• **Child: PO** 45-65 mg/kg/day elemental calcium (112.5-162.5 mg/kg/day calcium carbonate) in 4 divided doses

• **Neonate: PO** 50-150 mg/kg/day elemental calcium (125-375 mg/kg/day in 4-6 divided doses, max 1 g/day)

Supplementation

• **Child: PO** 45-65 mg/kg/day

Hyperphosphatemia (Acetate)

• **Adult: PO** 1334 mg with meals

Heartburn, dyspepsia, hyperacidity (OTC)

• **Adult:** PO 1-2 tablets q2hr, max 9 tablets/24 hr (Alka-Mints); chew 2-4 tablets q1hr prn, max 16 tablets (Tums regular strength); chew 2-4 tablets q1hr prn, max 10 tablets (Tums E-X)

Available forms: Calcium carbonate: chewable tablets 350, 420, 450, 500, 750, 1000, 1250 mg; tablets 500, 600, 650, 667, 1000, 1250, 1500 mg; **gum** 300, 450, 500 mg; **suspension** 1250 mg/5 mL; **capsules** 1250 mg; **powder** 6.5 g/packet

Administer:

PO route

• 1 g calcium carbonate = 400 mg elemental calcium = 10 mmol calcium = 20 mEq calcium

• Do not give enteric-coated within 1 hr of calcium carbonate

• **For ulcer treatment** (adjunct): give 1 and 3 hr after meals and at bedtime

• **For a phosphate binder:** give 1 hr after each meal or snack and at bedtime

• **For supplement:** give 1-1½ hr after meals; avoid oxalic acid foods (spinach, rhubarb), phytic acid (brans, cereals), or phosphorus (milk, dairy), may decrease calcium absorption

• **Suspension:** shake well; use calibrated measuring device

• Laxatives or stool softeners if constipation occurs

SIDE EFFECTS

GI: *Constipation,* anorexia, nausea, vomiting, diarrhea

GU: Calculi, hypercalciuria

PHARMACOKINETICS

⅓ of dose absorbed by small intestine, excreted in feces and urine, crosses placenta, must have adequate vitamin D for absorption

INTERACTIONS

Increase: digoxin toxicity—hypercalcemia

Increase: plasma levels of quiNIDine, amphetamines

Increase: hypercalcemia—thiazide diuretics, calcium supplements

Decrease: levels of salicylates, calcium channel blockers, ketoconazole, iron salts, tetracyclines, fluoroquinolones, phenytoin, etidronate, risedronate, atenolol PO, thyroid hormones

Drug/Food

Decrease: calcium supplement effect—cereal, spinach

Drug/Lab Test

Decrease: phosphates

False increase: chloride

False positive: benzodiazepines

False decrease: magnesium, oxalate, lipase

NURSING CONSIDERATIONS

Assess:

• Calcium (serum, urine), serum calcium should be 8.5-10.5 mg/dL, correct or use ionized calcium in low albumin or acid/base disorders, monitor weekly if used to treat electrolyte imbalances or use a daily supplement; urine calcium should be 150 mg/day, monitor weekly; serum phosphate

• **Milk-alkali syndrome:** nausea, vomiting, disorientation, headache

• Constipation; increase bulk in the diet if needed

• **Hypercalcemia:** headache, nausea, vomiting, confusion

• **Hypocalcemia:** paresthesia, twitching, colic, dysrhythmias, Chvostek's sign, Trousseau's sign

• Those taking digoxin for toxicity; monitor frequently

• Antacid—for abdominal pain; heartburn; indigestion before, after administration

Evaluate:

• Therapeutic response: absence of pain, decreased acidity; decreased hyperphosphatemia with renal failure

Teach patient/family:

• To increase fluids to 2 L unless contraindicated; to add bulk, liquids to diet for constipation; to notify prescriber of constipation

• Not to switch antacids unless directed by prescriber; not to use as antacid for >2 wk without approval by prescriber

• That therapeutic dose recommendations are figured as elemental calcium

• To avoid excessive use of alcohol, caffeine, tobacco

- To avoid spinach, cereals, dairy products in large amounts, other foods high in oxalates before taking the product; may interfere with absorption of calcium
- To take enteric product within 1 hr of calcium carbonate
- To take on regular schedule
- Pregnancy/breastfeeding: Notify prescriber if planned or suspected, hypocalcemia/hypercalcemia causes severe reactions
- To maintain vitamin D levels

CALCIUM SALTS

calcium acetate (Rx)
Calphron, PhosLo, Phoslyra
calcium chloride (Rx)
calcium citrate (OTC)
Citracal, Cal-C-Cap
calcium gluconate (Rx)
calcium lactate (Rx)
Cal-Lac

Func. class.: Electrolyte replacement—calcium product

ACTION: Calcium needed for maintenance of nervous, muscular, skeletal function; enzyme reactions; normal cardiac contractility; coagulation of blood; affects secretory activity of endocrine, exocrine glands

USES: Prevention and treatment of hypocalcemia, hypermagnesemia, hypoparathyroidism, neonatal tetany, cardiac toxicity caused by hyperkalemia, lead colic, hyperphosphatemia, vitamin D deficiency, osteoporosis prophylaxis, calcium antagonist toxicity (calcium channel blocker toxicity)
Unlabeled uses: Electrolyte abnormalities in cardiac arrest, CPR

CONTRAINDICATIONS
Hypercalcemia, digoxin toxicity, ventricular fibrillation, renal calculi
Precautions: Pregnancy, breastfeeding, children, respiratory/renal disease, cor pulmonale, digitalized patient, respiratory failure, diarrhea, dehydration

DOSAGE AND ROUTES
Acute hypocalcemia
- **Adult: IV** 7-14 mEq **for tetany** 4.5-16 mEq
- **Child/infant: IV** 1-7 mEq **for tetany** 0.5-0.7 mEq/kg tid-qid

For nutritional supplementation
PO (any oral calcium salt; dosage expressed as elemental calcium)
- **Adult: PO** 1-2 g mg/day
- **Child: PO** 45-65 mg/kg/day

Available forms: Calcium chloride: injection 10% (1.36 mEq); **calcium citrate:** tablets 250 mg; **calcium gluconate:** tablets 500, 650, 975, 1 g; injection 10% (0.45 mEq); **calcium lactate:** tablets 325, 500, 650 mg; **calcium acetate:** oral solution, caps, tablets 667 mg (169 mg calcium)
Administer:
PO route (only acetate, carbonate, citrate, lactate, phosphate)
- Give in 3-4 divided doses with or 1 hr after meals, follow with full glass of water; if using as phosphate binder in renal dialysis, do not follow with water, do not give oral medications within 1 hr of oral calcium; **chewable tablet:** chew thoroughly; **effervescent tablet:** dissolve in full glass of water; **oral powder:** mix and give with food; **oral solution:** give before meals; **oral suspension:** shake well
- Store at room temperature
IV route
- Warm to room temperature
- Undiluted or diluted with equal amounts of NS to a 5% solution for injection, give 0.5-1 mL/min, give slowly, rapid administration may cause cardiac arrest
- Through small-bore needle into large vein, do not use scalp vein; if extravasation occurs, necrosis will result (IV)
- Remain recumbent ½ hr after IV dose, drop in B/P may result

Calcium chloride
Y-site compatibilities: Acyclovir, alemtuzumab, alfentanil, amikacin, aminocaproic acid, aminophylline, amiodarone, anidulafungin, argatroban, arsenic trioxide, ascorbic acid injection, asparaginase, atenolol,

atracurium, atropine, azithromycin, aztreonam, benztropine, bivalirudin, bleomycin, bumetanide, buprenorphine, butorphanol, calcium gluconate, CARBOplatin, carmustine, caspofungin acetate, cefotaxime, cefOTEtan, cefOXitin, ceftaroline, ceftizoxime, chloramphenicol, chlorothiazide, chlorpheniramine, chlorproMAZINE, cimetidine, CISplatin, clindamycin, cloxacillin, colistimethate, cyanocobalamin, cyclophosphamide, cycloSPORINE, cytarabine, DACTINomycin, DAPTOmycin, DAUNOrubicin, dexmedetomidine, dexrazoxane, digoxin, diltiaZEM, diphenhydrAMINE, DOBUTamine, DOCEtaxel, dolasetron, DOPamine, doxacurium, doxapram, DOXOrubicin, doxycycline, edetate calcium disodium, enalaprilat, ePHEDrine, EPINEPHrine, epiRUBicin, epoetin alfa, eptifibatide, ergonovine, ertapenem, erythromycin, esmolol, etoposide, etoposide phosphate, famotidine, fenoldopam, fentaNYL, fluconazole, fludarabine, furosemide, gallamine, gallium, ganciclovir, gatifloxacin, gemcitabine, gentamicin, glycopyrrolate, granisetron, heparin sodium, HYDROmorphone, hydrOXYzine, IDArubicin, ifosfamide, inamrinone, insulin (regular), irinotecan, isoproterenol, kanamycin, labetalol, lactated Ringer's, lepirudin, leucovorin, lidocaine, lincomycin, linezolid, LORazepam, mannitol, meperidine, mephentermine, mesna, methohexital, methotrexate, methyldopate, metoclopramide, metoprolol, metroNIDAZOLE, micafungin, midazolam, milrinone, minocycline, mitoMYcin, mitoXANTRONE, mivacurium, morphine, moxifloxacin, multiple vitamins injection, mycophenolate mofetil, nafcillin, nalbuphine, nalorphine, naloxone, nesiritide, niCARDipine, nitroglycerin, nitroprusside, norepinephrine, octreotide, ondansetron, oxytocin, PACLitaxel (solvent/surfactant), pancuronium, papaverine, penicillin G potassium/sodium, pentazocine, PENTobarbital, PHENobarbital, phentolamine, phenylephrine, phytonadione, piperacillin, piperacillin-tazobactam, polymyxin B, potassium, potassium chloride, procainamide, prochlorperazine, promazine, promethazine, propranolol, protamine, pyridoxine, quinupristin-dalfopristin, raNITIdine, Ringer's injection, rocuronium, streptomycin, succinylcholine, SUFentanil, tacrolimus, teniposide, theophylline, thiamine, thiotepa, ticarcillin-clavulanate, tigecycline, tirofiban, TNA (3-in-1), tobramycin, tolazoline, topotecan, trimetaphan, tubocurarine, urokinase, vancomycin, vasopressin, vecuronium, verapamil, vinBLAStine, vinCRIStine, vinorelbine, voriconazole

Calcium gluconate

Y-site compatibilities: Acyclovir, aldesleukin, alemtuzumab, alfentanil, allopurinol, amifostine, amikacin, aminocaproic acid, aminophylline, amiodarone, anidulafungin, argatroban, arsenic trioxide, ascorbic acid injection, asparaginase, atenolol, atracurium, atropine, azaTHIOprine, azithromycin, aztreonam, benztropine, bivalirudin, bleomycin, bumetanide, buprenorphine, butorphanol, calcium chloride, CARBOplatin, carmustine, caspofungin, ceFAZolin, cefepime, cefoperazone, cefotaxime, cefoTEtan, cefOXitin, ceftaroline, cefTAZidime, ceftizoxime, cefuroxime, chloramphenicol sodium succinate, chlorothiazide, chlorpheniramine, chlorproMAZINE, cimetidine, ciprofloxacin, cisatracurium, CISplatin, cladribine, clindamycin, cloxacillin, codeine, colistimethate, cyanocobalamin, cyclophosphamide, cycloSPORINE, cytarabine, DACTINomycin, DAPTOmycin, DAUNOrubicin liposome, DAUNOrubicin, dexmedetomidine, dexrazoxane, digoxin, diltiaZEM, dimenhyDRINATE, diphenhydrAMINE, DOBUTamine, DOCEtaxel, dolasetron, DOPamine, doripenem, doxacurium, doxapram, DOXOrubicin, DOXOrubicin liposomal, doxycycline, edetate calcium disodium, enalaprilat, ePHEDrine, EPINEPHrine, epiRUBicin, epoetin alfa, eptifibatide, ergonovine, ertapenem, erythromycin, esmolol, etoposide, etoposide phosphate, famotidine, fenoldopam, fentaNYL, filgrastim, fludarabine, fluorouracil, folic acid (as sodium salt), furosemide, gallamine, gallium, ganciclovir, gatifloxacin, gemcitabine, gentamicin, glycopyrrolate, granisetron, heparin sodium, HYDROmorphone, hydrOXYzine, IDArubicin, ifosfamide, insulin (regular), irinotecan, isoproterenol, kanamycin, ketamine, labetalol, lactated Ringer's injection, lepirudin, leucovorin, levoFLOXacin, lidocaine, lincomycin, linezolid, LORazepam, magnesium sulfate, mannitol, melphalan, meperidine, mephentermine, mesna, methohexital, methotrexate, methyldopate, metoclopramide, metoprolol, metroNIDAZOLE, micafungin, midazolam, milrinone, mitoMYcin, mitoXANTRONE, mivacurium, morphine, moxifloxacin, multiple vitamins injection, nafcillin, nalbuphine, nalorphine, naloxone, nesiritide, netilmicin, niCARdipine, nitroglycerin, nitroprusside, norepinephrine, octreotide, ondansetron, oritavancin, oxaliplatin, oxytocin, PACLitaxel (solvent/surfactant), palonosetron, pancuronium, papaverine, penicillin G potassium/sodium, pentamidine, pentazocine, PENTobarbital, PHENobarbital, phentolamine, phenylephrine, phytonadione, piperacillin, polymyxin B, potassium acetate/chloride, procainamide, prochlorperazine, promazine, promethazine, propofol, propranolol, protamine, pyridoxine, quiNIDine, raNITIdine, remifentanil, Ringer's, riTUXimab, rocuronium, sargramostim, sodium acetate, streptomycin, succinylcholine, SUFentanil, tacrolimus, telavancin, teniposide, theophylline, thiamine, thiotepa, ticarcillin, ticarcillin-clavulanate, tigecycline, tirofiban, TNA (3-in-1), tobramycin, tolazoline, TPN (2-in-1), trastuzumab, trimetaphan, tubocurarine, urokinase, vancomycin, vasopressin, vecuronium, verapamil, vinBLAStine, vinCRIStine, vinorelbine, vitamin B complex with C, voriconazole

SIDE EFFECTS
CV: Hypotension, bradycardia, dysrhythmias; cardiac arrest (IV)
GI: Vomiting, nausea, constipation
GU: Hypercalciuria, renal calculi
META: Hypercalcemia
INTEG: Pain, burning at IV site, severe venous thrombosis, necrosis, extravasation

PHARMACOKINETICS
Crosses placenta, enters breast milk, excreted via urine and feces, half-life unknown, protein binding 40%-50%

PO: Onset, peak, duration unknown, absorption from GI tract
IV: Onset immediate, duration ½-2 hr

INTERACTIONS
Increase: milk-alkali syndrome—antacids
Increase: dysrhythmias—digoxin glycosides
Increase: toxicity—verapamil, dilTIAzem
Increase: hypercalcemia—thiazide diuretics
Decrease: absorption of fluoroquinolones, tetracyclines, iron salts, phenytoin, thyroid hormones when calcium is taken PO
Decrease: effects of atenolol—verapamil
Drug/Herb
Increase: action/side effects—lily of the valley, pheasant's eye, shark cartilage, squill
Drug/Food
Decrease: calcium absorption—cereal, spinach
Drug/Lab Test
Increase: calcium

NURSING CONSIDERATIONS
Assess:
• **Antacid:** monitor for heartburn relief
• **ECG** for decreased QT and T wave inversion: hypercalcemia, product should be reduced or discontinued, consider cardiac monitoring
• Calcium levels during treatment (8.5-11.5 g/dL is normal level); urine calcium if hypercalciuria occurs
• Cardiac status: rate, rhythm, CVP (PWP, PAWP if being monitored directly)
• **Hypocalcemia:** muscle twitching, paresthesia, dysrhythmias, laryngospasm
• **Digoxin therapy:** monitor frequently; an increase in calcium increases digoxin toxicity risk
• Store at room temperature
Evaluate:
• Therapeutic response: decreased twitching, paresthesias, muscle spasms; absence of tremors, seizures, dysrhythmias, dyspnea, laryngospasm; negative Chvostek's sign, negative Trousseau's sign
Teach patient/family:
• To increase fluids to 2 L/day unless contraindicated; to add bulk to diet for constipation; to notify prescriber of constipation

• Not to switch antacids unless directed by prescriber; not to use as antacid for >2 wk without approval by prescriber
• That therapeutic dose recommendations are figured as elemental calcium
• To avoid excessive use of alcohol, caffeine, tobacco

---

canagliflozin (Rx)
(kan′a-gli-floe′zin)

Invokana

Func. class.: Oral antidiabetic
Chem. class.: Sodium-glucose co-transporter 2 (SGLT2) inhibitor

---

Combination products
Invokamet: canagliflozin/metformin 50 mg/500 mg, 50 mg/1000 mg, 150 mg/500 mg, 150 mg/1000 mg

ACTION: Blocks glucose reabsorption by the kidney, increases glucose excretion, lowers blood glucose concentrations by inhibiting proximal renal tubular sodium glucose transporter 2 (SGLT2)

USES: Type 2 diabetes mellitus, with diet and exercise; may use in combination; to reduce CV events in type 2 diabetes mellitus with CV disease

CONTRAINDICATIONS
Dialysis, renal failure, hypersensitivity, breastfeeding, diabetic ketoacidosis
Precautions: Pregnancy, children, renal/hepatic disease, hypothyroidism, hyperglycemia, hypotension, pituitary insufficiency, type 1 diabetes mellitus, malnutrition, fever, dehydration, adrenal insufficiency, geriatric patients

Black Box Warning: Lower limb amputation

DOSAGE AND ROUTES
Type 2 diabetes mellitus with diet and exercise
• **Adult: PO** 100 mg/day, may increase to 300 mg/day if needed
Reduction of CV
Risk in diabetes mellitus and to reduce risk of ESKD, doubling of serum creatinine, reduction of HF in hospitalizations, CV death in diabetic neuropathy with albuminuria ≥300 mg/day

• **Adult: PO** 100 mg daily in AM before meal, may increase to 300 mg/day if needed
Renal dose
• **Adult: PO** eGFR 30-59 mL/min/1.73 m^2, max 100 mg/day; <30 mL/min/1.73 m^2 do not use
Available forms: Tablets 100, 300 mg
Administer:
PO route
• Once daily with first meal of the day
• Correct volume depletion prior to use
• Adjust dose in times of stress, surgery, trauma
• Store at room temperature

SIDE EFFECTS
CV: Hypotension, orthostatic hypotension
GI: Pancreatitis, nausea, vomiting, dehydration
GU: Cystitis, candidiasis, urinary frequency, polydipsia, polyuria, renal impairment, UTI, genital fungal infections
INTEG: Photosensitivity, rash, pruritus
META: Hypercholesterolemia, lipidemia, hypoglycemia, hyperkalemia, hypermagnesemia, hyperphosphatemia, hypersensitivity, ketoacidosis
MISC: Bone fractures

PHARMACOKINETICS
99% protein binding, metabolized by UGT1A9, UGT2B4, excreted 33% in urine, peak 1-2 hr, half-life 10.6-13 hr depending on dose

INTERACTIONS
Increase: hypoglycemia—sulfonylureas, insulin, MAOIs, salicylates, fibric acid derivatives, bile acid sequestrants, ACE inhibitors, angiotensin II receptor antagonists, beta-blockers, SSRIs; monitor for hypoglycemia, monitor blood glucose closely, dosage may need to be decreased
Increase: hyperkalemia—potassium-sparing diuretics, ACE inhibitors, ARBs, monitor potassium regularly
Antihypertensives, loop diuretics: Increased hypotension, monitor B/P loop diuretics
SSRIs (fluoxetine): Increased canaglifloxacin level, may need dose reduction

Increase or decrease: glycemic control—androgens, lithium, bortezomib, quinolones; monitor for glycemic control
Decrease: effect hyperglycemia—digestive enzymes, intestinal absorbents, thiazide diuretics, loop diuretics, corticosteroids, estrogen, progestins, oral contraceptives, sympathomimetics, isoniazid, phenothiazines; protease inhibitors, atypical antipsychotics, carbonic anhydrase inhibitors, cycloSPORINE, tacrolimus, baclofen, UGT inducers (PHENobarbital, phenytoin, rifAMPin, ritonavir); dose may need to be increased based on eGFR
Drug/Lab
Increase: urine glucose, potassium, lipids, cholesterol, magnesium phosphate, uric acid, serum creatinine
Decrease: serum glucose, eGFR
Drug/Herb
Decrease: canagliflozin level—St. John's wort

NURSING CONSIDERATIONS
Assess:
• **Hypoglycemia** (weakness, hunger, dizziness, tremors, anxiety, tachycardia, sweating), hyperglycemia; even though product does not cause hypoglycemia, if patient is on sulfonylureas or insulin, hypoglycemia may be additive; if hypoglycemia occurs, treat with dextrose, or, if severe, with IV glucagon
• **Ketoacidosis:** monitor for increased ketone levels; may occur with any glucose level, more common in those with severe illnesses
• **Necrotizing fasciitis (perineum):** requires immediate surgery
• **Volume depletion:** monitor for orthostatic hypotension, weakness, dizziness; may occur after beginning treatment; correct volume depletion before starting treatment
• For stress, surgery, or other trauma that may require a change in dose
• A1c q3mo; monitor serum glucose 1 hr PP throughout treatment; serum cholesterol, serum creatinine/BUN, serum electrolytes
• **Hyperkalemia (renal disease):** monitor potassium closely
• **Bone fractures:** monitor bone density, other conditions that may lead to bone fractures; fractures may occur within 3 mo of starting therapy

• **Renal impairment:** monitor more frequently in those with renal disease; increased creatinine, BUN, eGFR may be decreased

Black Box Warning: Lower limb amputation: Increased risk of amputation; monitor wound and feet closely for complications, provide foot care

• Monitor electrolytes, LDL, cholesterol and correct as needed
• **Fungal infections:** usually in those with other infections
• **Pregnancy/breastfeeding:** identify whether pregnancy is planned or suspected or if breastfeeding, use only if clearly needed not to use in second/third trimester, do not breastfeed
Evaluate:
• Therapeutic response: improved signs/symptoms of diabetes mellitus (decreased polyuria, polydipsia, polyphagia); clear sensorium, absence of dizziness, stable gait
Teach patient/family:
• The symptoms of hypo/hyperglycemia, what to do about each
• That medication must be taken as prescribed; explain consequences of discontinuing abruptly; that insulin may need to be used for stress, including trauma, fever, surgery, to take as soon as remembered if dose is missed unless close to next dose, then skip and take at next scheduled dose, do not double
• To avoid OTC medications and herbal supplements unless discussed with health care professional
• That diabetes is a lifelong illness; that the diet and exercise regimen must be followed; that this product is not a cure
• To carry emergency ID and glucose source
• That blood glucose monitoring is required to assess product effect
• **Renal injury:** edema in extremities decreased, dark urine, seek care immediately
• **Necrotizing fasciitis:** signs/symptoms of high temperature, genital swelling, pain, redness, seek care immediately

- **Hypersensitivity:** to notify prescriber immediately of itching, hives, rash, swelling of face/lips

Black Box Warning: Lower limb amputation risk: Inspect feet; monitor for new ulcerations, wounds; educate about foot care, to report injury to limbs, sores

- **Ketoacidosis:** to notify prescriber immediately of nausea, vomiting, lack of appetite, sleepiness, difficulty breathing
- **Yeast infections (women/men):** That yeast infections can occur with this product (women, vaginal; men, penile); to report discharge, itching, swelling
- **UTI:** to report immediately burning, pain on urination, hematuria, back pain, decreased urine
- **Pregnancy/breastfeeding:** Not to breastfeed; to advise prescriber if pregnancy is planned or suspected

candesartan (Rx)

(can-deh-sar'tan)

Atacand

Func. class.: Antihypertensive

Chem. class.: Angiotensin II receptor (type AT$_1$) antagonist

ACTION: Blocks the vasoconstrictor and aldosterone-secreting effects of angiotensin II; selectively blocks the binding of angiotensin II to the AT$_1$ receptor found in tissues

USES: Hypertension, alone or in combination; diabetic nephropathy in hypertension and type 2 diabetes

CONTRAINDICATIONS

Hypersensitivity, child GFR <30 mL/min/1.73 m^2, child <1 yr

Black Box Warning: Pregnancy

Precautions: Breastfeeding, children, geriatric patients, hypersensitivity to ACE inhibitors, volume/sodium depletion, renal/hepatic impairment, renal artery stenosis, hypotension, electrolyte abnormalities

DOSAGE AND ROUTES
Hypertension

- **Adult: PO** single agent 16 mg/day initially in patients who are not volume depleted, range 8-32 mg/day, with diuretic or volume depletion 8-32 mg/day as single dose or divided bid
- **Adolescent and child ≥6 yr and weight >50 kg: PO** 8-16 mg/day or divided bid, adjust to B/P; usual range 4-32 mg/day, max 32 mg/day
- **Child ≥6 yr, weight <50 kg: PO** 2-16 mg/day divided 1-2 doses, max 16 mg/day
- **Child ≥1 yr and <6 yr: PO** 0.2 mg/kg/day in 1 dose or in 2 divided doses, adjust to B/P, max 0.4 mg/kg/day

Heart failure (Class II to IV)

- **Adult: PO** 4 mg/day, double ≥2 wk, target dose 32 mg/day

Renal/hepatic disease

- **Adult: PO** ≤8 mg/day for severe renal disease/moderate hepatic disease; adjust dose as needed

Available forms: Tablets 4, 8, 16, 32 mg

Administer:
- Without regard to meals
- Oral liquid (compounded): shake well, do not freeze, use opened within 30 days

SIDE EFFECTS

CNS: *Dizziness,* fatigue, headache, syncope, insomnia

CV: Chest pain, peripheral edema, hypotension, palpitations

EENT: Sinusitis, rhinitis, pharyngitis

GI: *Diarrhea,* nausea, abdominal pain, vomiting

GU: Renal dysfunction

MS: Arthralgia, back pain, myalgia

SYST: Angioedema, hypersensitivity reactions

PHARMACOKINETICS

Onset unknown, peak 3-4 hr, protein binding 90%, half-life 9-12 hr, duration 24 hr, extensively metabolized, excreted in urine (33%) and feces (67%)

INTERACTIONS
Increase: lithium level—lithium
Increase: hyperkalemia—potassium, potassium-sparing diuretics, ACE inhibitors
Increase: hypotension—ACE inhibitors, beta-blockers, calcium channel blockers, alpha-blockers, MAOIs, diuretics
Decrease: hypotensive effect—COX-2 inhibitors, NSAIDs
Drug/Food
Potassium salt substitutes: increased hyperkalemia
Drug/Herb
Increase: antihypertensive effect—hawthorn
Decrease: antihypertensive effect—ephedra
Drug/Lab
Increase: albumin, ALT/AST, potassium, serum creatinine

NURSING CONSIDERATIONS
Assess
• **Hypotension:** B/P, pulse; note rate, rhythm, quality; notify prescriber of significant changes, if hypotension is significant, have patient lie down, effect of product may take 2 wk
• **Electrolytes:** potassium, sodium, calcium; baselines of renal/hepatic studies before therapy begins
• **Hydration:** skin turgor, dryness of mucous membranes, correct volume depletion
• **Blood studies:** BUN, creatinine, LFTs baseline, all may be increased
• **Serious hypersensitivity reaction:** angioedema, anaphylaxis: facial swelling, difficulty breathing (rare)
• **Hyperkalemia:** more common with other diuretics
• Response and adverse reactions, especially with renal disease; diuretic may be added
• **Heart failure:** monitor for jugular venous distention, weight, peripheral edema, dyspnea, crackles

Black Box Warning: Pregnancy/breast-feeding: This product can cause fetal death when given during pregnancy; do not breastfeed

Evaluate:
• Therapeutic response: decreased B/P, decreased heart failure–related complications, death

Teach patient/family:
• To notify prescriber of mouth sores, fever, swelling of hands or feet, irregular heartbeat, chest pain
• That excessive perspiration, dehydration, vomiting, diarrhea may lead to fall in B/P; to consult prescriber if these occur
• To avoid all OTC medications unless approved by prescriber; to inform all health care providers of use, full effect 4 wk, onset 2 wk; that product may be taken with or without meals; to store at room temperature, to comply with dosage schedule, even if feeling better
• To use proper technique for obtaining B/P; to understand acceptable parameters; to rise slowly to sitting or standing position to minimize orthostatic hypotension; that product may cause dizziness, fainting, light headedness
• To continue to follow other requirements, no smoking, lose weight, exercise
• To limit potassium foods or salt substitutes/supplements containing potassium unless discussed with health care professional

cangrelor (Rx)
(kan′grel-or)
Kengreal
Func. class.: Platelet aggregation inhibitor
Chem. class.: ADP receptor antagonist

ACTION: A direct competitive inhibitor of a platelet receptor, prevents further signaling and platelet activation, results in inhibition of platelet activation and aggregation, does not require hepatic conversion to an active metabolite

USES: For use as an adjunct to percutaneous coronary intervention (PCI) for myocardial infarction prophylaxis, repeat coronary revascularization, and stent thrombosis in patients who have not been treated with a P2Y12 platelet inhibitor and are not being given a glycoprotein IIb/IIIa inhibitor

Side effects: *italics* = common; red = life-threatening

CONTRAINDICATIONS

Hypersensitivity, active bleeding

Precautions: Pregnancy, breastfeeding, children, increased bleeding risk, neutropenia, agranulocytosis, renal disease

DOSAGE AND ROUTES
Adjunct to PCI

• **Adult: IV BOLUS** 30 mcg/kg as a single dose, then follow immediately by 4 mcg/kg/min continuous IV infusion; the bolus should be given before PCI and maintenance infusion should be continued for ≥2 hr or for the duration of PCI, whichever is longer; use ticagrelor, prasugrel, or clopidogrel to maintain platelet inhibition

Available forms: Lyophilized powder for injection 50 mg

Administer:

• Visually inspect parenteral products for particulate matter and discoloration before use, use IV only

• **Reconstitution:** Reconstitute by adding 5 mL sterile water for injection to a 50-mg vial, swirl until dissolved, do not shake, allow foam to settle, solution should be clear and colorless to pale yellow; withdraw contents of reconstituted 50-mg vial and add to 250-mL bag of 0.9% sodium chloride injection or dextrose 5% injection resulting in a final infusion concentration of 200 mcg/mL; usually, 1 bag should be sufficient for most patients for ≥2 hr of dosing; those weighing >100 kg will require a minimum of 2 bags

• Use diluted product immediately. When stored at room temperature, diluted product stable for ≤12 hr in dextrose 5% injection and 24 hr in 0.9% sodium chloride injection, use a dedicated line

• Bolus injection should be administered rapidly (<1 min). The bolus volume may be withdrawn from the diluted infusion bag and given by IV push or using an infusion pump

• Ensure the bolus dose is completely administered prior to start of PCI

• Start the continuous IV infusion immediately after administration of the bolus; use infusion pump for the continuous IV infusion

SIDE EFFECTS

CNS: Intracranial bleeding
GI: GI bleeding
GU: Hematuria
HEMA: Bleeding
RESP: Wheezing, dyspnea, bronchospasm
SYST: Anaphylaxis, angioedema

PHARMACOKINETICS

Half-life 3-6 min; plasma protein binding 97%; effect on platelets 2 min, excreted in urine

INTERACTIONS

Do not give clopidogrel or prasugrel until infusion is discontinued

Increase: effect of warfarin, platelet inhibitors

NURSING CONSIDERATIONS
Assess:

• **Bleeding:** intracranial, retroperitoneal, other frank bleeding, after completion of infusion, platelet inhibition decreases rapidly within 1 hr; monitor Hct/HB

• **Hypersensitivity:** identify if patient has a known cangrelor hypersensitivity

• **Severe renal impairment:** decreased renal function may occur in severe renal impairment, CCr >30 mL/min; no dosage change is required

• **Pregnancy/breastfeeding:** identify whether the patient is pregnant or breastfeeding; it is not known whether product is excreted in breast milk, no well-controlled studies

Evaluate:

• Therapeutic response: platelet inhibition during PCI

Teach patient/family:

• Use and expected results

• **Pregnancy/breastfeeding:** to inform prescriber if pregnancy is planned or suspected, or if breastfeeding

• **Bleeding:** to report bleeding immediately (blood in stools, urine, gums, bruising)

• **Hypersensitivity:** to report immediately any difficulty breathing; hives; swelling of face, lips, mouth

cannabidiol (Rx)

(ka-na'bi-dye-ole)

Epidiolex

Func. class.: Anticonvulsant

USES: Seizures associated with Lennox-Gastaut syndrome or Dravet syndrome or tuberous sclerosis complex

CONTRAINDICATIONS

Hypersensitivity to this product or sesame seed oil

Precautions: Abrupt discontinuation, breastfeeding, depression, driving or operating machinery, hepatic disease, pregnancy, suicidal ideation

DOSAGE AND ROUTES

• **Adult/adolescent/child ≥2 yr: PO** Initially, 2.5 mg/kg bid; after 1 wk may increase to 5 mg/kg bid, may increase weekly by 2.5 mg/kg bid, max 10 mg/kg bid

• **Available forms:** Oral solution 100 mg/mL

⚠ HIGH ALERT

capecitabine (Rx)

(cap-eh-sit'ah-bean)

Xeloda

Func. class.: Antineoplastic, antimetabolite

Chem. class.: Pyrimidine carbamate

Do not confuse:

Xeloda/Xenical

ACTION: Competes with physiologic substrate of DNA synthesis, thereby interfering with cell replication in the S phase of cell cycle (before mitosis); also interferes with RNA and protein synthesis; product is converted to 5-FU

USES: PACLitaxel- and anthracycline-resistant metastatic breast, colorectal cancer when 5-FU monotherapy is preferred; treatment of colorectal cancer patients who have undergone complete resection of their primary tumors

Unlabeled uses: Breast cancer (HER-2 negative) (adjuvant), pancreatic cancer (adjuvant locally advanced)

CONTRAINDICATIONS

Pregnancy, hypersensitivity to 5-FU, infants, severe renal impairment (CCr <30 mL/min)

Precautions: Breastfeeding, children, infections, radiation therapy, anticoagulation, geriatric patients, renal/hepatic/cardiac disease, ☞ DPD deficiency

Black Box Warning: Anticoagulant therapy

DOSAGE AND ROUTES

Breast cancer alone or with DOCEtaxel; metastatic colorectal cancer when fluoropyrimidine alone is preferred; Dukes Stage C colon cancer after resection when fluoropyrimidine alone is preferred

Adult: PO 2500 mg/m²/day divided q12hr after a meal × 2 wk, repeat q3wk; **Dukes C colon cancer** 8 cycles (24 wk), max 5600 mg/day

Renal dose

• **Adult: PO** CCr 30-50 mL/min, decrease initial dose to 75% of usual dose; CCr <30 mL/min, contraindicated

Primary breast cancer (adjuvant therapy) in those with HER-2 negative who have residual invasive disease containing an anthracycline or/and taxane (unlabeled)

• **Adult: PO** 1250 mg/m² bid on days 1 to 14 of a 21-day cycle × 6-8 cycles

Pancreatic adenocarcinoma (adjuvant) after rescetion (unlabeled)

• **Adult: PO** 1660 mg/m² divided bid on day 1-21 q28 days with gemcitabine × 6 cycles 8-12 wk after resection

Pancreatic cancer (locally advanced or metastatic) (unlabeled)

Adult: PO 1250 mg/m² bid on days 1-14 of a 3-wk cycle or 830 mg/m² bid with gemcitabine on days 1-21 of a 4-wk cycle

Available forms: Tablets 150, 500 mg
Administer:
• Swallow whole, take with water within 30 min of a meal
• Use cytotoxic handling procedures
• Do not double dose if missed

SIDE EFFECTS

CNS: Dizziness, *headache, paresthesia, fatigue,* insomnia
CV: Venous thrombosis, edema, chest pain
GI: *Nausea, vomiting, anorexia, diarrhea, stomatitis, abdominal pain, constipation, dyspepsia,* hyperbilirubinemia, hepatitis
HEMA: Neutropenia, lymphopenia, thrombocytopenia, anemia
INTEG: *Dermatitis,* nail disorders, alopecia, rash
OTHER: *Eye irritation, edema,* limb pain, *pyrexia,* dehydration, renal impairment, Stevens-Johnson syndrome
RESP: *Cough, dyspnea,* pulmonary embolism

PHARMACOKINETICS

Readily absorbed, peak 1½ hr, food decreases absorption, extensively metabolized in the liver, elimination half-life 45 min

INTERACTIONS

Increase: toxicity—leucovorin fosphenytoin; monitor for toxicity
Increase: capecitabine levels—antacids (aluminum, magnesium)
Increase: phenytoin level—phenytoin; monitor phenytoin level

> **Black Box Warning: Increase:** bleeding risk—anticoagulants, NSAIDs, salicylates, platelet inhibitors, thrombolytics; monitor PT and INR

Decrease: capecitabine effect—allopurinol; avoid using together

Drug/Food
Increase: absorption; give within 30 min of a meal
Drug/Lab Test
Increase: bilirubin
Decrease: HB/Hct/RBC, neutrophils, platelets, WBC

NURSING CONSIDERATIONS
Assess:
• **Bone marrow suppression,** CBC (RBC, Hct, HB), differential, platelet count weekly; withhold product if WBC is <1000/mm³, platelet count is <50,000/mm³, or RBC, Hct, HB low; notify prescriber of these results; frequently monitor INR in those receiving warfarin concurrently
• Renal studies: BUN; serum uric acid; urine CCr; electrolytes before, during therapy
• Infection: monitor temperature q4hr; fever may indicate beginning infection; no rectal temperatures
• Hepatic studies prior to, during therapy: bilirubin, ALT, AST, alkaline phophatase as needed or monthly

> **Black Box Warning: Bleeding:** hematuria, heme-positive stools, bruising or petechiae of mucosa or orifices q8hr; monitor INR and PT in those taking coumarin-derivative anticoagulants; adjustment of dose may be needed , those >60 at higher risk of bleeding; dose may need to be decreased

• Dyspnea, crackles, unproductive cough, chest pain, tachypnea, fatigue, increased pulse, pallor, lethargy; personality changes with high doses
• **Hand and foot syndrome/Stevens-Johnson syndrome:** paresthesia, tingling, painful/painless swelling, blistering, erythema with severe pain of hands or feet, toxicity is divided into grade 1, 2, 3; if grade 2 or 3, product should be discontinued until grade 1
• **GI toxicity:** severe diarrhea (multiple times/day or at night), nausea, vomiting, stomatitis, fever; adjust dose, stop treatment if severe

• Buccal cavity q8hr for dryness, sores, ulceration, white patches, oral pain, bleeding, dysphagia
• Fluid, electrolytes may need to be given; elderly patients are at greater risk of GI symptoms, dehydration
• Rinsing of mouth tid-qid with water, club soda; brushing of teeth bid-tid with soft brush or cotton-tipped applicators for stomatitis; use unwaxed dental floss
Evaluate:
• Therapeutic response: decreased tumor size, spread of malignancy
Teach patient/family:
• To avoid foods with citric acid, hot temperature, or rough texture if stomatitis is present; to take with water within 30 min of end of meal; not to take if dose is missed
• How to take (on for 14 days then 7 days off, then start a new cycle); do not crush, cut
• Not to double dose if dose is missed
• To immediately report severe diarrhea, vomiting, stomatitis, fever of more than 100° F (37.8° C), hand and foot syndrome, anorexia; stop taking product
• To report bleeding in those taking anticoagulants
• **To report signs of infection:** increased temperature, sore throat, flulike symptoms, to avoid crowds, persons with known infections; signs of **anemia:** fatigue, headache, faintness, shortness of breath, irritability; **bleeding;** to avoid use of razors, commercial mouthwash
• To use OTC antidiarrheals for mild diarrhea (4-6 stools/day or diarrhea at night)
• **Pregnancy/breastfeeding:** to notify prescriber if pregnancy is planned or suspected; to avoid pregnancy while taking this product, use adequate contraception during and for 6 mo after last dose; males should use contraception during and for 3 mo after last dose if partner is of child bearing potential; not to breastfeed
• That continuing exams and blood work will be needed

caplacizumab-yhdp (Rx)
(kap′luh-sih′-zoo-mab)
Cablivi
Func. class.: Hematologic agent

USES: Acquired thrombotic thrombocytopenia purpura (aTTP), in combination with plasma exchange and immunosuppressive therapy

CONTRAINDICATIONS
Hyper-sensitivity

DOSAGE AND ROUTES
• **Adult: IV** 11 mg once at least 15 min before plasma exchange on the first day of treatment (initial dose); **SUBCUT** 11 mg daily starting after the completion of plasma exchange on day 1 and continuing for 30 days after the last daily plasma exchange; treatment may be extended for a maximum of 28 days after the initial treatment (maintenance dose)
Available forms: Single-dose vial 11 mg

capmatinib (Rx)
(kap-ma′ti-nib)
Tabrecta
Func. class.: Antineoplastic

USES: Treatment of metastatic non–small-cell lung cancer with a mutation of mesenchymal-epithelial transition (MET) exon 14 skipping

CONTRAINDICATIONS
Hyper-sensitivity, pregnancy, breastfeeding

DOSAGE AND ROUTES
Adult: PO 400 mg bid, continue until disease progression or unacceptable toxicity
Available forms: Tablet 150, 250 mg

captopril (Rx)

(kap′toe-pril)

Func. class.: Antihypertensive

Chem. class.: Angiotensin-converting enzyme (ACE) inhibitor

Combinations: Captopril/hydrochlorothiazide: 25 mg/15 mg, 25 mg/25 mg, 50 mg/15 mg, 50 mg/25 mg

Do not confuse:
captopril/carvedilol

ACTION: Selectively suppresses renin-angiotensin-aldosterone system; inhibits ACE; prevents conversion of angiotensin I to angiotensin II

USES: Hypertension, HF, left ventricular dysfunction after MI, diabetic nephropathy, proteinuria

Unlabeled uses: Acute MI, hypertensive emergency/urgency, scleroderma renal crisis (SRC)

CONTRAINDICATIONS

Breast-feeding, children, hypersensitivity, heart block, potassium-sparing diuretics, bilateral renal artery stenosis, ACE inhibitors, ACE inhibitor–induced angioedema

Black Box Warning: Pregnancy

Precautions: Dialysis patients, hypovolemia, leukemia, scleroderma, SLE, blood dyscrasias, HF, diabetes mellitus, thyroid/renal/hepatic disease, ⚫ African descent, pregnancy first trimester, collagen vascular disease, hyperkalemia, hyponatremia

DOSAGE AND ROUTES

Hypertension

• **Adult:** PO initial dose: 12.5-25 mg bid-tid; may increase to 50 mg bid-tid at 1-2 wk intervals; usual range: 25-150 mg bid-tid; max 450 mg/day

• **Child (unlabeled):** PO 0.3-0.5 mg/kg/dose, may titrate up to 6 mg/kg/day in 2-4 divided doses

• **Infant (unlabeled):** PO 0.15-0.3 mg/kg/dose initially, max 6 mg/kg/day

• **Neonate (unlabeled):** PO 0.01-0.1 mg/kg/dose, may increase as needed

Heart failure

• **Adult:** PO 25 mg bid; may increase to 50 mg tid; after 14 days, may increase to 150 mg tid if needed

• **Adolescent (unlabeled):** PO 6.25-12.5 mg q8-12hr titrated up to max 50-75 mg/dose

• **Child (unlabeled):** PO 0.1-2 mg/kg/dose q6-12hr, max 6 mg/kg/day

• **Infant (unlabeled):** PO 0.15-0.3 mg/kg/dose, max 6 mg/kg/day in 1-4 divided doses

• **Neonate (unlabeled):** PO 0.05-0.1 mg/kg q8-24hr titrate to 0.5 mg/kg q6-24hr, max 2 mg/kg/day

Diabetic nephropathy

• **Adult:** PO 25 mg tid

Renal dose

• **Adult:** PO CCr 10-50 mL/min, decrease dose by 25%; CCr <10 mL/min, decrease dose by 50%

Left ventricular dysfunction/acute MI (unlabeled) or post-MI

• **Adult:** PO 6.25-12.5 mg tid, increase to 25 mg tid gradually

Hypertensive emergency/urgency (unlabeled)

• **Adult:** PO 25 mg, may repeat q30min

Available forms: Tablets 12.5, 25, 50, 100 mg

Administer:

• Store in tight container at 86° F (30° C) or less

• 1 hr prior to or 2 hr after meals

• Correct volume depletion before starting treatment

• **Oral solution:** May crush 25-mg tablet, dissolve in 50-100 mL water; give within ½ hr; make sure tablet completely dissolved

SIDE EFFECTS

CNS: Fever, chills, dizziness, drowsiness, fatigue, headache, insomnia, weakness

CV: *Hypotension,* postural hypotension, *tachycardia,* angina

GI: Loss of taste, increased LFTs

GU: Impotence, dysuria, nocturia, proteinuria, nephrotic syndrome, acute reversible renal failure, polyuria, oliguria, urinary frequency

HEMA: Neutropenia, agranulocytosis, pancytopenia, thrombocytopenia, anemia

INTEG: Rash, pruritus
MISC: Angioedema, hyperkalemia
RESP: Bronchospasm, *dyspnea, cough*

PHARMACOKINETICS

Peak 1 hr; duration 2-6 hr; half-life <2 hr, increased in renal disease; metabolized by liver (metabolites); excreted in urine; crosses placenta; excreted in breast milk, small amounts; protein binding 25%-30%

INTERACTIONS

• Do not use with potassium-sparing diuretics, sympathomimetics, potassium supplements

Increase: possible toxicity—lithium, digoxin; monitor individual drug levels
Increase: hyperkalemia—aliskiren
Increase: hypoglycemia—insulin, oral antidiabetics; monitor blood glucose
Increase: hypotension—diuretics, other antihypertensives, acute alcohol ingestion, MAOIs
Decrease: captopril effect—antacids, COX-2 inhibitors, NSAIDs, salicylates

Drug/Herb
Increase: antihypertensive effect—hawthorn
Decrease: antihypertensive effect—black licorice, ephedra

Drug/Food
Decrease: absorption of captopril

Drug/Lab Test
Increase: AST, ALT, alkaline phosphatase, bilirubin, uric acid, potassium
Decrease: platelets, WBC, RBC, HB/Hct
False positive: urine acetone
Positive: ANA titer

NURSING CONSIDERATIONS
Assess:

• **Blood dyscrasias:** blood studies: decreased platelets; CBC with differential at baseline, q2wk and periodically during 1 yr; if neutrophils <1000/mm^3, discontinue treatment (recommended with collagen-vascular or renal disease)
• **Hypertension:** B/P, pulse rates at baseline, frequently; notify prescriber of significant changes
• **Heart failure:** dyspnea, jugular venous distention, weight gain, edema, rales/crackles in lungs, increased B/P

• **Renal studies:** protein, BUN, creatinine electrolytes, watch for raised levels, if increased dose may need to be reduced
• **Angioedema/allergic reaction:** rash, fever, pruritus, urticaria; discontinue product if antihistamines fail to help; swelling of lips, mouth, face; difficulty breathing/swallowing (angioedema); provide supportive care; discontinue product
• Monitor AST, ALT, alkaline phosphatase, glucose, urine protein, bilirubin, uric acid baseline and periodically
• **Cough:** monitor for development of dry cough unexplained by other illness; notify prescriber
• Black patients may require higher dose and have higher incidence of angioedema

Renal disease/collagen vascular disorder (SLE, scleroderma): leukocytes, differential baseline and q2wk × 3 mo and periodically thereafter

Black Box Warning: **Pregnancy/breastfeeding:** Discontinue ACE inhibitors when pregnancy is detected; monitor fetal development regularly; do not breastfeed

Evaluate:

• Therapeutic response: decrease in B/P with hypertension; decreased edema, moist crackles (HF); decreased diabetic nephropathy symptoms

Teach patient/family:

• To take 1 hr prior to or 2 hr after meals; not to discontinue product abruptly; if dose is missed, take as soon as remembered but not if almost time for next dose; not to double doses, advise patient to tell all persons associated with care that product is being used
• Not to use OTC products (cough, cold, or allergy) unless directed by prescriber; to avoid salt substitutes, high-potassium or high-sodium foods
• To adhere to dosage schedule, even if feeling better
• To use cautiously in hot weather, make sure fluids are adequate
• To rise slowly to sitting or standing position to minimize orthostatic hypotension

- To notify prescriber of fever, swelling of hands or feet, irregular heartbeat, chest pain, signs of angioedema, rash, hoarseness, difficulty breathing
- **Infection:** to report fever, sore throat, flulike symptoms, other signs of infection
- That excessive perspiration, dehydration, vomiting, diarrhea may lead to fall in B/P; to consult prescriber if these occur
- That dizziness, fainting, light headedness may occur during first few days of therapy; to avoid activities that require concentration
- How to take B/P and when to notify prescriber
- **Diabetes:** to monitor blood glucose often, hypoglycemia

Black Box Warning: Pregnancy/breastfeeding: to notify if pregnancy is planned or suspected; not to breastfeed, contraception should be used, if pregnancy occurs, discontinue medication

carbachol ophthalmic
See Appendix B

carBAMazepine (Rx)

(kar-ba-maz'e-peen)

Carbatrol, Carnexiv, Epitol, Equetro, Tegretol CR, TEGretol, TEGretol-XR

Func. class.: Anticonvulsant
Chem. class.: Iminostilbene derivative

Do not confuse:

carBAMazepine/OXcarbazepine
TEGretol/Tegrotol XR/Tequin/TRENtal

ACTION: Exact mechanism unknown; appears to decrease polysynaptic responses and block posttetanic potentiation

USES: Tonic-clonic, complex-partial, mixed seizures; trigeminal neuralgia; bipolar disorder
Unlabeled uses: Neurogenic pain

CONTRAINDICATIONS

Pregnancy, hypersensitivity to carBAMazepine or tricyclics, MAOI therapy, bone marrow suppression

Precautions: Breastfeeding, children <6 yr, glaucoma, AV or bundle branch block, cardiac/renal/hepatic disease, psychosis, alcoholism, hepatic porphyria

Black Box Warning: Hematologic disease, ✇ Asian patients or those with positive HLA-B 1502 or HLA-A 3101 alleles, agranulocytosis, leukopenia, neutropenia, thrombocytopenia

DOSAGE AND ROUTES—NTI
General tonic/clonic and complex partial seizures, mixed seizure patterns

- **Adult and child >12 yr: PO** 200 mg bid, may be increased by 200 mg/day in weekly intervals, give in divided doses q6-8hr; maintenance 800-1200 mg/day, max 1600 mg/day (adult); max child 12-15 yr 1000 mg/day; max child >15 yr 1200 mg/day; **EXTENDED RELEASE** give bid; rectal administration of **ORAL SUSPENSION** 200 mg/10 mL or 6 mg/kg as a single dose
- **Child 6-12 yr: PO** tablets 100 mg bid or **extended release** 50 mg qid; may increase by <100 mg weekly; max 1000 mg/day, usual dose 15-30 mg/kg/day
- **Child <6 yr: PO** 10-20 mg/kg/day in 2-3 divided doses or 4 divided doses (suspension), may increase every wk, do not use extended release, max 35 mg/kg/day

Diabetic neuropathy (unlabeled)

- **Adult: PO** 100 mg bid or 50 mg qid, titrate to 600-800 mg/day

Acute mania and mixed episodes in bipolar I disorder

Adult: PO 100-400 mg/day in divided doses, increase by 200 mg q1-4days to desired response

- **Adult: PO** (Equetro only) 200 mg bid, increase by 200 mg/day until response, max 1600 mg/day

Trigeminal neuralgia

- **Adult: PO** 100 mg bid with meals; may increase 100 mg q12hr until pain subsides, max 1200 mg/day; maintenance 200-400

mg bid; suspension: 50 mg qid with meals, increase by 50 mg qid until response
Available forms: Chewable tablets 100, 200 mg; tablets 100, 200, 300, 400 mg; extended-release tablets (XR) 100, 200, 400 mg; oral suspension 100 mg/5 mL; extended-release capsules 100, 200, 300 mg
Administer:

PO route
• When converting from tablets to oral suspension, give same amount/day, or regular release to extended release same amount
• Do not crush, chew extended-release tablet; extended-release capsule may be opened and beads sprinkled over food; patient should chew chewable tablet, not swallow it whole
• With food, milk to decrease GI symptoms
Suspension: Turn off NG/enteral feeding 15 min prior to and hold for 15 min after
• Mix an equal amount of water, D_5W, 0.9% NaCl when giving by NG tube; flush tube with 15-30 mL, do not give at same time as other liquid products or diluents
• Shake oral suspension before use
• Store at room temperature

SIDE EFFECTS
CNS: *Drowsiness,* dizziness, fatigue, headache, suicidal thoughts/behaviors
CV: Hypertension, AV block, hypotension
EENT: Dry mouth, blurred vision, diplopia, nystagmus
ENDO: SIADH (geriatric patients)
GI: *Nausea,* anorexia, increased hepatic enzymes, pancreatitis, hepatotoxicity
GU: Retention, increased BUN, renal dysfunction
HEMA: Thrombocytopenia, leukopenia, agranulocytosis, aplastic anemia, eosinophilia, lymphadenopathy
INTEG: *Rash,* Stevens-Johnson syndrome, urticaria, photosensitivity, toxic epidermal necrolysis, DRESS, alopecia, pruritus
RESP: Pulmonary hypersensitivity (fever, dyspnea, pneumonitis)

PHARMACOKINETICS
Onset slow; peak 4-5 hr (PO), 1.5 hr (suspension) metabolized by liver; excreted in urine, feces; crosses placenta, blood-brain barrier; excreted in breast milk; half-life 6-12 hr; protein binding 76%; metabolized by CYP3A4

INTERACTIONS
Increase: CNS toxicity—lithium; avoid concurrent use
Fatal reaction: MAOIs; do not use within 14 days of beginning carBAMazepine
• Do not use with nonnucleoside reverse transcriptase inhibitors (NNRTIs), nefazodone
Increase: carBAMazepine levels—CYP3A inhibitors (cimetidine, clarithromycin, danazol, dilTIAzem, erythromycin, FLUoxetine, fluvoxaMINE, isoniazid, valproic acid, verapamil, voriconazole), SSRIs, tricyclics; adjust dose if needed, or do not use together
Increase: effects of desmopressin, lithium, lypressin, vasopressin
Decrease: carBAMazepine effect—CYP1A2, CYP2C9 substrates
Decrease: effect of CYP3A inducers
Decrease: effects of benzodiazepines, doxycycline, felbamate, haloperidol, oral contraceptives, PHENobarbital, phenytoin, primidone, theophylline, thyroid hormones, warfarin; adjust dose as needed
Decrease: carBAMazepine levels—CYP3A4 inducers (CISplatin, darunavir, delavirdine, DOXOrubicin, felbamate, nefazodone, OXcarbazepine, PHENobarbital, phenytoin, primidone, rifAMPin, theophylline); monitor carBAMazepine effectiveness

Drug/Herb
Decrease: carBAMazepine metabolism, increased levels—echinacea
Decrease: anticonvulsant effect—St. John's wort

Drug/Food
Increase: peak concentration of carBAMazepine—grapefruit juice; avoid use

Drug/Lab Test
Decrease: serum calcium, sodium
Increase: cholesterol

NURSING CONSIDERATIONS
Assess:

Black Box Warning: Asian patients for serious skin reaction; genetic test for HLA-B1502 allele prior to administration; these patients may develop toxic epidermal necrolysis, Stevens-Johnson syndrome, DRESS; may be fatal

- **Seizures:** character, location, duration, intensity, frequency, presence of aura, in mixed seizure disorder, worsening of symptoms may occur
- **Trigeminal neuralgia:** facial pain, including location, duration, intensity, character, activity that stimulates pain
- **Renal studies:** urinalysis, BUN, urine creatinine q3mo
- **Bipolar disorder:** assess for symptoms at baseline and during treatment
- **DRESS:** fever, lymphadenopathy with multiorgan involvement, including liver, kidney, cardiac; discontinue carBAMazepine

Black Box Warning: Bone marrow depression: blood studies: CBC reticulocyte counts every week for 4 wk, then q3-6mo if on long-term therapy; if myelosuppression occurs, product should be discontinued; blood dyscrasias: fever, sore throat, bruising, rash, jaundice, agranulocytosis, and aplastic anemia may occur

- Blood studies: ALT, AST, bilirubin; serum calcium, may be decreased and lead to osteoporosis; cholesterol periodically
- Drug levels during initial treatment or when changing dose; should remain at 4-12 mcg/mL; anorexia may indicate increased blood levels
- **Mental status:** mood, sensorium, affect, behavioral changes, **suicidal thoughts/behaviors;** if mental status changes, notify prescriber
- **Eye problems:** need for ophthalmic examinations prior to during, after treatment (slit lamp, funduscopy, tonometry)
- **Allergic reaction:** purpura, red, raised rash; if these occur, product should be discontinued; increased risk if past hypersensitivity to hydantoins
- **Toxicity:** bone marrow depression, nausea, vomiting, ataxia, diplopia, CV collapse
- Hard candy, gum, frequent rinsing for dry mouth
- **Beers:** avoid use in older adults unless safer alternative is unavailable; ataxia, impaired psychomotor function may occur

Evaluate:
- Therapeutic response: decreased seizure activity; document on patient's chart

Teach patient/family:
- To carry emergency ID stating patient's name, products taken, condition, prescriber's name, and phone number
- To avoid driving, other activities that require alertness usually for the first 3 days of treatment; dizziness, drowsiness may occur
- Not to discontinue medication quickly after long-term use; seizures may occur
- To immediately report chills, rash, light-colored stools, dark urine, yellowing of skin and eyes, abdominal pain, sore throat, mouth ulcers, bruising, blurred vision, dizziness, skin rash, fever
- That urine may turn pink to brown
- Not to use with grapefruit juice; to take on an empty stomach; that toxicity may occur
- That ophthalmic examinations will be needed; to report changes in vision
- **Pregnancy/breastfeeding:** to notify health care provider if pregnancy is planned or suspected; not to breastfeed; that if pregnant, patient should register with American Antiepileptic Drug Pregnancy Registry (888-233-2334), to use nonhormonal contraceptive

⚠ HIGH ALERT

CARBOplatin (Rx)

(kar-boe-pla´-tin)
Paraplatin
Func. class.: Antineoplastic alkylating agent
Chem. class.: Platinum coordination compound

Do not confuse:
CARBOplatin/CISplatin

ACTION: Produces interstrand DNA cross-links and, to a lesser extent, DNA-protein cross-links; activity is not cell-cycle–phase specific

USES: Advanced ovarian cancer in combination with other agents; palliative treatment of ovarian carcinoma recurrent after treatment with other antineoplastic agents

CONTRAINDICATIONS
Pregnancy, breastfeeding, hypersensitivity, significant bleeding, aluminum products used to prepare or administer CARBOplatin

Black Box Warning: Severe bone marrow depression, platinum compound hypersensitivity (anaphylaxis)

Precautions: Geriatric patients, radiation therapy within 1 mo, other cancer chemotherapy within 1 mo, renal/hepatic disease, hearing impairment, infection

Black Box Warning: Anemia, chemotherapy-induced nausea/vomiting; requires a specialized care setting and an experienced clinician

DOSAGE AND ROUTES
Advanced ovarian cancer:
• **Adults: IV:** For patients with previously untreated ovarian cancer, 300 mg/m² on day 1 in combination with cyclophosphamide (600 mg/m² IV on day 1), repeated q4wk × 6 cycles. For patients with recurrent ovarian cancer, give CARBOplatin 360 mg/m² on day 1, repeated q4wk
ALL with ifosfamide, etoposide, rituximab (unlabeled):
• **Adults ≤21: IV:** CARBOplatin 635 mg/m² on day 3 with ifosfamide 3000 mg/m²/day IV on days 3, 4, 5 (each dose mixed with mesna 600 mg/m² IV, then mesna 600 mg/m² IV over 15 min at 3, 6, 9, and 12 hr after the start of ifosfamide) and etoposide 100 mg/m²/day IV on days 3, 4, 5, repeated each cycle. Rituximab 375 mg/m² IV on days 1 and 3 of cycles 1 and 2 and on day 3 only of cycle 3. Treatment was given up to a maximum of 3 cycles. Colony-stimulating factors were initiated on day 6 of each cycle, and intrathecal chemotherapy was also given as appropriate
Relapsed Wilms tumor with etoposide and ifosfamide (unlabeled):
• **Adults ≤21 yr, adolescents, and children: IV:** Ifosfamide 1800 mg/m²/day

× 5 days (on days 0, 1, 2, 3, 4), CARBOplatin 400 mg/m²/day IV × 2 days (on days 0, 1), and etoposide 100 mg/m²/day IV × 5 days (on days 0, 1, 2, 3, 4), repeated q21day
Neuroblastoma with etoposide, cyclophosphamide, and DOXOrubicin (unlabeled):
• **Infants/children: IV:** In cycles 1 and 7: CARBOplatin 560 mg/m² on day 1 (18 mg/kg/day in children <12 kg) plus etoposide 120 mg/m²/day IV on days 1, 2, 3 (4 mg/kg/day in children <12 kg). Cycles 2 and 6: CARRBOplatin 560 mg/m² on day 1 (18 mg/kg/day <12 kg) plus cyclophosphamide 1000 mg/m² IV on day 1 (33 mg/kg/day in children <12 kg) and DOXOrubicin 30 mg/m² IV on day 1 (1 mg/kg/day in children <12 kg). Cycles 3 and 5: Cyclophosphamide 1000 mg/m² IV on day 1 (33 mg/kg/day in children <12 kg) plus etoposide 120 mg/m²/day IV on days 1, 2, 3 (4 mg/kg/day in children <12 kg). Cycle 4: CARBOplatin 560 mg/m² IV on day 1 (18 mg/kg/day in children <12 kg) plus etoposide 120 mg/m²/day IV on days 1, 2, 3 (4 mg/kg/day in children <12 kg) and DOXOrubicin 30 mg/m² IV on day 1 (1 mg/kg/day in children <12 kg). Cycle 8: Cyclophosphamide 1000 mg/m² IV on day 1 (33 mg/kg/day in children <12 kg) plus DOXOrubicin 30 mg/m² IV on day 1 (1 mg/kg/day in children <12 kg). All cycles given at 3-wk intervals. Patients given an additional 4 cycles. Patients with unfavorable biologic features received 8 cycles
Renal dose
Adult: (single agent) **IV INF** CCr 41-59 mL/min 250 mg/m²; CCr 16-40 mL/min 200 mg mg/m²; do not use if CCr <15 mL/min
Available forms: Solution for injection 10 mg/mL (50 mg/5 mL, 150 mg/15 mL, 450 mg/45 mL, 600 mg/60 mL)
Administer:

Black Box Warning: Give antiemetic 30-60 min prior to product and prn for vomiting

IV route
• Do not use needles or IV administration sets that contain aluminum;

may cause precipitate or loss of potency

• Use cytotoxic handling procedures

• Store protected from light at room temperature; reconstituted vials stable for 24 hr at room temperature, solutions further diluted in D₅W or NS are stable for 8 hr at room temperature. Paraplatin multidose (10 mg/mL) vials stable for up to 14 days after entry into vial

• **Reconstitute** CARBOplatin 50, 150, or 450 mg with 5, 15, or 45 mL, respectively, of sterile water for injection, D₅W, or NaCl (10 mg/mL); then further **dilute** with the same solution to 0.5-4 mg/mL; **give** over 15 min-1 hr (intermittent INFUSION)

• **Continuous IV INFUSION** give over 24 hr; max dose based on (GFR = 125 mg/mL)

Solution compatibilities: D₅/0.2% NaCl, D₅/0.45% NaCl, D₅/0.9% NaCl, 0.9% NaCl, D₅W, sterile water for injection

Y-site compatibilities: Acyclovir, alfentanil, allopurinol, amifostine, amikacin, aminocaproic acid, aminophylline, amiodarone, amphotericin B lipid complex, amphotericin B liposome, ampicillin, ampicillin-sulbactam, anidulafungin, atenolol, atracurium, azithromycin, aztreonam, bivalirudin, bleomycin, bumetanide, buprenorphine, butorphanol, calcium chloride/gluconate, caspofungin, ceFAZolin, cefepime, cefotaxime, cefoTEtan, cefOXitin, cefTAZidime, ceftizoxime, cefTRIAXone, cefuroxime, cimetidine, ciprofloxacin, cisatracurium, CISplatin, cladribine, clindamycin, codeine, cyclophosphamide, cycloSPORINE, cytarabine, DAPTOmycin, DAUNOrubicin, dexamethasone, dexmedetomidine, dexrazoxane, digoxin, diltiaZEM, diphenhydrAMINE, DOBUTamine, DOCEtaxel, DOPamine, doripenem, doxacurium, DOXOrubicin, DOXOrubicin liposomal, doxycycline, droperidol, enalaprilat, ePHEDrine, EPINEPHrine, epiRUBicin, ertapenem, erythromycin, esmolol, etoposide, famotidine, fenoldopam, fentaNYL, filgrastim, fluconazole, fludarabine, fluorouracil, foscarnet, fosphenytoin, furosemide, ganciclovir, gatifloxacin, gemcitabine, gentamicin, granisetron, haloperidol, heparin, hydrocortisone, HYDROmorphone, hydrOXYzine, IDArubicin, ifosfamide, imipenem-cilastatin, inamrinone, insulin (regular), irinotecan, isoproterenol, ketorolac, labetalol, levoFLOXacin, levorphanol, lidocaine, linezolid injection, LORazepam, magnesium sulfate, mannitol, melphalan, meperidine, meropenem, mesna, methohexital, methotrexate, methylPREDNISolone, metoclopramide, metoprolol, metroNIDAZOLE, micafungin, midazolam, milrinone, minocycline, mitoXANTRONE, mivacurium, morphine, nafcillin, nalbuphine, naloxone, nesiritide, niCARdipine, nitroglycerin, nitroprusside, norepinephrine, octreotide, ofloxacin, ondansetron, oxaliplatin, PACLitaxel, palonosetron, pamidronate, pancuronium, pantoprazole, PEMEtrexed, pentamidine, PENTobarbital, PHENobarbital, phenylephrine, piperacillin, piperacillin-tazobactam, potassium chloride, potassium phosphates, prochlorperazine, promethazine, propofol, propranolol, raNITIdine, remifentanil, riTUXimab, rocuronium, sargramostim, sodium acetate, sodium bicarbonate, sodium phosphates, succinylcholine, SUFentanil, sulfamethoxazole-trimethoprim, tacrolimus, teniposide, theophylline, thiotepa, ticarcillin, ticarcillin-clavulanate, tigecycline, tirofiban, TNA, tobramycin, topotecan, TPN, trastuzumab, trimethobenzamide, vancomycin, vasopressin, vecuronium, verapamil, vinBLAStine, vinCRIStine, vinorelbine, voriconazole, zidovudine

SIDE EFFECTS

CNS: Central neurotoxicity, *peripheral neuropathy,* dizziness, confusion

CV: Cardiac abnormalities (fatal CV events), stroke, HF, embolism

EENT: Tinnitus, hearing loss

GU: Nephrotoxicity

GI: *Severe nausea, vomiting,* diarrhea, weight loss, mucositis, anorexia, constipation, taste change

HEMA: Thrombocytopenia, leukopenia, neutropenia, anemia
INTEG: Dermatitis, rash
META: Hypomagnesemia, hypocalcemia, hypokalemia, hyponatremia, hyperuricemia
SYST: Anaphylaxis, hypersensitivity

PHARMACOKINETICS
Initial half-life 2-6 hr, postdistribution half-life 2½-6 hr, not bound to plasma proteins, excreted by the kidneys

INTERACTIONS
• Do not use with or within 3 mo of live virus vaccines
Increase: nephrotoxicity or ototoxicity—aminoglycosides, amphotericin B
Increase: toxicity—radiation, bone marrow suppressants; monitor for blood counts often
Increase: myelosuppression—myelosuppressives
Decrease: phenytoin levels; monitor levels
Drug/Lab Test
Increase: AST, BUN, alkaline phosphatase, bilirubin, creatinine
Decrease: platelets, neutrophils, WBC, RBC, HB/Hct, calcium, potassium, magnesium, phosphate

NURSING CONSIDERATIONS
Assess:

Black Box Warning: To be used only in a specialized care setting by a person experienced in the use of chemotherapeutic products

Black Box Warning: Bone marrow depression: CBC, differential, platelet count weekly; withhold product if neutrophil count is <2000/mm³ or platelet count is <100,000/mm³; notify prescriber of results; calcium, magnesium, phosphate, potassium, sodium, uric acid, CCr, bilirubin; CCr <60 mL/min may be responsible for increased bone marrow suppression; assess frequently for infection and treat active infection before use

Black Box Warning: Nausea/vomiting: may occur a few hours after administration; antiemetics are used; give fluids, food as tolerated

• **Vitals:** B/P, pulse, respiration often during infusion
• **Bleeding:** Avoid IM injections, shaving with razor if platelets <50,000/mm³
• **Renal studies:** BUN, creatinine, serum uric acid; urine CCr prior to, during therapy; I&O ratio; report fall in urine output to <30 mL/hr
• Hepatic studies prior to, during therapy (bilirubin, AST, ALT, LDH) as needed or monthly; jaundice of skin, sclera; dark urine, clay-colored stools, itchy skin, abdominal pain, fever, diarrhea

Black Box Warning: Anaphylaxis: hypotension, rash, pruritus, wheezing, tachycardia may occur within a few minutes of use; notify prescriber after discontinuing; resuscitation equipment, corticosteroids, EPINEPHrine should be available

• **Peripheral neuropathy:** may be increased in geriatric patients
• **Beers:** use with caution in older adults; may exacerbate or cause syndrome of inappropriate antidiuretic hormone secretion or hyponatremia
Evaluate:
• Therapeutic response: decreasing size of tumor, spread of malignancy
Teach patient/family:
• To report ringing/roaring in the ears; numbness, tingling in face, extremities; weight gain
• **Pregnancy/breastfeeding:** that impotence or amenorrhea can occur; that this is reversible after treatment is discontinued; to notify prescriber if pregnancy is suspected or planned; that contraception should be used if patient is of child-bearing potential; not to breastfeed during treatment
• To avoid OTC products with aspirin, NSAIDs, alcohol; not to receive live virus vaccines during treatment or for 3 mo after completion of treatment
• To notify prescriber immediately of fever, fatigue, sore throat, bleeding, bruising, chills, back pain, dyspnea,

tingling in extremities, blood in stools, urine, emesis
• To avoid crowds, persons with known infections; to avoid the use of razors, stiff-bristle toothbrushes

---

⚠ HIGH ALERT

carfilzomib (Rx)

(car-fil'zoe-mib)

Kyprolis

Func. class.: Antineoplastic biologic response modifier

Chem. class.: Signal transduction inhibitor (STI)

ACTION: Antiproliferative and pro-apoptotic activity

USES: Multiple myeloma in those who have received ≥2 therapies (including bortezomib and immunomodulatory agents)

CONTRAINDICATIONS
Pregnancy, hypersensitivity

DOSAGE AND ROUTES
• **Adult: IV** 20 mg/m^2 over 2-10 min on days 1, 2, 8, 9, 15, 16, then 12-day rest (days 17-28), then may increase to 27 mg/m^2 on days 1, 2, 8, 9, 15, 16 repeated every 28 days
• Refer to package insert for dosage adjustments for treatment-related toxicity

Available forms: Powder for injection 10, 30, 60 mg in single-dose vials

---

cariprazine (Rx)

(kar-ip'ra-zeen)

Vraylar

Func. class.: Antipsychotic, atypical

Do not confuse:
Vraylar/Valchlor

ACTION: May act on central dopamine and serotonin receptors

USES: Schizophrenia, manic or mixed episodes with bipolar I, unipolar depressive disorder, depressive episodes in bipolar I disorder

CONTRAINDICATIONS
Hypersensitivity, pregnancy

Precautions: Breastfeeding, orthostatic hypotension, opioids, tardive dyskinesia, seizures, CV disease, leukopenia, neutropenia, children, severe hepatic/renal disease

Black Box Warning: Children, dementia-related psychosis, suicidal ideation

DOSAGE AND ROUTES
Schizophrenia
• **Adult: PO** 1.5 mg on day 1, then may increase to 3 mg daily on day 2, may increase by either 1.5 mg or 3 mg to a max 6 mg daily
Unipolar, augmentation of antidepressant (unlabeled)
• **Adult: PO** 1.5 mg once daily, initially. May increase to 3 mg PO once daily on day 15 based on response/tolerability. Max: 3 mg/day
Depressive episodes in bipolar I disorder
• **Adult:** 1.5 mg daily, then may increase to 3 mg daily on day 15, max 3 mg/day
Adult: PO starting a strong CYP3A4 inhibitor while on a stable dose of this drug: Reduce the current dose of this drug by 50%; **initiating this drug while receiving a strong CYP3A4 inhibitor:** 1.5 mg daily on days 1 and 3, with no dose given on day 2; starting on day 4, 1.5 mg daily, max 3 mg/day; **withdrawing a strong CYP3A4 inhibitor while on this drug:** May need dose increase
Available forms: Capsules 1.5 mg, 3 mg, 4.5 mg, 6 mg
Administer
• Protect from light (3 mg and 4.5 mg)
• May give without regard to meals

SIDE EFFECTS
CNS: EPS, headache, fatigue, fever, dizziness, agitation, insomnia, restlessness, suicidal thoughts/behaviors
CV: Hypertension, tachycardia

GI: Nausea, vomiting, constipation, diarrhea, dry mouth, abdominal pain, weight gain, anorexia
GU: UTI
EENT: Blurred vision, dental pain, nasopharyngitis
MS: Back pain, arthralgia
INTEG: Rash, pruritus, urticaria, SJS, NMS
RESP: Cough

PHARMACOKINETICS
Onset unknown, peak 3-6 hr, duration unknown, half-life 48-96 hr, 1 day to 21 days metabolite

INTERACTIONS
Increase: CNS depression: CNS depressants, opioids
Increase: cariprazine effect: CYP3A4 inhibitors
Decrease: effect of cariprazine: dopamine agonists
Increase or decrease: cariprazine effect: CYP3A4 inducers
Drug/Herb
Increase: cariprazine side effects: kava kava
Decrease: cariprazine effect: St. John's wort
Drug/Food
Increase: cariprazine effect: grapefruit juice, avoid using together
Drug/Lab
Increase: LFTs, CK
Decrease: WBC

NURSING CONSIDERATIONS
Assess:
• **Vitals:** monitor B/P, pulse, respirations, check for orthostatic hypotension
• **Mental status:** assess mood, LOC, behavior, orientation, suicidal thoughts/behaviors, hallucinations, delusions
• **Hypersensitivity:** monitor for rash; pruritis; urticaria; edema of face, tongue, lips, throat; trouble breathing; if these occur, stop medication and contact emergency services
• **NMS:** elevated CK, hyperpyrexia, rigidity, delirium, renal failure, rhabdomyolysis, provide immediate medical intervention
• **Seizures:** monitor for seizures in those with underlying seizure disorders
• **EPS:** monitor for tardive dystonia (males), tardive dyskinesia (elderly females), may need to be discontinued, assess for involuntary movements

• **Blood studies:** monitor lipids, triglycerides, blood glucose, A1c, CBC, serum creatinine, pregnancy test, serum electrolytes, serum prolactin, thyroid function tests baseline and periodically
• **Hyperpyrexia:** monitor for overheating, dehydration, strenuous exercise
• **Pregnancy/breastfeeding:** Do not use in pregnancy, if pregnant, enroll in the National Registry for Atypical Antipsychotics (866-961-2388), effects in breastfeeding are unknown

Black Box Warning: **Suicidal ideation:** monitor for thoughts, behaviors in young adults, adolescents, and children

Black Box Warning: **Dementia-related psychosis:** do not use in these patients

Evaluate:
• Therapeutic response: decrease in symptoms of schizophrenia, depression, bipolar disorder
Teach patient/family:
• The need for continued follow-up
• To report hypersensitivity including rash, itching
• To avoid overheating, dehydration, strenuous exercise, make sure enough fluid is taken
• The signs of EPS and when to notify the provider
• To notify the provider of the signs of NMS, if seizures occur
• To rise slowly from lying or sitting to minimize orthostatic hypotension
• To notify provider if pregnancy is planned or suspected or if breastfeeding
• To avoid using with grapefruit juice
• To avoid driving or other hazardous tasks until results are known
• To discuss all OTC/Rx/herbs/supplements used with prescriber

Black Box Warning: Discuss the risks of taking opioids with benzodiazepines, to seek emergency services for severe sleepiness, stupor, slow breathing, or coma

---

Side effects: *italics* = common; red = life-threatening

carisoprodol (Rx)

(kar-eye-soe-proe'dole)

Soma

Func. class.: Skeletal muscle relaxant, central acting

Chem. class.: Meprobamate congener

Controlled Substance Schedule IV

Do not confuse:
Soma/Soma Compound

ACTION: Depresses CNS by blocking interneuronal activity in descending reticular formation, spinal cord, thereby producing sedation and possibly altering pain perception

USES: Relieving pain, stiffness with musculoskeletal disorders

CONTRAINDICATIONS

Hypersensitivity to these products or carbamates, intermittent porphyria
Precautions: Pregnancy, breastfeeding, geriatric patients, Asian patients, renal/hepatic disease, substance abuse, seizure disorder, CNS depression, abrupt discontinuation

DOSAGE AND ROUTES

• **Adult/adolescent ≥16 yr: PO** 250-350 mg qid, max 3 wk of use
Available forms: Tablets 250, 350 mg
Administer:
• With meals for GI symptoms
• For short term (2-3 wk), potential for habituation
• Store in tight container at room temperature

SIDE EFFECTS

CNS: *Dizziness, weakness, drowsiness,* headache, insomnia, irritability
CV: Postural hypotension, tachycardia
GI: *Nausea,* vomiting, hiccups, epigastric discomfort
HEMA: Eosinophilia, leukopenia
INTEG: Rash, facial flushing, erythema multiforme
RESP: Asthmatic attacks
SYST: Angioedema, anaphylaxis

PHARMACOKINETICS

PO: Onset ½ hr; peak 4 hr; duration 4-6 hr; extensively metabolized by liver, substrate of CYP2C19, some Asians, Blacks, Whites are poor metabolizers; excreted in urine; crosses placenta; excreted in breast milk (large amounts); half-life 8 hr

INTERACTIONS

• Do not use together with meprobamate
Increase: CNS depression—alcohol, tricyclics, barbiturates, sedatives, hypnotics; avoid concurrent use
Increase: CNS depression, addiction: opiates
Increase: carisoprodol metabolite, decreasing carisoprodol effect—CYP2C19 inhibitors (FLUoxetine, fluvoxaMINE, isoniazid, modafinil)
Decrease: carisoprodol metabolism, increasing carisoprodol effect—CYP219 inducers (rifAMPin)
Drug/Herb
Increase: CNS depression—kava, valerian
Increase: metabolism of carisoprodol—St. John's wort
Drug/Lab Test
Increase: eosinophils
Increase: RBC, WBC, platelets

NURSING CONSIDERATIONS
Assess:
• **Pain,** stiffness, mobility, activities of daily living at baseline and throughout treatment
• **Idiosyncratic reaction:** (weakness, dizziness, blurred vision, confusion, euphoria), anaphylaxis within a few minutes or hours of first to fourth dose, withhold and notify prescriber, usually seen in poor CYP2C19 metabolizers
• **Allergic reactions:** rash, fever, respiratory distress, anaphylaxis, angioedema
• **CNS depression:** dizziness, drowsiness, psychiatric symptoms, abuse potential
• **Abrupt discontinuation:** withdrawal reactions do occur but may be mild, dependence may occur
• **Beers:** avoid in older adults; may cause sedation, anticholinergic effects; may decrease urinary flow, cause retention (men)

Evaluate:
• Therapeutic response: decreased pain, spasticity; increased ROM

Teach patient/family:
• There is a high incidence of dependence when using this product
• To avoid hazardous activities if drowsiness, dizziness occur; not to drive while taking product; to avoid rapid position changes, postural hypotension occurs, not to use for >2-3 wk
• To avoid using OTC medications (cough preparations, antihistamines) unless directed by prescriber; not to take with alcohol, other CNS depressants; that there is a high incidence of dependence when using this product
• **Idiosyncratic reaction:** to report weakness, dizziness, blurred vision, confusion, euphoria; if these occur, to withhold product and call prescriber
• **To report allergic reaction immediately:** rash, swelling of tongue/lips, hives, dyspnea
• To take with food or milk for GI symptoms
• Do not take with opiates with CNS depressants, benzodiazepine, alcohol
• **Pregnancy/breastfeeding:** If pregnancy is planned or suspected or if breastfeeding

TREATMENT OF OVERDOSE:
Dialysis, lavage

⚠ HIGH ALERT

carmustine (Rx)
(kar-mus′teen)
BiCNU, Gliadel
Func. class.: Antineoplastic alkylating agent
Chem. class.: Nitrosourea

ACTION: Alkylates DNA, RNA; able to inhibit enzymes that allow for the synthesis of amino acids in proteins; activity is not cell-cycle–phase specific

USES: Brain tumors such as glioblastoma, medulloblastoma, brainstem glioma, astrocytoma, ependymoma, metastatic brain tumors; multiple myeloma (with predniSONE), non-Hodgkin's disease, Hodgkin's disease, other lymphomas; GI, breast, bronchogenic, renal carcinomas; wafer, as adjunct to surgery/radiation for patients newly diagnosed with high-grade malignant glioma

Unlabeled uses: Ablation, mycosis fungoides, stem cell transplant preparation

CONTRAINDICATIONS
Pregnancy, breastfeeding, hypersensitivity, leukopenia, thrombocytopenia

Precautions: Dental disease, extravasation, females, infection, secondary malignancy, thrombocytopenia, renal disease

Black Box Warning: Bone marrow suppression, pulmonary fibrosis, bleeding, infection

DOSAGE AND ROUTES
• **Adult: IV** 75-100 mg/m² over 1-2 hr × 2 days or 150-200 mg/m² × 1 dose q6-8wk or 40-75 mg/m²/day × 5 days q6wk **INTRACAVITARY** up to 8 wafers inserted into resection cavity

Nadir dose
• **Adult: IV** Reduce dose by 30% (WBC nadir) 2000-3000 mm³ (platelet nadir) 25,000-75,000 mm³; reduce dose by 50% (WBC nadir) <2000 mm³ (platelet nadir) <25,000 mm³

Stem cell transplant/bone marrow ablation (unlabeled)
• **Adult: IV** 450-600 mg/m² as a single dose or 2 divided doses q12hr at a rate of no more than 3 mg/m²/min

Available forms: Powder for injection 100 mg; wafer 7.7 mg (intracavitary)

Administer:
• Store reconstituted solution in refrigerator for 24 hr or at room temperature for 8 hr; protect from light
• Blood transfusions, RBC colony-stimulating factors to counter anemia
• Antiemetic, serotonin antagonists, dexamethasone

• All medications PO, if possible; avoid IM injection if platelets are <100,000/mm^3

Black Box Warning: Carmustine should not be given at full dose until platelets >100,000/mm^3 and WBC >4000/mm^2

Wafer route
• Use cytotoxic handling procedures
• If wafers are broken into several pieces, they should not be used
• Foil pouches may be kept at room temperature for 6 hr if unopened

Intermittent IV INFUSION route
• Use cytotoxic handling procedures; do not use if an oil film appears on vial (decomposition), use gloves
• Do not use with PVC IV tubing, do not admix
• After **diluting** 100 mg product/3 mL ethyl alcohol (provided); dilute with 27 mL of sterile water for injection; then, **further dilute** with 100-500 mL 0.9% NaCl or D$_5$W, **give** 250 mL over ≥2 min, reduce rate if discomfort is felt; use only glass containers, protect from light
• **Flush** IV line after carmustine with 10 mL 0.9% NaCl to prevent irritation at site

Y-site compatibilities: Amifostine, amphotericin B lipid complex, amphotericin B liposome, anidulafungin, aztreonam, bivalirudin, bleomycin, caspofungin, cefepime, codeine, DAPTOmycin, dexmedetomidine, DOCEtaxel, ertapenem, etoposide, fenoldopam, filgrastim, fludarabine, gemcitabine, granisetron, levoFLOXacin, melphalan, meperidine, mitoXANTRONE, nesiritide, octreotide, ondansetron, PACLitaxel, palonosetron, pamidronate, pantoprazole, PEMEtrexed, piperacillin-tazobactam, riTUXimab, sargramostim, sodium acetate, tacrolimus, teniposide, thiotepa, tigecycline, tirofiban, trastuzumab, vinCRIStine, vinorelbine, voriconazole

SIDE EFFECTS
GI: *Nausea, vomiting, anorexia, stomatitis,* hepatotoxicity
GU: *Azotemia,* renal failure
HEMA: Thrombocytopenia, leukopenia, myelosuppression, anemia

INTEG: Pain, burning, hyperpigmentation at injection site, alopecia
RESP: Fibrosis, pulmonary infiltrate
SYST: Secondary malignant neoplastic disease

PHARMACOKINETICS
Degraded within 15 min; crosses blood-brain barrier; 70% excreted in urine within 96 hr; 10% excreted as CO_2, fate of 20% is unknown

INTERACTIONS
Increase: bleeding risk—aspirin, anticoagulants, platelet inhibitors
Increase: myelosuppression—myelosuppressive agents, cimetidine
Increase: toxicity—other antineoplastics, radiation, cimetidine
Increase: adverse reactions, decreased antibody reaction—live vaccines
Decrease: effects of digoxin, phenytoins
Drug/Lab Test
Increase: bilirubin, prolactin, uric acid, LFTs
Decrease: platelets, WBC, neutrophils, Hct

NURSING CONSIDERATIONS
Assess:

Black Box Warning: Bone marrow suppression: CBC, differential, platelet count weekly; withhold product if WBC is <4000 or platelet count is <100,000; notify prescriber of results, a lower dose may be needed

• Hepatic studies: AST, ALT, bilirubin; monitor regularly; hepatotoxicity occurs rarely
• **Pregnancy/breastfeeding:** identify if pregnancy is planned or suspected, or if breastfeeding; do not use in pregnancy, breastfeeding; contraception should be used

Black Box Warning: Pulmonary fibrosis/infiltrate: pulmonary function tests; chest x-ray films before, during therapy; chest film q2wk during treatment; monitor for dyspnea, cough, pulmonary fibrosis; infiltrate occurs after high doses or several low-dose courses (>1400 mg/m^2 cumulative dose), may occur months or years after treatment

Black Box Warning: Only to be used by an experienced clinician in cases of cancer, immune suppression

• Renal studies: BUN, serum uric acid; urine CCr before, during therapy; I&O ratio; report fall in urine output of 30 mL/hr, may use allopurinol for hyperuricemia with increased fluids
• Monitor for cold, cough, fever (may indicate beginning infection)
• **Bleeding:** hematuria, guaiac, bruising, petechiae, mucosa, orifices q8hr
• Rinsing of mouth tid-qid with water or club soda; use of sponge brush for stomatitis
• Warm compresses at injection site for inflammation; reduce flow rate if patient complains of burning at infusion site
Evaluate:
• Therapeutic response: decreasing size of tumor, spread of malignancy
Teach patient/family:

Black Box Warning: To report any changes in breathing or coughing; to avoid smoking

• To avoid foods with citric acid, hot temperature, or rough texture if stomatitis is present; to report any bleeding, white spots, ulceration in mouth to prescriber; to examine mouth daily
• To avoid aspirin, ibuprofen, razors, commercial mouthwash
• To report signs of anemia (fatigue, irritability, shortness of breath, faintness); to report signs of infection (sore throat, fever); pulmonary toxicity can occur up to 15 yr after treatment
• Not to receive live vaccines during treatment
• That infusion can be painful to veins and that product contains ethanol
• To report chest pain
• **Pregnancy/breastfeeding:** to use contraception during treatment; not to breastfeed, discuss product impairing fertility

carteolol (ophthalmic) (Rx)

(kar′tee-oh-lol)
Func. class.: Antiglaucoma, beta-blocker

USES: Treatment of chronic open-angle glaucoma and ocular hypertension

CONTRAINDICATIONS
Hypersensitivity, AV block, heart failure, bradycardia, sick sinus syndrome
Precautions: Abrupt discontinuation, children, pregnancy, breastfeeding, COPD, depression, diabetes mellitus, myasthenia gravis, hyperthyroidism, pulmonary disease, angle-closure glaucoma

DOSAGE AND ROUTES
• **Adult:** Instill 1 drop in the affected eye(s) bid
Available forms: Opthalmic solution 1%

▲ HIGH ALERT

carvedilol (Rx)

(kar-ved′i-lole)
Coreg, Coreg CR
Func. class.: Antihypertensive, alpha-/beta-adrenergic blocker

Do not confuse:
carvedilol/captopril

ACTION: A mixture of nonselective alpha-/beta-adrenergic blocking activity; decreases cardiac output, exercise-induced tachycardia, reflex orthostatic tachycardia; causes vasodilation, reduction in peripheral vascular resistance

USES: Essential hypertension alone or in combination with other antihypertensives, HF, LV dysfunction after MI, cardiomyopathy
Unlabeled uses: Angina, pediatric patients, atrial fibrillation/flutter

CONTRAINDICATIONS

Hyper-sensitivity, asthma, class IV decompensated cardiac failure, second- or third-degree heart block, cardiogenic shock, severe bradycardia, pulmonary edema, severe hepatic disease, sick sinus symptoms

Precautions: Pregnancy, breastfeeding, children, geriatric patients, cardiac failure, hepatic injury, peripheral vascular disease, anesthesia, major surgery, diabetes mellitus, thyrotoxicosis, emphysema, chronic bronchitis, renal disease, abrupt discontinuation

DOSAGE AND ROUTES
Hypertension
- **Adult: PO** 6.25 mg bid × 7-14 days; may increase to 25 mg bid; max 50 mg/day; **EXTENDED RELEASE** capsule 20 mg/day, may double after 7-14 days to 40 mg/day, max 80 mg/day

Heart failure
- **Adult: PO** 3.125 mg bid × 2 wk; may increase to give 6.25 mg bid × 2 wk, then double q2wk to max dose of 25 mg bid <85 kg or 50 mg bid >85 kg; **EXTENDED RELEASE** capsules (Coreg CR) 10 mg/day × 2 wk, increase to 20, 40, 80 mg/day over successive intervals of 2 wk

Postmyocardial infarction
Left ventricular dysfunction
- **Adult: PO** 6.25 mg bid × 2 wk; titrate upward as tolerated q2wk; may increase to 12.5 mg bid, then titrate to 25 mg bid; **PO EXTENDED RELEASE** 20 mg daily; titrate upward after 3-10 days, increase to 40 mg daily; max 80 mg/day

Available forms: Tablets 3.125, 6.25, 12.5, 25 mg; extended-release capsule 10, 20, 40, 80 mg

Administer:
- With food to minimize orthostatic hypotension; regular tablets may be crushed or swallowed whole; give extended release every AM with food; do not break, crush, chew extended-release capsule; separate alcohol (including OTC products that contain ethanol) by ≥2 hr; capsules may be opened and sprinkled over applesauce
- Take apical pulse before use; notify prescriber if <50 bpm and hold dose
- Use extended-release product in the morning
- Conversion from immediate release to extended release: 3.125 mg bid is 10 mg daily; 6.25 mg bid is 20 mg daily; 12.5 mg bid is 40 mg daily; 25 mg bid is 80 mg daily
- Do not discontinue before surgery

SIDE EFFECTS

CNS: *Dizziness, fatigue, weakness,* somnolence, insomnia, ataxia, drowsiness, memory loss, paresthesia, vertigo, depression
CV: Bradycardia, *postural hypotension,* HF, pulmonary edema
GI: *Diarrhea,* abdominal pain, constipation, nausea, vomiting
GU: Decreased libido, *impotence*
INTEG: Rash, Stevens-Johnson syndrome, toxic epidermal necrolysis
MISC: Pruritus, *hyperglycemia,* weight gain, anaphylaxis, angioedema, lupus-like syndrome
RESP: Dyspnea, bronchospasm
EENT: Blurred vision, floppy iris syndrome, dry eyes

PHARMACOKINETICS

Peak 1-2 hr; duration 7-9 hr; extended release onset 30 min, peak 5 hr, readily and extensively absorbed PO; >98% protein binding; extensively metabolized (CYP2D6, CYP2C9) by liver; excreted through bile into feces; half-life 7-10 hr with increases in geriatric patients, hepatic disease; some individuals may be poor metabolizers

INTERACTIONS

Increase: conduction disturbances—calcium channel blockers
Increase: carvedilol level—CYP2D6 inhibitors (FLUoxetine, quiNIDine)
Increase: bradycardia, hypotension—levodopa, MAOIs
Increase: hypoglycemia—antidiabetic agents, monitor blood glucose level, dosage of antidiabetics may need to be decreased
Increase: concentrations of digoxin, cycloSPORINE, CYP2D6 inhibitors (FLUoxetine, quiNIDine)
Increase: toxicity of carvedilol—cimetidine, other antihypertensives, nitrates, acute alcohol ingestion; monitor for toxicity

Anesthetics; general: increased myocardial depression

Decrease: heart rate, B/P—cloNIDine; monitor B/P, pulse frequently

Decrease: carvedilol levels—rifAMPin, NSAIDs, thyroid medications; monitor B/P

Drug/Herb

Increase: antihypertensive effect—hawthorn

Decrease: antihypertensive effect—ephedra (ma huang)

Drug/Lab Test

Increase: blood glucose, BUN, potassium, triglycerides, uric acid, bilirubin, cholesterol, creatinine, LFTs, ANA titer

Decrease: sodium, HDL

NURSING CONSIDERATIONS
Assess:

• **Hypertension:** B/P when beginning treatment, periodically thereafter; pulse: note rate, rhythm, quality; apical/radial pulse before administration; in those with lower heart rate (<55 bpm) dose may need to be lowered; notify prescriber of significant changes; identify orthostatic hypotension when patient rises

• **Heart failure:** edema in feet, legs daily; fluid overload: dyspnea, weight gain, jugular venous distention, fatigue, crackles, monitor I&O

Evaluate:

• Therapeutic response: decreased B/P with hypertension; decreased anginal pain

Teach patient/family:

• To comply with dosage schedule even if feeling better; that improvement may take several weeks; not to crush, chew capsules; to take extended-release product with food

• To rise slowly to sitting or standing position to minimize orthostatic hypotension

• To report slow pulse, dizziness, confusion, depression, fever, weight gain, SOB, cold extremities, rash, sore throat, bleeding, bruising

• To weigh, take pulse, B/P at home; to advise if weight gain of >2 lb/day or 5 lb/wk and when to notify prescriber

• Not to discontinue product abruptly; to taper over 1-2 wk; life-threatening dysrhythmias may occur

• To avoid hazardous activities until stabilized on medication; dizziness may occur

• To carry emergency ID with product name, prescriber information at all times

• To inform all health care providers of products, supplements taken; to avoid all OTC medications unless approved by prescriber

• Inform patient may be sensitive to cold

• That product may mask hypoglycemia, thyroid symptoms; if diabetic, check glucose carefully

• **Pregnancy/breastfeeding:** to notify provider if pregnancy is planned or suspected; to avoid breastfeeding

caspofungin (Rx)
(cas-po-fun′gin)

Cancidas

Func. class.: Antifungal, systemic

Chem. class.: Echinocandin

ACTION: Inhibits an essential component in fungal cell walls; causes direct damage to fungal cell wall

USES: Treatment of invasive aspergillosis and candidemia that has not responded to other treatment, including peritonitis, intraabdominal abscesses; susceptible species: *Aspergillus flavus, A. fumigatus, A. terreus, Candida albicans, C. glabrata, C. krusei, C. lusitaniae, C. parapsilosis, C. tropicalis,* esophageal candidiasis; empiric therapy for presumed fungal infection in febrile, neutropenic patients

Unlabeled uses: *Aspergillus niger,* fungal infections in premature neonates, neonates, infants, children <2 yr

CONTRAINDICATIONS
Hyper-sensitivity

Precautions: Pregnancy, breastfeeding, children, geriatric patients, severe hepatic disease

DOSAGE AND ROUTES
Invasive aspergillosis

• **Adult:** IV loading dose 70 mg on day 1, then 50 mg/day maintenance dose, depending on condition; max 70 mg/day; if receiving rifAMPin, carBAMazepine, dexamethasone, phenytoin, use 70 mg daily

- **Adolescent/child/infant ≥3 mo: IV INFUSION** 70 mg/m² loading dose, then 50 mg/m²/day; max 70 mg/day
- **Neonate and infant <3 mo (unlabeled): IV** 25 mg/m²/day

Esophageal candidiasis

- **Adult: IV** 70 mg loading dose then 50 mg × 14-21 days over 1 hr
- **Child 3 mo-17 yr:** IV 70 mg/m² loading dose over 1 hr, day 1, then 50 mg/m²/day

Hepatic dose

- **Adult: IV** (Child-Pugh 7-9, class B) loading dose 70 mg, then 35 mg/day
- **Child 3 mo-17 yr: IV** 70 mg/m² loading dose, then 50 mg/m² daily; max 70 mg/m²

Available forms: Powder for injection 50, 70 mg (single-use vials)

Administer:

- Do not mix or confuse with other medications; do not use dextrose-containing products to dilute; do not give as bolus

Intermittent IV INFUSION route

- Allow vial to warm to room temperature
- May administer loading dose on day 1
- **Reconstitute** 50-mg vial or 70-mg vial with 10.8 mL 0.9% NaCl, sterile water for injection, or bacteriostatic water for injection (5 mg/mL or [50-mg vial] 7 mg/mL [70-mg vial]), respectively; **swirl** to dissolve, withdraw 10 mL reconstituted solution, and **further dilute** with 250 mL 0.9% NaCl, 0.45% NaCl, 0.225% NaCl, LR, 50 mg dose/100 mL (volume restriction); **run** over 1 hr or more
- Store at room temperature for up to 24 hr or refrigerated for 48 hr; store reconstituted solution at room temperature for 1 hr before preparation of solution for administration
- **Incompatibilities:** Do not admix with dextrose products
- Monitor for injection site reactions

SIDE EFFECTS

CNS: Dizziness, *headache,* fever, chills
CV: Sinus tachycardia, hypertension
GI: Abdominal pain, *nausea, anorexia, vomiting, diarrhea, increased AST/ALT, alkaline phosphatase*
GU: Renal failure
HEMA: Thrombophlebitis, vasculitis, anemia
INTEG: *Rash, pruritus, injection site pain*
META: Hypokalemia
MS: Myalgia
RESP: Acute respiratory distress syndrome (ARDS), pleural effusions
SYST: Anaphylaxis, histamine-related reactions, Stevens-Johnson syndrome, toxic epidermal necrolysis, angioedema

PHARMACOKINETICS

Metabolized in liver to inactive metabolites; excretion in feces, urine; half-life 9-11 hr; protein binding 97%

INTERACTIONS

Increase: caspofungin levels, hepatic toxicity—cycloSPORINE; avoid concurrent use

Decrease: levels of tacrolimus, sirolimus
Decrease: caspofungin levels—carBAMazepine, dexamethasone, efavirenz, nelfinavir, nevirapine, phenytoin, rifAMPin; caspofungin dose may need to be increased

Drug/Lab Test

Increase: AST, ALT, RBC, eosinophils, glucose, bilirubin, alkaline phosphatase, serum creatinine
Decrease: Hct/HB, WBC, potassium, magnesium

NURSING CONSIDERATIONS

Assess:

- **Infection:** clearing of cultures during treatment; obtain culture at baseline, throughout treatment; product may be started as soon as culture is taken (esophageal candidiasis); monitor cultures during hematopoietic stem cell transplantation (HSCT) for prevention of *Candida* infections
- Blood studies prior to, during treatment: bilirubin, AST, ALT, alkaline phosphatase, as needed; obtain baseline renal studies; CBC with differential, serum potassium
- **Hypersensitivity:** rash, pruritus, facial swelling; also for phlebitis; anaphylaxis (rare)
- GI symptoms: frequency of stools, cramping; if severe diarrhea occurs, electrolytes may need to be given
- **Pregnancy/breastfeeding:** no well-controlled studies; use in pregnancy only if benefits outweigh fetal risk; excreted in breast milk, use cautiously in breastfeeding

Evaluate:

- Therapeutic response: decreased symptoms of *Candida, Aspergillus* infections

---

Teach patient/family:
• To inform prescriber of renal/hepatic disease
• To report bleeding, phlebitis, facial swelling, wheezing, difficulty breathing, itching, rash, hives, increasing warmth, flushing; anaphylaxis can occur
• **Pregnancy/breastfeeding:** to notify prescriber if pregnancy is suspected or planned; to use cautiously in breastfeeding

---

cefaclor
See cephalosporins—second generation
cefadroxil
See cephalosporins—first generation
ceFAZolin
See cephalosporins—first generation
cefdinir
See cephalosporins—third generation
cefditoren pivoxil
See cephalosporins—third generation
cefepime
See cephalosporins—third generation
cefixime
See cephalosporins—third generation
cefotaxime
See cephalosporins—third generation
cefoTEtan
See cephalosporins—second generation
cefOXitin
See cephalosporins—second generation
cefpodoxime
See cephalosporins—third generation
cefprozil
See cephalosporins—second generation
cefTAZidime
See cephalosporins—third generation
ceftibuten
See cephalosporins—third generation
ceftizoxime
See cephalosporins—third generation
cefTRIAXone
See cephalosporins—third generation
cefuroxime
See cephalosporins—second generation

---

ceftaroline (Rx)
(sef-tar′oh-leen)
Teflaro
Func. class.: Antiinfective-cephalosporin derivative (fifth generation)

C

USES: Acute bacterial skin/skin structure infections (ABSSI), bacterial community-acquired pneumonia

CONTRAINDICATIONS
Cephalosporin hypersensitivity
Precautions: Child/infant/neonate, breastfeeding, elderly patients, antimicrobial resistance, carbapenem/penicillin hypersensitivity, coagulopathy, colitis, dialysis, diarrhea, GI disease, hypoprothrombinemia, IBS, pregnancy, pseudomembranous colitis, renal disease, ulcerative colitis, viral infection, vitamin K deficiency

DOSAGE AND ROUTES
• **Adult: IV** 600 mg q12hr × 5-14 days (skin/skin-structure infections) or × 5-7 days (bacterial community-acquired pneumonia)
• **Child 2-17 yr and >33 kg: IV** 400 mg q8hr or 600 mg q12hr; **2-17 yr and <33 kg;** 12 mg/kg q8hr
• **Child 2 mo to <2 yr: IV** 8 mg/kg q8hr
Renal dose
• **Adult: IV** CCr >30-≤50 mL/min, 400 mg q12hr; CCr ≥15-≤30 mL/min, 300 mg q12hr; CCr <15 mL/min, 200 mg q12hr, includes hemodialysis

⚠ HIGH ALERT

celecoxib (Rx)
(sel-eh-cox′ib)
CeleBREX
Func. class.: Nonsteroidal antiinflammatory, antirheumatic
Chem. class.: COX-2 inhibitor

Combinations: Seglentis: celecoxib/traMADol 56 mg/44 mg

Do not confuse:
CeleBREX/CeleXA/Cerebyx

Side effects: *italics* = common; red = life-threatening

ACTION: Inhibits prostaglandin synthesis by selectively inhibiting cyclooxygenase-2 (COX-2), an enzyme needed for biosynthesis

USES: Acute, chronic rheumatoid arthritis, osteoarthritis, acute pain, primary dysmenorrhea, ankylosing spondylitis, juvenile rheumatoid arthritis (JRA); acute migraine (Elyxyb)

CONTRAINDICATIONS

Pregnancy; hypersensitivity to salicylates, iodides, other NSAIDs, sulfonamides; for perioperative pain in CABG

Precautions: Breastfeeding, children <18 yr, geriatric patients, bleeding, GI/renal/hepatic/cardiac disorders, PVD, hypertension, severe dehydration, asthma, sulfa allergy, peptic ulcer disease, MI, stroke

Black Box Warning: GI bleeding/perforation, thromboembolism

DOSAGE AND ROUTES
Acute pain/primary dysmenorrhea
• **Adult:** PO 400 mg initially, then 200 mg if needed on first day, then 200 mg bid as needed on subsequent days; start with ½ dose for poor CYP2C9 metabolizers
Osteoarthritis
• **Adult:** PO 200 mg/day as a single dose or 100 mg bid
Rheumatoid arthritis
• **Adult:** PO 100-200 mg bid; start with ½ dose for poor CYP2C9 metabolizers
Ankylosing spondylitis
• **Adult:** PO 200 mg/day or in divided doses (bid)
Juvenile rheumatoid arthritis (JRA)
• **Adolescent/child ≥2 yr (>25 kg):** PO 100 mg bid
• **Child ≥2 yr (10-25 kg):** PO 50 mg bid
Migraine
• **Adult:** PO 120 mg (4.8 mL)
Hepatic disease
• **Adult:** PO (Child-Pugh B) reduce dose by 50%; (Child-Pugh C) do not use
Available forms: Capsules 50, 100, 200, 400 mg; oral solution 25 mg/mL

Administer:
• Do not break, crush, chew, or dissolve capsules; give with a full glass of water to enhance absorption; capsules may be opened into applesauce or soft food, ingest immediately with water
• With food, milk to decrease gastric symptoms (with higher doses [400 mg bid]); do not increase dose

SIDE EFFECTS
CNS: *Fatigue, nervousness,* insomnia, headache
CV: Stroke, MI, HF, hypertension, fluid retention
GI: Nausea, anorexia, dry mouth, GI bleeding/ulceration
INTEG: Serious (sometimes fatal) Stevens-Johnson syndrome, toxic epidermal necrolysis, exfoliative dermatitis, rash

PHARMACOKINETICS
Well absorbed, crosses placenta, metabolized by CYP2C9 in liver, some patients may be poor metabolizers; very little excreted by kidneys/in feces, peak 3 hr, half-life 11 hr, protein binding ~97%

INTERACTIONS
Increase: bleeding risk—anticoagulants, SNRIs, SSRIs, antiplatelets, thrombolytics, salicylates, alcohol
Increase: adverse reactions—glucocorticoids, NSAIDs, aspirin
Increase: toxicity—lithium
Increase: celecoxib blood level—CYP2C9 inhibitors (fluconazole)
Decrease: effect of aspirin, ACE inhibitors, thiazide diuretics, furosemide
Drug/Lab Test
Increase: ALT, AST, BUN, cholesterol, glucose, potassium, sodium
Decrease: glucose, sodium, WBC, platelets

NURSING CONSIDERATIONS
Assess
• **Pain** of rheumatoid arthritis, osteoarthritis; check ROM, inflammation of joints, characteristics of pain, baseline and periodically

Black Box Warning: For cardiac disease that may be worse after taking product; MI, stroke; do not use with coronary artery bypass graft (CABG)

• CBC during therapy; watch for decreasing platelets; if low, therapy may need to be discontinued, restarted after hematologic recovery; LFTs, serum creatinine/BUN
• **For blood dyscrasias (thrombocytopenia):** bruising, fatigue, bleeding, poor healing

Black Box Warning: GI toxicity: black, tarry stools; abdominal pain; monitor stool guaiac

• **Serious skin disorders:** Stevens-Johnson syndrome, toxic epidermal necrolysis; may be fatal, treat symptomatically; may recur after therapy is discontinued; if severe, may require discontinuing
• **Beers:** Avoid use in older adults; may increase risk of kidney injury, exacerbate heart failure, increase fluid retention
Evaluate:
• Therapeutic response: decreased pain, inflammation in arthritic conditions; decreased number of polyps
Teach patient/family:

Black Box Warning: Not to exceed recommended dose; to notify prescriber immediately of chest pain, skin eruptions; to stop product if these occur

• To check with prescriber to determine when product should be discontinued before surgery
• That product must be continued for prescribed time to be effective; to avoid other NSAIDs, aspirin, sulfonamides

Black Box Warning: To notify prescriber immediately of GI symptoms: black, tarry stools; cramping or rash; edema of extremities; weight gain or hepatotoxicity: nausea; pruritus; yellowing skin, eyes; lethargy; itching, upper abdominal pain

• To report bleeding, bruising, fatigue, malaise because blood abnormalities do occur

• **Pregnancy/breastfeeding:** to report if pregnancy is planned or suspected; avoid use in breastfeeding; not to use during pregnancy, breastfeeding; those who are pregnant should register at the Organization of Teratology of Information Specialists Autoimmune Diseases in Pregnancy Study (877-311-8972)

⚠ HIGH ALERT

cemiplimab-rwlc (Rx)
(seh-mip'lih-mab)
Libtayo
Func. class.: Antineoplastic—monoclonal antibody
Chem. class.: Programmed death receptor-1 (PD-1)/PD-L1

ACTION: Binds to the programmed death receptor-1 (PD-1) found on T cells. Blocking the PD-1/PD-L1 pathway improves the antitumor immune response by reducing immunosuppressive signals

USES: Squamous cell skin carcinoma in patients who are not candidates for curative surgery/radiation

CONTRAINDICATIONS
Hypersensitivity, pregnancy, breastfeeding
Precautions: Adrenal insufficiency, autoimmune disease, colitis, contraception requirements, Crohn's disease, hepatitis, hyperthyroidism, immune-mediated reactions, infusion-related reactions, organ transplant, pneumonitis, pregnancy testing, renal impairment, reproductive risk, serious rash, type 1 diabetes mellitus, ulcerative colitis

DOSAGE AND ROUTES
• **Adult: IV** 350 mg over 30 min q3wk until disease progression
Available forms: Injection 350 mg/7 mL (50 mg/mL) single-dose vial
Administer
IV INFUSION route
• Visually inspect for particulate matter and discoloration before use; product is

clear to slightly opalescent, colorless to pale yellow and may contain trace amounts of translucent to white particles

• Do not shake vial

Dilution:

• Withdraw 7 mL and dilute with normal saline or D$_5$W (1 mg/mL to 20 mg/mL) mix by gentle inversion, do not shake

• Discard any unused portion

• **Storage:** Store unopened vial in refrigerator, protect from light, store at room temperature (up to 77° F [25° C]) for up to 8 hr or refrigerated (36° F-46° F [2° C-8° C]) for up to 24 hr from time of dilution. Do not freeze

• If refrigerated, allow to warm to room temperature

• Give diluted solution over 30 min through a sterile, in-line or add-on 0.2- to 0.5-micron filter

SIDE EFFECTS

CNS: Fatigue, asthenia

EENT: Immune-mediated optic nephritis

ENDO: Immune-mediated hypophysitis, immune-mediated hypothyroidism/hyperthyroidism, immune-mediated type 1 diabetes mellitus

GI: Anorexia, nausea, vomiting, abdominal pain, constipation, diarrhea, immune-mediated colitis, immune-mediated hepatitis

GU: Immune-mediated nephritis

HEMA: Anemia

INTEG: Rash, pruritus, infusion-related reactions

MS: Immune-mediated rhabdomyolysis, back pain, myalgia, MS pain

RESP: Immune-mediated pneumonitis

PHARMACOKINETICS

Onset, peak, duration unknown; half-life 19 days

INTERACTION

None known

NURSING CONSIDERATIONS

Assess:

• **Immune-mediated pneumonitis:** shortness of breath, chest pain, new or worsening cough periodically; if present, obtain x-ray; withhold until grade ≤1; usually treated with corticosteroids

• **Immune-mediated colitis:** severe diarrhea or abdominal pain, blood or mucus in stool. Therapy may need to be interrupted or discontinued based on severity; corticosteroids may be used; permanently discontinue if grade 4 toxicity

• **Immune-mediated hepatitis:** jaundice of skin/eyes, severe nausea/vomiting; obtain liver function tests prior to starting and periodically during therapy; if hepatitis occurs, therapy may need to be interrupted or discontinued based on severity of the toxicity; corticosteroids may be given

• **Infusion-related reactions:** fever, pruritus, wheezing, rigors; if severe grade 3 or 4, discontinue permanently

• **Immune-mediated dermatologic reactions:** erythema multiforme, Stevens-Johnson syndrome, toxic epidermal necrolysis have occurred with similar products; interrupt or discontinue in patients who develop severe skin toxicity; provide corticosteroids followed by a 1-mo taper, starting when the toxicity resolves to grade ≤1

• **Immune-mediated hypophysitis:** continual headache, weakness, fatigue, blurred vision, dizziness; provide corticosteroids for grade 2; if severe (grade 3), withhold or discontinue until toxicity resolves to grade ≤1; permanently discontinue for grade 4

• **Immune-mediated nephritis:** monitor serum creatinine and BUN baseline and periodically; corticosteroids may be used for grade ≥2 nephritis; withhold for grade 2, resume when recovery is grade ≤1; discontinue for grade 4

• Blood glucose baseline and periodically; may cause hyperglycemia

• Thyroid function test baseline and periodically; may cause hypo/hyperthyroidism; corticosteroids may be used for grade 3 hypothyroidism; withhold product for severe grade 3, permanently discontinue for grade 4

• **Pregnancy/breastfeeding:** product should not be used in pregnancy and for 4 mo after last dose or breastfeeding and for 4 mo after last dose; perform pregnancy test in all women of childbearing potential

Evaluate:
• Therapeutic response: decreased spread of skin cancer

Teach patient/family:
• That product treats a type of skin cancer by working with your immune system
• To notify prescriber immediately of new or worsening cough, shortness of breath, chest pain, diarrhea; stools that are black, tarry, sticky, or have blood or mucus; abdominal pain, yellowing of skin/eyes, severe nausea/vomiting, bleeding or bruising more easily, unusual headaches, rapid heartbeat, increased sweating, extreme tiredness, weight gain/weight loss, dizziness/fainting, feeling hungrier or thirstier than usual, hair loss, feeling cold, constipation, skin rash with blisters
• To inform health care provider of all Rx, OTC, vitamins, and herbal products taken and not to take others without prescriber's approval
• That blood work and regular exams will be needed throughout treatment
• **Pregnancy/breastfeeding:** to inform health care provider if pregnancy is planned or suspected. That product should not be used in pregnancy or breastfeeding. That a pregnancy test is required before treatment begins and that a nonhormonal form of contraception will be needed to prevent pregnancy during treatment and for 4 mo after treatment ends. Not to breastfeed during treatment or for 4 mo after last dose

cephalexin
See cephalosporins—first generation

CEPHALOSPORINS— FIRST GENERATION

cefadroxil (Rx)
(sef-a-drox′ill)
ceFAZolin (Rx)
(sef-a′zoe-lin)
cephalexin (Rx)
(sef-a-lex′in)
Keflex, Panixine ✦
Func. class.: Antiinfective
Chem. class.: Cephalosporin (first generation)

ACTION: Inhibits bacterial cell wall synthesis; renders cell wall osmotically unstable, leads to cell death; lysis mediated by cell wall autolytic enzymes

USES: cefadroxil: gram-negative bacilli: *Escherichia coli, Proteus mirabilis, Klebsiella* (UTI only); gram-positive organisms: *Streptococcus pneumoniae, Streptococcus pyogenes, Staphylococcus aureus;* upper, lower respiratory tract; urinary tract, skin infections; otitis media; tonsillitis; UTIs
ceFAZolin: gram-negative bacilli: *Haemophilus influenzae, Escherichia coli, Proteus mirabilis, Klebsiella pneumoniae;* gram-positive organisms: *Staphylococcus aureus/epidermidis;* upper, lower respiratory tract; urinary tract, skin infections; bone, joint, biliary, genital infections; endocarditis, surgical prophylaxis, septicemia; *Streptococcus* sp.
cephalexin: gram-negative bacilli: *Haemophilus influenzae, Escherichia coli, Proteus mirabilis, Klebsiella pneumoniae;* gram-positive organisms: *Streptococcus pneumoniae, Streptococcus pyogenes, Streptococcus agalactiae, Staphylococcus aureus;* upper, lower respiratory tract; urinary tract, skin, bone infections; otitis media

CONTRAINDICATIONS
Hypersensitivity to cephalosporins, infants <1 mo

Precautions: Pregnancy, breastfeeding, hypersensitivity to penicillins, renal disease

DOSAGE AND ROUTES
cefadroxil
UTI
• **Adult:** PO 1-2 g/day or divided q12hr; loading dose of 1 g initially
• **Child:** PO 30 mg/kg/day in divided doses bid, max 2 g/day
Catheter-related bloodstream infections
• **Adult:** IV 2 g q8h
Renal dose
• **Adult:** PO CCr 25-50 mL/min, 1 g, then 500 mg q12hr; CCr 10-24 mL/min, 1 g, then 500 mg q24hr; CCr <10 mL/min, 1 g, then 500 mg q36hr

Available forms: Capsules 500 mg; tablets 1 g; oral suspension 250, 500 mg/5 mL
ceFAZolin
Surgical prophylaxis
• **Adult:** IM/IV <120 kg 1-2 g; >120 kg 3 g 30-60 min before surgery, then 0.5-1 g q6-8hr × 24 hr. Cefazolin surgical prophylaxis dosing can be 1-2 gm if patient is <120 kg, recommended 3 gm if patient is 120 kg or more.
Life-threatening infections
• **Adult:** IM/IV 1-2 g q6-8hr; max 12 g/day
• **Child >1 mo:** IM/IV 75-100 mg/kg/day in 3-4 divided doses; max 6 g/day
Mild/moderate infections
• **Adult:** IM/IV 250 mg-1 g q8hr, max 12 g/day
• **Child >1 mo:** IM/IV 50 mg/kg in 3-4 equal doses, max 6 g/day, or 2 g as a single dose
Renal dose
• **Adult:** IM/IV after loading dose, CCr 35-54 mL/min, dose q8hr; CCr 10-34 mL/min, 50% of dose q12hr; CCr <10 mL/min, 50% of dose q18-24hr
• **Child:** IM/IV CCr >70 mL/min, no dosage adjustment; CCr 40-70 mL/min after loading dose, reduce dose to 7.5-30 mg/kg q12hr; CCr 20-39 mL/min, give 3.125-12.5 mg/kg after loading dose q12hr; CCr 5-19 mL/min, 2.5-10 mg/kg after loading dose q24hr

Available forms: Powder for injection 500 mg, 1, 10, 20 g/vial; premixed infusion 500 mg, 1 g/50 mL, 500 mg/50 mL vial

cephalexin
Moderate infections
• **Adult:** PO 250-500 mg q6hr, max 4 g/day
• **Child:** PO 25-100 mg/kg/day in 4 equal doses, max 4 g/day
Moderate skin infections
• **Adult:** PO 500 mg q12hr
Severe infections
• **Adult:** PO 500 mg-1 g q6hr, max 4 g
• **Child:** PO 50-100 mg/kg/day in 4 equal doses, max 4 g/day
Renal dose
• **Adult:** PO CCr 10-40 mL/min, 250-500 mg then 250-500 mg q8-12hr; CCr <10 mL/min, 250-500 mg, then 250 mg q12-24hr

Available forms: Capsules 250, 500, 750 mg; tablets 250, 500 mg; oral suspension 125, 250 mg/5 mL
Administer:
cefadroxil
• For prescribed time to ensure organism death, prevent superinfection
• With food if needed for GI symptoms
• Shake suspension, refrigerate, discard after 2 wk
• Identify allergies before use
• After C&S specimen is obtained

ceFAZolin
• Obtain C&S specimen before use
• Identify allergies before use
IV route
• Check for irritation, extravasation often; dilute in 2 mL/500 mg or 2.5 mL/1 g sterile water for injection, inject over 3-5 min; may be further diluted with 50-100 mL of NS, D_5W solution, run over 10 min-1 hr by Y-tube or 3-way stopcock
• After C&S completed

Y-site compatibilities: Acyclovir, alfentanil, allopurinol, alprostadil, amifostine, amikacin, aminocaproic acid, aminophylline, amphotericin B liposome, anidulafungin, ascorbic acid injection, atenolol, atracurium, atropine, aztreonam, benztropine, bivalirudin, bleomycin, bumetanide, buprenorphine, butorphanol, calcium gluconate, CARBOplatin, cefamandole, cefmetazole, cefonicid, cefoTEtan, cefOXitin, cefpirome, cefTAZidime, ceftizoxime, cefTRIAXone, cefuroxime, chloramphenicol, cimetidine, CISplatin, clindamycin, codeine, cyanocobalamin, cyclophosphamide, cycloSPORINE, cytarabine, DACTINomycin, DAPTOmycin, dexamethasone, dexmedetomidine, digoxin, diltiaZEM, DOCEtaxel, doxacurium, doxapram, DOXOrubicin liposomal, enalaprilat, ePHEDrine, EPINEPHrine, epirubicin, epoetin alfa, eptifibatide, esmolol, etoposide, fenoldopam, fentaNYL, filgrastim, fluconazole, fludarabine, fluorouracil, folic acid (as sodium salt), foscarnet, furosemide, gallium, gatifloxacin, gemcitabine, gentamicin, glycopyrrolate, granisetron, heparin, hydrocortisone, hydrOXYzine, IDArubicin, ifosfamide, imipenem-cilastatin, indomethacin, insulin (regular), irinotecan, isoproterenol, ketorolac, lidocaine, linezolid, LORazepam, LR's injection, mannitol, mechlorethamine, melphalan, meperidine, methotrexate, methyldopate, methylPREDNISolone, metoclopramide, metoprolol, metroNIDAZOLE, miconazole, midazolam, milrinone, morphine, moxalactam, multiple vitamins injection, nafcillin, nalbuphine, naloxone, nesiritide, niCARdipine, nitroglycerin, nitroprusside, norepinephrine, octreotide, ondansetron, oxacillin, oxaliplatin, oxytocin, PACLitaxel, palonosetron, pamidronate, pancuronium, pantoprazole, penicillin G potassium/sodium, peritoneal dialysis solution, perphenazine, PHENobarbital, phenylephrine, phytonadione, piperacillin, Plasma-Lyte M in dextrose 5%, polymyxin B, potassium chloride, procainamide, propofol, propranolol, raNITIdine, remifentanil, Ringer's injection, ritodrine, riTUXimab, sargramostim,

sodium acetate, sodium bicarbonate, succinylcholine, SUFentanil, tacrolimus, teniposide, tenoxicam, theophylline, thiamine, thiotepa, ticarcillin, ticarcillin-clavulanate, tigecycline, tirofiban, TNA, tolazoline, trastuzumab, trimetaphan, urokinase, vasopressin, vecuronium, verapamil, vinCRIStine, vitamin B complex with C, voriconazole, warfarin, zoledronic acid

cephalexin

• Shake suspension, refrigerate, discard after 2 wk; use calibrated oral syringe, spoon, or measuring cup
• With food if needed for GI symptoms
• After C&S specimen is obtained
• Identify allergies before use

SIDE EFFECTS

CNS: Headache, dizziness, weakness, paresthesia, fever, chills, confusion, fatigue, hallucinations, seizures (with high doses)
GI: Nausea, vomiting, *diarrhea, anorexia,* abdominal pain, *Clostridium difficile-associated diarrhea (CDAD)*
GU: Vaginitis, pruritus, candidiasis
HEMA: Thrombocytopenia, anemia, neutropenia, eosinophilia, hemolytic anemia
INTEG: Rash, urticaria, dermatitis, injection site reactions
SYST: Anaphylaxis, serum sickness, superinfection, Stevens-Johnson syndrome

PHARMACOKINETICS
cefadroxil: Peak 1-1½ hr, duration 12-24 hr, half-life 1-2 hr, 20% bound by plasma proteins, crosses placenta, excreted in breast milk
ceFAZolin
IV: Onset 10 min, peak infusion's end, duration 6-12 hr, eliminated unchanged in urine, 75%-85% protein bound
IM: Peak 1-2 hr, duration 6-12 hr, half-life 1½-2 hr
cephalexin: Peak 1 hr, duration 6-12 hr, half-life 30-72 min, 5%-15% bound by plasma proteins, 80%-100% eliminated unchanged in urine, crosses placenta, excreted in breast milk

INTERACTIONS
Increase: toxicity—aminoglycosides, loop diuretics, probenecid

Drug/Lab Test
Increase: AST, ALT, alkaline phosphatase, LDH, BUN, creatinine, bilirubin
False positive: urinary protein, direct Coombs' test, urine glucose
Interference: cross-matching

NURSING CONSIDERATIONS
Assess:
• **Infection:** characteristics of wounds, sputum, urine, stools, WBC >10,000/mm^3, earache, fever; obtain baseline and periodically during treatment; obtain C&S before treatment starts, may start treatment before results are received
• Cross-sensitivity to penicillin and other cephalosporins; hypersensitivity reaction may occur
• **Nephrotoxicity:** increased BUN, creatinine; urine output: if decreasing, notify prescriber
• Blood studies: AST, ALT, CBC, Hct, bilirubin, LDH, alkaline phosphatase, Coombs' test monthly if patient is on long-term therapy
• **CDAD:** bowel pattern daily; if severe diarrhea occurs, product should be discontinued
• **Anaphylaxis:** rash, urticaria, pruritus, chills, fever, joint pain; angioedema; may occur a few days after therapy begins; discontinue product, notify prescriber immediately, keep emergency equipment nearby
• **Stevens-Johnson syndrome, toxic epidermal necrolysis:** painful, red rash; flulike symptoms, discontinue product, do not restart
• **Overgrowth of infection:** perineal itching, fever, malaise, redness, pain, swelling, drainage, rash, diarrhea, change in cough, sputum

Evaluate:
• Therapeutic response: decreased symptoms of infection, negative C&S

Teach patient/family:
• To take all medication prescribed for length of time ordered; take missed dose as soon as remembered, unless close to next dose; do not double dose; use calibrated device for syrup, liquid, suspension
• To report vaginal itching; loose, foul-smelling stools; furry tongue occurs; may indicate superinfection
• To report immediately rash, flulike symptoms, blisters, stop product
• Diarrhea with mucus, blood (may indicate **CDAD**)

TREATMENT OF ANAPHYLAXIS: EPINEPHrine, antihistamines; resuscitate if needed

---

CEPHALOSPORINS— SECOND GENERATION

cefaclor (Rx)
(sef'a-klor)
cefoTEtan (Rx)
(sef'oh-tee-tan)
Cefotan
cefOXitin (Rx)
(se-fox'i-tin)
cefprozil (Rx)
(sef-proe'zill)
cefuroxime (Rx)
(sef-yoor-ox'eem)
Func. class.: Antiinfective
Chem. class.: Cephalosporin (second generation)

Do not confuse:
cefaclor/cephalexin
Cefotan/Ceftin
cefprozil/ceFAZolin/cefuroxime

ACTION: Inhibits bacterial cell wall synthesis, renders cell wall osmotically unstable, leads to cell death by binding to cell wall membrane

USES: cefaclor: gram-negative bacilli: *Haemophilus influenzae, Escherichia coli, Proteus mirabilis, Klebsiella;* gram-positive organisms: *Streptococcus*

---

pneumoniae, Streptococcus pyogenes, Staphylococcus aureus; respiratory tract, urinary tract, skin, infections; otitis media

cefoTETan: gram-negative organisms: *Haemophilus influenzae, Escherichia coli, Enterobacter aerogenes, Proteus mirabilis, Klebsiella, Citrobacter, Salmonella, Shigella, Acinetobacter, Bacteroides fragilis, Neisseria, Serratia;* gram-positive organisms: *Streptococcus pneumoniae, Streptococcus pyogenes, Staphylococcus aureus;* lower, serious respiratory tract, urinary tract, skin, bone, joint, gynecologic, gonococcal, intraabdominal infections

cefOXitin: gram-negative bacilli: *Haemophilus influenzae, Escherichia coli, Proteus, Klebsiella, Bacteroides fragilis, Neisseria gonorrhoeae;* gram-positive organisms: *Streptococcus pneumoniae, Streptococcus pyogenes, Staphylococcus aureus;* anaerobes including *Clostridium;* lower respiratory tract, urinary tract, skin, bone, gynecologic, gonococcal infections; septicemia, peritonitis

cefprozil: pharyngitis/tonsillitis; otitis media; secondary bacterial infection of acute bronchitis; acute bacterial exacerbation of chronic bronchitis; uncomplicated skin and skin structure infections; acute sinusitis

cefuroxime: gram-negative bacilli: *Haemophilus influenzae, Escherichia coli, Neisseria, Proteus mirabilis, Klebsiella;* gram-positive organisms: *Streptococcus pneumoniae, Streptococcus pyogenes, Staphylococcus aureus;* serious lower respiratory tract, urinary tract, skin, bone, joint, gonococcal infections; septicemia, meningitis, surgery prophylaxis

CONTRAINDICATIONS

Hypersensitivity to cephalosporins or related antibiotics; seizures

Precautions: Pregnancy, breastfeeding, children, GI/renal disease, diabetes mellitus, coagulopathy, pseudomembranous colitis

DOSAGE AND ROUTES
cefaclor
• **Adult:** PO 250-500 mg q8hr, extended release 500 mg q12hr; max 1.5 g/day (capsule, oral suspension); 1 g/day (extended release)
• **Child >1 mo:** PO 20-40 mg/kg/day in divided doses q8hr or total daily dose may be divided and given q12hr, max 1 g/day
Available forms: Capsules 250, 500 mg; oral suspension 125, 250, 375 mg/5 mL; extended-release tablet 375, 500 mg

cefoTETan
• **Adult:** IM/IV 1-3 g q12hr × 5-10 days
Renal dose
• **Adult:** IM/IV CCr 30-50 mL/min 1-2 g, then 1-2 g q8-12hr; CCr 10-29 mL/min 1-2 g, then 1-2 g q12-24hr; CCr 5-9 mL/min 1-2 g, then 0.5-1 g q12-24hr; CCr<5 mL/min 1-2 g, then 0.5-1 g q24-48hr
Perioperative prophylaxis
• **Adult:** IV 1-2 g ½-1 hr before surgery
Available forms: Injection 1, 2, 10 g; premixed 1 g/50 mL D_5W, 2 g/50 mL D_5W

cefOXitin
Perioperative prophylaxis
• **Adult:** IV 2 g 30-60 min prior to surgery, then 2g q6hr × 24 hr
• **Child/infant >3 mo:** IV/30-40 mg/kg 30-60 min prior to surgery then 30-40 mg/kg q6hr × 24 hr
Renal dose
• **Adult:** IM/IV after loading dose, CCr 30-50 mL/min, 1-2 g q8-12hr; CCr 10-29 mL/min, 1-2 g q12-24hr; CCr <10 mL/min, 0.5-1 g q12-24hr
Severe infections
• **Adult:** IM/IV 2 g q4hr
• **Child ≥3 mo:** IM/IV 80-160 mg/kg/day divided q4-6hr; max 12 g/day
Available forms: Powder for injection 1, 2 g; premixed 1 g/50 mL D_5W, 2 g/50 mL D_5W

cefprozil
Upper respiratory infections
• **Adult:** PO 500 mg q24hr × 10 days
Otitis media
• **Child 6 mo-12 yr:** PO 15 mg/kg q12hr × 10 days

Side effects: *italics* = common; red = life-threatening

Lower respiratory infections
- **Adult:** PO 500 mg q12hr × 10 days

Skin/skin structure infections
- **Adult/child ≥13 yr:** PO 250-500 mg q12hr × 10 days

Child 2-12 yr: PO 20 mg/kg q24hr × 10 days, max adult dose

Renal dose
- **Adult:** PO CCr <30 mL/min, 50% of dose

Available forms: Tablets 250, 500 mg; suspension 125, 250 mg/5 mL

cefuroxime

- **Adult/child:** PO 250 mg q12hr; may increase to 500 mg q12hr for serious infections
- **Adult:** IM/IV 750 mg-1.5 g q8hr for 5-10 days

Urinary tract infections
- **Adult:** PO 250 mg q12hr × 7-10 days

Otitis media
- **Child >3 mo-12 yr:** PO 250 mg q12hr × 10 days

Surgical prophylaxis
- **Adult:** IV 1.5 g ½-1 hr before surgery

Severe infections
- **Adult:** IM/IV 1.5 g q6hr; may give up to 3 g q8hr for bacterial meningitis
- **Child >3 mo:** IM/IV 50-100 mg/kg/day or IM in divided doses q6-8hr

Uncomplicated gonorrhea
- **Adult:** IM 1 g as single dose in 2 separate sites with oral probenecid

Early Lyme disease
Adult/child ≥13 yr: PO 500 mg q12hr × 20 days

Renal dose
- Dosage reduction indicated with severe renal impairment (CCr <20 mL/min)

Available forms: Tablets 125, 250, 500 mg; solution for injection 1.5 g/50 mL, 750 mg/50 mL; suspension 125, 250 mg/5 mL

Administer:
- Do not break, crush, or chew extended-release tablets or capsules
- On an empty stomach 1 hr before or 2 hr after a meal

cefaclor

- Identify allergies before use
- Obtain C&S specimen before use
- Shake suspension, refrigerate, discard after 2 wk

- For 10-14 days to ensure organism death, prevent superinfection
- With food if needed for GI symptoms
- After C&S completed
- Swallow extended release whole

cefoTEtan

- Identify allergies before use
- Obtain C&S specimen before use

Direct IV route
- IV direct after diluting 1 g/10 mL sterile water for injection, give over 3-5 min

Intermittent IV infusion route
- May be diluted further with 50-100 mL NS or D$_5$W; shake; run over ½-1 hr by Y-tube or 3-way stopcock; discontinue primary infusion during administration
- May be stored 96 hr refrigerated or 24 hr at room temperature

Y-site compatibilities: Allopurinol, amifostine, aztreonam, diltiazem, famotidine, filgrastim, fluconazole, fludarabine, heparin, insulin (regular), melphalan, meperidine, morphine, PACLitaxel, remifentanil, sargramostim, tacrolimus, teniposide, theophylline, thiotepa

cefOXitin

IV route
Direct IV route
- After diluting 1 g/10 mL or more D$_5$W, NS, give over 3-5 min

Intermittent IV infusion route may be diluted further with 50-100 mL NS or D$_5$W; run over ½-1 hr by Y-tube or 3-way stopcock; discontinue primary infusion during administration

Continuous infusion route give by continuous infusion at prescribed rate; may store 96 hr refrigerated or 24 hr at room temperature
- After C&S completed

Y-site compatibilities: Acyclovir, amifostine, amphotericin B cholesteryl sulfate complex, aztreonam, cyclophosphamide, diltiazem, DOXOrubicin liposome, famotidine, fluconazole, foscarnet, HYDROmorphone, magnesium sulfate, meperidine, morphine, ondansetron, perphenazine, remifentanil, teniposide, thiotepa

cefprozil
PO route
- Without regard to meals
- Identify allergies before use
- Obtain C&S specimen before use, may start product before results are received
- Refrigerate/shake suspension before use; discard after 14 days

cefuroxime
PO route
- Identify allergies before use
- Obtain C&S specimen before use, may start product before results are received
- With food if needed for GI symptoms

Y-site compatibilities: Acyclovir, allopurinol, amifostine, atracurium, aztreonam, cyclophosphamide, diltiazem, famotidine, fludarabine, foscarnet, HYDROmorphone, melphalan, meperidine, morphine, ondansetron, pancuronium, perphenazine, remifentanil, sargramostim, tacrolimus, teniposide, thiotepa, vecuronium

SIDE EFFECTS
CNS: Dizziness, headache, seizures
GI: *Diarrhea*, nausea, vomiting, anorexia, CDAD
HEMA: Leukopenia, thrombocytopenia, agranulocytosis, neutropenia, eosinophilia, hemolytic anemia
INTEG: Rash, urticaria, dermatitis, Stevens-Johnson syndrome, IV site reactions
SYST: Anaphylaxis, serum sickness, superinfection

PHARMACOKINETICS
cefaclor
PO: Peak ½-1 hr, half-life 36-54 min, 25% bound by plasma proteins, 60%-85% eliminated unchanged in urine, crosses placenta, excreted in breast milk (low concentrations)
cefoTEtan
IM/IV: Peak 1½-3 hr, half-life hr, 75%-90% protein binding, 50%-80% eliminated unchanged in urine, crosses placenta, excreted in breast milk
cefOXitin
Half-life ½-1 hr; 65%-80% protein binding 90%-100%; eliminated unchanged in urine;

crosses placenta, blood-brain barrier; eliminated in breast milk; not metabolized
IM: Peak 15-30 min
IV: Peak infusion's end, duration 6-8 hr
cefprozil
PO: Peak 1.5 hr, protein binding 36%, half-life 1.3 hr (normal renal function), 2 hr (hepatic disease), 5½-6 hr (end-stage renal disease), extensively metabolized to an active metabolite, eliminated in urine 60%
cefuroxime
Peak **PO** 2 hr, **IM** 45 min, **IV** 2-3 min, 66% excreted unchanged in urine, half-life 1-2 hr in normal renal function

INTERACTIONS
Increase: effect/toxicity—aminoglycosides, probenecid
Increase: bleeding risk (cefoTEtan)—anticoagulants, thrombolytics, NSAIDs, antiplatelets
Decrease: absorption of cephalosporin—antacids
Drug/Lab Test
False increase: creatinine (serum urine), urinary 17-KS
False positive: urinary protein, direct Coombs' test, urine glucose testing (Clinitest)
Interference: cross-matching

NURSING CONSIDERATIONS
Assess:
- I&O ratio
- Blood studies: AST, ALT, CBC, Hct, bilirubin, LDH, alkaline phosphatase, Coombs' test monthly if patient is on long-term therapy
- Electrolytes: potassium, sodium, chlorine monthly if patient is on long-term therapy
- *Clostridium difficile*–associated **diarrhea (CDAD):** bowel pattern daily; if severe diarrhea occurs, product should be discontinued
- **Anaphylaxis:** rash, flushing, urticaria, pruritus, dyspnea; discontinue product, notify prescriber, have emergency equipment available; cross-sensitivity may occur with penicillins or other beta-lactam antibiotics
- **Bleeding:** ecchymosis, bleeding gums, hematuria, stool guaiac daily

• **Overgrowth of infection:** perineal itching, fever, malaise, redness, pain, swelling, drainage, rash, diarrhea, change in cough, sputum

Evaluate:

• Therapeutic response: negative C&S, decreased symptoms of infections

Teach patient/family:

• To complete full course of product therapy; to take missed dose as soon as remembered unless close to next dose, do not double dose; to use calibrated device for syrup, liquid suspension

• To report diarrhea with mucus, blood CDAD; symptoms of hypersensitivity, stools may change to red color

TREATMENT OF ANAPHY-LAXIS: EPINEPHrine, antihistamines; resuscitate if needed

---

CEPHALOSPORINS— THIRD/FOURTH GENERATION

cefdinir (Rx)
(sef′dih-ner)
cefditoren (Rx)
(sef-dit′oh-ren)
Spectracef
cefepime (Rx) (fourth generation)
(sef′e-peem)
Maxipime
cefixime (Rx)
(sef-icks′ime)
Suprax
cefotaxime (Rx)
(sef-oh-taks′eem)
cefpodoxime (Rx)
(sef-poe-docks′eem)
cefTAZidime (Rx)
(sef′tay-zi-deem)
Fortaz, Tazicef
cefTRIAXone (Rx)
(sef-try-ax′one)
Func. class.: Broad-spectrum anti-infective
Chem. class.: Cephalosporin (third generation)

Do not confuse:
cefTAZidime/ceftizoxime

ACTION: Inhibits bacterial cell wall synthesis, renders cell wall osmotically unstable, leads to cell death

USES: cefdinir: community-acquired pneumonia, otitis media, sinusitis, pharyngitis, skin and skin structure infections, acute exacerbations of chronic bronchitis, pneumonia, tonsillitis, *Citrobacter diversus, Escherichia coli, Klebsiella pneumoniae, Proteus mirabilis, Staphylococcus epidermidis, Streptococcus agalactiae* (group B), viridans streptococci alpha, *Haemophilus influenzae, Haemophilus parainfluenzae, Moraxella catarrhalis;* gram-positive organisms: *Streptococcus pneumoniae, Streptococcus pyogenes, Staphylococcus aureus* (MSSA)

cefditoren pivoxil: acute bacterial exacerbations of chronic bronchitis caused by *Haemophilus influenzae, Haemophilus parainfluenzae, Streptococcus pneumoniae, Moraxella catarrhalis;* pharyngitis/tonsillitis caused by *Streptococcus pyogenes;* uncomplicated skin and skin structure infections caused by *Staphylococcus aureus, Streptococcus pyogenes;* community-acquired pneumonia, viridans streptococci

cefixime: uncomplicated UTI *(Escherichia coli, Proteus mirabilis),* pharyngitis and tonsillitis *(Streptococcus pyogenes),* otitis media *(Haemophilus influenzae), Moraxella catarrhalis,* acute bronchitis and acute exacerbations of chronic bronchitis *(Streptococcus pneumoniae, H. influenzae),* uncomplicated gonorrhea

cefotaxime: *Haemophilus influenzae, Haemophilus parainfluenzae, Escherichia coli, Enterococcus faecalis, Neisseria gonorrhoeae, Neisseria meningitidis, Proteus mirabilis, Klebsiella, Citrobacter, Serratia, Salmonella, Shigella, Pseudomonas; Streptococcus pneumoniae, Streptococcus pyogenes, Staphylococcus aureus;* serious lower respiratory tract, urinary tract, skin, bone, gonococcal infections; bacteremia, septicemia, meningitis, skin, skin structure infections; CNS infections; perioperative prophylaxis, intraabdominal infections, PID, UTI, ventriculitis

cefpodoxime: *Bacteroides, Neisseria gonorrhoeae, Haemophilus influenzae, Escherichia coli, Proteus mirabilis, Klebsiella;* gram-positive organisms: *Streptococcus pneumoniae, Streptococcus pyogenes, Staphylococcus aureus;* upper and lower respiratory tract, urinary tract, skin infections; otitis media; sexually transmitted diseases

cefTAZidime: *Haemophilus influenzae, Escherichia coli, Enterobacter aerogenes, Pseudomonas aeruginosa, Proteus mirabilis, Klebsiella, Citrobacter, Enterobacter, Salmonella, Shigella, Acinetobacter, Bacteroides fragilis, Neisseria, Serratia; Streptococcus pneumoniae, Streptococcus pyogenes, Staphylococcus aureus;* serious lower respiratory tract, urinary tract, skin, gynecologic, bone, joint, intraabdominal infections; septicemia, meningitis

ceftibuten: pharyngitis/tonsillitis, otitis media, secondary bacterial infection of acute bronchitis

cefTRIAXone: gram-negative bacilli: *Haemophilus influenzae, Escherichia coli, Enterobacter aerogenes, Proteus mirabilis, Klebsiella, Citrobacter, Enterobacter, Salmonella, Shigella, Acinetobacter, Bacteroides fragilis, Neisseria, Serratia;* gram-positive organisms: *Streptococcus pneumoniae, Streptococcus pyogenes, Staphylococcus aureus;* serious lower respiratory tract, urinary tract, skin, gonococcal, intraabdominal infections; septicemia, meningitis, bone, joint infections; otitis media; PID

CONTRAINDICATIONS

Hypersensitivity to cephalosporins, infants <1 mo

Precautions: Pregnancy, breastfeeding, children, hypersensitivity to penicillins, GI/renal disease, geriatric patients, pseudomembranous colitis, viral infection, vitamin K deficiencies, diabetes

DOSAGE AND ROUTES
cefdinir

Uncomplicated skin and skin structure infections/community-acquired pneumonia
• **Adult and child ≥13 yr: PO** 300 mg q12hr × 10 days or 600 mg q24hr

• **Child 6 mo-12 yr: PO** 7 mg/kg q12hr or 14 mg/kg q24hr × 10 days

Acute exacerbations of chronic bronchitis/acute maxillary sinusitis
• **Adult and child ≥13 yr: PO** 300 mg q12hr or 600 mg q24hr × 10 days

Pharyngitis/tonsillitis
• **Adult and child ≥13 yr: PO** 300 mg q12hr or 600 mg q24hr × 10 days

• **Child 6 mo-12 yr: PO** 7 mg/kg q12hr × 5-10 days or 14 mg/kg q24hr × 10 days

Renal dose
• **Adult/child >13 yr: PO** CCr <30 mL/min, 300 mg/day (adult); 7 mg/kg/day (child 6 mo-12 yr)

Available forms: Capsules 300 mg; suspension 125 mg, 250 mg/5 mL

cefditoren
• **Adult: PO** 200-400 mg bid × 10-14 days

Renal dose
• **Adult: PO** CCr 30-49 mL/min, max 200 mg bid; CCr <30 mL/min, max 200 mg daily

Available forms: Tablets 200, 400 mg

cefepime

Febrile neutropenia
• **Adult/adolescent >16 yr/child ≥40 kg: IV** 2 g q8hr × 7 days or until neutropenia resolves

• **Infant ≥2 mo/child/adolescent ≤16 yr and ≤40 kg: IV** 50 mg/kg/dose q8hr × 7 days or until neutropenia resolves

Urinary tract infections (mild to moderate)
• **Adult/adolescent >16 yr: IV/IM** 0.5-1 g q12hr × 7-10 days

Urinary tract infections (severe)
• **Adult/adolescent >16 yr/ IV** 2 g q12hr × 10 days

Pneumonia (moderate to severe)
• **Adult: IV** 1-2 g q 8-12hr × 10 days
• **Infant 2-11 mo/child/adolescent: IV** 50 mg/kg/dose q12hr (max: 2 g/dose) × 10 days
• **Infant 1 mo (unlabeled): IV** 50 mg/kg/dose q12hr
• **Neonates ≥36 wk gestation (unlabeled): IV** 50 mg/kg/dose q12hr
• **Neonates <36 wk gestation (unlabeled): IV** 30 mg/kg/dose q12hr

C

Complicated intraabdominal infections (peritonitis), biliary tract infections (cholangitis, cholecystitis)

- **Adults/adolescents 17 yr: IV** 2 g q12hr with metronidazole × 7-10 days; for infections caused by *Pseudomonas aeruginosa*, 2 g q8hr
- **Infants/child/adolescent 13-16 yr (unlabeled): IV** 50 mg/kg/dose q12hr (max: 2 g/dose) with metronidazole × 7-10 days; for infections caused by *Pseudomonas aeruginosa*, 50 mg/kg/dose q8hr (max: 2 g/dose)
- **Neonates ≥36 wk gestation (unlabeled): IV** 50 mg/kg/dose q12hr with metronidazole × 7-10 days
- **Neonates <36 wk gestation (unlabeled): IV** 30 mg/kg/dose q12hr with metronidazole × 7-10 days

Available forms: Powder for injection 500 mg, 1, 2 g; 1 g/50 mL, 2 g/100 mL

Moderate-severe skin/structure infections due to Staphylococcus aureus or Streptococcus pyogenes or for diabetic foot ulcer (unlabeled)

cefixime

- **Adult/adolescent/child >12 yr old >45 kg: PO** 400 mg/day divided q12-24hr
- **Child ≤45 kg/infant ≥6 mo: PO** 8 mg/kg/day divided q12-24hr

Renal dose

- **Adult: PO** CCr 21-59 mL/min, give 65% of dose; CCr <20 mL/min, give 50% of dose

Available forms: Powder for oral suspension 100 mg/5 mL, 200 mg/5 mL, 500 mg/mL; chewable tablets 100, 200 mg; capsules 400 mg

cefotaxime

- **Adult/adolescent/child ≥50 kg: IV/IM (uncomplicated infections)** 1 g q12hr, **(moderate-severe infection)** 1-2 g q8hr, **(severe infections)** 2 g q6-8hr, **(life-threatening infections)** 2 g q4hr, max 12 g/day
- **Adolescent/child <50 kg and infants: IV/IM** 50-180 mg/kg/day divided q6-8hr, max 2 g/dose; **(severe infections)** 200-225 mg/kg/day divided q4-6hr, max 12 g
- **Neonate >7 days: IV/IM** 50 mg/kg/dose q8-12hr

Uncomplicated gonorrhea

- **Adult: IM** 500 mg as a single dose

Rectal gonorrhea

Adult: Men IM 1 g as a single dose
Adult: Women IM 500 mg as a single dose

Renal dose

- **Adult: IM** CCr <20 mL/min 50% dose reduction

Available forms: Powder for injection 500 mg, 1, 2, 10 g; injection 1, 2 g premixed frozen

cefpodoxime

Pneumonia

- **Adult/child >12 yr: PO** 200 mg q12hr × 14 days

Chronic bronchitis

- **Adult/child ≥12 yr: PO** 200 mg q12hr × 10 days

Uncomplicated gonorrhea

- **Adult/child ≥12 yr: PO** 200 mg as a single dose

Acute maxillary sinusitis

- **Adult/child ≥12 yr: PO** 200 mg q12hr × 10 days
- **Child 2 mo-12 yr: PO** 5 mg/kg q12hr × 10-14 days

Skin and skin structure

- **Adult/child >12 yr: PO** 400 mg q12hr × 7-14 days

Pharyngitis and tonsillitis

- **Adult/child >12 yr: PO** 100 mg q12hr × 5-10 days
- **Child 5 mo-12 yr: PO** 5 mg/kg q12hr (max 100 mg/dose or 200 mg/day) × 5-10 days

Uncomplicated UTI

- **Adult/child >12 yr: PO** 100 mg q12hr × 7 days; dosing interval increased with severe renal impairment

Acute otitis media

- **Child 2 mo-12 yr: PO** 5 mg/kg q12hr × 5 days

Available forms: Tablets 100, 200 mg; granules for suspension 50 mg, 100 mg/5 mL

cefTAZidime

- **Adult/child >12 yr: IV/IM** 1-2 g q8hr
- **Child: IV/IM** 30-50 mg/kg q8hr, max 6 g/day
- **Neonate: IV/IM** 30-50 mg/kg q8-12hr

Renal dose

- **Adult: IM/IV** CCr 31-50 mL/min 1 g q12hr; CCr 16-30 mL/min 1 g q24hr; CCr 6-15 mL/min 1-g loading dose, then 0.5 g q24hr; CCr <5 mL/min 1-g loading dose, then 0.5 g q48hr

Available forms: Injection 500 mg, 1, 2, 6 g/vial

cefTRIAXone

UTI, lower respiratory infections, bone joint, skin/skin structure infections

• **Adult/child >12 yr: IM/IV** 1-2 g/day, max 4 g/24 hr
• **Child ≤12 yr: IM/IV** 50-75 mg/kg/day in equal doses q12-24hr

Uncomplicated gonorrhea

• **Adult:** 250 mg **IM** as single dose with azithromycin 1 g single dose or doxycycline 100 mg bid × 7 days
• Reduce dosage in severe renal impairment (CCr <10 mL/min)

Meningitis

• **Adult: IV** 4 g/day divided every 12 to 24 hr × 7-21 days
• **Child: IV/IM** 100 mg/kg/day × 7-14 days

Available forms: Injection 250, 500 mg, 1, 2; infusion 1,2 g/50 mL

Administer

cefdinir

• Oral suspension after adding 39 mL water to the 60-mL bottle or 65 mL water to the 120-mL bottle; discard unused portion after 10 days; give without regard to food, do not give within 2 hr of antacids, iron supplements
• After C&S completed

cefditoren

• For 10-14 days to ensure organism death, prevent superinfection
• With food; do not give with antacids
• After C&S completed

cefepime

Intermittent IV INFUSION route

• IV after diluting in 50-100 mL or more D₅W, NS; give over 30 min
• For 7-10 days to ensure organism death, prevent superinfection

Y-site compatibilities: DOXOrubicin liposome

cefixime

• For 10-14 days to ensure organism death, prevent superinfection
• Without regard to food
• Chew tablets before swallowing

cefotaxime

IV route

• IV after **diluting** 1 g/10 mL D₅W, NS, sterile water for injection, **give** over 3-5 min by Y-tube or 3-way stopcock; may be **diluted further** with 50-100 mL NS or D₅W; **run** over ½-1 hr; discontinue primary infusion during administration; may be **diluted** in larger volume of solution, given as a continuous infusion
• For 10-14 days to ensure organism death, prevent superinfection
• Thaw frozen container at room temperature or refrigeration; do not force thaw by immersion or microwave; visually inspect container for leaks

Y-site compatibilities: Acyclovir, alfentanil, alprostadil, amifostine, amikacin, aminocaproic acid, aminophylline, anidulafungin, ascorbic acid injection, atenolol, atracurium, atropine, aztreonam, benztropine, bivalirudin, bleomycin, bumetanide, buprenorphine, butorphanol, caffeine, calcium chloride/gluconate, CARBOplatin, cefamandole, cefmetazole, cefonicid, cefoperazone, cefoTEtan, cefOXitin, cefTAZidime (L-arginine), cefTRIAXone sodium, cefuroxime, cimetidine, CISplatin, clindamycin, codeine, cyanocobalamin, cyclophosphamide, cycloSPORINE, cytarabine, DACTINomycin, DAPTOmycin, dexamethasone, dexmedetomidine, digoxin, diltiaZEM, DOCEtaxel, DOPamine, doxacurium, doxycycline, enalaprilat, ePHEDrine, EPINEPHrine, epiRUBicin, epoetin alfa, eptifibatide, erythromycin, esmolol, etoposide, famotidine, fenoldopam, fentaNYL, fludarabine, fluorouracil, folic acid, furosemide, gatifloxacin, gentamicin, glycopyrrolate, granisetron, heparin, hydrocortisone, HYDROmorphone, ifosfamide, imipenem-cilastatin, insulin (regular), isoproterenol, ketorolac, lidocaine, linezolid, LORazepam, LR, magnesium sulfate, mannitol, mechlorethamine, melphalan, meperidine, metaraminol, methicillin, methotrexate, methoxamine, methyldopate, metoclopramide, metoprolol, metroNIDAZOLE, mezlocillin, miconazole, midazolam, milrinone, minocycline, mitoXANTRONE, morphine, moxalactam, multiple vitamins, mycophenolate, nafcillin, nalbuphine, naloxone, nesiritide, netilmicin, nitroglycerin, nitroprusside, norepinephrine, normal saline, octreotide, ofloxacin, ondansetron, ornidazole, oxacillin, oxaliplatin, oxytocin, PACLitaxel, palonosetron, pamidronate, pancuronium, pantoprazole, papaverine, pefloxacin, PEMEtrexed, penicillin G potassium/sodium, pentamidine, pentazocine, PENTobarbital, peritoneal dialysis solution, perphenazine, PHENobarbital, phenylephrine, phenytoin, phytonadione, piperacillin, polymyxin B, potassium chloride, procainamide, prochlorperazine, promethazine, propofol, propranolol, protamine, pyridoxine, quiNIDine, quinupristin, raNITIdine, remifentanil, Ringer's injection, ritodrine, riTUXimab, rocuronium, sargramostim, sodium acetate/bicarbonate, sodium fusidate, sodium lactate, succinylcholine, SUFentanil, sulfamethoxazole-trimethoprim, tacrolimus, teniposide, theophylline, thiamine, thiotepa, ticarcillin, ticarcillin-clavulanate, tigecycline, tirofiban, TNA, tobramycin, tolazoline, TPN, trastuzumab, trimetaphan, urokinase, vancomycin, vasopressin, vecuronium, verapamil, vinorelbine, voriconazole

cefpodoxime

• Do not break, crush, or chew tablets due to taste
• For 10-14 days to ensure organism death, prevent superinfection
• With food for better absorption; do not give within 2 hr of antacids, H_2-receptor antagonists
• Shake suspension well, refrigerate, discard after 2 wk

cefTAZidime

IM route
• **Fortaz, vials:** reconstitute 500 mg or 1 g with 1.5 or 3 mL, respectively, of sterile or bacteriostatic water for injection or 0.5%-1% lidocaine (approx 280 mg/mL)
• **Tazicef vials:** reconstitute 1 g/3 mL sterile water for injection (approx 280 mg/mL)
• **Withdraw** dose while making sure needle remains in vial; **ensure** no CO_2 bubbles present; **inject** deeply in large muscle mass, **aspirate** before injection

IV route
• Visually inspect for particulate matter, discoloration, if possible

• **Fortaz, Tazicef packs: reconstitute** 1 or 2 g/100 mL sterile water for injection or other compatible IV solution (10 or 20 mg/mL, respectively); reconstitution is done in 2 stages: first, **inject** 10 mL of the diluent into the pack and **shake** well to dissolve and become clear; CO_2 pressure inside container will occur, **insert** vent needle to release pressure; **add** remaining diluents, **remove** vent needle
• **Fortaz, Tazicef vials: reconstitute** 500 mg, 1 g, 2 g with 5, 10 mL, respectively, of sterile water for injection or other compatible IV solution (100, 95-100, or 170-180 mg/mL, respectively); **shake** well to dissolve
• **Fortaz, ADD-Vantage vials (for IV only): reconstitute** 1 or 2 g with NS, ½ NS, D_5W in either 50- or 100-mL flexible diluent container; to release CO_2 pressure, **insert** vent needle after dissolving, **remove** vent before using

Direct intermittent IV INFUSION route
• **Vials: withdraw** dose while making sure needle remains in solution; make sure there are no CO_2 bubbles in syringe before injection; **inject** directly over 3-5 min or slowly into tubing of a free-flowing compatible IV solution

Intermittent IV INFUSION route
• **Vials: withdraw** dose while making sure needle opening remains in solution; make sure there are no CO_2 bubbles in syringe before injection; infusion packs and ADD-Vantage systems ready for infusion after reconstitution, **infuse** over 15-30 min

Y-site compatibilities: Acyclovir, alfentanil, allopurinol, amifostine, amikacin, aminocaproic acid, aminophylline, amphotericin B lipid complex, anakinra, anidulafungin, atenolol, atropine sulfate, aztreonam, benztropine, bivalirudin, bleomycin, bumetanide, buprenorphine, butorphanol, calcium gluconate, CARBOplatin, cefamandole, ceFAZolin, cefonicid, cefoperazone, cefoTEtan, cefOXitin, cefTAZidime, ceftizoxime, cefTRIAXone, cefuroxime, cephalothin, cephapirin, cimetidine, ciprofloxacin, CISplatin, clindamycin, codeine, cyanocobalamin, cyclophosphamide, cycloSPORINE, cytarabine, DACTINomycin, DAPTOmycin, dexamethasone, dexmedetomidine, digoxin, diltiaZEM, DOCEtaxel, DOPamine, doxacurium, doxapram, enalaprilat, ePHEDrine, EPINEPHrine, epoetin alfa, eptifibatide, esmolol, etoposide, famotidine, fenoldopam, fentaNYL, filgrastim, fludarabine, fluorouracil, folic acid, foscarnet, furosemide, gallium, gatifloxacin, gemcitabine, gentamicin, glycopyrrolate, granisetron, heparin, HYDROmorphone, ifosfamide, imipenem-cilastatin, indomethacin, insulin (regular), irinotecan, isepamicin, isoproterenol, isosorbide, ketamine, ketorolac, labetalol, levoFLOXacin, lidocaine, linezolid, LORazepam, LR, magnesium sulfate, mannitol, mechlorethamine, melphalan, meperidine, metaraminol, methicillin, methotrexate, methoxamine, methyldopate, methylPREDNISolone, metoclopramide, metoprolol, metroNIDAZOLE, miconazole, milrinone, morphine, moxalactam, multiple vitamins inj, nafcillin, nalbuphine, PACLitaxel, raNITIdine, remifentanil, tacrolimus, teniposide, theophylline, thiotepa, vinorelbine, zidovudine

cefTRIAXone

• For 7-14 days to ensure organism death, prevent superinfection
• **IM** inject deeply in large muscle mass
IV route
• **IV** after **reconstituting** 250 mg/2.4 mL, 500 mg/4.8 mL, 1 g/9.6 mL, 2 g/19.2 mL D₅W, water for injection, 0.9% NaCl; **further dilute** with 50-100 mL (40 mg/mL) NS, D₅W, D₁₀W; shake; **run** over ½ hr
• Do not mix with calcium salts

Y-site compatibilities: Acetaminophen, acyclovir, alfentanil, allopurinol, amifostine, amikacin, aminocaproic acid, aminophylline, amiodarone, amphotericin B liposome, anidulafungin, argatroban, atenolol, atracurium, atropine, aztreonam, benztropine, bivalirudin, bleomycin, bumetanide, buprenorphine, butorphanol, CARBOplatin, cefamandole, ceFAZolin, cefmetazole, cefonicid, cefoperazone, cefoTAXime, cefoTEtan, cefOXitin, cefTAZidime, ceftizoxime, cefuroxime, cephalothin, cephapirin, cimetidine, cisatracurium, CISplatin, codeine, cyanocobalamin, cyclophosphamide, cycloSPORINE, cytarabine, DACTINomycin, DAPTOmycin, dexamethasone, dexmedetomidine, digoxin, diltiaZEM, DOCEtaxel, DOPamine, doxacurium, DOXOrubicin liposomal, doxycycline, drotrecogin alfa, enalaprilat, ePHEDrine, EPINEPHrine, epoetin alfa, eptifibatide, erythromycin, esmolol, etoposide, fenoldopam, fludarabine, fluorouracil, folic acid, foscarnet, furosemide, gallium, gatifloxacin, gemcitabine, gentamicin, glycopyrrolate, granisetron, heparin, hydrocortisone, HYDROmorphone, ifosfamide, indomethacin, insulin (regular), isoproterenol, ketorolac, lansoprazole, levoFLOXacin, lidocaine, linezolid, LORazepam, mannitol, mechlorethamine, melphalan, meperidine, metARAMinol, methicillin, methotrexate, methoxamine, methyldopate, methylPREDNISolone, metoclopramide, metoprolol, metroNIDAZOLE, mezlocillin, miconazole, midazolam, milrinone, morphine, moxalactam, multiple vitamins injection, nafcillin, nalbuphine, naloxone, nesiritide, netilmicin, nitroglycerin, nitroprusside, norepinephrine, octreotide, oxacillin, oxaliplatin, oxytocin, PACLitaxel, palonosetron, pamidronate, pancuronium, pantoprazole, PEMEtrexed, penicillin G potassium/sodium, PHENobarbital, phenylephrine, phytonadione, piperacillin, polymyxin B, potassium chloride, procainamide, propofol, propranolol, pyridoxine, raNITIdine, remifentanil, ritodrine, riTUXimab, rocuronium, sargramostim, sodium acetate/bicarbonate, succinylcholine, SUFentanil, tacrolimus, teniposide, theophylline, thiamine, thiotepa, ticarcillin, ticarcillin-clavulanate, tigecycline, tirofiban, tolazoline, trastuzumab, trimetaphan, urokinase, vasopressin, vecuronium, verapamil, vinCRIStine, voriconazole, warfarin, zidovudine

SIDE EFFECTS

CNS: Headache, dizziness, seizures

GI: *Nausea, vomiting, diarrhea, anorexia,* abdominal pain, CDAD; cholestasis (cefotaxime)

GU: Renal failure

HEMA: Thrombocytopenia, agranulocytosis, neutropenia, lymphocytosis, eosinophilia, pancytopenia, hemolytic anemia

INTEG: Rash, urticaria, dermatitis, injection site reaction

MS: Arthralgia (cefditoren)

SYST: Anaphylaxis, serum sickness, Stevens-Johnson syndrome, toxic epidermal necrolysis

PHARMACOKINETICS

cefdinir

Unchanged in urine; crosses placenta, blood-brain barrier; eliminated in breast milk, not metabolized; 60%-70% protein binding, half-life 1.7 hr

cefditoren

Well absorbed when broken down (prodrug), wide distribution, half-life 100 min, onset rapid, peak 1.5-3 hr, duration 12 hr, 88% protein binding

cefepime

Peak 79 min; half-life 2 hr; 20% bound by plasma proteins; 90% excreted unchanged in urine; crosses placenta, blood-brain barrier; excreted in breast milk, not metabolized

cefixime

PO: Peak 2-8 hr, half-life 3-4 hr, 65%-70% protein binding, 50% eliminated unchanged in urine, crosses placenta, excreted in breast milk

cefotaxime

Half-life 1 hr, 35%-65% is bound by plasma proteins, 40%-65% is eliminated unchanged in urine in 24 hr, 25% metabolized in the liver to active metabolites, excreted in breast milk (small amounts)

IM: Onset 30 min

IV: Onset 5 min

cefpodoxime

Half-life 1-1.5 hr, 13%-38% bound by plasma proteins, 30% eliminated unchanged in urine in 8 hr, crosses placenta, excreted in breast milk

cefTAZidime

IM/IV: Half-life 1½-2 hr, 10% bound by plasma proteins, 80% eliminated unchanged in urine, crosses placenta, excreted in breast milk

cefTRIAXone

Half-life 6-9 hr, 58%-96% eliminated unchanged in urine, crosses placenta, excreted in breast milk

IM: Peak 1½-4 hr

IV: Peak 30 min

INTERACTIONS

Many products should not be used with calcium salts (mixed or administered) or H_2 blocker antacids (PO)

Increase: bleeding—anticoagulants, thrombolytics, NSAIDs (ceftriaxone)

Increase: toxicity—aminoglycosides, furosemide loop diuretics, probenecid

Decrease: absorption of cefdinir—iron

Drug/Food

Decrease: absorption—iron-rich cereal, infant formula

Drug/Lab Test

Increase: ALT, AST, alkaline phosphatase, LDH, bilirubin, BUN, creatinine

False increase: creatinine (serum urine), urinary 17-KS

False positive: urinary protein, direct Coombs' test, urine glucose

Interference: cross-matching

NURSING CONSIDERATIONS

Assess:

• **Infection:** characteristics of wounds, sputum, urine, stool, WBC >10,000/mm³, fever; obtain baseline and periodically during treatment

• Cross-sensitivity to penicillin, other cephalosporins; hypersensitivity reaction may occur

• Obtain C&S prior to treatment, may start treatment before results are received

• Blood studies: AST, ALT, CBC, Hct, bilirubin, LDH, alkaline phosphatase, Coombs' test monthly if patient is on long-term therapy

• Electrolytes: potassium, sodium, chloride monthly if patient is on long-term therapy

• **CDAD:** bowel pattern daily; if severe diarrhea occurs, product should be discontinued

- IV site for extravasation, phlebitis
- **Anaphylaxis:** rash, urticaria, pruritus, chills, fever, joint pain, angioedema; may occur a few days after therapy begins
- **Serious skin disorders:** Rash, blisters; toxic epidermal necrolysis, Stevens-Johnson syndrome may occur
- **Overgrowth of infection:** perineal itching, fever, malaise, redness, pain, swelling, drainage, rash, diarrhea, change in cough, sputum

Evaluate:
- Therapeutic response: decreased symptoms of infection; negative C&S

Teach patient/family:
- If diabetic, to check blood glucose
- To report sore throat, bruising, bleeding, joint pain, may indicate **blood dyscrasias (rare)**; diarrhea with mucus, blood, may indicate **CDAD**
- To complete full course of treatment, to take missed dose as soon as remembered unless close to next dose, do not double dose; to use calibrated device for suspension
- May turn stools red

TREATMENT OF ANAPHYLAXIS: EPINEPHrine, antihistamines; resuscitate if needed

---

ceritinib (Rx)
(cerr-ah-tin′ib)
Zykadia
Func. class.: Antineoplastic—miscellaneous

USES: Anaplastic lymphoma kinase (ALK)–positive metastatic non–small-cell lung cancer (NSCLC) in patients who have progressed on or are intolerant to crizotinib

CONTRAINDICATIONS
Pregnancy, hypersensitivity, QT prolongation
Precautions: Breastfeeding, children, geriatric patients, cardiac/hepatic disease, GI bleeding, bone marrow suppression, infection, diarrhea, hyperglycemia, diabetes mellitus, nausea/vomiting,

pancreatitis, pneumonitis, QT prolongation, torsades de pointes, bradycardia, cardiac arrhythmias, electrolyte imbalances, corticosteroid therapy

DOSAGE AND ROUTES
- **Adult: PO** 450 mg daily on an empty stomach until disease progression or unacceptable toxicity. Decrease dose by 1/3, round to nearest 150 mg with strong 3A4 inhibitors or inducers

Available forms: Capsules 150 mg

---

cephradine
See cephalosporins—first generation

⚠ HIGH ALERT

certolizumab (Rx)
(ser′tue-liz′oo-mab)
Cimzia
Func. class.: GI antiinflammatory antirheumatic
Chem. class.: Anti-tissue necrosis factor (anti-TNF) agent, DMARDs

ACTION: Monoclonal antibody that neutralizes the activity of tumor necrosis factor α (TNF-α) found in Crohn's disease; decreases infiltration of inflammatory cells

USES: Crohn's disease (moderate to severe) that has not responded to conventional therapy, rheumatoid arthritis (moderate to severe), psoriatic arthritis, ankylosing spondylitis, moderate-severe plaque psoriasis in those that are candidates for systemic/phototherapy, nonradiographic axial spondyloarthritis with signs of inflammation
Unlabeled uses: Fistulizing Crohn's disease

CONTRAINDICATIONS
Influenza, IV administration, sepsis, hypersensitivity

Side effects: *italics* = common; red = life-threatening

Precautions: Pregnancy, breastfeeding, children, geriatric patients, AIDS, coagulopathy, diabetes, fungal infection, heart failure, hepatitis, human antichimeric antibody, immunosuppression, leukopenia, MS, cancer, neurologic/renal disease, surgery, thrombocytopenia, TB, vaccinations

> **Black Box Warning:** Infection, neoplastic disease in children

DOSAGE AND ROUTES
Crohn's disease (moderate to severe)
• **Adult: SUBCUT** 400 mg given as 2 injections at wk 0, 2, 4; if clinical response occurs, give 400 mg q4wk
RA (moderate to severe)/ankylosing spondylitis/psoriatic arthritis
• **Adult: SUBCUT** 400 mg (as 2 injections of 200 mg) once, then repeat at wk 2 and 4; maintenance, 200 mg q2wk or 400 mg q4wk
Moderate-severe plaque psoriasis
• **Adult: SUBCUT** 400 mg (as two 200-mg injections) every other wk
• **Adult <90 kg: SUBCUT** 400 mg (as two 200-mg injections) at wk 0, 2, 4, then 200 mg every other wk
Available forms: Solution for injection 200 mg/mL; prefilled syringe 400-mg kit
Administer:
SUBCUT route
• **TB testing:** Required prior use, should be done baseline, periodically, use in TB or active infection is contraindicated
• Give by SUBCUT injection only
• **Reconstitution:** Allow to warm to room temperature; add 1 mL sterile water for injection to each vial; 2 vials will be needed for patients with Crohn's disease
• Gently swirl; do not shake; full reconstitution may take up to 30 min; reconstituted product may remain at room temperature for up to 2 hr or refrigerated up to 24 hr
• If reconstituted product has been refrigerated, allow to warm to room temperature
• Use 2 syringes and two 20G needles

• Withdraw reconstituted solution from each vial into separate syringes; each will contain 200 mg; switch 20G to 23G needle; inject into 2 separate sites in abdomen or thigh
• Store in refrigerator; do not freeze

SIDE EFFECTS
CNS: Anxiety, bipolar disorder, suicidal ideation
CV: Heart failure, MI, cardiac dysrhythmia, angina, stroke, thrombophlebitis, hypertension
GI: Abdominal pain
HEMA: Anemia, pancytopenia
INTEG: *Rash, urticaria,* angioedema
MISC: Anaphylaxis, antibody formation, arthralgia, bleeding, infection, lupus-like symptoms, lymphadenopathy, malignancies, serum sickness
RESP: Upper respiratory tract infection, cough

PHARMACOKINETICS
Peak 54-171 hr, half-life 14 days

INTERACTIONS
• Do not administer live vaccines, toxoids concurrently
Increase: possible infections—abatacept, adalimumab, anakinra, etanercept, immunosuppressive agents, inFLIXimab, rilonacept; do not use concurrently
Increase: immunosuppressant toxicity—pimecrolimus, tofacitinib, tocilzumab

NURSING CONSIDERATIONS
Assess:
• Antinuclear antibody test (ANA), hepatitis B serology, CBC with differential, blood dyscrasias
• **Rheumatoid arthritis/ankylosing spondylitis:** pain, range of motion baseline and during treatment
• **Crohn's disease:** nausea, vomiting, abdominal pain, hepatitis, increased LFTs
• CV status: B/P, pulse, chest pain
• **Allergic reaction, anaphylaxis:** rash, dermatitis, urticaria, dyspnea, hypotension, fever, chills; discontinue if severe; administer EPINEPHrine, corticosteroids, antihistamines; assess for allergies to murine proteins prior to starting therapy

Black Box Warning: Fungal infection: fever, weight loss, diaphoresis, fatigue, dyspnea; discontinue if infection occurs; do not administer to patients with active infection

Black Box Warning: Identify TB, risk for HBV before beginning treatment; TB test should be obtained; if present, TB should be treated prior to certolizumab treatment

Hepatitis B virus: Carriers of HBV should be monitored; those at risk for HBV should be evaluated prior to use

Black Box Warning: Do not use in children; lymphoma may occur

Evaluate:
• Therapeutic response: absence of fever, mucus in stools; decreased inflammation in joints, ability to move without pain
Teach patient/family:
• Not to breastfeed while taking this product
• To notify prescriber of GI symptoms, hypersensitivity reactions, infections, fluid retention; redness, pain, swelling at injection site
• Not to operate machinery, drive if dizziness, vertigo occur
• Not to receive live virus vaccines while taking this product
• How to inject medications if given prefilled syringes for home use
• To discuss with provider all OTC, Rx, herbals, supplements taken
• To seek emergency services for anaphylaxis, angioedema, hypersensitivity
• To report immediately rash; itching; swollen lips, tongue, face
• To discuss possible secondary malignancy

Black Box Warning: Infection: To report immediately increased temperature, trouble breathing, cough or other flulike symptoms

• **Pregnancy/breastfeeding:** Those pregnant should enroll in the Mother to Baby Autoimmune Disease Study (877-311-8972)

cetirizine (Rx, OTC)
(se-teer′i-zeen)
Quzyttir, ZyrTEC, ZyrTEC Children's Allergy
Func. class.: Antihistamine (second generation, peripherally selective)
Chem. class.: Piperazine, H$_1$-histamine antagonist

Combinations: Cetrizine/pseudoephedrine 5 mg/120 mg Zyrtec D 12 Hour
Do not confuse:
cetirizine/sertraline/stavudine
ZyrTEC/Xanax/Zantac/Zocor/ZyPREXA/Zerit

ACTION: Acts on blood vessels, GI, respiratory system by competing with histamine for H$_1$-receptor site; decreases allergic response by blocking pharmacologic effects of histamine; minimal anticholinergic, sedative action

USES: Rhinitis, allergy symptoms, chronic idiopathic urticaria
Unlabeled uses: Asthma, atopic dermatitis

CONTRAINDICATIONS
Breastfeeding, newborn or premature infants, hypersensitivity to this product or hydrOXYzine, severe hepatic disease
Precautions: Pregnancy, children, geriatric patients, respiratory disease, angle-closure glaucoma, prostatic hypertrophy, bladder neck obstruction, asthma

DOSAGE AND ROUTES
• **Adult and child ≥6 yr: PO** 5-10 mg/day
• **Child 2-5 yr: PO** 2.5 mg/day, may increase to 5 mg/day or 2.5 mg bid
• **Child 1-2 yr: PO** 2.5 mg/day, may increase to 2.5 mg q12hr
• **Geriatric: PO** 5 mg/day, may increase to 10 mg/day
Renal dose/hemodialysis dose
• **Adult: PO** CCr 11-31 mL/min, 5 mg/day
Hepatic dose
• **Adult: PO** 5 mg daily
• **Child 6-11 yr: PO** 2.5 mg daily
Acute urticaria
Adults: IV 10 mg once every 24 hr as needed
Children and adolescents 12 yr and older: IV 10 mg IV once every 24 hr as needed

Children 6-11 yr: IV 5 mg or 10 mg (depending on symptom severity) once every 24 hr as needed

Children 1-5 yr: IV 2.5 mg IV once every 24 hr as needed

Infants 6 mo and older: IV 2.5 mg once every 24 hr as needed

Available forms: Tablets 5, 10 mg; syrup 5 mg/5 mL, chewable tablets 5, 10 mg; oral disintegrating tablet 10 mg; capsules 10 mg; solution for injection 10 mg/mL

Administer:
• Without regard to meals
• Store in tight, light-resistant container
• **Chewable tablets:** chew before swallowing; may use with or without water
• **Syrup:** use calibrated measuring device
• **IV push route:** give undiluted over 1-2 min; do not use if precipitate is present

SIDE EFFECTS
CNS: *Headache, drowsiness,* sedation, *fatigue*
EENT: Pharyngitis, dry mouth
INTEG: Rash, eczema
RESP: Pharyngitis

PHARMACOKINETICS
Absorption rapid; onset ½ hr; peak 1-2 hr; duration 24 hr; protein binding 93%; half-life 8.3 hr, decreased in children, increased in renal/hepatic disease

INTERACTIONS
Increase: CNS depression—alcohol, opiates, sedative/hypnotics, other CNS depressants
Increase: anticholinergic/sedative effect—MAOIs

Drug/Lab Test
False negative: skin allergy tests

NURSING CONSIDERATIONS
Assess:
• **Allergy symptoms:** pruritus, urticaria, watering eyes at baseline and during treatment
• Respiratory status: rate, rhythm, increase in bronchial secretions, wheezing, chest tightness
Evaluate:
• Therapeutic response: absence of running or congested nose, rashes
Teach patient/family:
• About all aspects of product use; to notify prescriber if confusion, sedation, or hypotension occurs

• To avoid driving, other hazardous activity if drowsiness occurs; to take at night, as drowsiness may occur, especially in children
• To avoid alcohol, other CNS depressants, OTC antihistamines
• **Pregnancy/breastfeeding:** Inform patient to discuss with health care provider if pregnancy is planned or suspected or if breastfeeding
• To avoid exposure to sunlight; burns may occur
• To use sugarless gum, candy, frequent sips of water to minimize dry mouth

TREATMENT OF OVERDOSE:
Administer diazePAM, vasopressors, phenytoin IV

⚠ HIGH ALERT

cetrorelix (Rx)
(set-roe-ree′lix)
Cetrotide
Func. class.: Gonadotropin-releasing hormone antagonist
Chem. class.: Synthetic decapeptide

USES: For inhibition of premature LH surges in women undergoing controlled ovarian hyperstimulation

CONTRAINDICATIONS
Pregnancy, breastfeeding, hypersensitivity, latex allergy, renal disease, KRA5 mutation

DOSAGE AND ROUTES
Single-dose regimen
• **Adult:** SUBCUT 3 mg when serum estradiol level at appropriate stimulation response, usually on stimulation day 7; if hCG not given within 4 days after injection of 3 mg cetrorelix, give 0.25 mg daily until day of hCG administration
Multiple-dose regimen
• **Adult:** SUBCUT 0.25 mg given on stimulation day 5 (either morning or evening) or 6 (morning) and continued daily until day hCG is given
Available forms: Powder for injection 0.25 mg

⚠ HIGH ALERT

cetuximab (Rx)

(se-tux'i-mab)

Erbitux

Func. class.: Antineoplastic—miscellaneous

Chem. class.: Epidermal growth factor receptor inhibitor

ACTION: Not fully understood; binds to ⬥ K-RAS wild-type epidermal growth factor receptors (EGFRs); inhibits phosphorylation and activation of receptor-associated kinase, thereby resulting in inhibition of cell growth

USES: *And* for the treatment of previously treated metastatic colorectal cancer (mCRC) in patients with a BRAF V600E mutation, in combination with encorafenib

CONTRAINDICATIONS

Hypersensitivity to this product, murine proteins, ⬥ RAS-mutant metastatic colorectal cancer or unknown RAS mutation

Precautions: Pregnancy, breastfeeding, children, geriatric patients; CV/renal/hepatic disease; ocular or pulmonary disorders, arrhythmias, CAD, radiation/platinum-based therapy, respiratory arrest

Black Box Warning: Infusion-related reactions, cardiac arrest

DOSAGE AND ROUTES

Treatment of previously treated metastatic colorectal cancer (mCRC) in patients with a BRAF V600E mutation, in combination with encorafenib

Adults: IV 400 mg/m^2 over 120 min on day 1 followed by weekly infusions of cetuximab 250 mg/m^2 over 60 min in combination with encorafenib until disease progression or unacceptable toxicity

Available forms: Solution for injection 2 mg/mL

Administer:

• Premedicate with diphenhydramine 50 mg 30-60 min before first dose; use during infusion for reactions

Intermittent IV INFUSION route

• Use cytoxic handling procedures

• By IV infusion only; do not give by IV push or bolus; do not shake or dilute

• Do not dilute with other products

• Store refrigerated at 36° F-46° F (2.2° C to 7.7° C), discard unused portions

• **Infusion pump:** fill Erbitux into sterile evacuated container/bag, repeat until calculated volume is put into the container; use new needle for each vial; give through in-line filter (low protein binding 0.22 micrometer); prime before starting infusion, max rate 5 mL/min; flush line at end of infusion with 0.9% NaCl

• **Syringe pump:** use in-line filter (low protein binding 0.22 micrometer); connect infusion line, start infusion after priming; repeat until calculated volume given

• Use new needle and filter for each vial, max 5 mL/min rate; use 0.9% NaCl to flush line after infusion

• Do not piggyback

• Observe patient for adverse reactions for 1 hr after infusion

Black Box Warning: Infusion reactions (bronchospasm, stridor, urticaria, hypotension, MI): if mild (grade 1 or 2), reduce all doses by 50%; if severe (grade 3 or 4), permanently discontinue; monitor for at least 1 hr after completion of therapy; reactions usually occur during first dose; have emergency equipment nearby

SIDE EFFECTS

CNS: *Headache, insomnia, depression,* aseptic meningitis

CV: Cardiac arrest

GI: *Nausea, diarrhea, vomiting, anorexia, mouth ulceration, dehydration, constipation, abdominal pain*

HEMA: Leukopenia, anemia, neutropenia

INTEG: Rash, pruritus, acne, toxic epidermal necrolysis, angioedema, acute infusion reactions, other skin toxicities

MISC: *Conjunctivitis,* hypomagnesemia

Side effects: *italics* = common; red = life-threatening

RESP: Interstitial lung disease, *cough, dyspnea*, pulmonary embolus, respiratory arrest

SYST: Anaphylaxis, sepsis, infection, mucosal inflammation, Stevens-Johnson syndrome, toxic epidermal necrolysis

PHARMACOKINETICS
Half-life 114 hr, steady state by third weekly infusion

INTERACTIONS
Drug/Lab Test
Increase: LFTs
Decrease: Hb, neutrophils, calcium, magnesium, potassium

NURSING CONSIDERATIONS
Assess:
• **Pulmonary changes:** lung sounds, cough, dyspnea; interstitial lung disease may occur, may be fatal; discontinue therapy if confirmed

Black Box Warning: **Cardiac arrest:** monitor electrolytes; in those undergoing radiation therapy, electrolytes may be decreased; monitor cardiac patients who receive this product and radiation therapy or platinum-based therapy with 5-FU (head, neck cancer)

• **Serious hypersensitivity reactions:** toxic epidermal necrosis, angioedema, anaphylaxis, Stevens-Johnson syndrome; have emergency equipment nearby with epinephrine, corticosteroids, bronchodilators
• Monitor serum calcium, magnesium, potassium during and for 8 wk after treatment; low levels may occur from a few days to several months after treatment
• **GI symptoms:** frequency of stools, dehydration, abdominal pain, stomatitis
• ⚘ **K-RAS mutations** with metastatic colorectal carcinoma; if K-RAS mutation on codon 12 or 13 detected, patient should not receive anti-EGFR antibody therapy
Evaluate:
• Therapeutic response: decreased growth, spread of EGFR-expressing metastatic colorectal, head/neck carcinoma
Teach patient/family:
• About the reason for treatment, expected results

• To wear sunscreen and hats to limit sun exposure during and for 2 mo after last dose; sun exposure can exacerbate any skin reactions
• To avoid crowds, persons with known infections
• **Pregnancy/breastfeeding: To report adverse reactions immediately:** shortness of breath, severe abdominal pain, skin eruptions; to use contraception (both female and male) during treatment and for 2 mo after treatment; not to breastfeed during treatment and for 2 mo after treatment

---

chlordiazePOXIDE (Rx)
(klor-dye-az-e-pox'ide)
Func. class.: Antianxiety
Chem. class.: Benzodiazepine, long-acting

Controlled Substance Schedule IV

USES: Short-term management of anxiety, acute alcohol withdrawal, preoperatively for relaxation

CONTRAINDICATIONS
Pregnancy, breastfeeding, children <6 yr, hypersensitivity to benzodiazepines, closed-angle glaucoma, psychosis
Precautions: Geriatric patients, debilitated, renal/hepatic disease, suicidal ideation, abrupt discontinuation, respiratory depression, Parkinson's disease, myasthenia gravis

DOSAGE AND ROUTES
Mild anxiety
• **Adult: PO** 5-10 mg tid-qid
• **Geriatric: PO** 5 mg bid initially, increase as needed
• **Child >6 yr: PO** 5 mg bid-qid, max 10 mg bid-tid
Severe anxiety
• **Adult: PO** 20-25 mg 3-4 times per day, max 100 mg/day
Preoperatively
• **Adult: PO** 5-10 mg tid-qid on day before surgery
Alcohol withdrawal
• **Adult: PO** 50-100 mg q4-6hr prn, max 300 mg/day

Renal disease
• **Adult: PO** CCr <10 mL/min, give 50% dose
Available forms: Capsules 5, 10, 25 mg

---

chlordiazepoxide/ amitriptyline (Rx)
Func. class.: Antianxiety, benzodiazepine

Controlled Substance Schedule IV

USES: Severe depression

CONTRAINDICATIONS
Hyper-sensitivity

Black Box Warning: Children, opioid use

Dosage and Routes
Adult: PO 10 mg chlordiazepoxide/25 mg amitriptyline 3-6 times per day
Available forms: Tablets chlordiazepoxide 5 mg/amitriptyline 12.5 mg; 10 mg/amitriptyline 25 mg

---

chloroquine (Rx)
(klor'oh-kwin)
Func. class.: Antimalarial, antiprotozoal
Chem. class.: Synthetic 4-amino-quinoline derivative

ACTION: Inhibits parasite replication, transcription of DNA to RNA by forming complexes with DNA of parasite

USES: Malaria of *Plasmodium vivax, P. malariae, P. ovale, P. falciparum* (some strains); amebiasis
Unlabeled uses: Discoid lupus erythematosus, polymorphous light eruption, rheumatoid arthritis, ulcerative colitis

CONTRAINDICATIONS
Hypersensitivity, retinal field changes
Precautions: Pregnancy, breastfeeding, children, blood dyscrasias, severe GI/neurologic/cardiac disease, alcoholism, hepatic disease, G6PD deficiency, psoriasis, eczema, seizures, preexisting auditory damage, torsades de pointes, infection

DOSAGE AND ROUTES
Acute malaria attacks
• **Adult: PO** 1000 mg (600-mg base), then 500 mg (300-mg base) in 6-8 hr, then 500 mg (300-mg base) daily × 2 days for a total of 2.5 g (1.5-g base) in 3 days
• **Adult/adolescent of low body weight, child/infant: PO** 16.5 mg (10-mg base)/kg, max 600-mg base, then 8.3 mg (5-mg base)/kg, max 300-mg base 6 hr after first dose, then 8.3 mg (5-mg base)/kg, max 300-mg base 24 hr after first dose, then 8.3 mg (5-mg base)/kg, max 300-mg base 36 hr after first dose
Malaria prophylaxis (in areas with chloroquine-sensitive *P. falciparum*)
• **Adult: PO** 500 mg (300-mg base) weekly on same day of each week starting 2 wk prior to travel and for 8 wk after leaving
Extraintestinal amebiasis
• **Adult: PO** 1 g (600-mg base) daily × 2 days, then 500 mg (300-mg base) for ≥2-3 wk
• **Child (unlabeled): PO** 16.6 mg (10-mg base)/kg (max 300-mg base) daily × 2-3 wk
Available forms: Tablets 250 mg (150-mg base), 500 mg (300-mg base) phosphate
Administer:
• Product in mg or base; they are different
PO route
• Prior to or after meals at same time each day to maintain product level
• Store in tight, light-resistant container at room temperature; keep injection in cool environment

SIDE EFFECTS
CNS: Headache, stimulation, fatigue, seizures, psychosis, hallucinations, insomnia
CV: Hypotension, heart block, asystole with syncope, ECG changes, cardiomyopathy
EENT: *Blurred vision, corneal changes, retinal changes, difficulty focusing,* tinnitus, vertigo, deafness, photophobia, corneal edema

Side effects: *italics* = common; red = life-threatening

GI: *Nausea, vomiting, anorexia,* diarrhea, cramps
HEMA: Thrombocytopenia, agranulocytosis, hemolytic anemia, leukopenia
INTEG: Pruritus, pigmentary changes, skin eruptions, lichen-planus–like eruptions, eczema, exfoliative dermatitis

PHARMACOKINETICS
Metabolized in liver; excreted in urine, feces, breast milk; crosses placenta
PO: Peak 1-3 hr, half-life 3-5 days

INTERACTIONS
• Reduced oral clearance and metabolism of chloroquine, cimetidine
Increase: QT prolongation, torsades de pointes—class IA, III antidysrhythmics
Increase: effects—2D6 inhibitors (amiodarone, chlorpheniramine, FLUoxetine, haloperidol, ritonavir, PARoxetine, terbinafine, ticlopidine); CYP3A4 inhibitors (diltiaZEM, verapamil, itraconazole, ketoconazole, erythromycin, doxycycline, clarithromycin)
Decrease: action of chloroquine—magnesium, aluminum compounds, kaolin; do not use concurrently
Decrease: effects of ampicillin, rabies vaccine (ID)
Drug/Lab Test
Decrease: HB, platelets, WBC

NURSING CONSIDERATIONS
Assess:
• **Infection:** resistance is common; not to be used for *P. falciparum* acquired in areas of resistance or where prophylaxis has failed
• Ophthalmic test if long-term treatment or dosage of >150 mg/day, baseline and periodically
• Screen for G6PD deficiency; identify risk of hemolysis
• Blood studies: LFTs; CBC, as blood dyscrasias occur, stop if severe dyscrasias occur; monitor for malaise, fever, bruising, bleeding (rare)
• **ECG** during therapy; watch for depression of T waves, widening of QRS complex in those with QT prolongation
• **Allergic reactions:** pruritus, rash, urticaria

• **For ototoxicity** (tinnitus, vertigo, change in hearing); audiometric testing should be done prior to, after treatment
• **For toxicity:** blurring vision; difficulty focusing; headache; dizziness; decreased knee, ankle reflexes; seizures; CV collapse; product should be discontinued immediately and IV fluids given
Evaluate:
• Therapeutic response: decreased symptoms of infection
Teach patient/family:
• To take with meals or immediately after meals
• To use sunglasses in bright sunlight to decrease photophobia
• That urine may turn rust or brown color
• To report hearing, visual problems; fever, fatigue, bruising, bleeding (may indicate blood dyscrasias)
• To keep away from pets, children; overdose is fatal
• **Pregnancy/breastfeeding:** to avoid use in pregnancy unless suppression of malaria is needed and benefits outweigh fetal risk; do not use in breastfeeding

TREATMENT OF OVERDOSE:
• Administer barbiturate (ultra-short-acting), vasopressor; tracheostomy may be necessary

chlorproMAZINE (Rx)
(klor-proe′ma-zeen)
Func. class.: Antipsychotic/antiemetic

Do not confuse:
chlorproMAZINE/chlorproPAMIDE/
prochlorperazine

USES: Psychotic disorders, mania, schizophrenia, anxiety, intractable hiccups in adults, nausea, vomiting; preoperatively for relaxation; acute intermittent porphyria, behavioral problems in children, nonpsychotic, demented patients, Tourette's syndrome

CONTRAINDICATIONS
Children <6 mo, hypersensitivity, circulatory collapse, liver damage, cerebral

arteriosclerosis, coronary disease, coma

Precautions: Pregnancy, breastfeeding, geriatric patients, seizure disorders, hypertension, hepatic/cardiac disease, prostatic enlargement, Parkinson's disease, pulmonary disease, severe hypo/hypertension, blood dyscrasias, brain damage, bone marrow depression, alcohol/barbiturate withdrawal, closed-angle glaucoma

Black Box Warning: Dementia; increased mortality in geriatric patients with dementia-related psychosis

DOSAGE AND ROUTES
Psychosis
• **Adult: PO** 10-50 mg q1-4hr initially then increase up to 2 g/day if necessary; **IM** 10-50 mg q1-4hr, usual dose 300-800 mg/day
• **Geriatric: PO** 10-25 mg daily-bid, increase by 10-25 mg/day q4-7days, max 800 mg/day
• **Child >6 mo: PO/IM** 0.56 mg/kg q4-6hr
Nausea and vomiting
• **Adult: PO** 10-25 mg q4-6hr prn; **IM** 12.5-25 mg q3hr prn, then 25-50 mg q6-8 hr prn if no hypotension, max 400 mg/day; **IV** 25-50 mg daily-qid
• **Child ≥6 mo: PO** 0.55 mg/kg q4-6hr; **IM** q6-8hr; **IM** ≤5 yr or ≤22.7 kg, 40 mg; max **IM** 5-10 yr or 22.7-45.5 kg, 75 mg
Intractable hiccups/acute intermittent porphyria
• **Adult: PO** 25-50 mg tid-qid; **IM** 25-50 mg (only if **PO** dose does not work); **IV** 25-50 mg in 500-1000 mL NS (only for severe hiccups)
Available forms: Tablets 10, 25, 50, 100, 200 mg; injection 25 mg/mL

cholestyramine (Rx)
(koe-less-tir′a-meen)
Prevalite
Func. class.: Antilipemic
Chem. class.: Bile acid sequestrant

ACTION: Adsorbs, combines with bile acids to form insoluble complex that is excreted through feces; loss of bile acids lowers LDL, cholesterol levels

USES: Primary hypercholesterolemia (esp. type IIa/IIb hyperlipoproteinemia), pruritus associated with biliary obstruction

CONTRAINDICATIONS
Hypersensitivity; complete biliary obstruction; hyperlipidemia III, IV, V
Precautions: Pregnancy, breastfeeding, children, PKU, renal disease, coagulopathy

DOSAGE AND ROUTES
• **Adult: PO** 4 g/day or bid, max 24 g/day
• **Child: PO** 240 mg/kg/day in 3 divided doses with food or drink, max 8 g/day titrated up over several weeks to decrease GI effects
Available forms: Powder for suspension 4 g cholestyramine/packet or scoop; tablet 1 g
Administer:
• Product daily or bid; give all other medications 1 hr prior to or 4-6 hr after cholestyramine to avoid poor absorption
• Product mixed with applesauce or stirred into beverage (2-6 oz), let stand for 2 min; do not take dry, avoid inhaling powder, avoid GI tube administration, take with food
• Supplemental doses of vitamin A, D, K if levels are low
• Doses are expressed in anhydrous cholestyramine resin; amount of resin varies with each product

SIDE EFFECTS
CNS: Headache, dizziness, drowsiness, vertigo, tinnitus, anxiety
GI: *Constipation, abdominal pain, nausea,* fecal impaction, hemorrhoids, flatulence, vomiting, steatorrhea, peptic ulcer
HEMA: Bleeding, increased PT
INTEG: Rash, irritation of perianal area, tongue, skin
META: Decreased vitamin A, D, K, red cell folate content; hyperchloremic acidosis

Side effects: *italics* = common; red = life-threatening

MS: Muscle, joint pain

PHARMACOKINETICS
PO: Excreted in feces, LDL lowered within 4-7 days, serum cholesterol lowered within 1 mo, duration 2-4 wk

INTERACTIONS
Decrease: absorption of warfarin, thiazides, cardiac glycosides, propranolol, corticosteroids, iron, thyroid hormones, acetaminophen, amiodarone, penicillin G, tetracyclines, clofibrate, gemfibrozil, oral vancomycin, glipiZIDE; vitamin A, D, E, K

Drug/Lab Test
Increase: AST, ALT, alkaline phosphatase
Decrease: sodium, potassium

NURSING CONSIDERATIONS
Assess:
• Cardiac glycoside level if both products administered, may need to adjust dose of cardiac glycoside if this product is increased or decreased
• For signs of vitamin A, D, K deficiency
• **Hypercholesterolemia:** fasting LDL, HDL, total cholesterol, triglyceride levels, electrolytes if receiving extended therapy; diet history
• **Pruritus:** for signs of itching
• Bowel pattern daily; increase bulk, water in diet for constipation; diarrhea may also occur
• **Pregnancy/breastfeeding:** no well-controlled studies; may decrease vitamin absorption (fat-soluble); use only if benefits outweigh fetal risks; cautious use in breastfeeding, vitamins may be decreased

Evaluate:
• Therapeutic response: decreased LDL, cholesterol level (hyperlipidemia); diarrhea, pruritus (excess bile acids)

Teach patient/family:
• **About the symptoms of hypoprothrombinemia:** bleeding mucous membranes, dark tarry stools, hematuria, petechiae; report immediately
• To take with food, never use dry
• That PKU patients should avoid Questran Light (contains aspartame and phenylalanine)
• About the importance of compliance

• That risk factors should be decreased: high-fat diet, smoking, alcohol consumption, absence of exercise
• That GI side effects will resolve with continued use

ciclesonide (inhalation/ intranasal) (Rx)
(si-cleh'son-ide)
Alvesco, Omnaris, Zetonna
Func. class.: Corticosteroid

ACTION: Inhibits inflammation in asthma by inhibiting leukotrienes

USES: Prevention of asthma during maintenance treatment, perennial/seasonal allergic rhinitis

CONTRAINDICATIONS
Hypersensitivity, nasal septic ulcers, nasal surgery, nasal trauma
Precautions: Children, TB, immunosuppression

DOSAGE AND ROUTES
Prevention of asthma (Alvesco)
• **Adult and child ≥12 yr in those previously taking bronchodilators alone: INH** 80 mcg bid, increase to max of 160 mcg bid after 4 wk, if needed
• **Adult and child ≥12 in those previously taking inhaled corticosteroids: INH** 80 mcg bid, increase to 320 mcg bid after 4 wk if needed
• **Adult and child ≥12 yr in those previously taking oral corticosteroids: INH** 320 mcg bid

Perennial allergic rhinitis
• **Adult and child ≥12 yr: Nasal** 2 sprays in each nostril daily (Omnaris) or 1 actuation (Zetonna) in each nostril daily

Seasonal allergic rhinitis
• **Adult and child ≥12 yr: Nasal** 1 actuation (Zetonna) in each nostril daily
• **Adult and child ≥6 yr: Nasal** 2 sprays (Omnaris) in each nostril daily

Available forms: Nasal aerosol solution 37 mcg/metered spray; **nasal suspension** 50 mcg/metered spray; **oral inhalation aerosol** 80 mcg, 160 mcg

C

Administer:
- Prime the inhaler before the initial use by releasing 3 sprays into the air away from the face and other people
- If the inhaler is not used for more than 10 consecutive days, it should be primed by releasing 3 sprays into the air
- The canister contains a dose counter. The inhaler should be discarded after the counter reads zero; although the canister is still operational and may contain medication, the accuracy of medication delivery cannot be assured
- When the dose indicator shows a red zone, approximately 20 inhalations are left, and a refill is required
- Instruct patient on proper inhalation technique
- To avoid the spread of infection, do not use the inhaler for more than 1 person

Intranasal inhalation administration Omnaris:
- For intranasal use only
- Before the first use, shake the inhaler gently and prime the pump by actuating 8 times
- If not used in 4 consecutive days, shake gently and prime with 1 spray or until fine mist appears
- Product should be discarded after 120 sprays following initial priming, or 4 mo after removal from pouch
- Blow nose gently if needed. Insert spray tip into nostril, and close the other nostril with finger. With head slightly tilted forward and bottle upright, press pump quickly and firmly while inhaling through nose. Avoid spraying into eyes and directly onto the nasal septum. After administration, wipe the applicator tip with a clean tissue and replace dust cap. If applicator is clogged or needs further cleaning, remove nasal applicator and rinse with warm water
- Dry and replace applicator and prime the unit with 1 spray or until a fine mist appears, then replace cap. To avoid the spread of infection, do not use the container for more than 1 person.

Zetonna:
- For intranasal use only

- Before the first use or if not used in 10 consecutive days, shake the inhaler gently and prime the pump by actuating 3 times
- Product should be discarded after 60 sprays following initial priming, or when the dose indicator reads zero
- Clean the nose piece weekly by wiping with a clean, dry tissue or cloth; do not wash or put any part of the canister or applicator in water
- Blow nose gently if needed. Insert spray tip into nostril, and close the other nostril with finger. With head slightly tilted back and bottle upright, press pump quickly and firmly while inhaling through nose. Avoid spraying into eyes and directly onto the nasal septum. To avoid the spread of infection, do not use the container for more than 1 person

Inhalation route
- Rinse mouth after use

Intranasal route
- Shake gently (Omnaris) before first use, then prime spraying 8 times, re-prime with 1 spray if not used for 4 days
- Before first use (Zetonna), prime spraying 3 times, reprime with 3 sprays if not used for 10 days

SIDE EFFECTS

CNS: *Headache*
EENT: *Ear pain, sinusitis, nasal congestion, nosebleed*
META: *Growth retardation if used long-term*
MS: *Arthralgia, back pain*

PHARMACOKINETICS

INH: onset >4 wk, peak 1 hr, duration unknown
Nasal: onset 1-2 days, peak 1-5 wk, unknown

INTERACTIONS

Increase: hyperglycemia—ceritinib
Increase: effect of desmopressin, avoid using together
Increase: effect of CYP3A4 inhibitors

NURSING CONSIDERATIONS
Assess:

• **Nasal condition:** assess for dryness, discharge, sneezing, cough
• **Anaphylaxis, angioedema (assess for rash, trouble breathing):** discontinue treatment and notify provider immediately
• **HPA suppression:** monitor children for growth suppression in long-term therapy

Patient/family education:

• Teach patient to take as prescribed, not to skip or double doses
• Teach patient and caregiver how to use
• Advise patient to discuss with provider all OTC, Rx, herbs, supplements taken
• Advise patient to notify provider if pregnancy is planned or suspected, or if breastfeeding
• Inform patient that continuing follow-up exams may be needed

---

cidofovir (Rx)
(si-doh-foh´veer)

Func. class.: Antiviral
Chem. class.: Nucleotide analog

ACTION: Suppresses cytomegalovirus (CMV) replication by selective inhibition of viral DNA synthesis

USES: CMV retinitis in patients with HIV; used with probenecid

CONTRAINDICATIONS

Hypersensitivity to this product, probenecid, sulfa products; direct intraocular injection; proteinuria, renal disease/failure

Precautions: Pregnancy, breastfeeding, children <6 mo, geriatric patients, pre-existing cytopenias, renal function impairment, platelet count <25,000/mm^3, dehydration

Black Box Warning: Neutropenia, infertility, secondary malignancy, pregnancy, nephrotoxicity, use only for CMV retinitis (AIDS)

DOSAGE AND ROUTES

• **Adult: IV INFUSION** Induction: 5 mg/kg over 1 hr weekly × 2 wk; maintenance: 5 mg/kg over 1 hr every other week, give with probenecid

Renal dose

• **Adult: IV** CCr ≤55 mL/min, do not use; CCr increase of 0.3-0.4 mg/dL above baseline, decrease dose to 3 mg/kg; CCr increase of ≥0.5 mg/dL above baseline or ≥2+ proteinuria, discontinue

Available forms: Injection 75 mg/mL
Administer:

Black Box Warning: Use cytotoxic handling procedures

• Allow to warm to room temperature
• If product comes in contact with skin, wash with soap and water immediately
• If zidovudine is used, reduce dose to 50% on cidofovir treatment days

Intermittent IV INFUSION route

• **Dilute** in 100 mL 0.9% saline solution before administration; **give** probenecid PO 2 g 3 hr prior to the cidofovir infusion and 1 g at 2 and 8 hr after ending the cidofovir infusion; **give** 1 L of 0.9% saline solution IV with each INFUSION of cidofovir, give saline INFUSION over 1-2 hr period immediately prior to cidofovir; patient should be given a second L if the patient can tolerate the fluid load (second L given at time of cidofovir or immediately afterward, should be given over 1-3 hr)
• **Give** slowly; do not give by bolus IV, SUBCUT injection
• Use diluted solution within 24 hr, do not freeze; do not use solution with particulate matter or discoloration
• Do not admix

SIDE EFFECTS

CNS: *Fever, chills,* coma, confusion, abnormal thoughts, *dizziness,* bizarre dreams, *headache,* psychosis, tremors, somnolence, paresthesia, *amnesia, anxiety, insomnia,* seizures

CV: Dysrhythmias, hypo/hypertension

EENT: Retinal detachment with CMV retinitis

GI: Abnormal LFTs, *nausea, vomiting, anorexia, diarrhea,* abdominal pain, hemorrhage
GU: Hematuria, increased creatinine, BUN, nephrotoxicity
HEMA: Granulocytopenia, thrombocytopenia, irreversible neutropenia, anemia, eosinophilia
INTEG: *Rash, alopecia, pruritus, acne,* urticaria, pain at injection site, phlebitis
RESP: Dyspnea

PHARMACOKINETICS
Terminal half-life 2.6 hr

INTERACTIONS

Black Box Warning: **Nephrotoxicity:** amphotericin B, foscarnet, aminoglycosides, pentamidine IV, NSAIDs, salicylates; wait 7 days after use to begin cidofovir

Drug/Lab
Increase: ALT, AST, alkaline phosphatase, glucose, cholesterol, BUN, creatinine, urine protein
Decrease: neutrophils, platelets, calcium, potassium

NURSING CONSIDERATIONS
Assess:
• Culture prior to initiating treatment; cultures of blood, urine, and throat may all be taken; CMV not confirmed by this method; diagnosis made by ophthalmic exam

Black Box Warning: Renal, hepatic, increased hemopoietic studies, BUN; serum creatinine, AST, ALT, creatinine, CCr, A-G ratio, baseline and drip treatment, blood counts q2wk; watch for decreasing granulocytes, HB; if low, discontinue and restart after recovery; blood transfusions may be required, renal failure can occur, Fanconi syndrome

• **For GI symptoms:** severe nausea, vomiting, diarrhea; severe symptoms may necessitate discontinuing product
• **Electrolytes and minerals:** calcium, phosphorus, magnesium, sodium, potassium; watch closely for tetany during first administration

Black Box Warning: **Blood dyscrasias** (anemia, granulocytopenia); bruising, fatigue, bleeding, poor healing; leukopenia, neutropenia, thrombocytopenia: WBCs, platelets q2days during 2×/day dosing and every week thereafter; check for leukopenias with daily WBC count in prior leukopenia, with other nucleoside analogs, or for leukopenia counts <1000 cells/mm^3 at start of treatment

• **Allergic reactions:** flushing, rash, urticaria, pruritus
• Monitor serum creatinine or CCr at least q2wk; give only to those with creatinine levels ≤1.5 mg/dL, CCr >55 mL/min, urine protein <100 mg/dL

Black Box Warning: **Pregnancy/breastfeeding:** may cause fetal harm; use only if benefits outweigh fetal risk; do not use in breastfeeding; use contraception during and for 1 mo after last dose; males should use barrier method during and for 90 days after last dose

Evaluate:
• Therapeutic response: decreased symptoms of CMV
Teach patient/family:
• To notify prescriber if sore throat, swollen lymph nodes, malaise, fever occur; may indicate other infections
• To report perioral tingling, numbness in extremities, paresthesias; report rash immediately, mental/vision changes, urinary problems, abnormal bleeding
• That serious product interactions may occur if OTC products are ingested; check with prescriber
• That product is not a cure but will control symptoms
• That regular ophthalmic exams, renal studies must be continued
• That major toxicities may necessitate discontinuing product
• To use contraception during treatment, that infertility may occur, and that men

should use barrier contraception for 90 days after treatment

TREATMENT OF OVERDOSE:
Discontinue product; use hemodialysis; increase hydration

⚠ HIGH ALERT

cilostazol (Rx)
(sih-los'tah-zol)
Func. class.: Platelet aggregation inhibitor
Chem. class.: Quinolinone derivative

ACTION: Multifactorial effects (antithrombotic, antiplatelet vasodilation)

USES: Intermittent claudication associated with PVD

CONTRAINDICATIONS
Hypersensitivity, acute MI, active bleeding conditions, hemostatic conditions

> **Black Box Warning:** HF

Precautions: Pregnancy, breastfeeding, children, geriatric patients, previous hepatic disease, cardiac/renal disease, increased bleeding risk, low platelet count, platelet dysfunction, smoking

DOSAGE AND ROUTES
• **Adult: PO** 100 mg bid or 50 mg bid if using products that inhibit CYP3A4 and CYP2C19
Available forms: Tablets 50, 100 mg
Administer:
• Give bid 30 min prior to or 2 hr after meals with a full glass of water; do not give with grapefruit juice

SIDE EFFECTS
CNS: *Dizziness, headache*
CV: *Palpitations, tachycardia,* postural hypotension, chest pain
GI: *Nausea,* vomiting, *diarrhea,* GI discomfort, colitis, cholelithiasis, ulcer, esophagitis, gastritis, anorexia, *flatulence, dyspepsia*

INTEG: *Rash,* Stevens-Johnson syndrome
RESP: *Cough, pharyngitis, rhinitis*

PHARMACOKINETICS
95%-98% protein binding; metabolism: hepatic extensively by CYP3A4, 2C19 enzymes (active metabolite); excreted in urine (74%), feces (20%); half-life 11-13 hr

INTERACTIONS
Increase: bleeding tendencies—anticoagulants, NSAIDs, thrombolytics, abciximab, eptifibatide, tirofiban, ticlopidine
Increase: cilostazol levels—CYP3A4, CYP2C19 inhibitors; dilTIAZem, erythromycin, clarithromycin, verapamil, protease inhibitors, omeprazole; exercise caution when coadministering with fluvoxaMINE, FLUoxetine, ketoconazole, isoniazid, gemfibrozil, omeprazole, itraconazole, voriconazole, fluconazole; reduce dose to 50 mg bid
Decrease: cilostazol levels—CYP3A4 inducers

> **Black Box Warning: Decrease:** survival rates—when used with phosphodiesterase III inhibitors (milrinone) in those with heart failure class III, IV

Drug/Herb
Decrease: action—chamomile, coenzyme Q10, feverfew, garlic, ginger, ginkgo biloba, flax, goldenseal, St. John's wort
Drug/Food
• Do not use with grapefruit juice; toxicity may occur
Increase: cilostazol action—fatty meal; avoid giving with food

NURSING CONSIDERATIONS
Assess:

> **Black Box Warning:** For underlying CV disease because CV risk is great; for CV lesions with repeated oral administration; do not administer to patients with HF of any severity; for severe headache, signs of toxicity

• Blood studies: CBC q2wk, Hct, HB, PT

- **Beers:** avoid in older adults; may promote fluid retention and/or exacerbate heart failure

Evaluate:

- Therapeutic response: improved walking distance, duration; decreased pain

Teach patient/family:

- To avoid hazardous activities until effect is known; dizziness may occur
- To report any unusual bleeding
- To report side effects such as diarrhea, skin rashes, subcutaneous bleeding
- That effects may take 2-4 wk; treatment of up to 12 wk may be required for necessary effect
- That reading the patient package insert is necessary
- That it is best to discontinue tobacco use, not to use grapefruit juice
- That there are many drug and herb interactions; to obtain approval from prescriber before use

---

cimetidine (OTC, Rx)

(sye-met'i-deen)

Tagamet HB

Func. class.: H₂-histamine receptor antagonist

Chem. class.: Imidazole derivative

ACTION: Inhibits histamine at H₂-receptor site in the gastric parietal cells, which inhibits gastric acid secretion

USES: Short-term treatment of duodenal and gastric ulcers and maintenance; management of GERD (PO) and Zollinger-Ellison syndrome; prevention of upper GI bleeding; prevent, relieve heartburn, acid indigestion

CONTRAINDICATIONS

Hypersensitivity to this product, H₂ blockers, benzyl alcohol

Precautions: Pregnancy, breastfeeding, children <16 yr, geriatric patients, organic brain syndrome, renal/hepatic disease

DOSAGE AND ROUTES
Short-term treatment of active ulcers

- **Adult/adolescents ≥16 yr:** PO 300 mg qid × 8-12 wk or 400 mg bid × 8 wk
- **Child:** PO 20-40 mg/kg/day, divided q6hr

Prophylaxis of duodenal ulcer

- **Adult and child >16 yr:** PO 400 mg at bedtime or 300 mg bid

GERD

- **Adult:** PO 800-1600 mg/day in divided doses × up to 12 wk

Hypersecretory conditions (Zollinger-Ellison syndrome)

- **Adult:** PO 300-600 mg q6hr; max 2400 mg/day

Heartburn

- **Adult/child ≥12 yr:** PO 200 mg up to bid, may use before eating, max 400 mg/day, max daily use up to 2 wk

Renal disease

- **Adult:** PO CCr <30 mL/min, 300 mg q12hr

Available forms: Tablets 100, 300, 400, 800 mg; oral liquid 300 mg/5 mL

Administer:

PO route

- With meals for prolonged product effect; antacids 1 hr prior to or 1 hr after cimetidine

SIDE EFFECTS

CNS: *Confusion, headache,* depression, dizziness, psychosis

CV: Bradycardia, tachycardia, dysrhythmias

GI: *Diarrhea,* abdominal cramps

GU: Gynecomastia, galactorrhea, impotence, increase in BUN, creatinine

INTEG: Urticaria, rash

RESP: Pneumonia

PHARMACOKINETICS

Half-life 1½-2 hr; 30%-40% metabolized by liver, excreted in urine (unchanged), crosses placenta, enters breast milk

PO: Onset 30 min, peak 45-90 min; duration 4-5 hr, well absorbed

---

INTERACTIONS

Increase: toxicity due to CYP450 pathway—benzodiazepines, beta-blockers, calcium channel blockers, carBAMazepine, chloroquine, lidocaine, metroNIDAZOLE, moricizine, phenytoin, quiNIDine, quiNINE, sulfonylureas, theophylline, tricyclics, valproic acid, warfarin

Increase: bone marrow suppression—carmustine

Decrease: absorption of cimetidine—antacids, sucralfate

Decrease: absorption—ketoconazole, itraconazole

Drug/Lab Test

Increase: alkaline phosphatase, AST, creatinine, prolactin

False positive: gastroccult, hemoccult tests

False negative: TB skin tests

NURSING CONSIDERATIONS

Assess:

• **Ulcer symptoms:** epigastric pain, duration, intensity; aggravating, ameliorating factors; blood in stools; emesis

• **Beers:** avoid in older adults with delirium or at high risk for delirium, adverse CNS reactions

Evaluate:

• Therapeutic response: decreased pain in abdomen; healing of ulcers; absence of gastroesophageal reflux; gastric pH of 5

Teach patient/family:

• That gynecomastia, impotence may occur, are reversible

• To avoid driving, other hazardous activities until stabilized on this medication; drowsiness or dizziness may occur

• To avoid OTC preparations: aspirin; cough, cold preparations; condition may worsen; OTC therapy is used for short term (2 wk)

• Not to smoke because smoking decreases effectiveness of product

• That product must be taken exactly as prescribed and continued for prescribed time to be effective; not to double dose; if taking OTC, not to take maximum dose >2 wk unless directed by prescriber

• To report diarrhea, black tarry stools, sore throat, rash, dizziness, confusion, delirium to prescriber

• To use increased fluids, bulk in diet to decrease constipation

• **Pregnancy/breastfeeding:** to report if pregnancy is planned or suspected or if breastfeeding, avoid breastfeeding

---

cinacalcet (Rx)

(sin-a-kal'set)

Sensipar

Func. class.: Hyperparathyroidism agent, calcium receptor agonist

Chem. class.: Polypeptide hormone

ACTION: Directly lowers PTH levels by increasing sensitivity of calcium-sensing receptors to extracellular calcium

USES: Hypercalcemia with parathyroid carcinoma, secondary hyperparathyroidism with chronic kidney disease for patient on dialysis, primary hyperparathyroidism

CONTRAINDICATIONS

Hypersensitivity, hypocalcemia

Precautions: Pregnancy, breastfeeding, children, seizure disorders, hepatic disease

DOSAGE AND ROUTES

Parathyroid carcinoma

• **Adult: PO** 30 mg bid, titrate q2-4wk, with sequential doses of 30 mg bid, 60 mg bid, 90 mg bid, 90 mg tid-qid to normalize calcium levels

Secondary hyperparathyroidism

• **Adult: PO** 30 mg/day, titrate no more frequently than q2-4wk with sequential doses of 30, 60, 90, 120, 180 mg/day

Primary hyperparathyroidism

• **Adult: PO** 30 mg bid, titrate q2-4wk to target calcium levels

Available forms: Tablets 30, 60, 90 mg

Administer:

• Swallow tablets whole; do not break, crush, or chew; use with food or right after a meal

• Can be used alone or in combination with vitamin D sterols, phosphate binders

• Storage at <77° F (25° C)

Chronic kidney disease: Titrate q2-4wk to target iPTH consistent with National Kidney Foundation–Kidney Disease Outcomes Quality Initiative (NKF-K/DOQI) for chronic kidney disease patient on dialysis of 150-300 pg/mL; if iPTH <150-300 pg/mL, reduce dose of cinacalcet and/or vitamin D sterols or discontinue treatment

SIDE EFFECTS

CNS: Dizziness, asthenia, seizures, paresthesia, fatigue, headache
CV: Dysrhythmia hypotension
GI: Nausea, diarrhea, vomiting, anorexia, constipation
MISC: Infection, dehydration, hypercalcemia, anemia, hypocalcemia
MS: Myalgia, bone fractures binding

PHARMACOKINETICS

93%-97% plasma; proteins metabolized by CYP3A4, 2D6, 1A2; half-life 30-40 hr; renal excretion of metabolites (80% renal, 15% in feces)

INTERACTIONS

Increase: cinacalcet levels—CYP3A4 inhibitors (ketoconazole, erythromycin, itraconazole), dose may need to be reduced
Increase: levels of CYP2D6 inhibitors (flecainide, vinBLAStine, thioridazine, tricyclics)
Drug/Food
Increase: action by high-fat meal

NURSING CONSIDERATIONS
Assess:

• **Hypocalcemia:** cramping, seizures, tetany, myalgia, paresthesia; calcium, phosphorous within 1 wk and iPTH 1-4 wk after initiation or dosage adjustment when maintenance established; measure calcium, phosphorus monthly; iPTH q1-3mo, target range 150-300 pg/mL for iPTH level; biochemical markers of bone formation/resorption; radiologic evidence of fracture; serum testosterone
• **Renal disease (without dialysis):** these patients should not receive treatment with this product; high risk of hypocalcemia
• Liver studies in those with liver disease
• If calcium <8.4 mg/dL, do not start; if calcium is 7.5-8.4 mg/dL, give calcium-containing phosphate binders, vitamin D sterols to increase calcium; if calcium <7.5 mg/dL or if symptoms of hypocalcemia continue and vitamin D cannot be increased, withhold until calcium reaches 8.0 mg/dL, symptoms resolve, start product at next lowest dose
• **Pregnancy/breastfeeding:** no well-controlled studies, use only if benefits outweigh fetal risk; those who are pregnant should enroll in Amgen's Pregnancy Surveillance Program (800-772-6436); discontinue breastfeeding or product, it is unknown if excreted in breast milk
Evaluate:
• Therapeutic response: calcium levels 9-10 mg/dL, decreasing symptoms of hypercalcemia
Teach patient/family:
• To take with food or shortly after a meal; to take tablets whole, not to take any other meds, supplements without prescriber approval
• **Hypocalcemia:** to report cramping, seizures, muscle pain, tingling, tetany immediately
• To continue exams and lab work

ciprofloxacin (Rx)
(sip-ro-floks′a-sin)
Cipro
Func. class.: Antiinfective—broad spectrum
Chem. class.: Fluoroquinolone

Do not confuse:
ciprofloxacin/cephalexin

ACTION: Interferes with conversion of intermediate DNA fragments into high-molecular-weight DNA in bacteria; DNA gyrase inhibitor

USES: Infection caused by susceptible *Escherichia coli, Enterobacter cloacae, Proteus mirabilis, Klebsiella pneumoniae, Proteus vulgaris, Citrobacter freundii, Serratia marcescens, Pseudomonas aeruginosa, Staphylococcus aureus, Staphylococcus epidermidis, Enterobacter, Campylobacter*

jejuni, Salmonella, Streptococcus pyogenes, Bacillus anthracias; chronic bacterial prostatitis, acute sinusitis, postexposure inhalation anthrax, infectious diarrhea, typhoid fever, complicated intraabdominal infections, nosocomial pneumonia, urinary tract infections, plague

CONTRAINDICATIONS

Hypersensitivity to quinolones

Precautions: Pregnancy, breastfeeding, children, geriatric patients, renal disease, seizure disorder, stroke, CV disease, hepatic disease, QT prolongation, hypokalemia, colitis

Black Box Warning: Tendon pain/rupture, tendinitis, myasthenia gravis, nephrotoxicity

DOSAGE AND ROUTES
Uncomplicated urinary tract infections

• **Adult: PO** 250 mg q12hr × 3 days or **XL** 500 mg q24hr × 3 days

Mild-moderate UTI

• **Adult: PO** 250 mg q12hr or **IV** 200 mg q12hr × 7-14 days

Complicated/severe urinary tract infections

• **Adult: PO** 500 mg q12hr or **XL** 1000 mg q24hr × 7-14 days; **IV** 400 mg q12hr
• **Child/adolescent: PO** 10-20 mg/kg/ dose q12hr × 10-21 days; not first choice in pediatric patients due to high incidence of adverse reactions

Respiratory, bone, skin, joint infections (mild-moderate)

• **Adult: PO** 500-750 mg q12hr × 7-14 days; **IV** 400 mg q12hr

Nosocomial pneumonia

• **Adult: IV** 400 mg q8hr × 10-14 days

Intraabdominal infections, complicated

• **Adult: PO** 500 mg q12hr × 7-14 days; **IV** 400 mg q12hr × 7-14 days, usually given with metroNIDAZOLE

Acute sinusitis, mild/moderate

• **Adult: PO** 500 mg q12hr × 10 days; **IV** 400 mg q12hr × 10 days

Inhalational anthrax (postexposure)

• **Adult: PO** 500 mg q12hr × 60 days; **IV** 400 mg q12hr × 60 days
• **Child: PO** 15 mg/kg/dose q12hr × 60 days, max 500 mg/dose; **IV** 10 mg/kg q12hr, max 400 mg/dose

Plague

• **Adult: IV** 400 mg q8-12hr or 500-750 mg q12hr × 14 days
• **Child 1-17 yr: IV** 10 mg/kg or **PO** 15 mg/kg q8-12hr × 10-21 days

Infectious diarrhea

• **Adult: PO** 500-750 mg q12hr × 5-7 days

Chronic bacterial prostatitis

• **Adult: PO** 500 mg q12hr × 28 days; **IV** 400 mg q12hr × 28 days

Renal disease

• **Adult:** CCr 30-50 mL/min, **PO** 250-500 mg q12hr; CCr 5-29 mL/min, **PO** 250-500 mg q18hr, **IV** 200-400 mg q18-24hr

Available forms: Tablets 100, 250, 500, 750 mg; extended-release tablets (XR) 500, 1000 mg; injection 200 mg/100 mL D_5W; 400 mg/200 mL D_5W; injection 200, 400 mg; oral suspension 250 mg, 500 mg/5 mL

Administer:

• Obtain C&S before use, may give first dose before results are received
• Use caution when giving with antidysrhythmics IA, III

PO route

• Do not break, crush, chew XR (extended release) product, use adequate fluids to prevent stalluria
• Regular release and extended release are not interchangeable
• 2 hr prior to or 6 hr after antacids, zinc, iron, calcium
• Do not give oral suspension by GI tube
• Use adequate fluids to prevent crystalluria

IV route

• Over 1 hr as an infusion, comes in premixed plastic infusion container or diluted 20- or 40-mL vial to a final concentration of 0.5-2 mg/mL of NS or D_5W; give through Y-tube or 3-way stopcock, diluted vials can be stored for 14 days at room temperature or refrigerator; do not freeze

Y-site compatibilities: Amifostine, anakinra, anidulafungin, argatroban, arsenic, atenolol, aztreonam, bivalirudin, bleomycin, calcium gluconate, CARBOplatin, caspofungin, cefTAZidime, cisatracurium, CISplatin, clarithromycin, codeine, cytarabine, DACTINomycin, DAPTOmycin, dexmedetomidine, digoxin, diltiaZEM, diphenhydrAMINE, DOBUTamine, DOCEtaxel, doripenem, DOPamine, doxacurium, DOXOrubicin, epiRUBicin, eptifibatide, ertapenem, etoposide, fenoldopam, fludarabine, gallium, gemcitabine, gentamicin, granisetron, HYDROmorphone, hydrOXYzine, IDArubicin, ifosfamide, irinotecan, lidocaine, linezolid, LORazepam, LR, mechlorethamine, meperidine, methotrexate, metoclopramide, metroNIDAZOLE, midazolam, midodrine, milrinone, mitoXANTRONE, mycophenolate, nesiritide, octreotide, ondansetron, oxaliplatin, oxytocin, PACLitaxel, palonosetron, pamidronate, pancuronium, piperacillin, potassium acetate/chloride, promethazine, raNITIdine, remifentanil, rocuronium, sodium chloride, tacrolimus, teniposide, thiotepa, tigecycline, tirofiban, TNA, tobramycin, trastuzumab, vasopressin, vecuronium, verapamil, vinCRIStine, vinorelbine, voriconazole

SIDE EFFECTS
CNS: *Headache,* dizziness, fatigue, insomnia, depression, *restlessness,* seizures, suicidal ideation, pseudotumor cerebri, confusion, hallucinations
GI: *Nausea, diarrhea,* increased ALT/AST, flatulence, *vomiting,* abdominal pain, pancreatitis, hepatotoxicity, CDAD
GU: Vaginitis
INTEG: *Rash,* pruritus, urticaria, photosensitivity, toxic epidermal necrolysis, injection site reactions
MISC: Anaphylaxis, Stevens-Johnson syndrome, QT prolongation, pseudotumor cerebri
MS: Arthralgia, tendon rupture
META: Hypo- and hyperglycemia

PHARMACOKINETICS
PO: Peak 1-2 hr; half-life 4 hr; excreted in urine as active product, metabolites 35%-40%, 20%-40% protein binding

INTERACTIONS

Black Box Warning: Increase: tendinitis, tendon rupture—corticosteroids

Increase: nephrotoxicity—cycloSPORINE
Increase: ciprofloxacin levels—probenecid; monitor for toxicity
Increase: levels of theophylline, warfarin; monitor blood levels, reduce dose
Increase: hypoglycemia risk—antidiabetics
Increase: QT prolongation—astemizole, droperidol, class IA/III antidysrhythmics, tricyclics, tetracyclines, local anesthetics, phenothiazines, haloperidol, risperiDONE, sertindole, ziprasidone, alfuzosin, arsenic trioxide, beta-agonists, chloroquine, cloZAPine, cyclobenzapine, dasatinib, dolasetron, droperidol, flecainide, halogenated anesthetics, lapatinib, levomethadyl, macrolides, methadone, octreotide, ondansetron, paliperidone, palonosetron, pentamidine, propafenone, ranolazine, SUNitinib, tacrolimus, terfenadine, vardenafil, vorinostat; less likely than other quinolones
Decrease: ciprofloxacin absorption—antacids that contain magnesium, aluminum; zinc, iron, sucralfate, enteral feedings, calcium, sevelamer
Drug/Food
Increase: effect of caffeine
Decrease: absorption—dairy products, food
Drug/Lab Test
Increase: AST, ALT, BUN, creatinine, LDH, bilirubin, alkaline phosphatase, glucose, proteinuria, albuminuria
Decrease: WBC, glucose

NURSING CONSIDERATIONS
Assess:
• **Infection:** WBC, temperature before treatment, periodically
• **QT prolongation:** monitor for changes in QTc if taking other products that increase QT

Black Box Warning: Myasthenia gravis: avoid use in these patients, increases muscle weakness

• **CNS symptoms:** headache, dizziness, fatigue, insomnia, depression, seizures
• Renal, hepatic studies: BUN, creatinine, AST, ALT
• I&O ratio, urine pH <5.5 is ideal, to prevent crystalluria

Black Box Warning: Tendinitis, tendon rupture: discontinue at first sign of tendon pain, inflammation; increased in those >60 yr, those taking corticosteroids, organ transplants and children

• **Anaphylaxis:** fever, flushing, rash, urticaria, pruritus, dyspnea; discontinue immediately, have emergency equipment nearby
• **Pseudotumor cerebri:** may occur at excessive doses
• **Hepatotoxicity:** report immediately dark urine, jaundice, pruritus, clay-colored stools
• Limited intake of alkaline foods, products: milk, dairy products, alkaline antacids, sodium bicarbonate; caffeine intake if excessive cardiac or CNS stimulation
• Increase fluids to 3 L/day to avoid crystallization in kidneys
• **Clostridium difficile–associated diarrhea (CDAD):** monitor for diarrhea, abdominal pain, cramps, fever, bloody stools; usually occurs several weeks after completion of therapy; report to prescriber immediately
• **Pregnancy/breastfeeding:** no well-controlled studies; use in pregnancy only if benefits outweigh fetal risk; excreted in breast milk, discontinue breastfeeding or discontinue product
Evaluate:
• Therapeutic response: decreased pain, frequency, urgency, C&S; absence of infection
Teach patient/family:
• Not to take any products that contain magnesium, calcium (such as antacids), iron, aluminum with this product or 2 hr before, 6 hr after product; to drink fluids to prevent crystals in urine; not to crush, chew the extended-release product

Black Box Warning: To report tendon pain, chest pain, palpitations

• To complete full course of product therapy; not to double or miss doses
• To notify prescriber if rash occurs; discontinue product
• To notify prescriber if pregnancy is planned or suspected; not to breastfeed
• **Suicidal thoughts/behaviors:** To report immediately, suicidal thoughts, behaviors
• To contact prescriber if taking theophylline, warfarin
• That extended-release and regular-release products are not interchangeable
• Not to add or stop products without prescriber's approval
• To use calibrated measuring device for suspension

ciprofloxacin (ophthalmic) (Rx)

(sip-roe-flox′a-sin)

Ciloxan

Func. class.: Ophthalmic antiinfective

Do not confuse:
ciprofloxacin/gatifloxacin/levoFLOXAcin/moxifloxacin/ofloxacin

USES: Corneal ulcers, bacterial conjunctivitis

CONTRAINDICATIONS

Hypersensitivity to this product or fluoroquinolones
Precautions: Pregnancy, breastfeeding

DOSAGE AND ROUTES
Bacterial conjunctivitis
• **Adult/adolescent/child ≥1 yr: Ophthalmic (solution):** 1-2 drops in affected eye(s) every 2 hr while awake × 2 days, then every 4 hr while awake for the next 5 days
• **Adult/adolescent/child ≥2 yr: Ophthalmic (ointment):** ½-inch ribbon to conjunctival sac tid × 2 days, then ½ inch bid for next 5 days

Ophthalmic infection associated with corneal ulcer

• **Adult/adolescent/child ≥1 yr: Ophthalmic (solution):** 2 drops in affected eye(s) every 15 min × 6 hr, then every 30 min for the remainder of the first day; for the second day, 2 drops every hr; for days 3-14, 2 drops every 4 hr

---

⚠ HIGH ALERT

cisatracurium (Rx)

(sis-ah-trah-kyoo´ree-um)

Nimbex

Func. class.: Skeletal muscle relaxant
Chem. class.: Nondepolarizing neuromuscular blocker

ACTION: Antagonizes acetylcholine by binding to cholinergic receptors on the motor end plate, resulting in neuromuscular blockade

USES: To maintain neuromuscular blockade during mechanical ventilation and as an adjunct to general anesthesia

CONTRAINDICATIONS

Hypersensitivity

Precautions: Pregnancy, breastfeeding, children, benzyl alcohol hypersensitivity, electrolyte imbalances, long-term use in ICU, trauma, or burns, dehydration, metabolic alkalosis, respiratory acidosis, myopathy, myasthenia gravis

DOSAGE AND ROUTES
Endotracheal intubation

• **Adult/adolescent (healthy):** IV 0.15-0.2 mg/kg, 1 time; CABG surgery with induced hypothermia use 50% of dose
• **Adult with myasthenia gravis:** IV use peripheral nerve stimulator monitoring and an initial dose ≤0.02 mg/kg
• **Child 2-12 yr:** IV 0.1-0.15 mg/kg over 5-10 sec during either halothane or opioid anesthesia
• **Infant/child ≤23 mo:** IV 0.15 mg/kg over 5-10 sec during either halothane or opioid anesthesia

To maintain neuromuscular blockade during prolonged surgical procedures:

• **Adult/adolescent/child ≥2 yr (healthy):** IV maintenance dose 0.03 mg/kg; maintenance dosing is generally required 40-50 min after an initial dose of 0.15 mg/kg IV or 50-60 min after an initial dose of 0.2 mg/kg; the need for maintenance doses should be determined by clinical criteria; max 0.02 mg/kg/min (neuromuscular disease)

Available forms: Injection solution 2, 10 mg/mL

Administer:
IV route
• Visually inspect for particulate matter and discoloration before use
• Only experienced clinicians, familiar with the use of neuromuscular blocking drugs, should administer or supervise the use of this product
• Use by rapid IV injection or by continuous IV infusion

IV INFUSION route
• Inject IV over 5-10 sec

Continuous IV INFUSION route
• Dilute with NS, D₅W, or D₅NS (0.1-0.4 mg/mL); adjust the rate of infusion according to peripheral nerve stimulation
• The amount of infusion solution required per minute depends on the concentration of cisatracurium in the infusion solution, the desired dose of cisatracurium, and the patient's weight
• Store Nimbex injection diluted to 0.1 mg/mL either under refrigeration or at room temperature for 24 hr; dilutions to 0.1 mg/mL or 0.2 mg/mL in D₅W/LR injection may be stored under refrigeration for 24 hr
• Not an analgesic, treat pain with other agents

SIDE EFFECTS

CV: Bradycardia, *flushing,* hypotension
RESP: *Apnea,* bronchospasm, prolonged neuromuscular block

PHARMACOKINETICS

Onset 2 min, peak 3-5 min, duration 25-44 min, half-life 22-30 min

---

INTERACTIONS

Increase: neuromuscular blockade—aminoglycosides, clindamycin, lithium, local anesthetics, magnesium salts, colistin, colistimethate, procainamide, quiNIDine, tetracyclines, bacitracin, capreomycin, polymyxin B, vancomycin; amphotericin B, CISplatin, corticosteroids, loop/thiazide diuretics (if hypokalemia is present)

Decrease: neuromuscular blockade—carBAMazepine, phenytoin; dose of cisatracurium may need to be increased

NURSING CONSIDERATIONS
Assess:

• **Neuromuscular function:** use nerve stimulator to monitor neuromuscular function; if no response, stop until response; not to be used for rapid-sequence endotracheal intubation

• **Sedation/pain:** those undergoing neuromuscular blockage (paralytics) must receive treatment with sedative and pain control before and during therapy

• **Electrolytes:** electrolytes and acid-base balance may be altered

• **Malignant hyperthermia:** those with a family history of malignant hyperthermia should not receive this product or it should be used cautiously

• **Pregnancy/breastfeeding:** no well-controlled studies; use in pregnancy only if benefits outweigh fetal risk; use caution in breastfeeding; excretion is unknown

Evaluate:

• Maintenance of neuromuscular blockade

Teach patient/family:

• Reason for product and expected results

⚠ HIGH ALERT

CISplatin (Rx)

(sis′pla-tin)
Func. class.: Antineoplastic alkylating agent
Chem. class.: Platinum complex

Do not confuse:
CISplatin/CARBOplatin

ACTION: Alkylates DNA, RNA; inhibits enzymes that allow for the synthesis of amino acids in proteins; activity not cell cycle–phase specific

USES: Advanced bladder cancer; adjunct in metastatic testicular cancer; adjunct in metastatic ovarian cancer, head and neck, lung cancer

CONTRAINDICATIONS
Pregnancy, breastfeeding

Black Box Warning: Bone marrow suppression, platinum compound hypersensitivity

Precautions: Geriatric patients, vaccination, infections, extravasation, peripheral neuropathy, radiation therapy

Black Box Warning: Chemotherapy-induced nausea/vomiting, children, nephrotoxicity, ototoxicity; requires a specialized care setting and an experienced clinician, peripheral neuropathy

DOSAGE AND ROUTES
Dosage protocols may vary
Metastatic testicular cancer
• **Adult: IV** 20 mg/m^2/day × 5 days, repeat q3wk for 2 cycles or more, depending on response
Advanced bladder cancer
• **Adult: IV** 50-70 mg/m^2 q3-4wk, use 50 mg/m^2 q4wk in those who have been pretreated with radiation/other antineoplastics
Metastatic ovarian cancer
• **Adult: IV** 100 mg/m^2 q4wk or 75-100 mg/m^2 q3wk with cyclophosphamide
Hodgkin's/non-Hodgkin's lymphoma (unlabeled)
• **Adult/child: IV INFUSION** 100 mg/m^2 24 hr continuous infusion day 1 of 4-day regimen with cytarabine/dexamethasone q3-4wk
Gastric cancer (unlabeled)
• **Adult: IV** 75 mg/m^2 on day 1 with DOCEtaxel 75 mg/m^2 and fluorouracil 750 mg/m^2 on days 1-5, q21days
Available forms: Injection 1 mg/mL

Administer:
IV route
• Do not use aluminum equipment during any preparation or administration, will form precipitate; do not refrigerate unopened powder or solution; protect from sunlight
• Prepare in biologic cabinet using gown, gloves, mask; do not allow product to come in contact with skin; use soap and water if contact occurs; use cytotoxic handling procedures
• Do not use with neuromuscular blockers, fatal
• Hydrate patient with 1-2 L 0.9% NaCl over 8-12 hr before treatment

Black Box Warning: Use EPINEPHrine, antihistamines, corticosteroids immediately for hypersensitivity reaction

• Antiemetic 30-60 min prior to product and prn; allopurinol to maintain uric acid levels, alkalinization of urine; diuretic (furosemide 40 mg IV) or mannitol after infusion
Intermittent IV INFUSION route
• Check solution for particulate and color, do not use if present or if discolored
• **Dilute** 10 mg/10 mL or 50 mg/50 mL sterile water for injection, withdraw prescribed dose; **dilute** ½ dose with 1000 mL D₅0.2NaCl, D₅0.45NaCl with 37.5 g mannitol; IV INFUSION is **given** over 3-4 hr; use a 0.45-µm filter; total dose 2 L over 6-8 hr; check site for irritation, phlebitis
• **For extravasation (vesicant):** Use 4 mL sodium thiosulfate 10%/6 mL sterile water, inject 1-4 mL through current line
Continuous IV INFUSION route
• **Give** over 24 hr × 5 days

Y-site compatibilities: Acyclovir, alfentanil, allopurinol, amikacin, aminophylline, amiodarone, ampicillin, ampicillin-sulbactam, anidulafungin, atenolol, atracurium, azithromycin, aztreonam, bivalirudin, bleomycin, bumetanide, buprenorphine, butorphanol, calcium chloride/gluconate, carmustine, caspofungin, ceFAZolin, cefoperazone, cefotaxime, cefoTEtan, cefOXitin, cefTAZidime, ceftizoxime, cefTRIAXone, cefuroxime, chlorproMAZINE, cimetidine, ciprofloxacin, cisatracurium, cladribine, clindamycin, codeine, cyclophosphamide, cycloSPORINE, cytarabine, DACTINomycin, DAPTOmycin, DAUNOrubicin, dexamethasone, dexmedetomidine, dexrazoxane, digoxin, diltiaZEM, diphenhydrAMINE, DOBUTamine, DOCEtaxel, DOPamine, doripenem, doxacurium, DOXOrubicin, DOXOrubicin liposomal, doxycycline, droperidol, enalaprilat, ePHEDrine, EPINEPHrine, epiRUBicin, ertapenem, erythromycin, esmolol, etoposide, famotidine, fenoldopam, fentaNYL, filgrastim, fluconazole, fludarabine, fluorouracil, foscarnet, fosphenytoin, furosemide, ganciclovir, gatifloxacin, gemcitabine, gentamicin, glycopyrrolate, granisetron, haloperidol, heparin, hydrocortisone, HYDROmorphone, IDArubicin, ifosfamide, imipenem-cilastatin, inamrinone, indomethacin, irinotecan, isoproterenol, ketorolac, labetalol, leucovorin, levoFLOXacin, levorphanol, lidocaine, linezolid, LORazepam, magnesium sulfate, mannitol, melphalan, meperidine, meropenem, methohexital, methotrexate, methylPREDNISolone, metoclopramide, metoprolol, metroNIDAZOLE, midazolam, milrinone, minocycline, mitoMYcin, mitoXANTRONE, mivacurium, nafcillin, naloxone, nesiritide, niCARdipine, nitroglycerin, nitroprusside, norepinephrine, octreotide, ofloxacin, ondansetron, oxaliplatin, PACLitaxel, palonosetron, pamidronate, pancuronium, PEMEtrexed, pentamidine, pentazocine, PENTobarbital, PHENobarbital, phenylephrine, phenytoin, piperacillin, polymyxin B, potassium chloride/phosphates, procainamide, prochlorperazine, promethazine, propofol, propranolol, quiNIDine, quinupristin-dalfopristin, raNITIdine, remifentanil, riTUXimab, sargramostim, sodium acetate/bicarbonate/phosphates, succinylcholine, SUFentanil, sulfamethoxazole-trimethoprim, tacrolimus, teniposide, theophylline, thiopental, ticarcillin, ticarcillin-clavulanate, tigecycline, tirofiban, TNA, tobramycin, topotecan, trastuzumab, vancomycin, vasopressin, vecuronium, verapamil, vinBLAStine, vinCRIStine, vinorelbine, voriconazole, zidovudine, zoledronic acid

---

Side effects: *italics* = common; red = life-threatening

SIDE EFFECTS

CNS: Seizures, *peripheral neuropathy*
EENT: *Tinnitus, hearing loss, vestibular toxicity,* blurred vision, altered color perception
GI: *Severe nausea, vomiting, diarrhea, weight loss,* hepatotoxicity
GU: Renal tubular damage, *renal insufficiency,* sterility
HEMA: Thrombocytopenia, leukopenia, pancytopenia, *anemia*
INTEG: *Alopecia,* dermatitis
META: *Hypomagnesemia, hypocalcemia, hypokalemia*
RESP: Fibrosis
SYST: Anaphylaxis

PHARMACOKINETICS

Absorption complete, metabolized in liver, excreted in urine, half-life 30-90 min, accumulates in body tissues for several months, enters breast milk

INTERACTIONS

Increase: bleeding risk—aspirin, NSAIDs, alcohol
Increase: myelosuppression—myelosuppressive agents, radiation
Increase: nephrotoxicity—aminoglycosides, loop diuretics, salicylates
Decrease: effects of phenytoin
Decrease: antibody response—live virus vaccines
Decrease: potassium, magnesium levels—loop diuretics

Drug/Lab Test
Increase: uric acid, BUN, creatinine
Decrease: CCr, calcium, phosphate, potassium, magnesium
Positive: Coombs' test

NURSING CONSIDERATIONS
Assess:
• Monitor vital signs often during infusion

Black Box Warning: Bone marrow depression: CBC, differential, platelet count weekly; withhold product if WBC is <4000 or platelet count is <100,000; notify prescriber of results

Black Box Warning: Renal toxicity: BUN, creatinine, serum uric acid, urine CCr prior to, electrolytes during therapy; dose should not be given if BUN <25 mg/dL; creatinine <1.5 mg/dL; I&O ratio; report fall in urine output of <30 mL/hr; toxicity is cumulative; withhold until renal function returns to normal

Black Box Warning: Anaphylaxis: wheezing, tachycardia, facial swelling, fainting; discontinue product, report to prescriber; resuscitation equipment should be nearby, may occur within minutes; often EPINEPHrine, corticosteroids, antihistamines may alleviate symptoms

• **Infection:** monitor temperature; may indicate beginning infection; report signs of infection, cough, sore throat, fever
• **Hepatotoxicity:** report jaundice, dark urine, clay-colored stools, pruritus, abdominal pain
• Hepatic studies prior to, during therapy (bilirubin, AST, ALT, LDH) as needed
• **Bleeding:** hematuria, guaiac, bruising, petechiae, mucosa, or orifices q8hr; obtain prescription for viscous lidocaine (Xylocaine)

Black Box Warning: Ototoxicity: more common in genetic variants TPMT 3B and 3C in children; use audiometric testing baseline and prior to each dose; tinnitus or loss of high-frequency sounds is usually first indication of ototoxicity

• Comprehensive oral hygiene
• **RPLS:** Headache, change in eyesight, confusion, seizures, increased B/P, usually occurs a few hours up to a year after treatment starts, discontinue treatment
• **Hyperuricemia in lymphoma:** increase fluid intake to 2-3 L/day to prevent urate deposits, calculi formation, promote elimination of product; usually occurs between 3-5 days after a dose, may use allopurinol
Evaluate:
• Therapeutic response: decreased tumor size, spread of malignancy
Teach patient/family:
• **To report signs of infection:** increased temperature, sore throat, flulike symptoms
• **To report signs of anemia:** fatigue, headache, faintness, SOB, irritability

- To report bleeding, bruising, petechiae; to avoid use of razors, commercial mouthwash; to avoid aspirin, ibuprofen, NSAIDs, alcohol; may cause GI bleeding
- That impotence or amenorrhea can occur but is reversible after discontinuing treatment

Black Box Warning: Ototoxicity: to report loss of hearing, ringing, or roaring in the ears

- To maintain adequate fluids; to report decreased urine output, flank pain
- That hair may be lost during treatment; a wig or hairpiece may make patient feel better; that new hair may be different in color, texture
- To report numbness, tingling in face or extremities; poor hearing; joint pain, swelling
- Not to receive vaccinations during treatment
- **Pregnancy/breastfeeding:** to use contraception during treatment and for 4 mo after treatment; that product may cause infertility; not to breastfeed

---

citalopram (Rx)
(sigh-tal'oh-pram)
CeleXA
Func. class.: Antidepressant
Chem. class.: Selective serotonin reuptake inhibitor (SSRI)

Do not confuse:
CeleXA/CeleBREX/Cerebyx/ZyPREXA

ACTION: Inhibits CNS neuron uptake of serotonin but not of norepinephrine; weak inhibitor of CYP450 enzyme system, thus making it more appealing than other products

USES: Major depressive disorder
Unlabeled uses: Obsessive-compulsive disorder in adolescents

CONTRAINDICATIONS
Hypersensitivity

Precautions: Pregnancy, breastfeeding, geriatric patients, renal/hepatic disease, seizure disorder, hypersensitivity to escitalopram, bradycardia, recent MI, abrupt discontinuation, QT prolongation

Black Box Warning: Children, suicidal ideation

DOSAGE AND ROUTES
Depression
- **Adult: PO** 20 mg/day AM or PM, may increase if needed to 40 mg/day after 1 wk; ⚕ poor metabolizers of CYP2C19 or use of CYP2C19 inhibitors or ≥60 yr max 20 mg/day
Hepatic dose/geriatric
- **Adult: PO** 20 mg/day
OCD (unlabeled)
- **Adult: PO** 20-60 mg/day
Available forms: Tablets 10, 20, 40 mg; oral solution 10 mg/5 mL
Administer:
- With food or milk for GI symptoms
- Crushed if patient is unable to swallow medication whole
- Dosages at bedtime if oversedation occurs during the day; may take entire dose at bedtime
- Do not give within 14 days of MAOIs
- Store at room temperature; do not freeze

SIDE EFFECTS
CNS: *Headache, insomnia, drowsiness, anxiety, tremor, dizziness, fatigue, sedation, poor concentration,* seizures, suicidal attempts, neuroleptic malignant–like syndrome reactions
CV: Tachycardia, QT prolongation, orthostatic hypotension, torsades de pointes
EENT: Visual changes
GI: *Nausea, diarrhea, dry mouth, anorexia, dyspepsia, vomiting, flatulence, decreased appetite*
GU: *Dysmenorrhea, decreased libido,* amenorrhea, impotence
INTEG: *Sweating, rash, pruritus,* photosensitivity
MS: Arthritis, myalgia

Side effects: *italics* = common; red = life-threatening

RESP: *Infection, cough, dyspnea*
SYST: Hyponatremia (geriatric patients), serotonin syndrome

PHARMACOKINETICS

Metabolized in liver by CYP3A4, ✎ⓍⒾ CYP2C19, some individuals are poor metabolizers; excreted in urine; steady state 1 wk; peak 4 hr; half-life 35 hr

INTERACTIONS

Increase fatal reactions: do not use within 14 days of MAOIs
Increase: QTc interval—dofetilide, halofantrine, probucol, pimozide, quinolones, ziprasidone; do not use together
Increase: serotonin syndrome—serotonin receptor agonists, SSRIs, traMADol, lithium, MAOIs, traZODone, SNRIs (venlafaxine, DULoxetine), linezolid, methylene blue, tricyclics, fentaNYL, busPIRone, triptans, cyclobenzaprine
Increase: bleeding risk—NSAIDs, salicylates, thrombolytics, anticoagulants, antiplatelets
Increase: CNS effects—barbiturates, sedative/hypnotics, other CNS depressants
Increase: citalopram levels—macrolides, azole antifungals
Increase: plasma levels of beta-blockers
Decrease: citalopram levels—carBAMazepine, cloNIDine

Drug/Herb
Increase: serotonin syndrome—St. John's wort, SAM-e; fatal reaction may occur; do not use concurrently
Increase: CNS stimulation—yohimbe

Drug/Lab Test
Increase: serum bilirubin, blood glucose, alkaline phosphatase
Decrease: VMA, 5-HIAA
False increase: urinary catecholamines

NURSING CONSIDERATIONS
Assess:

Black Box Warning: Suicide: mood, sensorium, affect, suicidal tendencies, increase in psychiatric symptoms, depression, panic; risk for suicide is greater in children and those ≤24 yr; these patients should be evaluated weekly × 4 wk and then q3wk × 4 wk, give only a small amount of product

- **Serotonin syndrome:** increased heart rate, sweating, dilated pupils, tremors, twitching, hyperthermia, agitation, hyperreflexia, nausea, vomiting, diarrhea, coma, hallucinations; may be worse in those taking SSRIs, SNRIs, triptans, traZODone, traMADol, cyclobenzaprine, linezolid
- **QT prolongation:** Flattening T-wave, bundle branch block, AV block
- B/P lying, standing, pulse q4hr; if systolic B/P drops 20 mm Hg, hold product, notify prescriber; take vital signs q4hr in patients with CV disease
- Weight weekly; appetite may decrease or increase with product
- **Torsades de pointes, QT prolongation:** is dose-dependent; ECG for flattening of T wave, bundle branch, AV block, dysrhythmias in cardiac patients
- Alcohol consumption; if alcohol is consumed, hold dose until AM
- **Sexual dysfunction:** erectile dysfunction, decreased libido
- **Beers:** avoid in older adults unless safer alternative is unavailable; may cause ataxia, impaired psychomotor function
- **Pregnancy/breastfeeding:** no well-controlled studies; use in pregnancy only if benefits outweigh fetal risk; excreted in breast milk, discontinue breastfeeding or discontinue product

Evaluate:
- Therapeutic response: decreased depression

Teach patient/family:
- That therapeutic effect may take 4-6 wk; that patient may have increased anxiety first 5-7 days of therapy; not to discontinue abruptly
- To use caution when driving, performing other activities that require alertness because of drowsiness, dizziness, blurred vision; to report signs, symptoms of bleeding
- To use sunscreen, protective clothing to prevent photosensitivity
- To avoid alcohol, other CNS depressants

Black Box Warning: Suicide: that suicidal ideas, behavior may occur in children or young adults, to watch closely for suicidal thoughts, behaviors, notify prescriber immediately

• **About the effects of serotonin syndrome:** nausea/vomiting, tremors; if symptoms occur, to discontinue immediately, notify prescriber

---

clarithromycin (Rx)
(klare-ith'row-my-sin)
Func. class.: Antiinfective
Chem. class.: Macrolide

ACTION: Binds to 50S ribosomal subunits of susceptible bacteria and suppresses protein synthesis

USES: Mild to moderate infections of the upper and lower respiratory tract, uncomplicated skin and skin structure infections caused by *Streptococcus pneumoniae, Mycoplasma pneumoniae, Legionella pneumophila, Moraxella catarrhalis, Neisseria gonorrhoeae, Corynebacterium diphtheriae, Listeria monocytogenes, Haemophilus influenzae, Streptococcus pyogenes, Staphylococcus aureus, Mycobacterium avium* complex (MAC); complex infection in AIDS patients; *Mycobacterium avium intracellulare, Helicobacter pylori* in combination with omeprazole, *H. parainfluenzae*

CONTRAINDICATIONS
Hypersensitivity to this product or macrolide antibiotics, torsades de pointes, QT prolongation
Precautions: Pregnancy, breastfeeding, geriatric patients, renal/hepatic disease, heart disease

DOSAGE AND ROUTES
Acute exacerbation of chronic bronchitis
• **Adult: PO** 250-500 mg q12hr × 7-14 days or 1000 mg/day × 7 days (XL)
Pharyngitis/tonsillitis
• **Adult: PO** 250 mg q12hr × 10 days

Community-acquired pneumonia
• **Adult: PO** 250 mg q12hr × 7-14 days or 1000 mg/day × 7 days (XL)
Endocarditis prophylaxis
• **Adult: PO** 500 mg 1 hr prior to procedure
• **Child: PO** 15 mg/kg 1 hr prior to procedure
MAC prophylaxis/treatment
• **Adult: PO** 500 mg bid; will require an additional antiinfective for active infection
H. pylori infection
• **Adult: PO** 500 mg with 30 mg lansoprazole and 1 g amoxicillin together q12hr × 10-14 days or 500 mg with omeprazole 20 mg and 1 g amoxicillin together q12hr × 10 days or 500 mg q8hr and omeprazole 40 mg daily × 14 days, continue omeprazole for 14 more days
Acute maxillary sinusitis
• **Adult: PO** 500 mg q12hr × 14 days
Acute otitis media
• **Child: PO** 7.5 mg/kg q12hr × 10 days, max 500 mg/dose for MAC
Renal dose
• **Adult/child: PO** CCr 30-60 mL/min decrease dose by 50% if using with ritonavir; <30 mL/min, reduce dose by 50%, if used with ritonavir reduce by 75%
Available forms: Tablets 250, 500 mg; oral suspension 125 mg/5 mL, 250 mg/5 mL; extended-release tablet (XL) 500 mg
Administer:
• Do not break, crush, or chew extended release
• Adequate intake of fluids (2 L) during diarrhea episodes
• q12hr to maintain serum levels
• Store at room temperature
• **Suspension:** Shake well, store at room temperature, discard after 2 wk
• **Extended release:** Give with food

SIDE EFFECTS
CV: Ventricular dysrhythmias, QT prolongation, torsades de pointes

---

GI: *Nausea, vomiting, diarrhea,* hepatotoxicity, *abdominal pain,* anorexia, *abnormal taste,* CDAD, pancreatitis

INTEG: Rash, urticaria, pruritus, Stevens-Johnson syndrome, toxic epidermal necrolysis, angioedema

MISC: *Headache,* hearing loss

PHARMACOKINETICS

Regular release: peak 2-2.5 hr; duration 12 hr; extended release: peak 5-7 hr; half-life 5-7 hr; metabolized by liver; excreted in bile, feces; possible inhibition of P-glycoprotein, protein binding 70%

INTERACTIONS

Increase: levels, toxicity—ALPRAZolam, benzodiazepines, busPIRone, carBAMazepine, cycloSPORINE, digoxin, disopyramide, ergots, felodipine, fluconazole, omeprazole, tacrolimus, theophylline, antidiabetics, midazolam, triazolam

Increase: atorvastatin, pravastatin

Increase: myopathy, rhabdomyolysis risk—lovastatin, simvastatin; do not use concurrently

Increase: action, risk for toxicity—all products metabolized by CYP3A enzyme system

Increase: levels of sildenafil, tadalafil, vardenafil

Increase: effect of calcium channel blockers

Increase: QT prolongation—class IA, III antidysrhythmics, quinidines, procainamide, dofetilide, sotalol, amiodarone, or other products that prolong QT

Increase or decrease action: zidovudine

Drug/Food
Do not use with grapefruit juice

Drug/Herb
Decrease: clarithromycin effect—St. John's wort

Drug/Lab Test
Increase: AST, ALT, BUN, creatinine, LDH, total bilirubin, INR, PT

NURSING CONSIDERATIONS
Assess:
• **Infection:** wound characteristics, urine, stool, sputum, WBC, temperature; C&S prior to product therapy; product may be given as soon as culture is taken; C&S may be repeated after treatment

• **Bleeding:** check INR if anticoagulants are taken

• **Hypersensitivity:** allergies before treatment, reaction to each medication

• **Heart failure:** increased risk of heart-related disease and death in some patients; use caution in those with increased CV risk, and weigh benefits and risk

• **QT prolongation, ventricular dysrhythmias:** monitor ECG, cardiac status in those with underlying cardiac abnormalities

• ***Clostridium difficile*–associated diarrhea (CDAD):** monitor for diarrhea, cramping, blood in stools, fever; report immediately to prescriber; may start up to several weeks after conclusion of treatment

• **Serious skin reaction:** Stevens-Johnson syndrome, toxic epidermal necrolysis; product should be discontinued immediately; may occur after therapy is concluded

• **Pregnancy/breastfeeding:** no well-controlled studies; use in pregnancy only if benefits outweigh fetal risk; excreted in breast milk, use caution in breastfeeding

Evaluate:
• Therapeutic response: C&S negative for infection, prevention of endocarditis

Teach patient/family:
• To take with full glass of water; may give with food to decrease GI symptoms; to take extended release with food

• To report sore throat, fever, fatigue; may indicate superinfection

• To notify prescriber of diarrhea, dark urine, pale stools, yellow discoloration of eyes or skin, severe abdominal pain

• To take at evenly spaced intervals; to complete dosage regimen; to notify prescribers of all products used

• To notify prescriber if pregnancy is suspected or planned or if breastfeeding

TREATMENT OF HYPERSEN-SITIVITY: Withdraw product, maintain airway, administer EPINEPHrine, aminophylline, O₂, IV corticosteroids

clevidipine (Rx)

(klev-id'i-peen)

Cleviprex

Func. class.: Calcium channel blocker (L-type)

Chem. class.: Dihydropyridine

ACTION: L-type calcium channels mediate the influx of calcium during depolarization in arterial smooth muscle; reduces mean arterial B/P by decreasing systemic vascular resistance

USES: Reduction of B/P when oral therapy is not feasible

CONTRAINDICATIONS

Hypersensitivity to this product, eggs, soya lecithin; defective lipid metabolism; severe aortic stenosis, pancreatitis

Precautions: Pregnancy, labor, breastfeeding, children <18 yr, heart failure, hyperlipidemia, chronic hypertension, pheochromocytoma

DOSAGE AND ROUTES

• **Adult: CONTINUOUS IV** 1-2 mg/hr; dose may be doubled q90sec initially; as B/P reaches goal, adjust dose less frequently (q5-10min) with smaller increases in dose; most patients require 4-6 mg/hr, max 32 mg/hr; no more than 1000 mL should be infused per 24-hr period due to lipid load restrictions

Available forms: Single-dose vial 50, 100 mL (0.5 mg/mL)

Administer:

Intermittent IV INFUSION route

• Do not give through same line as other medications; do not dilute, do not filter

• Gently invert several times before use; do not use if discolored or if particulate matter is present

• Give through central or peripheral line at 1-2 mg/hr; use infusion device

• Store vials in refrigerator; do not freeze; leave vials in carton until use; product is photosensitive, but protection from light during administration is not required

Solution compatibilities: water for injection, 0.9% NaCl, D₅W/0.9% NaCl, D₅/LR, LR, 10% amino acid

SIDE EFFECTS

CNS: Headache

CV: *Reflex tachycardia, hypotension,* rebound hypertension, atrial fibrillation

GI: Nausea, vomiting

MS: Arthralgia

GU: Acute renal failure

PHARMACOKINETICS

Onset 2-4 min; half-life initially 1 min, terminal 15 min; metabolized via esterases in blood, extravascular tissues; excreted in urine 63%-74%, feces 7%-22%; protein binding >99%

NURSING CONSIDERATIONS

Assess:

• **Cardiac status:** Monitor B/P, pulse, respiration, ECG; some patients have developed severe angina, acute MI if obstructive CAD is severe; if not transitioned to other antihypertensive therapies after clevidipine infusion, patients should be monitored ≥8 hr for rebound hypertension; monitor for rebound hypertension after product stoppage

• **Pregnancy/breastfeeding:** no well-controlled studies; use in pregnancy only if benefits outweigh fetal risk; excretion is unknown, use cautiously in breastfeeding

Evaluate:

• Therapeutic response: decreased B/P

Teach patient/family:

• To notify prescriber immediately if neurologic symptoms, visual changes, or symptoms of HF occur

- To inform the patient of reason for product, expected result
- To continue follow-up for hypertension in patients with hypertension
- To notify prescriber if pregnancy is planned or suspected, or if breastfeeding

clindamycin (Rx)

(klin-da-my´sin)

Cleocin, Cleocin T, Clinda-Derm, Clindagel, Clindesse, Clindets, Dalacin T ✤, Evolin, Dalacin C ✤

Func. class.: Antiinfective— miscellaneous
Chem. class.: Lincomycin derivative

ACTION: Binds to 50S subunit of bacterial ribosomes, suppresses protein synthesis

USES: Skin, skin structure, respiratory tract infections; septicemia; intra-abdominal infections; endocarditis prophylaxis; infections caused by staphylococci, streptococci, *Rickettsia, Fusobacterium, Actinomyces, Peptococcus, Bacteroides, Pneumocystis jiroveci*

CONTRAINDICATIONS

Hypersensitivity to this product or lincomycin, tartrazine dye; ulcerative colitis/enteritis

Black Box Warning: Pseudomembranous colitis

Precautions: Pregnancy, breastfeeding, GI/hepatic disease, asthma, allergy, diarrhea

DOSAGE AND ROUTES
Most infections
- **Adult: PO** 150-450 mg q6hr, max 2700 mg/day; **IM/IV** 1.2-2.7 g/day in 2-4 divided doses, max 4800 mg/day severe infections
- **Child >1 mo: PO** 8-25 mg/kg/day in divided doses q6-8hr; **IM/IV** 20-40 mg/kg/day in 3-4 equal divided doses q6-8hr

- **Neonate: IM/IV** 15-20 mg/kg/day divided doses q6-8hr
PID
- **Adult: IV** 900 mg q8hr plus gentamicin
Bacterial endocarditis prophylaxis
- **Adult: PO/IV** 600 mg 1 hr (PO), 30 min (IV) prior to procedure
Bacterial vaginosis
- **Adult/adolescent:** Vaginal: (Clindamax) 1 applicator (5 g) at bedtime × 3-7 day; (Clindesse) 1 applicator (5 g) single dose or 1 suppository (100 mg) at bedtime × 3 nights

Available forms: Capsules 75, 150, 300 mg; granules for oral solution 75 mg/5 mL; injection infusion in D₅W 300 mg, 600 mg, 900 mg/16 mL; injection 150 mg/mL, 300 mg/2 mL, 600 mg/4 mL, 900 mg/6 mL; topical: foam/gel, lotion, solution 1%, cream 2%; **vaginal:** cream 2%; **vaginal suppositories** 100 mg
Administer:
- In equal intervals around the clock to maintain blood levels
- Obtain C&S prior to use, may start product before results are received
PO route
- Do not break, crush, chew capsules
- Orally with at least 8 oz of water
Oral solution
- Do not refrigerate reconstituted product; store at room temperature ≤2 wk
Vaginal route
- Use applicator supplied
- Partner is not treated
Topical route
- Do not get in eyes, mouth cuts
IM route
- IM deep injection; rotate sites; do not give >600 mg in single IM injection
IV route
- Visually inspect parenteral products for particulate matter and discoloration prior to use
- **Vials:** dilute 300- and 600-mg doses with 50 mL of a compatible diluent; dilute 900-mg doses with 50-100 mL of a compatible diluent; dilute 1200-mg doses with 100 mL of a compatible diluent, final concentration max 18 mg/mL

- **ADD-vantage vials:** dilute 600- and 900-mg ADD-vantage containers with 50 or 100 mL, respectively, of NS or D$_5$W
- **Storage:** when diluted in D$_5$W, NS, or LR, solutions with concentrations of 6, 9, or 12 mg/mL are stable for 16 days at room temperature or 32 days under refrigeration when stored in glass bottles or minibags; when diluted in D$_5$W, solutions with a concentration of 18 mg/mL are stable for 16 days at room temperature

Intermittent IV infusion route

- Infuse over at least 10-60 min, infusion rates max 30 mg/min and ≤1.2 g should be infused in a 1-hr period
- Infuse 300-mg doses over 10 min; 600-mg doses over 20 min, 900-mg doses over 30 min, and 1200-mg doses over 40 min

Continuous IV infusion route

- Give first dose rapidly, then follow with continuous infusion
- Rate is based on desired serum clindamycin levels
- To maintain serum concentrations above 4 mcg/mL, use a rapid infusion rate of 10 mg/min for 30 min and a maintenance rate of 0.75 mg/min; to maintain serum concentrations above 5 mcg/mL, use a rapid infusion rate of 15 mg/min for 30 min and a maintenance rate of 1 mg/min; to maintain serum concentrations above 5 mcg/mL, use a rapid infusion rate of 20 mg/min for 30 min and a maintenance rate of 1.25 mg/min

Y-site compatibilities: Acyclovir, alfentanil, amifostine, amikacin, aminocaproic acid, aminophylline, amiodarone, amphotericin B cholesteryl, amphotericin B lipid complex, amsacrine, anakinra, anidulafungin, ascorbic acid injection, atenolol, atracurium, atropine, aztreonam, benztropine, bivalirudin, bleomycin, bumetanide, buprenorphine, butorphanol, calcium chloride/gluconate, CARBOplatin, cefamandole, ceFAZolin, cefmetazole, cefonicid, cefoperazone, cefotaxime, cefoTEtan, cefOXitin, cefpirome, cefTAZidime, ceftizoxime, ceftobiprole, cefuroxime, cephalothin, cephapirin, chloramphenicol, cimetidine, cisatracurium, CISplatin, codeine, cyanocobalamin, cyclophosphamide, cycloSPORINE, cytarabine, DACTINomycin, DAPTOmycin, dexamethasone, dexmedetomidine, digoxin, diltiaZEM, diphenhydrAMINE, DOCEtaxel, DOPamine, doxacurium, DOXOrubicin liposomal, doxycycline, enalaprilat, ePHEDrine, EPINEPHrine, epirubicin, epoetin alfa, eptifibatide, esmolol, etoposide, famotidine, fenoldopam, fentaNYL, fludarabine, fluorouracil, folic acid, foscarnet, furosemide, gatifloxacin, gemcitabine, gemtuzumab, gentamicin, glycopyrrolate, granisetron, heparin, hydrocortisone, HYDROmorphone, ifosfamide, imipenem-cilastatin, indomethacin, insulin (regular), irinotecan, isoproterenol, ketorolac, levoFLOXacin, lidocaine, linezolid, LORazepam, LR, magnesium sulfate, mannitol, mechlorethamine, melphalan, meperidine, metaraminol, methicillin, methotrexate, methoxamine, methyldopate, methylPREDNISolone, metoclopramide, metoprolol, metroNIDAZOLE, mezlocillin, miconazole, milrinone, morphine, moxalactam, multiple vitamins injection, nafcillin, nalbuphine, naloxone, nesiritide, netilmicin, niCARdipine, nitroglycerin, nitroprusside, norepinephrine, octreotide, ondansetron, oxacillin, oxaliplatin, oxytocin, PACLitaxel, palonosetron, pamidronate, pancuronium, pantoprazole, PEMEtrexed, penicillin G potassium/sodium, pentazocine, perphenazine, PHENobarbital, phenylephrine, phytonadione, piperacillin, piperacillin-tazobactam, potassium chloride, procainamide, propofol, propranolol, protamine, pyridoxine, raNITIdine, remifentanil, Ringer's, ritodrine, riTUXimab, rocuronium, sargramostim, sodium acetate/bicarbonate, succinylcholine, SUFentanil, tacrolimus, teniposide, theophylline, thiamine, thiotepa, ticarcillin, ticarcillin-clavulanate, tigecycline, tirofiban, TNA, tobramycin, tolazoline, TPN, trimetaphan, urokinase, vancomycin, vasopressin, vecuronium, verapamil, vinCRIStine, vinorelbine, vitamin B complex/C, voriconazole, zidovudine, zoledronic acid

SIDE EFFECTS

GI: *Nausea, vomiting, abdominal pain, diarrhea,* CDAD, anorexia

CV: Dysrrthmias, hypotension
INTEG: Rash, urticaria, pruritus, abscess at inj site
SYST: Stevens-Johnson syndrome, exfoliative dermatitis
MISC: Candidiasis

PHARMACOKINETICS
PO: Peak 45 min, duration 6-8 hr
IM: Peak 3 hr (adult), 1 hr (child); duration 8-12 hr; half-life 2½ hr; metabolized in liver by CYP3A4; excreted in urine, bile, feces as inactive metabolites; crosses placenta; excreted in breast milk, protein binding 94%

INTERACTIONS
• May block clindamycin effect: erythromycin; avoid using together
Increase: neuromuscular blockade—neuromuscular blockers
Decrease: absorption—kaolin/pectin
Drug/Lab Test
Increase: alkaline phosphatase, bilirubin, CPK, AST, ALT

NURSING CONSIDERATIONS
Assess:
• **Infection:** C&S prior to product therapy; product may be given as soon as culture is taken; monitor appearances of wounds, sputum, stools, urine baseline and periodically

Black Box Warning: CDAD: bowel pattern prior to, during treatment; if severe diarrhea occurs, product should be discontinued; may occur several weeks after therapy is terminated; use this product in serious infections only

• **Labs:** platelets, WBCs may be decreased
• **Serious skin reactions:** Stevens-Johnson syndrome, exfoliative dermatitis (monitor for rash); discontinue at first appearance of rash, may occur after conclusion of therapy
• **Pregnancy/breastfeeding:** no well-controlled studies; use in pregnancy only if benefits outweigh fetal risk; excreted in breast milk, not recommended if breastfeeding
Evaluate:
• Therapeutic response: negative C&S

Teach patient/family:
• To take oral product with full glass of water; that antiperistaltic products may worsen diarrhea
• About all aspects of product therapy; to complete entire course of medication to ensure organism death (10-14 days); culture may be taken after medication course completed
• To report sore throat, fever, fatigue; may indicate **superinfection**
• To take with food to reduce GI symptoms

Black Box Warning: To notify nurse or prescriber of diarrhea with pus, mucus, rash

• Teach patient not to miss or double doses, take missed dose as soon as remembered unless almost time for next dose
• **CDAD:** Advise patient to notify health care provider immediately if diarrhea, fever, cramping, or blood in stools occurs, not to self-treat
• Teach patient IV infusion may result in metal taste
• **Vaginal:** Teach patient not to engage in sexual intercourse while using this product; to be inserted high in vagina, to remain lying down for ≥30 min
• **Topical:** Advise patient to notify health care provider of dry skin, not to wash area for ≥30 min after application

TREATMENT OF HYPERSENSITIVITY:
• Withdraw product; maintain airway; administer EPINEPHrine, O_2, IV corticosteroids

---

clindamycin (topical, vaginal) (Rx)
(klin-da-mye′sin)
Cleocin, Cleocin-T, Clindacin-P, Clindagel, ClindaMax, Clindasol ♣, Clinda-T ♣, Clindesse, Clindets, Dalacin ♣, Evoclin
Func. class.: Topical antiinfective
Chem. class.: Lincosamide derivative

ACTION: Antibacterial activity results from inhibition of protein synthesis; bacteriostatic

USES: For the treatment of acne vulgaris; treatment of bacterial vaginosis and anaerobic bacteria

CONTRAINDICATIONS

Hypersensitivity to this product or lincomycin, history of antibiotic-associated colitis or ulcerative colitis

Precautions: Breastfeeding, children <12 yr

DOSAGE AND ROUTES
Acne vulgaris

• **Adult/adolescent: TOPICAL** (gel, lotion, solution) Apply a thin film of 1% to affected areas bid; **TOPICAL (foam)** Apply 1% topical foam to affected areas once daily; if there is no improvement after 6-8 wk or if the condition worsens, discontinue treatment; **TOPICAL** (medicated pledgets). Use a pledget to apply a thin film to the affected area bid

Bacterial vaginosis and anaerobic bacteria

Nonpregnant adult/adolescent/post-menarchal females: Intravaginal cream: one applicatorful (100 mg clindamycin/5 g cream) intravaginally, preferably at bedtime, for 3 or 7 consecutive days in nonpregnant women and for 7 consecutive days in pregnant women; Clindesse is administered as a single dose at any time of the day

• **Intravaginal ovules/suppositories:** 1 ovule (100-mg clindamycin) inserted intravaginally at bedtime for 3 days

Available forms: Topical gel, foam, lotion, pledget, solution 1%; vaginal cream 2%, vaginal suppositories 100 mg

Administer:
Topical route

• Improvement occurs after 6 wk but can require 8-12 wk

• Topical skin products are not for intravaginal therapy and are for external use only; do not use skin products near the eyes, nose, or mouth

• Wash hands prior to and after use; wash affected area and gently pat dry

Cream/ointment/lotion: Shake well before use (lotion); apply a thin film to the cleansed affected area; massage gently into affected areas

Foam formulations: Do not dispense foam directly onto hands or face; the warmth of the skin will cause the foam to melt; apply directly into the cap or onto a cool surface; gently massage into the affected areas

Solution formulations: Shake well prior to use; apply a thin film to the cleansed affected area; massage gently into affected areas; if using a solution-soaked pledget, may use more than 1 pledget per application as needed; use only once and then discard

Intravaginal route: Only use dosage formulations specified for intravaginal use

Suppository: Unwrap vaginal ovule (suppository) before insertion; use applicator(s) supplied by the manufacturer

Cream: Use applicator(s) supplied by the manufacturer

SIDE EFFECTS

GU: Colitis, *diarrhea*, overgrowth, vaginitis, vaginal moniliasis, UTI

INTEG: Redness, burning, dermatitis, rash, pruritus

NURSING CONSIDERATIONS
Assess:

• Contact prescriber immediately if severe diarrhea, stomach cramps/pain, or bloody stools occur

Infection: Assess for number of lesions, severity in acne, itching in vaginosis

Evaluate:

• Decreased lesions in acne, infection in vaginosis

Teach patient/family:
Topical route

• That improvement occurs after 6 wk but can require 8-12 wk

• That topical products are not for intravaginal therapy and are for external use only; not to use skin products near the eyes, nose, or mouth

• To wash hands prior to and after use; to wash affected area and gently pat dry

---

Side effects: *italics* = common; red = life-threatening

- **Cream/ointment/lotion:** to shake well prior to use; **lotion:** to apply a thin film to the cleansed affected area and massage gently into affected area
- **Foam formulations:** not to dispense foam directly onto hands or face; use fingertips and gently massage into the affected areas
- **Solution formulations:** to shake well; to apply a thin film to the cleansed affected area and massage gently into affected areas; if using a solution-soaked pledget, may use more than one pledget per application as needed; each pledget should be used only once and then discarded

Intravaginal route

- To use only dosage formulations specified for intravaginal use; not to ingest
- **Suppository:** to unwrap vaginal ovule (suppository) before insertion; to use applicator(s) supplied by the manufacturer
- **Cream:** to use applicator(s) supplied by the manufacturer

---

clobazam (Rx)

Kloe′ba-zam

Onfi, Sympazan

Func. class.: Anticoagulant

Chem. class.: Benzodiazepine

Controlled Substance Schedule IV

ACTION: Potentates the GABA system by binding at the benzodiazepine site

USES: Adjunctive treatment of seizures associated with Lennox-Gastaut syndrome

CONTRAINDICATIONS

Hyper-sensitivity, breastfeeding

Precautions: Abrupt discontinuation, dependency, drug abuse, depression, suicidal thoughts/behaviors, CNS depressants, opiates

DOSAGE AND ROUTES

- **Adult and child ≥2 yr and >30 kg:** PO 5 mg bid × 6 days; on day 7, increase to 10 bid; on day 14, increase to 20 mg bid as needed, max 40 mg/day

- **Adult and child ≥2 yr and <30 kg:** PO 5 mg daily × 6 days, then day 7 increase to 5 mg bid, then day 14 increase to 10 mg bid as tolerated, max 20 mg/day

Hepatic dose, poor CYP2C19 metabolizers, elderly

- **Adult:** PO 5 mg daily × 7 days, then titrate to half the recommended dose

Available forms: Tablets 10, 20 mg; oral suspension 2.5 mg/mL; oral film 5 mg, 10 mg, 20 mg

Administer:

- May crush, break and give with soft food, may give without regard to food
- Shake oral suspension prior to use
- Apply oral film to tongue immediately after opening, do not use with liquids
- Not to discontinue abruptly, taper on weekly basis by 10 mg

SIDE EFFECTS

CNS: *Fatigue, sedation, hyperactivity, insomnia, lethargy*

GI: *Vomiting, nausea, constipation*

GU: *UTI*

META: *Increased/decreased appetite*

RESP: *URI, pneumonia, cough*

PHARMACOKINETICS

Onset rapid, peak 1-4 hr, duration unknown, half-life 36-82 hr

INTERACTIONS

Increase: sedation: CNS depressants, avoid using together

Increase: sedation, respiratory depression: opioids

Increase: clobazam effect: CYP2C19 inhibitors, alcohol

Decrease: effect of hormonal contraceptives, use alternative contraception

NURSING CONSIDERATIONS

Assess:

- **Hypersensitive reactions, and Stevens-Johnson syndrome, toxic epidermal necrolysis:** rashes, blistering/swelling of mouth, may occur anytime, but more common during the first 2 mo of use
- **Suicidal thoughts/behaviors:** monitor for depression, change in behaviors, thoughts, mood

• **Opioids, CNS depression use:** monitor for severe respiratory depression, avoid using together; monitor for abuse, dependence
• **Pregnancy/breastfeeding:** to avoid use in pregnancy, if pregnant, enroll in North American AED Pregnancy Registry (888-238-2334), not to breastfeed

Evaluate:
• Therapeutic response: decreasing seizures without serious reactions

Patient/family teaching:
• To use caution in driving, other hazardous activities until response is known
• To discuss with providers the use of this product and all others taken
• **Pregnancy/breastfeeding:** to report if pregnancy is planned or suspected, or if breastfeeding or if using hormonal contraceptives, use alternative contraceptive
• How to use suspension and film
• Not to use suspension after 90 days, discard
• **Suicidal thoughts/behaviors:** to have patient or family members, caregivers to report suicidal thought/behaviors, depression, change in mood
• Not to discontinue abruptly

---

clobetasol (Rx)

(kloe-bay′ta-sol)

Clobex, Clodan, Dermovate, Impoyz, Olux, Olux-E, Temovate, Temovate-E

Func. class.: Corticosteroid, topical

ACTION: Crosses cell membrane to attach to receptors to decrease inflammation, itching

USES: Inflammation/itching in corticosteroid-responsive dermatoses on the skin/scalp

CONTRAINDICATIONS

Hypersensitivity, use of some preparations on face, axilla, groin; monotherapy for primary bacterial infections
Precautions: Pregnancy, breastfeeding, children <12 yr

DOSAGE AND ROUTES

• **Adult: TOPICAL** Apply to affected areas bid (shampoo: daily up to 4×/wk)
Available forms: Gel, lotion, ointment, cream, shampoo, solution, spray, foam 0.05%

Administer:
Topical route
• Do not use with occlusive dressings
• Treatment should be limited to 2 wk
• **Cream/ointment/lotion:** using gloves, apply sparingly in a thin film and rub gently into the cleansed, slightly moist affected area
• **Gel:** using gloves, apply sparingly in a thin film and rub gently into the cleansed, slightly moist affected area
• **Scalp foam:** invert can and dispense foam onto a saucer or other cool surface; do not dispense directly onto hands; pick up small amounts of foam with fingers and gently massage into affected area until foam disappears; repeat until entire affected scalp area is treated
• **Shampoo:** apply onto dry scalp in thin film, leave lather on scalp for 15 min, rinse off

SIDE EFFECTS

GU: Glycosuria
INTEG: Burning, folliculitis, pruritus, dermatitis, irritation, erythema, hypertrichosis, acne
MISC: Hyperglycemia, HPA axis suppression

NURSING CONSIDERATIONS
Assess:
• Skin reactions: burning, pruritus, folliculitis, dermatitis
• **Beers:** avoid in older adults with delirium or with high risk for delirium; may induce or worsen delirium
Evaluate:
• Therapeutic response: decrease in itching, inflammation on the skin, scalp
Teach patient/family:
Topical route
• Not to use with occlusive dressings
• That treatment should be limited to 2 wk
• **Cream/ointment/lotion:** to apply sparingly in a thin film and rub gently into the cleansed affected area

Side effects: *italics* = common; red = life-threatening

• **Gel:** to apply sparingly in a thin film and rub gently into the cleansed, slightly moist affected area

• **Scalp foam:** to invert can and dispense a small amount of foam onto a saucer or other cool surface; not to dispense onto hands; to pick up small amounts and gently massage into affected area until foam disappears; repeat until affected scalp area is treated

clomiPHENE (Rx)

(kloe'mi-feen)

Func. class.: Ovulation stimulant

Do not confuse:
clomiPHENE/clomiPRAMINE

USES: Female infertility (ovulatory failure)

CONTRAINDICATIONS

Pregnancy, hypersensitivity, hepatic disease, undiagnosed uterine bleeding, uncontrolled thyroid or adrenal dysfunction, intracranial lesion, ovarian cysts, endometrial carcinoma

Precautions: Hypertension, depression, seizures, diabetes mellitus, abnormal ovarian enlargement, ovarian hyperstimulation

DOSAGE AND ROUTES

• **Adult: PO** 50 mg/day × 5 days or 50 mg/day beginning on day 5 of menstrual cycle, may increase to 100 mg daily × 5 days with next cycle; may be repeated until conception occurs or max 6 cycles of therapy

Available forms: Tablets 50 mg

clomiPRAMINE (Rx)

(kloe-mip'ra-meen)

Anafranil

Func. class.: Antidepressant, tricyclic

Chem. class.: Tertiary amine

Do not confuse:
clomiPRAMINE/clomiPHENE

USES: Obsessive-compulsive disorder

CONTRAINDICATIONS

Hypersensitivity to this product, carBAMazepine, tricyclics, immediate post-MI, MAOI therapy

Precautions: Pregnancy, breastfeeding, geriatric patients, seizures, cardiac disease, glaucoma, prostatic hypertrophy, urinary retention

Black Box Warning: Children, suicidal ideation

DOSAGE AND ROUTES

Obsessive-compulsive disorder

• **Adult: PO** 25 mg at bedtime, increase gradually over 4 wk to 75-250 mg/day in divided doses

• **Child 10-18 yr: PO** 25 mg/day, gradually increase over 2 wk; max 3 mg/kg/day or 200 mg/day, whichever is smaller

Available forms: Capsules 25, 50, 75 mg

⚠ HIGH ALERT

clonazePAM (Rx)

(kloe-na'zi-pam)

KlonoPIN, Rivotril ✦

Func. class.: Anticonvulsant

Chem. class.: Benzodiazepine derivative

Controlled Substance Schedule IV

Do not confuse:
clonazePAM/LORazepam/cloNIDine
KlonoPIN

ACTION: Inhibits spike, wave formation during absence seizures (petit mal); decreases amplitude, frequency, duration, spread of discharge during minor motor seizures

USES: Absence, atypical absence, akinetic, myoclonic seizures; Lennox-Gastaut syndrome, panic disorder

CONTRAINDICATIONS

Pregnancy, hypersensitivity to benzodiazepines, acute closed-angle glaucoma, psychosis, severe hepatic disease

Precautions: Breastfeeding, geriatric patients, open-angle glaucoma, chronic

respiratory   disease,   renal/hepatic
disease

Black Box Warning: Coadministration
with other CNS depressants, especially
opiates

DOSAGE AND ROUTES
**Lennox-Gastaut syndrome/atypical
absence seizures/akinetic and
myclonic seizures**
• **Adult: PO** up to 1.5 mg/day in 3 divided
doses; may be increased 0.5-1 mg q3days
until desired response, max 20 mg/day
• **Geriatric: PO** 0.25 daily-bid initially,
increase by 0.25/day q7-14days as needed
• **Child ≤10 yr or ≤30 kg: PO** initial
0.01-0.03 mg/kg/day in divided doses
q8hr, max 0.05 mg/kg/day; may be increased 0.25-0.5 mg q3days until desired
response, max 0.1-0.2 mg/kg/day
Panic disorder
• **Adult: PO** 0.25 mg bid, increase to 1
mg daily after 3 days, max 4 mg/day
Available forms: Tablets 0.5, 1, 2 mg;
orally disintegrating tablets 0.125, 0.25,
0.5, 1, 2 mg
Administer:
PO route
• With food, milk for GI symptoms
• **Orally disintegrating tablets:** open
pouch by peeling back foil on blister pack
(do not push tablet through foil), place on
tongue, allow to dissolve; may be swallowed with/without water
• Store at room temperature

SIDE EFFECTS
CNS: *Drowsiness,* dizziness, confusion,
behavioral changes, tremors, insomnia,
headache, suicidal tendencies, slurred
speech, fatigue
CV: Palpitations, bradycardia
EENT: *Nystagmus, diplopia*
GI: *Nausea, constipation,* anorexia,
diarrhea
GU: Dysuria, enuresis, nocturia, reten-
tion, libido changes
HEMA: Anemia, thrombocytopenia,
leukopenia
INTEG: Rash

RESP: Congestion, respiratory depression

PHARMACOKINETICS
PO: Peak 1-2 hr, metabolized by liver,
excreted in urine, half-life 18-50 hr,
duration 6-12 hr, protein binding 85%

INTERACTIONS
Increase: clonazePAM effects—CYP3A4
inhibitors (azoles, cimetidine, clarithromycin, diltiazem, erythromycin, FLUoxetine), oral contraceptives; adjust dosage

Black Box Warning: Increase: CNS
depression—alcohol, barbiturates, opiates,
antidepressants, other anticonvulsants,
general anesthetics, hypnotics, sedatives

Decrease: clonazePAM effect—CYP3A4
inducers (carBAMazepine, PHENobarbital, phenytoin); monitor effect
Drug/Herb

Black Box Warning: Increase: CNS depression—kava, chamomile, valerian

Increase: clonazePAM effect—ginkgo,
melatonin
Decrease: clonazePAM effect—ginseng,
St. John's wort
Drug/Lab Test
Increase: AST, alkaline phosphatase,
bilirubin
Decrease: platelets, WBC, thyroid uptake
123I, 131IV

NURSING CONSIDERATIONS
Assess:
• **Seizures:** monitor duration, type, intensity, with/without aura
• Blood studies: RBC, Hct, HB, reticulocyte counts periodically
• Hepatic studies: ALT, AST, bilirubin,
creatinine
• **Abrupt discontinuation:** do not discontinue abruptly; seizures may increase
• Signs of physical withdrawal if medication suddenly discontinued
• **Mental status:** mood, sensorium, affect, oversedation, behavioral changes,
suicidal thoughts/behaviors; if mental
status changes, notify prescriber

Side effects: *italics* = common; red = life-threatening

• **Allergic reaction:** red, raised rash; product should be discontinued
• **Blood dyscrasias:** fever, sore throat, bruising, rash, jaundice
• **Toxicity:** bone marrow depression, nausea, vomiting, ataxia, diplopia, CV collapse; drug levels during initial treatment (therapeutic 20-80 ng/mL)

> **Black Box Warning: Coadministration with other CNS depressants, especially opioids:** increased risk of sedation causing death with benzodiazepines and opioids

• **Beers:** may be appropriate in older adults for seizure disorders, rapid eye movement sleep disorder, benzodiazepine/ethanol withdrawal; avoid in those with delirium or at high risk of delirium
Evaluate:
• Therapeutic response: decreased seizure activity
Teach patient/family:
• To carry emergency ID bracelet stating name, products taken, condition, prescriber's name, phone number
• About potential drug tolerance, withdrawal symptoms
• To continue with follow-up exams, lab work

> **Black Box Warning: Coadministration with other CNS depressants, especially opioids:** to avoid driving, other activities that require alertness

• To take as prescribed, not to skip or take double doses, provide "Medication Guide"
• To avoid driving and other hazardous activities until response is known
• **ODT:** open when ready to use, peel foil back with dry hands, place on tongue to dissolve
• To avoid alcohol, other CNS depressants; increased sedation may occur
• Not to discontinue medication quickly after long-term use; to taper off over several weeks
• To notify prescriber of yellowing of skin/eyes, clay-colored stools, bleeding,

fever, extreme fatigue, sore throat, suicidal thoughts/behaviors
• **Pregnancy/breastfeeding:** to notify prescriber if pregnancy is planned or suspected or if breastfeeding, to register with North American Antiepileptic Drug Pregnancy Registry (888-233-2334) if pregnant, not to use during pregnancy/breastfeeding

TREATMENT OF OVERDOSE:
Lavage, flumazenil, monitor electrolytes, VS, administer vasopressors, sodium bicarbonate

---

cloNIDine (Rx)
(klon´i-deen)
Catapres, Catapres-TTS, Duraclon, Kapvay, Nexiclon XR
Func. class.: Antihypertensive
Chem. class.: Central alpha-adrenergic agonist

Do not confuse:
cloNIDine/KlonoPIN/clonazePAM

ACTION: Inhibits sympathetic vasomotor center in CNS, which reduces impulses in sympathetic nervous system; B/P, pulse rate, cardiac output are decreased; prevents pain signal transmission in CNS by alpha-adrenergic receptor stimulation of the spinal cord

USES: Mild to moderate hypertension, used alone or in combination; severe pain in cancer patients (epidural), attention-deficit/hyperactivity disorder (ADHD)

CONTRAINDICATIONS
Hypersensitivity; (epidural) bleeding disorders, anticoagulants
Precautions: Pregnancy, breastfeeding, children <12 yr (transdermal), geriatric patients, noncompliant patients, MI (recent), diabetes mellitus, chronic renal failure, Raynaud's disease, thyroid disease, depression, COPD, asthma, pheochromocytoma

> **Black Box Warning:** Labor (epidermal cloNIDine)

DOSAGE AND ROUTES
Hypertension
• **Adult: PO** 0.1 mg bid then increase by 0.1-0.2 mg/day at weekly intervals until desired response; max 2.4 mg; range 0.2-0.6 mg/day in divided doses or **TRANSDERMAL** q7days, start 0.1 mg and adjust q1-2wk; Nexiclon XR 0.17 mg q day, then increase by 0.09 mg/day q wk, to 0.2-0.6 mg/day in divided doses
• **Geriatric: PO** 0.1 mg at bedtime; may increase gradually
• **Child: PO** 5-10 mcg/kg/day in divided doses q8-12hr, max 0.9 mg/day
Severe pain
• **Adult: CONTINUOUS EPIDURAL INFUSION** 30 mcg/hr
• **Child: CONTINUOUS EPIDURAL INFUSION** 0.5 mcg/kg/hr, then titrate to response
ADHD (Kapvay)
• **Adolescent/child ≥6 yr: PO** 0.1 mg PO once daily at bedtime, initially, may increase by 0.1 mg/day weekly up to 0.4 mg/day; extended release 0.1 mg at bedtime, increase dose by 0.1 mg/day up to 0.4 mg/day

Available forms: Tablets 0.1, 0.2, 0.3 mg; transdermal 0.1, 0.2, 0.3 mg/24 hr injection for epidural 100 mcg/mL; injection for epidural use; concentrate 500 mcg/mL extended-release tablet 0.1 mg; tablets, scored extended release 0.17, 0.26

Administer:
• Store patches in cool environment, tablets in tight container
PO route
• Give last dose at bedtime
• Do not crush, cut, chew, or break extended-release tablets; Kapvay is not interchangeable with other products
Transdermal route
• Once weekly; apply to site without hair; best absorption over chest or upper arm; rotate sites; clean site before application; apply firmly, especially around edges; may secure with adhesive tape if loose; fold sticky sides together and discard
• Should be removed before MRI

Epidural route
• Used for severe cancer pain
• May be used with opiates
• Use only if familiar with epidural infusion devices

Black Box Warning: Dilute 500 mcg/mL with 0.9% NaCl (100 mcg/mL)

Black Box Warning: Do not use for labor, postpartum pain management

SIDE EFFECTS
CNS: *Drowsiness,* nightmares, anxiety, depression, hallucinations, syncope, dizziness
CV: *Orthostatic hypotension,* HF, ECG abnormalities, sinus tachycardia
EENT: Taste change, dry eyes
ENDO: Hyperglycemia
GI: *Nausea, vomiting,* constipation, *dry mouth*
GU: Impotence, urinary retention, decreased libido
INTEG: *Rash,* pruritus, excoriation (transdermal patches)
MISC: Withdrawal symptoms

PHARMACOKINETICS
PO: Onset ½ to 1 hr, peak 2-4 hr, duration 8-12 hr, half-life 6-12 hr
TRANSDERMAL: Onset 3 days; duration 1 wk; metabolized by liver (metabolites); excreted in urine (45% unchanged, inactive metabolites), feces; crosses blood-brain barrier; excreted in breast milk

INTERACTIONS
Increase: bradycardia, verapamil, dilTIA-Zem
Life-threatening elevations of B/P: tricyclics, beta-blockers
Increase: CNS depression—opiates, sedatives, hypnotics, anesthetics, alcohol
Increase: hypotensive effects—diuretics, other antihypertensive nitrates
Increase: bradycardia—amphetamines, beta-blockers, digoxin, dilTIAZem, MAO inhibitors, verapamil
Decrease: hypotensive effects—tricyclics, MAOIs, appetite suppressants, amphetamines, prazosin, antipsychotics

Side effects: *italics* = common; red = life-threatening

Decrease: effect of levodopa

Drug/Herb

Increase: antihypertensive effect—hawthorn

Decrease: antihypertensive effect—ephedra, ginseng

Drug/Lab Test

Increase: blood glucose

Decrease: VMA, urinary catecholamines, aldosterone

Positive: Coombs' test

NURSING CONSIDERATIONS

Assess:

• **Hypertension:** B/P, pulse; report significant changes

• **Allergic reaction:** rash, fever, pruritus, urticaria; product should be discontinued if antihistamines fail to help

• **HF:** edema, dyspnea, wet crackles, B/P, more common in geriatric patients

• **ADHD:** B/P, pulse, palpitations, syncope

• **Beers:** avoid as first-line in older adults; high risk of CNS effects, bradycardia, orthostatic hypotension

Black Box Warning: Pregnancy/breast-feeding: do not use for labor/epidural; excreted in breast milk, discontinue breastfeeding or product

Evaluate:

• Therapeutic response: decrease in B/P with hypertension, decrease in withdrawal symptoms (opioid), decrease in pain

Teach patient/family:

• To avoid hazardous activities and driving until response is known, product may cause drowsiness

• To notify all health care providers of medication use

• Not to discontinue product abruptly or **withdrawal symptoms** may occur: anxiety, increased B/P, headache, insomnia, increased pulse, tremors, nausea, sweating; to comply with dosage schedule even if feeling better

• Not to use OTC (cough, cold, or allergy), alcohol, or CNS depressant products unless directed by prescriber

• To rise slowly to sitting or standing position to minimize orthostatic hypotension, especially among geriatric patients

• To notify prescriber of mouth sores, sore throat, fever, swelling of hands or feet, irregular heartbeat, chest pain, signs of **angioedema**

• About excessive perspiration, dehydration, vomiting; diarrhea may lead to fall in B/P; consult prescriber if these occur; that product may cause dizziness, fainting; that light headedness may occur during first few days of therapy

• That product may cause dry mouth; to use hard candy, saliva product, sugarless gum, or frequent rinsing of mouth

• Not to skip or stop product unless directed by prescriber; tolerance may develop with long-term use

• **Transdermal:** how to use patch; that patch comes in 2 parts: product patch and overlay to keep patch in place; not to trim or cut; that response may take 2-3 days, if switching from tablets to patch, to taper tablets to avoid withdrawal; to remove for MRI; can use during bathing, swimming

TREATMENT OF OVERDOSE: Supportive treatment; administer tolazoline, atropine, DOPamine prn

⚠ HIGH ALERT

clopidogrel (Rx)

(klo-pid'oh-grel)

Plavix

Func. class.: Platelet aggregation inhibitor

Chem. class.: Thienopyridine derivative

Do not confuse:

Plavix/Paxil

ACTION: Inhibits ADP-induced platelet aggregation

USES: Reducing the risk of stroke, MI, vascular death, peripheral arterial disease in high-risk patients, acute coronary syndrome, transient ischemic attack (TIA), unstable angina

CONTRAINDICATIONS

Hypersensitivity, active bleeding

Precautions: Pregnancy, breastfeeding, children, previous hepatic disease, increased bleeding risk, neutropenia, agranulocytosis, renal disease, ⚕☞ Asian/Black/Caucasian patients

Black Box Warning: ⚕☞ CYP2C19 allele (poor metabolizers)

DOSAGE AND ROUTES
Recent MI, stroke, peripheral arterial disease, TIA
• **Adult: PO** 75 mg/day with/without aspirin

Acute MI (ST-segment elevation, MI)
• **Adult: PO** 75 mg/day with aspirin 75-325 mg/day; with or without loading dose or thrombolytics; those >75 yr no loading dose should be given; continue this product for 2 wk to <1 yr with aspirin 81 mg indefinitely

Acute coronary syndrome
• **Adult: PO** loading dose 300 mg, then 75 mg/day with aspirin

Available forms: Tablets 75, 300 mg

Administer:
• Without regard to food
• Should be discontinued 5 days prior to elective surgery if an antiplatelet action is not desired

SIDE EFFECTS
CNS: Headache, dizziness, depression
CV: Edema, hypertension, chest pain
GI: Diarrhea, constipation, GI discomfort
HEMA: Bleeding (major/minor from any site), neutropenia, aplastic anemia, agranulocytosis, thrombotic thrombocytopenic purpura
INTEG: Rash, pruritus, anaphylaxis
MISC: Fatigue, intracranial hemorrhage, toxic epidermal necrolysis, Stevens-Johnson syndrome, flulike syndrome
MS: Arthralgia
RESP: Bronchospasm

PHARMACOKINETICS
Rapidly absorbed; metabolized by liver (CYP3A4, CYP2B6, CYP1A2, CYP2C8); excreted in urine, feces; half-life 6 hr; protein binding 95%; effect on platelets after 3-7 days

INTERACTIONS

Black Box Warning: ⚕☞ Avoid use with CYP2C19 inhibitors (omeprazole, esomeprazole)

CYP2C8 substrates (repaglinide): Increased level of CYP2C8 substrates, avoid using together
Increase: bleeding risk—anticoagulants, aspirin, NSAIDs, abciximab, eptifibatide, tirofiban, thrombolytics, ticlopidine, SSRIs, treprostinil, rifampin, SNRIs, prasugrel, monitor closely
Increase: action of some NSAIDs, phenytoin, TOLBUTamide, tamoxifen, torsemide, fluvastatin, warfarin, monitor closely
Decrease: clopidogrel effect—proton pump inhibitors (PPIs)
Decrease: CYP3A4 inhibitors/substrates—atorvastatin, simvastatin, cerivastatin

Drug/Food
Grapefruit juice: may decrease antiplatelet effect

Drug/Herb
Increase: clopidogrel effect—feverfew, fish oil, omega-3 fatty acid, garlic, ginger, ginkgo biloba, green tea, horse chestnut
Decrease: clopidogrel effect—bilberry, saw palmetto

Drug/Lab Test
Increase: AST, ALT, bilirubin, uric acid, total cholesterol, nonprotein nitrogen (NPN)

NURSING CONSIDERATIONS
Assess:
• **Thrombotic/thrombocytic purpura:** fever, thrombocytopenia, hemolytic anemia, neurologic changes, treat immediately

Black Box Warning: ⚕☞ **CYP2C19 allele (poor metabolizers):** consider using another antiplatelet product; higher CV reaction occurs after acute coronary syndrome or PCI; tests are available to determine CYP2C19 allele

• Hepatic studies: AST, ALT, bilirubin, creatinine (long-term therapy)
• Blood studies: CBC, differential, Hct, HB, PT, cholesterol (long-term therapy);

thrombocytopenia, neutropenia are rare

• **Hypersensitivity:** rash, angioedema may occur

Evaluate:

• Therapeutic response: absence of stroke, MI

Teach patient/family:

• That blood work will be necessary during treatment (CBC, LFTs)

• To report any unusual bruising, bleeding to prescriber; that it may take longer to stop bleeding

• To take without regard to food

• To tell all health care providers that clopidogrel is being used; may be held for 5 days before surgery, restart as soon as possible

• **Hypersensitivity:** To report immediately rash, pruritus

• **Pregnancy/breastfeeding:** to notify provider if pregnancy is planned or suspected or if breastfeeding; do not breastfeed, use cautiously in pregnancy

---

clotrimazole (topical, vaginal, oral) (OTC)

(kloe-trim′a-zole)

Canesten ✦, Clotrimaderm ✦, Cruex, Desenex Gyne-Lotrimin, Lotrimin, Lotrimin AF, Trivagizole 3

Func. class.: Topical antifungal
Chem. class.: Imidazole derivative

Do not confuse:
clotrimazole/miconazole/clobetasol

ACTION: Antifungal activity results from altering cell wall permeability

USES: Vulvovaginal, oropharyngeal candidiasis; topical fungal infections, prevention of oropharyngeal candidiasis in immunocompromised

CONTRAINDICATIONS

Hypersensitivity, ophthalmic use
Precautions: Hepatic impairment (oral)

DOSAGE AND ROUTES

Tinea corporis, cruris, pedis, versicolor; candidiasis

• **Adult/child ≥2 yr: TOPICAL** apply to affected area and rub into area AM/PM × 2-4 wk

Vulvovaginal candidiasis

• **Adult/child ≥12 yr: VAG CREAM** 1 applicator at bedtime × 3 days (2%) or 7 days (1%)

Oropharyngeal candidiasis

• **Adult/child ≥3 yr: LOZENGE** 1 PO dissolved 5×/day × 2 wk or adults 1 lozenge dissolved tid (prevention)

Oropharyngeal candidiasis prevention in immunocompromised

• **Adult: PO:** Lozenge dissolve tid

Available forms: Topical cream, solution, 1%; vaginal cream 1%, 2%; lozenges, troches 10 mg

Administer:

Topical route

• Topical skin products are not for intravaginal therapy and are for external use only; do not use skin products near the eyes, nose, or mouth

• Wash hands prior to and after use; wash affected area and gently pat dry

• **Cream/solution:** apply to the cleansed affected area; massage gently into affected areas

PO route

• **Troches:** allow to dissolve; do not chew or swallow whole

Intravaginal route

• Only use dosage formulations specified for intravaginal use; intravaginal dosage forms are not for topical therapy; do not ingest

• **Cream:** use applicator(s) supplied by the manufacturer

SIDE EFFECTS

GI: Nausea, vomiting
GU: Vaginal burning, irritation
INTEG: Burning, peeling, rash, pruritus

PHARMACOKINETICS

PO duration 3 hr

INTERACTIONS

Drug/Lab Test
Increase: LFTs

NURSING CONSIDERATIONS
Assess:
• **Allergic reaction:** assess for hypersensitivity; product might need to be discontinued
• **Infection:** assess for severity of infection, itching
• Hepatic function studies periodically if using oral troches
Evaluate:
• Decreased infection, itching
Teach patient/family:
Topical route:
• That topical skin products are not for intravaginal therapy and are for external use only; do not use skin products near the eyes, nose, or mouth; do not use occlusive dressings
• To wash hands prior to and after use; wash affected area and gently pat dry
• **Cream:** to shake well before use; apply a thin film to the cleansed affected area; massage gently into affected areas
PO route:
• **Troches:** allow to dissolve; do not chew or swallow whole
• **Cream:** to use applicator(s) supplied by the manufacturer

---

cloZAPine (Rx)
(kloz′a-peen)

Clozaril, FazaClo ODT, Versacloz
Func. class.: Antipsychotic
Chem. class.: Tricyclic dibenzodiazepine derivative

Do not confuse:
Clozaril/Colazal
cloZAPine/cloNIDine/clofazimine/clonazePAM/KlonoPIN

ACTION: Interferes with DOPamine receptor binding with lack of EPS; also acts as an adrenergic, cholinergic, histaminergic, serotonergic antagonist

USES: Management of psychotic symptoms for schizophrenic patients for whom other antipsychotics have failed; recurrent suicidal behavior

CONTRAINDICATIONS
Hypersensitivity, severe granulocytopenia (WBC <3500 before therapy), coma, ileus
Precautions: Pregnancy, breastfeeding, children <16 yr, geriatric patients; CV, pulmonary, cardiac, renal, hepatic disease; seizures, prostatic enlargement, closed-angle glaucoma, stroke

> **Black Box Warning:** Bone marrow suppression, hypotension, myocarditis, orthostatic hypotension, geriatric patients with dementia-related psychosis, seizures, syncope

DOSAGE AND ROUTES
• **Adult: PO** 12.5 mg daily or bid; may increase by 25-50 mg/day over 2 wk; dose >500 mg requires 3 divided doses; do not increase dose more than 2×/wk; max 900 mg/day; if dose is to be discontinued, taper over 1-2 wk
Available forms: Tablets 25, 50, 100, 200 mg; orally disintegrating tablets 12.5, 25, 100, 150, 200 mg; oral suspension 50 mg/mL
Administer:
• May be taken with or without food
• Patient-specific registration required before administration (cloZAPine REMS program); if WBC <3500 cells/mm^3 or ANC <2000 cells/mm^3, therapy should not be started; may only dispense the 7-, 14-, 28-day supply upon receipt of lab report that is appropriate
• Check to confirm PO medication swallowed; monitor for hoarding or giving of medication to other patients, if hospitalized; avoid giving patient >7 days' worth of medication if outpatient
• Store in tight, light-resistant container
• **Orally disintegrating tablet:** do not push through foil; leave in foil blister until ready to take, peel back foil, place tablet in mouth; allow to dissolve, swallow; water is not needed
• **Oral suspension:** shake before using; use oral syringe and syringe adapter

SIDE EFFECTS
CNS: Neuroleptic malignant syndrome, *sedation, dizziness, headache,* seizures, *insomnia,* dystonia

---

CV: *Tachycardia, hypo/hypertension,* orthostatic hypotension, mitral valve incompetence, myocarditis, ventricular dysrrthmias
EENT: *Blurred vision*
GI: *Drooling or excessive salivation, constipation, nausea, abdominal discomfort, vomiting,* anorexia, *dry mouth, dyspepsia,* hepatotoxicity, GI obstruction, paralytic ileus, intestinal ischemia
GU: *Urinary abnormalities,* incontinence
HEMA: Leukopenia, agranulocytosis
RESP: Dyspnea, pulmonary embolism
SYST: Death among geriatric patients with dementia, aggravation of diabetes mellitus

PHARMACOKINETICS

Bioavailability 27%-47%; 97% protein bound; completely metabolized by liver enzymes involved in metabolism ⚕CYP1A2, 2D6, 3A4; excreted in urine (50%), feces (30%) (metabolites); half-life 8-12 hr

INTERACTIONS

Increase: CNS depression—CNS depressants, psychoactives, alcohol, antihistamines, opioids, sedative/hypnotics
Increase: cloZAPine level—caffeine, citalopram, FLUoxetine, sertraline, ritonavir, risperiDONE, CYP1A2 inhibitors (fluvoxaMINE), CYP3A4 inhibitors (ketoconazole, erythromycin), CYP2D6 inhibitors
Increase: plasma concentration—warfarin, digoxin, other highly protein-bound products
Increase: QT prolongation—beta-blockers, class IA/III antidysrhythmias, and other drugs that increase QT
Increase: hypotension, respiratory, cardiac arrest, collapse—benzodiazepines
Increase: bone marrow suppression—antineoplastics, radiation therapy
Increase: seizures—lithium
Decrease: cloZAPine level—CYP1A2 inducers (carBAMazepine, omeprazole, rifAMPin); PHENobarbital; CYP3A4 inducers

Drug/Herb
Decrease: cloZAPine action—St. John's wort

Drug/Lab Test
Increase: cholesterol, blood glucose, triglycerides
Decrease: WBC, ANC

NURSING CONSIDERATIONS
Assess:

Black Box Warning: Myocarditis: if suspected, discontinue use; myocarditis usually occurs during first month of treatment; dyspnea, fever, palpitations, ECG changes

Black Box Warning: Seizures: usually occur with higher doses >600 mg/day or dosage change >100 mg/day; do not use in uncontrolled seizure disorder; use cautiously in those with a predisposition to seizures

• AIMS assessment, blood glucose, CBC differential, glycosylated hemoglobin A1c, LFTs, neurologic function, pregnancy test, serum creatinine, electrolytes, lipid profile, prolactin, thyroid function tests, weight

Black Box Warning: Bone marrow depression: bilirubin, CBC, LFTs monthly; discontinue treatment if WBC <3000-3500/mm^3 or ANC <1500/mm^3; test weekly; may resume when normal; if WBC <2000/mm^3 or ANC <1000/mm^3, discontinue; if agranulocytosis develops, never restart product

• Affect, orientation, LOC, reflexes, gait, coordination, sleep pattern disturbances
• **GI status:** Monitor for nausea, vomiting, abdominal pain, paralytic ileus may occur; if constipated add fluids, bulk in diet, some patients may require laxatives
• **Respiratory status:** Monitor respirations, check for dyspnea, chest pain, may indicate PE

Black Box Warning: Hypotension, bradycardia, syncope: B/P standing and lying; take pulse, respirations q4hr during initial treatment; establish baseline prior to starting treatment; report drops of 30 mm Hg; dizziness, faintness, palpitations, tachycardia on rising

• **Extrapyramidal symptoms:** including akathisia (inability to sit still, no pattern to movements), tardive dyskinesia (bizarre movements of the jaw, mouth, tongue, extremities), pseudoparkinsonism (rigidity, tremors, pill rolling, shuffling gait)

• **Neuroleptic malignant syndrome:** tachycardia, seizures, fever, dyspnea, diaphoresis, increased/decreased B/P; notify prescriber immediately

• **Beers:** avoid in older adults except for schizophrenia, bipolar disorder; increased risk of stroke and cognitive decline

• **Pregnancy/breastfeeding:** no well-controlled studies; use in pregnancy only if benefits outweigh fetal risk; excreted in breast milk; discontinue breastfeeding or discontinue product; EPS may be present in neonates exposed to this product during third trimester

Evaluate:

• Therapeutic response: decrease in emotional excitement, hallucinations, delusions, paranoia, reorganization of patterns of thought, speech

Teach patient/family:

• About symptoms of agranulocytosis and need for blood tests weekly for 6 mo, then q2wk; to report flulike symptoms

• That orthostatic hypotension often occurs; to rise gradually from sitting or lying position; to avoid hot tubs, hot showers, tub baths; hypotension may occur

• To avoid abrupt withdrawal of this product because EPS may result; that product should be withdrawn over 1-2 wk

• To avoid OTC preparations (cough, hay fever, cold) unless approved by prescriber because serious product interactions may occur; to avoid use with alcohol or CNS depressants, increased drowsiness may occur

• About compliance with product regimen

Black Box Warning: To report sore throat, malaise, fever, bleeding, mouth sores; if these occur, CBC should be drawn and product discontinued

• That heat stroke may occur in hot weather; to take extra precautions to stay cool

• To avoid driving, other hazardous activities; seizures may occur

• To notify prescriber if pregnant or if pregnancy is intended; not to breastfeed

TREATMENT OF OVERDOSE: Lavage; provide an airway; do not induce vomiting

---

⚠ HIGH ALERT

cobimetinib (Rx)

(koe-bi-me′ti-nib)

Cotellic

Func. class.: Antineoplastic

USES: Orphan drug. For the treatment of unresectable or metastatic melanoma in patients with a BRAF V600E or V600K mutation, in combination with vemurafenib

CONTRAINDICATIONS
Hypersensitivity

DOSAGE AND ROUTES

• **Adult: PO** 60 mg (three 20-mg tablets) daily × 21 days, in combination with vemurafenib 960 mg bid × 28 days; repeat cycle q28days until disease progression or unacceptable toxicity

Available forms: Tablets 20 mg

⚠ HIGH ALERT

codeine (Rx)

(koe′deen)

Func. class.: Opiate analgesic, antitussive

Chem. class.: Opiate, phenanthrene derivative

Controlled Substance Schedule II, III, IV, V (depends on content)

Do not confuse:
codeine/Lodine/iodine

ACTION: Depresses pain impulse transmission at the spinal cord level by interacting with opioid receptors; decreases cough reflex, GI motility

USES: Mild to moderate pain

CONTRAINDICATIONS
Breastfeeding, hypersensitivity to opiates, respiratory depression, increased intracranial pressure, seizure disorders, severe respiratory disorders

---

Side effects: *italics* = common; red = life-threatening

Black Box Warning: Children recovering from tonsillectomy/adenoidectomy who are ultrarapid metabolizers; respiratory depression

Precautions: Pregnancy, geriatric patients, cardiac dysrhythmias, prostatic hypertrophy, bowel impaction

Black Box Warning: Accidental exposure, coadministration with other CNS depressants, including opioids

DOSAGE AND ROUTES
Pain
• **Adult: PO** 15-60 mg q4hr, max 360 mg/day
• **Child 6-17 yr (unlabeled): PO** 0.5 to 1 mg/kg/dose, max: 60 mg/dose every 4 hours as needed
Renal disease
• **Adult: PO** CCr 10-50 mL/min, 75% of dose; CCr <10 mL/min, 50% of dose
Available forms: Tablets 15, 30 mg; injection 15, 30, 60 mg/mL; oral solution 25 mg/5 mL ✖
Administer:
• Discontinue gradually after long-term use, use stool softener, laxative for constipation
• Store in light-resistant container at room temperature

SIDE EFFECTS
CNS: *Drowsiness, sedation,* dizziness, dependency, headache, confusion
CV: Bradycardia, palpitations, orthostatic hypotension
GI: *Nausea, vomiting, anorexia, constipation,* dry mouth
GU: Urinary retention
INTEG: Flushing, rash, sweating
RESP: Respiratory depression

PHARMACOKINETICS
Bioavailability 60%-90%; peak ½-1 hr; duration 4-6 hr; metabolized by liver ✖ (CYP3A4 to morphine); excreted by kidneys, in breast milk; crosses placenta; half-life 3 hr; protein binding 7%; ✖ altered codeine metabolism occurs in different ethnic groups

PO: Onset 30-60 min

INTERACTIONS
Linezolid, methylene blue, mirtazapine, traMADol, traZODone; increased serotonin syndrome

Black Box Warning: Increase: CNS depression—alcohol, antihistamines, antidepressants, opiates, sedative/hypnotics, antipsychotics, skeletal muscle relaxants; monitor response

SSRIs, SNRIs, MAOIs, TCAs, 5-HT3 receptor antagonists: Increased serotonin syndrome
Drug/Herb
Increase: CNS depression—chamomile, kava, valerian
Drug/Lab Test
Increase: lipase, amylase
Decrease: opioid effect—opioid antagonists

NURSING CONSIDERATIONS
Assess:
• **Pain:** intensity; type; location; aggravating, alleviating factors; need for pain medication, tolerance; use pain scoring
• I&O ratio; check for decreasing output; may indicate urinary retention, especially among geriatric patients
• GI function: nausea, vomiting, constipation
• **Cough:** type, duration, ability to raise secretion for productive cough; do not use to suppress productive cough
• CNS changes, dizziness, drowsiness, hallucinations, euphoria, LOC, pupil reaction
• Allergic reactions: rash, urticaria
• B/P, pulse respirations baseline and periodically

Black Box Warning: Monitor for tolerance, addiction, abuse

Black Box Warning: Children (tonsillectomy/adenoidectomy and are ultrarapid metabolizers): deaths have occurred; use is contraindicated

Black Box Warning: Respiratory dysfunction: respiratory depression, character, rate, rhythm; notify prescriber if respirations are <10/min, shallow; obstructive sleep apnea (children) (tonsillectomy/adenoidectomy)

✖ Canada only   ✖ Genetic warning

• **Beers:** avoid in older adults unless safer alternative is unavailable; may cause ataxia, impaired psychomotor function

Evaluate:

• Therapeutic response: decrease in pain, absence of grimacing, decreased cough, decreased diarrhea

Teach patient/family:

• To report any symptoms of CNS changes, allergic reactions

• That physical dependency may result after extended periods, product should be used short term

• To change position slowly; orthostatic hypotension may occur

• To avoid hazardous activities if drowsiness or dizziness occurs

Black Box Warning: To avoid alcohol, other CNS depressants unless directed by prescriber

• To increase fiber, water in diet to help avoid constipation

• **Pregnancy/breastfeeding:** to notify prescriber if pregnancy is planned or suspected; infants born to those using opioids are at risk of neonatal opiate withdrawal; not to breastfeed

TREATMENT OF OVERDOSE: Naloxone 0.4-mg ampule diluted in 10 mL 0.9% NaCl and given by direct IV push, 0.02 mg q2min (adult)

colchicine (Rx)

(kol′chih-seen)

ColciGel, Colcrys, Gloperba, Mitigare

Func. class.: Antigout agent

Chem. class.: Alkaloid

Do not confuse:

colchicine/Cortrosyn

ACTION: Inhibits microtubule formation of lactic acid in leukocytes, which decreases phagocytosis and inflammation in joints

USES: Gout, gouty arthritis (prevention, treatment); to arrest the progression of neurologic disability in those with MS, Mediterranean fever

Unlabeled uses: Bechet syndrome with arthritis, cutaneous lesions or mucocutaneous ulcers, acute and recurrent pericarditis with NSAIDs, or aspirin

CONTRAINDICATIONS

Serious GI, severe cardiac/renal/hepatic disorders, hypersensitivity

Precautions: Pregnancy (PO), breastfeeding, children, geriatric patients, blood dyscrasias, hepatic disease

DOSAGE AND ROUTES

Gout prevention

• **Adult: PO** 0.6-1.2 mg/day in 1-2 divided doses, depending on severity

Gout treatment

• **Adult: PO** 1.2 mg initially, then 0.6 mg 1 hr later (1.8 mg); *for those on strong CYP3A4 inhibitor* (during past 14 days), 0.6 mg initially, then 0.3 mg 1 hr later

Mediterranean fever

• **Adult on no interacting products: PO** 1.2-2.4 mg/day in 1-2 divided doses; **strong CYP3A4 inhibitors; P-glycoprotein inhibitors within 14 days:** max 0.6 mg/day in 1-2 divided doses; **moderate CYP3A4 inhibitors within 14 days:** max 1.2 mg/day in 1-2 divided doses

• **Adolescent: PO** 1.2-2.4 mg/day in 1-2 divided doses, titrate by 0.3 mg/day

• **Child >6-12 yr: PO** 0.9-1.8 mg/day in 1-2 divided doses

• **Child 4-6 yr: PO** 0.3-1.8 mg/day in 1-2 divided doses

Bechet syndrome (unlabeled)

• **Adult: PO:** 1.2-1.8 mg/day in divided doses

Pericarditis (unlabeled)

• **Adult 18-17 yr: PO:** ≥70 kg 0.5-0.6 mg bid; <70 kg 0.5-0.6 mg daily for 3 mo

• **Adults >70 yr and ≥70 kg: PO** 0.25-0.3 mg twice daily; <70 kg 0.25-0.3 mg once daily for 3 mo

Renal dose

• **Adult: PO** CCr <30 mL/min, for acute gout, do not repeat course for 2 wk; for familial Mediterranean fever, 0.3 mg daily, increase cautiously

Available forms: Tablets 0.6 mg; oral solution 0.6 mg/5 mL; capsules 0.6 mg; oral solution 0.6 mg/5 mL

Administer:

PO route

• Without regard to food

• Cumulative doses ≤4 mg, renal patients ≤2 mg

SIDE EFFECTS

GI: *Nausea, vomiting, anorexia,* cramps

HEMA: Agranulocytosis, thrombocytopenia, aplastic anemia, pancytopenia

MISC: Alopecia, peripheral neuritis

PHARMACOKINETICS

PO: Peak ½-2 hr, half-life 30 hr, deacetylates in liver, excreted in feces (metabolites/active product)

INTERACTIONS

Increase: colchicine level/toxicity—moderate/strong CYP3A4 inhibitors (atazanavir, clarithromycin, indinavir, itraconazole, ketoconazole, ritonavir, nefazodone, nelfinavir, saquinavir, telithromycin), P-glycoprotein inhibitors; reduce dose

Increase: GI effects—NSAIDs, ethanol

Increase: bone marrow depression—radiation, bone marrow depressants, cycloSPORINE

Increase: rhabdomyolysis HMG-CoA reductase inhibitors—digoxin

Decrease: action of vitamin B_{12}; may cause reversible malabsorption

Drug/Food

Increase: colchicine level—grapefruit juice, avoid using together

Drug/Lab Test

Increase: alkaline phosphatase, AST

Decrease: platelets, WBC, granulocytes

False positive: urine HB

Interference: urinary 17-hydroxycorticosteroids

NURSING CONSIDERATIONS

Assess:

• **Gout:** relief of pain, uric acid levels decreasing; monitor response to treatment q1hr

• **Familial Mediterranean fever:** chest pain, fever, joint pain, red lesions baseline and during treatment

• I&O ratio; observe for decrease in urinary output

• CBC; platelets; reticulocytes before, during therapy (q3mo); may cause aplastic anemia, agranulocytosis, decreased platelets in those on long-term therapy

• **Toxicity:** weakness, abdominal pain, nausea, vomiting, diarrhea; product should be discontinued, report symptoms immediately

• **Beers:** reduce dose in older adults; monitor for adverse reactions

• **Pregnancy/breastfeeding:** no well-controlled studies; use in pregnancy only if benefits outweigh fetal risk; neonatal codeine withdrawal may occur; don't use in labor (premature infant); excreted in breast milk, avoid breastfeeding

Evaluate:

• Therapeutic response: decreased stone formation, decreased pain in kidney region, absence of hematuria, decreased pain in joints, reduced familial Mediterranean fever episodes

Teach patient/family:

• To avoid alcohol, OTC preparations that contain alcohol

• To report any pain, redness, hard areas, usually in legs; rash, sore throat, fever, bleeding, bruising, weakness, numbness, tingling, nausea, vomiting, abdominal pain, muscle pain, weakness

• To avoid grapefruit and juice, may increase colchicine level

• About the importance of complying with medical regimen (diet, weight loss, product therapy); about the possibility of bone marrow depression occurring; not to double or skip doses; during acute attacks other products may be needed

• To advise all providers of product use; that surgery may increase the possibility of acute gout symptoms

TREATMENT OF OVERDOSE:

D/C medication; may need opioids to treat diarrhea

colesevelam (Rx)

(koe-leh-seve'eh-lam)

Lodalis ✤, WelChol

Func. class.: Antilipemic
Chem. class.: Bile acid sequestrant

ACTION: Adsorbs, combines with bile acids to form insoluble complex excreted through feces; loss of bile acids lowers cholesterol levels

USES: Elevated LDL cholesterol, alone or in combination with HMG-COA reductase inhibitor; type 2 diabetes (adjunct)

CONTRAINDICATIONS

Hypersensitivity, bowel disease, primary biliary cirrhosis, triglycerides >500 mg/dL, bowel obstruction, pancreatitis, biliary obstruction, dysphagia, fat-soluble vitamin deficiency

Precautions: Pregnancy, breastfeeding, children

DOSAGE AND ROUTES

Hyperlipidemia

• **Adult: PO** three 625-mg tablets bid with meals or 6 tablets daily with meal; may increase to 7 tablets if needed (monotherapy); 3 tablets bid with meals or 6 tablets daily with meal given with an HMG-CoA reductase inhibitor (combination)

Type 2 diabetes

• **Adult and geriatric: PO** approx 3.8 g (6 tablets)/day or approx 1.9 g (3 tablets) bid

Available forms: Tablets 625 mg; granules for oral suspension 3.75 g/packet

Administer:

• Swallow tablets whole; do not break, crush, or chew

• Give product daily or bid with meals; give all other medications 4 hr before colesevelam; with liquid to avoid poor absorption

• **Granules for oral suspension:** empty contents of packet into a cup/glass, add ½-1 cup (4-8 oz) of water, fruit juice, diet soda; stir well before drinking

SIDE EFFECTS

CNS: Headache, fatigue
ENDO: Hypoglycemia
CV: Hypertension
GI: *Constipation, nausea,* flatulence, hypertriglyceridemia

PHARMACOKINETICS

Excreted in feces, peak response 2 wk

INTERACTIONS

Decrease: absorption of—diltiaZEM, gemfibrozil, mycophenolate, phenytoin, propranolol, warfarin, thiazides, digoxin, penicillin G, tetracyclines, corticosteroids, iron, thyroid, fat-soluble vitamins, glyBURIDE, fluoroquinolones

Decrease: action of—oral contraceptives, give ≥4 hr prior to colesevelam

Drug/Lab Test

Increase: LFTs

NURSING CONSIDERATIONS

Assess:

• Cardiac glycoside level if used with an HMG-CoA

• **Hypercholesterolemia:** fasting LDL, HDL, total cholesterol, triglyceride levels baseline and q4-6wk after initiation of treatment and periodically, electrolytes if on extended therapy; monitor BUN/creatinine, take diet history

• Bowel pattern daily; increase bulk, water in diet for constipation

• **Diabetes:** hypoglycemia (weakness, hunger, dizziness, diaphoresis) can result from use of this product, monitor blood glucose, A1c

Evaluate:

• Therapeutic response: decreased total cholesterol level, LDL cholesterol, apolipoproteins

Teach patient/family:

• About the importance of compliance; timing of dose 4 hr after other meds

• **Hypercholesterolemia:** That risk factors should be decreased: high-fat diet, smoking, alcohol consumption, absence of exercise

• To take with meal and fluids

• To discuss with health care professional all OTC, herbals, supplements, to use oral contraceptive at least 4 hr prior to this product

• Diabetes: to monitor glucose
• **Pregnancy/breastfeeding:** to notify prescriber if pregnancy is planned or suspected or if breastfeeding; that insulin may be used in diabetes during pregnancy; to use another form of contraception other than oral contraceptives

---

collagenase clostridium histolyticum-aaes (Rx)
(kol'la-je-nase)
Xiaflex
Func. class.: Enzyme

USES: Treatment of adults with Dupuytren's contracture with a palpable cord; treatment of adult men with Peyronie's disease with a palpable plaque/curvature deformity of at least 30 degrees

CONTRAINDICATIONS
Hyper-sensitivity, pregnancy, breastfeeding

DOSAGE AND ROUTES
Dupuytren's contracture
Adult: Intralesional: Inject 0.58 mg per cord affecting a metacarpophalangeal (MP) joint or a proximal interphalangeal (PIP) joint. If contracture persists, finger extension procedure should be performed 24 to 72 hr following injection
Peyronie's disease
Adult male: Intralesional Inject 0.58 mg into a Peyronie's plaque; repeat 1 to 3 days later. Perform a penile modeling procedure 1-3 days after second injection. Use a second treatment cycle (two 0.58-mg injections and a penile modeling procedure) in 6 wk if needed (max 4 cycles)
Available forms: Capsules 25, 50, 75 mg

---

conivaptan (Rx)
(kon-ih-vap'tan)
Vaprisol
Func. class.: Vasopressin receptor antagonist

ACTION: Dual arginine vasopressin (AVP) antagonist with affinity for V_{1A}, V_2 receptors; level of AVP in circulating blood is critical for regulation of water, electrolyte balance and is usually elevated in euvolemic/hypervolemic hyponatremia

USES: Euvolemia hyponatremia in hospitalized patients; not indicated for HF, hypervolemic hyponatremia
Unlabeled uses: Increased intracranial pressure

CONTRAINDICATIONS
Hypersensitivity, hypovolemia
Precautions: Pregnancy, breastfeeding, orthostatic disease, renal disease, heart failure, rapid correction of serum sodium

DOSAGE AND ROUTES
• **Adult: IV INFUSION** loading dose 20 mg given over 30 min then CONT INFUSION of 20 mg over 24 hr; after day 1, give 20 mg/24 hr for an additional 1-3 days; can be titrated up to 40 mg/day if serum sodium is not rising at desired rate; max time 4 days
Hepatic/renal dose
• **Adult: IV** Child-Pugh A-C or CCr 30-60 mL/min: give IV loading dose over 10 min then **CONTINUOUS IV INFUSION** 10 mg over 24 hr × 2-4 days
Available forms: Injection (premixed) 0.2 mg/mL in 100 mL D_5W
Administer:
Intermittent IV Infusion
• Premixed, do not need dilution (0.2 mg/mL)
Continuous IV INFUSION route
• Give over 24 hr or 40 mg/24 hr

SIDE EFFECTS
CNS: Headache, confusion, insomnia
CV: Hypo/hypertension, *orthostatic hypotension*
GI: Nausea, vomiting, constipation, dry mouth
GU: Hematuria, infertility (women), polyuria
INTEG: Erythema, injection site reaction
META: Dehydration, hypokalemia, hypomagnesemia, hyponatremia
MISC: Oral candidiasis

PHARMACOKINETICS
Protein binding 99%, metabolized by
CYP3A4, half-life 5 hr

INTERACTIONS
Increase: effect of—CYP3A4 substrates
(alfuzosin, ARIPiprazole, bexarotene, bortezomib, bosentan, bupivacaine, buprenorphine, carBAMazepine, cevimeline, cilostazol, cinacalcet, clopidogrel, colchicine,
cyclobenzaprine, dapsone, darifenacin,
disopyramide, DOCEtaxel, donepezil, DOXO-
rubicin, dutasteride, eletriptan, eplerenone,
ergots, erlotinib, eszopiclone, ethinyl estradiol, ethosuximide, etoposide, fentaNYL,
galantamine, gefitinib, ifosfamide, irinotecan, lidocaine, loperamide, loratadine,
mefloquine, methadone, modafinil, PACLitaxel, paricalcitrol, pimozide, praziquantel,
quiNIDine, quiNINE, ramelteon, repaglinide,
rifabutin, sibutramine, sildenafil, sirolimus,
SUFentanil, SUNItinib, tacrolimus, tamoxifen, teniposide, testosterone, tiaGABine, tinidazole, trimetrexate, vardenafil, vinca alkaloids, ziprasidone, zolpidem, zonisamide);
do not use concurrently

NURSING CONSIDERATIONS
Assess:
• Renal, hepatic function
• **Sodium levels/volume status:** monitor serum sodium levels q2-3hr until
stable; overly rapid correction of sodium
concentration (>12 mEq/L per 24 hr) may
result in osmotic demyelination syndrome
• Neurologic status: confusion, headache
• **Injection site reactions:** redness, inflammation, pain; if these occur, product
needs to be discontinued
• CV status: atrial fibrillation, hypo/hy-
pertension, orthostatic hypotension; monitor B/P, pulse baseline and periodically
• Monitor other electrolytes (magnesium
and potassium)
• **Pregnancy/breastfeeding:** no well-
controlled studies; use in pregnancy only if
benefits outweigh fetal risk, may cause
fetal harm; discontinue breastfeeding or
discontinue product; excretion is unknown
Evaluate:
• Therapeutic response: correction of
serum sodium levels

Teach patient/family:
• To report neurologic changes: headache, insomnia, confusion
• About administration procedure and
expected results
• To report injection site pain, redness,
swelling

CONTRACEPTIVES, HORMONAL

Monophasic, Oral

ethinyl estradiol/ desogestrel (Rx)
Apri-28, EnsKyce, Isibloom,
Kalliga, Reclipsen, Solia,
Emoquette
ethinyl estradiol/ drospirenone (Rx)
Beyaz, Gianvi, Loryna, Nikki,
Safyral, Syeda, Yaela, Zarah,
Yasmin, Yaz, Ocella
ethinyl estradiol/ ethynodiol (Rx)
Kelnor, Lo-Mamorede, Malmorede,
Zovia 1/35-28, Zovia 1/50-28
ethinyl estradiol/ levonorgestrel (Rx)
Aviane-28, Altavera, Aubra,
Chateal, Falmina, Kurvelo,
Marlissa, Vienva, Lessina,
Levora, Lutera, Sronyx
ethinyl estradiol/ norethindrone (Rx)
Alyacen 1/35, Briellyn, Dasetta,
Generess Fe, Larin 1/20, Larin Fe
1.5/30, Junel 1/20, Junel 1.5/30,
Loestrin 1.5/30, Loestrin 1/20,
Nortrel 1/35
ethinyl estradiol/ norgestimate (Rx)
Estarylla, Milli, Mono-Linyah,
MonoNessa, Previfem, Sprintec

ethinyl estradiol/
norgestrel (Rx)
Cryselle, Elinest, Low-Ogestrel
mestranol/
norethindrone (Rx)
Necon 1/50

Biphasic, Oral

ethinyl estradiol/
norethindrone (Rx)

Triphasic, Oral

ethinyl estradiol/
desogestrel (Rx)
Azurette, Bekyree, Cyclessa,
Kariva, Kimidess, Pimtrea,
Viorele
ethinyl estradiol/
norethindrone (Rx)
Nortrel 7/7/7, Tri-Norinyl-28
ethinyl estradiol/
norgestimate (Rx)
Ortho Tri-Cyclen, Tri-Estarylla,
Tri-Linyah
ethinyl estradiol/
levonorgestrel (Rx)
Enpresse, Levonest

Four-Phasic Oral
Estradiol/valerate/
dienogest
Natazia

Extended Cycle, Oral

ethinyl estradiol/
levonorgestrel (Rx)
Amethia, Amethia Lo, Amethyst,
Ashlyna, Camrese, Camrese Lo,
Daysee, Dolishale, Iclevia,
Introvale, Jaimiess, Jolessa,
LoSeasonique, Quartette,
Quasense, Seasonale,
Seasonique, Setlakin,
Simpesse

Progestin, Oral

norethindrone (Rx)
Errin, Jencycla, Nora-BE, Camila,
Jolivette
norgestrel (OTC)
Opill

Progressive Estrogen, Oral

ethinyl estradiol/
norethindrone acetate (Rx)
Estrostep, Estrostep Fe

Emergency

levonorgestrel (Rx)
Athentia Next, Fallback Solo,
Plan B, Logilia
Ulipristal
Ella
medroxyPROGESTER-
one (Rx)
Depo-SubQ, Depo-Provera,
Provera 104

Intrauterine

levonorgestrel (Rx)
Kyleena, Liltta, Mirena, Skyla

Implant

etonogestrel (Rx)
Nexplanon

Vaginal Ring

ethinyl estradiol/
etonogestrel (Rx)
Elu Ring, NuvaRing

Transdermal

ethinyl estradiol/
norelgestromin (Rx)
Onsura, Xulane
ethinyl estradiol
levonorgestral
Twirla

ACTION: Prevents ovulation by suppressing FSH and LH; *monophasic:* estrogen/progestin (fixed dose) used during a 21-day cycle; ovulation is inhibited by suppression of FSH and LH; thickness of cervical mucus and endometrial lining prevents pregnancy; *biphasic:* ovulation is inhibited by suppression of FSH and LH; alteration of cervical mucus, endometrial lining prevents pregnancy; *triphasic:* ovulation is inhibited by suppression of FSH and LH; change of cervical mucus, endometrial lining prevents pregnancy; variable doses of estrogen/progestin combinations may be similar to natural hormonal fluctuations; *extended cycle:* estrogen/progestin continuous for 84 days, off for 7 days, results in 4 menstrual periods/yr; *progressive estrogen:* constant progestin with 3 progressive doses of estrogen; *progestin-only pill, implant, intrauterine:* change of cervical mucus and endometrial lining prevents pregnancy; ovulation may be suppressed

USES: To prevent pregnancy, regulation of menstrual cycle, treatment of acne in women >14 yr for whom other treatment has failed, emergency contraception; *injection:* inhibits gonadotropin secretion, ovulation, follicular maturation; *emergency:* inhibits ovulation and fertilization, decreases transport of sperm and egg from fallopian tube to uterus; *vaginal ring, transdermal:* inhibits ovulation, prevents sperm entry into uterus; *antiacne:* may decrease sex hormone binding globulin, results in decreased testosterone

CONTRAINDICATIONS

Pregnancy, breastfeeding, women ≥40 yr, reproductive cancer, thrombophlebitis, MI, hepatic tumors, hepatic disease, CAD, CVA, breast cancer, jaundice, stroke, vaginal bleeding

Precautions: Depression, hypertension, renal disease, seizure disorders, lupus erythematosus, rheumatic disease, migraine headache, amenorrhea, irregular menses, gallbladder disease, diabetes mellitus, heavy smoking, acute mononucleosis, sickle cell disease

Black Box Warning: Tobacco smoking

DOSAGE AND ROUTES
Monophasic
• **Adult: PO** Take first tablet on Sunday after start of menses × 21 days; skip 7 days, then repeat cycle; may contain 7 placebo tablets when 1 tablet is taken daily
Biphasic
• **Adult: PO** Take 10 days of small progestin, then large progestin; estrogen is the same during cycle; skip 7 days, then repeat cycle; may contain 7 placebo tablets when 1 tablet is taken daily
Triphasic
• **Adult: PO** Estrogen dose remains constant; progestin changes throughout 21-day cycle; some products contain 28 tablets per month
Four-phasic
Adult: PO Give in 4 phases: 1st: more estrogen, no progestin; 2nd/3rd: lower estrogen, increasing progestin; 4th: low estrogen
Extended cycle
• **Adult: PO** Start taking on first day of menses; continue for 84 days of active tablets, then 7 days of placebo; repeat cycle
Progestin
• **Adult: PO** Start on first day of menses, then daily and continuously
Progressive estrogen
• **Adult: PO** Progestin dose remains constant; estrogen increases q7days throughout 21-day cycle; may include 7 placebo tablets for 28-day cycle
Emergency
• **Adult/adolescent: PO** Give within 72 hr of intercourse, repeat 12 hr later; **Plan B** 1 tablet, then 1 tablet 12 hr later; **Preven** 2 tablets, then 2 tablets 12 hr later; **Ovral** 2 white tablets; **Lo/Ovral (unlabeled)** 4 white tablets; **Levlen, Nordette** 4 orange tablets; **Triphasil, Tri-Levlen** 4 yellow tablets
Injectable
• **Adult: IM (Depo-Provera)** 150 mg within 5 days of start of menses or within 5 days postpartum (must not be breastfeeding); if breastfeeding, give 6 wk postpartum, repeat q3mo
Intrauterine
• **Adult: INTRAUTERINE** To be inserted using the levonorgestrel-releasing intrauterine system (LRIS) by those trained

Side effects: *italics* = common; red = life-threatening

in procedure; inserted into uterine cavity within 7 days of the onset of menstruation; use should not exceed 5 yr per implant

Vaginal ring

• **Adult: VAG** Insert 1 ring on or prior to day 5 of cycle; leave in place 3 wk; remove for 1 wk, then repeat

Transdermal

• **Adult: TD** Apply patch within 7 days of menses; change weekly × 3 wk; no patch wk 4; repeat cycle

Implant

• **Adult: SUBDERMAL** In inner side of upper arm on days 1-5 of menses, replace q3yr

Acne

• **Adult: PO (Ortho Tri-Cyclen)** Take daily × 21 days, off 7 days

Administer:

• PO with food for GI symptoms; give at same time each day

• Subdermal implant of 6 capsules effective for 5 yr, then should be removed

• IM injection deep in large muscle mass after shaking suspension; ensure patient not pregnant if injections are 2 wk or more apart

SIDE EFFECTS

CNS: Depression, fatigue, dizziness, nervousness, anxiety, headache

CV: Increased B/P, cerebral hemorrhage, thrombosis, pulmonary embolism, fluid retention, edema, MI

EENT: Optic neuritis, retinal thrombosis, cataracts

ENDO: Decreased glucose tolerance, increased TBG, PBI, T_4, T_3, temporary infertility

GI: *Nausea,* vomiting, cramps, diarrhea, bloating, constipation, change in appetite, cholestatic jaundice, weight change

GU: Breakthrough bleeding, amenorrhea, spotting, dysmenorrhea, galactorrhea, endocervical hyperplasia, vaginitis, cystitis-like syndrome, breast changes

HEMA: Increased fibrinogen, clotting factor

INTEG: *Chloasma, melasma,* acne, rash, urticaria, erythema, pruritus, hirsutism, alopecia, photosensitivity

PHARMACOKINETICS

Excreted in breast milk

INTERACTIONS

Decrease: oral contraceptives' effectiveness—anticonvulsants, rifAMPin, analgesics, antibiotics, antihistamines, griseofulvin

Decrease: oral anticoagulants' action

Drug/Herb

Altered action: black cohosh

Decrease: oral contraceptives' effect—saw palmetto, St. John's wort

Drug/Food

Increase: peak level—grapefruit juice

Drug/Lab Test

Increase: PT; clotting factors VII, VIII, IX, X; TBG, PBI, T_4, platelet aggregability, BSP, triglycerides, bilirubin, AST, ALT

Decrease: T_3, antithrombin III, folate, metyrapone test, GTT, 17-OHCS

NURSING CONSIDERATIONS

Assess:

• Glucose, thyroid function, LFTs, B/P

• Reproductive changes: changes in breasts, tumors; positive Pap smear; product should be discontinued

Evaluate:

• Therapeutic response: absence of pregnancy, endometriosis, hypermenorrhea

Teach patient/family:

• To use sunscreen or avoid sunlight; photosensitivity can occur

• To take at same time each day to ensure equal product level

• To report GI symptoms that occur after 4 mo

• **Pregnancy/breastfeeding:** to use another birth control method during first 3 wk of oral contraceptive use; to avoid use in breastfeeding; many antibiotics interfere with oral contraceptives

• To take another tablet as soon as possible if one is missed

• That, after product is discontinued, pregnancy may not occur for several months

• To report abdominal pain, change in vision, shortness of breath, change in menstrual flow, spotting, breakthrough bleeding, breast lumps, swelling, headache, severe leg pain

- That continuing medical care is needed: Pap smear and gynecologic examinations q12mo
- To notify health care providers and dentists of oral contraceptive use; many antibiotics interfere with oral contraceptive effect

Black Box Warning: Do not smoke; increased risk of CV side effects

copanlisib (Rx)
(koh-pan′-lih-sib)
Aliqopa
Func. class.: Antineoplastic biologic response modifiers

USES: For the treatment of non-Hodgkin's lymphoma

CONTRAINDICATIONS
Pregnancy, hypersensitivity
Precautions: Breastfeeding, contraception requirements, children, diabetes mellitus, diarrhea, geriatric patients, hepatic/pulmonary disease, hyperglycemia, hypertension, infertility, male-mediated teratogenicity, neutropenia, pneumonitis, bone marrow suppression, infection, reproductive risk, serious rash, thrombocytopenia

DOSAGE AND ROUTES
Relapsed follicular lymphoma
- **Adult:** IV 60 mg over 1 hr on days 1, 8, and 15 repeated q28days until disease progression; reduce dose to 45 mg if using with strong CYP3A4 inhibitor
Available forms: Injection, lyophilized 60-mg single-dose vials

crisaborole (Rx)
(kris′a-bor-ole)
Eucrisa
Func. class.: Dermatologic agent
Chem. class.: Phosphodiesterase 4 enzyme inhibitor

ACTION: Increases intracellular cyclic adenosine monophosphate (cAMP) levels in the skin

USES: Mild to moderate atopic dermatitis

CONTRAINDICATIONS
Hypersensitivity
Precautions: Children, pregnancy, breastfeeding

DOSAGE AND ROUTES
- **Adult/child ≥2 yr: TOPICAL;** Apply ointment bid in a thin film to cover area
Available forms: Topical ointment 2%
Administer:
Topical route:
- For external use only; store at room temperature
- Tube should be tightly closed
- Apply only to affected areas

SIDE EFFECTS
INTEG: Burning, stinging, application site pain

PHARMACOKINETICS
97% protein bound, excreted renally

INTERACTIONS
None known

NURSING CONSIDERATIONS
Assess:
- **Contact dermatitis:** for redness, itching, inflammation; assess if these symptoms are relieved after application
- **Hypersensitivity:** for pruritus, inflammation, rash; if present, product should be discontinued
- **Pregnancy/breastfeeding:** no adverse reactions in animal studies, no human studies available; consider benefits to mother and infant if breastfeeding; product is systemically absorbed
Evaluate:
- Therapeutic response: decreasing redness, itching, inflammation
Teach patient/family:
- **Contact dermatitis:** to identify whether symptoms are relieved after application;

to apply a thin film and wash hands after use; to use externally only

• **Hypersensitivity:** to report immediately itching, inflammation, rash; if present, product should be discontinued

• **Pregnancy/breastfeeding:** to advise prescriber if pregnant or planning to get pregnant, or if breastfeeding; effects are unknown

---

crizotinib (Rx)
(kriz-oh′ti-nib)
Xalkori
Func. class.: Antineoplastic

USES: ⟐ Locally advanced or metastatic non–small-cell lung cancer (NSCLC) that is anaplastic lymphoma kinase (ALK)-positive as detected by an FDA-approved test, ⟐ relapsed or refractory systemic anaplastic large cell lymphoma positive for ALK

CONTRAINDICATIONS
Pregnancy, breastfeeding, hypersensitivity, concurrent use of strong CYP3A4 inducers/inhibitors
Precautions: Neonates, infants, children, adolescents, pneumonitis, severe hepatic disease, congenital long QT syndrome, severe renal impairment, end-stage renal disease, vision disorders

DOSAGE AND ROUTES
• **Adult: PO** 250 mg bid; continue as long as beneficial; if CCr <30 mL/min use 250 mg daily

Available forms: Capsules 200, 300 mg

---

crofelemer (Rx)
(kroe-fel′e-mer)
Mytesi
Func. class.: Antidiarrheal
Chem. class.: Red sap of *Croton lechleri* plant

ACTION: Blocks chloride channel and high-volume water loss in diarrhea

USES: Noninfectious diarrhea in those with HIV/AIDS using antiretrovirals

CONTRAINDICATIONS
Hypersensitivity
Precautions: Pregnancy, ⟐ breastfeeding, Black patients, children/adolescents, GI disease, infection, malabsorption syndrome, pancreatitis

DOSAGE AND ROUTES
• **Adult: PO** 125 mg bid
Available forms: Delayed-release tablets 125 mg
Administer:
• Do not break, crush, or chew
• Without regard to meals

SIDE EFFECTS
CNS: Dizziness, depression
GI: Nausea, constipation, abdominal pain, anorexia, flatulence, hemorrhoids
INTEG: Acne vulgaris, contact dermatitis
MISC: Arthralgia, cough, increased urinary frequency

INTERACTIONS
Increase: serious constipation, bowel obstruction—alosetron (IBS)
Increase: constipation—may occur with antimuscarinics, opiate agonists

NURSING CONSIDERATIONS
Assess:
• Stools: volume, color, characteristic, frequency; bowel pattern before protein rebound constipation
• Electrolytes (K, Na, Cl), hydration status
• Monitor effect in Black patients; may be less effective
Evaluate: Therapeutic response: decreased diarrhea
Teach patient/family:
• To avoid OTC products unless directed by prescriber
• If drowsiness occurs, not to operate machinery

crotamiton
(kroe-tam´-ih-tuhn)

Crotan, Eurax (Rx)
Func. class.: Scabicide/pediculicide

USES: Scabies, lice

CONTRAINDICATIONS
Hypersensitivity; raw, inflamed skin

DOSAGE AND ROUTES
• **Adult: TOPICAL** After routine bath, apply over the entire body from the chin to the soles; do not apply to the face or head; repeat in 24 hr; patient may take a cleansing bath 48 hr after the second dose
Treatment of pruritus
• **Adult: TOPICAL** Apply topically by massaging gently into affected area until medication is completely absorbed; repeat if needed
Available forms: Lotion, cream 10%

cyanocobalamin (vitamin B$_{12}$) (OTC, Rx)
(sye-an-oh-koe-bal´a-min)

Nascobal, Rubramin PC
hydroxocobalamin (OTC, Rx)

CytoKit
Func. class.: Vitamin B$_{12}$, water-soluble vitamin

ACTION: Needed for adequate nerve functioning, protein and carbohydrate metabolism, normal growth, RBC development, cell reproduction

USES: Vitamin B$_{12}$ deficiency, pernicious anemia, Vitamin B$_{12}$ malabsorption syndrome, Schilling test, increased requirements with pregnancy, thyrotoxicosis, hemolytic anemia, hemorrhage, renal/hepatic disease, nutritional supplementation

CONTRAINDICATIONS
Hypersensitivity to this product, cobalt, benzyl alcohol, optic nerve atrophy

Precautions: Pregnancy, breastfeeding, children, renal/hepatic disease, folic acid/iron deficiency anemia, infection

DOSAGE AND ROUTES
cyanocobalamin
• **Adult: PO** Up to 1000 mcg/day **SUB-CUT/IM** 30-100 mcg/day × 1 wk, then 100-200 mcg/mo
Schilling test
• **Adult/child: IM** 1000 mcg in 1 dose
• **Child: PO** up to 1000 mcg/day **SUB-CUT/IM** 30-50 mcg/day × 2 wk, then 100 mcg/mo; **NASAL** 500 mcg weekly

hydroxocobalamin
• **Adult: SUBCUT/IM** 30-50 mcg/day × 5-10 days, then 100-200 mcg/mo
• **Child: SUBCUT/IM** 30-50 mcg/day × 5-10 days, then 30-50 mcg/mo
Available forms: *Cyanocobalamin:* tablets 50, 100, 250, 500, 1000, 5000 mcg; extended-release tablets 1000 mcg; lozenges 100, 250, 500 mcg; nasal 500 mcg/spray; injection 100, 1000 mcg/mL; *hydroxocobalamin:* injection 1000 mcg/mL, powder for injection 5 g/vial
Administer:
PO route
• With fruit juice to disguise taste; immediately after mixing
• With meals if possible for better absorption; large doses should not be used because most is excreted
• Protect from light, heat
IM route
• By IM injection for pernicious anemia for life unless contraindicated
Intranasal route
• Avoid use within 1 hr of hot fluids, food, no priming needed
IV route
• IV route not recommended but may be admixed in TPN solution
Additive compatibilities: Ascorbic acid, chloramphenicol, hydrocortisone, vitamin B/C
Solution compatibilities: Dextrose/Ringer's or LR combinations, dextrose/saline combinations, D$_5$W, D$_{10}$W, 0.45% NaCl, Ringer's or LR solution
Y-site compatibilities: Alfentanil, amikacin, aminophylline, ascorbic acid, atracurium,

---

Side effects: *italics* = common; red = life-threatening

atropine, azaTHIOprine, aztreonam, benztropine, bretylium, bumetanide, buprenorphine, butorphanol, calcium chloride/gluconate, ceFAZolin, cefmetazole, cefonicid, cefotaxime, cefoTEtan, cefOXitin, cefTAZidime, ceftizoxime, cefTRIAXone, cefuroxime, chloramphenicol, chlorproMAZINE, cimetidine, clindamycin, dexamethasone, digoxin, diphenhydrAMINE, DOBUTamine, DOPamine, doxycycline, enalaprilat, ePHEDrine, EPINEPHrine, epoetin alfa, erythromycin, esmolol, famotidine, fentaNYL, fluconazole, folic acid, furosemide, ganciclovir, gentamicin, glycopyrrolate, heparin, hydrocortisone, hydrOXYzine, imipenem-cilastatin, indomethacin, insulin (regular), isoproterenol hydrochloride, ketorolac, labetalol, lidocaine, magnesium, mannitol, meperidine, methoxamine, methyldopate, methylPREDNISolone, metoclopramide, metoprolol, miconazole, midazolam, minocycline, morphine, moxalactam, multiple vitamins injection, nafcillin, nalbuphine, naloxone, netilmicin, nitroglycerin, nitroprusside, norepinephrine, ondansetron, oxacillin, oxytocin, papaverine, penicillin G potassium/sodium, pentamidine, pentazocine, PENTobarbital, PHENobarbital, phentolamine, phenylephrine, phytonadione, piperacillin, polymyxin B, potassium chloride, procainamide, prochlorperazine, promethazine, propranolol, protamine, pyridoxine, quiNIDine, raNITIdine, ritodrine, sodium bicarbonate, succinylcholine, SUFentanil, theophylline, thiamine, ticarcillin, ticarcillin-clavulanate, tobramycin, tolazoline, trimetaphan, urokinase, vancomycin, vasopressin, verapamil, vitamin B complex with C

SIDE EFFECTS

CNS: Flushing, optic nerve atrophy
CV: HF, peripheral vascular thrombosis, pulmonary edema
GI: *Diarrhea*
INTEG: Itching, rash, pain at injection site
META: Hypokalemia
SYST: Anaphylactic shock

PHARMACOKINETICS

Gastric intrinsic factor must be present for absorption to occur; stored in liver, kidneys, stomach; 50%-90% excreted in urine; crosses placenta; excreted in breast milk

INTERACTIONS

Increase: absorption—predniSONE
Decrease: absorption—aminoglycosides, anticonvulsants, colchicine, chloramphenicol, aminosalicylic acid, potassium preparations, cimetidine
Drug/Herb
Decrease: vitamin B_{12} absorption—goldenseal
Drug/Lab Test
False positive: intrinsic factor

NURSING CONSIDERATIONS
Assess:
- For vitamin B_{12} deficiency: red, beefy tongue; psychosis; pallor; neuropathy, ataxia, positive Romberg
- GI function: diarrhea, constipation
- Potassium levels during treatment in megaloblastic anemia; q6mo in pernicious anemia; folic acid, plasma vitamin B_{12} (after 1 wk), reticulocyte counts
- Nutritional status: egg yolks, fish, organ meats, dairy products, clams, oysters: good sources of vitamin B_{12}
- For pulmonary edema, worsening of HF in cardiac patients
Evaluate:
- Therapeutic response: decreased anorexia, dyspnea on exertion, palpitations, paresthesias, psychosis, visual disturbances
Teach patient/family:
- That treatment must continue for life for pernicious anemia
- To eat a well-balanced diet
- To avoid contact with persons with infection; that infections are common

TREATMENT OF OVERDOSE:
Discontinue product

---

cyclobenzaprine (Rx)
(sye-kloe-ben′za-preen)
Amrix, Fexmid
Func. class.: Skeletal muscle relaxant, central acting
Chem. class.: Tricyclic amine salt

ACTION: Reduces tonic muscle activity at the brainstem; may be related to antidepressant effects

USES: Adjunct for relief of muscle spasm and pain in musculoskeletal conditions

CONTRAINDICATIONS
Acute recovery phase of MI, dysrhythmias, heart block, HF, hypersensitivity, intermittent porphyria, thyroid disease, QT prolongation, within 14 days of MAOIs
Precautions: Pregnancy, breastfeeding, geriatric patients, renal/hepatic disease, addictive personality, CV disease, child <15 yr

DOSAGE AND ROUTES
Muscloskeletal disorders
• **Adult/adolescent ≥15 yr: PO** 5 mg tid × 1 wk, max 30 mg/day × 3 wk
• **Adult: EXTENDED RELEASE** 15 mg/day, max 30 mg/day × 3 wk
• **Geriatric: PO** 5 mg tid
Hepatic dose
• **Adult (mild hepatic disease): PO** 5 mg, titrate slowly
Available forms: Tablets 5, 7.5, 10 mg; extended-release tablets 15, 30 mg
Administer:
• Without regard to meals, give with food for GI symptoms
• Do not crush, break, chew extended-release tablets
• Store in tight container at room temperature

SIDE EFFECTS
CNS: *Dizziness, weakness, drowsiness,* headache, insomnia, confusion, nervousness, fatigue
CV: Postural hypotension, dysrhythmias
EENT: Diplopia, temporary loss of vision, blurred vision, dry mouth
GI: *Nausea,* dry mouth, constipation
GU: Urinary retention
INTEG: Rash

PHARMACOKINETICS
PO: Onset 1 hr, peak 3-8 hr, duration 12-24 hr, half-life 1-3 days, 32 hr extended release, metabolized by liver, excreted in urine, crosses placenta, excreted in breast milk

INTERACTIONS
• Do not use within 14 days of MAOIs, traMADol
Increase: QT interval—Class IA/III antidysrhythmics and other products that increase QT interval
Increase: serotonin syndrome—SSRIs, SNRIs, tricyclics, triptans, fentaNYL, busPIRone, traMADol, traZODone
Increase: CNS depression—alcohol, tricyclics, opiates, barbiturates, sedatives, hypnotics
Drug/Herb
Increase: CNS depression—kava, chamomile, hops, valerian

NURSING CONSIDERATIONS
Assess:
• **Serotonin syndrome:** If using with SSRIs, SNRIs, monitor closely; if syndrome occurs, discontinue both products immediately, hallucinations, nausea, vomiting, diarrhea, tachycardia, hyperthermia
• **Pain:** location, duration, mobility, stiffness at baseline, periodically
• **Allergic reactions**: rash, fever, respiratory distress
• Severe weakness, numbness in extremities
• Assistance with ambulation if dizziness, drowsiness occurs, especially for geriatric patients
• **Beers:** avoid use in older adults; anticholinergic effects
• **Pregnancy/breastfeeding:** no well-controlled studies; use only if clearly needed; use cautiously in breastfeeding
Evaluate:
• Therapeutic response: decreased pain, spasticity; relief of muscle spasms of acute, painful musculoskeletal conditions generally short-term; long-term therapy seldom warranted
Teach patient/family:
• Not to discontinue medication abruptly; that insomnia, nausea, headache, spasticity, tachycardia will occur; that product should be tapered off over 1-2 wk
• Not to take with alcohol, other CNS depressants or MAOIs
• To avoid hazardous activities if drowsiness, dizziness occurs

Side effects: *italics* = common; red = life-threatening

- To avoid using OTC medication (cough preparations, antihistamines) unless directed by prescriber
- To use gum, frequent sips of water for dry mouth
- To notify prescriber of serotonin syndrome
- To report feeling of fullness of bladder, inability to void adequate amounts
- To use fluids, bulk in diet to prevent constipation

TREATMENT OF OVERDOSE: Use anticonvulsants if indicated; monitor cardiac function

---

cyclopentolate ophthalmic
See Appendix B

⚠ HIGH ALERT

cyclophosphamide (Rx)
(sye-kloe-foss'fa-mide)
Procytox ✤
Func. class.: Antineoplastic alkylating agent
Chem. class.: Nitrogen mustard

Do not confuse:
cyclophosphamide/cycloSPORINE

ACTION: Alkylates DNA; is responsible for cross-linking DNA strands; activity is not cell-cycle–phase specific

USES: Hodgkin's disease, lymphomas, leukemia; cancer of female reproductive tract, breast, multiple myeloma; neuroblastoma; retinoblastoma; Ewing's sarcoma; nephrotic syndrome

CONTRAINDICATIONS
Pregnancy, hypersensitivity, prostatic hypertrophy, bladder neck obstruction
Precautions: Radiation therapy, cardiac disease, anemia, dysrhythmias, child, dental disease/work, dialysis, geriatric patients, heart failure, hematuria,

infections, leukopenia QT prolongation, secondary malignancy surgery, tumor lysis syndrome, vaccinations, breastfeeding, severely depressed bone marrow function

DOSAGE AND ROUTES
Acute lymphocytic leukemia (ALL)
- **Adult/adolescent/child:** IV Total doses of IV 300-1500 mg/m² have been incorporated into induction, intensification, consolidation regimens, possibly using vinCRIStine, predniSONE, or others; **PO** 1-5 mg/kg/day depending on response
Neuroblastoma
- **Adult/child:** IV For induction, 40-50 mg/kg in divided doses over 2-5 days or 10-15 mg/kg q7-10days, 3-5 mg/kg 2×/wk or 1-5 mg/kg daily
- **Child and infant:** PO 150 mg/m²/day, days 1-7 with DOXOrubicin (IV 35 mg/m² on day 8) q21days × 5 cycles
- **Child:** IV 70 mg/kg/day with hydration on days 1, 2 with DOXOrubicin and vinCRIStine q21days for courses 1, 2, 4, 6 alternating with CISplatin and etoposide q21days for courses 3, 5, 7
Breast cancer
- **Adult:** PO 100-200 mg/m²/day or 2 mg/kg/day × 4-14 days; IV 500-1000 mg/m² on day 1 in combination with fluorouracil and methotrexate or DOXOrubicin or DOXOrubicin alone, also cyclophosphamide 600 mg/m²; may be given dose-dense on day 1 of q14days with DOXOrubicin (60 mg/m²) with growth-factor support
Operable node-positive breast cancer IV (TAC regimen)
- **Adult:** IV 500 mg/m² with DOXOrubicin (50 mg/m² IV), then DOCEtaxel (75 mg/m²) IV given 1 hr later q3wk × 6 cycles
Nephrotic syndrome
- **Child:** PO 2 mg/kg daily × 60-90 days, cumulative dose 168 mg/kg
Available forms: Powder for injection ✤ 200, 500 mg, 1, 2 g/vials; capsules 25, 50 mg
Administer:
- Use cytotoxic handling procedures

- In AM so product can be eliminated before bedtime
- Fluids IV or PO prior to chemotherapy to hydrate patient
- Antacid prior to oral agent; give after evening meal, before bedtime
- Antiemetic 30-60 min before product and prn
- Allopurinol or sodium bicarbonate to maintain uric acid levels, alkalinization of urine

PO route
- Take on empty stomach; do not crush, break, chew capsules; wash hands immediately if in contact with capsules
- May be taken as a single dose or divided doses
- Take in AM or afternoon, avoid evening
- Store in tight container at room temperature

Direct IV route
- Reconstitute with NS only 100 mg/5 mL, swirl, inject slowly

Intermittent IV INFUSION route
- Use cytotoxic handling procedures
- IV after diluting 100 mg/5 mL, 0.9% NaCl of sterile water or bacteriostatic water; shake; let stand until clear; may be further diluted in ≤250 mL D$_5$/NS, 0.45% NaCl; give 100 mg or less/min (2 mg/mL)
- Use 21, 23, 25G needle; check site for irritation, phlebitis

Y-site compatibilities: Acyclovir, alfentanil, allopurinol, amifostine, amikacin, aminocaproic acid, aminophylline, amiodarone, amphotericin B lipid complex, amphotericin B liposome, ampicillin, ampicillin-sulbactam, anidulafungin, atenolol, atracurium, azlocillin, aztreonam, bivalirudin, bleomycin, bumetanide, buprenorphine, butorphanol, calcium chloride/gluconate, CARBOplatin, caspofungin, cefamandole, ceFAZolin, cefepime, cefoperazone, cefotaxime, cefoTEtan, cefOXitin, cefTAZidime, ceftizoxime, cefTRIAXone, cefuroxime, chloramphenicol, chlorproMAZINE, cimetidine, ciprofloxacin, cisatracurium, CISplatin, cladribine, clindamycin, codeine, cycloSPORINE, cytarabine, DACTINomycin, DAPTOmycin, DAUNOrubicin, dexamethasone, dexmedetomidine, dexrazoxane, digoxin, diltiaZEM, diphenhydrAMINE, DOBUTamine, DOCEtaxel, dolasetron, DOPamine, doripenem, doxacurium, DOXOrubicin, DOXOrubicin liposomal, doxycycline, droperidol, enalaprilat, ePHEDrine, EPINEPHrine, epiRUBicin, ertapenem, erythromycin, esmolol, etoposide, famotidine, fenoldopam, fentaNYL, filgrastim, fluconazole, fludarabine, fluorouracil, foscarnet, fosphenytoin, furosemide, gallium, ganciclovir, gatifloxacin, gemcitabine, gentamicin, granisetron, haloperidol, heparin, hydrocortisone, HYDROmorphone, hydrOXYzine, IDArubicin, imipenemcilastatin, inamrinone, insulin (regular), irinotecan, isoproterenol, kanamycin, ketorolac, labetalol, leucovorin, levoFLOXacin, levorphanol, lidocaine, linezolid, LORazepam, magnesium sulfate, mannitol, melphalan, meperidine, meropenem, mesna, methohexital, methotrexate, methylPREDNISolone, metoclopramide, metoprolol, metroNIDAZOLE, midazolam, milrinone, minocycline, mitoMYcin, mitoXANTRONE, mivacurium, morphine, nafcillin, nalbuphine, naloxone, nesiritide, nitroglycerin, nitroprusside, norepinephrine, octreotide, ondansetron, oxacillin, oxaliplatin, PACLitaxel, palonosetron, pamidronate, pancuronium, pantoprazole, PEMEtrexed, penicillin G potassium, pentamidine, PENTobarbital, PHENobarbital, phenylephrine, piperacillin, piperacillin-tazobactam, potassium chloride/phosphates, procainamide, prochlorperazine, promethazine, propofol, propranolol, quinupristin-dalfopristin, raNITIdine, rapacuronium, remifentanil, riTUXimab, rocuronium, sargramostim, sodium acetate/bicarbonate/phosphates, succinylcholine, SUFentanil, sulfamethoxazole-trimethoprim, tacrolimus, teniposide, theophylline, thiopental, thiotepa, ticarcillin, ticarcillin-clavulanate, tigecycline, tirofiban, TNA, tobramycin, topotecan, TPN, trastuzumab, vancomycin, vasopressin, vecuronium, verapamil, vinBLAStine, vinCRIStine, vinorelbine, voriconazole, zidovudine, zoledronic acid

SIDE EFFECTS
CV: Cardiotoxicity (high doses), myocardial fibrosis, hypotension
ENDO: SIADH, gonadal suppression
GI: *Nausea, vomiting, weight loss,* anorexia
GU: Hemorrhagic cystitis, *hematuria*
HEMA: Thrombocytopenia, leukopenia, myelosuppression
INTEG: *Alopecia*
META: Hyperuricemia
MISC: Secondary neoplasms
RESP: Pulmonary fibrosis, interstitial pneumonia

PHARMACOKINETICS
Metabolized by liver, excreted in urine, half-life 4-6½ hr, 50% bound to plasma proteins

INTERACTIONS
Increase: neuromuscular blockade—succinylcholine
Increase: action of warfarin
Increase: bone marrow depression—other antineoplastics, radiation, allopurinol, thiazides
Decrease: digoxin levels—digoxin
Decrease: cyclophosphamide effect
Decrease: antibody response—live virus vaccines
Drug/Herb
Increase: toxicity—St. John's wort
Drug/Lab Test
Increase: uric acid
False positive: Pap smear
False negative: PPD, mumps, *Candida, Trichophyton,* Pap smear

NURSING CONSIDERATIONS
Assess:
• **Hemorrhagic cystitis; renal studies:** BUN, serum uric acid, urine CCr prior to, during therapy; I&O ratio; report fall in urine output <30 mL/hr; provide increased fluid intake to 3 L/day (adults)
• **Bone marrow depression:** CBC, differential, platelet count baseline, weekly; withhold product if WBC is <2500 or platelet count is <75,000; notify prescriber.

Assess for hematuria, guaiac, bruising or petechiae, mucosa or orifices q8hr
• **Pulmonary fibrosis/interstitial pneumonia:** pulmonary function tests, chest x-ray films prior to, during therapy; chest film should be obtained q2wk during treatment; monitor for dyspnea, rales/crackles, edema
• **Hepatotoxicity:** hepatic studies prior to, during therapy (bilirubin, AST, ALT, LDH), as needed; jaundice of skin, sclera; dark urine, clay-colored stools; itchy skin; abdominal pain; fever; diarrhea
• Unproductive cough, chest pain, tachypnea
• Buccal cavity q8hr for dryness, sores or ulceration, white patches, oral pain, bleeding, dysphagia; obtain prescription for viscous lidocaine (Xylocaine); provide rinsing of mouth tid-qid with water, club soda; brushing of teeth bid-tid with soft brush or cotton-tipped applicators for stomatitis; use unwaxed dental floss
• Increase fluid intake to 2-3 L/day to prevent urate deposits, calculi formation, reduce incidence of hemorrhagic cystitis
• Warm compresses at injection site for inflammation
• **Beers:** avoid in older adults; delirium, dementia may occur; avoid in men due to decrease in urine flow, retention
Evaluate:
• Therapeutic response: decreased tumor size, spread of malignancy; nephrotic syndrome
Teach patient/family:
• To take adequate fluids (3 L/day, adults) to eliminate product
• That amenorrhea can occur and may last up to 1 yr after therapy but is reversible after stopping treatment
• To report any changes in breathing or coughing
• To avoid foods with citric acid, hot temperature, or rough texture; that skin, fingernails may become darker
• **To report signs of infection:** increased temperature, sore throat, flulike symptoms
• **To report signs of anemia:** fatigue, headache, faintness, SOB, irritability

• To report bleeding (bruising, hematuria, petechiae); to avoid the use of razors, commercial mouthwash
• To avoid the use of aspirin products, ibuprofen
• To avoid vaccinations during therapy
• About proper handling and disposal of chemotherapy drugs
• **Pregnancy/breastfeeding:** to use reliable contraception during treatment and for 1 yr after treatment (women); men should use condoms during and for 4 mo following treatment; not to breastfeed

cycloSPORINE (Rx)

(sye′kloe-spor-een)

Gengraf, Neoral, SandIMMUNE
Func. class.: Immunosuppressant, antirheumatic (DMARD)
Chem. class.: Fungus-derived peptide

Do not confuse:
cycloSPORINE/cycloSERINE/cyclophosphamide

ACTION: Produces immunosuppression by inhibiting T lymphocytes

USES: Organ transplants (liver, kidney, heart) to prevent rejection (GVHD), rheumatoid arthritis, psoriasis

CONTRAINDICATIONS
Breastfeeding, hypersensitivity to polyoxyethylated castor oil (injection only); psoriasis or RA in renal disease (Neoral/Gengraf); Gengraf/Neoral used with PUVA/UVB, methotrexate, coal tar; ocular infections

Black Box Warning: Uncontrolled malignant hypertension

Precautions: Pregnancy, geriatric patients, severe hepatic disease

Black Box Warning: Immunosuppression, nephrotoxicity, skin cancer; requires a specialized care setting and experienced clinician; infections; new primary malignancy (lymphoma, skin cancer)

DOSAGE AND ROUTES—NTI
Prevention of transplant rejection (nonmodified) (Sandimmune)
• **Adult/child: PO** 15 mg/kg 4-12 hr prior to surgery, daily for 2 wk, reduce dosage by 2.5 mg/kg/wk to 5-10 mg/kg/day; **IV** 5-6 mg/kg 4-12 hr prior to surgery, daily, switch to **PO** form as soon as possible
Prevention of transplant rejection (modified) (Neoral)
• **Adult/child: PO** 4-12 mg/kg/day divided q12hr, depends on organ transplanted
Rheumatoid arthritis (Neoral/Gengraf)
• **Adult: PO** 2.5 mg/kg/day divided bid, may increase 0.5-0.75 mg/kg/day after 8-12 wk, max 4 mg/kg/day; decrease dose by 25% in HTN
Psoriasis (Neoral/Gengraf)
• **Adult: PO** 2.5 mg/kg/day divided bid, × 4 wk, then increase by 0.5 mg/kg/day q2wk, max 4 mg/kg/day; decrease dose by 25% in HTN
Autoimmune diseases (Sandimmune)
• **Adult/child: PO** 1-3 mg/kg/day
Available forms: Oral solution 100 mg/mL; soft gel capsule 25, 50, 100 mg; injection 50 mg/mL
Administer:
PO route
• Some brands are not interchangeable
• Do not break, crush, or chew capsules
• Use pipette provided to draw up oral solution; may mix with milk or juice; wipe pipette, do not wash (Neoral)
• For several days prior to transplant surgery; give at same time of day
• With corticosteroids
• With meals for GI upset or in chocolate milk, milk, or orange juice (SandIMMUNE)
Rheumatoid arthritis
• Give Neoral or Gengraf 2.5 mg/kg/day divided bid; may use with salicylates, NSAIDs, PO corticosteroids
• Always give the daily dose of Neoral/Gengraf in 2 divided doses on consistent schedule

Side effects: *italics* = common; red = life-threatening

Rejection prevention

• Give initial SandIMMUNE PO dose 4-12 hr prior to transplantation as a single dose of 15 mg/kg, continue the single daily dose for 1-2 wk, then taper 5%/wk to a maintenance dose of 5-10 mg/kg/day

Intermittent IV INFUSION route

• After diluting each 50 mg/20-100 mL of 0.9% NaCl or D_5W (2.5 mg/mL), run over 2-6 hr, use an infusion pump

Continuous IV INFUSION route

• May run over 24 hr

• **For SandIMMUNE parenteral,** give ⅓ of PO dose, initial dose 4-12 hr before transplantation as a single IV dose 5-6 mg/kg/day, continue the single daily dose until PO can be used

Y-site compatibilities: Abciximab, alatrofloxacin, alfentanil, amikacin, aminocaproic acid, aminophylline, amphotericin B lipid complex, anidulafungin, argatroban, ascorbic acid injection, atenolol, atracurium, atropine, azaTHIOprine, aztreonam, benztropine, bivalirudin, bleomycin, bretylium, bumetanide, buprenorphine, butorphanol, calcium chloride/gluconate, CARBOplatin, carmustine, caspofungin, ceFAZolin, cefmetazole, cefonicid, cefotaxime, cefoTEtan, cefOXitin, cefTAZidime, ceftizoxime, cefTRIAXone, cefuroxime, chloramphenicol, chlorproMAZINE, cimetidine, ciprofloxacin, CISplatin, clindamycin, codeine, cyanocobalamin, cyclophosphamide, cytarabine, DACTINomycin, DAPTOmycin, DAUNOrubicin, dexamethasone, dexmedetomidine, digoxin, diltiaZEM, diphenhydrAMINE, DOBUTamine, DOCEtaxel, DOPamine, doripenem, doxacurium, DOXOrubicin, doxycycline, enalaprilat, ePHEDrine, EPINEPHrine, epiRUBicin, epoetin alfa, eptifibatide, ertapenem, erythromycin, esmolol, etoposide, famotidine, fenoldopam, fentaNYL, fluconazole, fludarabine, fluorouracil, folic acid, furosemide, gallium, ganciclovir, gatifloxacin, gemcitabine, gentamicin, glycopyrrolate, granisetron, heparin, hydrocortisone, HYDROmorphone, hydrOXYzine, ifosfamide, imipenem-cilastatin, indomethacin, irinotecan, isoproterenol, ketorolac, labetalol, lansoprazole, levoFLOXacin, lidocaine, linezolid, LORazepam, mannitol, mechlorethamine, meperidine, meropenem, methotrexate, methyldopate, methylPREDNISolone, metoclopramide, metoprolol, metroNIDAZOLE, micafungin, miconazole, midazolam, milrinone, minocycline, mitoXANTRONE, morphine, multiple vitamins injection, nafcillin, naloxone, nesiritide, netilmicin, nitroglycerin, nitroprusside, norepinephrine, octreotide, ondansetron, oxacillin, oxaliplatin, oxytocin, PACLitaxel, palonosetron, pamidronate, pancuronium, pantoprazole, papaverine, PEMEtrexed, penicillin G potassium/sodium, pentamidine, pentazocine, phentolamine, phenylephrine, phytonadione, piperacillin, piperacillin-tazobactam, polymyxin B, potassium acetate/chloride, procainamide, prochlorperazine, promethazine, propofol, propranolol, protamine, pyridoxine, quiNIDine, quinupristin-dalfopristin, raNITIdine, ritodrine, sargramostim, sodium acetate/bicarbonate, succinylcholine, SUFentanil, tacrolimus, teniposide, theophylline, thiamine, thiotepa, ticarcillin, ticarcillin-clavulanate, tigecycline, tirofiban, tobramycin, trimetaphan, urokinase, vancomycin, vasopressin, vecuronium, verapamil, vinCRIStine, vinorelbine, zoledronic acid

SIDE EFFECTS

CNS: *Tremors, headache,* seizures, progressive multifocal leukoencephalopathy, confusion, migraine, paresthesia

GI: Nausea, vomiting, diarrhea, *oral candida, gum hyperplasia,* hepatotoxicity, pancreatitis

GU: Nephrotoxicity

INTEG: Rash, acne, *hirsutism*

META: Hyperkalemia, hypomagnesemia, hyperlipidemia, hyperuricemia

MISC: *Infection,* gingival hyperplasia, hypersensitivity, malignancy

PHARMACOKINETICS

Peak 4 hr; highly protein bound; half-life (biphasic) 1.2 hr, 25 hr; metabolized in liver; excreted in feces, 6% in urine; crosses placenta; excreted in breast milk

INTERACTIONS

Increase: action, toxicity of cycloSPO-RINE—allopurinol, amiodarone, amphotericin B, androgens, azole antifungals, beta-blockers, bromocriptine, calcium channel blockers, carvedilol, cimetidine, colchicine, corticosteroids, fluoroquinolones, foscarnet, imipenem-cilastatin, macrolides, metoclopramide, oral contraceptives, NSAIDs, melphalan, SSRIs

Increase: effects of aliskiren, digoxin, etoposide, HMG-CoA reductase inhibitors, methotrexate, potassium-sparing diuretics, sirolimus, tacrolimus

Increase: action, toxicity of—digoxin, colchicine

Increase: hyperkalemia—potassium-sparing diuretics, potassium supplements, ACE inhibitors

Increase: renal dysfunction—aminoglycosides, ciprofloxacin, NSAIDs, fibric acid derivatives, vancomycin, melphalan, ketoconazole

Decrease: cycloSPORINE action—anticonvulsants, nafcillin, orlistat, PHENobarbital, phenytoin, rifamycins, sulfamethoxazole-trimethoprim, terbinafine, ticlopidine

Decrease: antibody reaction—live virus vaccines

Drug/Herb

Decrease: immunosuppression—echinacea, melatonin; do not use together

Decrease: cycloSPORINE levels—St. John's wort; do not use together

Drug/Food

Slowed metabolism of product—grapefruit juice, food

NURSING CONSIDERATIONS
Assess:

Black Box Warning: Nephrotoxicity: BUN, creatinine at least monthly during treatment, 3 mo after treatment; nephrotoxicity increases with increasing doses and duration of treatment

• Product blood level during treatment 12 hr after dose, toxic >400 ng/mL

• Hepatic studies: alkaline phosphatase, AST, ALT, bilirubin; **hepatotoxicity:** dark urine, jaundice, itching, light-colored stools; product should be discontinued

• Serum lipids, magnesium, potassium, cycloSPORINE blood concentrations, therapeutic cycloSPORINE range: 100-400 mg/mL

• **Posterior reversible encephalopathy:** impaired cognition, seizures, visual changes including blindness, loss of motor function, movement disorders, and psychiatric changes; dosage reduction or discontinuation may be needed

• **Progressive multifocal leukoencephalopathy (PML):** apathy, confusion, cognitive changes; may be fatal, withhold dose, notify prescriber immediately

• **Immunosuppression/infection:** bacterial, viral, protozoal, and fungal infections are common; assess for signs of infection often

• **Nephrotoxicity:** Increased with increased doses and duration

• **Psoriasis:** Lesions baseline and during treatment

• **RA:** Pain, ROM, ADLs baseline and during treatment

Black Box Warning: Requires a specialized care setting and experienced clinician: product must be given in a facility equipped with adequate laboratory and supportive medical services

Black Box Warning: New primary malignancy: lymphoma, skin cancer; increased risk in psoriasis with use of PUVA or UVB therapy, methotrexate, other immunosuppressives, coal tar or radiation; these patients may be at increased risk of skin cancer also

Evaluate:

• Therapeutic response: absence of rejection; decreased pain in rheumatoid arthritis, decreased lesions in psoriasis

Teach patient/family:

• To report fever, chills, sore throat, fatigue since serious infections may occur; tremors, bleeding gums, increased B/P

• To take at same time of day, every day; not to skip doses or double dose; not to use with grapefruit juice or receive vaccines; that there are many drug interactions; not to add new products without approval of prescriber

Black Box Warning: To limit UV exposure

• That treatment is lifelong to prevent rejection; to identify signs of rejection
• To report severe diarrhea because drug loss and rejection may result
• **About the signs of nephrotoxicity:** increased B/P; tremors of the hands; changes in gums; increased hair on body, face
• To continue with all lab work and follow-up appointments
• That types of products are not interchangeable
• Not to wash syringe/container with water; variation in dose may result
• To notify prescriber of all medications, herbal products, supplements that are taken
• **Pregnancy/breastfeeding:** to use contraceptive measures during treatment, for 12 wk after ending therapy; to notify prescriber if pregnancy is planned or suspected; no well-controlled studies; use only if benefits outweigh risks; discontinue breastfeeding or product

---

⚠ HIGH ALERT

cytarabine (Rx)

(sye-tare′a-been)

Cytosar ✤

Func. class.: Antineoplastic, antimetabolite

Chem. class.: Pyrimidine nucleoside analog

Do not confuse:
Cytosar/Cytoxan/Cytovene

ACTION: Competes with physiologic substrate of DNA synthesis, thus interfering with cell replication in the S phase of the cell cycle (before mitosis)

USES: Acute myelocytic leukemia, acute nonlymphocytic leukemia, chronic myelocytic leukemia; lymphomatous meningitis (intrathecal/intraventricular)

Unlabeled uses: Hodgkin's/non-Hodgkin's lymphoma, malignant meningitis, mantle cell lymphoma

CONTRAINDICATIONS

Pregnancy, hypersensitivity

Precautions: Breastfeeding, children, renal/hepatic disease, tumor lysis syndrome, infection, hyperkalemia, hyperphosphatemia, hyperuricemia, hypocalcemia

Black Box Warning: Bone marrow suppression, arachnoiditis, abdominal pain, nausea/vomiting of chemotherapy, diarrhea, hepatotoxicity; requires a specialized care setting and experienced clinician, oral ulceration

DOSAGE AND ROUTES

Regimens will vary

Acute myelogenous leukemia (AML)
• **Adult:** CONTINUOUS IV INFUSION 100 mg/m²/day × 7 days q2wk as single agent or 2-6 mg/kg/day (100-200 mg/m²/day) as a single dose or 2-3 divided doses for 5-10 days until remission, used in combination; maintenance 70-200 mg/m²/day for 2-5 days monthly; **SUBCUT/IM** maintenance 100 mg/m²/day × 5 days q28days

Meningeal leukemia
• **Adult/child:** INTRATHECAL 5-75 mg/m², frequency varies

Acute promyelocytic leukemia (unlabeled)
Adult: CONTINUOUS IV 200 mg/m² by continuous infusion × 7 days starting on day 3 of therapy with daunorubicin and tretinoin

Renal dose
• **Adult:** IV CCr ≤60 mL/min, serum creatinine 1.5-1.9 mg/dL or increase of 0.5-1.2 mg/dL from baseline: reduce to 1 g/m²/dose; serum creatinine ≥2 mg/dL or change from baseline serum creatinine was 1.2 mg/dL: reduce to 100 mg/m²/day

Available forms: Solution for injection 20 mg/mL, 100 mg/mL

Administer:
• Antiemetic 30-60 min prior to product and prn
• Allopurinol to maintain uric acid levels and alkalinization of the urine

IV route
• Use cytotoxic handling precautions

Direct IV route
• Give undiluted, give by direct IV over 1-3 min through free-flowing tubing (IV)

Intermittent IV INFUSION route
• Dilute in 50-100 mL NS or D$_5$W, given over 30 min to 24 hr, depending on dose

Continuous IV INFUSION route
• May also be given by continuous infusion

Y-site compatibilities: Acyclovir, alfentanil, amifostine, amikacin, aminocaproic acid, aminophylline, amphotericin B lipid complex, amphotericin B liposome, ampicillin, ampicillin-sulbactam, amsacrine, anidulafungin, atenolol, atracurium, azithromycin, aztreonam, bivalirudin, bleomycin, bumetanide, buprenorphine, butorphanol, calcium chloride/gluconate, CARBOplatin, ceFAZolin, cefepime, cefotaxime, cefoTEtan, cefOXitin, cefTAZidime, ceftizoxime, cefTRIAXone, cefuroxime, chlorproMAZINE, cimetidine, ciprofloxacin, cisatracurium, CISplatin, cladribine, clindamycin, codeine, cyclophosphamide, cycloSPORINE, DAUNOrubicin, dexamethasone, dexmedetomidine, dexrazoxane, digoxin, diltiaZEM, diphenhydrAMINE, DOBUTamine, DOCEtaxel, dolasetron, DOPamine, doxacurium, DOXOrubicin, DOXOrubicin liposomal, doxycycline, droperidol, enalaprilat, ePHEDrine, EPINEPHrine, ertapenem, erythromycin, esmolol, etoposide, famotidine, fenoldopam, fentaNYL, filgrastim, fluconazole, fludarabine, foscarnet, fosphenytoin, furosemide, gatifloxacin, gemcitabine, gemtuzumab, gentamicin, granisetron, haloperidol, heparin, hydrocortisone, HYDROmorphone, hydrOXYzine, IDArubicin, ifosfamide, imipenem-cilastatin, inamrinone, insulin (regular), irinotecan, isoproterenol, ketorolac, labetalol, leucovorin, levoFLOXacin, levorphanol, lidocaine, linezolid, LORazepam, magnesium sulfate, mannitol, melphalan, meperidine, meropenem, mesna, methohexital, methotrexate, methylPREDNISolone, metoclopramide, metoprolol, metroNIDAZOLE, midazolam, milrinone, minocycline, mitoXANTRONE, mivacurium, morphine, nalbuphine, naloxone, nesiritide, niCARdipine, nitroglycerin, nitroprusside, norepinephrine, octreotide, ofloxacin, ondansetron, oxaliplatin, PACLitaxel, palonosetron, pamidronate, pancuronium, pantoprazole, PEMEtrexed, pentamidine, PENTobarbital, PHENobarbital, phenylephrine, piperacillin, piperacillin-tazobactam, potassium chloride/phosphates, procainamide, prochlorperazine, promethazine, propofol, propranolol, quinupristin-dalfopristin, raNITIdine, rapacuronium, remifentanil, riTUXimab, rocuronium, sargramostim, sodium acetate/bicarbonate/phosphates, succinylcholine, SUFentanil, sulfamethoxazole-trimethoprim, tacrolimus, teniposide, theophylline, thiopental, thiotepa, ticarcillin, ticarcillin-clavulanate, tigecycline, tirofiban, TNA, tobramycin, trastuzumab, trimethobenzamide, vancomycin, vasopressin, vecuronium, verapamil, vinCRIStine, vinorelbine, voriconazole, zidovudine, zoledronic acid

SIDE EFFECTS

CNS: Dizziness, headache, confusion, drowsiness, chemical arachnoiditis (IT)
CV: Edema
EENT: Conjunctivitis, visual changes
GI: *Nausea, vomiting, anorexia, diarrhea, stomatitis,* hepatotoxicity, abdominal pain, GI ulceration (high dose)
GU: Urinary retention, renal dysfunction
HEMA: Thrombophlebitis, bleeding, thrombocytopenia, leukopenia, myelosuppression, anemia
INTEG: *Rash*
META: Hyperuricemia
RESP: Dyspnea, pulmonary edema (high doses)
SYST: Anaphylaxis, tumor lysis syndrome
Cytarabine syndrome: *Fever,* myalgia, bone pain, chest pain, *rash,* conjunctivitis, malaise (6-12 hr after administration)

PHARMACOKINETICS

INTRATHECAL: Half-life 100-236 hr; metabolized in liver; excreted in urine

---

Side effects: *italics* = common; red = life-threatening

(primarily inactive metabolite); crosses blood-brain barrier, placenta

IV/SUBCUT: Distribution half-life 10 min, elimination half-life 1-3 hr

INTERACTIONS

• Do not use with live virus vaccines
• Do not use within 24 hr of chemotherapy—sargramostim, GM-CSF, filgrastim, G-CSF

Increase: toxicity—immunosuppressants, methotrexate, flucytosine, radiation, or other antineoplastics

Increase: bleeding risk—anticoagulants, platelet inhibitors, salicylates, thrombolytics, NSAIDs

Decrease: effects of oral digoxin, gentamicin

NURSING CONSIDERATIONS
Assess:

Black Box Warning: Bone marrow suppression: CBC (RBC, Hct, HB), differential, platelet count weekly; withhold product if WBC is <1000/mm³, platelet count is <50,000/mm³, or RBC, Hct, HB are low; notify prescriber of these results; assess for bleeding: hematuria, heme-positive stools, bruising or petechiae, mucosa, or orifices q8hr

• Renal studies: BUN, serum uric acid, urine CCr, electrolytes prior to and during therapy
• I&O ratio; report fall in urine output to <30 mL/hr
• Monitor temperature; fever may indicate beginning infection; no rectal temperatures

Black Box Warning: Hepatotoxicity: hepatic studies prior to and during therapy: bilirubin, ALT, AST, alkaline phosphatase, as needed or monthly; check for jaundice of skin, sclera; dark urine; clay-colored stools; pruritus; abdominal pain; fever; diarrhea

• Serum uric acid during therapy
• **For anaphylaxis:** rash, pruritus, facial swelling, dyspnea; resuscitation equipment should be nearby

Black Box Warning: Chemical arachnoiditis (IT): headache, nausea, vomiting, fever; neck rigidity/pain, meningism, CSF pleocytosis; may be decreased by dexamethasone

• **Cytarabine syndrome** 6-12 hr after infusion: fever, myalgia, bone pain, chest pain, rash, conjunctivitis, malaise; corticosteroids may be ordered
• Dyspnea, crackles, unproductive cough, chest pain, tachypnea, fatigue, increased pulse, pallor, lethargy; personality changes, with high doses; pulmonary edema may be fatal (rare)
• Buccal cavity q8hr for dryness, sores or ulceration, white patches, oral pain, bleeding, dysphagia
• Local irritation, pain, burning, discoloration at injection site
• GI symptoms: frequency of stools, cramping; antispasmodic may be used
• Increased fluid intake to 2-3 L/day to prevent urate deposits and calculi formation unless contraindicated
• Rinsing of mouth tid-qid with water, club soda; brushing of teeth bid-tid with soft brush or cotton-tipped applicators for stomatitis; use unwaxed dental floss

Evaluate:
• Therapeutic response: improvement of hematologic parameters, decrease in size, spread of tumor

Teach patient/family:
• To report any coughing, chest pain, changes in breathing; may indicate beginning pneumonia, pulmonary edema
• **Stomatitis:** To avoid foods with citric acid, hot temperature, or rough texture if stomatitis is present; use sponge brush and rinse with water after each meal; to report stomatitis: any bleeding, white spots, ulcerations in mouth; to examine mouth daily, report any symptoms
• To report signs of infection: increased temperature, sore throat, flulike symptoms; to avoid crowds, persons with infections
• To report signs of **anemia:** fatigue, headache, faintness, SOB, irritability

• To report bleeding; to avoid use of razors, commercial mouthwash, salicylates, NSAIDs, anticoagulants

• To use thrombocytopenia precautions

• To take fluids to 3 L/day to prevent renal damage

• To avoid receiving vaccines during treatment

• That fever, headache, nausea, vomiting are likely to occur

• **Pregnancy/breastfeeding:** to use reliable contraception during treatment and for 4 mo thereafter; not to breastfeed

dabigatran (Rx)

(da-bye-gat′ran)

Pradaxa

Func. class.: Anticoagulant
Chem. class.: Direct thrombin inhibitor

Do not confuse:
dabigatran/vigabatrin, Pradaxa/Plavix

ACTION: Direct thrombin inhibitor that inhibits both free and clot-bound thrombin; prevents thrombin-induced platelet aggregation and thrombus formation by preventing conversion of fibrinogen to fibrin

USES: Stroke/systemic embolism prophylaxis with nonvalvular atrial fibrillation, DVT, pulmonary embolism in hip replacement

CONTRAINDICATIONS

Hypersensitivity, active bleeding, prosthetic heart valves, use with P-gp inducers
Precautions: Pregnancy, labor, obstetric delivery, children, geriatric patients, abrupt discontinuation, anticoagulant therapy, renal disease, surgery

> **Black Box Warning:** Abrupt discontinuation, epidural/spinal anesthesia, lumbar puncture

DOSAGE AND ROUTES
Stroke prophylaxis, atrial fibrillation, and DVT/PE prophylaxis
• **Adult: PO** 150 mg bid
For conversion from an alternative anticoagulant to dabigatran
• When converting from warfarin to dabigatran, discontinue warfarin and initiate dabigatran when the INR is <2.0; when converting from a parenteral anticoagulant to dabigatran, initiate dabigatran 0-2 hr prior to the time of the next scheduled anticoagulant dose or at the time of discontinuation of a continuously administered anticoagulant (IV unfractionated heparin)
For conversion from dabigatran to warfarin
• **Adult:** CCr >50 mL/min, start warfarin 3 days prior to discontinuing dabigatran; CCr 31-50 mL/min, start warfarin 2 days prior to discontinuing dabigatran; CCr 15-

30 mL/min, start warfarin 1 day prior to discontinuing dabigatran
For conversion from dabigatran to parenteral anticoagulants
• **Adult: PO** discontinue dabigatran; start parenteral anticoagulant 12 hr (CCr ≥30 mL/min) or 24 hr (CCr <30 mL/min) after the last dabigatran dose
Deep venous thrombus (DVT)/ pulmonary embolism (PE) prophylaxis
• **Adult: PO** 220 mg or 150 mg/day × 28-35 days, starting with ½ dose 1-4 hr after surgery **(knee replacement);** 110 mg on first day 1-4 hr after surgery, hemostasis achieved, then 220 mg daily × 28-35 days; those previously treated 150 mg bid **(hip replacement)**
DVT/PE/treated with a parenteral anticoagulant × 5-10 days
• **Adult: PO** 150 mg bid
Renal dose
• **Adult: PO** CCr 15-30 mL/min, 75 mg bid (for reduction in stroke risk and systemic embolism in nonvalvular atrial fibrillation)
Available forms: Capsules 75, 110, 150 mg; pellets/granules 20, 30, 40, 50, 110, 150 mg
Administer:
• Do not interchange capsules with granules/pellets
• Prior to surgery, discontinue product; restart after surgery is completed
• Do not crush, break, chew, or empty contents of capsule
• Without regard to food
• Store in original package at room temperature until time of use; discard after 30 days; protect from moisture
• **Pellets:** mix in 2 tsp (10 mL) of mashed bananas or apple sauce, or have patient swallow with apple juice; don't mix with dairy products, do not use in feeding tube
• Do not interchange capsules with pellets, swallow capsules whole with water

SIDE EFFECTS
GI: Abdominal pain, dyspepsia, esophagitis, gastritis, diarrhea
HEMA: Bleeding (any site)
SYST: Anaphylaxis (rare), angioedema

PHARMACOKINETICS
Protein binding 35%, half-life 12-17 hr (extended in renal disease), onset unknown, peak 1-2 hr, duration unknown, high-fat meal delays peak

INTERACTIONS
Increase: bleeding risk—amiodarone, other anticoagulants, clopidogrel, ketoconazole, quiNIDine, thrombolytics, verapamil, monitor frequently

P-gp inhibitors: dose should be reduced to 150 mg/day (75 mg bid) in those wit CCr 30-50 mL/min

Decrease: dabigatran effect—rifAMPin; avoid concurrent use

Decrease: dabigatran effect—P-glycoprotein inducers (carBAMazepine, rifAMPin, tipranavir)

Drug/Herb
Decrease: dabigatran—St. John's wort
Drug/Lab Test
Increase: thrombin time, aPTT, ECT

NURSING CONSIDERATIONS
Assess:
• **Stroke:** facial palsy, weakness, headache, blurred vision, speaking difficulty
• **DVT/PE:** Pain in calf, swelling, or behind knee, trouble breathing, chest pain, lightheadedness
• **Bleeding:** blood in urine or emesis, dark tarry stools, lower back pain; caution with arterial/venous punctures, catheters, NG tubes; monitor vital signs frequently; elderly patients more prone to serious bleeding, monitor aPTT, ecarin clotting time baseline and during treatment

Black Box Warning: Premature discontinuation: risk of thrombosis/MI/emboli: swelling, pain, redness, difficulty breathing, chest pain, tachypnea, cough, coughing up blood, cyanosis

• **Postthrombotic syndrome:** pain, heaviness, itching/tingling, swelling, varicose veins, brownish/reddish skin discoloration, ulcers; use of ambulation, compression stockings, adequate anticoagulation can prevent this syndrome

• **Surgery:** discontinue 24-48 hr prior to surgery in those with CCr ≥50 mL/min, 72-96 hr in those with CCr <50 mL/min; longer times may be needed in major surgery; restart after surgery, spinal epidural catheter

Black Box Warning: Epidural/spinal anesthesia, lumbar puncture: risk of hematoma that may cause permanent paralysis; indwelling epidural catheters and products that cause coagulation changes (NSAIDs, anticoagulants) may increase the risk of paralysis

Black Box Warning: Do not discontinue abruptly

• **Pregnancy/breastfeeding:** no well-controlled studies; bleeding may occur if used during pregnancy; discontinue breastfeeding or product, unknown if excreted in breast milk
Evaluate:
• Therapeutic response: decreased thrombus formation/extension, absence of emboli, postthrombotic effects
Teach patient/family:
• About the purpose and expected results; to take at same time of day; not to skip or double doses; if dose is missed, to take as soon as remembered if on the same day; do not administer if <6 hr before next dose; to store in original container, protect from moisture
• To take without regard to food; to swallow capsule whole, not to open; to take with a full glass of water, mix pellets/granules with 2 tsp of soft foods, do not mix with dairy, do not use in feeding tube
• To notify all providers that this product is being used; to check with prescriber about when to discontinue
• **Bleeding:** to report any bleeding or bruising, including blood in stool, emesis, urine; nosebleeds

Black Box Warning: Neurologic changes: to notify prescriber immediately of bowel or bladder changes, numbness in lower extremities, midline back pain

• Not to use any other OTC products, herbs without prescriber approval
• That lab tests may be required during treatment

---

dabrafenib (Rx)

(da-braf'e-nib)

Tafinlar

Func. class.: Antineoplastic
Chem. class.: Signal transduction inhibitor, kinase inhibitor

---

ACTION: Inhibits kinase, inhibitor against mutated forms 🔬ᴏᴇ of BRAF kinases in melanoma cells

USES: 🔬ᴏᴇ Unresectable or metastatic BRAF V600E-mutated malignant melanoma or V600K-mutated melanoma in combination with tramatinib; locally advanced thyroid cancer (BRAF V600E); metastatic non–small cell lung cancer (BRAF V 600E) with trametinib; adjuvant treatment in melanoma (BRAF V600E or V600K) and node involvement

CONTRAINDICATIONS

Pregnancy, hypersensitivity, use with CYP2C8, CYP3A4 inhibitors or inducers, breastfeeding

Precautions: Children, infection, dehydration, diabetes mellitus, fever, G6PD deficiency, hemolytic anemia, hyperglycemia, hypotension, infertility, iritis, renal failure, secondary malignancy, BRAF wild-type melanoma, hepatic disease (moderate-severe), renal disease (moderate-severe)

DOSAGE AND ROUTES

• **Adult: PO** 150 mg q12hr until disease progression; avoid strong CYP3A4/CYP2C8 inhibitors or inducers

Available forms: Capsules 50, 75 mg

Administer:

PO route

• Obtain testing for genetic evidence of BRAF V60E or K
• Swallow whole; do not open, crush, chew capsules

• If dose is missed, take within 6 hr of missed dose; if >6 hr have passed, skip dose
• Space doses q12hr
• Take at least 1 hr prior to or 2 hr after a meal

SIDE EFFECTS

CNS: Headache, fever, fatigue
GI: Pancreatitis
INTEG: Rash, alopecia, DRESS, SJS
MISC: Myalgia
OTHER: Hyperglycemia, hypophosphatemia, hyponatremia, new primary malignancy, hand/foot syndrome
CV: Cardiomyopathy, HF, thromboembolism
EENT: Uveitis, retinal detachment
ENDO: *Hyperglycemia*

PHARMACOKINETICS

Protein binding 99.7%, half-life 8 hr (dabrafenib), 10 hr, 21-22 hr metabolites, excreted 71% (feces), 23% (urine)

INTERACTIONS

Altered: dabrafenib concentrations—CYP3A4 inhibitors (ketoconazole, itraconazole, erythromycin, clarithromycin)
Decrease: dabrafenib concentrations—CYP3A4 inducers (dexamethasone, phenytoin, carBAMazepine, rifAMPin, PHENobarbital), antacids, proton pump inhibitors
Decrease: effect of CYP3A4, CYP2C9 substrates

Drug/Herb
Decrease: dabrafenib concentrations—St. John's wort

Drug/Food Test
Increase: dabrafenib effect—grapefruit juice; avoid use while taking product

NURSING CONSIDERATIONS

Assess:

• **New primary malignancy:** perform a dermatologic evaluation before therapy, q2mo while on therapy, and for up to 6 mo after discontinuing, hold for grades 2-4 skin toxicity, may continue at lower dose if resolved, if not, discontinue, do not restart

---

- **Serious fever and febrile reaction:** hypotension, rigors/chills, dehydration, renal failure; fever occurs when given with trametinib. Interruption of therapy, a dose reduction, or permanent therapy discontinuation may be needed. Monitor for signs and symptoms of infection. If severe, monitor renal function (BUN/serum creatinine) during and after and give antipyretics when therapy is resumed. In a febrile reaction that does not resolve within 3 days, give corticosteroids (predniSONE 10 mg/day PO) for at least 5 days; ensure that there is no evidence of active infection prior to starting corticosteroids
- **Hyperglycemia:** Monitor serum glucose levels at baseline and as clinically indicated
- **Uveitis, iritis, and iridocyclitis:** steroid and mydriatic ophthalmic drops may provide relief for these conditions. Monitor for visual signs and symptoms of uveitis (blurred vision, photophobia, and eye pain). Continue at the same dose in iritis. Hold for mild or moderate uveitis that does not respond to ocular therapy, severe uveitis, or iridocyclitis; initiate treatment as indicated. Permanently discontinue in those who develop persistent grade 2 or higher uveitis that lasts longer than 6 wk
- **Bleeding:** major intracranial bleeding/GI bleeding can occur when used with trametinib. Monitor for signs of bleeding (frank blood; blood in stools, urine, vomit); evaluate any fall in hematocrit, hypotension, grade 3 bleeding, hold product; grade 4, discontinue
- **Cardiomyopathy:** a decrease in left ventricular ejection fraction (LVEF) ≥10% from baseline and below the lower limit of normal (LLN) was higher when given in combination with trametinib. Obtain an ECG or MUGA prior to starting combination therapy, 1 mo after starting dabrafenib, and then q2-3mo during treatment. Hold dabrafenib for symptomatic CHF or LVEF below the LLN with an absolute decrease of >20% from baseline. Resume at the same dose if LVEF improves to the institutional LLN and an absolute decrease of 10% or less from baseline

- **Palmar-plantar erythrodysesthesia syndrome (hand and foot syndrome):** may occur when given with trametinib, usually within 37 days; hospitalization may be required due to a secondary infection of the skin. Interruption of therapy, a dose reduction, or permanent therapy discontinuation may be needed in those who develop severe skin toxicity

Evaluate:
- Therapeutic response: decrease in melanoma, ATC, NSCLC progression

Teach patient/family:
- To notify prescriber of new lesions
- To notify providers of all OTC, Rx, herbal products taken
- To take as prescribed 1 hr prior to or 2 hr after meals, to take a missed dose at least 6 hr before next dose
- To report adverse reactions immediately
- About reason for treatment, expected results
- Advise patients to report symptoms of severe hyperglycemia (excessive thirst, increased urinary frequency)
- Advise that other malignancies are possible
- **Pregnancy:** to use effective nonhormonal contraception during treatment and for at least 30 days after discontinuing treatment; not to breastfeed

---

⚠ HIGH ALERT

dacarbazine (Rx)
(da-kar′ba-zeen)
Func. class.: Antineoplastic alkylating agent
Chem. class.: Cytotoxic triazine

Do not confuse:
dacarbazine/procarbazine

ACTION: Alkylates DNA, RNA; inhibits DNA, RNA synthesis; also responsible for breakage, cross-linking of DNA strands; activity is not cell-cycle–phase specific

USES: Hodgkin's disease, malignant melanoma
Unlabeled uses: Metastatic soft tissue sarcoma in combination with other agents

CONTRAINDICATIONS
Breastfeeding, hypersensitivity
Precautions: Renal disease, infection

Black Box Warning: Pregnancy first trimester, radiation therapy, hepatic disease, bone marrow suppression, secondary malignancy, requires an experienced clinician

DOSAGE AND ROUTES
Metastatic malignant melanoma
• **Adult: IV** 2-4.5 mg/kg/day × 10 days or 100-250 mg/m^2/day × 5 days; repeat q3-4wk depending on response
Hodgkin's lymphoma
• **Adult: IV** 150 mg/m^2/day × 5 days with other agents, repeat q4wk; or 375 mg/m^2 on days 1 and 15 when given in combination, repeat q15days
Soft tissue sarcoma (unlabeled)
• **Adult/child: IV** 250 mg/m^2/day as continuous infusion × 4 days q21days
Available forms: Powder for injection 100-, 200-, 500-mg vials
Administer:
• Antiemetic 30-60 min prior to giving product to prevent vomiting, nausea; vomiting may subside after several doses, nausea/vomiting may be severe and last several hours
• Antibiotics for prophylaxis of infection
IV route
• Use cytotoxic handling precautions
• Clarify all orders, double-check original order; may be fatal if wrong dose is given
Direct IV route
• After diluting 100 mg/9.9 or 200 mg/19.7 mL of sterile water for injection (10 mg/mL), give by slow direct IV over 2-3 min
Intermittent IV INFUSION route
• Further dilute in 50-250 mL D$_5$W or NS for injection, given as an infusion over ½-1 hr
• Watch for extravasation; stop infusion, notify prescriber, provide treatment as to protocol
• Store in light-resistant container in a dry area (vials); reconstituted solutions can be stored at ≤8 hr at room temperature or 24 hr refrigerated

Y-site compatibilities: Amifostine, anidulafungin, atenolol, aztreonam, bivalirudin, bleomycin, caspofungin, DAPTOmycin, dexmedetomidine, DOCEtaxel, DOXOrubicin, ertapenem, etoposide, fenoldopam, filgrastim, fludarabine, gemtuzumab, granisetron, levofloxacin, mechlorethamine, melphalan, nesiritide, octreotide, ondansetron, oxaliplatin, PACLitaxel, palonosetron, pamidronate, quinupristin-dalfopristin, sargramostim, teniposide, thiotepa, tigecycline, tirofiban, vinorelbine, voriconazole, zoledronic acid

SIDE EFFECTS
GI: *Nausea, anorexia, vomiting,* hepatotoxicity, diarrhea, hepatic necrosis
HEMA: Thrombocytopenia, leukopenia, anemia
INTEG: *Alopecia,* dermatitis, pain at injection site, photosensitivity; severe sun reactions (high doses)
MISC: Flulike symptoms, malaise, fever, myalgia, hypotension
SYST: Anaphylaxis, new primary malignancy

PHARMACOKINETICS
Metabolized by liver; excreted in urine; half-life 5 hr; onset, peak, duration unknown

INTERACTIONS

Black Box Warning: Increased: toxicity, bone marrow suppression: bone marrow suppressants, radiation, other antineoplastics

Increase: adverse reaction, decrease antibody reaction—live virus vaccines, do not use together, complete all needed vaccines ≥2 wk prior to first dose
Drug/Lab Test
Increase: BUN, AST, ALT
Decrease: platelets, WBC, RBC

NURSING CONSIDERATIONS
Assess:

Black Box Warning: Bone marrow suppression: monitor CBC, differential, platelet count weekly; notify prescriber of results, allow blood counts to rise to normal prior to use

- **Vitals:** Monitor baseline and periodically
- Monitor temperature, may indicate beginning infection, I&O, for nausea, appetite

Black Box Warning: New primary malignancy: assess for new malignancy that may occur with this product

- **Bleeding:** hematuria, guaiac, bruising, petechiae of mucosa or orifices q8hr
- Effects of alopecia on body image; discuss feelings about body changes

Black Box Warning: Hepatotoxicity/hepatic necrosis: assess for jaundice of skin, sclera; dark urine; clay-colored stools; itchy skin; abdominal pain; fever; diarrhea; monitor hepatic studies prior to, during therapy (bilirubin, AST, ALT, LDH) as needed or monthly

- Inflammation of mucosa, breaks in skin
- IV site for irritation, redness, pain; if infiltration occurs, discontinue, restart at new site
- **Hypersensitivity reactions, anaphylaxis:** discontinue product, administer meds for anaphylaxis
- Increased fluid intake to 2-3 L/day to prevent urate deposits, calculi formation

Black Box Warning: Product must be administered by those experienced in the use of cancer chemotherapy

Evaluate:
- Therapeutic response: decreased tumor size, spread of malignancy

Teach patient/family:
- That patient should avoid prolonged exposure to sun, wear sunscreen
- That hair may be lost during treatment; that a wig or hairpiece may make the patient feel better; that new hair may be different in color, texture
- To report signs of **infection:** fever, sore throat, flulike symptoms; **hepatic symptoms:** yellowing of eyes, clay-colored stools
- To report signs of **anemia:** fatigue, headache, faintness, SOB, irritability

- To report bleeding; to avoid use of razors, commercial mouthwash
- To avoid aspirin products or ibuprofen

Black Box Warning: Pregnancy/breastfeeding: to notify prescriber if pregnancy is planned or suspected; to use reliable contraceptives during and for several months after therapy; not to breastfeed, contraindicated in first trimester

dalbavancin (Rx)

(dal-ba-van´sin)

Dalvance, Xydalba ✦

Func. class.: Antiinfective
Chem. class.: Glycopeptide

ACTION: Binds to the bacterial cell walls, inhibiting their synthesis

USES: Treatment of acute bacterial skin and skin structure infections due to gram-positive organisms (cellulitis, major abscess, wound infections); *Enterococcus faecalis, Enterococcus faecium, Staphylococcus aureus* (MRSA), *Staphylococcus aureus* (MSSA), *Streptococcus agalactiae* (group B streptococci), *Streptococcus anginosus, Streptococcus constellatus, Streptococcus dysgalactiae, Streptococcus intermedius, Streptococcus pyogenes* (group A beta-hemolytic streptococci)

CONTRAINDICATIONS

Hyper-sensitivity

Precautions: Antimicrobial resistance, breastfeeding, infusion-related reactions, pregnancy, CDAD, ulcerative colitis, vancomycin or glycopeptide hypersensitivity, viral infection, elderly, children, hepatic disease, CCr <30 mL/min (no dialysis)

DOSAGE AND ROUTES

- **Adult:** IV 1500 mg once; or 1000 mg once, then 500 mg **IV** 1 wk later
- **Child 6-18 yr:** IV CCr ≥30 mL/min/1.73 m² 18 mg/kg/max 1500 as a single dose
- **Child birth to 6 yr:** IV CCr ≥30 mL/min/1.73 m²: 22.5 mg/kg, max 1500 as a single dose

---

Side effects: *italics* = common; red = life-threatening

Renal dose
• **Adult:** IV CCr <30 mL/min 1125 mg as a single dose or 750 mg once then 375 mg 1 wk later

Available forms: Injection 500 mg/vial (single use)

Administer:

IV INFUSION route
• Visually inspect parenteral products for particulate matter and discoloration
• **Reconstitution:** Reconstitute each 500 mg/25 mL (20 mg/mL) sterile water for injection or D_5W; to avoid foaming, alternate between gentle swirling and inversion until completely dissolved, do not shake; further dilution is required
• **Storage:** Refrigerate or store at room temperature. Do not freeze. The total time from reconstitution to dilution to use max 48 hr
• **Dilution:** Transfer the dose of reconstituted solution from the vial(s) to an IV bag or bottle containing D_5W (1-5 mg/mL), discard unused product

Intermittent IV INFUSION
• Give over 30 min, do not infuse with other medications or electrolytes, saline-based infusion solutions may cause precipitation and should not be used; if a common IV line is being used to administer other drugs, the line should be flushed prior to and after each dose

SIDE EFFECTS

CNS: Dizziness, headache, flushing
GI: Nausea, CDAD, abdominal pain, diarrhea, vomiting
RESP: Bronchospasm
SYST: Red man syndrome, hypersensitivity reactions
GU: Mycotic vulvovaginal infections
ENDO: Hypoglycemia
INTEG: Rash, urticaria, infusion-related reactions, pruritus, petechiae, phlebitis

PHARMACOKINETICS

Protein binding 93%, primarily to albumin, excreted in feces and urine, metabolism decreased in renal disease, half-life 8 days, peak infusion's end, duration 1 wk

INTERACTIONS
None known

NURSING CONSIDERATIONS

Assess:
• Monitor CBC with differential, LFTs
• BUN/creatinine; lower dose may be required in severe renal disease
• **CDAD:** monitor for bowel pattern daily; if severe diarrhea occurs, product should be discontinued, may occur ≥8 wk after last dose
• **Infection:** B/P, pulse, temperature, characteristics of urine, stools, sputum baseline and during treatment, make sure use is for a bacterial infection
• **Anaphylaxis:** rash, urticaria, pruritus, wheezing; may occur a few days after administration
• **Infusion site reactions:** monitor for reactions, discontinue if present
• **Red man–like syndrome:** assess for flushing, rash over upper torso and neck; may occur after a few minutes of infusion; may be treated with antihistamines and a slower infusion, usually caused by too rapid an infusion

Evaluate:
• Therapeutic response: decreased symptoms of infection, negative C&S

Teach patient/family:
• To report allergic reactions to this product, vancomycin, or other glycopeptides
• That product is used for bacterial infections only
• To report sore throat, bruising, bleeding, joint pain **(blood dyscrasias)**; diarrhea with mucus, blood **(CDAD)**; rash, pruritus, wheezing **(hypersensitivity reactions)**
• **Pregnancy/breastfeeding:** to notify health care professional if pregnancy is planned or suspected or if breastfeeding
• To notify prescriber of all OTC, prescription medications, and herbals used

dalfampridine (Rx)

(dal-fam′pri-deen)

Ampyra, Fampyra ✦

Func. class.: Neurologic agent—multiple sclerosis

Chem. class.: Broad-spectrum potassium channel blocker

USES: For improved walking in patients with multiple sclerosis

CONTRAINDICATIONS

Renal failure (CCr <50 mL/min), seizures

Precautions: Pregnancy, breastfeeding, geriatric patients, renal disease

DOSAGE AND ROUTES

• **Adult: PO** 10 mg q12hr

Renal dose

• **Adult: PO** CCr 51-80 mL/min, no dosage adjustment needed but seizure risk unknown; CCr ≤50 mL/min, do not use

Available forms: Extended-release tablets 10 mg

⚠ HIGH ALERT

dalteparin (Rx)

(dahl′ta-pear-in)

Fragmin

Func. class.: Anticoagulant

Chem. class.: Low-molecular-weight heparin

ACTION: Inhibits factor Xa/IIa (thrombin), resulting in anticoagulation

USES: Unstable angina/non–Q-wave MI; prevention/treatment of deep venous thrombosis in abdominal surgery, hip replacement, or in those with restricted mobility during acute illness, pulmonary embolism, reduced recurrence of VTE in pediatrics

Unlabeled uses: VTE prophylaxis in gynecologic surgery

CONTRAINDICATIONS

Hypersensitivity to this product, heparin, or pork products; active major bleeding, hemophilia, leukemia with bleeding, thrombocytopenic purpura, cerebrovascular hemorrhage, cerebral aneurysm; those undergoing regional anesthesia for unstable angina, non–Q-wave MI, dalteparin-induced thrombocytopenia

Precautions: Hypersensitivity to benzyl alcohol, pregnancy, breastfeeding, children, recent childbirth, geriatric patients; hepatic disease; severe renal disease; blood dyscrasias; bacterial endocarditis; acute nephritis; uncontrolled hypertension; recent brain, spine, eye surgery; congenital or acquired disorders; severe cardiac disease; peptic ulcer disease; hemorrhagic stroke; history of HIT; pericarditis; pericardial effusion; recent lumbar puncture; vasculitis; other diseases in which bleeding is possible

Black Box Warning: Epidural/spinal anesthesia, lumbar puncture

DOSAGE AND ROUTES

DVT/pulmonary embolism (cancer-associated venous thrombosis)

• **Adult: SUBCUT** 200 IU/kg daily during first mo (max single dose 18,000 IU), then 150 IU/kg daily for mo 2-6 (max single dose 18,000 IU), use prefilled syringe that is closest to calculated dose; if platelets are 50,000-100,000/mm³, reduce dose by 2500 units until platelets ≥100,000 mm³; if platelets <50,000/mm³, discontinue until >50,000/mm³

Hip replacement surgery/DVT prophylaxis

• **Adult: SUBCUT** 2500 IU 2 hr prior to surgery and second dose in the evening on the day of surgery (4-8 hr postop), then 5000 IU **SUBCUT** first postop day and daily × 5-10 days

Unstable angina/non–Q-wave MI

• **Adult: SUBCUT** 120 IU/kg q12hr × 5-8 days, max 10,000 IU q12hr × 5-8 days with concurrent aspirin; continue until stable

DVT, prophylaxis for abdominal surgery

• **Adult: SUBCUT** 2500 IU 1-2 hr prior to surgery; repeat daily × 5-10 days; for high-risk patients, >3400 IU should be used

DVT prophylaxis in patients with severely restricted mobility due to acute illness

---

Side effects: *italics* = common; red = life-threatening

Adult: SUBCUT 5000 IU daily × 12-14 days
VTE in pediatrics. See manufacturer's information
Renal dose
• **Adult: SUBCUT** cancer patient with CCr <30 mL/min, monitor and adjust based on anti–factor Xa during extended treatment
VTE prophylaxis in gynecologic surgery (unlabeled)
• **Adults: SUBCUT** 2500 IU daily starting 1-2 hr prior to surgery then daily
Available forms: Prefilled syringes, 2500, 5000 IU/0.2 mL; 7500 IU/0.3 mL; 10,000 IU/mL, 12,500 IU/0.5 mL, 15,000 IU/0.6 mL, 18,000 IU/0.72 mL, 95,000 IU/3.8 mL

Administer:
• Cannot be used interchangeably (unit for unit) with unfractionated heparin or other LMWHs
• Do not give IM or IV product route; approved is SUBCUT only; do not mix with other injections or solutions
• Have patient sit or lie down; SUBCUT injection may be 2 inches from umbilicus in a U-shape, upper outer side of thigh, or upper outer quadrangle of the buttocks; rotate injection sites
• Change injection site daily; use at same time of day

SIDE EFFECTS
CNS: Intracranial bleeding, fever
HEMA: Thrombocytopenia, DIC
GU: Hematuria
INTEG: Skin necrosis, injection site reaction
SYST: Hypersensitivity, hemorrhage, anaphylaxis

PHARMACOKINETICS
87% absorbed, excreted by kidneys, elimination half-life 2-2.3 hr, peak 2-4 hr, onset 1-2 hr, duration up to 24 hr

INTERACTIONS
Increase: bleeding risk—aspirin, oral anticoagulants, platelet inhibitors, NSAIDs, salicylates, thrombolytics, some cephalosporins, SSRIs; cautious use
Drug/Herb
Increase: bleeding risk— angelica, capsicum, chamomile, dandelion, dan shen, feverfew, garlic, ginger, ginkgo, horse chestnut, avoid using together
Drug/Lab Test
Increase: AST, ALT
Decrease: platelets

NURSING CONSIDERATIONS
Assess:
• **Blood studies** (Hct/HB, CBC, platelets, anti-Xa,) during treatment because bleeding can occur
• **Bleeding:** bleeding gums, petechiae, ecchymosis, black tarry stools, hematuria, epistaxis; decrease in Hct, B/P may indicate bleeding, possible hemorrhage; notify prescriber immediately; product should be discontinued

Black Box Warning: Epidural/spinal anesthesia: neurologic impairment may occur frequently when neuraxial anesthesia has been used; spinal/epidural hematomas may occur with paralysis; numbness in lower extremities; bowel, bladder changes; back pain; notify prescriber immediately; those at greatest risk are taking products that cause increased bleeding risk

• **Hypersensitivity:** fever, skin rash, urticaria; notify prescriber immediately
• Needed dosage change q1-2wk; dose may need to be decreased if bleeding occurs
• **Pregnancy/breastfeeding:** no well-controlled studies; use only if clearly needed; LMWH does not cross placenta; benefits and risk must be weighed with provider; if used, discontinue 24 hr prior to induction or cesarean delivery; use of multidose vials containing benzyl alcohol is contraindicated; use caution in breastfeeding
Evaluate:
• Therapeutic response: absence of DVT/PE, prevention of complication (unstable angina, non-Q-wave MI)
Teach patient/family:
• To avoid OTC preparations that contain aspirin, other anticoagulants unless approved by prescriber; serious product interactions may occur
• To use soft-bristle toothbrush to avoid bleeding gums; to avoid contact sports; to use electric razor; to avoid IM injections

• **Bleeding:** to report any signs of bleeding (gums, under skin, urine, stools), unusual bruising

TREATMENT OF OVERDOSE:
Protamine sulfate 1% given IV; 1 mg protamine/100 anti-Xa international units of dalteparin given

---

⚠ HIGH ALERT

dantrolene (Rx)
(dan'troe-leen)

Dantrium, Revonto, Ryanodex
Func. class.: Skeletal muscle relaxant, direct acting
Chem. class.: Hydantoin

USES: Spasticity in multiple sclerosis, stroke, spinal cord injury, cerebral palsy, malignant hyperthermia

CONTRAINDICATIONS
Hypersensitivity, hepatic disease, hepatitis
Precautions: Pregnancy, breastfeeding, geriatric patients, peptic ulcer disease, cardiac/renal/hepatic disease, stroke, seizure disorder, diabetes mellitus, ALS, COPD, MS, mannitol/gelatin hypersensitivity, labor, lactase deficiency, extravasation

Black Box Warning: Hepatotoxicity

DOSAGE AND ROUTES
Spasticity
• **Adult: PO** 25 mg daily × 7 days, then 25 mg tid × 7 days, then 50 mg tid × 7 days, then 100 mg tid (max 100 mg qid); if no further benefit is observed at the next higher dose, decrease dosage to the previous dose; stop if no benefit seen within 45 days
• **Child: PO** 0.5 mg/kg daily × 7 days, then 0.5 mg/kg tid × 7 days, then 1 mg/kg tid × 7 days, then 2 mg/kg tid; max 100 mg qid, if no further benefit is observed at the next higher dose, decrease dosage to the previous dose; stop if no benefit is seen in 45 days

Prevention of malignant hyperthermia
• **Adult/child: PO** 4-8 mg/kg/day in 3-4 divided doses × 1-3 days prior to procedure, give last dose 4 hr preop; **IV** 2.5 mg/kg prior to anesthesia
Malignant hyperthermia
• **Adult/child: IV** 1-2.5 mg/kg, may repeat to total dose of 10 mg/kg; **PO** 4-8 mg/kg/day in 4 divided doses × 1-3 days
Neuroleptic malignant syndrome (unlabeled)
• **Adult: PO** 75-600 mg/day in divided doses; **IV** 1 to 2.5 mg/kg/dose once, initially. May continue 1 to 2.5 mg/kg/dose q6hr or 0.25 mg/kg/hr continuous IV infusion for 48 to 72 hr
Available forms: Capsules 25, 50, 100 mg; injection 20 mg/vial, 250 mg/vial

---

⚠ HIGH ALERT

dapagliflozin (Rx)
(dap'a-gli-floe'zin)

Farxiga
Func. class.: Oral antidiabetic
Chem. class.: Sodium-glucose co-transporter 2 (SGLT 2) inhibitor

---

ACTION: Blocks reabsorption of glucose by the kidney, increases glucose excretion, lowers blood glucose concentrations

USES: Type 2 diabetes mellitus, with diet and exercise

CONTRAINDICATIONS
Dialysis, renal failure (eGFR <30 mL/min/1.73 m^2) or ESRD (dialysis), hypersensitivity, breastfeeding, diabetic ketoacidosis, active bladder cancer
Precautions: Pregnancy, children, renal/hepatic disease, hypothyroidism, hyperglycemia, hypotension, bladder cancer, hypercholesterolemia, pituitary insufficiency, type 1 diabetes mellitus, malnutrition, fever, dehydration, adrenal insufficiency, geriatrics, genital fungal infections, hypoglycemia

---

DOSAGE AND ROUTES
Type 2 diabetes mellitus in combination with diet and exercise
- **Adult: PO** 5 mg daily, increase dose to 10 mg daily in those who require additional glycemic control

Reduction of HF hospitalizations in type 2 diabetes mellitus and established cardiovascular (CV) disease or multiple CV risk factors
- **Adult: PO** 10 mg once daily

HF with reduced ejection fraction (NYHA class II to IV) to reduce the risk of cardiovascular death and hospitalization for HF
- **Adult: PO** 10 mg once daily

Chronic kidney disease to reduce the risk of sustained eGFR decline, end-stage kidney disease, CV death, and hospitalization for HF in those at risk of disease progression
- **Adult: PO** 10 mg once daily

Renal dose
- **Adult: PO** eGFR ≥45 mL/min/1.73 m^2 no change, eGFR <45 mL/min, do not use

Available forms: Tablets 5, 10 mg
Administer:
PO route
- Once daily in AM without regard to food
- Store at room temperature

SIDE EFFECTS
GI: Pancreatitis, constipation, nausea
GU: Cystitis, candidiasis, urinary frequency, polydipsia, polyuria, increased serum creatinine; renal impairment/failure; infections
INTEG: Photosensitivity, rash, pruritus
META: Hypercholesterolemia, lipidemia, hypoglycemia, hyperkalemia, hypomagnesemia, hypo/hyperphosphatemia
MISC: Bone fractures, hypotension; dehydration; orthostatic hypotension; hypersensitivity; new bladder cancer

PHARMACOKINETICS
91% protein binding, primary excretion in urine, half-life 12.9 hr; primarily metabolized by O-glucuronidation by UGT1A9; minor CYP3A4; Cmax is less than 2 hr

INTERACTIONS
Increase: hypoglycemia—sulfonylureas, insulin, MAOIs, salicylates, fibric acid derivatives, bile acid sequestrates, ACE inhibitors, angiotensin II receptor antagonists, beta-blockers; adjust antidiabetics
Increase or decrease: glycemic control—androgens, lithium, bortezomib, quinolones
Decrease: effect, hyperglycemia—digestive enzymes, intestinal absorbents, thiazide diuretics, loop diuretics, corticosteroids, estrogen, progestins, oral contraceptives, sympathomimetics, isoniazid, phenothiazines, protease inhibitors, atypical antipsychotics, carbonic anhydrase inhibitors, cycloSPORINE, tacrolimus, baclofen

Drug/Lab Test
Increase: Hct, LDL
Decrease: eGFR

NURSING CONSIDERATIONS
Assess:
- **Hypoglycemia** (weakness, hunger, dizziness, tremors, anxiety, tachycardia, sweating) when used with other agents even though product does not cause hypoglycemia; if patient is on sulfonylureas or insulin, hypoglycemia may be additive; if hypoglycemia occurs, treat with dextrose or, if severe, with IV glucagon; monitor HbA1c, lipid panel, blood glucose, BUN, creatinine; if renal function is reduced, discontinue; monitor volume status, B/P, usually in those with eGFR <60 mL/min/1.73m^2; more frequent in those with poor renal function
- **Necrotizing fasciitis of the perineum:** may occur in both females and males and require surgical intervention; assess perineum for swelling, pain, fever; if present, discontinue and start antibiotics
- **Bone fracture risk:** avoid use in those at increased risk of fractures; renal impairment increases fracture risk
- **Mycotic infections:** increased risk of mycotic infections, especially genital;

caution in those with previous infections or in uncircumcised males
• **Hypersensitivity:** discontinue immediately
• **Ketoacidosis:** increased urine/serum ketone levels, may occur without increased glucose levels; may occur more frequently in those with reduced intake of food, fluids, or in serious conditions
• **Renal function:** baseline and periodically; discontinue if renal function is reduced; assess for signs of UTIs (serious)
• **Pregnancy/breastfeeding:** avoid use in pregnancy; do not breastfeed
Evaluate:
• Therapeutic response: improved signs/symptoms of diabetes mellitus (decreased polyuria, polydipsia, polyphagia); clear sensorium, absence of dizziness, stable gait; HbA1c WNL
Teach patient/family:
• The symptoms of hypo/hyperglycemia, what to do about each
• That medication must be taken as prescribed; explain consequences of discontinuing medication abruptly; that insulin may need to be used for stress, including trauma, fever, surgery
• To avoid OTC medications and herbal supplements unless approved by health care provider
• That diabetes is a lifelong illness; that the diet and exercise regimen must be followed; that this product is not a cure
• To carry emergency ID and glucose source
• That blood glucose monitoring and periodic lab tests are required to assess product effect
• That GI side effects may occur
• That there is a risk of renal impairment, dehydration, and bladder cancer
• To report immediately fever, itching, change in urine output, light headedness or feeling faint, other signs of UTI
• To ensure adequate fluid intake to avoid dehydration and/or hypotension; to report symptoms to provider
• **Necrotizing fasciitis of the perineum:** Teach patient to report immediately pain, swelling of perineum, fever

• **Candidiasis (yeast infection):** Have patient report itching, discharge, inflammation, redness, burning; discuss dietary ways of preventing
• **Ketoacidosis:** to report immediately confusion, abdominal pain, fatigue, trouble breathing, nausea, vomiting, food intolerance

⚠ HIGH ALERT

dapagliflozin/saxagliptin (Rx)
(dap′a-gli-floe′zin/sax-a-glip′tin)
Qtern
Func. class.: Oral antidiabetic
Chem. class.: Sodium-glucose cotransporter 2 (SGLT-2) inhibitor/dipeptidyl peptidase-4 (DPP-4) inhibitor antidiabetics

USES: Type 2 diabetes mellitus, with diet and exercise

CONTRAINDICATIONS
Dialysis, renal failure, hypersensitivity, breastfeeding, diabetic ketoacidosis
Precautions: Pregnancy, children, renal/hepatic disease, hypothyroidism, hyperglycemia, hypotension, bladder cancer, hypercholesterolemia, pituitary insufficiency, type 1 diabetes mellitus, malnutrition, fever, dehydration, adrenal insufficiency, geriatrics, genital fungal infections, hypoglycemia

DOSAGE AND ROUTES
Type 2 diabetes mellitus
• **Adult: PO** 10 mg dapagliflozin and 5 mg saxagliptin once daily, taken in the morning, with or without food
Renal dose
• **Adult: PO** eGFR 45 mL/min/1.73 m² or more: no change; eGFR <45 mL/min/1.73 m²: do not start in these patients. In patients currently taking the product, discontinue when eGFR is persistently <60 mL/min/1.73 m²; eGFR <45 mL/min/1.73 m²: do not use
Available forms: Tablets 10 mg, 5 mg

DAPTOmycin (Rx)

(dap'toe-mye-sin)

Cubicin Cubicin RF

Func. class.: Antiinfective—miscellaneous
Chem. class.: Lipopeptide

ACTION: Binds to the bacterial membrane and results in a rapid depolarization of the membrane potential, leading to inhibition of DNA, RNA, and protein synthesis

USES: Bacteremia, endocarditis, UTI, complicated skin, skin structure infections caused by *Staphylococcus aureus* (MRSA, MSSA) including methicillin-resistant strains, *Streptococcus agalactiae, Streptococcus dysgalactiae, Enterococcus faecalis* (vancomycin-susceptible strains), *Streptococcus pyogenes* (group A beta-hemolytic), *Staphylococcus aureus, Staphylococcus epidermidis, Corynebacterium jeikeium, Staphylococcus haemolyticus*

CONTRAINDICATIONS

Hyper-sensitivity

Precautions: Pregnancy, breastfeeding, children, geriatric patients, GI/renal disease, myopathy, ulcerative/CDAD, rhabdomyolysis, eosinophilic pneumonia

DOSAGE AND ROUTES
Complicated skin and skin structure infections

• **Adult: IV INFUSION** 4 mg/kg over ½ hr diluted in 0.9% NaCl, give q24hr × 7-14 days; some indications may use up to 6 mg/kg
• **Child/Adolescent 12 to 17 yr: IV** 5 mg/kg/dose q24hr for up to 14 days
• **Child 7-11 yr: IV** 7 mg/kg/dose q24hr for up to 14 days
• **Child 2-6 yr: IV** 9 mg/kg/dose q24hr for up to 14 days
• **Child 1 year: IV** 10 mg/kg/dose q24hr for up to 14 days

Staphylococcus aureus bacteremia, right-sided infective endocarditis

• **Adult: IV INFUSION** 6 mg/kg daily × 2-6 wk, up to 8-10 mg/kg daily; treatment failures should use another agent

Renal dose

• **Adult: IV INFUSION** CCr <30 mL/min, hemodialysis, CAPD 4 mg/kg q48hr, 6 mg/kg q48hr (bacteremia)

Bacteremia caused by *S. aureus* in children with normal renal function

• **Child 12-17 yr: IV INFUSION** 7 mg/kg q24hr for up to 42 days
• **Child 7-11 yr: IV INFUSION** 9 mg/kg q24hr up to 42 days
• **Child 1-6 yr: IV INFUSION** 12 mg/kg q24hr up to 42 days

Available forms: Lyophilized powder for injection 500 mg/vial; powder for IV infusion 350 mg/vial

Administer:
IV route

• Cubicin RF and Cubicin have different reconstitution and storage methods
• For IV use only; use a 21-gauge or smaller needle for all transfers
• Do not admix
• Cubicin RF is compatible with 0.9% NaCl injection, sterile water for injection, and bacteriostatic water for injection; Cubicin is compatible with 0.9% NaCl injection and LR injection
• Do not use with ReadyMED elastomeric infusion pumps
• Visually inspect for particulate matter and discoloration prior to use

Cubicin RF preparation
Reconstitution

• Reconstitute a 500-mg vial/10 mL of sterile water for injection or bacteriostatic water for injection (50 mg/mL)
• Do NOT reconstitute with saline products
• Transfer the 10 mL of sterile water for injection or bacteriostatic water for injection through the center of the rubber stopper. Point the transfer needle against the inside wall of the vial
• Prior to use, rotate or swirl the vial for a few minutes
• Vials are not preserved and are for single-use only
• *Storage (Vials):* Vials reconstituted with sterile water for injection can be stored for 1 day at room temperature, and vials reconstituted with bacteriostatic water for

injection can be stored for 2 days at room temperature. Vials reconstituted with either solution can be stored for 3 days under refrigeration at 36° F to 46° F (2° C to 8° C)

• *Storage (Syringes):* Solutions reconstituted with sterile water for injection are stable in polypropylene syringes with an elastomeric plunger stopper for 1 day at room temperature, and solutions reconstituted with bacteriostatic water for injection are stable in this type of syringe for 2 days at room temperature. Solutions reconstituted with sterile water for injection and bacteriostatic water for injection are stable in this syringe for 3 days and 5 days, respectively, under refrigeration

Dilution:
• **Adults/child 7-17 yr:** Further dilute in 50 mL of 0.9% sodium chloride injection
• **Child 1 to 6 yr:** Further dilute in 25 mL of 0.9% sodium chloride injection

Cubicin preparation
Reconstitution
• To minimize foaming, avoid vigorous agitation or shaking of the vial during or after reconstitution
• Reconstitute the vial with 0.9% NaCl for injection according to the manufacturer's instructions (50 mg/mL)
• Transfer the appropriate volume of 0.9% sodium chloride for injection through the center of the rubber stopper. Point the transfer needle against the inside wall of the vial
• Ensure that all the powder is wetted by gently rotating the vial. Allow the wetted product to stand undisturbed for 10 min. Gently rotate or swirl the vial contents for a few minutes, as needed, to obtain a completely reconstituted solution
• Vials are not preserved and are for single-use only
• **Storage:** The reconstituted solution is stable in the vial for 12 hr at room temperature and up to 48 hr if stored under refrigeration at 35° F to 46° F (2° C to 8° C)

Dilution:
• **Adults/child 7-17 yr:** Further dilute in 50 mL of 0.9% NaCl
• **Child 1-6 yr:** Further dilute in 25 mL of 0.9% NaCl

• **Storage:** Diluted solutions are stable for 12 hr at room temperature or 48 hr under refrigeration

Cubicin RF and Cubicin administration:
• Do not use IV push in children
IV push:
• Give via slow IV push over 2 min
Intermittent IV Infusion:
• **Adult/child 7-17 yr:** Give over 30 min
• **Child 1-6 yr:** Give over 60 min
• If the same IV line is used for sequential infusion of different drugs, flush the line with a compatible IV solution prior to and after daptomycin administration

Y-site compatibilities: Alfentanil, amifostine, amikacin, aminocaproic acid, aminophylline, amiodarone, amphotericin B liposome, ampicillin, ampicillin-sulbactam, argatroban, arsenic trioxide, atenolol, atracurium, azithromycin, aztreonam, bivalirudin, bleomycin, bumetanide, buprenorphine, busulfan, butorphanol, calcium chloride/gluconate, CARBOplatin, carmustine, caspofungin, ceFAZolin, cefepime, cefotaxime, cefoTEtan, cefOXitin, cefTAZidime, ceftizoxime, cefTRIAXone, cefuroxime, chloramphenicol, chlorproMAZINE, cimetidine, ciprofloxacin, cisatracurium, CISplatin, clindamycin, cyclophosphamide, cycloSPORINE, dacarbazine, DACTINomycin, DAUNOrubicin, dexamethasone, dexmedetomidine, dexrazoxane, diazepam, digoxin, diltiazem, diphenhydrAMINE, DOBUTamine, DOCEtaxel, DOPamine, doripenem, doxacurium, DOXOrubicin, DOXOrubicin liposomal, doxycycline, droperidol, enalaprilat, ePHEDrine, EPINEPHrine, epirubicin, eptifibatide, ertapenem, erythromycin, esmolol, etoposide, famotidine, fenoldopam, fentaNYL, fluconazole, fludarabine, fluorouracil, foscarnet, fosphenytoin, furosemide, ganciclovir, gentamicin, glycopyrrolate, granisetron, haloperidol, heparin, hydrALAZINE, hydrocortisone, HYDROmorphone, hydrOXYzine, IDArubicin, ifosfamide, inamrinone, insulin (regular), irinotecan, isoproterenol, ketorolac, labetalol, lepirudin, leucovorin, levofloxacin, lidocaine, linezolid, LORazepam, magnesium sulfate, mannitol, mechlorethamine, melphalan, meperidine, meropenem, mesna, metaraminol, methyldopate, methyl-PREDNISolone, metoclopramide, metoprolol, midazolam, milrinone, mitoXANtrone, mivacurium, morphine, moxifloxacin, mycophenolate mofetil, nafcillin, nalbuphine, naloxone, niCARdipine, nitroprusside, norepinephrine, octreotide, ondansetron, oxaliplatin, oxytocin, PACLitaxel, palonosetron, pamidronate, pancuronium, PEMEtrexed, pentamidine, PHENobarbital, phenylephrine, piperacillin-tazobactam, polymyxin B, potassium acetate/chloride/phosphates, procainamide, prochlorperazine, promethazine, propranolol, quinupristin-dalfopristin, ranitidine, rocuronium, sodium acetate/bicarbonate/citrate/phosphates, succinylcholine, sulfamethoxazole-trimethoprim, tacrolimus, teniposide, theophylline, thiotepa, ticarcillin, ticarcillin-clavulanate, tigecycline, tirofiban, tobramycin, topotecan, trimethobenzamide, vasopressin, vecuronium, verapamil, vinBLAStine, vinCRIStine, vinorelbine, voriconazole, zidovudine, zoledronic acid

SIDE EFFECTS
CNS: Headache, insomnia, dizziness
CV: Hypo/hypertension
GI: Nausea, constipation, diarrhea, vomiting, dyspepsia, CDAD, abdominal pain
GU: Nephrotoxicity
HEMA: Anemia
INTEG: Rash, pruritus, injection site reactions
MS: Rhabdomyolysis
RESP: Cough, eosinophilic pneumonia, dyspnea
SYST: Anaphylaxis, DRESS, Stevens-Johnson syndrome, angioedema

PHARMACOKINETICS
Site of metabolism unknown, protein binding 92%, half-life 8.1 hr, 78% excreted unchanged (urine), excreted in breast milk, peak infusion's end, duration 24 hr

INTERACTIONS
• May alter anticoagulant levels—warfarin; monitor PT, INR
Increase: myopathy—HMG-CoA reductase inhibitors

Drug/Lab Test
Increase: CK, AST, ALT, BUN, creatinine, albumin, LDH
Increase/Decrease: glucose
Decrease: alkaline phosphatase, magnesium, phosphate, bicarbonate, Hb/Hct

NURSING CONSIDERATIONS
Assess:
• **Eosinophilic pneumonia:** assess for dyspnea, fever, cough, shortness of breath; if left untreated, can lead to respiratory failure and death
• **DRESS:** Assess for swelling, rash, fever, may lead to organ involvement, discontinue product
• **Nephrotoxicity:** any patient with compromised renal system; toxicity may occur; BUN, creatinine
• **Rhabdomyolysis:** check for myopathy, CPK >1000 U/L (>5 × ULN), discontinue product, muscle pain, weakness; caution if concomitant HMG-CoA reductase inhibitor therapy, consider discontinuation of therapy
• **Bowel function:** assess for diarrhea, fever, abdominal pain; report to prescriber; CDAD may occur
• Monitor I&O ratio: report hematuria, oliguria; nephrotoxicity may occur
• B/P during administration; hypotension/hypertension may occur
• Signs of infection
• **Pregnancy/breastfeeding:** Identify whether pregnancy is planned or suspected; avoid use in pregnancy or breastfeeding, lack of controlled studies
Evaluate:
• Therapeutic response: negative culture, resolution of infection
Teach patient/family:
• About allergies prior to treatment, reaction to each medication
• To report sore throat, fever, fatigue; could indicate superinfection; diarrhea; muscle weakness, pain, shortness of breath
• To avoid driving, hazardous activities until response is known; may cause dizziness
• To avoid breastfeeding, use in pregnancy

D

daratumumab (Rx)

(dar′a-toom-ue-mab)

Darzalex Faspro

Func. class.: Antineoplastic

Chem. class.: Monoclonal antibody

ACTION: Binds to CD38, thereby inducing apoptosis in tumor cells

USES: For the treatment of multiple myeloma in patients who have received at least 3 prior therapies including a proteasome inhibitor (PI) and an immunomodulatory agent or who are double refractory to a PI and an immunomodulatory agent

CONTRAINDICATIONS

Hypersensitivity

DOSAGE AND ROUTES

• **Adult:** IV 16 mg/kg (actual body weight) weekly on wk 1 to 8 (8 doses), 16 mg/kg every other week on wk 9 to 24 (8 doses), and then 16 mg/kg q4wk starting on wk 25 until disease progression; premedicate 1-3 hr prior to infusion with corticosteroid, oral antipyretic, oral or IV antihistamine

Available forms: Injection 100 mg/5 mL, 400 mg/mL in single-dose vials

Administer

• Visually inspect for particulate matter and discoloration prior to use, solution in single-dose vials is colorless to pale yellow

• Premedication 1-3 hr prior to each infusion with acetaminophen 650-1000 mg PO, diphenhydramine 25-50 mg IV/PO, dexamethasone 20 mg

• If a dose is missed, give as soon as possible and adjust the dosing schedule to maintain the treatment interval

• Initial dilution volume and/or infusion rate differ for first, second, and subsequent infusions; the maximum infusion rate is 200 mL/hr

• Withdraw the needed amount (mL) from the 20-mg/mL vials for the calculated dose (use actual body weight); discard any unused portion left in the vial

• For the first infusion (wk 1), dilute the calculated amount in 0.9% NaCl injection to a total infusion bag volume of 1000 mL for a single-dose infusion (16 mg/kg) or 500 mL for split-dose infusions (8 mg/kg). For subsequent infusions, dilute the calculated amount in 0.9% NaCl injection to a total infusion bag volume of 500 mL. Following a single-dose infusion (16 mg/kg), reduce the total infusion bag volume to 500 mL only if there were no grade 1 or higher infusion reactions during the previous week

• Gently invert the bag to mix, do not shake

• Infusion bags/containers must be made of polyvinylchloride (PVC), polypropylene (PP), polyethylene (PE), or polyolefin blend

• *Storage of admixture:* Store at room temperature 59° F to 77° F (15° C to 25° C) for up to 15 hr (includes infusion time) or for up to 24 hr refrigerated 36° F to 46° F (2° C to 8° C), protect from light; allow refrigerated admixtures to warm to room temperature prior to use

• Administer using an infusion-set fitted with a flow regulator and with an inline, sterile, nonpyrogenic, low-protein-binding polyethersulfone filter (pore size of 0.2 or 0.22 micrometer); polyurethane, polybutadiene (PBD), PVC, PP, or PE administration sets must be used

• Do not infuse other drugs concomitantly in the same IV line

• Administer the diluted infusion intravenously at the appropriate infusion rate as follows: ***Week 1 infusion(s):*** start at 50 mL/hr, increase by 50 mL/hr hourly to a max 200 mL/hr; ***Week 2 infusion (following a single 16-mg/kg dose infusion only):*** start at 50 mL/hr, increase by 50 mL/hr hourly to max 200 mL/hr; ***Subsequent infusions:*** start at 100 mL/hr, increase by 50 mL/hr hourly to max 200 mL/hr if there were no grade 1 or higher infusion reactions during the previous week

• Discard unused product

SIDE EFFECTS
CNS: Fever, headache, fatigue, chills
GI: Nausea, vomiting, diarrhea, constipation, anorexia
CV: Hypertension
RESP: Cough, dyspnea, URI, pneumonia
HEMA: Thrombocytopenia, neutropenia, lymphopenia, anemia
EENT: Nasal congestion
MS: Arthralgia, back pain
MISC: Infusion site reactions, herpes zoster reactivation

PHARMACOKINETICS
Onset, peak, duration unknown; half-life 9-27 days

INTERACTIONS
None known
Drug/Lab Test
Decrease: platelets, RBCs, neutrophils, lymphocytes

NURSING CONSIDERATIONS
Assess:
• **Hypersensitivity/bronchospasm:** premedicate prior to infusion to prevent hypersensitivity and bronchospasm, have emergency equipment nearby, reactions may occur for up to 4 hr after conclusion of infusion
• **Thrombocytopenia, neutropenia, lymphopenia:** monitor CBC, platelets periodically; type and cross for blood transfusions prior to infusion, type and cross-match may not be accurate after using product
• **Pregnancy/breastfeeding:** not to use during pregnancy, response is unknown, use contraception during and for 3 mo after last dose; secretion in breast milk is unknown
• **Herpes zoster reactivation:** use antivirals 1 wk prior to infusion and continue for 3 mo after conclusion of therapy
Evaluate:
• Therapeutic response: Slowly, prevention of growth in multiple myeloma
Teach patient/family:
• That bloodwork and continuing labs will be needed
• To report immediately change in breathing, tight chest, wheezing, itching, chills, nausea, vomiting
• To report to all providers the use of this product

• Pregnancy/breastfeeding: To report if pregnancy is planned or suspected or if breastfeeding

daratumumab/hyaluronidase-fihj (Rx)
(dar'a-toom'ue-mab/hye'al-ureon' i-dase)
Darzalex
Func. class.: Antineoplastic

USES:
Multiple myeloma

CONTRAINDICATIONS
Hypersensitivity, pregnancy, breastfeeding

DOSAGE AND ROUTES
Multiple myeloma (newly diagnosed)
Adult: SUBCUT with lenalidomide and dexamethasone in those ineligible for autologous stem cell transplant: Wk 1-8: daratumumab 1800 mg/hyaluronidase 30,000 units weekly × 8 doses; wk 9-24: daratumumab 1800 mg/hyaluronidase 30,000 units q2wk × 8 doses; wk 25 and thereafter: daratumumab 1800 mg/hyaluronidase 30,000 units q4wk until disease progression or unacceptable toxicity
Adult: SUBCUT with bortezomib, melphalan, predniSONE; in those ineligible for autologous stem cell transplant: wk 1-6: daratumumab 1800 mg/hyaluronidase 30,000 units weekly × 6 doses; wk 7-54: daratumumab 1800 mg/hyaluronidase 30,000 units q3wk × 16 doses; wk 55 and thereafter: daratumumab 1800 mg/hyaluronidase 30,000 units q4wk until disease progression or unacceptable toxicity
Available forms: solution for injection 1800 units-30,000 units/15 mL

⚠ HIGH ALERT

darbepoetin alfa (Rx)
(dar'bee-poh'eh-tin)
Aranesp
Func. class.: Colony-stimulating factor
Chem. class.: Recombinant human erythropoietin

ACTION: Stimulates erythropoiesis by the same mechanism as endogenous erythropoietin; in response to hypoxia, erythropoietin is produced in the kidney and released into the bloodstream, where it interacts with progenitor stem cells to increase red cell production

USES: Anemia associated with chronic renal failure in patients on and not on dialysis and anemia in nonmyeloid malignancies for patients receiving coadministered chemotherapy

CONTRAINDICATIONS
Hypersensitivity to hamster protein products, human albumin, polysorbate 80; uncontrolled hypertension; red cell aplasia
Precautions: Pregnancy, breastfeeding, children, seizure disorder, porphyria, hypertension, sickle cell disease; vitamin B_{12}, folate deficiency; chronic renal failure, dialysis; latex hypersensitivity, CABG, angina, anemia

> **Black Box Warning:** HB >11 g/dL, neoplastic disease, MI, stroke, thromboembolic disease

DOSAGE AND ROUTES
Correction of anemia in chronic renal failure
• **Adult:** SUBCUT/IV For those on dialysis 0.45 mcg/kg as a single injection; every week, or 0.75 mcg/kg q2wk; **for those not on dialysis** 0.45 mcg/kg q4wk titrate, max target Hb of 11 g/dL
• **Child:** IV/SUBCUT 0.45 mcg/kg qwk or 0.75 mcg/kg q2wk (no dialysis)
Anemia due to chemotherapy
• **Adult:** SUBCUT 2.25 mcg/kg/wk or 500 mcg q3wk, start only if Hb <10 g/dL and 2 more months of chemotherapy
Epoetin alfa to darbepoetin conversion
• **Adult:** SUBCUT/IV (epoetin alfa <2500 units/wk) 6.25 mcg/wk; (epoetin alfa 2500-4999 units/wk) 12.5 mcg/wk; (epoetin alfa 5000-10,999 units/wk) 25 mcg/wk; (epoetin alfa 11,000-17,999 units/wk) 40 mcg/wk; (epoetin alfa 18,000-33,999 units/wk) 60 mcg/wk; (epoetin alfa 34,000-89,999 units/wk) 100 mcg/wk; (epoetin alfa >90,000 units/wk) 200 mcg/wk

Available forms: Sol for injection 25, 40, 60, 100, 150, 200, 300, 500 mcg/mL
Administer:
• Transfusions may still be required for anemia, use iron supplements with this product
SUBCUT route
• Do not give intradermally
• Identify latex allergy
• Don't shake, protect from light
IV route
• Without shaking; check for discoloration, particulate matter, do not use if present; do not dilute, do not mix with other products or solutions, discard unused portion
• IV given direct undiluted or bolus into IV tubing or venous line after completion of dialysis; watch for clotting of line
• Adjust dosage every month or more
• Store refrigerated, do not freeze; protect from light

SIDE EFFECTS
CNS: Seizures, headache, dizziness, stroke
CV: *Hypo/hypertension,* cardiac arrest, *angina pectoris,* HF, acute MI, dysrhythmias, chest pain, edema
GI: *Diarrhea, vomiting, nausea, abdominal pain, constipation*
HEMA: Red cell aplasia
MISC: *Infection, fatigue, fever*
MS: *Bone pain, myalgia, limb pain, back pain, arthralgia*
RESP: *Dyspnea, cough, bronchitis*
SYST: Allergic reactions, anaphylaxis

PHARMACOKINETICS
IV: Onset of increased reticulocyte count 2-6 wk; distributed to vascular space; absorption slow and rate limiting; terminal half-life 49 hr (SUBCUT), 21 hr (IV); peak 34 hr; increased Hb levels not observed until 2-6 wk

INTERACTIONS
Increase: darbepoetin alfa effect—androgens

Drug/Lab Test
Increase: WBC, platelets, Hb
Decrease: bleeding time

NURSING CONSIDERATIONS
Assess:

• Symptoms of **anemia:** fatigue, dyspnea, pallor

• **Serious allergic reactions:** rash, urticaria; if anaphylaxis occurs, stop product, administer emergency treatment (rare)

Black Box Warning: Increased risk of death if hemoglobin >11 g/dL: monitor Hb prior to and weekly × 4 wk or after change in dose and then often after target range has been reached; a rise >1g/dL over 2 wk may increase risks; reduce dose, keep Hb <10 g/dL in chronic kidney disease

Black Box Warning: Renal studies: urinalysis, protein, blood, BUN, creatinine, electrolytes; monitor dialysis shunts; during dialysis, heparin may need to be increased; those with renal dysfunction may be at greater risk of death. Keep Hb <10 g/dL in chronic kidney disease

Black Box Warning: Blood studies: ferritin, transferrin monthly; transferrin saturation ≥20%, ferritin ≥100 ng/mL; Hb 2×/wk until stabilized in target range (30%-33%), then at regular intervals; those with endogenous erythropoietin levels of <500 units/L respond to this agent; iron stores should be corrected prior to beginning therapy; if there is lack of response, obtain folic acid, iron, vitamin B_{12} levels

Black Box Warning: Neoplastic disease: breast, non–small-cell lung, head and neck, lymphoid, or cervical cancers, increased tumor progression; use lowest dose to avoid RBC transfusion

• B/P: check for rising B/P as Hb rises; antihypertensives may be needed

Black Box Warning: CV status: hypertension may occur rapidly, leading to **hypertensive encephalopathy;** Hb >11 g/dL may lead to stroke, MI, death; do not administer

• I&O; report drop in output to <50 mL/hr

• **Seizures:** if Hb is increased by 1 g/dL within 2 wk, institute seizure precautions, decrease dose

• CNS symptoms: sweating, pain in long bones

• **Dialysis patients:** thrill, bruit of shunts; monitor for circulation impairment

• **Pregnancy/breastfeeding:** Those who become pregnant should register with Amgen's Pregnancy Surveillance Program (800-772-6436), may cause fetal harm
Evaluate:

• Therapeutic response: increase in reticulocyte count, Hb/Hct; increased appetite, enhanced sense of well-being
Teach patient/family:

• To avoid driving or hazardous activity during beginning of treatment

• To monitor B/P, Hb, max Hb 11 g/dL

• To take iron supplements, vitamin B_{12}, folic acid as directed

Black Box Warning: To report to prescriber any chest pain, SOB, swelling/pain in legs, confusion, inability to speak; to comply with treatment regimen

• That menses and fertility may return; to use contraception

• About home administration procedures, if appropriate

• **Seizures:** discuss injury prevention in those who are prone to seizures, may occur if Hb is increased too rapidly, to report immediately if seizures occur

• **Chronic renal failure:** that product does not cure condition, that other treatment regimens should be followed

---

darifenacin (Rx)
(da-ree-fen'ah-sin)
Enablex
Func. class.: Antispasmodic/GU anticholinergic
Chem. class.: M3 selective receptor antagonist

Do not confuse:
Enablex/Effexor XR

ACTION: Bladder smooth muscle relaxation by decreasing the action of muscarinic receptors, thereby relieving overactive bladder

USES: Urge incontinence, frequency, urgency in overactive bladder

CONTRAINDICATIONS
Hypersensitivity, urinary retention, narrow-angle glaucoma (uncontrolled)
Precautions: Severe hepatic disease (Child-Pugh C), GI/GU obstruction, controlled narrow-angle glaucoma, ulcerative colitis, myasthenia gravis, moderate hepatic disease (Child-Pugh B), elderly

DOSAGE AND ROUTES
Urge incontinence
• **Adult: PO** 7.5 mg/day, initially; may increase to 15 mg/day after 14 days if needed
With CYP3A4 inhibitor
• **Adult: PO** max 7.5 mg/day
Hepatic dosage
• **Adult: PO** (Child-Pugh B) max 7.5 mg/day; do not use in severe hepatic disease
Available forms: Tablets, extended release 7.5, 15 mg
Administer:
• Without regard to meals; do not crush, break, chew extended-release tablets
• Store at room temperature

SIDE EFFECTS
CNS: Dizziness, headache, confusion, hallucinations, drowsiness
EENT: Blurred vision, dry eyes
GI: Constipation, dry mouth, nausea, dyspepsia
INTEG: Rash, pruritus, skin drying
MISC: Angioedema, flulike symptoms

PHARMACOKINETICS
Peak 7 hr, half-life 12-19 hr, extensively metabolized by CYP2D6, less metabolism in poor metabolizers; some metabolism by CYP3A4, protein binding 98%, duration 24 hr

INTERACTIONS
Increase: level of—digoxin
Increase: anticholinergic effect—anticholinergics
Increase: darifenacin level—CYP3A4 (ketoconazole, itraconazole, ritonavir), max 7.5 mg/day

Increase: levels of—drugs metabolized by CYP2D6 (flecainide, tricyclics)

NURSING CONSIDERATIONS
Assess:
• **Urinary function:** urgency, frequency, retention, incontinence in bladder outflow obstruction
• **Anticholinergic effects (CNS):** headache, confusion after dosage change
• **Bowel pattern:** constipation, abdominal pain, increase fluids, bulk in diet if constipation occurs
• **Pregnancy/breastfeeding:** no well-controlled studies; use only if benefit outweighs fetal risk; cautious use in breastfeeding, excretion is unknown
Evaluate:
• Therapeutic response: decreasing urgency, frequency of urination
Teach patient/family:
• To take without regard to meals; not to crush, break, chew extended-release tablets; not to use other products unless approved by prescriber
• Not to double or skip doses, provide "Patient Information" and ask to read
• To discuss with provider all OTC, Rx, herbals, supplements used
• To store at room temperature
• To avoid breastfeeding; to notify prescriber if pregnancy is planned or suspected
• About anticholinergic symptoms (dry mouth, constipation, dry eyes, heat prostration); not to become overheated
• To avoid hazardous activities until reaction is known; dizziness, blurred vision can occur
• **Angioedema:** to report facial swelling, difficulty swallowing, or large tongue

darunavir/cobicistat/emtricitabine/tenofovir alafenamide (Rx)
(da-roo'na-veer/koe-bik'i-stat/emtrye-sye'ta-been/ten-oh-fohveer)
Symtuza
Func. class.: Antiretroviral, pharmacoenhancers
Chem. class.: Protease inhibitors, enzyme inhibitors NRTI

ACTION:
- **Darunavir:** Inhibits HIV protease needed for replication
- **Cobicistat:** Enhances elvitegravir
- **Emtricitabine:** Inhibits viral reverse transcriptase and acts as a DNA chain terminator
- **Tenofovir:** Inhibits viral reverse transcriptase and acts as a DNA chain terminator

Therapeutic outcome: Improvement in CD4, HIV RNC counts; decreasing signs and symptoms of HIV

USES:
HIV in treatment-naïve patients and certain virologically stable (HIV RNA <50 copies/mL) treatment-experienced patients

PHARMACOKINETICS
Absorption: darunavir: unknown; **cobicistat:** unknown; **emtricitabine:** rapid and extensively; **tenofovir:** a prodrug bioavailability is increased with a high-fat meal
Distribution: darunavir: protein binding 95%, unknown; **cobicistat:** protein binding 97%-98%, unknown; **emtricitabine:** unknown; **tenofovir:** unknown
Metabolism: darunavir: by CYP3A4; **cobicistat:** by CYP3A4; **emtricitabine:** metabolized by oxidation to 3′-sulfoxide diastereomer (approximately 9% of dose) and via conjugation with glucuronic acid to 2′-O-glucuronide; **tenofovir:** undergoes phosphorylation to its active metabolite
Excretion: darunavir: 41% (feces), 8% (urine); **cobicistat:** 86% (feces), 8% (urine); **emtricitabine:** excreted renally (86%) and via feces (14%); **tenofovir:** eliminated by a combination of glomerular filtration and active renal tubular secretion, 70%-80% excreted unchanged in urine by 72 hr
Half-life: darunavir: 9.4 hr; **cobicistat:** 3.5 hr; **emtricitabine:** 10 hr; **tenofovir:** 30 min

PHARMACODYNAMICS
Onset: Unknown
Peak: darunavir: 3 hr; **cobicistat:** 3 hr; **emtricitabine:** 1-2 hr; **tenofovir:** 2 hr
Duration: 24 hr

CONTRAINDICATIONS
Hypersensitivity, CCr <30 mL/min, severe hepatic disease
Precautions:: Alcoholism, autoimmune disease, bone fractures, breastfeeding, children, depression, females, Graves' disease, Guillain-Barré syndrome, hepatic disease, hepatitis, hepatitis B and HIV coinfection, hepatitis C and HIV coinfection, hepatomegaly, Hispanic patients, HIV resistance, hypercholesterolemia, hyperlipidemia, hypertriglyceridemia, hypophosphatemia, immune reconstitution syndrome, lactic acidosis, obesity, osteomalacia, osteoporosis, pregnancy, renal failure, renal impairment, serious rash, suicidal ideation, torsades de pointes

Black Box Warning: Hepatitis B exacerbation, hepatotoxicity

DOSAGE AND ROUTES
HIV infection in antiretroviral treatment-naïve patients
Adults/child ≥40 kg: PO: One tablet (darunavir 800 mg; cobicistat 150 mg; emtricitabine 200 mg; tenofovir 10 mg) q day
Available forms: Tablet 800-150-200-10 mg

ADVERSE EFFECTS
CNS: *Headache,* abnormal dreams, *depression,* dizziness, *insomnia,* neuropathy, paresthesia, asthenia, suicide, fatigue, drowsiness
GI: Nausea, vomiting, anorexia, diarrhea, abdominal pain, dyspepsia, hepatomegaly with stenosis (may be fatal), hyperbilirubinemia, hypercholesterolemia, pancreatitis
GU: Glomerulonephritis (membranous/mesangial proliferative)
INTEG: *Rash,* skin discoloration
MS: Arthralgia, myalgia, rhabdomyolysis
RESP: Cough
SYST: Change in body fat distribution, lactic acidosis

INTERACTIONS
Individual drugs
Efavirenz, lamivudine: Do not use with, treatment duplication will occur

Drug classifications

CYP3A4 inhibitors (aldesleukin IL-2, amiodarone, aprepitant, atazanavir, basiliximab, boceprevir, bromocriptine, chloramphenicol, clarithromycin, conivaptan, danazol, dalfopristin, darunavir, dasatinib, delavirdine, dilTIAzem, dronedarone, efavirenz, erythromycin, ethinyl estradiol, fluconazole, fluoxetine, FLUvoxamine, fosamprenavir, fosaprepitant, imatinib, indinavir, isoniazid, itraconazole, ketoconazole, lanreotide, lapatinib, miconazole, nefazodone, nelfinavir, nicardipine, octreotide, posaconazole, quinine, ranolazine, rifAXIMin, tamoxifen, telaprevir, telithromycin, tipranavir, troleandomycin, verapamil, voriconazole, zafirlukast): increased level interferons: decreased emtricitabine level

Drug/food

Increased: Adverse reactions: grapefruit juice

Drug/lab test

Increased: AST/ALT, amylase, bilirubin, CK, glucose, lipase

Decreased: Neutrophils

NURSING CONSIDERATIONS
Assessment:

• **HIV infection:** Assess symptoms of HIV, including opportunistic infections, before and during treatment, some may be life threatening; monitor plasma CD4+, CD8 cell counts, serum beta-2 microglobulin, serum ICD 24 antigen levels, treatment failures occur more often in those with baseline HIV-1 RNA concentrations >100,000 copies/mL than in those <100,000 copies/mL; monitor blood glucose, CBC with differential, serum cholesterol, lipid panel

Black Box Warning: **Hepatotoxicity/ lactic acidosis:** Monitor hepatitis B serology, LFTs, plasma hepatitis C RNA, lactic acidosis levels. If lab reports confirm these conditions, discontinue product. More common in females or those who are overweight. Avoid use in alcoholism

• **Pregnancy:** Obtain pregnancy testing before use, hepatitis B exacerbation; those with coexisting HBV and HIV infections who discontinue emtricitabine or tenofovir may experience severe acute hepatitis B exacerbation, with some cases resulting in hepatic decompensation and hepatic failure

• Patients coinfected with HBV and HIV who discontinue this product should have transaminase concentrations monitored q6wk for the first 3 mo and q3-6mo thereafter

• Resumption of anti–hepatitis B treatment may be required. For patients who refuse a fully suppressive antiretroviral regimen but still require treatment for HBV, consider 48 wk of peginterferon alfa; do not administer HIV-active medications in the absence

• Periodically monitor serum bilirubin (total and direct), serum creatinine, urinalysis, LFTs, amylase, lipase

Patient problems:

• Infection (uses)

• Risk for injury (adverse reactions)

• Nonadherence (teaching)

Implementation:

• Antiretroviral drug resistance testing (preferably genotypic testing) is recommended before use in treatment-naïve patients and before changing therapy for treatment failure

• For adults, treatment is recommended in all patients to reduce the risk of disease progression and to prevent the transmission of HIV, including perinatal transmission and transmission to sexual partners

• For pregnant women, therapy should begin immediately after HIV diagnosis, as early maternal viral suppression is associated with lower risk of perinatal infection

• Avoid use of tenofovir-containing regimens in those with renal disease and osteoporosis

• Don't use with other antiretrovirals

Teach patient/family:

• That hepatitis and HIV coinfected patients should avoid consuming alcohol; offer vaccinations against hepatitis A/ hepatitis B as appropriate

• That GI complaints resolve after 2-3 wk of treatment

- To report suspected or planned pregnancy, not to breastfeed
- To take at the same time of day to maintain blood level; not to crush, break, or chew
- That product controls the symptoms of HIV but does not cure, that patient is still able to infect others, that other products may be necessary to prevent other infections
- **Lactic acidosis:** To notify prescriber of fatigue, muscle aches/pains, abdominal pain, difficulty breathing, nausea, vomiting, change in heart rhythm

Black Box Warning: Hepatotoxicity: To notify prescriber of dark urine, yellowing skin or eyes, clay-colored stools, anorexia, nausea, vomiting

- **Suicide:** To report severe depression, suicidal ideation to prescriber immediately

Evaluate:
- Improvement in CD4, HIV RNC counts, decreasing signs and symptoms of HIV

---

dasatinib (Rx)

(da-si′ti-nib)

Sprycel

Func. class.: Antineoplastic—miscellaneous

Chem. class.: Protein-tyrosine kinase inhibitor

USES: Treatment of accelerated, chronic blast phase CML or acute lymphoblastic leukemia (ALL); chronic phase CML with resistance or intolerance to prior therapy; ✖ Philadelphia chromosome–positive CML in chronic phase

CONTRAINDICATIONS

Pregnancy, hypersensitivity

DOSAGE AND ROUTES

Accelerated or myeloid/lymphoid blast phase CML with resistance/intolerance to prior therapy
- **Adult: PO** 140 mg daily titrated up to 180 mg daily in those resistant to therapy

Chronic phase CML with resistance/intolerance to prior therapy
- **Adult: PO** 100 mg daily either AM or PM

Dosage reduction for those taking a strong CYP3A4 inhibitor
- **Adult: PO** 20-40 mg daily

Available forms: Tablets 20, 50, 70, 80, 100, 140 mg

---

dasiglucagon

(das-i-gloo′ka-gon)

Zegalogue

Func. class.: Antihypoglycemic

Chem. class.: Glucagon receptor agonist

ACTION: Increases blood glucose concentration by activating hepatic glucagon receptors, thereby stimulating glycogen breakdown and release of glucose from the liver. Hepatic stores of glycogen are necessary for dasiglucagon to produce an antihypoglycemic effect

Therapeutic outcome: Blood glucose levels WNL

USES:

To treat severe hypoglycemia in those with diabetes

PHARMACOKINETICS

Absorption: Unknown

Distribution: Unknown

Metabolism: Proteolytic degradation pathways in blood, liver, and kidney

Excretion: Unknown

Half-life: 30 min

PHARMACODYNAMICS

Onset: Unknown

Peak: 35 min

Duration: Unknown

CONTRAINDICATIONS

Insulinoma, pheochromocytoma, hypersensitivity

Precautions: Latex allergy, breastfeeding, adrenal insufficiency, pregnancy, malnutrition

DOSAGE AND ROUTES

Severe hypoglycemia in patients with diabetes mellitus

Adults/child ≥6 yr: SUBCUT 0.6 mg; if no response after 15 min, may give an additional dose; IV dextrose must be given if the patient fails to respond to glucagon. Once the patient has responded to treatment, give oral carbohydrates to prevent recurrence of hypoglycemia

Available forms: Injection: 0.6 mg/0.6 mL single-dose injector; 0.6 mg/0.6 mL single-dose prefilled syringe

SIDE EFFECTS
CNS: Headache
GI: Nausea, vomiting, diarrhea
CV: Hyper-/hypotension, bradycardia, orthostatic hypotension
INTEG: Injection site reaction
MISC: Hypersensitivity

INTERACTIONS
Anticholinergics: Increased GI adverse reactions
Beta blockers: Increased B/P and HR
Indomethacin: Decreased action of dasiglucagon
Warfarin: Increased anticoagulant effect, monitor closely
Administer:
SUBCUT route
• Give by SUBCUT injection only, do not give IM or IV
• Visually inspect parenteral products for particulate matter and discoloration prior to use
• Available as an autoinjector or as a prefilled syringe. Keep in the red protective case until ready for use
• The inside of the gray cap of the autoinjector device and the inside of the gray needle cover of the prefilled syringe contain dry natural rubber, which may cause allergic reactions in people with latex allergy
• Inject into the outer upper arm, front or back of the thigh, lower abdomen (at least 2 inches from the belly button), or buttocks
• Roll back any clothing to expose bare skin; do not inject through clothes
• After injection:
  • Roll the unconscious person on to their side to prevent choking

• Call for emergency medical help right away. Even if the injection helps the person to wake up, still call for emergency medical help right away
• If the person does not respond after 15 min, another dose may be given, if available
• Once the person is able to safely consume food or drink, give the person a fast-acting source of sugar (fruit juice) and a long-acting source of sugar (crackers with cheese or peanut butter)
• Replace the used autoinjector or prefilled syringe right away so the patient will have a new one in case it is needed

SUBCUT autoinjector (Zegalogue Single-dose Autoinjector)
• Choose injection site and expose the skin
• Hold the red protective case upright with the gray lid on top and pull the gray cap straight off. Carefully remove the autoinjector from the red protective case without dropping it
• Pull the gray cap straight off the autoinjector device. Do not put hand or fingers anywhere near the yellow needle guard
• Push the autoinjector straight down on the patient's skin until the yellow needle guard is fully pressed down; you may hear the first "click." Keep holding the injector down and slowly count to 10 seconds; during this time, the medicine window will turn red and you may hear a second "click." Check that the medicine window is red to ensure that the full dose has been given
• Remove the autoinjector from the skin by lifting it straight up. The yellow needle guard will cover the needle and lock, preventing an accidental needle stick injury
• Place the used autoinjector in an FDA-cleared sharps disposal container right away; do not dispose of injectors in household trash

SUBCUT prefilled syringe (Zegalogue Single-Use Prefilled Syringe)
• Choose injection site, hold the red protective case upright with the gray lid on top and pull the gray cap straight off. Carefully remove the prefilled syringe from the red protective case without dropping it
• Gently pinch the skin and insert the entire needle into the skin at a 45-degree angle
• After inserting the needle, release the pinched skin and slowly press the plunger rod all the way down until the syringe is empty and the plunger rod stops
• After the plunger rod stops and the injection is complete, carefully remove the needle from the injection site
• Place the used syringe in an FDA-cleared sharps disposal container right away; do not dispose of loose needles or syringes in household trash

NURSING CONSIDERATIONS
Assess:
• **Hypoglycemia:** Determine reaction to be severe hypoglycemia, monitor blood glucose
• **Hypersensitivity:** Identify hypersensitivity (difficulty breathing, hypotension)
Patient problems:
• Risk of injury (uses)
Teach patient/family:
• Instruct the patient and/or caregiver to read the "Instructions for Use."
• Teach patient and caregiver the signs and symptoms of hypoglycemia (vision change, sleepiness, dizziness, hunger, anxiety, confusion)
• Hypersensitivity: Teach patient to seek emergency services for serious hypersensitivity reactions
• Teach patient and/or caregiver how to use product and dispose of equipment
• Teach patient when conscious to consume sugar or fruit juice, then a longer-duration carbohydrate
Evaluate:
• Positive therapeutic outcome
• Conscious, blood glucose WNL

⚠ HIGH ALERT

DAUNOrubicin (Rx)
(daw-noe-roo'bi-sin)
Cerubidine ✤

Func. class.: Antineoplastic, antibiotic
Chem. class.: Anthracycline glycoside

USES: Acute lymphocytic leukemia (ALL), acute myelogenous leukemia (AML)

CONTRAINDICATIONS
Pregnancy, breastfeeding, hypersensitivity, systemic infections, cardiac disease, bone marrow depression

Black Box Warning: IM/SUBCUT use

Precautions: Tumor lysis syndrome, MI, infection, thrombocytopenia, renal/hepatic disease; gout

Black Box Warning: Bone marrow suppression, cardiac disease, extravasation, renal failure, hepatic disease; requires a specialized care setting and an experienced clinician

DOSAGE AND ROUTES
• **Adult <60 yr:** IV 45 mg/m^2/day × 3 days, first cycle, then 2 days second cycle
• **Adult ≥60 yr:** IV 30 mg/m^2/day × 3 days, then 2 days of subsequent courses in combination, max 400-600 mg/m^2 total cumulative dose
• **Child ≥2 yr:** IV 25 mg/m^2/day depending on cycle weekly in combination; **<2 yr or BSA <0.5** determine on mg/m^2/kg basis
Available forms: Injection 5 mg/mL

⚠ HIGH ALERT

DAUNOrubicin/cytarabine (Rx)
(daw-noe-roo'bi-sin/sye-tare'a-been)
Vyxeos
Func. class.: Antineoplastic

USES: For the treatment of newly diagnosed therapy-related AML or AML with myelodysplasia-related changes

DOSAGE AND ROUTES
• **Adult: IV first induction,** 44 mg/m²
daunorubicin liposomal and 100 mg/
m² cytarabine liposomal over 90 min
on days 1, 3, and 5; patients who do not
achieve a response may receive a second induction. **Second induction**
(given 2-5 wk after first induction cycle), 44 mg/m² daunorubicin liposomal and 100 mg/m² cytarabine liposomal on days 1 and 3. **Consolidation
therapy** (given 5-8 wk after start of the
last induction), 29 mg/m² daunorubicin liposomal and 65 mg/m² cytarabine
liposomal on days 1 and 3. Patients
without disease progression or unacceptable toxicity should receive a second cycle of consolidation therapy
given 5-8 wk after the start of the previous consolidation
Available forms: Injection (lyophilized
cake) 44 mg daunorubicin/100 mg
cytarbine (single-dose vial)

daxibotulinumtoxin A-lanm (Rx)
Daxxify
Func. class.: Muscle relaxant

USES: Temporary improvement in
moderate to severe glabellar (frown)
lines

DOSAGE AND ROUTES

Black Box Warning: Distant spread of
toxin effects

Adults: IM 40 units administered in 5
equal aliquots of 8 units each: 2 injections in each corrugator muscle and 1
injection in the procerus muscle. Do not
administer more frequently than every
3 mo
Available forms: Injection 50 units,
100 units

decitabine/cedazuridine (Rx)
(de-sye′ta-been/sed′az-ure′i-deen)
Inqovi
Func. class.: Antineoplastic, antimetabolite

USES: Treatment of myelodysplastic
syndromes (MDSs)

CONTRAINDICATIONS
Hypersensitivity

DOSAGE AND ROUTES
• **Adult: PO** 35 mg decitabine/100 mg
cedazuridine daily × 5 days of each 28-day
cycle, complete at least 4 cycles
Available forms: Tablets 35-100 mg

deferasirox (Rx)
(def-a′sir-ox)
Exjade, Jadence ✦, Jadenu,
Jadenu Sprinkle
Func. class.: Heavy-metal chelating
agent

USES: Chronic iron overload, transfusion hemosiderosis

CONTRAINDICATIONS
Breastfeeding, children, hypersensitivity,
severe renal/hepatic disease, GI hemorrhage

Black Box Warning: Renal failure, GI
bleeding/perforation, hepatotoxicity,
nephrotoxicity

DOSAGE AND ROUTES
• **Adult and child >2 yr: PO** (Jadenu) Estimated GFR >60 mL/min/1.73 m²: Initial, 14
mg/kg orally once daily; adjust in increments
of 3.5 or 7 mg/kg every 3-6 mo based on
clinical response and goals; use lowest effective dose to provide a trend in decreasing
ferritin; if not adequately controlled with
21 mg/kg/day (e.g., serum ferritin levels
persistently >2500 mcg/L and not decreas-

ing over time), may increase to a max of 28 mg/kg/day; consider dose reduction if serum ferritin falls below 1000 mcg/L at 2 consecutive visits (especially if dose is >17.5 mg/kg/day); if serum ferritin falls below 500 mcg/L, interrupt therapy and monitor monthly (Exjade) Estimated GFR >60 mL/min/1.73 m². Initial, 20 mg/kg orally once daily; adjust in increments of 5 or 10 mg/kg every 3-6 mo based on clinical response and goals; use lowest effective dose to provide a trend in decreasing ferritin; max 40 mg/kg

Available forms: Tablets 90, 180, 360 mg; oral suspension tablets 125, 250, 500 mg; sprinkles 90, 180, 360 mg

---

⚠ HIGH ALERT

degarelix (Rx)
(day-gah-rel'iks)

Firmagon

Func. class.: Antineoplastic
Chem. class.: GnRH-receptor antagonist

ACTION: Reduces release of gonadotropins and testicular steroidogenesis by reversibly binding to GnRH receptors

USES: Advanced prostate cancer

CONTRAINDICATIONS
Hypersensitivity, QT prolongation, osteoporosis, severe hepatic/renal disease, pregnancy, breastfeeding

Precautions: CV disease, electrolyte abnormalities, geriatric patients

DOSAGE AND ROUTES
• **Adult (male): SUBCUT** 240 mg given as two 120-mg injections (40 mg/mL concentrations); maintenance 80 mg (20 mg/mL concentration) every 28 days, starting 28 days after first dose

Available forms: Injection 80-, 120-mg vial

Administer:
• Do not give IV, SUBCUT only
• Use double gloves, gown, aseptic technique during preparation and administration, all safe handling procedures

• Keep vials vertical; do not shake the vials; give reconstituted drug within 1 hr after addition of sterile water for injection

Reconstitution of 120-mg vial (240-mg dose *only*):
• Use two 120-mg vials; repeat for each 120-mg vial: draw up 3 mL of sterile water for injection with a 2-inch, 21-G needle; do not use bacteriostatic water for injection; inject the sterile water slowly, swirl gently; reconstitution can take up to 15 min; avoid turning the vial upside down; repeat with a new vial, needle, and syringe for the second 120-mg dose (total dose = 240 mg)

Reconstitution of 80-mg vial:
• Use 4.2 mL of sterile water for injection with a 2-inch, 21-G needle; do not use bacteriostatic water for injection; inject the sterile water slowly into vial containing 80 mg; swirl gently; reconstitution can take up to 15 min; withdraw 4 mL (20 mg/mL); avoid turning vial upside down during withdrawal

SUBCUT injection:
• Exchange the reconstitution needle with a 1.25-inch, 27-G needle; remove air bubbles; give in the abdominal region; rotate injection site periodically; use area not exposed to pressure; grasp aspirate before injection; inject the dose SUBCUT; when giving the loading dose of two 120-mg doses, the second dose should be injected at a different site

SIDE EFFECTS
CNS: Chills, dizziness, fatigue, fever, headache, insomnia
CV: Increased QT prolongation, hypotension, hot flashes, hypertension
GI: Diarrhea, constipation, nausea
GU: ED, UTI, gynecomastia, testicular atrophy
INTEG: Injection site reactions, pain at site, redness, swelling
MS: Back pain, decreased bone density
SYST: Hypersensitivity, anaphylaxis, angioedema

PHARMACOKINETICS
Peak 2 days, duration 50 days, half-life 53 days

INTERACTIONS
Increase: QT prolongation—class IA/III antidysrhythmics, methyldopa, metoclopramide, reserpine, avoid using together

Drug/Lab Test
Increase: PSA, LFTs, GGT
Decrease: bone density test

NURSING CONSIDERATIONS
Assess:
• Monitor HbA1c, lipids, B/P prior to initiation and 3-6 mo after
• **QT prolongation:** more common in those taking class IA/III antidysrhythmics, heart failure, congenital long QT syndrome; monitor cardiac status at baseline and often thereafter, include ECG periodically
• **Anaphylaxis, angioedema (rash, trouble breathing):** discontinue treatment and do not restart in serious reactions; assess for rash, dyspnea, wheezing, facial swelling
• Liver function studies, PSA, GGT that may be elevated; bone density that may be decreased; electrolytes; if PSA is elevated, monitor testosterone levels
Evaluate:
• Therapeutic response: decreasing spread, size of tumor
Teach patient/family:
• To notify all prescribers of cardiac disease or use of all cardiac products, irregular pulse, heartbeat
• Side effects and adverse reactions that may occur
• Injection technique if patient/family will be giving product (provide patient information)

---

delafloxacin (Rx)
(dela-flox′-a-sin)
Baxdela
Func. class.: Antiinfective
Chem. class.: Fluoroquinolone

ACTION: Inhibits bacterial DNA gyrase

USES: For the treatment of acute bacterial skin and skin structure infections

DOSAGE AND ROUTES
• **Adult: PO** 450 mg q12hr × 5-14 days
• **Adult: IV** 300 mg q12hr × 5-14 days
Renal dose: Adult (eGFR 15-29 mL/min/1.73 m²) no change: PO 200 mg q12hr IV then switch to 450 mg PO

Available forms: Injection 300 mg in single-dose vials; tablets 450 mg

CONTRAINDICATIONS
Hypersensitivity to this product or fluoroquinolones, tendon rupture, aortic aneurysm, renal failure, myasthenia gravis, children
Precautions: Pregnancy, breastfeeding, renal disease, CDAD, elderly, transplants, RA, psychiatric disorders
Administer
PO route
• Take without regard to meals, give ≥2 hr prior to or 6 hr after any antacid, multivitamin, or other medication that contains divalent or trivalent cations
• If a dose is missed, take it as soon as possible up to 8 hr prior to the next scheduled dose. If less than 8 hr before next dose, wait until the next scheduled dose
IV route
• Reconstitute the 300-mg vial/10.5 mL of 5% dextrose for injection or 0.9% sodium chloride for injection 300 mg/12 mL (25 mg/mL)
• Shake vigorously until dissolved
• The reconstituted vial must be further diluted
• *Storage:* Reconstituted vials refrigerated at 36° F to 46° F (2° C to 8° C) or at room temperature of 68° F to 77° F (20° C to 25° C) for up to 24 hr. Do not freeze
• Withdraw the needed volume of reconstituted solution per dose, 12 mL for a 300-mg dose and 8 mL for a 200-mg dose
• Dilute the reconstituted solution to a total volume of 250 mL using either 5% dextrose for injection or 0.9% sodium chloride for injection to achieve a concentration of 1.2 mg/mL
• *Storage:* Diluted solutions may be kept refrigerated at 36° F to 46° F (2° C to 8° C) or at room temperature of 68° F to 77° F (20° C to 25° C) for up to 24 hr. Do not freeze
Intermittent IV infusion
• Infuse over 60 min
• Do not administer with any solution containing multivalent cations through the same IV line
• Do not admix with other medications. Flush lines with 5% dextrose for injection or 0.9% sodium chloride for injection prior to and after each infusion if using common IV line

Side effects: *italics* = common; red = life-threatening

SIDE EFFECTS

CNS: Headache, dizziness, insomnia, anxiety, paresthesia, unusual dreams
CV: Palpitations, sinus tachycardia, hyper/hypotension, flushing, bradycardia
GI: Nausea, vomiting, anorexia, abdominal pain, CDAD
GU: Vaginal candidiasis, renal dysfunction, renal failure
EENT: Blurred vision, tinnitus, oral candidiasis
META: Hypo/hyperglycemia
MS: Myalgia
INTEG: Infusion site reactions
MISC: Hypersensitivity, fungal infections

PHARMACOKINETICS

PO: Onset unknown, peak 1 hr, duration unknown
IV: Onset unknown, peak 1 hr, duration unknown
Half-life PO 4-8½ hr, IV 3.7 hr

INTERACTIONS

Increase: Infection risk—corticosteroids
Decrease: Delafloxacin level—antacids, didanosine
Drug/Lab: Increase: LFTs, CK, alkaline phosphatase, blood glucose
Decrease: Blood glucose

NURSING CONSIDERATIONS

Assess:
• C&S prior to starting treatment, may begin treatment before results are received
• **Infection:** monitor WBC, temperature, vital signs, baseline and periodically

Black Box Warning: **Myasthenia gravis:** avoid use in these patients, muscle weakness

Black Box Warning: **Tendonitis, rupture:** monitor for tenderness, weakness, inflammation of tendons, muscles, discontinue at first signs, increased in those >60 yr or taking corticosteroids

Black Box Warning: **Peripheral neuropathy:** monitor for tingling, burning, pain of extremities

• **CDAD:** Monitor for diarrhea with blood, mucus, abdominal pain, stop product immediately
• **Hypersensitivity:** Assess for rash, pruritus, discontinue immediately
• **Psychiatric disorders:** Assess for hallucinations, psychosis, paranoia, delusions, suicidal thought/behaviors
• **CNS symptoms:** Headache, dizziness, fatigue, insomnia
• Monitor renal, hepatic studies: LFTs, BUN, creatinine

Evaluate:
• Therapeutic response
• C&S negative, decreasing signs or symptoms of infection

Teach patient/family:
• Teach the patient continuing follow-ups and lab work will be needed
• To report diarrhea with blood or mucous, abdominal pain, fever, stop product immediately
• To report if pregnancy is planned or suspected or if breastfeeding
• To report rash, itching, headache, dizziness, fatigue, insomnia
• To report injection site pain, redness, burning

Black Box Warning: To report muscle tenderness, weakness, inflammation to stop immediately

---

⚠ HIGH ALERT

denosumab (Rx)

(den-oh′sue-mab)
Prolia, Xgeva
Func. class.: Bone resorption inhibitor
Chem. class.: Monoclonal antibody, bone resorption

ACTION: Neutralizes activity of receptor activator nuclear factor kappa-B ligand (RANKL) by binding and blocking its interaction with cell-surface receptors; use of a RANKL inhibitor may reduce bone turnover and decrease tumor burden

USES: Prolia: Osteoporosis in postmenopausal women or men at high risk for fractures; increase bone mass in men who are receiving androgen deprivation therapy for prostate cancer and women receiving aromatase inhibitor therapy for breast cancer at high risk for fractures; **Xgeva:** prevention of skeletal-related events in bone metastases from solid tumors

CONTRAINDICATIONS
Hypersensitivity, hypocalcemia, pregnancy
Precautions: Breastfeeding, child/infant/neonate, anemia, coagulopathy, diabetes mellitus, dialysis, eczema, hypoparathyroidism, immunosuppression, latex hypersensitivity, malabsorption syndrome, neoplastic disease, pancreatitis, parathyroid disease, dental/renal/thyroid disease, TB, vitamin D deficiency

DOSAGE AND ROUTES
Osteoporosis in men and postmenopausal osteoporosis (Prolia)
• **Adults:** SUBCUT (Prolia) 60 mg q6mo with 1000 mg of calcium and ≥400 units of vitamin D daily
Hypercalcemia of malignancy that is refractory to bisphosphonate therapy:
• **Adults:** SUBCUT (Xgeva) 120 mg on days 1, 8, and 15, then 120 mg q4wk beginning on day 29
Bone metastases from solid tumors (Xgeva)
• **Adult:** SUBCUT 120 mg q4wk, max 120 mg q4wk
Giant cell tumor (bone) (Xgeva)
• **Adult:** SUBCUT (Xgeva) 120 mg on days 1, 8, and 15, then 120 mg q4wk beginning on day 29
Available forms: Solution for injection 60 mg/mL (Prolia); 120 mg/1.7 mL (Xgeva)
Administer:
SUBCUT route
• Calcium 1000 mg and vitamin D 400 IU should be given daily
• Give acetaminophen prior to and for 72 hr after to decrease pain
• Do not use if particulate matter or discoloration is present; solution is clear

and colorless to slightly yellow with small white/opalescent particles; remove from refrigerator and allow to warm to room temperature (15-30 min)
• **Use of prefilled syringe with needle safety guard:** leave green guard in original position until after use; remove and discard needle cap immediately before injection; give by SUBCUT injection in upper arm/thigh or abdomen; after injection, point needle away from people and slide green guard over needle
• **Use of single-use vials:** use 27-G needle; give in upper arm/thigh or abdomen; do not reinsert needle in vial; discard supplies as appropriate
• Store and use out of direct sunlight/heat; do not freeze; use within 14 days after removal from refrigerator; store unopened containers in refrigerator, those with latex allergy should not touch gray needle cap on Prolia

SIDE EFFECTS
CNS: Headache, vertigo, fatigue, insomnia
CV: Angina, atrial fibrillation
GI: Abdominal pain, constipation, *diarrhea,* flatulence, GERD, *vomiting, nausea,* pancreatitis
GU: Cystitis
HEMA: Anemia
INTEG: Dermatitis, pruritus
META: Hypercholesterolemia, hypocalcemia, hypophosphatemia
MS: Back, bone pain; MS pain, myalgia, osteonecrosis of the jaw
RESP: Cough, *dyspnea*
SYST: Infection, secondary malignancy, anaphylaxis

PHARMACOKINETICS
Half-life 25.4 days, bioavailability 62%, max serum concentration 3-21 days

INTERACTIONS
Increase: infection, possible—immunosuppressives (except cytarabine liposomal), corticosteroids
Drug/Lab Test
Increase: cholesterol

Decrease: calcium, phosphate

NURSING CONSIDERATIONS
Assess:

• **Acute phase reaction:** fever, myalgia, headache, flulike symptoms for 72 hr after injection; usually resolves after 72 hr

• **Blood tests:** serum calcium, creatinine, BUN, magnesium, phosphate; provide adequate calcium, vitamin D, magnesium

• **Hypocalcemia (may be fatal):** paresthesia, twitching, laryngospasm, Chvostek's and Trousseau's signs; preexisting hypocalcemia should be corrected before treatment; patient with vitamin D deficiency may require higher doses of vitamin D

• **Hypercalcemia:** nausea, vomiting, anorexia, weakness, thirst, constipation, dysrhythmias

• **Dental status:** correct dental complications prior to product use; good oral hygiene should be maintained; if dental work is to be performed, antiinfectives should be given to prevent osteonecrosis of the jaw

• **Infection:** do not start treatment in patients with active infections; infections should be resolved first

• **Pregnancy:** identify whether pregnancy is planned or suspected; women who become pregnant should enroll in Amgen's Pregnancy Surveillance Program (800-772-6436); do not use in pregnancy, breastfeeding

Evaluate:

• Therapeutic response: increased/maintained bone density, decreased calcium levels

Teach patient/family:

• To report hypercalcemic relapse: nausea, vomiting, bone pain, thirst

• To notify prescriber immediately if rash, infection, cramps, twitching occur

• To continue with dietary recommendations, including additional Ca 1000 mg/day and vitamin D ≥400 units (Prolia product labeling)

• That product must be continued or fractures may occur

• To use acetaminophen prior to and for 72 hr after injection to lessen bone pain

• About the purpose of this product and its expected results

• To avoid OTC, Rx medications, and herbs and supplements unless approved by prescriber

• To exercise regularly, stop smoking, and avoid alcohol to maintain bone health

• To inform all health care providers of product use; to avoid dental procedures/surgery if possible; to practice good oral hygiene

• That lab tests and follow-up exams will be required

• **Pregnancy/breastfeeding:** not to use during pregnancy and breastfeeding; to notify prescriber if pregnancy is planned, suspected; to use contraception during and for (Xgeva) 5 mo after completion of therapy; that males should use contraception if partner is pregnant

---

deoxycholic acid (Rx)

(dee-ox′-i-koe′-lik as′-id)

Belkyra ✦, Kybella

Func. class.: Cytolytic agent

USES: For improvement in the appearance of moderate to severe convexity or fullness associated with submental fat

CONTRAINDICATIONS
Infection

DOSAGE AND ROUTES

• **Adult:** SUBCUT 0.2 mL per injection site. A single treatment consists of up to a max of 50 injections (10 mL total dose), with each injection spaced 1 cm apart. Up to 6 single treatments may be given at intervals of no less than 1 mo. Injections are made into the subcutaneous fat of the submental region, between the dermis and the platysma

---

Available forms: Injection 10 mg/mL (2-mL single-use vials)

---

desipramine (Rx)

(dess-ip′ra-meen)

Func. class.: Antidepressant, tricyclic
Chem. class.: Dibenzazepine, secondary amine

Do not confuse:
desipramine/disopyramide

ACTION: Blocks reuptake of norepinephrine, serotonin into nerve endings, thereby increasing action of norepinephrine, serotonin in nerve cells

USES: Depression

Unlabeled uses: Anxiety, insomnia, chronic pain conditions

CONTRAINDICATIONS
Hypersensitivity to tricyclics, carBAMazepine, angle-closure glaucoma, acute MI, MAOIs, QT prolongation
Precautions: Pregnancy, breastfeeding, geriatric patients, severe depression, increased intraocular pressure, seizure disorder, CV disease, urinary retention, cardiac dysrhythmias, cardiac conduction disturbances, family history of sudden death, prostatic hypertrophy, thyroid disease

Black Box Warning: Children <18 yr, suicidal patients

DOSAGE AND ROUTES
Depression
• **Adult: PO** 50-75 mg/day in 1-4 divided doses; titrate by 25-50 mg weekly up to 300 mg/day in single or divided doses (inpatient), 200 mg/day (outpatient)
• **Geriatric: PO** 25 mg/day at bedtime, titrate weekly; may increase to 150 mg/day
• **Adolescent: PO** 25-50 mg/day in divided doses; max 150 mg/day
• **Child 6-12 yr: PO** 1-3 mg/kg/day in divided doses; max 5 mg/kg/day
Available forms: Tablets 10, 25, 50, 75, 100, 150 mg

Administer:
• Increased fluids, bulk in diet for constipation, especially in geriatric patients; with food or milk for GI symptoms; crushed if patient is unable to swallow medication whole; without regard for food
• Dosage at bedtime if oversedation occurs during day; may take entire dose at bedtime; geriatric patients may not tolerate once-daily dosing

SIDE EFFECTS
CNS: *Dizziness, drowsiness,* confusion, headache, fatigue, anxiety, tremors, stimulation, weakness, insomnia, nightmares, EPS (geriatric patients), increased psychiatric symptoms, paresthenia, suicidal ideation, impaired memory, seizures, serotonin syndrome
CV: *Orthostatic hypotension,* ECG changes, *tachycardia, hypertension,* palpitations
EENT: *Blurred vision,* tinnitus, mydriasis, ophthalmoplegia
ENDO: SIADH
GI: *Diarrhea, dry mouth,* nausea, vomiting, paralytic ileus, increased appetite, cramps, epigastric distress, jaundice, hepatitis, stomatitis, constipation, weight gain
GU: *Retention,* dereased libido
HEMA: Agranulocytosis, thrombocytopenia, eosinophilia, leukopenia
INTEG: Rash, urticaria, sweating, pruritus, photosensitivity

PHARMACOKINETICS
Well absorbed, widely distributed, protein binding 92%, extensively metabolized in the liver ✇ (CYP2D6) to active metabolite of imipramine; ✇ some patients are poor metabolizers; half-life 15-60 hr

INTERACTIONS
Increase: serotonin syndrome, neuroleptic malignant syndrome—SSRIs, SNRIs, serotonin-receptor agonists, other tricyclic antidepressants
Increase: CNS depression—alcohol, barbiturates, opioids, CNS depressants, skeletal muscle relaxants

---

Increase: desipramine level—cimetidine, dilTIAZem, fluvoxaMINE, FLUoxetine, PARoxetine, sertraline, verapamil

Increase: life-threatening B/P elevations—cloNIDine; do not use concurrently

Increase: hypertension—EPINEPHrine, norepinephrine

Increase: hyperpyrexia, seizures, excitation; do not use within 14 days of MAOIs

Increase: QT interval—tricyclics, SUNItinib, vorinostat, ziprasidone, gatifloxacin, levoFLOXacin, moxifloxacin, sparfloxacin, class IA/III antidysrhythmics, linezolid, methylene blue

Drug/Herb

Increase: serotonin syndrome—St. John's wort, SAM-e, yohimbe; avoid concurrent use

Increase: CNS depression—kava, valerian

Drug/Lab Test

Increase: serum bilirubin, blood glucose, alkaline phosphatase, LFTs

NURSING CONSIDERATIONS
Assess:

• **Pain (unlabeled):** characteristics, including locations, intensity, alleviating factors, prior to and periodically

• **CV:** B/P (lying, standing), pulse; if systolic B/P drops 20 mm Hg, hold product, notify prescriber; take VS, ECG in cardiac patients

• **Hepatic studies:** AST, ALT, bilirubin; thyroid function studies; monitor blood glucose and cholesterol in those who are overweight

• Weight weekly, BMI initially and periodically; appetite may increase with product

• **EPS** primarily in geriatric patients: rigidity, dystonia, akathisia

• **Seizure activity** in those with a history of seizures; may be prior to cardiac events

Black Box Warning: Depression: monitor mental status: mood, sensorium, affect, **suicidal tendencies,** increase in psychiatric symptoms (depression, panic); this product is not indicated for children; monitor mental status baseline and during first few months of treatment, suicidal thoughts/behaviors are more common in children/young adults

• Urinary retention, constipation; constipation most likely in children

• **Withdrawal symptoms:** headache, nausea, vomiting, muscle pain, weakness; not usual unless product discontinued abruptly

• **Beers:** avoid in older adults with delirium or at high risk for delirium; assess for confusion; highly anticholinergic

• **Pregnancy/breastfeeding:** no well-controlled studies, use only if benefit outweighs fetal risk; avoid breastfeeding, excretion is unknown

Evaluate:

• Therapeutic response: decreased depression

Teach patient/family:

• That therapeutic effects may take 2-3 wk

Black Box Warning: That suicidal thoughts/behaviors may occur; to notify prescriber immediately

• To use caution when driving, performing other activities requiring alertness because of drowsiness, dizziness, blurred vision

• To avoid alcohol, other CNS depressants

• Not to discontinue medication abruptly after long-term use because this may cause nausea, headache, malaise

• To wear sunscreen or large hat because photosensitivity occurs

TREATMENT OF OVERDOSE:
ECG monitoring; lavage; administer anticonvulsant

desloratadine (Rx)
(des'lor-at'ah-deen)
Aerius ✦, Aerius Kids ✦, Allergy Control ✦ Clarinex, Clarinex RediTabs
Func. class.: Antihistamine, second generation
Chem. class.: Selective histamine (H$_1$)-receptor antagonist

ACTION: Binds to peripheral histamine receptors, thus providing antihistamine action without sedation

USES: Seasonal/perennial allergic rhinitis, chronic idiopathic urticaria, pruritus

CONTRAINDICATIONS
Hypersensitivity, infants/neonates
Precautions: Pregnancy, breastfeeding, child, asthma, renal/hepatic impairment, phenylketonuria

DOSAGE AND ROUTES
- **Adult and child ≥12 yr: PO** 5 mg/day
- **Child 6-11 yr: PO** 2.5 mg/day
- **Child 2-5 yr: PO** 1.25 mg/day
- **Child 6-11 mo: PO** 1 mg/day (urticaria only)

Hepatic/renal dose
- **Adult: PO** 5 mg every other day

Available forms: Tablets 5 mg; orally disintegrating tablets 2.5, 5 mg (RediTabs); oral solution 0.5 mg/mL
Administer:
- Without regard to meals
- Do not remove RediTabs from blister until ready to use
- RediTabs directly on tongue; may take with or without water
- Use calibrated device for syrup

SIDE EFFECTS
CNS: Sedation (more common with increased doses), headache, psychomotor hyperactivity, seizures, fatigue, dizziness
GI: Hepatitis, nausea, dry mouth
MISC: Flulike symptoms, pharyngitis, myalgias

PHARMACOKINETICS
Onset antihistamine effect 1 hr, peak 1½ hr, elimination half-life 8½-28 hr, metabolized in liver to active metabolites, excreted in urine

INTERACTIONS
Increase: CNS depression (rare)—alcohol, opiates, sedative/hypnotics, H₁ blockers, antipsychotics, tricyclic antidepressants, anxiolytics
Increase: desloratadine—nilotinib, etravirine

NURSING CONSIDERATIONS
Assess:
- **Allergy:** hives, rash, rhinitis; monitor respiratory status; stop product 4 days prior to antigen skin test

- **Pregnancy/breastfeeding:** identify whether pregnancy is planned or suspected; use only if benefits outweigh fetal risk; avoid breastfeeding, excretion unknown
Evaluate:
- Therapeutic response: absence of running or congested nose, other allergy symptoms
Teach patient/family:
- To avoid driving, other hazardous activities if drowsiness occurs; to use caution until product's effects are known
- That product may cause photosensitivity; to use sunscreen or stay out of the sun to prevent burns
- Not to exceed max dose, to take without regard to meals
- To use RediTab by removing from pack and allowing to dissolve on tongue, without regard to water

desmopressin (Rx)
(des-moe-press'in)
DDAVP, Nocdurna ✦, Octostim ✦, Stimate
Func. class.: Pituitary hormone
Chem. class.: Synthetic antidiuretic hormone

ACTION: Promotes reabsorption of water by action on renal tubular epithelium; causes smooth muscle constriction, increase in plasma factor VIII levels, which increases platelet aggregation, thereby resulting in vasopressor effect; similar to vasopressin

USES: Hemophilia A, von Willebrand's disease type 1, nonnephrogenic diabetes insipidus, symptoms of polyuria/polydipsia caused by pituitary dysfunction, nocturnal enuresis, nocturia
Unlabeled uses: Uremic bleeding

CONTRAINDICATIONS
Hypersensitivity, nephrogenic diabetes insipidus, severe renal disease, loop diuretics or systemic/inhaled glucocorticosteroids (nocturia)

Black Box Warning: Hyponatremia

Precautions: Pregnancy, breastfeeding, coronary artery disease, hypertension, cystic fibrosis, thrombus, electrolyte imbalances, male infertility

DOSAGE AND ROUTES

• **PO** is 10-20× greater effect than nasal
• **Child:** Evening dose is 2× higher than daytime to provide sufficient antidiuresis during the night

Primary nocturnal enuresis

• **Adult/child ≥6 yr: PO** 200 mcg at bedtime, max 0.6 mg at bedtime; **INTRANASAL** 0.2 ml at bedtime, half in each nostril

Diabetes insipidus

• **Adult: INTRANASAL** 10-40 mcg in divided doses (1-4 sprays with pump); **PO** Initially 0.05 mg bid, adjust based on diurnal pattern of response; usual range (0.1-1.2 mg)/day in 2-3 divided doses **IV/SUBCUT** 2-4 mcg/day or **SUBCUT** in 2 divided doses
• **Child 3 mo to 12 yr: INTRANASAL** 5-30 mcg/day in divided doses

Hemophilia/von Willebrand's disease

• **Adult/child >3 mo: IV** 0.3 mcg/kg in 0.9% NaCl over 15-30 min; may repeat if needed, max 20 mcg/dose
• **Adult/child >11 mo: NASAL SPRAY** 300 mcg (1 spray in each nostril); give 2 hr prior to surgery

Antihemorrhagic

• **Adult/child >3 mo: IV/SUBCUT** 0.2-0.4 mcg/kg/dose max 20 mcg/dose
• **Adult/child ≥50 kg: INTRANASAL** 1 spray in 1 nostril
• **Adult/child >50 kg: INTRANASAL** 1 spray in each nostril

Nocturia

• **Adult 50-64 yr: INTRANASAL** 1 spray in 1 nostril 30 min before going to bed (not at increased risk for hyponatremia); **women SL** 27.7 mcg 1 hr prior to bedtime with no water; **men** 55.3 mcg 1 hr prior to bedtime with no water

Uremic bleeding (unlabeled)

• **Adult: SUBCUT/IV** 0.3-0.4 mcg/kg as a single injection

Available forms: Injection 4 mcg/mL, tablets 0.1, 0.2 mg; nasal spray pump (DDAVP) 10 mcg/spray (0.1 mg/mL); nasal spray (Stimate) 1.5 mg/mL (150 mcg/dose); tablets (SL) 27.7, 55.3 mcg

Administer:

PO route

• Store at room temperature

SL: Keep under tongue to dissolve; limit fluids at night 1 hr prior to 8 hr after use, avoid caffeine/alcohol before bed

SUBCUT route

• Rotate sites

Nasal route

• DDAVP and Stimate are not interchangeable
• Prime before first dose (press down 4 times), pump stays primed for 1 wk; to reprime, press down 1 time
• **Nocturia:** do not shake bottle, prime by pumping 5 times into the air away from the face; if not used for >3 days, reprime with 2 actuations, have patient blow nose, tilt head back slightly, close nostril, inhale while pumping 1 time, wipe applicator and replace cap

Direct IV route

• Undiluted over 1 min for diabetes insipidus

Intermittent IV INFUSION route

• Diluted single dose/50 mL of 0.9% NaCl **(adult and child >10 kg)**, single dose/10 mL in **child <10 kg**; give as IV infusion over 15-30 min; monitor B/P and pulse during infusion
• Store in refrigerator

SIDE EFFECTS

CNS: Drowsiness, headache, lethargy, flushing, seizures
CV: Increased B/P, palpitations, tachycardia
EENT: Nasal irritation, congestion, rhinitis
GI: Nausea, heartburn, cramps
GU: Vulval pain
META: Hyponatremia, hyponatremia-induced seizures
SYST: Anaphylaxis (IV)

PHARMACOKINETICS

PO: Onset 1 hr, peak 4-7 hr
INTRANASAL: Onset 1 hr; peak 1-4 hr; duration 8-20 hr

IV: Onset 1 min, peak ½ hr, duration >3 hr
Half-life 1.4-3.8 hr (eGFR >50 mL/min/1.73m^2) (PO)

INTERACTIONS

Increase: adverse reactions—carBAMazepine, chlorproPAMIDE, clofibrate, SSRIs, lamotrigine

Black Box Warning: **Increase:** hyponatremia—loop diuretics, inhaled glucocorticosteroids, do not use together in nocturia

Increase: pressor effect—pressor products, monitor
Decrease: antidiuretic action—lithium, alcohol, demeclocycline, heparin, large doses of EPINEPHrine

NURSING CONSIDERATIONS
Assess:
• Pulse, B/P when giving IV or SUBCUT
• Renal studies: BUN/creatinine, serum sodium, urine osmolality, I&O ratio, weight daily; check for edema in extremities; if water retention severe, diuretic may be prescribed
• **Water intoxication:** lethargy, behavioral changes, disorientation, neuromuscular excitability
• **Intranasal use:** nausea, congestion, cramps, headache; usually decreased with decreased dose; for nasal mucosa changes: congestion, edema, discharge, scarring (nasal route)
• For severe allergic reaction, including anaphylaxis (IV route); notify prescriber, discontinue use
• **Nocturnal enuresis:** identify how often enuresis is occurring; avoid use in those prone to water intoxication or sodium depletion

Black Box Warning: **Hyponatremia:** assess for conditions that can cause hyponatremia (fluid/electrolyte imbalances, loop diuretics/inhaled glucocorticosteroids, severe diarrhea, infections); monitor sodium levels baseline, 7 days, 30 days after start of treatment (nocturia)

• **Diabetes insipidus:** urine volume/osmolality and plasma osmolality; monitor for dry skin, poor turgor, thirst (dehydration)
• **Hemophilia/von Willebrand's disease:** factor VIII coagulant activity, bleeding time prior to using for hemostasis; assess for bleeding, frank and occult
• **Pregnancy/breastfeeding:** no well-controlled studies; use only if benefit outweighs fetal risk; use caution in breastfeeding, excretion is unknown
• **Beers:** avoid for treatment of nocturia or nocturnal polyuria; high risk of hyponatremia
Evaluate:
• Therapeutic response: absence of severe thirst, decreased urine output, decreased osmolality
Teach patient/family:
• About the proper technique for nasal instillation: to insert tube into nostril to instill product, clear nasal passage before use
• To avoid OTC products (cough, hay fever) because these preparations may contain EPINEPHrine, decrease product response; not to use with alcohol because adverse reactions may occur
• To wear emergency ID specifying therapy
• That if dose is missed, to take when remembered up to 1 hr prior to next dose; not to double dose; to avoid fluids from 1 hr to up to 8 hr after PO dose
• To report upper respiratory infection, nasal congestion to prescriber
• How to use SUBCUT, rotate sites

---

desonide topical
See Appendix B

---

desoximetasone (Rx)
(dess-ox'ee-met'ah-sone)
Topicort, Topicort Spray
Func. class.: Corticosteroid, topical

ACTION: Crosses cell membrane to attach to receptors to decrease inflammation, itching; inhibits multiple inflammatory cytokines

USES: Inflammation/itching of corticosteroid-responsive dermatoses on the skin; spray—plaque psoriasis

CONTRAINDICATIONS

Hypersensitivity, use of some preparations on face, axilla, groin, intertriginous areas; monotherapy in primary bacterial infection, TB

Precautions: Pregnancy, breastfeeding, children, skin infections, Cushing's syndrome

DOSAGE AND ROUTES

Dermatosis (except spray)
• **Adult/child >10 yr:** Apply to affected areas 2 times/day

Plaque psoriasis (spray)
Adult: Spray, apply to affected areas, rub gently bid for ≤4 wk

Available forms: Cream 0.05%, 0.25%; ointment 0.05%, 0.25%; gel 0.05%; spray 0.25%

Administer:
Topical route
• Do not use with occlusive dressings
• **Cream/ointment/lotion:** apply sparingly in a thin film and rub gently into the cleansed affected area
• **Gel:** apply sparingly in a thin film and rub gently into the cleansed affected area
• **Spray:** discard after 30 days; keep away from heat/flame; store at room temperature

SIDE EFFECTS

INTEG: Burning, folliculitis, pruritus, dermatitis, maceration
MISC: Hyperglycemia, glycosuria, systemic absorption, hypothalamic-pituitary-adrenal (HPA) axis suppression, Cushing's syndrome

NURSING CONSIDERATIONS

Assess:
• Skin reactions: burning, pruritus, folliculitis, dermatitis
• **Systemic absorption:** HPA suppression and possible adrenocortical insufficiency after stopping treatment
• **Pregnancy/breastfeeding:** if pregnancy is planned or suspected; no well-controlled studies; use only if benefit outweighs fetal risk; caution use in breastfeeding; do not apply to breast

Evaluate:
• Decrease in itching, inflammation on the skin

Teach patient/family:
Topical route
• Not to use with occlusive dressings
• **Cream/ointment/lotion:** apply sparingly in a thin film and rub gently into the cleansed affected area
• **Gel:** apply sparingly in a thin film and rub gently into the cleansed affected area
• **Spray:** discard after 30 days; keep away from heat/flame; store at room temperature

---

desvenlafaxine (Rx)

Khedezla, Pristiq
Func. class.: Antidepressant
Chem. class.: Serotonin-receptor norepinephrine reuptake inhibitor (SNRI)

Do not confuse:
Pristiq/Prilosec

ACTION: May work by blocking the central presynaptic reuptake of 5-HT and NE, resulting in an increased sustained level of these neurotransmitters

USES: Major depressive disorder
Unlabeled uses: Vasomotor symptoms (hot flashes) associated with menopause

CONTRAINDICATIONS

Hypersensitivity to this product or venlafaxine, MAOI therapy

Precautions: CNS depression, abrupt discontinuation, hypertension, hepatic/renal disease, hyponatremia, geriatric patients, pregnancy, labor and delivery, breastfeeding, angina, bleeding, cardiac dysrhythmias, MI, stroke, mania, hypovolemia, dehydration, increased intraocular pressure, anticoagulant therapy, bipolar disorder

Black Box Warning: Children, suicidal ideation

DOSAGE AND ROUTES
Major depressive disorder
• **Adult: PO** Initially, 50 mg/day; max 400 mg/day with adjustments as needed
Reduction of hot flash frequency/severity in women with natural or medically induced menopause (unlabeled)
• **Adult: PO** 25-150 mg/day, max 200 mg/day
Renal/hepatic dose
• **Adult: PO** CCr 30-50 mL/min 50 mg daily; CCr <30 mL/min or end-stage renal disease 50 mg every other day; moderate to severe hepatic disease, max 100 mg/day
Available forms: Extended-release tablets 25, 50, 100 mg
Administer:
• Without regard to food; food may minimize GI symptoms
• Extended-release tablet: do not crush, break, or chew
• Store at room temperature

SIDE EFFECTS
CNS: *Dizziness,* drowsiness, *headache,* tremor, paresthesias, asthenia, suicidal thoughts/behaviors, seizures, fatigue, chills, yawning, hot flashes, flushing, *irritability, insomnia, anxiety, abnormal dreams, fatigue*
CV: Palpitations, sinus tachycardia, increased B/P, orthostatic hypotension
EENT: Blurred vision, mydriasis, tinnitus, bruxism
GI: *Nausea,* xerostomia, *diarrhea,* constipation, vomiting, anorexia, weight loss, dysgeusia, hypercholesterolemia, hypertriglyceridemia
GU: Urinary retention/hesitancy, orgasm dysfunction, decreased libido, impotence, proteinuria
HEMA: Impaired platelet aggregation
INTEG: Photosensitivity, hyperhidrosis, diaphoresis, rash
SYST: Serotonin syndrome, neuroleptic malignant syndrome–like symptoms, toxic epidermal necrolysis, Stevens-Johnson syndrome, erythema multiforme, angioedema; neonatal abstinence syndrome (fetal exposure)

PHARMACOKINETICS
Protein binding 30%, elimination half-life 11 hr; elimination half-life is increased (hepatic/renal disease)

INTERACTIONS
Increase: serotonin syndrome, neuroleptic malignant syndrome–like reactions—SSRIs, other SNRIs, serotonin receptor agonists (almotriptan, eletriptan, frovatriptan, naratriptan, rizatriptan, SUMAtriptan, ZOLMitriptan), tricyclics, traZODone, sibutramine, ergots, lithium, nefazodone, meperidine, phentermine, MAOIs, dextromethorphan, linezolid, promethazine, methylphenidate, dexmethylphenidate, mirtazapine, pentazocine, tryptophan, methylene blue IV; do not administer concurrently
Increase: bleeding risk—salicylates, thrombolytics, NSAIDs, platelet inhibitors, anticoagulants
Increase: CNS depression—alcohol, opioids, antihistamines, sedatives/hypnotics
Increase: hallucinations, delusions, disorientation—zolpidem
Drug/Herb
Increase: desvenlafaxine action—kava, valerian
Drug/Lab Test
Increase: cholesterol, triglycerides
False positive: amphetamine, phencyclidine
Decrease: sodium

NURSING CONSIDERATIONS
Assess:

Black Box Warning: Suicidal thoughts/behaviors: mental status and mood; identify suicidal ideation, more frequently during beginning treatment and dosage changes, assess for increasing depression, change in mood, activity, altered sleep habits, impaired focus; risk is increased in children, young adults

• **Serious skin reactions:** assess during and after treatment; discontinue product immediately if rash develops
• **Serotonin syndrome, neuroleptic malignant syndrome–like symptoms:** assess

for nausea/vomiting, sedation, dizziness, diaphoresis (sweating), facial flush, hallucinations, mental status changes, myoclonia, restlessness, shivering, elevated B/P, hyperthermia, muscle rigidity, autonomic instability, mental status changes; if serotonin syndrome occurs, discontinue desvenlafaxine and any other serotonergic agents

• Monitor B/P baseline and periodically during treatment, lipid levels, signs of glaucoma

• Appetite and nutritional intake; weight loss is common, change diet as needed to support weight, weigh weekly

• **Sexual dysfunction:** Monitor sexual dysfunction baseline and throughout treatment, decreased libido and delayed or absent orgasm may occur

• **Bleeding:** Monitor for bruising, bleeding, hematoma, petechiae

• **Angle closure glaucoma:** Monitor IOP in those at risk for glaucoma

• **Labs:** Sodium, lipids baseline and periodically during therapy

• **Pregnancy/breastfeeding:** no well-controlled studies; use only if benefit outweighs fetal risk; discontinue breastfeeding or product, excreted in breast milk, women using antidepressants during pregnancy should register with the national pregnancy registry for antidepressants: 844-405-6185

Evaluate:

• Decreased depression, increased sense of well-being, renewed interest in activities

Teach patient/family:

• To take as directed, not to double or skip doses; if a dose is missed, take as soon as remembered unless close to next dose; do not discontinue abruptly, decrease gradually

Black Box Warning: To report immediately suicidal thoughts/behaviors; have family members look for symptoms of suicidal ideation

• Not to operate machinery or engage in hazardous activities until reaction is known, may cause dizziness, drowsiness

• To avoid all other products unless approved by prescriber

• To report if pregnancy is planned or suspected or if breastfeeding

• **Serious skin reactions:** to report immediately allergic reactions, including rash, hives, difficulty breathing, or swelling of face, lips

• **Serotonin syndrome, neuroleptic malignant syndrome:** to report immediately nausea/vomiting, sedation, dizziness, sweating, facial flush

• That continuing follow-up exams will be needed; that low sodium levels may occur, to watch for headache, confusion, weakness

• Advise patient to discuss with health care provider all Rx, OTC, herbals, supplements taken

• Advise patient to notify health care provider of rashes, itching, trouble breathing

• Discuss with patients possible sexual dysfunction

---

deucravacitinib (Rx)
(doo-krav-a-sih-ti-nib)
Sotyktu
Func. class.: Systemic antipsoriasis agent
Chem. class.: Tyrosine kinase 2 (TYK2) inhibitor

ACTION: Mediates multiple cytokine pathways and also pairs with JAK2 to transmit signals through activation of signal transducers and activators of transcription (STATs). By binding to TYK2, deucravacitinib stabilizes an inhibitory interaction between the regulatory and catalytic domains of the enzyme

USES: Moderate to severe plaque psoriasis

CONTRAINDICATIONS
Hypersensitivity

Precautions: Pregnancy, children, geriatric patients, breastfeeding, cardiac/hepatic/neoplastic disease, HF, hepatitis B carriers, infections, MI, stroke, rhabdomyolysis, thromboembolism, immunosuppression

DOSAGE AND ROUTES
Plaque psoriasis
Adult: PO 6 mg once daily
Available forms: Tablet 6 mg
Administer:
PO route
• Swallow whole; do not cut, break, crush
• Give without regard to food

SIDE EFFECTS
EENT: Sinusitis, rhinitis, stomatitis, oral ulceration
INTEG: *Rash,* angioedema, severe hypersensitivity reactions
MS: Rhabdomyolysis
MISC: Infection, increased cancer risk

PHARMACOKINETICS
Protein binding 90%, terminal half-life 10 hr, peak 2-3 hr, metabolized by CYP1A2, CYP2B6, CYP2D6, CES2, and UGT1A9. The drug is also a substrate for the transporters P-gp, BCRP, and OCT1, an inhibitor of BCRP and OATP1B3

INTERACTIONS
Do not give concurrently with live virus vaccines; immunizations should be brought up to date before treatment
Drug/Lab Test: Increase: ALT, cholesterol, lipids

NURSING CONSIDERATIONS
Assess:
• **Plaque psoriasis:** Improvement in raised, red, inflamed lesions; dry skin with cracking and bleeding; itching, burning, or painful skin; silvery, scaly plaques; pitted nails or separation from the nail bed
• Monitor serum triglycerides
• Infections (fever, flulike symptoms, dyspnea, change in urination, redness/swelling around any wounds), stop treatment if some serious infections occur, may be fatal; patients with active infections should not be started on this product
• May reactivate hepatitis B in chronic carriers, may be fatal; monitor hepatitis B serology, plasma hepatitis C RNA, LFTs; watch for reactivation in these individuals
• Latent TB before therapy; obtain TB test; if positive, treat before starting this product
• Neoplastic disease (lymphomas/leukemia): monitor for primary cancers
• Pregnancy/breastfeeding: identify if pregnancy is planned or suspected, effects in pregnancy or breastfeeding are unknown
Evaluate:
• Therapeutic response: improvement in symptoms of plaque psoriasis
Teach patient/family:
• The reason for the medication and expected result
• Not to take any live virus vaccines during, bring up to date before treatment
• Treatment and to read the "medication guide"
• To report signs of infection, allergic reaction, TB, immediately
• To advise all health care professionals of Rx, OTC, herbals, supplements taken
• To do regular skin assessments and report changes to provider
• That rhabdomyolysis may occur, to report muscle pain, weakness, especially with fever
• That continuing laboratory exams will be needed
• Pregnancy/breastfeeding: to advise health care professional if pregnancy is planned or suspected or if breastfeeding

---

deutetrabenazine (Rx)
(du-tet-ra-BEN-a-zeen)
Austedo
Func. class.: Central monoamine-depleting agent

USES: For the treatment of chorea associated with Huntington's disease and tardive dyskinesia

CONTRAINDICATIONS
Hypersensitivity, hepatic disease, MAOIs

Black Box Warning: Suicidal ideation

DOSAGE AND ROUTES
• **Adult (treatment naïve; not switching from tetrabenazine): PO** Initially, 6 mg/bid; increase at weekly intervals by increments of 6 mg/day to a max of 48 mg/day; doses >12 mg should be divided throughout the day
• **Adult (switching from tetrabenazine): PO** Discontinue tetrabenazine and start deutetrabenazine the next day. Use 6 mg/day for patients taking tetrabenazine 12.5 mg/day
Available forms: Tablets 6, 9, 12 mg

---

dexamethasone (Rx)
(dex-ah-meth'a-sone)
Decadron, Hemady
dexamethasone sodium phosphate (Rx)
Func. class.: Corticosteroid, synthetic
Chem. class.: Glucocorticoid, long acting

ACTION: Decreases inflammation by suppression of migration of polymorphonuclear leukocytes, fibroblasts, reversal of increased capillary permeability and lysosomal stabilization, suppresses normal immune response, no mineralocorticoid effects

USES: Inflammation, allergies, neoplasms, cerebral edema, septic shock, collagen disorders, dexamethasone suppression test for Cushing syndrome, adrenocortical insufficiency, TB, meningitis, acute exacerbations of MS

CONTRAINDICATIONS
Hypersensitivity to corticosteroids, sulfites, or benzyl alcohol; fungal infections, abrupt discontinuation, coagulopathy, ulcerative colitis, seizure disorders

Precautions: Pregnancy, breastfeeding, diabetes mellitus, osteoporosis, seizure disorders, ulcerative colitis, HF, myasthenia gravis, renal disease, peptic ulcer, esophagitis, recent MI, hypertension, TB, active hepatitis, psychosis, sulfite hypersensitivity, thromboembolic disorders

DOSAGE AND ROUTES
Inflammatory condition/neoplasias
• **Adult: PO** 0.75-9 mg/day in divided doses q6-12hr or phosphate **IM** 0.5-9 mg/day divided q6-12hr
• **Child: PO** 0.024-0.34 mg/kg/day in divided doses q6-12hr
Anaphylactic shock
• **Adult: IV** (phosphate) single dose 1-6 mg/kg or **IV** 40 mg q2-6hr as needed up to 72 hr
Airway edema/extubation
• **Adult: PO/IM/IV** 0.5-2 mg/kg/day divided q6hr; use 24 hr before extubation and use for 24 hr after extubation
Chemotherapy-induced vomiting
• **Adult: PO/IV** 10-20 mg 15-30 min prior to chemotherapy or 10 mg q12hr on each treatment day
• **Child: IV** 5-20 mg 15-30 min prior to chemotherapy
Cerebral edema
• **Adult: IV** (phosphate) 10 mg, then 4-6 mg **IM** q6hr × 2-4 days, then taper over 1 wk
• **Child:** loading dose 1-2 mg/kg **(PO/IM/IV)**, then 1-1.5 mg/kg/day, max 16 mg/day divided q4-6hr for 2-4 days, then taper down weekly
Cushing syndrome (suppression test)
Adult: PO 0.5 mg q6hr × 48 hr (after determining 24-hr 17 hydroxycorticosteroids urine level); repeat urine collection to determine levels during 24 hr or 1 mg at 11 PM and draw plasma cortisol at 8 AM next morning
Palliative management of recurrent or inoperable brain tumors
• **Adult: IM/IV** 2 mg bid-tid (maintenance)
Adrenocortical insufficiency
• **Adult: PO** 0.75-9 mg/day in divided doses

- **Child: PO** 0.03-0.3 mg/kg/day in 2-4 divided doses

Intraarticular/intralesional

Adult: PO 0.2-6 mg daily to q3days, depends on condition

Available forms: Tablets 0.5, 0.75, 1, 1.5, 2, 4, 6 mg; oral solution 0.5 mg/5 mL; elixir 0.5 mg/5 mL, oral concentrate 1 mg/mL; injection 4 mg/mL, 10 mg/mL

Administer:

PO route

- Titrated dose; use lowest effective dose
- With food or milk to decrease GI symptoms, give once daily in AM for less toxicity, fewer adverse reactions
- Use concentrated PO solution using calibrated dropper supplied, discard after 90 days
- Use concentrated PO solution mixed in liquid or soft food like applesauce, use immediately

IM route

- IM injection deeply in large muscle mass; rotate sites; avoid deltoid; use 21-G needle
- In 1 dose in AM to prevent adrenal suppression; avoid SUBCUT administration, may damage tissue

Intra-articular/intralesional route

- Use rarely, as injections may damage joints

Direct IV route (sodium phosphate)

- Undiluted direct over ≥1 min

Intermittent IV INFUSION route

- Diluted with 0.9% NaCl or D₅W, give as IV infusion at prescribed rate

Continuous IV infusion

- Change IV solution q24hr

Y-site compatibilities: Acetaminophen, acyclovir, alfentanil, allopurinol, amifostine, amikacin, aminocaproic acid, aminophylline, amphotericin B cholesteryl, amphotericin B lipid complex, amphotericin B liposome, amsacrine, anidulafungin, argatroban, ascorbic acid injection, atenolol, atracurium, atropine, aztreonam, benztropine, bivalirudin, bleomycin, bumetanide, buprenorphine, butorphanol, caffeine, CARBOplatin, carmustine, ceFAZolin, cefepime, cefmetazole, cefonicid, cefotaxime, cefoTEtan, cefOXitin, cefpirome, ceftaroline, cefTAZidime, ceftizoxime, cefTRIAXone, chloramphenicol, cimetidine, cisatracurium, CISplatin, cladribine, clindamycin, codeine, cyanocobalamin, cyclophosphamide, cycloSPORINE, cytarabine, DACTINomycin, DAPTOmycin, DAUNORubicin, dexmedetomidine, digoxin, diltiazem, DOCEtaxel, DOPamine, doripenem, doxacurium, DOXOrubicin, DOXOrubicin liposomal, enalaprilat, ePHEDrine, EPINEPHrine, epoetin alfa, eptifibatide, ertapenem, etoposide, etoposide phosphate, famotidine, fentaNYL, filgrastim, fluconazole, fludarabine, fluorouracil, folic acid, fosaprepitant, foscarnet, furosemide, ganciclovir, gatifloxacin, gemcitabine, glycopyrrolate, granisetron, heparin, hydrocortisone, HYDROmorphone, ifosfamide, imipenem-cilastatin, indomethacin, insulin (regular), irinotecan, isoproterenol, ketorolac, lansoprazole, leucovorin, levofloxacin, lidocaine, linezolid, liposome, LORazepam, LR, mannitol, mechlorethamine, melphalan, meropenem, metaraminol, methadone, methicillin, methoxamine, methyldopate, methylPREDNISolone, metoclopramide, metoprolol, metroNIDAZOLE, mezlocillin, miconazole, milrinone, morphine, multiple vitamins injection, nafcillin, nalbuphine, naloxone, nitroglycerin, nitroprusside, norepinephrine, octreotide, ondansetron, oxacillin, oxaliplatin, oxyCODONE, oxytocin, PACLitaxel, palonosetron, pamidronate, pancuronium, PEMEtrexed, penicillin G potassium/sodium, PENTobarbital, PHENobarbital, phenylephrine, phytonadione, piperacillin, piperacillin-tazobactam, potassium chloride, procainamide, propofol, propranolol, pyridoxine, ranitidine, remifentanil, Ringer's, ritodrine, riTUXimab, sargramostim, sodium acetate/bicarbonate, succinylcholine, SUFentanil, tacrolimus, telavancin, teniposide, theophylline, thiamine, thiotepa, ticarcillin, ticarcillin-clavulanate, tigecycline, tirofiban, TNA, tolazoline, topotecan, trastuzumab, urokinase, vancomycin, vasopressin, vecuronium, verapamil, vinCRIStine, vinorelbine, vitamin B complex/C, voriconazole, zidovudine, zoledronic acid

SIDE EFFECTS
CNS: *Depression,* headache, mood changes, euphoria, pseudotumor cerebi, seizures
CV: *Hypertension*
EENT: Increased intraocular pressure, cataracts
ENDO: HPA suppression, hyperglycemia, sodium, fluid retention, pheochromocytoma
GI: *Nausea,* peptic ulceration, vomiting, weight gain
INTEG: Acne, poor wound healing, ecchymosis, petechiae, hirsutism
META: Hypokalemia, fluid retention, hypokalemic alkalosis
MS: Fractures, osteoporosis, weakness, arthralgia, myopathy

PHARMACOKINETICS
Half-life 1-2 days
PO: Onset 1 hr, peak 1-2 hr, duration 2½ days
IM: Onset 1 hr, peak 1 hr, duration 2 days-3 wk
IV: Onset 1 hr, peak 1 hr, duration varies

INTERACTIONS
Increase: toxicity—cycloSPORINE, monitor closely
Increase: side effects—alcohol, salicylates, amphotericin B, digoxin, cycloSPORINE, diuretics, NSAIDs, monitor closely
Increase: dexamethasone action—salicylates, estrogens, hormonal contraceptives, ketoconazole, macrolide antiinfectives, NSAIDs
Increase: tendinitis, tendon rupture risk—quinolones
Decrease: effect of—antidiabetics, insulin dose may need to be increased
Decrease: dexamethasone action—cholestyramine, colestipol, barbiturates, rifAMPin, phenytoin, theophylline, antacids, bosentan, carBAMazepine
Decrease: anticoagulant effect—anticonvulsants, antidiabetics, isoniazid, toxoids, anticholinesterases, salicylates
Decrease: potassium levels—thiazide/loop diuretics, amphotericin B
Decrease: antibody response—vaccines, avoid using concurrently
Drug/Herb
Decrease: dexamethasone action—echinacea, avoid using together

Drug/Lab Test
Increase: cholesterol, sodium, blood glucose
Decrease: calcium, potassium, T_4, T_3, thyroid ^{131}I uptake test
False negative: skin allergy tests

NURSING CONSIDERATIONS
Assess:
• **Labs:** Obtain pregnancy test before use with Hemady, confirm negative, potassium, blood, urine glucose while receiving long-term therapy; hypo/hyperglycemia, weight daily; notify prescriber of weekly gain >5 lb, B/P, pulse; notify prescriber of chest pain
• I&O ratio; be alert for decreasing urinary output, increasing edema
• **Cerebral edema:** LOC and headache, baseline and periodically
• **Adrenal insufficiency:** weight loss, nausea, vomiting, anorexia, confusion, decreased B/P, baseline and periodically
• **Epidural injections (unlabeled):** may cause rare events (vision loss, paralysis, stroke, death)
• **Cushingoid symptoms:** assess for buffalo hump, moon face, increased B/P; monitor plasma cortisol levels during long-term therapy (normal: 138-635 nmol/L SI units when drawn at 8 AM); prolonged use can cause cushingoid symptoms
• **Infection:** fever, WBC even after withdrawal of medication; product masks infection
• **Potassium depletion:** paresthesias, fatigue, nausea, vomiting, depression, polyuria, dysrhythmias, weakness
• Edema, hypertension, cardiac symptoms
• **Mental status:** affect, mood, behavioral changes, aggression
• **Abrupt withdrawal:** acute adrenal insufficiency and death may occur following abrupt discontinuation of systemic therapy; withdraw gradually
• **Child:** Monitor growth during treatment, growth may be slowed
• **Pregnancy/breastfeeding:** no well-controlled studies; use only if benefit outweighs fetal risk; discontinue breastfeeding or product

Evaluate:
• Therapeutic response: decreased inflammation

Teach patient/family:
• To carry medical alert ID as corticosteroid user at all times
• To contact prescriber if surgery, trauma, stress occurs because dose may need to be adjusted
• To notify prescriber if therapeutic response decreases because dosage adjustment may be needed
• To take with food or milk
• That bruising may occur easily
• That if on long-term therapy, a high-protein diet may be needed
• Not to discontinue abruptly because **adrenal crisis** can result
• **About symptoms of adrenal insufficiency:** nausea, anorexia, fatigue, dizziness, dyspnea, weakness, joint pain, hypertension
• To avoid OTC products: salicylates, alcohol in cough products, cold preparations unless directed by prescriber
• About all aspects of product usage, including cushingoid symptoms; to notify health care provider of infection
• To avoid exposure to chickenpox or measles, persons with infection
• **Body image:** Explore ways of coping with body changes
• Advise patient to inform health care provider if pregnancy is suspected or if breastfeeding; if using Hemady to use contraception during and for 1 mo after last dose, not to breastfeed during or for 2 wk after last dose

---

dexamethasone (ophthalmic) (Rx)

(dex-a-meth′a-sone)

Dextenza, Dexycu, Maxidex, Ozurdex

Func. class.: Ophthalmic antiinflammatory

Chem. class.: Corticosteroid

Do not confuse:
dexamethasone/desoximetasone

ACTION: Exact mechanism of antiinflammatory action unknown; inhibits multiple inflammatory cytokines; decreases inflammation, collagen deposits, capillary dilation, edema

USES: Treatment of corticosteroid-responsive ophthalmic disorders

CONTRAINDICATIONS

Hypersensitivity to this product or sulfites, ocular TB, acute herpes simplex (superficial), fungal/viral infections of the eye, posterior lens capsule rupture

Precautions: Corneal infected abrasions, glaucoma, pregnancy, breastfeeding, migration of intravitreal implant risk, children

DOSAGE AND ROUTES

Corticosteroid-responsive ophthalmic disorders
• **Adult:** Instill 1 or 2 drops of 0.1% ophthalmic solution or suspension every hour during the day and every 2 hr at night; reduce application to every 4 hr after response occurs

Available forms: Ophthalmic solution, suspension 0.1%; implant, intravitreal (0.7 mg); insert, opthalmic 0.4 mg; intraocular suspension 9%

Administer:
• For ophthalmic use only
• Instruct patient on proper instillation of eye ointment or solution; do not touch the tip of the dropper to the eye, fingertips, or other surface; wait ≥15 min before inserting soft contact lens

SIDE EFFECTS

EENT: Burning, stinging, poor vision, corneal ulcerations, increased IOP, optic nerve damage

NURSING CONSIDERATIONS

Assess:
• **Corneal effects:** ulcerations, infections can worsen with this product

Evaluate:
• Decreased corneal inflammation

Side effects: *italics* = common; red = life-threatening

Teach patient/family:
- How to use products
- Not to share with others or use for other conditions
- To notify prescriber immediately if vision changes or if condition worsens
- To take as prescribed

---

dexlansoprazole (Rx)

(dex-lan-so-prey′zole)

Dexilant

Func. class.: Antiulcer, proton pump inhibitor

Chem. class.: Benzimidazole

ACTION: Suppresses gastric secretion by inhibiting hydrogen/potassium ATPase enzyme system in gastric parietal cell; characterized as gastric acid pump inhibitor because it blocks final step of acid production

USES: Gastroesophageal reflux disease (GERD), severe erosive esophagitis, heartburn

CONTRAINDICATIONS

Hyper-sensitivity

Precautions: Pregnancy, breastfeeding, children, proton-pump hypersensitivity, gastric cancer, hepatic disease, vitamin B_{12} deficiency, colitis

DOSAGE AND ROUTES
Erosive esophagitis
- **Adult: PO** 60 mg daily for up to 8 wk; maintenance: **PO** 30 mg daily for up to 6 mo
GERD
- **Adult: PO** 30 mg daily × 4 wk
Hepatic disease
- **Adult: PO** (Child-Pugh B): max 30 mg/day; Child-Pugh C
Available forms: Delayed-release capsules 30, 60 mg
Administer:
- Swallow capsules whole; do not crush, chew capsules; capsules may be opened, contents sprinkled on food, use immediately; do not chew contents of capsule; give without regard to food

SIDE EFFECTS
CNS: Headache, dizziness, confusion, agitation, amnesia, depression, anxiety, seizures, insomnia, migraine
CV: Chest pain, angina, bradycardia, palpitations, CVA, hypertension, MI
EENT: Tinnitus
GI: Diarrhea, abdominal pain, vomiting, nausea, constipation, flatulence, colitis, dysgeusia, CDAD
HEMA: Anemia, neutropenia, thrombocytopenia, pernicious anemia, thrombosis
INTEG: Rash, urticaria, pruritus
META: Gout
MS: Arthralgia, mylagia
RESP: Upper respiratory infections, cough, epistaxis, dyspnea, pneumonia
SYST: Anaphylaxis, Stevens-Johnson syndrome, toxic epidermal necrolysis, exfoliative dermatitis

PHARMACOKINETICS
Absorption 57%-64%; half-life 1-2 hr; protein binding 96.1%-98.8%; extensively metabolized in liver ✨ by CYP2C19/CYP3A4; excreted in urine, feces; clearance decreased in geriatric patients, renal/hepatic impairment; peak 4 hr

INTERACTIONS
Increase: dexlansoprazole effect—CYP2C19, 3A4 inhibitors (fluvoxaMINE, voriconazole)
Decrease: dexlansoprazole absorption—sucralfate
Decrease: absorption of ketoconazole, itraconazole, iron, delavirdine, ampicillin, calcium carbonate
Drug/Herb
Decrease: dexlansoprazole effect—St. John's wort
Drug/Lab Test
Increase: LFTs, bilirubin, creatinine, glucose, lipids
Decrease: platelets, magnesium

NURSING CONSIDERATIONS
Assess:
- **CDAD (rare):** diarrhea, abdominal cramps, fever; report to prescriber promptly
- **Hepatotoxicity (rare):** hepatitis, jaundice; monitor hepatic studies (AST,

ALT, alkaline phosphatate) if hepatic adverse reactions occur

• **Hypomagnesemia:** usually 3 mo to 1 yr after beginning therapy; monitor magnesium level, assess for irregular heartbeats, muscle spasms; in children, fatigue, upset stomach, dizziness; magnesium supplement may be used

• **Anaphylaxis (rare), serious skin disorders:** require emergency intervention

• **Beers:** avoid scheduled use >8 wk in older adults who are at high risk for erosive esophagitis, pathologic hypersecretory conditions

• **Pregnancy/breastfeeding:** no well-controlled studies; use only if benefit outweighs fetal risk; avoid breastfeeding, excretion is unknown

Evaluate:

• Therapeutic response: absence of epigastric pain, swelling, fullness; healing of erosive esophagitis

Teach patient/family:

• **CDAD:** to report to prescriber at once abdominal cramps, bloody diarrhea, fever

• That diabetic patient should know that hypoglycemia may occur

• To avoid hazardous activities; dizziness may occur

• To avoid alcohol, salicylates, ibuprofen; may cause GI irritation

• To report allergic reactions, symptoms of low magnesium levels

• To notify prescriber if pregnancy is planned or suspected; not to breastfeed

• To swallow capsule whole, not to chew, crush; to report all products being used to prescriber

---

dexmethylphenidate (Rx)

(dex′meth-ul-fen′ih-dayt)

Focalin, Focalin XR

Func. class.: Central nervous system (CNS) stimulant, psychostimulant

Controlled Substance Schedule II

Do not confuse:
dexmethylphenidate/methylphenidate

ACTION: Increases release of norepinephrine and DOPamine into the extraneuronal space; also blocks the reuptake of norepinephrine and DOPamine into the presynaptic neuron; mode of action for treating attention-deficit/hyperactivity disorder (ADHD) is unknown

USES: ADHD

CONTRAINDICATIONS

Hypersensitivity to methylphenidate, anxiety, history of Gilles de la Tourette's syndrome, tics, glaucoma, concurrent treatment with MAOIs or within 14 days of discontinuing treatment with MAOIs

Precautions: Pregnancy, hypertension, depression, seizures, CV disorders, breastfeeding, child <6 yr, geriatric patients, psychosis, thyrotoxicosis

Black Box Warning: Substance abuse, alcoholism

DOSAGE AND ROUTES

• **Adult/adolescent/child ≥6 yr: (immediate release)** PO 2.5 mg bid with doses at least 4 hr apart, gradually increase to a maximum of 20 mg/day (10 mg bid); for those taking methylphenidate, use ½ of methylphenidate dose initially, then increase as needed to a max of 20 mg/day

• **Adolescent/child ≥6 yr: EXTENDED RELEASE** 5 mg/day, (not taking methylphenidate/dexmethylphenidate) may adjust to 20 mg/day in 5-mg increments, max 30 mg/day

• **Adult: PO EXTENDED RELEASE** 10 mg/day, may adjust to 20 mg/day in 10-mg increments, max 40 mg/day

Available forms: Tablets 2.5, 5, 10 mg; extended-release capsules 5, 10, 15, 20, 25, 30, 35, 40 mg

Administer:

• Twice daily at least 4 hr apart; extended release once a day; in the morning, extended-release capsule may be opened and contents sprinkled onto applesauce and consumed without chewing

• Without regard to meals

• Do not break, crush, or chew extended-release product

• Med guide should be provided by dispenser

SIDE EFFECTS

CNS: Dizziness, headache, drowsiness, nervousness, insomnia, toxic psychosis, neuroleptic malignant syndrome (rare), Tourette's syndrome

CV: Palpitations, B/P changes, angina, dysrhythmias, tachycardia, MI, stroke

GI: *Nausea, anorexia,* abnormal hepatic function, hepatic coma, *abdominal pain*

HEMA: Leukopenia, anemia, thrombocytopenic purpura

INTEG: Exfoliative dermatitis, urticaria, rash, erythema multiforme

MISC: *Fever,* arthralgia, scalp hair loss, rhabdomyolysis

PHARMACOKINETICS

Readily absorbed, elimination half-life 2.2 hr, metabolized by liver, excreted by kidneys

PO: Peak 1½ hr, onset ½-1 hr

PO-ER: Onset unknown, peak 4 hr

INTERACTIONS

Increase: hypertensive crisis—MAOIs or within 14 days of MAOIs, vasopressors

Increase: sympathomimetic effect—decongestants, vasoconstrictors

Increase: effects of anticonvulsants, tricyclics, SSRIs, coumarin

Increase: serious adverse reactions with clonidine, other centrally acting alpha-2 agonists, avoid concurrent use

Decrease: effects of antihypertensives, monitor B/P

Decrease: metabolism of anticoagulants, phenytoins, barbiturates, TCAs, dose adjustment may be needed

Drug/Herb

Synergistic effect—melatonin

NURSING CONSIDERATIONS

Assess:

Black Box Warning: Assess for substance abuse, past or current; psychotic episodes may occur, especially with parenteral abuse; avoid use in a history of substance abuse or alcoholism, as dependence may occur

• **Toxicity:** rhabdomyolysis, headache, flushing, vomiting, agitation, tachycardia, tremor, euphoria, hallucinations, hyperreflexia

• VS, B/P; may reverse antihypertensives; check patients with cardiac disease more often for increased B/P

• CBC, differential platelet counts during long-term therapy, urinalysis; with diabetes: blood glucose, urine glucose; insulin changes may have to be made because eating will decrease

• Height, growth rate q3mo in children; growth rate may be decreased; weight loss, anorexia may occur

• Mental status: mood, sensorium, affect, stimulation, insomnia, aggressiveness, hostility

• **Withdrawal symptoms:** headache, nausea, vomiting, muscle pain, weakness

• Appetite, sleep, speech patterns

• For attention span, decreased hyperactivity in persons with ADHD

• **Pregnancy/breastfeeding:** no well-controlled studies; use only if benefit outweighs fetal risk; avoid breastfeeding, excretion is unknown

Evaluate:

• Therapeutic response: decreased hyperactivity or ability to stay awake

Teach patient/family:

• To decrease caffeine consumption (coffee, tea, cola, chocolate); may increase irritability, stimulation

• To take early in day to prevent insomnia; not to take more than prescribed, dependence may occur

• To avoid OTC preparations unless approved by prescriber; to avoid alcohol ingestion

• To taper off product over several weeks to avoid depression, increased sleeping, lethargy

• To report weight loss; anorexia may occur

• To avoid hazardous activities until stabilized on medication

• To get needed rest; patients will feel more tired at end of day

• To notify all health care workers, including school nurse, of medication and schedule

• About information, instructions provided in patient information section

• To notify prescriber if pregnancy is planned or suspected; to avoid breastfeeding
• **To report toxicity immediately:** vomiting, agitation, tremor, hyperreflexia, euphoria, confusion, hallucinations, flushing, headache, tachycardia, rhabdomyolysis

TREATMENT OF OVERDOSE:
Administer fluids; hemodialysis: or peritoneal dialysis; antihypertensive for increased B/P; administer short-acting barbiturate prior to lavage

dextroamphetamine (Rx)
(dex-troe-am-fet′a-meen)
Dexedrine, ProCentra, Zenzedi
Func. class.: Cerebral stimulant
Chem. class.: Amphetamine

Controlled Substance Schedule II

ACTION: Increases release of norepinephrine, DOPamine in cerebral cortex to reticular activating system

USES: Narcolepsy, attention-deficit/hyperactivity disorder (ADHD)

CONTRAINDICATIONS
Hypersensitivity to sympathomimetic amines, hyperthyroidism, glaucoma, severe arteriosclerosis

Black Box Warning: Substance abuse

Precautions: Pregnancy, breastfeeding, children <3 yr, depression, Gilles de la Tourette's disorder, cardiomyopathy, bipolar disorder, abrupt discontinuation, acute MI; benzyl alcohol, salicylate hypersensitivity; hypercortisolism, obesity, psychosis, seizure disorder, hypertension, anxiety, anorexia nervosa, tartrazine dye hypersensitivity

Black Box Warning: Symptomatic cardiac disease

DOSAGE AND ROUTES
Narcolepsy
• **Adult: PO** 5 mg bid, titrate daily dose by no more than 10 mg/wk, max 60 mg/day

• **Child 6-12 yr: PO** 5 mg/day, titrate daily dose by no more than 5 mg/day at weekly intervals, max 40 mg/day
ADHD
• **Adult: PO** 5-60 mg/day daily or divided bid, max 40 mg/day
• **Child 3-5 yr: PO** 2.5 mg/day increasing by 2.5 mg/day at weekly intervals, max 40 mg/day
• **Child >6-12 yr: PO** 5 mg daily-bid increasing by 5 mg/day at weekly intervals, max 40 mg/day

Available forms: Tablets 2.5, 5, 7.5, 10, 15, 20, 30 mg; oral solution 5 mg/5 mL; extended-release capsules 5, 10, 15 mg
Administer:
• At least 6 hr prior to bedtime to avoid sleeplessness
• Use calibrated measuring device for oral solution
• Store all forms at room temperature

SIDE EFFECTS
CNS: *Hyperactivity, insomnia, restlessness, talkativeness,* dizziness, headache, chills, stimulation, dysphoria, irritability, aggressiveness, tremor, dependence, addiction
CV: *Palpitations, tachycardia,* hypertension, decrease in heart rate, dysrhythmias
GI: *Anorexia,* dry mouth, diarrhea, constipation, weight loss, metallic taste
GU: Impotence, change in libido
INTEG: Urticaria
MISC: Rhabdomyolysis

PHARMACOKINETICS
Onset 30-60 min, peak 2 hr, duration 4 hr; extended release onset 1 hr, peak 2 hr, duration 8 hr; metabolized by liver; urine excretion pH dependent; crosses placenta, breast milk; half-life 6-8 hr (child), 10-12 hr (adult)

INTERACTIONS
Increase: hypertensive crisis: MAOIs or within 14 days of MAOIs
Increase: serotonin syndrome, neuroleptic malignant syndrome: SSRIs, SNRIs, serotonin-receptor agonists; do not use concurrently
Increase: dextroamphetamine effect—acetaZOLAMIDE

Side effects: *italics* = common; red = life-threatening

Increase: CNS effect—haloperidol, tricyclics, phenothiazines

Decrease: absorption of barbiturates, phenytoin

Decrease: dextroamphetamine effect—ascorbic acid, ammonium chloride

Decrease: effect of adrenergic blockers, antidiabetics, antihypertensives, antihistamines

Drug/Herb

Serotonin syndrome—St. John's wort

Decrease: stimulant effect—eucalyptus

Drug/Food

Increase: amine effect—caffeine (cola, coffee, tea [green/black])

Decrease: effect—fruit juice (oral solution)

Drug/Lab Test

Increase: plasma corticosteroids, urinary steroids

NURSING CONSIDERATIONS
Assess:

Black Box Warning: Cardiac disease: VS, B/P; product may reverse antihypertensives; check patients with cardiac disease often

Black Box Warning: Substance abuse: use for prolonged periods may lead to dependence; sudden death or serious CV events can occur from misuse; chronic intoxication (insomnia, irritability, personality changes)

• CBC, urinalysis; with diabetes: blood glucose, urine glucose; insulin changes may be required because eating will decrease

• Height, growth rate in children (growth rate may be decreased), weight

• **Toxicity:** symptoms may vary in children; anxiety, headache, flushing, vomiting, rhabdomyolysis, tremor, hyperreflexia, confusion, euphoria, tachycardia

• **ADHD:** change in behavior, growth retardation in children

• Mental status: mood, sensorium, affect, stimulation, insomnia, irritability

• Tolerance or dependency: increased amount may be used to get same effect; will develop after long-term use

• **Pregnancy/breastfeeding:** no well-controlled studies; use only if benefit outweighs fetal risk; infants may show withdrawal and low birth weight, avoid breastfeeding, excreted in breast milk

Evaluate:

• Therapeutic response: increased CNS stimulation, except in ADHD, decreased drowsiness

Teach patient/family:

• To take before meals (obesity)

• To decrease caffeine consumption (coffee, tea, cola, chocolate); may increase irritability, stimulation

• To avoid OTC preparations unless approved by prescriber; to avoid alcohol ingestion; to avoid fruit juice at same time as solution, effect is decreased

• To tell parents that change in behavior may occur in beginning treatment, irritability, hostility

• **Seizures:** that those with a seizure disorder may have decreased seizure threshold

• To taper product over several weeks; depression, increased sleeping, lethargy may occur

• To avoid hazardous activities until stabilized on medication

• To get needed rest; patient will feel more tired at end of day

TREATMENT OF OVERDOSE:
Administer fluids, hemodialysis; antihypertensive for increased B/P, ammonium chloride for increased excretion

dextroamphetamine sulfate/dextroamphetamine saccharate/ amphetamine aspartate/amphetamine sulfate (Rx)

Adderall XR, Mydayis

Func. class.: CNS stimulant

Chem. class.: Amphetamine

Controlled Substance Schedule II

ACTION: Causes the release of DOPamine and norepinephrine in the brain

USES: Narcolepsy, ADHD

CONTRAINDICATIONS

Hypersensitivity to sympathomimetic amines, hyperthyroidism, glaucoma, severe arteriosclerosis

Black Box Warning: Substance abuse

Precautions: Pregnancy, breastfeeding, children <3 yr, depression, Tourette's syndrome, cardiomyopathy, bipolar disorder, abrupt discontinuation, acute MI, benzyl alcohol, salicylate hypersensitivity, hypercortisolism, obesity, psychosis, seizure disorder, hypertension, anxiety, anorexia nervosa

DOSAGE AND ROUTES
ADHD

Adults: PO (immediate-release Adderall) Initially, 5 mg daily or bid. If divided doses are required, give first dose upon awakening and the subsequent doses (1 or 2) at 4- to 6-hr intervals. Titrate by no more than 5 mg/day at weekly intervals to the minimum effective dose; doses greater than 60 mg/day are not usually needed

Child/adolescent ≥6 yr: PO (immediate-release Adderall): 5 mg daily or bid. May titrate daily dose in 5-mg increments at weekly intervals to minimum effective dose. Daily dose may be given in 1 to 3 divided doses at 4- to 6-hr intervals, 40 mg daily

Child 3-5 yr: (immediate-release Adderall) PO: 2.5 mg daily in the morning. May titrate daily dose in 2.5-mg increments at weekly intervals to minimum effective dose. Daily dose may be given in 1 to 3 divided doses at 4- to 6-hr intervals

Adults: PO (extended-release capsules – Adderall XR) When initiating treatment for the first time or switching from another ADHD medication, the recommended dose is 20 mg daily upon awakening

Adolescents: PO (extended-release capsules – Adderall XR) 10 mg daily in the morning for both initial therapy and when converting to extended-release amphetamine, dextroamphetamine from another stimulant medication. May titrate to 20 mg daily after 1 wk if ADHD symptoms are not adequately controlled

Child 6-12 yr: PO (extended-release capsules – Adderall XR) 5 to 10 mg daily in the morning for initial treatment. If converting to extended-release (ER) amphetamine, dextroamphetamine from a different stimulant medication, begin with 10 mg daily. May titrate daily dose in 5- to 10-mg increments at weekly intervals to the minimum effective dose. Max: 40 mg/day PO ER capsules

Adults: PO (extended-release capsules – Mydayis) Initially, 12.5 mg daily in the morning upon awakening; take consistently with or without food. Initial doses of 25 mg daily may be considered for some patients. Dose may be increased by 12.5-mg increments no sooner than weekly. Max: 50 mg/day

Adolescent ≥13 yr: PO Initially, 12.5 mg daily in the morning upon awakening; take consistently with or without food. Dose may be increased by 12.5-mg increments no sooner than weekly. Max: 25 mg/day

Narcolepsy

Adult/adolescent/child ≥12 yr: PO (immediate-release tablets – Adderall): 10 mg daily in the morning. If divided doses are required, give first dose upon awakening and the subsequent doses (1 or 2) at 4- to 6-hr intervals. Titrate by no more than 10 mg/day at weekly intervals to the minimum effective dose. Maximum: 60 mg/day

Child 6-11 yr: PO (immediate-release tablets – Adderall): 5 mg daily in the morning. Titrate daily dose in 5-mg increments at weekly intervals to minimum effective dose. Daily dose may be given in 1 to 3 divided doses at 4- to 6-hour intervals. Max: 60 mg/day

Available forms: Many products, check with manufacturer

Administer

• At least 6 hr prior to bedtime to avoid sleeplessness

- Use calibrated measuring device for oral solution
- Store all products at room temperature

SIDE EFFECTS

CNS: Hyperactivity, insomnia, restlessness, talkativeness, dizziness, headache, chills, stimulation, dysphoria, irritability, aggressiveness, tremor, dependence, addiction

CV: Palpitations, tachycardia, hypertension, decrease in heart rate, dysrhythmias

GI: Anorexia, dry mouth, diarrhea, constipation, weight loss, metallic taste

GU: Impotence, change in libido

INTEG: Urticaria

MISC: Rhabdomyolysis

PHARMACOKINETICS

Immediate release: Onset unknown, peak 3 hr, duration 4-6 hr
Extended release: Onset unknown, peak 7-8 hr, duration unknown
Half-life immediate release 9-14 hr; extended release 10-14 hr

INTERACTIONS

Increase: Hypertensive crisis risk—MAOIs or within 14 days of MAOIs

Increase: Serotonin syndrome, neuroleptic malignant syndrome—SSRIs, SNRIs, serotonin-receptor agonists; do not use concurrently

Increase: Amphetamine effect—acetaZOLAMIDE

Increase: CNS effect—haloperidol, tricyclics, phenothiazines

Decrease: absorption of barbiturates, phenytoin

Decrease: dextroamphetamine effect—ascorbic acid, ammonium chloride

Decrease: effect of—adrenergic blockers, antidiabetics, antihypertensives, antihistamines

Drug/Herb

Serotonin syndrome—St. John's wort

Decrease: stimulant effect—eucalyptus

Drug/Food

Increase: amine effect—caffeine (cola, coffee, tea)

Drug/Lab

Increase: plasma corticosteroids, urinary steroids

NURSING CONSIDERATIONS
Assess:

Black Box Warning: Cardiac disease: VS, B/P product may reverse antihypertensives, check patients with cardiac disease often

Black Box Warning: Substance abuse: use for prolonged periods may lead to dependence; sudden death or serious CV events can occur from misuse, chronic intoxication (insomnia, irritability, personality changes)

- CBC, urinalysis; with diabetes blood glucose, urine glucose; insulin changes may be required because eating will decrease
- Height, growth rate in children (growth rate may be decreased), weight
- Toxicity: symptoms may vary in children; anxiety, headache, flushing, vomiting, rhabdomyolysis, tremor, hyperreflexia, confusion, euphoria, tachycardia
- ADHD: change in behavior, growth retardation in children
- Mental status: mood, sensorium, affect, stimulation, insomnia, irritability
- Tolerance or dependency: increased amount may be used to get same effect; will develop after long-term use
- Pregnancy/breastfeeding: no well-controlled studies; use only if benefit outweighs fetal risk; avoid breastfeeding, excreted in breast milk

Evaluate:
- Therapeutic response: decreased CNS stimulation (ADHD); decreased drowsiness (narcolepsy)

Teach patient/family:
- To decrease caffeine consumption; may increase irritability, stimulation
- To avoid OTC products unless discussed with provider
- To tell parents that change in behavior may occur at beginning treatment; irritability, hostility
- Seizures: that those with a seizure disorder may have decreased seizure threshold

• To taper product over several weeks; depression, increased sleeping, lethargy may occur

• To get needed rest; patient will feel more tired at end of day

---

dextromethorphan (OTC)

(dex-troe-meth-or'fan)

Balminil ✦, Benylin DM ✦, Bronchophan Forte DM ✦, Delsym 12-Hour, ElixSure Cough, Koffex ✦, Robitussin, Robitussin Cough with Honey, Robitussin Long Acting Strength, Scot-Tussin Diabetes CF, Triaminic Long Acting Cough, Vicks Formula 44

Func. class.: Antitussive, nonopioid
Chem. class.: Levorphanol derivative

ACTION: Depresses cough center in medulla by direct effect

USES: Nonproductive cough caused by colds or inhaled irritants

CONTRAINDICATIONS

Hypersensitivity, MAOIs, SSRIs
Precautions: Pregnancy, fever, hepatic disease, asthma/emphysema, chronic cough, child <4 yr, breastfeeding

DOSAGE AND ROUTES

• **Adult/child ≥12 yr:** PO 10-20 mg q4hr or 30 mg q6-8hr, max 120 mg/day; **SUS REL LIQ** 60 mg q12hr, max 120 mg/day

• **Child 6-11 yr:** PO 5-10 mg q4hr; **SUS REL LIQ** 30 mg bid, **LOZ** 5-10 mg q1-4hr; max 60 mg/day

• **Child 4-5 yr:** PO 2.5-7.5 mg q4-8hr, max 30 mg/day; **SUS REL LIQ** 15 mg bid
Available forms: Liquid, extended release, 15 mg/5 mL, 30 mg/5 mL; gel capsules 5, 15 mg; capsules 15 mg; extended-release suspension: 30 mg/5 mL; lozenges 5 mg; ✦ solution 3 mg/mL; 7.5 mg/5 mL, 10 mg/5 mL, 15 mg/5 mL; strips, orally disintegrating 7.5 mg

Administer:
• **Extended-release suspension:** shake well, use calibrated measuring device
• Decreased dose for geriatric patients; metabolism may be slowed

SIDE EFFECTS

CNS: *Dizziness,* sedation, confusion, ataxia, fatigue
GI: *Nausea*

PHARMACOKINETICS

PO: Onset 15-30 min, duration 3-6 hr
SUS: Duration 12 hr
Half-life 11 hr, metabolized by the liver, excreted via kidneys

INTERACTIONS

• Do not give with MAOIs or within 2 wk of MAOIs; avoid furazolidone, linezolid, procarbazine (MAOI activity)
Increase: CNS depression—alcohol, antidepressants, antihistamines, opioids, sedative/hypnotics
Increase: adverse reactions—amiodarone, quiNIDine, serotonin receptor agonist, sibutramine, SSRI

NURSING CONSIDERATIONS

Assess:
• **Cough:** type, frequency, character, lung sounds, sputum
• Increase fluids to liquefy secretions, unless contraindicated
• **Pregnancy/breastfeeding:** no well-controlled studies; use only if benefit outweighs fetal risk; avoid breastfeeding
Evaluate:
• Therapeutic response: absence of cough
Teach patient/family:
• To avoid driving, other hazardous activities until stabilized on medication
• To avoid smoking, smoke-filled rooms, perfumes, dust, environmental pollutants, cleaners that increase cough
• To avoid alcohol, CNS depressants
• To notify prescriber if cough persists over a few days
• Not to use if breastfeeding or in child <4 yr

Side effects: *italics* = common; red = life-threatening

⚠ HIGH ALERT

diazePAM (Rx)

(dye-az´-e-pam)

Diastat, Diastat Acudial, Valium, Valtoco

Func. class.: Antianxiety, anticonvulsant, skeletal muscle relaxant, central acting

Chem. class.: Benzodiazepine, long-acting

Controlled Substance Schedule IV

Do not confuse:
diazePAM/Ditropan/LORazepam

ACTION: Potentiates the actions of GABA, especially in the limbic system, reticular formation; enhances presympathetic inhibition, inhibits spinal polysynaptic afferent paths

USES: Anxiety, acute alcohol withdrawal, adjunct for seizure disorders; preoperatively as a relaxant for skeletal muscle relaxation; rectally for acute repetitive seizures

CONTRAINDICATIONS

Pregnancy, hypersensitivity to benzodiazepines, closed-angle glaucoma, coma, myasthenia gravis, ethanol intoxication, hepatic disease, sleep apnea

Precautions: Breastfeeding, children <6 mo, geriatric patients, debilitation, renal disease, asthma, bipolar disorder, COPD, CNS depression, labor, Parkinson's disease, neutropenia, psychosis, seizures, substance abuse, smoking

Black Box Warning: Coadministration with other CNS depressants, respiratory depression

DOSAGE AND ROUTES
Anxiety/seizure disorders

• **Adult: PO** 2-10 mg bid-qid; **IM/IV** 2-5 mg q3-4hr

• **Geriatric: PO** 2-2.5 mg daily-bid, increase slowly as needed

• **Child >6 mo: PO** 1-2.5 mg tid/qid; **IM/IV** 0.04-0.3 mg/kg/dose q2-4hr, max 0.6 mg/kg in an 8-hr period

Precardioversion
• **Adult: IV** 5-15 mg 5-10 min precardioversion

Preendoscopy
• **Adult: IV** 2.5-20 mg; **IM** 5-10 mg ½ hr preendoscopy

Pediatric conscious sedation for procedures
Child >6 mo: PO 0.2-0.3 mg/kg, max 10 mg/dose, 45-60 min prior to procedure

Muscle relaxation
• **Adult: PO** 2-10 mg tid-qid or **EXTENDED RELEASE** 15-30 mg/day; **IV/IM** 5-10 mg, repeat in 2-4 hr

Tetanic muscle spasms
• **Adult: IV/IM** 10 mg, then 10 mg in 3-4 hr
• **Child >5 yr: IM/IV** 5-10 mg q3-4hr prn
• **Infant >30 days: IM/IV** 1-2 mg q3-4hr prn

Status epilepticus
• **Adult: IV/IM** 5-10 mg, 2 mg/min, may repeat q10-15min, max 30 mg; may repeat in 2-4 hr if seizures reappear
• **Child >5 yr: IM** 1 mg q2-5min; **IV** 1 mg slowly
• **Child 1 mo-5 yr: IV** 0.2-0.5 mg slowly; **IM** 0.2-0.5 mg slowly q2-5min up to 5 mg, may repeat in 2-4 hr prn

Seizures other than status epilepticus
• **Adult: RECT** 0.2 mg/kg, may repeat in 4-12 hr
• **Child 6-11 yr: RECT** 0.3 mg/kg, may repeat in 4-12 hr
• **Child 2-5 yr: RECT** 0.5 mg/kg, may repeat in 4-12 hr

Febrile seizure prophylaxis
• **Child >1 mo:** PO 1 mg/kg/day divided q8hr when fever starts, continue for 24 hr after fever is relieved

Alcohol withdrawal
• **Adult: IV** 10 mg initially, then 5-10 mg q3-4hr prn

Epilepsy cluster seizures
Adult: Nasal spray 0.2 mg/kg or 0.3 mg/kg, depending on the patient's age and weight

Available forms: Tablets 2, 5, 10 mg; injection 5 mg/mL; oral solution 5 mg/5 mL, rectal 2.5 (pediatric), 10, 20 mg, twin packs; extended-release capsule 15 mg, rectal gel; nasal spray 5 mg in 0.1 mL

Administer:
PO route
• With food or milk for GI symptoms; crushed if patient is unable to swallow medication whole
• Reduce opioid dose by ⅓ if given concomitantly with diazepam
• **Concentrate:** use calibrated dropper only; mix with water, juice, pudding, applesauce; to be consumed immediately
Rectal route
• Do not use more than 5×/mo or for an episode q5days (Diastat)
Nasal route
• Do not prime
• Place patient on side or back
• Remove from blister pack
• Insert nozzle in nostril, press plunger to deliver dose, remove
IM route
• Painful, use deltoid if used this route
Direct IV route
• Have emergency equipment nearby
• Observe for several hours after IV; if used in combination with opioids, decrease opioid dose
• Into large vein; give IV 5 mg or less/1 min or total dose over 3 min or more (children, infants); continuous infusion is not recommended; inject as close to vein insertion as possible; do not dilute or mix with other products

SIDE EFFECTS
CNS: *Dizziness, drowsiness,* headache, hangover, slurred speech, paradoxical excitation
CV: Hypotension, tachycardia
EENT: *Blurred vision*
GI: Constipation, nausea, vomiting, diarrhea, weight gain
INTEG: Rash, dermatitis, itching, phlebitis (IV), venous thrombosis
RESP: Respiratory depression
MISC: Psychological/physical dependency, tolerance, neutropenia

PHARMACOKINETICS
Metabolized by liver via CYP2C19, CYP3A4; 15%-20% of Asian patients and up to 5% of White and Black patients are poor metabolizers; excreted by kidneys; crosses placenta; excreted in breast milk; crosses the blood-brain barrier; half-life 1-12 days; more reliable by mouth; 99% protein binding
PO: Rapidly absorbed, onset ½ hr, peak 2 hr, duration up to 24 hr
IM: Onset 15-30 min, duration 1-1½ hr, absorption slow and erratic
RECT: Peak 1.5 hr
IV: Onset immediate, duration 15 min-1 hr

INTERACTIONS
Increase: diazepam effect—amiodarone, protease inhibitors, dilTIAZem, cimetidine, clarithromycin, dalfopristin-quinupristin, delavirdine, disulfiram, efavirenz, erythromycin, fluconazole, fluvoxaMINE, imatinib, itraconazole, ketoconazole, IV miconazole, nefazodone, niCARdipine, ranolazine, troleandomycin, valproic acid, verapamil, voriconazole, zafirlukast, zileuton; monitor for increased sedation
Increase: toxicity—barbiturates, SSRIs, cimetidine, CNS depressants, valproic acid, CYP3A4 inhibitors
Increase: CNS depression—CNS depressants, alcohol; monitor for increased sedation
Decrease: diazePAM metabolism—oral contraceptives, valproic acid, disulfiram, isoniazid, propranolol
Decrease: diazePAM effect—CYP3A4 inducers (rifAMPin, barbiturates, carBAMazepine, ethotoin, phenytoin, fosphenytoin), smoking
Drug/Herb
Increase: CNS depression—kava, chamomile, valerian
Drug/Lab Test
Increase: AST/ALT, alkaline phosphatase

NURSING CONSIDERATIONS
Assess:
• **CV:** B/P (lying, standing), pulse; if systolic B/P drops 20 mm Hg, hold product, notify prescriber
• **Blood studies:** CBC during long-term therapy; blood dyscrasias (rare); hepatic

studies: AST, ALT, bilirubin, creatinine, LDH, alkaline phosphatase

• **IV site:** frequently, watch for phlebitis

• **Degree of anxiety:** what precipitates anxiety and whether product controls symptoms

• **Alcohol withdrawal symptoms,** including hallucinations (visual, auditory), delirium, irritability, agitation, fine to coarse tremors

• Seizure control and type, duration, intensity of seizures

• For muscle spasms; pain relief

Black Box Warning: Avoid coadministration with other CNS depressants; do not use with opioids

Black Box Warning: Respiratory depression: monitor for respiratory depression, respirations q5-15 min if given IV

• IV site for thrombosis or phlebitis, which may occur rapidly

• **Mental status:** mood, sensorium, affect, sleeping pattern, drowsiness, dizziness, suicidal tendencies

• **Physical dependency, withdrawal symptoms:** headache, nausea, vomiting, muscle pain, weakness after long-term, high-dose use

• **MS spasm:** assess for swelling, mobility, identify location, duration, type of pain/spasm

• **Beers:** avoid use in older adults; may be appropriate for seizures, sleep disorders, benzodiazepine/ethanol withdrawal, severe anxiety disorders

• **Pregnancy/breastfeeding:** use in pregnancy not recommended; do not breastfeed, excretion in breast milk

Evaluate:

• Therapeutic response: decreased anxiety, restlessness, insomnia; seizure, muscle spasm control; amnesia related to procedure or surgery

Teach patient/family:

• That product may be taken with food

• That product not to be used for everyday stress or for >4 mo unless directed by prescriber; to take no more than prescribed amount; that product may be habit forming, review package insert with patient

• To avoid OTC preparations unless approved by prescriber

• To avoid driving, activities that require alertness; drowsiness may occur

• To avoid alcohol, other psychotropic medications unless directed by prescriber; that smoking may decrease diazePAM effect by increasing diazePAM metabolism

• Not to discontinue medication abruptly after long-term use; to gradually taper

• To rise slowly or fainting may occur, especially in geriatric patients

• That drowsiness may worsen at beginning of treatment

• To notify prescriber if pregnancy is planned or suspected; to avoid breastfeeding

TREATMENT OF OVERDOSE: Lavage, VS, supportive care, flumazenil

---

dibucaine topical
See Appendix B

---

diclofenac (Rx)
(dye-kloe′fen-ak)
diclofenac epolamine (Rx)
diclofenac potassium (Rx)
Cambia, Zipsor
diclofenac sodium (Rx)
Dyloject 37
Func. class.: Nonsteroidal antiinflammatory products (NSAIDs), nonopioid analgesic
Chem. class.: Phenylacetic acid

Do not confuse:
Cataflam/Catapres

ACTION: Inhibits COX-1, COX-2 by blocking arachidonate, resulting in analgesic, antiinflammatory, antipyretic effects

---

USES: Acute, chronic RA; osteoarthritis; ankylosing spondylitis; analgesia; primary dysmenorrhea; patch: mild to moderate pain

CONTRAINDICATIONS

Hypersensitivity to aspirin, iodides, other NSAIDs, bovine protein, asthma, serious CV disease; eczema, exfoliative dermatitis, skin abrasions (gel, patch); treatment of perioperative pain in CABG surgery
Precautions: Pregnancy, breastfeeding, children, bleeding disorders, GI disorders, cardiac disorders, hypersensitivity to other antiinflammatory agents, CCr <30 mL/min, accidental exposure, acute bronchospasm, hypersensitivity to benzyl alcohol

Black Box Warning: GI bleeding/perforation, MI, stroke

DOSAGE AND ROUTES
Osteoarthritis
• **Adult: PO** (diclofenac potassium/delayed-release diclofenac sodium) 50 mg bid-tid, max 150 mg/day; **DELAYED RELEASE** 50 mg bid-tid or 75 mg bid, max 150 mg/day; **EXTENDED RELEASE** (extended-release diclofenac sodium) 100 mg daily, max 150 mg/day; **TOPICAL GEL** 1% 4 g for each of lower extremities qid, max 16 g/day; 2 g for each of upper extremities qid, max 8 g/day; **TOPICAL SOL** apply 40 drops to each affected knee qid; apply 10 drops at a time, spread over entire knee
Rheumatoid arthritis
• **Adult: PO** (diclofenac potassium/delayed-release diclofenac sodium) 50 mg tid-qid, max 200 mg/day; **DELAYED RELEASE** 50 mg tid-qid or 75 mg bid, max 200 mg/day; **EXTENDED RELEASE** (extended-release diclofenac sodium) 100 mg daily, may increase to 200 mg/day, max 200 mg/day
Ankylosing spondylitis
• **Adult: PO DELAYED RELEASE** (delayed-release diclofenac sodium) 25 mg qid and 25 mg at bedtime, max 125 mg/day
Acute migraine with/without aura
• **Adult: PO** (powder for oral solution) 50 mg as a single dose, mix contents of packet in 1-2 oz water

Mild to moderate pain
• **Adult: PO** (diclofenac potassium) 25 mg qid
Dysmenorrhea or nonrheumatic inflammatory conditions
• **Adult: PO** (diclofenac potassium) 50 mg tid or 100 mg initially, then 50 mg tid, max 200 mg first day, then 150 mg/day, immediate release only
Pain of strains/sprains
• **Adult: TOPICAL PATCH** apply patch to area bid
Actinic keratosis
• **Adult: TOPICAL GEL** apply to area bid
Hepatic dose
• **Adult: PO** Moderate to severe hepatic impairment: use not recommended
Renal dose
• **Avoid:** Use of topical gel, patch, solution, potassium oral tablet for advanced renal disease

Available forms: Epolamine: topical patch 1.3%; **potassium:** tablets 50 mg; tablets, liquid filled 25 mg; oral powder for solution 50 mg; **sodium:** delayed-release tablets (enteric-coated) 25, 50, 75 mg; Pennsaid: extended-release tablets, 100 mg
Administer:
PO route
• Do not break, crush, or chew enteric products
• Take with a full glass of water to enhance absorption, remain upright for ½ hr; if dose is missed, take as soon as remembered within 2 hr if taking 1-2×/day; do not double doses
• Allow 6 hr between use with another NSAID
• Store at room temperature
Powder:
• Mix powder in 30-60 mL water only
• Mix solution; have patient drink immediately
• Powder (Cambia) and Zorvolex may be less effective if taken with food; Zorvolex capsules are not interchangeable with other formulations of oral product
Topical patch route
• Wash hands before handling patch
• Remove and release liner prior to administration

- Use only on normal, intact skin
- Remove before bath, shower, swimming; do not use heat or occlusive dressings
- Discard removed patch in trash away from children, pets
- Store at room temperature

Topical gel route
- Apply to intact skin; do not use heat or occlusive dressings
- Use only for osteoarthritis, mild to moderate pain
- Store at room temperature, avoid heat, do not freeze

Topical solution route
- Apply to clean, dry skin
- Wait until dry before applying clothing, other creams/lotions
- Wait ≥30 min after use before bathing, swimming
- Store at room temperature

SIDE EFFECTS
CNS: *Dizziness, headache*
CV: HF, MI, stroke, edema
EENT: Tinnitus
GI: Nausea, anorexia, vomiting, diarrhea, constipation, flatulence, GI bleeding, hepatotoxicity
GU: Nephrotoxicity: hematuria
HEMA: Anemia, blood dyscrasias
INTEG: Rash, pruritus, photosensitivity
SYST: Anaphylaxis, Stevens-Johnson syndrome, exfoliative dermatitis, toxic epidermal necrolysis

PHARMACOKINETICS
PO: Peak 2-3 hr; **TOPICAL Patch:** Peak 12 hr; elimination half-life 1-2 hr, patch 12 hr, 99% bound to plasma proteins, metabolized in liver to metabolite, excreted in urine

INTERACTIONS
- Need for dosage adjustment: antidiabetics
Increase: hyperkalemia—potassium-sparing diuretics
Increase: anticoagulant effect—anticoagulants, NSAIDs, platelet inhibitors, salicylates, thrombolytics, SSRIs
Increase: toxicity—phenytoin, lithium, cycloSPORINE, methotrexate, digoxin, lithium, cidofovir

Increase: GI side effects—aspirin, other NSAIDs, bisphosphonates, corticosteroids
Decrease: antihypertensive effect—beta-blockers, diuretics, ACE inhibitors
Decrease: effect of diuretics
Drug/Herb
Increase: bleeding risk—garlic, ginger, ginkgo; monitor for bleeding

NURSING CONSIDERATIONS
Assess:
- **CABG:** do not use oral, topical, gel, patch in perioperative pain in coronary artery bypass graft surgery for 10-14 days

> **Black Box Warning: Stroke/MI:** may increase HF and hypertension; increased CV thrombotic events, which may be fatal; those with CV disease may be at greater risk

- **Pain:** location, character, aggravating/alleviating factors, ROM prior to and 1 hr after dose
- **Actinic keratosis:** check lesions prior to use and periodically
- LFTs (may be elevated), uric acid (may be decreased—serum; increased—urine) periodically; also BUN, creatinine, electrolytes (may be elevated)
- **Serious skin disorders/anaphylaxis:** if rash develops, discontinue immediately, may be fatal; patients with asthma, aspirin hypersensitivity, nasal polyps may develop hypersensitivity
- **GI bleed:** Increased risk for peptic/duodenal ulceration, perforation, obstruction, GI bleeding
- **Blood dyscrasias (thrombocytopenia):** Bruising, fatigue, bleeding, poor healing; blood counts during therapy; watch for decreasing platelets; if low, therapy may need to be discontinued and restarted after hematologic recovery; check stool guaiac
- **Beers:** avoid chronic use in older adults unless other alternatives are ineffective; increased risk of GI bleeding
- **Pregnancy/breastfeeding:** use only if benefit outweighs fetal risks <30 wk, do not use after 30 wk; discontinue breastfeeding, excretion is unknown

Evaluate:
• Therapeutic response: decreased inflammation in joints, after cataract surgery
Teach patient/family:
• That product must be continued for prescribed time to be effective; to contact prescriber prior to surgery regarding when to discontinue this product
• To report bleeding, bruising, fatigue, malaise; **blood dyscrasias** do occur
• To notify prescriber immediately, stop product if rash occurs
• To avoid aspirin, alcoholic beverages, NSAIDs, or other OTC medications unless approved by prescriber
• To take with food, milk, or antacids to avoid GI upset; to swallow whole
• To use caution when driving; drowsiness, dizziness may occur
• To report **hepatotoxicity:** flulike symptoms, nausea, vomiting, jaundice, pruritus, lethargy
• To use sunscreen to prevent photosensitivity
• To notify all providers of product use
• To notify prescriber if pregnancy is planned or suspected
• **Stroke/MI:** to notify prescriber immediately, seek medical attention if chest pain, slurred speech, weakness, shortness of breath occur
• **Gel:** to use dosing card to measure; not to apply where cosmetics, sunscreen have been applied
• **Transdermal:** not to use in water (swimming/bathing); to use only on intact skin; not to cover with occlusive dressing; to apply adhesive tape or mesh sleeve if patch begins to peel off

---

diclofenac ophthalmic
See Appendix B

---

dicyclomine (Rx)
(dye-sye′kloe-meen)
Bentyl, Protylol ✦
Func. class.: Gastrointestinal anticholinergic, antispasmodic

ACTION:
Inhibits acetylcholine on receptors, decreases GI motility

USES: IBS

CONTRAINDICATIONS
Hypersensitivity to anticholinergics, closed-angle glaucoma, GI obstruction, myasthenia gravis, paralytic ileus, GI atony, toxic megacolon, dementia

DOSAGE AND ROUTES
• **Adult: PO** 10-20 mg tid-qid, max 160 mg/day; **IM** 10-20 mg q6hr; max 1-2 days
• **Child >2 yr: PO** 10 mg tid-qid
• **Child 6 mo-2 yr: PO** 5 mg tid-qid

Available forms: Capsules 10 mg; 20 mg; syrup 10 mg/mL; injection 10 mg/mL
Administer:
PO route
• Protect from light/heat
• **Children:** Syrup should be diluted with equal volume of water before use
IM route
• Aspirate prior to use
• Do not give IV, SUBCUT

SIDE EFFECTS
CNS: Headache, dizziness, fever, insomnia, drowsiness, confusion, numbness, excitement, restlessness
GI: Dry mouth, thirst, constipation, nausea, vomiting, distention, paralytic ileus
GU: Urinary hesitancy/urgency, ED
EENT: Blurred vision, increased IOP, photophobia
INTEG: Rash, urticaria, allergic reaction
MISC: Heat stroke

PHARMACOKINETICS
Onset unknown, peak 1-1½, duration unknown, half-life 1.8 hr

INTERACTIONS
Increase: side effects—antihistamines, antiparkinson agents, phenothiazines, TCAs, avoid using together
Decrease: dicyclomine effect—antacids, use antacids 1 hr prior to product
Decrease: effect of anticoagulants—anticoagulants

Side effects: *italics* = common; red = life-threatening

Decrease: effect of motility agents

NURSING CONSIDERATIONS
Assess:
• **IBS symptoms:** assess for constipation/diarrhea or both, abdominal pain, bloating, gas. Identify if product is lessening symptoms
• **Pregnancy/breastfeeding:** used in pregnancy to decrease nausea/vomiting; do not breastfeed
• **Anticholinergic effects:** Monitor for dry mouth, constipation, dizziness
• **CNS changes:** Assess for dizziness, drowsiness; caution against driving or other hazardous activities until response is known
• **Pregnancy/breastfeeding:** Use in pregnancy only if clearly needed, do not breastfeed
Evaluate:
• Therapeutic response
• Decreasing abdominal pain, bloating, gas, diarrhea/constipation
Teach patient/family:
• To report anticholinergic effects
• Not to drive or perform other hazardous activities until response is known
• Pregnancy/breastfeeding: do not breastfeed

---

didanosine (Rx)
(dye-dan'oh-seen)
Videx EC ✦
Func. class.: Antiretroviral
Chem. class.: Nucleoside reverse transcriptase inhibitor (NRTI)

ACTION: Nucleoside analog incorporating into cellular DNA by viral reverse transcriptase, thereby terminating the cellular DNA chain

USES: HIV-1 infection in combination with at least 2 other antiretrovirals

CONTRAINDICATIONS
Hypersensitivity, lactic acidosis, pancreatitis, phenylketonuria

Precautions: Pregnancy, breastfeeding, children, renal disease, sodium-restricted diets, elevated amylase, preexisting peripheral neuropathy, hyperuricemia, gout, HF, noncirrhotic portal hypertension

Black Box Warning: Hepatic disease, lactic acidosis, pancreatitis

DOSAGE AND ROUTES
• **Adult/adolescent/child ≥6 yr and ≥60 kg: PO DELAYED-RELEASE CAPSULE** 400 mg/day; if used with tenofovir, reduce to 250 mg/day
• **Adult/adolescent/child ≥6 yr and 25 kg to <60 kg: PO DELAYED-RELEASE CAPSULE** 250 mg/day; if used with tenofovir, reduce to 200 mg/day
• **Adolescent 20 kg to <25 kg: PO DELAYED-RELEASE CAPSULE** 200 mg/day
• **Adult ≥60 kg: PO ORAL SOLUTION** 200 mg bid or 400 mg/day; if used with tenofovir, reduce to 250 mg/day
• **Adult <60 kg: PO ORAL SOLUTION** 125 mg bid or 250 mg/day; if used with tenofovir, reduce to 200 mg/day
• **Adolescent/child/infant >8 mo: PO ORAL SOLUTION** 120 mg/m^2 every 12 hr, max adult dosing
• **Infant <8 mo/neonate ≥2 wk: PO ORAL SOLUTION** 100 mg/m^2 every 12 hr for up to 3 mo
Renal dose
• **Adult: PO** CrCl ≥60 mL/min: No change
• **Adult/adolescent ≥60 kg: PO** CCr 30-59 mL/min: reduce oral solution to 100 mg 12 hr or 200 mg every 24 hr; reduce extended-release capsules to 200 mg/day; CCr 10-29 mL/min: reduce oral solution to 150 mg every 24 hr; reduce extended-release capsules to 125 mg/day; CCr <10 mL/min: reduce oral solution to 100 mg every 24 hr; reduce extended-release capsules to 125 mg/day
• **Adult/adolescent <60 kg: PO** CCr 30-59 mL/min: reduce oral solution to 75 mg every 12 hr or to 150 mg every 24 hr; reduce extended-release capsules to 125 mg/day; CCr 10-29 mL/min: reduce oral solution to 100 mg every 24 hr; reduce extended-re-

lease capsules to 125 mg/day; CCr <10 mL/min: reduce oral solution to 75 mg every 24 hr; extended-release capsules are not recommended

Available forms: Powder for oral solution 10 mg/mL; delayed-release capsules 125, 200, 250, 400 mg

Administer:
• Pediatric: powder for oral solution after preparation by pharmacist; dilution required using purified USP water, then antacid (10 mg/mL), refrigerate, shake before use
• On an empty stomach ≥30 min prior to or 2 hr after meals
• Adjust dose with renal impairment
• Store tablets, capsules in tightly closed bottle at room temperature; store oral solution after dissolving at room temperature ≤4 hr

SIDE EFFECTS

CNS: Peripheral neuropathy, seizures, confusion, *anxiety,* hypertonia, abnormal thinking, asthenia, *insomnia,* CNS depression, pain, dizziness, chills, fever
CV: Hypertension, vasodilation, dysrhythmia, syncope, HF, palpitation
EENT: Ear pain, otitis, photophobia, visual impairment, retinal depigmentation, optic neuritis
GI: Pancreatitis, *diarrhea, nausea,* vomiting, *abdominal pain,* constipation, stomatitis, dyspepsia, liver abnormalities, flatulence, taste perversion, dry mouth, oral thrush, melena, increased ALT/AST, alkaline phosphatase, amylase, hepatic failure, noncirrhotic portal hypertension
GU: Increased bilirubin, uric acid
HEMA: Leukopenia, granulocytopenia, thrombocytopenia, anemia
INTEG: *Rash, pruritus,* alopecia, ecchymosis, hemorrhage, petechiae, sweating
MS: Myalgia, arthritis, myopathy, muscular atrophy
RESP: Cough, pneumonia, dyspnea, asthma, epistaxis, hypoventilation, sinusitis
SYST: Lactic acidosis, anaphylaxis

PHARMACOKINETICS

PO: Peak 0.67 hr, delayed release 2 hr; half-life 1½ hr, child 1 hr; extensive metabolism; administration within 5 min of food will decrease absorption (50%); excreted in urine, feces

INTERACTIONS

Increase: didanosine level—allopurinol, tenofovir
Increase: side effects from magnesium, aluminum antacids
Increase: pancreatitis risk—stavudine

Black Box Warning: Increase: fatal acetic acidosis: Stavudine (pregnancy), do not use together

Decrease: absorption—ketoconazole, dapsone
Decrease: concentrations of fluoroquinolones, other antiretrovirals, itraconazole, tetracyclines

Black Box Warning: Increase: fatal lactic acidosis—stavudine, tenofovir, other antiretrovirals; do not use together

Do not use with these products PO: gatifloxacin, gemifloxacin, levoFLOXacin, moxifloxacin, norfloxacin
Drug/Food
Any food decreases rate of absorption 50%; do not use with food
Do not use with acidic juices

NURSING CONSIDERATIONS
Assess:

Black Box Warning: Pancreatitis: do not use in those with symptoms of pancreatitis; may be dose related in advanced HIV, alcoholism, history of pancreatitis

• **Peripheral neuropathy:** tingling or pain in hands and feet, distal numbness; onset usually occurs 2-6 mo after beginning treatment; may persist if product not discontinued

Black Box Warning: Lactic acidosis, severe hepatomegaly, pancreatitis: abdominal pain, nausea, vomiting, elevated hepatic enzymes; product should be discontinued because condition can be fatal

• Children by dilated retinal exam q6mo may be considered to rule out retinal depigmentation
• CBC, differential, platelet count monthly; notify prescriber of results; alkaline phosphatase, monitor amylase; viral load, CD4 count
• **Renal studies:** BUN, serum uric acid, urine CCr prior to, during therapy
• Temperature may indicate beginning infection
• **Hepatic studies** prior to, during therapy (bilirubin, AST, ALT) as needed, monthly
• Cleanup of powdered products; use wet mop or damp sponge

Black Box Warning: Pregnancy/breastfeeding: identify if pregnancy is planned or suspected; product is not recommended in initial treatment due to toxicity; do not breastfeed; enroll in the Antiretroviral Pregnancy Registry (800-258-4263); do not use with stavudine

Evaluate:
• Therapeutic response: absence of infection; symptoms of HIV
Teach patient/family:

Black Box Warning: Pancreatitis: to report immediately abdominal pain, diarrhea, nausea, vomiting

• To report numbness, tingling in extremities
• To take on an empty stomach; not to take dapsone at same time as ddI; not to mix powder with fruit juice; to chew tablets or crush and dissolve in water; to drink powder immediately after mixing

• To report signs of **infection:** increased temperature, sore throat, flulike symptoms; other infections and complications may still occur
• To report signs of **anemia:** fatigue, headache, faintness, SOB, irritability
• To report **bleeding;** to avoid use of razors, commercial mouthwash
• That product does not cure symptoms, only controls them; that infection of others may occur via sex or blood

Black Box Warning: Pregnancy/breastfeeding: identify if pregnancy is planned or suspected, do not use with stavudine, fatal lactic acidosis may occur

difelikefalin (RX)
(dye-fel-i-KEF-a-lin)
Korsuva
Func. class.: Selective opioid receptor agonist

USES: Chronic kidney disease–associated pruritus

DOSAGE AND ROUTES
• **Adult IV** 0.5 mcg/kg at the end of each hemodialysis treatment
Available forms: Injection: 65 mcg/1.3 mL (50 mcg/mL)

difluprednate (ophthalmic) (Rx)
(die-flu′pred-nate)
Durezol
Func. class.: Ophthalmic antiinflammatory
Chem. class.: Corticosteroid

USES: For the treatment of postoperative ocular pain and postoperative ocular inflammation; for the treatment of endogenous anterior uveitis

CONTRAINDICATIONS
Hypersensitivity to this product, glycerin, polysorbate, ocular TB, acute herpes simplex (superficial), fungal/viral infections of the eye
Precautions: Pregnancy, breastfeeding, children, corneal infected abrasions, glaucoma

DOSAGE AND ROUTES
Postoperative ocular pain, inflammation
• **Adult/geriatric/adolescents/children/infants: OPHTH** Instill 1 drop into the conjunctival sac of the affected eye(s) qid beginning 24 hr after surgery; continue giving 4×/day for the first 2 wk of the postoperative period, then administer bid × 1 wk; at the end of the third week, taper dosage based on response
Endogenous anterior uveitis
• **Adult: OPHTH** Instill 1 drop into the conjunctival sac of the affected eye(s) qid × 14 days, followed by tapering based on response

⚠ HIGH ALERT

digoxin (Rx) NTI
(di-jox′in)
Digitek, Digox, Lanoxin, Lanoxin Pediatric, Toloxin ✤
Func. class.: Cardiac glycoside, inotropic, antidysrhythmic
Chem. class.: Digoxin preparation

Do not confuse:
Lanoxin/Lasix/Lonox/Lomotil/Xanax/naloxone

ACTION: Inhibits the sodium-potassium ATPase pump, which makes more calcium available for contractile proteins, thereby resulting in increased cardiac output (positive inotropic effect); increases force of contractions; decreases heart rate (negative chronotropic effect); decreases AV conduction speed

USES: Heart failure, atrial fibrillation/flutter, paroxysmal supraventricular tachycardia (PSVT) treatment/prophylaxis

CONTRAINDICATIONS
Hypersensitivity to digoxin, ventricular fibrillation, ventricular tachycardia
Precautions: Pregnancy, breastfeeding, geriatric patients, renal disease, acute MI, AV block, severe respiratory disease, hypothyroidism, sinus nodal disease, hypokalemia, carotid sinus syndrome, second- or third-degree heart block, electrolyte disturbances, hypertension, cor pulmonale, Wolff-Parkinson-White syndrome

DOSAGE AND ROUTES—NTI
• Digitalization may be done either by rapid digitalization with a loading dose over days or gradual digitalization with slow titration over weeks
• Digoxin injection is often used first to achieve rapid digitalization, then switched to PO dosing for maintenance
• Total loading dose (rapid, IV) is divided and administered 50% of dose over 5 min, then 25% at 4-8 hr after initial dose, and last 25% at 8-16 hr after first dose
Heart failure
• Target serum level ≤1.3 nmol/L
Optional loading dose
• **Adult: IV/PO** 10 mcg/kg lean body weight
Maintenance dose
• **Adult: PO** 0.0625-0.125 mg daily (usual max, 0.25 daily)
• **Older adult: PO** 0.0625-0.125 mg daily (usual max, 0.125 mg daily)
Atrial fibrillation
• Target serum level 1.3-2.6 nmol/L
Optional loading dose
• **Adult: IV/PO** 10 mcg/kg lean body weight Adult dosages/body weight
Maintenance dose
• **Adult: PO** 0.125-0.25 mg daily (usual max 0.25 mg daily)
Child: 2-5 yr: 10-15 mcg/kg: 5-10 yr: 7-10 mcg/kg; >10 yr 3-5 mcg/kg

Digitalization and maintenance doses (digoxin IV and digoxin oral solution) in children

Age	Oral Digitalizing Dose (mcg/kg)	IV Digitalizing Dose (mcg/kg)	Daily maintenance dose PO/IV (mcg/kg)	Clinical Notes
Premature	20-30	15-25	20%-30% of digitalizing dose	Divided daily dosing
Full Term	25-35	20-30	25%-35% of digitalizing dose	
1-24 mo	35-60	30-50		
2-5 yr	30-40	25-35		
5-10 yr	20-35	15-30		
Over 10 yr	10-15	8-12		Adult dosages/ body weight

Available forms: Pediatric elixir 0.05 mg/mL; tablets 0.0625, 0.125, 0.25 mg; injection 0.25 mg/mL; pediatric injection 0.1 mg/mL

Administer:
• Serum levels should be drawn just prior to the next scheduled dose or within 6-8 hr after the last dose
• Apical heart rate (BPM) must be assessed prior to administering dose; follow agency protocol for minimum BPM for administering digoxin (usually 60 BPM)

PO route
• Bioavailability varies among different oral dosage forms and different brands; changing from one preparation to another might require dosage adjustments
• Digitalization may be done either by rapid digitalization with a loading dose over days or gradual digitization with slow titration over weeks
• Digoxin injection is often used first to achieve rapid digitalization, then switched to PO dosing for maintenance

• Total loading dose (rapid, IV) is divided and administered: 50% of dose over 5 min, then 25% at 4-8 hr after initial dose, and last 25% at 8-16 hr after first dose
• **All dosage forms:** may be administered without regard to meals
• **Tablet:** may be crushed and administered with food or fluids
• **Pediatric elixir:** administer using a calibrated measuring device

Injectable
• When changing from PO to IM/IV, use 20%-25% less
• IV is preferred over IM because it is less painful and more rapid action
• PO should replace parenteral therapy as soon as possible
• Visually inspect parenteral products for particulate matter and discoloration prior to use

IM route
• Do not administer >2 mL at any one IM injection site
• Inject deeply into gluteal muscle, then massage area

IV route
• Monitor ECG during and for 6 hr after IV use; watch for dysrhythmias or bradycardia; notify prescriber
• May be given undiluted or each 1 mL may be diluted in 4 mL of sterile water for injection, NS, D_5W, or LR; diluent volumes <4 mL will cause precipitation; use diluted solutions immediately
• Inject over ≥5 min via Y-site or 3-way stopcock; in patients with pulmonary edema, administer over 10-15 min; to avoid inadvertent overdosage, do not flush the syringe following administration
• Check for potency and check site for redness, inflammation, infiltration; tissue sloughing can occur

Y-site compatibilities: Acyclovir, alfentanil, amikacin, aminocaproic acid, aminophylline, amphotericin B lipid complex, anidulafungin, ascorbic acid injection, atenolol, atracurium, atropine, aztreonam, benztropine, bivalirudin, bleomycin, bumetanide, buprenorphine, butorphanol, calcium chloride/gluconate, CARBOplatin, ceFAZolin, cefonicid, cefotaxime, cefoTEtan, cefOXitin, cefTAZidime, ceftizoxime, cefTRIAXone, cefuroxime, chloramphenicol, chlorproMAZINE, cimetidine, ciprofloxacin, cisatracurium, CISplatin, clindamycin, codeine, cyanocobalamin, cyclophosphamide, cycloSPORINE, cytarabine, DACTINomycin, DAPTOmycin, dexamethasone, dexmedetomidine, diltiazem, diphenhydrAMINE, DOBUTamine, DOCEtaxel, DOPamine, doripenem, doxacurium, doxycycline, enalaprilat, ePHEDrine, EPINEPHrine, epirubicin, epoetin alfa, eptifibatide, ertapenem, erythromycin, esmolol, etoposide, famotidine, fenoldopam, fentaNYL, fludarabine, fluorouracil, folic acid, furosemide, ganciclovir, gatifloxacin, gemcitabine, gentamicin, glycopyrrolate, granisetron, heparin, hydrocortisone, HYDROmorphone, hydrOXYzine, ifosfamide, imipenemcilastatin, indomethacin, irinotecan, isoproterenol, ketorolac, labetalol, levofloxacin, lidocaine, linezolid, LORazepam, LR, magnesium sulfate, mannitol, mechlorethamine, meperidine, meropenem, methicillin, methotrexate, methyldopate, methylPREDNISolone, metoclopramide, metoprolol, metroNIDAZOLE, mezlocillin, miconazole, midazolam, milrinone, morphine, multiple vitamins injection, mycophenolate mofetil, nafcillin, nalbuphine, naloxone, nesiritide, metilmicin, nitroglycerin, nitroprusside, norepinephrine, octreotide, ondansetron, oxacillin, oxaliplatin, oxytocin, palonosetron, pamidronate, pancuronium, pantoprazole, papaverine, PEMEtrexed, penicillin G potassium/sodium, pentazocine, PENTobarbital, PHENobarbital, phenylephrine, phytonadione, piperacillin, piperacillin-tazobactam, polymyxin B, potassium chloride, procainamide, prochlorperazine, promethazine, propranolol, protamine, pyridoxine, quiNIDine, ranitidine, remifentanil, Ringer's, ritodrine, riTUXimab, rocuronium, sodium acetate/bicarbonate, succinylcholine, SUFentanil, tacrolimus, teniposide, theophylline, thiamine, thiotepa, ticarcillin, ticarcillin-clavulanate, tigecycline, tirofiban, TNA, tobramycin, tolazoline, TPN, trastuzumab, trimetaphan, urokinase, vancomycin, vasopressin, vecuronium, verapamil, vinCRIStine, vinorelbine, vitamin B complex, voriconazole, zoledronic acid

SIDE EFFECTS

CNS: *Headache*, drowsiness, apathy, confusion, disorientation, fatigue, depression, hallucinations

CV: Dysrhythmias, *hypotension*, bradycardia, AV block

EENT: Blurred vision, yellow-green halos, photophobia, diplopia

GI: Nausea, vomiting, anorexia, abdominal pain, diarrhea

PHARMACOKINETICS

Half-life 30-40 hr, excreted in urine, protein binding 20%-30%

PO: Onset ½-2 hr, peak 2-6 hr, duration 3-4 days

IV: Onset 5-30 min, peak 1-4 hr, duration variable

INTERACTIONS

Increase: toxicity—azole antifungals, macrolides, tetracyclines, ritonavir; monitor for toxicity

Increase: hypercalcemia, hypomagnesemia, digoxin toxicity—thiazides, parenteral calcium; monitor electrolytes

Increase: hypokalemia, digoxin toxicity—diuretics, amphotericin B, carbenicillin, ticarcillin, corticosteroids

Increase: digoxin levels—propantheline, quiNIDine, verapamil, amiodarone, anticholinergics, dilTIAZem, NIFEdipine, indomethacin

Increase: bradycardia—beta-adrenergic blockers, antidysrhythmics

Increase: cardiac dysrhythmia risk—sympathomimetics

Decrease: digoxin absorption—antacids, kaolin/pectin, cholestyramine, metoclopramide

Decrease: digoxin level—thyroid agents, cholestyramine, colestipol, metoclopramide, aMILoride

Drug/Food

Decrease: digoxin effect- high-fiber food, separate by ≥2 hr

Decrease: GI absorption—flaxseed, psyllium

Drug/Herb

Increase: cardiac effects—foxglove, goldenseal, hawthorn, rue

Decrease: product effect—St. John's wort

Drug/Lab Test

Increase: CPK

NURSING CONSIDERATIONS

Assess:

• Apical pulse for 1 min prior to giving product; if pulse <60 in adult or <90 in infant, take again in 1 hr; if <60 in adult, notify health care provider; note rate, rhythm, character; monitor ECG continuously during parenteral loading dose; monitor I&O, daily weight; check for edema

• **Labs:** electrolytes: potassium, sodium, chloride, magnesium, calcium; renal function studies: BUN, creatinine; blood studies: ALT, AST, bilirubin, Hct, Hb before initiating treatment and periodically thereafter; monitor for decrease or increase in potassium

• Monitor product levels; therapeutic level 0.5-2 ng/mL, draw ≥6-8 hr after last dose, optimally 12-24 hr after a dose

• **Beers:** avoid dosage >0.125 mg/dL in atrial fibrillation, heart failure in older adults; decreased renal clearance may lead to toxicity

• **Pregnancy/breastfeeding:** no well-controlled studies; use only if clearly needed; excreted in breast milk (small amounts), may breastfeed

Evaluate:

• Therapeutic response: decrease in heart failure, dysrhythmias; serum digoxin level (0.5-2 ng/mL)

Teach patient/family:

• Not to stop product abruptly; about all aspects of product; to take exactly as ordered; how to monitor heart rate

• To avoid OTC medications, herbal remedies because many adverse product interactions may occur; not to take antacid within 2 hr of this product

• To notify prescriber of loss of appetite, lower stomach pain, diarrhea, weakness, drowsiness, headache, blurred or yellow vision, rash, depression, toxicity

• About the toxic symptoms of this product; when to notify prescriber

• To maintain a sodium-restricted diet as ordered

• To use one brand consistently, to keep in original container

• To notify prescriber if pregnancy is planned or suspected

• To carry ID stating condition treated, products taken

• How to take pulse, when to notify prescriber

• **Pregnancy/breastfeeding:** Advise patient to notify health care provider if pregnancy is planned or suspected or if breastfeeding; neonates may show symptoms of toxicity

TREATMENT OF OVERDOSE:

Discontinue product; give potassium; monitor ECG; give adrenergic-blocking agent, digoxin immune FAB

---

digoxin immune FAB (Rx)

(di-jox′in im-myoon′ FAB)

DigiFab

Func. class.: Antidote—digoxin specific

USES: Life-threatening digoxin toxicity

CONTRAINDICATIONS

Mild digoxin toxicity, hypersensitivity to this product, papain or ovine protein

DOSAGE AND ROUTES

1 (40 mg) DigiFab binds 0.5 mg digoxin

Digoxin toxicity (known amount) (tablets, oral solution, IM)

• **Adult and child:** IV dose (mg) = dose ingested (mg) × 0.8/1000 × 38- or 40-mg vial

Toxicity (known amount) (capsule, IV)

• **Adult and child:** IV dose = dose ingested (mg)/0.5 × 38- or 40-mg vial

Toxicity (known amount) by serum digoxin concentrations (SDCs)

• **Adult and child:** IV SDC (ng/mL) × kg of weight/100 × 38- or 40-mg vial

---

Digoxin toxicity (unknown amount)
• Adult and child >20 kg: **IV** 228 mg (6 vials)
• Infant and child <20 kg: **IV** 38 mg (1 vial)
Acute ingestion
• Adult: **IV** 380 mg (10 vials)
Life-threatening ingestion
• Adult: **IV** 760 mg (20 vials)
Skin test
• Adult: **ID** 0.1 mL of 1:100 dilution, check after 20 min

> **⚠ HIGH ALERT**

dilTIAZem (Rx)

(dil-tye′a-zem)

Cardizem, Cardizem CD, Cardizem LA, Cartia XT, Dilt-XR, Matzim LA, Taztia XT, Tiadylt ER, Tiazac

Func. class.: Calcium channel blocker, antiarrhythmic class IV, antihypertensive
Chem. class.: Benzothiazepine

ACTION: Inhibits calcium ion influx across cell membrane during cardiac depolarization; produces relaxation of coronary vascular smooth muscle, dilates coronary arteries, slows SA/AV node conduction times, dilates peripheral arteries

USES: PO angina pectoris due to coronary artery spasm, hypertension, improvement in exercise tolerance (chronic stable angina), **IV** atrial fibrillation, flutter, paroxysmal supraventricular tachycardia

CONTRAINDICATIONS

Sick sinus syndrome, AV heart block, hypotension <90 mm Hg systolic, acute MI, pulmonary congestion, cardiogenic shock
Precautions: Pregnancy, breastfeeding, children, geriatric patients, HF, aortic stenosis, bradycardia, GERD, hepatic disease, hiatal hernia, ventricular dysfunction

DOSAGE AND ROUTES
Prinzmetal's or variant angina, chronic stable angina
• **Adult:** **PO** 30 mg qid, increasing dose gradually to 180-360 mg/day in divided doses or **EXTENDED RELEASE** (LA, CD, XT, XR products) 180-360 mg/day, max 480-540 mg/day, depending on brand
Atrial fibrillation/flutter, paroxysmal supraventricular tachycardia
• **Adult:** **IV BOLUS** 0.25 mg/kg over 2 min initially, then 0.35 mg/kg may be given after 15 min; if no response, may give **CONTINUOUS INFUSION** 5-15 mg/hr for up to 24 hr
Hypertension
• **Adult:** **PO** 30 mg tid, increase to max 480 mg/day; **EXTENDED RELEASE** 120-240 mg daily, max 540 mg/day; **SUSTAINED RELEASE** 60 mg bid, max 360 mg/day
Rapid ventricular rate secondary to dysrhythmias (unlabeled)
• **Adolescent/child/infant >7 mo:** **IV BOLUS** 0.25 mg/kg over 5 min, then **CONTINUOUS IV INFUSION** 0.11 mg/kg/hr
Exercise tolerance in chronic stable angina (Cardizem LA) Adult PO extended release 180 mg daily, increase q7-14days, max 360 mg
Available forms: Tablets 30, 60, 90, 120 mg; extended-release tablets 120, 180, 240, 300, 360, 420 mg; extended-release capsules 60, 90, 120, 180, 240, 300, 360, 420 mg; injection 5 mg/mL (5, 10 mL); powder for injection 100 mg
Administer:
PO route
• Not all products are interchangeable
• CCBs should be used cautiously in those prone to excessive hypotension with acute cerebral interactions, hemorrhage, edema, severely raised intracranial pressure or cerebrovascular insufficiency, or with outflow obstruction of the left ventricle (aortic stenosis)
• Store at room temperature
• **Cardizem LA** extended-release tablet 24 hr: give daily, either AM or PM, without regard to meals

- **Tiazac, Tiztia XT:** give daily without regard to meals
- **Conventional regular-release tablet:** give before meals, at bedtime
- **Cardizem CD or equivalent (Cartia XT):** generic extended-release capsule 24 hr: give daily, without regard to meals
- May crush, sprinkle regular tablet on applesauce for administration

Direct IV route

- IV undiluted over 2 min, 5 mg/mL

Continuous IV INFUSION route

- Diluted 125 mg/100 mL, 250 mg/250 mL of D₅W, 0.9% NaCl, D₅/0.45% NaCl, give 10 mg/hr, may increase by 5 mg/hr to 15 mg/hr, continue infusion up to 24 hr max

Y-site compatibilities: Albumin, amikacin, amphotericin B, aztreonam, bumetanide, ceFAZolin, cefotaxime, cefoTEtan, cefOXitin, cefTAZidime, cefTRIAXone, cefuroxime, cimetidine, ciprofloxacin, clindamycin, digoxin, DOBUTamine, DOPamine, doxycycline, EPINEPHrine, erythromycin, esmolol, fentaNYL, fluconazole, gentamicin, hetastarch, HYDROmorphone, imipenem-cilastatin, labetalol, lidocaine, LORazepam, meperidine, metoclopramide, metroNIDAZOLE, midazolam, milrinone, morphine, multivitamins, niCARdipine, nitroglycerin, norepinephrine, oxacillin, penicillin G potassium, pentamidine, piperacillin, potassium chloride, potassium phosphates, ranitidine, sodium nitroprusside, theophylline, ticarcillin, ticarcillin/clavulanate, tobramycin, trimethoprim-sulfamethoxazole, vancomycin, vecuronium

SIDE EFFECTS

CNS: Tremor, paresthesia
CV: Dysrhythmia, *edema*, HF, bradycardia, hypotension, palpitations
GI: *Nausea*, vomiting, diarrhea, *constipation*
GU: Nocturia, polyuria, sexual dysfunction, dysuria
INTEG: *Rash*, flushing, photosensitivity, burning, pruritus, Stevens-Johnson syndrome, sweating
RESP: Rhinitis, dyspnea, pharyngitis, cough
EENT: Blurred vision, epistaxis, tinnitus
ENDO: Hyperglycemia, gynecomastia
HEMA: Anemia, leukopenia, thrombocytopenia
MS: Stiffness, muscle cramps
MISC: Gingival hyperplasia

PHARMACOKINETICS

Onset 30-60 min; peak 2-3 hr immediate release, 10-14 hr extended release, 11-18 hr sustained release; half-life 3½-9 hr; metabolized by liver; excreted in urine (96% as metabolites)

INTERACTIONS

Increase: effect, toxicity—theophylline, lithium
Increase: effects of β-blockers, digoxin, lithium, carBAMazepine, cycloSPORINE, anesthetics, HMG-CoA reductase inhibitors, benzodiazepines, methylPREDNISolone; monitor for increased action of each product
Increase: AV node slowing—cimetidine, ranitidine; monitor closely
Decrease: antihypertensive effect—NSAIDs, phenobarbital, phenytoin

Drug/Food
Increase: dilTIAZem effect—grapefruit juice; avoid use

NURSING CONSIDERATIONS
Assess:

- **HF:** dyspnea, weight gain, edema, jugular venous distention, rales; monitor I&O ratios daily, weight
- **Angina:** location, duration, alleviating factors, activity when pain starts
- **Dysrhythmias:** cardiac status: B/P, pulse, respiration, ECG and intervals PR, QRS, QT; if systolic B/P <90 mm Hg or HR <50 BPM, hold dose, notify prescriber; monitor B/P, ECG continuously if using IV; report bradycardia, have emergency equipment nearby
- Monitor if refills are being purchased
- Monitor digoxin levels if taking both products, digoxin toxicity is more common

- Potassium baseline and periodically; LFTs, renal studies
- Stevens-Johnson syndrome: assess for rash, fever, fatigue, mouth blistering; discontinue product immediately if severe
- **Beers:** avoid extended-release capsule in older adults; promotes fluid retention, exacerbates heart failure
- **Pregnancy/breastfeeding:** identify whether pregnancy is planned or suspected or if breastfeeding; no well-controlled studies; use only if benefit outweighs fetal risk; discontinue breastfeeding or product, excreted in breast milk

Evaluate:
- Therapeutic response: decreased anginal pain, decreased B/P, increased exercise tolerance

Teach patient/family:
- How to take pulse, B/P before taking product; that a record or graph should be kept
- To avoid hazardous activities until stabilized on product, dizziness is no longer a problem
- To limit caffeine consumption; to avoid grapefruit juice
- To discuss OTC, Rx, herbals, supplements with provider
- About the importance of complying with all areas of medical regimen: diet, exercise, stress reduction, product therapy
- To report dizziness, SOB, palpitations, rash, nausea, headache, swelling of face, hands
- Not to discontinue abruptly
- To use sunscreen, protective clothing to prevent photosensitivity
- To rise or change positions slowly, orthostatic hypotension may occur
- **Angina:** To discuss other therapy, including nitrates, beta-blockers and when to take
- To use good oral hygiene and teeth cleaning, gingival hyperplasia occurs
- **Pregnancy/breastfeeding:** to avoid pregnancy and breastfeeding

TREATMENT OF OVERDOSE: Atropine for AV block, vasopressor for hypotension

dimenhyDRINATE (OTC, Rx)
(dye-men-hye′dri-nate)
Dramamine, Driminate, GoodSense Motion Sickness, Gravol ✦
Func. class.: Antiemetic, antihistamine, anticholinergic
Chem. class.: H_1-receptor antagonist, ethanolamine derivative

Do not confuse:
dimenhydrinate/diphenhydramine

USES: Motion sickness, nausea, vomiting, vertigo

CONTRAINDICATIONS
Hypersensitivity, infants, neonates, tartrazine dye hypersensitivity
Precautions: Pregnancy, breastfeeding, children, geriatric patients, cardiac dysrhythmias, asthma, prostatic hypertrophy, bladder-neck obstruction, closed-angle glaucoma, stenosing peptic ulcer, pyloroduodenal obstruction

DOSAGE AND ROUTES
- **Adult: PO** 50-100 mg q4hr; max 400 mg/24 hr; **IM/IV** 50 mg q4hr as needed (Canada only)
- **Child 6-12 yr: PO** 25-50 mg q6-8hr prn, max 150 mg/day
- **Child 2-5 yr: PO** 12.5-25 mg q6-8hr, max 75 mg/day

dimethyl fumarate (Rx)
(dye-meth′il fue′ma-rate)
Tecfidera
Func. class.: MS agent

USES: Relapsing multiple sclerosis

CONTRAINDICATIONS
Hypersensitivity
Precautions: Pregnancy, breastfeeding, immunosuppression, infertility, male-mediated teratogenicity

DOSAGE AND ROUTES
• **Adult: PO** 120 mg bid × 7 days, may increase to 240 mg bid for maintenance
Available forms: Delayed-release capsule 120, 240 mg

---

dinoprostone (Rx)
(dye-noe-prost'one)
Cervidil, Prepidil
Func. class.: Oxytocic, abortifacient
Chem. class.: Prostaglandin E$_2$

USES: Cervical ripening

CONTRAINDICATIONS
Hypersensitivity, C-section, surgery, fetal distress, multiparity, vaginal bleeding, cephalopelvic disproportion
Precautions: Pregnancy, cardiac disease, asthma, anemia, jaundice, diabetes mellitus, seizure disorders, hypertension, glaucoma, uterine fibrosis, cervical stenosis, pelvic surgery, pelvic inflammatory disease, respiratory disease

Black Box Warning: Requires a specialized setting and an experienced clinician

DOSAGE AND ROUTES
Cervical ripening
• **Adult: Vaginal GEL** 0.5 mg vaginal gel placed in cervical canal, may repeat after 6 hr, max 1.5 mg/24 hr; vaginal insert 10 mg high in vagina, remove at onset of active labor or within 12 hr
Available forms: Vaginal gel 0.5 mg/3 g; vaginal insert 10 mg

---

diphenhydrAMINE (OTC, Rx)
(dye-fen-hye'dra-meen)
Aler-Dryl, Allergy Childrens, Allergy Relief Childrens, Allergy Relief, Anti-Hist Allergy, Aurodryl Allergy Childrens, Banophen, Benadryl Allergy Childrens, Benadryl Allergy, Complete Allergy Relief, Di-Phen, Diphen, Diphenhist, Genahist, Geri-Dryl, GoodSense Allergy Relief, GoodSense Sleep Aid, M-Dryl, Naramin, Nighttime Sleep Aid, Nytol Maximum Strength, Nytol, Ormir, PediaCare Childrens Allergy, Pharbedryl, Siladryl Allergy, Simply Sleep, Sleep Tabs, Tetra-Formula Nighttime Sleep, Total Allergy Medicine, Total Allergy, ZzzQuil
Func. class.: Antihistamine (first generation, nonselective)
Chem. class.: Ethanolamine derivative, H$_1$-receptor antagonist

---

Do not confuse:
diphenhydrAMINE/dicyclomine/dimenhyDRINATE

ACTION: Acts on blood vessels, GI, respiratory system by competing with histamine for H$_1$-receptor site; decreases allergic response by blocking histamine

USES: Allergy symptoms, rhinitis, motion sickness, antiparkinsonism, nighttime sedation, infant colic, nonproductive cough, insomnia in children

CONTRAINDICATIONS
Hypersensitivity to H$_1$-receptor antagonist, neonates
Precautions: Pregnancy, breastfeeding, children <6 yr, increased intraocular pressure, cardiac/renal disease, hypertension, bronchial asthma, seizure disorder, stenosed peptic ulcers, hyperthyroidism, prostatic hypertrophy, bladder neck obstruction

DOSAGE AND ROUTES
Antihistamine/antiemetic/antivertigenia
• **Adult/child >12 yr: PO** 25-50 mg q4-6hr, max 400 mg/day; **IM/IV** 10-50 mg, max 300 mg/day
• **Child 6-12 yr: PO** 12.5 to 25 mg q4-6hr as needed. Max: 150 mg per 24 hs for OTC
• **Infant/Child IV/IM** 1 to 2 mg/kg/dose (Max: 50 mg/dose) Iq 4 to 8 hr as needed, up to 5 mg/kg/day (Max: 200 mg/day)
Nighttime sleep aid
• **Adult and child ≥12 yr: PO** 25-50 mg at bedtime

Antitussive (syrup only)

• **Adult and child >12 yr: PO** 25 mg q4hr, max 150 mg/24 hr
• **Child 6-12 yr: PO** 12.5 mg q4hr, max 75 mg/24 hr

Motion sickness

• **Adult: IM/IV** 10-50 mg, max 25 mg/min; doses up to 100 mg/dose may be used; **PO** 25-50 mg q4-6hr

Available forms: Capsules 25, 50 mg; tablets 25, 50 mg; chewable tablets 12.5 mg; elixir 12.5 mg/5 mL; syrup 12.5 mg/5 mL; injection 50 mg/mL

Administer:

• Avoid use in children <6 yr; death has occurred; overdose has occurred with topical gel taken orally (adult/child)
• With meals for GI symptoms; absorption rate may slightly decrease
• At bedtime only if using for sleep aid

IM route

• Deep IM in large muscle; rotate site

Direct IV route

• Undiluted; give 25 mg/min or less

Intermittent IV INFUSION route

• Dilute with 0.9% NaCl, 0.45% NaCl, D_5W, 0.9% NaCl, $D_{10}W$, LR, Ringer's; infuse at ≤25 mg/min

Y-site compatibilities: Acetaminophen, aldesleukin, alfentanil hydrochloride, amifostine, amikacin sulfate, aminocaproic acid, amphotericin B lipid complex (Abelcet), amphotericin B liposome (AmBisome), amsacrine, anidulafungin, argatroban, ascorbic acid injection, atenolol, atracurium besylate, atropine sulfate, azithromycin, benztropine mesylate, bivalirudin, bleomycin, bumetanide, buprenorphine, butorphanol, calcium chloride/gluconate, CARBOplatin, caspofungin, cefTAZidime, ceftizoxime, chlorproMAZINE, cimetidine, ciprofloxacin, cisatracurium, CISplatin, cladribine, clindamycin, codeine, cyanocobalamin, cyclophosphamide, cycloSPORINE, cytarabine, DACTINomycin, DAPTOmycin, digoxin, diltiazem, DOBUTamine, DOCEtaxel, DOPamine, doripenem, doxacurium, DOXOrubicin, DOXOrubicin liposomal, doxycycline, enalaprilat, ePHEDrine, EPINEPHrine, epirubicin, epoetin alfa, eptifibatide, ertapenem, erythromycin, esmolol, etoposide, famotidine, fenoldopam, fentaNYL, filgrastim, fluconazole, fludarabine, folic acid, gallium, gatifloxacin, gemcitabine, gemtuzumab, gentamicin, glycopyrrolate, granisetron, HYDROmorphone, hydrOXYzine, IDArubicin, ifosfamide, imipenem-cilastatin, irinotecan, isoproterenol, labetalol, levofloxacin, lidocaine, linezolid, LORazepam, LR, magnesium sulfate, mannitol, mechlorethamine, melphalan, meperidine, meropenem, metaraminol, methadone, methicillin, methotrexate, methoxamine, methyldopate, metoclopramide, metoprolol, metroNIDAZOLE, miconazole, midazolam, minocycline, mitoXANtrone, morphine, multiple vitamins injection, mycophenolate, nalbuphine, naloxone, nesiritide, netilmicin, nitroglycerin, norepinephrine, octreotide, ondansetron, oxaliplatin, oxytocin, PACLitaxel, palonosetron, pamidronate, pancuronium, papaverine, PEMEtrexed, penicillin G potassium/sodium, pentamidine, pentazocine, phenylephrine, phytonadione, piperacillin, piperacillin-tazobactam, polymyxin B, potassium chloride, procainamide, prochlorperazine, promethazine, propofol, propranolol, protamine, pyridoxine, quiNIDine, quinupristin-dalfopristin, ranitidine, remifentanil, Ringer's, ritodrine, riTUXimab, rocuronium, sargramostim, sodium acetate, succinylcholine, SUFentanil, tacrolimus, teniposide, theophylline, thiamine, thiotepa, ticarcillin, ticarcillin-clavulanate, tigecycline, tirofiban, TNA, tobramycin, tolazoline, TPN, trastuzumab, trimetaphan, urokinase, vancomycin, vasopressin, vecuronium, verapamil, vinCRIStine, vinorelbine, vitamin B complex/C, voriconazole, zoledronic acid

SIDE EFFECTS

CNS: *Dizziness, drowsiness,* confusion, headache, seizures
CV: Hypotension, palpitations
EENT: Blurred vision, tinnitus, nasal stuffiness
GI: Nausea, anorexia, diarrhea
GU: *Retention,* dysuria, frequency
HEMA: Thrombocytopenia, agranulocytosis, hemolytic anemia
INTEG: Photosensitivity, rash
MISC: Anaphylaxis

Side effects: *italics* = common; red = life-threatening

RESP: Increased thick secretions, wheezing, chest tightness

PHARMACOKINETICS
Metabolized in liver, excreted by kidneys, crosses placenta, excreted in breast milk, half-life 2-4 hr
PO: Peak 2-4 hr, duration 4-8 hr
IM: Onset ½ hr, peak 2-4 hr, duration 4-8 hr
IV: Onset immediate, duration 4-8 hr

INTERACTIONS
Increase: CNS depression—barbiturates, opiates, hypnotics, tricyclics, alcohol
Increase: diphenhydrAMINE effect—MAOIs
Drug/Herb
Increase: CNS depression—chamomile, kava, valerian
Drug/Lab Test
False negative: skin allergy tests

NURSING CONSIDERATIONS
Assess:
• Urinary retention, frequency, dysuria; product should be discontinued
• CBC during long-term therapy; blood dyscrasias may occur
• Respiratory status: rate, rhythm, increase in bronchial secretions, wheezing, chest tightness
• **EPS:** If using for dystonic reactions, assess type of involuntary movement and evaluate response to medication
• **Cough:** Characteristics (type, frequency, thickness of secretions); evaluate response to this medication, increase fluids to 2L/day unless contraindicated
• **Anaphylaxis:** used for this rash, throat tightness, have emergency equipment nearby
• Store in tight container at room temperature
• **Pregnancy/breastfeeding:** no well-controlled studies; use only if benefit outweighs fetal risk; avoid breastfeeding, excreted in breast milk
Evaluate:
• Therapeutic response: absence of running or congested nose or rashes, improved sleep

Teach patient/family:
• About all aspects of product use; to notify prescriber of confusion, sedation, hypotension
• To avoid driving, other hazardous activity if drowsiness occurs
• That photosensitivity may occur, use sunscreen, protective clothing
• To avoid concurrent use of alcohol, other CNS depressants
• To use hard candy, gum, frequent rinsing of mouth for dryness
• Product should be discontinued 4 days before skin allergy tests
• Not to use for sedation in child <4 yr, deaths have occurred
• **Pregnancy/breastfeeding:** To report if pregnancy is planned or suspected or if breastfeeding, avoid if breastfeeding

TREATMENT OF OVERDOSE:
Administer diazePAM, vasopressors, phenytoin IV

---

diphenoxylate/atropine (Rx)
(dye-fen-ox′ee-late/a′troe-peen)
Lomotil, Lonox
difenoxin/atropine (Rx)
(dye-fen-ox′in/a′troe-peen)
Motofen
Func. class.: Antidiarrheal
Chem. class.: Phenylpiperidine derivative opiate agonist

Controlled Substance Schedule V
diphenoxylate/atropine
Controlled Substance Schedule **IV**
difenoxin/atropine

USES: Acute nonspecific and acute exacerbations of chronic functional diarrhea

CONTRAINDICATIONS
Children <2 yr, hypersensitivity, CDAD, severe electrolyte imbalances, diarrhea associated with organisms that penetrate intestinal mucosa

DOSAGE AND ROUTES
Diphenoxylate/atropine
• **Adult:** PO 5 mg qid titrated to patient response needed, max 8 tablets/day
• **Child 2-12 yr:** PO (liquid only) 0.3-0.4 mg/kg/day in 4 divided doses
Difenoxin/atropine
• **Adult:** PO 2 tablets, then 1 tablet after each loose stool or q3-4hr prn, max 8 tablets/day
Available forms: Diphenoxylate/atropine 2.5 mg/0.025 mg/5 mL solution, tablet; difenoxin/atropine tablet 1 mg/0.025 mg

---

dipyridamole (Rx)
(dye-peer-id'a-mole)
Persantine ✤
Func. class.: Coronary vasodilator, antiplatelet agent
Chem. class.: Nonnitrate

ACTION: Inhibits adenosine uptake, which produces coronary vasodilation; increases oxygen saturation in coronary tissues, coronary blood flow; acts on small resistance vessels with little effect on vascular resistance; may increase development of collateral circulation; decreases platelet aggregation by the inhibition of phosphodiesterase (an enzyme)

USES: Prevention of transient ischemic attacks, inhibition of platelet adhesion to prevent myocardial reinfarction, thromboembolism, with warfarin in prosthetic heart valves, prevention of coronary bypass graft occlusion with aspirin; IV form used to evaluate CAD; used as alternative to exercise with thallium myocardial perfusion imaging to evaluate CAD
Unlabeled uses: Cardiomyopathy, MI prophylaxis, proteinuria, TIA, valvular heart disease

CONTRAINDICATIONS
Hypersensitivity
Precautions: Pregnancy, breastfeeding, hypotension, unstable angina, asthma, hepatic disease, labor

DOSAGE AND ROUTES
Inhibition of platelet adhesion
• **Adult:** PO 75-100 mg qid in combination with warfarin, 75 mg qid with aspirin
Thallium myocardial perfusion imaging
• **Adult:** IV 570 mcg/kg, max 60 mg/day
TIA with aspirin (unlabeled)
• **Adult:** PO 225-400 mg/day max 400 mg/day
Available forms: Tablets 25, 50, 75 mg; injection 10 mg/2 mL
Administer:
PO route
• On empty stomach: 1 hr before meals or 2 hr after; give with 8 oz water for better absorption
• Store at room temperature
IV route
• IV after diluting to at least 1:2 ratio using D_5W, 0.45% NaCl, or 0.9% NaCl to a total volume of 20-50 mL; give over 4 min; do not give undiluted
• Inject thallium 201 within 5 min after product infusion
• Do not admix

SIDE EFFECTS
CNS: *Headache, dizziness, weakness, fainting, syncope;* IV: transient cerebral ischemia, weakness
CV: *Postural hypotension;* IV: MI
GI: *Nausea, vomiting,* anorexia, diarrhea
INTEG: *Rash,* flushing

PHARMACOKINETICS
PO: Peak 75 min; **IV** peak 2 min, therapeutic response may take several months, metabolized in liver, excreted in bile, undergoes enterohepatic recirculation, protein binding 91%-99%, terminal half-life 12 hr

INTERACTIONS
• Prevention of coronary vasodilation: theophylline, other xanthines; do not use together, causes a false-negative thallium imaging result
Increase: digoxin effect—digoxin
Increase: bleeding risk—NSAIDs, cefoTEtan, valproic acid, salicylates,

sulfinpyrazole, anticoagulants, thrombolytics; monitor for bleeding
Increase: adenosine effects
Increase: myasthenia gravis effects—cholinesterase inhibitors

NURSING CONSIDERATIONS
Assess:
• B/P, pulse during treatment until stable; take B/P lying, standing; orthostatic hypotension is common
• Cardiac status: chest pain; what aggravates, ameliorates condition
• **Pregnancy/breastfeeding:** no well-controlled studies, use only if clearly needed; cautious use in breastfeeding, excreted in breast milk
Evaluate:
• Therapeutic response: decreased platelet adhesion
Teach patient/family:
• That medication is not a cure; may have to be taken continuously in evenly spaced doses only as directed
• To avoid hazardous activities until stabilized on medication; dizziness may occur
• To rise slowly from sitting or lying to prevent orthostatic hypotension
• Not to use alcohol or OTC medications unless approved by prescriber
• About cardiac stress testing, expectations

---

diroximel (Rx)
(dye-rox′i-mel)
Vumerity
Func. class.: MS agent

USES: Relapsing multiple sclerosis

CONTRAINDICATIONS
Hypersensitivity

DOSAGE AND ROUTES
• **Adults:** PO 231 mg bid for 7 days, then increase to 462 mg bid
Available forms: Delayed-release capsule 231 mg

DOBUTamine (Rx)
(doe-byoo′ta-meen)
Func. class.: Adrenergic direct-acting β_1-agonist, cardiac stimulant
Chem. class.: Catecholamine

Do not confuse:
DOBUTamine/DOPamine

ACTION: Causes increased contractility, increased cardiac output without marked increase in heart rate by acting on β_1-receptors in heart; minor α and β_2 effects

USES: HF (<48 hr treatment) due to organic heart disease or cardiac surgery
Unlabeled uses: Cardiogenic shock in children; congenital heart disease in children undergoing cardiac catheterization

CONTRAINDICATIONS
Hypersensitivity to this product or bisulfites, idiopathic hypertrophic subaortic stenosis
Precautions: Pregnancy, breastfeeding, children, hypertension, CAD, MI, hypovolemia, dysrhythmias, sulfite hypersensitivity, renal failure, geriatric patients

DOSAGE AND ROUTES
• **Adult and child:** IV INFUSION 0.5-1 mcg/kg/min; titrate to 2-20 mcg/kg/min, may increase to 40 mcg/kg/min if needed
Available forms: Injection 12.5 mg/mL; premixed infusion 250 mg/mL, 500 mg/500 mL, 500 mg/250 mL, 1000 mg/250 mL
Administer:
Injectable
• Visually inspect parenteral products for particulate matter and discoloration prior to administration whenever solution and container permit
• Store reconstituted solution for 24 hr if refrigerated
IV route
• Must be diluted prior to administration
• Infuse into a large vein
Dilution
• Concentrate for injection must be diluted with ≥50 mL of a compatible IV

---

solution, dilute 500 mg (40 mL) in 210 mL D$_5$W or NS (withdraw 40 mL from a 250-mL bag) to produce a final concentration of 2000 mcg/mL; or 1000 mg (80 mL) in 170 mL D$_5$W or NS (withdraw 80 mL from a 250-mL bag) to produce a final concentration of 4000 mcg/mL; max 5000 mcg/mL and should be adjusted according to the patient's fluid requirements

Infusion

• Continuous: Use a controlled-infusion device

• Premixed bags in D$_5$W solutions can be a pink color that increases with time

• Do not give DOBUTamine simultaneously with solutions containing sodium bicarbonate or strong alkaline solutions (incompatible)

• Infusion should be started at a low rate and titrated frequently to reach the optimal dosage; titrate to B/P, urine flow, frequency of ectopic activity, heart rate, and measurements of cardiac output, central venous pressure, and/or pulmonary capillary wedge pressure

Y-site compatibilities: Alfentanil, alprostadil, amifostine, amikacin, aminocaproic acid, amiodarone, anidulafungin, argatroban, ascorbic acid injection, atenolol, atracurium, atropine, aztreonam, benztropine, bleomycin, bumetanide, buprenorphine, butorphanol, calcium chloride/gluconate, CARBOplatin, caspofungin, chlorproMAZINE, cimetidine, ciprofloxacin, cisatracurium, CISplatin, cladribine, clarithromycin, cloNIDine, codeine, cyanocobalamin, cyclophosphamide, cycloSPORINE, cytarabine, DACTINomycin, DAPTOmycin, dexmedetomidine, digoxin, diltiazem, diphenhydrAMINE, DOCEtaxel, DOPamine, doripenem, doxacurium, DOXOrubicin, DOXOrubicin liposomal, doxycycline, enalaprilat, ePHEDrine, EPINEPHrine, epirubicin, epoetin alfa, eptifibatide, erythromycin, esmolol, etoposide, famotidine, fenoldopam, fentaNYL, fluconazole, fludarabine, gatifloxacin, gemcitabine, gentamicin, glycopyrrolate, granisetron, HYDROmorphone, hydrOXYzine, IDArubicin, ifosfamide, irinotecan, isoproterenol, labetalol, levofloxacin, lidocaine, linezolid, LORazepam, LR, magnesium sulfate, mannitol, mechlorethamine, meperidine, meropenem, metaraminol, methoxamine, methyldopate, methylPREDNISolone, metoclopramide, metoprolol, metroNIDAZOLE, miconazole, milrinone, minocycline, mitoXANtrone, morphine, multiple vitamins injection, mycophenolate mofetil, nafcillin, nalbuphine, naloxone, netilmicin, niCARdipine, nitroglycerin, norepinephrine, octreotide, ondansetron, oxaliplatin, oxytocin, PACLitaxel, palonosetron, pamidronate, pancuronium, papaverine, pentamidine, pentazocine, phenylephrine, polymyxin B, potassium chloride, procainamide, prochlorperazine, promethazine, propofol, propranolol, protamine, pyridoxine, quiNIDine, ranitidine, remifentanil, Ringer's, ritodrine, riTUXimab, rocuronium, sodium acetate, succinylcholine, SUFentanil, tacrolimus, temocillin, teniposide, theophylline, thiamine, thiotepa, tigecycline, tirofiban, TNA, tobramycin, tolazoline, TPN, trastuzumab, trimetaphan, urokinase, vancomycin, vasopressin, vecuronium, verapamil, vinCRIStine, vinorelbine, voriconazole, zidovudine, zoledronic acid

SIDE EFFECTS

CNS: *Anxiety,* headache, dizziness, fatigue

CV: Palpitations, tachycardia, hypo/hypertension, PVCs, angina

ENDO: Hypokalemia

GI: Heartburn, nausea, vomiting

MS: Muscle cramps (leg)

RESP: Dyspnea

PHARMACOKINETICS

IV: Onset 1-2 min, peak 10 min, half-life 2 min, metabolized in liver (inactive metabolites), excreted in urine

INTERACTIONS

Increase: severe hypertension—guanethidine

Increase: dysrhythmias—general anesthetics

Increase: pressor effect, dysrhythmias—atomoxetine, COMT inhibitors, tricyclics, MAOIs, oxytocics

Decrease: DOBUTamine action—other beta-blockers

NURSING CONSIDERATIONS
Assess:
• **Hypovolemia:** if present, correct first; administer any cardiac glycoside before DOBUTamine
• **Oxygenation/perfusion deficit:** check B/P, chest pain, dizziness, loss of consciousness
• **Heart failure:** S_3 gallop, dyspnea, neck venous distention, bibasilar crackles in patients with HF, cardiomyopathy; palpate peripheral pulses, report if extremities become cold or mottled or if peripheral pulses decrease
• **ECG** during administration continuously; if B/P increases, product is decreased; CVP or PCWP, cardiac output during infusion; report changes, may induce ectopic rhythms
• Serum electrolytes, urine output; correct before use
• **Sulfite sensitivity,** which may be life threatening
• **Pregnancy/breastfeeding:** no well-controlled studies; use only if benefit outweighs fetal risk; cautious use in breastfeeding, excretion is unknown
Evaluate:
• Therapeutic response: increased B/P with stabilization, increased urine output
Teach patient/family:
• About the reason for product administration
• To report shortness of breath, chest pain, numbness of extremities, headache, IV site discomfort, exercise intolerance, inability to complete ADLs

TREATMENT OF OVERDOSE:
Administer a β_1-adrenergic blocker; reduce IV or discontinue, ensure oxygenation/ventilation; for severe tachydysrhythmias (ventricular), give lidocaine or propranolol

---

⚠ HIGH ALERT

DOCEtaxel (Rx)
(doe-se-tax′el)
Taxotere
Func. class.: Antineoplastic—miscellaneous
Chem. class.: Taxane

Do not confuse:
Taxotere/Taxol

ACTION: Inhibits reorganization of microtubule network needed for interphase and mitotic cellular functions; also causes abnormal bundles of microtubules during cell cycle and multiple esters of microtubules during mitosis

USES: Locally advanced or metastatic breast cancer, non–small-cell lung cancer, androgen-independent metastatic prostate cancer, postsurgery operable node-positive breast cancer, induction treatment of locally advanced squamous cell carcinoma of the head and neck, gastric adenocarcinoma

CONTRAINDICATIONS
Pregnancy, breastfeeding, hypersensitivity to this product or PACLitaxel, bilirubin exceeding ULN, ALT/AST >1.5× upper limit and alkaline phosphatase >2.5× upper limit

Black Box Warning: Other products with polysorbate 80, neutropenia of <1500/mm³

Precautions: Children, cardiovascular disease, pulmonary disorders, bone marrow depression, herpes zoster, pleural effusion, reproductive potential (female/male)

Black Box Warning: Edema, hepatic disease, lung cancer, taxane hypersensitivity

DOSAGE AND ROUTES:
• Other regimens are used
Breast cancer
• **Adult:** IV 60-100 mg/m² given over 1 hr q3wk; if neutrophil count is <500

cells/mm^3 for >1 wk, reduce dose by 25%

Operable node-positive breast cancer, adjuvant
• **Adult: IV** (TAC regimen) 75 mg/m^2 1 hr after DOXOrubicin 50 mg/m^2 and cyclophosphamide 500 mg/m^2 q3wk × 6 cycles

Locally advanced or metastatic non–small-cell lung cancer after failure of CISplatin chemotherapy
• **Adult: IV** 75 mg/m^2 over 1 hr q3wk; if neutrophil count is <500 cells/mm^3 for >1 wk, reduce dose to 55 mg/m^2; if patient develops grade 3 peripheral neuropathy, stop product

Androgen-independent metastatic prostate cancer
• **Adult: IV** 75 mg/m^2 given over 1 hr q3wk with 5 mg predniSONE **PO** bid continuously; give dexamethasone 8 mg **PO** at 12 hr, 3 hr, and 1 hr prior to DOCEtaxel; if neutrophil count is <500 cells/mm^3 for more than 1 wk or other toxicities occur, reduce dose to 60 mg/m^2

Squamous cell carcinoma of head and neck
• **Adult: IV** 75 mg/m^2 over 1 hr, then CISplatin 75 mg/m^2 over 1 hr on day 1, then 5FU 750 mg/m^2/day as a **CONTINUOUS INFUSION** × 5 days, repeat cycle q3wk × 4 cycles

Gastric adenocarcinoma
• **Adult: IV** 75 mg/m^2 q3wk with cisplatin and fluorouracil

Available forms: Injection 10 mg/mL, 20 mg/0.5 mL, 20 mg/mL, 80 mg/2 mL, 80 mg/4 mL; 20, 80 mg powder for injection/vial

Administer:
• Premedicate with dexamethasone 8 mg **PO** bid × 3 days starting 1 day prior to treatment
• Antiemetic 30-60 min prior to product and prn
• Confirmation that dexamethasone was given 8 mg bid × 3 days starting 1 day prior to infusion; for prostate cancer give 8 mg 12 hr, 3 hr, and 1 hr prior to infusion
• Store prepared solution up to 27 hr in refrigerator

Intermittent IV INFUSION route
• Use cytotoxic handling procedures
• Use non-PVC bag and use non-DEHP tubing
• Double-check all orders and products; errors can be fatal
• Solution is yellow to brown, do not use if particulate is present
• Allow vials to warm to room temperature; withdraw all diluent, inject in vial of DOCEtaxel; rotate gently to mix; allow to stand to decrease foaming, then withdraw the required amount (10 mg/mL), inject in 250 mL of 0.9% NaCl, D$_5$W; mix gently; give over 1 hr

Y-site compatibilities: Acyclovir, alfentanil, allopurinol, amifostine, amikacin, aminocaproic acid, aminophylline, amiodarone, amphotericin B lipid complex, ampicillin, ampicillin-sulbactam, anidulafungin, atenolol, atracurium, azithromycin, aztreonam, bivalirudin, bleomycin, bumetanide, buprenorphine, busulfan, butorphanol, calcium chloride/gluconate, CARBOplatin, carmustine, caspofungin, ceFAZolin, cefepime, cefonicid, cefotaxime, cefoTEtan, cefOXitin, cefTAZidime, ceftizoxime, cefTRIAXone, cefuroxime, chloramphenicol, chlorproMAZINE, cimetidine, ciprofloxacin, cisatracurium, CISplatin, clindamycin, codeine, cyclophosphamide, cycloSPORINE, cytarabine, dacarbazine, DACTINomycin, DAPTOmycin, dexamethasone, dexmedetomidine, dexrazoxane, diazepam, digoxin, diltiazem, diphenhydrAMINE, DOBUTamine, DOPamine, doripenem, doxacurium, DOXOrubicin HCl, doxycycline, droperidol, enalaprilat, ePHEDrine, EPINEPHrine, epirubicin, ertapenem, erythromycin, esmolol, etoposide, famotidine, fenoldopam, fentaNYL, fluconazole, fludarabine, fluorouracil, foscarnet, fosphenytoin, furosemide, ganciclovir, gatifloxacin, gemcitabine, gentamicin, glycopyrrolate, granisetron, haloperidol, heparin, hydrALAZINE, hydrocortisone, HYDROmorphone, hydrOXYzine, ifosfamide, imipenem-cilastatin, inamrinone, insulin (regular), irinotecan, isoproterenol, ketorolac, labetalol, leucovorin, levofloxacin, levorphanol, lidocaine, linezolid, LORazepam, LR, magnesium sulfate, mannitol, meperidine, meropenem, mesna, methotrexate, methyldopa, metoclopramide, metoprolol, metroNIDAZOLE, midazolam, milrinone, minocycline, mitoXANtrone, mivacurium, morphine, nafcillin, naloxone, nesiritide, netilmicin, niCARdipine, nitroglycerin, nitroprusside, norepinephrine, octreotide, ofloxacin, ondansetron, oxaliplatin, palonosetron, pamidronate, pancuronium, pantoprazole, PEMEtrexed, pentamidine, pentazocine, PENTobarbital, PHENobarbital, phenylephrine, piperacillin, piperacillin-tazobactam, polymyxin B, potassium chloride/phosphates, procainamide, prochlorperazine, promethazine, propranolol, quiNIDine, quinupristin-dalfopristin, ranitidine, remifentanil, riTUXimab, rocuronium, sodium acetate/bicarbonate/phosphates, succinylcholine, SUFentanil, sulfamethoxazole-trimethoprim, tacrolimus, teniposide, theophylline, thiopental, thiotepa, ticarcillin, ticarcillin-clavulanate, tigecycline, tirofiban, tobramycin, tolazoline, trastuzumab, trimethobenzamide, vancomycin, vasopressin, vecuronium, verapamil, vinCRIStine, vinorelbine, voriconazole, zidovudine, zoledronic acid

SIDE EFFECTS
EENT: Altered hearing, cystoid macular edema
CNS: Seizures, fatigue, weakness
CV: *Fluid retention, peripheral edema*
GI: *Nausea, vomiting, diarrhea,* hepatotoxicity, stomatitis
HEMA: Leukopenia, thrombocytopenia, anemia
INTEG: *Alopecia,* nail changes, rash, skin eruptions
MISC: Secondary malignancy, Stevens-Johnson syndrome
MS: *Arthralgia, myalgia,* back pain, weakness
NEURO: *Peripheral neuropathy*
RESP: Dyspnea, pulmonary edema, fibrosis, embolism, acute respiratory distress syndrome, interstitial lung disease
SYST: Hypersensitivity reactions

PHARMACOKINETICS
Metabolized in liver, excreted in feces, half-life 11.1 hr, peak 5-9 days, duration 1 wk

INTERACTIONS
Increase: Docetaxel effect—CYP3A inhibitors: anastrozole (high doses), aprepitant, fosaprepitant, clarithromycin, conivaptan, delavirdine, efavirenz (induces or inhibits), erythromycin, fluconazole, FLUoxetine, fluvoxaMINE, imatinib, itraconazole, ketoconazole, nefazodone, voriconazole, and others
Increase: modified effect of docetaxel CYP3A inducers: barbiturates, bosentan, carBAMazepine, nevirapine, phenytoin, fosphenytoin, rifabutin, rifampin, rifapentine
Increase: myelosuppression—other antineoplastics, radiation
Decrease: immune response—live virus vaccines

NURSING CONSIDERATIONS
Assess:

Black Box Warning: Neutropenia: CBC, differential, platelet count prior to treatment and weekly; withhold product if WBC is <1500/mm^3 or platelet count is <100,000/mm^3; notify prescriber, nadir 8 days

Black Box Warning: DOCEtaxel, polysorbate 80 hypersensitivity: contraindicated; some products may contain polysorbate 80

Black Box Warning: Edema: oral corticosteroids should be given as premedication; assess for fluid retention; may be severe, is usually dose related

Black Box Warning: Lung cancer: increased mortality in those with increased LFTs and a history of platinum-based products

Black Box Warning: Hepatic disease: hepatic studies prior to each cycle (bilirubin, AST, ALT, LDH); check for jaundiced skin and sclera, dark urine, clay-colored stools, itchy skin, abdominal pain, fever, diarrhea, if LFTs are >5x upper limit discontinue

- **Neurosensory changes:** confusion, paresthesias, peripheral neuropathy, dysesthesia, pain, weakness; if severe, product should be discontinued or pyridoxine used
- VS during first hour of infusion, check IV site for signs of infiltration

Black Box Warning: Hypersensitivity reactions, anaphylaxis, including hypotension, dyspnea, angioedema, generalized urticaria; discontinue infusion immediately, usually during first or second dose; mild reactions can be treated by slowing infusion, treating symptomatically; do not re-treat in those with severe reactions

- **Bone marrow depression/bleeding:** hematuria, guaiac, bruising or petechiae, mucosa or orifices q8hr; obtain prescription for viscous lidocaine (Xylocaine); avoid invasive procedures, avoid IM injections, rectal temps if platelets are low
- Effects of alopecia on body image; discuss feelings about body changes
- **MS symptoms:** Pain in joints, muscles, can usually be relieved with NSAIDs
- **Tumor lysis syndrome:** Correct dehydration, treat high uric acid levels; monitor for renal impairment, hyperuricemia, bulky tumor baseline and periodically —Assess for alcoholism, alcohol is in injection products, do not use in these individuals if possible
- **Pregnancy/breastfeeding:** Obtain a pregnancy test in females of reproductive potential before starting therapy, use adequate contraception during and for 2 mo after last dose, males with female partner of reproductive potential use effective contraception during and for 4 mo after last dose; do not breastfeed during and for 1 wk after last dose

Evaluate:
- Therapeutic response: decreased tumor size, spread of malignancy

Teach patient/family:
- To report signs of infection: fever, sore throat, flulike symptoms
- To report signs of anemia: fatigue, headache, faintness, SOB, irritability

- To report bleeding; to avoid use of razors, commercial mouthwash
- To avoid use of aspirin, ibuprofen, alcohol
- That hair may be lost during treatment; that a wig or hairpiece may make patient feel better; that new hair may be different in color and texture
- Not to drive until effects are known, dizziness, drowsiness may occur
- That pain in muscles and joints 2-5 days after infusion is common
- To avoid receiving vaccinations while taking product
- **Pregnancy/breastfeeding:** to use barrier contraception during and for several months after treatment; to avoid breastfeeding

docosanol topical
See Appendix B

docusate calcium (OTC)
(dok′yoo-sate cal′see-um)
docusate sodium (OTC)
Colace, Diocto, DOK, Enemeez, Selax ♣, Silace
Func. class.: Laxative, emollient; stool softener
Chem. class.: Anionic surfactant

Do not confuse:
Colace/Cozaar
Dulcolax (docusate)/Dulcolax (bisacodyl)

ACTION: Increases water, fat penetration in intestine; allows for easier passage of stool

USES: Prevention of dry, hard stools

CONTRAINDICATIONS
Hypersensitivity, obstruction, fecal impaction, nausea/vomiting
Precautions: Pregnancy, breastfeeding

DOSAGE AND ROUTES
- **Adult/child 12-17 yr: PO** 50-300 mg/day in divided doses (sodium) or 240 mg daily (calcium); **Rectal** (283 mg docusate sodium enema); 1 to 3 rectal enemas per day as needed

Available forms: *Calcium:* 240 mg; *sodium:* capsules 50, 100, 250 mg; tablets 100 mg; syrup 20 mg/5 mL; liquid 50 mg/5 mL, enema 283 mg/5 mL

Administer:
• Swallow tablets whole; do not break, crush, or chew
• Oral solution: diluted in milk, fruit juice to decrease bitter taste
• In morning or evening (oral dose)
• Store in cool environment; do not freeze

SIDE EFFECTS
EENT: Bitter taste, throat irritation
GI: Nausea, anorexia, cramps, diarrhea
INTEG: Rash

PHARMACOKINETICS
Onset 12-72 hr (PO), 2-15 min (rectal)

INTERACTIONS
Toxicity: mineral oil
Drug/Herb
Increase: laxative action—flax, senna

NURSING CONSIDERATIONS
Assess:
• **Cause of constipation;** identify whether fluids, bulk, or exercise is missing from lifestyle; constipating products
• Cramping, rectal bleeding, nausea, vomiting; if these occur, product should be discontinued
• **Pregnancy/breastfeeding:** low risk of fetal harm in pregnancy, breastfeeding
Evaluate:
• Therapeutic response: decrease in constipation
Teach patient/family:
• That normal bowel movements do not always occur daily
• Not to use in presence of abdominal pain, nausea, vomiting
• To notify prescriber if constipation is unrelieved or if symptoms of electrolyte imbalance occur: muscle cramps, pain, weakness, dizziness, excessive thirst
• That product may take up to 3 days to soften stools

• To take oral preparations with a full glass of water (unless on fluid restrictions) and to increase fluid intake

---

⚠ HIGH ALERT

dofetilide (Rx)
Tikosyn
Func. class.: Antidysrhythmic (Class III)

ACTION: Blocks cardiac ion channel carrying the rapid component of delayed potassium current; no effect on sodium channels

USES: Atrial fibrillation, flutter, maintenance of normal sinus rhythm

CONTRAINDICATIONS
Children, hypersensitivity, digoxin toxicity, aortic stenosis, pulmonary hypertension, severe renal disease, QT prolongation, torsades de pointes, renal failure
Precautions: Pregnancy, breastfeeding, AV block, bradycardia, electrolyte imbalance, renal disease

Black Box Warning: Arrhythmias, ventricular arrhythmias/tachycardia; requires an experienced clinician in specialized care setting

DOSAGE AND ROUTES
Adult: PO 500 mcg bid initially; maintenance 250 mcg bid, max 500 mcg bid; adjust dose based on QT and renal function
Renal dose
• **Adult:** PO CCr >60 mL/min, 500 mcg bid; CCr 40-60 mL/min, 250 mcg bid; CCr 20-39 mL/min, 125 mcg bid; CCr <20 mL/min, do not use
Available forms: Capsules 125, 250, 500 mcg
Administer:
• Physician and pharmacy must be registered to use product
• With patient hospitalized for ≥3 days

Black Box Warning: Step 1: Assess cardiac conduction: Prior to first dose, the QTc interval must be determined using an average of 5-10 beats; if the QTc interval is >440 msec (or >500 msec in ventricular conduction abnormalities), do not use; if baseline heart rate is <60 BPM, then the QT interval should be used

Black Box Warning: Step 2: Assess renal function: Prior to first dose, determine renal function using the Cockcroft-Gault equation, use actual body weight to calculate creatinine clearance

Black Box Warning: Step 3: Adjust starting dose according to renal function: Refer to the renal dose section above to determine the appropriate initial dosage

Black Box Warning: Step 4: ECG monitoring: Begin continuous ECG monitoring starting with the first dose

Black Box Warning: Step 5: Dosage adjustments: Approximately 2-3 hr after the first dose, determine the QTc interval; if the QTc interval has increased by >15% (compared to baseline), or if the QTc interval is >500 msec (>550 msec in patients with ventricular conduction abnormalities), the initial dosage should be reduced by half as follows:
• Decrease an initial dose of 500 mcg bid to 250 mcg bid
• Decrease an initial dose of 250 mcg bid to 125 mcg bid
• Decrease an initial dose of 125 mcg bid to 125 mcg/day

Black Box Warning: Step 6: Reassess QTc interval: Reassess the QTc interval 2-3 hr after each subsequent dose; if the QTc interval lengthens to >500 msec (or >550 msec in patients with ventricular conduction abnormalities), discontinue

Black Box Warning: Step 7: ECG monitoring: Monitor continuous ECG for a minimum of 3 days or for 12 hr after conversion to normal sinus rhythm, whichever is greater

SIDE EFFECTS
CNS: *Dizziness,* headache, stroke
CV: QT prolongation, torsades de pointes, ventricular dysrhythmias, chest pain
GI: *Nausea,* diarrhea

PHARMACOKINETICS
Well absorbed, max plasma concentrations 2-3 hr, steady state 2-3 days, half-life 10 hr, metabolized by liver, excreted by kidneys, peak 3 hr, duration up to 24 hr

INTERACTIONS
• Do not use with cimetidine, ketoconazole, verapamil, prochlorperazine, trimethoprim-sulfamethoxazole, megestrol, hydroCHLOROthiazide
Increase: QT prolongation, torsades de pointes—class IA/III antidysrhythmics, arsenic trioxide, chloroquine, clarithromycin, droperidol, erythromycin, halofantrine, haloperidol, methadone, pentamidine, some phenothiazines, ziprasidone, ciprofloxacin
Increase: hypokalemia—potassium-depleting diuretics
Increase: toxicity—aMILoride metFORMIN, entecavir, lamiVUDine, memantine, triamterene, procainamide, trospium
Increase: dofetilide levels—antiretroviral protease inhibitors
Increase: dysrhythmias—CYP3A4 inhibitors (SSRIs, macrolides, azoles, protease inhibitors, amiodarone, diltiazem, quinine)
Drug/Food
Do not use with grapefruit juice

NURSING CONSIDERATIONS
Assess:
• AF patients should receive anticoagulation prior to cardioversion

Black Box Warning: Dysrhythmias: 3 days of continuous ECG monitoring, monitoring of CCr are required when starting or restarting medication; have cardiac resuscitation equipment nearby

• Cardiac status: rate, rhythm, character, continuously; B/P
• **Severe renal impairment CCr <20 mL/min:** do not use for mild to moderate renal disease; monitor BUN/creatinine; adjust dose based on creatinine clearance

• **Pregnancy/breastfeeding:** no well-controlled studies; use only if benefit outweighs fetal risk; avoid breastfeeding, excretion is unknown

Evaluate:

• Therapeutic response: control of atrial fibrillation, normal sinus rhythm

Teach patient/family:

• To make position changes slowly; orthostatic hypotension may occur

• To notify prescriber if fast heartbeats with fainting or dizziness occur

• To notify all prescribers of all medications, supplements taken

• That if dose is missed, not to double; to take next dose at usual time

• To avoid breastfeeding

---

dolasetron (Rx)

(do-la'se-tron)

Anzemet

Func. class.: Antiemetic

Chem. class.: 5-HT3 receptor antagonist

Do not confuse:

Anzemet/Avandamet

ACTION: Prevents nausea, vomiting by blocking serotonin peripherally, centrally, and in the small intestine

USES: Prevention of chemotherapy-induced and postoperative nausea, vomiting

CONTRAINDICATIONS

Hypersensitivity

Precautions: Pregnancy, breastfeeding, children, geriatric patients, hypokalemia, electrolyte imbalances; granisetron/ondansetron/palonosetron hypersensitivity, QT prolongation

DOSAGE AND ROUTES

Prevention of cancer chemotherapy nausea/vomiting

• **Adult: PO** 100 mg 1 hr prior to chemotherapy

• **Child 2-16 yr: PO** 1.8 mg/kg given 1 hr prior to chemotherapy, max 100 mg

Available forms: Tablets 50, 100 mg

Administer:

PO route

• Do not mix product for oral administration in apple or apple-grape juice until immediately prior to administration; diluted product can be kept for 2 hr at room temperature

• Store at room temperature 48 hr after dilution

SIDE EFFECTS

CNS: *Headache,* dizziness, fatigue, drowsiness, serotonin syndrome

CV: Dysrhythmias, ECG changes, hypo/hypertension, tachycardia, bradycardia; ventricular tachycardia/fibrillation, QT prolongation, torsades de pointes, cardiac arrest (IV)

GI: *Diarrhea,* constipation, increased AST/ALT, abdominal pain, anorexia

GU: Urinary retention, oliguria

MISC: Rash, bronchospasm

PHARMACOKINETICS

Well absorbed, metabolized to active metabolite, half-life of active metabolite 8 hr, max concentrations after 1 hr

INTERACTIONS

Increase: dysrhythmias—antidysrhythmics

Increase: dolasetron levels—cimetidine

Increase: QT prolongation—thiazide/loop diuretics, antidysrhythmics (class IA, III), arsenic trioxide, chloroquine, clarithromycin, droperidol, erythromycin, halofantrine, haloperidol, methadone, pentamidine, some phenothiazines, ziprasidone; occurs at higher dose of dolasetron

Decrease: dolasetron levels—rifAMPin

NURSING CONSIDERATIONS

Assess:

• **Hypersensitivity reaction:** rash, bronchospasm

• Nausea, vomiting, prior to and after use

• **Cardiac conduction conditions:** monitor ECG, electrolyte imbalances, dysrhythmias, heart rate

• **QT prolongation:** QRS, PR prolongation; do not use in those with congenital long QT syndrome, hypokalemia, hypomagnesemia, complete heart block (unless a pacemaker is in place), correct electrolytes prior to use, monitor ECG in elderly patients, renal cardiac disease

• **Serotonin syndrome:** usually when combined with SSRIs, SNRIs, MAOIs
• **Pregnancy/breastfeeding:** no well-controlled studies; use only if clearly needed, cautious use in breastfeeding, excretion is unknown

Evaluate:
• Therapeutic response: absence of nausea, vomiting during cancer chemotherapy

Teach patient/family:
• To report diarrhea, constipation, nausea, vomiting, rash; or changes in respirations, heart rate, nausea, vomiting
• May cause headache; use analgesic

⚠ HIGH ALERT

dolutegravir (Rx)
(doe-loo-teg′ra-vir)
Tivicay, Tivicay PD
Func. class.: Antiretroviral

ACTION: Inhibits catalytic activity of HIV integrase, which is an HIV-encoded enzyme needed for replication

USES: HIV in combination with other antiretrovirals

CONTRAINDICATIONS
Breastfeeding, hypersensitivity
Precautions: Pregnancy, children, geriatric patients, hepatic disease, immune reconstitution syndrome, hepatitis, antimicrobial resistance, lactase deficiency

DOSAGE AND ROUTES
• **Adult and child ≥12 yr and ≥40 kg (treatment naïve or treatment experienced but integrase strand transfer inhibitor naïve): PO** 50 mg daily; if given with efavirenz, fosamprenavir/ritonavir, tipranavir/ritonavir, or rifAMPin, give 50 mg bid
Infant/child 3 to <14 kg: PO soluble tablets for oral suspension (Tivicay PD): 3-<6 kg: 5 mg daily; 6-<10 kg: 15 mg daily; 10-<14 kg: 20 mg daily
Infant/child/adolescent ≥14 kg: PO soluble tablets for oral suspension (Tivicay PD): 14-<20 kg: 25 mg daily; ≥20 kg: 30 mg daily; **tablets (Tivicay): 14-<20 kg:** 40 mg daily; **≥20 kg:** 50 mg daily
INSTI-experienced with any INSTI-associated resistance mutation or clinically suspected INSTI resistance Children and adolescents weighing ≥40 kg: PO tablets (Tivicay): 50 mg bid

Available forms: Tablets 10, 25, 50 mg; dispersible tab 5 mg
Administer:
• May give without regard to meals, with 8 oz of water
• Store at room temperature
• Give 2 hr prior to or 6 hr after cation-containing antacids or laxatives, sucralfate, oral iron, oral calcium, or buffered products

SIDE EFFECTS
CNS: Fatigue, headache, insomnia
GI: Nausea, vomiting, diarrhea, hepatotoxicity
INTEG: Rash, pruritus
META: Hyperglycemia
SYST: Immune reconstitution syndrome
GU: Renal dysfunction

PHARMACOKINETICS
Peak 2-3 hr, steady state 5 days, half-life 14 hr, 98% protein binding, metabolized in the liver, excreted in feces 53%, urine 31%

INTERACTIONS
Decrease: effect of dolutegravir—antacids, laxatives/sucralfate, oral iron, oral calcium, buffered products
Decrease: levels—rifAMPin efavirenz, tenofovir, tipranavir/ritonavir

Drug/Herb

Avoid concurrent use with St. John's wort

NURSING CONSIDERATIONS
Assess:

• **HIV infection:** CD4, T-cell count, plasma HIV RNA, viral load; resistance testing prior to treatment, at treatment failure

• Drug resistance testing prior to use in treatment-naïve patients

• **Immune reconstitution syndrome,** usually during initial phase of treatment; may need antiinfective prior to starting

• **Infection:** monitor for opportunistic or other infection

• Monitor total HDL/LDL cholesterol baseline and periodically; all may be elevated

• **Pregnancy/breastfeeding:** all HIV-positive women should receive antiretroviral therapy, report pregnancy to the Antiretroviral Pregnancy Registry (800-258-4263); avoid breastfeeding, excretion unknown; glucose screening should be performed at 24-48 wk gestation, confirm gestation age in each trimester by ultrasound

Evaluate:

• Therapeutic response: improvement in cell counts, T-cell counts

Teach patient/family:

• To take as prescribed; if dose is missed, to take as soon as remembered up to 1 hr prior to next dose; not to double dose; not to share with others

• That sexual partners need to be told that patient has HIV; that product does not cure infection, just controls symptoms, does not prevent infecting others

• To report sore throat, fever, fatigue (may indicate infection)

• That continued follow-up and lab work will be needed

• That fat accumulation/redistribution may occur

• To notify prescriber if pregnancy is planned or suspected; to avoid breastfeeding and to continue follow-up exams and lab work

dolutegravir/lamivudine
(doe-loo-teg'ra-vir/la-mi'vyoo-deen)

Dovato

Func. class.: Antiretroviral/antiviral
Chem. class.: INST/NRTI

ACTION: Dolutegravir/lamivudine is active against infections caused by human immunodeficiency virus type 1 (HIV-1). Lamivudine is a nucleoside analog that works by inhibiting HIV reverse transcriptase, while dolutegravir works by inhibiting the catalytic activity of HIV integrase

USES: HIV-1 infection in adults

CONTRAINDICATIONS
Hypersensitivity

Precautions: Alcoholism, autoimmune disease, bone fractures, breastfeeding, children, depression, females, Graves' disease, Guillain-Barré syndrome, hepatic disease, hepatitis, hepatitis B and HIV coinfection, hepatitis C and HIV coinfection, hepatomegaly, HIV resistance, hypercholesterolemia, hyperlipidemia, hypertriglyceridemia, hypophosphatemia, immune reconstitution syndrome, lactic acidosis, obesity, osteomalacia, osteoporosis, pregnancy, renal failure, renal impairment, serious rash, suicidal ideation, torsades de pointes

Black Box Warning: Hepatitis B exacerbation, hepatotoxicity

DOSAGE AND ROUTES
Adults: PO One tablet (50 mg dolutegravir; 300 mg lamivudine) daily
Available forms: Tablet 50 mg-300 mg
Administer:

• Give without regard to food

• During coadministration with carBAMazepine or rifAMPin, the dolutegravir dose needs to be increased to 50 mg bid; add 50 mg/day of dolutegravir (separated by 12 hr from dolutegravir; lamivudine) should be given

• Avoid use in treatment-experienced patients and in patients with known substitutions associated with resistance to dolutegravir or lamivudine
• Do not use within 2 hr prior to or 6 hr after iron or calcium supplement
• Do not use within 2 hr prior to or 6 hr after antacids, laxatives, or other medicines that contain aluminum, magnesium, sucralfate, or buffered medicines
• Admixtures are stable for ≥24 hr at room temperature

SIDE EFFECTS

CNS: *Headache,* abnormal dreams, *depression, dizziness, insomnia,* neuropathy, paresthesia, asthenia, fatigue, drowsiness
GI: *Nausea, vomiting, anorexia, diarrhea, abdominal pain, dyspepsia,* hepatomegaly with stenosis (may be fatal), hyperbilirubinemia, hypercholesterolemia, pancreatitis
GU: Glomerulonephritis membranous/mesangial **proliferative**
INTEG: *Rash,* skin discoloration
MS: *Arthralgia, myalgia,* rhabdomyolysis
RESP: Cough
SYST: *Change in body fat distribution,* lactic acidosis

PHARMACOKINETICS

• **Lamivudine:** 36% protein binding, half-life is 13 to 19 hr
• **Dolutegravir:** 99% protein binding, metabolism occurs via UDP-glucuronosyltransferase (UGT)1A1 (major) and by the hepatic isoenzyme CYP3A (minor), half-life 14 hr, 53% excreted unchanged in the feces, urine excretion 31%

INTERACTIONS

Increased level: CYP3A4 inhibitors (aldesleukin IL-2, amiodarone, aprepitant, atazanavir, basiliximab, boceprevir, bromocriptine, chloramphenicol, clarithromycin, conivaptan, danazol, dalfopristin, darunavir, dasatinib, delavirdine, diltiazem, dronedarone, efavirenz, erythromycin, ethinyl estradiol, fluconazole, fluoxetine, fluvoxamine, fosamprenavir, fosaprepitant, imatinib, indinavir, isoniazid, itraconazole, ketoconazole, lanreotide, lapatinib, micon-

azole, nefazodone, nelfinavir, nicardipine, octreotide, posaconazole, quinine, ranolazine, rifaximin, tamoxifen, telaprevir, telithromycin, tipranavir, troleandomycin, verapamil, voriconazole, zafirlukast)
Increased: metformin
Increased: dofetilide, coadministration is contraindicated
Decrease: dolutegravir-carbamazepine, rifAMPin, an additional dolutegravir 50-mg dose should be taken
Decrease: dolutegravir-oxcarbazepine, phenytoin, phenobarbital; avoid coadministration

Drug/Lab Test
Increased: AST/ALT, amylase, bilirubin, CK, glucose, lipase
Decrease: neutrophils

NURSING CONSIDERATIONS
Assess:
• **HIV infection:** Assess symptoms of HIV, including opportunistic infections, prior to and during treatment, some may be life threatening; monitor plasma CD4+, CD8 cell counts, serum beta-2 microglobulin, serum antigen levels, treatment failures occur more often in those with baseline HIV-1 RNA concentrations <100,000 copies/mL than in those <100,000 copies/mL; monitor blood glucose, CBC with differential, serum cholesterol, lipid panel

Black Box Warning: **Hepatotoxicity/ lactic acidosis:** Monitor hepatitis B serology, LFTs, plasma hepatitis C RNA, lactic acidosis levels. If lab reports confirm these conditions, discontinue product. More common in females or those who are overweight. Avoid use in alcoholism

• Patients coinfected with HBV and HIV who discontinue this product should have transaminase concentrations monitored q6wk for the first 3 mo and q3-6 mo thereafter.
• Resumption of anti–hepatitis B treatment may be required. For patients who refuse a fully suppressive antiretroviral regimen but still require treatment for HBV, consider 48 wk of peginterferon alfa;

do not administer HIV-active medications in the absence

• Periodically monitor serum bilirubin (total and direct), serum creatinine, urinalysis, LFTs, amylase, lipase

• Pregnancy: obtain pregnancy testing prior to use; hepatitis B exacerbation: those with coexisting HBV and HIV infections who discontinue this product may experience severe acute hepatitis B exacerbation with some cases resulting in hepatic decompensation and hepatic failure

Evaluate

• **Therapeutic response:** Improvement in CD4, HIV RNC counts, decreasing signs and symptoms of HIV

Teach patient/family

• That hepatitis and HIV coinfected patients should avoid consuming alcohol; offer vaccinations against hepatitis A/hepatitis B as appropriate

• That GI complaints resolve after 2-3 wk of treatment

• To report suspected or planned pregnancy, not to breastfeed. Instruct mothers with HIV-1 infection not to breastfeed because HIV-1 can be passed to the baby in the breast milk, inform patients that there is an antiretroviral pregnancy registry to monitor fetal outcomes

• To take at the same time of day to maintain blood level; not to crush, break, or chew

• That product controls the symptoms of HIV but does not cure, that patient is still able to infect others, that other products may be necessary to prevent other infections

• **Lactic acidosis:** to notify prescriber of fatigue, muscle aches/pains, abdominal pain, difficulty breathing, nausea, vomiting, change in heart rhythm

---

Black Box Warning: Hepatotoxicity: To notify prescriber of dark urine, yellowing skin or eyes, clay-colored stools, anorexia, nausea, vomiting

---

• Discuss with provider all Rx, OTC, herbs and supplements taken, as there are many drug interactions

• **Immune reconstitution syndrome:** advise patients to inform their health care provider immediately of any signs and symptoms of infection, as inflammation from previous infection may occur

• Instruct patients that if they miss a dose, to take it as soon as they remember, not to double their next dose or take more than the prescribed dose

---

dolutegravir/rilpivirine (Rx)

(doe-loo-teg′ra-vir/ril-pi-vir′een)

Juluca

Func. class.: Antiretroviral/antiviral

Chem. class.: INST/NRTI

ACTION:

Rilpivirine is a nucleoside analog that inhibits HIV reverse transcriptase; dolutegravir inhibits the catalytic activity of HIV integrase

USES:

HIV-1 infection in adults

CONTRAINDICATIONS

Hypersensitivity

Precautions: Alcoholism, autoimmune disease, bone fractures, breastfeeding, children, depression, females, Graves disease, Guillain-Barré syndrome, hepatic disease, hepatitis, hepatitis B and HIV coinfection, hepatitis C and HIV coinfection, hepatomegaly, HIV resistance, hypercholesterolemia, hyperlipidemia, hypertriglyceridemia, hypophosphatemia, immune reconstitution syndrome, lactic acidosis, obesity, osteomalacia, osteoporosis, pregnancy, renal failure, renal impairment, serious rash, suicidal ideation, torsades de pointes

---

Black Box Warning: Hepatitis B exacerbation, hepatotoxicity

DOSAGE AND ROUTES

Adults: PO 1 tablet 50 mg dolutegravir; 25 mg rilpivirine daily

---

Available forms: Tablet 50 mg dolutegravir, 25 mg rilpviirine
Administer:
• Give without regard to food
• During coadministration with carBAMazepine or rifAMPin, the dolutegravir dose needs to be increased to 50 mg bid; add 50 mg/day of dolutegravir (separated by 12 hr from dolutegravir; lamivudine) should be given
• Avoid use in treatment-experienced patients and in patients with known substitutions associated with resistance to dolutegravir or lamivudine
• Do not use within 2 hr prior to or 6 hr after iron or calcium supplement
• Do not use within 2 hr prior to or 6 hr after antacids, laxatives, or other medicines that contain aluminum, magnesium, sucralfate, or buffered medicines
• Admixtures are stable for at least 24 hr at room temperature under normal room fluorescent light in Baxter Viaflex PVC infusion containers

SIDE EFFECTS

CNS: Headache, abnormal dreams, depression, dizziness, insomnia, neuropathy, paresthesia, asthenia, fatigue, drowsiness
GI: Nausea, vomiting, anorexia, diarrhea, abdominal pain, dyspepsia **hepatomegaly with stenosis (may be fatal)**, hyperbilirubinemia, hypercholesterolemia, **pancreatitis**
GU: Glomerulonephritis membranous/mesangial proliferative
INTEG: Rash, skin discoloration
MS: Arthralgia, myalgia, **rhabdomyolysis**
RESP: Cough
SYST: Change in body fat distribution, lactic acidosis

PHARMACOKINETICS

• **Rilpivirine:** Onset unknown, peak 4 hr, duration unknown, half-life 50 hr
• **Dolutegravir:** 99% protein binding, metabolism occurs via UDP-glucuronosyltransferase (UGT)1A1 (major) and by the hepatic isoenzyme CYP3A (minor), half-life 14 hr, 53% excreted unchanged in the feces, urine excretion 31%

INTERACTIONS

Decreased levels, virologic resistance-CYP3A4 inhibitors (aldesleukin IL-2, amiodarone, aprepitant, atazanavir, basiliximab, boceprevir, bromocriptine, chloramphenicol, clarithromycin, conivaptan, danazol, dalfopristin, darunavir, dasatinib, delavirdine, dilTIAZem, dronedarone, efavirenz, erythromycin, ethinyl estradiol, fluconazole, fluoxetine, fluvoxamine, fosamprenavir, fosaprepitant, imatinib, indinavir, isoniazid, itraconazole, ketoconazole, lanreotide, lapatinib, miconazole, nefazodone, nelfinavir, nicardipine, octreotide, posaconazole, quinine, ranolazine, rifAXIMin, tamoxifen, telaprevir, telithromycin, tipranavir, troleandomycin, verapamil, voriconazole, zafirlukast)
Increased: metFORMIN
Increased: dofetilide, coadministration is contraindicated
Decrease: dolutegravir—carBAMazepine, rifAMPin, an additional dolutegravir 50-mg dose should be taken
Decrease: dolutegravir—OXcarbazepine, phenytoin, phenobarbital, avoid coadministration
Drug/Lab Test:
Increase: AST/ALT, amylase, bilirubin, CK, glucose, lipase
Decrease: neutrophils

NURSING CONSIDERATIONS
Assess:
• **HIV infection:** Assess symptoms of HIV, including opportunistic infections, prior to and during treatment, some may be life threatening; monitor plasma CD4+, CD8 cell counts, serum beta-2 microglobulin, serum antigen levels, treatment failures occur more often in those with baseline HIV-1 RNA concentrations <100,000 copies/mL than in those <100,000 copies/mL; monitor blood glucose, CBC with differential, serum cholesterol, lipid panel

Black Box Warning: Hepatotoxicity/lactic acidosis: Monitor hepatitis B serology, LFTs, plasma hepatitis C RNA, lactic acidosis levels. If lab reports confirm these conditions, discontinue product. More common in females or those who are overweight. Avoid use in alcoholism

Side effects: *italics* = common; red = life-threatening

- Patients coinfected with HBV and HIV who discontinue this product should have transaminase concentrations monitored q6wk for the first 3 mo, and q3-6 mo thereafter
- Resumption of anti–hepatitis B treatment may be required
- Periodically monitor serum bilirubin (total and direct), serum creatinine, urinalysis, LFTs, amylase, lipase
- **Pregnancy:** Obtain pregnancy testing prior to use; hepatitis B exacerbation: those with coexisting HBV and HIV infections who discontinue this product may experience severe acute hepatitis B exacerbation with some cases resulting in hepatic decompensation and hepatic failure

Evaluate:
- Therapeutic response: improvement in CD4, HIV RNC counts, decreasing signs and symptoms of HIV

Teach patient/family:
- That hepatitis and HIV coinfected patients should avoid consuming alcohol; offer vaccinations against hepatitis A/hepatitis B as appropriate
- That GI complaints resolve after 2-3 wk of treatment
- To report suspected or planned pregnancy, not to breastfeed. Instruct mothers with HIV-1 infection not to breastfeed because HIV-1 can be passed to the baby in the breast milk, inform patients that there is an antiretroviral pregnancy registry to monitor fetal outcomes
- To take at the same time of day to maintain blood level; not to crush, break, or chew
- That product controls the symptoms of HIV but does not cure, that patient is still able to infect others, that other products may be necessary to prevent other infections
- **Lactic acidosis:** to notify prescriber of fatigue, muscle aches/pains, abdominal pain, difficulty breathing, nausea, vomiting, change in heart rhythm

Black Box Warning: Hepatotoxicity: to notify prescriber of dark urine, yellowing skin or eyes, clay-colored stools, anorexia, nausea, vomiting

- Discuss with provider all Rx, OTC, herbs, and supplements taken, as there are many drug interactions
- **Immune reconstitution syndrome:** Advise patients to inform their health care provider immediately of any signs and symptoms of infection, as inflammation from previous infection may occur
- Instruct patients that if they miss a dose, to take it as soon as they remember, not to double their next dose or take more than the prescribed dose

donepezil (Rx)
(doe-nep′i-zill)
Aricept, Aricept ODT
Func. class.: Anti-Alzheimer's agent
Chem. class.: Reversible cholinesterase inhibitor

Do not confuse:
Aricept/Aciphex/Azilect

ACTION: Elevates acetylcholine concentrations (cerebral cortex) by slowing degradation of acetylcholine released in cholinergic neurons; does not alter underlying dementia

USES: Mild to severe dementia with Alzheimer's disease

CONTRAINDICATIONS
Hypersensitivity to this product or piperidine derivatives
Precautions: Pregnancy, breastfeeding, children, sick sinus syndrome, history of ulcers, GI bleeding, hepatic disease, bladder obstruction, asthma, seizures, COPD, abrupt discontinuation, AV block, GI obstruction, Parkinson's disease, surgery

DOSAGE AND ROUTES
- **Adult: PO** 5 mg/day at bedtime; may increase to 10 mg/day after 4-6 wk, may increase to 23 mg/day after 3 mo of 10 mg/day (moderate to severe)
Available forms: Tablets 5, 10, 23, mg; tablets ODT 5, 10 mg

Administer:
• Give between meals, may give with meals for GI symptoms
• Allow ODT to dissolve on tongue, then drink water
• Do not chew, crush, break

SIDE EFFECTS

CNS: Dizziness, *insomnia, headache,* fatigue, abnormal dreams, syncope, seizures, drowsiness, agitation, depression, confusion, hallucinations
CV: Atrial fibrillation, hypo/hypertension
GI: *Nausea, vomiting,* anorexia, *diarrhea,* abdominal pain, weight gain
GU: Urinary frequency
INTEG: Rash, flushing, diaphoresis, bruising
MS: Cramps, arthritis, arthralgia, back pain

PHARMACOKINETICS

Well absorbed PO; metabolized by CYP2D6, CYP3A4; half-life 10-hr single dose, 70-hr multiple doses; protein binding 96%

INTERACTIONS

Increase: donepezil effects—CYP2D6, CYP3A4 inhibitors
Increase: synergistic effect—succinylcholine, cholinesterase inhibitors, cholinergic agonists
Increase: GI bleeding—NSAIDs
Decrease: donepezil effects—CYP2D6, CYP3A4 inducers
Decrease: action of anticholinergics
Increase: QT prolongation—dofetilide, dronedarone, grepafloxacin, mesoridazine, pimozide, probucol, sparfloxacin, ziprasidone; do not use concurrently
Decrease: donepezil effect—carBAMazepine, dexamethasone, phenytoin, PHENobarbital, rifAMPin
Drug/Herb
Decrease: donepezil—St. John's wort
Drug/Lab
Increase: CK

NURSING CONSIDERATIONS

Assess:
• **Alzheimer's disease:** ADLs, memory, language, confusion baseline and during treatment

• B/P: hypo/hypertension, heart rate, ECG, QT
• Mental status: affect, mood, behavioral changes, depression, complete neurologic status
• GI status: nausea, vomiting, anorexia, diarrhea; monitor weight, active/occult GI bleeding
• GU status: urinary frequency, incontinence, I&O
• **Beers:** avoid use in older adults; increases risk of hypotension/bradycardia
• **Pregnancy/breastfeeding:** no well-controlled studies; use only if benefit outweighs fetal risk; avoid breastfeeding, excretion is unknown
Evaluate:
• Therapeutic response: decrease in confusion; improved mood, memory
Teach patient/family:
• To report side effects: twitching, nausea, vomiting, sweating, dizziness; indicates cholinergic crisis or overdose
• That continuing follow-up will be needed
• To use product exactly as prescribed, not to use with other products unless approved by prescriber
• To notify prescriber of nausea, vomiting, diarrhea (dose increase or beginning treatment), or rash
• Not to increase or abruptly decrease dose; serious side effects may result
• That product is not a cure, relieves symptoms
• To report if pregnancy is planned or suspected; to avoid breastfeeding

> **⚠ HIGH ALERT**

DOPamine (Rx)
(dope′a-meen)
Func. class.: Adrenergic
Chem. class.: Catecholamine

Do not confuse:
DOPamine/DOBUTamine

ACTION: Causes increased cardiac output; acts on β_1- and α-receptors, causing vasoconstriction in blood vessels; low dose causes renal and mesenteric vasodilation; β_1 stimulation produces inotropic effects with increased cardiac output

USES: Shock, increased perfusion, hypotension, cardiogenic/septic shock

CONTRAINDICATIONS
Hypersensitivity, ventricular fibrillation, tachydysrhythmias, pheochromocytoma, hypovolemia

Precautions: Pregnancy, breastfeeding, geriatric patients, arterial embolism, peripheral vascular disease, sulfite hypersensitivity, acute MI

> **Black Box Warning:** Extravasation

DOSAGE AND ROUTES
Shock
• **Adult: IV INFUSION** 2-5 mcg/kg/min, titrate upward in 5-10 mcg/kg/min increments, max 50 mcg/kg/min; titrate to patient's response

Bradycardia (unlabeled)
• **Adult: IV** 2-10 mcg/kg/min, titrate as needed

Available forms: Injection 40 mg, 80 mg, 160 mg/mL; concentrations for IV infusion 0.8, 1.6, 3.2 mg/mL in 250, 500 mL D_5W

Administer:
• Correct volume depletion prior to use
• Store reconstituted solution for up to 24 hr if refrigerated
• Do not use discolored solution; protect from light

IV route
• IV after diluting 200-400 mg/250-500 mL of D_5W, $D_50.45\%NaCl$, $D_50.9\%NaCl$, D_5LR, LR; use large vein
• After reconstituting, use infusion pump; give at rate of 0.5-5 mcg/kg/min, increase by 1-4 mcg/kg/min at 10-30 min intervals until desired response, titrate as needed, decrease infusion gradually

> **Black Box Warning: Extravasation:** if extravasation occurs, stop infusion; may inject area with phentolamine 10 mg/15 mL of NS

Y-site compatibilities: Alfentanil, alprostadil, amifostine, amikacin, aminocaproic acid, aminophylline, amiodarone, anidulafungin, argatroban, ascorbic acid injection, atenolol, atracurium, atropine, aztreonam, benztropine, bivalirudin, bleomycin, bumetanide, buprenorphine, butorphanol, calcium chloride/gluconate, CARBOplatin, caspofungin, cefmetazole, cefonicid, cefotaxime, cefoTEtan, cefOXitin, cefTAZidime, ceftizoxime, cefTRIAXone, cefuroxime, chlorproMAZINE, cimetidine, ciprofloxacin, cisatracurium, CISplatin, cladribine, clarithromycin, clindamycin, cloNIDine, codeine, cyanocobalamin, cyclophosphamide, cycloSPORINE, cytarabine, DACTINomycin, DAPTOmycin, dexamethasone, dexmedetomidine, digoxin, diltiazem, diphenhydrAMINE, DOBUTamine, DOCEtaxel, doripenem, doxacurium, DOXOrubicin, DOXOrubicin liposomal, doxycycline, droperidol, enalaprilat, ePHEDrine, EPINEPHrine, epirubicin, epoetin alfa, eptifibatide, ertapenem, erythromycin, esmolol, etoposide, famotidine, fenoldopam, fentaNYL, fluconazole, fludarabine, fluorouracil, folic acid, foscarnet, gatifloxacin, gemcitabine, gemtuzumab, gentamicin, glycopyrrolate, granisetron, heparin, hydrocortisone, HYDROmorphone, hydrOXYzine, IDArubicin, ifosfamide, imipenem-cilastatin, irinotecan, isoproterenol, ketorolac, labetalol, levofloxacin, lidocaine, linezolid, LORazepam, LR, magnesium sulfate, mannitol, mechlorethamine, meperidine, methicillin, methyldopate, methylPREDNISolone, metoclopramide, metoprolol, metroNIDAZOLE, micafungin, miconazole, midazolam, milrinone, minocycline, mitoXANtrone, morphine, multiple vitamins injection, mycophenolate, nafcillin, nalbuphine, naloxone, netilmicin, niCARdipine, nitroglycerin, nitroprusside, norepinephrine, octreotide, ondansetron, oxacillin, oxaliplatin, oxytocin, PACLitaxel, palonosetron, pamidronate, pancuronium, pantoprazole, papaverine, PEMEtrexed, penicillin G potassium/sodium, pentamidine, pentazocine, PENTobarbital, PHENobarbital, phenylephrine, phytonadione, piperacillin, piperacillin-tazobactam, polymyxin B, potassium chloride, procainamide, prochlorperazine, promethazine, propofol, propranolol, protamine, pyridoxine, quiNIDine, ranitidine, remifentanil, Ringer's, ritodrine, riTUXimab, rocuronium, sargramostim, sodium acetate, succinylcholine, SUFentanil, tacrolimus, temocillin, teniposide, theophylline, thiamine, thiotepa, ticarcillin, ticarcillin-clavulanate, tigecycline, tirofiban, TNA, tobramycin, tolazoline, TPN, trastuzumab, trimetaphan, urokinase, vancomycin, vasopressin, vecuronium, verapamil, vinCRIStine, vinorelbine, vitamin B complex/C, voriconazole, warfarin, zidovudine, zoledronic acid

SIDE EFFECTS

CNS: *Headache,* anxiety
CV: *Palpitations, angina,* wide QRS complex, peripheral vasoconstriction, hypotension
GI: *Nausea, vomiting, diarrhea*
INTEG: Necrosis, tissue sloughing with extravasation
RESP: Dyspnea

PHARMACOKINETICS

IV: Onset 5 min; duration <10 min; metabolized in liver, kidney, plasma; excreted in urine (metabolites); half-life 2 min

INTERACTIONS

• Do not use within 2 wk of MAOIs; hypertensive crisis may result
Increase: bradycardia, hypotension—phenytoin
Increase: dysrhythmias—general anesthetics
Increase: severe hypertension—ergots
Increase: B/P—oxytocics
Increase: pressor effect—tricyclics, MAOIs
Decrease: DOPamine action—beta-/alpha-blockers
Drug/Lab Test
Increase: urinary catecholamine, serum glucose

NURSING CONSIDERATIONS
Assess:
• Hypovolemia; if present, correct first
• **Oxygenation/perfusion   deficit:** check B/P, chest pain, dizziness, loss of consciousness

• **Heart failure:** S$_3$ gallop, dyspnea, neck venous distention, bibasilar crackles in patients with HF, cardiomyopathy, palpate peripheral pulses
• I&O ratio: if urine output decreases without decrease in B/P, product may need to be reduced
• **ECG** during administration continuously; if B/P increases, product should be decreased; PCWP, CVP during infusion
• B/P, pulse q5min
• Paresthesias and coldness of extremities; peripheral blood flow may decrease
• **Pregnancy/breastfeeding:** no well-controlled studies; use only if benefit outweighs fetal risk, may cause toxicity; avoid use in breastfeeding, excretion is unknown
Evaluate:
• Therapeutic response: increased B/P with stabilization; increased urine output
Teach patient/family:
• About the reason for product administration
• To report immediately chest pain, shortness of breath, numbness/tingling of extremities
• To report immediately pain, burning, redness at IV site

TREATMENT OF OVERDOSE:
Discontinue IV, may give a short-acting alpha-adrenergic blocker

---

doravirine (Rx)
(dor'a-vir'een)
Pifeltro
Func. class.: Antiviral
Chem. class.: Nonnucleoside reverse transcriptase inhibitor (NNRTI)

USES: Human immunodeficiency virus (HIV) infection in antiretroviral-naive adults in combination with other antiretrovirals

CONTRAINDICATIONS
Hypersensitivity

DOSAGE AND ROUTES
• **Adult: PO** 100 mg daily; when given with rifabutin 100 mg q12hr

---

doravirine/lamivudine/ tenofovir (Rx)
(dor′a-vir′een/lam-i-voo′deen/ ten-oh-foh′veer)

Delstrigo
Func. class.: Antiretroviral
Chem. class.: Nonnucleoside reverse transcriptase inhibitor (NNRTI), nucleoside reverse transcriptase inhibitor (NRTI)

USES: Human immunodeficiency virus (HIV) infection in antiretroviral-naive adults

CONTRAINDICATIONS
Hypersensitivity
Precautions: Alcoholism, autoimmune disorders, bipolar disease, breastfeeding, children, depression, driving or operating hazardous machinery, geriatric patients, Graves' disease, Guillain-Barré syndrome, hepatic disease, hepatitis B and HIV coinfection, hepatitis C and HIV coinfection, HIV resistance, immune reconstitution syndrome, pregnancy, psychosis, substance abuse

Black Box Warning: Hepatitis B exacerbation

DOSAGE AND ROUTES
• **Adult: PO** 1 tablet (doravirine 100 mg; lamivudine 300 mg; tenofovir disoproxil fumarate 300 mg) daily

Concurrent treatment with rifabutin
• **Adult: PO** 1 tablet (doravirine 100 mg; lamivudine 300 mg; tenofovir disoproxil fumarate 300 mg) daily, then 12 hr later, give an additional 100 mg of doravirine by mouth each day of rifabutin concurrent therapy

---

dorzolamide (Rx) (ophthalmic)
(dor-zole′ah-mide)

Trusopt
Func. class.: Antiglaucoma
Chem. class.: Carbonic anhydrase inhibitor

USES: For the treatment of elevated intraocular pressure in patients with ocular hypertension or open-angle glaucoma

CONTRAINDICATIONS
Hypersensitivity
Precautions: Hypersensitivity to sulfonamides, hepatic/renal disease, angle-closure glaucoma, electrolyte disturbances

DOSAGE AND ROUTES
• **Adult/adolescent/child/infant/neonate ≥1 wk: Ophthalmic** Instill 1 drop of a 2% solution into the affected eye(s) tid

---

dostarlimab-gxly (Rx)
(dos-TAR-li-mab-gxly)

Jemperli
Func. class.: Antineoplastic, misc
Chem. class.: PD-1 blocking antibody

ACTION: Binds PD-1 ligands to the PD-1 receptor found on T cells, inhibits T-cell proliferation and cytokine production

USES: Endometrial cancer, solid tumors

CONTRAINDICATIONS
Hypersensitivity, pregnancy, breastfeeding
Precautions: Immune-mediated adverse reactions, pneumonitis, respiratory disorders

DOSAGE AND ROUTES

- **Adult: : IV INF** dose 1 through dose 4: 500 mg q3wk; then dose 5 onwards 1000 mg q6wk, give over 30 min

Available forms: Injection 500-mg/10-mL (50 mg/mL) single-dose vial

Administer:

- Visually inspect the solution for particulate matter and discoloration; the solution is clear to slightly opalescent, colorless to yellow
- Discard the vial if visible particles are observed
- Do not shake
- Discard the vial if visible particles are observed
- For the 500-mg dose, withdraw 10 mL of product and dilute in an IV infusion bag with 0.9% Sodium Chloride Injection USP or 5% Dextrose Injection USP (2-10 mg/mL; max 250 mL). Compatible infusion bags are polyolefin, ethylene vinyl acetate, or polyvinyl chloride with DEHP
- For the 1000-mg dose, withdraw 10 mL from each of 2 vials (withdraw 20 mL total) and dilute in an IV bag containing 0.9% Sodium Chloride Injection USP or 5% Dextrose Injection USP (4-10 mg/mL; max 250 mL)
- Mix by gentle inversion; do not shake
- Discard unused portion
- Storage: protect from light; store prepared solution at room temperature for up to 6 hr from the time of preparation until the end of infusion or refrigerated at 2° C-8° C (36°F-46°F) for up to 24 hr from time of preparation until end of infusion, allow the diluted solution to come to room temperature before use; do not freeze
- Give over 30 min through an IV line using tubing made of polyvinyl chloride or platinum-cured silicon; fittings made of polyvinyl chloride or polycarbonate; and a sterile, nonpyrogenic, low-protein-binding, 0.2-micron, in-line or add-on filter
- Do not admix or run drugs through the same infusion line

SIDE EFFECTS

CNS: Fatigue, asthenia, neurologic toxicities

GI: Diarrhea, nausea, vomiting, constipation, hepatitis, colitis

INTEG: Infusion-related reactions

CV: Myocarditis

GU: Nephritis

RESP: Pneumonitis

INTERACTIONS

None known

Lab/Drug Test

Increase: alkaline phosphatase

Decrease: lymphocytes, sodium, albumin

PHARMACOKINETICS

Half-life 23.5 days

NURSING CONSIDERATIONS

Assess:

- **Severe and fatal immune-mediated adverse reactions:** During and after last dose. Monitor for symptoms/signs that may be immune-mediated adverse reactions. Monitor LFTs, creatinine, and thyroid function tests baseline and periodically during treatment. In cases of suspected immune-mediated adverse reactions
- **Transplant-related complications:** Closely monitor for febrile syndrome, GVHD, may be fatal
- **Pregnancy/breastfeeding:** Do not use in pregnancy or breastfeeding, verify pregnancy status in those of reproductive potential before starting therapy, use effective contraception during and for 4 mo after last dose
- Infusion-related reactions: Assess for burning, redness, inflammation at the site; interrupt or slow infusion or discontinue if severe

Evaluate:

- Therapeutic response
- Decreasing spread of endometrial cancer, solid tumors.

Teach patient/family:

- **Pregnancy/breastfeeding:** Not to use in pregnancy and breastfeeding, a pregnancy test will be obtained before starting treatment in those of pregnancy potential, use effective contraception during and for 4 mo after last dose

---

doxazosin (Rx)

(dox-ay′zoe-sin)

Cardura, Cardura XL

Func. class.: Peripheral α$_1$-adrenergic receptor blocker

Chem. class.: Quinazoline

Do not confuse:

Cardura/Coumadin/Cardene/Ridaura

ACTION: Dilates peripheral blood vessels, lowers peripheral resistance; reduction in B/P results from peripheral α$_1$-adrenergic receptors being blocked

USES: Hypertension, urinary outflow obstruction, symptoms of benign prostatic hyperplasia

CONTRAINDICATIONS

Hypersensitivity to quinazolines

Precautions: Pregnancy, breastfeeding, children, hepatic disease, geriatric patients

DOSAGE AND ROUTES

BPH

• **Adult: PO** 1 mg/day at bedtime; increase in stepwise manner to 2, 4, 8 mg/day as needed at 1-2 wk intervals, max 8 mg; extended-release tablet (Cardura XL) 4 mg daily with breakfast, adjust dose q3-4wk, up to 8 mg daily

Hypertension

• **Adult: PO** 1 mg/day at bedtime, increasing gradually up to 16 mg/day if required; usual range 4-16 mg/day

• **Geriatric: PO** 0.5 mg nightly, gradually increase

Available forms: Tablets 1, 2, 4, 8 mg; extended-release tablets 4, 8 mg

Administer:

• Store in tight container at room temperature

• **Tablets:** may be broken, crushed, or chewed; if chewed, will be bitter; do not break, crush, chew XL tablets

• **Immediate-release tablet:** without regard to meals; **extended-release tablets:** give with breakfast; when switching from immediate release to extended release, the final evening dose of immediate release should not be taken

SIDE EFFECTS

CNS: *Dizziness, headache,* drowsiness, anxiety, depression, *vertigo,* weakness, fatigue

CV: Palpitations, *orthostatic hypotension,* tachycardia, *edema,* dysrhythmias, chest pain

EENT: Epistaxis, tinnitus, dry mouth, red sclera, pharyngitis, rhinitis, blurred vision

GI: *Nausea,* vomiting, diarrhea, constipation, abdominal pain, hepatitis

GU: Priapism, impotence, decreased libido

RESP: Dyspnea

PHARMACOKINETICS

PO: Onset 2 hr, peak 2-3 hr, duration up to 24 hr, half-life 22 hr, metabolized in liver, excreted via bile/feces (<63%) and in urine (9%), extensively protein bound (98%)

INTERACTIONS

Increase: hypotensive effects—alcohol, other antihypertensives, nitrates, PDE-5 inhibitors, CYP3A4 inhibitors, monitor B/P

Decrease: hypotensive effects—NSAIDs, estrogens, sympathomimetics

Drug/Herb

Decrease: Ma huang

Drug/Lab

Decrease: WBCs, neutrophils

NURSING CONSIDERATIONS

Assess:

• **Hypertension:** B/P (lying, standing), pulse 2-6 hr after each dose, with each increase; postural effects may occur, crackles, dyspnea, orthopnea with increased B/P; increased pulse; jugular venous distention during beginning treatment

• **BPH:** urinary pattern changes (hesitancy, dribbling, incomplete bladder emptying, dysuria, urgency, nocturia, urgency incontinence, intermittency) before and during treatment

• I&O, weight daily; edema in feet, legs daily

• **Pregnancy/breastfeeding:** no well-controlled studies; use only if clearly needed; use caution in breastfeeding (immediate release), avoid use with extended release

Evaluate:
• Therapeutic response: decreased B/P; decreased symptoms of BPH

Teach patient/family:
• That fainting occasionally occurs after first dose; not to drive, operate machinery for 4 hr after first dose, after dosage increase; to take first dose at bedtime; may take 1-2 wk to respond with BPH
• To rise slowly from sitting position
• To comply with hypertension regimen: low-sodium diet, exercise, weight reduction, stress management; not to smoke
• How to take B/P, to check at least once/wk
• For male to notify prescriber of erection >4 hr or priapism
• To notify all health care providers of all Rx and OTC medications and herbal supplements; not to add any products unless approved by prescriber
• To avoid hazardous activities until response is known; dizziness or drowsiness may occur
• To continue to take product even if feeling better; to take at same time each day, not to double doses

TREATMENT OF OVERDOSE:
Administer volume expanders or vasopressors; discontinue product; place patient in supine position

⚠ HIGH ALERT

doxepin (Rx)
(dox′e-pin)
Sinequan ✦, Silenor
Func. class.: Antidepressant, tricyclic, antihistamine (topical)
Chem. class.: Dibenzoxepine, tertiary amine

Do not confuse:
Sinequan/Seroquel/Saquinavir/Singulair/Zonegran

ACTION: Blocks reuptake of norepinephrine, serotonin into nerve endings, increasing action of norepinephrine, serotonin in nerve cells

USES: Major depression, anxiety; *topical:* lichen simplex, atopic dermatitis, eczema, insomnia, migraine prophylaxis
Unlabeled uses: Topical pruritus

CONTRAINDICATIONS
Hypersensitivity to tricyclics, urinary retention, closed-angle glaucoma, prostatic hypertrophy, acute recovery from MI
Precautions: Pregnancy, breastfeeding, geriatric patients, seizures

Black Box Warning: Children, suicidal patients

DOSAGE AND ROUTES
Depression/anxiety
• **Adult: PO** 50-75 mg/day, may increase to 300 mg/day for severely ill; give in divided doses if >150 mg/day
• **Geriatric: PO** 25-50 mg at bedtime, increase weekly by 25-50 mg to desired dose, max 150 mg/day
Pruritus
• **Adult: PO** 10 mg at bedtime, may increase to 25 mg at bedtime; **TOPICAL** apply thin film qid at least 3 hr apart
Insomnia (Silenor)
• **Adult: PO** 6 mg 30 min prior to bedtime, 3 mg may be sufficient, max 6 mg/night
Available forms: Capsules 10, 25, 50, 75, 100, 150 mg; oral concentrations 10 mg/mL; tablets (Silenor) 3, 6 mg
Administer:
• **Oral concentrations:** should be diluted with 120 mL water; milk; or orange, grapefruit, tomato, prune, or pineapple juice; do not mix with grape juice
• Increased fluids, bulk in diet for constipation
• With food, milk for GI symptoms; do not give with carbonated beverages

• Dosage at bedtime to avoid oversedation during day; may take entire dose at bedtime; geriatric patients may not tolerate daily dosing

• Gum, hard candy, or frequent sips of water for dry mouth

• Store in tight container protected from direct sunlight

SIDE EFFECTS
CNS: *Dizziness, drowsiness,* confusion, headache, anxiety, tremors, stimulation, weakness, insomnia, nightmares, EPS (geriatric patients), increased psychiatric symptoms, paresthesia, suicidal ideation
CV: *Orthostatic hypotension, ECG changes, tachycardia,* hypertension, palpitations, dysrhythmias
EENT: *Blurred vision,* tinnitus, mydriasis, ophthalmoplegia, glossitis
GI: *Diarrhea, dry mouth,* nausea, vomiting, paralytic ileus, increased appetite, cramps, epigastric distress, jaundice, hepatitis, stomatitis, constipation
GU: *Urinary retention,* acute renal failure
HEMA: Agranulocytosis, thrombocytopenia, eosinophilia, leukopenia, pancytopenia, purpuric disorder
INTEG: Rash, urticaria, sweating, pruritus, photosensitivity

PHARMACOKINETICS
PO: Peak 2 hr, metabolized in liver by CYP2C19/CYP2D6, which exert genetic polymorphism; Asians, Black patients may be poor metabolizers; excreted by kidneys, crosses placenta, excreted in breast milk, half-life 8-24 hr

INTERACTIONS
Increase: hyperpyretic crisis, seizures, hypertensive episode—MAOIs
Increase: hypertensive action—EPINEPHrine, norepinephrine
Increase: hypertensive crisis—cloNIDine; do not use together
Increase: doxepin effect—cimetidine, FLUoxetine, fluvoxaMINE, PARoxetine, sertraline

Increase: CNS depression—barbiturates, benzodiazepines, sedative/hypnotics, alcohol, other CNS depressants
Increase: QT interval—class IC/III antiarrhythmics (propafenone, flecainide), quinolones
Increase: serotonin syndrome, toxicity—SSRIs, SNRIs, serotonin-receptor agonists, triptans
Increase: anticholinergic effects—anticholinergics
Drug/Herb
Serotonin syndrome: St. John's wort; avoid using together
Drug/Lab Test
Increase: serum bilirubin, blood glucose, alkaline phosphatase, LFTs

NURSING CONSIDERATIONS
Assess:
• B/P (lying, standing), pulse q4hr; if systolic B/P drops 20 mm Hg, hold product, notify prescriber; VS q4hr in patients with CV disease
• Blood studies: CBC, leukocytes, differential, cardiac enzymes if patient is receiving long-term therapy
• Hepatic studies: AST, ALT, bilirubin
• Weight weekly; appetite may increase with product
• **ECG** for flattening of T wave, bundle branch block, AV block, dysrhythmias in cardiac patients; product should be discontinued gradually several days prior to surgery
• **EPS** primarily in geriatric patients: rigidity, dystonia, akathisia
• **Depression:** mood, sensorium, affect, suicidal tendencies, increase in psychiatric symptoms; assess often during initial treatment; restrict the amount of the product given to the patient
• **Chronic pain:** location, severity, type prior to and during treatment, alleviating/aggravating factors
• **Sexual dysfunction:** decreased libido and erectile dysfunction may occur
• Urinary retention, constipation; constipation most likely in children, geriatric patients

• **Withdrawal symptoms:** headache, nausea, vomiting, muscle pain, weakness; not usual unless product is discontinued abruptly

• Alcohol consumption; if alcohol is consumed, hold dose until morning

• Assistance with ambulation during beginning therapy because drowsiness/dizziness occurs; safety measures primarily for geriatric patients

• **Serotonin syndrome:** nausea, vomiting, diarrhea, agitation, hallucinations, hyperthermia, incoordination; may occur when used with other products known to cause serotonin syndrome

• **Beers:** avoid use in older adults; highly anticholinergic, sedating; causes orthostatic hypotension, may cause delirium

• **Pregnancy/breastfeeding:** no well-controlled studies; use only if benefit outweighs fetal risk; use caution in breastfeeding, excreted in breast milk

Evaluate:

• Therapeutic response: decreased anxiety, depression

Teach patient/family:

• That therapeutic effect (depression) may take 2-3 wk, antianxiety effects sooner

• To use caution when driving, during other activities requiring alertness because of drowsiness, dizziness, blurred vision

• To avoid alcohol, other CNS depressants; may potentiate effects; not to take other products unless approved by prescriber

• Not to discontinue medication abruptly after long-term use; may cause nausea, headache, malaise

• To wear sunscreen or large hat; photosensitivity occurs

• That clinical worsening and suicide may occur, usually in children, young adults ≤24 yr

• To immediately report urinary retention

TREATMENT OF OVERDOSE:

ECG monitoring; lavage, administer anticonvulsant, sodium bicarbonate

⚠ HIGH ALERT

DOXOrubicin (Rx)

(dox-oh-roo′bi-sin)

Adriamycin ✦

Func. class.: Antineoplastic, antibiotic

Chem. class.: Anthracycline glycoside

Do not confuse:

DOXOrubicin/DOXOrubicin liposomal/DAUNOrubicin

ACTION: Inhibits DNA synthesis primarily; replication is decreased by binding to DNA, which causes strand splitting; active throughout entire cell cycle; a vesicant

USES: Wilms' tumor; bladder, breast, lung, ovarian, stomach, thyroid cancer; Hodgkin's/non-Hodgkin's disease; acute lymphoblastic leukemia; myeloblastic leukemia; neuroblastomas; soft tissue/bone sarcomas

CONTRAINDICATIONS

Pregnancy, breastfeeding, hypersensitivity, systemic infections, cardiac disorders, severe myelosuppression, lifetime dose of 550 mg/m^2, hepatic disease

Precautions: Accidental exposure, cardiac disease, dental work, electrolyte imbalance, infection, hyperuricemia

Black Box Warning: Bone marrow suppression, extravasation, heart failure, secondary malignancy; requires an experienced clinician, IM/SUBCUT use

DOSAGE AND ROUTES

Any regimen may be used

• **Adult: IV** 60-75 mg/m^2 every 3 wk, or 25-30 mg/m^2 daily × 2-3 days, repeat q3-4wk or 20 mg/m^2/wk, or may be used in combination with other antineoplastics with 40-75 mg/m^2 every 21-28 days, max cumulative dose 550 mg/m^2 or 450 mg/m^2 if prior DAUNOrubicin, cyclophosphamide, mediastinal XRT

• **Child: IV** 30 mg/m^2/day × 3 days q4wk

Hepatic dose
• **Adult: IV** Bilirubin 1.2-3 mg/dL, give 50% of dose; bilirubin 3.1-5 mg/dL, give 25% of dose

Renal dose
• **Adult: IV** CCr <10 mL/min give 75% of dose

Available forms: Powder for injection 10, 20, 50 mg/vial; solution for injection 2 mg/mL

Administer:

IV route
• Give antiemetic 30-60 min prior to product to prevent vomiting
• Give allopurinol or sodium bicarbonate to maintain uric acid levels, alkalinization of urine
• **Use cytotoxic handling procedures:** inspect for particulate and discoloration prior to use

Black Box Warning: Do not give IM, SUBCUT

Black Box Warning: If extravasation occurs, stop infusion and complete via another vein, preferably in another limb, use dexrazoxane topically

• Aluminum needles may be used during administration; avoid aluminum during storage
• Rapid injection can cause facial flushing or erythema along the vein

Reconstitution:
• To avoid risks with reconstitution, the commercially available injection may be used; there are still risks involved in handling the injection
• Do not use diluents containing preservatives to reconstitute powder for injection
• Reconstitute 10, 20, 50, 100 mg of DOXOrubicin with 5, 10, 25, 50 mL, respectively, of nonbacteriostatic NS injection (2 mg/mL), shake until completely dissolved; use reconstituted solution within 24 hr; do not expose to sunlight

• **IV injection**
Inject reconstituted solution over >3-5 min via Y-site into a free-flowing IV infusion of NS or D$_5$W; a butterfly needle inserted into a large vein is preferred
• Increase fluid intake to 2-3 L/day to prevent urate, calculi formation
• Store at room temperature for 24 hr after reconstituting

Intermittent IV infusion
• May mix in 100-250 mL of 0.9% NaCl, give over 30-60 min

Y-site compatibilities: Alemtuzumab, alfentanil, amifostine, amikacin, anidulafungin, argatroban, aztreonam, bivalirudin, bleomycin, bumetanide, buprenorphine, butorphanol, calcium chloride/gluconate, CARBOplatin, carmustine, caspofungin, ceftizoxime, chlorproMAZINE, cimetidine, ciprofloxacin, CISplatin, cladribine, clindamycin, cyclophosphamide, cycloSPORINE, cytarabine, DACTINomycin, DAPTOmycin, dexamethasone, diltiazem, diphenhydrAMINE, DOBUTamine, DOCEtaxel, dolasetron, DOPamine, doripenem, doxycycline, droperidol, enalaprilat, ePHEDrine, EPINEPHrine, erythromycin, esmolol, etoposide, etoposide phosphate, famotidine, fenoldopam, fentaNYL, filgrastim, fluconazole, fludarabine, gemcitabine, gentamicin, granisetron, haloperidol, hydrocortisone, HYDROmorphone, ifosfamide, imipenem cilastatin, inamrinone, isoproterenol, ketorolac, labetalol, leucovorin, levorphanol, lidocaine, linezolid, LORazepam, mannitol, mechlorethamine, melphalan, meperidine, mesna, methotrexate, metoclopramide, metoprolol, metroNIDAZOLE, midazolam, milrinone, mitoMYcin, morphine, nalbuphine, naloxone, nesiritide, niCARdipine, nitroglycerin, nitroprusside, octreotide, ofloxacin, ondansetron, oxaliplatin, PACLitaxel, palonosetron, pancuronium, phenylephrine, potassium chloride, procainamide, prochlorperazine, promethazine, propranolol, quinupristin-dalfopristin, ranitidine, sargramostim, sodium acetate, tacrolimus, teniposide, theophylline, thiotepa, ticarcillin/clavulanate, tigecycline, tirofiban, tobramycin, topotecan, trastuzumab, trimethobenzamide, vancomycin, vaso-pressin, vecuronium, verapamil, vin-BLAStine, vinCRIStine, vinorelbine, zidovudine, zoledronic acid

SIDE EFFECTS

CV: Increased B/P, sinus tachycardia, PVCs, chest pain, bradycardia, extrasystoles, irreversible cardiomyopathy, acute left ventricular failure

GI: *Nausea, vomiting,* anorexia, *mucositis,* hepatotoxicity

GU: Impotence, sterility, amenorrhea, gynecomastia, hyperuricemia, urine discoloration

HEMA: Thrombocytopenia, leukopenia, anemia

RESP: Recall pneumonitis

INTEG: *Rash,* necrosis at injection site, dermatitis, reversible *alopecia,* cellulitis, thrombophlebitis at injection site, radiation recall

SYST: Anaphylaxis, secondary malignancy

PHARMACOKINETICS

Half-life 30 min, terminal 16.5 hr; metabolized by liver; crosses placenta; excreted in urine, bile, breast milk

INTERACTIONS

Increase: life-threatening dysrhythmias—posaconazole, fluconazole; do not use together

Increase: toxicity-CYP2D6 inhibitors, CYP3A4 inhibitors, P-glycoprotein inhibitors, avoid using together

Increase: QT prolongation—other drugs that increase QT prolongation

Increase: neutropenia, thrombocytopenia—progesterone

Increase: cardiomyopathy—calcium-channel blockers

Increase: toxicity—other antineoplastics, cycloSPORINE, radiation, mercaptopurine

Increase: hemorrhagic cystitis risk, cardiac toxicity—cyclophosphamide

Increase: effect of phenytoin, fosphenytoin

Increase: DOXOrubicin effect—streptozocin

Decrease: DOXOrubicin effect—PHENobarbital

Decrease: antibody response—live virus vaccine

Decrease: effect of CYP2D6 inducers, CYP3A4 inducers, P-glycoprotein inducers, avoid using together

Decrease: clearance of DOXOrubicin—PACLitaxel

Drug/Lab Test
Increase: uric acid

NURSING CONSIDERATIONS
Assess:

Black Box Warning: Bone marrow depression: CBC, differential, platelet count weekly; withhold or reduce dose of product if WBC is <1500/mm³ or platelet count is <50,000/mm³; notify prescriber of these results

• **Renal studies:** BUN, serum uric acid, urine CCr, electrolytes prior to, during therapy
• **I&O ratio:** report fall in urine output to <30 mL/hr
• **Monitor temperature:** fever might indicate beginning infection
• **Hepatotoxicity:** hepatic studies prior to, during therapy: bilirubin, AST, ALT, alkaline phosphatase as needed or monthly; check for jaundice of skin and sclera, dark urine, clay-colored stools, itchy skin, abdominal pain, fever, diarrhea

Black Box Warning: Dysrhythmias: ECG; watch for ST-T wave changes, low QRS and T, possible dysrhythmias (sinus tachycardia, heart block, PVCs), ejection fraction prior to treatment, signs of irreversible cardiomyopathy, can occur up to 6 mo after treatment begins

• Bleeding: hematuria, guaiac, bruising, petechiae of mucosa or orifices every 8 hr
• Effects of alopecia on body image; discuss feelings about body changes; almost total alopecia is expected
• Buccal cavity every 8 hr for dryness, sores, ulceration, white patches, oral pain, bleeding, dysphagia
• Alkalosis if severe vomiting is present

Side effects: *italics* = common; red = life-threatening

Black Box Warning: Secondary malignancy: assess for AML and MDS, which may occur

Black Box Warning: Extravasation: local irritation, pain, burning at injection site; a vesicant; if extravasation occurs, stop drug, restart at another site, apply ice, elevate extremity to reduce swelling; if resolution does not occur, surgical debridement may be required

• GI symptoms: frequency of stools, cramping
• Rinsing of mouth tid-qid with water, club soda; brushing of teeth bid-tid with soft brush or cotton-tipped applicators for stomatitis; use unwaxed dental floss
Evaluate:
• Therapeutic response: decreased tumor size, spread of malignancy
Teach patient/family:
• To add 2-3 L of fluids unless contraindicated prior to and for 24-48 hr after to decrease possible hemorrhagic cystitis
• To report any complaints, side effects to nurse or prescriber
• That hair may be lost during treatment; that wig or hairpiece might make patient feel better; that new hair might be different in color, texture
• That continuing follow-up and lab work will be needed
• To notify health care professional of trouble breathing; swelling of hands, feet; increase in weight; change in heart rate
• That body fluids should not be handled unless protective equipment is used
• To discuss OTC, Rx, herbals, supplements with health care professional
• To avoid foods with citric acid, hot temperature, or rough texture
• To report any bleeding, white spots, ulcerations in mouth to prescriber; to examine mouth daily
• That urine, other body fluids may be red-orange for 48 hr
• To avoid crowds and persons with infections when granulocyte count is low
• To avoid vaccinations

• **Pregnancy/breastfeeding:** that barrier contraceptive measures are recommended during therapy and for 4 mo after ending therapy; to avoid breastfeeding

---

⚠ HIGH ALERT

DOXOrubicin liposomal (Rx)
(dox-oh-roo′bi-sin)
Caelyx ✦, Doxil, Myocet ✦
Func. class.: Antineoplastic, antibiotic
Chem. class.: Anthracycline glycoside

Do not confuse:
DOXOrubicin/DOXOrubicin liposomal/DAUNOrubicin

ACTION: Inhibits DNA synthesis primarily; replication is decreased by binding to DNA, which causes strand splitting; active throughout entire cell cycle; a vesicant

USES: AIDS-related Kaposi's sarcoma, multiple myeloma, metastatic ovarian carcinoma, multiple myeloma, refractory metastatic breast cancer

CONTRAINDICATIONS
Pregnancy, breastfeeding, hypersensitivity
Precautions: Children, infection, leukopenia, stomatitis, thrombocytopenia, systemic infections, cardiac disorders

Black Box Warning: Cardiotoxicity, infusion reactions, myelosuppression, hepatic disease

DOSAGE AND ROUTES
Max lifetime cumulative dose 550 mg/m²; 400 mg/m² for those who have received other cardiotoxics or mediastinal radiation
Kaposi's sarcoma
• **Adult: IV** 20 mg/m² every 3 wk
Multiple myeloma
• **Adult: IV** 30 mg/m² IV infusion on day 4 every 3 wk plus bortezomib 1.3 mg/m²/dose IV bolus on days 1, 4, 8, 11 of each cycle; give DOXOrubicin liposomal after bortezomib receipt on day 4; administer up

to 8 treatment cycles or until disease progression or unacceptable toxicity occurs
Ovarian cancer
• **Adult: IV** 50 mg/m² q4wk
Refractory metastatic breast cancer
• **Adult: IV** 50 mg/m² q4wk
Hematologic toxicity in patients with ovarian cancer or HIV-related Kaposi's sarcoma
Grade 1 (ANC of 1500-1900/mm³, platelets ≥75,000/mm³): No dose reduction; **grade 2 (ANC of 1000-1499/mm³, platelets ≥50,000/mm³ and <75,000/mm³:** Wait until ANC ≥1500 cells/mm³ and platelets ≥75,000 cells/mm³; redose with no dose reduction; **grade 3 (ANC of 500-999/mm³, platelets ≥25,000/mm³ and <50,000/mm³):** Wait until ANC ≥1500 cells/mm³ and platelets ≥75,000 cells/mm³; redose with no dose reduction; **grade 4 (ANC <500/mm³, platelets <25,000/mm³):** Wait until ANC ≥1500 cells/mm³ and platelets ≥75,000 cells/mm³; reduce dose by 25% or continue with full dose with colony-stimulating factor
Available forms: Liposomal dispersion for injection: 2 mg/mL
Administer:
• Use cytotoxic protocol according to agency policy
• Prepared liposomal DOXOrubicin is translucent, red liposomal dispersion; visually inspect for particulate matter and discoloration prior to use
• Pegylated liposomal DOXOrubicin (Doxil) is for IV INFUSION use only and should not be given IM/SUBCUT; give under the supervision of a physician who is experienced in cancer chemotherapy

Black Box Warning: Care should be taken to avoid extravasation because the drug is irritating to extravascular tissue

• Premedication with antiemetics is recommended
IV route
• **Reconstitution (Doxil):** Dilute the appropriate dose, not to exceed 90 mg/250 mL D₅W; do not mix with any other diluent, drugs, or bacteriostatic agent; use aseptic technique; product contains no preservative or bacteriostatic agent; diluted solution must be refrigerated and used within 24 hr
• **IV INFUSION (Doxil):** Do not administer as a bolus injection or an undiluted solution; rapid injection can increase the risk of an infusion-related reaction

• An acute infusion reaction can occur during the first infusion and is usually resolved by slowing the rate of infusion; most patients can tolerate subsequent infusions

• **Rate:** Infuse at an initial rate of 1 mg/min; if no infusion-related action, the rate can be increased to complete the infusion over 1 hr; do not filter
• Give antiemetic 30-60 min prior to product to prevent vomiting
• Use allopurinol or sodium bicarbonate to maintain uric acid levels, alkalinization of urine
• Avoid mixing with other products
• Increase fluid intake to 2-3 L/day to prevent urate, calculi formation
• Store refrigerated for 24 hr after reconstituting

SIDE EFFECTS
CNS: Paresthesias, headache, depression, insomnia, fatigue, fever
CV: Chest pain, decreased B/P, cardiomyopathy, heart failure, dysrhythmias, tachycardia
EENT: Optic neuritis, rhinitis, pharyngitis, stomatitis
GI: *Nausea, vomiting,* anorexia, *mucositis,* hepatotoxicity, abdominal pain
HEMA: Thrombocytopenia, leukopenia, anemia, secondary malignancy
INTEG: *Rash,* necrosis at injection site, dermatitis, *reversible alopecia,* exfoliative dermatitis, palmar-plantar erythrodysesthesia, thrombophlebitis at injection site
RESP: Dyspnea, cough, respiratory infections

Side effects: *italics* = common; red = life-threatening

PHARMACOKINETICS

Half-life 55 hr; metabolized by liver; crosses placenta; excreted in urine, bile, breast milk

INTERACTIONS

Increase: life-threatening dysrhythmias—posaconazole, fluconazole; do not use together

Increase: QT prolongation—other drugs that increase QT prolongation

Increase: neutropenia, thrombocytopenia—progesterone

Increase: cardiomyopathy—calcium channel blockers

Increase: toxicity—other antineoplastics, cycloSPORINE, radiation, mercaptopurine

Increase: hemorrhagic cystitis risk, cardiac toxicity—cyclophosphamide

Increase: effect of—phenytoin, fosphenytoin

Increase: DOXOrubicin effect—streptozocin

Decrease: DOXOrubicin effect—PHENobarbital

Decrease: antibody response—live virus vaccine

Decrease: antineoplastic effect—hematopoietic progenitor cells; do not use 24 hr prior to or after treatment

Decrease: clearance of DOXOrubicin—PACLitaxel

Drug/Lab Test

Increase: uric acid

NURSING CONSIDERATIONS
Assess:

Black Box Warning: Bone marrow depression: CBC, differential, platelet count weekly; withhold product if WBC is <4000/mm^3 or platelet count is <75,000/mm^3; notify prescriber of these results

• Renal studies: BUN; serum uric acid; urine CCr; electrolytes prior to, during therapy
• I&O ratio: report fall in urine output to <30 mL/hr
• **Hepatotoxicity:** Hepatic studies prior to, during therapy: bilirubin, AST, ALT, alkaline phosphatase as needed or monthly; check for jaundice of skin and sclera, dark urine, clay-colored stools, itchy skin, abdominal pain, fever, diarrhea

Black Box Warning: Dysrhythmias: ECG: watch for ST-T wave changes, low QRS and T, possible dysrhythmias (sinus tachycardia, heart block, PVCs), ejection fraction prior to treatment, signs of irreversible cardiomyopathy, can occur up to 6 mo after treatment begins

• Bleeding: hematuria, guaiac, bruising, petechiae of mucosa or orifices every 8 hr
• Effects of alopecia on body image; discuss feelings about body changes; almost total alopecia is expected
• Buccal cavity every 8 hr for dryness, sores, ulceration, white patches, oral pain, bleeding, dysphagia
• **Secondary malignancy:** assess for acute myelogenous leukemia and oral cancer

Black Box Warning: Extravasation: local irritation, pain, burning at injection site; a vesicant; if extravasation occurs, stop drug, restart at another site, apply ice, elevate extremity to reduce swelling; if resolution does not occur, surgical debridement may be required

• GI symptoms: frequency of stools, cramping
• Rinsing of mouth tid-qid with water, club soda; brushing of teeth bid-tid with soft brush or cotton-tipped applicators for stomatitis; use unwaxed dental floss

Evaluate:
• Therapeutic response: decreased tumor size, spread of malignancy

Teach patient/family:
• To add 2-3 L of fluids unless contraindicated prior to and for 24-48 hr after to decrease possible **hemorrhagic cystitis**
• To report any complaints, side effects to nurse or prescriber
• That hair may be lost during treatment; that wig or hairpiece might make

patient feel better; that new hair may be different in color, texture
• To avoid foods with citric acid, hot temperature, or rough texture
• To report any bleeding, white spots, ulcerations in mouth to prescriber; to examine mouth daily
• That urine, other body fluids may be red-orange for 48 hr
• To avoid crowds and persons with infections when granulocyte count is low
• To avoid vaccinations because reactions can occur; to avoid alcohol
• **Pregnancy/breastfeeding:** that barrier contraceptive measures are recommended during therapy and for 4 mo after therapy ends including males of child-bearing potential; fertility may be impaired and may be permanent; to avoid breastfeeding

doxycycline (Rx)
(dox-i-sye′kleen)
doxycycline hyclate (Rx)
Atridox, Acticlate, Doryx, Doxy MPC, Monodox, Vibramycin
doxycycline monohydrate (Rx)
Adoxa, Apprilon ✤, Oracea, Vibramycin
Func. class.: Antiinfective
Chem. class.: Tetracycline

Do not confuse:
doxycycline/doxepin/dicyclomine
Oracea/Orencia

ACTION: Inhibits protein synthesis, phosphorylation in microorganisms by binding to 30S ribosomal subunits; bacteriostatic

USES: *Acinetobacter* sp., *Actinomyces israelii, Bacillus anthracis, Bacteroides* sp., *Balantidium coli, Bartonella bacilliformis, Borrelia recurrentis, Brucella* sp., *Campylobacter fetus, Chlamydia psittaci, Chlamydia trachomatis, Clostridium* sp., *Entamoeba histolytica,*

Enterobacter aerogenes, Enterococcus sp., *Escherichia coli, Francisella tularensis, Fusobacterium fusiforme, Haemophilus ducreyi, Haemophilus influenzae* (beta-lactamase negative), *Haemophilus influenzae* (beta-lactamase positive), *Klebsiella granulomatis, Klebsiella* sp., *Leptospira* sp., *Listeria monocytogenes, Mycoplasma pneumoniae, Neisseria gonorrhoeae, Neisseria meningitidis, Orientia tsutsugamushi, Plasmodium falciparum, Propionibacterium acnes, Rickettsia akari, Rickettsia prowazekii, Rickettsii, Shigella* sp., *Staphylococcus aureus* (MSSA), *Streptococcus pneumoniae, Streptococcus pyogenes* (group A beta-hemolytic streptococci), *Streptococcus* sp., *Treponema pallidum, Treponema pertenue, Ureaplasma urealyticum, Vibrio cholerae,* viridans streptococci, *Yersinia pestis;* syphilis, gonorrhea, lymphogranuloma venereum, uncommon gram-negative/gram-positive organisms, malaria prophylaxis
Unlabeled uses: Enterocolitis, biliary tract, intraabdominal infections; epididymitis *(Chlamydia trachomatis);* chronic prostatitis *(Ureaplasma urealyticum);* traveler's diarrhea (enterotoxigenic *Escherichia coli*); Legionnaire's disease *(Legionella pneumophila);* Lyme disease *(Borrelia burgdorferi),* Lyme disease (erythema migrans); Lyme arthritis; Lyme carditis; pleural effusion; malaria (chloroquine-resistant *Plasmodium falciparum*); pelvic inflammatory disease (PID), tubo-ovarian abscess in combination; acute dental infection, dentoalveolar infection, endodontic infection; aggressive juvenile periodontitis, plaque prophylaxis *(Yersinia pestis);* tularemia prophylaxis *(Francisella tularensis);* Bancroft's filariasis (elephantiasis) *(Wuchereria bancrofti);* melioidosis due to *Burkholderia pseudomallei;* leptospirosis *(Leptospira* sp) infection prophylaxis for gynecologic procedures/surgical infection prophylaxis hysterosalpingogram or chromotubation/induced abortion/dilation and

evacuation; methicillin-resistant *Staphylococcus aureus* (MRSA)–associated bone and joint infections

CONTRAINDICATIONS

Pregnancy, children <8 yr, hypersensitivity to tetracyclines, esophageal ulceration

Precautions: Breastfeeding, hepatic disease, CDAD, ulcerative colitis, sulfite hypersensitivity, excessive sunlight

DOSAGE AND ROUTES
Most infections

• **Adult:** PO/IV 100 mg q12hr on day 1, then 100 mg/day; **IV** 200 mg in 1-2 infusions on day 1, then 100-200 mg/day

• **Child >8 yr, ≥45 kg:** PO 100 mg q12hr on day 1, then 100 mg daily; severe infections 100 mg q12hr; **IV** 200 mg on day 1, then 100-200 mg daily, give 200 mg dose as 1 or 2 infusions

• **Child >8 yr, ≤45 kg:** PO 2.2 mg/kg q12hr on day 1, then 2.2 mg/kg daily, severe infections 2.2 mg/kg q12hr; **IV** 4.4 mg/kg divided on day 1, then 2.2-4.4 mg/kg daily in 1 to 2 divided doses

Gonorrhea in patients allergic to penicillin

• **Adult:** PO 100 mg q12hr × 7 days or 300 mg followed 1 hr later by another 300 mg

Malaria prophylaxis

• **Adult:** PO 100 mg/day 1-2 days prior to travel, daily during travel, and for 4 wk after return

• **Adolescent/child ≥8 yr** PO 2 mg/kg/day (up to 100 mg/day), 2.4 mg/kg Doryxm PC begin 1-2 days prior to travel, continue for 4 wk after return

C. trachomatis

• **Adult:** PO 100 mg bid × 7 days

Syphilis (early)

• **Adult:** PO 100 mg bid × 14 days or 120 mg Doryx MPC bid × 14 days

Primary/secondary syphilis (allergic to penicillin)

Adult: PO 300 mg daily divided × 14 days

Anthrax, postexposure

• **Adult and child >8 yr** IV 100 mg q12hr; change to **PO** when able × 60 days

• **Adolescent/child ≥8 yr and <45 kg:** PO 2.2 mg/kg q12hr × 60 days; **IV** 100

mg q12hr, change to **PO** when able × 60 days total

Lyme disease

• **Adult/adolescent/child ≥8 yr:** PO 100 mg bid × 10-21 days

Periodontitis

• **Adult:** 20 mg bid after scaling and root planing for ≤9 mo; give close to mealtime AM or PM

Pleural effusion (unlabeled)

• **Adult:** INTRACAVITARY 500 mg diluted with 250 mL 0.9% NaCl given by chest tube lavage and drainage

Available forms: Capsule 40 mg; suspension 50 mg/5 mL; capsule 20, 50, 100 mg; delayed-release tablets 75, 100, 150 mg; delayed-release capsule 75, 100 mg; injection 42.5, 100, 200 mg; tablets 20, 100 mg; capsules 50, 100, 150 mg; tablets 50, 75, 100 mg; oral suspension 25 mg/5 mL

Administer:
PO route

• Do not break, crush, or chew capsules; may crush tablets and mix with food

• On empty stomach or with full glass of water 2 hr prior to or after meals; avoid dairy products, antacids, laxatives, iron-containing products; if these must be taken, give 2 hr prior to or after product; avoid giving oral products within 1 hr of bedtime, esophageal ulceration may occur

• **Delayed-release capsule:** Swallow whole or open and sprinkle on applesauce

• **Suspension:** Shake well, use calibrated device, may give with food/milk for GI irritation, store at room temperature, discard after 14 days

Intermittent IV INFUSION route

• After diluting 100 mg or less/10 mL or 200 mg/20 mL of sterile water or NS for injection, each 100 mg must be further diluted with 100-1000 mL of NaCl, D₅W, Ringer's, LR, D₅LR, Normosol-M, Normosol-R in D₅W; run 100 mg or less over 1-4 hr; infusion must be completed in 6 hr when diluted in LR solution or 12 hr with other solution; protect from light, heat

• Avoid rapid use, extravasation may occur

• Store in tight, light-resistant container at room temperature; IV stable for 12 hr at room temperature, 72 hr refrigerated; discard if precipitate forms

Y-site compatibilities: Acyclovir, alemtuzumab, alfentanil, amifostine, amikacin, aminophylline, amiodarone, anidulafungin, ascorbic acid, atracurium, atropine, aztreonam, bivalirudin, bumetanide, buprenorphine, butorphanol, calcium chloride/gluconate, CARBOplatin, caspofungin, cefonicid, cefotaxime, cefTRIAXone, chlorproMAZINE, cimetidine, cisatracurium, CISplatin, clindamycin, codeine, cyanocobalamin, cyclophosphamide, cycloSPORINE, cytarabine, DACTINomycin, DAPTOmycin, dexmedetomidine, digoxin, diltiazem, diphenhydrAMINE, DOBUTamine, DOCEtaxel, DOPamine, doxacurium, DOXOrubicin, enalaprilat, ePHEDrine, EPINEPHrine, epirubicin, epoetin alfa, eptifibatide, ertapenem, esmolol, etoposide, etoposide phosphate, famotidine, fenoldopam, fentaNYL, filgrastim, fluconazole, fludarabine, gemcitabine, gemtuzumab, gentamicin, glycopyrrolate, granisetron, HYDROmorphone, IDArubicin, ifosfamide, imipenem/cilastatin, insulin, isoproterenol, labetalol, levofloxacin, lidocaine, linezolid, LORazepam, magnesium sulfate, mannitol, mechlorethamine, melphalan, meperidine, methyldopate, metoclopramide, metoprolol, metroNIDAZOLE, miconazole, midazolam, milrinone, mitoXANtrone, morphine, multivitamins, nalbuphine, naloxone, nesiritide, netilmicin, nitroglycerin, nitroprusside, norepinephrine, octreotide, ondansetron, oxaliplatin, oxytocin, PACLitaxel, pancuronium, pantoprazole, papaverine, pentamidine, pentazocine, perphenazine, phentolamine, phenylephrine, phytonadione, potassium chloride, procainamide, prochlorperazine, promethazine, propofol, propranolol, protamine, pyridoxime, quinupristin/dalfopristin, ranitidine, remifentanil, ritodrine, riTUXimab, rocuronium, sargramostim, sodium acetate, succinylcholine, SUFentanil, tacrolimus, telavancin, teniposide, theophylline, thiamine, thiotepa, tirofiban, tobramycin, tolazoline, TPN (2 in 1), trastuzumab, trimetaphan, urokinase, vancomycin, vasopressin, vecuronium, verapamil, vinCRIStine, vinorelbine, voriconazole, zoledronic acid

SIDE EFFECTS

CNS: Fever, headache
CV: Pericarditis
EENT: Dysphagia, glossitis, decreased calcification of deciduous teeth, oral candidiasis, tooth discoloration
GI: *Nausea, abdominal pain, vomiting, diarrhea,* anorexia, enterocolitis, hepatotoxicity, flatulence, abdominal cramps, gastric burning, stomatitis, CDAD
GU: *Increased BUN*
HEMA: Eosinophilia, neutropenia, thrombocytopenia, hemolytic anemia
INTEG: *Rash, urticaria, photosensitivity, increased pigmentation,* exfoliative dermatitis, pruritus, phlebitis, injection site reaction, DRESS
MS: Bone growth retardation (<8 yr old), muscle, joint pain
RESP: Cough
SYST: Stevens-Johnson syndrome, angioedema, anaphylaxis, toxic epidermal necrolysis

PHARMACOKINETICS

PO: Well absorbed, widely distributed; peak 1½-4 hr; half-life 1 day; excreted in urine, feces, bile; 90% protein bound; crosses placenta; enters breast milk

INTERACTIONS

Increase: effect of—anticoagulants, digoxin, methotrexate
Decrease: doxycycline effect—antacids, NaHCO₃, dairy products, alkali products, iron, kaolin/pectin, barbiturates, carBAMazepine, phenytoin, cimetidine sucralfate, cholestyramine, colestipol, rifAMPin, bismuth; iron, magnesium, zinc, calcium, aluminum salts, sevelamer
Decrease: effects—penicillins, oral contraceptives, digoxin

Drug/Lab Test
Increase: BUN, alkaline phosphatase, bilirubin, amylase, ALT, AST, eosinophils, WBC
Decrease: Hb
False increase: urinary catecholamines

NURSING CONSIDERATIONS
Assess:
- I&O ratio
- Blood studies: PT, CBC, AST, ALT, BUN, creatinine
- Signs of infection
- **Allergic reactions:** rash, itching, pruritus, angioedema, discontinue, do not restart
- Nausea, vomiting, diarrhea; administer antiemetic, antacids as ordered
- **Overgrowth of infection:** fever, malaise, redness, pain, swelling, drainage, perineal itching, diarrhea, changes in cough or sputum
- IV site for phlebitis/thrombosis; product is highly irritating
- After C&S is obtained, do not wait for results
- **DRESS:** rash, fever, facial swelling, lymphadenopathy; discontinue
- **Labs:** hepatic and renal studies, CBC, baseline and periodically
- **CDAD** bowel pattern daily (diarrhea, fever, blood in stools) may occur several weeks to months after treatment
- **Pregnancy/breastfeeding:** no well-controlled studies; may affect skeletal development, do not use in second half of pregnancy unless benefit outweighs fetal risk; discontinue breastfeeding or product, excreted in small amounts in breast milk

Evaluate:
- Therapeutic response: decreased temperature, absence of lesions, negative C&S

Teach patient/family:
- To avoid sun because burns may occur; that sunscreen does not seem to decrease photosensitivity
- That all prescribed medication must be taken to prevent superinfection; not to use outdated products because Fanconi syndrome may occur (reversible nephrotoxicity)
- That if children ≤8 yr old are undergoing tooth development, teeth may be permanently discolored
- Not to use with antacids, iron products, H₂ blockers, sevelamer, calcium (milk), magnesium, zinc
- To take with full glass of water; if nausea occurs, take with food
- Inform patient to wear sunscreen, protective clothing to prevent burns
- **Pregnancy/breastfeeding:** advise patient to notify health care provider if pregnancy is planned or suspected; to use nonhormonal contraception during and to next menstrual period, crosses placental barrier; avoid breastfeeding

---

doxylamine/pyridoxine (Rx)
(docks-ill'ah-meen/peer-reh-dock'seen)
Diclegis, Bonjesta, Diclectin/B6 ✦
Func. class.: Antiemetic
Chem. class.: Antihistamine/vitamin B_6

ACTION:
Unknown, may act by anticholinergic effect

USES:
Nausea and vomiting of pregnancy in women who do not respond to other treatment

CONTRAINDICATIONS
Hypersensitivity to this product or ethanolamine derivatives, antihistamines, MAOIs, lactation
Precautions:
Angle closure glaucoma, urinary bladder neck obstruction, increase IOP, stenosing peptic ulcer

DOSAGE AND ROUTES
- **Adult pregnant females: PO** 2 tablets (on an empty stomach) at bedtime, on day 1; if dose controls symptoms the next day, continue regimen. If symptoms persist on the afternoon of day 2, continue 2 tablets at bedtime, then take 3 tablets starting on day 3 (1 tablet in AM and 2 tablets at bedtime); if symptoms are controlled, continue regimen. If symptoms persist, on day 4, take 4 tablets (1 tablet in AM, 1 tablet midafternoon, and 2 tablets at bedtime); max 4 tablets/day. Use only as needed

Available forms: Tablets extended release: doxylamine 20 mg/pyridoxine 20 mg; tablets delayed release: doxylamine 10 mg/pyridoxine 10 mg; doxylamine 20 mg/pyridoxine 20 mg

Administer

• Give whole on empty stomach with 8 oz of water

• Take as prescribed, do not double or miss doses

• Store at room temperature, protect from light

SIDE EFFECTS

CNS: Somnolence, dizziness, drowsiness

PHARMACOKINETICS

Doxylamine: Onset unknown, peak 1.7-8 hr, duration unknown; **pyridoxine:** Onset unknown, peak ½-4.7 hr; half-life: doxylamine: 12½ hr, pyridoxine: ½ hr

INTERACTIONS

Increase: CNS depression—CNS depressants, MAOIs, alcohol, avoid using together

Increase: anticholinergic effect—MAOIs

Drug/Food

Decrease: effect by food

NURSING CONSIDERATIONS

Assess:

• **Anticholinergic effects:** monitor for dry mouth, constipation, dizziness

• **CNS changes:** Assess for dizziness, drowsiness, and somnolence; caution against driving or other hazardous activities until response is known

• **Pregnancy/breastfeeding:** Used in pregnancy to decrease nausea/vomiting; do not breastfeed

Evaluate:

• Therapeutic response

• Decreasing nausea/vomiting of pregnancy

Teach patient/family:

• To report anticholinergic effects

• Not to drive or perform other hazardous activities until response is known

• Pregnancy/breastfeeding: Do not breastfeed

⚠ *HIGH ALERT*

dronedarone (Rx)

(droe-ned′a-rone)

Multaq

Func. class.: Antidysrhythmic (class III)

Chem. class.: Iodinated benzofuran derivative

ACTION: Prolongs duration of action potential and effective refractory period, noncompetitive alpha- and beta-adrenergic inhibition; increases PR and QT intervals, decreases sinus rate, decreases peripheral vascular resistance

USES: To reduce hospitalization for atrial fibrillation

CONTRAINDICATIONS

Pregnancy, breastfeeding; second, third-degree AV block; bradycardia, severe sinus node dysfunction, hypersensitivity, heart failure, hepatic disease, QT prolongation, aminodarone-induced lung/liver toxicity

Black Box Warning: NYHA Class IV heart failure or Class II-III with recent decompensation requiring hospitalization, permanent atrial fibrillation (cannot restore sinus rhythm)

Precautions: Children, geriatric patients, ⁿ⁰ꙮ Asian patients, females, electrolyte imbalances, atrial fibrillation/flutter

DOSAGE AND ROUTES

• **Adult: PO** 400 mg bid; discontinue class I, III antidysrhythmics or strong CYP3A4 inhibitors prior to beginning treatment; max 800 mg/day; severe hepatic disease

Available forms: Tablets 400 mg

Administer:

PO route

• Give bid with morning, evening meals

• Do not double if missed, skip

• Give medication guide; should be dispensed with each prescription, refill

---

SIDE EFFECTS
CNS: Weakness
CV: *Bradycardia,* heart failure, QT prolongation, torsades de pointes, atrial flutter
GI: Nausea, vomiting, diarrhea, abdominal pain, severe hepatic injury, hepatic failure
INTEG: Rash, photosensitivity, anaphylaxis, angioedema
RESP: Interstitial pneumonitis, pulmonary fibrosis

PHARMACOKINETICS
Peak 3-6 hr, half-life 13-19 hr, metabolized by liver, by CYP3A excreted in feces (84%), via kidneys (6%), protein binding >98%

INTERACTIONS
Increase: dronedarone levels—CYP3A inhibitors/2D6 inhibitors
Decrease: dronedarone levels—3A/2D6 inducers
Increase: bradycardia—beta-blockers, calcium channel blockers
Increase: levels of cycloSPORINE, dextromethorphan, digoxin, disopyramide, flecainide, methotrexate, phenytoin, procainamide, quiNIDine, theophylline
Increase: anticoagulant effects—dabigatran, warfarin
Drug/Herb
Increase: anticoagulant effect—yohimbine
Decrease: dronedarone effect—St. John's wort, avoid using together
Drug/Food:
Increase: dronedarone effect—grapefruit; avoid use
Drug/Lab Test
Increase: T4, creatinine, LFTs, bilirubin
Decrease: potassium, magnesium

NURSING CONSIDERATIONS
Assess:

Black Box Warning: NYHA Class IV heart failure or symptomatic heart failure with recent decomposition requiring hospitalization doubles risk of death

• **ECG** to determine product effectiveness; measure PR, QRS, QT intervals; check for PVCs, other dysrhythmias, B/P continuously for hypo/hypertension; report dysrhythmias, slowing heart rate
• Serum creatinine, potassium, magnesium
• I&O ratio; electrolytes (potassium, creatinine, magnesium)
• Dehydration or hypovolemia
• Rebound hypertension after 1-2 hr
• Cardiac rate; respiration: rate, rhythm, character; chest pain; start with patient hospitalized and monitored up to 1 wk
• **Pregnancy/breastfeeding:** do not use in pregnancy, breastfeeding
Evaluate:
• Therapeutic response: maintenance of normal heart rhythm following atrial fibrillation, flutter
Teach patient/family:
• To take this product as directed in AM, PM with meals; to avoid missed doses; not to use with grapefruit juice; to avoid all other products without approval of provider
• To immediately report weight gain, edema, difficulty breathing, fatigue, peripheral edema
• **Pregnancy/breastfeeding:** to use effective contraception during treatment; not to breastfeed

TREATMENT OF OVERDOSE:
O₂, artificial ventilation, ECG, administer DOPamine for circulatory depression

---

droxidopa (Rx)
(drox′-i-doe′-pa)
Northera
Func. class.: Cardiovascular agent, vasopressor

ACTION: A synthetic amino acid precursor of norepinephrine. It is used to increase blood pressure with symptomatic neurogenic orthostatic hypotension caused by primary autonomic failure (Parkinson's disease, multiple system atrophy, and pure autonomic failure), dopamine beta-hydroxylase deficiency, or nondiabetic autonomic neuropathy

USES: Symptomatic neurogenic orthostatic hypotension

CONTRAINDICATIONS
Hypersensitivity

Precautions: Angina, breastfeeding, cardiac arrhythmias, cardiac disease, children, coronary artery disease, heart disease, hyperthermia, infants, mental status changes, myocardial infarction, neonates, pregnancy, salicylate/tartrazine dye hypersensitivity

Black Box Warning: Supine hypertension

DOSAGE AND ROUTES
• **Adult: PO** 100 mg tid: upon arising in the morning, at midday, and in the late afternoon at least 3 hr prior to bedtime; titrate to response, by 100 mg tid q24-48 hr up to a dose of 600 mg **PO** tid, max 1800 mg/day
Available forms: Capsules 100, 200, 300 mg
Administer:

Black Box Warning: Give tid at the following times: upon arising in the morning, at midday, and in the late afternoon at least 3 hr prior to bedtime (to reduce the potential for supine hypertension during sleep)

• Use without regard to food, but should be taken consistently in regard to food to ensure consistent absorption
• Swallow capsules whole

SIDE EFFECTS
CNS: Headache, dizziness, fatigue
CV: Supine hypertension, arrhythmia exacerbation, chest pain
MISC: Urinary tract infection, neuroleptic malignant syndrome

PHARMACOKINETICS
Peak 3-4 hr

INTERACTIONS
Increase: droxidopa effects—carbidopa, serotonin receptor agonists, sympathomimetics
Increase: hypertensive crisis—MAOIs

NURSING CONSIDERATIONS
Assess:

Black Box Warning: **Supine hypertension:** monitor supine B/P prior to and at every dosage increase; assess response periodically. Advise to elevate the head of the bed when resting or sleeping to lessen the risk for supine hypertension. B/P should be monitored in supine position and in the recommended head-elevated sleeping position. Reduce or discontinue if supine hypertension persists

• **Neuroleptic malignant syndrome:** hyperthermia, severe extrapyramidal dysfunction, alterations in consciousness, mental status changes, and autonomic instability (tachycardia, blood pressure fluctuations, diaphoresis). In those with Parkinson's disease, this condition may occur with abrupt reduction of products with dopaminergic properties
• **Arrhythmia exacerbation:** exacerbation of existing ischemic cardiac disease (coronary artery disease, angina, myocardial infarction, HF); consider the potential risk prior to initiating therapy; if chest pain occurs during use, assess cardiac status
• **Pregnancy/breastfeeding:** no well-controlled studies in pregnancy, breastfeeding
Evaluate:
• **Therapeutic response:** increased B/P
Teach patient/family:

Black Box Warning: Instruct patients to rest and sleep in an upper-body-elevated position and to monitor B/P (to reduce the potential for supine hypertension); to take ≥3 hr prior to bedtime

• To take consistently with or without food
• Not to double doses

⚠ HIGH ALERT

dulaglutide (Rx)
(doo-la-gloo'-tide)
Trulicity
Func. class.: Antidiabetic
Chem. class.: Human glucagon–like peptide-1 (GLP-1) receptor agonist

---

Side effects: *italics* = common; red = life-threatening

ACTION: Binds and activates known human glucagon-like peptide-1 (GLP-1) receptor agonist, mimics natural physiology for self-regulating glycemic control

USES: Type 2 diabetes mellitus, once-weekly dosing with diet and exercise

CONTRAINDICATIONS
Hypersensitivity

> **Black Box Warning:** Medullary thyroid carcinoma, multiple endocrine neoplasia syndrome type 2 (MEN-2), thyroid cancer

Precautions: Pregnancy, breastfeeding, children, geriatric patients, severe renal/hepatic/GI disease, pancreatitis, vitamin D deficiency, burns, colitis, diarrhea, fever, GI bleeding/perforation/obstruction, ileus, infection, CDAD, thyroid disease, trauma, surgery, type 1 diabetes mellitus, tobacco smoking, vomiting

DOSAGE AND ROUTES
• **Adult: SUBCUT** 0.75 mg weekly, may increase to 1.5 mg weekly if needed, may increase to 3 mg q wk after 1.5 mg q wk × 4 wk

Available forms: Solution for SUBCUT injection 0.75 mg/0.5 mL, 1.5 mg/0.5 mL, 3 mg/0.5 mL, 4.5 mg/0.5 mL, 3 mg/0.5 mL, 4.5 mg/0.5 mL

Administer:
SUBCUT route

• Do not use as first-line therapy for those who have inadequate glycemic control on diet and exercise
• Administer the dose at any time of day, with or without meals
• If a dose is missed, take as soon as remembered, as long as the next dose is due at least 3 days later; if it is more than 3 days after the missed dose, wait until the next regularly scheduled dose
• Give SUBCUT only, do not give IV or IM, inject into the thigh, abdomen, or upper arm, rotate sites with each injection to prevent lipodystrophy
• Properly dispose of the pen or syringe
• Store in refrigerator for unopened pen; may store at room temperature after opening for up to 30 days, do not freeze

• When using concomitantly with insulin, give as separate injections. Never mix them together. The two injections may be injected in the same body region, but not adjacent to each other
• Part of pen is glass; if dropped on a hard surface, do not use

SIDE EFFECTS
CNS: Fatigue
ENDO: Hypoglycemia, thyroid C-cell tumors
GI: *Nausea, vomiting,* diarrhea, anorexia, gastroesophageal reflux, pancreatitis, flatulence, *abdominal pain,* constipation
SYST: Secondary malignancy
INTEG: Injection site reactions, rash, urticaria, hypersensitivity (anaphylaxis, angioedema)
GU: Renal failure

PHARMACOKINETICS
Peak 24-72 hr, half-life 5 days, metabolized by catabolism

INTERACTIONS
Increase: hypoglycemia—ACE inhibitors, disopyramide, sulfonylureas, androgens, fibric acid derivatives, alcohol
Increase: hyperglycemia—phenothiazines, corticosteroids, anabolic steroids
Decrease: effect of dulaglutide—niacin, dextrothyroxine, thiazide diuretics, triamterene, estrogens, progestins, oral contraceptives, MAOIs

NURSING CONSIDERATIONS
Assess:
• **Diabetes:** fasting blood glucose, A1c levels (check twice a year or quarterly in those with therapy changes or uncontrolled disease), postprandial glucose during treatment to determine diabetes control; hypo/hyperglycemic reaction that can occur soon after meals; for severe hypoglycemia, give IV D50W, then IV dextrose solution
• **Pancreatitis:** severe abdominal pain, with or without vomiting; product should be discontinued
• Nausea, vomiting, diarrhea, ability to tolerate product, may cause dehydration

• **Pregnancy/breastfeeding:** no well-controlled studies; use only if benefit outweighs fetal risk; avoid breastfeeding, excretion is unknown

Evaluate:

• Therapeutic response: decrease in polyuria, polydipsia, polyphagia, clear sensorium, improving A1c, weight; absence of dizziness, stable gait

Teach patient/family:

• About the symptoms of hypo/hyperglycemia, what to do about each; to have glucagon emergency kit available; to carry a glucose source (candy, sugar cube) to treat hypoglycemia

---

DULoxetine (Rx)

(do-lox′e-teen)

Cymbalta, Drizalma

Func. class.: Antidepressant

Chem. class.: Serotonin-norepinephrine reuptake inhibitor (SNRI)

Do not confuse:

Cymbalta/Symbyax
duloxetine/fluoxetine/paroxetine/
Dexilant

ACTION: May potentiate serotonergic, noradrenergic activity in the CNS; in studies, DULoxetine is a potent inhibitor of neuronal serotonin and norepinephrine reuptake

USES: Major depressive disorder (MDD), neuropathic pain associated with diabetic neuropathy, generalized anxiety disorder, fibromyalgia, chronic low back pain, osteoarthritis pain

CONTRAINDICATIONS

Alcohol intoxication, alcoholism, closed-angle glaucoma, hepatic disease, hepatitis, jaundice, hypersensitivity

Precautions: Pregnancy, breastfeeding, geriatric patients, mania, hypertension, renal/cardiac disease, seizures, increased intraocular pressure, anorexia nervosa, bleeding, dehydration, diabetes, hyponatremia, hypotension, hypovolemia, orthostatic hypotension, abrupt product withdrawal

Black Box Warning: Children, suicidal ideation

DOSAGE AND ROUTES

Major depressive disorder

• **Adult: PO** 40-60 mg/day as single dose or 2 divided doses

Diabetic neuropathy

• **Adult: PO** 60 mg/day

Generalized anxiety disorder

• **Adult: PO** 60 mg/day, may start with 30 mg/day × 1 wk, then increase to 60 mg/day; maintenance 60-120 mg/day

Fibromyalgia

• **Adult: PO** 30 mg/day × 1 wk, then 60 mg/day

Musculoskeletal pain

• **Adult: PO** 60 mg/day or 30 mg/day × 1 wk, then 60 mg/day

Renal dose

• **Adult: PO** Start with 20 mg, gradually increase; avoid use in severe renal disease

Hepatic disease (mild, moderate, severe): Avoid use

Available forms: Capsules delayed release 20, 30, 40, 60 mg

Administer:

• Swallow capsules whole; do not break, crush, or chew; do not sprinkle on food or mix with liquid

• Without regard to food

• Store in tight container at room temperature; do not freeze

SIDE EFFECTS

CNS: Insomnia, anxiety, dizziness, tremor, somnolence, fatigue, decreased appetite, decreased weight, agitation, diaphoresis, hallucinations, neuroleptic malignant–like syndrome reaction, aggression, seizures, *headache*, abnormal dreams, flushing, hot flashes, chills

CV: Thrombophlebitis, peripheral edema, hypertension, palpitations, supraventricular dysrhythmia, orthostatic hypotension

EENT: *Abnormal vision*

ENDO: Hypo/hyperglycemia, SIADH

GI: Constipation, diarrhea, dysphagia, *nausea*, vomiting, anorexia, dry mouth, colitis, gastritis, abdominal pain, hepatic failure

Side effects: *italics* = common; red = life-threatening

GU: Abnormal ejaculation, urinary hesitation/retention/frequency, ejaculation delayed, erectile dysfunction, gynecologic bleeding

INTEG: Photosensitivity, bruising, sweating, Stevens-Johnson syndrome

MS: Gait disturbance, muscle spasm, restless legs syndrome, myalgia

SYST: Anaphylaxis, angioedema, serotonin syndrome, Stevens-Johnson syndrome

PHARMACOKINETICS

Well absorbed; extensively metabolized ⚕ (CYP2D6, CYP1A2) in the liver to an active metabolite; 70% of product recovered in urine, 20% in feces; 90% protein binding; elimination half-life 9.2-19.1 hr

INTERACTIONS

• Do not use with linezolid or methylene blue IV

• **Narrow therapeutic index:** CYP2D6 extensively metabolized products (flecainide, phenothiazines, propafenone, tricyclics, thioridazine)

• Hyperthermia, rigidity, rapid fluctuations of vital signs, mental status changes, neuroleptic malignant syndrome—MAOIs; coadministration contraindicated within 14 days of MAOI use

Increase: CNS depression—opioids, antihistamines, sedative/hypnotics

Increase: serotonin syndrome, neuroleptic malignant syndrome—SSRIs, serotonin-receptor agonists, tricyclics, traZODone, amphetamines, triptans

Increase: bleeding risk—anticoagulants, antiplatelets, salicylates, NSAIDs

Increase: action of DULoxetine—CYP1A2 inhibitors (fluvoxamine, quinolone antiinfectives); CYP2D6 inhibitors (FLUoxetine, quiNIDine, PARoxetine)

Drug/Herb

Increase: serotonin syndrome—St. John's wort; avoid using together

Increase: CNS depression—kava, valerian

Drug/Lab Test

Increase: ALT, bilirubin—alcohol

Increase: blood glucose

NURSING CONSIDERATIONS

Assess:

Black Box Warning: Depression: mood, sensorium, affect, **suicidal tendencies,** increase in psychiatric symptoms, depression, panic; monitor children weekly face to face during first 4 wk or dosage change, then every other week for next 4 wk, then at 12 wk

• **Vitals:** B/P lying, standing; pulse q4hr; if systolic B/P drops 20 mm Hg, hold product, notify prescriber; take VS q4hr in patients with CV disease

• **Hypo/hyperglycemia:** assess for each during treatment and before dosing

• Hepatic studies: AST, ALT, bilirubin

• Weight weekly; weight loss or gain; appetite may increase; peripheral edema may occur

• **Withdrawal symptoms:** headache, nausea, vomiting, muscle pain, weakness; not common unless product is discontinued abruptly

• Malignant neuroleptic–like syndrome reaction

• **Serotonin syndrome:** nausea/vomiting, dizziness, facial flush, shivering, sweating, discontinue if present, do not restart

• **Sexual dysfunction:** ejaculation dysfunction, erectile dysfunction, decreased libido, orgasm dysfunction

• Assistance with ambulation during beginning therapy; drowsiness, dizziness occur

• **Beers:** use with caution in older adults; may exacerbate or cause SIADH

• **Pregnancy/breastfeeding:** no well-controlled studies; use only if benefit outweighs fetal risk, complications in late third trimester have occurred; pregnancy should be registered with the Cymbalta Pregnancy Registry (866-814-6975); excreted in breast milk

Evaluate:

• Therapeutic response: decreased depression

Teach patient/family:

• To use sugarless gum, hard candy, frequent sips of water for dry mouth

• To report urinary retention; about signs and symptoms of bleeding (GI bleeding, nosebleed, ecchymoses, bruising)
• To use with caution when driving, performing other activities requiring alertness because of drowsiness, dizziness, blurred vision
• To avoid alcohol ingestion, MAOIs, other CNS depressants
• To notify prescriber of nausea, vomiting, dizziness, facial flushing, shivering, sweating, confusion, hallucinations, incordination; may indicate serotonin syndrome
• Not to discontinue medication quickly after long-term use; may cause nausea, headache, malaise; taper

Black Box Warning: That clinical worsening and suicide risk may occur

• To wear sunscreen or large hat; photosensitivity may occur
• To notify prescriber if pregnancy is planned or suspected, or if breastfeeding
• Improvement may occur in 4-8 wk or in up to 12 wk (geriatric patients)

dupilumab (Rx)
(doo-pil'-ue-mab)
Dupixent
Func. class.: Dermatologicals

USES: Moderate to severe atopic dermatitis in patients whose disease is not adequately controlled with topical therapies or when those therapies are not advised, add-on maintenance in moderate-severe asthma with eosinophils, phenotype, or oral corticosteroid–dependent asthma; add-on maintenance treatment of poorly controlled chronic rhinosinusitis with nasal polyps

DOSAGE AND ROUTES
Atopic dermatitis
• **Adult/child 6-17 yr ≥60 kg: SUBCUT** Initially, 600 mg (administered as two

300-mg injections); maintenance dosing: 300 mg every other week
• **Child 6-17 yr 30-<60 kg yr SUBCUT** Initially, 400 mg (two 200-mg injections), then 200 mg every other week

Asthma
• **Adult/ child ≥12 yr:** SUBCUT Loading, 400 mg (two 200-mg injections) followed by 200 mg every other week or an initial loading dose of 600 mg (two 300-mg injections) followed by 300 mg every other week
Available forms: Injection: 300-mg/2-mL single-dose syringes

⚠ HIGH ALERT

durvalumab (Rx)
(dur-val'-yoo-mab)
Imfinzi
Func. class.: Antineoplastic monoclonal antibody

ACTION: A human IgG1 kappa (IgG1k) monoclonal antibody, produced in Chinese hamster ovary; inhibits its programmed death ligand interactions

USES: For the treatment of locally advanced non-small cell lung cancer (NSCLC); extensive stage small cell lung cancer in combination with etoposide and either CARBOplatin or CISplatin

CONTRAINDICATIONS
Pregnancy, hypersensitivity
Precautions: Adrenal insufficiency, aseptic meningitis, autoimmune disease, breastfeeding, colitis, contraception requirements, Crohn's disease, diabetes mellitus, diarrhea, hemolytic anemia, hepatic disease, hepatitis, hypophysitis, hypopituitarism, IBS, infusion-related reactions, keratitis, myocarditis, organ transplant, pneumonitis, pulmonary disease, reproductive risk,

serious rash, SLE, thyroid disease, ulcerative colitis, uveitis

DOSAGE AND ROUTES

Consolidation treatment of locally advanced or unresectable non–small-cell lung cancer (NSCLC)

• **Adult:** IV INF 10 mg/kg, beginning 1-42 days after the last radiation dose, q2wk until disease progression or unacceptable toxicity, for up to 12 mo

Extensive small cell lung cancer

• **Adult >30 kg:** IV INF 1500 mg prior to chemotherapy on same day; q3wk × 4 cycles, then 1500 mg q4wk (single agent)
Adult <30 kg: IV INF 20 mg/kg before chemotherapy on the same day q3wk × 4 cycles, then q4wk (single agent)

Renal dose

• **Mild to moderate renal impairment (CCr ≥30 mL/min):** no change
• **Severe renal impairment (CCr 15-29 mL/min):** unknown

Available forms: Powder for injection 120 mg/2.4 mL, 500 mg/10 mL

Administer:

IV route

• Follow cytotoxic handling procedures
• Visually inspect for particulate matter and discoloration, product should be clear to opalescent, colorless to slightly yellow, free from particles. Discard if solution is cloudy or discolored or if particles are observed
• Do not shake

Preparation:

• Withdraw the required volume of drug and transfer into an IV container containing 0.9% sodium chloride injection or 5% dextrose injection to prepare an infusion with a final concentration ranging from 1 mg/mL to 15 mg/mL
• Mix diluted solution by gentle inversion. Do not shake
• Discard partially used or empty vials of durvalumab

Storage of diluted solution:

• Does not contain a preservative; give immediately after preparation

• If storage of diluted solution is necessary, the total time from vial puncture to the start of administration should be <24 hr if refrigerated 36° F-46° F (2° C-8° C), or <4 hr at room temperature up to 77° F (up to 25° C). Do not freeze

IV Infusion:

• Give diluted over 60 min through an IV line using a low protein-binding 0.2- or 0.22-micron in-line filter
• Do not admix or give other products through the same line

SIDE EFFECTS

CNS: Fatigue, fever
GI: Nausea, diarrhea, constipation, anorexia, abdominal pain, colitis
HEMA: Anemia, hemolytic anemia, lymphopenia
RESP: Cough, dyspnea
META: Hyponatremia, hyperbilirubinemia, hypercalcemia, hypermagnesium, hypoalbuminemia
ENDO: Hyperglycemia, hyperthyroidism, hypothyroidism
MISC: Infection, peripheral edema, musculoskeletal pain, rash, antibody formation, aseptic meningitis, dehydration, infusion reactions, keratitis, myocarditis, uveitis

PHARMACOKINETICS

Steady state 16 wk, half-life 17 days

INTERACTIONS

None known

Drug/Lab Test

Increase: LFTs, blood glucose, serum creatinine/BUN, thyroid function tests
Decrease: thyroid function tests

NURSING CONSIDERATIONS

Assess:

• Monitor baseline and periodically blood glucose, LFTs, serum creatinine/BUN
• **Serious infection:** may be fatal; monitor for signs and symptoms of infection; use prophylactic anti-infectives as appropriate.
• **Pregnancy/breastfeeding:** product can cause fetal harm; females of reproductive potential should avoid becoming pregnant during and for 3 mo after final

dose; obtain a pregnancy test prior to starting product; do not breastfeed during and for at least 3 mo after last dose

• **Immune-mediated pneumonitis or interstitial lung disease (ILD):** may be fatal; monitor for signs or symptoms (new or worsening chest pain or shortness of breath) of pneumonitis. If pneumonitis is suspected, obtain a chest x-ray; an interruption or discontinuation of therapy and treatment with high-dose corticosteroids (followed by a steroid taper) may be necessary. The median time to onset of immune-mediated pneumonitis was 55.5 days (range, 24 to 423 days)

• **Immune-mediated hepatitis:** may be fatal; monitor for abnormal liver tests prior to each cycle of treatment; interruption or discontinuation of therapy may be needed with high-dose corticosteroids (followed by a steroid taper). The median time to onset of immune-mediated hepatitis was 51.5 days (range, 15 to 312 days)

• **Diarrhea and immune-mediated colitis:** monitor for signs and symptoms of colitis (diarrhea or severe abdominal pain). Treatment with antidiarrheal agents and high-dose corticosteroids (followed by a steroid taper), along with an interruption or discontinuation of therapy, may be necessary. The median time to onset of immune-mediated colitis was 73 days (range, 13 to 345 days). Use with caution in those with inflammatory bowel disease such as ulcerative colitis or Crohn's disease

• **Thyroid disease/disorders (hypothyroidism/hyperthyroidism):** monitor thyroid function tests (TFTs) at baseline and periodically during treatment. Asymptomatic patients with abnormal TFTs can receive treatment; manage these patients with hormone replacement and symptomatic management as needed. The median time to onset of hypothyroidism was 42 days (range, 15 to 239 days), and the median time to first onset of hyperthyroidism was 43 days (range, 14-71 days)

• **Immune-mediated adrenal insufficiency and hypophysitis/hypopituitarism:** monitor for signs and symptoms of adrenal insufficiency (hypotension, decreased cortisol level, fatigue, weakness, and weight loss) and hypophysitis (decreased pituitary hormone levels, pituitary gland inflammation, severe intractable headache, and vision impairment) during and after treatment. An interruption of therapy, treatment with high-dose corticosteroids, and hormone replacement may be necessary

• **Immune-mediated nephritis:** monitor renal function at baseline and prior to each cycle of treatment. No initial dose adjustment is recommended in patients with renal dysfunction; use with caution in patients with renal disease or renal impairment. If immune-mediated nephritis occurs, an interruption or discontinuation of therapy may be needed with treatment with high-dose corticosteroids

• **Immune-mediated reactions (aseptic meningitis, hemolytic anemia, immune thrombocytopenic purpura, myocarditis, myositis) and ocular inflammatory toxicity (uveitis and keratitis):** monitor for signs and symptoms of immune-mediated reactions; confirm etiology or exclude other causes. Therapy may need to be temporarily withheld or permanently discontinued; administer corticosteroids as needed

• **Severe infusion-related reactions:** monitor signs and symptoms of an infusion-related reaction. Interrupt or slow the rate of infusion in those with mild or moderate infusion reactions. Permanently discontinue in those with grade 3 or 4 infusion reactions

Evaluate:
• Therapeutic response: lack of disease progression

Teach patient/family:
• To report adverse reactions immediately; to report diarrhea, hepatic, flu-like symptoms, cough, trouble breathing, rash
• About reason for treatment, expected results
• **Pregnancy/breastfeeding:** to notify provider if pregnancy is planned or sus-

pected; to use effective contraception during treatment and for 3 mo after discontinuing treatment; do not breastfeed during or for 3 mo after final dose

---

dutasteride (Rx)

(doo-tass'ter-ide)

Avodart

Func. class.: Androgen inhibitor

Chem. class.: Synthetic 5α-reductase inhibitor, 4-azasteroid compound

---

ACTION: Inhibits both type 1 and type 2 forms of a steroid enzyme that converts testosterone to 5α-dihydrotestosterone (DHT), which is responsible for the initial growth of prostatic tissue

USES: Treatment of benign prostatic hyperplasia (BPH) in men with an enlarged prostate gland; may be used in combination with tamsulosin

CONTRAINDICATIONS

Pregnancy, breastfeeding, women, children, hypersensitivity

Precautions: Hepatic disease

DOSAGE AND ROUTES

Benign prostatic hyperplasia (BPH)

• **Adult:** PO 0.5 mg/day; may use without tamsulosin

Available form: Capsules 0.5 mg

Administer:

• Swallow capsules whole; do not break, crush, chew

• Without regard to meals

SIDE EFFECTS

GU: Decreased libido, impotence, gynecomastia, ejaculation disorders (rare), mastalgia, teratogenesis

INTEG: Serious skin infections

PHARMACOKINETICS

Peak 2-3 hr, protein binding 99%, metabolized in liver by CYP3A4, excreted in feces, half-life 5 wk at steady state

INTERACTIONS

Increase: dutasteride concentrations—ritonavir, ketoconazole, verapamil, dilTIAZem, cimetidine, ciprofloxacin, antiretroviral protease inhibitors, or other products metabolized by CYP3A4

Drug/Lab Test

Decrease: PSA

NURSING CONSIDERATIONS

Assess:

• **For decreasing symptoms of BPH:** decreasing urinary retention, frequency, urgency, nocturia

• PSA levels baseline and at 3 mo, 3-mo level becomes new baseline; double PSA level and compared with normal levels in those untreated; urinary obstruction; determine the absence of urinary or prostate cancer prior to starting treatment

• Blood studies: ALT, AST, bilirubin, CBC with differential, serum creatinine, serum electrolytes

Evaluate:

• Therapeutic response: decreasing symptoms of BPH; decreased urinary retention, frequency, urgency, nocturia

Teach patient/family:

• To read patient information leaflet prior to starting therapy; to reread it upon prescription renewal

• To notify prescriber if therapeutic response decreases, if edema occurs

• Not to discontinue product abruptly

• About changes in sex characteristics, gynecomastia, breast hardness; that decreased libido decreases after 6 mo

• That men taking dutasteride should not donate blood for at least 6 mo after last dose to prevent blood administration to pregnant female

• That ejaculate volume may decrease during treatment; that product rarely interferes with sexual function

• That product should not be used or handled by breastfeeding women

• To swallow whole; do not crush, chew, or open capsules

• That product may increase risk for developing high-grade prostate cancer

• To report signs/symptoms of urinary obstruction or decreased urinary flow after starting therapy; to monitor for obstructive uropathy

---

- That continuing exams and blood counts will be needed
- **Pregnancy/breastfeeding:** do not use in pregnancy/breastfeeding; not indicated for women; that capsules should not be handled by a woman who is pregnant or who may become pregnant because product can be absorbed through skin; that product should not be used or handled by breastfeeding women

dutasteride/tamsulosin (Rx)
Jalyn
Func. class.: BPH agent

USES: BPH

CONTRAINDICATIONS
Hypersensitivity

DOSAGE AND ROUTES
- **Adult men:** PO 1 capsule daily, 30 min after a meal

Available forms: Capsules 0.5 mg dutasteride/0.4 mg tamsulosin

duvelisib (Rx)
(doo´-veh-lih´-sib)
Copiktra
Func. class.: Antineoplastic, kinase inhibitor

USES: Relapsed/refractory CLL, SLL, follicular lymphoma in those who have received at least 2 prior therapies

CONTRAINDICATIONS
Hypersensitvity

Black Box Warning: Colitis, diarrhea, infection, pneumonitis

DOSAGE AND ROUTES
- **Adult:** PO 25 mg bid
Available forms: Capsules 15, 25 mg

ecallantide (Rx)

(ee-kal′an-tide)

Kalbitor

Func. class.: Hematologic agent
Chem. class.: Kallikrein inhibitor

USES: Acute attacks of hereditary angioedema (≥12 yr)

CONTRAINDICATIONS

Hypersensitivity to the drug or its components

Black Box Warning: Anaphylaxis (usually within first hour after dosing)

DOSAGE AND ROUTES

• **Adult/adolescent ≥12 yr: SUBCUT** 30 mg given as three 10-mg injections; give additional 30-mg dose within 24 hr if attack persists

Available forms: Injection 10-mg/mL vials

econazole (Rx)

(ee-koe′na-zole)

Ecoza, Ecostatin ✦, Zolpak

Func. class.: Topical antifungal
Chem. class.: Imidazole derivative

USES: Tinea corporis, cruris, pedis, versicolor; cutaneous candidiasis

CONTRAINDICATIONS

Hypersensitivity
Precautions: Pregnancy

DOSAGE AND ROUTES

Tinea corporis, cruris, pedis, versicolor

• **Adult/child: TOPICAL** rub into affected areas daily × 2 wk, or × 4 wk (pedis)

Cutaneous candidiasis

• **Adult/child:** rub into affected areas bid × 2 wk

Available forms: Cream, foam 1%

econazole topical

See Appendix B

eculizumab (Rx)

eck-u-liz′uh-mob

Solaris

Func. class.: Monoclonal antibody

USES: Hemolysis in paroxysmal nocturnal hemoglobinuria (PNH), atypical hemolytic-uremic syndrome (aHUS) to prevent complement-mediated thrombotic microangiopathy

CONTRAINDICATIONS

Hypersensitivity

Black Box Warning: Life-threatening and fatal meningococcal infections

DOSAGE AND ROUTES

Hemolysis in paroxysmal nocturnal hemoglobinuria (PNH):

• **Adult: IV INF** 600 mg q7days × 4 wk, then 900 mg week 5, then 900 mg q14days

Atypical hemolytic-uremic syndrome (aHUS) to prevent complement-mediated thrombotic microangiopathy

• **Adult: IV INF** 900 mg q7days × 4 wk, then 1200 mg week 5, then 1200 mg q14days

• **Child/adolescent ≥40 kg:** 900 mg q7days × 4 wk, then 1200 mg week 5, then 1200 mg q14days

• **Child/adolescent 30-39 kg:** 600 mg q7days × 4 wk, then 900 mg on wk 5 and then 900 mg q14days

• **Child/adolescent 20-29 kg:** 600 mg q7days × 3 wk, then 600 mg q14days

• **Child/adolescents 10-19 kg: IV INF** 600 mg single dose, then after 7 days 300 mg, then 300 mg q14days

• **Infant/child >2 mo and 5-9 kg IV INF:** 300 mg q7days × 2 wk, then 300 mg q21days

Anti-acetylcholine antibody-positive generalized myasthenia gravis
• Adult: IV INF 900 mg q7days × 4 wk, then 1200 mg week 5, then 1200 mg q14days, usually for 12 wk
Anti-aquaporin-4 (AQP4) antibody-positive neuromyelitis optica spectrum disorder (NMOSD)
• Adult: IV INF 900 mg q7days for the first 4 wk, then 1200 mg week 5, then 1200 mg q14days
Available forms: Injection 100 mg/mL (300-mg single-use vial)

---

edaravone (Rx)
(e-dar′-a-vone)
Radicava
Func. class.: CNS agents (ALS)

USES: Amyotrophic lateral sclerosis

DOSAGE AND ROUTES
• Adult: IV: 60 mg/day × 14 days then a 14-day drug-free period for an initial treatment cycle. For subsequent cycles, give × 10 days out of 14-day periods followed by 14-day drug-free periods
Available forms: Injection 30 mg/100 mL premixed bags

---

edetate calcium disodium (Rx)
(ee′de-tate)
Calcium Disodium Versenate
Func. class.: Heavy metal antagonist (antidote, chelating agent)

USES: Lead poisoning, acute lead encephalopathy

CONTRAINDICATIONS
Hypersensitivity, anuria, poisoning of other metals, severe renal disease, hepatitis

Black Box Warning: Child <3 yr, increased ICP, encephalopathy

DOSAGE AND ROUTES
Lead mobilization test (lead toxicity 25-45 mcg/dL)
• Adult/adolescent: IV INFUSION 500 mg/m² over 1 hr or IM
• Child: IV INFUSION 500 mg/m², max 1 g, over 1 hr or IM as single dose or 2 divided doses
Acute lead encephalopathy (blood levels >70 mcg/dL)
• Adult/adolescent/child/infant: IM/IV 1500 mg/m² as IV INFUSION over 12-24 hr in combination with dimercaprol IM, give first dose ≥4 hr after initial dimercaprol, when urine flow established
Available forms: Injection 200 mg/mL

---

efavirenz (Rx)
(ef-ah-veer′enz)
Sustiva
Func. class.: Antiretroviral
Chem. class.: Nonnucleoside reverse transcriptase inhibitor (NNRTI)

ACTION: Binds directly to reverse transcriptase and blocks RNA, DNA polymerase, thus causing a disruption of the enzyme's site

USES: HIV-1 in combination with at least 2 other antivirals
Unlabeled uses: HIV prophylaxis

CONTRAINDICATIONS
Pregnancy, hypersensitivity, moderate/severe hepatic disease
Precautions: Breastfeeding, children <3 yr, renal/hepatic disease, myelosuppression, depression, seizures

DOSAGE AND ROUTES

- **Adult and child ≥3 mo and ≥40 kg: PO** 600 mg/day at bedtime
- **Child ≥3 mo, 32.5-39.9 kg: PO** 400 mg/day at bedtime
- **Child ≥3 mo, 25-32.4 kg: PO** 350 mg/day at bedtime
- **Child ≥3 mo, 20-24.9 kg: PO** 300 mg/day at bedtime
- **Child ≥3 mo, 15-19.9 kg: PO** 250 mg/day at bedtime
- **Child ≥3 mo, 7.5-14.9 kg: PO** 200 mg/day at bedtime
- **Child ≥3 mo, 5-<7.5 kg: PO** 150 mg/day at bedtime
- **Child ≥3 mo, 3.5-<5 kg: PO** 100 mg/day at bedtime

Taking with vorconazole
Adult: PO 400 mg q12h and efavirenz 300 mg q day

Available forms: Capsules 50-, 200-mg; 600-mg tablets

Administer:
- Give on empty stomach; give at bedtime to decrease CNS side effects
- Capsules may be opened, added to grape jelly to disguise peppery taste or sprinkled on food, may be mixed in formula, do not cut/break tablets

SIDE EFFECTS

CNS: Fatigue, impaired cognition, insomnia, abnormal dreams, depression, headache, dizziness, anxiety, drowsiness, odd feeling, suicidal thoughts/behaviors

GI: *Diarrhea,* abdominal pain, *nausea,* vomiting, hepatotoxicity

GU: Hematuria, kidney stones

HEMA: Neutropenia

INTEG: Rash, Stevens-Johnson syndrome, toxic epidermal necrolysis, exfoliative dermatitis

SYST: Immune reconstitution syndrome

MISC: Fat accumulation/redistribution

ENDO: Hyperlipidemia

CV: QT prolongation

PHARMACOKINETICS

Peak 3-5 hr, duration up to 24 hr, well absorbed, metabolized by liver; half-life 40-76 hr; >99% protein binding, excreted in urine, feces; concentrations higher in females and ✍ in those of African, Asian, and Hispanic descent

INTERACTIONS

- Avoid use with boceprevir, delavirdine, rilpivirine; dosage change may be needed if given with telaprevir
- Do not give together with benzodiazepines, ergots, midazolam, triazolam, pimozide

Increase: CNS depression—alcohol, antidepressants, antihistamines, opioids

Increase: levels of both products—ritonavir, estrogens, anticonvulsants

Increase: levels of warfarin, statins (except pravastatin, fluvastatin)

Decrease: levels of indinavir, amprenavir, lopinavir, oral contraceptives, ketoconazole, itraconazole, posaconazole, voriconazole, saquinavir, cyclosporine, tacrolimus, sirolimus, buPROPion, sertraline

Decrease: metabolism of CYP2B6 inhibitors, CYP2C19 substrates, CYP3A4 substrates

Decrease: efavirenz metabolism—CYP3A4 inhibitors (conivaptan, ambrisentan, SORAfenib)

Decrease: efavirenz effect—CYP3A4 inducers (carBAMazepine, rifamycins)

Drug/herb
Decrease: efavirenz level—St. John's wort; do not use together

Drug/food
Increase: absorption—high-fat foods

Drug/lab
Increase: ALT, AST, glucose, amylase
Decrease: neutrophils
False positive: cannabinoids

NURSING CONSIDERATIONS

Assess:
- **HIV:** monitor CBC with differential, plasma HIV RNA, absolute CD4+/CD8+ cell counts/%, serum β_2 microglobulin, serum ICD+24 antigen levels, cholesterol, hepatic enzymes, blood

glucose, pregnancy test, bilirubin, urinalysis

- **Psychiatric/behavioral reactions:** Assess for suicidal thoughts/behaviors, poor concentration, dizziness, inability to sleep, usually resolves after 4 wk, give at bedtime
- Bowel pattern prior to, during treatment; if severe abdominal pain with bleeding occurs, product should be discontinued; monitor hydration
- **QT prolongation:** Monitor those taking drugs that increase QT or those with cardiac diagnosis
- **Immune reconstitution syndrome:** Monitor those using multiple antiretrovirals
- **Serious skin reactions:** Stevens-Johnson syndrome, toxic epidermal necrolysis, usually occurs during first 2 wk, mild rash may resolve within 30 days; severe skin reactions including blistering, fever, product should be discontinued immediately and corticosteroids started
- **Signs of toxicity:** severe nausea/vomiting, maculopapular rash
- **Hepatotoxicity:** LFTs in those with liver disease, hold if LFTs are moderately elevated; if severe or if LFTs increase after product is restarted, discontinue permanently
- **Pregnancy/breastfeeding:** rule out pregnancy prior to starting treatment; use contraception, oral/nonhormonal contraceptives are decreased, use barrier methods also. Avoid use in first trimester (particular caution in first 8 wk of pregnancy) and in females of childbearing potential. Register pregnant women with Antiretroviral Pregnancy Registry (800-258-4263), do not breastfeed

Evaluate:
- Therapeutic response: increased CD4 cell counts; decreased viral load; slowing progression of HIV

Teach patient/family:
- To take as prescribed; if dose is missed, to take as soon as remembered; not to double dose; to take with water, juice; to take on empty stomach at bedtime; to take at same time of day; not to break tablets; to use with other antiretrovirals

- To make sure health care provider knows all medications, supplements, OTC products taken
- To notify health care provider if severe rash occurs; that adverse reactions (rash, dizziness, abnormal dreams, insomnia) lessen after 1 mo, not to stop taking
- To avoid hazardous activities if dizziness, drowsiness occur
- That product does not cure disease but controls symptoms; that HIV can be transmitted to others even while taking this product; to continue with safe-sex practices, that opportunistic infections can occur
- To report all adverse reactions, insomnia, poor concentration, but usually are less in 2-4 wk
- That CNS side effects of feeling "stoned" or "drunk" usually abate in several months
- **Pregnancy/breastfeeding:** Identify if pregnancy is planned or suspected or if breastfeeding; not to breastfeed or become pregnant if taking this product; to use nonhormonal contraception because serious birth defects have occurred, to use barrier method for ≥12 wk after last dose

efavirenz/lamivudine/tenofovir (Rx)

(ef-ah-veer′enz/lam-i-voo′deen/ten-oh-foh′veer)

Symfi, Symfi Lo

Func. class.: Antiretroviral

USES: Human immunodeficiency virus (HIV) infection

CONTRAINDICATIONS
Hypersensitivity

Black Box Warning: Hepatitis B exacerbation

DOSAGE AND ROUTES
- **Adult/adolescent/child ≥35 kg: PO** (Symfi Lo) 1 tablet (efavirenz 400 mg; lamivudine 300 mg; tenofovir 300 mg) on an empty stomach daily at bedtime

• **Adult/adolescent/child ≥40 kg: PO** (Symfi) 1 tablet (efavirenz 600 mg; lamivudine 300 mg; tenofovir 300 mg) on an empty stomach daily at bedtime

Available forms: Tablets 400-300-300 mg; 600-300-300 mg

---

efavirenz/emtricitabine/ tenofovir (Rx)
Atripla
Func. class.: Antiretroviral

USES: HIV

CONTRAINDICATIONS
Hypersensitivity

Black Box Warning: Hepatitis B exacerbation

DOSAGE AND ROUTES
HIV:
• **Adults ≥40 kg : PO** 1 tablet (efavirenz 600 mg, emtricitabine 200 mg, tenofovir 300 mg) daily at bedtime, may be used alone or with other antiretrovirals
• **Child/adolescent ≥40 kg: PO** 1 tablet (efavirenz 600 mg, emtricitabine 200 mg, tenofovir 300 mg) daily at bedtime, may be used alone or with other antiretrovirals

Available forms: Tablet 600-200-300 mg

---

efinaconazole topical
See Appendix B

---

eflapegrastim (Rx)
(ef'la-peg'ra-stim)
Rolvedon
Func. class.: Hemopoietic agent
Chem. class.: Granulocyte colony stimulating factor

ACTION: Stimulates proliferation and differentiation of neutrophils

USES: For chemotherapy-induced neutropenia prophylaxis, to decrease the incidence of febrile neutropenia, in patients with nonmyeloid malignancies receiving myelosuppressive anticancer drugs

CONTRAINDICATIONS
Hypersensitivity to this product, other granulocyte colony stimulating factors, *Escherichia coli* proteins
Precautions: Pregnancy, breastfeeding, myeloid malignancies, sickle cell disease, leukocytosis, splenic rupture, allergic-type reaction

DOSAGE AND ROUTES
Adults: SUBCUT 13.2 mg once per chemotherapy cycle; administer approximately 24 hr after chemotherapy.
Available forms: Solution for injection 13.2 mg/0.6 mL
Administer:
SUBCUT route
• Using single-use vials; after dose is withdrawn, do not reenter vial
• Inspect solution for discoloration, particulates; if present, do not use
• Allow the prefilled syringe to reach room temperature for 30 min prior to use
• Give entire contents of prefilled syringe
• Do not administer during the period 14 days prior to and 24 hr after cytotoxic chemotherapy
• Store in refrigerator; do not freeze; may store at room temperature up to 12 hr; avoid shaking, protect from light

SIDE EFFECTS
CNS: Fever, fatigue, headache, dizziness, insomnia, peripheral edema
GI: Splenic rupture
HEMA: Leukocytosis
INTEG: Alopecia
MISC: Chest pain, hyperuricemia, anaphylaxis, capillary leak syndrome
GU: Glomerulonephritis
MS: Skeletal pain
RESP: Respiratory distress syndrome

PHARMACOKINETICS
Half-life: 15-80 hr; 20-38 hr (children), Tmax 25 hr

INTERACTIONS
• Do not use product concomitantly, 2 wk prior to, or 24 hr after administration of cytotoxic chemotherapy
• Do not use abemaciclib for ≥48 hr after last dose of this product, if required
• Avoid use of eflapegrastim for 21 days after betibeglogene autotemcel infusion

NURSING CONSIDERATIONS
Assess:
• Allergic reactions, anaphylaxis: rash, urticaria; discontinue product, have emergency equipment nearby
• ARDS: dyspnea, fever, tachypnea, occasionally confusion; obtain ABGs, chest x-ray; product may need to be discontinued
• Bone pain: give mild analgesics
• Blood studies: CBC with differential, platelet count before treatment, 2× weekly; neutrophil counts may be increased for 2 days after therapy
• B/P, respirations, pulse prior to and during therapy
• Pregnancy/breastfeeding: use only if benefits outweigh fetal risk, possible major birth defects; cautious use in breastfeeding, excretion unknown
Evaluate:
• Therapeutic response: absence of infection
Teach patient/family:
• To notify prescriber immediately of allergic reaction, trouble breathing, abdominal pain
• To notify provider if dose is missed
• To notify provider if pregnancy is planned or suspected or if breastfeeding

elagolix (Rx)
(el′a-goe′lix)

Orilissa

Func. class.: Gonadotropin-releasing hormone (GnRH) receptor antagonist

ACTION: Suppresses the pituitary, decreases estradiol, progesterone, and other hormones

USES: Moderate to severe pain associated with endometriosis, including endometriosis-related dyspareunia

CONTRAINDICATIONS
Hypersensitivity, osteoporosis, pregnancy

DOSAGE AND ROUTES
• **Moderate-severe pain of endometriosis, not dyspareunia**
Adult female: PO Initiate at 150 mg daily; max duration 24 mo
• **Moderate-severe pain of endometriosis with dyspareunia**
Adult female: PO 200 mg bid, max duration 6 mo
Hepatic dose
Adult female: PO Child-Pugh B 150 mg daily, max 6 mo (all uses)

Available forms: Tablets 200, 300 mg
Administer
• Complete pregnancy test prior to use, or use within 7 days of start of menses
• Give without regard to food, at same time of day
• If dose is missed, give on same day and then start normal dosing
• Store at room temperature

SIDE EFFECTS
CNS: Headache, depression, anxiety, mood/behavior changes, dizziness, insomnia, excitability
GI: Nausea, constipation, diarrhea, abdominal pain, increased LFTs
GU: Decreased libido, amenorrhea
MS: Arthralgia, bone loss, myalgia
MISC: Hypersensitivity

PHARMACOKINETICS
Onset unknown, peak 1 hr, duration unknown
Half-life 4-6 hr

INTERACTIONS

Increase: elagolix effect—CYP3A4 inhibitors

Decrease: elagolix effect—CYP3A4 inducers, midazolam, hormonal contraceptives, strong OATP1B1 inhibitors

Decrease: effect of—CYP3A4 substrates

Drug/lab

Increase: LFTs, triglycerides, cholesterol, LDL, HDL

NURSING CONSIDERATIONS
Assess:
- **Endometriosis:** assess for pain and pain associated with dyspareunia prior to starting product and after use
- **Suicidal ideation:** assess for depression, change in mood, product may need to be discontinued
- **Bone density:** monitor for fractures, osteoporosis, obtain bone density test
- Monitor LFTs baseline and periodically

Evaluate:
- Therapeutic response: decreasing pain in endometriosis

Teach patient/family:
- **Pregnancy/breastfeeding:** identify if pregnancy is planned or suspected, do not use in pregnancy, consider risks in breastfeeding, hormonal contraceptives with estrogen will reduce the product's effectiveness
- **Suicidal thoughts/behaviors:** advise caretakers, family, patient to notify provider immediately of depression, change in mood, suicidal thoughts, behaviors
- If dose is missed, take as soon as remembered, then continue with regular dosing
- Report yellowing eyes, skin, clay-colored stool, dark urine, nausea, vomiting, which may signal liver injury
- That the product will change menses
- **Bone density:** advise patient bone loss may occur, that bone density test may be required, to supplement with calcium and vitamin D to prevent bone loss if prescribed

---

elbasvir/grazoprevir (Rx)
(el'bas-vir/graz-oh'pre-vir)

Zepatier

Func. class.: Antiviral

USES: Chronic HCV genotypes 1 or 4 ✎⃝

CONTRAINDICATIONS
Hypersensitivity

Black Box Warning: Reactivation of HBV

DOSAGE AND ROUTES
Chronic HCV genotypes 1 or 4
- **Adult:** 1 tablet daily, may give with or without ribavirin

Hepatic dose
- **Adult:** PO do not use in severe hepatic disease

Available forms: Tablets 50-100 mg

---

eletriptan (Rx)
(el-ee-trip'tan)

Relpax

Func. class.: Antimigraine agent, abortive
Chem. class.: 5-HT$_1$-1B/1D receptor agonist, triptan

ACTION: Binds selectively to the vascular 5-HT$_1$-receptor subtype; causes vasoconstriction in cranial arteries

USES: Acute treatment of migraine with/without aura

CONTRAINDICATIONS
Hypersen-sitivity, coronary artery vasospasm, peripheral vascular disease, hemiplegic/basilar migraine, uncontrolled hypertension; ischemic bowel, heart disease; severe renal/hepatic disease, acute MI, stroke, angina, postmenopausal women, men >40 yr; risk factors of CAD, MI, or other cardiac disease; hypercholesterolemia, obesity, diabetes

---

Precautions: Pregnancy, breastfeeding, children, geriatric patients, impaired renal/hepatic function

DOSAGE AND ROUTES
• **Adult: PO** 20 or 40 mg, may increase if needed, max 40 mg (single dose); may repeat in 2 hr if headache improves but returns, max 80 mg/24 hr
Available forms: Tablets 20, 40 mg
Administer:
• Swallow tablets whole; do not break, crush, or chew; use with 8 oz of water, without regard to food
• At beginning of headache; if headache returns, repeat dose after 2 hr if first dose is ineffective; treat no more than 3 headaches per 30 days

SIDE EFFECTS
CNS: *Dizziness,* headache, anxiety, paresthesia, asthenia, somnolence, flushing, fatigue, hot/cold sensation, chills, vertigo, hypertonia, seizures, serotonin syndrome
CV: Chest pain, palpitations, hypertension, MI, sinus tachycardia, stroke, ventricular fibrillation/tachycardia, atrial fibrillation, AV block, bradycardia, chest pressure syndrome, coronary vasospasm
GI: Nausea, dry mouth, vomiting
MS: *Weakness,* back pain
RESP: Chest tightness, pressure

PHARMACOKINETICS
Onset of pain relief ½ hr, peak 1½-2 hr, half-life 4 hr, metabolized in the liver, 70% excreted in urine and feces

INTERACTIONS
Increase: eletriptan effect—CYP3A4 inhibitors (clarithromycin, erythromycin, itraconazole, ketoconazole, nelfinavir, ritonavir), propranolol; avoid use within 72 hr of these products
Increase: serotonin syndrome—SSRIs, SNRIs, serotonin-receptor agonists, linezolid, MAOIs, TCAs, methylene blue
Increase: vasospastic reactions—ergots, ergot-similar products; avoid use within 24 hr of these products
Do not use with other 5-HT antagonists

NURSING CONSIDERATIONS
Assess:
• **Migraine:** pain location, character, intensity, nausea, vomiting, aura; quiet, calm environment with decreased stimulation from noise, bright light, excessive talking
• **CV:** B/P; signs, symptoms of coronary vasospasms, geriatric patients may be at higher risk
• Tingling, hot sensation, burning, feeling of pressure, numbness, flushing
• Stress level, activity, recreation, coping mechanisms
• **Neurologic status:** LOC, blurring vision, nausea, vomiting, tingling in extremities preceding headache
• Ingestion of tyramine foods (pickled products, beer, wine, aged cheese), food additives, preservatives, colorings, artificial sweeteners, chocolate, caffeine, which may precipitate these types of headaches
• Patients with CAD risk factors; first dose should be administered in prescriber's office or medical facility
• Determine whether CYP3A4 inhibitors or other ergot-type products have been given
Evaluate:
• Therapeutic response: decrease in frequency, severity of migraine
Teach patient/family:
• To avoid driving or hazardous activity if dizziness occurs
• To report chest pain, neck or jaw pain
• To take whole with full glass of water
• To take when migraine is starting; a second dose may be used if headache returns
• To use contraception while taking product; to inform prescriber if pregnant or intending to become pregnant
• To provide dark, quiet environment

- That product does not prevent or reduce number of migraine attacks
- To use product only short term

elexacaftor/tezacaftor/ivacaftor and ivacaftor (Rx)
(el-ex-a-kaf'tor/tez-a-kaf'tor/eye-va-kaf'tor)

Trikafta

Func. Class.: Metabolic

USES: Cystic fibrosis (CF) with at least 1 *F508del* mutation in the cystic fibrosis transmembrane conductance regulator (CFTR) gene

CONTRAINDICATIONS
Hypersensitivity

DOSAGE AND ROUTES
Cystic fibrosis (CF) with at least one *F508del* mutation in the cystic fibrosis transmembrane conductance regulator (CFTR) gene:
- **Adult/adolescent ≥12 yr: PO** 2 tablets (elexacaftor 100 mg/tezacaftor 50 mg/ivacaftor 75 mg) in the morning and 1 tablet ivacaftor 150 mg in the evening 12 hr apart and given with fat-containing food

Hepatic dose:
- **Adult/adolescent ≥12 yr: PO moderate impairment (Child-Pugh class B):** 2 tablets containing elexacaftor 100 mg/tezacaftor 50 mg/ivacaftor 75 mg PO once daily; NO ivacaftor 150-mg dose. Use with caution; this drug has not been studied in patients with moderate impairment; **severe impairment (Child-Pugh class C):** Do not use

Available forms: Tablets 100-50-75 mg with ivacaftor 150 mg

⚠ HIGH ALERT

elotuzumab (Rx)
(El-oh-tooz'ue-mab)

Empliciti

Func. class.: Antineoplastic

Chem. class.: Monoclonal antibody

ACTION: A humanized IgG1 monoclonal antibody that binds to the signaling lymphocytic activation molecule family member 7 (SLAMF7), a cell surface glycoprotein receptor, and activates natural killer (NK) cell–mediated antibody-dependent cellular cytotoxicity of SLAMF7-expressing myeloma cells

USES: Multiple myeloma in patients who have received 1 to 3 prior therapies, in combination with lenalidomide and dexamethasone

CONTRAINDICATIONS
Hypersensitivity, breastfeeding, hepatotoxicity, infection, infusion-related reactions, new primary malignancy, pregnancy
Precautions: Hepatic disease

DOSAGE AND ROUTES
Multiple myeloma in patients who have received 1 to 3 prior therapies, in combination with lenalidomide and dexamethasone
- **Adult: IV** 10 mg/kg weekly on cycles 1 and 2 (on days 1, 8, 15, and 22), then q2wk (on days 1 and 15), give in combination with lenalidomide 25 mg daily on days 1 through 21 and dexamethasone 28 mg PO (taken 3 to 24 hr prior to elotuzumab) on days 1, 8, 15, and 22 on cycles 1 and 2 and on days 1 and 15 of subsequent cycles; give dexamethasone 40 mg PO on days 8

and 22 of cycles 3 and beyond. Repeat treatment cycles q28 days until disease progression

Multiple myeloma in patients who have received at least 2 prior therapies including lenalidomide and a proteasome inhibitor, in combination with pomalidomide and dexamethasone

• **Adult:** IV 10 mg/kg weekly on cycles 1 and 2 (on days 1, 8, 15, and 22), then 20 mg/kg IV q4wk (on day 1) starting on cycle 3, give in combination with pomalidomide 4 mg PO daily on days 1 through 21 and PO dexamethasone (age 75 yr or less, 28 mg; age over 75 yr, 8 mg) at 3 to 24 hr prior to elotuzumab on days 1, 8, 15, and 22 on cycles 1 and 2 and on day 1 of subsequent cycles, give PO dexamethasone (age 75 yr or less, 40 mg; age over 75 yr, 20 mg) at 3 to 24 hr prior to elotuzumab on days 8, 15, and 22 of cycles 3 and beyond. Repeat treatment cycles q28days until disease progression

Available forms: Injection 300, 400 mg in single-dose vials

Administer:

IV route

• Visually inspect parenteral products for particulate matter and discoloration prior to use

• Premedication with acetaminophen PO, an IV/PO H1-blocker (diphenhydramine), an IV/PO H2-blocker, and IV dexamethasone is required prior to each infusion; hold therapy for grade 2 or higher infusion-related reactions

• Do not mix with other drugs or infuse with other drugs through the same IV line

• Calculate the appropriate dose and reconstitute (using an 18-gauge or smaller needle) the 300-mg vial with 13 mL of sterile water for injection and the 400-mg vial with 17 mL of sterile water for injection

• Following reconstitution, each vial contains overfill to allow for a maximum withdrawal of 12 mL for the 300-mg vial and 16 mL for the 400-mg vial; the final vial concentration is 25 mg/mL

• Swirl the solution by rotating the vial; invert the vial a few times to dissolve the powder

• The lyophilized powder should dissolve within 10 min; allow the reconstituted solution to stand for 5 to 10 min after all powder is dissolved

• Withdraw the needed amount (mL) from the elotuzumab 25-mg/mL vials; do not exceed a maximum withdrawal of 12 mL for the 300-mg vial and of 16 mL for the 400-mg vial; discard any unused portion

• Add the calculated amount of elotuzumab to an infusion bag made of polyvinyl chloride or polyolefin and then add enough 0.9% NaCl for injection or 5% dextrose injection so that the final diluted admixture concentration is between 1 and 6 mg/mL

• Do NOT exceed 5 mL/kg of patient weight at any given dose

• *Storage following dilution:* The diluted admixture may be stored for up to 24 hr when refrigerated 36° F to 46° F (2° C to 8° C) and protected from light; a maximum of 8 hr (of the total 24 hr) may be at room temperature 68° F to 77° F (20° C to 25° C)

• Administer the diluted admixture using an infusion set and a sterile, nonpyrogenic, low-protein-binding filter (pore size of 0.2 to 1.2 micrometer); use an automated infusion pump

• **For the 10-mg/kg dose,** give the diluted infusion IV at the appropriate infusion rate as follows:

Cycle 1, dose 1: start at 0.5 mL/min for 30 min, increase to 1 mL/min for 30 min, then increase to a maximum rate of 2 mL/min

Cycle 1, dose 2: start at 3 mL/min for 30 min, then increase to a maximum rate of 4 mL/min

Cycle 1, doses 3 and 4, and all subsequent cycles: 5 mL/min; do not exceed this rate

• **For the 20 mg/kg dose,** administer the diluted infusion intravenously at the appropriate infusion rate as follows:

Dose 1: Start at 3 mL/min for 30 min, then increase to a maximum rate of 4 mL/min

Dose 2 and all subsequent doses: 5 mL/min; do not exceed this rate
• Up titration of the infusion rate may be considered only in the absence of infusion reactions
• Complete the infusion within 24 hr from reconstitution

PHARMACOKINETICS
Onset, peak, duration unknown; half-life unknown

INTERACTIONS
Palifermin: should not be administered within 24 hr prior to, during infusion of, or within 24 hr after administration of antineoplastic agents
Increased risk of developing severe hematologic and renal toxicity: Penicillamine: Do not use together
Decrease immunologic response to tuberculin purified protein derivative (PPD): Tuberculin Purified Protein Derivative, PPD

NURSING CONSIDERATIONS
Assess:
• **Hypersensitivity:** Assess for rash, throat tightness, dyspnea, stop infusion immediately
• **Infections:** Assess for fever, flulike symptoms, may be fatal, treat as needed
• **New primary malignancy:** Monitor for new malignancies
• **Infusion reactions:** Assess for infusion reactions: redness, inflammation, burning at site within 24 hr of infusion, chills, fever; stop infusion, treat as needed, monitor VS
• **Pregnancy/breastfeeding:** Do not use in pregnancy or breastfeeding. Males and females should use contraception if of reproductive potential
Evaluate:
• **Therapeutic response:** decreasing symptoms and spread of multiple myeloma
Teach patient/family:
• **Hypersensitivity:** teach patient to report immediately rash, throat tightness, dyspnea
• **Infections:** teach patient to report fever, flulike symptoms, may be fatal

• **New primary malignancy:** teach patient to report any new malignancies
• **Infusion reactions:** teach patient to report infusion reactions: redness, inflammation, burning at site within 24 hr of infusion
• **Pregnancy/breastfeeding:** identify if pregnancy is planned or suspected. Do not use in pregnancy or breastfeeding. Males and females should use contraception if of reproductive potential

---

eltrombopag (Rx)
(ell-trom-bow'pag)
Promacta
Func. class.: Hematopoietic

USES: Thrombocytopenia in chronic immune thrombocytopenic purpura when unresponsive to other treatment, chronic hepatitis C–associated thrombocytopenia

CONTRAINDICATIONS
Hypersensitivity

Black Box Warning: Hepatotoxicity

DOSAGE AND ROUTES
• **Adult: PO** 50 mg/day, adjust dosage to maintain platelets at $\geq 50 \times 10^9$, max 75 mg/day; 25 mg/day chronic hepatitis C; ✵ East Asian descent, reduce dose to 25 mg daily
Available forms: Powder for oral suspension packets 12.5, 25 mg; tablets 12.5, 25, 50, 75 mg

---

eluxadoline (Rx)
(el-ux-ad'oh-leen)
Viberzi
Func. class.: GI agent

ACTION: Acts locally, reducing abdominal pain of IBS, works on the μ-opioid receptor

USES: Irritable bowel syndrome with diarrhea

CONTRAINDICATIONS
Hypersensitivity, alcoholism, GI/biliary obstruction, constipation, pancreatitis

DOSAGE AND ROUTES
• **Adult:** PO 100 mg bid with food. Decrease to 75 mg bid with food in those who are receiving an OATP1B1 inhibitor; do not use in those without a gallbladder
Renal dose
Adult: PO CCr <60 mL/min: reduce to 75 mg bid with food
Hepatic dose
Adult: PO Child-Pugh Class A or B: reduce to 75 mg bid with food; Child-Pugh Class C: Do not use

Available forms: Tablets 75, 100 mg
Administer
• Give with food
• Give as prescribed, do not double, if a dose is missed, give at next regular scheduled dose
• Store at room temperature

SIDE EFFECT
CNS: Headache, dizziness, insomnia, drowsiness, drunk feeling
GI: Constipation, nausea, vomiting, distention, increased LFTs
EENT: Nasopharyngitis
INTEG: Rash
RESP: URI, asthma

PHARMACOKINETICS: Onset unknown, peak 1½ hr, duration unknown, half-life 3.7-6 hr

INTERACTIONS
Increase: CYP3A4 substrate (narrow therapeutic index) effect
Increase: constipation risk—anticholinergics
Increase: eluxadoline effect—OATP1B1 inhibitors, CYP3A4 inhibitors

NURSING CONSIDERATIONS
Assess:
• **IBS symptoms:** assess for constipation/diarrhea or both, abdominal pain, bloating, gas. Identify if product is lessening symptoms; monitor AST/ALT, serum lipase, BUN/creatinine
• **CNS changes:** assess for dizziness, drowsiness; caution against driving or other hazardous activities until response is known, usually with hepatic impairment
• **Spasm:** epigastric pain, may radiate to back, may have increased LFTs
• **Pregnancy/breastfeeding:** unknown as to fetal risk, use cautiously in breastfeeding
Evaluate:
• Therapeutic response
• Decreasing abdominal pain, bloating, gas, diarrhea/constipation
Teach patient/family:
• **Severe constipation:** avoid using with other products that cause constipation; if severe constipation occurs, stop drug, notify prescriber, avoid using
• **Pancreatitis:** usually with increased alcohol use, severe abdominal pain, nausea, vomiting, discontinue immediately
• Not to drive or perform other hazardous activities until response is known
• **Pregnancy/breastfeeding:** identify if pregnancy is planned or suspected
• **Spasm:** to notify provider of increasing epigastric pain that radiates to back
• To take missed dose at prescribed time, do not double or skip doses

elvitegravir/cobicistat/ emtricitabine/tenofovir disoproxil fumarate (Rx)
(el-vye-teg´gra-veer/koe-bik´i-stat/ em-tra-sye´tah-ben/ten-oh-foh´veer)
Stribild
elvitegravir/cobicistat/ emtricitabine/tenofovir alafenamide
Genvoya
Func. class.: Antiretrovirals

ACTION: Elvitegravir: Inhibits the activity of HIV integrase, which is one of three HIV-encoded enzymes required for viral replication

Cobicistat: An inhibitor of CYP3A enzymes

Emtricitabine: A synthetic nucleoside analog of cytidine, inhibits the activity of HIV-1 reverse transcriptase (RT) by competing with the natural substrate into viral DNA, resulting in chain termination

Tenofovir disoproxil fumarate: Inhibits viral reverse transcriptase.

USES: HIV in treatment-naive patients

CONTRAINDICATIONS

Hypersensitivity, CCr <50 mL/min, severe hepatic disease

PRECAUTIONS

Pregnancy, obesity, osteoporosis, renal disease, Hispanic patients immune reconstitution syndrome

Black Box Warning: Hepatitis B/HIV combination, hepatitis B exacerbation

DOSAGE AND ROUTES

Stribild
• **Adult/child ≥12 yr, ≥35 kg, CCr ≥70 mL/min: PO** 1 tablet daily with food

Renal dose
• **Adult: PO** do not use in CCr <50 mL/min

Genvoya
• **Adult/child ≥12 yr, ≥35 kg: PO** 1 tablet daily with food

Available forms: Stribild: Tablet 150 mg: elvitegravir-150 mg, cobicistat-200 mg, emtricitabine-300 mg, tenofovir disoproxil; **Genvoya:** tablet 150 mg elvitegravir, 150 mg cobicistat, 200 mg emtricitabine, 10 mg tenofovir alafenamide

Administer
• Administer tablet with food
• Don't use with other antiretrovirals

SIDE EFFECTS

GI: Abdominal pain, diarrhea, dyspepsia, flatulence, hepatic decompensation, hepatic failure, hepatitis B exacerbation, hepatomegaly, nausea, vomiting, weight gain, pancreatitis, increased LFTs

CNS: Anxiety, depression, dizziness, fatigue, headache, insomnia, paresthesias, peripheral neuropathy, suicidal ideation, fever

INTEG: Angioedema, rash, pruritis, skin discoloration/hyperpigmentation

MS: Arthralgia, back pain, bone fractures, bone pain, myalgia, myopathy, rhabdomyolysis

RESP: Cough, dyspnea, pharyngitis, rhinitis, sinusitis

GU: Glycosuria, hematuria, proteinuria, renal failure, Fanconi syndrome

META: Hyperamylasemia, hyperbilirubinemia, hypercholesterolemia, hyperglycemia, hyperlipidemia, hypertriglyceridemia, hypoglycemia, hypokalemia, hypophosphatemia

HEMA: Neutropenia

MISC: Infection, lactic acidosis, myasthenia, steatosis

PHARMACOKINETICS

Elvitegravir: Onset unknown, peak 4 hr, duration unknown, half-life 13 hr

Cobicistat: Onset unknown, peak 3 hr, duration unknown, half-life 4 hr

Emtricitabine: Onset unknown, peak 3 hr, duration unknown, half-life 10 hr

Tenofovir disoproxil fumarate: Onset unknown, peak 2 hr, duration unknown, half-life 12-18 hr

INTERACTIONS

Decrease: elvitegravir levels—antacids

Increase: alfa1 adrenoreceptor antagonists (alfuzosin)

Decrease: elvitegravir, cobicistat levels with analeptics (modafinil)

Increase: antiarrhythmic levels (amiodarone, bepridil, digoxin, disopyramide, flecainide, systemic lidocaine, propafenone, quiNIDine)

Increase: antibacterials (clarithromycin, telithromycin), cobicistat

Increase or Decrease: anticoagulants (warfarin) levels possible

Increase: anticonvulsants (carBAMazepine, OXcarbazepine, phenobarbital, phenytoin, clomazepam, ethosuximide), cobicistat, tenofovir, alafenamide

Increase: Antidepressants (SSRI paroxetine, tricyclic antidepressants [TCAs], amatriptyline, desipramine, imipramine, nortriptyline, buPROPion; traZODone)

Increase: antifungals (itraconazole, ketoconazole, voriconazole)

Increase: antigout (colchicine)

Decrease: elvitegrvir, cobicistat, tenofovir, alafenamide

Increase: rifabutim with antimicrobacterial (rifabutim, rifAMPin, rifapentine)

Increase: levels of antipsychotic (quetiapine)

Increase: levels of benzodiazepine (diazePAM, lorazePAM, midazolam, triazolam)

Increase: levels of beta-blockers (metoprolol, timolol)

Increase: levels of calcium channel blockers (amLODIPine, dilTIAZem, felodipine, nicardipine, nifedipine, verapamil)

Decrease: levels of elvitegravir, cobicistat with corticosteroids (dexamethasome)

Increase: levels of corticosteroids (betamethasone, budesonide, dexamethasone, fluticasone, mometasone, triamcinolone)

Increase: levels of endothelin receptor antagonists (bosentan)

Increase: levels of ergot derivatives (dihydroergotamine, ergonovine, ergotamine, methylergonovine)

Increase: levels of GI motility agents (cisapride)

Increase: levels of HCV antivirals (tenofovir, elbasvir, grazoprevir, alafenamide)

Increase: levels of HMG-CoA reductase inhibitors

Increase: drospirenone, norgesimate

Decrease: ethinyl estradiol

Increase: levels of immunosuppressants, tenofovir alafenamide

Drug/lab

Increase: AST/ALT, amylase, bilirubin, CK, glucose, lipase, total cholesterol, triglycerides

Decrease: neutrophils, potassium, phosphate

NURSING CONSIDERATIONS
Assess:
• **HIV:** monitor for infections and improvement in symptoms of HIV

• Renal/hepatic function tests: AST, ALT, bilirubin, amylase, lipase, triglycerides periodically during treatment

• Lactic acidosis, severe hepatomegaly with steatosis: if lab reports confirm these conditions, discontinue treatment; may be fatal; more common in females or those who are overweight; monitor lactic acid levels, LFTs

> **Black Box Warning: Hepatotoxicity:** do not use in risk factors such as alcoholism; discontinue if hepatotoxicity occurs

• Carefully evaluate drug interactions before starting therapy

• **Hepatitis B & HIV coinfection (unlabeled);** perform HBV screening in any patient who has HIV; avoid single-drug treatments in HBV

• **Pregnancy/breastfeeding:** use if clearly needed; register pregnant women in the Antiretroviral Pregnancy Registry at 800-258-4263; to reduce the risk of postnatal transmission, HIV-infected mothers are advised to avoid breastfeeding

Evaluate:
• Therapeutic response: decreased signs, symptoms of HIV; decreased viral load, increased CD4 counts

Teach patient/family:
• That GI complaints resolve after 3-4 wk of treatment

• That product must be taken at same time of day to maintain blood level; solution and capsule are not interchangeable; that if dose is missed, to take as soon as remembered; not to double doses; not to share with others

• That product will control symptoms but is not a cure for HIV; patient still infectious, may pass HIV virus on to others; that other products may be necessary to prevent other infections; to practice safe sex and use a condom; not to share needles or donate blood

• That changes in body fat distribution may occur

• **Lactic acidosis:** to notify prescriber immediately if fatigue, muscle aches/pains, abdominal pain, difficulty breathing, nausea, vomiting, change in heart rhythm occur

> **Black Box Warning: Hepatotoxicity:** to notify prescriber of dark urine, yellowing of skin/eyes, clay-colored stools, anorexia, nausea, vomiting product

---

Side effects: *italics* = common; red = life-threatening

• To report planned or suspected pregnancy; not to breastfeed while taking

emapalumab-lzsg (Rx)
(em-a-pal′ue-mab)
Gamifant
Func. class.: Immunomodulator
Chem. class.: Monoclonal antibody

USES: Treatment of primary hemophagocytic lymphohistiocytosis (HLH) with refractory, recurrent, or progressive disease or intolerance with conventional HLH therapy

CONTRAINDICATIONS
Hypersensitivity

DOSAGE AND ROUTES
• **Adults/children:** IV 1 mg/kg/dose over 1 hr twice per week (every 3 to 4 days). A dose increase on day 3 (to 3 mg/kg/dose), days 6 to 8 (to 6 mg/kg/dose), and day 9 onwards (to 10 mg/kg/dose) may be needed
Available forms: Injection 10 mg/2 mL, 50 mg/mL, 100 mg/mL single dose

emedastine ophthalmic
See Appendix B

emicizumab-kxwh (Rx)
(em′i-siz′ue-mab)
Hemlibra
Func. class.: Antibody IgG4

USES:
For routine bleeding prophylaxis to prevent or reduce the frequency of bleeding episodes in patients with hemophilia A (congenital factor VIII deficiency) with or without factor VIII inhibitors

CONTRAINDICATIONS
Hypersensitivity

DOSAGE AND ROUTES
• **Adult and child:** SUBCUT: 3 mg/kg/dose weekly for the first 4 wk, then a maintenance dose of 1.5 mg/kg/dose, weekly, 3 mg/kg/dose weekly every 2 wk, or 6 mg/kg/dose q4wk
Available forms:
Injection 30 mg/mL, 60 mg/0.4 mL, 105 mg/0.7 mL, 150 mg/mL single dose

empagliflozin (Rx)
(em-pa-gli-floe′zin)
Jardiance
Func. class.: Antidiabetic
Chem. class.: Sodium-glucose cotransporter 2 (SGLT2) inhibitor

ACTION: An inhibitor of sodium-glucose cotransporter 2 (SGLT2), the transporter responsible for reabsorbing the majority of glucose filtered by the tubular lumen in the kidney

USES: Type 2 diabetes mellitus with diet and exercise to reduce CV death in diabetes mellitus

CONTRAINDICATIONS
Hypersensitivity, dialysis, renal failure
Precautions: Adrenal insufficiency, breastfeeding, children, dehydration, diabetic ketoacidosis, fever, geriatric patients, hypercholesterolemia, hypercortisolism, hyperglycemia, hyperthyroidism, hypoglycemia, hypotension, hypothyroidism, hypovolemia, malnutrition, pituitary insufficiency, pregnancy, renal impairment, type 1 diabetes mellitus, vaginitis

DOSAGE AND ROUTES
Type 2 diabetes with CV disease
• **Adult:** PO 10 mg q day, may increase to 25 mg q day
HF with reduced ejection fraction
• **Adult:** PO 10 mg q day
Renal dose
• **Adult:** PO GFR <30 (DM), 20 (HF) mL/min do not use
Type 2 diabetes
• **Adult:** PO 10 mg daily, may increase to 25 mg daily
Available forms: Tablets 10, 25 mg
Administer:
• Give every day without regard to food in the AM

• Store at room temperature, protect from moisture

SIDE EFFECTS
MS: Arthralgia
ENDO: Hypercholesterolemia, hyperlipidemia, hypoglycemia (in combination)
CV: Hypotension, orthostatic hypotension
GU: Increased urinary frequency, nocturia, polyuria, cystitis, dehydration, diuresis, UTI
GI: Nausea
CNS: Syncope
HEMA: Increased Hct
RESP: URI
MISC: Infection, ketoacidosis, URI

PHARMACOKINETICS
Protein binding 82.6%, terminal elimination half-life 12.4 hr, peak 1.5 hr

INTERACTIONS
Increase: hypoglycemic effect—angiotensin II receptor antagonists, angiotensin-converting enzyme (ACE) inhibitors, loop diuretics, thiazide diuretics, fluoxetine, olanzapine, beta-blockers, other antidiabetics, octreotide, fibric acid derivatives, MAOIs type A
Increase/Decrease: hypoglycemic effect—clonidine, androgens, bortezomib, lithium, alcohol, sulfonamides
Decrease: hypoglycemic effect—phenothiazines, typical antipsychotics, baclofen, carbonic anhydrase inhibitors, estrogens, progestins, oral contraceptives, dextrothyroxine, glucagon, corticosteroids, fenfluramine, dexfenfluramine, phenytoin, fosphenytoin, ethotoin, salicylates, cycloSPORINE, tacrolimus, tobacco
Drug/herb/Supplements
Increase: hypoglycemia—chromium, horse chestnut
Increase/Decrease: hypoglycemia—niacin
Decrease: hypoglycemia—green tea
Drug/lab
Increase: HCT, creatinine
Decrease: GFR

NURSING CONSIDERATIONS
Assess:
• **Diabetes:** monitor blood glucose, glycosylated hemoglobin A1c (HbA1c), serum cholesterol profile, serum creatinine/BUN, assess for polydipsia, other products taken by patient; assess for hypoglycemia, headache, drowsiness, hunger, weakness, sweating; have sugar source available
• **Ketoacidosis:** if patient has volume depletion, dehydration, discontinue, give insulin, glucose source
• **Renal studies:** monitor serum creatinine eGFR baseline and periodically avoid in those with eGFR <45 mL/min/1.73 m^2
• **UTI:** treat with anti-infective
• **Pregnancy/breastfeeding:** use if benefits outweigh risk to fetus; no well-controlled studies; do not breastfeed
Evaluate:
• Therapeutic response: decreasing blood glucose, A1c
Teach patient/family:
• How to check blood glucose; to continue with diet and exercise changes; to avoid smoking, alcohol
• That frequent blood glucose, HbA1c, BUN/creatinine will be needed
• To avoid other products unless approved by prescriber
• To take in the AM, without regard to food; that if dose is missed, to take when remembered, do not double dose; to read "medication guide" provided; that product controls symptoms but does not cure diabetes
• To follow medical regimen including diet, exercise, and weight loss
• Teach how to take blood glucose, urine ketones readings and how often
• **Hypoglycemia:** to report rapid heartbeat, dizziness, weakness; that lab testing will be needed, including blood glucose monitoring, and that a dosage change may be needed; to carry a sugar source at all times; review signs and symptoms of hypoglycemia and hyperglycemia and what to do about each
• **Hypotension:** to report vision changes, dizziness, fatigue; B/P should be checked regularly, stress adequate hydration
• **Ketoacidosis:** to report nausea, vomiting, abdominal pain, confusion, sleepiness
• **Infections:** (usually UTIs) to report burning; cloudy, foul-smelling urine; fever; back pain; antibiotics will be needed; and

to report symptoms of mycotic infections, including foul-smelling vaginal discharge or penile discharge and redness; UTI: burning/stinging on urination, frequency
• **Pregnancy/breastfeeding:** to report if pregnancy is planned or suspected; not to breastfeed

empagliflozin/ metformin (Rx)

(em′pa-gli-floe′zin/met-for′min)

Synjardy, Synjardy XR

Func. class.: Antidiabetic

Chem. class.: Biguanide; sodium-glucose cotransporter 2 (SGLT2) inhibitor

USES: Type 2 diabetes mellitus

CONTRAINDICATIONS

Hypersensitivity, diabetic ketoacidosis, dialysis, metabolic acidosis, radiographic contrast administration, renal failure

Black Box Warning: Lactic acidosis

Precautions: Pregnancy, geriatric patients, severe renal/hepatic/GI disease, pancreatitis, vitamin D deficiency, acidemia, acute heart failure, acute myocardial infarction, alcoholism, balanitis, breastfeeding, burns, cardiac disease, children, dehydration, diarrhea, ethanol intoxication, fever, gastroparesis, hypercholesterolemia, hypercortisolism, hyperglycemia, hyperthyroidism, hypoglycemia, hypotension, hypovolemia, hypoxemia, infection, malnutrition, pernicious anemia, pituitary insufficiency, polycystic ovary syndrome, sepsis, surgery, trauma, type 1 diabetes mellitus, vaginitis, vomiting

DOSAGE AND ROUTES

• **Adult: PO** bid with meals; individualize. In geriatric patients, use lowest effective dose. Max in normal renal function is empagliflozin 25 mg/day and metformin 2000 mg/day; correct volume depletion prior to initiation of treatment

• **Patients currently treated with empagliflozin:** metformin 500 mg with a similar total daily dose of empagliflozin; increase gradually to reduce the GI side effects
• **Patients currently treated with metformin:** empagliflozin 5 mg/dose with a similar total daily dose of metformin. Patients taking an evening dose of metformin XR should check with their provider about when to take their last dose prior to starting empagliflozin/ metformin
• **Patients already treated with both empagliflozin and metformin:** use the same doses of each component per day, then divide the daily doses to bid dosing with meals
Renal dose:
• **Adult: PO** eGFR ≥45 mL/min/1.73 m^2, no change; eGFR <45 mL/min/1.73 m^2, do not use
Available forms: Tablets 5 mg/1000 mg, 12.5 mg/1000 mg; extended-release tablets 5 mg/1000 mg, 12.5 mg/1000 mg

emtricitabine (Rx)

(em-tri-sit′uh-bean)

Emtriva

Func. class.: Antiretroviral

Chem. class.: Nucleoside reverse transcriptase inhibitor (NRTI)

ACTION: A synthetic nucleoside analog of cytosine; inhibits replication of HIV virus by competing with the natural substrate and then becoming incorporated into cellular DNA by viral reverse transcriptase, thereby terminating the cellular DNA chain

USES: HIV-1 infection with other antiretrovirals
Unlabeled uses: HBV infection with HIV, HIV prophylaxis

CONTRAINDICATIONS

Hyper-sensitivity
Precautions: Pregnancy, breastfeeding, children, geriatric patients, renal disease, lactic acidosis

Black Box Warning: Hepatic insufficiency, chronic hepatitis B virus (HBV)

DOSAGE AND ROUTES
HIV-1 infection with other antiretrovirals
• **Adult:** PO Capsules 200 mg/day; oral solution 240 mg (24 mL)/day
• **Adolescent/child >33 kg: PO** Capsules 200 mg/day; **child 3 mo-17 yr:** oral solution 6 mg/kg/day, max 240 mg (24 mL)
• **Infants <3 mo: PO oral solution** 3 mg/kg daily, do not use capsules
Renal dose
• **Adult: PO** Capsules CCr 30-49 mL/min, 200 mg q48hr; oral solution 120 mg q24hr; capsules CCr 15-29 mL/min, 200 mg q72hr; oral solution 80 mg q24hr; capsules CCr <15 mL/min, 200 mg q96hr; oral solution 60 mg q24hr
Available forms: Capsules 200 mg; oral solution 10 mg/mL
Administer:
• Give without regard to meals
• Refrigerate oral solution, if stored at room temperature, discard after 3 mo
• Oral capsules and solution not interchangeable
• Store capsules at 77° F (25° C); oral solution refrigerated, use within 3 mo

SIDE EFFECTS
CNS: *Headache,* abnormal dreams, *depression,* dizziness, *insomnia,* neuropathy, paresthesia, *asthenia,* weakness
GI: *Nausea, vomiting, diarrhea, anorexia,* abdominal pain, dyspepsia, hepatomegaly with steatosis (may be fatal)
INTEG: *Rash,* skin discoloration
MS: Arthralgia, myalgia
RESP: *Cough*
SYST: Change in body fat distribution, lactic acidosis, immune reconstitution syndrome

PHARMACOKINETICS
Rapidly, extensively absorbed; peak 1-2 hr; protein binding <4%; excreted unchanged in urine (86%), feces (14%); half-life 10 hr

INTERACTIONS
Decrease: emtricitabine level—interferons, orlistat; avoid using together
Complex interactions—ribavirin, cautious use

Drug/lab
Increase: AST/ALT, glucose, amylase, bilirubin, CK, lipase
Decrease: neutrophils

NURSING CONSIDERATIONS
Assess:
• **HIV:** monitor for infections and improvement in symptoms of HIV
• **Renal/hepatic function tests:** AST, ALT, bilirubin, amylase, lipase, triglycerides periodically during treatment
• **Lactic acidosis, severe hepatomegaly with steatosis:** if lab reports confirm these conditions, discontinue treatment; may be fatal; more common in females or those who are overweight; monitor lactic acid levels, LFTs
• **Immune reconstitution syndrome:** often occurs in response to opportunistic infections

Black Box Warning: Hepatotoxicity: do not use in those with risk factors such as alcoholism; discontinue if hepatotoxicity occurs

• **Hepatitis B and HIV coinfection (unlabeled);** perform HBV screening in any patient who has HIV to ensure appropriate treatment; avoid single-drug treatments in HBV
• **Pregnancy/breastfeeding:** use if clearly needed; register pregnant women in the Antiretroviral Pregnancy Registry at 800-258-4263; to reduce the risk of postnatal transmission, HIV-infected mothers are advised to avoid breastfeeding
Evaluate:
• Therapeutic response: decreased signs, symptoms of HIV; decreased viral load, increased CD4 counts
Teach patient/family:
• That GI complaints resolve after 3-4 wk of treatment
• That product must be taken at same time of day to maintain blood level; that solution and capsule are not interchangeable; that if dose is missed, to take as soon as remembered; not to double doses; not to share with others, refrigerate oral solution

---

Side effects: *italics* = common; red = life-threatening

• That product will control symptoms but is not a cure for HIV; patient still infectious, may pass HIV virus on to others; that other products may be necessary to prevent other infections; to practice safe sex and use a condom; not to share needles or donate blood

• That changes in body fat distribution may occur

• **Lactic acidosis:** to notify prescriber immediately if fatigue, muscle aches/pains, abdominal pain, difficulty breathing, nausea, vomiting, change in heart rhythm occur

Black Box Warning: Hepatotoxicity: to notify prescriber of dark urine, yellowing of skin/eyes, clay-colored stools, anorexia, nausea, vomiting

• To report planned or suspected pregnancy; not to breastfeed while taking product

emtricitabine/rilpivirine/ tenofovir alafenamide (Rx)

Odefsey
Func. class.: Antiretrovirals

USES: HIV in antiretroviral treatment-naive patients with HIV-1 RNA concentrations 100,000 copies/mL or less at treatment initiation and certain virologically stable (HIV-1 RNA <50 copies/mL) treatment-experienced patients

CONTRAINDICATIONS
Hypersensitivity

Black Box Warning: Hepatitis B exacerbation

DOSAGE AND ROUTES
HIV in antiretroviral treatment-naive patients with HIV-1 RNA concentrations 100,000 copies/mL or less at treatment initiation and certain virologically stable (HIV-1 RNA <50 copies/mL) treatment-experienced patients

• **Adults/child >12 yr; ≥35 kg: PO** 1 tablet (200 mg emtricitabine; 25 mg rilpivirine; 25 mg tenofovir alafenamide) daily
Available forms: Tablets 200-25-25 mg

emtricitabine/rilpivirine/ tenofovir disoproxil fumarate (Rx)

(em-tri-sit′uh-bean/ril-pi-vir′een/ ten-oh-foh′veer)

Complera
Func. class.: Antiretroviral
Chem. class.: Nucleoside reverse transcriptase inhibitor (NRTI)

ACTION:
• **Emtricitabine:** inhibits viral reverse transcriptase and is active both on HIV-1 and HBV
• **Tenofovir:** inhibits viral reverse transcriptase and acts as a DNA chain terminator
• **Rilpivirine:** inhibits HIV-1 reverse transcriptase; it does not compete for binding, nor does it require phosphorylation to be active

USES: HIV in treatment-naive patients with HIV RNA ≤100,000 copies/mL at initiation and certain virologically stable (HIV RNA <50 copies/mL) treatment-experienced patients

CONTRAINDICATIONS
Hypersensitivity, hepatotoxicity, lactic acidosis

Black Box Warning: Hepatitis B exacerbation

Precautions: Alcoholism, autoimmune disease, bone fractures, breastfeeding, children, depression, females, Graves' disease, Guillain-Barré syndrome, hepatic disease, hepatitis, hepatitis B and HIV coinfection, hepatitis C and HIV coinfection, hepatomegaly, HIV resistance, hypercholesterolemia, hyperlipidemia, hypertriglyceridemia, hypophosphatemia, immune reconstitution syndrome, obesity, osteomalacia, osteoporosis, pregnancy, QT prolongation, renal failure, renal impairment, serious rash, suicidal ideation, torsades de pointes

DOSAGE AND ROUTES

• **Adult/adolescent/child >12 yr and weighing ≥35 kg:** PO 1 tablet (200 mg emtricitabine; 25 mg rilpivirine; 300 mg tenofovir) daily. Coadministration with rifabutin, the rilpivirine dose needs to be increased to 50 mg/day; give an additional 25 mg/day of rilpivirine with a meal

HIV prophylaxis after occupational exposure to HIV (unlabeled)

• **Adult:** PO 1 tablet (200 mg emtricitabine; 25 mg rilpivirine; 300 mg tenofovir disoproxil fumarate) daily × 28 days

Renal dose

• **Adult:** PO CCr <50 mL/min: not recommended

Available forms: Tablet 200-25-300 mg

Administer:

• Give with a meal

• Antiretroviral drug resistance testing (preferably genotypic testing) before use in treatment-naive patients and before changing therapy for treatment failure

• For pregnant women, therapy should begin immediately after HIV diagnosis

• Prior to initiating, identify virologic failures; failures occurred more frequently in those with baseline HIV RNA concentrations >100,000 copies; CD4 counts <200 cells/mm^3

• Avoid use of tenofovir-containing regimens in those with renal disease and osteoporosis

SIDE EFFECTS

CNS: *Headache,* abnormal dreams, *depression,* dizziness, *insomnia,* neuropathy, paresthesia, suicide, fatigue, drowsiness

GI: *Nausea, vomiting, anorexia, diarrhea, abdominal pain, dyspepsia,* hepatomegaly with stenosis (may be fatal), pancreatitis

INTEG: *Rash,* skin discoloration

MS: Arthralgia, myalgia, rhabdomyolysis

GU: Glomerulonephritis membranous/mesangioproliferative

SYST: Change in body fat distribution, lactic acidosis

PHARMACOKINETICS

• **Emtricitabine:** protein binding <4%, metabolized via oxidation half-life 10 hr, excreted renally (86%) and via feces (14%); peak 1-2 hr

• **Tenofovir:** protein binding <0.7%, undergoes phosphorylation, eliminated by a combination of glomerular filtration and active renal tubular secretion, 70%-80% excreted unchanged in urine half-life 17 hr, bioavailability is increased with a high-fat meal

• **Rilpivirine:** protein binding 99.7% to albumin, metabolism via oxidation by CYP3A system, half-life 50 hr, excretion 85% feces, 6.1% urine, peak 4-5 hr

INTERACTIONS

• Do not use with efavirenz, lamiVUDine; treatment duplication

Increase: rilpivirine level—CYP3A4 inhibitors (delavirdine, efavirenz, darunavir, tipranavir, atazanavir, fosamprenavir, indinavir, nelfinavir, aldesleukin IL-2, amiodarone, aprepitant, basiliximab, boceprevir, bromocriptine, chloramphenicol, clarithromycin, conivaptan, danazol, dalfopristin, dasatinib, diltiazem, dronedarone, erythromycin, ethinyl estradiol, fluconazole, FLUoxetine, fluvoxamine, fosaprepitant, imatinib, isoniazid, itraconazole, ketoconazole, lantreotide, lapatinib, miconazole, nefazodone, nicardipine, octreotide, posaconazole, quinine, ranolazine, rifAXIMin, tamoxifen, telaprevir, telithromycin, troleandomycin, verapamil, voriconazole, zafirlukast)

Decrease: emtricitabine level—interferons

Increase: QT prolongation—class IA/III antidysrhythmics, some phenothiazines, beta-agonists, local anesthetics, tricyclics, haloperidol, chloroquine, droperidol, pentamidine; CYP3A4 inhibitors (amiodarone, clarithromycin, erythromycin, telithromycin, troleandomycin), arsenic trioxide; CYP3A4 substrates (methadone, pimozide, QUEtiapine, quiNIDine, risperiDONE, ziprasidone)

Increase: rilpivirine adverse reactions, fungal infections—fluconazole, voriconazole

Decrease: rilpivirine effect, treatment failure—CYP3A4 inducers (rifAMPin, rifapentine, rifabutin, primadone, phenytoin, PHENobarbital, nevirapine, nafcillin, modafinil, griseofulvin, etravirine, efavirenz, barbiturates, bexarotene, bosentan, carBAMazepine, enzalutamide, dexamethasone), proton pump inhibitors

Drug/lab

Increase: AST/ALT, glucose, amylase, bilirubin, lipase, CK

Decrease: neutrophils

NURSING CONSIDERATIONS

Assess:

• **HIV infection:** assess symptoms of HIV, including opportunistic infections, prior to and during treatment, some may be life-threatening; monitor plasma CD4+, CD8 cell counts, serum beta-2 microglobulin, serum ICD+24 antigen levels, treatment failures occur more often in those with baseline HIV-1 RNA concentrations >100,000 copies/mL than in those <100,000 copies/mL; monitor blood glucose, CBC with differential, serum cholesterol, lipid panel

• **Hepatotoxicity/lactic acidosis:** monitor hepatitis B serology, LFTs, plasma hepatitis C RNA, lactic acidosis levels. If lab reports confirm these conditions, discontinue product. More common in females or those who are overweight. Avoid use in alcoholism

• **Pregnancy/breastfeeding:** obtain pregnancy testing before use

Black Box Warning: Hepatitis B exacerbation: those with coexisting HBV and HIV infections who discontinue emtricitabine or tenofovir may experience severe acute hepatitis B exacerbation and hepatic decompensation and hepatic failure. Those coinfected with HBV and HIV who discontinue this product, monitor LFTs q6wk for the first 3 mo and q3-6mo thereafter. Resumption of anti–hepatitis B treatment may be required

• Monitor serum bilirubin (total and direct), serum creatinine, urinalysis, LFTs, amylase, lipase, periodically

Evaluate:

• Improvement in CD4, HIV RNA counts, decreasing signs and symptoms of HIV

TEACH PATIENT/FAMILY:

• That hepatitis and HIV coinfected patients should avoid consuming alcohol; offer vaccinations against hepatitis A and hepatitis B as appropriate

• That GI complaints resolve after 2-3 wk of treatment

• To take at the same time of day to maintain blood level; not to crush, break, or chew

• That product controls the symptoms of HIV but does not cure; patient is still able to infect others, that other products may be necessary to prevent other infections

• **Lactic acidosis:** to notify prescriber if fatigue, muscle aches/pains, abdominal pain, difficulty breathing, nausea, vomiting, change in heart rhythm occur

• **Hepatotoxicity:** to notify prescriber of dark urine, yellowing skin or eyes, clay-colored stools, anorexia, nausea, vomiting

• **Suicide:** to report severe depression, suicidal ideation to prescriber immediately

• To report suspected or planned pregnancy, not to breastfeed

---

emtricitabine/tenofovir alafenamide fumarate (Rx)

(em-tri-sit′uh-bean/ten-oh-foh′veer)

Descovy

Func. class.: Antiretroviral
Chem. class.: Nucleoside reverse transcriptase inhibitor (NRTI)

ACTION:

• **Emtricitabine:** inhibits viral reverse transcriptase and is active both on HIV-1 and HBV

• **Tenofovir:** inhibits viral reverse transcriptase and acts as a DNA chain terminator

USES: Human immunodeficiency virus (HIV) infection used in combination with other antiretrovirals

CONTRAINDICATIONS

Hypersensitivity, CCr <30 mL/min

Precautions:

Black Box Warning: Hepatitis B exacerbation

Alcoholism, autoimmune disease, bone fractures, breastfeeding, children, depression, females, Graves' disease, Guillain-Barré syndrome, hepatic disease, hepatitis, hepatitis B and HIV coinfection, hepatitis C and HIV coinfection, hepatomegaly, HIV resistance, hypercholesterolemia, hyperlipidemia, hypertriglyceridemia, hypophosphatemia, immune reconstitution syndrome, obesity, osteomalacia, osteoporosis, pregnancy, QT prolongation, renal failure, renal impairment, serious rash, suicidal ideation, torsades de pointes, hepatotoxicity, lactic acidosis

DOSAGE AND ROUTES

• **Adult/adolescent/child ≥12 yr and weighing ≥35 kg: PO** 1 tablet (200 mg emtricitabine; 25 mg tenofovir) daily
Available forms: Tablets 200 mg emtricitabine; 25 mg tenofovir
Administer:
• Antiretroviral drug resistance testing (preferably genotypic testing) is recommended prior to use in treatment-naive patients and prior to changing therapy for treatment failure
• For adults, use in all patients to reduce the risk of disease progression and to prevent the transmission of HIV, including perinatal transmission and transmission to sexual partners
• For pregnant women, therapy should begin immediately after HIV diagnosis

• Avoid use of tenofovir-containing regimens in those with renal disease and osteoporosis

SIDE EFFECTS

CNS: Weakness
GI: *Nausea,* hepatomegaly with stenosis (may be fatal), hepatic failure/decompensation, hepatitis
MS: Myalgia, bone pain, osteopenia, osteoporosis
GU: Breast enlargement, renal failure
SYST: Change in body fat distribution, lactic acidosis, Fanconi syndrome
META: Hypercholesterolemia, hypertriglyceridemia, hypophosphatemia

PHARMACOKINETICS

• **Emtricitabine:** protein binding <4%, metabolized via oxidation, half-life 10 hr, excreted renally (86%) and via feces (14%); peak 1-2 hr
• **Tenofovir:** protein binding <0.7%, undergoes phosphorylation to its active metabolite, eliminated by glomerular filtration and active renal tubular secretion, 70%-80% excreted unchanged in urine by 72 hr; half-life 17 hr, bioavailability is increased with a high-fat meal

INTERACTIONS

• Do not use with efavirenz, lamiVUDine; treatment duplication
Decrease: emtricitabine level—interferons
Increase: QT prolongation—class IA/III antidysrhythmics, some phenothiazines, beta-agonists, local anesthetics, tricyclics, haloperidol, chloroquine, droperidol, pentamidine; CYP3A4 inhibitors (amiodarone, clarithromycin, erythromycin, telithromycin, troleandomycin), arsenic trioxide; CYP3A4 substrates (methadone, pimozide, QUEtiapine, quiNIDine, risperiDONE, ziprasidone)

NURSING CONSIDERATIONS

Assess:

• **HIV infection:** assess symptoms of HIV, including opportunistic infections, prior to and during treatment, some may be life-threatening; monitor plasma CD4+, CD8 cell counts, serum beta-2 microglobulin; treatment failures occur more often in those with baseline HIV-1 RNA concentrations >100,000 copies/mL than in those <100,000 copies/mL; monitor blood glucose, CBC with differential, serum cholesterol, lipid panel

• **Hepatotoxicity/lactic acidosis:** monitor hepatitis B serology, LFTs, plasma hepatitis C RNA, lactic acidosis levels. If lab reports confirm these conditions, discontinue product. More common in females or those who are overweight. Avoid use in alcoholism

Black Box Warning: Hepatitis B exacerbation: those with coexisting HBV and HIV infections who discontinue emtricitabine or tenofovir may experience severe acute hepatitis B exacerbation with hepatic decompensation/failure. Those coinfected with HBV and HIV who discontinue this product, monitor LFTs q6wk × the first 3 mo and q3-6mo. Resumption of anti–hepatitis B treatment may be required

• Monitor serum bilirubin (total and direct), serum creatinine, urinalysis, LFTs, amylase, lipase periodically
• **Pregnancy/breastfeeding:**   obtain pregnancy testing prior to use
Evaluate:
• Improvement in CD4, HIV, RNC counts, decreasing signs and symptoms of HIV
Teach patient/family:
• That hepatitis and HIV coinfected patients should avoid consuming alcohol; offer vaccinations against hepatitis A and hepatitis B as needed
• That GI complaints resolve after 2-3 wk of treatment
• To take at the same time of day to maintain blood level; not to crush, break, or chew
• That product controls the symptoms of HIV but does not cure; that patient is still able to infect others, that other products may be necessary to prevent other infections
• **Lactic acidosis:** to notify prescriber if fatigue, muscle aches/pains, abdominal pain, difficulty breathing, nausea, vomiting, change in heart rhythm occur
• **Hepatotoxicity:** to notify prescriber of dark urine, yellowing skin or eyes, clay-colored stools, anorexia, nausea, vomiting
• To report suspected or planned pregnancy, not to breastfeed

emtricitabine/tenofovir disoproxil fumarate (Rx)

Truvada
Func. class.: Antiretroviral

USES:
HIV

CONTRAINDICATIONS
Hypersensitivity

DOSAGE AND ROUTES
• **Adult:** PO emtricitabine 200 mg; tenofovir DF 300 mg daily
• **Adult/children and adolescent ≥35 kg:** PO 1 tablet (emtricitabine 200 mg; tenofovir DF 300 mg) daily
• **Children and adolescent 28 to 34 kg:** PO 1 tablet (emtricitabine 167 mg; tenofovir DF 250 mg) daily
• **Children 22 to 27 kg:** PO 1 tablet (emtricitabine 133 mg; tenofovir DF 200 mg) daily
• **Children 17 to 21 kg:** PO 1 tablet (emtricitabine 100 mg; tenofovir DF 150 mg) daily
For HIV pre-exposure prophylaxis in high-risk patients without HIV to reduce the risk of sexually acquired HIV-1

enalapril/enalaprilat (Rx)
(e-nal′a-pril/e-nal′a-pril-at)
Epaned, Vasotec
Func. class.: Antihypertensive
Chem. class.: Angiotensin-converting enzyme (ACE) inhibitor

USES: Hypertension, HF, left ventricular dysfunction

CONTRAINDICATIONS
Hypersensitivity, history of angioedema, ACE inhibitors

Black Box Warning: Pregnancy second/third trimester

Precautions: Breastfeeding, renal disease, hyperkalemia, hepatic failure, dehydration, bilateral renal artery/aortic stenosis

DOSAGE AND ROUTES
Hypertension
• **Adult: PO** 2.5-5 mg/day, may increase or decrease to desired response, range 10-40 mg/day in 1-2 divided doses; **IV** 0.625-1.25 mg/0.625 mg with diuretics q6hr over 5 min
• **Child: PO** 0.08 mg/kg/day, max 5 mg, in 1-2 divided doses, max 0.6 mg/kg/day
• **Child: IV** 5-10 mcg/kg/dose q8-24hr
Heart failure
• **Adult: PO** 2.5-20 mg/day in 2 divided doses, max 40 mg/day in divided doses
Left ventricular cardiac dysfunction, asymptomatic
• **Adult: PO** 2.5 mg bid, titrate to max 10 mg bid, as tolerated; diuretic dose may require adjustment; monitor for ≥2 hr for hypotension
Renal disease
• **Adult: PO** 2.5 mg/day (CCr <30 mL/min), increase gradually; **IV** CCr >30 mL/min, 1.25 mg q6hr; CCr <30 mL/min, 0.625 mg as one-time dose, increase as per B/P
• **Child >1 mo: PO/IV** CCr <30 mL/min contraindicated

Hypertensive emergency/urgency (unlabeled)
• **Adult: IV** 1.25-5 mg q6hr
Available forms: Enalapril: tablets 2.5, 5, 10, 20 mg; oral solution 1 mg/mL; enalaprilat: injection 1.25 mg/mL

enalapril/hydrochlorothiazide (Rx)
Vaseretic
Func. class.: Antihypertensive/diuretic

USES: Hypertension

CONTRAINDICATIONS
Hypersensitivity

Black Box Warning: Pregnancy

DOSAGE AND ROUTES
• **Adult: PO** 1 tablet (10/25 mg), may increase after 2-3 wk
Available forms: Tablets 5-12.5 mg, 10-25 mg

⚠ HIGH ALERT

enasidenib (Rx)
(en′-a-sid′-a-nib)
IDHIFA
Func. class.: Antineoplastic, isocitrate dehydrogonase-2 inhibitor

USES: Relapsed or refractory acute myeloid leukemia (AML) with ☞ IDH2 mutation

DOSAGE AND ROUTES

Black Box Warning: Differentiation syndrome

• **Adult: PO:** 100 mg/day until disease progression. Treat those without disease progression for a minimum of 6 mo to allow time for clinical response
Available forms: Tablets 50, 100 mg

enfuvirtide (Rx)
(en-fyoo′vir-tide)
Fuzeon
Func. class.: Antiretroviral
Chem. class.: Fusion inhibitor

ACTION: Inhibitor of the fusion of HIV-1 with CD4+ cells

USES: Treatment of HIV-1 infection in combination with other antiretrovirals in those who are treatment experienced only
Unlabeled uses: HIV prophylaxis after occupational exposure

CONTRAINDICATIONS
Breastfeeding, hypersensitivity
Precautions: Pregnancy, children <6 yr, liver disease, myelosuppression, infections

DOSAGE AND ROUTES
HIV-1 with other antiretrovirals
• **Adult:** SUBCUT 90 mg (1 mL) bid
• **Child ≥11 kg:** SUBCUT 2 mg/kg bid, max 90 mg bid
HIV prophylaxis (unlabeled)
• **Adult:** SUBCUT 90 mg bid added to PEP regimen
Available forms: Powder for injection, lyophilized 108 mg (90 mg/mL when reconstituted)
Administer:
SUBCUT route
• **Reconstitute** vial with 1.1 mL sterile water for injection; tap and roll to mix; allow to stand until completely dissolved, may take up to 45 min; after dissolved, immediately **inject** or refrigerate up to 24 hr
• Do not mix with other medications
• **SUBCUT:** Give bid, rotate sites; preferred sites: upper arm, anterior thigh, abdomen
• Discard unused product
• **Storage:** Use reconstituted product within 24 hr, refrigerated, let product come to room temperature prior to injecting

SIDE EFFECTS
CNS: Anxiety, peripheral neuropathy, taste disturbance, Guillain-Barré syndrome, insomnia, depression, fatigue, peripheral neuropathy

GI: Nausea, abdominal pain, anorexia, constipation, pancreatitis, dry mouth, weight loss
GU: Glomerulonephritis, renal failure
HEMA: Thrombocytopenia, neutropenia
INTEG: *Injection site reactions, skin papilloma*
MISC: Influenza, cough, conjunctivitis, lymphadenopathy, myalgia, hyperglycemia, bacterial pneumonia, rhinitis, fatigue, hypersensitivity

PHARMACOKINETICS
Peak 8 hr, terminal half-life 3.8 hr, well absorbed, undergoes catabolism, 92% protein binding

INTERACTIONS
Decrease: enfuvirtide effect—orlistat, avoid using together
Drug/lab
Increase: LFTs, lipase, CK, triglycerides
Decrease: Hb
Drug/Drug
Increase: effect of either product—protease inhibitor

NURSING CONSIDERATIONS
Assess:
• **Signs of infection, injection site reactions:** use analgesics; bacterial pneumonia may occur if blood counts are low or viral load is high or low CD4 counts, IV drug user, lung disease, smoker
• **Peripheral neuropathy:** may occur and last for several months, where nerves are close to the skin those with coagulation disorders are at greater risk
• **Glomerulonephritis/renal failure:** BUN, creatinine, renal failure may occur
• Bowel pattern prior to, during treatment; if severe abdominal pain or constipation occurs, notify prescriber; monitor hydration
• **Hypersensitivity:** skin eruptions, rash, urticaria, itching; assess allergies prior to treatment, reaction to each medication; may occur quickly or later after continued use, stop product, do not restart

- **Pneumonia:** those with low CD4 count or increased viral load are more susceptible
- **Immune reconstitution syndrome:** with combination theory
- **HIV:** CBC, blood chemistry, plasma HIV RNA, absolute CD4+/CD8+ cell counts/%, serum β_2 microglobulin, serum ICD+24 antigen levels, cholesterol
- **Injection site reactions:** monitor for pain, redness, swelling at site, treat as needed
- **Pregnancy/breastfeeding:** identify if pregnancy is planned or suspected, if breastfeeding; if pregnant, register with the Antiretroviral Pregnancy Registry (800-258-4263), do not breastfeed

Evaluate:
- Therapeutic response: increased CD4 cell counts; decreased viral load; slowing progression of HIV-1 infection

Teach patient/family:
- That pneumonia may occur; to contact prescriber if cough, fever occur
- That hypersensitive reactions may occur; rash, pruritus; to stop product, contact prescriber
- That product is not a cure for HIV-1 infection but controls symptoms; HIV-1 can still be transmitted to others; that product is to be used in combination only with other antiretrovirals
- How to prepare and give using SUBCUT injection, watch for site reactions, rotate sites; if more information is needed, call 877-438-9366
- To notify prescriber if pregnancy is suspected; not to breastfeed, to register with the Antiretroviral Pregnancy Registry (800-258-4263)

⚠ HIGH ALERT

enoxaparin (Rx)

(ee-nox′a-par-in)

Lovenox

Func. class.: Anticoagulant, antithrombotic

Chem. class.: Low-molecular-weight heparin (LMWH)

Do not confuse:
enoxaparin/enoxacin
Lovenox/Lotronex

ACTION: Binds to antithrombin III inactivating factors Xa/IIa, thereby resulting in a higher ratio of anti–factor Xa to IIa

USES: Prevention of DVT (inpatient or outpatient), PE (inpatient) in hip and knee replacement, abdominal surgery at risk for thrombosis; unstable angina, acute MI, coronary artery thrombosis

Unlabeled uses: Antiphospholipid antibody syndrome, arterial thromboembolism prophylaxis, cerebral thromboembolism, percutaneous coronary intervention

CONTRAINDICATIONS

Hypersensitivity to this product, heparin, pork; active major bleeding, hemophilia, leukemia with bleeding, thrombocytopenic purpura, heparin-induced thrombocytopenia

Precautions: Pregnancy, breastfeeding, children, geriatric patients, low-weight men (<57 kg), women (<45 kg), severe renal/hepatic disease, severe hypertension, subacute bacterial endocarditis, acute nephritis, recent burn, spinal surgery, indwelling catheters, hypersensitivity to benzyl alcohol

> **Black Box Warning:** Lumbar puncture, aneurysm, coagulopathy, epidural anesthesia, spinal anesthesia

DOSAGE AND ROUTES

DVT prevention prior to hip or knee surgery
- **Adult:** SUBCUT 30 mg bid given 12-24 hr postop for 7-10 days

DVT prevention prior to hip replacement
- **Adult:** SUBCUT 40 mg/day started 9-12 hr preop or 30 mg q12hr started 12-24 hr postop

DVT prophylaxis prior to abdominal surgery
- **Adult:** SUBCUT 40 mg/day starting 24 hr prior to surgery × 7-12 days

---

Side effects: *italics* = common; red = life-threatening

Treatment of DVT or PE

• **Adult: SUBCUT** 1 mg/kg q12hr (without PE, outpatient); 1 mg/kg q12hr or 1.5 mg/kg/day (with or without PE, inpatient); warfarin should be started within 72 hr, continued ≥5 days until INR is 2-3 (at least 3 days)

DVT prophylaxis in patients with restricted mobility due to acute illness

• **Adult: SUBCUT** 40 mg q24hr × 6-11 days

Prevention of ischemic complications in unstable angina or non–Q-wave MI/non-ST

• **Adult <75 yr: SUBCUT/IV** loading bolus 30 mg plus 1 mg **SUBCUT** then 1 mg/kg q12hr until stable with aspirin 100-325 mg/day

• **Adults >75 yr: SUBCUT/IV** do not give initial bolus, **SUBCUT** 0.75 mg/kg q12hr, max 75 mg for first two doses

Acute MI with ST-segment elevation

• **Adult/geriatric <75 yr: IV/SUBCUT** 30 mg **IV BOLUS** plus 1 mg/kg **SUBCUT**, then 1 mg/kg **SUBCUT** q12hr, max 100 mg for first 2 doses only

• **Geriatric ≥75 yr: SUBCUT** 0.75 mg/kg q12hr, max 75 mg for first 2 doses only

Renal dose

• **Adult: SUBCUT** CCr <30 mL/min: 30 mg daily **(thrombosis prophylaxis in abdominal surgery, hip or knee replacement surgery, during acute illness);** 1 mg/kg daily **(concurrently with aspirin to treat unstable angina or non-Q-wave MI);** 1 mg/kg daily **(STEMI in those ≥75 yr),** 30 mg IV bolus plus 1 mg/kg SC, then 1 mg/kg daily **(STEMI in those <75 yr),** or 1 mg/kg daily **(concurrently with warfarin for inpatient or outpatient treatment of acute deep vein thrombosis with or without pulmonary embolism)**

Available forms: Prefilled syringes 30 mg/0.3 mL, 40 mg/0.4 mL; graduated prefilled syringes 60 mg/0.6 mL, 80 mg/0.8 mL, 100 mg/1 mL, 120 mg/0.8 mL, 150 mg/mL

Administer:

• Only after screening patient for bleeding disorders

• Do not mix with other products or infusion fluids

• Only this product when ordered; not interchangeable with heparin or other LMWHs

• At same time each day to maintain steady blood levels

• Avoid all IM injections that may cause bleeding

• Prepare in a sterile environment using aseptic technique

SUBCUT route

• Do not give IM; begin 1 hr prior to surgery; do not aspirate; rotate sites; do not expel bubble from syringe before administration

• To recumbent patient, give SUBCUT; rotate injection sites (left/right anterolateral, left/right posterolateral abdominal wall)

• Insert whole length of needle into skin fold held with thumb and forefinger

• If withdrawing from multidose vial, use TB syringe for proper measurement

• Prefilled syringes (30, 40 mg) not graduated; do not use for partial doses

• Do not administer if particulate is present; do not use products with benzyl alcohol in pregnant women

Direct IV route

• Use multidose vial for IV administration; use TB syringe, other graduated syringe to measure dose; give IV BOLUS through IV line, flush prior to and after

• Dilution may be stored for up to 4 wk in glass vial at room temperature, up to 2 wk in TB syringes with rubber stoppers at room temperature or refrigerated

SIDE EFFECTS

CNS: Fever, confusion, dizziness, headache

GI: Nausea, vomiting, constipation

HEMA: Hemorrhage from any site, hypochromic anemia, thrombocytopenia, bleeding

INTEG: Ecchymosis, injection site hematoma, alopecia, pruritus, rash

META: Hyperkalemia in renal failure

MS: Osteoporosis

SYST: Edema, peripheral edema, angioedema, anaphylaxis

PHARMACOKINETICS

SUBCUT: 90% absorbed, maximum antithrombin activity (3-5 hr), duration 12 hr half-life 4½ hr, excreted in urine

INTERACTIONS

Increase: enoxaparin action—anticoagulants, salicylates, NSAIDs, antiplatelets, thrombolytics, RU-486, SSRIs; monitor INR/PT
Drug/lab
Increase: AST, ALT
Decrease: platelet count
Drug/herb
Increase: bleeding risk—feverfew, garlic, ginger, ginkgo, green tea, horse chestnut

NURSING CONSIDERATIONS
Assess:

• Monitor anti—factor Xa activity in chronic therapy (renal disease)
• Blood studies (Hct/Hb, CBC, coagulation studies, platelets [for HIT], occult blood in stools), anti–factor Xa (should be checked 4 hr after injection); thrombocytopenia may occur; PT, PTT is not needed in those with adequate coagulation; discontinue use and notify prescriber if platelets <100,000/mm^3
• Renal studies: BUN/creatinine baseline and periodically
• **Bleeding:** gums, petechiae, ecchymosis, black tarry stools, hematuria; notify prescriber
• **Anaphylaxis, angioedema:** monitor for rash; swelling of face, lips, tongue; dyspnea; stop product, initiate emergency procedures
• **Neurologic status:** those with epidural catheters are at greater chance for impairments
• Injection site reactions: inflammation, redness, hematomas

Black Box Warning: **Neurologic symptoms** in patients who have received spinal anesthesia, may develop spinal hematoma; those who have had trauma, spinal surgery are at greater risk

• **Beers:** reduce dose in older adults; increased bleeding risk, or if CCr <30 mL/min
• **Pregnancy/breastfeeding:** do not use in multidose vials, benzyl alcohol is present; do not breastfeed
Evaluate:
• Therapeutic response: prevention of DVT/PE

Teach patient/family:

• Black Box Warning: **Spinal anesthesia:** to report numbness, weakness in lower extremities

• To use soft-bristle toothbrush to avoid bleeding gums; to use electric razor
• To report any signs of bleeding: gums, under skin, urine, stools; do not rub injection site, easy bruising
• To report dizziness, rash, breathing changes
• To teach how to use SUBCUT form
• To have patient discuss all products taken with all prescribers and health care providers
• To avoid OTC products containing aspirin, NSAIDs unless approved by prescriber; not to start any Rx, OTC, supplements, or herbal products unless approved by prescriber

---

entacapone (Rx)
(en′ta-kah-pone)
Comtan
Func. class.: Antiparkinson agent
Chem. class.: COMT inhibitor

USES: Parkinson's disease for those experiencing end-of-dose, decreased effect as adjunct to levodopa/carbidopa

CONTRAINDICATIONS
Hypersensitivity

DOSAGE AND ROUTES
• **Adult: PO** 200 mg given with carbidopa/levodopa, max 1600 mg/day; may allow for 25% dosage reduction in levodopa therapy
Available forms: Tablets 200 mg

---

entecavir (Rx)
(en-te′ka-veer)
Baraclude
Func. class.: Antiviral
Chem. class.: Nucleoside analog

ACTION: Inhibits hepatitis B virus DNA polymerase by competing with natural substrates and by causing DNA termination after its incorporation into viral DNA; causes viral DNA death

USES: Chronic hepatitis B (HBV) with active viral replication and either persistent elevations in AST or ALT or histologically active disease

CONTRAINDICATIONS
Hyper-sensitivity

Precautions: Pregnancy, breastfeeding, children <2 yr, geriatric patients, severe renal disease, liver transplant

> **Black Box Warning:** Hepatic disease, hepatitis, HIV, lactic acidosis

DOSAGE AND ROUTES
Chronic hepatitis B (nucleoside treatment naive)
• **Adult and adolescent ≥16 yr: PO** tablet 0.5 mg/day
• **Adult: PO** (solution) 0.5 mg daily; **Child/adolescent ≥2 yr >30 kg:** 0.5 mg (10 mL) daily; **Child ≥2 yr, 27 to 30 kg:** 0.45 mg (9 mL) daily; **Child ≥2 yr, 24 to 26 kg:** 0.4 mg (8 mL) daily; **Child ≥2 yr, 21 to 23 kg:** 0.35 mg (7 mL) daily; **Child ≥2 yr, 18 to 20 kg:** 0.3 mg (6 mL) daily; **Child ≥2 yr, 15 to 17 kg:** 0.25 mg (5 mL) daily; **Child ≥2 yr, 12 to 14 kg:** 0.2 mg (4 mL) daily; **Child ≥2 yr,** 0.15 mg (3 mL) daily

Chronic hepatitis B with compensated liver disease
• **Adult/adolescent ≥16 yr: PO** tablet 1 mg/day; lamivudine resistance, 0.5 mg q day
• **Adult: PO** (solution) 1 mg/day; **Child/adolescent ≥2 yr, >30 kg:** 1 mg (20 mL) daily; **Child ≥2 yr, 27 to 30 kg:** 0.9 mg (18 mL) daily; **Child ≥2 yr, 24 to 26 kg:** 0.8 mg (16 mL) daily; **Child ≥2 yr, 21 to 23 kg:** 0.7 mg (14 mL) daily; **Child ≥2 yr, 18 to 20 kg:** 0.6 mg (12 mL) daily; **Child ≥2 yr, 15 to 17 kg:** 0.5 mg (10 mL) daily; **Child ≥2 yr, 12 to 14 kg:** 0.4 mg (8 mL) daily; **Child ≥2 yr, 10 to 11 kg:** 0.3 mg (6 mL) daily

Renal dose
• **Adult/child >16 yr: PO** CCr ≥50 mL/min, 0.5 mg/day; CCr 30-49 mL/min, 0.25 mg/day, 0.5 mg/day or 1 mg q48hr for lamiVUDine-refractory patient; CCr 10-29 mL/min, 0.15/day or 1 mg q72hr for lami-VUDine-refractory patient; CCr <10 mL/min, 0.05 mg/day, 0.1 mg/day or 1 mg q7day for lamiVUDine-refractory patient
• **Child 2-<16 yr: PO** (dosage based on weight) **10-11 kg:** 0.15 mg once daily (0.3 mg once daily if history of lami-VUDine resistance) **>11-14 kg:** 0.2 mg once daily (0.4 mg once daily if history of lamiVUDine resistance) **>14-17 kg:** 0.25 mg once daily (0.5 mg once daily if history of lamiVUDine resistance) **>17-20 kg:** 0.3 mg once daily (0.6 mg once daily if history of lamiVUDine resistance) **>20-23 kg:** 0.35 mg once daily (0.7 mg once daily if history of lamiVUDine resistance) **>23-26 kg:** 0.4 mg once daily (0.8 mg once daily if history of lamiVUDine resistance) **>26-30 kg:** 0.45 mg once daily (0.9 mg once daily if history of lamiVUDine resistance) **>30 kg:** 0.5 mg once daily (1 mg once daily if history of lamiVUDine resistance)

Available forms: Tablets, film coated 0.5, 1 mg; oral solution 0.05 mg/mL

Administer:
• After hemodialysis
• By mouth on empty stomach 2 hr prior to or after food
• Store at room temperature
• **Oral solution:** use calibrated oral dosing spoon provided; may be used interchangeably with tablets, do not dilute

SIDE EFFECTS
CNS: *Headache,* fatigue, dizziness, insomnia
ENDO: Hyperglycemia
GI: *Dyspepsia,* nausea, vomiting, diarrhea, elevated liver function enzymes
INTEG: Alopecia, rash
SYST: Lactic acidosis, severe hepatomegaly with steatosis

PHARMACOKINETICS
Peak 0.5-1.5 hr, steady-state 6-10 days, 100% bioavailability, extensively distributed to tissues, protein binding

13%, terminal half-life 128-149 hr duration up to 24 hr, excreted unchanged (62%-73%) via kidneys

INTERACTIONS
Drug/food
Decrease: absorption—high-fat meal
Drug/lab
Increase: ALT, AST, total bilirubin, amylase, lipase, creatinine, blood glucose, urine glucose
Decrease: platelets, albumin

NURSING CONSIDERATIONS
Assess:
• **For nephrotoxicity:** increasing CCr, BUN

Black Box Warning: For HIV prior to beginning treatment because HIV resistance may occur in chronic hepatitis B patients; monitor HIV RNA; don't use in those with HIV and HBV unless receiving antiretroviral treatment for both

Black Box Warning: For lactic acidosis and severe hepatomegaly with stenosis; increased serum lactate, increased hepatic enzymes; discontinue if present, discontinue if signs occur; may be fatal

• Geriatric patients more carefully; may develop renal, cardiac symptoms more rapidly

Black Box Warning: For exacerbations of hepatitis (jaundice, pruritus, fatigue), anorexia after discontinuing treatment, and for several months monitor LFTs

• **Pregnancy/breastfeeding:** use if clearly needed; register pregnant women at the Antiretroviral Pregnancy Registry at 800-258-4263; to reduce risk of postnatal transmission, HIV-infected mothers are advised to avoid breastfeeding
Evaluate:
• Therapeutic response: decreased symptoms of chronic hepatitis B, improving LFTs
Teach patient/family:
• Not to take with food; to take 2 hr prior to or after meals

• To take exactly as prescribed, to read the "Patient Information," to take missed dose when remembered unless close to time of next dose; that compliance with dosage schedule is required; not to share product
• Not to stop medication without approval of prescriber
• That optimal duration of treatment is unknown
• To avoid use with other medications, supplements unless approved by prescriber
• To notify prescriber of decreased urinary output, blood in urine

Black Box Warning: Symptoms of lactic acidosis: muscle pain, severe tiredness, weakness, trouble breathing, stomach pain with nausea/vomiting, coldness in arms/legs, fast/irregular heartbeat, dizziness

Black Box Warning: Symptoms of hepatotoxicity: eyes/skin turning yellow, dark urine, light-colored bowel movements, no appetite for days, nausea, stomach pain; may be worsened after discontinuing treatment

• That product does not cure but lowers amount of HBV in body
• That product does not stop spread of HBV to others by sex, sharing needles, or being exposed to blood
• Not to breastfeed; to notify prescriber if pregnancy is planned or suspected
• Not to operate machinery until effect is known, dizziness may occur
• That regular follow-up and lab tests will be needed

> ## ⚠ HIGH ALERT
>
> ## entrectinib (Rx)
> (en-trek′tih-nib)
> Rozlytrek
> *Func. class.:* Antineoplastic orphan drug
> *Chem. class.:* Tyrosine kinase ROS1 inhibitor, tropomyosin receptor kinase (TRK) inhibitor

USES: ROS1-positive non–small-cell lung cancer and NTRK gene fusion–positive solid tumors

Side effects: *italics* = common; red = life-threatening

CONTRAINDICATIONS

Hypersensitivity, pregnancy, breastfeeding

DOSAGE AND ROUTES

• **Adult: PO** 600 mg daily until disease progression or unacceptable toxicity

Available forms: Capsule 100, 200 mg

enzalutamide (Rx)

(en-zal-u'ta-mide)

Xtandi

Func. class.: Antineoplastic hormone
Chem. class.: Nonsteroidal antiandrogen

USES: Metastatic, castration-resistant prostate cancer in those who have received DOCEtaxel

CONTRAINDICATIONS

Pregnancy, women, hypersensitivity

DOSAGE AND ROUTES

• **Adult: PO** 160 mg (4 × 40-mg caps) daily. If a patient experiences a grade 3 or higher toxicity or an intolerable adverse effect, withhold dosing for 1 wk or until symptoms improve to grade 2 or less, then resume at the same or a reduced dosage (120 or 80 mg), if warranted

• The concomitant use of strong CYP2C8 give 80 mg once daily; CYP3A4 inducers 240 mg daily

Available forms: Capsules 40 mg

ephedrine (Rx)

(e-FED-rin)

Rezipres

Func. class.: Antihypertensive, alpha and beta agonist

USES: Hypotension in anesthesia

DOSAGE AND ROUTES

• **Adult: IV BOLUS** 4.7 mg-9.4 mg, give additional boluses as needed, max total doses 47 mg

Available forms: Solution for IV bolus 47 mg/mL, 47 mg/5 mL (9.4 mg/mL), 23.5 mg/5 mL (4.7 mg/mL)

epinastine (ophthalmic) (Rx)

(ep-ih-nas'teen)

Func. class.: Antihistamine (ophthalmic)
Chem. class.: Histamine 1 receptor antagonist/mast cell stabilizer

ACTION: A topically active, direct H_1-receptor antagonist and mast cell stabilizer; by reducing these inflammatory mediators, it relieves the ocular pruritus associated with allergic conjunctivitis

USES: Prevention of ocular pruritus associated with signs and symptoms of allergic conjunctivitis

CONTRAINDICATIONS

Hyper-sensitivity

Precautions: Pregnancy, breastfeeding, children, contact lenses

DOSAGE AND ROUTES

• **Adult/child ≥3 yr: OPHTH** Instill 1 drop in each eye bid

Available forms: Ophthalmic solution 0.5%

Administer:

Ophthalmic route

• For topical ophthalmic use only

• The preservative benzalkonium chloride may be absorbed by soft contact lenses; wait ≥10 min after instilling the ophthalmic solution before inserting contact lenses; contact lenses should not be worn if eye is red

• Do not share ophthalmic drops with others

• Keep bottle tightly closed when not in use

• Treatment should be continued throughout the period of exposure (i.e., until the pollen season is over or until exposure to the offending allergen is terminated), even when symptoms are absent

SIDE EFFECTS

EENT: Ocular irritation, folliculosis, hyperemia, ocular pruritus

MISC: Infection (including cold symptoms and upper respiratory infections), headache, rhinitis, sinusitis, increased cough, pharyngitis

PHARMACOKINETICS
Onset 3-5 min, peak 2 hr, duration 8 hr

NURSING CONSIDERATIONS
Assess:
• Eyes: for itching, redness, use of soft or hard contact lenses
Evaluate:
• Therapeutic response: absence of redness, itching in the eyes
Teach patient/family:
Ophthalmic route
• Product is for topical ophthalmic use only
• Wash hands prior to and after use; tilt the head back slightly and pull the lower eyelid down with the index finger; squeeze the prescribed number of drops into the conjunctival sac and gently close eyes for 1-2 min; do not blink
• Do not touch the tip of the dropper to the eye, fingertips, or other surface
• Wait ≥10 min after instilling the ophthalmic solution before inserting contact lenses; contact lenses should not be worn if eye is red
• Keep bottle tightly closed when not in use
• Do not share ophthalmic drops with others
• Remove contact lenses prior to use because the preservative benzalkonium chloride may be absorbed by soft contact lenses; product should not be used to treat contact lens–related irritation

---

⚠ HIGH ALERT

ePINEPHrine (Rx)
(ep-i-nef′rin)
Adrenalin, Adrenaclick 🍁, Auvi-Q, Anapen 🍁, Anapen Jr. 🍁, EpiPen, EpiPen Jr., Symjepi
Func. class.: Bronchodilator nonselective adrenergic agonist, vasopressor
Chem. class.: Catecholamine

Do not confuse:
EPINEPHrine/ePHEDrine/norepinephrine

ACTION: β_1- and β_2-agonist causing increased levels of cAMP, thereby producing bronchodilation, cardiac, and CNS stimulation; high doses cause vasoconstriction via alpha-receptors; low doses can cause vasodilation via β_2-vascular receptors

USES: Acute asthmatic attacks, hemostasis, bronchospasm, anaphylaxis, allergic reactions, cardiac arrest, adjunct in anesthesia, shock
Unlabeled uses: Bradycardia, chloroquine overdose

CONTRAINDICATIONS
Hypersensitivity to sympathomimetics, sulfites, closed-angle glaucoma, non-anaphylactic shock during general anesthesia
Precautions: Pregnancy, breastfeeding, cardiac disorders, hyperthyroidism, diabetes mellitus, prostatic hypertrophy, hypertension, organic brain syndrome, local anesthesia of certain areas, labor, cardiac dilation, coronary insufficiency, cerebral arteriosclerosis, organic heart disease

DOSAGE AND ROUTES
Anaphylaxis/severe asthma exacerbation
• **Adult: IM/SUBCUT** 0.3-0.5 mg, may repeat q10-15min (anaphylaxis) or q20min-4 hr (asthma)
• **Child 15-30 kg IM/SUBCUT** 0.01-0.15 mg/kg, repeat q5-10min as needed
• **Child 7.5-15 kg: IM/SUBCUT** 0.1 mg/kg, repeat q5-10min as needed
Hypotension-associated septic shock
• **Adult: IV infusion** 0.05-2 mcg/kg/min, titrate to desired mean arterial pressure, adjust q10-15min by 0.05-0.2 mcg/kg/min, decrease gradually to withdraw
Severe anaphylaxis
• **Adult: IV** 0.1-0.25 mg q5-15min, then 1-4 mcg/min continuous infusion if needed

---

Side effects: *italics* = common; red = life-threatening

• **Child: IV** ≤0.1 mcg/kg/min, then 0.1 mcg/kg/min continuous infusion if needed

Severe allergic reactions type I
• **Adult/child ≥30 kg: IM** 0.3 mg (EpiPen/EpiPen 2-Pak)
• **Child <30 kg: IM** 0.15 mg (EpiPen Jr/EpiPen Jr 2-Pak)

CPR (ACLS)
• **Adult: IV** 1 mg q3-5min
• **Child: IV/intraosseus** 0.01 mg/kg repeat q3-5min until circulation returns

Bradycardia (ACLS)
• **Adult: IV** 2-10 mcg/min

Bradycardia/pulseless arrest (PALS)
• **Child: IV** 0.01 mg/kg may repeat q3-5min, may increase to 0.1-0.2 mg/kg if needed

Asthma (unlabeled)
• **Adult/child >12 yr: IM/SUBCUT** 0.01 mg/kg divided into 3 doses (0.3-0.5 mg) q20min as needed, (only use 1 mg/mL concentration)

Available forms: Nasal spray (solution) 1 mg/mL; **solution for injection** 1 mg/mL (1:1000); 0.1 mg/mL (1:10,000); inhaled vapor (solution) 0.22 mg/actuation; pressurized inhalation (solution) 0.22 mg/actuation; solution for injection 0.15 mg/0.15 mL autoinjector, 0.3 mg/0.3 mL autoinjector, 0.15 mg/0.3 mL

Administer:
• Increased dose of insulin for diabetic patients if glucose is elevated
• Check for correct concentrations, route, dosage prior to administering
• Give SUBCUT, IM, intraosseously, IV; suspensions are for SUBCUT use only; do not give IV
• Visually inspect parenteral products for particulate matter and discoloration prior to use; do not use solutions that are pinkish to brownish or that contain a precipitate
• Avoid extravasation during parenteral administration; if extravasation occurs, infiltrate the affected area with phentolamine diluted in NS

• Death has occurred from drug errors; make sure the right concentration is used
• Store reconstituted solution refrigerated ≤24 hr

Inhalation route
• Place in nebulizer (10 drops of a 1% base solution)
• Dilute racepinephrine 2.25% solution

IM route
• Give in the deltoid or anterior thigh (vastus lateralis); do not administer into the gluteal muscle, may give through clothing in emergency

SUBCUT route
• Inject, taking care not to inject intradermally; massage injection site well after use to enhance absorption and to decrease local vasoconstriction; injection can cause tissue irritation

Intraosseous INFUSION route (unlabeled)
• During CPR, the same EPINEPHrine dosage may be given via the intraosseous route when IV access is not available

Intracardiac route
• Intracardiac route should be reserved for extreme emergencies; intracardiac injection should only be performed by properly trained medical personnel

Endotracheal route
• Per the ACLS or PALS guidelines, the EPINEPHrine parenteral product is administered via endotracheal (ET) route; ET administration should only be used if access to IV or intraosseous routes is not possible
• **Adult:** Dilute dose in 5-10 mL of NS or sterile distilled water; administer via ET tube; endotracheal absorption of EPINEPHrine may be improved by diluting with water instead of NS
• **Child:** After dose administration, flush the ET tube with a minimum of 5 mL NS

E

Direct IV INJ route

• 1:10,000 solution can be given directly without diluting: dilute 1:1000 (1 mg/0.9 mL) 0.9% NaCL (1:1000 solution)

• Inject EPINEPHrine directly into a vein over 5-10 min for adults or 1-3 min for children; may be given IV push in cardiac arrest

• In neonates, may administer via the umbilical vein

During adult cardiopulmonary resuscitation (CPR):

• Resuscitation drugs may be given IV by bolus injection into a peripheral vein, followed by an injection of 20 mL IV fluid; elevate the extremity for 10-20 sec to facilitate drug delivery to the central circulation

Continuous IV INFUSION route

• Dilute 1 mg EPINEPHrine in 250 or 500 mL of a compatible IV infusion solution to provide a concentration of 4 or 2 mcg/mL, respectively; give into a large vein, if possible; more concentrated solutions (16-32 mcg/mL) may be used in fluid-restricted patients when administered through a central line

Y-site compatibilities: Alfentanil, amikacin, amiodarone, amphotericin B liposome, anidulafungin, ascorbic acid, atracurium, atropine, aztreonam, benztropine, bivalirudin, bleomycin, bumetanide, buprenorphine, butorphanol, calcium chloride/gluconate, CARBOplatin, caspofungin, ceFAZolin, cefotaxime, cefoTEtan, cefOXitin, cefTAZidime, ceftizoxime, cefTRIAXone, cefuroxime, chloramphenicol, chlorproMAZINE, cimetidine, cisatracurium, CISplatin, clindamycin, cyanocobalamin, cyclophosphamide, cycloSPORINE, cytarabine, DACTINomycin, DAPTOmycin, dexamethasone, dexmedetomidine, digoxin, diltiazem, diphenhydrAMINE, DOBUTamine, DOCEtaxel, DOPamine, DOXOrubicin, doxycycline, enalaprilat, epirubicin, epoetin alfa, ertapenem, erythromycin, esmolol, etoposide, etoposide phosphate, famotidine, fenoldopam, fentaNYL, fluconazole, fludarabine, folic acid, furosemide, gemcitabine, gentamicin, glycopyrrolate, granisetron, heparin, hydrocortisone, HYDROmorphone,

ifosfamide, imipenem-cilastatin, isoproterenol, ketorolac, labetalol, levofloxacin, lidocaine, linezolid, LORazepam, magnesium sulfate, mannitol, mechlorethamine, meperidine, metaraminol, methicillin, methotrexate, methoxamine, methyldopa, methylPREDNISolone, metoclopramide, metoprolol, metroNIDAZOLE, midazolam, milrinone, minocycline, mitoXANtrone, morphine, multiple vitamins, nafcillin, nalbuphine, naloxone, niCARdipine, nitroglycerin, nitroprusside, norepinephrine, octreotide, ondansetron, oxacillin, oxaliplatin, oxytocin, PACLitaxel, palonosetron, pancuronium, pantoprazole, PEMEtrexed, penicillin G potassium, pentamidine, pentazocine, phentolamine, phenylephrine, phytonadione, piperacillin/tazobactam, potassium chloride, procainamide, prochlorperazine, promethazine, propofol, propranolol, protamine, pyridoxime, quinupristin/dalfopristin, ranitidine, remifentanil, ritodrine, rocuronium, sodium acetate, streptomycin, succinylcholine, SUFentanil, tacrolimus, teniposide, theophylline, thiamine, thiotepa, ticarcillin/clavulanate, tigecycline, tirofiban, tobramycin, tolazoline, trimethaphan, urokinase, vancomycin, vasopressin, vecuronium, verapamil, vinCRIStine, vinorelbine, vitamin B complex with C, voriconazole, warfarin, zoledronic acid

SIDE EFFECTS

CNS: *Tremors, anxiety,* insomnia, headache, *dizziness,* confusion, hallucinations, weakness, drowsiness
CV: *Palpitations, tachycardia,* hypertension, dysrhythmias, increased T wave
GI: *Anorexia, nausea, vomiting*
MISC: Sweating, dry eyes
RESP: *Dyspnea,* paradoxical bronchospasm (inhalation)
META: Hypoglycemia

PHARMACOKINETICS

Crosses placenta, metabolized in liver
IM: 6-10 min, duration 1-4 hr
SUBCUT: Onset 5-10 min, duration 20 min-4 hr
IV: Onset immediate, peak 20 min, duration 1-4 hr
INH: Onset 1-5 min, duration 1-3 hr

INTERACTIONS

• Do not use with MAOIs or tricyclics; hypertensive crisis may occur

• **Toxicity:** other sympathomimetics

Decrease: hypertensive effects—beta-adrenergic blockers, stop beta-blocker 3 days prior to starting product

Increase: hypotension—alpha-blockers

Increase: cardiac effects—antihistamines, thyroid replacement hormones

Increase: dysrhythmias—cardiac glycosides

Drug/herb

Increased stimulation: coffee, tea, guarana, yerba maté

NURSING CONSIDERATIONS

Assess:

• **Asthma:** auscultate lungs, pulse, B/P, respirations, sputum (color, character); monitor pulmonary function studies before and during treatment

• **Shock:** monitor for hypovolemia before use

• **Vasopressor:** ECG during administration continuously; if B/P increases, decrease dose; B/P, pulse q5min after parenteral route; CVP, ISVR, PCWP during infusion if possible; inadvertent high arterial B/P can result in angina, aortic rupture, cerebral hemorrhage

• **Injection site:** tissue sloughing; administer phentolamine 5 mg with NS 10-15 mL, use within 12 hr of infiltration

• **Sulfite sensitivity;** may be life-threatening

• Cardiac status, I&O; blood glucose in diabetes

• **Labs:** monitor pulmonary function tests baseline and periodically

• **Allergic reactions, bronchospasms** (swelling of face/lips/eyelids, rash, difficulty breathing): withhold dose, notify prescriber

Evaluate:

• **Therapeutic response:** increased B/P with stabilization or ease of breathing, relief of bronchospasm

Teach patient/family:

• About the reason for product administration

• **Inhalation:** to rinse mouth after use to prevent dryness after inhalation, not to spray near eyes, teach correct use

• To take exactly as prescribed. If on scheduled regimen, take missed dose as soon as remembered. Space remaining doses evenly. Do not double doses. To contact prescriber immediately if shortness of breath is not relieved or diaphoresis, dizziness, or chest pain occurs

• To consult prescriber prior to taking any OTC, Rx medications, supplements or herbals

• To use bronchodilator prior to using other products

• To maintain adequate fluid intake (2000-3000 mL/day) to help liquefy secretions

• To notify prescriber if pregnancy is planned or suspected or if breastfeeding

• **Autoinjector:** how to use for anaphylaxis; remove cap, place injector end tip on thigh at 90-degree angle, hold 10 sec, remove

• **Pregnancy/breastfeeding:** identify if pregnancy is planned or suspected or if breastfeeding

TREATMENT OF OVERDOSE:

Administer alpha-blocker and beta-blocker

EPINEPHrine nasal agent

See Appendix B

⚠ HIGH ALERT

epirubicin (Rx)

(ep-ih-roo′bi-sin)

Ellence, Pharmorubicin ✦

Func. class.: Antineoplastic, antibiotic

Chem. class.: Anthracycline

Do not confuse:

epirubicin/eribulin

ACTION: Inhibits DNA synthesis primarily; replication is decreased by binding to DNA, which causes strand splitting; maximum cytotoxic effects at S and for G_2 phases; a vesicant

USES: Adjuvant therapy for breast cancer with axillary node involvement after resection

Unlabeled uses: Used in combination for treatment of advanced forms of cancer: bladder, gastric, head and neck, hepatocellular, lung, ovarian, multiple myeloma, soft tissue sarcoma

CONTRAINDICATIONS
Pregnancy, breastfeeding; hypersensitivity to product, anthracyclines, anthracenediones; baseline neutrophil count <1500 cells/mm^3, severe myocardial insufficiency, recent MI, heart failure, cardiomyopathy

Black Box Warning: Severe hepatic disease, IM/SUBCUT use

Precautions: Children, geriatric patients, cardiac/renal/hepatic disease, accidental exposure, angina, dental disease, herpes, hyperkalemia, hyperphosphatemia, hypertension, hyperuricemia, hypocalcemia, infection, infertility, tumor lysis syndrome, ventricular dysfunction, previous anthracycline use

Black Box Warning: Bone marrow depression (severe), heart failure, extravasation, secondary malignancy, requires an experienced clinician

DOSAGE AND ROUTES
• **Adult:** IV 100 mg/m^2 on day 1 with fluorouracil and cyclophosphamide (FEC regimen) every 21 days × 6 cycles or 60 mg/m^2 on days 1 and 8 with oral cyclophosphamide and fluorouracil every 28 days × 6 cycles

Dosage adjustments based on hematologic and nonhematologic toxicities
• **Nadir platelet counts <50,000/mm^3, absolute neutrophil counts (ANC) <250/mm^3, neutropenic fever, or grades 3/4 nonhematologic toxicities:** Day 1 dose in subsequent cycles should be reduced by 25% of the previous dose
• **For patients receiving divided-dose epirubicin (days 1 and 8):** Day 8 dose should be reduced by 25% of the day 1 dose if the platelet counts are 75,000-100,000/mm^3 and the ANC is 1000-1499/mm^3; if day 8 platelet counts are <75,000/mm^3, ANC <1000/mm^3, or grade 3/4 nonhematologic toxicity has occurred, omit the day 8 dose

Hepatic dose
• **Adult:** IV Bilirubin 1.2-3 mg/dL or AST 2-4 × normal upper limit, 50% of starting dose; bilirubin >3-5 mg/dL or AST >4 × normal upper limit, 25% of starting dose

Available forms: Solution for injection 2 mg/mL (250 mg/25 mL, 200 mg/100 mL)

Administer:
• Antiemetic 30-60 min prior to product to prevent vomiting

Black Box Warning: To be used by a clinician experienced in giving cytotoxic products

Black Box Warning: Do not use IM/SUBCUT, severe tissue necrosis, give IV only, a vesicant; if extravasation occurs, stop and complete via another vein, preferably in another limb; avoid infusion into veins over joints or in extremities with compromised venous or lymphatic drainage

• Rapid injection can cause facial flushing or erythema along the vein; avoid administration time of <3 min
• Product should be given to those with neutrophils ≥1500/mm^3, platelet count ≥100,000/mm^3, and nonhematologic toxicities recovered to ≤grade 1
• When refrigerated, the preservative-free, ready-to-use solution can form a gelled product and will return to solution after 2-4 hr at room temperature
• Visually inspect for particulate matter and discoloration prior to use

IV route
• Double-check dose and product; fatalities have occurred with wrong dose or product
• Give anti-infectives prior to use of this product
• Use cytotoxic handling procedures; pregnant women must not handle product

Side effects: *italics* = common; red = life-threatening

• Reconstitute 50 mg and 200 mg powder for injection vials with 25 mL and 100 mL, respectively, of sterile water for injection (2 mg/mL); shake vigorously for up to 4 min; reconstituted solutions are stable for 24 hr when stored refrigerated and protected from light or at room temperature in normal light

• Solution can be further diluted with sterile water for injection

IV INJ route

• Give doses of 100-120 mg/m² into tubing of a freely flowing 0.9% sodium chloride (NS) or D₅W IV infusion over 15-20 min; the infusion time may be decreased proportionally in those who require lower doses; infusion times <3 min are not recommended

• Direct injection into the vein is not recommended because of the risk of extravasation; avoid use with any solution of alkaline pH because hydrolysis will occur

IV INFUSION route

• Dilute dose in 0.9% sodium chloride (NS) or D₅W, infuse over 30-60 min, avoid use with any solution of alkaline pH because hydrolysis will occur

Y-site compatibilities: Alemtuzumab, alfentanil, amifostine, amikacin, aminocaproic acid, anidulafungin, argatroban, atracurium, aztreonam, bivalirudin, bleomycin, bumetanide, buprenorphine, butorphanol, calcium chloride/gluconate, CARBOplatin, caspofungin, ceFAZolin, cefotaxime, ceftizoxime, chlorproMAZINE, cimetidine, ciprofloxacin, cisatracurium, CISplatin, clindamycin, cyclophosphamide, cycloSPORINE, DAPTOmycin, dexrazoxane, digoxin, diltiazem, diphenhydrAMINE, DOBUTamine, DOCEtaxel, dolasetron, DOPamine, doxacurium, doxycycline, droperidol, enalaprilat, ePHEDrine, EPINEPHrine, ertapenem, erythromycin, etoposide, famotidine, fenoldopam, fentaNYL, fluconazole, gatifloxacin, gemcitabine, gentamicin, granisetron, haloperidol, hydrocortisone, HYDROmorphone, hydrOXYzine, ifosfamide, imipenem-cilastatin, inamrinone, insulin (regular), isoproterenol, labetalol, levofloxacin, levorphanol, lidocaine, linezolid, LORazepam, mannitol, meperidine, mesna, methotrexate, metoclopramide, metoprolol, metroNIDAZOLE, midazolam, milrinone, minocycline, mitoMYcin, mivacurium, morphine, moxifloxacin, nalbuphine, naloxone, nesiritide, niCARdipine, nitroglycerin, nitroprusside, norepinephrine, octreotide, ofloxacin, ondansetron, oxaliplatin, PACLitaxel, palonosetron, pamidronate, pancuronium, pentamidine, pentazocine, phenylephrine, potassium chloride, procainamide, prochlorperazine, promethazine, propranolol, quinupristin-dalfopristin, ranitidine, remifentanil, rocuronium, sodium acetate, succinylcholine, SUFentanil, tacrolimus, teniposide, theophylline, thiotepa, tigecycline, tirofiban, tobramycin, trimethobenzamide, vancomycin, vasopressin, vecuronium, verapamil, vinBLAStine, vinCRIStine, vinorelbine, voriconazole, zidovudine, zoledronic acid

SIDE EFFECTS

CV: Increased B/P, sinus tachycardia, PVCs, chest pain, bradycardia, extrasystoles, cardiomyopathy

GI: *Nausea, vomiting, anorexia, mucositis, diarrhea*

GU: *Amenorrhea, hot flashes, hyperuricemia, red urine*

HEMA: Thrombocytopenia, leukopenia, anemia, neutropenia, secondary AML

INTEG: *Rash,* necrosis, *pain at injection site, reversible alopecia*

MISC: *Infection, febrile neutropenia, lethargy, fever, conjunctivitis,* tumor lysis syndrome

PHARMACOKINETICS

Triphasic pattern of elimination; half-life 3 min, 1 hr, 30 hr; metabolized by liver, extensively; crosses placenta; widely distributed to RBCs, excreted in urine, bile, breast milk

INTERACTIONS

• Give epiRUBicin prior to PACLitaxel if both are given

Increase: toxicity—other antineoplastics or radiation, cimetidine

Increase: ventricular dysfunction, HF—trastuzumab

Increase: heart failure—calcium channel blockers

Decrease: antibody response—live virus vaccine

NURSING CONSIDERATIONS
Assess:

Black Box Warning: Bone marrow depression (severe): CBC, differential, platelet count weekly; withhold product if baseline neutrophil ≤1500/mm³; leukocyte nadir occurs 10-14 days after administration, recovery by day 21; notify prescriber of results; assess for bleeding: hematuria, guaiac, bruising, or petechiae, or mucosa, orifices

• **Infection:** treat prior to receiving this product if regimens >120 mg/m², prophylactic antibiotics should be given (trimethoprim-sulfamethoxazole or a quinolone)

• Blood, urine uric acid levels; swelling, joint pain primarily in extremities; patient should be well hydrated to prevent urate deposits

• Renal disease: BUN, serum uric acid, urine CCr, electrolytes prior to, during therapy; I&O ratio; report fall in urine output to <30 mL/hr; dosage adjustment needed if serum creatinine >5 mg/dL

• Increase fluid intake to 2-3 L/day to prevent urate, calculi formation

Black Box Warning: Hepatic studies prior to, during therapy: bilirubin, AST, ALT, alkaline phosphatase as needed or monthly

Black Box Warning: Heart failure: B/P, pulse, character, rhythm, rate, ABGs, ECG, LVEF, MUGA scan, or ECHO; watch for ST-T wave changes, low QRS and T, possible dysrhythmias (sinus tachycardia, heart block, PVCs); identify cumulative amount of anthracycline received (lifetime); reactions that follow may be delayed; assess for dyspnea, tachycardia, peripheral edema, rales/crackles, ascites

• Effects of alopecia on body image; discuss feelings about body changes

Black Box Warning: Extravasation (vesicant): local irritation, pain, burning, necrosis at injection site; discontinue and start at another site.

• **Stomatitis:** oral mucosa for ulceration, burning, bleeding; may lead to inability to eat and swallow

• GI symptoms: frequency of stools, cramping

• **Pregnancy/breastfeeding:** Women of reproductive potential should avoid becoming pregnant during therapy and should be advised to use effective contraceptive methods. If a woman becomes pregnant during therapy, she should be advised of the potential risks to the fetus. There is potential for male-mediated teratogenicity. Men with sexual partners of reproductive potential should use effective contraceptive methods during and after therapy. Men or women who receive this product may have a risk of infertility. Women treated may develop irreversible amenorrhea or premature menopause; discontinue breastfeeding or discontinue product

Evaluate:

• Therapeutic response: decreased tumor size, spread of malignancy

Teach patient/family:

• That hair may be lost during treatment; that wig or hairpiece may make patient feel better; that new hair may be different in color, texture; new hair growth occurs in ≤3 mo after treatment

• To avoid crowds, persons with infections when granulocyte count is low

• To avoid vaccinations because reactions may occur; to avoid cimetidine during therapy

• That urine may appear red for 2 days

• To avoid OTC medications, supplements unless approved by prescriber

Black Box Warning: That irreversible myocardial damage, leukopenia, menopause may occur

• To report rapid heartbeat, trouble breathing, fever, nausea, vomiting, oral sores

• To report pain at site immediately

• **Pregnancy/breastfeeding:** that contraceptive measures are recommended during therapy and for 4 mo thereafter for men and women; not to breastfeed

---

eplerenone (Rx)
(ep-ler-ee′known)

Inspra

Func. class.: Antihypertensive
Chem. class.: Selective aldosterone receptor antagonist

Do not confuse:
Inspra/Spiriva

ACTION: Binds to mineralocorticoid receptor and blocks the binding of aldosterone, a component of the renin-angiotensin-aldosterone system (RAAS)

USES: Hypertension, alone or in combination with thiazide diuretics, HF, post-MI

CONTRAINDICATIONS
Hypersensitivity; increased serum creatinine >2 mg/dL (male), >1.8 mg/dL (female); potassium >5.5 mEq/L, type 2 diabetes with microalbuminuria, hepatic disease, CCr <30 mL/min; CCr <50 mL/min in hypertension
Precautions: Pregnancy, breastfeeding, children, geriatric patients, impaired renal/hepatic function, hyperkalemia

DOSAGE AND ROUTES
Hypertension
• **Adult:** PO 50 mg/day initially, may increase to 50 mg bid after 4 wk, max 100 mg/day; 25 mg/day max if patient is taking CYP3A4 inhibitors
HF or post-MI
• **Adult:** PO 25 mg/day initially, may increase to 50 mg/day max after 4 wk
Renal dose
• **Adult:** PO CCr <30 mL/min: contraindicated; CCr <50 mL/min for HTN: contraindicated; CCr 30-49 mL/min for HF: 25 mg every other day, max 25 mg daily

Dosage adjustments for those receiving moderate CYP3A4 inhibitors
• Potassium level <5 mEq/L, increase from 25 mg every other day to 25 mg daily, or increase dose from 25 mg daily to 50 mg daily; potassium level 5 to 5.4 mEq/L no adjustment; potassium level 5.5 to 5.9 mEq/L, decrease dose from 50 mg to 25 mg, or decrease dose from 25 mg daily to 25 mg every other day; if dose was 25 mg every other day, withhold dose; if potassium is >6 mEq/L, withhold; may restart drug at 25 mg every other day when potassium level is <5.5 mEq/L
Available forms: Tablets 25, 50 mg
Administer:
• Without regard to food
• Do not use salt substitutes containing potassium
• Store in tight container at ≤86° F (30° C)

SIDE EFFECTS
CNS: Headache, *dizziness, fatigue*
CV: Angina, MI
GI: Increased GGT, *diarrhea,* abdominal pain, increased ALT
GU: Gynecomastia, mastodynia (males), abnormal vaginal bleeding
META: *Hyperkalemia,* hyponatremia, hypercholesteremia, hypertriglyceridemia, increased uric acid
RESP: *Cough*

PHARMACOKINETICS
Peak 1½ hr; serum protein binding 50%; half-life 4-6 hr; metabolized in liver by CYP3A4; excreted in urine <5%, feces

INTERACTIONS
Increase: hyperkalemia—ACE inhibitors, angiotensin II antagonists, NSAIDs, potassium supplements, potassium-sparing diuretics; do not use together
Increase: serum levels of lithium; monitor lithium level
Increase: eplerenone levels—erythromycin, fluconazole, verapamil; reduce dose of eplerenone
Increase: levels of eplerenone—CYP3A4 inhibitors (ketoconazole, itraconazole, saquinavir, clarithromycin, imatinib, nelfinavir,

nefazodone, ritonavir, troleandomycin); do not use concurrently or reduce dose of eplerenone

Decrease: antihypertensive effect—NSAIDs
Drug/herb
Decrease: antihypertensive effect—ephedra, St. John's wort
Drug/food
Grapefruit, grapefruit juice—increase product level by 25%
Do not use salt substitutes containing potassium
Drug/lab
Increase: BUN, creatinine, potassium, cholesterol, lipids, uric acid, ALT, BUN, GGT
Decrease: sodium

NURSING CONSIDERATIONS
Assess:
• **Hypertension:** B/P at peak/trough level of product, orthostatic hypotension, syncope when used with diuretic; monitor lithium level in those also taking lithium; those on CYP3A4 inhibitor should monitor potassium at baseline, within first week, at 1 mo, and more often in diabetes, renal disease
• **Renal studies:** protein, BUN, creatinine; LFTs, uric acid may be increased; contraindicated in CCr <30 mL/min
• **Potassium levels;** hyperkalemia may occur
• **Pregnancy/breastfeeding:** use in pregnancy only if clearly needed; may be excreted in breast milk; do not breastfeed
Evaluate:
• Therapeutic response: decreased B/P
Teach patient/family:
• Not to discontinue product abruptly
• Not to use OTC products (cough, cold, allergy) unless directed by prescriber; not to use salt substitutes containing potassium without consulting prescriber
• To comply with dosage schedule, even if feeling better
• That product may cause dizziness, fainting, light headedness; may occur during first few days of therapy
• How to take B/P and about normal readings for age group

⚠ HIGH ALERT

epoetin alfa (Rx)
(ee-poe'e-tin)
Epogen, Eprex ✦, Procrit
epoetin alfa epbx (Rx)
Retacrit
Func. class.: Antianemic, erythropoiesis-stimulating agent
Chem. class.: Amino acid polypeptide

ACTION: Erythropoietin is a factor controlling the rate of red cell production; product is developed by recombinant DNA technology

USES: Anemia caused by reduced endogenous erythropoietin production, in end-stage renal disease; to correct hemostatic defect in uremia; anemia due to AZT treatment in patients with HIV or those receiving chemotherapy; reduction of allogenic blood transfusion in surgery patients
Unlabeled uses: Anemia in premature preterm infants, anemia due to ribavirin and interferon-alfa therapy in hepatitic C

CONTRAINDICATIONS
Hypersensitivity to mammalian-cell–derived products, human albumin; uncontrolled hypertension
Precautions: Pregnancy, breastfeeding, children <1 mo, seizure disorder; multidose preserved formulation contains benzyl alcohol and should not be used in premature infants; porphyria, CV disease, hemodialysis, latex allergy, hypertension, history of CABG

Black Box Warning: HB >11 g/dL, surgery, neoplastic disease

DOSAGE AND ROUTES
Anemia due to chronic kidney disease to decrease the need for red blood cell transfusion
• **Adult:** IV/SUBCUT 50-100 units/kg/dose or 3 times weekly initially; for patients on dialysis, administer IV. For patients on dialysis, initiate treatment when hemoglobin (Hgb) is less than 10 g/dL

• **Adolescents 17 years: IV/SUBCUT** 50-100 units/kg/dose 3 times weekly initially; for patients on dialysis, administer IV. For patients on dialysis, initiate treatment when hemoglobin (Hgb) is less than 10 g/dL. If Hgb approaches or exceeds 11 g/dL, reduce or interrupt the dose

• **Infants, children, and adolescents 1 mo to 16 yr:** 50 units/kg/dose IV or SUBCUT 3 times weekly initially; for patients on dialysis, administer IV. Initiate treatment when hemoglobin (Hgb) is less than 10 g/dL. If Hgb approaches or exceeds 12 g/dL, reduce or interrupt the dose

To reduce the need for allogeneic red blood cell transfusions in patients with perioperative hemoglobin more than 10 g/dL to 13 g/dL scheduled to undergo elective, noncardiac, nonvascular surgery who are at high risk for perioperative blood loss and who are NOT willing to donate autologous blood preoperatively

• **Adult: SUBCUT** 300 units/kg/day for 10 days prior to surgery, on the day of surgery, and for 4 days after surgery (15 days total) plus deep vein thrombosis (DVT) prophylaxis

Zidovudine-induced anemia in HIV-infected patients with circulating endogenous erythropoietin concentrations of 500 mUnits/mL or less who are receiving a dose of zidovudine of 4200 mg/week or less

• **Adult: SUBCUT/IV** Initially, 100 units/kg/dose 3 times weekly. If Hgb does not increase after 8 wk, increase by 50-100 units/kg/dose at 4- to 8-wk intervals until Hgb is at a concentration to avoid RBC transfusions or a dose of 300 units/kg is reached. If the Hgb is more than 12 g/dL, withhold epoetin and once Hgb is less than 11 g/dL, resume at a dose 25% below the previous dose.

Anemia in nonmyeloid malignancies where the anemia is due to the effect of chemotherapy and at least 2 additional mo of chemotherapy are planned

• **Adult: SUBCUT** 150 units/kg/dose 3 times weekly or 40,000 units once weekly only when the hemoglobin (Hgb) is less than 10 g/dL and only until the chemotherapy course is completed. Adjust the dose to maintain the lowest Hgb concentration sufficient to avoid RBC transfusions

• **Children and adolescent 5-17 yr: IV** 600 units/kg/dose weekly only when the hemoglobin (Hgb) is less than 10 g/dL and only until the chemotherapy course is completed. Adjust the dose to maintain the lowest Hgb concentration sufficient to avoid RBC transfusions

To reduce the need for allogeneic red blood cell transfusions in patients with perioperative hemoglobin more than 10 g/dL to 13 g/dL scheduled to undergo elective, noncardiac, nonvascular surgery who are at high risk for perioperative blood loss and who are NOT willing to donate autologous blood preoperatively

• **Adult: SUBCUT** 300 units/kg/day for 10 days prior to surgery, on the day of surgery, and for 4 days after surgery (15 days total) plus deep vein thrombosis (DVT) prophylaxis

Available forms: Injection 2000, 3000, 4000, 10,000, 20,000, 40,000 units/mL

Administer:

• Use 1 single-use vial/dose, once syringe has entered single-dose vial, sterility cannot be guaranteed, do not administer with other product, multidose vials can be stored in refrigerator up to 21 days once opened, do not use if discolored or particulates are present

SUBCUT route

• Before injecting, preservative-free, single-dose formulation may be admixed using 0.9% NaCl with benzyl alcohol 0.9% at a 1:1 ratio to reduce injection site discomfort, store solution in refrigerator, protect from light

Direct IV route

• Additional heparin to lower chance of clots

• By direct injection or bolus into IV tubing or venous line at end of dialysis; do not shake vial; can use undiluted or diluted in 0.9% NaCl (1000-40,000 U/mL); give over ≥1 min

---

• Decrease dose by 25% if Hb increases by 1 g/dL in 2 wk; increase dose if Hb does not increase by 5-6 pts after 8 wk of therapy; suggested target Hb range 30%-36%

Solution compatibilities: Do not dilute or administer with other solutions

SIDE EFFECTS
CNS: Seizures, coldness, sweating, headache, fatigue, dizziness
CV: *Hypertension,* hypertensive encephalopathy, HF, edema, DVT, MI, stroke
INTEG: Pruritus, rash, injection site reaction
MISC: Iron deficiency
MS: Bone pain, arthralgia, myalgia
RESP: Cough

PHARMACOKINETICS
IV: Metabolized in body, extent of metabolism unknown, onset of increased reticulocyte count 2-6 wk, peak immediate
Subcut: Peak 5-24 hr

INTERACTIONS
Need for increased heparin during hemodialysis

NURSING CONSIDERATIONS
Assess:
• Renal studies: urinalysis, protein, blood, BUN, creatinine; I&O, electrolytes, report drop in output <50 mL/hr

Black Box Warning: Blood studies: ferritin, transferrin, serum iron monthly; transferrin sat ≥20%, ferritin ≥100 ng/mL; Hct 2×/wk until stabilized in target range (30%-36%) then at regular intervals; those with endogenous erythropoietin levels of <500 units/L respond to product; monitor Hct 2×/wk with chronic renal failure; patients treated with zidovudine or patients with cancer should be monitored weekly, then periodically after stabilization; death may occur with Hb >12 g/dL; monitor for blood clots

• B/P; check for rising B/P as Hct rises, antihypertensives may be needed; hypertension may occur rapidly, leading to hypertensive encephalopathy, use of antihypertensive may be needed

• CNS symptoms: coldness, sweating, pain in long bones; for seizures if Hct is increased within 2 wk by 4 points
• Hypersensitivity reactions: skin rashes, urticaria (rare), antibody development does not occur
• **Pure cell aplasia (PRCA)** in absence of other causes; evaluate by testing sera for recombinant erythropoietin antibodies; any loss of response to epoetin should be evaluated
• Dialysis patients: thrill, bruit of shunts; monitor for circulation impairment
• **Chemotherapy anemia:** Begin only if Hb ≥10 g/dL and 2 more months of chemotherapy is planned
• **Seizures:** place patient on seizure precautions if increase of 1 g/dL Hct in any 2-wk period, increased B/P; more common in chronic renal failure during the first 90 days of treatment
• **Pregnancy/breastfeeding:** product should be used during pregnancy only when benefits outweigh fetal risk. Multidose vials are contraindicated due to the use of benzyl alcohol as a preservative; it is not known whether epoetin alfa is distributed into breast milk
Evaluate:
• Therapeutic response: increase in reticulocyte count in 2-6 wk, Hb/Hct WNL
Teach patient/family:
• How to take B/P, have patient read the "Medication Guide"; a form must be signed before each cycle
• To avoid driving or hazardous activities during beginning of treatment
• To take iron supplements, vitamin B_{12}, folic acid as directed
• To report immediately chest pain; pain in calves; confusion; inability to speak; numbness in face, arm, leg
• **Chronic renal failure (anemia):** product does not cure condition, to maintain prescribed diet, medications, dialysis follow-up appointments
• **Pregnancy/breastfeeding:** to report if pregnancy is planned or suspected or if breastfeeding
• The reason for treatment, expected results, to notify health care professional of use

⚠ HIGH ALERT

eptifibatide (Rx)
(ep-tih-fib'ah-tide)
Func. class.: Antiplatelet agent
Chem. class.: Glycoprotein IIb/IIIa
inhibitor

ACTION: Platelet glycoprotein antagonist; this agent reversibly prevents fibrinogen, von Willebrand's factor from binding to the glycoprotein IIb/IIIa receptor, thus inhibiting platelet aggregation

USES: Acute coronary syndrome including those undergoing percutaneous coronary intervention (PCI)

CONTRAINDICATIONS
Hypersensitivity, active internal bleeding; recent history of bleeding, stroke within 30 days or any hemorrhagic stroke; major surgery with severe trauma, severe hypertension, current or planned use of another parenteral GP IIb/IIIa inhibitor, dependence on renal dialysis, coagulopathy, AV malformation, aneurysm
Precautions: Pregnancy, breastfeeding, children, geriatric patients, bleeding, impaired renal function

DOSAGE AND ROUTES
Acute coronary syndrome
• **Adult: IV BOLUS** 180 mcg/kg as soon as diagnosed, max 22.6 mg, then **IV CONTINUOUS** 2 mcg/kg/min until discharge or CABG; in CABG discontinue ≥2-4 hr prior to procedure; max infusion rate 15 mg/hr
PCI in patients without acute coronary syndrome
• **Adult: IV BOLUS** 180 mcg/kg given immediately prior to PCI, then 2 mcg/kg/min × 18 hr **CONTINUOUS IV INFUSION** and a second 180-mcg/kg bolus by 10 min after first bolus; continue infusion for up to 18-24 hr, minimum 12 hr; max infusion rate 15 mg/hr
Renal dose
• **Adult: IV** maintenance CCr <50 mL/min, 1 mcg/kg/min, max rate 7.5 mg/hr; CCr <10 mL/min, contraindicated

Available forms: Solution for injection 2 mg/mL (10 mL), 0.75 mg/mL (100 mL)
Administer:
• Aspirin may be given with this product; check for bleeding
• D/C heparin prior to removing femoral artery sheath, after PCI
• Do not give discolored solutions, those with particulates; discard unused amount, protect from light
• Discontinue product prior to CABG
Direct IV route
• After withdrawing bolus dose from 20 mg/10 mL (2 mg/mL) vial, give IV push over 1-2 min
Continuous IV INFUSION route
• Follow bolus dose with continuous infusion using pump; give product undiluted directly from 100-mL vial, spike 100-mL vial with vented infusion set, use caution when centering spike on circle of stopper top, refrigerate vials, or may store vials ≤2 mo at room temperature

Y-site compatibilities: Alfentanil, alteplase, amikacin, aminophylline, amphotericin B lipid complex, amphotericin B liposome, ampicillin, ampicillin-sulbactam, anidulafungin, argatroban, atenolol, atracurium, atropine, azithromycin, aztreonam, bivalirudin, bumetanide, buprenorphine, butorphanol, calcium chloride/gluconate, ceFAZolin, cefepime, cefotaxime, cefoTEtan, cefOXitin, cefTAZidime, ceftizoxime, cefTRIAXone, cefuroxime, cimetidine, ciprofloxacin, cisatracurium, clindamycin, cycloSPORINE, DAPTOmycin, dexamethasone, D₅/NaCl 0.9%, diazepam, dilTIAZem, diphenhydrAMINE, DOBUTamine, dolasetron, DOPamine, doxycycline, droperidol, enalaprilat, ePHEDrine, EPINEPHrine, ertapenem, erythromycin, esmolol, famotidine, fentaNYL, fluconazole, fosphenytoin, ganciclovir, gatifloxacin, gentamicin, granisetron, haloperidol, heparin, hydrocortisone, HYDROmorphone, hydrOXYzine, imipenem-cilastatin, inamrinone, isoproterenol, ketorolac, labetalol, leucovorin, levofloxacin, levorphanol, lidocaine, linezolid, LORazepam, magnesium sulfate, mannitol, meperidine, meropenem, methylPREDNISolone, metoclopramide, metoprolol, metroNIDAZOLE, micafungin, midazolam, milrinone, minocycline, mivacurium, morphine, nalbuphine, naloxone, niCARdipine, nitroglycerin, nitroprusside, NS, octreotide, ofloxacin, ondansetron, oxytocin, palonosetron, pancuronium, PEMEtrexed, PENTobarbital, PHENobarbital, phenylephrine, piperacillin, piperacillintazobactam, potassium chloride/phosphates, procainamide, prochlorperazine, promethazine, propranolol, ranitidine, remifentanil, rocuronium, sodium bicarbonate/phosphates, succinylcholine, SUFentanil, sulfamethoxazole-trimethoprim, teniposide, theophylline, ticarcillin, ticarcillin-clavulanate, tigecycline, tirofiban, tobramycin, trimethobenzamide, vancomycin, vecuronium, verapamil, zidovudine, zoledronic acid

SIDE EFFECTS
CV: Stroke, hypotension
GU: Hematuria
HEMA: Thrombocytopenia, platelet dysfunction
SYST: Major/minor bleeding from any site, anaphylaxis

PHARMACOKINETICS
Onset within 1 hr, protein binding 25%, half-life 1.5-2 hr, steady-state 4-6 hr, metabolism limited, excretion via kidneys

INTERACTIONS
• Do not give with glycoprotein inhibitors IIb, IIIa
Increase: bleeding—aspirin, heparin, NSAIDs, anticoagulants, ticlopidine, clopidogrel, dipyridamole, thrombolytics, valproate, abciximab, SSRIs, SNRIs
Drug/herb
Increase: bleeding risk—feverfew, garlic, ginger, ginkgo, ginseng

NURSING CONSIDERATIONS
Assess:
• **Renal disease:** reduce dose if CCr >50; contraindicated in dialysis
• **Thrombocytopenia:** platelets, Hb, Hct, creatinine, APTT baseline within 6 hr of loading dose, daily therafter, patients undergoing PCI should have ACT monitored; maintain APTT 50-70 sec unless PCI to be performed; during PCI, ACT should be 200-300 sec; if

platelets drop <100,000/mm³, obtain additional platelet counts; if thrombocytopenia is confirmed, discontinue product; draw Hct, Hb, serum creatinine, arterial sheath should be removed unless aPTT is >45 sec
• **Bleeding:** gums, bruising, ecchymosis, petechiae; from GI, GU tract, cardiac cath sites, IM injection sites, if platelets are <100,000 discontinue
• **Labs:** Hct, HB, platelets, serum creatinine, ACT, PT, aPTT baseline in PCI patients
• **Pregnancy/breastfeeding:** use in pregnancy only if clearly needed; it is not known if product is excreted in breast milk; consider risks and benefits
Evaluate:
• Therapeutic response: decreased mortality in MI patients
Teach patient/family:
• About reason for medication and expected results
• To report bruising, bleeding, chest pain immediately
• Not to use other Rx, OTC products or supplements without prescriber approval
• **Pregnancy/breastfeeding:** To notify health care provider if pregnancy is planned or suspected or if breastfeeding

eptinezumab-jjmr (Rx)
(ep′ti-nez′ue-mab)
Vyepti
Func. class.: Antimigraine agent
Chem. class.: Calcitonin gene–related peptide receptor antagonist

ACTION: A humanized monoclonal antibody, binds to calcitonin gene–related peptide ligand and blocks binding to the receptor

USES: Prevention of migraine

CONTRAINDICATIONS
Serious hypersensitivity
Precautions: Pregnancy, breastfeeding, child

DOSAGE AND ROUTES
Migraine prophylaxis
• **Adult: IV:** 100 mg q3mo; may use 300 mg q3mo

Available forms: solution, preservative free 100 mg/mL (1 mL)
Administer:
Intermittent IV infusion
- Contains polysorbate 80
- Dilute in 100 mL NS; infusion bags must be made of polyvinyl chloride, polyethylene, polyolefin; mix by gentle inverting; do not shake, discard unused portion; 100-mg dose: Withdraw 1 mL eptinezumab/100 mL NS (1 mg/mL); 300-mg dose: Withdraw 1 mL eptinezumab from 3 vials/100 mL NS (3 mg/mL)
- Run over 30 min using an infusion set with a 0.2 or 0.22 micron in-line or add-on sterile filter; do not give IV push/bolus
- Do not admix or infuse other medications in same infusion set
- After infusion, flush line with 20 mL NS
- Store intact vial at 2° C to 8° C (36° F to 46° F), protect from light, do not freeze; diluted solution may be stored at room temperature, infuse within 8 hr

SIDE EFFECTS
MISC: Antibody development
RESP: Nasopharyngitis
CNS: Fatigue
GI: Nausea
INTEG: Hypersensitivity, angioedema

PHARMACOKINETICS: Onset 1 day, peak infusion's end, duration unknown, half-life 27 days

INTERACTIONS
None known

NURSING CONSIDERATIONS
Assess:
- **Migraine:** Baseline and periodically, presence of aura, nausea/vomiting
- Assess for hypersensitivity, dyspnea; reaction may be delayed, discontinue if these occur
Evaluate:
- Therapeutic response: Prevention of migraine
Teach patient/family:
- Reason for product and expected result
- Identify if pregnancy is planned or suspected

---

eravacycline (Rx)
(er'a-va-sye'kleen)
Xerava
Func. class.: Antibiotic—tetracycline
Chem. class.: Synthetic fluorocycline

ACTION: Disrupts bacterial protein synthesis by binding to the 30S ribosomal subunit and preventing the incorporation of amino acid residues into elongating peptide chains

USES: Complicated intraabdominal infections caused by *Bacteroides caccae, Bacteroides fragilis, Bacteroides ovatus, Bacteroides thetaiotaomicron, Bacteroides uniformis, Bacteroides vulgatus, Citrobacter freundii, Citrobacter koseri, Clostridium perfringens, Enterobacter aerogenes, Enterobacter cloacae, Enterococcus faecalis, Enterococcus faecium, Escherichia coli, Klebsiella oxytoca, Klebsiella pneumoniae, Parabacteroides distasonis, Staphylococcus aureus* (MRSA), *Staphylococcus aureus* (MSSA), *Streptococcus anginosus, Streptococcus salivarius*

CONTRAINDICATIONS
Hypersensitivity to this product or tetracyclines
Precautions: Breastfeeding, children, colitis, diarrhea, geriatric patients, GI/hepatic disease, increased intracranial pressure, inflammatory bowel disease/ulcerative colitis, papilledema, pregnancy, CDAD, UV exposure

DOSAGE AND ROUTES
- **Adult:** IV 1 mg/kg q12hr × 4-14 days
Available forms: Powder for injection 50 mg
Administer:
Intermittent IV INFUSION route
- Visually inspect for particulate matter and discoloration prior to use; reconstituted solution is clear, pale yellow to orange
- **Reconstitution:** Reconstitute each vial with 5 mL of sterile water for injec-

tion to a concentration of 10 mg/mL; swirl until powder has dissolved; avoid shaking or rapid movement. Do not give reconstituted solution by direct injection

• **Dilution:** Withdraw the full or partial reconstituted content from each vial and add it into a 0.9% sodium chloride for injection infusion bag to a concentration of 0.3 mg/mL (within a range of 0.2-0.6 mg/mL). Do not shake

• **Storage:** Diluted solution must be infused within 6 hr if stored at room temperature 77° F (max 25° C) or within 24 hr if stored refrigerated at 36° F-46° F (2° C-8° C). Do not freeze

Intermittent IV infusion

• Infuse through a dedicated IV line or by Y-site. If the same IV line is used for sequential infusion of several drugs, flush the line prior to and after infusion with 0.9% sodium chloride for injection. Give over 60 min; assess IV site frequently

SIDE EFFECTS

CV: Hypotension
EENT: Tooth discoloration
GI: Nausea, vomiting, diarrhea, pancreatitis, *Clostridium difficile*
HEMA: Thrombosis
INTEG: Rash
RESP: Pleural effusion
SYST: Anaphylaxis, wound dehiscence

PHARMACOKINETICS

Metabolized primarily by CYP3A4- and FMO-mediated oxidation, excretion 47% feces, 34% urine, half-life 20 hr

INTERACTIONS

Increase: anticoagulation—anticoagulants; anticoagulant may need dosage reduction
Increase: eravacycline effect—strong CYP3A inducers (clarithromycin, telithromycin, nefazodone, itraconazole, ketoconazole, atazanavir, darunavir, indinavir, lopinavir, nelfinavir, ritonavir, saquinavir, tipranavir)
Decrease: eravacycline effect—strong CYP3A inducers (carBAMazepine, rifAMPin)

NURSING CONSIDERATIONS

Assess:

• **Infection:** fever, condition of wound, pain, vital signs, urine, stools; monitor WBC for increased levels indicating continued infection; obtain C&S prior to starting treatment, may start product prior to receiving results

• **Bowel function:** diarrhea with mucus, blood; may indicate CDAD (*Clostridium difficile*–associated disease); report to health care provider immediately; may occur several weeks after last dose

• **Wound dehiscence:** fever, inflammation, bleeding, pain, wound opening; report any of these signs immediately

• **Anaphylaxis:** rash, dyspnea, swelling of lips/tongue; discontinue product; if severe, EPINEPHrine is usually given; if allergic reaction is mild, discontinuing product and giving diphenhydramine may be sufficient

• **Tooth discoloration:** may occur if used in second or third trimester of pregnancy or in children <8 yr

Teach patient/family:

• To inform health care provider of all OTC, Rx, herbal and supplemental products taken; not to change medication without prescriber's approval

• **Pregnancy/breastfeeding:** to inform health care provider if pregnancy is planned or suspected, or if breastfeeding; that this product may cause permanent tooth discoloration and reversible inhibition of bone growth when used in the second and third trimesters of pregnancy; not to breastfeed during and for 4 days after last dose

• **Allergic reactions:** to identify allergies; that allergic reactions, including serious ones, could occur and that serious reactions require immediate treatment. Ask patient about any previous allergies

• **Diarrhea:** to report watery and bloody stools (with or without stomach cramps and fever), which may be a serious intestinal infection, even 2 or more mo after last dose

• That this product is used only to treat bacterial infections; to take all of the medication even if feeling better; not to skip doses or fail to complete the full course of therapy

---

erdafitinib (Rx)

(er′-duh-fih′-tih-nib)

Balversa

Func. class.: Antineoplastic-kinase inhibitor

Chem. class.: Fibroblast growth factor receptor (FGFR) inhibitors

---

ACTION: Inhibits the enzymatic activity of FGFR1, FGFR2, FGFR3, and FGFR4

USES: Locally advanced or metastatic urothelial carcinoma

DOSAGE AND ROUTES
• **Adult: PO** 8 mg daily; after 14 to 21 days of treatment, increase to 9 mg daily if serum phosphate level is <5.5 mg/dL and there are no ocular disorders or grade 2 or higher adverse reactions; continue treatment until disease progression or unacceptable toxicity

Available forms: Tablets 3, 4, 5 mg

Administer:
• Swallow tablets whole, with or without food
• If vomiting occurs, do not replace the dose; the next dose should be taken the next day
• If a dose is missed, it can be taken as soon as possible on the same day; do not take extra tablets to make up for the missed dose; resume the regular daily schedule on the next day

SIDE EFFECTS
GI: Abdominal pain, nausea, vomiting, anorexia, constipation, diarrhea

CNS: Fatigue, fever

EENT: Stomatitis, blurred vision, retinal detachment

INTEG: Rash, nail discoloration

META: Hyperglycemia, hyper-hypophosphatemia, hypomagnesemia, hyponatremia, hypoalbuminemia

HEMA: Leukopenia, anemia, thrombocytopenia

SYST: Infection

PHARMACOKINETICS
99.8% protein bound to alpha-1-acid glycoprotein; half-life 59 hr; 69% excreted in feces (19% unchanged) and 19% in urine (13% unchanged), metabolized by CYP2C9 (39%) and CYP3A4 (20%); an inhibitor of OCT2; peak 2.5 hr

INTERACTIONS
Avoid use with CYP3A4 inducers, inhibitors

NURSING CONSIDERATIONS
Assess:
• **Ocular disease:** Provide dry eye prophylaxis with ocular demulcents as needed; perform monthly ophthalmologic examinations during the first 4 months of treatment and every 3 months thereafter, and urgently at any time for visual disturbance; examinations should include an assessment of visual acuity, slit-lamp examination, fundoscopy, and optical coherence tomography; an interruption of therapy, discontinuation of therapy, or dose reduction may be necessary for ocular adverse reactions
• **Infection:** Assess for infection (fever, flulike symptoms)
• Avoid coadministration with agents that alter serum phosphate levels prior to the initial dose increase period (days 14 to 21); monitor phosphate levels monthly for hyperphosphatemia and follow dose modification guidelines when required; in patients with hyperphosphatemia, restrict phosphate intake to 600 to 800 mg daily; if serum phosphate is >7 mg/dL, consider adding an oral phosphate binder until the serum phosphate level returns to less than 5.5 mg/dL
• **Pregnancy/breastfeeding:** Pregnancy should be avoided during and for at least 1 mo after the last dose; obtain pregnancy testing before use

---

Evaluate:
• Therapeutic response: decreased progression of cancer

Teach patient/family:
• About the reproductive risk and contraception requirements during treatment; men with female partners of reproductive potential should also use effective contraception during treatment and for 1 mo after the last dose; not to breastfeed during and for 1 mo after last dose
• Ophthalmic examinations will be needed periodically

---

erenumab (Rx)

(e-ren′ue-mab)

Aimovig

Func. class.: CNS analgesic; antimigraine agent

Chem. class.: IgG2 monoclonal antibody

ACTION: A human immunoglobulin G2 (IgG2) monoclonal antibody that binds to the calcitonin gene-related peptide (CGRP) receptor. CGRP is involved in migraine pathophysiology

USES: For the preventive treatment of migraine in adults

CONTRAINDICATIONS

Hypersensitivity

Precautions: Breastfeeding, latex hypersensitivity, pregnancy

DOSAGE AND ROUTES

• **Adult: SUBCUT** 70 mg monthly, may use 140 mg monthly if needed

Available forms: SureClick 70 mg/mL autoinjector solution for injection; solution for injection single-use 70 mg/mL prefilled syringe

Administer:

Injectable administration

• Visually inspect for particulate matter and discoloration prior to use; do not use if solution is cloudy or discolored or contains flakes or particles; product should be a clear to opalescent, colorless to light yellow solution

Subcutaneous route

• Product is intended for patient self-administration
• Prior to use allow to warm to room temperature for at least 30 min, protected from direct sunlight
• Do not shake
• Clean injection site on the abdomen, thigh, or upper arm with an alcohol wipe; allow skin to dry
• Do not leave cap off the autoinjector or prefilled syringe for more than 5 min; product will dry out
• Do not inject into areas where skin is tender, bruised, red, or hard
• If using the same body area for the 2 separate injections needed for the 140-mg dose, ensure that the second injection is not at same location
• **Storage:** After removing the product from the refrigerator, it can be stored at room temperature between 68° F and 77° F (20° C and 25° C) for up to 7 days. Do not return to the refrigerator after room temperature

Single-dose, prefilled SureClick autoinjector

• When ready to inject, press the purple start button; a click will be heard, and the window will turn yellow

Single-dose prefilled syringe

• Using slow, constant pressure, push the plunger rod all the way down with thumb until the prefilled syringe stops moving
• When finished, release thumb, and gently lift syringe off skin

SIDE EFFECTS

MISC: Antibody formation, injection site reaction, erythema

PHARMACOKINETICS

SUBCUT route: Peak 6 days, bioavailability 82%, half-life 28 days

INTERACTIONS

None known

NURSING CONSIDERATIONS
Assess

• **Hypersensitivity:** rash, dyspnea, swelling of face, anaphylaxis/angioedema may occur up to a wk or more after dosing, if severe, discontinue and contact emergency services

• **Migraines:** time of day, aggravating and ameliorating effects, auras or halos, sensitivity to light, noise, diet

• **Pregnancy/breastfeeding:** data are lacking

Evaluate:

• Therapeutic response: decrease in severity and number of migraines

Teach patient/family

• To read the FDA-approved patient labeling (Patient Information and Instructions for Use)

• Proper SUBCUT administration technique, including aseptic technique, and how to use the single-dose prefilled autoinjector or single-dose prefilled syringe

• To read and follow the Instructions for Use with each use of Aimovig

• That if the 140-mg once-monthly dosage is prescribed, to administer it as 2 separate SUBCUT injections of 70 mg each

• **Latex sensitivity:** that the needle shield within the white cap of the Aimovig prefilled autoinjector and the gray needle cap of the Aimovig prefilled syringe contain dry natural rubber (a derivative of latex), which may cause allergic reactions in individuals sensitive to latex

---

ergotamine/caffeine (Rx)

Cafergot, Migergot
Func. class.: Ergot

USES: Prevention/treatment of vascular headache

DOSAGE AND ROUTES

• **Adult: PO** 2 tablets at beginning of headache, then 1 tablet q30 min, max 6 tablets per headache, max 10 tablets per wk; **suppository** 1 at beginning of headache, then another dose in 1 hr, max 2 suppositories/headache, max 5 suppositories/wk

Available forms: Tablets 1 mg-100 mg

⚠ HIGH ALERT

eriBULin (Rx)
(er´i-bu´lin)

Halaven
Func. class.: Antineoplastics—non-taxane
Chem. class.: Microtubule inhibitor

ACTION: Potent antimitotic agent, different from taxanes, vinca alkaloids, epothilones; blocks cell progression during G2-M phase; inhibits the growth phase of microtubules and sequesters tubules, leading to the disruption of mitotic spindles and apoptotic cell death

USES: Metastatic breast cancer in patients who have received at least 2 chemotherapy regimens

CONTRAINDICATIONS
Hypersensitivity, pregnancy
Precautions: Breastfeeding, neonates, infants, children, bradycardia, electrolyte imbalances, heart failure, hypokalemia, hypomagnesemia, infertility, neutropenia, peripheral neuropathy, QT prolongation, hepatic/renal disease

DOSAGE AND ROUTES

• **Adult: IV** 1.4 mg/m^2 over 2-5 min on days 1 and 8, repeat q21days

• **Recommendations for dose delay:** for ANC <1000/mm^3, platelets <75,000/mm^3, or grade 3 or 4 nonhematologic toxicities: do not administer; the day 8 dose may be delayed a maximum of 1 wk; for the day 8 dose, if toxicities do not resolve to ≤ grade 2 by day 15: omit the dose; for the day 8 dose, if toxicities resolve or improve to ≤ grade 2 by day 15: administer eriBULin at reduced dose (see later), initiate the next cycle no sooner than 2 wk later

• **Dose adjustments for hematologic toxicity:** ANC <500/mm^3 for >7 days or ANC <1000/mm^3 with fever or infection: permanently reduce dose to 1.1 mg/m^2; platelets <25,000/mm^3 or <50,000/mm^3

---

requiring transfusion: permanently reduce dose to 1.1 mg/m^2; if day 8 of previous cycle omitted or delayed: permanently reduce dose to 1.1 mg/m^2; while receiving 1.1 mg/m^2, if recurrence of hematologic event occurs, or if day 8 of previous cycle omitted or delayed: permanently reduce dose to 0.7 mg/m^2; while receiving 0.7 mg/m^2, if recurrence of hematologic event occurs, or if day 8 of previous cycle omitted or delayed: discontinue

Available forms: Solution for injection 1 mg/2 mL

Administer:

IV direct, intermittent route

• Visually inspect for particulate matter, discoloration; withdraw amount (0.5 mg/mL) from single-use vial, give undiluted over 2-5 min or diluted in 100 mL 0.9% NaCl and give as intermittent infusion; do not give through line with dextrose or any other product

• Store at room temperature for 4 hr or 24 hr refrigerated

SIDE EFFECTS

CNS: Depression, dizziness, *fatigue,* fever, headache, insomnia, *peripheral neuropathy*

CV: QT prolongation, peripheral edema

GI: Abdominal pain, anorexia, constipation, diarrhea, dyspepsia, nausea, vomiting, weight loss

HEMA: Anemia, neutropenia, thrombocytopenia

INTEG: *Alopecia,* rash, stomatitis, infusion-related reactions

META: Hypokalemia

MS: Arthralgia, myalgia, bone/back pain

RESP: Cough, dyspnea

SYST: Infection

PHARMACOKINETICS

Protein binding 49%-65%; inhibits CYP3A4; excreted in feces 82%; urine 9%; elimination half-life 40 hr; increased levels in hepatic/renal disease

INTERACTIONS

Increase: QT prolongation—arsenic trioxide, bepridil, chloroquine, certain phenothiazines (chlorproMAZINE, mesoridazine,

thioridazine), clarithromycin, class IA antiarrhythmics (disopyramide, procainamide, quiNIDine), class III antiarrhythmics (amiodarone, bretylium, dofetilide, ibutilide, sotalol), dextromethorphan; quiNIDine, dronedarone, droperidol, erythromycin, halofantrine, haloperidol, levomethadyl, methadone, pentamidine, pimozide, posaconazole, probucol, propafenone, saquinavir, sparfloxacin, troleandomycin, and ziprasidone; also to a lesser degree abarelix, alfuzosin, amoxapine, apomorphine, artemether; lumefantrine, asenapine, beta-agonists, ofloxacin, cloZAPine, cyclobenzaprine, dasatinib, dolasetron, flecainide, gatifloxacin, gemifloxacin, halogenated anesthetics, iloperidone, lapatinib, levoFLOXacin, local anesthetics, lopinavir; ritonavir, magnesium sulfate; potassium sulfate; sodium sulfate, maprotiline, mefloquine, moxifloxacin, nilotinib, norfloxacin, octreotide, ciprofloxacin, OLANZapine, ondansetron, paliperidone, palonosetron, some phenothiazines (fluPHENAZine, perphenazine, prochlorperazine, trifluoperazine), QUEtiapine, ranolazine, risperiDONE, sertindole, SUNItinib, tacrolimus, telavancin, telithromycin, tetrabenazine, tricyclic antidepressants, venlafaxine, vardenafil, vorinostat

Increase: adverse reactions—live virus vaccines; do not use together

NURSING CONSIDERATIONS

Assess:

• **Peripheral neuropathy:** pain, numbness in extremities

• **Infection:** increased temperature, sore throat, flulike symptoms

• **Electrolyte imbalances:** correct prior to administration; monitor during therapy

• **QT prolongation:** assess for drug interactions that may occur; monitor ECG, heart rate

• **Bone marrow depression:** CBC, differential, serum creatinine, BUN, electrolytes, LFTs at baseline, periodically; increased AST/ALT >3 × ULN or total bilirubin >1.5 × ULN involves greater chance of grade 4 or febrile neutropenia

Side effects: *italics* = common; red = life-threatening

• **Pregnancy/breastfeeding:** may cause fetal harm; do not use in pregnancy or breastfeeding

Teach patient/family:
• **Infection:** to notify prescriber of increased temperature, sore throat, fatigue, flulike symptoms
• **QT prolongation:** to report extra heartbeats

Peripheral neuropathy:
• To report tingling, pain in extremities
• About reason for product and expected results
• To avoid other medications, supplements unless approved by provider; serious drug interactions may occur
• About hair loss, use of wig or hairpiece
• To notify prescriber if pregnancy is planned or suspected; to use contraception during treatment; to avoid breastfeeding

⚠ HIGH ALERT

erlotinib (Rx)
(er-loe′tye-nib)
Tarceva
Func. class.: Antineoplastic—miscellaneous
Chem. class.: Epidermal growth factor receptor inhibitor

ACTION: Not fully understood; inhibits intracellular phosphorylation of cell-surface receptors associated with epidermal growth factor receptors

USES: Non–small-cell lung cancer (NSCLC) including ☜ EGFR exon 19 deletions or exon 21 substitution mutations, pancreatic cancer

CONTRAINDICATIONS
Pregnancy, breastfeeding
Precautions: Children, geriatric patients, ocular/pulmonary/renal/hepatic disorders, diverticulitis

DOSAGE AND ROUTES
Non–small-cell lung cancer (NSCLC), maintenance, after failure of at least one chemotherapy regimen
• **Adult: PO** 150 mg/day
Pancreatic cancer
• **Adult: PO** 100 mg/day in combination with gemcitabine 1000 mg/m² cycle 1, days 1, 8, 15, 22, 29, 36, 43 of 8-wk cycle; cycle 2 and subsequent cycles, days 1, 8, 15 of 4-wk cycle, used with gemcitabine
CYP3A4 inducers concurrently (rifAMPin, phenytoin)
• Increase dose by 50 mg q2wk (max 450 mg/day)
CYP3A4 inhibitors (atazanavir, clarithromycin, indinavir, itraconazole, ketoconazole, telithromycin, ritonavir, saquinavir, troleandomycin, nelfinavir) or CYP3A4 and CYP1A2 inhibitors concurrently (ciprofloxacin)
• Decrease dose by 50 mg as needed
Available forms: Tablets 25, 100, 150 mg
Administer:
• 1 hr prior to or 2 hr after food; at same time of day

SIDE EFFECTS
CNS: CVA, anxiety, depression, headache, rigors, insomnia
CV: MI/ischemia
EENT: Ocular changes, *conjunctivitis, eye pain,* hypertrichosis
GI: *Nausea, diarrhea, vomiting, anorexia, mouth ulceration,* hepatic failure, GI perforation
GU: Renal impairment/failure
HEMA: Deep vein thrombosis, bleeding
INTEG: *Rash,* Stevens-Johnson–like skin reaction, toxic epidermal necrolysis
MISC: *Fatigue, infection*
RESP: Interstitial lung disease, *cough, dyspnea*
SYST: Hepatorenal syndrome

PHARMACOKINETICS
Slowly absorbed (60%); peak 3-7 hr; duration up to 24 hr; excreted in feces (86%), urine (<4%); metabolized by CYP3A4; half-life 36 hr; protein binding 93%; inhibits tyrosine kinase, which is a factor in epidermal growth factor receptor (EGFR)

INTERACTIONS

Increase: GI bleeding, may be fatal—warfarin, NSAIDs

Increase: erlotinib concentrations—CYP3A4 inhibitors (ketoconazole, itraconazole, erythromycin, clarithromycin, telithromycin)

Increase: plasma concentrations of warfarin, metoprolol

Increase: myopathy—HMG-CoA reductase inhibitors

Decrease: erlotinib levels—CYP3A4 inducers (phenytoin, rifAMPin, carBAMazepine, PHENobarbital), proton pump inhibitors

Drug/herb

Decrease: erlotinib levels—St. John's wort

Drug/Smoking

Decrease: erlotinib level; dose may need to be increased

Drug/food

Increase: effect of erlotinib—grapefruit juice

Drug/lab

Increase: INR, PT, AST, ALT, bilirubin

NURSING CONSIDERATIONS

Assess:

• **Serious skin toxicities:** toxic epidermal necrolysis, Stevens-Johnson syndrome; check for rash, blistering; discontinue treatment, may need corticosteroids, antiinfectives

• **MI/ischemia, CVA** in patients with pancreatic cancer

• **Pulmonary changes:** lung sounds, cough, dyspnea; interstitial lung disease may occur, may be fatal; discontinue therapy if confirmed

• **Ocular changes:** eye irritation, corneal erosion/ulcer, aberrant eyelash growth, discontinue if ulcers are present in the cornea, hold for keratitis (grade 3 or 4)

• **GI symptoms:** frequency of stools; if diarrhea is poorly tolerated, therapy may be discontinued for ≤14 days, monitor for dehydration; fluid status during period of vomiting and diarrhea, may use antidiarrheal

• Blood studies: INR, LFTs, PT; elevated INR and hemorrhage are increased when used with warfarin

• **Hepatic failure:** interrupt if severe changes to liver function occur (total bilirubin >3× ULN and/or transaminases >5× ULN when normal pretreatment LFTs)

• **GI perforation/bleeding:** some cases have been fatal; usually occurs in those using NSAIDs, taxanes, or in those with diverticulitis or peptic ulcer disease; discontinue if these occur

• **Pregnancy/breastfeeding:** do not use in pregnancy or for 1 mo after last dose; do not breastfeed during or for 2 wk after final dose

Evaluate:

• Therapeutic response: decrease in NSCLC cells, pancreatic cancer cells

Teach patient/family:

• **To report adverse reactions immediately:** SOB, severe abdominal pain, persistent diarrhea or vomiting, ocular changes, skin eruptions (face, upper chest/back)

• About reason for treatment, expected results; to take on empty stomach 1 hr prior to or 2 hr after meals

• To use sunscreen, protective clothing to prevent sunburn

• To avoid use with other products, herbs, supplements unless approved by provider, not to use with grapefruit or grapefruit juice

• To avoid smoking; decreases effect of this product

• **Pregnancy/breastfeeding:** To use reliable contraception during treatment; to avoid breastfeeding

---

ertapenem (Rx)

(er-tah-pen′em)

INVanz

Func. class.: Antiinfective—miscellaneous

Chem. class.: Carbapenem

Do not confuse:

INVanz/AVINza

ACTION: Interferes with cell-wall replication of susceptible organisms; bactericidal

USES: *Bacteroides distasonis, Bacteroides fragilis, Bacteroides ovatus, Bacteroides thetaiotaomicron, Bacteroides uniformis, Bacteroides vulgatus, Citrobacter freundii, Citrobacter koseri, Clostridium clostridioforme, Clostridium perfringens, Enterobacter aerogenes, Enterobacter cloacae, Escherichia coli, Eubacterium lentum, Fusobacterium sp., Haemophilus influenzae* (beta-lactamase negative), *Haemophilus influenzae* (beta-lactamase positive), *Haemophilus parainfluenzae, Klebsiella oxytoca, Klebsiella pneumoniae, Moraxella catarrhalis, Morganella morganii, Peptostreptococcus sp., Porphyromonas asaccharolytica, Prevotella bivia, Proteus mirabilis, Proteus vulgaris, Providencia rettgeri, Providencia stuartii, Serratia marcescens, Staphylococcus aureus* (MSSA), *Staphylococcus epidermidis, Streptococcus agalactiae* (group B streptococci), *Streptococcus pneumoniae, Streptococcus pyogenes* (group A beta-hemolytic streptococci); bacteremia, community-acquired pneumonia, diabetic foot ulcer, endometritis, GYN/intraabdominal skin/skin structure/urinary tract infections, surgical infection prophylaxis

CONTRAINDICATIONS
Hypersensitivity to this product, its components, amide-type local anesthetics (IM only); anaphylactic reactions to beta-lactams, other carbapenems
Precautions: Pregnancy, breastfeeding, children, geriatric patients, GI/renal/hepatic disease, seizures

DOSAGE AND ROUTES
• **Adult/child ≥13 yr: IM/IV** 1 g/day × 14 days (IV), 7 days (IM)
• **Infant/child 3 mo-12 yr: IM/IV** 15 mg/kg q12hr (max 1 g/day) × 5-14 days
Renal dose
• **Adult: IM/IV** CCr ≤30 mL/min 500 mg daily

Available form: Powder, lyophilized, 1 g/vial
Administer:
IM route
• Reconstitute 1-g vial of ertapenem with 3.2 mL of 1% lidocaine HCl injection (without EPINEPHrine) (280 mg/mL), agitate; the IM reconstituted formulation is not for IV use
• IM may be used as an alternative to IV administration in the treatment of infections where IM therapy is appropriate; only give via IM injection × 7 days
• **For a 1-g dose:** immediately withdraw the contents of the vial and inject deeply into a large muscle, aspirate prior to injection to avoid injection into a blood vessel
• **For a dose <1 g (for pediatric patients 3 mo-12 yr):** immediately withdraw a volume equal to 15 mg/kg (max 1 g/day) and inject deeply into a large muscle, aspirate prior to injection to avoid injecting into a blood vessel; use the reconstituted IM solution within 1 hr after preparation
IV route
• Visually inspect for particulate matter and discoloration prior to use, may be colorless to pale yellow; do not mix with other products; dextrose solutions are not compatible
• **1-g vial:** For each gram reconstitute with 10 mL of either NS injection, sterile water for injection, or bacteriostatic water for injection to 100 mg/mL, shake
• **1 g dose:** Immediately transfer contents of the reconstituted vial to 50 mL of NS injection; for a dose <1 g (pediatric patients 3 mo-12 yr): from the reconstituted vial, immediately withdraw a volume equal to 15 mg/kg of body weight (max 1 g/day) and dilute in NS injection to a concentration of 20 mg/mL or less
Intermittent IV INFUSION route
• Complete the infusion within 6 hr of reconstitution, infuse over 30 min; do not co-infuse with other medications
• The reconstituted IV solution may be stored at room temperature if used within 6 hr, or store under refrigeration

for 24 hr and use within 4 hours after removal from refrigeration; do not freeze

Y-site compatibilities: Acyclovir, alfentanil, amifostine, amikacin, aminocaproic acid, aminophylline, amphotericin B lipid complex, amphotericin B liposome, argatroban, arsenic trioxide, atenolol, atracurium, azithromycin, aztreonam, bivalirudin, bleomycin, bumetanide, buprenorphine, busulfan, butorphanol, calcium chloride/gluconate, CARBOplatin, carmustine, chloramphenicol, cimetidine, ciprofloxacin, cisatracurium, CISplatin, cyclophosphamide, cycloSPORINE, cytarabine, dacarbazine, DACTINomycin, DAPTOmycin, dexamethasone, dexmedetomidine, dexrazoxane, digoxin, diltiazem, diphenhydrAMINE, DOCEtaxel, dolasetron, DOPamine, doxacurium, doxycycline, enalaprilat, ePHEDrine, EPINEPHrine, eptifibatide, erythromycin, esmolol, etoposide, etoposide phosphate, famotidine, fenoldopam, fluconazole, fludarabine, fluorouracil, foscarnet, fosphenytoin, furosemide, ganciclovir, gatifloxacin, gemcitabine, gemtuzumab, gentamicin, glycopyrrolate, granisetron, haloperidol, heparin, hydrocortisone, HYDROmorphone, ifosfamide, inamrinone, insulin (regular), irinotecan, isoproterenol, ketorolac, labetalol, lepirudin, leucovorin, levofloxacin, lidocaine, linezolid, LORazepam, magnesium sulfate, mannitol, mechlorethamine, melphalan, meperidine, mesna, metaraminol, methotrexate, methyldopate, methylPREDNISolone, metoclopramide, metroNIDAZOLE, milrinone, mitoMYcin, mivacurium, morphine, moxifloxacin, nalbuphine, naloxone, nesiritide, nitroglycerin, nitroprusside, norepinephrine, octreotide, oxaliplatin, oxytocin, PACLitaxel, pamidronate, pancuronium, pantoprazole, PEMEtrexed, PENTobarbital, PHENobarbital, phentolamine, phenylephrine, polymyxin B, potassium acetate/chloride/phosphates, procainamide, propranolol, ranitidine, remifentanil, rocuronium, sodium acetate/bicarbonate/phosphates, streptozocin, succinylcholine, SUFentanil, sulfamethoxazole-trimethoprim, tacrolimus, telavancin, teniposide, theophylline, thiotepa, tigecycline, tirofiban, tobramycin, trimethobenzamide, vancomycin, vasopressin, vecuronium, vinBLAStine, vinCRIStine, vinorelbine, voriconazole, zidovudine, zoledronic acid

SIDE EFFECTS

CNS: Insomnia, seizures, dizziness, *headache,* agitation, confusion, somnolence, disorientation, edema, hypotension
CV: Tachycardia, seizures
GI: *Diarrhea, nausea, vomiting,* CDAD, abdominal pain
GU: *Vaginitis,* dysuria
INTEG: *Rash,* pain at injection site, *phlebitis/thrombophlebitis,* erythema at injection site, dermatitis
RESP: Dyspnea, cough, pharyngitis, crackles, respiratory distress
SYST: Anaphylaxis, angioedema

PHARMACOKINETICS

IV: Onset immediate; peak dose dependent; **IM:** Peak 2.3 hr half-life 4 hr; metabolized by liver; excreted in urine, feces, breast milk

INTERACTIONS

Increase: ertapenem levels—probenecid; do not coadminister
Decrease: effect of valproic acid; monitor valproic acid level, seizure control
Drug/lab
Increase: hepatic enzymes, albumin, alkaline phosphatase, bilirubin, creatinine, PT
Decrease: Hct, WBC

NURSING CONSIDERATIONS
Assess:
• **Renal disease:** lower dose may be required
• **CNS symptoms:** for confusion, seizures; may increase seizure risk
• **CDAD:** bowel pattern, abdominal pain, mucus or blood in stools daily; if severe diarrhea occurs, product should be discontinued
• For infection: temperature, sputum, characteristics of wound, monitor WBC prior to, during, after treatment
• **Allergic reactions, anaphylaxis;** rash, urticaria, pruritus; may occur a few days

---

after therapy begins; sensitivity to carbapenem antibiotics, other beta-lactam antibiotics, penicillins; have emergency equipment, epinephrine close by

• **Overgrowth of infection:** perineal itching, fever, malaise, redness, pain, swelling, drainage, rash, diarrhea, change in cough or sputum

• **Pregnancy/breastfeeding:** use only when clearly needed; use caution in breastfeeding

Evaluate:

• Therapeutic response: negative C&S; absence of signs, symptoms of infection

Teach patient/family:

• **CDAD:** to report severe diarrhea, CNS side effects

• **To report overgrowth of infection:** black, furry tongue; vaginal itching; foul-smelling stools

• **Pregancy/breastfeeding:** identify if pregnancy is planned or suspected or if breastfeeding to avoid breastfeeding; product is excreted in breast milk

TREATMENT OF OVERDOSE:

EPINEPHrine, antihistamines; resuscitate if needed (anaphylaxis)

---

ertugliflozin (Rx)

(er-too-gli-floe′-zin)

Steglatro

Func. class.: Antidiabetic

Chem. class.: Sodium-glucose cotransporter 2 inhibitors

ACTION:

An inhibitor of sodium-glucose cotransporter 2 (SGLT2), the transporter responsible for reabsorbing most of the glucose filtered by the tubular lumen in the kidney

USES:
For the treatment of type 2 diabetes mellitus

DOSAGE AND ROUTES

For type 2 diabetes mellitus in combination with diet and exercise

• **Adult: PO** 5 mg/day in the morning, with or without food; max 15 mg/day

Renal dose

• **Adult: PO** CCr 30-60 mL/min/ 1.73 m^2, avoid use

Available forms: Tablets 5 mg, 15 mg

Administer:

• Administer daily in the morning, with or without food

CONTRAINDICATIONS

Hypersensitivity, severe renal disease

Precautions: Adrenal insufficiency, balanitis, breastfeeding, burns, children, dehydration, diabetic ketoacidosis, dialysis, fever, geriatric, hepatic disease, hypercholesterolemia, hypercortisolism, hyperglycemia, hyperthyroidism, hypoglycemia, hypotension, hypothyroidism, hypovolemia, infants, infection, lower limb amputation, malnutrition, pituitary insufficiency, pregnancy, pyelonephritis, renal disease, surgery, tissue necrosis, trauma, type 1 diabetes mellitus, UTI, vaginitis

SIDE EFFECTS

MS: Back pain

GU: Diuresis, dysuria, increased urinary frequency/urgency, nocturia, polyuria, renal failure, vaginitis, cystitis, dehydration

CNS: Headache, syncope

META: Hypercholesterolemia, hyperlipidemia, hyperphosphatemia, hypoglycemia, diabetic ketoacidosis

CV: Hypotension, hypovolemia, orthostatic hypotension

MISC: Infection, lower limb amputation, necrotizing fasciitis, orthostatic hypotension, pharyngitis, polydipsia, tissue necrosis, weight loss, candidiasis

PHARMACOKINETICS

Onset unknown, peak 1-2 hr, duration unknown, half-life 18.5 hr

INTERACTIONS

Increase: hypoglycemia—insulin, antidiabetes

Increase: urinary injury—ACE inhibitors, diuretics, NSAIDs, ARBs

Drug/lab

Increase: LDL, cholesterol, Hb, serum creatinine, phosphate

Interference: Urine glucose, 1,5-AG assay

NURSING CONSIDERATIONS

Assess:

• Hypoglycemia (weakness, hunger, dizziness, tremors, anxiety, tachycardia, sweating), hyperglycemia; even though product does not cause hypoglycemia, if patient is on sulfonylureas or insulin, hypoglycemia may be additive; if hypoglycemia occurs, treat with dextrose, or, if severe, with IV glucagon

• **Ketoacidosis:** monitor for increased ketone levels; may occur with any glucose level, more common in those with severe illnesses

• **Volume depletion:** monitor for orthostatic hypotension, weakness, dizziness; may occur after beginning treatment; correct volume depletion prior to starting treatment

• For stress, surgery, or other trauma that may require a change in dose

• **Diabetes:** A1c q3mo; monitor serum glucose 1 hr PP throughout treatment; serum cholesterol, serum creatinine/BUN, serum electrolytes

• **Bone fractures:** monitor bone density, other conditions that may lead to bone fractures; fractures may occur within 3 mo of starting therapy

• **Renal impairment:** monitor more frequently in those with renal disease; increased creatinine, eGFR may be decreased, BUN may occur

Black Box Warning: Lower limb amputation: increased risk of amputation; monitor wound and feet closely for complications

• **Pregnancy/breastfeeding:** identify whether pregnancy is planned or suspected or if breastfeeding

Evaluate:

• Therapeutic response: improved signs/symptoms of diabetes mellitus (decreased polyuria, polydipsia, polyphagia); clear sensorium, absence of dizziness, stable gait

Teach patient/family:

• The symptoms of hypo/hyperglycemia, what to do about each

• That medication must be taken as prescribed; explain consequences of discontinuing medication abruptly; that insulin may need to be used for stress, including trauma, fever, surgery; to take as soon as remembered if dose is missed unless close to next dose, then skip and take at next scheduled dose, do not double doses

• To avoid OTC medications and herbal supplements unless discussed with health care professional

• That diabetes is a lifelong illness; that the diet and exercise regimen must be followed; that this product is not a cure

• To carry emergency ID and glucose source

• That blood glucose monitoring is required to assess product effect

• **Hypersensitivity:** to notify prescriber immediately of itching, hives, rash, swelling of face/lips

Black Box Warning: Lower limb amputation risk: inspect feet; monitor for new ulcerations, wounds; educate about foot care

• **Ketoacidosis:** to notify prescriber immediately of nausea, vomiting, lack of appetite, sleepiness, difficulty breathing

• **Yeast infections (women/men):** that yeast infections can occur with this product (women, vaginal; men, penile); to report discharge, itching, swelling

• **Pregnancy/breastfeeding:** not to breastfeed; to advise prescriber if pregnancy is planned or suspected

ertugliflozin/
metformin (Rx)

(er-too-gli-floe′zin/met-for′min)

Segluromet

Func. class.: Antidiabetics
Chem. class.: Sodium-glucose
cotransporter 2 (SGLT2) inhibitor

ACTION:
An inhibitor of sodium-glucose cotransporter 2 (SGLT2), the transporter
responsible for reabsorbing most of the
glucose filtered by the tubular lumen in
the kidney

Uses: Treatment of type 2 diabetes mellitus in combination with diet and exercise

CONTRAINDICATIONS
Hypersensitivity, severe renal disease

Black Box Warning: Lactic acidosis

Precautions: Adrenal insufficiency, balanitis, breast feeding, burns, children,
dehydration, diabetic ketoacidosis, dialysis, fever, geriatric, hepatic disease, hypercholesterolemia, hypercortisolism, hyperglycemia, hyperthyroidism, hypoglycemia,
hypotension, hypothyroidism, hypovolemia, infants, infection, lower limb amputation, malnutrition, pituitary insufficiency,
pregnancy, pyelonephritis, renal disease,
surgery, tissue necrosis, trauma, type 1
diabetes mellitus, UTI, vaginitis

DOSAGE AND ROUTES
Adult: PO Individualize the starting dose.
Take ertugliflozin/metformin bid with
meals. **Max:** ertugliflozin 7.5 mg/metfor-
min 1000 mg bid with meals. **Those taking ertugliflofloxacin:** Initiate at current
dose of ertugliflozin in combination with
metformin 500 mg given bid with meals;
increase gradually to reduce the GI side
effects due to metformin. **Those taking
metformin:** Initiate at ertugliflozin 2.5 mg/
metformin (either 500 mg or 1000 mg)
given bid with meals, using whichever metformin dose is the same or closest to the
current metformin dose. **Those taking
both:** Switch to the combination product
using the same daily doses of each component, divided and given bid with meals

Available forms: Tablets ertugliflozin
2.5 mg and metformin hydrochloride
500 mg, ertugliflozin 7.5 mg and metformin hydrochloride 500 mg, ertugliflozin
2.5 mg and metformin hydrochloride
1000 mg, ertugliflozin 7.5 mg and metformin hydrochloride 1000 mg

Administer:
• Administer daily in the morning, with
or without food

SIDE EFFECTS
MS: Back pain
GU: Diuresis, dysuria, increased urinary
frequency/urgency, nocturia, polyuria,
renal failure, vaginitis, cystitis, dehydration
CNS: Headache syncope
META: Hypercholesterolemia, hyperlipidemia, hyperphosphatemia, hypoglycemia, diabetic ketoacidosis
CV: Hypotension, hypovolemia
MISC: Infection, lower limb amputation,
necrotizing fasciitis, orthostatic hypotension, pharyngitis, polydipsia, tissue
necrosis, weight loss, candidiasis, lactic
acidosis

PHARMACOKINETICS
Ertugliflozin: Onset unknown, peak 1-2
hr, duration unknown, half-life 18.5 hr
Metformin: Onset unknown, peak 2-3
hr, duration unknown

INTERACTIONS
Increase: hypoglycemia—insulin, antidiabetes
Increase: urinary injury—ACE inhibitors, diuretics, NSAIDs

NURSING CONSIDERATIONS
Assess:
• Hypoglycemia (weakness, hunger,
dizziness, tremors, anxiety, tachycardia,
sweating), hyperglycemia; even though
product does not cause hypoglycemia, if
patient is on sulfonylureas or insulin,
hypoglycemia may be additive; if
hypoglycemia occurs, treat with dextrose, or, if severe, with IV glucagon

E

• **Ketoacidosis:** monitor for increased ketone levels; may occur with any glucose level, more common in those with severe illnesses
• **Volume depletion:** monitor for orthostatic hypotension, weakness, dizziness; may occur after beginning treatment; correct volume depletion before starting treatment
• For stress, surgery, or other trauma that may require a change in dose
• A1c q3mo; monitor serum glucose 1 hr PP throughout treatment; serum cholesterol, serum creatinine/BUN, serum electrolytes
• **Bone fractures:** monitor bone density, other conditions that may lead to bone fractures; fractures may occur within 3 mo of starting therapy
• **Renal impairment:** monitor more frequently in those with renal disease; increased creatinine, eGFR may be decreased, BUN may occur

Black Box Warning: Lactic acidosis: hypothermia, dysrrhythmias, death

• Lower limb amputation: Increased risk of amputation; monitor wound and feet closely for complications
• **Pregnancy/breastfeeding:** identify whether pregnancy is planned or suspected or if breastfeeding
Evaluate:
• Therapeutic response: improved signs/symptoms of diabetes mellitus (decreased polyuria, polydipsia, polyphagia); clear sensorium, absence of dizziness, stable gait
Teach patient/family:
• The symptoms of hypo/hyperglycemia, what to do about each
• That medication must be taken as prescribed; explain consequences of discontinuing medication abruptly; that insulin may need to be used for stress, including trauma, fever, surgery; to take as soon as remembered if dose is missed unless close to next dose, then skip and take at next scheduled dose, do not double
• To avoid OTC medications and herbal supplements unless discussed with health care professional
• That diabetes is a lifelong illness; that the diet and exercise regimen must be followed; that this product is not a cure
• To carry emergency ID and glucose source
• That blood glucose monitoring is required to assess product effect
• **Hypersensitivity:** to notify prescriber immediately of itching, hives, rash, swelling of face/lips
• Lower limb amputation risk: Inspect feet; monitor for new ulcerations, wounds; educate about foot care
• **Ketoacidosis:** to notify prescriber immediately of nausea, vomiting, lack of appetite, sleepiness, difficulty breathing
• **Yeast infections (women/men):** That yeast infections can occur with this product (women, vaginal; men, penile); to report discharge, itching, swelling
• **Pregnancy/breastfeeding:** Not to breastfeed; to advise prescriber if pregnancy is planned or suspected

Black Box Warning: Lactic acidosis: to discontinue immediately if symptoms of lactic acidosis occur: myalgia, change in heart rhythm, feeling cold, hyperventilation, report immediately

ertugliflozin/ sitagliptin (Rx)
(er-too-gli-floe′zin/sit-a-glip′tin)
Steglujan
Func. class.: Antidiabetics
Chem. class.: Sodium-glucose cotransporter 2 (SGLT 2) inhibitor

ACTION:

An inhibitor of sodium-glucose co-transporter 2 (SGLT2), the transporter responsible for reabsorbing most of the glucose filtered by the tubular lumen in the kidney

USES:

Treatment of type 2 diabetes mellitus in combination with diet and exercise

CONTRAINDICATIONS

Hypersensitivity, severe renal disease
Precautions: Adrenal insufficiency, balanitis, breastfeeding, burns, children, dehydration, diabetic ketoacidosis, dialysis, fever, geriatric, hepatic disease, hypercholesterolemia, hypercortisolism, hyperglycemia, hyperthyroidism, hypoglycemia, hypotension, hypothyroidism, hypovolemia, infants, infection, lower limb amputation, malnutrition, pituitary insufficiency, pregnancy, pyelonephritis, renal disease, surgery, tissue necrosis, trauma, type 1 diabetes mellitus, UTI, vaginitis

DOSAGE AND ROUTES

• **Adult: PO** Initial: ertugliflozin 5 mg/sitagliptin 100 mg daily; if further glycemic control is needed, dose may be increased to ertugliflozin 15 mg/sitagliptin 100 mg daily (max: ertugliflozin 15 mg/sitagliptin 100 mg/day)
Available forms: Tablets: Ertugliflozin 5 mg and sitagliptin 100 mg, ertugliflozin 15 mg and sitagliptin 100 mg
Administer:
• Administer daily in the morning, with or without food
• If dose is missed, give as soon as remembered; if close to next dose, skip
• Store at room temperature

SIDE EFFECTS

MS: Back pain
GU: Diuresis, dysuria, increased urinary frequency/urgency, nocturia, polyuria, renal failure, vaginitis, cystitis, dehydration

CNS: Headache, syncope
META: Hypercholesterolemia, hyperlipidemia, hyperphosphatemia, hypoglycemia, diabetic ketoacidosis
CV: Hypotension, hypovolemia
MISC: Infection, lower limb amputation, necrotizing fasciitis, orthostatic hypotension, pharyngitis, polydipsia, tissue necrosis, weight loss, candidiasis

PHARMACOKINETICS

Ertugliflozin: Onset unknown, peak 1-2 hr, duration unknown, half-life 18.5 hr
Sitagliptin: Onset rapid, peak 1-4 hr, duration unknown, half-life 12.4 hr

INTERACTIONS

Increase: hypoglycemia: insulin, antidiabetes
Increase: urinary injury: ACE inhibitors, diuretics, NSAIDs, ARBs
Increase: levels of digoxin
Drug/lab
Increase: LDL, cholesterol, phosphate, Hb, serum creatinine
Interference: Urine glucose, 1,5-AG assay

NURSING CONSIDERATIONS

Assess:
• **Hypoglycemia** (weakness, hunger, dizziness, tremors, anxiety, tachycardia, sweating), hyperglycemia; even though product does not cause hypoglycemia, if patient is on sulfonylureas or insulin, hypoglycemia may be additive; if hypoglycemia occurs, treat with dextrose, or, if severe, with IV glucagon
• **Ketoacidosis:** Monitor for increased ketone levels; may occur with any glucose level, more common in those with severe illnesses
• **Volume depletion:** Monitor for orthostatic hypotension, weakness, dizziness; may occur after beginning treatment; correct volume depletion prior to starting treatment
• For stress, surgery, or other trauma that may require a change in dose
• **Diabetes:** A1c q3mo; monitor serum glucose 1 hr PP throughout treatment;

serum cholesterol, serum creatinine/BUN, serum electrolytes

• **Bone fractures:** Monitor bone density, other conditions that may lead to bone fractures; fractures may occur within 3 mo of starting therapy

• **Renal impairment:** Monitor more frequently in those with renal disease; increased creatinine, eGFR may be decreased, BUN may occur

Lower limb amputation: Increased risk of amputation; monitor wound and feet closely for complications

• **Pregnancy/breastfeeding:** identify whether pregnancy is planned or suspected or if breastfeeding

Evaluate: Therapeutic response: improved signs/symptoms of diabetes mellitus (decreased polyuria, polydipsia, polyphagia); clear sensorium, absence of dizziness, stable gait

Teach patient/family:

• The symptoms of hypo/hyperglycemia, what to do about each

• That medication must be taken as prescribed; explain consequences of discontinuing medication abruptly; that insulin may need to be used for stress, including trauma, fever, surgery, to take as soon as remembered if dose is missed unless close to next dose, then skip and take at next scheduled dose, do not double dose

• To avoid OTC medications and herbal supplements unless discussed with health care professional

• That diabetes is a lifelong illness; that the diet and exercise regimen must be followed; that this product is not a cure

• To carry emergency ID and glucose source

• That blood glucose monitoring is required to assess product effect

• **Hypersensitivity:** to notify prescriber immediately of itching, hives, rash, swelling of face/lips

Lower limb amputation risk: Inspect feet; monitor for new ulcerations, wounds; educate about foot care

• **Ketoacidosis:** to notify prescriber immediately of nausea, vomiting, lack of appetite, sleepiness, difficulty breathing

• **Yeast infections (women/men):** that yeast infections can occur with this product (women, vaginal; men, penile); to report discharge, itching, swelling

• **Pregnancy/breastfeeding:** Not to breastfeed; to advise prescriber if pregnancy is planned or suspected

E

erythromycin (ophthalmic) (Rx)

(e-rith´roe-mye´sin)

Func. class.: Ophthalmic antiinfective
Chem. class.: Macrolide

ACTION: Inhibits protein synthesis, thereby decreasing bacterial replication

USES: Conjunctivitis, eye infections, prevention of ophthalmic neonatorum

CONTRAINDICATIONS

Hyper-sensitivity to this product or macrolides

Precautions: Pregnancy, breastfeeding

DOSAGE AND ROUTES

Bacterial conjunctivitis

• **Adult/adolescent/child: TOPICAL** apply 1 cm of ointment directly to the eye up to 6 times a day × 7-10 days depending on severity of infection

Prevention of ophthalmic neonatorum

• **Neonate: TOPICAL** apply 1-cm ribbon of ointment to lower conjunctival sac of each eye once after birth

Administer:

Ophthalmic route

• Apply ribbon of ointment directly to the eye; for ophthalmic use only

Available forms: ointment/ophthalmic 0.5%

SIDE EFFECTS

EENT: Hypersensitivity, irritation, redness

PHARMACOKINETICS

Unknown

NURSING CONSIDERATIONS
Assess:
• **Allergic reaction:** assess for hypersensitivity; discontinue product
Evaluate:
• Decreased ophthalmic infection
Teach patient/family:
Ophthalmic route:
• Apply ribbon of ointment directly to the eye; for ophthalmic use only

---

erythromycin base (Rx)
(eh-rith-roh-my'sin)
Ery-Tab
erythromycin ethylsuccinate (Rx)
E.E.S., Ery Ped
erythromycin lactobionate (Rx)
Erythrocin
erythromycin stearate (Rx)
Erythrocin Stearate
erythromycin (topical) (Rx)
AKne-Mycin, Erygel
Func. class.: Antiinfective
Chem. class.: Macrolide

Do not confuse:
erythromycin/azithromycin

ACTION: Binds to 50S ribosomal subunits of susceptible bacteria and suppresses protein synthesis

USES: Mild to moderate respiratory tract, skin, soft tissue infections caused by *Bordetella pertussis, Borrelia burgdorferi, Chlamydia trachomatis; Corynebacterium diphtheriae, Haemophilus influenzae* (when used with sulfonamides); *Legionella pneumophila,* Legionnaire's disease, *Listeria monocytogenes; Mycoplasma pneumoniae, Streptococcus pneumoniae,* syphilis: *Treponema pallidum; Staphylococcus* sp.
Unlabeled uses: Bartonellosis, burn wound infection, chancroid, cholera, diabetic gastroparesis, endocarditis prophylaxis, gastroenteritis, granuloma inguinale, Lyme disease, tetanus

CONTRAINDICATIONS
Hypersensitivity, preexisting hepatic disease (estolate)
Precautions: Pregnancy, breastfeeding, geriatric patients, hepatic disease, GI disease, QT prolongation, seizure disorder, myasthenia gravis

DOSAGE AND ROUTES
Most infections
• **Adults PO (base, stearate):** 250 mg q6hr or 333 mg q8hr or 500 mg q12hr; (ethylsuccinate) 400 mg q6hr or 800 mg q12hr; IV 250 mg-500 mg q6hr
• **Child >1 mo: PO (base, ethylsuccinate)** 30-50 mg/kg/day divided q6-8hr, max 2 g/day **(base),** max 3.2 g/day **(ethylsuccinate);** 30-50 mg/kg/day divided q6hr, max 2 g/day (stearate); IV 15-50 mg/kg/day divided q6hr, max 4 g/day
• **Neonates: PO (ethylsuccinate)** 20-50 mg/kg/day divided q6-8hr
Available forms: *Base:* enteric-coated tablets 250, 333, 500 mg; film-coated tablets 250, 500 mg; enteric-coated capsules 250, 333 mg; *stearate:* film-coated tablets 250 mg; *ethylsuccinate:* granules for oral suspension 200, 400 mg/5 mL; powder for injection 500 mg, 1 g (lactobionate), 1 g (as glucceptate)
Administer:
• Do not break, crush, or chew time-released capsule or tablet; chew only chewable tablets; enteric-coated tablets may be given with food
• Do not give by IM or IV push
• Oral product with full glass of water; do not give with fruit juice
• Give 1 hr prior to or 2 hr after meals
• Store at room temperature; store suspension in refrigerator

---

- Adequate intake of fluids (2 L) during diarrhea episodes

IV route

- After **reconstituting** 500 mg or less/10 mL sterile water without preservatives, dilute further in 100-250 mL of 0.9% NaCl, LR, Normosol-R; may be **further diluted** to 1 mg/mL and **given** as continuous infusion; run 1 g or less/100 mL over ½-1 hr; continuous infusion over 6 hr, may require buffers to neutralize pH if dilution is <250 mL, use infusion pump

Lactobionate

Y-site compatibilities: Acyclovir, alfentanil, amikacin, aminocaproic acid, aminophylline, amiodarone, anidulafungin, argatroban, atenolol, atosiban, atracurium, atropine, azaTHIOprine, benztropine, bivalirudin, bleomycin, bumetanide, buprenorphine, butorphanol, calcium chloride/gluconate, CARBOplatin, caspofungin, cefotaxime, cefTRIAXone, cefuroxime, chlorproMAZINE, cimetidine, CISplatin, cyanocobalamin, cyclophosphamide, cycloSPORINE, cytarabine, DACTINomycin, DAPTOmycin, dexmedetomidine, digoxin, diltiazem, diphenhydrAMINE, DOBUTamine, DOCEtaxel, DOPamine, doxacurium, doxapram, DOXOrubicin, enalaprilat, ePHEDrine, EPINEPHrine, epirubicin, epoetin alfa, eptifibatide, ertapenem, esmolol, etoposide, famotidine, fenoldopam, fentaNYL, fluconazole, fludarabine, fluorouracil, folic acid, foscarnet, gatifloxacin, gemcitabine, gentamicin, glycopyrrolate, granisetron, hydrocortisone, HYDROmorphone, hydrOXYzine, IDArubicin, ifosfamide, imipenem-cilastatin, insulin (regular), irinotecan, isoproterenol, labetalol, levofloxacin, lidocaine, LORazepam, LR, mannitol, mechlorethamine, meperidine, methicillin, methotrexate, methoxamine, methyldopate, methylPREDNISolone, metoclopramide, metroNIDAZOLE, miconazole, midazolam, milrinone, mitoXANtrone, morphine, multiple vitamins injection, mycophenolate, nafcillin, nalbuphine, naloxone, nesiritide, netilmicin, niCARdipine, nitroglycerin, norepinephrine, octreotide, ondansetron, oxacillin, oxaliplatin, oxytocin, PACLitaxel, palonosetron, pamidronate, pancuronium, papaverine, pentamidine, pentazocine, perphenazine, phenylephrine, phytonadione, piperacillin, piperacillin-tazobactam, polymyxin B, procainamide, prochlorperazine, promethazine, propranolol, protamine, pyridoxine, quiNIDine, ranitidine, Ringer's, ritodrine, sodium acetate/bicarbonate, succinylcholine, SUFentanil, tacrolimus, temocillin, teniposide, theophylline, thiamine, thiotepa, tigecycline, tirofiban, TNA, tobramycin, tolazoline, TPN, trimetaphan, urokinase, vancomycin, vasopressin, vecuronium, verapamil, vinCRIStine, vinorelbine, vitamin B complex/C, voriconazole, zidovudine, zoledronic acid

SIDE EFFECTS

CNS: Seizures

CV: Dysrhythmias, QT prolongation

GI: *Nausea, vomiting, diarrhea,* hepatotoxicity, abdominal pain, stomatitis, heartburn, anorexia, CDAD, esophagitis

GU: *Vaginitis, moniliasis*

INTEG: Rash, urticaria, pruritus, thrombophlebitis, injection site reactions (IV site)

SYST: Anaphylaxis

PHARMACOKINETICS

Peak 1-4 hr (base); ½-2½ hr (ethylsuccinate); half-life 1-2 hr, neonates 2 hr; metabolized in liver; excreted in bile, feces; protein binding 75%-90%; inhibitor of CYP3A4 and P-glycoprotein

INTERACTIONS

- Serious dysrhythmias—diltiaZEM, itraconazole, ketoconazole, nefazodone, pimozide, protease inhibitors, verapamil; do not use together

Increase: QT prolongation—products that increase QT prolongation

Increase: action, toxicity of alfentanil, ALPRAZolam, bromocriptine, busPIRone, carBAMazepine, cilostazol, clindamycin, cloZAPine, cycloSPORINE, diazePAM, digoxin, disopyramide, ergots, felodipine,

---

Side effects: *italics* = common; red = life-threatening

HMG-CoA reductase inhibitors, ibrutinib methylPREDNISolone, midazolam, quiNIDine, rifabutin, sildenafil, tacrolimus, tadalafil, theophylline, triazolam, vardenafil, vinBLAStine, warfarin

Decrease: erythromycin effect—rifabutin, rifAMPin, rifapentine

Drug/lab

Increase: AST/ALT

Decrease: folate assay

False increase: 17-OHCS/17-KS

Drug/food

Decrease: erythromycin metabolism—grapefruit juice; avoid using together

NURSING CONSIDERATIONS
Assess:

• **Infection:** temperature, characteristics of wounds, urine, stools, sputum, WBCs at baseline and periodically

• I&O ratio; report hematuria, oliguria in renal disease

• Hepatic studies: AST, ALT if patient is receiving long-term therapy

• Hearing at baseline and after treatment

• Renal studies: urinalysis, protein, blood

• C&S prior to product therapy; product may be given as soon as culture is taken; C&S may be repeated after treatment

• **CDAD:** diarrhea with blood, mucus; abdominal pain, fever; product should be discontinued immediately, notify prescriber

• **Anaphylaxis:** generalized hives; itching; flushing; swelling of lips, tongue, throat; wheezing; have emergency equipment nearby

• **QT prolongation:** may occur (IV >15 mg/min); those with electrolyte imbalances, congenital QT prolongation, elderly at greater risk; correct electrolyte imbalances prior to treatment, ECG

• **Pregnancy/breastfeeding:** use only if clearly needed; use other form of erythromycin, avoid estolate salt; use caution

in breastfeeding, product appears in breast milk

Evaluate:

• Therapeutic response: decreased symptoms of infection

Teach patient/family:

• To notify nurse of diarrhea stools, dark urine, pale stools, jaundice of eyes or skin, severe abdominal pain

• To take at evenly spaced intervals; to complete dosage regimen; to take without food

• To avoid use with other products unless approved by prescriber

TREATMENT OF HYPERSENSITIVITY: Withdraw product; maintain airway; administer EPINEPHrine, aminophylline, O_2, IV corticosteroids

---

erythromycin (topical) (Rx)

(e-rith-roe-mye´sin)

Akne-mycin, Ery-sol ♣

Func. class.: Topical antiinfective, anti-acne

Chem. class.: Macrolide

ACTION: Antibacterial activity results from inhibition of protein synthesis; bacteriostatic

USES: Treatment of acne vulgaris

CONTRAINDICATIONS
Hypersensitivity, children

DOSAGE AND ROUTES
Acne vulgaris

• **Adult/adolescent:** TOPICAL Apply to affected areas bid, AM, PM

Available forms: Topical gel, ointment, pledget, solution 2%

Administer:

Topical route

• For external use only; do not use skin products near the eyes, nose, or mouth

---

• Wash hands prior to and after use. Wash affected area and gently pat dry before using
• **Gel/ointment/pledget/solution:** Apply to the cleansed affected area. Massage gently into affected areas
• Each pledget should be used once and discarded

SIDE EFFECTS
INTEG: Burning, rash, pruritus, peeling, irritation

NURSING CONSIDERATIONS
Assess:
• **Allergic reaction:** assess for hypersensitivity; may need to discontinue product
• **Infection:** assess for number of lesions, severity in acne
Evaluate:
• Decreased lesions in acne
Teach patient/family:
Topical route:
• That product is for external use only; do not use skin products near the eyes, nose, or mouth
• To wash hands prior to and after use; wash affected area and gently pat dry before using
• **Gel/pledget/solution/ointment/lotion:**
• To apply to the cleansed affected area; to massage gently into affected areas
• That each pledget should be used once and discarded

---

escitalopram (Rx)
(es-sit-tal′oh-pram)
Cipralex ✤, Lexapro
Func. class.: Antidepressant, SSRI (selective serotonin reuptake inhibitor)

Do not confuse:
Lexapro/Loxitane

ACTION: Inhibits CNS neuron uptake of serotonin but not of norepinephrine

USES: General anxiety disorder; major depressive disorder in adults/adolescents
Unlabeled uses: Panic disorder, social phobia, hot flashes related to menopause

CONTRAINDICATIONS
Hypersensitivity to this product, citalopram, MAOIs
Precautions: Pregnancy, breastfeeding, geriatric patients, renal/hepatic disease, history of seizures, abrupt discontinuation, bleeding, anticoagulants

Black Box Warning: Children/adolescents ≤12 yr, suicidal ideation

DOSAGE AND ROUTES
• **Adult/adolescent: PO** 10 mg/day; after 1 wk, dose may be increased to 20 mg/day PM
Hepatic dose/geriatric
• **Adult/child ≤12 yr:** PO 10 mg/day
Hot flashes related to menopause (unlabeled)
• **Adult: PO** 10-20 mg/day × 8 wk
Available forms: Tablets 5, 10, 20 mg; oral solution 5 mg (as base)/5 mL (contains sorbitol)
Administer:
• With food or milk for GI symptoms, give with full glass of water once a day in the AM
• Crushed if patient is unable to swallow medication whole; scored tablets can be cut
• Dosage at bedtime if oversedation occurs during the day
• Gum, hard candy, frequent sips of water for dry mouth
• **Oral solution:** measure with calibrated device
• Store at room temperature; do not freeze

SIDE EFFECTS
CNS: *Insomnia,* suicidal ideation, *drowsiness, anxiety, tremor, dizziness, fatigue, sedation, abnormal dreams,* neuroleptic malignant–like syndrome
CV: Postural hypotension
GI: *Nausea, diarrhea, dry mouth, anorexia, constipation, taste changes,* hepatitis

GU: *Decreased libido,* impotence, ejaculation disorder
INTEG: *Sweating, rash, pruritus*
SYST: Serotonin syndrome, Stevens-Johnson syndrome

PHARMACOKINETICS

PO: Metabolized in liver; excreted in urine; 56% protein binding; metabolized by CYP2C19, CYP 3A4, half-life 27-32 hr; half-life increased by 50% in geriatric patients

INTERACTIONS

• Paradoxical worsening of OCD: busPI-Rone
Increase: serotonin syndrome—tryptophan, amphetamines, busPIRone, lithium, amantadine, bromocriptine, SSRIs, SNRIs, serotonin-receptor agonists, traMADol, trazodone, tricyclic antidepressants, linezolid, methylene blue
• Do not use pimozide, MAOIs with or 14 days prior to escitalopram
Increase: CNS depression—alcohol, antidepressants, opioids, sedatives
Increase: side effects of escitalopram—highly protein-bound products
Increase: levels or toxicity of carBAMazepine, lithium, warfarin, phenytoin, antipsychotics, antidysrhythmics
Increase: levels of tricyclics, phenothiazines, haloperidol, diazePAM
Increase: bleeding risk—NSAIDs, salicylates, anticoagulants, SSRIs, platelet inhibitors
Drug/herb
SAMe, St. John's wort: do not use together; serotonin syndrome may occur
Increase: CNS effect—kava, valerian
Drug/food
Grapefruit juice—increased escitalopram effect
Drug/lab
Increase: serum bilirubin, blood glucose, alkaline phosphatase
Decrease: VMA, 5-HIAA, sodium
False increase: urinary catecholamines

NURSING CONSIDERATIONS
Assess:

Black Box Warning: Mental status: mood, sensorium, affect, **suicidal tendencies,** increase in psychiatric symptoms, depression, panic; not approved for use in children <12 yr, provide a limited amount of product, continuing follow-ups should be weekly × 4 wk, q3wk × next 4 wk

• Appetite with bulimia nervosa, weight daily; increase nutritious foods in diet, watch for bingeing and vomiting
• **Allergic reactions:** itching, rash, urticaria; product should be discontinued, may need to give antihistamine
• B/P (lying/standing), pulse q4hr; if systolic B/P drops 20 mm Hg, hold product, notify prescriber
• **Serotonin syndrome:** nausea, vomiting, sedation, dizziness, sweating, facial flushing, mental changes, shivering, increased B/P; discontinue product, notify prescriber
• Weight weekly; appetite may decrease with product
• Alcohol consumption; if alcohol is consumed, hold dose until AM
• **Sexual dysfunction:** ejaculation dysfunction, erectile dysfunction, decreased libido, orgasm dysfunction, priapism
• Assistance with ambulation during therapy, since drowsiness, dizziness occur; safety measures primarily for geriatric patients
• **Pregnancy/breastfeeding:** use only if benefit outweighs risk to fetus; if used during pregnancy, taper in third trimester; use cautiously in breastfeeding, excreted in breast milk
Evaluate:
• Therapeutic response: decreased depression
Teach patient/family:
• That therapeutic effect may take 1-4 wk, may have increased anxiety for first 5-7 days, do not abruptly discontinue

---

- **Serotonin syndrome:** to report immediately nausea, vomiting, sedation, dizziness, sweating, facial flushing, mental changes, shivering
- To use caution when driving, performing other activities requiring alertness because drowsiness, dizziness, blurred vision may occur
- To avoid alcohol, other CNS depressants; to avoid all OTC, herbals, supplement products unless approved by prescriber, to take without regard to meals
- To change positions slowly; orthostatic hypotension may occur

Black Box Warning: That clinical worsening of depression and suicide risk may occur, especially in adolescents and young adults, increased depression, thoughts of dying

- To use medication guide provided
- To notify prescriber if pregnant or planning to become pregnant or if breastfeeding, discuss sexual dysfunction

esketamine (Rx)

(es-ket′-a-meen)

Spravato nasal spray

Func. class.: Antidepressant

Chem. class.: Augmentation agent

Controlled Substance: Schedule III

ACTION: Noncompetitively blocks the NMDA receptor, which is an ionotropic glutamate receptor; mechanism of action for antidepressant effect is unknown; however, the activity on NMDA receptors may be responsible for both the therapeutic and the adverse psychiatric effects

USES: Treatment-resistant depression in adults with an oral antidepressant

CONTRAINDICATIONS

Aneurysm, arteriovenous malformation, intracranial bleeding, ketamine hypersensitivity

Precautions:

Alcoholism, breastfeeding, cardiac disease, cerebrovascular disease, coadministration with other CNS depressants, driving or operating machinery, encephalopathy, geriatrics, hepatic disease, hypertension, hypertensive crisis, loss of consciousness, pregnancy, psychosis, schizophrenia

Black Box Warning: Children, CNS depression, dissociation, requires a specialized care setting, substance abuse, suicidal ideation

DOSAGE AND ROUTES

Adult: NASAL INDUCTION PHASE: On day 1, give 56 mg; for subsequent doses during wk 1 through 4, give 56 mg or 84 mg twice weekly; use 2 devices for the 56-mg dose and 3 devices for the 84-mg dose with a 5-min rest between use of each device; **MAINTENANCE PHASE:** During wk 5 through 8, give 56 mg or 84 mg weekly; during wk 9 and thereafter, give 56 mg or 84 mg q2wk or weekly

Available forms: Nasal spray 56, 84 dose kit

Administer:

Nasal route

- Must be given under the direct supervision of a health care provider and including a supervised postadministration observation
- Each device contains 28 mg; use 2 devices for a 56-mg dose and 3 devices for an 84-mg dose with a 5-min rest between use of each device
- To prevent loss of medication, do not prime the device before use
- During and after use at each treatment session, observe the patient for at least 2 hr until the patient is safe to leave
- Assess B/P prior to use; if baseline B/P >140 mm Hg systolic or >90 mm Hg diastolic, do not use if an increase in B/P or intracranial pressure poses a serious risk
- Reassess B/P about 40 min after dosing and subsequently as clinically indicated; if B/P is decreasing and the patient appears clinically stable for at least 2 hr, the patient may be discharged at the end

of the post-dose monitoring period; if not, continue to monitor

• Because of the potential for drug-induced nausea and vomiting, advise patients to avoid food for at least 2 hr prior to use and avoid liquids at least 30 min prior to administration

• Patients requiring a nasal corticosteroid or nasal decongestant on dosing day should use these at least 1 hr before receiving this product

• If treatment sessions are missed and there is a worsening of depression symptoms, consider returning to the previous dosing schedule

SIDE EFFECTS

CNS: Anxiety, dissociation, drowsiness, dizziness, headache, vertigo, dependence, impaired cognition, hallucinations, confusion, lethargy, suicidal ideation
CV: Hypertension, hypertensive crisis
GI: Nausea

PHARMACOKINETICS

Primarily metabolized to noresketamine, the active metabolite, by CYP2B6 and CYP3A4 and to a lesser extent by CYP2C9 and CYP2C19; noresketamine is metabolized by CYP-dependent pathways and metabolism occurs through glucuronidation; elimination is biphasic, with a rapid decline for the initial 2-4 hr and a mean terminal half-life 7-12 hr; elimination of the metabolite is also biphasic, 4 hr and a terminal half-life of 8 hr; metabolites are excreted in urine (78%) and feces (2%); bioavailability 48%; peak 20-40 min

INTERACTIONS

Black Box Warning: Increased: CNS depression, other CNS depressants—do not use together

Black Box Warning: Increased: sedation, B/P, MAOIs, psychostimulants—do not use together

NURSING CONSIDERATIONS
Assess

Black Box Warning: Dissociation: monitor B/P baseline and 40 min after use, then periodically for at least 2 hr after each treatment session, then provide an assessment to determine when the patient is stable and ready to leave the health care setting; special care is needed with those with schizophrenia

Black Box Warning: Substance abuse: monitor for signs of abuse or dependence; physical dependence has been reported with prolonged use of ketamine; withdrawal symptoms of ketamine include craving, fatigue, poor appetite, anxiety

Black Box Warning: Suicidal ideation: behaviors should be closely monitored during treatment, more frequently during first few months; consider changing the therapeutic regimen, including the discontinuation of esketamine and/or the concurrent oral antidepressant, in patients with worsening of depression or emergent suicidality

Evaluate
• Therapeutic response: decreasing depression

Teach patient/family:

Black Box Warning: Suicidal ideation: teach family members or caregivers to monitor for changes in behavior and to alert the health care provider if such behaviors occur

Black Box Warning: CNS depression: tell health care provider about all the Rx, OTC, vitamins, and herbal supplements used, not to use with other CNS depressants unless discussed with health care provider

• Prior to use instruct patients not to engage in potentially hazardous activities (driving, operating heavy machinery), until the next day after a restful sleep

HOW TO USE:
• **Step 1:** Instruct patient to blow nose before the first device use only; confirm the required number of devices (56 mg = 2 devices; 84 mg = 3 devices)
• **Step 2:** Check expiration date; peel blister and remove device; do not prime the device—this will cause loss of medication; ensure that the indicator on the device shows 2 green dots; give device to patient
• **Step 3:** Instruct patient to hold device with thumb gently supporting but not pressing the plunger as shown in the product labeling; patient should recline head at about 45 degrees during administration to keep medication in nose
• **Step 4:** Instruct patient to insert tip straight into the first nostril; the nose rest should touch the skin between the nostrils; close the opposite nostril; breathe in through nose while pushing plunger all the way up until it stops; sniff gently after spraying to keep medication inside nose; switch hands to insert tip into the second nostril; repeat steps to deliver second spray
• **Step 5:** After administration is complete, take the device from the patient; check that indicator on device shows no green dots; if green dot remains, have patient spray again into the second nostril. Instruct patient to rest comfortably (preferably semi-reclined) for 5 min after each device; if liquid drips out, dab nose with a tissue; DO NOT blow nose
• If a second device is required, ensure a 5-min waiting period prior to use to allow medication from first device to be absorbed
• **Pregnancy/breastfeeding:** Identify if pregnancy is planned or suspected or if breastfeeding; if patient is pregnant, she should register with the National Pregnancy Registry for Antidepressants online at https://womensmentalhealth.org/clinical-and-research-programs/pregnancyregistry/antidepressants/ or by calling 844-405-6185

eslicarbazepine (Rx)
(es′lye-kar-bay′ze-peen)
Aptiom
Func. class.: Anticonvulsant
Chem. class.: Carboxamide derivative

ACTION: Exact mechanism unknown; a voltage-gated sodium-channel blocker inhibits repetitive neuronal firing

USES: Partial seizures, adjunctive treatment

CONTRAINDICATIONS
Hypersensitivity to this product or OXcarbazepine
Precautions: Breastfeeding, abrupt discontinuation, depression, driving/operating machinery, ethanol intoxication, hepatic disease, renal disease, hyponatremia, suicidal ideation, pregnancy

DOSAGE AND ROUTES
• **Adult: PO** 400 mg daily; after 1 wk, increase wk of 400 to 600 mg based on clinical response y to 800 to 1,600 mg qd
Renal dose
• **Adult: PO** CCr <50 mL/min 200 mg daily; after 2 wk, increase to 400 mg daily, max 800 mg daily
Available forms: Tablets 200, 400, 600, 800 mg
Administer:
• May be taken without regard to food
• May be crushed or whole
• Store at room temperature

SIDE EFFECTS
CNS: Drowsiness, dizziness, amnesia, depression, insomnia, lethargy, memory impairment, confusion, fatigue, headache, speech disturbance, suicidal thoughts/behaviors, tremors
CV: Hypertension, peripheral edema
EENT: Blurred vision, nystagmus, diplopia
GI: Nausea, constipation, diarrhea, hypercholesterolemia/hypertriglyceridemia, vomiting, hepatotoxicity
GU: Cystitis

INTEG: Rash, Stevens-Johnson syndrome, toxic epidermal necrolysis, anaphylaxis, angioedema
META: Hyponatremia
RESP: Cough

PHARMACOKINETICS
Peak 1-4 hr; metabolized by liver; moderate CYP2C19 inhibitor; weak/moderate CYP3A4 inducer; steady-state 4-5 days; excreted in urine, feces; half-life 13-20 hr; protein binding <40%

INTERACTIONS
Decrease: effects of bedaquiline, boceprevir, bosutinib, cabozantinib, cobicistat, elvitegravir, emtricitabine, crizotinib, cycloSPORINE, dronedarone, erlotinib, fosamprenavir, galantamine, gefitinib, HYDROcodone, maraviroc, oxyCODONE, paliperidone, perampanel, pimozide, praziquantel, QUEtiapine, ranolazine, rilpivirine
Decrease: eslicarbazepine effect—CYP1A2, CYP2C19 substrates
Decrease: effect of CYP3A inducers

NURSING CONSIDERATIONS
Assess:
• **Hyponatremia:** nausea, vomiting, increased seizures, headache, weakness, confusion, irritability
• **Seizures:** character, location, duration, intensity, frequency, presence of aura
• **Hepatic studies:** ALT, AST, bilirubin; sodium

Black Box Warning: Mental status: mood, sensorium, affect, behavioral changes, suicidal thoughts/behaviors; if mental status changes, notify prescriber

• Eye problems: need for ophthalmic examinations prior to, during, after treatment (slit lamp, fundoscopy, tonometry)
• **Allergic reaction:** purpura; red, raised rash; if these occur, product should be discontinued
• **Beers:** avoid in older adults unless safer alternative is unavailable; may cause ataxia, impaired psychomotor function

• **Pregnancy/breastfeeding:** use in pregnancy only if benefits outweigh risks to fetus. Patient should enroll in North American Antiepileptic Drug (NAAED) Pregnancy Registry (888-233-2334; www.aedpregnancyregistry.org). Product is present in breast milk; consider benefits of breastfeeding, risk of potential infant drug exposure, and risk of an untreated or inadequately treated condition
Evaluate:
• Therapeutic response: decreased seizure activity; document on patient's chart
Teach patient/family:
• To carry emergency ID stating patient's name, products taken, condition, prescriber's name, and phone number
• To avoid driving, other activities that require alertness, usually for the first 3 days of treatment
• Not to discontinue medication quickly after long-term use
• **Pregnancy:** to notify prescriber if pregnancy is planned or suspected; to use additional contraceptives if using hormonal contraceptives; to avoid breastfeeding
• Not to abruptly discontinue drug
• To report signs of decreased renal function, dizziness, increased cholesterol, ocular toxicity, suicide risk, skin rashes
• To take with or without food; that tablet can be crushed
• To report increased seizures, headache, nausea, vomiting, weakness, confusion, irritability (hyponatremia)

⚠ HIGH ALERT

esmolol (Rx)
(ez'moe-lole)
Brevibloc
Func. class.: Beta-adrenergic blocker (antidysrhythmic II)

Do not confuse:
Brevibloc/Brevital

ACTION: Competitively blocks stimulation of β_1-adrenergic receptors in the myocardium; produces negative chronotropic, inotropic activity (decreases rate of SA node discharge, increases recovery time), slows conduction of AV node, decreases heart rate, decreases O_2 consumption in myocardium; also decreases renin-aldosterone-angiotensin system at high doses; inhibits β_2-receptors in bronchial system at higher doses

USES: Supraventricular tachycardia, noncompensatory sinus tachycardia, intraoperative and postoperative tachycardia and hypertension, atrial fibrillation/flutter

CONTRAINDICATIONS
Second- or third-degree heart block; cardiogenic shock, HF, cardiac failure, hypersensitivity, severe bradycardia
Precautions: Pregnancy, breastfeeding, geriatric patients, hypotension, peripheral vascular disease, diabetes, hypoglycemia, thyrotoxicosis, renal disease, atrial fibrillation, bronchospasms, hyperthyroidism, myasthenia gravis, asthma, COPD, CV disease, pheochromocytoma, abrupt discontinuation

DOSAGE AND ROUTES
Atrial fibrillation/flutter
• **Adult:** IV loading dose 500 mcg/kg/min over 1 min; maintenance 50 mcg/kg/min for 4 min; if no response after 5 min, give second loading dose, then increase infusion to 100 mcg/kg/min for 4 min; if no response, repeat loading dose, then increase maintenance infusion by 50 mcg/kg/min (max of 300 mcg/kg/min); titrate to patient response
• **Child:** IV total loading dose of 600 mcg/kg over 2 min, maintenance **IV INFUSION** 200 mcg/kg/min, titrate upward by 50-100 mcg/kg/min q5-10min until B/P, heart rate reduced by >10%
Perioperative hypertension/tachycardia
• **Adult:** IV immediate control 80 mg, 1000 mcg/kg (bolus) over 30 seconds, then 150 mcg/kg/min, adjust to response,

max 300 mcg/kg/min, perioperative hypertension, 200 mcg/kg/min (tachycardia)
Available forms: Injection 10 mg/mL, 10 mg/mL in 250-mL bag, 20 mg/mL in 100-mL bag
Administer:
• Do not discontinue product suddenly
• Store protected from light, moisture, in cool environment
IV route
• Check that correct concentration is being given
IV direct route
• 10 mg/mL injection solution needs no dilution, may be used as an IV loading dose using a handheld syringe
Continuous IV INFUSION route
• Ready-to-use bags of premixed isotonic solution of 10 mg/mL and 20 mg/mL available in 100-, 250-mL bags; use controlled infusion device, central line preferred; rate is based on patient's weight

Y-site compatibilities: Amikacin, aminophylline, amiodarone, atracurium, butorphanol, calcium chloride, ceFAZolin, cefTAZidime, ceftizoxime, chloramphenicol, cimetidine, cisatracurium, clindamycin, diltiazem, DOPamine, enalaprilat, erythromycin, famotidine, fentaNYL, gentamicin, insulin (regular), labetalol, magnesium sulfate, methyldopate, metroNIDAZOLE, midazolam, morphine, nitroglycerin, nitroprusside, norepinephrine, pancuronium, penicillin G potassium, piperacillin, polymyxin B, potassium chloride, potassium phosphate, propofol, ranitidine, remifentanil, streptomycin, tacrolimus, tobramycin, trimethoprim-sulfamethoxazole, vancomycin, vecuronium, voriconazole, zoledronic acid

SIDE EFFECTS
CNS: Confusion, drowsiness, weakness, dizziness, fatigue, headache
CV: Hypotension, peripheral ischemia
GI: *Nausea,* vomiting, anorexia
INTEG: *Inflammation at site,* sweating

PHARMACOKINETICS
Onset very rapid, duration short, half-life 9 min, metabolized by hydrolysis of ester linkage, excreted via kidneys

INTERACTIONS

- Avoid use with MAOIs, Sotalol

Increase: effect of antidiabetics

Increase: possible fatal B/P increase—clonidine

Increase: potentiate suppressive effects of dilTIAZem, verapamil

Increase: antihypertensive effect—general anesthetics

Increase: digoxin levels—digoxin

Increase: alpha-adrenergic stimulation—ePHEDrine, EPINEPHrine, amphetamine, norepinephrine, phenylephrine, pseudo-ePHEDrine

Decrease: action of thyroid hormones

Decrease: action of esmolol—thyroid hormone, salicylates

Drug/herb

Increase: beta-blocking effect—hawthorn

Decrease: antihypertensive effect—ephedra

Drug/lab

Interference: glucose/insulin tolerance test

NURSING CONSIDERATIONS

Assess:

- **Heart failure:** I&O ratio, weight daily, jugular venous distention, weight gain, crackles, edema
- **Dysrhythmias:** B/P, pulse; note rate, rhythm, quality; rapid changes can cause shock; if systolic <100 or diastolic <60, notify prescriber before giving product; ECG continuously during infusion, hypotension common, if severe, slow or stop infusion
- **Infusion site:** monitor infusion site during infusion; do not use butterfly if irritation occurs; stop and start at another site
- **Bronchospasm:** breath sounds, respiratory pattern
- **Pregnancy/breastfeeding:** use only if benefit outweighs risk to fetus; use in the last trimester or labor or obstetric delivery has resulted in fetal bradycardia; not known if excreted in breast milk

Evaluate:

- Therapeutic response: lower B/P immediately, lower heart rate

Teach patient/family:

- Not to drive or perform other hazardous activities if drowsiness occurs
- To change positions slowly to prevent orthostatic hypotension
- About reason for use; expected results
- To notify prescriber if chest pain, SOB, wheezing, hypotension, bradycardia, pain, swelling at IV site occurs
- **Pregnancy/breastfeeding:** identify if pregnancy is planned or suspected

TREATMENT OF OVERDOSE: Discontinue product; IV glucagon if needed

---

esomeprazole (Rx)

(es'oh-mep'rah-zohl)

NexIUM, NexIUM 24HR, NexIUM I.V.

Func. class.: Antiulcer

Chem. class.: Proton pump inhibitor, benzimidazole

Combination: esomeprazole/naproxen 20 mg/375 mg, 20 mg/500 mg

Do not confuse:
esomeprazole/omeprazole

ACTION: Suppresses gastric secretions by inhibiting hydrogen/potassium ATPase enzyme system in gastric parietal cell; characterized as gastric acid pump inhibitor because it blocks the final step of acid production

USES: Gastroesophageal reflux disease (GERD), adult/child/infant; severe erosive esophagitis, adult/child; treatment of active duodenal ulcers in combination with anti-infectives for *Helicobacter pylori* infection; long-term use for hypersecretory conditions

CONTRAINDICATIONS

Hypersensitivity to proton pump inhibitors (PPIs)

Precautions: Pregnancy, breastfeeding, children, geriatric patients, hypomagnesemia, osteoporosis

DOSAGE AND ROUTES

Active duodenal ulcers associated with *H. pylori*

- **Adult: PO** 40 mg/day × 10-14 days in combination with clarithromycin 500 mg bid × 10 days and amoxicillin 1000 mg bid × 10 days

GERD/erosive esophagitis
• **Adult: PO** 20 or 40 mg/day × 4-8 wk; no adjustment needed in renal/liver failure, geriatric patients; **IV** 20 or 40 mg/day up to 10 days
• **Adolescent and child 12-17 yr: PO** 20 or 40 mg/day 1 hr prior to meals for ≤8 wk
• **Child 1-11 yr and ≥20 kg: PO** 10-20 mg/day 1 hr prior to meals for ≤8 wk
• **Infant ≥1 mo: IV** 0.5 mg/kg over 10-30 min
• **Infant 1-11 mo (>7.5-12 kg): PO** 10 mg daily × up to 6 wk
• **Infant 1-11 mo (>5-7.5 kg): PO** 5 mg daily × up to 6 wk
• **Infant 1-11 mo (3-5 kg): PO** 2.5 mg daily × up to 6 wk

Gastric ulcer prophylaxis, NSAID-associated gastropathy
• **Adult: PO** 20-40 mg/day up to 6 mo

Zollinger-Ellison syndrome
• **Adult: PO** 40 mg bid, up to 240 mg/day

Dyspepsia (unlabeled)
Adult: PO 20 mg daily in the morning before eating for 14 days

Hepatic dose
• **Adult: PO/IV** max 20 mg/day (severe hepatic disease)

Available forms: Delayed-release capsules 20, 40 mg; powder for IV injection 20, 40 mg/vial; delayed-release powder for oral suspension 2.5, 5, 10, 20, 40 mg

Administer:
PO route
• Swallow capsules whole; do not crush or chew; capsule may be opened and sprinkled over Tbsp of applesauce
• Same time daily, 1 hr before meal
• **Oral suspension (delayed release):** empty contents of packet into container with 1 Tbsp of water, let stand 2-3 min to thicken, restir, give within 30 min of mixing; any residual product should be flushed with more water, taken immediately
• **NG tube (delayed-release oral suspension):** add 50 mL water to contents of packet in syringe, shake, leave 2-3 min to thicken, shake, inject through NG tube within 30 min, make sure granules are dissolved

IV, direct route
• Reconstitute each vial with 5 mL 0.9% NaCl, D₅W, LR; give over 3 min
Intermittent IV INFUSION route
• Dilute reconstituted solution to 50 mL, give over 30 min, do not admix, flush line with D₅W, 0.9% NaCl, LR after infusion
Continuous IV route
• Use 2 (40-mg vials) with 5 mL of 0.9% NaCL for 80-mg loading dose, further dilute in 100 mL 0.9% NaCL give over 30 min, then infusion at 8 mg/hr

Y-site compatibility: Ceftaroline, fentanyl, furosemide, regular insulin, nitroglycerin

SIDE EFFECTS
CNS: *Headache, dizziness*
GI: *Diarrhea, flatulence,* abdominal pain, constipation, dry mouth, hepatic failure, hepatitis, microscopic colitis, *Clostridium difficile*–associated diarrhea (CDAD)
INTEG: *Rash,* dry skin
GU: Nephritis
MISC: Fractures, SLE, vitamin B₁₂ deficiency
SYST: Stevens-Johnson syndrome, toxic epidermal necrolysis, exfoliative dermatitis

PHARMACOKINETICS
Well absorbed 90%; protein binding 97%; extensively metabolized in liver (CYP2C19); terminal half-life 1-1.5 hr; eliminated in urine as metabolites and in feces; in geriatric patients, elimination rate decreased, bioavailability increased

INTERACTIONS
Increase: effect, toxicity of diazePAM, digoxin, penicillins, saquinavir, cilostazol, cloZAPine, those drugs metabolized by CYP2C19
Increase: effect of methotrexate, tacrolimus, warfarin
Decrease: effect—atazanavir, nelfinavir, dapsone, iron, itraconazole, ketoconazole, indinavir, calcium carbonate, vitamin B₁₂, clopidogrel, iron salts, mycophenolate
Drug/lab
Interference: sodium, HB, WBC, platelets, magnesium
False-positive: CgA

NURSING CONSIDERATIONS
Assess:

• **GI system:** bowel sounds, abdomen for pain, swelling, anorexia, bloody stools; CDAD may occur

• **Hepatic failure, hepatitis:** AST, ALT, alkaline phosphatase at baseline and periodically during treatment

• **Serious skin disorders:** Stevens-Johnson syndrome, toxic epidermal necrolysis, exfoliative dermatitis

• **CDAD:** Monitor for diarrhea with blood, abdominal pain, this product may increase risk of CDAD

• **Vitamin B$_{12}$ deficiency:** In those on long-term treatment >3 yr, women and young adults

• **Acute tubulointerstitial nephritis:** Monitor for rash, fever, arthralgia, nausea, vomiting; change in renal studies

• **Pregnancy/breastfeeding:** use only if benefits clearly outweigh risks to fetus; do not breastfeed

Evaluate:

• Therapeutic response: absence of epigastric pain, swelling, fullness, decreased GERD

Teach patient/family:

• To report severe diarrhea, abdominal pain, black tarry stools, rash; product may have to be discontinued

• That hypoglycemia may occur if diabetic

• To avoid hazardous activities; dizziness may occur

• To notify provider if pregnancy is planned or suspected or if breastfeeding

• To avoid alcohol, salicylates, NSAIDs; may cause GI irritation

• To take ≥1 hr prior to meal; not to crush, chew delayed-release product; if missed, to take as soon as remembered if not almost time for next dose; to take full course prescribed; to read "Patient Information"

• That if capsule is unable to be swallowed whole, contents may be mixed with a Tbsp of applesauce

• To notify provider of all OTC, Rx, or herbal products taken

• **Hypomagnesemia:** to notify prescriber of dizziness, fast heartbeat, tremors, weakness, spasm, cramps

---

estradiol (Rx)
(es-tra-dye´ole)
Estrace
estradiol cypionate (Rx)
Depo-Estradiol
estradiol gel (Rx)
Divigel, Elestrin, Estrogel
estradiol spray (Rx)
Evamist
estradiol topical emulsion (Rx)
Estrasorb
estradiol transdermal system (Rx)
Alora, Climara, Minivelle, Vivelle-Dot
estradiol vaginal ring (Rx)
Estring, Femring
estradiol vaginal tablet (Rx)
Vagifem
estradiol valerate (Rx)
Delestrogen
Func. class.: Estrogen, progestins

ACTION: Needed for adequate functioning of female reproductive system; affects release of pituitary gonadotropins; inhibits ovulation; adequate calcium use in bone

USES: Vasomotor symptoms (menopause), inoperable breast cancer (selected cases), prostatic cancer, atrophic vaginitis, kraurosis vulvae, hypogonadism, primary ovarian failure, prevention of osteoporosis, castration

CONTRAINDICATIONS
Pregnancy, breastfeeding, reproductive cancer, genital bleeding (abnormal, undiagnosed), protein S or C deficiency, antithrombin deficiency, angioedema, MI, stroke

---

Black Box Warning: Breast/endometrial cancer, thromboembolic disorders, MI, stroke

Precautions: Hypertension, asthma, blood dyscrasias, gallbladder/bone/renal/ hepatic disease, HF, diabetes mellitus, depression, migraine headache, seizure disorders, family history of cancer of breast or reproductive tract, smoking, uterine fibroids, vaginal irritation/infection, history of angioedema, cardiac disease

Black Box Warning: dementia, accidental exposure pets/children (topical)

DOSAGE AND ROUTES
Hormone replacement/menopause symptoms
• **Adult: TRANSDERMAL** 1 patch delivering 0.025, 0.0375, 0.05, 0.075, or 0.1 mg/day 2×/wk (Alora, Estraderm, Vivelle-Dot); 1 patch delivering 0.025, 0.0375, 0.05, 0.06, 0.075, or 0.1 mg/day replace q7days (Climara); **GEL** apply entire unit-dose packet to 5 × 7-inch area of upper thigh/day, alternate thighs; **SPRAY** (Evamist) 1 spray to inner surface of forearm/day in AM
Menopause/hypogonadism/ castration/ovarian failure
• **Adult: PO** 0.5-2 mg/day, 3 wk on, 1 wk off or continuously; **IM** (cypionate) 1-5 mg q3-4wk; (valerate) 10-20 mg q4wk
• **Adult: TOPICAL** (Estraderm) 0.05 mg/24 hr applied 2×/wk; (Climara) 0.05 mg/hr applied 1×/wk in cyclic regimen; women with hysterectomy may use continuously
Postmenopausal osteoporosis, prophylaxis
• **Adult female: PO** 0.5 mg/day × 23 days of a 28-day cycle; **TRANSDERMAL** (Alora, Minivelle, Vivelle-Dot) 0.025 mg/day applied to skin 2×/wk; adjust as needed based on clinical response, bone mineral density; **TRANSDERMAL** (Climara) 0.025 mg/day applied to skin weekly
Prostatic cancer (inoperable)
• **Adult: IM** (valerate) 30 mg q1-2wk; **PO** (oral estradiol) 1-2 mg bid-tid
Breast cancer (palliative treatment)
• **Adult: PO** 10 mg tid × 3 mo or longer

Atrophic vaginitis/kraurosis vulvae
• **Adult: VAG CREAM** 2-4 g/day × 1-2 wk, then 1 g 1-3×/wk cycled; **VAG TABLET** 1/day × 2 wk, maintenance 1 tab 2×/wk; **VAG RING** inserted, left in place continuously for 3 mo
Vasomotor symptoms
• **Adult: TOPICAL** after cleaning and drying skin on left thigh, calf, rub in contents of pouch using both hands until completely absorbed; wash hands
Available forms: *Estradiol:* tablets 0.5, 1, 2 mg; *valerate:* injection 10, 20, 40 mg/ mL; *transdermal:* 0.014, 0.025, 0.0375, 0.05, 0.075, 0.1 mg/24 hr release rate; *vag cream:* 100 mcg/g; *vag tablet:* 10 mcg; *vag ring:* 2 mg/90 days; *topical emulsion:* 2.5 mg; *gel* (Divigel) 0.06%, 0.1%; *spray* (Evamist) 1.53 mg/actuation
Administer:
• Titrated dose; use lowest effective dose
• IM inject deeply in large muscle mass
PO route
• With food or milk to decrease GI symptoms
Transdermal route
• May contain aluminum or other metals in backing of patch, can overheat in MRI scan and burn patients
• Apply to trunk of body 2×/wk; press firmly, hold in place for 10 sec to ensure good contact; do not apply to breasts
• On intermittent cycle schedule: 3 wk on, then 1 wk off; if patch falls off, reapply
Topical route
• Use Evamist daily; spray to inner upper arm; may increase to 2-3×/day based on response; allow to dry for 2 min, avoid secondary exposure to children, pets, caregivers
Vaginal route
• Use a new applicator daily, provided

SIDE EFFECTS
CNS: Dizziness, headache, migraines, depression, seizures
CV: Hypertension, thrombophlebitis, edema, thromboembolism, stroke, pulmonary embolism, MI, chest pain
EENT: Contact lens intolerance, increased myopia, astigmatism, throat swelling, eyelid edema

---

Side effects: *italics* = common; red = life-threatening

GI: *Nausea,* vomiting, diarrhea, anorexia, pancreatitis, cramps, constipation, increased appetite, increased weight, cholestatic jaundice, hepatic adenoma
GU: Amenorrhea, cervical erosion, breakthrough bleeding, dysmenorrhea, vaginal candidiasis, breast changes, *gynecomastia, testicular atrophy, impotence,* increased risk of breast cancer, endometrial cancer, changes in libido; toxic shock, vaginal wall ulceration/erosion (vag ring)
INTEG: Rash, urticaria, acne, hirsutism, alopecia, oily skin, seborrhea, purpura, erythema, pruritus, melasma; site irritation (transdermal)
META: Folic acid deficiency, hypercalcemia, hyperglycemia

PHARMACOKINETICS
PO/INJECTION/TRANSDERMAL: Degraded in liver, excreted in urine, crosses placenta, excreted in breast milk

INTERACTIONS
Increase: action of corticosteroids, tricyclics
Increase: toxicity—cycloSPORINE, dantrolene
Decrease: action of anticoagulants, oral hypoglycemics, tamoxifen
Decrease: estradiol action—anticonvulsants, barbiturates, phenylbutazone, rifAMPin, calcium
Drug/herb
Altered estrogen effect: black cohosh, DHEA
Decrease: estrogen effect—saw palmetto, St. John's wort
Drug/food
Increase: estrogen level—grapefruit juice
Drug/lab
Increase: BSP retention test, PBI, T_4, serum sodium, platelet aggregation, thyroxine-binding globulin (TBG), prothrombin; factors VII, VIII, IX, X; triglycerides
Decrease: serum folate, serum triglyceride, T_3 resin uptake test, glucose tolerance test, antithrombin III, pregnanediol, metyrapone test
False positive: LE prep, ANA

NURSING CONSIDERATIONS
Assess:

Black Box Warning: For previous breast/endometrial cancer, thromboembolic disorders, MI, stroke, dementia; use adequate screening for these conditions, estrogen increases the risk

• Blood glucose of diabetic patient; hyperglycemia may occur
• Weight daily; notify prescriber of weekly weight gain >5 lb; if increase, diuretic may be ordered
• B/P q4hr; watch for increase caused by water and sodium retention
• I&O ratio; decreasing urinary output, increasing edema, report changes
• Hepatic studies, including AST, ALT, bilirubin, alkaline phosphatase at baseline, periodically; periodic folic acid level
• Hypertension, cardiac symptoms, jaundice, hypercalcemia
• Mental status: affect, mood, behavioral changes, aggression
• Female patient for intact uterus; if so, progesterone should be added to estrogen therapy to decrease risk of endometrial cancer
• **Beers:** avoid oral and topical patch in older adults; evidence of carcinogenic potential (breast, endometrial)
• **Pregnancy/breastfeeding:** do not use in pregnancy; estrogens decrease milk production; use only if needed
Evaluate:
• Therapeutic response: reversal of menopause symptoms; decrease in tumor size in prostatic, breast cancer
Teach patient/family:
• To weigh weekly; to report gain >5 lb
• To report breast lumps, vaginal bleeding, edema, jaundice, dark urine, clay-colored stools, dyspnea, headache, blurred vision, abdominal pain, numbness or stiffness in legs, chest pain; tenderness, redness, and swelling in extremities; males to report impotence, gynecomastia; to report dermal rash with transdermal patch
• To avoid grapefruit or grapefruit juice (PO)

• That smoking increases CV conditions; encourage to stop
• To notify prescriber if pregnancy is planned or suspected; not to become pregnant when using estrogen
• To report changes in blood glucose if diabetic

⚠ HIGH ALERT

estrogens, conjugated (Rx)
Cenestin, Premarin, C.E.S. ✦
estrogens, conjugated synthetic B (Rx)
Enjuvia
Func. class.: Estrogen, hormone

Do not confuse:
Premarin/Provera
Enjuvia/Januvia

ACTION: Needed for adequate functioning of female reproductive system; affects release of pituitary gonadotropins, inhibits ovulation; adequate calcium use in bone

USES: Vasomotor symptoms (menopause), inoperable breast cancer, prostatic cancer, abnormal uterine bleeding, hypogonadism, primary ovarian failure, prevention of osteoporosis, castration, atrophic vaginitis
Unlabeled uses: Hyperparathyroidism, infertility

CONTRAINDICATIONS
Pregnancy, breastfeeding, thromboembolic disorders, reproductive cancer, genital bleeding (abnormal, undiagnosed), hypersensitivity, MI, stroke, thrombophlebitis

Black Box Warning: Endometrial, breast cancer, thromboembolic diseases

Precautions: Hypertension, asthma, blood dyscrasias, HF, diabetes mellitus, depression, migraine headache, seizure disorders, gallbladder/bone/hepatic/renal disease, family history of cancer of breast or reproductive tract, smoking, hypothyroidism, obesity, SLE

Black Box Warning: Dementia

DOSAGE AND ROUTES
Estrogens conjugated
Vasomotor symptoms (menopause)
• **Adult: PO** 0.3-1.25 mg/day 3 wk on, 1 wk off
Prevention of osteoporosis
• **Adult: PO** 0.3 mg/day or in cycle
Atrophic vaginitis
• **Adult: VAG CREAM** 0.5 g/day × 21 days, off 7 days, repeat
Prostatic cancer
• **Adult: PO** 1.25-2.5 mg tid
Advanced inoperable breast cancer
• **Adult: PO** 10 mg tid × ≥3 mo
Abnormal uterine bleeding
• **Adult: IV/IM** 25 mg q6-12hr
Castration/primary ovarian failure
• **Adult: PO** 1.25 mg/day 3 wk on, 1 wk off
Hypogonadism
• **Adult: PO** 0.3 or 0.625 mg daily (3 wk on, 1 wk off), adjust to response

Estrogens conjugated synthetic B
Vasomotor symptoms (menopause)
• **Adult: PO** 0.625 mg/day initially; may increase based on response
Dyspareunia (moderate to severe); menopausal-cyclic regimen:
• **Adult: INTRAVAGINALLY** 0.5 g daily × 21 days, then off 7 days; continuous regimen **INTRAVAGINALLY** 0.5 g bid
Available forms: Tablets 0.3, 0.45, 0.625, 0.9, 1.25, 2.5 mg; injection 25 mg/vial; vag cream 0.625 mg/g; *synthetic B:* tablets 0.625, 1.25 mg
Administer:
Titrated dose; use lowest effective dose
PO route
• Give with or immediately after food to reduce nausea
IM route
• Reconstitute after withdrawing 5 mL of air from container, inject sterile diluent on vial side, rotate to dissolve; give injection deep in large muscle mass, aspirate before injection
Vaginal route
• Use applicator provided, wash after use

Side effects: *italics* = common; red = life-threatening

○ **Direct IV route** ○────────

• IV, after reconstituting as for IM, inject into distal port of running IV line of D₅W, 0.9% NaCl at ≤5 mg/min

Y-site compatibilities: Heparin, hydrocortisone, potassium chloride, vitamin B/C

SIDE EFFECTS

CNS: Dizziness, headache, migraine, depression, seizures, mood disturbances
CV: Hypertension, thrombophlebitis, edema, thromboembolism, stroke, pulmonary embolism, MI, chest pain
EENT: Contact lens intolerance, increased myopia, astigmatism
GI: *Nausea,* vomiting, diarrhea, anorexia, pancreatitis, cramps, constipation, increased appetite, cholestatic jaundice, hepatic adenoma, weight gain/loss
GU: Amenorrhea, cervical erosion, breakthrough bleeding, dysmenorrhea, vaginal candidiasis, breast changes, *gynecomastia, testicular atrophy, impotence,* increased risk of breast cancer, endometrial cancer, libido changes
INTEG: Rash, urticaria, acne, hirsutism, alopecia, oily skin, seborrhea, purpura, melasma
META: Folic acid deficiency, hypercalcemia, hyperglycemia

PHARMACOKINETICS

PO/IM/IV: Degraded in liver, excreted in urine, crosses placenta, excreted in breast milk

INTERACTIONS

Increase: toxicity—cycloSPORINE, dantrolene
Increase: action of corticosteroids
Decrease: action of estrogens—anticonvulsants, barbiturates, phenylbutazone, rifAMPin, bosentan
Decrease: action of anticoagulants, oral hypoglycemics, tamoxifen, thyroid, tricyclics
Drug/food
Increase: estrogen level—grapefruit juice
Drug/lab
Increase: T₄, serum sodium, platelet aggregation, thyroxine-binding globulin (TBG), prothrombin; factors VII, VIII, IX, X; triglycerides

Decrease: serum folate, serum triglyceride, T₃ resin uptake test, glucose tolerance test, antithrombin III, metyrapone test
False positive: LE prep, antinuclear antibodies

NURSING CONSIDERATIONS
Assess:

Black Box Warning: Breast, endometrial cancer: estrogens should not be used in known, suspected, or history of these disorders

Black Box Warning: Stroke, thromboembolic disease of MI: should not be used in these conditions or known protein C deficiency, protein S deficiency, or antithrombin deficiency

• Blood glucose if diabetic patient; hyperglycemia may occur
• Weight daily; notify prescriber of weekly weight gain >5 lb; if increase, diuretic may be ordered; check for edema; B/P baseline and periodically
• Hepatic studies: AST, ALT, bilirubin, alkaline phosphatase
• Hypertension, cardiac symptoms, jaundice, hypercalcemia
• Mental status: affect, mood, behavioral changes, aggression
• Female patient for intact uterus; if so, progesterone should be added to estrogen therapy to decrease risk of endometrial cancer; abnormal uterine bleeding, breast exam; Pap smear
• **Use lowest dose/shortest time period:** estrogen therapy should be limited to the shortest duration of therapy and lowest effective dose; individualize risks and benefits with each patient
• **Beers:** avoid oral and topical patch in older adults; evidence of carcinogenic potential (breast, endometrial)
• **Pregnancy/breastfeeding:** do not use in pregnancy; estrogens decrease milk production; use only if clearly needed
Evaluate:
• Therapeutic response: absence of breast engorgement, reversal of menopause symptoms, decrease in tumor size with prostatic cancer

Teach patient/family:
• To avoid breastfeeding; product is excreted in breast milk
• To weigh weekly; to report gain >5 lb

Black Box Warning: To report breast lumps, vaginal bleeding, edema, jaundice, dark urine, clay-colored stools, dyspnea, headache, blurred vision, abdominal pain; leg pain and redness, numbness or stiffness; chest pain; males to report impotence or gynecomastia

• To avoid sunlight or wear sunscreen; burns may occur
• To notify prescriber if pregnancy is suspected
• That vasomotor symptoms improve in 2 wk, max relief in 8 wk

⚠ HIGH ALERT

eszopiclone (Rx)
(es-zop′i-klone)
Lunesta
Func. class.: Sedative/hypnotic, nonbenzodiazepine
Chem. class.: Cyclopyrrolone
Controlled Substance Schedule IV

Do not confuse:
Lunesta/Neulasta

ACTION: Interacts with GABA receptors

USES: Insomnia

CONTRAINDICATIONS
Hypersensitivity
Precautions: Pregnancy, breastfeeding, children, geriatric patients, severe hepatic disease, abrupt discontinuation, COPD, depression, labor, sleep apnea, substance abuse, suicidal ideation, ethanol intoxication

DOSAGE AND ROUTES
• **Adult: PO** 1 mg immediately before bed, may increase to 2-3 mg if needed, max 3 mg nightly
Hepatic dose/CYP3A4 inhibitors
• **Adult: PO** 1 mg immediately before bed with severe hepatic disease, max 2 mg/day

Available forms: Tablets 1, 2, 3 mg
Administer:
• Do not break, crush, or chew tablet
• Immediately prior to bedtime; avoid use with food; for short-term use only
• If dose is missed, wait to take until next scheduled time prior to bed the next day

SIDE EFFECTS
CNS: Worsening depression, hallucinations, headache, *daytime drowsiness,* suicidal thoughts/actions, migraine, restlessness, anxiety, sleep driving, sleepwalking
CV: Peripheral edema, chest pain
GI: *Dry mouth,* bitter taste (dysgeusia)
GU: Gynecomastia, dysmenorrhea
INTEG: Rash, angioedema

PHARMACOKINETICS
Onset rapid; peak 1 hr; duration 6 hr; extensively metabolized in the liver by CYP3A4, CYP2E1; excreted via kidneys; half-life 6 hr, geriatric patients 9 hr, protein binding 52%-59%

INTERACTIONS
Increase: CNS depression—CNS depressants
Increase: toxicity due to decreased eszopiclone elimination—CYP3A4 inhibitors (clarithromycin, itraconazole, ketoconazole, nefazodone, nelfinavir, ritonavir, troleandomycin, SSRIs)
Decrease: eszopiclone effect—CYP3A4 inducers (dexamethasone, barbiturates, carBAMazepine, OXcarbazepine, phenytoin, fosphenytoin, ethotoin)
Drug/food
Decrease: product action—food
Drug/herb
Decrease: eszopiclone effect—St. John's wort

NURSING CONSIDERATIONS
Assess:
• **Sleep pattern:** ability to go to sleep, stay asleep, early morning awakenings, conservative methods used
• For abuse of this product, other products
• **Anaphylaxis, angioedema:** monitor during first dose

Side effects: *italics* = common; red = life-threatening

- **CNS depression/suicidal thoughts, behaviors:** assess for these symptoms
- Alternative methods to improve sleep: reading, quiet environment, warm bath, milk
- Assistance with ambulation; night light, call bell within reach
- **Beers:** avoid in older adults with delirium or at high risk for delirium
- **Pregnancy/breastfeeding:** identify whether pregnancy is planned or suspected; avoid breastfeeding

Evaluate:
- Therapeutic response: ability to fall asleep and stay asleep throughout the night

Teach patient/family:
- That daytime drowsiness may occur; not to engage in hazardous activities until effect is known; that memory problems may occur
- That all other medications and supplements should be avoided unless approved by prescriber; to avoid alcohol
- To notify prescriber if pregnancy is suspected or planned
- To avoid use after a high-fat meal
- To swallow tablet whole
- To notify prescriber of facial swelling, rash, complex sleep disorders (sleep driving, sleep eating), change in thinking or behavior
- That tolerance and dependence may occur after extended use
- To take immediately prior to going to bed
- To be aware of CNS depression and suicidal thoughts/behaviors, report at once

etanercept (Rx)

(eh-tan´er-sept)

Enbrel, Enbrel SureClick, Erelzi, Eticovo

Func. class.: Antirheumatic agent (disease modifying) (DMARD)

Chem. class.: Anti-TNF agent

ACTION: Binds tumor necrosis factor (TNF), which is involved in immune and inflammatory reactions

USES: Acute, chronic rheumatoid arthritis that has not responded to other disease-modifying agents, polyarticular course of juvenile rheumatoid arthritis (JRA), ankylosing spondylitis, plaque psoriasis, psoriatic arthritis

Unlabeled uses: Crohn's disease; plaque psoriasis (child ≥4 yr)

CONTRAINDICATIONS

Sepsis

Precautions: Pregnancy, breastfeeding, children <4 yr, geriatric patients, malignancies, HF, seizures, multiple sclerosis, latex hypersensitivity

> **Black Box Warning:** Infection, lymphoma, neoplastic disease, TB

DOSAGE AND ROUTES

RA/ankylosing spondylitis
- **Adult:** SUBCUT 50 mg/wk or 25 mg 2×/wk, 3-4 days apart
- **Child 2-17 yr:** SUBCUT 0.8 mg/kg/wk, max 50 mg/wk

Plaque psoriasis
- **Adult:** SUBCUT 50 mg (Enbrel) 2×/wk × 3 mo, then 50 mg weekly maintenance or 50 mg (Erelzi) 2×/wk × 3 mo, then weekly
- **Child ≥4 yr and ≥63 kg:** SUBCUT 50 mg q wk
- **Child ≥4 yr and <63 kg:** SUBCUT (Enbrel or Eticoro) 0.8 mg/kg q wk
- **Child ≥2 yr and ≥63 kg:** SUBCUT 50 mg q wk
- **Child ≥2 yr and <63 kg:** SUBCUT 0.8 mg/kg q wk

Psoriatic arthritis (Enbrel only)
- **Adult:** SUBCUT 50 mg weekly

Available forms: Powder for injection 25 mg; injection 50 mg/mL; autoinjector, single use

Administer:
- May be administered by the patient or a caregiver
- The needle caps on the prefilled syringe and on the SureClick autoinjector contain dry natural rubber (latex) and should not be handled by persons sensitive to this product

Injectable route
• Inspect for particulate matter and discoloration prior to use, solution should be clear and colorless, small white particles may be seen in the autoinjector or prefilled syringe

Subcut route
• Injection sites include front of the thigh, abdomen except the 2 inches around the navel, or outer area of the upper arm; rotate injection sites; do not administer where skin is tender, bruised, red, or hard

• Do not mix or transfer the contents of one vial into another vial; do not filter reconstituted product during preparation or administration; do not add other medications to solutions containing etanercept; ONLY use the supplied diluent

• A vial adapter is supplied when reconstituting the powder; the adapter should not be used if multiple doses are to be withdrawn

• If the vial will be used for multiple doses, use a 25-gauge needle for reconstituting and withdrawing

• Use as soon as possible after reconstitution; place reconstituted vials for multiple doses in the refrigerator at 36° F-46° F (2° C-8° C) within 4 hr of reconstitution; may be stored up to 14 days; do not freeze

Use of the SureClick autoinjector
• Warm to room temperature, do not shake; immediately prior to use, remove the needle shield by pulling it straight off

Use of the prefilled syringe
• **Single-use:** warm to room temperature, do not shake; remove the needle shield

SIDE EFFECTS
CNS: *Headache,* asthenia, dizziness, seizures
CV: Heart failure
GI: Abdominal pain, dyspepsia, vomiting, hepatitis, diarrhea
HEMA: Pancytopenia, anemia, thrombocytopenia, leukopenia, neutropenia
INTEG: Rash, *injection site reaction,* keratoderma blenorrhagicum
RESP: *Pharyngitis, cough, URI, non-URI,* sinusitis, *rhinitis*
SYST: Serious infections, sepsis, death, malignancies, Stevens-Johnson syndrome, reactivation of hepatitis B virus, lupus-like syndrome

PHARMACOKINETICS
Elimination half-life 102 hr, 60% absorbed (SUBCUT)

INTERACTIONS
Increase: neutropenia—sulfaSALAzine
• Do not give concurrently with live virus vaccines; immunizations should be brought up to date before treatment
• Avoid use with anakinra, cyclophosphamide, rilonacept

Drug/lab
Increase: LFTs

NURSING CONSIDERATIONS
Assess:
• **RA:** pain, stiffness, ROM, swelling of joints prior to, during, after treatment

Black Box Warning: Secondary malignancy: assess for lymphoma and other neoplastic diseases in children and adolescents; avoid use in those with a history of malignancy

• For injection site pain, swelling; usually occurs after 2 injections (4-5 days)

Black Box Warning: Infection: patients using immunosuppressives, corticosteroids, methotrexate at greater risk; assess for fever, discontinue in serious infection; do not use in active infection; obtain TB testing prior to use; TB must be treated prior to use

• **Fungal infections:** Monitor for weight loss, sweating, cough, fever, serious illness, may occur after travel to areas with serious fungal infections
• **Labs:** Monitor CBC/differential baseline and periodically, if blood dyscrasias occur, discontinue
• **Hypersensitivity:** to this product, latex needle cap, benzyl alcohol; usual reactions to product last 3-5 days
• **Pregnancy/breastfeeding:** use only if clearly needed; use cautiously in breastfeeding; enroll in pregnancy surveillance program, Amgen (800-772-6436)

Evaluate:
• Therapeutic response: decreased inflammation, pain in joints

---

Side effects: *italics* = common; red = life-threatening

Teach patient/family:
• That product must be continued for prescribed time to be effective
• To use caution when driving; dizziness may occur
• Not to receive live vaccinations during treatment
• About self-administration if appropriate: injection should be made in thigh, abdomen, upper arm; rotate sites at least 1 inch from previous site, check for injection reactions that last 3-5 days
• To notify prescriber of possible infection (upper respiratory, other)

ethacrynate (Rx)

(eth-uh-KRIH′nayt)

Edecrin

Func. class.: Diuretic
Chem. class.: Loop diuretic

ACTIONS:

Primarily acts to inhibit the reabsorption of sodium and chloride in the ascending limb of the loop of Henle

USES:

Treatment of peripheral edema (idiopathic edema, lymphedema, or edema secondary to ascites, heart failure, or nephrotic syndrome)

CONTRAINDICATIONS

Hypersensitivity, acute myocardial infarction, anuria, breastfeeding, heart failure, pregnancy, renal failure
Precautions: Acid/base imbalance, breastfeeding, children, dehydration, diabetes mellitus, diarrhea, electrolyte imbalance, geriatric, gout, hearing impairment, hepatic disease, hepatic encephalopathy, hyperaldosteronism, hyperglycemia, hyperuricemia, hypocalcemia, hypochloremia, hypokalemia, hypomagnesemia, hypotension, hypovolemia, infants, metabolic alkalosis, orthostatic hypotension, pancreatitis, pregnancy, renal disease, renal failure, sympathectomy, syncope, systemic lupus erythematosus (SLE), ventricular arrhythmias

DOSAGE AND ROUTES

• **Adult: PO** initially, 50 to 100 mg/day divided once or twice daily. May increase by 25 to 50 mg/day, max dosage is 200 mg bid; **IV** initially, 50 mg or 0.5 to 1 mg/kg, usually 1 dose is sufficient, single doses more than 100 mg IV are not recommended
• **Children and adolescent: PO** initially, 0.5-1 mg/kg q6-12hr, may increase up to 3 mg/kg/day, 400 mg max adjust dosage at intervals of 2 to 3 days
• **Children and adolescent (unlabeled): IV** 1 to 2 mg/kg/dose q8-12hr, usual Max: 50 mg/dose
Available forms: Tablets 25 mg; injection 50 mg/vial
Administer
PO route
• Administer after meals
IV route
• Do not administer SUBCUT or IM because of local pain and irritation
• Reconstitute vial containing ethacrynate sodium equivalent to 50 mg of ethacrynic acid by adding 50 mL of 5% dextrose injection or 0.9% sodium chloride injection. The resulting IV solution contains the equivalent of 1 mg/mL of ethacrynic acid. If 5% dextrose injection with a pH ≤5 is used, a hazy or opalescent solution may develop and should not be used
• Infuse slowly IV over 20-30 min through freely running IV infusion or inject directly over several min

SIDE EFFECTS

CNS: Headache, confusion, fatigue, anxiety, vertigo, syncope
GI: Anorexia, GI bleeding, diarrhea, jaundice, nausea, pancreatitis, vomiting, increased LFTs
HEMA: Agranulocytosis, thrombocytopenia, neutropenia
GU: Azotemia, hematuria, polyuria, oliguria
EENT: Blurred vision, hearing loss
CV: Orthostatic hypotension, hypovolemia, tinnitus
META: Hyperglycemia, hyperuricemia, hypocalcemia, hypochloremia, hypokalemia, hypomagnesemia, hyponatremia
MISC: Fever, chills, injection site reaction, muscle cramps, rash

PHARMACOKINETICS
PO: Onset 30 min, peak 2 hr, duration 6-8 hr
IV: Onset rapid, peak 15-30 min, duration 2 hr
Half-life: 2-4 hr

INTERACTIONS
Increase: ototoxic effect—aminoglycosides, antibiotics, CISplatin
Increase: hypotension—antihypertensives
Increase: digoxin toxicity—cardiac glycosides, monitor drug level of digoxin
Increase: diuresis—thiazides
Increase: toxicity—lithium
Decrease: hypoglycemic effects—antidiabetics
Decrease: diuresis—NSAIDs
Drug/herb
Increase: effect—hawthorn, horse chestnut
Decrease: effect of bumetanide—ginseng, ephedra
Drug/lab
Increase: glucose
Decrease: chloride, potassium, sodium, calcium, phosphorus

NURSING CONSIDERATIONS
Assess:
• For tinnitus, hearing loss, ear pain; obtain audiometric testing for long-term IV treatment

Black Box Warning: Dehydration: weight, I&O daily to determine fluid loss; if urinary output decreases or azotemia occurs, product should be discontinued; safest dosage schedule is alternate days

• B/P lying, standing; postural hypotension may occur

Black Box Warning: Fluid and electrolyte depletion: potassium, sodium, calcium; include BUN, blood glucose, CBC, serum creatinine, blood pH, ABGs, uric acid, calcium, magnesium; severe electrolyte depletion should be corrected prior to starting treatment

• Blood glucose if patient is diabetic; blood uric acid levels in those with gout
• Improvement in edema of feet, legs, sacral area daily if medication is being used for HF
• **Signs of metabolic alkalosis:** drowsiness, restlessness
• **Hypokalemia:** postural hypotension, malaise, fatigue, tachycardia, leg cramps, weakness
• Rashes, temperature elevation daily
• Confusion, especially in geriatric patients; take safety precautions if needed
• Digoxin toxicity in patients taking digoxin products: anorexia, nausea, vomiting, confusion, paresthesia, muscle cramps; lithium toxicity in those taking lithium
• **Beers:** use cautiously in older adults; may cause or exacerbate syndrome of inappropriate antidiuretic hormone secretion
Evaluate:
• Therapeutic response: decreased edema, B/P
Teach patient/family:
• To increase fluid intake to 2-3 L/day unless contraindicated; to take potassium supplement; to rise slowly from lying or sitting position
• **To recognize adverse reactions:** muscle cramps, weakness, nausea, dizziness, edema, weight gain
• To take with food, milk for GI symptoms; to avoid alcohol
• To take early in day to prevent nocturia; if another dose is needed, take after noon, not to double or miss dose
• To take B/P, pulse, weight weekly
• That orthostatic hypotension may occur, to avoid rising rapidly
• To continue other medical regimens
• **Pregnancy/breastfeeding:** to report if pregnancy is planned or suspected or if breastfeeding
• That continuing exams and blood work will be needed
• To notify other health care professionals of condition being treated, medications taken

TREATMENT OF OVERDOSE
Lavage if taken orally; monitor electrolytes; administer dextrose in saline; monitor hydration, CV, renal status

---

ethambutol (Rx)
(e-tham′byoo-tole)
Etibi ✦, Myambutol
Func. class.: Antitubercular
Chem. class.: Diisopropylethylene diamide derivative

ACTION: Inhibits RNA synthesis, decreases tubercle bacilli replication

USES: Pulmonary TB as an adjunct, other mycobacterial infections

CONTRAINDICATIONS
Children <13 yr, hypersensitivity, optic neuritis
Precautions: Pregnancy, breastfeeding, renal disease, diabetic retinopathy, cataracts, ocular defects, hepatic and hematopoietic disorders

DOSAGE AND ROUTES
• **Adult/child >13 yr: PO** 15-25 mg/kg/day as single dose (treatment naive) or 25 mg/kg daily (treatment experienced)
Renal disease
• **Adult: PO** CCr 10-50 mL/min, dose q24-36hr; CCr <10 mL/min, dose q48hr
Retreatment
• **Adult: PO** 25 mg/kg/day as single dose × 2 mo with at least 1 other product, then decrease to 15 mg/kg/day as single dose, max 2.5 g/day
• **Child: PO** 15 mg/kg/day
Available forms: Tablets 100, 400 mg
Administer:
• With meals to decrease GI symptoms
• Antiemetic if vomiting occurs
• After C&S completed; monthly to detect resistance
• 4 hr between this product and antacids

SIDE EFFECTS
CNS: *Headache, confusion,* fever, malaise, dizziness, *disorientation,* hallucinations, peripheral neuropathy

EENT: Blurred vision, optic neuritis, photophobia, decreased visual acuity
GI: *Abdominal distress, anorexia, nausea, vomiting*
INTEG: Dermatitis, pruritus, toxic epidermal necrolysis, erythema multiforme
META: *Elevated uric acid, acute gout,* impaired hepatic function
MISC: Thrombocytopenia, joint pain, anaphylaxis

PHARMACOKINETICS
Peak 2-4 hr, half-life 3 hr, metabolized in liver, excreted in urine (unchanged product/inactive metabolites, unchanged product in feces)

INTERACTIONS
• Delayed absorption of ethambutol: aluminum salts, separate by 4 hr
• Neurotoxicity: other neurotoxics

NURSING CONSIDERATIONS
Assess:
• **TB:** Obtain C&S tests including sputum tests before initiating treatment; monitor monthly to detect resistance; lung sounds, amount and characteristics of sputum baseline and periodically
• Hepatic studies weekly × 2 wk, then q2mo: ALT, AST, bilirubin; decreased appetite, jaundice, dark urine, fatigue
• Signs of anemia: Hct, Hb, fatigue
• **Mental status often:** affect, mood, behavioral changes; psychosis may occur
• C&S, including sputum, prior to treatment
• **Visual status:** decreased acuity, altered color perception
• **Serious skin reactions:** toxic epidermal necrolysis
• **Pregnancy/breastfeeding:** use only if benefit outweighs risk to fetus; product appears in breast milk
Evaluate:
• Therapeutic response: decreased symptoms of TB, decrease in acid-fast bacteria, improving chest x-ray

Teach patient/family:
- To avoid alcohol products
- That compliance with dosage schedule, duration is necessary
- That scheduled appointments must be kept or relapse may occur
- To report to prescriber any visual changes; rash; hot, swollen, painful joints; numbness, tingling of extremities

⚠ HIGH ALERT

etoposide (Rx)
(e-toe-poe′side)
VePesid ✦

etoposide phosphate (Rx)
Etopophos
Func. class.: Antineoplastic—miscellaneous
Chem. class.: Semisynthetic podophyllotoxin

ACTION: Inhibits cells from entering mitosis, depresses DNA/RNA synthesis, cell-cycle–specific S and G_2; binds to a complex of DNA and topoisomerase II, leading to DNA strand breaks

USES: Testicular cancer, small cell lung cancer
Unlabeled uses: Leukemias (ALL, AML), desmoid tumor, gastric/ovarian cancer, bone marrow ablation, Hodgkin's/non-Hodgkin's lymphoma, malignant glioma, neuroblastoma, stem cell transplant preparation, trophoblastic disease

CONTRAINDICATIONS
Pregnancy, breastfeeding, hypersensitivity
Precautions: Children, renal/hepatic disease, gout, neutropenia, thrombocytopenia, infection, bleeding

Black Box Warning: Bone marrow depression, bleeding, infection; requires an experienced clinician

DOSAGE AND ROUTES
Testicular cancer
- **Adult:** IV 100 mg/m²/day on days 1, 2 in combination with bleomycin and CISplatin (BEP) or 100 mg/m²/day on days 1, 3, 5, repeat q3-4wk
Small cell lung carcinoma first-line treatment with CISplatin
- **Adult:** IV 50 mg/m²/day over 5 min-3.5 hr 5 days of a 21-day cycle
Renal dose
- **Adult:** IV CCr 45-60 mL/min, reduce dose by 15%; CCr 30-44 mL/min, reduce dose by 20%; CCr <30 mL/min, reduce dose by 25%
Hepatic dose
- **Adult:** IV/PO total bilirubin 1.5-2.9 mg/dL: reduce dose by 50%; total bilirubin 3-5 mg/dL: reduce dose by 75%; total bilirubin >5 mg/dL: hold

Available forms: Injection 20 mg/mL; 100 mg powder for injection, capsules 50 mg
Administer:
- Antiemetic 30-60 min prior to product and prn to prevent vomiting
Urate nephropathy
- Allopurinol, aggressive alkalinization to maintain uric acid levels
- Antispasmodic, EPINEPHrine, corticosteroids, antihistamines for reactions
PO route
- Give without regard to food
- Increase fluid intake to 2-3 L/day to prevent urate deposits, calculi formation
- Refrigerate oral product; do not freeze
IV route
- Do not use acrylic or ABS plastic devices; may crack, leak
Intermittent IV INFUSION route (etoposide)
- Use cytotoxic handling procedures, use Luer-Lok fittings to prevent leakage
- After **diluting** 5-mL vial with 100 mg/250 mL or more D₅W or NaCl to 0.2-0.4 mg/mL, **infuse** over 30-60 min

Y-site compatibilities: Acyclovir, alfentanil, allopurinol, amifostine, amikacin, aminocaproic acid, aminophylline, amiodarone, amphotericin B colloidal, amphotericin B lipid complex, amphotericin B liposome, ampicillin, ampicillin-sulbactam, anidulafungin, atenolol, atracurium, aztreonam, bivalirudin, bleomycin, bumetanide, buprenorphine, butorphanol, calcium chloride/gluconate, CARBOplatin, caspofungin, ceFAZolin, cefotaxime, cefoTEtan, cefOXitin, cefTAZidime, ceftizoxime, cefTRIAXone, cefuroxime, chloramphenicol, chlorproMAZINE, cimetidine, ciprofloxacin, cisatracurium, CISplatin, cladribine, clindamycin, codeine, cyclophosphamide, cycloSPORINE, cytarabine, DACTINomycin, DAPTOmycin, DAUNOrubicin, dexamethasone, dexmedetomidine, dexrazoxane, digoxin, dilTIAZem, diphenhydrAMINE, DOBUTamine, DOCEtaxel, DOPamine, doxacurium, DOXOrubicin, DOXOrubicin liposomal, doxycycline, droperidol, enalaprilat, ePHEDrine, EPINEPHrine, epirubicin, ertapenem, erythromycin, esmolol, famotidine, fenoldopam, fentaNYL, floxuridine, fluconazole, fludarabine, fluorouracil, foscarnet, fosphenytoin, furosemide, ganciclovir, gatifloxacin, gemcitabine, gentamicin, glycopyrrolate, granisetron, haloperidol, heparin, hydrALAZINE, hydrocortisone, HYDROmorphone, hydrOXYzine, ifosfamide, imipenem-cilastatin, inamrinone, insulin (regular), irinotecan, isoproterenol, ketorolac, labetalol, lansoprazole, leucovorin, levofloxacin, levorphanol, lidocaine, linezolid, LORazepam, magnesium sulfate, mannitol, mechlorethamine, melphalan, meperidine, meropenem, mesna, methohexital, methotrexate, methyldopate, methylPREDNISolone, metoclopramide, metoprolol, metroNIDAZOLE, micafungin, midazolam, milrinone, minocycline, mitoXANtrone, mivacurium, morphine, nafcillin, nalbuphine, naloxone, nesiritide, nitroglycerin, nitroprusside, norepinephrine, NS, octreotide, ofloxacin, ondansetron, oxaliplatin, PACLitaxel, palonosetron, pamidronate, pancuronium, PEMEtrexed, pentamidine, pentazocine, PENTobarbital, PHENobarbital, phenylephrine, piperacillin, piperacillin-tazobactam, polymyxin B, potassium chloride/phosphates, procainamide, prochlorperazine, promethazine, propranolol, quinupristin-dalfopristin, ranitidine, remifentanil, rocuronium, sargramostim, sodium acetate/bicarbonate/phosphates, succinylcholine, SUFentanil, sulfamethoxazole-trimethoprim, tacrolimus, teniposide, theophylline, thiotepa, ticarcillin, ticarcillin-clavulanate, tigecycline, tirofiban, tobramycin, topotecan, trimethobenzamide, vancomycin, vasopressin, vecuronium, verapamil, vinBLAStine, vinCRIStine, vinorelbine, voriconazole, zidovudine, zoledronic acid

Intermittent IV INFUSION route (etoposide phosphate)
- **Reconstitute** each vial with 5 or 10 mL of D_5W, 0.9% NaCl for concentrations of 20 mg/mL or 10 mg/mL, respectively; may give diluted or undiluted to concentrations of as little as 0.1 mg/mL, **give over 5-10 min**

Y-site compatibilities: Acyclovir, alfentanil, amifostine, amikacin, aminocaproic acid, aminophylline, amiodarone, ampicillin, ampicillin-sulbactam, anidulafungin, atenolol, atracurium, aztreonam, bivalirudin, bleomycin, bumetanide, buprenorphine, butorphanol, calcium acetate/chloride/gluconate, CARBOplatin, carmustine, caspofungin, ceFAZolin, cefonicid, cefoperazone, cefotaxime, cefoTEtan, cefOXitin, cefTAZidime, ceftizoxime, cefTRIAXone, cefuroxime, chloramphenicol, cimetidine, ciprofloxacin, cisatracurium, CISplatin, clindamycin, codeine, cyclophosphamide, cycloSPORINE, cytarabine, dacarbazine, DACTINomycin, DAPTOmycin, DAUNOrubicin, dexamethasone, digoxin, diltiazem, diphenhydrAMINE, DOBUTamine, DOCEtaxel, DOPamine, doripenem, doxacurium, DOXOrubicin, HCL/liposome, doxycycline, enalaprilat, ePHEDrine, EPINEPHrine, epirubicin, ertapenem, erythromycin, esmolol, famotidine, fenoldopam, fentaNYL, floxuridine, fluconazole, fludarabine, fluorouracil, foscarnet, fosphenytoin, furosemide, ganciclovir, gatifloxacin, gemcitabine, gentamicin, glycopyrrolate, granisetron, haloperidol, heparin, hydrALAZINE, hydrocortisone, HYDROmorphone, hydrOXYzine, IDArubicin, ifosfamide, inamrinone, insulin (regular), irinotecan, isoproterenol, ketorolac, labetalol, leucovorin, levofloxacin, levorphanol, lidocaine, linezolid, LORazepam, magnesium sulfate, mannitol, mechlorethamine, meperidine, meropenem, mesna, metaraminol, methotrexate, methyldopate, metoclopramide, metoprolol, metroNIDAZOLE, midazolam, milrinone, minocycline, mitoXANtrone, mivacurium, morphine, nafcillin, nalbuphine, naloxone, nesiritide, netilmicin, nitroglycerin, nitroprusside, norepinephrine, octreotide, ofloxacin, ondansetron, oxaliplatin, PACLitaxel, palonosetron, pamidronate, pancuronium, PEMEtrexed, pentamidine, pentazocine, PENTobarbital, PHENobarbital, phenylephrine, piperacillin, piperacillin-tazobactam, plicamycin, polymyxin B, potassium chloride/phosphates, procainamide, promethazine, propranolol, quiNIDine, quinupristin-dalfopristin, ranitidine, remifentanil, riTUXimab, rocuronium, sodium acetate/bicarbonate/phosphates, streptozocin, succinylcholine, SUFentanil, sulfamethoxazole-trimethoprim, tacrolimus, teniposide, theophylline, thiopental, thiotepa, ticarcillin, ticarcillin-clavulanate, tigecycline, tirofiban, tobramycin, tolazoline, trastuzumab, trimethobenzamide, vancomycin, vasopressin, vecuronium, verapamil, vinBLAStine, vinCRIStine, vinorelbine, voriconazole, zidovudine, zoledronic acid

SIDE EFFECTS

CNS: Headache, *fever,* peripheral neuropathy, paresthesias, confusion, chills, fever
CV: *Hypotension,* MI, dysrhythmias
GI: *Nausea, vomiting, anorexia,* hepatotoxicity, dyspepsia, diarrhea, constipation
GU: Nephrotoxicity

HEMA: Thrombocytopenia, leukopenia, myelosuppression, anemia
INTEG: *Rash, alopecia,* phlebitis at IV site, Stevens-Johnson syndrome
RESP: Bronchospasm
SYST: Anaphylaxis,   secondary malignancy

PHARMACOKINETICS
Half-life ½-2 hr (initial), terminal 5¼ hr, metabolized in liver, excreted in urine, feces, crosses placental barrier, protein binding 95%

INTERACTIONS
Increase: bone marrow depression—other antineoplastics, radiation, immunosuppressives
Increase: adverse reactions—live virus vaccines, toxoids
Increase: effect of etoposide, toxicity—voriconazole, conivaptan, cycloSPORINE, imatinib,   nilotinib,   etravirine, telithromycin
Increase: risk of bleeding—anticoagulants, NSAIDs, platelet inhibitors, thrombolytics, salicylate
Decrease: etoposide effect—sargramostim, filgrastim, separate by ≥24 hr
Drug/food
Decreased oral etoposide—grapefruit juice
Drug/lab
Decrease: platelets, RBC, WBC, neutrophils, Hb, calcium, phosphate
Increase: uric acid, potassium

NURSING CONSIDERATIONS
Assess:

Black Box Warning: Bone marrow depression: CBC, differential, platelet count weekly; withhold product if WBC is <500/mm^3 or platelet count is <50,000/mm^3; notify prescriber, treatment should be delayed

• **Nephrotoxicity:** BUN; serum uric acid; urine CCr; electrolytes prior to, during therapy; I&O ratio; report fall in urine output to <30 mL/hr; check B/P bid, report any significant decrease

Black Box Warning: **Infection:** monitor temperature, fever may indicate beginning infection; treat active infection before treatment

• **Hepatotoxicity:** hepatic studies prior to, during therapy (bilirubin, AST, ALT, LDH) as needed or monthly; monitor jaundice of skin and sclera, dark urine, clay-colored stools, itchy skin, abdominal pain, fever, diarrhea

Black Box Warning: **Bleeding:** hematuria, guaiac stools, bruising or petechiae, mucosa or orifices q8hr

• Effects of alopecia on body image; discuss feelings about body changes
• B/P q15min during infusion; if systolic reading <90 mm Hg, discontinue infusion, notify prescriber
• Buccal cavity q8hr for dryness, sores or ulceration, white patches, oral pain, bleeding, dysphagia
• **Injection site reaction:** monitor site closely for infiltration
• Local irritation, pain, burning, discoloration at injection site
• **Symptoms indicating severe allergic reaction:** rash, pruritus, urticaria, purpuric skin lesions, itching, flushing, restlessness, coughing, difficulty breathing
• **Frequency of stools, characteristics:** cramping, acidosis
• **Signs of dehydration:** rapid respirations, poor skin turgor, decreased urine output, dry skin, restlessness, weakness
• **Geriatric patients:** increased alopecia, GI effects, infection, nephrotoxicity, myelosuppression

Black Box Warning: An experienced clinician knowledgeable in the use of cytotoxic products

• **Pregnancy/breastfeeding:** do not use in pregnancy, breastfeeding unless benefits to mother outweigh risk to fetus

Evaluate:
• **Therapeutic response:** decreased tumor size, spread of malignancy
Teach patient/family:
• To report any changes in breathing or coughing
• That hair may be lost during treatment; that a wig or hairpiece may make patient feel better; that new hair may be different in color, texture
• That metallic taste may occur
• **Infection:** to report symptoms of infection (fever, sore throat); to avoid crowds, persons with known infections
• To avoid immunizations
• **Pregnancy/breastfeeding:** to notify prescriber if pregnancy is planned or suspected; to use reliable contraception during and for several months after therapy; to avoid breastfeeding
• To take as prescribed (PO), not to double dose
• To report signs of infection (flu-like symptoms, fever, fatigue, sore throat)
• To check B/P, hypotension occurs

---

etravirine (Rx)

(e-tra'veer-een)

Intelence

Func. class.: Antiretroviral
Chem. class.: Nonnucleoside reverse transcriptase inhibitor (NNRTI)

ACTION: Binds directly to reverse transcriptase, thus blocking the RNA- and DNA-dependent DNA polymerase action and causing a disruption of the enzyme's catalytic site

USES: In combination with other antiretroviral agents for HIV infection in treatment-experienced patients with evidence of HIV replication despite ongoing antiretroviral therapy

---

CONTRAINDICATIONS

Breastfeeding, hypersensitivity

Precautions: Pregnancy, children, geriatric patients, impaired hepatic function, antimicrobial resistance, hepatitis, hypercholesterolemia, hypertriglycerides, immune reconstitution syndrome

DOSAGE AND ROUTES

- **Adult/child/adolescent ≥6 yr, ≥30 kg:** PO 200 mg bid
- **Child/adolescent ≥6 yr, 25 to 29 kg:** PO 150 mg bid
- **Child/adolescent ≥6 yr, 20 to 24 kg:** PO 125 mg bid
- **Child/adolescent ≥6 yr, 16 to 19 kg:** PO 100 mg bid

Available forms: Tablets 25, 100, 200 mg
Administer:

- In combination with other antiretrovirals with food or after a meal
- Tablets may be dispersed in ≥5 mL of water; once dispersed, stir well, give immediately, rinse glass, have patient drink to ensure all medication taken
- Store in cool environment; protect from light

SIDE EFFECTS

CNS: *Headache, insomnia,* amnesia, anxiety, confusion, fatigue, nightmares, peripheral neuropathy, seizures, stroke, tremor
CV: Atrial fibrillation, hypertension, MI
EENT: Blurred vision
GI: *Nausea, vomiting, diarrhea, anorexia,* abdominal pain, increased AST/ALT, constipation, flatulence, gastritis, GERD, hematemesis, hepatitis, hepatomegaly, pancreatitis
GU: Renal failure
HEMA: Hemolytic anemia, neutropenia, thrombocytopenia, anemia
INTEG: *Rash,* erythema multiforme, angioedema, Stevens-Johnson syndrome
MS: Rhabdomyolysis
OTHER: Diabetes mellitus, gynecomastia, hyperamylasemia, hypercholesterolemia, hyperglycemia, hyperlipidemia
RESP: Dyspnea, bronchospasm
SYST: DRESS

PHARMACOKINETICS

99.9% plasma protein binding; metabolized by CYP3A4, 2C9, 2C19; half-life 21-61 hr; excreted in feces

INTERACTIONS

- Do not use concurrently with atazanavir, carBAMazepine, delavirdine, fosamprenavir, fosphenytoin, phenytoin, PHENobarbital, rifapentine, rifAMPin, tipranavir, rilpivirine
- Altered effect of cycloSPORINE, tacrolimus, sirolimus

Increase: myopathy, rhabdomyolysis—HMG-CoA reductase inhibitors
Increase: etravirine levels—CYP3A4 inhibitors (fluconazole, itraconazole, ketoconazole, lopinavir, posaconazole, ritonavir, voriconazole)
Increase: withdrawal symptoms—methadone
Increase: levels of diazePAM, rifAMPin, voriconazole, warfarin
Decrease: levels of CYP3A4 inducers (amiodarone, atazanavir, clarithromycin, flecainide, fosamprenavir, lidocaine, mexiletine, propafenone, quiNIDine, sildenafil, tadalafil, vardenafil)
Decrease: etravirine levels—darunavir, dexamethasone, disopyramide, efavirenz, nevirapine, ritonavir, saquinavir, tipranavir

Drug/herb
Decrease: etravirine—St. John's wort

NURSING CONSIDERATIONS

Assess:

- **Symptoms of HIV, possible infections:** increased temperature
- **HIV:** monitor viral load, CD4 counts, plasma HIV RNA during treatment; watch for decreasing granulocytes, Hb; if low, therapy may have to be discontinued and restarted after hematologic recovery; blood transfusions may be required; cholesterol/lipid profile
- **Fatal hypersensitivity reactions:** fever, rash, nausea, vomiting, fatigue, cough, dyspnea, diarrhea, abdominal discomfort; treatment should be discontinued and not restarted; incidence of rash may be worse in women

E

- **Blood dyscrasias (anemia, granulo-cytopenia):** bruising, fatigue, bleeding, poor healing
- **Renal failure:** BUN; serum uric acid; CCr prior to, during therapy; may be elevated throughout treatment
- **Hepatitis/pancreatitis:** hepatic studies prior to and during therapy: bilirubin, AST, ALT, amylase, alkaline phosphatase, creatine phosphokinase, creatinine, monthly
- **Pregnancy/breastfeeding:** use only if benefits outweigh risk; enroll pregnant patients in the Antretroviral Pregnancy Registry (800-258-4263); do not breastfeed

Evaluate:
- Therapeutic response: increased CD4 count, decreased viral load

Teach patient/family:
- That product is not a cure but will control symptoms; that patient is still infective, may pass AIDS virus to others
- To notify prescriber of sore throat, swollen lymph nodes, malaise, fever; other infections may occur; to stop product and notify prescriber immediately if skin rash, fever, cough, SOB, GI symptoms occur; to advise all health care providers that allergic reaction has occurred with etravirine
- That follow-up visits must be continued, since serious toxicity may occur; blood counts must be performed
- To use contraception during treatment; that patient is still able to transmit disease
- About information on medication guide and warning card; discuss points on guide
- That other products may be necessary to prevent other infections
- To take medication after a meal

⚠ HIGH ALERT

everolimus (Rx)
(e-ve-ro'li-mus)

Afinitor, Afinitor Disperz, Zortress
Func. class.: Antineoplastic—miscellaneous
Chem. class.: Kinase inhibitor

Do not confuse:
everolimus/sirolimus/tacrolimus/temsirolimus

ACTION: Proliferation signal inhibitor that inhibits mammalian target of rapamycin (mTOR); this pathway is dysregulated in cancer

USES: Renal cell cancer in those with failed treatment with SORAfenib or SUNItinib kidney transplant rejection prophylaxis with cycloSPORINE, subependymal giant cell astrocytoma, progressive pancreatic neuroendocrine tumor (PNET) with unresectable locally advanced/metastatic disease, breast cancer hormone receptor–positive/HER-2 negative, renal angiomyolipoma, tuberous sclerosis complex, liver transplant rejection prophylaxis

CONTRAINDICATIONS
Breastfeeding; hypersensitivity to this product, Rapamune, Torisel, pregnancy, CYP3A4 inhibitors, severe hepatic disease, breast cancer, functional carcinoid tumors

Precautions: Children, renal/hepatic disease, diabetes mellitus, hyperlipidemia, pleural effusion

> **Black Box Warning:** Immunosuppression, infection, renal artery thrombosis, renal impairment, renal vein thrombosis, neoplastic disease, heart transplant

DOSAGE AND ROUTES
Prophylaxis (Zortress)
- **Adult:** PO 0.75 mg q12hr with cycloSPORINE in combination with basiliximab, corticosteroids, reduced doses of cycloSPORINE

Liver transplant rejection prophylaxis
- **Adult:** PO 1 mg bid starting at least 30 days after transplant in combination with reduced-dose tacrolimus and corticosteroids

Advanced renal cancer (Afinitor)
- **Adult:** PO 10 mg daily as long as clinically beneficial; with strong 3A4 in-

ducers 10 mg daily, then may increase by 5-mg increments to 20 mg daily

Progressive neuroendocrine tumor (PNET) (Afinitor only)

• **Adult: PO** 10 mg daily, reduce dose to 5 mg daily if intolerable adverse reactions occur

Subependymal giant-cell astrocytoma (SEGA) (Afinitor only)

• **Adult/adolescent/child:** 4.5 mg/m^2 daily, then titrate to a target trough of 5-15 ng/mL

Hepatic dose

• **Adult:** PO (Child-Pugh A) Afinitor: 7.5 mg/day; (Child-Pugh B) Afinitor: 5 mg/day, Zortress: 0.75 mg/day divided q12hr; (Child-Pugh C) Afinitor: 2.5 mg/day

Available forms: Tablets 0.25, 0.5, 0.75 mg (Zortress); 2.5, 5, 7.5, 10 mg (Afinitor); tablets for oral suspension 2, 3, 5 mg (Afinitor Disperg)

Administer:

Follow procedure for proper handling of antineoplastics

• Swallow tablets whole with a full glass of water; do not chew, crush, or break

• **Afinitor:** take at same time of day; if unable to swallow, consistently with or without food, disperse in 30 mL of water

• **Zortress:** must take consistently with/without food, give at same time of day q12hr with cycloSPORINE

• Store protected from light at room temperature

Afinitor adjustments for toxicity

Noninfectious pneumonitis

• **Grade 1:** asymptomatic with radiographic findings only: no dosage change

• **Grade 2:** symptomatic but no interference with activities of daily living (ADLs): consider withholding therapy, resume Afinitor at a lower dosage when symptoms improve to ≤grade 1; discontinue Afinitor if symptoms do not improve within 4 wk

• **Grade 3:** symptomatic and interfering with ADL and oxygen therapy indicated: hold therapy; consider resuming Afinitor at a lower dosage when symptoms improve to ≤grade 1; consider discontinuing Afinitor if grade 3 toxicity recurs

• **Grade 4:** life-threatening and ventilator support indicated: discontinue therapy

Stomatitis

• **Grade 1:** minimum symptoms and normal diet: no dosage adjustment required

• **Grade 2:** symptomatic but can eat and swallow modified diet: hold therapy until symptoms improve to ≤grade 1 and resume Afinitor at the same dosage; if grade 2 toxicity recurs, hold therapy and resume Afinitor at a lower dosage when symptoms improve to ≤grade 1

• **Grade 3:** symptomatic and unable to adequately eat or hydrate orally: hold therapy; resume Afinitor at a lower dosage when symptoms improve to ≤grade 1

• **Grade 4:** symptomatic and life-threatening: discontinue therapy

Other nonhematologic toxicity (excluding metabolic events)

• **Grade 1:** no dosage adjustment required if toxicity is tolerable

• **Grade 2:** no dosage adjustment required if toxicity is tolerable; if toxicity is intolerable, hold therapy until symptoms improve to ≤grade 1 and resume Afinitor at the same dosage; if grade 2 toxicity recurs, hold therapy and resume Afinitor at a lower dosage when symptoms improve to ≤grade 1

• **Grade 3:** hold therapy; consider resuming Afinitor at a lower dosage when symptoms improve to ≤grade 1; if grade 3 toxicity recurs, consider discontinuing therapy

• **Grade 4:** discontinue Afinitor therapy

Metabolic events (hyperglycemia, dyslipidemia)

• **Grade 1 or 2:** no dose adjustment required

• **Grade 3:** temporarily withhold therapy; resume Afinitor at a lower dosage

• **Grade 4:** discontinue Afinitor therapy

• **Afinitor Disperz (oral suspension):** wear gloves when preparing, use 10-mL syringe and place dose in syringe, do not crush, break, using 5-mL water and 4-mL air draw into syringe with dose, wait a few minutes until in suspension after use, use same amount of water and air, swirl, give contents

SIDE EFFECTS

CNS: *Headache, insomnia, paresthesia,* chills, fever, seizure, personality changes, insomnia, dizziness, weakness, fatigue

CV: *Hypertension, peripheral edema*

EENT: Blurred vision, photophobia, eyelid edema, epistaxis, sinusitis, cataracts, conjunctivitis

GI: Nausea, vomiting, diarrhea, constipation, stomatitis, anorexia, abdominal pain, dysgeusia, hepatic artery thrombosis

GU: Renal failure, UTI, infertility

HEMA: Anemia, leukopenia, thrombocytopenia, hemolytic uremic syndrome, thrombotic microangiopathy, thrombotic thrombocytopenia, purpura

INTEG: *Rash, acne,* leukocytoclastic vasculitis

META: Hyperglycemia, increased creatinine, *hyperlipidemia,* hypophosphatemia, weight loss, hypertriglyceridemia

RESP: Pleural effusion

SYST: Angioedema, anaphylaxis, lymphoma

PHARMACOKINETICS

Rapidly, well absorbed; peak 1-2 hr; protein binding 74%; extensively metabolized by CYP3A4 enzyme system, P-gp; half-life 30 hr; reduced by high-fat meal; excreted in feces (80%), urine (5%)

INTERACTIONS

Black Box Warning: Increase: nephrotoxicity—immunosuppressants

Increase: everolimus effect—CYP3A4 inhibitors (strong, moderate), antifungals, calcium channel blockers, cimetidine, danazol, erythromycin, cycloSPORINE, HIV-protease inhibitors

Decrease: everolimus effect—CYP3A4 inducers, carBAMazepine, PHENobarbital, phenytoin, rifamycin, rifapentine

Decrease: effect of live vaccines

Drug/herb

St. John's wort: may decrease effect of everolimus

Drug/food

Alters bioavailability; use consistently with/without food; do not use with grapefruit juice

Drug/lab

Increase: bilirubin, calcium, cholesterol, glucose, potassium, lipids, phosphate, triglycerides, uric acid

Decrease: calcium, glucose, potassium, magnesium, phosphate

NURSING CONSIDERATIONS

Assess:

• **Lipid profile:** cholesterol, triglycerides, lipid-lowering agent may be needed; blood glucose

Black Box Warning: Immunosuppression: CBC with differential during treatment monthly; if leukocytes <3000/mm^3 or platelets <100,000/mm^3, product should be discontinued or reduced; decreased hemoglobin level may indicate bone marrow suppression

• **Hepatic/renal studies:** AST, ALT, amylase, bilirubin, creatinine, phosphate, and for hepatotoxicity: dark urine, jaundice, itching, light-colored stools; product should be discontinued

• **Pneumonitis:** continuing cough, dyspnea, pleural effusion baseline and during treatment, use corticosteroids if needed, if severe, reduce dose or discontinue

Black Box Warning: Infection: bacterial fungal infections can occur and are more common with combination immunosuppression therapy; assess for fever, cough, dyspnea, fatigue

Black Box Warning: May result in graft loss within 30 days after transplantation

• Obtain everolimus blood levels in kidney transplant, hepatic disease, CYP3A4 inducers, inhibitors

• **Pregnancy/breastfeeding:** avoid in pregnancy; use adequate contraception during and for 12 wk after final dose; report exposure to the National Transplant Pregnancy Registry (877-955-6877); do not breastfeed

Evaluate:
• Therapeutic response: decreased spread of tumor; prevention of transplant rejection

Teach patient/family:

Black Box Warning: To report fever, rash, severe diarrhea, chills, sore throat, fatigue; serious infections may occur; to report clay-colored stools, cramping (hepatotoxicity)

Black Box Warning: To avoid crowds, persons with known infections to reduce risk for infection

• Not to use with grapefruit juice
• To avoid individuals recently vaccinated with live vaccines; children may require accelerated vaccine schedule before treatment
• That frequent lab tests are required
• That product may decrease male, female fertility
• That drinking alcohol is not recommended
• To take consistently with or without food
• To report vision changes, weight gain, edema, shortness of breath, impaired wound healing
• **Pregnancy:** to notify prescriber if pregnancy is planned or suspected; to use contraception prior to, during, and 12 wk after product discontinued; to avoid breastfeeding

evolocumab (Rx)

(e′-voe-lok′-ue-mab)

Repatha

Func. class.: Antilipemic
Chem. class.: Proprotein convertase subtilisin/kexin type 9 (PCSK9) inhibitor

ACTION: Binds to low-density lipoproteins, a human monoclonal antibody (IgG1)

USES: Heterozygous, familial hypercholesterolemia, atherosclerotic disease

CONTRAINDICATIONS
Hypersensitivity
Precautions: Pregnancy, breastfeeding, latex sensitivity

DOSAGE AND ROUTES
Primary hyperlipidemia with established clinical atherosclerosis:
• **Adult: SUBCUT** 140 mg q2wk or 420 mg monthly
Homozygous familial hypercholesterolemia:
• **Adult/adolescent: SUBCUT** 420 mg monthly
Heterozygous familial hypercholesterolemia
Child ≥10 yr: SUBCUT 140 mg q2wk or 420 mg q mo
Disorder of CV system, secondary prophylaxis and primary hypercholesterolemia, alone or in combination with other lipid-lowering therapies
• **Adult: SUBCUT** 140 mg q2wk or 420 mg monthly
Available forms: Autoinjector 140 mg/mL, solutions for injection 120 mg/mL, 140 mg/mL
Administer:
• Visually inspect for particulate matter and discoloration; solution is clear, colorless to pale yellow
SUBCUT route
Prefilled syringe or SureClick autoinjector
• If stored in the refrigerator, warm to room temperature for ≥30 min prior to use. Do not shake
• Give into areas of the abdomen (except for a 2-inch area around the umbilicus), thigh, or upper arm that are not tender, bruised, red, or indurated
• To use the 420-mg dose, give 3 injections consecutively within 30 min
• Rotate the site with each injection
• Do not administer with other injectable drugs at the same injection site

Prefilled syringe administration
• Do not pick up or pull the prefilled syringe by the plunger rod or gray needle cap. Hold the syringe by the barrel
• Pull the gray needle cap off. It is normal to see a drop of solution at the end of the needle. Do not remove any air bubbles in the syringe
• Pinch the skin injection site to create a firm surface approximately 2 inches wide. Hold the pinch, and insert the needle into the skin using a 45- to 90-degree angle
• Push the plunger rod all the way down until the syringe is empty
• When done, release the plunger and gently lift the syringe off skin

SureClick autoinjector administration
• Do not remove the orange cap until you are ready to inject
• Pull the orange cap off
• Firmly push down onto the skin when ready to inject; press the gray button. A click should be heard. Keep pushing on the skin and then lift the thumb. The injection could take about 15 sec

SIDE EFFECTS
CV: Hypertension
MS: *Myalgia, back pain, muscle spasms*
INTEG: Pruritus, injection site reaction, erythema, rash

PHARMACOKINETICS
Absorption 40%, distribution extensive, metabolism liver (CYP3A4), excretion urine, feces; onset 4 hr, peak 3-7 days; half-life 2-3 days

INTERACTIONS
None known
Drug/lab
Increase: LFTs
Decrease: cholesterol

NURSING CONSIDERATIONS
Assess:
• **Hypercholesterolemia:** diet history: fat content, lipid levels (triglycerides, LDL, HDL, cholesterol); LFTs at baseline, periodically during treatment

• **Hypersensitivity:** Monitor for rash, itching; also latex allergy; injector contains latex
• **Pregnancy/breastfeeding:** no well-controlled studies; use only if benefits outweigh fetal risk; cautious use in breastfeeding, excretion is unknown
Evaluate:
• Therapeutic response: decreased cholesterol, LDL; increased HDL
Teach patient/family:
• That compliance is needed
• That risk factors should be decreased: high-fat diet, smoking, alcohol consumption, absence of exercise
• To notify prescriber if pregnancy suspected, planned, or if breastfeeding
• To report confusion, injection site reactions

exemestane (Rx)
(ex-em′eh-stane)
Aromasin
Func. class.: Antineoplastic
Chem. class.: Aromatase inhibitor

USES: Advanced breast carcinoma not responsive to other therapy (postmenopausal), estrogen receptor–positive early breast cancer that has received tamoxifen

CONTRAINDICATIONS
Pregnancy, breastfeeding, premenopausal women, hypersensitivity

DOSAGE AND ROUTES
• **Adult: PO** 25 mg/day after meals; may need 50 mg/day if taken with a potent CYP3A4 inducer
Available forms: Tablets 25 mg

⚠ HIGH ALERT

exenatide (Rx)
(ex-en′a-tide)
Bydureon BCise, Byetta
Func. class.: Antidiabetic
Chem. class.: Incretin mimetic

ACTION: Binds and activates known human GLP-1 receptor, mimics natural physiology for self-regulating glycemic control

USES: Type 2 diabetes mellitus given in combination with metFORMIN, a sulfonylurea, thiazolidinedione, insulin glargine

CONTRAINDICATIONS
Hypersensitivity

Black Box Warning: Medullary thyroid carcinoma, multiple endocrine neoplasia syndrome type 2 (MEN-2), thyroid cancer

Precautions: Pregnancy, geriatric patients, severe renal/hepatic/GI disease, pancreatitis, vit D deficiency

DOSAGE AND ROUTES
• **Adult: SUBCUT** 5 mcg bid 1 hr prior to morning and evening meal; may increase to 10 mcg bid after 1 mo; extended release **SUBCUT (Bydureon)** 2 mg q7days
Renal dose
• **Adult:** PO CCr 30-50 mL/min, use caution when increasing dose
Available forms: Injection 5, 10 mcg pen; extended-release powder for suspension for injection 2 mg; Injection: 2 mg/dose single-dose pen
Administer:
Store in refrigerator for unopened pen; may store at room temperature after opening for up to 30 days
SUBCUT route (regular release—Byetta)
• May be used as monotherapy or combined with other products
• SUBCUT only, do not give IV/IM
• Pen needles must be purchased separately, compatible; prime prior to use; inject into thigh, abdomen, upper arm; rotate sites
• Product 1 hr prior to meals, approximately 6 hr apart; if patient is NPO, may need to hold dose to prevent hypoglycemia
• If added to insulin glargine, insulin, or detemir, a dosage reduction in these products may be required
SUBCUT route (extended release—Bydureon)

• Give every 7 days (weekly); the dose can be given at any time of day without regard to meals
• Available as a single-dose tray containing a vial of 2 mg, a prefilled syringe delivering 0.65 mL diluent, a vial connector, and 2 custom needles (23G × 5/16′) specific to this delivery system (one is a spare needle); do not substitute needles or any other components
• Inject immediately after the white to off-white powder is suspended in the diluent and transferred to the syringe
• Inject SUBCUT into the thigh, abdomen, or upper arm, rotate sites to prevent lipodystrophy

SIDE EFFECTS
CNS: *Headache, dizziness,* feeling jittery, restlessness, weakness
ENDO: Hypoglycemia, thyroid hyperplasia
GI: Nausea, vomiting, diarrhea, dyspepsia, anorexia, gastroesophageal reflux, weight loss, pancreatitis
SYST: Angioedema, anaphylaxis
INTEG: Serious injection site reactions (cellulitis, abscess, skin necrosis)

PHARMACOKINETICS
Absorption well, immediate release: peak 2.1 hr, elimination by glomerular filtration, half-life 2.4 hr; extended release: peak 2 wk

INTERACTIONS
• May decrease effect of acetaminophen
• Do not use with erythromycin, metoclopramide
Increase: hypoglycemia—ACE inhibitors, disopyramide, sulfonylureas, androgens, fibric acid derivatives, alcohol
Increase: hyperglycemia—phenothiazines, corticosteroids, anabolic steroids
Decrease: action of digoxin, lovastatin, acetaminophen (elixir)
Decrease: efficacy—niacin, dextrothyroxine, thiazide diuretics, triamterene, estrogens, progestins, oral contraceptives, MAOIs

NURSING CONSIDERATIONS
Assess:

• Fasting blood glucose, A1c levels, postprandial glucose during treatment to determine diabetes control

• **Pancreatitis:** severe abdominal pain with or without vomiting, product should be discontinued

> **Black Box Warning:** Increased risk of thyroid tumors (medullary C-cell tumors)

• **Anaphylaxis, angioedema:** product should be discontinued immediately

• Renal studies: urinalysis, creatinine

• Hypo/hyperglycemic reaction that can occur soon after meals; for severe hypoglycemia, give IV $D_{50}W$, then IV dextrose solution

• Nausea, vomiting, diarrhea, ability to tolerate product, may cause dehydration

• **Pregnancy/breastfeeding:** use only if benefits clearly outweigh risks; if pregnant, enroll in the Exenatide Pregnancy Registry (800-633-9081); do not breastfeed

Evaluate:

• Therapeutic response: decrease in polyuria, polydipsia, polyphagia, clear sensorium, improving A1c, weight; absence of dizziness, stable gait

Teach patient/family:

• About the symptoms of hypo/hyperglycemia, what to do about each; to have glucagon emergency kit available; to carry a glucose source (candy, sugar cube) to treat hypoglycemia

• That product must be continued on a daily or weekly basis (extended release); about consequences of discontinuing product abruptly

• That diabetes is a lifelong illness; that product will not cure disease; to carry emergency ID with prescriber and medication information

• To continue weight control, dietary restrictions, exercise, hygiene

• That regular blood glucose monitoring and A1c testing are needed

• To notify prescriber if pregnant or intending to become pregnant

• About the importance of reading "Information for the Patient" and "Pen User Manual"; about self-injection

• **Pancreatitis:** if severe abdominal pain with or without vomiting occurs, seek medical attention immediately

• To review injection procedure; to store product in refrigerator, room temperature after first use; discard 30 days after first use; do not freeze; to protect from light (Byetta)

---

ezetimibe (Rx)

(ehz-eh-tim′bee)

Ezetrol ♣, Zetia

Func. class.: Antilipemic; cholesterol absorption inhibitor

ACTION: Inhibits absorption of cholesterol by the small intestine, causes reduced hepatic cholesterol stores

USES: Hypercholesterolemia, homozygous familial hypercholesterolemia (HoFH), homozygous sitosterolemia

CONTRAINDICATIONS

Hypersensitivity, severe hepatic disease

Precautions: Pregnancy, breastfeeding, children, hepatic disease

DOSAGE AND ROUTES

• **Adult/adolescent/child >10 yr: PO** 10 mg/day

Available forms: Tablets 10 mg

Administer:

• Without regard to meals

• Separate by ≥2 hr prior to or ≥4 hr after bile acid sequestrant, may use with HMG-CoA reductase inhibitors

SIDE EFFECTS

CNS: Fatigue, dizziness, headache

GI: Diarrhea, abdominal pain

MISC: Chest pain

MS: *Myalgias, arthralgias,* back pain, myopathy, rhabdomyolysis

RESP: Pharyngitis, sinusitis, cough, *URI*

EENT: Sinusitis, nasopharyngitis

SYST: Angioedema

PHARMACOKINETICS
Absorption variable, metabolized in small intestine, liver; excreted in feces 78%, urine 11%; peak 4-12 hr; half-life 22 hr

INTERACTIONS
Increase: action of ezetimibe—fibric acid derivatives, cycloSPORINE
Decrease: action of ezetimibe—antacids, bile acid sequestrants
Drug/lab
Increase: LFTs

NURSING CONSIDERATIONS
Assess:
• **Hypercholestrolemia:** diet history: fat content, lipid levels (triglycerides, LDL, HDL, cholesterol); LFTs at baseline, periodically during treatment
• **Myopathy/rhabdomyolysis:** increased CPK, myalgia, muscle cramps, musculoskeletal pain, lethargy, fatigue, fever; more common when combined with statins
• **Pregnancy/breastfeeding:** do not use in pregnancy, breastfeeding
Evaluate:
• Therapeutic response: decreased cholesterol, LDL; increased HDL
Teach patient/family:
• That compliance is needed

• That risk factors should be decreased: high-fat diet, smoking, alcohol consumption, absence of exercise
• To notify prescriber if pregnancy suspected, planned, or if breastfeeding
• To notify prescriber if unexplained weakness, muscle pain present
• To notify prescriber of dietary/herbal supplements

ezetimibe/simvastatin (Rx)
(ehz-eh-tim′bee/sim′va-sta-tin)
Vytorin
Func. class.: Antilipemic; cholesterol absorption inhibitor

USES: Hypercholesterolemia, homozygous familial hypercholesterolemia (HoFH), homozygous sitosterolemia

CONTRAINDICATIONS
Hypersensitivity, severe hepatic disease
Precautions: Pregnancy, breastfeeding, children, hepatic disease

DOSAGE AND ROUTES
• **Adult: PO** 1 tablet/day in the evening
Available forms: Tablets 10-10, 10-20, 10-40, 10-80

factor IX complex (Rx)
Profilnine, Profilnine SD
factor IX, human (Rx)
Alphanine SD, Mononine
factor IX, recombinant (Rx)
Alprolix, BeneFIX, Ixinity, Rixubis
Func. class.: Clotting factor

USES: Factor IX deficiency (hemophilia B [Christmas disease])

DOSAGE AND ROUTES
• **Adult:** IV Individualized, check manufacturer's guidelines
Available forms: Injection

factor Xa (Rx)
Andexxa
Func. class.: Antidote

USES: For rivaroxaban reversal and apixaban reversal in patients with life-threatening or uncontrolled bleeding

CONTRAINDICATIONS
None

DOSAGE AND ROUTES
Dose based on specific factor Xa inhibitor, dose of factor Xa inhibitor, and time since the patient's last dose of factor Xa inhibitor
• **Adult:** IV For rivaroxaban ≤10 mg or apixaban ≤5 mg within 8 hr or unknown timing of last dose or for any dose of rivaroxaban or apixaban at 8 hr or more since timing of last dose, 400 mg **IV BOL** at 30 mg/min then 4 mg/min **CONT IV INFUSION** for up to 120 min
• **Adult:** IV For rivaroxaban >10 mg, apixaban >5 mg, or unknown dose of either drug within 8 hr of timing of last dose, 800 mg **IV BOL** at 30 mg/min followed by 8 mg/min **CONT IV INFUSION** for up to 120 min. Resume anticoagulant therapy as soon as medically appropriate after factor Xa treatment
Available forms: Powder for injection 100, 200 mg

famciclovir (Rx)
(fam-cy'clo-veer)
Func. class.: Antiviral
Chem. class.: Guanosine nucleoside

ACTION: Inhibits DNA polymerase and viral DNA synthesis by conversion of this guanosine nucleoside to penciclovir

USES: Treatment of acute herpes zoster (shingles), genital herpes; recurrent mucocutaneous herpes simplex virus (HSV) in patients with HIV; initial episodes of herpes genitalis; herpes labialis in the immunocompromised, herpes labialis prophylaxis
Unlabeled uses: Herpes simplex virus, varicella infection (chickenpox) in HIV

CONTRAINDICATIONS
Hypersensitivity to this product, penciclovir, acyclovir, ganciclovir, valacyclovir, valganciclovir
Precautions: Pregnancy, breastfeeding, renal disease, lactose intolerance, child, geriatrics

DOSAGE AND ROUTES
Acute herpes zoster (shingles)
• **Adult:** PO 500 mg q8hr for 7 days
Renal dose
• **Adult:** PO CCr 40-59 mL/min, 500 mg q12hr; CCr 20-39 mL/min, 500 mg q24hr; CCr <20 mL/min, 250 mg q24hr
Suppression of recurrent herpes simplex
• **Adult:** PO 250 mg q12hr up to 1 yr
Renal dose
• **Adult:** PO CCr 20-39 mL/min, 125 mg q12hr × 5 days; CCr <20 mL/min, 125 mg q24hr × 5 days
Recurrent herpes labialis (cold sores)
• **Adult:** PO 1500-mg single dose
Renal impairment: recurrent herpes labialis
• **Adult:** PO CCr ≥60 mL/min, usual dose; CCr 40-59 mL/min, 750 mg as a single dose; CCr 20-39 mL/min, 500 mg as single dose; CCr <20 mL/min, 250 mg as a

single dose; hemodialysis, 250 mg as a single dose following dialysis

Recurrent mucocutaneous orolabial genital herpes simplex infections in HIV
• **Adult: PO** 500 mg bid × 7 days

Renal impairment: recurrent orolabial or genital herpes in HIV-infected patients
• **Adult: PO** CCr ≥40 mL/min, usual dose; CCr 20-39 mL/min, 500 mg q24hr; CCr <20 mL/min, 250 mg q24hr; hemodialysis, 250 mg following each dialysis

Recurrent genital herpes simplex
• **Adult: PO** 1000 mg bid on a single day

Renal dose
• **Adult: PO** CCr 40-59 mL/min, 500 mg q12hr × 1 day; CCr 20-39 mL/min, 500 mg as a single dose; CCr <20 mL/min, 250 mg as a single dose

Chickenpox (unlabeled)
• **Adult: PO** 500 mg q8hr × 7 days, preferably within 48 hr of onset

Available forms: Tabs 125, 250, 500 mg
Administer:
• Without regard to meals
• As soon as diagnosed; for herpes zoster within 72 hr

SIDE EFFECTS

CNS: *Headache, fatigue, dizziness,* paresthesia, somnolence, fever, seizures
GI: Nausea, vomiting, diarrhea, constipation, abdominal pain, anorexia
GU: Decreased sperm count
INTEG: *Pruritus,* vasculitis
MS: Back pain, arthralgia
RESP: Pharyngitis, sinusitis
SYST: Anaphylaxis

PHARMACOKINETICS

Bioavailability 77%, 20% protein binding, 73% excreted via kidneys, half-life 2-3 hr, peak 1 hr, duration 12 hr

INTERACTIONS

Increase: effect of famciclovir—probenecid
Decrease: effect of zoster, varicella virus vaccine

Drug/Lab
Increase: LFTs

NURSING CONSIDERATIONS
Assess:
• **Herpes zoster:** severity of the breakout; burning, itching, pain, which are early symptoms of herpes infection; assess daily during therapy
• Monitor CBC, LFTs test if on long-term treatment
• **Acute renal failure:** usually in high dose or in those >65 yr; urine CCr; BUN before and during treatment if decreased renal function; dose may have to be lowered; hepatic studies: LFTs
• Bowel pattern before, during treatment; diarrhea may occur
• Postherpetic neuralgia during and after treatment
• **Pregnancy/breastfeeding:** use only if benefits outweigh fetal risk; pregnant patients

Evaluate:
• **Therapeutic response:** decreased size, spread of lesions

Teach patient/family:
• How to recognize beginning infection (pain, itching, tingling), use product within 48 hr of rash/urticaria
• How to prevent spread of infection; that this medication does not prevent spread to others; that condoms should be used; that until crusting of lesions has taken place, not to be around those who have not had the chickenpox vaccine or those who are immunocompromised
• About the reason for medication, expected results; that product must be taken for whole course of treatment; if lactose intolerant, to notify prescriber before use
• That women with genital herpes should have yearly Pap smears; that cervical cancer is more likely
• To avoid driving or other hazardous activities until results are known; dizziness may occur

Hypersensitivity/anaphylaxis: To report rash, difficulty breathing, swelling of face
Pregnancy/breastfeeding: Report if pregnancy is planned or suspected or if breastfeeding; if pregnant, enroll in Novartis Adverse Event Reporting System (888-669-6682); male fertility may be affected

F

Side effects: *italics* = common; red = life-threatening

famotidine (otc, Rx)

(fa-moe′ti-deen)

Pepcid, Pepcid AC, Zantac
Func. class.: Antiulcer agent
Chem class.: H₂-histamine receptor antagonist

ACTION: Competitively inhibits histamine at histamine H₂-receptor site, thus decreasing gastric secretion while pepsin remains at a stable level

USES: Short-term treatment of duodenal ulcer, maintenance therapy for duodenal ulcer, Zollinger-Ellison syndrome, multiple endocrine adenomas, gastric ulcers; gastroesophageal reflux disease, heartburn
Unlabeled uses: GI disorders in those taking NSAIDs; urticaria; prevention of stress ulcers, aspiration pneumonitis

CONTRAINDICATIONS

Hypersensitivity
Precautions: Pregnancy, breastfeeding, children <12 yr, geriatric patients, severe renal/hepatic disease

DOSAGE AND ROUTES
Short-term treatment of benign gastric ulcer
- **Adult/child ≥40 kg: PO** 40 mg/day at bedtime × 4-8 wk, then 20 mg/day at bedtime if needed (maintenance); **IV** 20 mg q12hr if unable to take **PO**
- **Child 1-16 yr: PO/IV** 0.25 mg/kg/dose q12hr, max 40 mg/day

Short-term treatment of duodenal ulcer
- **Adult/child ≥40 kg: PO** 40 mg at bedtime or 20 mg bid; maintenance 20 mg daily at bedtime for up to 8 wk

Pathologic hypersecretory conditions
- **Adult: PO** 20 mg q6hr; may give up to 160 mg q6hr if needed; **IV** 20 mg q6hr if unable to take **PO**

GERD
- **Adult/child ≥40 kg: PO** 20 mg bid for up to 6 wk; 20-40 mg bid up to 12 wk (with ulcerative esophagitis)

- **Child 1-16 yr: PO** 0.5 mg/kg bid, max 40 mg bid
- **Child 3 mo-<1 yr: PO** 0.5 mg/kg/dose bid ≤8 wk
- **Child <3 mo: PO** 0.5 mg/kg/dose daily, may increase to 1 mg/kg/day ≤8 wk

Heartburn relief/prevention (OTC)
- **Adult/child >12 yr: PO** 10 mg with water for relief or take 15 min-1 hr before eating for prevention

Renal dose
- **Adult: PO** CCr <50 mL/min give ½ dose or increase interval to q36-48h

Available forms: Tabs 10, 20, 40 mg; powder for oral susp 40 mg/5 mL; inj 0.4 mg/mL premixed in normal saline, 10 mg/mL, 20 mg/50 mL; tabs chewable 10, 20 mg
Administer:
- Store in cool environment (oral); IV sol stable for 48 hr at room temperature; do not use discolored sol; discard unused oral sol after 1 mo

PO route
- After shaking oral suspension
- Give with meals and at bedtime
- Separate antacids by (1 hr), sucralfate (2 hr)
- Use at bedtime for once-a-day dosing
- Store suspension room temperature, discard after 30 days
- Protect tablets from light

Direct IV route
- After diluting 2 mL of product (10 mg/mL) in 0.9% NaCl to total volume of 5-10 mL; inject over 2 min to prevent hypotension

Intermittent IV INFUSION route
- After diluting 20 mg (2 mL) of product in 100 mL of LR, 0.9% NaCl, D₅W, D₁₀W; run over 15-30 min, stable for 48 hr after dilution refrigerated

Y-site compatibilities: Acyclovir, alfentanil, allopurinol, amifostine, amikacin, aminocaproic acid, aminophylline, amiodarone, amphotericin B lipid complex, amphotericin B liposome, amsacrine, anakinra, anidulafungin, ascorbic acid injection, atenolol, atracurium, atropine, aztreonam, benztropine, bivalirudin, bleomycin, bumetanide, buprenorphine, butorphanol, calcium chloride/gluconate,

CARBOplatin, caspofungin, cefonicid, cefotaxime, cefTAZidime, cefuroxime, chlorproMAZINE, cimetidine, cisatracurium, CISplatin, cladribine, clindamycin, codeine, cyanocobalamin, cyclophosphamide, cycloSPORINE, cytarabine, DACTINomycin, DAPTOmycin, dexamethasone, dexmedetomidine, digoxin, diltiazem, diphenhydrAMINE, DOBUTamine, DOCEtaxel, DOPamine, doripenem, doxacurium, DOXOrubicin, DOXOrubicin liposomal, doxycycline, droperidol, enalaprilat, ePHEDrine, EPINEPHrine, epirubicin, epoetin alfa, eptifibatide, ertapenem, erythromycin, esmolol, etoposide, fenoldopam, fentaNYL, filgrastim, fluconazole, fludarabine, fluorouracil, folic acid, gatifloxacin, gemcitabine, gentamicin, glycopyrrolate, granisetron, heparin, hydrocortisone, HYDROmorphone, hydrOXYzine, IDArubicin, ifosfamide, imipenem-cilastatin, irinotecan, isoproterenol, ketorolac, labetalol, levofloxacin, lidocaine, linezolid, LORazepam, LR, magnesium sulfate, mannitol, mechlorethamine, melphalan, meperidine, metaraminol, methicillin, methotrexate, methoxamine, methyldopate, methylPREDNISolone, metoclopramide, metoprolol, metroNIDAZOLE, miconazole, midazolam, milrinone, mitoXANtrone, morphine, moxalactam, multiple vitamins injection, mycophenolate, nafcillin, nalbuphine, naloxone, nesiritide, netilmicin, niCARdipine, nitroglycerin, nitroprusside, norepinephrine, 0.9% NaCl, octreotide, ondansetron, oxacillin, oxaliplatin, oxytocin, PACLitaxel, palonosetron, pamidronate, pancuronium, papaverine, PEMEtrexed, penicillin G potassium/sodium, pentamidine, pentazocine, PENTobarbital, perphenazine, PHENobarbital, phenylephrine, phytonadione, polymyxin B, potassium chloride/phosphates, procainamide, prochlorperazine, promethazine, propofol, propranolol, protamine, pyridoxine, quiNIDine, ranitidine, remifentanil, Ringer's, ritodrine, riTUXimab, sargramostim, sodium acetate/bicarbonate, succinylcholine, SUFentanil, tacrolimus, teniposide, theophylline, thiamine, thiotepa, ticarcillin, ticarcillin-clavulanate, tigecycline, tirofiban, TNA, tobramycin, tolazoline, TPN, trastuzumab, trimetaphan, urokinase, vancomycin, vasopressin, vecuronium, verapamil, vinCRIStine, vinorelbine, voriconazole, zoledronic acid

SIDE EFFECTS
CNS: *Headache, dizziness,* paresthesia, depression, anxiety, somnolence, insomnia, fever, seizures in renal disease
CV: Dysrhythmias, QT prolongation (impaired renal functioning)
EENT: Taste change, tinnitus, orbital edema
GI: *Constipation,* nausea, vomiting, anorexia, cramps, abnormal hepatic enzymes, diarrhea
INTEG: Rash, toxic epidermal necrolysis, Stevens-Johnson syndrome
MS: Myalgia, arthralgia
RESP: Pneumonia

PHARMACOKINETICS
Protein binding 15%-20%, metabolized in liver 30% (active metabolites), 70% excreted by kidneys, half-life 2½-3½ hr
PO: Onset 60 min, duration 12 hr, peak 1-3 hr, absorption 50%
IV: Onset 60 min, peak 1-4 hr, duration 8-12 hr

INTERACTIONS
Decrease: absorption—ketoconazole, itraconazole, cefpodoxime, cefditoren cefuroxime, delaviridine
Decrease: famotidine absorption—antacids
Drug/Lab Test
Increase: LFTs, BUN, creatinine
False negative: Skin tests
False positive: Urine protein

NURSING CONSIDERATIONS
Assess:
• **Ulcers:** epigastric pain, adominal pain, frank or occult blood in emesis, stools
• **Renal function:** patients with decreased renal function are at risk for prolonged QT
• Intragastric pH, serum creatinine/BUN baseline and periodically
• For bleeding, hematuria, hematuresis, occult blood in stools; abdominal pain
• Increase in bulk and fluids in diet to prevent constipation
• **Beers:** avoid in older adults with delirium or at high risk for delirium; may induce or worsen the condition; assess for confusion

• **Pregnancy/breastfeeding:** cautious use in pregnancy, breastfeeding; excreted in breast milk

Evaluate:

• **Therapeutic response:** decreased abdominal pain, healing of duodenal ulcers, decreased gastroesophageal reflux

Teach patient/family:

• That product must be continued for prescribed time in prescribed method to be effective; not to double dose; do not take for extended periods of time, risk of B_{12} malabsorption

• About possibility of decreased libido; that this is reversible after discontinuing therapy

• To avoid irritating foods, alcohol, aspirin, NSAIDs, extreme-temperature foods that may irritate GI system

• That smoking should be avoided because it diminishes effectiveness of product

• To avoid tasks requiring alertness because dizziness, drowsiness may occur

---

fam-trastuzumab deruxtecan-nxki (Rx)

Enhertu

Func. class.: Antineoplastic, *HER2*-directed antibody

USES: *HER2*-positive metastatic breast cancer

CONTRAINDICATIONS

Hypersensitivity

DOSAGE AND ROUTES

Adult: intermittent IV infusion

5.4 mg/kg once q3wk (21-day cycle) until disease progression or unacceptable toxicity

Available forms: Solution reconstituted IV 100 mg

---

faricimab-svoa (Rx)

(far′lK′i′mab)

Vabysmo

Func. class.: Ophthalmic

Chem. class.: Selective vascular endothelial growth factor antagonist

---

ACTION: Binds to receptor-binding site of active forms of vascular endothelial growth factor A (VEGF-A), which causes angiogenesis and cell proliferation

USES: Age-related macular degeneration (neovascular) (wet), macular edema after retinal vein occlusion (RVO), diabetic macular edema

CONTRAINDICATIONS

Hypersensitivity, ocular infections

Precautions: Pregnancy, breastfeeding, children, retinal detachment, increased intraocular pressure

DOSAGE AND ROUTES

Neovascular (wet) age-related macular degeneration (nAMD)

• **Adult: INTRAVITREAL** 6 mg every 4 wk (approximately every 28 +/− 7 days) for the first 4 doses, then perform optical coherence tomography and visual acuity evaluations 8 and 12 wk after the fourth dose. Based on the results of these evaluations, subsequent 6-mg intravitreal injections may be given using 1 of the following 3 regimens: (1) wk 28 and 44; (2) wk 24, 36, 48; or (3) wk 20, 28, 36, 44

Available forms: Solution for injection 120 mg/mL

Administer:

• By ophthalmologist via intravitreal injection using adequate anesthesia

• Gather supplies needed, kit containing the faricimab single-use glass vial and single-use 5-micron blunt, 18-gauge × 1.5-inch transfer filter needle; sterile 1-mL Luer-Lok syringe with 0.05-mL dose mark; sterile 30-gauge × 0.5-inch injection needle. Note: A 30-gauge needle is recommended to avoid increased injection force; alcohol swab; remove from refrigerator, allow to come to room temperature

SIDE EFFECTS

EENT: Blepharitis, cataract, conjunctival hemorrhage/hyperemia, detachment of retinal pigment epithelium, dry eye, irritation/pain in eye, visual impairment, vitreous floaters, ocular infection

---

PHARMACOKINETICS
Elimination half-life 7.5 days, peak 2 days

INTERACTIONS
None known

NURSING CONSIDERATIONS
Assess:
• Eye changes: redness; sensitivity to light, vision change; increased intraocular pressure change; report infection to ophthalmologist immediately, complete procedure with anesthesia and antibiotic prior to use, check perfusion of optic nerve after use
• Hypersensitivity: monitor for inflammation
Evaluate:
• **Therapeutic response:** prevention of increasing macular degeneration
Teach patient/family:
• If eye becomes red, sensitive to light, painful, or if there is a change in vision, to seek immediate care from ophthalmologist
• About reason for treatment, expected results; that product is injected into the eye, an anesthetic will be used

febuxostat (Rx)
(feb-ux´oh-stat)
Uloric
Func. class.: Antigout drug, antihyperuricemic
Chem. class.: Xanthene oxidase inhibitor

ACTION: Inhibits the enzyme xanthine oxidase, thereby reducing uric acid synthesis; more selective for xanthine oxidase than allopurinol

USES: Chronic gout, hyperuricemia

CONTRAINDICATIONS
Hypersensitivity
Precautions: Pregnancy, breastfeeding, children, renal/hepatic/cardiac/neoplastic disease, stroke, MI, organ transplant, Lesch-Nyhan syndrome

Black Box Warning: CV mortality

DOSAGE AND ROUTES
• **Adult:** PO 40 mg daily, may increase to 80 mg daily if uric acid levels are >6 mg/dL after 2 wk of therapy
Renal dose
• **Adult:** PO CCr <30 mL/min 40 mg/day
Available forms: Tabs 40, 80 mg
Administer:
PO route
• Without regard to meals or antacids; may crush and add to foods or fluids
• Only use in patients unable to take allopurinol or if allopurinol is ineffective

SIDE EFFECTS
CNS: Dizziness, weakness, flushing
GI: *Nausea*, vomiting, diarrhea, constipation, hepatitis
EENT: Cataracts, retinopathy, epistaxis
HEMA: Thrombocytopenia, anemia, leukopenia, bone marrow suppression
INTEG: Rash, DRESS, SJS, TEN
MISC: Arthralgia, gout flare

PHARMACOKINETICS
Peak 1-1.5 hr, duration up to 24 hr; metabolized extensively in the liver, excreted in feces, urine; half-life 5-8 hr; protein binding 99.2%; max lowering of uric acid 2 wk

INTERACTIONS
Increase: toxicity—azaTHIOprine, didanosine, mercaptopurine; do not use together
Increase: xanthine nephropathy, calculi—rasburicase, antineoplastics
Drug/Lab
Increase: LFTs, alkaline phosphatase, serum cholesterol, triglycerides, amylase, BUN, creatinine, aPTT, PT, CPK, creatine
Decrease: Hct/HB, RBC, platelets, lymphocytes, neutrophils, TSH, blood glucose

NURSING CONSIDERATIONS
Assess:
• **Hyperuricemia:** uric acid levels q2wk; uric acid levels should be ≤6 mg/dL, flares may occur during first 6 wk of treatment
• **Hepatic studies** before use, then 2, 4 mo and then periodically; assess for fatigue, anorexia, right upper abdominal discomfort, dark urine, jaundice
• **CV disease:** Avoid use in those with CV disease, deaths have occurred, monitor for MI, stroke

Side effects: *italics* = common; red = life-threatening

- **Renal disease:** I&O ratio; increase fluids to 2 L/day to prevent stone formation and toxicity

Black Box Warning: For rash, hypersensitivity reactions; discontinue immediately; may be fatal, more common in those allergic to allopurinol

- **Gout:** joint pain/swelling, may be relieved with NSAIDs for acute gouty attacks and gout flare (first 6 wk)
Evaluate:
- **Therapeutic response:** decreased pain in joints, decreased stone formation in kidneys, decreased uric acid levels
Teach patient/family:
- That tabs may be crushed
- To take as prescribed; if dose is missed, to take as soon as remembered; not to double dose
- To increase fluid intake to 2 L/day unless contraindicated
- To avoid alcohol, caffeine because they will increase uric acid levels

Black Box Warning: To report cardiovascular events to prescriber immediately (chest pain, dyspnea, slurred speech, weakness)

- To report serious skin reactions immediately
- **Pregnancy/breastfeeding:** To report to health care provider if pregnancy is planned or suspected or if breastfeeding
- **Gout:** that flares may occur during first 6 wk of treatment; continue and notify prescriber; NSAIDs or colchicine may be added to reduce the risk of flares

---

fedratinib
See Appendix B

---

felodipine (Rx)
(fe-loe´-di-peen)
Plendil ♣, Renedil ♣
Func. class.: Antihypertensive, calcium channel blocker, antianginal
Chem. class.: Dihydropyridine

ACTION: Inhibits calcium ion influx across cell membrane, resulting in the inhibition of the excitation and contraction of vascular smooth muscle

USES: Essential hypertension alone or with other antihypertensives
Unlabeled uses: Hypertension in adolescents and children, angina pectoris; Prinzmetal's angina (vasospastic)

CONTRAINDICATIONS
Hypersensitivity to this product or dihydropyridines, sick sinus syndrome, 2nd- or 3rd-degree heart block, hypotension <90 mm Hg systolic

Black Box Warning: CV death

Precautions: Pregnancy, breastfeeding, children, geriatric patients, HF, hepatic injury, renal disease, coronary artery disease

DOSAGE AND ROUTES
- **Adult:** PO 2.5-5 mg/day initially; usual range 2.5-10 mg/day; max 10 mg/day; do not adjust dosage at intervals of <2 wk
- **Geriatric:** PO 2.5 mg/day, max 10 mg/day
Hepatic disease
- **Adult:** PO 2.5-5 mg, max 10 mg/day
Hypertension in adolescent/child (unlabeled)
- **Adolescent/child:** PO 2.5 mg initially, titrate upward, max 10 mg/day
Available forms: Ext rel tabs 2.5, 5, 10 mg
Administer:
PO route
- Swallow whole; do not break, crush, or chew ext rel products
- Once daily with light meal; avoid grapefruit juice

SIDE EFFECTS
CNS: *Headache,* fatigue, drowsiness, dizziness, anxiety, depression, nervousness, insomnia, light-headedness, paresthesia, tinnitus, psychosis, somnolence, flushing
CV: Dysrhythmia, *edema,* HF, hypotension, palpitations, MI, pulmonary edema, tachycardia, syncope, AV block, angina
GI: Nausea, vomiting, diarrhea, gastric upset, constipation, dry mouth
GU: Nocturia, polyuria, sexual dysfunction, decreased libido
HEMA: Anemia

INTEG: Rash, pruritus, peripheral edema
MISC: Flushing, sexual difficulties, cough, nasal congestion, SOB, wheezing, epistaxis, respiratory infection, chest pain, angioedema, gingival hyperplasia, Stevens-Johnson syndrome

PHARMACOKINETICS
Onset 1 hr, peak 2.5-5 hr, highly protein bound >99%, metabolized in liver, 0.5% excreted unchanged in urine, elimination half-life 11-16 hr

INTERACTIONS
Increase: bradycardia, HF—β-blockers, digoxin, phenytoin, disopyramide
Increase: toxicity, hypotension—nitrates, alcohol, quiNIDine, zileuton, miconazole, dilTIAZem, delavirdine, quinupristin-dalfopristin, conivaptan, cycloSPORINE, cimetidine, clarithromycin, antiretroviral protease inhibitors, other antihypertensives, MAOIs, ketoconazole, erythromycin, itraconazole, propranolol
Decrease: antihypertensive effects—NSAIDs, carBAMazepine, barbiturates, phenytoin
Drug/Herb
Increase: antihypertensive effect—ginseng, ginkgo, hawthorn
Decrease: antihypertensive effect—ephedra, St. John's wort
Drug/Food
Increase: felodipine level—grapefruit juice

NURSING CONSIDERATIONS
Assess:

Black Box Warning: **CV status,** fluid volume status, I&O, weight daily; weight gain, crackles, dyspnea, edema, jugular venous distention, adequacy of pulses, moist mucous membranes; bilateral lung sounds, peripheral pitting edema; dehydration symptoms of decreasing output, thirst, hypotension, dry mouth, and mucous membranes should be reported

• Monitor ALT, AST, bilirubin often if elevated
• **Cardiac status:** B/P, pulse, respiration; ECG periodically during prolonged treatment
• **Angina pain:** location, duration, intensity; ameliorating, aggravating factors

• **Hypertension:** check for compliance, number of refills
• **Pregnancy/breastfeeding:** no well-controlled studies; use only if benefits outweigh fetal risk, may cause fetal harm; discontinue breastfeeding or product, excretion unknown
Evaluate:
• **Therapeutic response:** B/P, WNL, decreased anginal attacks, increased activity tolerance
Teach patient/family:
• To avoid hazardous activities until stabilized on product, dizziness no longer a problem
• To avoid OTC products, alcohol unless directed by prescriber; to limit caffeine consumption
• About the importance of complying with all areas of medical regimen: diet, exercise, stress reduction, product therapy
• That tablets may appear in stools but are insignificant

Black Box Warning: To report dyspnea, palpitations, irregular heartbeat, swelling of extremities, nausea, vomiting, severe dizziness, severe headache

• To change positions slowly to prevent orthostatic hypotension
• To obtain correct pulse; to contact prescriber if pulse <50 bpm
• To use good oral hygiene to prevent gingival hyperplasia
• Not to stop abruptly
• To avoid grapefruit juice

TREATMENT OF OVERDOSE:
Atropine for AV block, vasopressor for hypotension

---

fenofibrate (Rx)
(fen-oh-fee′brate)
Antara, Fenoglide, Lipidil Supra
🍁, Lipofen, TriCor, Trilipix
fenofibric acid (Rx)
Fibricor
Func. class.: Antilipemic
Chem. class.: Fibric acid derivative

Do not confuse:
Tricor/Tracleer

ACTION: Increases lipolysis and elimination of triglyceride-rich particles from plasma by activating lipoprotein lipase, resulting in changes in triglyceride size and composition of LDL, leading to rapid breakdown of LDL; mobilizes triglycerides from tissue; increases excretion of neutral sterols

USES: Hypercholesterolemia; types IV, V hyperlipidemia that do not respond to other treatment and that increase risk for pancreatitis; Fredrickson type IV, V hypertriglyceridemia

CONTRAINDICATIONS
Hypersensitivity, severe renal/hepatic disease, primary biliary cirrhosis, preexisting gallbladder disease, breastfeeding
Precautions: Pregnancy, geriatric patients, peptic ulcer, pancreatitis, renal/hepatic disease, diabetes mellitus

DOSAGE AND ROUTES
Hypertriglyceridemia
• **Adult: PO (Antara)** 43-130 mg/day; **(Fenoglide)** 40-120 mg/day; **(Tricor)** 48-145 mg/day; **(Lipofen)** 50-150 mg/day; (Fibricor) 35-105 mg/day, max 105 mg/day; 54-160 mg/day (Lofibral), 160 mg/day (Triglide), 30-90 mg/day (micronized fenofibrate)
Primary hypercholesterolemia/ mixed hyperlipidemia
• **Adult: PO (Antara)** 130 mg/day; **(Fenoglide)** 120 mg/day; **(Tricor)** 145 mg/day; (Fibricor) 105 mg/day, (Triplex) 135 mg/day; (Lipofen) 150 mg/day; Lofibral: 160 mg/day, Triglide: 160 mg/day, Micronized capsules: 90 mg/day or 200 mg/day depending on product
Renal dose (geriatric)
• **Adult: PO (Tricor)** CCr 30-80 mL/min, 48 mg/day; CCr <30 mL/min, contraindicated; Adult: PO CCr 30-80 mL/min, 50 mg/day **(Triglide, Lipofen),** 30 mg/day **(Antara),** CCr <30 mL/min, contraindicated **(Antara, Lipofen)**

Available forms: Cap: *Antara* 30, 90 mg; *Lipofen* 50, 150 mg; **Tab:** 43, 50, 67, 130, 134, 150, 200 mg; *TriCor* 48, 145 mg; *Fenoglide* 40, 120 mg; fenofibrate choline: **del rel caps** 45, 135 mg; **fenofibric acid:** tabs 35, 105 mg
Administer:
• Product with meals (Lipofen); Antara without regard to food; may increase q4-8wk; discontinue if there is not adequate response after 2 mo
• Caps must be swallowed whole
• Brands are not interchangeable
• Protect Lipofen, Triglide from light, moisture

SIDE EFFECTS
CNS: *Fatigue, dizziness,* headache, paresthesia, insomnia, depression
CV: Hypertension, angina, DVT, PE
GI: *Nausea, vomiting, dyspepsia,* flatulence, pancreatitis, cholelithiasis, diarrhea, constipation, hepatotoxicity
GU: *Polyuria*
INTEG: *Rash, pruritus,* DRESS, STS, TEN
MS: *Myalgias, arthralgias, myopathy, rhabdomyolysis*
RESP: Bronchitis, cough

PHARMACOKINETICS
Peak 2 wk, protein binding 99%, converted to fenofibric acid, metabolized in liver to fenofibric acid, excreted in urine (60%), feces (25%), half-life 20 hr

INTERACTIONS
Increase: myopathy, rhabdomyolysis—colchicine
• Avoid use with HMG-CoA reductase inhibitors; rhabdomyolysis may occur
Increase: anticoagulant effects—oral anticoagulants
Decrease: absorption of fenofibrate—bile acid sequestrants; give 1 hr prior to or ≥4 hr after bile acid sequestrant
Drug/Food
Increase: absorption
Drug/Lab Test
Increase: ALT, AST, BUN, CK, creatinine
Decrease: WBC, uric acid, HB, paradoxical effect in HDL

NURSING CONSIDERATIONS
Assess:
• **Hypercholesterolemia/hyperlipidemia diet history:** obtain a dietary history including fat content; lipid levels (triglyc-

erides, LDL, HDL, cholesterol); may cause a paradoxical decrease in HDL; LFTs at baseline, periodically during treatment, if >3 × ULN, discontinue; CPK if muscle pain occurs; CBC, Hct, HB, PT with anticoagulant therapy; serum bilirubin (total and direct)

• **Pancreatitis, cholelithiasis, renal failure, rhabdomyolysis** (when combined with HMG Co-A reductase inhibitors), myositis; product should be discontinued; assess often for muscle pain, weakness, fever

• **Severe skin reactions:** angioedema, anaphylaxis, monitor throughout treatment

• **Pregnancy/breastfeeding:** identify whether pregnancy is planned or suspected; do not breastfeed

Evaluate:

• **Therapeutic response:** decreased triglycerides, cholesterol levels

Teach patient/family:

• That compliance is needed; not to consume chipped or broken tabs (Triglide)

• That risk factors should be decreased: high-fat diet, smoking, alcohol consumption, absence of exercise

• To notify prescriber if pregnancy is suspected or planned; not to breastfeed during or for ≥5 days of last dose

• To notify prescriber of muscle pain, weakness, fever, fatigue, epigastric pain, yellowing of skin/eyes, fever

• To report signs/symptoms of DVT (swollen, warm extremity) or PE (shortness of breath, chest pain) to provider immediately

---

⚠ HIGH ALERT

fentaNYL (parenteral) (Rx) REMS
(fen´ta-nill)
fentaNYL transdermal (Rx)
Ionsys
fentaNYL nasal spray (Rx)
Lazanda

fentaNYL SL spray (Rx)
Subsys
fentaNYL buccal (Rx)
Fentora
fentaNYL lozenge (transmucosal) (Rx)
Actiq
fentanyl SL (Rx)
Abstral

Func. class.: Opioid analgesic
Chem. class.: Synthetic phenylpiperidine

Controlled Substance Schedule II

Do not confuse:
fentaNYL/sufentanil

ACTION: Inhibits ascending pain pathways in CNS, increases pain threshold, alters pain perception by binding to opiate receptors

USES: Controls moderate to severe pain; preoperatively; postoperatively; adjunct to general anesthetic, adjunct to regional anesthesia; **fentaNYL:** anesthesia as premedication, conscious sedation; **Actiq:** breakthrough cancer pain

CONTRAINDICATIONS
Hypersensitivity to opiates; myasthenia gravis

Black Box Warning: Headache, migraine (Actiq, Abstral, Fentora, Lazanda); emergency room use (Abstral, Lazanda); outpatient surgeries (Duragesic TD); opioid-naive patients, respiratory depression

Precautions: Pregnancy, breastfeeding, geriatric patients, increased intracranial pressure, seizure disorders, severe respiratory disorders, cardiac dysrhythmias

Black Box Warning: Accidental exposure, ambient temperature increase, fever, skin abrasion (TD patch), substance abuse, surgery, requires an experienced clinician

---

DOSAGE AND ROUTES

FentaNYL (parenteral)

Anesthetic (adjunct to regional anesthesia)

• **Adult: IV** 50-100 mcg/kg over 1-2 min

Anesthesia supplement to general anesthesia

• **Adult/child >12 yr: IM/IV** (low dose) 1-2 mcg/kg; **IV** (moderate dose) 2-20 mcg/kg; **IM/IV** (high dose) 20-50 mcg/kg, then 25 mcg to ½ initial loading dose as needed

Induction and maintenance of anesthesia

• **Child 2-12 yr: IV** 2-3 mcg/kg q1-2hr as needed

Preoperatively

• **Adult/child >12 yr: IM/IV** 50-100 mcg q30-60min before surgery

Postoperatively

• **Adult/child >12 yr: IM/IV** 50-100 mcg q1-2hr prn

Moderate/severe pain

• **Adult: IV/IM** 50-100 mcg q1-2hr; **nasal; 100 mcg spray in one nostril, titrate stepwise**

Actiq

• **Adult: TRANSMUCOSAL** 200 mcg; redose if needed 15 min after completion of 1st dose; do not give more than 2 doses during titration period, max 4 doses/day

Fentora

• **Adult: BUCCAL/SL** 100 mcg placed above rear molar between upper cheek and gum; a second 100 mcg dose, if needed, may be started 30 min after 1st dose

FentaNYL transdermal

• **Adult:** 25 mcg/hr; may increase until pain relief occurs; apply patch to flat surface on upper torso and wear for 72 hr; apply new patch on different site; may use 12.5 mcg/hr if <60 mg/day morphine equivalent

FentaNYL nasal spray

• **Adult:** 100 mcg (1 spray in 1 nostril), may retreat after ≥2 hr, titrate upward until adequate analgesia; treat a max of 4 episodes daily

FentaNYL SL spray

• **Adult:** 100 mcg sprayed under tongue, titrate stepwise carefully

Available forms: Inj 0.05 mg/mL; lozenges 100, 200, 300, 400, 600, 800, 1200, 1600 mcg; lozenges on a stick 200, 400, 600, 800, 1200, 1600 mcg; buccal tab 100, 200, 400, 600, 800 mcg; transdermal: patch 12, 25, 50, 75, 100 mcg/hr; SL spray 100, 200, 400, 600, 800, 1200, 1600 mcg/spray; nasal spray 100, 400 mcg/actuation

Administer:

• By inj (IM, IV); give slowly to prevent rigidity

• Overdose has been fatal when confusing products/dose; recheck both before using

• Must have emergency equipment available, opioid antagonists, O_2; to be used only by those appropriately trained; IV products to be used in OR, ER, ICU

Transmucosal route

• Remove foil just before administration; instruct patient to place product between cheek and lower gum, moving it back and forth and sucking, not chewing (Actiq); place above rear molar (Fentora); place film on the inside of the cheek; all products not used or only partially used should be flushed down the toilet; this product may be used SL

Transdermal route

• q72hr for continuous pain relief; dosage adjusted after at least 2 applications; apply to clean, dry skin and press firmly

• Give short-acting analgesics until patch takes effect (8-24 hr); when reducing dosage or switching to alternative IV treatment, withdraw gradually; serum levels drop gradually, give ½ the equianalgesic dose of new analgesic 12-18 hr after removal as ordered

SL spray

• Open blister package with scissors immediately prior to use; spray contents under tongue; dispose of unit by placing it into disposable bags provided; seal bag, discard into trash container out of reach of children

IV route

• IV undiluted by anesthesiologist or diluted with 5 mL or more sterile water or 0.9% NaCl given through Y-tube or 3-way stopcock at 0.1 mg or less/1-2 min. Muscular rigidity may occur with rapid IV administration

Y-site compatibilities: Abciximab, acyclovir, alfentanil, alemtuzumab alprostadil, amikacin, aminocaproic acid, aminophylline, amiodarone, amphotericin B cholesteryl, amphotericin B lipid complex, amphotericin B liposome, anidulafungin, argatroban, ascorbic acid injection, atenolol, atracurium, atropine, azaTHIOprine, aztreonam, benztropine, bivalirudin, bleomycin, bumetanide, buprenorphine, butorphanol, calcium chloride/gluconate, CARBOplatin, caspofungin, ceFAZolin, cefmetazole, cefonicid, cefotaxime, cefoTEtan, cefOXitin, cefTAZidime, ceftizoxime, ceftobiprole, cefTRIAXone, cefuroxime, cephalothin, chloramphenicol, chlorproMAZINE, cimetidine, cisatracurium, CISplatin, clindamycin, cloNIDine, cyanocobalamin, cyclophosphamide, cycloSPORINE, cytarabine, DACTINomycin, DAPTOmycin, dexamethasone, dexmedetomidine, digoxin, diltiazem, diphenhydrAMINE, DOBUTamine, DOCEtaxel, DOPamine, doripenem, doxacurium, doxapram, DOXOrubicin, doxycycline, enalaprilat, ePHEDrine, EPINEPHrine, epirubicin, epoetin alfa, eptifibatide, erythromycin, esmolol, etomidate, etoposide, famotidine, fenoldopam, fluconazole, fludarabine, fluorouracil, folic acid, furosemide, ganciclovir, gatifloxacin, gemcitabine, gentamicin, glycopyrrolate, granisetron, heparin, hydrocortisone, HYDROmorphone, hydrOXYzine, IDArubicin, ifosfamide, imipenem-cilastatin, inamrinone, insulin (regular), irinotecan, isoproterenol, ketorolac, labetalol, lansoprazole, levofloxacin, lidocaine, linezolid, LORazepam, LR, magnesium sulfate, mannitol, mechlorethamine, meperidine, metaraminol, methicillin, methotrexate, methotrimeprazine, methoxamine, methyldopate, methylPREDNISolone, metoclopramide, metoprolol, metroNIDAZOLE, mezlocillin, miconazole, midazolam, milrinone, minocycline, mitoXANtrone, mivacurium, morphine, moxalactam, multiple vitamins injection, mycophenolate, nafcillin, nalbuphine, naloxone, nesiritide, netilmicin, niCARdipine, nitroglycerin, nitroprusside, norepinephrine, octreotide, ondansetron, oxacillin, oxaliplatin, oxytocin, PACLitaxel, palonosetron, pamidronate, pancuronium, papaverine, PEMEtrexed, penicillin G potassium/sodium, pentamidine, pentazocine, PENTobarbital, PHENobarbital, phenylephrine, phytonadione, piperacillin, piperacillin-tazobactam, polymyxin B, potassium chloride, procainamide, prochlorperazine, promethazine, propofol, propranolol, protamine, pyridoxine, quiNIDine, quinupristin-dalfopristin, ranitidine, remifentanil, Ringer's, ritodrine, riTUXimab, rocuronium, sargramostim, scopolamine, sodium acetate/bicarbonate, succinylcholine, SUFentanil, tacrolimus, teniposide, theophylline, thiamine, thiopental, thiotepa, ticarcillin, ticarcillin-clavulanate, tigecycline, tirofiban, TNA, tobramycin, tolazoline, TPN, trastuzumab, trimetaphan, urokinase, vancomycin, vasopressin, vecuronium, verapamil, vinCRIStine, vinorelbine, vitamin B complex/C, voriconazole, zoledronic acid

SIDE EFFECTS
CNS: Dizziness, *delirium, euphoria, sedation, confusion, weakness, dizziness,* seizures
CV: *Bradycardia, arrest, hypo/hypertension,* DVT, PE
EENT: *Blurred vision, miosis*
GI: *Nausea, vomiting, constipation*
GU: Urinary retention
INTEG: Rash, diaphoresis
MS: Muscle rigidity
RESP: *Respiratory depression, arrest,* laryngospasm

PHARMACOKINETICS
Metabolized by liver, excreted by kidneys, crosses placenta, excreted in breast milk; half-life: IV, 2-4 hr; transdermal, 13-22 hr; transmucosal, 7 hr; buccal, 4-12 hr; 80% bound to plasma proteins
IM: Onset 7-15 min, peak 30 min, duration 1-2 hr
IV: Onset 1 min, peak 3-5 min, duration ½-1 hr
Intranasal: Onset 15-20 min, peak 25-30 min
Transdermal: Onset 12-24 hr, peak 1-3 days
Transmucosal: Onset 5-15 min, peak 30 min

INTERACTIONS

Black Box Warning: Increase: fentaNYL effect, fetal respiratory depression: CYP3A4 inhibitors (cycloSPORINE, ketoconazole, itraconazole, cimetidine, conivaptan, fluconazole, nefazodone, ranolazine), zafirlukast, zileuton

Increase: fatal reactions—MAOIs
Increase: hypotension—droperidol
Increase: CV depression—diazePAM
Increase: fentaNYL effect with other CNS depressants—alcohol, opioids, sedative/hypnotics, antipsychotics, skeletal muscle relaxants, protease inhibitors
Decrease: fentaNYL effect—CYP3A4 inducers (carBAMazepine, phenytoin, PHENobarbital, rifAMPin)
Drug/Herb
Increase: action of fentaNYL—St. John's wort
Decrease: effect of fentaNYL—echinacea
Drug/Lab Test
Increase: amylase, lipase

NURSING CONSIDERATIONS
Assess:

• VS after parenteral route; note muscle rigidity, drug history, hepatic/renal function tests
• CNS changes: dizziness, drowsiness, hallucinations, euphoria, LOC, pupil reaction
• Allergic reactions: rash, urticaria

Black Box Warning: Respiratory dysfunction: respiratory depression, character, rate, rhythm; notify prescriber if respirations are <10/min

Black Box Warning: Headache/migraine: Actiq, Fentora, Lazanda not to be used for this condition; Lazanda not to be used in ER; Duragesic TD not to be used for outpatient surgery patients

Black Box Warning: Apnea, respiratory arrest in opioid-naive patients: do not use Actiq, Duragesic, Fentora, Lazanda; opioid-tolerant patients are those using ≥60 mg/day oral morphine, ≥30 mg/day oxyCODONE PO, 8 mg/day HYDROmorphone, 25 mcg TD fentaNYL/hr

Black Box Warning: Pregnancy/breast-feeding: no well-controlled studies; use only if benefits outweigh fetal risk; if used for prolonged periods, neonatal withdrawal syndrome may occur; discontinue breast-feeding or product, excreted in breast milk

• **Beers:** avoid in older adults unless safer alternative is unavailable; may cause ataxia, impaired psychomotor function
Evaluate:
• **Therapeutic response:** induction of anesthesia, relief of breakthrough cancer pain, general pain relief
Teach patient/family:
• **About CNS changes:** physical dependence; not to use with alcohol, other CNS depressants

Black Box Warning: Accidental exposure: discuss the danger of children or pets ingesting or coming in contact with product; there are increasing numbers of fatal overdose with drugs laced with fentanyl, tests are available to identify illicit drugs for the presence of fentanyl

Transdermal route

Black Box Warning: Ambient temperature: that excessive heat may increase absorption; do not use with heating pads, electric blankets, heat/tanning lamps, saunas, hot tubs, heated waterbeds, when sunbathing, never cut patch in half

• That excessive perspiration may alter adhesiveness
• To dispose of patch by placing sticky sides together and flushing down toilet
• That patient may need to clip hair before applying to ensure adhesion
• May add first aid tape around the edges if there is a problem with adhesion, always remove old patch before applying new patch

ferric carboxymaltose (Rx)
Injectafer
ferric derisomaltose (Rx)
Monoferric
Func. class.: Hematinic
Chem. class.: Iron preparation

ACTION:
Releases iron stores needed for red blood cell development as well as energy and O_2 transport and use

USES:
Iron-deficiency anemia in those intolerant to PO iron and those with kidney disease not on dialysis

CONTRAINDICATIONS
Hemosiderosis/hemochromatosis
Precautions: Pregnancy, anemia, hepatic disease, vitamin D deficiency, hemoglobinopathy, hyperparathyroidism, hypophosphatemia

DOSAGE AND ROUTES
Ferric carboxymaltose
• **Adult ≥50 kg: IV** 750 mg on day 1, repeat after ≥7 days, may repeat if needed; **<50 kg: IV** 15 mg/kg on day 1, repeat after ≥7 days; max cumulative dose 1500 mg per course of treatment
Available forms: Injection 750 mg of elemental iron in 15-mL, single-dose vial
Ferric derisomaltose
• **Adult: IV infusion ≥50 kg:** 1000 mg as a single dose. Repeat dose if iron deficiency recurs; **≤50 kg:** 20 mg/kg/dose as a single dose. Repeat dose if iron deficiency recurs

Administer:
Ferric carboxymaltose
• Visually inspect for particulate matter and discoloration prior to use
• Give as an undiluted slow IV push or by continuous IV infusion
• Each vial is for single use only. Discard any unused portions; contains no preservatives
• Avoid extravasation since brown discoloration of the extravasation site may be long lasting. If extravasation occurs, discontinue administration at that site
IV push
• No dilution necessary. Administer at a rate of approximately 2 mL/min (100 mg/min)
Intermittent IV infusion
• Dilute up to 750 mg of iron in a maximum of 250 mL of sterile 0.9% NaCl and

infuse over at least 15 min. Do not dilute to concentrations less than 2 mg iron/mL in order to maintain stability
• Store at room temperature for 72 hr when added to an infusion bag containing 0.9% NaCl at concentrations ranging from 2 to 4 mg of iron per mL
Ferric derisomaltose
IV infusion route
• Visually inspect parenteral products for particulate matter and discoloration prior to use
• Withdraw appropriate volume of ferric derisomaltose and dilute in 100-500 mL of 0.9% NaCl injection. The final diluted concentration should be more than 1 mg/mL
• Each vial of ferric derisomaltose is for single dose only; discard unused portion
• Do not admix
• *Storage:* Following dilution in 0.9% NaCl injection, ferric derisomaltose may be stored at room temperature for up to 8 hr
• Give via IV infusion over 20 min

SIDE EFFECTS
GI: Nausea, constipation, vomiting
CNS: Dizziness, headache, chills, syncope
CV: Hyper/hypotension, flushing, tachycardia, chest pain
INTEG: Pruritus, injection site color change, rash

PHARMACOKINETICS
IV: Onset unknown, peak 15 min-1.2 hr, duration unknown

INTERACTIONS
Increase: nephrotoxicity—dimercaprol
Drug/Lab Test
Increase: LFTs GGT
False positive: Serum iron within 24 hr after use

NURSING CONSIDERATIONS
Assess:
• **Blood studies:** Hct, HB, serum phosphate, before treatment; iron studies (iron, transferrin, ferritin)
• **Elimination:** If constipation occurs, increase water, bulk, activity

• **Nutrition:** Amount of iron in diet (meat, dark green leafy vegetables, dried beans, dried fruits, eggs)

• **Hypersensitivity:** Assess allergic reaction to IV iron, usually within 30 min of injection, have emergency equipment available

• **Extravasation:** Check for injection site reactions during treatment

• **Pregnancy/breastfeeding:** No well-controlled studies; use only if benefits outweigh fetal risk; excreted in breast milk

Evaluate:

• **Therapeutic response:** improvement in Hct, HB, decreased fatigue, weakness

Teach patient/family:

• Not to take PO iron with this product
• To report signs of hypersensitivity

---

ferrous fumarate (Rx)

Ferretts, Ferrocite, Hemocyte

ferrous gluconate (Rx)

Ferate

ferrous sulfate (Rx)

Fer-In-Sol, Slow Iron ✚

ferrous sulfate, dried (Rx)

Feosol, Feratab, slow-release Iron

carbonyl iron (otc)

(kar′bo-nil)

ICAR, Feosol

iron dextran

DexFerrum, Dexiron ✚, Infeb Infuser

iron sucrose

Venofer

sodium ferric gluconate complex

Ferrlecit

iron polysaccharide (Rx)

Ferrex, IFEREX, Nu-Iron, Poly Iron

Func. class.: Hematinic
Chem. class.: Iron preparation

ACTION: Replaces iron stores needed for red blood cell development as well as energy and O_2 transport and use; fumarate contains 33% elemental iron; gluconate, 12%; sulfate, 20%; iron, 30%; ferrous sulfate exsiccated

USES: Iron-deficiency anemia, prophylaxis for iron deficiency in pregnancy, nutritional supplementation

CONTRAINDICATIONS

Thalassemia, hemosiderosis/hemochromatosis

Precautions: Pregnancy, anemia (long term), ulcerative colitis/regional enteritis, peptic ulcer disease, hemolytic anemia, cirrhosis, sulfite sensitivity

Black Box Warning: Accidental exposure

DOSAGE AND ROUTES

Fumarate

• **Adult:** PO 200-325 mg tid
• **Child:** PO 3 mg/kg/day (elemental iron) tid-qid
• **Infant:** PO 10-25 mg/day (elemental iron) in 3-4 divided doses, max 15 mg/day

Gluconate

• **Adult:** PO 50-100 mg elemental iron tid
• **Child:** PO 3 mg/kg/day in divided doses

Sulfate

• **Adult:** PO 0.75-1.5 g/day in divided doses
• **Child 6-12 yr:** PO 3 mg/kg/day in divided doses

Pregnancy

• **Adult:** PO 300-600 mg/day in divided doses

Iron polysaccharide

• **Adult:** PO 100-200 mg tid
• **Child:** PO 4-6 mg/kg/day in 3 divided doses (severe iron deficiency)

Iron sucrose

• **Adult:** IV 5 mL (100 mg of elemental iron) given during dialysis; most will need 1000 mg of elemental iron over 10 sequential dialysis sessions
• **Child >2 yr/adolescents:** IV 0.5 mg/kg by slow IV inj over 5 min (undiluted) or diluted in 25 mL of 0.9% NaCl, give over 5-60 min, max 100 mg every 2 wk × 12 wk

---

✚ Canada only   ⚕Rx Genetic warning

Hyperphosphatemia in chronic kidney disease

• **Adult: PO** 500 mg tid with meals

Available forms: Inj 20 mg/mL; chew tab 500 mg

sodium ferric gluconate complex

Adult: IV 10 mL (125 mg elemental iron), use dialysis 8 times to total dose of 1g

Child >6 yr: IV 0.12 mL/kg (max 125 mg/dose) use dialysis 8 times

Available forms: Fumarate: tabs 90, 150, 200, 300, 324, 325 mg; chewable tabs 100 mg; ext rel tabs 18 mg; **gluconate:** tabs 225, 240, 324, 325 mg; **sulfate:** tabs 195, 300, 325 mg; elixir 220 mg/5 mL; **dried:** tabs 200 mg; ext rel tabs 160 mg; ext rel caps 160 mg; **iron polysaccharide:** tabs 50 mg; caps 150 mg; sol 100 mg/5 mL; **iron dextran:** solution for injection 50 mg/mL; **iron sucrose:** aqueous complex for injection, 20 mg/mL; **sodium ferric gluconate complex** solution for injection 12.5 mg/mL (must be diluted)

Administer:

PO route

• Swallow tabs whole; do not break, crush, or chew unless labeled as chewable

• Between meals for best absorption; may give with juice; do not give with antacids or milk, delay at least 1 hr; if GI symptoms occur, give after meals even if absorption is decreased; eggs, milk products, chocolate, caffeine interfere with absorption

• Store in tight, light-resistant container

• **Liquid** through plastic straw to avoid discoloration of tooth enamel; dilute thoroughly

• At least 1 hr before bedtime; corrosion may occur in stomach; ferrous gluconate is less irritating to GI tract than ferrous sulfate

• For <6 mo for anemia

SIDE EFFECTS

GI: *Nausea, constipation, epigastric pain, black and red tarry stools,* vomiting, diarrhea

INTEG: Temporarily discolored tooth enamel and eyes

PHARMACOKINETICS

PO: Excreted in feces, urine, skin, breast milk; enters bloodstream; bound to transferrin; crosses placenta

INTERACTIONS

Increase: action of iron preparation—ascorbic acid, chloramphenicol

Decrease: absorption of penicillamine, levodopa, methyldopa, fluoroquinolones, L-thyroxine, tetracycline

Decrease: absorption of iron preparations—antacids, H$_2$-antagonists, proton pump inhibitors, cholestyramine, vit E

Drug/Food

Decrease: absorption—dairy products, caffeine, eggs

Drug/Lab Test

False positive: occult blood

NURSING CONSIDERATIONS

Assess:

• Blood studies: Hct, HB, reticulocytes, bilirubin before treatment, at least monthly; iron studies (iron, TIBC, ferritin); avoid use with blood transfusions, iron overload may occur

• **Toxicity:** nausea, vomiting, diarrhea (green then tarry stools), hematemesis, pallor, cyanosis, shock, coma

• Elimination: if constipation occurs, increase water, bulk, activity

• **Nutrition:** amount of iron in diet (meat, dark green leafy vegetables, dried beans, dried fruits, eggs)

• Cause of iron loss or anemia, including salicylates, sulfonamides, antimalarials, quiNIDine

• **Pregnancy/breastfeeding:** no well-controlled studies; use only if benefits outweigh fetal risk; excreted in breast milk

Evaluate:

• **Therapeutic response:** improvement in Hct, HB, reticulocytes; decreased fatigue, weakness

Teach patient/family:

• That iron will turn stools black or dark green, stain teeth

• **Accidental exposure:** to keep out of reach of children, pets; iron poisoning may occur if increased beyond recommended level

• Not to substitute 1 iron salt for another; that elemental iron content differs (e.g., 300 mg ferrous fumarate contains about 100 mg elemental iron; 300 mg ferrous gluconate contains only about 30 mg elemental iron)

• To avoid reclining position for 15-30 min after taking product to avoid esophageal corrosion

• To follow a diet high in iron; to avoid taking iron, dairy products, calcium supplements, and vit C together because they compete for absorption

TREATMENT OF OVERDOSE:
Induce vomiting; give eggs, milk until lavage can be done

ferumoxytol (Rx)
(fer-u-mox-y-tole)
Feraheme
Func. class.: Iron supplements

USES:
Treatment of iron-deficiency anemia in patients with chronic kidney disease or intolerance or unsatisfactory response to oral iron

CONTRAINDICATIONS
Hypersensitivity, hemosiderosis/hemochromatosis

Black Box Warning: Serious hypersensitivity reaction

DOSAGE AND ROUTES
• **Adults:** IV 510 mg followed by a second 510 mg IV dose 3 to 8 days later
Available forms: Solution, IV 51 mg/17 mL

fesoterodine (Rx)
(fess'oh-ter-oh-deen)
Toviaz
Func. class.: Overactive bladder product
Chem. class.: Muscarinic receptor antagonist

ACTION: Relaxes smooth muscles in urinary tract by inhibiting acetylcholine at postganglionic sites

USES: Overactive bladder (urinary frequency, urgency), urinary incontinence

CONTRAINDICATIONS
GI obstruction, ileus, pyloric stenosis, urinary retention, gastric retention, hypersensitivity, closed-angle glaucoma
Precautions: Pregnancy, breastfeeding, children, renal/hepatic disease, urinary tract obstruction, ambient temperature increase, autonomic neuropathy, constipation, contact lenses, hazardous activity, GERD, gastroparesis, myasthenia gravis, prostatic hypertrophy, toxic megacolon, ulcerative colitis, possible cross-sensitivity with tolterodine

DOSAGE AND ROUTES
Overactive bladder
• **Adult and geriatric:** PO EXT REL 4 mg/day, may increase to 8 mg/day, max 4 mg/day in those taking potent CYP3A4 inhibitors
Renal dose
• **Adult:** PO EXT REL CCr <30 mL/min, max 4 mg/day
Hepatic dose
Adult: Child-Pugh C: Not recommended
Neurogenic detrusor overactivity
Child ≥6 yr and >35 kg: PO 4 mg qday, increase to 8 mg qday after 1 wk; CYP3A4 inhibitors: max 4 mg/day
Child ≥6 yr and 25-35 kg: PO 4 mg qday, increase to 8 mg qday if needed; CYP3A4 inhibitors: do not use
Renal dose:
Child ≥6 yr and >35 kg: PO eGFR 15-29 mL/min/1.73 m^2, max 4 mg/day; eGFR <15 mL/min/1.73 m^2 or dialysis, do not use
Child ≥6 yr and 25-35 kg: PO eGFR 30-89 mL/min/1.73 m^2: max 4 mg/day; eGFR <30 mL/min/ 1.73 m^2 or dialysis, do not use
Available forms: EXT REL TABS 4, 8 mg
Administer:
• Do not break, crush, or chew ext rel product

- Give without regard to meals
- Store at room temperature; protect from moisture

SIDE EFFECTS
CNS: Insomnia, headache, dizziness
CV: Chest pain, angina, QT prolongation, peripheral edema
EENT: Xerophthalmia
GI: *Nausea, vomiting,* abdominal pain, constipation, dry mouth
GU: Dysuria, urinary retention, UTI
INTEG: Rash, angioedema
MISC: Peripheral edema, insomnia
MS: Back pain
RESP: Cough, URI
SYST: Infection

PHARMACOKINETICS
Peak 5 hr, duration up to 24 hr, rapidly absorbed, protein binding 50%, excreted in urine/feces, half-life 7 hr metabolized by the liver (CYP2D6, CYP344 converted to active metabolite)

INTERACTIONS
Increase: action of fesoterodine—CYP3A4 inhibitors (antiretroviral protease inhibitors, macrolide antiinfectives, azole antifungals), avoid use with doses >4 mg
Increase: anticholinergic effect—antimuscarinics, anticholinergics
Increase: urinary frequency—diuretics
Drug/Herb
Decrease: fesoterodine—caffeine, green tea, guarana
Drug/Food
Increase: fesoteradine level—grapefruit juice
Decrease: festerodine level—cola, coffee, tea
Drug/Lab
Increase: ALT, GGT

NURSING CONSIDERATIONS
Assess:
- **Urinary patterns:** distention, nocturia, frequency, urgency, incontinence
- **Allergic reactions:** angioedema; swelling of face, tongue, throat may occur anytime during treatment; have emergency equipment nearby

- **Pregnancy/breastfeeding:** no well-controlled studies; use only if benefits outweigh fetal risk
Evaluate:
- **Therapeutic response:** absence of urinary frequency, urgency, incontinence, increase in bladder capacity
Teach patient/family:
- To avoid increased temperature, may decrease sweating
- Not to drive or operate machinery until response is known
- To avoid alcohol; drowsiness may occur
- To report immediately allergic reactions including rash; swelling of mouth, face, lips; trouble breathing
- Not to drink liquids before bedtime
- About the importance of bladder maintenance
- Not to use new medications, herbs without prescriber approval

fexofenadine (Rx, OTC)
(fex-oh-fi′na-deen)
Allegra Allergy Childrens, Allegra Allergy, Allergy 24-HR, Allergy Relief, Allergy Relief/Indoor/Outdoor
Func. class.: Antihistamine—2nd generation
Chem. class.: Piperidine, peripherally selective

Combinations: Allegra D

ACTION: Acts on blood vessels, GI, respiratory system by competing with histamine for H_1-receptor site; decreases allergic response by blocking pharmacologic effects of histamine, less sedating

USES: Rhinitis, allergy symptoms, chronic idiopathic urticaria

CONTRAINDICATIONS
Breastfeeding, newborn or premature infants, hypersensitivity
Precautions: Pregnancy, children, geriatric patients, respiratory disease,

closed-angle glaucoma, prostatic hypertrophy, bladder neck obstruction, asthma, renal failure

DOSAGE AND ROUTES

• **Adult and child >12 yr: PO** 60 mg bid or 180 mg/day
• **Child 2-11 yr: PO** 30 mg bid
• **Child 6-11 yr: Susp PO** 30 mg bid
Renal dose
• **Adult and child ≥12 yr: PO** CCr <80 mL/min, 60 mg/day initial
• **Child 2-11 yr: PO** CCr <80 mL/min, 30 mg daily
Available forms: Tabs 30, 60 mg; Gel cap 180 mg; oral susp 6 mg/mL, orally disintegrating tab 30 mg; gel caps 180 mg
Administer:
• Without regard to meals; caps/tabs should not be given with or right before grapefruit, orange, or apple juice
• Store in tight, light-resistant container
• **Orally disintegrating tab:** allow to dissolve, swallow; do not remove from blister pack until time of administration
• **Oral susp:** shake well; use calibrated measuring device

SIDE EFFECTS

CNS: Headache, drowsiness, sedation, fatigue, blurred vision, paradoxical excitation in children or geriatric patients
GI: Dyspepsia, nausea
GU: Dysmenorrhea

PHARMACOKINETICS

Well absorbed; onset 1 hr; peak 2-3 hr; duration 12-24 hr; 80% excreted in urine; feces 11%, half-life 14.5 hr, increased in renal disease

INTERACTIONS

Decrease: fexofenadine effect—magnesium-aluminum–containing antacids
Drug/Food
Decrease: absorption of product—apple, orange, grapefruit juice
Drug/Lab Test
False negative: skin allergy tests

NURSING CONSIDERATIONS
Assess:

• **Allergy:** itchy, runny, watery eyes; congested nose; before and during treatment
• Bronchial secretions, lung sounds; increase fluids to 2000 mL/day unless contraindicated to decrease thickness of secretions
• **Pregnancy/breastfeeding:** no well-controlled studies; use only if benefits outweigh fetal risk
Evaluate:
• **Therapeutic response:** absence of running or congested nose or rashes
Teach patient/family:
• About all aspects of product use; to notify prescriber if confusion, sedation, hypotension occur
• To avoid driving, other hazardous activity if drowsiness occurs
• To avoid alcohol, other CNS depressants
• To take with water; avoid fruit juices as they may decrease effectiveness

---

fidaxomicin (Rx)
(fye-dax′oh-mye′sin)
Dificid
Func. class.: Antiinfective-macrolide

ACTION: Bactericidal against *Clostridium difficile;* inhibits RNA synthesis by inhibiting transcription of bacterial RNA polymerase; may act at the early stages of transcription

USES: *Clostridium difficile*–associated diarrhea

CONTRAINDICATIONS

Hypersensitivity
Precautions: Pregnancy, breastfeeding, children

DOSAGE AND ROUTES

• **Adult: PO** 200 mg bid × 10 days
Available forms: Tab 200 mg; granules for oral suspension 40 mg/mL
Administer:
• Without regard to food
• Store at room temperature (tablets) refrigerate (suspension)

• **Suspension:** Allow to stand 15 min before use, shake, use dosing syringe, suspension must be reconstituted with 130 mL purified water

SIDE EFFECTS
GI: Nausea, vomiting, abdominal pain, GI bleeding, intestinal obstruction
HEMA: Anemia, neutropenia
INTEG: Rash, pruritus

PHARMACOKINETICS
Half-life 12 hr, onset <1 hr, peak 1-5 hr, excreted in feces 92%, minimal absorption, substrate of PGP efflux transporter

INTERACTIONS
Drug/Lab Test
Increase: glucose, LFTs, alk phos
Decrease: fexofenadine sodium bicarbonate, platelets

NURSING CONSIDERATIONS
Assess:
• **CDAD:** for diarrhea, abdominal pain, fever, fatigue, anorexia, anemia, elevated WBC and low serum albumin; product may be used in place of vancomycin (PO); monitor CBC with differential and stool culture *(C. difficile)*, not to be used for systemic infection; obtain C&S before use; monitor glucose (diabetic patients); monitor fluid, electrolyte depletion
• **Hypersensitivity:** rash, pruritus; angioedema (rare)
• **Pregnancy/breastfeeding:** no well-controlled studies; use only if clearly needed; cautious use in breastfeeding, excretion unknown
Evaluate:
• **Positive therapeutic response:** resolution of *C. difficile*, decreased diarrhea
Teach patient/family:
• To report GI bleeding, severe abdominal pain
• To notify if pregnancy is planned or suspected or if breastfeeding
• To take as directed; must take all of medication
• May take without regard to food
• Advise patient if allergic to latex, not to handle, or use prefilled syringes

• **Allergic reactions:** Teach patient to report immediately to health care provider rash, trouble breathing, facial swelling, increased HR
• Teach patient to seek emergency services for left upper abdominal pain
• Advise patient that continuing labs and exams will be needed
• **Pregnancy/breastfeeding:** Advise patient to notify health care provider if pregnancy is planned or suspected or if breastfeeding

> ## ⚠ HIGH ALERT
> ### filgrastim (Rx)
> (fill-grass´stim)
> Grastofil ✿, Neupogen, Nivestym, Zarxio, Granix
> *Func. class.:* Biologic modifier
> *Chem. class.:* Granulocyte colony-stimulating factor

ACTION: Stimulates proliferation and differentiation of neutrophils

USES: To decrease infection in patients receiving antineoplastics that are myelosuppressive; to increase WBC in patients with product-induced neutropenia; bone marrow transplantation, acute radiation exposure
Unlabeled uses: Neutropenia with HIV infection, aplastic anemia, ganciclovir-induced neutropenia, zidovudine-induced neutropenia

CONTRAINDICATIONS
Hypersensitivity to proteins of *Escherichia coli*
Precautions: Pregnancy, breastfeeding, children, myeloid malignancies, radiation therapy, sepsis, sickle cell disease, chemotherapy, respiratory disease

DOSAGE AND ROUTES
After myelosuppressive chemotherapy (Neupogen, Nivestym, Zarxio)
• **Adult/child: IV/SUBCUT** 5 mcg/kg/day in a single dose × up to 14 days; may increase by 5 mcg/kg with each cycle

After myelosuppressive doses of radiation (Neupogen)

• **Adult/child >7 mo: SUBCUT** 10 mcg/kg/day, start as soon as possible after receiving ≥2 Gy

After bone marrow transplantation (Neupogen, Nivestym, Zarxio)

• **Adult: IV/SUBCUT** 10 mcg/kg/day as **INFUSION (IV)** over 4 hr or 24 hr; begin 24 hr after chemotherapy and 24 hr after bone marrow transplantation

Peripheral blood progenitor cell collection/therapy (Neupogen, Nivestym, Zarxios)

• **Adult:** 10 mcg/kg/day as bolus or **CONT INFUSION** × ≥4 days before leukapheresis, continue to last leukapheresis; may alter dose if WBC >100,000 cells/mm^3

Severe neutropenia (chronic) (Neupogen, Nivestym, Zarxios)

• **Adult: SUBCUT** 5 mcg/kg daily

Neonatal neutropenia

• **Neonate: IV/SUBCUT** 5-10 mcg/day × 3-5 days

Available forms: Inj 300 mcg/mL, 480 mcg/1.6 mL; vials 300 mcg/0.5 mL, 480 mcg/0.8 mL

Administer:

• Given by SUBCUT inj, short IV infusion, or continuous SC or IV infusion

• Avoid use within 24 hr before or after chemotherapy

• Do not shake commercial single-dose vials before withdrawing the dose; if the vial is shaken and froth or bubbles form, allow the vial to stand undisturbed for a few minutes until the froth or bubbles dissipate

• Before injection, filgrastim may be allowed to reach room temperature for a maximum of 24 hr; any vial or syringe exposed to room temperature for more than 24 hr should be discarded

• Visually inspect for particulate matter and discoloration before use

• Store in refrigerator; do not freeze; may store at room temperature up to 24 hr

SUBCUT route

• **SUBCUT inj:** no dilution is necessary; inject by rapid subcut inj, taking care not to inject intradermally; inject into abdomen, upper outer buttock, upper outer arms, rotate sites

• **SUBCUT continuous infusion:** infuse subcut at a rate not to exceed 2 mL/hr (after bone transplant)

IV route

• May be diluted with 5% dextrose; do not dilute with NS; product can precipitate

• May be diluted to concentrations 5-15 mcg/mL; should be protected from adsorption to plastic by the addition of albumin to a final albumin concentration of 2 mg/mL; do not dilute filgrastim to a concentration <5 mcg/mL

• **IV infusion:** infuse IV over 15-30 min or as a continuous infusion, chemotherapy after bone transplant over 4-24 hr

Y-site compatibilities: Acyclovir, allopurinol, amikacin, aminophylline, ampicillin, ampicillin/sulbactam, aztreonam, bleomycin, bumetanide, buprenorphine, butorphanol, calcium gluconate, CARBOplatin, carmustine, ceFAZolin, cefoTEtan, cefTAZidime, chlorproMAZINE, cimetidine, CISplatin, cyclophosphamide, cytarabine, dacarbazine, DAUNOrubicin, dexamethasone, diphenhydrAMINE, DOXOrubicin, doxycycline, droperidol, enalaprilat, famotidine, floxuridine, fluconazole, fludarabine, gallium, ganciclovir, granisetron, haloperidol, hydrocortisone, HYDROmorphone, hydrOXYzine, IDArubicin, ifosfamide, leucovorin, LORazepam, mechlorethamine, melphalan, meperidine, mesna, methotrexate, metoclopramide, miconazole, minocycline, mitoXANtrone, morphine, nalbuphine, netilmicin, ondansetron, plicamycin, potassium chloride, promethazine, ranitidine, sodium bicarbonate, streptozocin, ticarcillin, ticarcillin/clavulanate, tobramycin, trimethoprimsulfamethoxazole, vancomycin, vinBLAStine, vinCRIStine, vinorelbine, zidovudine

SIDE EFFECTS

CNS: Fever, headache

GI: *Nausea,* vomiting, diarrhea, mucositis, anorexia, splenic rupture

HEMA: Thrombocytopenia, excessive leukocytosis
INTEG: Alopecia, exacerbation of skin conditions, urticaria, cutaneous vasculitis, allergic reactions
MS: Osteoporosis, skeletal pain
OTHER: Chest pain, hypotension
RESP: Acute respiratory distress syndrome, wheezing, alveolar hemorrhage

PHARMACOKINETICS
SUBCUT: Onset 5-60 min, peak 2-8 hr, duration up to 1 wk
IV: Onset 5-60 min, peak 24 hr, duration up to 1 wk

INTERACTIONS
Increase: adverse reactions—do not use this product concomitantly with antineoplastics, lithium
Drug/Lab Test
Increase: uric acid, LDH, alk phos, WBC

NURSING CONSIDERATIONS
Assess:
• **Labs:** CBC, platelet count before treatment and twice weekly; neutrophil counts drop by 50% if filgrastim is discontinued the next day
• **Vitals:** B/P, respirations, pulse before and during therapy
• Bone pain; give mild analgesics: loratadine 10 mg before filgrastim may help
• **Respiratory distress syndrome:** fever, dyspnea; withhold product if these occur
• **Allergic reactions:** rash, wheezing, facial edema, dyspnea; may occur within 30 min of use; give antihistamines, steroids bronchodilators, and EPINEPHrine if needed
• **Splenic rupture:** severe left upper abdominal pain
• **Pregnancy/breastfeeding:** may cause fetal harm; if used in pregnancy, enroll in Amgen's Surveillance Program, 800-772-6436
Evaluate:
• **Therapeutic response:** absence of infection, improved outcome in bone marrow transplantation, improved neutropenia counts in chronic neutropenia
Teach patient/family:
• About the technique for self-administration: dose, side effects, disposal of containers and needles; provide instruction sheet
• That bone pain is common

---

finasteride (Rx)
(fin-ass´te-ride)
Propecia, Proscar
Func. class.: Hormone, androgen inhibitor, hair stimulant
Chem. class.: 5-α-Reductase inhibitor

Combinations:
Finasteride 5 mg/tadalafil 5 mg (Entadafi)

Do not confuse:
finasteride/furosemide
Proscar/Prograf/Provera

ACTION: Inhibits 5-α-reductase and reduction in DHT; DHT induces androgenic effects by binding to androgen receptors in the cell nuclei of the prostate gland, liver, skin; prevents development of BPH

USES: Symptomatic benign prostatic hyperplasia (Proscar); male-pattern baldness (Propecia)

CONTRAINDICATIONS
Pregnancy, breastfeeding, children, women who are pregnant or who may become pregnant should not handle tabs, hypersensitivity
Precautions: Large residual urinary volume, severely diminished urinary flow, hepatic function abnormalities

DOSAGE AND ROUTES
BPH
• **Adult: PO** 5 mg/day (Proscar)
Male-pattern baldness
• **Adult: PO** 1 mg/day for 3 mo or more for results (Propecia)
Available forms: Tabs (Propecia) 1 mg, (Proscar) 5 mg
Administer:
• Without regard to meals
• For a minimum of 6 mo; not all patients will respond
• Store <86° F (30° C); protect from light; keep container tightly closed

---

Side effects: *italics* = common; red = life-threatening

SIDE EFFECTS

GU: Impotence, decreased libido, decreased volume of ejaculate, sexual dysfunction, gynecomastia
INTEG: Rash
MISC: Breast tenderness, secondary malignancy, angioedema

PHARMACOKINETICS

Bioavailability 63%; readily absorbed from GI tract; protein binding 90%; metabolized in the liver; excreted in urine (metabolites) 39%, feces (57%); crosses blood-brain barrier; peak 1-2 hr; duration 24 hr

INTERACTIONS

Drug/Lab Test
Decrease: PSA levels

NURSING CONSIDERATIONS

Assess:
• **BPH:** urinary patterns, residual urinary volume, severely diminished urinary flow
• PSA levels and exclusion of prostate/urinary cancer before initiating therapy and periodically thereafter; PSA levels may be altered by this product
• Hepatic studies before treatment; extensively metabolized in liver
• **Pregnancy/breastfeeding:** not to be used in females; do not use in pregnancy/breastfeeding
Evaluate:
• **Therapeutic response:** increased urinary flow; decreased postvoiding dribbling, frequency, nocturia; hair growth within 3-6 mo; regression of prostate size
Teach patient/family:
• That volume of ejaculate may be decreased during treatment; that impotence and decreased libido may also occur and may continue after discontinuing treatment
• That Propecia results may not occur for 3 mo
• That Proscar results may not occur for 6-12 mo
• Advise patient to take as directed, not to skip or double doses, up to 12 mo may be required
• Inform patient that reading the "Patient Package Insert" is necessary

• Advise patient to notify health care provider of breast tenderness, pain, discharge
• Teach patient that continuing labs and exams will be needed
• That pregnant women or women who may become pregnant should not touch crushed tabs or come into contact with the semen of a patient taking this product; that product may adversely affect developing male fetus

---

finerenone (Rx)

(fin-ER-e-none)
Kerendia
Func. class.: Nonsteroidal, mineralo-corticoid antagonist

USES: Chronic kidney disease associated with type 2 diabetes

DOSAGES AND ROUTES

• **Adult: PO** 10 or 20 mg daily based on eGFR
Available forms: Tabs 10, 20 mg

---

fingolimod (Rx)

(fin-gol′i-mod) (fin-go′li-mod)
Gilenya
Func. class.: Immunosuppressant, anti-MS agent
Chem. class.: Sphingosine 1-phosphate receptor modulator

ACTION: Binds with high affinity to sphingosine 1-phosphate receptors; blocks lymphocyte egress to lymph nodes, thereby reducing the number of peripheral blood lymphocytes; may reduce lymphocyte migration into the CNS

USES: To reduce frequency of exacerbation, to delay physical disability of relapsing forms of MS

CONTRAINDICATIONS

Hypersensitivity
Precautions: Pregnancy, breastfeeding, neonates/infants/children, AIDS, asthma,

---

AV block, bradycardia, cardiac disease, COPD, diabetes mellitus, dysrhythmias, heart failure, hepatic disease, HIV, hypertension, immunosuppression, leukemia, lymphoma, QT prolongation, respiratory insufficiency, sick sinus syndrome, syncope, uveitis

DOSAGE AND ROUTES
• **Adult/child ≥10 yr and >40 kg: PO** 0.5 mg/day
Child ≥10 yr and ≤40 kg: 0.25 mg daily
Hepatic dose
• **Adult: PO** Child-Pugh C, total score >10: closely monitor, fingolimod exposure is doubled
Available forms: Caps 0.25, 0.5 mg; ODT 0.25 mg
Administer:
PO route
• Watch patient for 6 hr after initial dose or if product not given for >2 wk for development of bradycardia
• Give without regard to food
• Store at room temperature, protect from moisture

SIDE EFFECTS
CNS: Asthenia, depression, fatigue, headache, dizziness, progressive multifocal leukoencephalopathy, migraine, paresthesias, stroke
CV: AV block, bradycardia, chest pain, hypertension, palpitations, QT prolongation
EENT: Blurred vision, vision impairment, ocular pain, macular edema
GI: Abdominal pain, anorexia, diarrhea, jaundice, vomiting, weight loss, hepatotoxicity
HEMA: Leukopenia, lymphopenia, neutropenia
INTEG: Alopecia, pruritus
MS: Back pain
RESP: Dyspnea, cough
SYST: Infection, influenza, secondary malignancy

PHARMACOKINETICS
Protein binding (99.7%), distributed to RBCs (86%), steady-state 1-2 mo, metabolized by CYP4F2 and CYP2D6 to a lesser extent, terminal half-life 6-9 days, excreted in urine (81% inactive metabolites), peak 12-16 hr

INTERACTIONS
Increase: risk of heart block, serious bradycardia—β-blockers, calcium channel blockers, digoxin; avoid if possible
Increase: immunosuppression—antineoplastics, immunosuppressants, immune-modulating therapies
Increase: fingolimod effect—ketoconazole
Increase: infection risk—live vaccines
Decrease: effect of—inactive vaccines, toxoids
Increase: risk of torsades de pointes—Class Ia/III antidysrhythmics

NURSING CONSIDERATIONS
Assess:
• **Multiple sclerosis:** improving paresthesia; muscle weakness; clonus; muscle spasms; difficulty with moving; difficulty with coordination of balance, speech, swallowing, vision problems, fatigue; prevention of increasing disability
• **Vision:** opthalmologic exam baseline and periodically
• **Labs:** baseline: CBC, LFTs, serum bilirubin, ophthalmologic exam, antibodies to VZV; if there is no history of chickenpox or no vaccination, may give VZV vaccination to antibody-negative patient before giving product, postpone for 1 mo after vaccination; obtain ECG for evidence of bradycardia, AV block; monitor pulmonary function tests periodically
• **Progressive multifocal leukoencephalopathy (PML):** confusion, apathy, dizziness, unstable gait; may be fatal, discontinue product, contact prescriber, MRIs may be ordered q6mo
• **Bradycardia:** monitor for ≥6 hr after beginning dose, ECG before and after 1st dose, if heart rate <45 bpm or new heart block (2nd degree) occurs, do not use until resolved
• **Infections:** fever, chills, nausea, vomiting, fatigue, sore throat; monitor during and for up to 2 mo after last dose
• Monitor for QT prolongation
• **Hypersensitivity:** may include angioedema

Side effects: *italics* = common; red = life-threatening

• **Pregnancy/breastfeeding:** use only if benefits outweigh fetal risk, may cause fetal harm; contraception should be used during and for 2 mo after final dose; enroll in Gilenya Pregnancy Registry (877-598-7237) if pregnant; discontinue breastfeeding or product, excretion unknown

Evaluate:

• **Therapeutic response:** improved symptoms of multiple sclerosis and prevention of increasing disability

Teach patient/family:

• About use of product and expected results; provide med guide to patient

• That continuing follow-up exams and laboratory tests will be required on a regular basis

• **Vaccines:** not to receive any live attenuated vaccines during and for ≥2 mo after last dose

• **Malignancy:** Use sunscreen, protective clothing; may cause melanoma basal cell carcinoma

• **Liver dysfunction:** to report jaundice, nausea, vomiting, anorexia, abdominal pain, fatigue, dark urine

• **Cardiac changes:** to report chest pain, palpitations

• **Infection:** Teach patient to report flu-like symptoms, nausea, vomiting, headache, fever

• **PML:** Teach patient to report confusion, seizures, vision change, headache, weakness, apathy, dizziness

• **Hypersensitvity:** Teach patient to report rash, itching, trouble breathing, swelling of face

• **Pregnancy/breastfeeding:** To use contraception during and for 2 mo after conclusion of treatment

fish oil triglycerides emulsion (Rx)

(fish oyl try-glyc′e-rides)

Omegaven

Func. class.: Nutritional supplement—essential fatty acid

USES: A source of calories and fatty acids in pediatric patients with parenteral nutrition–associated cholestasis (PNAC)

CONTRAINDICATIONS

Hypersensitivity to this product or fish or eggs, severe hemorrhagic disorders due to a potential effect on platelet aggregation, severe hyperlipidemia, or severe disorders of lipid metabolism characterized by hypertriglyceridemia (serum triglyceride concentrations greater than 1000 mg/dL)

DOSAGE AND ROUTES

• **Child:** IV infusion 1 g/kg/day is the recommended and maximum daily dose, do not exceed 0.05 mL/min for the first 15-30 min of the infusion, max rate 1.5 mL/kg/hr

Available forms: injection 2 g/50 mL, 10 g/100-mL single dose

⚠ HIGH ALERT

flecainide (Rx)

(flek-ay′nide)

Tambocor ♦

Func. class.: Antidysrhythmic (Class IC)

Chem. class.: Benzamide derivative

ACTION: Decreases conduction in all parts of the heart, with greatest effect on the His-Purkinje system, which stabilizes cardiac membrane

USES: Life-threatening ventricular dysrhythmias, sustained ventricular tachycardia, supraventricular tachydysrhythmias, paroxysmal atrial fibrillation/flutter associated with disabling symptoms

CONTRAINDICATIONS

Hypersensitivity, AV bundle branch block, cardiogenic shock

Precautions: Pregnancy, breastfeeding, children, geriatric patients, renal/

hepatic disease, HF, respiratory depression, myasthenia gravis, electrolyte abnormalities, atrial fibrillation, sick sinus syndrome, torsades de pointes, MI, bundle branch block, QT prolongation

Black Box Warning: Cardiac arrhythmias, atrial fibrillation, MI

DOSAGE AND ROUTES
PSVT/PAT
• **Adult: PO** 50 mg q12hr; may increase q4days by 50 mg q12hr to desired response, max 300 mg/day
Life-threatening ventricular dysrhythmias
• **Adult: PO** 100 mg q12hr; may increase by 50 mg q12hr q4days, max 400 mg/day
Renal dose
• **Adult: PO** CCr <35 mL/min, 100 mg daily or 50 mg bid initially
Available forms: Tabs 50, 100, 150 mg
Administer:
PO route
• Reduced dosage as soon as dysrhythmia is controlled
• May give with meals for GI upset
• May adjust dose q4days
• Adjust dosage at intervals of ≥4 days (approximate plateau effects); however, longer intervals are needed in patients with renal or hepatic impairment
• Frequent serum drug concentration monitoring is required for patients with severe renal (CrCl <35 mL/min) or hepatic disease and may also be helpful in patients with HF or in patients with moderate renal disease
• Monitoring of flecainide serum concentrations is strongly recommended in patients receiving amiodarone therapy

SIDE EFFECTS
CNS: *Headache, dizziness,* involuntary movement, confusion, psychosis, restlessness, irritability, paresthesias, ataxia, flushing, somnolence, depression, anxiety, malaise, fatigue, asthenia, tremors
CV: *Hypotension, bradycardia,* angina, PVCs, heart block, cardiovascular collapse, arrest, dysrhythmias, HF, fatal ventricular tachycardia, palpitations, QT prolongation, torsades de pointes
EENT: Tinnitus, *blurred vision,* hearing loss, corneal deposits, dry eyes
GI: Nausea, vomiting, anorexia, constipation, abdominal pain, flatulence, change in taste, diarrhea
GU: Impotence, decreased libido, polyuria, urinary retention
HEMA: Leukopenia, thrombocytopenia
INTEG: Rash, urticaria, edema, swelling
RESP: Dyspnea, respiratory depression

PHARMACOKINETICS
Peak 3 hr, half-life 12-27 hr, metabolized by liver, excreted unchanged by kidneys (10%), excreted in breast milk

INTERACTIONS
Increase: QT prolongation—class IA/III antidysrhythmics, some phenothiazines, β-agonists, local anesthetics, tricyclics, haloperidol, chloroquine, droperidol, pentamidine; CYP3A4 inhibitors (amiodarone, clarithromycin, erythromycin, telithromycin, troleandomycin), arsenic trioxide, levomethadyl; CYP3A4 substrates (methadone, pimozide, QUEtiapine, quiNIDine, risperiDONE, ziprasidone)
Increase: of both products—propranolol
Increase: CV depressant action—β-blockers, disopyramide, verapamil
Increase: flecainide level—amiodarone, cimetidine, ritonavir
Increase: digoxin level—digoxin
Increase or decrease: effect—urinary, alkalinizing agents, acidifying agents
Drug/Herb
Do not use with hawthorn
Drug/Lab Test
Increase: CPK

NURSING CONSIDERATIONS
Assess:

Black Box Warning: HF, cardiogenic shock, LVEF <30%: should not be used in these conditions

Black Box Warning: Atrial fibrillation: avoid use; risk of ventricular dysrhythmias; use only in life-threatening dysrhythmias

---

Side effects: *italics* = common; red = life-threatening

F

Black Box Warning: Cardiac dysrhythmias: discontinue in those with prolonged QRS >180 ms or prolonged PR >300 ms, monitor for QT prolongation, monitor ECG before and during treatment

• **Electrolyte imbalances:** hypo/hyperkalemia before administration; correct electrolytes before use
• **CNS effects:** dizziness, confusion, psychosis, paresthesias, seizures; product should be discontinued
• **Monitor renal studies:** BUN, creatinine
• **Flecainide level:** monitor level in those with HF or renal failure; peak, trough
• **Pregnancy/breastfeeding:** no well-controlled studies; use only if benefits outweigh fetal risk; discontinue breastfeeding or product, excreted in breast milk
Evaluate:
• **Therapeutic response:** decreased dysrhythmias
Teach patient/family:
• To change position slowly from lying or sitting to standing to minimize orthostatic hypotension
• To take as prescribed; not to skip or double dose, to take missed dose as soon as remembered within 6 hr of next dose
• To avoid hazardous activities that require alertness until response is known
• To carry emergency ID with disorder, medications taken
• To notify all health care providers of treatment, that follow-up will be needed
• To report new or worsening cardiac symptoms (chest pain, trouble breathing, sweating)

TREATMENT OF OVERDOSE: O_2, artificial ventilation, ECG, DOPamine for circulatory depression, diazePAM or thiopental for seizures, treat ventricular dysrhythmias

---

flibanserin (Rx)
(flib-an´ser-in)
Addyi
Func. class.: Sexual dysfunction agent

USES: For the treatment of acquired, generalized hypoactive sexual desire disorder (HSDD) (also known as female sexual interest/arousal disorder)

CONTRAINDICATIONS
Hypersensitivity, hepatic disease, pregnancy, breastfeeding

DOSAGE AND ROUTES
• **Adult premenopausal females: PO** 100 mg once daily at bedtime. Discontinue after 8 wk if no improvement
Available forms: Tabs 100 mg

---

fluconazole (Rx)
(floo-kon´a-zole)
Canesoral ✦, Diflucan, Diflucan One
Func. class.: Antifungal, systemic; azole

Do not confuse:
Diflucan/Diprivan

ACTION: Inhibits fungal sterols, causes direct damage to fungal membrane phospholipids

USES: Oropharyngeal candidiasis, chronic mucocutaneous candidiasis; systemic, vaginal, urinary candidiasis; cryptococcal meningitis; prevention of candidiasis in bone marrow transplant in those who receive chemotherapy and/or radiation therapy; cystitis, fungal prophylaxis, peritonitis, pneumonia, pyelonephritis

CONTRAINDICATIONS
Hypersensitivity to this product or azoles, pregnancy
Precautions: Breastfeeding, renal/hepatic disease, torsades de pointes

DOSAGE AND ROUTES
Vulvovaginal candidiasis
• **Adult: PO** 150 mg as a single dose; **prevention of recurrence (unlabeled)** 100-200 mg wk for 6 mon for non-HIV patients, 150 mg/wk for HIV patients
Serious fungal infections
• **Adult: PO/IV** Most serious CNS infections 400-1200 mg daily

- **Child:** PO/IV 6-12 mg/kg/day; max 400-800 mg/day depending on indication
- **Neonates <14 days, 30-36 wk gestation:** PO/IV same as child except q48hr

Oropharyngeal candidiasis

- **Adult:** PO/IV 200 mg initially, then 100 mg/day for ≥2 wk, max 600 mg/day
- **Child >14 days:** PO/IV 6 mg/kg; max 200 mg initially, then 3 mg/kg/day; max 100 mg for ≥2 wk
- **Neonate <14 days, 30-36 wk gestation:** PO/IV 6 mg/kg/dose once, then 3 mg/kg/dose once daily

Esophageal candidiasis

- **Adult:** PO/IV 200 mg on 1st day, then 100 mg daily × ≥3 wk and for ≥2 wk after resolution of symptoms
- **Child >14 days:** PO/IV 6 mg/kg; max 400 mg on 1st day, then 3-6 mg/kg/day, max 400 mg × ≥3 wk and for ≥2 wk after resolution of symptoms, max 400 mg/day or 12 mg/kg PO
- **Neonate:** PO/IV 6 mg/kg q 24-48hr

Cryptococcal meningitis

- **Adult:** PO/IV 400 mg on 1st day, then 200 mg/day × 10-12 wk after CSF culture negative, suppressive therapy 200 mg/day
- **Child/infant/neonate ≥14 days:** PO/IV 12 mg/kg on 1st day, then 6-12 mg/kg daily × 10-12 wk after CSF culture negative, max 600 mg/day, suppressive therapy 6 mg/kg/day
- **Neonate 0-14 days (unlabeled):** PO 10 to 12 mg/kg/dose q day X 8 wk after the initial 2-wk course of induction therapy, followed by 6 mg/kg/dose q day X 6 to 12 mo

Prevention of candidiasis in bone marrow transplant

- **Adult:** PO/IV 400 mg/day, those anticipated to have neutrophils <500/mm^3, start several days before anticipated onset of neutropenia and continue for 7 days after rise of neutrophils >1000/mm^3
- **Adolescents+:** PO 3 to 6 mg/kg/dose (Max: 400 mg/dose) q day
- **Child >14 days:** PO/IV 10-12 mg/kg/day, max 600 mg/day

Renal disease

- **Adult:** PO/IV CCr ≤50 mL/min, after loading dose, give 50% of usual dose; hemodialysis give 100% of usual dose after dialysis treatment, give dose as per CCr on non-dialysis days

Available forms: Tabs 50, 100, 150, 200 mg; inj 2 mg/mL (100 mg/50 mL, 200 mg/100 mL, 400 mg/200 mL); powder for oral susp 10 mg/mL, 40 mg/mL

Administer:

PO route

- Shake oral susp before each use, use within 2 wk

Intermittent IV INFUSION route

- Premixed solutions are ready to use, run at ≤200 mg/hr
- Use infusion pump; check for extravasation and necrosis q2hr
- Do not use if cloudy or precipitated
- Do not admix; do not refrigerate
- Store protected from moisture and light; diluted sol stable 24 hr; do not freeze

Y-site compatibilities: Acyclovir, aldesleukin, alfentanil, allopurinol, amifostine, amikacin, aminocaproic acid, aminophylline, amiodarone, anidulafungin, ascorbic acid injection, atenolol, atracurium, atropine, azaTHIOprine, aztreonam, benztropine, bivalirudin, bleomycin, bumetanide, buprenorphine, butorphanol, calcium chloride, CARBOplatin, caspofungin, ceFAZolin, cefepime, cefmetazole, cefonicid, cefoTEtan, cefOXitin, cefpirome, cefTAZidime, ceftizoxime, ceftobiprole, cephalothin, cephapirin, chlorproMAZINE, cimetidine, cisatracurium, CISplatin, codeine, cyanocobalamin, cyclophosphamide, cycloSPORINE, cytarabine, DACTINomycin, DAPTOmycin, dexamethasone, diltiazem, dimenhyDRINATE, diphenhydrAMINE, DOBUTamine, DOCEtaxel, DOPamine, doripenem, doxacurium, DOXOrubicin, DOXOrubicin liposomal, doxycycline, droperidol, drotrecogin alfa, enalaprilat, ePHEDrine, EPINEPHrine, epirubicin, epoetin alfa, eptifibatide, ertapenem, erythromycin, esmolol, etoposide, famotidine, fenoldopam, fentaNYL, filgrastim, fludarabine, fluorouracil, folic acid, foscarnet, gallium, ganciclovir, gatifloxacin, gemcitabine, gentamicin, glycopyrrolate, granisetron, heparin, hydrocortisone, HYDROmorphone, IDArubicin, ifosfamide, IV immune globulin, inamrinone, indomethacin, insulin (regular), irinotecan, isoproterenol, ketorolac, labetalol, lansoprazole, leucovorin, levofloxacin, lidocaine, linezolid, LORazepam, LR, magnesium sulfate, mannitol, mechlorethamine, melphalan, meperidine, meropenem, metaraminol, methicillin, methotrexate, methoxamine, methyldopate, methylPREDNISolone, metoclopramide, metoprolol, metroNIDAZOLE, mezlocillin, miconazole, midazolam, milrinone, minocycline, mitoXANtrone, morphine, moxalactam, multiple vitamins injection, mycophenolate, nafcillin, nalbuphine, naloxone, nesiritide, nitroglycerin, nitroprusside, norepinephrine, octreotide, ondansetron, oxacillin, oxaliplatin, oxytocin, PACLitaxel, palonosetron, pamidronate, pancuronium, papaverine, PEMEtrexed, penicillin G potassium/sodium, pentazocine, PENTobarbital, PHENobarbital, phenylephrine, phenytoin, phytonadione, piperacillin-tazobactam, polymyxin B, potassium chloride, procainamide, prochlorperazine, promethazine, propofol, propranolol, protamine, pyridoxine, quiNIDine, quinupristin-dalfopristin, ranitidine, remifentanil, Ringer's, ritodrine, riTUXimab, rocuronium, sargramostim, sodium acetate/bicarbonate, succinylcholine, SUFentanil, tacrolimus, temocillin, teniposide, theophylline, thiotepa, ticarcillin-clavulanate, tigecycline, tirofiban, TNA, tobramycin, tolazoline, TPN, trastuzumab, trimetaphan, urokinase, vancomycin, vasopressin, vecuronium, verapamil, vinCRIStine, vinorelbine, voriconazole, zidovudine, zoledronic acid

SIDE EFFECTS

CNS: *Headache,* seizures
CV: QT prolongation, torsades de pointes
GI: *Nausea, vomiting;* diarrhea; cramping; flatus; increased AST, ALT; hepatotoxicity; abdominal pain; cholestasis
HEMA: Agranulocytosis, eosinophilia, leukopenia, neutropenia, thrombocytopenia
INTEG: Stevens-Johnson syndrome, angioedema, anaphylaxis, exfoliative dermatitis, toxic epidermal necrolysis

PHARMACOKINETICS

Peak 1-2 hr, bioavailability (PO) >90%, widely distributed (peritoneum, CSF), excreted in breast milk, excreted unchanged in urine 80%, metabolized by CYP3A enzyme system at dose >200 mg/day, half-life 30 hr (adult); child 19-25 hr (PO); premature neonates (46-74 hr)

INTERACTIONS

Increase: hypoglycemia—oral sulfonylureas (glipiZIDE)
Increase: anticoagulation—warfarin
Increase: plasma concentrations/toxicity—cycloSPORINE, phenytoin, theophylline, rifabutin, tacrolimus, sirolimus, zidovudine, zolpidem
Increase: myopathy, rhabdomyolysis risk—HMG-CoA reductase inhibitors: lovastatin, simvastatin, avoid using together
Increase: effect of zidovudine, methadone, SUFentanil, alfentanil, buprenorphine, saquinavir, fentaNYL, ergots
Decrease: effect of calcium channel blockers
Decrease: fluconazole effect—proton pump inhibitors

Drug/Lab Test
Increase: alk phos, LFTs
Decrease: WBC, platelets

NURSING CONSIDERATIONS

Assess:
- **Infection:** clearing of CSF and other culture during treatment, obtain C&S baseline and throughout treatment, product may be started as soon as culture is taken
- **QT prolongation:** avoid with other products that cause QT prolongation
- **Hepatotoxicity:** monitor for increasing AST, ALT, baseline and periodically alk phos, bilirubin; for renal status: BUN, creatinine
- **Skin symptoms:** color, lesions, inj-site reactions; if lesions progress, stop product; monitor rash, usually appears after 2nd wk of treatment and disappears in 2 wk if continuing product
- **Pregnancy/breastfeeding:** birth defects may occur if used in 1st trimester; do not use in pregnancy, breastfeeding

Evaluate:

• **Therapeutic response:** decreasing oral candidiasis, fever, malaise, rash; negative C&S for infection organism

Teach patient/family:

• That long-term therapy may be needed to clear infection, not to add new medications, herbs without prescriber approval

• That medication may be taken with food to reduce GI effects

• To notify prescriber of nausea, vomiting, diarrhea, jaundice, anorexia, clay-colored stools, dark urine, skin rash, abdominal pain, fever, bruising, bleeding

• **Pregnancy/breastfeeding:** To use adequate contraception during and for 1 wk after last dose

---

⚠ HIGH ALERT

fludarabine (Rx)

(floo-dar′a-been)
Func. class.: Antineoplastic, antimetabolite
Chem. class.: Purine antagonist

ACTION: Inhibits DNA synthesis by inhibition of DNA polymerase and ribonucleotide reductase; also inhibits DNA primase and DNA ligase

USES: Chronic lymphocytic leukemia

CONTRAINDICATIONS
Pregnancy, breastfeeding, hypersensitivity

Black Box Warning: Hemolytic anemia, bone marrow suppression, coma, seizures, visual disturbances

DOSAGE AND ROUTES
Chronic lymphocytic leukemia (CLL), refractory or progressive
• **Adult:** IV 25 mg/m² once daily for 5 consecutive days q28days; continue for at least 3 additional cycles after maximal

response is achieved; PO (Canada only) 40 mg/m² once daily for 5 consecutive days q28days

Acute myeloid leukemia, newly diagnosed (Unlabeled)
• **Adult:** IV 30 mg/m²/day for 5 days (cytarabine ± G-CSF ± idarubicin (FA, FLAG, or FLAG-IDA regimens), followed by consolidation therapy

Acute myeloid leukemia, refractory or high/poor-risk patients (unlabeled)
• **Adult:** IV 30 mg/m²/day × 5 days (with cytarabine and filgrastim [FLAG regimen]), may repeat once for partial remission **or** 30 mg/m²/day for 5 days for 1 or 2 cycles (in combination with cytarabine, idarubicin, and filgrastim [FLAG-IDA regimen])

Hematopoietic stem cell transplant (allogeneic) myeloablative conditioning regimen (off-label use)
• **Adult:** IV 40 mg/m²/day for 4 days (with busulfan) beginning 6 days prior to transplantation

Hematopoietic stem cell transplant (allogeneic) reduced-intensity conditioning regimen (unlabeled)
• **Adult:** IV 30 mg/m²/day × 5 days (with melphalan and alemtuzumab) prior to transplant **or** 30 mg/m²/day for 6 days beginning 10 days prior to transplant **or** 30 mg/m²/day for 5 days beginning 6 days prior to transplant (with busulfan with or without antithymocyte globulin)

Hematopoietic stem cell transplant (allogeneic) nonmyeloablative conditioning regimen (unlabeled)
• **Adult:** IV 30 mg/m²/day × 3 doses beginning 5 days prior to transplant (with cyclophosphamide and rituximab) **or** 30 mg/m²/day for 3 doses beginning 4 days prior to transplant (with total body irradiation)

Available forms: Solution for injection 50 mg/2 mL (2 mL); powder for injection 50 mg/2 mL

Administer
IV route
• Reconstitute lyophilized powder with 2 mL SWFI to a concentration of 25 mg/mL

• Dilute in 100 to 125 mL D_5W or NS, give over 30 min (CLL)
• Store vials under refrigeration or at room temperature, as specified according to each manufacturer's labeling. Protect from light. Reconstituted solution or vials of the solution for injection that have been punctured (in use) should be used within 8 hr

PO route

• Tablet [Canadian product] give with or without food; swallow whole with water; do not chew, break, or crush
• Tablet [Canadian product]: Store at 15° C-30° C (59° F-86° F); keep in packaging until use

SIDE EFFECTS

CV: Edema, angina pectoris, cardiac arrhythmia, cardiac failure, CVA, MI, supraventricular tachycardia, DVT, phlebitis
CNS: Fatigue, cortical blindness, coma, paralysis, chills, paresthesia, malaise, headache, sleep disorder
INTEG: Rash, diaphoresis, alopecia, pruritus
GI: Nausea, vomiting, anorexia, diarrhea, GI hemorrhage, stomatitis, cholelithiasis, esophagitis, constipation, mucositis
GU: UTI, hematuria, dysuria
HEMA: Anemia, neutropenia, thrombocytopenia, bone marrow depression
EENT: Visual disturbance, hearing loss
RESP: Cough, pneumonia, dyspnea, URI, pharyngitis, hypersensitivity, pneumonitis, hemoptysis, sinusitis
MISC: Fever, infection, myalgia, hypersensitivity, hyperglycemia, TLS

PHARMACOKINETICS

Onset, peak, duration unknown; half-life 20 hr

INTERACTIONS

Increase: toxicity—other myelosuppressives
Increase: adverse reactions—live virus vaccines, bring up to date before treatment

Black Box Warning: **Increase:** pulmonary toxicity—pentostatin, do not use together

NURSING CONSIDERATIONS
Assess:

Black Box Warning: **Severe bone marrow suppression (anemia, thrombocytopenia, and neutropenia):** may be cumulative. Time to nadir 13 days (range: 3-25 days) for granulocytes and 16 days (range: 2-32 days) for platelets. Monitor those with bone marrow impairment closely for excess toxicity; may require dosage reductions

• **Autoimmune effects:** Instances of life-threatening and sometimes fatal autoimmune phenomena, such as hemolytic anemia, autoimmune thrombocytopenia/thrombocytopenic purpura, Evans syndrome, and acquired hemophilia, have been reported to occur after 1 or more cycles of treatment with fludarabine. Patients undergoing treatment should be evaluated and closely monitored for hemolysis

Black Box Warning: **Autoimmune effects:** May be life-threatening, hemolytic anemia, autoimmune thrombocytopenia/thrombocytopenic purpura, Evans syndrome, and acquired hemophilia, have been reported after 1 or more cycles, evaluate and closely monitored for hemolysis, corticosteroids may be needed

• **Tumor lysis syndrome:** Risk is increased in patients with large tumor burden prior to treatment. Hydration and prophylactic antihyperuricemic therapy may be used

Black Box Warning: **Neurotoxicity:** Higher-than-recommended doses (up to 96 mg/m²/day for 5-7 days) may cause severe neurologic toxicity (delayed blindness, coma, death); similar neurotoxicity (agitation, coma, confusion, seizure) has been reported (rare) with standard CLL doses (25 mg/m²/day for 5 days). Symptoms of neurotoxicity due to high doses appeared from 21-60 days following the last dose, neurotoxicity may occur as early as 7 days and up to 225 days

Black Box Warning: Combination with pentostatin: Do not use together, fatal pulmonary toxicity may occur

Black Box Warning: Experienced physician: Injection should be administered under the supervision of a qualified health care provider experienced in the use of antineoplastic therapy

• **PML:** PML (usually fatal) due to JC virus has been reported; most cases were in patients who had received prior and/or other concurrent chemotherapy. Onset may be a few weeks or may be delayed up to 1 yr. Evaluate any neurologic change promptly
• **Transfusion-associated graft-versus-host disease:** Patient should only receive irradiated blood products due to the potential for transfusion-related GVHD
• **Pregnancy/breastfeeding:** Not to be used in pregnancy or breastfeeding; effective contraception should be used by females and males during and for ≥6 mo after last dose
• Monitor CBC with differential, platelet count, AST, ALT, serum creatinine, serum albumin, uric acid; monitor for signs of infection, neurotoxicity, and tumor lysis syndrome
Evaluate:
• **Therapeutic response:** Inhibiting CLL
Teach patient/family:
• To report mouth irritation, mouth sores, muscle pain
• **PML:** To report confusion, depression, trouble with memory, behavioral changes, change in strength on one side is greater than the other, trouble speaking, change in balance, or vision changes
• **Bleeding:** To report vomiting blood or vomit that looks like coffee grounds or is black; coughing up blood; blood in the urine; black, red, or tarry stools; bleeding from the gums; abnormal vaginal bleeding; bruises without a reason or that get bigger; or any severe or persistent bleeding
• **Tumor lysis syndrome:** To report fast heartbeat or abnormal heartbeat; fainting; unable to pass urine; muscle weakness or cramps; nausea, vomiting, diarrhea or lack of appetite; or feeling fatigued

• To report shortness of breath or other trouble breathing, cough that is new or worse
• **Stevens-Johnson syndrome/toxic epidermal necrolysis:** To report red, swollen, blistered, or peeling skin (with or without fever); red or irritated eyes; or sores in mouth, throat, nose, or eyes
• **Signs of an allergic reaction:** To report rash; hives; itching; red, swollen, blistered, or peeling skin with or without fever; wheezing; tightness in the chest or throat; trouble breathing, swallowing, or talking; unusual hoarseness; or swelling of the mouth, face, lips, tongue, throat
• **Pregnancy/breastfeeding:** To report if pregnancy is planned or suspected or if breastfeeding; to use contraceptives (males and females taking product) during and for ≥6 mo after last dose

fludrocortisone (Rx)
(floo-droe-kor′ti-sone)
Func. class.: Corticosteroid, synthetic
Chem. class.: Mineralocorticoid

USES: Adrenal insufficiency, salt-losing adrenogenital syndrome, Addison's disease

CONTRAINDICATIONS
Children <2 yr, hypersensitivity

DOSAGE AND ROUTES
Adrenocortical insufficiency
• **Adult:** PO 100-200 mcg/day
• **Child:** PO 50-200 mcg/day
Available forms: Tabs 100 mcg (0.1 mg)

flumazenil (Rx)
(flu-maz′e-nill)
Func. class.: Antidote: benzodiazepine receptor antagonist
Chem. class.: Imidazobenzodiazepine derivative

Do not confuse:
flumazenil/influenza virus vaccine

ACTION: Antagonizes actions of benzodiazepines on CNS, competitively inhibits activity at benzodiazepine recognition site on GABA/benzodiazepine receptor complex

USES: Reversal of sedative effects of benzodiazepines

CONTRAINDICATIONS
Hypersensitivity to this product or benzodiazepines, serious cyclic antidepressant overdose, patients given benzodiazepine for control of life-threatening conditions
Precautions: Pregnancy, breastfeeding, children, geriatric patients, status epilepticus, head injury, labor/delivery, renal/hepatic disease, hypoventilation, panic disorder, drug and alcohol dependency, ambulatory patients, benzodiazepine dependence

Black Box Warning: Seizures

DOSAGE AND ROUTES
Reversal of conscious sedation or general anesthesia
• **Adult: IV** 0.2 mg over 15 sec; wait 45 sec, then 0.2 mg if consciousness does not occur; may be repeated at 60-sec intervals prn (max 3 mg/hr) or 1 mg/5 min
• **Child: IV** 10 mcg (0.01 mg)/kg; cumulative dose of 1 mg or less
Management of suspected benzodiazepine overdose
• **Adult: IV** 0.2 mg over 30 sec; wait 30 sec, then give 0.3 mg over 30 sec if consciousness does not occur; further doses of 0.5 mg can be given over 30 sec at intervals of 1 min up to cumulative dose of 3 mg
• **Child (unlabeled): IV** 10 mcg (0.01 mg/kg), cumulative dose of <1 mg
Available forms: Inj 0.1 mg/mL
Administer:
• Check airway and IV access before administration
• Use large vein

Direct IV route
• Give undiluted or diluted with 0.9% NaCl, D_5W, LR ($\leq$0.1 mg/mL); give over 15-30 sec into running IV, check for extravasation
• Stable for 24 hr if drawn into a syringe or mixed with other solutions

SIDE EFFECTS
CNS: Dizziness, agitation, emotional lability, confusion, seizures, somnolence, panic attacks
CV: Hypertension, palpitations, cutaneous vasodilation, dysrhythmias, bradycardia, tachycardia, chest pain
EENT: Abnormal vision, blurred vision, tinnitus
GI: Nausea, vomiting, hiccups
SYST: Headache, inj site pain, increased sweating, fatigue, rigors

PHARMACOKINETICS
Half-life 41-79 min (adult), 20-75 min (child), metabolized in liver, onset 1-2 min 50% protein binding (albumin)

INTERACTIONS
• Toxicity: mixed product overdosage
• Antagonize action of benzodiazepines, zaleplon, zolpidem

NURSING CONSIDERATIONS
Assess:
• **Cardiac and respiratory status** using continuous monitoring during and for $\geq$2 hr after completion

Black Box Warning: **Seizures:** protect from injury; most likely among those who are withdrawing from benzodiazepines; seizures are increased in head trauma

• **GI symptoms:** nausea, vomiting; place patient in side-lying position to prevent aspiration
• **Allergic reactions:** flushing, rash, urticaria, pruritus

Black Box Warning: **Seizures/benzodiazepine dependence:** do not use in those who have used these products for status epilepticus; use in intensive care setting cautiously, there may be unrecognized benzodiazepine dependence

Overdose type: after use and no response, consider another overdose
• **Pregnancy/breastfeeding:** no well-controlled studies; use only if benefits outweigh fetal risk; discontinue breastfeeding or product

Teach patient/family:
• Not to use with alcohol or other medications for at least 24 hr
• That sedation may occur after treatment
• To avoid hazardous activities, driving until effects are known
• That amnesia may continue

fluocinolone (Rx)
(floo-oh-sin′oh-lone)

Capex, Derma-Smoothe/FS Body, Derma-Smoothe/FS Scalp, Synalar, Synalar (Cream), Synalar (Ointment), Synalar TS
Func. class.: Corticosteroid

USES: **Body oil:** Moderate-severe atopic dermatitis in pediatric patients ≥3 mo; treatment of atopic dermatitis in adults. **Cream, ointment, topical solution:** Relief of inflammatory/pruritic corticosteroid-responsive dermatoses. **Scalp oil:** Psoriasis of the scalp in adults. **Shampoo:** seborrheic dermatitis of the scalp

DOSAGE AND ROUTES
Atopic dermatitis:
• **Topical:** Body oil: Apply thin film to affected area tid
Corticosteroid-responsive dermatoses:
• **Topical:** Cream, ointment, solution: Apply a thin layer to affected area bid to qid; may use occlusive dressing
Scalp psoriasis:
• **Topical:** Scalp oil: Massage thoroughly into wet or dampened hair/scalp; cover with shower cap. Leave on overnight (≥4 hr). Wash hair with shampoo and rinse well
Seborrheic dermatitis of the scalp:
• **Topical:** Shampoo: Apply no more than 1 ounce to scalp daily; work into lather and allow to remain on scalp for

about 5 min; remove from hair and scalp by rinsing well with water
Available forms: Cream 0.01%, 0.025%; oil 0.01%

fluocinolone topical
See Appendix B

fluocinonide (Rx)
(floo-oh-sin′oh-nide)

Lidex, Vance
Func. class.: Corticosteroid

USES: Dermatoses

DOSAGE AND ROUTES
• **Adult/child ≥12 yr: Topical** apply to clean area bid-qid
Available forms: Cream 0.05%, 0.1%; gel, ointment, topical solution 0.05%

fluorometholone ophthalmic
See Appendix B

⚠ HIGH ALERT

fluorouracil (Rx)
(flure-oh-yoor′a-sil)

Carac, Efudex, Fluoroplex, Tolak
Func. class.: Antineoplastic, antimetabolite
Chem. class.: Pyrimidine analog

ACTION: Inhibits DNA, RNA synthesis; interferes with cell replication by competitively inhibiting thymidylate production, specific for S phase of cell cycle

USES: **Systemic:** cancer of breast, colon, rectum, stomach, pancreas; **topical:** multiple actinic keratoses, superficial basal cell carcinomas

---

Unlabeled uses: Anal carcinoma, bladder cancer, cervical cancer, esophageal cancer, glaucoma surgery (adjunctive therapy), head and neck cancer, hepatobiliary cancer, pancreatic tumors, penile cancer, unknown primary cancer, vulvar cancer

CONTRAINDICATIONS

Pregnancy, breastfeeding, hypersensitivity, poor nutritional status, serious infections, dihydropyrimidine dehydrogenase deficiency ⏧⏧, bone marrow suppression

Precautions: Children, renal/hepatic disease, angina, stomatitis, diarrhea, sunlight exposure, vaccination, occlusive dressing, GI bleeding

> Black Box Warning: Requires an experienced clinician and a specialized care setting

DOSAGE AND ROUTES

Doses vary widely, based on actual body weight unless obese, then based on lean body weight

Colorectal cancer
• **Adult: IV Bolus** 400 mg/m² bolus on day 1, then **continuous IV infusion** 2400-3000 mg/m² over 46 hr q2wk (with leucovorin ± either oxaliplatin or irinotecan) or **IV Bolus** 500 mg/m² on days 1, 8, 15, 22, 29, and 36 (1 hr after the start of leucovorin) q8wk (with leucovorin) for 4 cycles

Gastric cancer
• **Adult: IV Continuous Infusion** 200-1000 mg/m²/day over 24 hr (as part of a platinum-containing regimen); the duration and frequency of each cycle vary based on the dose and regimen

Pancreatic cancer
• **Adult: IV Continuous Infusion** 2400 mg/m² over 46 hr q14days (with leucovorin, irinotecan, and oxaliplatin) for 24 wk

Breast cancer
• **Adult: IV** 500 mg/m² on days 1 and 8 every 28 days; CMF regimen: 600 mg/m² on days 1 and 8 every 28 days

Anal carcinoma (unlabeled)
• **Adult: IV Continuous Infusion** 1000 mg/m²/day days 1-4 and days 29-32 (with mitomycin and radiation therapy)

Bladder cancer, muscle invasive (unlabeled)
• **Adult: IV Continuous Infusion** 500 mg/m²/day during radiation therapy fractions 1-5 and 16-20 (with mitomycin and radiation therapy)

Cervical cancer (unlabeled)
• **Adult: IV Continuous Infusion** 1000 mg/m²/day days 1-4 (with cisplatin and radiation therapy) q3wk for 3 cycles

Esophageal cancer (unlabeled)
• **Adult: IV Continous Infusion** 1000 mg/m²/day days 1-4 and days 29-32 of a 35-day treatment cycle (preoperative chemoradiation; with cisplatin)

Glaucoma surgery, adjunctive therapy (unlabeled)
• **Adult: Ophthalmic:** Intraoperative topical application: Apply sponge soaked in fluorouracil 50 mg/mL for 5 min. Postoperative subconjunctival injection: 5 mg once daily for 10 days or 5 mg once daily for 1 wk, then every other day the next week for a total of 10 doses

Head and neck cancer, squamous cell (unlabeled)
• **Adult: IV Continuous Infusion** 1000 mg/m²/day days 1-4 q3wk (in combination with cisplatin) for at least 6 cycles or 1000 mg/m²/day days 1-4 q4wk (with carboplatin) or 600 mg/m²/day days 1-4, 22-25, and 43 to 46 (with carboplatin and radiation)

Actinic/solar keratoses
Adult: TOP (Carac) 1% cream qday; (efudex) 2% or 5% solution or cream to lesions bid × 2-4 wk; (Fluoroplex) 1% cream bid × 2-6 wk; (Tolak) 4% cream qday × up to 4 wk

Superficial basal cell carcinoma
Adult: TOP (Efudex) 5% cream/solution bid × 3-6 wk

Available forms: Inj 50 mg/mL; cream 0.5%, 1%, 4%, 5%; sol 2%, 5%

Administer:
Topical route
• The 1% strength is used on face; higher strengths are used on other parts of the body
• Wear gloves when applying; may use with a loose dressing; use plastic or wooden applicator, do not use occlusive dressings, may use gauze dressing
IV route
• Prepared in biologic cabinet using gloves, gown, mask; use cytotoxic handling procedures
• Double-check all dosage amounts, type of product to be used; fatalities have occurred
• Antiemetic 30-60 min before product to prevent vomiting, for several days thereafter
IV direct
• Undiluted; may inject through Y-tube or 3-way stopcock; give over 1-3 min; may be diluted in NS, D$_5$W and given as an **intermittent infusion;** use infusion in plastic containers; given over 2-8 hr; do not refrigerate/freeze; protect from light, discard unused portion, stable for 24 hr at room temperature; do not use discolored, cloudy solution; solution is pale yellow; for crystals, dissolve by warming slowly and shaking; let cool to body temperature before use

Y-site compatibilities: Acyclovir, alatrofloxacin, alfentanil, allopurinol, amifostine, amikacin, amphotericin B lipid complex, amphotericin B liposome, ampicillin, ampicillin-sulbactam, anidulafungin, argatroban, atenolol, atracurium, azithromycin, aztreonam, bivalirudin, bleomycin, bumetanide, butorphanol, calcium gluconate, CARBOplatin, ceFAZolin, cefepime, cefotaxime, cefoTEtan, cefOXitin, cefTAZidime, ceftizoxime, cefTRIAXone, cefuroxime, cimetidine, cisatracurium, CISplatin, clindamycin, codeine, cyclophosphamide, cycloSPORINE, DAPTOmycin, dexamethasone, digoxin, DOCEtaxel, DOPamine, doripenem, DOXOrubicin liposomal, enalaprilat, ePHEDrine, er-tapenem, erythromycin, esmolol, etoposide phosphate, famotidine, fenoldopam, fentaNYL, fluconazole, fludarabine, foscarnet, fosphenytoin, furosemide, ganciclovir, gatifloxacin, gemcitabine, gentamicin, granisetron, heparin, hydrocortisone, HYDROmorphone, ifosfamide, imipenem-cilastatin, inamrinone, isoproterenol, ketorolac, labetalol, leucovorin, levorphanol, lidocaine, linezolid, magnesium sulfate, mannitol, melphalan, meperidine, meropenem, mesna, methohexital, methotrexate, methylPREDNISolone, metoprolol, metroNIDAZOLE, milrinone, mitoMYcin, mitoXANtrone, morphine sulfate, nalbuphine, naloxone, nesiritide, nitroglycerin, nitroprusside, octreotide, ofloxacin, PACLitaxel, palonosetron, pamidronate, pancuronium, pantoprazole, PEMEtrexed, PENTobarbital, PHENobarbital, phenylephrine, piperacillin, piperacillin-tazobactam, potassium chloride/phosphates, procainamide, propofol, propranolol, ranitidine, remifentanil, riTUXimab, sargramostim, sodium acetate/bicarbonate/phosphates, succinylcholine, SUFentanil, sulfamethoxazole-trimethoprim, teniposide, theophylline, thiopental, thiotepa, ticarcillin, ticarcillin-clavulanate, tigecycline, tirofiban, tobramycin, trastuzumab, vasopressin, vecuronium, vinBLAStine, vinCRIStine, vitamin B complex/C, voriconazole, zidovudine, zoledronic acid

SIDE EFFECTS
Systemic use
CV: Cardiotoxicity

CNS: Malaise, acute cerebellar dysfunction

EENT: Light intolerance, lacrimation, visual changes

GI: *Anorexia, stomatitis,* diarrhea, nausea, vomiting, GI bleeding, enteritis, glossitis

HEMA: Thrombocytopenia, leukopenia, myelosuppression, anemia, agranulocytosis

INTEG: *Rash,* fever, photosensitivity, anaphylaxis, alopecia, hand-foot syndrome

---

Side effects: *italics* = common; red = life-threatening

PHARMACOKINETICS

Half-life 16 min (IV): metabolized in liver; excreted in lungs (60%-80%) urine; IV onset 1-9 days, peak 9-21 days (nadir), duration 30 days; top: onset 2-3 days, peak 2-6 wk, duration 1-2 mo; crosses blood-brain barrier (up to 15%)

INTERACTIONS

Increase: bleeding—anticoagulants, NSAIDs, platelet inhibitors, thrombolytics
Increase: toxicity—metroNIDAZOLE, irinotecan
Increase: toxicity, bone marrow depression—radiation or other antineoplastics, leucovorin
Decrease: antibody response—live virus vaccines
Decrease: effect of phenytoin
Drug/Lab Test
Increase: AST, ALT, LDH, serum bilirubin, Hct, HB, WBC, platelets, 5-HIAA
Decrease: albumin

NURSING CONSIDERATIONS
Assess:
• **Bone marrow suppression:** monitor daily during IV treatment: CBC, differential, platelet count daily (IV); withhold product if WBC is <3500/mm^3 or platelet count is <100,000/mm^3; notify prescriber of results; product should be discontinued; nadir of leukopenia within 2 wk, recovery 1 mo, if pretreatment of WBC is <2000/mm^3 or platelets <100,000/mm^3, delay until recovery of counts above this level; nadir usually 7-14 days, recovery 30 days
• **Vitals:** monitor baseline and often during infusion, occurs after 8-10 wk of treatment, hold if severe

> **Black Box Warning:** Use only with an experienced clinician in a specialized care setting, for cancer chemotherapy

• **Palmar-plantar erythrodysesthesia:** hand/foot tingling changing to pain, redness
• **Infiltration:** monitor frequently for pain, redness, inflammation at site; if present, stop infusion and start at new site, may use ice at site
• **Renal studies:** BUN, serum uric acid, urine CCr; electrolytes before, during therapy
• **Hepatic studies before, during therapy:** bilirubin, alk phos, AST, ALT, LDH before, during therapy
• **Bleeding:** hematuria, guaiac, bruising, petechiae, mucosa or orifices; avoid IM injections, rectal temperatures
• Inflammation of mucosa, breaks in skin; buccal cavity q8hr for dryness, sores or ulceration, white patches, oral pain, bleeding, dysphagia
• **Infection:** fever, chills, cough, sore throat; those with current infections should be treated before receiving 5-FU, the dose reduced or discontinued if infection occurs
• **Toxicity:** hemorrhage, severe vomiting, severe diarrhea, stomatitis, WBC <3500/mm^3, platelets <100,000/mm^3, notify prescriber
• **Cardiotoxicity:** Monitor for HF, angina, dysrrthmias that may lead to MI, if symptoms appear discontinue, do not restart
• **Hyperammonemic encephalopathy:** Monitor for confusion, dizziness, ataxia; withhold drug, provide products to lower ammonia
• **Acute cerebellar dysfunction:** dizziness, weakness, confusion, vision changes may occur during treatment and last after last dose
• **Topical:** check lesions and surrounding skin baseline and during treatment, document new areas of concern
• **Pregnancy:** identify pregnancy before starting therapy; do not use in pregnancy or breastfeeding; drug may cause fetal harm
Evaluate:
• **Therapeutic response:** decreased tumor size, spread of malignancy
Teach patient/family:
• To avoid crowds, persons with known infection
• To avoid foods with citric acid, hot temperature, or rough texture if stomatitis is present; to drink adequate fluids

- **To report stomatitis:** any bleeding, white spots, ulcerations in mouth; that patient should examine mouth daily, report symptoms; viscous lidocaine may be used; rinsing of mouth tid-qid with water, club soda; brushing of teeth bid-tid with soft brush or cotton-tipped applicator for stomatitis; use unwaxed dental floss, give ice chips for mucositis
- **To report signs of infection:** fever, sore throat, flulike symptoms
- **To report signs of anemia:** fatigue, headache, faintness, shortness of breath, irritability
- **To report bleeding:** to avoid razors, commercial mouthwash, IM inj if counts are low
- Not to use aspirin products or NSAIDs
- To use contraception during therapy (men and women); to avoid breastfeeding (topical use)
- Not to receive vaccinations during therapy
- To use sunscreen or stay out of the sun to prevent photosensitivity
- About hair loss; to explore use of wigs or other products until hair regrowth occurs
- **Topical:** to apply only to affected areas, being careful around mouth, nose, eyes; to avoid occlusive dressings; to wash hands after application
- **Pregnancy/breastfeeding:** Advise patient to discuss if pregnancy is planned or suspected or if breastfeeding; to use effective contraception during and for 3 mo after last dose, males with partners of childbearing potential should also use contraception for the specified time

fLUoxetine (Rx)

(floo-ox′eh-teen)

PROzac

Func. class.: Antidepressant, SSRI (selective serotonin reuptake inhibitor)

Do not confuse:

PROzac/PriLOSEC/Prograf/Provera
fluoxetine/duloxetine/loxitane/paroxetine

ACTION: Inhibits CNS neuron uptake of serotonin but not of norepinephrine

USES: Major depressive disorder, obsessive-compulsive disorder (OCD), bulimia nervosa, premenstrual dysphoric disorder (PMDD), panic disorder

Unlabeled uses: Binge eating disorder, body dysmorphic disorder, fibromyalgia, generalized anxiety disorder, posttraumatic stress disorder, premature ejaculation, selective mutism, social anxiety disorder

CONTRAINDICATIONS

Hypersensitivity, MAOI therapy

Precautions: Pregnancy, breastfeeding, geriatric patients, diabetes mellitus, narrow-angle glaucoma, cardiac malformations in infants (exposed to FLUoxetine in utero), osteoporosis, QT prolongation

Black Box Warning: Children, suicidal ideation

DOSAGE AND ROUTES

Depression/obsessive-compulsive disorder

- **Adult:** PO 20 mg/day in AM; after 4 wk, if no clinical improvement is noted, dose may be increased to 20 mg bid in AM, PM, max 80 mg/day
- **Geriatric:** PO 10 mg/day, increase as needed
- **Child 8-17 yr:** PO 10-20 mg/day, max 60 mg/day

Maintenance therapy for depression who are stabilized

Adult: PO del rel 90 mg qwk start 7 days after last daily dose of regular release 20 mg

Premenstrual dysphoric disorder

- **Adult:** PO 20 mg/day, may be taken daily 14 days before menses

Depressive episodes associated with bipolar I disorder

Adult: PO 20 mg/day with OLANZapine 5 mg/day, give in evening, may increase FLUoxetine to 50 mg/day and OLANZepine to 12.5 mg/day; max: 18 mg olanzapine with 75 mg fluoxetine/day

Child 10-17 yr: PO 20 mg with OLANZapine 2.5 mg qday in the evening

Treatment-resistant depression

Adult: PO 10 mg/day with OLANZepine 5 mg/day in the evening, may increase

FLUoxetine to 50 mg/day and OLANZapine to 20 mg/day

Bulimia nervosa

Adult: PO 60 mg qday in AM, may titrate to this dose over several days

Panic disorder

Adult: PO 10 mg qday × 1 wk, then increase to 20 mg as needed, max 60 mg/day

Available forms: 20, 40 mg; tabs 10, 20, 60 mg; oral sol 20 mg/5 mL; delayed release capsule 90 mg

Administer:

- Without regard to meals
- Crushed if patient is unable to swallow medication whole (tab only)
- Immediate-release product should be given in the AM unless sedation occurs
- Gum, hard candy, frequent sips of water for dry mouth
- Sarafem is used only for premenstrual dysphoric disorder
- Store at room temperature; do not freeze
- **Oral sol:** use oral syringe or calibrated measuring device

SIDE EFFECTS

CNS: *Headache, nervousness, insomnia, drowsiness, anxiety, tremor, dizziness, fatigue, sedation, poor concentration, abnormal dreams, agitation,* seizures, apathy, euphoria, hallucinations, delusions, psychosis, suicidal ideation, neuroleptic malignant syndrome–like reactions

CV: *Hot flashes, palpitations,* angina pectoris, hypertension, tachycardia, 1st-degree AV block, bradycardia, MI, thrombophlebitis, generalized edema, torsades de pointes

EENT: Visual changes, ear/eye pain, photophobia, tinnitus, increased intraocular pressure

GI: *Nausea, diarrhea, dry mouth, anorexia, dyspepsia, constipation,* taste changes, flatulence, decreased appetite

GU: *Dysmenorrhea, decreased libido, urinary frequency, UTI,* amenorrhea, cystitis, impotence, urine retention

HEMA: Hemorrhage

INTEG: *Sweating, rash, pruritus,* acne, alopecia, urticaria, angioedema, exfoliative dermatitis, Stevens-Johnson syndrome, toxic epidermal necrolysis

META: Hyponatremia

MS: *Pain,* arthritis, twitching

RESP: *Pharyngitis, cough, dyspnea, bronchitis,* asthma, hyperventilation, pneumonia

SYST: *Asthenia,* serotonin syndrome, flu-like symptoms, neonatal abstinence syndrome

PHARMACOKINETICS

PO: Peak 6-8 hr, metabolized in liver to norfluoxetine active metabolite by CYP2D6 isoenzyme, some patients may be poor metabolizers; excreted in urine, half-life 2-3 days, half-life 4-16 days, protein binding 94%

INTERACTIONS

Increase: serotonin syndrome—SSRIs, SNRIs, serotonin-receptor agonists, selegiline, busPIRone, tryptophan, phenothiazines, haloperidol, loxapine, thiothixene, tricyclics, linezolid, traZODone, traMADol, amphetamines, triptans, 5HT-1 agonists

Increase: QT prolongation—pimozide, thioridiazine, antidysrhythmics class III

Increase: bleeding risk—platelet inhibitors, thrombolytics, NSAIDs, salicylates, anticoagulants

- Do not use MAOIs, linezolid, methylene blue with or 14 days before FLUoxetine

Increase: levels or toxicity of carBAMazepine, lithium, digoxin, warfarin, phenytoin, diazepam, vinBLAStine, donepezil, antidiabetics, dorifenacin, paricalcitrol, budesonide, bosentan, thioridazine

Increase: CNS depression—alcohol, antidepressants, opioids, sedatives

Decrease: FLUoxetine effect—cyproheptadine

Drug/Herb

Do not use together; increased risk of serotonin syndrome: St. John's wort, SAM-e

Increase: CNS effect—hops, kava, lavender, valerian

NURSING CONSIDERATIONS
Assess:

Black Box Warning: Mental status: mood, sensorium, affect, suicidal tendencies (child/young adult), increase in psychiatric symptoms, depression, panic; monitor for seizures, seizure potential increased, Sarafem is not approved for children

• **Serotonin syndrome:** symptoms can occur anytime after first dose; nausea/vomiting, sedation, dizziness, diaphoresis, mental changes, elevated B/P; if these occur, product should be stopped, notify prescriber
• **QT prolongation:** may be more severe in those with history of QT prolongation; if thioridazine is being used, discontinue for 5 wk prior to using this product
• **Neuroleptic malignant syndrome:** fever, seizures, diaphoresis, dyspnea, hyper/hypotension; report immediately
• **Bulimia nervosa:** appetite, weight daily, increase nutritious foods in diet, watch for bingeing and vomiting
• Allergic reactions/serious skin reactions: angioedema, exfoliative dermatitis, Stevens-Johnson syndrome, toxic epidermal necrolysis, itching, rash, urticaria; product should be discontinued, may need to give antihistamine
• **Vitals:** B/P (lying/standing), pulse; if systolic B/P drops 20 mm Hg, hold product, notify prescriber; ECG for flattening of T wave, bundle branch, AV block, dysrhythmias in cardiac patients
• **Blood studies:** CBC, leukocytes, differential, cardiac enzymes if patient is receiving long-term therapy; check platelets; bleeding can occur, thyroid function, growth rate (children), weight
• **Hepatic studies:** AST, ALT, bilirubin, creatinine, weight weekly; appetite may decrease with product
• Safety measures, primarily for geriatric patients
• **Beers:** avoid use in older adults unless safer alternative is unavailable; may cause ataxia, impaired psychomotor function

• **Pregnancy/breastfeeding:** no well-controlled studies; use only if benefits outweigh fetal risk; not recommended in breastfeeding
Evaluate:
• **Therapeutic response:** decreased depression, symptoms of OCD, absence of suicidal thoughts decreased symptoms of PMDD
Teach patient/family:
• That therapeutic effect may take 1-4 wk, not to discontinue abruptly, that follow-up will be required
• To use caution when driving, performing other activities requiring alertness because of drowsiness, dizziness, blurred vision
• To avoid alcohol, other CNS depressants
• To notify prescriber if pregnant, planning to become pregnant, or breastfeeding
• To change positions slowly because orthostatic hypotension may occur
• To avoid all OTC products, herbals, supplements unless approved by prescriber
• To notify prescriber if allergic reactions occur (rash, trouble breathing, itching)

Black Box Warning: That suicidal thoughts/behaviors may occur in young adults, children, usually during early treatment, to report immediately

• That decreased libido, erectile dysfunction may occur and is reversible after discontinuing
• To notify prescriber of worsening symptoms, or if insomnia, anxiety, or depression continues
• **Serotonin syndrome:** to report fever, sweating, diarrhea, poor coordination, nausea/vomiting, sedation, flushing, mental changes

fluPHENAZine decanoate (Rx)
(floo-fen´a-zeen)
fluPHENAZine hydrochloride (Rx)
Func. class.: Antipsychotic
Chem. class.: Phenothiazine, piperazine

Side effects: *italics* = common; red = life-threatening

ACTION: Depresses cerebral cortex, hypothalamus, limbic system, which control activity and aggression; blocks neurotransmission produced by DOPamine at synapse; exhibits strong α-adrenergic and anticholinergic blocking action; mechanism for antipsychotic effects is unclear

USES: Schizophrenia

CONTRAINDICATIONS

Hypersensitivity, blood dyscrasias, coma, bone marrow depression
Precautions: Pregnancy, breastfeeding, children <12 yr, geriatric patients, seizure disorders, hypertension, cardiac/hepatic disease, abrupt discontinuation, accidental exposure, agranulocytosis, ambient temperature increase, angina, hypersensitivity to benzyl alcohol/parabens/sesame oil/tartrazine dye, QT prolongation, suicidal ideation, renal failure, Parkinson's disease, hypocalcemia, head trauma, prostatic hypertrophy, pulmonary disease, infection, ileus, chemotherapy, breast cancer

Black Box Warning: Increased mortality in elderly patients with dementia-related psychosis

DOSAGE AND ROUTES
Decanoate
• **Adult and child >12 yr: IM/SUBCUT** 12.5-25 mg q1-3wk, may increase slowly, max 100 mg/dose
HCl
• **Adult: PO** 2.5-10 mg in divided doses q6-8hr, max 40 mg/day; **IM** initially 1.25 mg, then 2.5-10 mg in divided doses q6-8hr
Available forms: *Decanoate:* inj 25, 100 ♣ mg/mL; *HCl:* tabs 1, 2.5, 5, 10 mg; inj 2.5 mg/mL; elixir 2.5 mg/5 mL; oral solution 5 mg/mL
Administer:
PO route
• Give with food, milk, or a full glass of water to minimize gastric irritation
• **Oral concentrate:** Give using a calibrated measuring device; dilute just before

use with 120-240 mL of water, saline, milk, 7-Up, carbonated orange beverage, or apricot, orange, pineapple, prune, tomato, or V-8 juice; do not mix with beverages containing caffeine (coffee, cola), tannics (tea), or pectinates (apple juice) or with other liquid medications; avoid spilling the solution on the skin and clothing
• **Oral elixir:** Give using a calibrated measuring device; avoid spilling the solution on the skin and clothing
Injectable routes
• Visually inspect for particulate matter and discoloration before use, slight yellow to amber color does not alter potency, markedly discolored solutions should be discarded, protect from light
IM route (fluPHENAZine HCl only)
• No dilution necessary; if irritation occurs, subsequent IM doses may be diluted with NS for injection or 2% procaine
• Inject slowly and deeply into the upper outer quadrant of the gluteal muscle using a dry syringe and needle, aspirate before injection
• Keep patient in a recumbent position ≥30 min following injection to minimize hypotensive effects
• Rotate the site of injection to avoid irritation or sterile abscess formation with repeat use
IM injection (fluPHENAZine decanoate)
• Use syringe and needle of at least 21-G, do not dilute
• Inject slowly and deeply into the upper outer quadrant of the gluteal muscle, aspirate
• Keep patient in a recumbent position for at least 30 min following the initial injection to minimize hypotensive effects; rotate the site of injection to avoid irritation or sterile abscess formation with repeat administration
SUBCUT injection route (fluPHENAZine decanoate)
• Use a dry syringe and a needle of at least 21-G, do not dilute
• Inject SUBCUT, taking care not to inject intradermally
• Keep patient in a recumbent position for at least 30 min following the initial injection to minimize hypotensive effects; rotate the injection sites

SIDE EFFECTS
CNS: *EPS: pseudoparkinsonism, akathisia, dystonia, tardive dyskinesia, drowsiness, headache,* seizures, neuroleptic malignant syndrome
CV: *Orthostatic hypotension,* hypertension, cardiac arrest, ECG changes, tachycardia
EENT: Blurred vision, glaucoma, dry eyes, nasal congestion
GI: *Dry mouth, nausea, vomiting, anorexia, constipation,* diarrhea, jaundice, weight gain, paralytic ileus, hepatitis, cholecystic jaundice
GU: Urinary retention, urinary frequency, enuresis, impotence, amenorrhea, gynecomastia
HEMA: Anemia, leukopenia, leukocytosis, agranulocytosis, aplastic anemia, thrombocytopenia
INTEG: *Rash,* photosensitivity, dermatitis, hyperpigmentation (long-term use)
RESP: Laryngospasm, dyspnea, respiratory depression

PHARMACOKINETICS
Metabolized by liver, excreted in urine (metabolites), crosses placenta, enters breast milk, protein binding >90%, not dialyzable
PO/IM (HCl): Onset 1 hr, peak 90-120 min, duration 6-8 hr, half-life 15 hr
IM/SUBCUT (decanoate): Onset 1-3 days; peak 1-2 days, duration over 4 wk, single-dose half-life 7-10 days, multiple dose 14.3 days

INTERACTIONS
Increase: QT prolongation, torsades de pointes (at higher doses)—amiodarone, arsenic trioxide, astemizole, dasatinib, disopyramide, dofetilide, droperidol, erythromycin, flecainide, gatifloxacin, ibutilide, levomethadyl, ondansetron, paliperidone, palonosetron, some antidepressants, vorinostat, ziprasidone, haloperidol, phenothiazines, ARIPiprazole, lurasidone
Increase: sedation—other CNS depressants, alcohol, barbiturate anesthetics, haloperidol, metyrosine, risperiDONE
Increase: toxicity—EPINEPHrine

Increase: anticholinergic effects—anticholinergics
Decrease: effects of levodopa, lithium
Decrease: fluPHENAZine effects—smoking, barbiturates
Drug/Lab Test
Increase: LFTs, cardiac enzymes, cholesterol, blood glucose, prolactin, bilirubin, cholinesterase
Decrease: hormones (blood and urine)
False positive: pregnancy tests, PKU urinary steroids, 17-OHCS

NURSING CONSIDERATIONS
Assess:
• **QT prolongation, torsades de pointes:** ECG for changes
• Bilirubin, CBC, LFTs monthly; ophthalmic exams periodically
• Urinalysis recommended before and during prolonged therapy
• Affect, orientation, LOC, reflexes, gait, coordination, sleep pattern disturbances
• B/P standing and lying; pulse and respirations q4hr during initial treatment; establish baseline before starting treatment; report drops of 30 mm Hg
• Dizziness, faintness, palpitations, tachycardia on rising
• **EPS** including akathisia (inability to sit still, no pattern to movements), tardive dyskinesia (bizarre movements of jaw, mouth, tongue, extremities), pseudoparkinsonism (rigidity, tremors, pill rolling, shuffling gait)
• **Anticholinergic effects:** constipation, urinary retention daily; if these occur, increase bulk, water in diet
• Supervised ambulation until stabilized on medication; do not involve patient in strenuous exercise; fainting possible; patient should not stand still for long periods

Black Box Warning: Beers: avoid in older adults except for schizophrenia, bipolar disorder, or short-term use as an antiemetic during chemotherapy; increased risk of stroke, cognitive decline, mortality

• **Pregnancy/breastfeeding:** no well-controlled studies; use only if benefits outweigh fetal risk; may cause EPS in infant if used during 3rd trimester; excreted in breast milk

Evaluate:

• **Therapeutic response:** decrease in emotional excitement; hallucinations; delusions; paranoia; reorganization of patterns of thought, speech

Teach patient/family:

• That orthostatic hypotension occurs often; to rise from sitting or lying position gradually; to avoid hazardous activities until stabilized on medication

• To avoid hot tubs, hot showers, tub baths because hypotension may occur; that in hot weather, heat stroke may occur; to take extra precautions to stay cool

• To avoid abrupt withdrawal of this product or EPS may result; that product should be withdrawn slowly

• To avoid OTC preparations (cough, hay fever, cold) unless approved by prescriber; that serious product interactions may occur; to avoid use with alcohol, CNS depressants; that increased drowsiness may occur

• To use a sunscreen to prevent burns

• About the importance of compliance with product regimen, follow-up, lab, ophthalmic exams

• About EPS; about the need for meticulous oral hygiene because oral candidiasis may occur

• To report sore throat, malaise, fever, bleeding, mouth sores; if these occur, CBC should be drawn, product discontinued

• That urine may turn pink to reddish brown

TREATMENT OF OVERDOSE:
Lavage; if orally ingested, provide an airway; *do not induce vomiting*

---

flurandrenolide topical
See Appendix B

---

flurbiprofen ophthalmic
See Appendix B

---

flutamide (Rx)
(floo′ta-mide)
Func. class.: Antineoplastic, hormone
Chem. class.: Antiandrogen

ACTION: Interferes with androgen uptake in the nucleus or androgen activity in target tissues; arrests tumor growth in androgen-sensitive tissue (i.e., prostate gland)

USES: Metastatic prostatic carcinoma, stage D_2 in combination with LHRH agonistic analogs (leuprolide), B_2-C in combination with goserelin and radiation

CONTRAINDICATIONS
Pregnancy, hypersensitivity

Black Box Warning: Severe hepatic disease

Precautions: G6PD deficiency, hemoglobinopathy, lactase deficiency, polycystic ovary syndrome, tobacco smoking

DOSAGE AND ROUTES
• **Adult: PO** 250 mg q8hr for a daily dosage of 750 mg

Available forms: Caps 125, 250 ✦ mg

Administer:
• Do not break, crush, chew caps
• Give without regard to food with a full glass of water
• Use cytotoxic handling procedures

SIDE EFFECTS
CNS: *Hot flashes,* drowsiness, confusion, depression, anxiety, paresthesia
GI: *Diarrhea, nausea, vomiting,* increased levels in hepatic studies, hepatitis, anorexia, hepatotoxicity, abdominal pain, cholestasis, **hepatic necrosis/failure hepatic necrosis/failure**
GU: *Decreased libido, impotence, gynecomastia*
HEMA: Hemolytic anemia, leukopenia, thrombocytopenia

INTEG: Irritation at site, rash, photosensitivity
MISC: Edema, neuromuscular and pulmonary symptoms, hypertension, secondary malignancy

PHARMACOKINETICS
Rapidly and completely absorbed; excreted in urine and feces as metabolites; half-life 6 hr, geriatric half-life 8 hr; 94% protein binding, peak 2 hr

INTERACTIONS
Increase: PT—warfarin
Decrease: flutamide action—LHRH analog (leuprolide)
Drug/Lab Test
Increase: LFTs, BUN, creatinine
Decrease: WBC, platelets

NURSING CONSIDERATIONS
Assess:

Black Box Warning: Severe hepatic disease: Monitor before start of therapy and monthly × 4 mo, AST, ALT, alk phos, which may be elevated; if LFTs elevated, product may need to be discontinued; monitor CBC, bilirubin, creatinine periodically

• CNS symptoms, including drowsiness, confusion, depression, anxiety
Evaluate:
• **Therapeutic response:** decrease in prostatic tumor size, decrease in spread of cancer
Teach patient/family:
• To report side effects: decreased libido, impotence, breast enlargement, hot flashes, diarrhea

Black Box Warning: Hepatotoxicity: to report nausea, vomiting, yellow eyes or skin, dark urine, clay-colored stools; hepatotoxicity may be the cause

• Notify of yellow, green urine discoloration
• Avoid sun exposure, tanning beds
• To use contraception during treatment; pregnancy category
• To use with full glass of water, without regard to food

fluticasone (Rx, OTC)
(floo-tic′a-sone)
Armon Air Digihaler, Arnuity, Ellipta, Flonase, Flonase Allergy Relief, Sensimist Allergy Relief, Flovent Diskus, Flovent HFA, Xhance
Func. class.: Steroidal anti-inflammatory, antiasthmatic
Chem. class.: Corticosteroid

Do not confuse:
Flonase/Flovent
ACTION: Decreases inflammation by inhibiting mast cells, macrophages, and leukotrienes; antiinflammatory and vasoconstrictor properties

USES: Prevention of chronic asthma during maintenance treatment in those requiring oral corticosteroids; nasal symptoms of seasonal/perennial, allergic/nonallergic rhinitis

CONTRAINDICATIONS
Hypersensitivity to this product or milk protein, primary treatment in status asthmaticus, acute bronchospasm
Precautions: Pregnancy, breastfeeding, active infections, glaucoma, diabetes, immunocompromised patients, Cushing syndrome

DOSAGE AND ROUTES
Prevention of chronic asthma
Flovent HFA
• **Adult/child ≥12 yr: INH** 88-440 mcg bid (in those previously taking bronchodilators alone); **INH** 88-220 mcg bid, max 440 mcg bid (in those previously taking inhaled corticosteroids); **INH** 440 mcg bid, max 880 mcg bid (in those previously taking oral corticosteroids)
• **Child 4-11 yr: INH** 88 mcg bid
Flovent Diskus
• **Adult/child ≥12 yr: INH** 100 mcg bid, max 500 mcg bid (in those previously taking bronchodilators alone); **INH** 100-

250 mcg bid, max 500 mcg bid (in those previously taking inhaled corticosteroids); **INH** 500-1000 mcg bid, max 1000 mcg bid (in those previously taking oral corticosteroids)

• **Child 4-11 yr: INH** Initially 50 mcg bid, max 100 mcg bid (in those previously taking bronchodilators alone or inhaled corticosteroids)

Arnuity Ellipta

• **Adult/child ≥12 yr: INH** 100 mcg via oral inhalation daily initially; may increase to 200 mcg/day after 2 wk; max 200 mcg/day

Seasonal, perennial allergic, nonallergic rhinitis

Flonase

• **Adult: NASAL** 2 sprays initially in each nostril daily or 1 spray bid; when controlled, lower to 1 spray in each nostril daily

• **Adolescent/child >4 yr: NASAL** 1 spray in each nostril daily, may increase to 2 sprays in each nostril daily; when controlled, lower to 1 spray in each nostril daily

Flonase Sensimist Allergy Relief (OTC)

Adult/child ≥12 yr: Nasal 110 mcg qday as 2 sprays in each nostril × 1 wk, then 1 or 2 sprays in each nostril qday × 2- 6 mo, determine future treatment after 6 mo

Child 2-11 yr: Nasal 1 spray in each nostril, use only until relief

Nasal polyps (Xhance)

Adult: Nasal 1 spray in each nostril bid, may increase to 2 sprays in each nostril bid

Available forms: Oral inhalation aerosol 44, 110, 220 mcg; oral inhalation powder 50, 100, 250 mcg; nasal spray 27.5 mcg/actuation, (propionate) 50 mcg/actuation, 27.5 mcg/spray (furoate); inhalation powder 100, 200 mcg/actuation (Arnuity Ellipta)

Administer:

• Give at 1-min intervals; if a bronchodilator aerosol spray is used, use bronchodilator first, wait 5-15 min, then use fluticasone

• Decrease dose to lowest effective dose after desired effect; decrease dose at 2-4 wk intervals

Inhalation route (aerosol)

• Shake well, prime before 1st use, release 4 sprays into air away from face, prime using 1 spray if not used for ≥7 days; when the counter reads 000, discard; clean mouthpiece daily in warm water, dry; do not share inhaler with others

• Child <4 yr requires a face mask with spacer/VHC device for delivery; allow 3-5 INH per actuation; do not use spacer with Flovent Diskus

Inhalation route: Powder for oral inhalation (Flovent Diskus)

• Fill in the "Pouch opened" and "Use by" dates in the blank lines on the label; the "Use by" date for Flovent Diskus 50 mcg is 6 wk from the date the pouch is opened; the "Use by" date for Diskus 100 mcg and 250 mcg is 2 mo from the date the pouch is opened

• After use, patient should rinse mouth with water and spit out the water, not swallow it

• To avoid the spread of infection, do not use the inhaler for more than one person

Intranasal

• Prime before first use

• Shake bottle gently before each use

• Rinse tip after use, dry with tissue

• Blow nose before use

SIDE EFFECTS

CNS: Fatigue, fever, headache, nervousness, dizziness, migraines

EENT: *Pharyngitis,* sinusitis, rhinitis, laryngitis, hoarseness, dry eyes, cataracts, nasal discharge, epistaxis, blurred vision

GI: Diarrhea, abdominal pain, nausea, vomiting, *oral candidiasis*

INTEG: Urticaria, dermatitis

META: Hyperglycemia, growth retardation in children, cushingoid features

MISC: Influenza, eosinophilic conditions, angioedema, Churg-Strauss syndrome, anaphylaxis, adrenal insufficiency (high doses), bone mineral density reduction

MS: Osteoporosis, muscle soreness, joint pain, arthralgia

RESP: *Upper respiratory infection,* dyspnea, cough, bronchitis, bronchospasm

PHARMACOKINETICS
Absorption 30% aerosol, 13.5% powder; protein binding 91%; metabolized in liver after absorption in lung; half-life 7-24 hr depending on product; <5% excreted in urine and feces
Oral INH: Onset 24 hr, peak several days, duration 1-2 wk
Intranasal: Onset 12 hr, peak several days

INTERACTIONS
Increase: fluticasone levels—CYP3A4 inhibitors (ketoconazole, itraconazole), darunavir, nelfinavir, ritonavir, amprenavir, fosamprenavir, atazanavir, delavirdine, saquinavir
Increase: cardiac toxicity—isoproterenol (asthma patients)

NURSING CONSIDERATIONS
Assess:
• **Respiratory status:** lung sounds, pulmonary function tests during, for several mo after change from systemic to inhalation corticosteroids
• Withdrawal symptoms from oral corticosteroids: depression, pain in joints, fatigue
• **Adrenal insufficiency:** nausea, weakness, fatigue, hypotension, hypoglycemia, anorexia; may occur when changing from systemic to inhalation corticosteroids; may be life-threatening; adrenal function tests periodically: hypothalamic–pituitary–adrenal axis suppression in long-term treatment
• Growth rate in children; blood glucose, serum potassium for all patients
• **Beers:** avoid use in older adults with delirium or at high risk of delirium; may worsen the condition
• **Pregnancy/breastfeeding:** use only if benefits outweigh fetal risk; use caution in breastfeeding, excretion unknown
Evaluate:
• **Therapeutic response:** decreased severity of asthma, COPD, allergies

Teach patient/family:
• To use bronchodilator 1st, before using inhalation, if taking both
• Not to use for acute asthmatic attack; acute asthma may require oral corticosteroids
• To avoid smoking, smoke-filled rooms, those with URIs, those not immunized against chickenpox or measles
• To rinse mouth after inhaled product to decrease risk of oral candidiasis
• To report immediately cushingoid symptoms: no appetite, nausea, weakness, fatigue, decreased B/P
• How to use, and when it may be empty
• To use medical ID identifying corticosteroid use

---

fluticasone (topical) (Rx)
(floo-tic′a-sone)
Cutivate
Func. class.: Corticosteroid, topical

Do not confuse:
fluticasone/mometasone/fludrocortisone

ACTION: Crosses cell membrane to attach to receptors to decrease inflammation, itching; inhibits multiple inflammatory cytokines

USES: Inflammation/itching of corticosteroid-responsive dermatoses on the skin

CONTRAINDICATIONS
Hypersensitivity to this product or milk protein, status asthmaticus, monotherapy in primary infections, Cushing syndrome, rosacea, perioral dermatitis, diabetes mellitus
Precautions: Pregnancy, children, breastfeeding, skin infections, skin atrophy

DOSAGE AND ROUTES
• **Adult:** Apply to affected areas bid (cream/ointment) or daily (lotion) × 4 wk
Available forms: Lotion, cream 0.05%, ointment 0.005%
Administer:
Topical route
• Do not use with occlusive dressings

• **Cream/ointment/lotion:** Apply sparingly in a thin film and rub gently into the cleansed affected area; wash hands, use gloves; avoid use on face, groin, underarms
• Reassess treatment after 2 uses

SIDE EFFECTS

INTEG: Burning, pruritus, dermatitis, hypertrichosis, hives, rash, xerosis, irritation, hyperpigmentation, miliaria
META: Hyperglycemia, glycosuria
MISC: HPA axis suppression, Cushing syndrome

PHARMACOKINETICS

Absorption 5% but variable; half-life 7 hr

INTERACTIONS

Drug/Lab
Increase: Blood glucose

NURSING CONSIDERATIONS

Assess:
• Skin reactions: burning, pruritus, dermatitis
Evaluate:
• Decreasing itching, inflammation on the skin
Teach patient/family:
Topical route:
• Not to use with occlusive dressings
• **Cream/ointment/lotion:** to apply sparingly in a thin film and rub gently into the cleansed affected area; avoid use on face, groin, underarms; wash hands; use gloves
• To reassess treatment after each use

---

fluticasone/salmeterol (Rx)

(floo-tic′a-sone/sal-mee′ter-ol)

Advair Diskus, Advair HFA, AirDuo Digihaler, AirDuo RespiClick 113/14, AirDuo RespiClick 232/14, AirDuo RespiClick 55/14, Wixela Inhub
Func. class.: Corticosteroid, long-acting/β₂-adrenergic agonist

---

ACTION: Decreased inflammation in inhibiting mast cells, macrophages and leukotrienes; antiinflammatory and vasoconstrictor properties relax bronchial smooth muscles

USES: Maintenance of asthma (long term), COPD

CONTRAINDICATIONS

Hypersensitivity, acute asthma/COPD episodes, severe hypersensitivity to milk proteins
Precautions: Pregnancy, breastfeeding, active infections, diabetes mellitus, glaucoma, immunosuppression, hyperthyroidism, Cushing syndrome, hypertension, QT prolongation, pheochromocytoma, seizures, MAOIs, other long-acting β₂-agonists, inhaled corticosteroid

Black Box Warning: Asthma-related deaths

DOSAGE AND ROUTES

Asthma maintenance
• **Adult/adolescent ≥12 yr: INH** 100 mcg fluticasone/50 mcg salmeterol (1 actuation) or 250 mcg fluticasone/50 mcg salmeterol (1 actuation) or 500 mcg fluticasone/50 mcg salmeterol (1 actuation) inhaled by mouth twice daily, approximately every 12 hr Max: 1,000 mcg fluticasone/100 mcg salmeterol/day; or 90 mcg fluticasone/42 mcg salmeterol (2 actuations of 45 mcg fluticasone/21 mcg salmeterol/actuation) or 230 mcg fluticasone/42 mcg salmeterol (2 actuations of 115 mcg fluticasone/21 mcg salmeterol/actuation) or 460 mcg fluticasone/42 mcg salmeterol (2 actuations of 230 mcg fluticasone/21 mcg salmeterol/actuation) inhaled by mouth twice daily, approximately q12hr. Max: 920 mcg fluticasone/84 mcg salmeterol/day
• **Child 4-11 yr: INH** 1 inhalation of fluticasone 100 mcg/salmeterol 50 mcg (Advair Diskus) q12hr, must be 12 hr apart
COPD
• **Adult: INH** 1 inhalation of Advair 250/50 Diskus q12hr, must be 12 hr apart
Available forms: Inhalation 100/50, 250/50, 500/50 mcg fluticasone/salmeterol; aerosol spray 45/21, 115/21, 230/21 mcg fluticasone/salmeterol
Administer:
Oral inhalation route

Powder for oral inhalation (Diskus):
• Most children <4 years of age do not generate sufficient inspiratory flow to activate dry powder inhalers
• Give with the Diskus device
• Mouth should be rinsed, spit out water
• Discard device after 1 mo or when counter reads 0 (whichever comes first)

HFA aerosol:
• Shake canister; prime the inhaler before first use with 4 sprays away from face or with 2 sprays (away from the face) if it has not been used for more than 4 wk, or after dropping; use spacer if unable to coordinate inhalation/activation
• Rinse mouth with water after use, clean mouthpiece at least every day; discard inhaler after 120 sprays or when the counter reads 000

Powder for inhalation (AirDuo RespiClick)
• Do not use a spacer or volume holding chamber
• Before using for the first time, check the dose counter window to ensure that the inhaler is full and the number "60" is in the window. The dose counter will count down each time the mouthpiece cap is opened and closed
• Following use, instruct patient to rinse mouth with water without swallowing
• Do not wash inhaler. If the mouthpiece needs cleaning, gently wipe it with a dry cloth or tissue
• When there are "20" doses left, the numbers on the dose counter will change to red; refill the prescription
• When the dose counter reaches "0," the background will change to solid red
• Throw away the inhaler 30 days after removing it from the foil pouch, when the counter displays "0," or after the expiration date, whichever comes first

SIDE EFFECTS
CNS: Fever, headache, nervousness, dizziness, migraines, insomnia, tremors, agitation, anxiety, depression, hyperactivity, irritability
EENT: Pharyngitis, sinusitis, rhinitis, laryngitis, hoarseness, dry eyes, cataracts, nasal discharge, epistaxis, hypersalivation, eye edema, dysphonia, conjunctivitis
GI: Diarrhea, abdominal pain, nausea, vomiting, oral candidiasis

GU: UTI
INTEG: Urticaria, dermatitis
META: Hyperglycemia, growth retardation in children, cushingoid features
MISC: Influenza, eosinophilic conditions, angioedema, Churg-Strauss syndrome, anaphylaxis, adrenal insufficiency (high doses), reduced bone mineral density, HPA axis suppression
MS: Osteoporosis, muscle soreness, joint pain, decreased growth velocity
RESP: Upper respiratory infection, dyspnea, cough, bronchitis, bronchospasm

PHARMACOKINETICS
Fluticasone: half-life 8 hr, peak 1-2 hr; salmeterol: half-life 5.5 hr, peak 5 min

INTERACTIONS
Increase: CNS stimulation—theophylline
Increase: fluticasone levels—CYP3A4 inhibitors (ketoconazole, itraconazole), darunavir, nelfinavir, ritonavir, amprenavir, fosamprenavir, atazanavir, delavirdine, saquinavir, MAOIs, linezolid
Increase: tendinitis, tendon rupture—quinolones
Increase: hypokalemia—loop diuretics, thiazides, theophylline

Drug/Lab Test
Increase: LFTs
Decrease: Potassium

NURSING CONSIDERATIONS
Assess:
• **Respiratory status:** vital capacity, forced expiratory volume, ABGs, lung sounds, heart rate/rhythm
• Withdrawal symptoms from oral corticosteroids: depression, pain in joints, fatigue
• **Adrenal insufficiency:** nausea, weakness, fatigue, hypotension, hypoglycemia, anorexia; can occur when changing from systemic to inhalation corticosteroids; may be life threatening; adrenal function tests periodically: hypothalamic–pituitary–adrenal axis suppression in long-term treatment
• Growth rate in children; blood glucose, serum potassium for all patients

Black Box Warning: Asthma-related deaths: if wheezing worsens and cannot be relieved during an acute attack, provide emergency response

• **Pregnancy/breastfeeding:** use only if benefits outweigh fetal risk; use caution in breastfeeding, excretion unknown

Evaluate:

• **Therapeutic response:** decreased severity of asthma

Teach patient/family:

• To use bronchodilator first, before using inhalation, if taking both; may use spacer or valved chamber

• Not to use for acute asthmatic attack; acute asthma might require oral corticosteroids; may use short-acting B$_2$ agonists for rescue

• To avoid smoking, smoke-filled rooms, those with URIs, those not immunized against chickenpox or measles

Black Box Warning: Asthma-related deaths: seek medical attention immediately if wheezing worsens and cannot be relieved during an acute attack

• To rinse mouth after inhaled product to reduce the risk of oral candidiasis; not to swallow

---

fluticasone/vilanterol (Rx)

(floo-tic′a-sone/vye-lan′ter-ol)

Breo Ellipta

Func. class.: Corticosteroid, long-acting/β-2-adrenergic agonists

Do not confuse:
Flonase/Flovent

ACTION:
Decreases inflammation by inhibiting mast cells, macrophages, and leukotrienes; anti-inflammatory and vasoconstrictor properties; vilanterol relaxes smooth muscles in the respiratory tract, inhibits mast cells

USES:
Asthma, COPD

CONTRAINDICATIONS
Hypersensitivity to this product or milk protein, primary treatment in status asthmaticus, acute bronchospasm

Precautions: Pregnancy, breastfeeding, active infections, glaucoma, diabetes, immunocompromised patients

DOSAGE AND ROUTES
Asthma

• **Adult:** INH 1 inhalation, 100 mcg fluticasone/vilanterol 25 mcg or 200 mcg fluticasone/vilanterol 25 mcg daily

Maintenance treatment of COPD

• **Adult:** 1 inhalation, 100 mcg fluticasone/vilanterol 25 mcg once daily

Available forms: Powder for inhalation Blister 100 mcg fluticasone/vilanterol 25 mcg, 200 mcg fluticasone/vilanterol 25 mcg

Administer:

• Give 1 inhalation in 24 hr

• Discard device 6 wk after it is removed from the foil tray or when the dose counter reads "0" (whichever comes first)

• Do not open the cover of the inhaler until ready for use; each time cover is opened, 1 dose of medicine is prepared

• Exhale fully before taking one long, steady, deep breath through the mouthpiece (do not breathe through nose); hold breath for 3 to 4 sec and exhale slowly and gently

• Patient should rinse mouth with water after inhalation and expectorate rinse solution

SIDE EFFECTS
CNS: Fatigue, fever, headache, dizziness
EENT: *Pharyngitis,* sinusitis, rhinitis, laryngitis
GI: Diarrhea, abdominal pain
MISC: Flulike symptoms
MS: Back pain, arthralgia
RESP: *Upper respiratory infection,* dyspnea, COPD, pneumonia, cough, bronchitis

PHARMACOKINETICS
Fluticasone: Onset unknown, peak 30-60 min, duration unknown
Vilanterol: Onset unknown, peak 10 min, duration unknown

INTERACTIONS
Increase: fluticasone levels—CYP3A4 inhibitors (ketoconazole, itraconazole),

---

darunavir, nelfinavir, ritonavir, amprenavir, fosamprenavir, atazanavir, delavirdine, saquinavir

Increase: cardiac toxicity—isoproterenol (asthma patients)

Increase: hypokalemia—thiazide and thiazide-like diuretics

Increase: adverse reactions—tricyclic antidepressants

NURSING CONSIDERATIONS
Assess:
• **Respiratory status:** lung sounds, pulmonary function tests during, for several months after change from systemic to inhalation corticosteroids
• Use a short-acting β-2 agonist
• **Pregnancy/breastfeeding:** use only if benefits outweigh fetal risk; use caution in breastfeeding, excretion unknown
Evaluate:
• **Therapeutic response:** decreased severity of asthma, COPD
Teach patient/family:
• Withdrawal symptoms from oral corticosteroids: depression, pain in joints, fatigue
• **Adrenal insufficiency:** nausea, weakness, fatigue, hypotension, hypoglycemia, anorexia; may occur when changing from systemic to inhalation corticosteroids; may be life-threatening; adrenal function tests periodically: hypothalamic–pituitary–adrenal axis suppression in long-term treatment
• Blood glucose, serum potassium for all patients
• **Beers:** avoid use in older adults with delirium or at high risk of delirium; may worsen the condition
• **Pregnancy/breastfeeding:** use only if benefits outweigh fetal risk; use caution in breastfeeding, excretion unknown
Teach patient/family:
• To use bronchodilator first, before using inhalation, if taking both
• Not to use for acute asthmatic attack; acute asthma may require oral corticosteroids
• To avoid smoking, smoke-filled rooms, those with URIs, those not immunized against chickenpox or measles

• To rinse mouth after inhaled product to decrease risk of oral candidiasis
• To report immediately cushingoid symptoms: no appetite, nausea, weakness, fatigue, decreased B/P
• How to use, and when it may be empty
• To use medical ID identifying corticosteroid use

fluvastatin (Rx)
(flu´vah-stay-tin)
Lescol XL
Func. class.: Antilipemic
Chem. class.: HMG-CoA reductase inhibitor

Do not confuse:
fluvastatin/FLUoxetine

ACTION: Inhibits HMG-CoA reductase enzyme, which reduces cholesterol synthesis

USES: As an adjunct for primary hypercholesterolemia (types Ia, Ib), coronary atherosclerosis in CAD; to reduce the risk for secondary prevention of coronary events in patients with CAD; as an adjunct to diet to reduce LDL, total cholesterol, apo B levels in heterozygous familial hypercholesterolemia (LDL-C ≥190 mg/dL or LDL-C ≥160 mg/dL) with history of premature CV disease

CONTRAINDICATIONS
Pregnancy, breastfeeding, hypersensitivity, active hepatic disease
Precautions: Previous hepatic disease, alcoholism, severe acute infections, trauma, hypotension, uncontrolled seizure disorders, severe metabolic disorders, electrolyte imbalance, myopathy, rhabdomyolysis

DOSAGE AND ROUTES
• **Adult:** PO 20-40 mg/day in PM initially, titrate up to 40 mg bid; or 80 mg/day (ext rel) dosage adjustments may be made at ≥4-wk intervals or ext rel 80 mg at bedtime

Side effects: *italics* = common; red = life-threatening

Heterozygous familial hypercholesterolemia

• **Adolescent ≥1 yr postmenarche (10-16 yr):** PO 20 mg daily at bedtime, may increase q6wk, max 40 mg bid (cap) or 80 mg (ext rel)

Renal dose

• **Adult: PO** Max 40 mg/day

Available forms: Caps 20, 40 mg; ext rel tab 80 mg

Administer:

• Do not break, crush, or chew ext rel tabs, use at any time of day (tab), in the evening (cap)

• Bile acid sequestrant should be given at least 2 hr before fluvastatin

• Give without regard to food

• Store at room temperature, protected from light

SIDE EFFECTS

CNS: Headache, dizziness, insomnia, confusion

EENT: Lens opacities

GI: *Abdominal pain, cramps, nausea, constipation, diarrhea, dyspepsia, flatus,* hepatic dysfunction, pancreatitis

HEMA: Thrombocytopenia, hemolytic anemia, leukopenia

INTEG: Rash, pruritus

MISC: Fatigue, influenza, photosensitivity

MS: Myalgia, myositis, rhabdomyolysis, *arthritis, arthralgia*

PHARMACOKINETICS

Peak response 3-4 wk, metabolized in liver, >98% protein bound, excreted primarily in feces, enters breast milk, half-life 1.9 hr, steady-state 4-5 wk

INTERACTIONS

Increase: effects of warfarin, digoxin, phenytoin; monitor closely

Increase: myopathy—cycloSPORINE, niacin, colchicine, protease inhibitors, fibric acid derivatives, erythromycin

Increase: effects of fluvastatin—alcohol, cimetidine, ranitidine, omeprazole, phenytoin, rifAMPin

Increase: adverse reactions—fluconazole, itraconazole, ketoconazole

Decrease: fluvastatin effect—cholestyramine, colestipol; separate by ≥4 hr

Drug/Herb

Increase: adverse reactions—red yeast rice

Drug/Lab Test

Increase: LFTs, CK

Decrease: platelets, WBC

NURSING CONSIDERATIONS

Assess:

• **Hypercholesterolemia:** diet history: fats, protein carbohydrate; nutritional analysis should see dietitian before treatment; fasting lipid profile (cholesterol, LDL, HDL, TG) before and q4-6wk, then q3-6mo when stable

• **Hepatotoxicity/pancreatitis:** monitor hepatic studies before, q12wk after dosage change, then q6mo; AST, ALT, LFTs may be increased

• Renal studies in patients with compromised renal system: BUN, I&O ratio, creatinine

• Myopathy, rhabdomyolysis: muscle pain, tenderness; obtain baseline CPK if elevated; if these occur, product should be discontinued

• **Pregnancy/breastfeeding:** do not use in pregnancy/breastfeeding

Evaluate:

• **Therapeutic response:** decrease in sLDL, VLDL, total cholesterol; increased HDL, decreased triglycerides, slowing of CAD

Teach patient/family:

• That blood work will be necessary during treatment; to take product as prescribed; that effect may take ≥4 wk

• To report severe GI symptoms, headache, muscle pain, weakness, tenderness

• That previously prescribed regimen will continue: low-cholesterol diet, exercise program, smoking cessation

• To report suspected pregnancy; not to use during pregnancy, breastfeeding

• To take without regard to meals; to take immediate-release product in the evening; separate by ≥4 hr from bile-acid product; not to cut, break, chew capsule

fluvoxaMINE (Rx)

(flu-vox´a-meen)

Luvox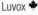

Func. class.: Antidepressant SSRI
(selective serotonin reuptake inhibitor)

Do not confuse:
FluvoxaMINE/FluPHENAZine/Flavoxate

ACTION: Inhibits CNS neuron uptake
of serotonin but not of norepinephrine

USES: Obsessive-compulsive disorder,
social phobia

CONTRAINDICATIONS

Hypersensitivity to this product, MAOIs,
SSRIs, methylene blue, linezolid, pimozide, alosetran, thioridazine
Precautions: Pregnancy, breastfeeding,
geriatric patients, hepatic/cardiac disease,
abrupt discontinuation, dehydration, ECT,
hyponatremia, hypovolemia, bipolar disorder, seizure disorder

> **Black Box Warning:** Children <8 yr, sui-
> cidal ideation

DOSAGE AND ROUTES
**Depression, OCD, social anxiety dis-
order**

• **Adult:** **PO** 50 mg at bedtime, increase
by 50 mg/day at 4-7 day intervals, max
300 mg/day; doses over 100 mg should
be divided; **EXT REL** 100 mg at
bedtime, may titrate upward by 50 mg/
wk, max 300 mg/day

• **Child 8-18 yr: PO** 25 mg at bedtime,
increase by 25 mg/day q4-7days, max
300 mg/day ≥12 yr; max 300 mg/day
8-11 yr (OCD), 200 mg (social anxiety
disorder); doses over 50 mg should be
divided

Hepatic dose/geriatric

• **Adult: PO** 25 mg at bedtime, may titrate
upward slowly

Available forms: Tabs 25, 50, 100 mg,
ext rel capsule 100,150 mg
Administer:

• With food, milk for GI symptoms

• When discontinuing, taper by 50%,
after 3 days taper by another 50% for 3
days, then discontinue

• Store at room temperature; do not
freeze

• **Immediate release:** give at bedtime;
doses >100 mg/day (or >50 mg/day in
those aged 8-17 yr) in 2 divided doses; if
doses are not equal, give larger dose at
bedtime

• **Ext rel:** give at bedtime; do not break,
crush, chew ext rel product

SIDE EFFECTS

CNS: *Headache, drowsiness, dizziness,
seizures,* sleep disorders, insomnia, suicidal ideation (children/adolescents),
neuroleptic malignant syndrome–like
reactions, *weakness,* neuroleptic malignant syndrome, tremors

CV: Palpitation, chest pain, syncope, nervousness, agitation

GI: *Nausea, anorexia, constipation,*
hepatotoxicity, *vomiting, diarrhea,* dry
mouth, altered taste

GU: *Decreased libido,* anorgasmia, uri-
nary frequency, priapism
INTEG: *Rash, sweating*
MS: Myalgia
SYST: Neonatal abstinence syndrome

PHARMACOKINETICS

Crosses blood-brain barrier, 77% protein
binding, metabolism by the liver, terminal half-life 15.6 hr, peak 2-8 hr

INTERACTIONS

Increase: CNS depression—alcohol, barbiturates, benzodiazepines, adjunct dose
Increase: effect of—ramelteon, thioridazine; do not use together
Increase: QT prolongation, death—
pimozide; do not use together
Increase: fluvoxaMINE, toxicity levels—
tricyclics, cloZAPine, alosetron, tiZANidine, thioridazine; do not use together
Increase: metabolism, decrease effects—
smoking
Increase: serotonin syndrome, neuroleptic malignant syndrome: SSRIs, SNRIs,
serotonin-receptor agonists, atypical

antipsychotics, traMADol, MAOIs, methylene blue, linezolid

Increase: bleeding risk—anticoagulants, NSAIDs, salicylates, thrombolytics

Decrease: metabolism, increase action of propranolol, diazePAM, lithium, theophylline, carBAMazepine, warfarin

Drug/Herb

Increase: CNS effect—kava, valerian, avoid using together

Increase: serotonin syndrome—tryptophan, St. John's wort; do not use together

NURSING CONSIDERATIONS
Assess:

Black Box Warning: **Suicidal thoughts/behaviors:** risk increases in children, young adults; this group needs to be monitored more closely, weekly × 4 wk, then every other wk × 4 wk, then at 12 wk; only small amounts should be given on each refill

• **Neuroleptic malignant syndrome:** high fever, confusion, rigid muscles, diaphoresis, tachypenia; notify prescriber immediately
• Hepatic studies: AST, ALT, bilirubin
• Mental status: mood, sensorium, affect, suicidal tendencies; increase in psychiatric symptoms: depression, panic, obsessive-compulsive symptoms
• Constipation; most likely in geriatric patients
• Growth rate (children), bone density (postmenopausal females), glucose (diabetes)
• **Serotonin syndrome:** agitation, hypothermia, hallucinations, tachycardia, nausea, vomiting, diarrhea, instability, changes in B/P
• **For toxicity:** nausea, vomiting, diarrhea, syncope, increased pulse, seizures
• **Beers:** avoid in older adults unless safer alternatives are unavailable; may cause ataxia, impaired motor function
• **Pregnancy/breastfeeding:** neonatal abstinence syndrome can occur; do not breastfeed if used in pregnancy, register patient with the National Pregnancy Registry for antidepressants (866-961-2388)

Evaluate:
• **Therapeutic response:** decrease in OCD, social phobia symptoms

Teach patient/family:
• That therapeutic effects may take 2-3 wk; not to discontinue abruptly
• To use caution when driving, performing other activities requiring alertness because drowsiness, dizziness may occur
• Not to use other CNS depressants, alcohol, barbiturates, benzodiazepines, St. John's wort, kava
• To notify prescriber of allergic reaction
• To increase bulk in diet if constipation occurs, especially in geriatric patients

Black Box Warning: That suicidal thoughts/behaviors may occur; that family health care providers should look closely for suicidal tendencies, especially during early therapy or in young adults, children

• **Serotonin syndrome:** to report immediately nausea, vomiting, diarrhea, agitation, instability, hallucinations
• To stop taking MAOIs at least 14 days before starting product

Pregnancy/breastfeeding: to avoid use in pregnancy; not to breastfeed

---

folic acid (vit B$_9$) (OTC)
(foe′lik a′sid)

FA-8, Folvite ✦

Func. class.: Vit B complex group, water-soluble vitamin

ACTION: Needed for erythropoiesis; increases RBC, WBC, platelet formation with megaloblastic anemias

USES: Megaloblastic or macrocytic anemia caused by folic acid deficiency; hepatic disease, alcoholism, hemolysis, intestinal obstruction, pregnancy to reduce risk for neural tube defects

Unlabeled uses: Methotrexate toxicity prophylaxis, in those receiving methotrexate for RA

CONTRAINDICATIONS
Hypersensitivity

Precautions: Pregnancy, anemias other than megaloblastic/macrocytic anemia, vit B$_{12}$ deficiency anemia, uncorrected pernicious anemia

DOSAGE AND ROUTES
RDA
- **Adult and child ≥14 yr: PO** 400 mcg
- **Adult (pregnant/lactating): PO** 600 mcg/day
- **Child 9-13 yr: PO** 300 mcg
- **Child 4-8 yr: PO** 200 mcg
- **Child 1-3 yr: PO** 150 mcg
- **Infant 6 mo-1 yr: PO** 80 mcg
- **Neonate/infant <6 mo: PO** 65 mcg

Megaloblastic/macrocytic anemia due to folic acid or nutritional deficiency
- **Pregnant/lactating: PO** 800-1000 mcg

Therapeutic dose
- **Adult and child: PO/IM/SUBCUT/IV** up to 1 mg/day (until blood counts are normal)

Maintenance dose
- **Adult and child >4 yr: PO/IM/SUB-CUT/IV** 0.4 mg/day
- **Pregnant and lactating: PO/IM/SUB-CUT/IV** 0.8-1 mg/day
- **Child <4 yr: PO/IM/SUBCUT/IV** up to 0.3 mg/day
- **Infant: PO/IM/SUBCUT/IV** up to 0.1 mg/day

Prevention of neural tube defects during pregnancy
- **Adult: PO** 0.6 mg/day

Prevention of megaloblastic anemia during pregnancy
- **Adult: PO/IM/SUBCUT** up to 1 mg/day during pregnancy

Tropical sprue
- **Adult: PO** 3-15 mg/day

Methotrexate toxicity (unlabeled)
- **Adult: PO/IM/SUBCUT** 1 mg daily or 5 mg weekly

Available forms: Tab: 400, 800 mcg; cap 0.8, 5, 20 mg; solution, injection 5 mg/mL (10 mL)

Administer:
SUBCUT route
- Do not inject intradermally

IM route
- Inject deeply in large muscle mass, aspirate

Direct IV route
- Direct undiluted ≤5 mg/1 min or more

Continuous IV INFUSION route
- May be added to most IV sol or TPN

Y-site compatibilities: Alfentanil, aminophylline, ascorbic acid injection, atracurium, atropine, azaTHIOprine, aztreonam, benztropine, bumetanide, calcium gluconate, ceFAZolin, cefonicid, cefotaxime, cefoTEtan, cefOXitin, cefTAZidime, ceftizoxime, cefTRIAXone, cefuroxime, chloramphenicol, cimetidine, clindamycin, cyanocobalamin, cycloSPORINE, dexamethasone, digoxin, diphenhydrAMINE, DOPamine, enalaprilat, ePHEDrine, EPINEPHrine, epoetin alfa, erythromycin, esmolol, famotidine, fentaNYL, fluconazole, furosemide, ganciclovir, glycopyrrolate, heparin, hydrocortisone, hydrOXYzine, imipenem-cilastatin, indomethacin, insulin (regular), ketorolac, labetalol, lidocaine, LR, magnesium sulfate, mannitol, meperidine, methicillin, methylPREDNISolone, metoclopramide, metoprolol, mezlocillin, midazolam, moxalactam, multiple vitamins injection, naloxone, nitroglycerin, nitroprusside, ondansetron, oxacillin, oxytocin, penicillin G potassium/sodium, PENTobarbital, PHENobarbital, phenylephrine, phytonadione, piperacillin, potassium chloride, procainamide, propranolol, ranitidine, Ringer's, ritodrine, sodium bicarbonate, succinylcholine, SUFentanil, theophylline, ticarcillin, ticarcillin-clavulanate, TPN, trimetaphan, urokinase, vancomycin, vasopressin

SIDE EFFECTS
CNS: Confusion, depression, excitability, irritability
GI: *Anorexia, nausea, bitter taste*
INTEG: *Pruritus, rash, erythema*
RESP: Bronchospasm
SYST: Anaphylaxis (rare)

PHARMACOKINETICS
PO: Peak ½-1 hr, bound to plasma proteins, excreted in breast milk, metabolized by liver, excreted in urine (small amounts)

INTERACTIONS
Increase: need for folic acid—estrogen, hydantoins, carBAMazepine, glucocorticoids
Decrease: folate levels—methotrexate, sulfonamides, sulfaSALAzine, trimethoprim
Decrease: phenytoin levels, fosphenytoin, may increase seizures

NURSING CONSIDERATIONS
Assess:
• **Megaloblastic anemia:** fatigue, dyspnea, weakness
• HB, Hct, reticulocyte count
• Nutritional status: bran, yeast, dried beans, nuts, fruits, fresh vegetables, asparagus
• Products currently taken: estrogen, carBAMazepine, methotrexate, trimethoprim, hydantoins; these products may cause increased folic acid use by the body and contribute to a deficiency if taking other neurotoxic products
• **Pregnancy/breastfeeding:** may be used in pregnancy/breastfeeding
Evaluate:
• **Therapeutic response:** increased weight, oriented, well-being; absence of fatigue; increase in reticulocyte count within 5 days of beginning treatment, absence of fetal neural tube defect
Teach patient/family:
• To take product exactly as prescribed; that periodic lab work is required
• To alter nutrition to include foods high in folic acid: organ meats, vegetables, fruit
• That urine will turn bright yellow
• To notify prescriber of allergic reaction
• To avoid breastfeeding

> **⚠ HIGH ALERT**
>
> ## fondaparinux (Rx)
> (fon-dah-pair´ih-nux)
> Arixtra
> *Func. class.:* Anticoagulant, antithrombotic
> *Chem. class.:* Synthetic, selective factor Xa inhibitor

Do not confuse:
Arixtra/Anti-Xa

ACTION: Inhibits factor Xa; neutralization of factor Xa interrupts blood coagulation and thrombin formation

USES: Prevention/treatment of deep venous thrombosis, PE in hip and knee replacement, hip fracture or abdominal surgery
Unlabeled uses: Acute symptomatic superficial vein thrombosis in the legs (≥5 cm length) HIT, prophylaxis of venous thromboembolism (major surgery for cancer)

CONTRAINDICATIONS
Hypersensitivity to this product; hemophilia, leukemia with bleeding, peptic ulcer disease, hemorrhagic stroke, surgery, thrombocytopenic purpura, weight <50 kg, severe renal disease (CCr <30 mL/min), active major bleeding, bacterial endocarditis
Precautions: Pregnancy, breastfeeding, children, geriatric patients, alcoholism, hepatic disease (severe), blood dyscrasias, heparin-induced thrombocytopenia, uncontrolled severe hypertension, acute nephritis, mild to moderate renal disease

> **Black Box Warning:** Spinal/epidural anesthesia, lumbar puncture

DOSAGE AND ROUTES
Deep venous thrombosis/PE
• **Adult <50 kg: SUBCUT** 5 mg/day × ≥5 days until INR 2-3; give warfarin within 72 hr of fondaparinux
• **Adult 50-100 kg: SUBCUT** 7.5 mg/day × ≥5 days until INR 2-3; give warfarin within 72 hr of fondaparinux
• **Adult >100 kg: SUBCUT** 10 mg/day × ≥5 days until INR 2-3; give warfarin within 72 hr of fondaparinux
Prevention of deep venous thrombosis in hip fracture, hip/knee replacement, abdominal surgery
• **Adult: SUBCUT** 2.5 mg/day given 6 hr after surgery; (hemostasis established) continue for 5-9 days; for hip surgery, up to 32 days; for abdominal surgery, up to 24 days

Acute symptomatic superficial leg vein thrombosis (unlabeled)
- **Adult:** SUBCUT 2.5 mg daily × 45 days

Available forms: Inj 2.5 mg/0.5 mL, 5 mg/0.4 mL, 7.5 mg/0.6 mL, 10 mg/0.8 mL prefilled syringes

Administer:
- Alone; do not mix with other products or solutions; cannot be used interchangeably (unit to unit) with other anticoagulants
- Only after screening patient for bleeding disorders

SUBCUT route
- SUBCUT only; do not give IM; do not give <6 hr after surgery
- Check for discolored sol or sol with particulate; if present, do not give
- Administer 6-8 hr after surgery; administer to recumbent patient, rotate inj sites (left/right anterolateral, left/right posterolateral abdominal wall)
- Wipe surface of inj site with alcohol swab, twist plunger cap and remove, remove rigid needle guard by pulling straight off needle; do not aspirate, do not expel air bubble from surface
- Insert whole length of needle into skinfold held with thumb and forefinger
- When product is injected, a soft click may be felt or heard
- Give at same time each day to maintain steady blood levels; observe inj site
- Avoid all IM inj that may cause bleeding
- Store at 77° F (25° C); do not freeze

SIDE EFFECTS
CNS: Confusion, headache, dizziness, *insomnia*

HEMA: *Anemia*, hematoma, thrombocytopenia, major bleeding (intracranial, cerebral, retroperitoneal hemorrhage), postoperative hemorrhage, heparin-induced thrombocytopenia

INTEG: Increased wound drainage, bullous eruption, local reaction—*rash*, pruritus, inj-site bleeding

META: Hypokalemia

PHARMACOKINETICS
Rapidly, completely absorbed; peak 3 hr, duration up to 24 hr; distributed primarily in blood; does not bind to plasma proteins except 94% to ATIII; eliminated unchanged in urine within 72 hr with normal renal function; half-life 17-21 hr

INTERACTIONS
Increase: bleeding risk—salicylates, NSAIDs, abciximab, eptifibatide, tirofiban, clopidogrel, dipyridamole, quiNIDine, valproic acid, some cephalosporins

Drug/Herb
Increase: bleeding risk—feverfew, garlic, ginger, ginkgo, ginseng, green tea, horse chestnut, kava

NURSING CONSIDERATIONS
Assess:

Black Box Warning: Monitor patients who have received epidural/spinal anesthesia or lumbar puncture for neurologic impairment, including spinal hematoma; may lead to permanent disability or paralysis

- Blood studies (CBC, anti-Xa, HB/Hct, prothrombin time, platelets, occult blood in stools); thrombocytopenia may occur; if platelets <100,000/mm^3, treatment should be discontinued; renal studies: BUN, creatinine; contraindicated in CCr <30 mL/min; use caution in CCr 30-50 mL/min
- For bleeding: gums, petechiae, ecchymosis, black tarry stools, hematuria; decreased Hct, notify prescriber
- For risk of hemorrhage if coadministering with other products that may cause bleeding
- For hypersensitivity: rash, fever, chills; notify prescriber
- **Beers:** Avoid in older adults; increased risk of bleeding, lower creatinine clearance
- **Pregnancy/breastfeeding:** use only if benefits outweigh fetal risk; cautious use in breastfeeding, excretion unknown

Evaluate:
- **Therapeutic response:** prevention of DVT

Teach patient/family:
- To use soft-bristle toothbrush to avoid bleeding gums; to use electric razor
- To report any signs of bleeding: gums, under skin, urine, stools

- To avoid OTC products containing aspirin, NSAIDs
- Method for SUBCUT injection if needed

---

formoterol (Rx)
(for-moh′ter-ahl)
Perforomist
Func. class.: Bronchodilator
Chem. class.: β-Adrenergic agonist

Do not confuse:
Formoterol/fluticasone
Foradil/Toradol

ACTION: Has β$_1$ and β$_2$ action; relaxes bronchial smooth muscle and dilates the trachea and main bronchi by increasing levels of cAMP, which relaxes smooth muscles; causes increased contractility and heart rate by acting on β-receptors in heart

USES: Maintenance, treatment of asthma, COPD; prevention of exercise-induced bronchospasm

CONTRAINDICATIONS
Hypersensitivity to sympathomimetics, monotherapy for asthma, COPD, status asthmaticus
Precautions: Pregnancy, geriatric patients, cardiac disorders, hyperthyroidism, diabetes mellitus, prostatic hypertrophy, hypertension, African descent, aneurysm, asthma-related death

DOSAGE AND ROUTES
Adult: NEB Perforomist solution: 20 mcg bid, max 40 mcg/day; Canada: Foradil: Dry powder inhaler: 12 mcg or 24 mcg bid, max 48 mcg/day
Available form: Inhalation solution: 20 mg/2-mL vial ✤
Administer:
- Store at room temperature; protect from heat, moisture

SIDE EFFECTS
CNS: *Tremors, anxiety,* insomnia, headache, dizziness, stimulation
CV: Palpitations, tachycardia, hypertension, chest pain
GI: Nausea, vomiting, xerostomia

RESP: Bronchial irritation, dryness of oropharynx, bronchospasms (overuse), infection, inflammatory reaction (child)

PHARMACOKINETICS
Bronchodilation: Onset 15 min; peak 1-3 hr; duration 12 hr; metabolized in liver, lungs, GI tract; half-life 10 hr

INTERACTIONS
Increase: serious dysrhythmias—MAOIs, tricyclics
Increase: hypokalemia—loop/thiazide diuretics
Increase: effects of both products—other sympathomimetics, thyroid hormones
Increase: QT prolongation—class IA/III antiarrhythmics, phenothiazines, pimozide, haloperidol, risperiDONE, sertindole, ziprasidone, amoxapine, arsenic trioxide, chloroquine, clarithromycin, dasatinib, dolasetron, droperidol, erythromycin, halofantrine, halogenated anesthetics, levomethadyl, maprotiline, methadone, some quinolones, ondansetron, paliperidone, palonosetron, pentamidine, probucol, ranolazine, SUNItinib, tricyclics, vorinostat
Decrease: action when used with β-blockers

NURSING CONSIDERATIONS
Assess:
- Respiratory function: B/P, pulse, lung sounds; note sputum color, character; respiratory function tests before, during treatment; be alert for bronchospasm, which may occur with this patient
- **Cardiac status:** hypertension, palpitations, tachycardia; if CV reactions occur, product may need to be discontinued
- For paresthesias, coldness of extremities; peripheral blood flow may decrease
- **Pregnancy/breastfeeding:** use only if benefits outweigh fetal risk; use caution in breastfeeding, excretion unknown
Evaluate:
- **Therapeutic response:** ease of breathing
Teach patient/family:
Asthma-related death, severe asthma exacerbations; if wheezing worsens and cannot be relieved during an acute asthma attack, immediate medical attention should be sought

- About correct use of inhaler/nebulizer (review package insert with patient); to avoid getting aerosol in eyes
- About all aspects of product; to avoid smoking, smoke-filled rooms, persons with respiratory infections; not to swallow caps

TREATMENT OF OVERDOSE: Administration of β-blocker

fosamprenavir (Rx)
(fos-am-pren′a-veer)
Lexiva, Telzir ✦
Func. class.: Antiretroviral
Chem. class.: Protease inhibitor

USES: HIV-1 infection in combination with antiretrovirals, not recommended for initial treatment

CONTRAINDICATIONS
Hypersensitivity to protease inhibitors

DOSAGE AND ROUTES
Therapy-naive patients
- **Adult: PO** 1400 mg bid without ritonavir or fosamprenavir 1400 mg/day with ritonavir 200 mg/day or fosamprenavir 700 mg bid and ritonavir 100 mg bid
- **Child >2 yr/adolescent, ≥20 kg: PO** 18 mg/kg (max: 700 mg) bid plus ritonavir 3 mg/kg (max: 100 mg) bid; 15 kg to <20 kg: 23 mg/kg bid plus ritonavir 3 mg/kg bid; 11 kg to <15 kg: 30 mg/kg/dose bid plus ritonavir 3 mg/kg/dose bid; <11 kg: 45 mg/kg/dose bid plus ritonavir 7 mg/kg/dose bid
Protease-experienced patients (PI)
- **Adult: PO** 700 mg bid and ritonavir 100 mg bid
- **Child/adolescent ≥20 kg: PO** 18 mg/kg bid with ritonavir 3 mg/kg bid
- **Child/adolescent 15 kg to <20 kg: PO** 23 mg/kg bid with ritonavir 3 mg/kg bid
- **Child/adolescent 11 kg to <15 kg: PO** 30 mg/kg bid with ritonavir 3 mg/kg bid
- **Child/adolescent <11 kg: PO** 45 mg/kg bid with ritonavir 7 mg bid

- **Infant ≥6 mo, 15 kg to <20 kg: PO** susp 23 mg/kg bid with ritonavir 3 mg/kg bid
- **Infant ≥6 mo, 11 kg to <15 kg: PO** susp 30 mg/kg bid with ritonavir 3 mg/kg bid
- **Infant ≥6 mo, <11 kg: PO** susp 45 mg/kg bid with ritonavir 7 mg/kg bid
Combination with efavirenz
- **Adult: PO** add another 100 mg/day of ritonavir for a total of 300 mg/day when all 3 products given
Hepatic dose
- **Adult: PO** (Child-Pugh 5-6) 700 mg bid without ritonavir (treatment-naive patients) or 700 mg bid with ritonavir 100 mg daily (treatment-naive or experienced patients); (Child-Pugh 7-9) 700 mg bid without ritonavir (treatment-naive patients) or 450 mg bid with ritonavir 100 mg daily (treatment-naive or experienced patients); (Child-Pugh 10-15) 350 mg bid without ritonavir (treatment-naive patients) or 300 mg bid with ritonavir 100 mg daily

foscarnet (Rx)
(foss-kar′net)
Foscavir
Func. class.: Antiviral
Chem. class.: Inorganic pyrophosphate organic analog

ACTION: Antiviral activity is produced by selective inhibition at the pyrophosphate binding site on virus-specific DNA polymerases and reverse transcriptases at concentrations that do not affect cellular DNA polymerases

USES: Treatment of CMV retinitis in patients with AIDS, treatment of acyclovir-resistant HSV infections

CONTRAINDICATIONS
Hypersensitivity, CCr <0.4 mL/min/kg
Precautions: Pregnancy, breastfeeding, children, geriatric patients, seizure disorders, severe anemia

Black Box Warning: Nephrotoxicity, electrolyte/mineral imbalances, seizures

DOSAGE AND ROUTES
Acyclovir-resistant HSV infections
• **Adult/adolescent (unlabeled): IV** 40 mg/kg every 8-12 hr × 2-3 wk or until lesions are healed, max 120 mg/kg/day
Cytomegalovirus (CMV) retinitis (AIDS)
• **Adult/adolescent: IV** 90 mg/kg every 12 hr or 60 mg/kg every 8 hr × 3 wk (or until symptomatic improvement); maintenance IV infusion 90-120 mg/kg over 2 hr daily, max 180 mg/kg/day (initial); 120 mg/kg/day (maintenance)
Available forms: Inj 6000 mg/250 mL, 12,000 mg/500 mL (24 mg/mL)
Administer:
• Increased fluids before and during product administration to induce diuresis, minimize renal toxicity
Intermittent IV INFUSION route
• Using infusion device at no more than 1 mg/kg/min; do not give by rapid or bolus IV; give by CVL or peripheral vein; standard 24 mg/mL sol may be used without dilution if using by CVL; dilute the 24 mg/mL sol to 12 mg/mL with D₅W or NS if using peripheral vein
• Manufacturer recommends product not be given with other medications in syringe or admixed

SIDE EFFECTS
CNS: *Fever,* dizziness, *headache,* seizures, *fatigue,* neuropathy, asthenia, encephalopathy, malaise, meningitis, *paresthesia,* depression, *confusion, anxiety*
CV: ECG abnormalities, 1st-degree AV block, nonspecific ST-T segment changes, cerebrovascular disorder, cardiomyopathy, cardiac arrest, atrial fibrillation, HF, sinus tachycardia
GI: *Nausea, vomiting, diarrhea, anorexia,* abdominal pain, pancreatitis
GU: Acute renal failure, decreased CCr, increased serum creatinine, azotemia, diabetes insipidus, renal tubular disorders
HEMA: *Anemia,* granulocytopenia, leukopenia, thrombocytopenia, thrombosis, neutropenia, lymphadenopathy
INTEG: *Rash,* sweating, pruritus, skin discoloration

RESP: *Coughing, dyspnea,* pneumonia, pulmonary infiltration, pneumothorax, hemoptysis
SYST: *Hypokalemia, hypocalcemia, hypomagnesemia;* hypophosphatemia

PHARMACOKINETICS
14%-17% protein bound, half-life 3 hr in normal renal function, 79%-92% excreted via kidneys, onset rapid, peak infusions end, duration up to 24 hr

INTERACTIONS
Black Box Warning: Increase: nephrotoxicity—acyclovir, cidofovir, CISplatin, gold compounds, tacrolimus, tenofovir, vancomycin, aminoglycosides, amphotericin B, NSAIDs, lithium, cycloSPORINE, pentamidine

Increase: hypocalcemia—pentamidine, calcium products (decreases ionized calcium)

NURSING CONSIDERATIONS
Assess:
HSV: characteristics of lesions baseline and daily during treatment

Black Box Warning: Renal tubular disorders: I&O ratio, urine pH, serum creatinine at baseline, 3×/wk during initial therapy then 2×/wk thereafter; CCr at baseline, throughout treatment; if CCr <0.4 mL/min/kg, discontinue; provide adequate hydration before and during infusion to prevent toxicity

• Blood counts q2wk; watch for decreasing granulocytes, HB; if low, therapy may have to be discontinued and restarted after hematologic recovery; blood transfusions may be required
• Lesions in HSV

Black Box Warning: Seizures: may be caused by alterations in minerals and electrolytes, monitor for seizures; monitor electrolytes and minerals (calcium, phosphate, magnesium, potassium) baseline and 2-3 times/wk during initial treatment and at least qwk maintenance; watch closely for tetany during 1st administration

- Electrolytes and minerals (calcium, phosphate, magnesium, potassium); watch closely for tetany during 1st administration
- **GI symptoms: nausea,** vomiting, diarrhea; severe symptoms may necessitate discontinuing product
- **Blood dyscrasias (anemia, granulocytopenia):** bruising, fatigue, bleeding, poor healing
- **Allergic reactions:** flushing, rash, urticaria, pruritus
CMV retinitis
- Culture (blood, urine, throat) should be performed before treatment; a negative culture does not rule out CMV. Ophthalmic exam should confirm diagnosis, another exam at conclusion of induction and q4wk during treatment. Monitor closely during therapy for tingling, numbness, paresthesias; if these occur, stop infusion, obtain lab sample for electrolytes
- **Pregnancy/breastfeeding:** use only if benefits outweigh fetal risk; do not breastfeed
Evaluate:
- **Therapeutic response:** improvement in CMV retinitis, healing of HSV lesions
Teach patient/family:
- To call prescriber if sore throat, swollen lymph nodes, malaise, fever occur, since other infections may occur
- To report perioral tingling, numbness in extremities, and paresthesias
- That serious product interactions may occur if OTC products are ingested; check first with prescriber
- That product is not a cure but will control symptoms

fosinopril (Rx)

(foss′in-oh-pril)
Func. class.: Antihypertensive
Chem. class.: Angiotensin-converting enzyme (ACE) inhibitor

ACTION: Selectively suppresses renin-angiotensin-aldosterone system; inhibits ACE; prevents conversion of angiotensin I to angiotensin II; results in dilation of arterial, venous vessels

USES: Hypertension, alone or in combination with thiazide diuretics, systolic HF
Unlabeled uses: Proteinuria in nondiabetic nephropathy

CONTRAINDICATIONS

Breastfeeding, children, hypersensitivity to ACE inhibitors, history of ACE-inhibitor–induced angioedema

Black Box Warning: Pregnancy

Precautions: Geriatric patients, impaired hepatic function, hypovolemia, blood dyscrasias, HF, COPD, asthma, angioedema, hyperkalemia, renal artery stenosis, renal disease, aortic stenosis, autoimmune disorders, collagen vascular disease, febrile illness, black patients

DOSAGE AND ROUTES
HF
- **Adult: PO** 10 mg/day, then up to 40 mg/day increased over several weeks; use lower dose for those diuresed before fosinopril, max 40 mg/day
Hypertension
- **Adult: PO** 5-10 mg/day initially, then 20-40 mg/day divided bid or daily, max 80 mg/day
- **Child >50 kg: PO** 5-10 mg daily, initially, max 40 mg/day
Available forms: Tabs 10, 20, 40 mg
Administer:
- May be taken without regard to meals
- Store in tight container at ≤86° F (30° C)

SIDE EFFECTS
CNS: *Headache, dizziness,* fatigue, syncope, stroke, insomnia, weakness
CV: MI, chest pain, angina, palpitations, flushing, *hypotension,* orthostatic hypotension, tachycardia
GI: *Nausea;* constipation; *vomiting;* diarrhea; hepatotoxicity; pancreatitis; red, dry mouth; abdominal pain
GU: Sexual dysfunction, urinary frequency, renal changes
HEMA: Decreased Hct, HB; eosinophilia, leukopenia, neutropenia, agranulocytosis

Side effects: *italics* = common; red = life-threatening

META: *Hyperkalemia*
INTEG: Rash, urticaria, photosensitivity, pruritus
RESP: *Cough,* bronchospasm
MS: Myalgia, arthralgia
SYST: Anaphylaxis, angioedema

PHARMACOKINETICS
Peak 3 hr, protein binding 99%, half-life 11.5-14 hr, metabolized by liver (metabolites excreted in urine, feces, 50%)

INTERACTIONS
Increase: hyperkalemia risk—potassium-sparing diuretics, potassium supplements
Increase: hypotension—diuretics, other antihypertensives, ganglionic blockers, adrenergic blockers, nitrates, acute alcohol ingestion
Increase: toxicity—vasodilators, hydrALAZINE, prazosin, potassium-sparing diuretics, sympathomimetics, digoxin, lithium, NSAIDs
Decrease: absorption—antacids
Decrease: antihypertensive effect—salicylates
Drug/Herb
Increase: antihypertensive effect—hawthorn
Decrease: antihypertensive effect—ephedra
Drug/Lab Test
Increase: AST, ALT, alk phos, glucose, bilirubin, uric acid, BUN, potassium
False positive: urine acetone
Positive: ANA titer

NURSING CONSIDERATIONS
Assess:
• **Hypertension:** B/P, orthostatic hypotension, syncope
HF: edema in feet, legs daily; weigh daily
• **Collagen vascular disease:** neutrophils, decreased platelets; obtain WBC with differential baseline and monthly × 6 mo, then q2-3mo × 1 yr; if neutrophils <1000/mm³, discontinue
Renal studies: protein, BUN, creatinine; increased levels may indicate nephrotic syndrome

• Baselines of renal, hepatic studies before therapy begins
• Potassium levels
• **Allergic reactions:** rash, fever, pruritus, urticaria; product should be discontinued if antihistamines fail to help; monitor for angioedema
• Supine position for severe hypotension

Black Box Warning: Pregnancy: identify pregnancy before starting therapy; do not use in pregnancy, breastfeeding

Evaluate:
• **Therapeutic response:** decrease in B/P; decreased signs, symptoms in HF; prevention of early death due to MI, stroke
Teach patient/family:
• Not to discontinue product abruptly; to take at same time of day
• Not to use OTC products (cough, cold, allergy) unless directed by prescriber; not to use salt substitutes containing potassium without consulting prescriber
• About the importance of complying with dosage schedule, even if feeling better
• To rise slowly to sitting or standing position to minimize orthostatic hypotension
• To notify prescriber of mouth sores, sore throat, fever, swelling of hands or feet, irregular heartbeat, chest pain, nonproductive cough
• To report excessive perspiration, dehydration, vomiting, diarrhea; may lead to fall in B/P
• That product may cause dizziness, fainting, light-headedness during first few days of therapy
• That product may cause skin rash or impaired perspiration
• How to take B/P; normal readings for age group

Black Box Warning: To notify prescriber if pregnancy is planned or suspected; to use contraception during treatment

TREATMENT OF OVERDOSE:
0.9% NaCl IV infusion, hemodialysis

---

fosinopril/
hydrochlorothiazide (Rx)
Func. class.: Antihypertensive

USES: Hypertension

DOSAGE:

Black Box Warning: Do not use in pregnancy

• **Adult:** 1 tablet per day in the AM
Available forms:
Tablets: 10 mg/12.5 mg, 20 mg/12.5 mg

---

fosphenytoin (Rx)
(foss-fen′i-toy-in)

Cerebyx, Sequient
Func. class.: Anticonvulsant
Chem. class.: Hydantoin, phosphate
phenytoin ester

ACTION: Inhibits spread of seizure activity in motor cortex by altering ion transport; increases AV conduction, prodrug of phenytoin

USES: Generalized tonic-clonic seizures, status epilepticus, partial seizures

CONTRAINDICATIONS
Pregnancy, hypersensitivity, bradycardia, SA and AV block, Stokes-Adams syndrome
Precautions: Breastfeeding, allergies, renal/hepatic disease, myocardial insufficiency, hypoalbuminemia, hypothyroidism, ✖ Asian patients positive for HLA-B 1502, abrupt discontinuation, agranulocytosis, alcoholism, carBAMazepine/barbiturate hypersensitivity, bone marrow suppression, CAD, geriatric patients, hemolytic anemia, hyponatremia, methemoglobinemia, myasthenia gravis, psychosis, suicidal ideation

Black Box Warning: Dysrhythmias, hypotension (rapid IV infusion)

DOSAGE AND ROUTES
All doses in PE (phenytoin sodium equivalent)

Status epilepticus
• **Adult/child:** IV 15-20 mg PE/kg
Nonemergency/maintenance dosing
• **Adult/adolescent >16 yr:** **IM/IV** 10-20 mg PE/kg; 4-6 mg PE/kg/day (maintenance)
Available forms: Inj 50-mg/mL vials
Administer:
Injectable routes
• Give IM/IV; the dosage, concentration, and infusion rate of fosphenytoin should always be expressed, prescribed, and dispensed in phenytoin sodium equivalents (PE); exercise extreme caution when preparing and administering fosphenytoin; the concentration and dosage should be carefully confirmed; fatal overdoses have occurred in children when the per mL concentration of the product (50 mg PE/mL) was misinterpreted as the total amount of drug in the vial
• Visually inspect for particulate matter and discoloration before use
IV INFUSION route
• Before infusion, dilute in 5% dextrose or 0.9% saline solution to a concentration ranging from 1.5 to 25 mg PE/mL

Black Box Warning: Because of the risk of hypotension, do not exceed recommended infusion rates; continuous monitoring of ECG, B/P, and respiratory function is recommended, especially throughout the period in which phenytoin concentrations peak (about 10-20 min after the end of the infusion)

• Loading doses should always be followed by maintenance doses of oral or parenteral phenytoin or parenteral fosphenytoin

Black Box Warning: **Adult:** IV Infuse at a max rate of 150 mg PE/min; **Elderly or debilitated adults:** IV Infuse at a max 3 mg PE/kg/min or 150 mg PE/min, whichever is less; **Child:** IV Infuse at a rate of 0.5-3 mg PE/kg/min or max 150 mg PE/min, whichever is less; **Infant/neonate:** IV Infuse at a rate max 0.5-3 mg PE/kg/min

---

Y-site compatibilities: Aminocaproic acid, amphotericin B lipid complex, amphotericin B liposome, anidulafungin, atenolol, bivalirudin, bleomycin, CARBOplatin, CISplatin, cyclophosphamide, cytarabine, DACTINomycin, DAPTOmycin, dexmedetomidine, diltiazem, DOCEtaxel, doxacurium, eptifibatide, ertapenem, etoposide, fludarabine, fluorouracil, gatifloxacin, gemcitabine, gemtuzumab, granisetron, ifosfamide, levofloxacin, linezolid, LORazepam, mechlorethamine, meperidine, methotrexate, metroNIDAZOLE, nesiritide, octreotide, oxaliplatin, oxytocin, PACLitaxel, palonosetron, pamidronate, pantoprazole, PEMEtrexed, PHENobarbital, piperacillin-tazobactam, rocuronium, sodium acetate, tacrolimus, teniposide, thiotepa, tigecycline, tirofiban, vinCRIStine, vinorelbine, voriconazole, zoledronic acid

SIDE EFFECTS

CNS: *Drowsiness,* dizziness, insomnia, paresthesias, depression, suicidal tendencies, aggression, headache, confusion, paresthesia, emotional lability, syncope, cerebral edema
CV: Hypo/hypertension, HF, shock, dysrhythmias
EENT: Nystagmus, diplopia, blurred vision
GI: Nausea, vomiting, diarrhea, constipation, anorexia, weight loss, hepatitis, jaundice, gingival hyperplasia
HEMA: Agranulocytosis, leukopenia, aplastic anemia, thrombocytopenia, megaloblastic anemia
INTEG: Rash, lupus erythematosus, Stevens-Johnson syndrome, hirsutism, hypersensitivity, pruritus
RESP: Bronchospasm, cough
SYST: Hyperglycemia, hypokalemia, ⍟⊙⍟ SJS/TEN ⍟⊙⍟ in Asian patients positive for HLA-B 1502; drug reaction with eosinophilia and systemic symptoms (DRESS), purple glove syndrome, anaphylaxis

PHARMACOKINETICS

Metabolized by liver, excreted by kidneys (minimal), protein binding 95%-99%, rapidly converted to phenytoin, distributed to CSF, tissue, crosses placenta; half-life 15 min; IM: onset unknown, peak 30 min, duration 24 hr, IV onset 15-45 min, peak 15-60 min, duration 24 hr

INTERACTIONS

Increase: fosphenytoin level—cimetidine, amiodarone, chloramphenicol, estrogens, H_2 antagonists, phenothiazines, salicylates, sulfonamides, tricyclics, CYP1A2 inhibitors
Decrease: fosphenytoin effects—alcohol (chronic use), antihistamines, antacids, traMADol, antineoplastics, rifAMPin, folic acid, carBAMazepine, theophylline, CYP1A2 inducers
Decrease: virologic response, resistance—delavirdine; do not use concurrently
Drug/Herb
Increase: anticonvulsant effect—ginkgo
Decrease: anticonvulsant effect—ginseng, valerian
Drug/Lab Test
Increase: glucose, alk phos
Decrease: dexamethasone, metyrapone test serum, PBI, urinary steroids, potassium

NURSING CONSIDERATIONS
Assess:

> **Black Box Warning: Rapid IV infusion:** risk of hypotension and dysrhythmias with rapid infusion rates

- Seizure activity, including type, location, duration, character; provide seizure precautions
- **Drug level:** target level 10-20 mcg/mL, toxic level 30-50 mcg/mL, wait >2 hr after dose before testing, 4 hr after IM dose; phenytoin blood levels are used for this product
- **Blood studies:** CBC, platelets q2wk until stabilized, then monthly × 12 mo, then q3mo; serum calcium, albumin, phosphorus, potassium
- **Mental status:** mood, sensorium, affect, memory (long, short), suicidal thoughts/behaviors
- **Serious skin reactions:** usually occurring within 28 days of treatment; if a rash develops, patient should be evaluated for DRESS

- **Pregnancy, breastfeeding:** do not use in pregnancy; birth defects have occurred; avoid breastfeeding
- **Renal studies:** urinalysis, BUN, urine creatinine
- **Hepatic studies:** ALT, AST, bilirubin, creatinine
- **Allergic reaction:** red, raised rash; product should be discontinued
- **Toxicity/bone marrow depression:** nausea, vomiting, ataxia, diplopia, cardiovascular collapse, slurred speech, confusion
- **Respiratory depression:** rate, depth, character of respirations
- **Blood dyscrasias:** fever, sore throat, bruising, rash, jaundice
- Continuous monitoring of ECG, B/P, respiratory function
- **Rash:** discontinue as soon as rash develops; serious adverse reactions such as Stevens-Johnson syndrome can occur

Evaluate:
- **Therapeutic response:** decrease in severity of seizures

Teach patient/family:
- About the reason for, expected outcomes of treatment
- Not to use machinery or engage in hazardous activity, since drowsiness, dizziness may occur
- To carry emergency ID denoting product use, name of prescriber
- To notify prescriber of rash, bleeding, bruising, slurred speech, jaundice of skin or eyes, joint pain, nausea, vomiting, severe headaches, depression, suicidal thoughts
- To keep all medical appointments, including those for lab work, physical assessment
- To notify prescriber if pregnancy is planned or suspected; not to use in pregnancy; to avoid breastfeeding
- To use contraception while using this product

---

fostamatinib (Rx)

(fos´-tuh-ma´-tih-nib)

Tavalisse

Func. class.: Antihemorrhagics

USES: Thrombocytopenia in chronic idiopathic thrombocytopenic purpura (ITP) in patients who have had an insufficient response to previous treatment

CONTRAINDICATIONS
Hypersensitivity

DOSAGE AND ROUTES
- **Adult: PO** 100 mg bid. If platelet count has not increased to at least 50×10^9/L after 1 mo, increase to 150 mg bid

---

fostemsavir (Rx)

(fos-tem´sa-vir)

Rukobia

Func. class.: Antiretroviral
Chem. class.: gp120 attachment inhibitor

ACTION: Binds to the HIV-1 protein glycoprotein 120 subunit, inhibits the interaction between the virus and cellular CD4 receptors, prevents attachment

USES: Treatment of HIV-1 infection with other antiretrovirals in multidrug-resistant HIV-1 infection

DOSAGE AND ROUTES
HIV-1 infection
Adult PO: 600 mg bid with other antiretrovirals
Available forms: Ext rel tablets 600 mg
Administer:
PO route
- Give without regard to food; swallow whole; do not chew, crush, split

CONTRAINDICATIONS
Breastfeeding, hypersensitivity, use of strong CYP3A inducers (enzalutamide, carbamazepine, phenytoin, rifampin, St. John's wort)

Precautions:
Pregnancy, infants, liver disease, myelosuppression, infections

SIDE EFFECTS
CNS: Fatigue, headache, dizziness, drowsiness, insomnia, abnormal dreams, peripheral neuropathy

CV: QT prolongation
GI: Nausea, vomiting, abdominal pain, diarrhea, dyspepsia, increased LFTs
META: Hyperbilirubinemia, hypercholesterolemia, hyperglycemia, hypertriglyceridemia
HEMA: Anemia, neutropenia
INTEG: Rash, pruritus

PHARMACOKINETICS
Onset unknown, peak 2 hr, duration unknown, protein binding 88.4%, half-life 11 hr

INTERACTIONS
Many drug interactions, refer to manufacturer's information

NURSING CONSIDERATIONS
Assess:
• **HIV:** CBC with differential, blood chemistry, blood glucose, plasma HIV RNA, absolute CD4+/CD8+ cell counts, serum ICD+24 antigen levels, cholesterol, serum bilirubin (total and direct), serum lipid profile, urinalysis baseline and periodically
• **Hepatotoxicity:** Monitor LFTs, signs of hepatotoxicity in HBV and/or HCV coinfection; continue with or start anti-HBV therapy in those coinfected with HBV
• Monitor for QT prolongation in those with a history of prolonged QT interval, preexisting cardiac disease, or those taking drugs known to cause torsades de pointes
• **Hepatitis B virus coinfection:** Use with caution; elevations in LFTs are more common in patients with HBV coinfection, which may be related to HBV reactivation. Monitor hepatitis B serology, plasma hepatitis C RNA
• **Peripheral neuropathy:** May occur and last for several months, where nerves are close to the skin
• Bowel pattern before, during treatment; if severe abdominal pain or constipation occurs, notify prescriber; monitor hydration
• **Hypersensitivity:** Skin eruptions, rash, urticaria, itching; assess allergies before treatment, reaction to each medication; may occur quickly or later after continued use
• **Immune reconstitution syndrome:** With combination therapy, patients may develop immune reconstitution syndrome

with inflammatory response to an opportunistic infection during initial HIV treatment or activation of autoimmune disorders (Graves disease, polymyositis, Guillain-Barre syndrome, autoimmune hepatitis)
• **Pregnancy/breastfeeding:** Identify if pregnancy is planned or suspected, or if breastfeeding; if pregnant, register with the Antiretroviral Pregnancy Registry, 800-258-4263, obtain a pregnancy test
Evaluate:
• **Therapeutic response:** Increased CD4 cell counts; decreased viral load; slowing progression of HIV-1 infection
Teach patient/family:
• That hypersensitive reactions may occur; rash, pruritus; to stop product, contact prescriber
• That product is not a cure for HIV-1 infection but controls symptoms; HIV-1 can still be transmitted to others; that product is to be used in combination only with other antiretrovirals
• To notify prescriber if pregnancy is suspected; not to breastfeed

fremanezumab (Rx)
(free-ma-nez'ue-mab)
Ajovy
Func. class.: Antimigraine agent
Chem. class.: Calcitonin gene-related peptide (CGRP) antagonist

ACTION: Binds to and antagonizes the calcitonin gene-related peptide (CGRP) receptor and antagonizes CGRP receptor function

USES: Migraine prophylaxis

CONTRAINDICATIONS
Hypersensitivity
Precautions: Breastfeeding, pregnancy

DOSAGE AND ROUTES
• **Adult:** SUBCUT 225 mg monthly or 675 mg q3mo
Available forms: 225 mg/1.5 mL prefilled syringe sol for injection

Administer:
SUBCUT route

• When switching between monthly and quarterly dosage options, give the first dose of the new regimen on the next scheduled date of administration

• Visually inspect for particulates, discoloration before use; do not use if solution is cloudy, discolored, or contains particles; product is clear to opalescent, colorless to slightly yellow

• Allow to sit at room temperature ≥30 min, protect from direct sunlight, do not shake

• Clean injection site on the abdomen, thigh, or upper arm with an alcohol wipe, and allow skin to dry

• Do not inject into areas where skin is tender, bruised, red, or hard. Avoid injecting directly into raised, thick, red, or scaly skin patch or lesion, or into areas with scars or stretch marks

• If using the same body area for the 3 separate injections needed for the 675-mg dose, do not use the same location used for the previous injection

• Do not coadminister with other injectable drugs at the same injection site

• If a dose is missed, give the next dose as soon as possible

• **Storage:** After removing from refrigerator, may be stored at room temperature up to 77° F (25° C) for ≤24 hr; discard if not used within 24 hr after removal from refrigerator

Single-dose prefilled syringe

• Pinch injection site skin firmly between thumb and fingers

• Hold, insert syringe at a 45- to 90-degree angle for administration

SIDE EFFECTS

INTEG: Injection site reaction, rash, urticaria, pruritus, erythema
MISC: Antibody formation

PHARMACOKINETICS
Half-life 31 days, peak 5-7 days

INTERACTIONS
None known

NURSING CONSIDERATIONS

Assess:

• **Migraine:** pain, location, intensity, duration, photophobia in the past; assess response to preventing migraine after use of this product

• Injection site reaction, rash, urticaria, pruritus, erythema; may indicate allergic reactions

• **Pregnancy/breastfeeding:** identify if pregnancy is planned or suspected, or if breastfeeding; no adequate studies are available

Evaluate:

• **Therapeutic response:** prevention of migraine

Teach patient/family:

• How to self-administer product

• Not to double, skip doses; when switching between monthly and quarterly dosage options, to give the first dose of the new regimen on the next scheduled date of administration

• To report injection site reaction, rash, itching; may indicate allergic reaction

---

frovatriptan (Rx)
(froh-vah-trip′tan)
Frova
Func. class.: Antimigraine agent
Chem. class.: 5-HT₁-Receptor agonist

ACTION: Binds selectively to the vascular 5-HT₁B, 5-HT₁D receptor subtypes; exerts antimigraine effect; binds to benzodiazepine receptor sites, causes vasoconstriction in cranium

USES: Acute treatment of migraine with/without aura

CONTRAINDICATIONS
Hypersensitivity, angina pectoris, history of MI, documented silent ischemia, Prinzmetal's angina, ischemic heart disease; concurrent ergotamine-containing preparations; uncontrolled hypertension; basilar or hemiplegic migraine; ischemic bowel disease; peripheral vascular

disease, severe hepatic disease, prophylactic migraine treatment

Precautions: Pregnancy, breastfeeding, children, geriatric patients, postmenopausal women, men >40 yr, risk factors for CAD, hypercholesterolemia, obesity, diabetes, impaired hepatic function, seizure disorder

DOSAGE AND ROUTES

• **Adult: PO** 2.5 mg; a 2nd dose may be taken after ≥2 hr; max 3 tabs (7.5 mg/day)

Available form: Tabs 2.5 mg

Administer:

• Swallow tabs whole; do not break, crush, or chew

• With fluids

• 2 days/wk or less; rebound headache may occur

SIDE EFFECTS

CNS: *Hot/cold sensation,* paresthesia, *dizziness,* headache, fatigue, insomnia, anxiety, somnolence, seizures

CV: *Flushing,* chest pain, palpitation, coronary artery vasospasm, MI, myocardial ischemia, ventricular tachycardia, ventricular fibrillation

GI: Dry mouth, dyspepsia, abdominal pain, diarrhea, vomiting, nausea

MS: Skeletal pain

PHARMACOKINETICS

Onset of pain relief 2-3 hr, terminal half-life 25-29 hr, protein binding 15%, metabolized in liver by CYP1A2

INTERACTIONS

Increase: frovatriptan levels—CYP1A2 inhibitors (cimetidine, ciprofloxacin, erythromycin), estrogen, propranolol, hormonal contraceptives

Increase: toxicity—SSRIs, other serotonin agonists (dextromethorphan, MAOIs, antidepressants)

NURSING CONSIDERATIONS

Assess:

• **Migraine symptoms:** aura, unable to view light; ingestion of tyramine-containing foods (pickled products, beer, wine, aged cheese), food additives, preservatives, colorings, artificial sweeteners, chocolate, caffeine, which may precipitate these types of headaches

• **Serious cardiac reactions:** may occur within a few hours of taking a 5-HT1 agent; dysrhythmias, ventricular tachycardia, ventricular fibrillation leading to death

• B/P; signs, symptoms of coronary vasospasms

• For stress level, activity, recreation, coping mechanisms

• Quiet, calm environment with decreased stimulation from noise, bright light, excessive talking

• **Serotonin syndrome:** agitation, confusion, diaphoresis, increased B/P, nausea, vomiting, diarrhea; product should be discontinued

• **Pregnancy/breastfeeding:** use only if benefit outweighs fetal risk; do not breastfeed, excretion unknown

Evaluate:

• **Therapeutic response:** decrease in frequency, severity of migraine

Teach patient/family:

• To report any side effects to prescriber

• To inform prescriber if pregnant or planning to become pregnant

• To consult prescriber if breastfeeding

• **Serious cardiac reactions:** to report immediately pain, chest tightness

• **Serotonin syndrome:** to report agitation, confusion, sweating, nausea, vomiting, diarrhea

• **Short-term use only:** That abortive migraine agents used >10 days/mo may lead to a worsening of headaches, medication overuse

---

⚠ HIGH ALERT

fulvestrant (Rx)

(full-vess′trant)

Faslodex

Func. class.: Antineoplastic

Chem. class.: Estrogen-receptor antagonist

ACTION: Inhibits cell division by competitive binding to cytoplasmic estrogen receptors, downregulates estrogen receptors

USES: Advanced breast carcinoma in estrogen-receptor-positive patients (usually postmenopausal)

CONTRAINDICATIONS
Pregnancy, breastfeeding, children, hypersensitivity

Precautions: Hepatic disease, jaundice, thrombocytopenia, biliary tract disease, coagulopathy

DOSAGE AND ROUTES
• **Adult: IM** 500 mg as 2-, 5-mL injections on days 1, 15, 29, and monthly thereafter

Available forms: Inj 50 mg/mL

Administer:

IM route

• IM 5 mL give one inj in each buttock slowly, over 1-2 min

• Antiemetic 30-60 min before product to prevent vomiting prn

• Store in refrigerator; protect from light

SIDE EFFECTS
CNS: *Headache,* depression, dizziness, insomnia, paresthesia, anxiety

GI: *Nausea, vomiting,* anorexia, constipation, diarrhea, abdominal pain, hepatitis, hepatic failure, hyperbilirubinemia

HEMA: Anemia

INTEG: *Rash,* sweating, *hot flashes,* inj site pain

MS: Bone pain, arthritis, back pain

RESP: Pharyngitis, dyspnea, cough

SYST: Angioedema

PHARMACOKINETICS
Half-life 40 days, metabolized by CYP3A4, excretion in feces 90%

INTERACTIONS
Increase: Bleeding—anticoagulants, do not use concurrently

Drug/Lab Test

Increase: LFTs

NURSING CONSIDERATIONS
Assess:

• For anticoagulant use

• For side effects; report to prescriber

• **Pregnancy/breastfeeding:** Obtain a pregnancy test within 7 days of first dose, have patient use contraception during and for 1 yr after last dose, do not breastfeed

Evaluate:

• **Therapeutic response:** decreased tumor size, spread of malignancy

Teach patient/family:

• To report any complaints, side effects to prescriber

• To report vaginal bleeding immediately

• That tumor flare (increase in size of tumor, increased bone pain) may occur, will subside rapidly; that analgesics may be taken for pain

• That premenopausal women must use mechanical birth control because ovulation may be induced; not to breastfeed

• To use contraception during and for 1 yr after last dose to prevent pregnancy

---

furosemide (Rx)
(fur-oh′se-mide)

Lasix

Func. class.: Loop diuretic

Chem. class.: Sulfonamide derivative

Do not confuse:

furosemide/torsemide

Lasix/Luvox/Lomotil/Lanoxin/Losec

ACTION: Inhibits reabsorption of sodium and chloride at proximal and distal tubule and in the loop of Henle

USES: Pulmonary edema; edema with HF, hepatic disease, nephrotic syndrome, ascites, hypertension

CONTRAINDICATIONS
Anuria

Precautions: Pregnancy, breastfeeding, diabetes mellitus, dehydration, severe renal disease, cirrhosis, ascites, hypersensitivity to sulfonamides/thiazides, infants, hypovolemia, electrolyte depletion, hypersensitivity

DOSAGE AND ROUTES

Acute pulmonary edema

• **Adult: IV** 40 mg slowly over 2 min, then 80 mg in 60-90 min if needed, max 200 mg/dose

Edema

• **Adult: PO** 20-80 mg/day in AM; may give another dose after 6 hr up to 600 mg/day; **IM/IV** 20-40 mg; increase by 20 mg q2hr until desired response

• **Child: PO/IM/IV** 1-2 mg/kg; may increase by 1-2 mg/kg q6-8hr up to 6 mg/kg

Hypertension

• **Adult: PO** 40 mg bid, adjust based on response

Available forms: Tabs 20, 40, 80 mg; oral sol 8 mg/mL, 10 mg/mL; inj 10 mg/mL

Administer:

• In AM to avoid interference with sleep if using product as diuretic

• Potassium replacement if potassium <3 mg/dL

PO route

• PO with food if nausea occurs; absorption may be decreased slightly; tabs may be crushed

IV route

• Undiluted; may be given through Y-tube, give ≤20 mg/min

Intermittent IV INFUSION route

• May be added to NS or D₅W; if large doses required and given as IV infusion, max 4 mg/min; use infusion pump

Y-site compatibilities: Acyclovir, alfentanil, allopurinol, alprostadil, amifostine, amikacin, aminocaproic acid, aminophylline, amphotericin B cholesteryl/lipid complex/liposome, anidulafungin, argatroban, ascorbic acid, atenolol, atropine, azaTHIOprine, aztreonam, bivalirudin, bleomycin, bumetanide, calcium chloride/gluconate, CARBOplatin, cefamandole, ceFAZolin, cefepime, cefonicid, cefotaxime, cefoTEtan, cefOXitin, cefTAZidime, ceftizoxime, ceftobiprole, cefTRIAXone, cefuroxime, chloramphenicol, CISplatin, cladribine, clindamycin, cyanocobalamin, cyclophosphamide, cycloSPORINE, cytarabine, DACTINomycin, DAPTOmycin, dexamethasone, dexmedetomidine, digoxin, DOCEtaxel, doripenem, doxacurium, DOXOrubicin liposome, enalaprilat, ePHEDrine, EPINEPHrine, etoposide, fentaNYL, fludarabine, fluorouracil, folic acid, foscarnet, gallium nitrate, ganciclovir, granisetron, heparin, hydrocortisone, HYDROmorphone, ifosfamide, imipenemcilastatin, indomethacin, insulin (regular), isosorbide, kanamycin, leucovorin, lidocaine, linezolid, LORazepam, LR, mannitol, mechlorethamine, melphalan, meropenem, methicillin, methotrexate, methylPREDNISolone, metoprolol, metroNIDAZOLE, mezlocillin, micafungin, miconazole, mitoMYcin, moxalactam, multiple vitamin injection, nafcillin, naloxone, nitroprusside, octreotide, oxacillin, oxaliplatin, oxytocin, PACLitaxel, palonosetron, pamidronate, pantoprazole, PEMEtrexed, penicillin G, PENTobarbital, PHENobarbital, phytonadione, piperacillin, piperacillin-tazobactam, potassium chloride, procainamide, propofol, propranolol, ranitidine, remifentanil, Ringer's, ritodrine, sargramostim, sodium acetate/bicarbonate, succinylcholine, SUFentanil, temocillin, teniposide, theophylline, thiopental, thiotepa, ticarcillin, ticarcillinclavulanate, tigecycline, tirofiban, TNA, tobramycin, urokinase, vit B/C, voriconazole, zoledronic acid

SIDE EFFECTS

CNS: Headache, fatigue, weakness, vertigo, paresthesias

CV: Orthostatic hypotension, chest pain, ECG changes, circulatory collapse

EENT: Loss of hearing, ear pain, tinnitus, blurred vision

ELECT: *Hypokalemia, hypochloremic alkalosis, hypomagnesemia, hyperuricemia, hypocalcemia, hyponatremia,* metabolic alkalosis

ENDO: *Hyperglycemia*

GI: *Nausea,* diarrhea, dry mouth, vomiting, anorexia, cramps, oral, gastric irritations, pancreatitis

GU: *Polyuria,* renal failure, glycosuria, bladder spasms

HEMA: Thrombocytopenia, agranulocytosis, leukopenia, neutropenia, anemia

INTEG: *Rash, pruritus,* purpura, sweating, photosensitivity, urticaria
MS: Cramps, stiffness
SYST: Toxic epidermal necrolysis, erythema multiforme, Stevens-Johnson syndrome

PHARMACOKINETICS
PO: Onset 1 hr, peak 1-2 hr, duration 6-8 hr, absorbed 70%
IV: Onset 5 min; peak ½ hr; duration 2 hr (metabolized by the liver 30%); excreted in urine, some as unchanged product, and feces; crosses placenta, enters breast milk; excreted in breast milk; half-life ½-1 hr, protein binding 90%-99%

INTERACTIONS
Increase: toxicity—lithium, nondepolarizing skeletal muscle relaxants, digoxin, salicylates, aminoglycosides, CISplatin
Increase: hypotensive action of antihypertensives, nitrates
Increase: ototoxicity—aminoglycosides, CISplatin, vancomycin
Increase: effects of anticoagulants, salicylates
Decrease: furosemide effect—probenecid
Drug/Lab Test
Interference: GTT
Increase: LDL

NURSING CONSIDERATIONS
Assess:
• **HF:** weight, I&O daily to determine fluid loss; effect of product may be decreased if used daily
• **Hypertension:** B/P lying, standing; postural hypotension may occur; assess for full risk in older adults, and implement fall prevention strategies
• **Metabolic alkalosis:** drowsiness, restlessness
• **Hypokalemia:** postural hypotension, malaise, fatigue, tachycardia, leg cramps, weakness; assess those who are also taking digoxin for digoxin toxicity due to hypokalemia
• Rashes, temperature elevation daily
• Confusion, especially in geriatric patients; take safety precautions if needed

• **Hearing,** including tinnitus and hearing loss, when giving high doses for extended periods or rapid infusion
• Rate, depth, rhythm of respiration; effect of exertion; lung sounds
• Electrolytes (potassium, sodium, chloride); include BUN, blood glucose, CBC, serum creatinine, blood pH, ABGs, uric acid
• Glucose in urine if patient diabetic
• Allergies to sulfonamides, thiazides
• **Serious rash:** monitor for skin rash often; Stevens-Johnson syndrome, toxic epidermal necrolysis, erythema multiforme may occur and are life threatening
• **Beers:** use with caution in older adults; may exacerbate or cause syndrome of inappropriate antidiuretic hormone secretion or hyponatremia; monitor sodium level closely when changing doses
• **Pregnancy/breastfeeding:** use only if benefit outweighs fetal risks; do not breastfeed, excretion unknown
Evaluate:
• **Therapeutic response:** improvement in edema of feet, legs, sacral area (HF); increased urine output, decreased B/P; decreased calcium levels (hypercalcemia)
Teach patient/family:
• To discuss the need for a high-potassium diet or potassium replacement with prescriber
• To rise slowly from lying or sitting position because orthostatic hypotension may occur; teach fall prevention strategies
• To recognize adverse reactions that may occur: muscle cramps, weakness, nausea, dizziness; teach diabetic patients to monitor blood glucose carefully; blood glucose levels can be elevated
• About the entire treatment regimen, including exercise, diet, stress relief for hypertension
• To contact prescriber if rash, cramps, nausea, dizziness, numbness, weakness occur
• To take with food or milk for GI symptoms
• To use sunscreen or protective clothing to prevent photosensitivity

• To take early in the day to prevent sleeplessness
• To avoid OTC medications unless directed by prescriber

TREATMENT OF OVERDOSE:
Lavage if taken orally; monitor electrolytes; administer dextrose in saline; monitor hydration, CV, renal status

gabapentin (Rx)

(gab´a-pen-tin)

Gralise, Gralise Starter, Horizant, Neurontin

Func. class.: Anticonvulsant

Chem. class.: GABA analogue

Do not confuse:

Neurontin/Noroxin/Motrin/Neoral

ACTION: Mechanism unknown; may increase seizure threshold; structurally similar to GABA but does not bind to GABAa or GABAb; gabapentin binding sites in neocortex, hippocampus

USES: Adjunct treatment of partial seizures, with/without generalization in patients >12 yr; adjunct for partial seizures in children 3-12 yr, postherpetic neuralgia, primary restless leg syndrome in adults, ALS, neuropathic pain

CONTRAINDICATIONS

Hypersensitivity to this product

Precautions: Pregnancy, breastfeeding, children <3 yr, geriatric patients, renal disease, hemodialysis, suicidal thoughts, depression

DOSAGE AND ROUTES

Adjunctive in partial seizures with or without secondary generalized tonic-clonic seizures (Neurontin only)

• **Adult/child >12 yr:** PO 300 mg tid; may titrate to 1800 mg/day in 3 divided doses

• **Child 3-12 yr:** PO 10-15 mg/kg/day in 3 divided doses initially titrate dose upward over approximately 3 days; if >5 yr old, use 25-35 mg/kg/day; if 3-4 yr old, 40 mg/kg/day divided in 3 doses

Postherpetic neuralgia (PHN)

• **Adult:** PO (IR) 300 mg on day 1, 600 mg/day divided bid on day 2, 900 mg/day on day 3 divided tid, may titrate to 3600 mg divided tid if needed; **EXT REL (Gralise only)** 300 mg on day 1, 600 mg on day 2, 900 mg on days 3-6, 1200 mg on days 7-10, 1500 mg on days 11-14, max 1800 mg/day divided, 1800

mg on day 15 and thereafter; **(Horizant only)** 600 mg in AM × 3 days, day 4 give 600 mg bid, max 1200 mg/day divided

Moderate to severe restless legs syndrome (RLS) (Horizant only)

• **Adult:** PO EXT REL 600 mg daily with food at about 5 PM; if dose missed, take next day at 5 PM

Neuropathic pain (immediate release)

• **Adult:** PO 1200-3600 mg/day in 3 divided doses, maintenance 300-1200 mg tid, max 3600 mg/day

Renal dose

• **Adult:** PO EXT REL tablets (Gralise tablets only): CCr 30-59 mL/min: 600-1800 mg/day as tolerated; CCr <30 mL/min: do not use; ext-rel tablets (Horizant tablets only) CCr 30-59 mL/min: for RLS, 300 mg/day, increase to 600 mg/day as needed, for PHN, 300 mg in the AM × 3 days, then increase to 300 mg bid, increase to 600 mg bid as needed; for dose tapering, reduce the maintenance dose to daily in the AM × 1 wk before discontinuing; CCr 15-29 mL/min: for RLS, 300 mg/day; for PHN, 300 mg PO on days 1 and 3, then 300 mg daily in the AM, increase to 300 mg bid as needed, for tapering, if dose is 300 mg bid, reduce to 300 mg daily in AM × 1 wk before discontinuation; if the dose is 300 mg daily, no taper is required; CCr <15 mL/min: for RLS and PHN, 300 mg every other day; for PHN, dose can be increased to 300 mg daily in AM; no dose taper is required

Available forms: Caps 100, 300, 400 mg; tablets 100, 300, 400, 600, 800 mg; oral sol 250 mg/5 mL; ext rel tab: 300, 600 mg

Administer:

• Do not crush or chew caps, ext rel tabs; caps may be opened and contents put in applesauce or dissolved in juice; scored tabs may be cut in half

• 2 hr apart when giving antacids

• Give without regard to meals (immediate release)

• Give with food (ext rel)

• Refrigerate oral solution

• Gradually withdraw over 7 days; abrupt withdrawal may precipitate seizures

• Beginning dose at bedtime to minimize daytime drowsiness

- **Oral sol:** measure with calibrated device, refrigerate
- **Ext rel:** give with food at about 5 PM (Gralise); bioavailability increased with food; swallow whole; do not interchange Gralise with Horizant
- Store at room temperature away from heat and light

SIDE EFFECTS

CNS: Dizziness, fatigue, somnolence, ataxia, amnesia, abnormal thinking, *depression;* **children 3-12 yr old,** emotional lability, aggression, thought disorder, hyperkinesia, hostility

CV: Vasodilation, peripheral edema

EENT: Dry mouth, blurred vision, *diplopia,* nystagmus; otitis media **(child 3-12 yr)**

GI: Constipation, weight gain, increased appetite, nausea, vomiting; diarrhea (Gralise)

GU: Impotence, *UTI*

HEMA: Leukopenia

INTEG: Pruritus, abrasion, acne vulgaris

META: Hyperglycemia

MS: Myalgia, back pain, gout

RESP: Cough, upper respiratory infection (child 3-12 yr)

SYST: Drug reaction with eosinophilia and systemic symptoms (DRESS); dehydration (child 3-12 yr)

PHARMACOKINETICS

Half-life 5-7 hr; immediate release peak 2 hr, ext rel peak 8 hr (Gralise); 5-7 hr (Horizant)

INTERACTIONS

Increase: CNS depression—alcohol, sedatives, opioids, antihistamines, all other CNS depressants; monitor for CNS depression

Increase: effect of—HYDROcodone; dosage reduction may be needed

Decrease: gabapentin levels—antacids, separate by 2 hr

Drug/Herb

Increased: CNS depression—chamomile, kava, valerian

Drug/Lab Test

Increase: glucose

Decrease: WBC

False positive: urinary protein using Ames N-Multistix SG dipstick

NURSING CONSIDERATIONS

Assess:

- **Seizures:** aura, location, duration, frequency, activity at onset; use seizure precautions if present
- **Pain:** location, duration, characteristics if using for chronic pain, migraine
- **Vision changes:** obtain testing baseline, during and after treatment
- **RLS:** restless leg syndrome characteristics baseline and periodically
- **Mental status:** mood, sensorium, affect, behavioral changes, **suicidal thoughts/behaviors;** if mental status changes, notify prescriber
- **Labs:** WBC, gabapentin level (therapeutic 5.9-21 mcg/mL, toxic >85 mcg/mL), serum creatinine/BUN, weight; monitor glucose in those with diabetes
- Drug reaction with eosinophilia and systemic symptoms
- Increased fluids, fiber in diet for constipation
- **Beers:** avoid in older adults unless safer alternative is unavailable; ataxia, impaired psychomotor function may occur
- **Pregnancy/breastfeeding:** use only if benefits outweigh fetal risk

Evaluate:

- **Therapeutic response:** decreased seizure activity; decrease in chronic pain; decreased RLS

Teach patient/family:

- To carry emergency ID stating patient's name, products taken, condition, prescriber's name and phone number
- To avoid driving, other activities that require alertness until response is known because dizziness, drowsiness may occur
- Not to discontinue medication quickly after long-term use; to taper over ≥1 wk because withdrawal-precipitated seizures may occur; not to double doses if dose is missed; to take if 2 hr or more before next dose
- To report changes in vision, diplopia, eye irritation to provider
- To avoid to use with alcohol, sedatives, opioids, antihistamines, or other products that cause dizziness/sleepiness
- To notify providers of use before surgery

• To take as prescribed; not to interchange formulations; that ext rel product should not be crushed or chewed, if tablet is to be broken in half, use within 28 days or discard
• To report suicidal thoughts or feelings, increased depression, panic attacks, hostility, confusion to provider
• Not to use within 2 hr of antacid, may take regular release without regard to meals; ext rel should be taken with food; doses interval should not be ≥12 hr
• To obtain emergency treatment for seizures or dizziness, cyanosis of extremities or lips, trouble breathing, unusual sleepiness
• To keep oral solution refrigerated
• To notify prescriber if pregnancy is planned or suspected; to avoid breastfeeding

galantamine (Rx)
(gah-lan′tah-meen)
Razadyne, Razadyne ER, Reminyl ✦
Func. class.: Anti-Alzheimer agent
Chem. class.: Centrally acting cholinesterase inhibitor

USES: Mild to moderate dementia of Alzheimer's disease, dementia with Lewy bodies

DOSAGE AND ROUTES
• **Adult:** PO 4 mg bid with morning and evening meals; after 4 wk or more, may increase to 8 mg bid; may increase to 12 mg bid after another 4 wk, usual dose 16-24 mg/day in 2 divided doses; **EXT REL** 8 mg/day in AM; may increase to 16 mg/day after 4 wk and 24 mg/day after another 4 wk
Hepatic dose
• **Adult:** PO Child-Pugh 7-9, max 16 mg/day; Child-Pugh 10-15, avoid use
Renal dose
• **Adult:** PO CCr 10-70 mL/min, max 16 mg/day; CCr <9 mL/min, avoid use

Available forms: Tabs 4, 8, 12 mg; ext rel caps 8, 16, 24 mg; oral sol 4 mg/mL
• To take with food to minimize side effects

galcanezumab-gnlm (Rx)
(gal-kuh-nezz′-you-mab)
Emgality
Func. class.: Antimigraine agent
Chem. class.: Calcitonin gene-related peptide (CGRP) antagonist

USES: Migraine prophylaxis, cluster headache

DOSAGE AND ROUTES
Migraine prevention
• **Adult:** SUBCUT 240 mg once as a loading dose, then 120 mg monthly
Episodic cluster headache
Adult: SUBCUT 300 mg (3 SUBCUT injections of 100 mg each) at the onset of the cluster period, and then monthly until the end of the cluster period

Available forms: Prefilled pen or prefilled syringe 120 mg/mL sol for inj

ganciclovir (Rx)
(gan-sye′kloe-vir)
Zirgan
Func. class.: Antiviral
Chem. class.: Synthetic nucleoside analog

ACTION: Inhibits replication of herpesviruses; competitively inhibits human CMV DNA polymerase and is incorporated, resulting in termination of DNA elongation

USES: Cytomegalovirus (CMV) retinitis in immunocompromised persons, including those with AIDS, after indirect ophthalmoscopy confirms diagnosis; prophylaxis for CMV in transplantation; ophthalmic: acute herpes keratitis

CONTRAINDICATIONS
Hypersensitivity to acyclovir, ganciclovir

Black Box Warning: Absolute neutrophil count <500/mm³, platelet count <25,000/mm³ (intravitreal)

Precautions: breastfeeding, children <6 mo, geriatric patients, preexisting cytopenias, renal function impairment, radiation therapy, hypersensitivity to famciclovir, penciclovir, valacyclovir, valganciclovir

Black Box Warning: Secondary malignancy, bone marrow suppression, anemia, infertility, neutropenia, pregnancy, male-mediated teratogenicity

DOSAGE AND ROUTES
Prevention of CMV
CMV retinitis in those mmunocompromised
• **Adult:** IV 5 mg/kg q12hr × 14-21 days, maintenance: 5 mg/kg × 7 days/wk or 6 mg/kg qday 5 times/wk
• **Adult/adolescent:** IV 5 mg/kg/dose over 1 hr q12hr × 1-2 wk, then 5 mg/kg/day 7 day/wk, or 6 mg/kg/day × 5 days/wk
Acute herpes keratitis
• **Adult/adolescent/child ≥2 yr: OPHTH** 1 drop in affected eye every 3 hr while awake until ulcer heals, then 1 drop tid × 7 days
Renal dose
• **Adult:** IV CCr 50-69 mL/min, reduce to 2.5 mg/kg q12hr (induction), 2.5 mg/kg q24hr (maintenance); **IV** CCr 25-49 mL/min, reduce to 2.5 mg/kg (induction); 1.25 mg/kg q24hr (maintenance); **IV** CCr 10-24 mL/min, reduce to 1.25 mg/kg q24hr (induction); 0.625 mg/kg q24hr (maintenance); **IV** CCr <10 mL/min, reduce to 1.25 mg/kg 3×/wk after hemodialysis (induction); 0.625 mg/kg 3×/wk after hemodialysis (maintenance)
Available forms: Injection 500 mg/vial, 500 mg/250 mL; ophth gel 0.15% (Zirgan)
Administer:
IV route
• Mixed in biologic cabinet using gown, gloves, mask; use cytotoxic handling procedures; do not use if particulate matter is present
Intermittent IV INFUSION route

• IV after reconstituting 500 mg/10 mL sterile water for inj (50 mg/mL), don't use bacteriostatic water with parabens; shake; further dilute in 50-250 mL D₅W, 0.9% NaCl, LR, Ringer's and run over 1 hr; use infusion pump, in-line filter, flush line well before and after product
• Do not give by bolus IV, IM, SUBCUT inj
• Use reconstituted sol within 24 hr; do not refrigerate or freeze

Y-site compatibilities: Allopurinol, amphotericin B cholesteryl, CISplatin, cyclophosphamide, DOXOrubicin liposome, enalaprilat, etoposide, filgrastim, fluconazole, gatifloxacin, granisetron, linezolid, melphalan, methotrexate, PACLitaxel, propofol, remifentanil, tacrolimus, teniposide, thiotepa

SIDE EFFECTS
CNS: *Fever,* chills, coma, *confusion,* abnormal thoughts, dizziness, bizarre dreams, *headache,* psychosis, tremors, somnolence, *paresthesia, weakness,* seizures, peripheral neuropathy
CV: Dysrhythmia, hypo/hypertension
EENT: Retinal detachment in CMV retinitis, ocular hypertension, ocular pain, conjunctival scarring, cataracts
GI: *Abnormal LFTs, nausea, vomiting, anorexia, diarrhea, abdominal pain,* hemorrhage, perforation, pancreatitis
GU: Hematuria, *increased creatinine,* BUN, infertility, decreased sperm count
HEMA: Granulocytopenia, thrombocytopenia, irreversible neutropenia, anemia, eosinophilia, pancytopenia
INTEG: *Rash,* alopecia, *pruritus,* urticaria, pain at site, phlebitis
RESP: Dyspnea, pneumonia

PHARMACOKINETICS
Half-life 3-4½ hr (IV); excreted by kidneys (unchanged); crosses blood-brain barrier, CSF, onset rapid, peak infusions end, duration up to 24 hr

INTERACTIONS
Increase: severe granulocytopenia—zidovudine, antineoplastics, radiation; do not give together

Increase: ganciclovir toxicity—adriamycin, amphotericin B, cycloSPORINE, dapsone, DOXOrubicin, flucytosine, pentamidine, probenecid, trimethoprim-sulfamethoxazole combinations, vinBLAStine, vinCRIStine, other nucleoside analogs, mycophenolate, tenofovir, tacrolimus, aminoglycosides, NSAIDs
Increase: seizures—imipenem/cilastatin
Increase: didanosine effect—didanosine
Drug/Lab Test
Increase: LFTs, creatinine, GCT
Decrease: Hb, WBC, platelets, neutrophils, granulocytes

NURSING CONSIDERATIONS
Assess:

Black Box Warning: **Secondary malignancy:** avoid direct contact with powder in caps/solution; if skin contact occurs, wash thoroughly with soap and water; do not get in the eyes

• **CMV retinitis:** Culture of blood, urine, and throat may be taken, CMV is not confirmed by this method; ophthalmic exam confirms this diagnosis, these exams should be done baseline, weekly (induction), q2wk (maintenance)
• **Infection:** Increased temperature, sore throat, chills, fever; report to prescriber

Black Box Warning: **Leukopenia/neutropenia/thrombocytopenia:** CBC, WBCs, platelets q2days during 2×/day dosing and then q1wk for leukopenia with daily WBC count in patients with prior leukopenia with other nucleoside analogs or for whom leukopenia counts are <1000 cells/mm³ at start of treatment

• Serum creatinine or CCr ≥q2wk, BUN; LFTs; ophthalmic exam
• For seizures, dysrhythmias
• **Infection:** Assess for flulike symptoms/fever, sore throat, coughing
• **Bleeding:** Assess for bleeding, thrombocytopenia, check gums, urine, emesis, avoid rectal temperature, vein punctures
• **Pregnancy/breastfeeding:** Not to be used in pregnancy, confirm by pregnancy test

Evaluate:
• **Therapeutic response:** decreased symptoms or prevention of CMV retinitis in transplant patients (if needed)
Teach patient/family:
• Not to wear contact lenses while using gel
• That product does not cure condition; that regular blood tests, ophthalmologic exams are necessary
• That major toxicities may necessitate discontinuing product

Black Box Warning: **Pregnancy:** use contraception during treatment (males/females) and that infertility may occur; males should use barrier contraception for 90 days after treatment; may cause reversible infertility at lower doses, irreversible infertility at higher doses; not to breastfeed (IV)

• **To report infection:** fever, chills, sore throat; blood dyscrasias: bruising, bleeding, petechiae; to avoid crowds, persons with respiratory infections
• To report itching, redness or eye pain (ophthalmic treatment)

ganciclovir ophthalmic
See Appendix B

gatifloxacin (Rx)
(ga-ti-floks'a-sin)
Zymar ✿, Zymaxid
Func. class.: Ophthalmic antiinfective
Chem. class.: Fluoroquinolone

USES: Bacterial conjunctivitis

DOSAGE AND ROUTES
Bacterial conjunctivitis
• Adult/adolescent/child ≥1 yr: **OPHTH SOL** (0.5% ophthalmic solution) 1 drop in affected eye(s) q2hr while awake (up to 8 times a day) for 1 day, then 1 drop 2-4 times a day while awake on days 2 through 7
Available forms: Ophthalmic solution 0.5%

Side effects: *italics* = common; red = life-threatening

> ⚠️ **HIGH ALERT**

gemcitabine (Rx)

(jem-sit′a-been)

Infugem

Func. class.: Antineoplastic—
miscellaneous

Chem. class.: Pyrimidine analog

ACTION: Exhibits antitumor activity by killing cells undergoing DNA synthesis (S phase) and blocking G1/S-phase boundary

USES: Adenocarcinoma of the pancreas (nonresectable stage II, III, or metastatic stage IV); in combination with CISplatin for inoperable, advanced, or metastatic non-small cell lung cancer; advanced breast cancer in combination with PACLitaxel; with CARBOplatin for ovarian cancer, pancreatic cancer, ovarian cancer, ovarian cancer relapse

Unlabeled uses: Bladder cancer, biliary tract cancer

CONTRAINDICATIONS

Pregnancy, breastfeeding, hypersensitivity

Precautions: Children, geriatric patients, myelosuppression, radiation therapy, renal/hepatic disease, accidental exposure, alcoholism, dental disease, infection

DOSAGE AND ROUTES
Breast cancer (metastatic)

• **Adult: IV:** 1250 mg/m^2 give over 30 min days 1 and 8 q21days (in combination with paclitaxel), adjust dose on platelets and AGC on days 1, 8 of cycle, obtain CBC/differential before each dose

Ovarian cancer (advanced)

• **Adult: IV:** 1000 mg/m^2 give over 30 min days 1 and 8; q21days (in combination with CARBOplatin); check CBC/differential platelets before each dose

Pancreatic cancer (adjuvant)

• **Adult: IV:** 1000 mg/m^2 on days 1, 8, 15 of 28-day cycle in combination with capecitabine × 6 cycles starting within 12 wk of pancreatic resection

Non-small cell lung cancer (inoperable, locally advanced, or metastatic)

• **Adult: IV:** 1000 mg/m^2 give over 30 min days 1, 8, and 15; q28days (in combination with CISplatin) or 1250 mg/m^2 give over 30 min days 1 and 8; q21 days (in combination with CISplatin)

Biliary tract cancer, advanced (unlabeled)

• **Adult: IV:** 1000 mg/m^2 over 30 min days 1 and 8; repeat cycle every 21 days (with CISplatin) or 1000 mg/m^2 over 30 min days 1 and 8; repeat cycle every 21 days (with capecitabine) or 1000 mg/m^2 infused at 10 mg/m^2/min every 2 wk (with oxaliplatin)

Bladder cancer (unlabeled)

• **Adult:** *Advanced or metastatic:* **IV:** 1000 mg/m^2 over 30 to 60 min days 1, 8, and 15; repeat cycle every 28 days (in combination with CISplatin) or 1000 mg/m^2 over 30 min days 1 and 8; repeat cycle every 21 days (with CARBOplatin) until disease progression or unacceptable toxicity; *transitional cell carcinoma (refractory):* Intravesicular instillation: 2000 mg (in 100 mL NS; retain for 1 hr) twice weekly for 3 wk; repeat cycle every 4 wk for at least 2 cycles

Available forms: solution for injection 200 mg (1- and 2-g vials); powder for injection 200 mg (1-g vial); injection 10 mg/mL

Administer:
Intermittent IV route

• Prepare in biologic cabinet using gown, mask, gloves; use cytotoxic handling procedures

• After reconstituting with 0.9% NaCl 5 mL/200-mg vial of product or 25 mL/1-g vial of product (38 mg/mL), shake; may be further diluted with 0.9% NaCl to concentrations as low as 0.1 mg/mL; discard unused portions, give over 30 min, do not admix

• Diluted solution stable at room temperature for 24 hr; do not refrigerate

• Infusion longer than 60 min increases toxicity; infusion-related reactions include hypotension, severe flulike symptoms, myelosuppression, asthenia

• **Bone marrow depression:** CBC, differential, platelet count before each dose; single agent: absolute granulocyte count

>1000/mm^3 and platelets >100,000/mm^3, give complete dose; absolute granulocyte count 500-999/mm^3, platelets 50,000-99,999/mm^3, give 75%; absolute granulocyte count <500/mm^3 or platelets <50,000/mm^3, do not give; combination with PACLitaxel for breast cancer: absolute granulocyte count >1200/mm^3 and platelets >75,000/mm^3, give complete dose; absolute granulocyte count 1000-1199/mm^3 or platelets 50,000-75,000/mm^3, give 75%; absolute granulocyte count 700-999/mm^3 or platelets ≥50,000/mm^3, give 50%; absolute granulocyte count <700/mm^3 or platelets <50,000/mm^3, do not give; combination with CARBOplatin for ovarian cancer: absolute granulocyte count >1500/mm^3 and platelet count >100,000/mm^3, give complete dose; absolute granulocyte count 1000-1499/mm^3 or platelets 75,000-99,000/mm^3, give 75%; absolute granulocyte count <1000/mm^3 or platelets <75,000/mm^3, do not give

Y-site compatibilities: Alemtuzumab, alfentanil, allopurinol, amifostine, amikacin, aminophylline, ampicillin, anidulafungin, argatroban, aztreonam, bivalirudin, bleomycin, bumetanide, butorphanol, calcium gluconate, caspofungin, cefOXitin, cefTAZidime, ceftizoxime, cefTRIAXone, chlorproMAZINE, cimetidine, ciprofloxacin, CISplatin, clindamycin, cyclophosphamide, cytarabine, DACTINomycin, DAUNOrubicin, diphenhydrAMINE, DOBUTamine, DOCEtaxel, DOPamine, DOXOrubicin, droperidol, enalaprilat, etoposide, famotidine, floxuridine, fluconazole, fludarabine, fluorouracil, gentamicin, granisetron, haloperidol, heparin, hydrocortisone, HYDROmorphone, IDArubicin, ifosfamide, leucovorin, linezolid, LORazepam, mannitol, meperidine, mesna, metoclopramide, metroNIDAZOLE, minocycline, mitoXANtrone, morphine, nalbuphine, ondansetron, PACLitaxel, promethazine, ranitidine, streptozocin, teniposide, thiotepa, ticarcillin, tigecycline, tobramycin, topotecan, trimethoprim/sulfamethoxazole, vancomycin, vinBLAStine, vinCRIStine, vinorelbine, voriconazole, zidovudine, zoledronic acid

SIDE EFFECTS
CNS: Posterior reversible encephalopathy syndrome (PRES)
CV: Dysrthymias, hypertension
ENDO: Hyperglycemia
GI: Diarrhea, *nausea, vomiting,* anorexia, constipation, stomatitis, diarrhea, hepatotoxicity
GU: *Proteinuria,* hematuria
HEMA: Leukopenia, anemia, neutropenia, thrombocytopenia
INTEG: Irritation at site, *rash, alopecia*
META: Hypocalcemia, hypokalemia, hypomagnesemia
RESP: Dyspnea, bronchospasm, pneumonitis
OTHER: *Fever,* hemorrhage, infection, flulike symptoms, paresthesia, *peripheral edema,* myalgia, capillary leak syndrome

PHARMACOKINETICS
Half-life 2.5-18 hr; crosses placenta; excretion: renal, 92%-98% peak 30 min

INTERACTIONS
Increase: bleeding—NSAIDs, anticoagulants
Increase: myelosuppression, diarrhea—other antineoplastics, radiation
Decrease: antibody response—live virus vaccines
Drug/Lab Test
Increase: BUN, AST, ALT, alk phos, bilirubin, creatinine
Decrease: Hb, WBC, neutrophils, platelets

NURSING CONSIDERATIONS
Assess:
• **Blood dyscrasias:** assess for bruising, bleeding, petechiae
• Renal, hepatic studies before and during treatment; may increase AST, ALT, alk phos, bilirubin, BUN, creatinine, calcium, potassium, glucose, magnesium, urine protein, monitor I&O
• Buccal cavity for dryness, sores, ulceration, white patches, oral pain, bleeding, dysphagia
• **Blood studies:** Monitor blood studies (neutrophils, platelets) often

G

- **PRES:** monitor for headache seizures, hypertension, vision changes, if confirmed with MRI, discontinue
- **Hepatotoxicity:** May be fatal, monitor LFTs, baseline and periodically, those with preexisting liver conditions are at a greater risk
- **Pulmonary toxicity:** May be fatal, may occur up to 2 wk after last dose, if dyspnea, bronchospasm occur, discontinue
- **Capillary leak syndrome:** hemoconcentration, decreased albumin, B/P; discontinue if these occur
- **Hemolytic uremic syndrome (HUS):** more frequent when given with bleomycin; assess renal function before use and periodically; anemia with microangiopathic hemolysis, elevated bilirubin or LDH, reticulocytosis, severe thrombocytopenia, or increases in BUN/creatinine (HUS); permanently discontinue if evidence of pulmonary toxicity, may occur ≤2 wk after last dose
- **Radiation therapy risks:** avoid radiation therapy 7 days before and 7 days after treatment; there is increased risk of life-threatening mucositis and toxicity at any time
- **Pregnancy/breastfeeding:** No controlled studies, avoid use in pregnancy, do not breastfeed

Evaluate:
- **Therapeutic response:** decrease in tumor size; decrease in spread of cancer; symptom relief

Teach patient/family:
- To avoid foods with citric acid, hot temperature, or rough texture if stomatitis is present; to drink adequate fluids; to avoid use with NSAIDs, alcohol, salicylates
- To report stomatitis and any bleeding, white spots, ulcerations in mouth; to examine mouth daily, report symptoms
- To report signs of anemia: fatigue, headache, faintness, SOB, irritability; hematuria, dysuria
- Not to receive vaccinations during treatment
- About possible hair loss and what can be done
- **Infection:** to report sore throat, fever, flulike symptoms immediately

- That continuing follow-up exams and lab work will be needed
- **Pregnancy/breastfeeding:** to use contraception during and for 4 mo after; do not breastfeed

gemfibrozil (Rx)
(jem-fi'broe-zil)
Lopid
Func. class.: Antilipemic
Chem. class.: Fibric acid derivative

Do not confuse:
gemfibrozil/gabapentin

ACTION: Inhibits biosynthesis of VLDL, decreases triglycerides, production in the liver increases HDL

USES: For use as an adjunct to diet for the treatment of hyperlipoproteinemia and for hypertriglyceridemia including type IV (elevated triglycerides, VLDL) and type V (elevated triglycerides, chylomicrons, VLDL) in patients who have significant risk of coronary artery disease or pancreatitis and who have not responded to diet

CONTRAINDICATIONS
Severe renal/hepatic disease, preexisting gallbladder disease, primary biliary cirrhosis, hypersensitivity, use with dasabuvir, repaglinide, or simvastatin
Precautions: Pregnancy, breastfeeding, renal disease, cholelithiasis, children

DOSAGE AND ROUTES
- **Adult:** PO 600 mg bid 30 min before AM, PM meal
Hepatic/renal dose
- Avoid use
Available forms: Tabs 600 mg; caps 300 mg ♥
Administer:
PO route
- 30 min before AM, PM meals
- Discontinue product if response does not occur within 3 mo

SIDE EFFECTS
CNS: Fatigue, vertigo, headache, paresthesia, dizziness

GI: *Dyspepsia, diarrhea, abdominal pain,* nausea, vomiting
HEMA: Leukopenia, anemia, eosinophilia, thrombocytopenia
INTEG: Rash, urticaria, pruritus
MS: Myopathy, rhabdomyolysis

PHARMACOKINETICS

Peak 1-2 hr; plasma protein binding >95%; half-life 1½ hr; 70% excreted in urine mostly unchanged; metabolized in liver (minimal)

INTERACTIONS

• Do not use with dasabuvir, repaglinide, simvastatin

Increase: hypoglycemic effect—sulfonylureas, repaglinide, metformin, glyburide, pioglitazone, other antidiabetic agents

Increase: myopathy—colchicine

Increase: anticoagulant effect—warfarin; monitor coagulation tests

Increase: nephrotoxicity—cyclosporine; monitor renal function

Increase: levels of CYP2C8, CYP2C9, CYP2C19; monitor for toxicities

Increase: risk of myositis, myalgia, rhabdomyolysis—HMG-CoA reductase inhibitors; avoid concurrent use

Decrease: effect of gemfibrozil—bile acid sequestrants, colestipol, separate by >2 hr

Decrease: level of cyclosporine

Drug/Lab Test
Increase: LFTs, CK, bilirubin, alkaline phosphatase
Decrease: HB, Hct, WBC, potassium, eosinophils, platelets

NURSING CONSIDERATIONS
Assess:

• **Hyperlipidemia:** diet history; fats, triglycerides, cholesterol; if lipids increase, product should be discontinued; LDL, VLDL baseline and periodically

• **Myopathy, rhabdomyolysis:** for muscle pain, tenderness; obtain baseline CPK; if elevated or if these occur, product should be discontinued; at greater risk if combined with HMG-CoA reductase inhibitors

• **Labs:** renal, hepatic studies, CBC, blood glucose if patient is receiving long-term therapy; if LFTs increase, therapy should be discontinued; monitor hematologic and hepatic functions

• Bowel pattern daily; watch for increasing diarrhea (common)

• **Pregnancy/breastfeeding:** use only if benefits outweigh fetal risk; do not breastfeed, excretion unknown

Evaluate:

• **Therapeutic response:** decreased cholesterol, triglyceride levels; HDL, cholesterol ratios improved

Teach patient/family:

• That compliance is needed for positive results; not to double or skip dose, to take missed dose as soon as remembered unless almost time for next dose

• To minimize risk factors: high-fat diet, smoking, alcohol consumption, absence of exercise

• To notify prescriber of diarrhea, nausea, vomiting, chills, fever, sore throat, muscle cramps, abdominal cramps, severe flatulence, tendon pain

• To avoid driving, hazardous activities if dizziness, blurred vision occur

gentamicin (Rx)

jen-ta-mye´sin
Func. class.: Antiinfective
Chem. class.: Aminoglycoside

Do not confuse:
gentamicin/kanamycin

ACTION: Interferes with protein synthesis in bacterial cell by binding to 30S ribosomal subunit, thus causing misreading of genetic code; inaccurate peptide sequence forms in protein chain, thereby causing bacterial death

USES: Severe systemic infections of CNS, respiratory, GI, urinary tract, bone, skin, soft tissues caused by susceptible strains of *Pseudomonas aeruginosa, Proteus, Klebsiella, Serratia, Escherichia coli, Enterobacter, Citrobacter, Staphylococcus, Shigella, Salmonella, Acinetobacter, Bacillus anthracis*

CONTRAINDICATIONS

Hypersensitivity to this product, other aminoglycosides

Side effects: *italics* = common; red = life-threatening

Precautions: Breastfeeding, neonates, geriatric patients, pseudomembranous colitis, sulfite hypersensitivity

> **Black Box Warning:** Myasthenia gravis, Parkinson's disease, infant botulism, tinnitus, nephrotoxicity, neurotoxicity, pregnancy

DOSAGE AND ROUTES
Severe systemic infections
- **Adult: IV INFUSION** 3-5 mg/kg/day in divided doses q8hr; **IM** 3-5 mg/kg/day in divided doses q8hr
- **Child: IM/IV** 2-2.5 mg/kg q8hr
- **Neonate and infant >1 wk: IM/IV** 2.5 mg/kg q8-12hr
- **Neonate <1 wk: IM/IV** 2.5 mg/kg q12hr

Renal dose: regular dosing
- **Adult: IM/IV CCr 70-100 mL/min,** reduce dose by multiplying maintenance dose by 0.85, give q8-12hr; **CCr 50-69 mL/min,** reduce as above, give q12hr; **CCr 25-49 mL/min,** reduce as above, give q24hr; **CCr <25 mL/min,** reduce as above, give based on serum concentrations, give doses after dialysis

Available forms: Inj 10, 40 mg/mL; premixed inj 60 mg/50 mL, 80 mg/50 mL, 80 mg/100 mL, 100 mg/50 mL, 100 mg/100 mL, 120 mg/100 mL

Administer:
- Obtain C&S before starting treatment, treatment may be started before results are received
- Draw for peak 1 hr after IM, 30 min after IV; draw trough before next dose, do not use heparin-coated tube for blood draw

IM route
- IM inj in large muscle mass; rotate inj sites
- Product in evenly spaced doses to maintain blood level

Intermittent IV INFUSION route
- After diluting in 50-200 mL NS, D$_5$W; decrease vol of diluent in child; maintain 0.1% sol run over ½-1 hr (adults) or up to 2 hr (children); flush IV line with NS, D$_5$W after administration

Y-site compatibilities: Alatrofloxacin, aldesleukin, alemtuzumab, alfentanil, alprostadil, amifostine, amikacin, aminocaproic acid, aminophylline, amiodarone, amsacrine, anidulafungin, argatroban, arsenic trioxide, ascorbic acid injection, asparaginase, atenolol, atracurium, atropine, aztreonam, benztropine, bivalirudin, bleomycin, bumetanide, buprenorphine, butorphanol, calcium chloride/gluconate, carboplatin, carmustine, caspofungin, cefamandole, ceFAZolin, cefepime, cefotaxime, cefOXitin, cefpirome, ceftaroline, cefTAZidime, ceftizoxime, ceftRIAXone, cefuroxime, chlorothiazide, chlorpheniramine, chlorproMAZINE, cimetidine, ciprofloxacin, cisatracurium, CISplatin, clarithromycin, clindamycin, cloxacillin, codeine, colistimethate, cyanocobalamin, cyclophosphamide, cycloSPORINE, cytarabine, DACTINomycin, DAPTOmycin, DAUNOrubicin citrate liposome, DAUNOrubicin hydrochloride, dexmedetomidine, dexrazoxane, digoxin, diltiazem, dimenhyDRINATE, diphenhydrAMINE, DOBUTamine, DOCEtaxel, dolasetron, DOPamine, doripenem, doxacurium, doxapram, DOXOrubicin hydrochloride, doxorubicin hydrochloride liposomal, doxycycline, edetate calcium disodium, edetate disodium, enalaprilat, ePHEDrine, EPINEPHrine, epirubicin, epoetin alfa, eptifibatide, ergonovine, ertapenem, erythromycin lactobionate, esmolol, etoposide, etoposide phosphate, famotidine, fenoldopam, fentaNYL, fluconazole, fludarabine, fluorouracil, foscarnet, gallamine, gallium, gatifloxacin, gemcitabine, glycopyrrolate, granisetron, HYDROmorphone, hydrOXYzine, ifosfamide, imipenem-cilastatin, irinotecan, isoproterenol, ketamine, ketorolac, labetalol, lactated Ringer's injection, lansoprazole, lepirudin, leucovorin, levofloxacin, lidocaine, lincomycin, linezolid, LORazepam, magnesium sulfate, mannitol, mechlorethamine, melphalan, meperidine, mephentermine sulfate, meropenem, mesna, metaraminol, methyldopate, methylPREDNISolone sodium succinate, metoclopramide, metoprolol, metroNIDAZOLE, midazolam, milrinone, minocycline, mitoXANtrone, mivacurium, morphine, multiple vitamins injection, mycophenolate mofetil, nafcillin, nalbuphine, nalorphine, naloxone, netilmicin, niCARdipine, nitroglycerin, nitroprusside, norepinephrine, octreotide, ondansetron, oritavancin, oxaliplatin, oxytocin, PACLitaxel (solvent/surfactant), palonosetron, pamidronate, pancuronium, papaverine, penicillin G potassium/sodium, pentazocine, perphenazine, PHENobarbital, phentolamine, phenylephrine, phytonadione, piperacillin, polymyxin B, posaconazole, potassium acetate/chloride, procainamide, prochlorperazine, promazine, promethazine, propranolol, protamine, pyridoxine, quiNIDine gluconate, ranitidine, remifentanil, Ringer's injection, riTUXimab, rocuronium, sargramostim, sodium acetate/bicarbonate/citrate, streptomycin, succinylcholine, SUFentanil, tacrolimus, telavancin, temocillin, teniposide, theophylline, thiamine, thiotepa, ticarcillin, ticarcillin-clavulanate, tigecycline, tirofiban, TNA (3-in-1), tobramycin, tolazoline, topotecan, TPN (2-in-1), trastuzumab, trimetaphan, tubocurarine, urokinase, vancomycin, vasopressin, vecuronium, verapamil, vinBLAStine, vinCRIStine, vinorelbine, vitamin B complex with C, voriconazole, zidovudine, zoledronic acid

SIDE EFFECTS

CNS: Confusion, depression, numbness, tremors, seizures, muscle twitching, neurotoxicity, dizziness, vertigo, encephalopathy, fever, headache, lethargy
CV: Hypo/hypertension, palpitations, edema
EENT: Ototoxicity, *deafness,* visual disturbances, tinnitus
GI: *Nausea, vomiting, anorexia;* increased ALT, AST, bilirubin; hepatomegaly, hepatic necrosis, splenomegaly
GU: Oliguria, hematuria, renal damage, azotemia, renal failure, nephrotoxicity, proteinuria
HEMA: Agranulocytosis, thrombocytopenia, leukopenia, eosinophilia, anemia

INTEG: *Rash,* burning, urticaria, dermatitis, alopecia, photosensitivity, anaphylaxis
MS: Twitching, myasthenia gravis–like symptoms
RESP: Apnea

PHARMACOKINETICS

Not metabolized, excreted unchanged in urine, crosses placental barrier
IM: Onset rapid, peak 30-60 min
IV: Onset immediate; peak 30-90 min; plasma half-life 1-2 hr, infants 6-7 hr; duration 6-8 hr

INTERACTIONS

• Do not use at the same time as or physically mix with penicillins, may inactivate gentamicin

Black Box Warning: Increase: ototoxicity, neurotoxicity, nephrotoxicity—other aminoglycosides, amphotericin B, polymyxin, vancomycin, ethacrynic acid, furosemide, mannitol, methoxyflurane, CISplatin, cephalosporins, penicillins, cidofovir, acyclovir, foscarnet, cycloSPORINE, tacrolimus, ganciclovir, zoledronic acid, pamidronate, monitor hearing

Increase: effects—nondepolarizing neuromuscular blockers, digoxin, entecavir, reduce dose or do not use together
Drug/Lab Test
Increase: LDH, AST, ALT, bilirubin, BUN, creatinine, eosinophils
Decrease: Hb, WBC, platelets, serum calcium/sodium/potassium/magnesium

NURSING CONSIDERATIONS
Assess:

Black Box Warning: Neurotoxicity: (myasthenia gravis, Parkinson's disease, infant botulism): monitor for paresthesias, tetany, positive Chvostek's/Trousseau's signs, confusion (adults), muscle weakness (infants); correct electrolyte imbalance

• Weight before treatment; calculation of dosage is usually based on ideal body weight but may be calculated on actual body weight

---

Side effects: *italics* = common; red = life-threatening

Black Box Warning: Nephrotoxicity: Monitor I&O ratio, urinalysis daily for proteinuria, cells, casts; report sudden change in urine output; urine pH if product is used for UTI; urine should be kept alkaline; urine for CCr testing, BUN, serum creatinine; lower dosage should be given with renal impairment (CCr <80 mL/min); toxicity is increased in patients with decreased renal function if high doses are given

• **Vitals:** VS during infusion; watch for hypotension, change in pulse
• IV site for thrombophlebitis, including pain, redness, swelling q30min, change site if needed; discontinue, apply warm compresses to site

Black Box Warning: Peak/trough levels: Serum peak drawn at 30-60 min after IV infusion or 60 min after IM inj and trough level drawn just before next dose; blood level should be 2-4 times bacteriostatic level; peak (8 mcg/mL), trough (1-2 mcg/mL), depending on type of infection (based on traditional dosing), prolonged peak levels >10 mcg/mL may lead to toxicity

Black Box Warning: Ototoxicity: Assess eighth cranial nerve dysfunction by audiometric testing; also ringing, roaring in ears, vertigo; assess hearing before, during, after treatment

• **Dehydration:** Monitor for high specific gravity, decrease in skin turgor, dry mucous membranes, dark urine
• **Superinfection:** fever, malaise, redness, pain, swelling, perineal itching, diarrhea, stomatitis, change in cough or sputum
• C&S before starting treatment to identify infecting organism
• **Vestibular dysfunction:** nausea, vomiting, dizziness, headache; product should be discontinued if severe
• Adequate fluids of 2-3 L/day unless contraindicated to prevent irritation of tubules

Black Box Warning: Pregnancy/breastfeeding: identify whether pregnancy is planned or suspected; do not use in pregnancy or breastfeeding, deafness may occur in neonates

Evaluate:
• **Therapeutic response:** absence of fever, draining wounds, negative C&S after treatment
Teach patient/family:
• To report headache, dizziness, symptoms of overgrowth of infection, renal impairment

Black Box Warning: Ototoxicity: to report loss of hearing; ringing, roaring in ears; feeling of fullness in head

• To drink adequate fluids
• To avoid hazardous activities until reaction is known

gentamicin (ophthalmic) (Rx)

(jen-ta-mye′sin)

Gentak, Garamycin ✦
Func. class.: Ophthalmic antiinfective
Chem. class.: Aminoglycoside

Do not confuse:
gentamicin/clindamycin/tobramycin/erythromycin/vancomycin

ACTION: Inhibits protein synthesis by binding of 30s ribosomal subunits, thereby decreasing bacterial replication

USES: External ocular infections

CONTRAINDICATIONS
Hypersensitivity to this product or amino-glycosides
Precautions: Pregnancy, breastfeeding, corneal healing, local redness/irritation

DOSAGE AND ROUTES
Ophthalmic (solution)
• **Adult/adolescent/child ≥1 mo: SOL** 1-2 drops in affected eye(s) every 4 hr while awake × 2 days, then every 4 hr; severe infections ≤2 drops every 1 hr

- **Ointment:** apply a small amount (½ in) to lower conjunctival sac bid or tid
Available forms: Ophthalmic ointment, ophthalmic solution 0.3%
Administer:
Ophthalmic route
- Commercially available ophthalmic solutions are not for injection subconjunctivally or into the anterior chamber of the eye
- Apply topically to the eye, taking care to avoid contamination
- Do not touch the tip of the dropper to the eye, fingertips, or other surface; wash hands before use
- Apply pressure to lacrimal sac for 1 min after instillation
- To apply the ointment, pull down gently on lower eyelid and apply a thin film of the ointment

SIDE EFFECTS
EENT: Burning, hypersensitivity, stinging, blurred vision, hyperemia, corneal ulcers

PHARMACOKINETICS
Unknown

NURSING CONSIDERATIONS
Assess:
- **Allergic reaction:** hypersensitivity, discontinue product
Evaluate:
- **Therapeutic response:** decreased ophthalmic infection
Teach patient/family:
Ophthalmic route
- To apply topically to the eye, taking care to avoid contamination; for ophthalmic use only
- Not to touch the tip of the dropper to the eye, fingertips, or other surface; to wash hands before use
- To apply pressure to lacrimal sac for 1 min after instillation
- To apply the ointment by pulling down gently on lower eyelid and applying a thin film of the ointment

gentamicin (topical) (Rx)
(jen-ta-mye′sin)
Func. class.: Topical antiinfective
Chem. class.: Aminoglycoside

Do not confuse:
gentamicin/clindamycin

ACTION: Antibacterial activity results from inhibition of protein synthesis; bactericidal

USES: Superficial infections

CONTRAINDICATIONS
Hypersensitivity to this product or other aminoglycosides
Precautions: Infections, local sensitivity

DOSAGE AND ROUTES
- **Adult/child >1 yr:** apply to affected areas tid-qid
Available forms: Topical cream, ointment 0.1%
Administer:
- For external use only; do not use skin products near the eyes, nose, or mouth
- Wash hands before and after use; wash affected area and gently pat dry
- **Cream/ointment:** Apply to the cleansed affected area, massage gently into affected areas

SIDE EFFECTS
INTEG: Rash, irritation, erythema, pruritus

PHARMACOKINETICS
Unknown

NURSING CONSIDERATIONS
Assess:
- **Allergic reaction:** hypersensitivity; product may need to be discontinued
- **Infection:** skin infection
Evaluate:
- **Therapeutic response:** decreased skin infection
Teach patient/family:
- To use for external use only; do not use skin products near the eyes, nose, or mouth
- To wash hands before and after use; wash affected area and gently pat dry
- **Cream/ointment:** to apply to the cleansed affected area and massage gently into affected areas

gilteritinib (Rx)

(gil´teh-rih´tih-nib)

Xospata

Func. class.: Antineoplastic
Chem. class.: Kinase inhibitor

USES: 🔆 Acute myeloid leukemia-relapsed or the treatment of relapsed or refractory FLT3 mutation–positive AML

DOSAGE AND ROUTES

• **Adult: PO** 120 mg daily for a minimum of 6 mo

Qtc interval increase: Interval >500 msec, stop treatment, when Qtc decreases to 30 msec (of baseline or ≤480 msec), restart at 80 mg/day

Available form: Tablet 40 mg

glasdegib (Rx)

(glass-deg´ib)

Daurismo

Func. class.: Antineoplastic
Chem. class.: Hedgehog pathway inhibitor

USES

Acute myeloid leukemia in combination

DOSAGE AND ROUTES

Adults ≥75 yr or with comorbidities: PO 100 mg once daily (in combination with subcutaneous low-dose cytarabine) for a minimum of 6 (28-day) cycles

Available forms: Tabs 25, 100 mg

Toxicity: Refer to manufacturer's information for dosage changes

---

⚠ HIGH ALERT

glatiramer (Rx)

(glah-tear´a-meer)

Copaxone, Glatopa, Glatect ✽
Func. class.: Multiple sclerosis agent
Chem. class.: Biologic response modifier

ACTION: Unknown; may modify the immune responses responsible for multiple sclerosis (MS) by serving as a decoy to locally generated autoantibodies

USES: Reduction of the frequency of relapses in patients with relapsing or remitting MS after first clinical episode with MRI results consistent with MS

CONTRAINDICATIONS

Hypersensitivity to this product or mannitol, IV use

Precautions: Pregnancy, breastfeeding, children <18 yr, immune disorders, renal disease, infection, vaccinations, geriatric patients

DOSAGE AND ROUTES

• 20 mg/mL and 40 mg/mL are not interchangeable

• **Adult: SUBCUT** 20 mg/day or 40 mg 3 × per wk, give ≥48 hr apart

Available forms: Inj premixed 20 mg/mL in single-use syringe; sol for inj 40 mg/mL

Administer:

SUBCUT route

• Refrigerate, allow to warm for 20 min; visually inspect for particulate or cloudiness; if present, discard; prefilled syringe contents are for single use; administer SUBCUT into hip, thigh, arm; discard unused portion; if refrigeration is unavailable, may store ≤1 mo at room temperature

• Use SUBCUT route only; do not give IM or IV, do not expel air bubble in prefilled syringe

• Give 40-mg dose on same 3 days of the week, must be 48 hr apart

SIDE EFFECTS

CNS: *Anxiety, hypertonia, tremor, vertigo,* speech disorder, *agitation,* confusion, flushing

CV: *Migraine, palpitations, syncope, tachycardia, vasodilation,* chest pain, hypertension

EENT: *Ear pain, blurred vision*

GI: *Nausea, vomiting, diarrhea, anorexia, gastroenteritis*

GU: *Urinary urgency, dysmenorrhea, vaginal moniliasis,* vaginal hemorrhage
HEMA: *Ecchymosis, lymphadenopathy*
INTEG: *Pruritus, rash, sweating, urticaria, erythema,* inj-site reaction
META: Edema, weight gain
MS: *Arthralgia, back pain, neck pain,* increased muscle tone
RESP: *Bronchitis, dyspnea, laryngismus, rhinitis,* laryngospasm

PHARMACOKINETICS
May be hydrolyzed locally, may reach regional lymph nodes

INTERACTIONS
Increase: serious infection—denosumab, natalizumab, roflumilast; avoid using together
Increase: hematologic toxicity (pancytopenia, thrombocytopenia)—leflunomide
• Avoid use with live virus vaccines
Increase: neutropenia effect—trastuzumab
Increase: immunosuppression—tofacitinib, avoid use
Drug/Herb
Decrease: glatiramer effect—echinacea, may need dosage change

NURSING CONSIDERATIONS
Assess:
• **CNS symptoms:** anxiety, confusion, vertigo
• **GI status:** diarrhea, abdominal pain/cramps, vomiting
• **CV status:** B/P, pulse, HR; tachycardia, palpitations, vasodilation, and chest pain may occur
• **Postinjection reactions:** Assess for chest pain, dyspnea, flushing, palpitations, usually resolve on their own, may occur quickly or several months after use; usually at least one episode of chest pain occurs 1 mo after start of therapy
• **Pregnancy/breastfeeding:** use only if clearly needed; no well-controlled studies; cautious use in breastfeeding
Evaluate:
• **Therapeutic response:** decreased symptoms of MS

Teach patient/family:
• With written, detailed instructions about product; provide initial and return demonstrations on inj procedure; give information about use and disposal of product, inj-site reaction (hives, rash, irritation, severe pain, flushing, chest pain)
• To notify prescribers of allergic reactions including itching, trouble breathing, chest pain, dizziness, sweating
• That irregular menses, dysmenorrhea, metrorrhagia, breast pain may occur; to use contraception during treatment
• To notify prescriber if pregnancy is suspected or if nursing
• Not to change dosing or stop taking product without advice of prescriber
• About immediate postinjection reaction: flushing, chest pain, palpitations, anxiety, dyspnea, laryngeal constriction, urticaria; does not usually require treatment, may occur months after beginning treatment
• To take as directed; not to stop product or change schedule; teach on self-injection technique
• That the 20 mg/mL and 40 mg/mL are not interchangeable

glecaprevir/pibrentasvir (Rx)
(glek-a′pre-vir/pi-brent′as-vir)
Mavyret, Maviret ✤
Func. class.: Antiviral
Chem. class.: HCV MS3/4A protease inhibitor/HCV NSSA inhibitor

Do not confuse:
Mavyret/Mavik

ACTION:
Glecaprevir is an inhibitor of hepatitis C virus (HCV) NS3/4A protease, necessary for the proteolytic cleavage of the HCV-encoded polyprotein and is essential for viral replication

Pibrentasvir is an inhibitor of HCV NS5A, essential for viral RNA replication

USES:
Chronic hepatitis C (HCV monoinfected or HCV/HIV coinfected patients), without cirrhosis or with compensated cirrhosis (Child-Pugh class A)

CONTRAINDICATIONS
Moderate or severe hepatic impairment (Child-Pugh class B or C); hepatic decompensation; coadministration with atazanavir or rifAMPin

Black Box Warning: HBV reactivation/exacerbation

PRECAUTIONS
Pregnancy, children, breastfeeding, immunosuppressants, chemotherapy

DOSAGE AND ROUTES
• **Adult/child >45 kg: PO** 3 tablets with food
• **Child 12-17: PO** 6 packets daily with food × 8 wk
• **Child 3-11 yr, >45 kg: PO** 6 packets daily with food × 8 wk
• **Child 3-11 yr, 30-44 kg: PO** 5 packets daily with food × 8 wk
• **Child 3-11 yr, 20-29 kg: PO** 4 packets daily with food × 8 wk
• **Child 3-11 yr, <20 kg: PO** 3 packets daily with food × 8 wk

Duration:
Therapy-naive: HCV genotype 1, 2, 3, 4, 5, 6: No cirrhosis: 8 wk; compensated cirrhosis (Child-Pugh A): 8 wk
Therapy-experienced: HCV genotype 1 (prior therapy with regimen containing an NS5A inhibitor without prior therapy with an NS3/4A protease inhibitor): No cirrhosis: 16 wk; compensated cirrhosis (Child-Pugh A): 16 wk
HCV genotype 1 (prior therapy with an NS3/4A protease inhibitor without prior therapy with an NS5A inhibitor): No cirrhosis: 12 wk; compensated cirrhosis (Child-Pugh A): 12 wk

HCV genotype 1, 2, 4, 5, 6 (prior therapy with PRS): No cirrhosis: 8 wk; compensated cirrhosis (Child-Pugh A): 12 wk

HCV genotype 3 (prior therapy with PRS): No cirrhosis: 16 wk; compensated cirrhosis (Child-Pugh A): 16 wk

Available forms: Tablet: glecaprevir 100 mg/pibrentasvir 40 mg; oral pellets 50 mg/20 mg

Administer:
• Give with food
• If dose is missed, give as soon as remembered if within 18 hr, then normal dosing; if >18 hr, skip
• Store at room temperature
• **Oral pellets:** take with food, may use soft food that will stick to pellets, do not crush or chew

PHARMACOKINETICS
Peak 5 hr, half-life: glecaprevir 6 hr; pibrentasvir 13 hr

INTERACTIONS
Increase: effect of—afatinib, aliskiren, alpelisib, asunaprevir, atorvastatin, betrixaban, bilastine, celiprolol, cladribine, CYP1A2 inhibitors, colchicine, dabigatran, dofetilide, doxorubicin, edoxaban, elagolix, digoxin, eluxadoline, etoposide, everolimus, grazoprevir, HMG-CoA reductase inhibitors
Increase: hypoglycemic effect—antidiabetics
Increase: effect of glecaprevir/pibrentasvir—atazanavir, cobicistat, cyclosporine, darunavir, P-glycoprotein inhibitors (except cyclosporine)
Decrease: effect of glecaprevir/pibrentasvir—carBAMazepine, CYP3A4 inducers, efavirenz, fosphenytoin, rifamycins
Increase: adverse reactions of glecaprevir/pibrentasvir—ethinyl
Drug/Herb
Decrease: effect of glecaprevir/pibrentasvir, avoid using together—St. John's Wort
Drug/Lab Test
Increase: bilirubin

NURSING CONSIDERATIONS
Assess:
• **Baseline (within 12 wk prior to starting antiviral therapy)** CBC, INR, hepatic function panel (albumin, total and direct bilirubin, ALT, AST, and alkaline phosphatase), and calculated GFR; repeat CBC, serum creatinine, calculated GFR, and LFTs panel after 4 wk of therapy and as clinically indicated
• **Baseline (at any time prior to starting therapy)** hepatitis C virus (HCV) genotype and subtype and quantitative HCV viral load; repeat quantitative HCV viral load testing (after 4 wk of therapy and at 12 wk after completion of therapy). If quantitative HCV viral load is detectable at treatment wk 4, repeat testing after 2 additional wk of treatment (treatment wk 6)

Black Box Warning: Hepatitis B surface antigen (HBsAg) and hepatitis B core antibody (anti-HBc) prior to initiation

Black Box Warning: Serologic evidence of hepatitis B virus (HBV) infection, monitor for clinical and laboratory signs of hepatitis flare or HBV reactivation during treatment and during post-treatment follow-up

• **Diabetes,** monitor blood glucose and for signs/symptoms of hypoglycemia
• Monitor for treatment failure; if decompensation occurs, discontinue treatment
• **Pregnancy/breastfeeding:** Avoid use in pregnancy and breastfeeding
Evaluate:
• **Therapeutic response:** hepatitis C RNA reduction
Teach patient/family:
• To report side effects to the prescriber
• To notify all providers of product use, many drug interactions; do not take with St. John's wort
• To take at the same time each day, to use for full course even if feeling better, to take missed doses when remembered on the same day; not to double doses
• That the product will not decrease transmission of infection in others

• **Pregnancy/breastfeeding:** To notify provider if pregnancy is planned or suspected, or if breastfeeding

⚠ HIGH ALERT

glimepiride (Rx)
(glye-me′pi-ride)
Amaryl
glipiZIDE (Rx)
(glip-i′zide)
Glucotrol, Glucotrol XL
Func. class.: Antidiabetic
Chem. class.: Sulfonylurea (2nd generation)

Do not confuse:
glipiZIDE/Glucotrol/glyBURIDE

ACTION: Causes functioning β-cells in pancreas to release insulin, leading to drop in blood glucose levels; may improve insulin binding to insulin receptors or increase the number of insulin receptors with prolonged administration; may also reduce basal hepatic glucose secretion; not effective if patient lacks functioning β-cells

USES: Type 2 diabetes mellitus

CONTRAINDICATIONS
Hypersensitivity to sulfonylureas/sulfonamides, type 1 diabetes, diabetic ketoacidosis
Precautions: Pregnancy, geriatric patients, cardiac disease, severe renal/hepatic disease, G6PD deficiency

DOSAGE AND ROUTES
glimepiride
• **Adult: PO** 1-2 mg/day with breakfast, then increase by ≤2 mg/day q1-2wk, max 8 mg/day
• **Geriatric: PO** 1 mg/day; may increase if needed
Renal/hepatic dose
• **Adult: PO** 1 mg/day with breakfast; may titrate upward as needed

glipiZIDE
• **Adult: PO** 5 mg initially before breakfast, then increase by 2.5-5 mg after several days to desired response; max 40 mg/day in divided doses; **PO** (XL) 5 mg/day with breakfast, may increase to 10 mg/day, max 20 mg/day
• **Geriatric: PO** 2.5 mg/day; may increase if needed
Hepatic disease
• **Adult: PO** 2.5 mg initially, then increase to desired response; max 40 mg/day in divided doses or 15 mg/dose
Available forms: *glimepiride:* tabs 1, 2, 4 mg; *glipiZIDE:* tabs, scored 5, 10 mg; ext rel tabs (XL) 2.5, 5, 10 mg
Administer:
• Do not break, crush, or chew ext rel tabs; may crush tabs and mix with fluids if unable to swallow whole
• **GlipiZIDE:** give product 30 min before meals (regular release); with breakfast (ext rel); **glimepiride:** with breakfast; if patient is NPO, may need to hold dose to prevent hypoglycemia
• Gradual conversion from other oral hypoglycemics to these products is not needed; insulin ≥20 units/day, convert using 25% reduction in insulin dose every day or every other day
• Store in tight, light-resistant container at room temperature

SIDE EFFECTS
CNS: *Headache, weakness, dizziness, drowsiness,* tinnitus, fatigue, vertigo
ENDO: Hypoglycemia
GI: Hepatotoxicity, cholestatic jaundice, nausea, vomiting, diarrhea, heartburn, weight gain
HEMA: Leukopenia, thrombocytopenia, agranulocytosis, aplastic anemia; increased AST, ALT, alk phos; pancytopenia, hemolytic anemia
INTEG: Rash, allergic reactions, pruritus, urticaria, eczema, photosensitivity, erythema, allergic vasculitis
SYST: Serious hypersensitivity

PHARMACOKINETICS
PO: Completely absorbed by GI route; **glipiZIDE:** onset 1-1½ hr, peak 2-3

hr, duration 12-24 hr, half-life 2-4 hr; **glimepiride:** peak 2-3 hr, half-life 5 hr; metabolized in liver, excreted in urine, 90%-95% plasma-protein bound

INTERACTIONS
• May mask symptoms of hypoglycemia: β-blockers
Increase: action of digoxin, glycosides, cyclosporine
Increase: hypoglycemic effects—insulin, MAOIs, cimetidine, chloramphenicol, guanethidine, methyldopa, NSAIDs, salicylates, probenecid, androgens, anticoagulants, clofibrate, fenfluramine, fluconazole, gemfibrozil, histamine H₂ antagonists, magnesium salts, phenylbutazone, sulfinpyrazone, sulfonamides, tricyclics, urinary acidifiers, clarithromycin, fibric acid derivatives, voriconazole; monitor blood glucose
Decrease: hypoglycemic effect—thiazide diuretics, rifAMPin, isoniazid, cholestyramine, diazoxide, hydantoins, urinary alkalinizers, charcoal, corticosteroids, colesevelam; monitor blood glucose
Drug/Herb
Increase: antidiabetic effect—garlic, horse chestnut
Decrease: hypoglycemic effect—green tea
Drug/Lab Test
Increase: AST, ALT, LDH, BUN, creatinine
Decrease: platelets, WBC, sodium

NURSING CONSIDERATIONS
Assess:
• **Hypo/hyperglycemic reaction** that can occur soon after meals; for severe hypoglycemia, give IV D₅₀W, then IV dextrose solution
• Blood glucose, A1c levels during treatment to determine diabetes control
• **Blood dyscrasias:** CBC at baseline and throughout treatment; report decreased blood count
• For allergy to sulfonamides, potential for cross-reactivity
• For renal, hepatic dysfunction: use dose reductions, or avoidance of use may be required; increased risk of hypoglycemia in hepatic failure

• **Pregnancy/breastfeeding:** identify whether pregnancy is planned or suspected; breastfed infant may be hypoglycemic; use only if benefits outweigh fetal risk

Evaluate:
• **Therapeutic response:** decrease in polyuria, polydipsia, polyphagia; clear sensorium; absence of dizziness; stable gait; improved serum glucose, A1c

Teach patient/family:
• Not to drink alcohol; about disulfiram reaction (nausea, headache, cramps, flushing, hypoglycemia)
• To report bleeding, bruising, weight gain, edema, SOB, weakness, sore throat, swelling in ankles, rash
• To check for symptoms of cholestatic jaundice: dark urine, pruritus, yellow sclera; prescriber should be notified
• About symptoms of hypo/hyperglycemia, what to do about each; to have glucagon emergency kit available; to carry sugar packets
• That product must be continued on daily basis; about consequences of discontinuing product abruptly; to take product in morning to prevent hypoglycemic reactions at night
• To use sunscreen or stay out of the sun, wear protective clothing (photosensitivity)
• To avoid OTC medications unless ordered by prescriber
• That diabetes is a lifelong illness; product will not cure disease
• That all food in diet plan must be eaten to prevent hypoglycemia; to continue weight control, dietary restrictions, exercise, hygiene
• To carry emergency ID with prescriber and medication information
• To test using blood glucose meter while taking this product
• That ext rel tab may appear in stool
• To notify prescribers of use prior to surgery
• Not to drive or engage in hazardous tasks until response is known, dizziness may occur
• That continuing follow-up exams and lab work will be needed

TREATMENT OF OVERDOSE: Use one of the following: glucose 25 g IV via dextrose 50% sol, 50 mL, 1 mg glucagon, oral carbohydrate depending on severity

glucagon (Rx)
(gloo′ka-gon)
Baqsimi GlucaGen Diagnostic, GlucaGen HypoKit, Glucagon Emergency, Gvoke HypoPen, Gvoke PFS
Func. class.: Antihypoglycemic

USES: Hypoglycemia, used to temporarily inhibit movement of GI tract as a diagnostic test

CONTRAINDICATIONS
Hypersensitivity, pheochromocytoma, insulinoma
Precautions: Pregnancy, breastfeeding, cardiac disease, adrenal insufficiency

DOSAGE AND ROUTES
Severe hypoglycemia

Glucagon Emergency Kit and GlucaGen HypoKit
• **Adult: IM/IV/SUBCUT:** 1 mg once, may repeat if response is delayed

GVOKE Auto-Injector/Prefilled Syringes
• **Adult: SUBCUT** 1 mg once, may repeat if response is delayed

Baqsimi
• **Adult: Nasal** 1 actuation (3 mg) into 1 nostril once, after 15 min if no response, may repeat

DIAGNOSTIC USE
GlucaGen Diagnostic
Relaxation of the stomach, duodenum, small bowel:
• **Adult: IV:** 0.2-0.5 mg before procedure; **IM:** 1 mg before procedure
Relaxation of the colon:
• **Adult IV:** 0.5-0.75 mg before procedure; **IM:** 1-2 mg before procedure
Available forms: Powder for injection 1-mg vial; solution for SUBCUT injection

G

Side effects: *italics* = common; red = life-threatening

0.5 mg/0.1 mL, 1 mg/0.2 mL; nasal powder 3 mg/device

⚠ HIGH ALERT

glyBURIDE (Rx)
(glye´byoor-ide)

DiaBeta ♣, Glynase PresTab
Func. class.: Antidiabetic
Chem. class.: Sulfonylurea (2nd generation)

Do not confuse:
glyBURIDE/Glucotrol/glipiZIDE

ACTION: Causes functioning β-cells in pancreas to release insulin, thereby leading to a drop in blood glucose levels

USES: Type 2 diabetes mellitus

CONTRAINDICATIONS
Hypersensitivity to sulfonylureas, type 1 diabetes, diabetic ketoacidosis, renal failure
Precautions: Pregnancy, geriatric patients, cardiac/thyroid disease, severe renal/hepatic disease, severe hypoglycemic reactions, sulfonamide/sulfonylurea hypersensitivity, G6PD deficiency

DOSAGE AND ROUTES
Nonmicronized
• **Adult: PO** 1.25-5 mg initially, then increase to desired response at weekly intervals up to 20 mg/day; may be given as a single or divided dose
• **Geriatric: PO** 1.25 mg initially, then increase to desired response; max 20 mg/day, maintenance 1.25-20 mg/day

Micronized
• **Adult: PO** 1.5-3 mg/day initially, may increase by 1.5 mg/wk, max 12 mg/day
• **Geriatric: PO** 0.75-3 mg/day, may increase by 1.5 mg/wk

To replace insulin
• **Adult: PO** if insulin was <40 U/day, switch directly; if insulin was <20 U/day, give 2.5-5 mg (or 1.5-3 mg micronized); if insulin was 20-40 U/day, give 5 mg (or 3 mg micronized); if insulin was >40 U/day,

give 5 mg (3 mg micronized) initially with 50% insulin dose, gradually taper insulin and increase glyBURIDE

Available forms: Tabs 1.25, 2.5, 5 mg (nonmicronized); 1.5, 3, 6 mg (micronized)

Administer:
• With breakfast as single or divided dose; hold dose if patient NPO to avoid hypoglycemia; take at same time each day
• Twice-daily dosing may be used if conventional doses >10 mg, micronized >6 mg
• Gradual conversion from other oral hypoglycemics to product is not needed
• Micronized glyBURIDE/nonmicronized glyBURIDE are not equivalent
• Store in tight container in cool environment

SIDE EFFECTS
CNS: *Headache, weakness,* paresthesia
ENDO: Hypoglycemia
GI: Nausea, hepatotoxicity, cholestatic jaundice, vomiting, diarrhea, weight gain
HEMA: Leukopenia, thrombocytopenia, agranulocytosis, aplastic anemia (rare)
INTEG: Rash, pruritus, photosensitivity, erythema
MISC: Angioedema, serious hypersensitivity

PHARMACOKINETICS
Completely absorbed; **Nonmicronized** onset 2 hr; peak 2-4 hr; duration 24 hr; **Micronized:** Onset 1 hr, peak 2-3 hr, duration <24 hr metabolized in liver; excreted in urine, feces (metabolites); crosses placenta; 99% plasma-protein bound

INTERACTIONS
Increase: masking symptoms of hypoglycemia—β-blockers; monitor blood glucose
Increase: level—digoxin
Increase: hypoglycemic effects—insulin, MAOIs, oral anticoagulants, chloramphenicol, NSAIDs, salicylates, probenecid, androgens, fluconazole, gemfibrozil, histamine H_2 antagonists, magnesium salts, phenylbutazone, sulfinpyrazone, sulfonamides, tricyclics, urinary acidifiers, β-blockers, clarithromycin, voriconazole; monitor blood glucose, use cautiously

---

Increase: triglyceride levels—colesevelam

Increase: action of—cycloSPORINE

Increase: hyperglycemia—alcohol

Decrease: both products' effects—diazoxide

Decrease: glyBURIDE action—thiazide diuretics, rifAMPin, carBAMazepine, glucagon, corticosteroids, monitor blood glucose

Drug/Herb

Increase: antidiabetic effect—garlic, horse chestnut

Decrease: hypoglycemic effect—green tea

Drug/Lab Test

Increase: AST, ALT, LDH, BUN, creatinine, alkaline phosphatase, cholesterol, ALP

Decrease: Hb, sodium, glucose, platelets, WBC

NURSING CONSIDERATIONS
Assess:

• Hypo/hyperglycemic reaction that can occur soon after meals; for severe hypoglycemia, give IV $D_{50}W$, then IV dextrose sol

• Blood glucose, A1c levels during treatment

• For allergy to sulfonamides, potential for cross-reactivity

• For renal, hepatic dysfunction: use dose reductions, or avoidance of use may be required; increased risk of hypoglycemia in hepatic failure

• **Blood dyscrasias:** CBC at baseline, throughout treatment; report decreased blood counts

• **Beers:** avoid in older adults; risk of severe prolonged hypoglycemia

• **Pregnancy/breastfeeding:** identify if pregnancy is planned or suspected; breastfed infant may be hypoglycemic; insulin should be used in pregnancy

Evaluate:

• **Therapeutic response:** decrease in polyuria, polydipsia, polyphagia; clear sensorium; absence of dizziness; stable gait; improved serum glucose, A1c

Teach patient/family:

• To check for symptoms of cholestatic jaundice: dark urine, pruritus, jaundiced sclera; if these occur, notify prescriber

• To use a blood glucose meter for testing while taking this product

• About the symptoms of hypo/hyperglycemia, what to do about each

• That product must be continued on a daily basis; about consequences of discontinuing product abruptly; that in times of stress, infection, surgery, trauma, a higher dose may be needed, also may require administration of insulin during these times

• To take product with breakfast or first meal of the day to prevent hypoglycemic reactions at night if taking once a day; if taking twice a day, not to take after last meal of the day

• To avoid OTC medications unless ordered by prescriber

• To report bleeding, bruising, weight gain, edema, shortness of breath, weakness, sore throat

• That diabetes is a lifelong illness; that product will not cure disease

• That all food included in diet plan must be eaten to prevent hypoglycemia; to have glucagon emergency kit, sugar packets always available

• To use sunscreen or stay out of the sun, wear protective clothing (photosensitivity)

• To carry an emergency ID with prescriber and medication information

• To notify prescribers of use prior to surgery

• To not drive or operate machinery until response is known, dizziness may occur

• That continuing follow-up exams and lab work will be needed

TREATMENT OF OVERDOSE:
Use one of the following: glucose 25 g IV via dextrose 50% sol, 1 mg glucagon, oral carbohydrate depending on severity

---

glycerin (OTC)
(glis´er-in)

Fleet Liquid Glycerin Supp,
Pedia-Lax

Func. class.: Laxative

USES: Constipation

DOSAGE AND ROUTES
Adult/child ≥6: RECT supp 1 daily as needed or as directed; enema 5-15 mL as needed

---

Child 2-6: **RECT supp** 1 daily; enema: 2 mL as needed

Available forms: Supp 1, 2 g; enema 5.4 g; enema (pediatric) 4 mL/applicator

---

golimumab (Rx)

(goal-lim′yu-mab)

Simponi, Simponi Aria ♣

Func. class.: Antirheumatic agent (disease modifying), immunomodulator

Chem. class.: Anti–tumor necrosis factor modifier

ACTION: Monoclonal antibody specific for human tumor necrosis factor (TNF); elevated levels of TNF are found in patients with rheumatoid arthritis

USES: Rheumatoid arthritis (RA), ankylosing spondylitis, psoriatic arthritis, ulcerative colitis

CONTRAINDICATIONS

Hypersensitivity, active infections

Precautions: Pregnancy, breastfeeding, children, geriatric patients, CNS demyelinating disease, Guillain-Barré syndrome, HF, hepatitis B carriers, blood dyscrasias, surgery, MS, neurologic disease, diabetes, immunosuppression

> **Black Box Warning:** TB; fungal, bacterial, viral infections, new primary malignancy

DOSAGE AND ROUTES
Rheumatoid arthritis

• **Adult: SUBCUT** 50 mg monthly; give with methotrexate; **IV (Simponi Aria only)** 2 mg/kg over 30 min, repeat 4 wk later, then q8wk give with methotrexate

Ulcerative colitis:

• **Adult: SUBCUT** 200 mg for 1 dose, then 100 mg in 2 wk, maintenance 100 mg q4wk starting at wk 6

Psoriatic arthritis

Adult: SUBCUT (Simponi) 50 mg qmo; IV (Simponia Aria) 2 mg/kg, then 4 wk after, then 2 mg/kg q8wk

Child ≥2 yr: IV (Simponia Aria) 80 mg/m², then 4 wk later, then 80 mg/m² q8wk

Available forms: Inj (SUBCUT) 50 mg/0.5 mL, 100 mg/mL prefilled syringe, SmartJect Auto Injector; inj (IV) 50-mg/4-mL single-use vial

Administer:
SUBCUT route

• Refrigerate, do not freeze; allow to warm to room temperature before using

• Visually inspect sol for particulate or discoloration; sol should be clear to slightly opalescent and colorless to slightly yellow; there may be tiny white particles; do not shake; rotate injection sites

• Use multiple injection sites for multiple injections

• Rotate injection sites, discard unused portions

SmartJect Autoinjector

• Allow the single-use prefilled autoinjector to reach room temperature for at least 30 min

• Immediately prior to use, remove cap. Inject within 5 min of cap removal. Do not put the cap back on

• Do not rub the injection site

• If the viewing window is not yellow, call 800-526-7736; do not give a second dose without talking with the prescribing health care provider

Prefilled syringe

• Allow the single-use prefilled syringe to reach room temperature for at least 30 min prior to use

• Immediately before use, remove the needle cover by pulling it straight off; do not twist off or recap. Inject within 5 min of needle cover removal

• Do not rub the injection site

• Properly dispose of the used prefilled syringe

IV route
(Simponi Aria)

• Calculate number of vials needed; do not shake; dilute total volume of product in NS to yield 100 mL for infusion; slowly add product, mix gently

• Infuse over 30 min, use infusion set with in-line, low–protein-binding filter (0.22 mm pore size)

• May store diluted solution for 4 hr

SIDE EFFECTS

CNS: Dizziness, paresthesia, CNS demyelinating disorder, weakness, Guillian-Barre syndrome, MS

CV: Hypertension, HF

GI: Hepatitis

HEMA: Agranulocytosis, aplastic anemia, leukopenia, polycythemia, thrombocytopenia, pancytopenia

INTEG: Psoriasis

MISC: Increased cancer risk; antibody development to this drug; risk for infection (TB, invasive fungal infections, other opportunistic infections), may be fatal; inj-site reactions, *anaphylaxis*

PHARMACOKINETICS

Half-life 2 wk, SUBCUT peak 2-7 days, IV peak 12 wk

INTERACTIONS

• Do not give concurrently with live vaccines or within 3 mo; immunizations should be brought up to date before treatment

• Dosage change may be needed: warfarin, cycloSPORINE, theophylline

Increase: infection—abatacept, etanercept, rilonacept, riTUXimab, adalimumab, anakinra, immunosuppressants, inFLIXimab; avoid concurrent use

Drug/Lab Test

Increase: LFTs

Decrease: platelets, WBC, neutrophils

Positive: ANA titer

NURSING CONSIDERATIONS

Assess:

• **Pain,** stiffness, ROM, swelling of joints during treatment

• Inj-site pain, swelling; usually occur after 2 inj (4-5 days)

Black Box Warning: **TB:** obtain TB skin test before starting treatment; treat latent TB before starting therapy; continue to monitor for TB even if TB test is negative

• **Blood dyscrasias:** CBC, differential before and periodically during treatment

Black Box Warning: **Infection:** fever, flulike symptoms, dyspnea, change in urination, redness/swelling around any wounds; stop treatment if present; some serious infections including sepsis may occur, may be fatal; patients with active infections should not be started on this product; obtain a chest x-ray, fungal serology, TB testing before starting treatment

• **HBV infection:** test for HBV before starting treatment; HBV can be fatal in HBV carriers; monitor LFTs; hepatitis B serology, may reactivate HBV

• **HF:** B/P, pulse, edema, SOB, may occur or worsen with treatment

• **Psoriasis:** may occur or worsen

Black Box Warning: **Neoplastic disease:** may occur in those <18 yr; avoid use in those with known malignancies; monitor for secondary malignancies during treatment

• **Anaphylaxis:** rash, dyspnea, wheezing, emergency equipment should be nearby, if present, discontinue product immediately

• **Pregnancy/breastfeeding:** use only if benefits outweigh fetal risk; do not breastfeed, excretion unknown

Evaluate:

• **Therapeutic response:** decreased inflammation, pain in joints, decreased joint destruction

Teach patient/family:

• About self-administration if appropriate: inj should be made in thigh, abdomen, upper arm; rotate sites at least 1 inch from old site; do not inject in areas that are bruised, red, hard

• That, if medication not taken when due, to inject next dose as soon as remembered and then the following dose as scheduled

• Not to receive any live virus vaccines during treatment

• To check skin often and report any growths

Black Box Warning: To report signs, symptoms of infection, allergic reaction, or lupuslike syndrome

• To notify prescriber if pregnancy is planned or suspected; not to breastfeed

G

goserelin (Rx)

(goe´se-rel-lin)

Zoladex

Func. class.: Gonadotropin-releasing hormone, antineoplastic (hormone)

Chem. class.: Synthetic decapeptide analog of LHRH

USES: Advanced and locally confined prostate cancer stage B2-C (10.8 mg), endometriosis, advanced breast cancer, endometrial thinning (3.6 mg)

DOSAGE AND ROUTES
Breast cancer
• **Adult: SUBCUT** 3.6 mg q28days or 10.8 mg q12wk into anterior abdominal wall below the navel

Endometrial thinning
• **Adult: SUBCUT** 3.6 mg 1-2 depots, 4 wk apart into anterior abdominal wall below the navel

Endometriosis
Adult: SUBCUT 3.6 mg q28days into anterior abdominal wall below the navel, max 6 mo

Advanced prostate cancer
Adult: SUBCUT 3.6 mg q28days or 10.8 mg q12wk into anterior abdominal wall below the navel

B2-C prostate cancer
Adult: SUBCUT 3.6 mg into anterior abdominal wall below navel 8 wk before radiotherapy, then after 28 days 10.8 mg or 3.6 mg 2 doses before and 2 doses q28days after radiotherapy

Available forms: Depot inj 3.6, 10.8 mg

granisetron (Rx)

(grane-iss´e-tron)

Sancuso, Sustol

Func. class.: Antiemetic

Chem. class.: 5-HT$_3$ receptor antagonist

ACTION: Prevents nausea, vomiting by blocking serotonin peripherally, centrally, and in the small intestine

USES: Prevention of nausea, vomiting associated with cancer chemotherapy, including high-dose CISplatin, radiation

Unlabeled uses: Acute nausea, vomiting after surgery

CONTRAINDICATIONS
Hypersensitivity to this product, benzyl alcohol

Precautions: Pregnancy, breastfeeding, children, geriatric patients, ondansetron/palonosetron/dolasetron hypersensitivity, cardiac dysrhythmias, cardiac/hepatic/GI disease, electrolyte imbalances

DOSAGE AND ROUTES
Prevention of nausea, vomiting in chemotherapy
• **Adult/child ≥2 yr: IV** 10 mcg/kg over 30 sec or over 5 min diluted and infused, 30 min before the start of cancer chemotherapy; **TD** apply 1 patch (3.1 mg/24 hr) to upper outer arm 24-48 hr before chemotherapy, patch may be worn up to 7 days
• **Adult: PO** 1 mg bid, give 1st dose 1 hr before chemotherapy and next dose 12 hr after 1st or 2 mg as a single dose anytime within 1 hr before chemotherapy

Nausea, vomiting in radiation therapy
• **Adult: PO** 2 mg/day 1 hr before radiation

Renal Dose
• **Adult: Subcut CCr 30-59 mL/min use only every 14 days**

Available forms: Inj 0.1 mg/mL; solution for injection, extended release 10 mg/0.4 mL; tab 1 mg; patch TD 3.1 mg/24 hr

Administer:
• Chemotherapy/radiation: given on day of chemotherapy or radiation

PO route
• Give dose 1 hr before chemotherapy/radiation and another 12 hr after 1st dose

Transdermal
• Apply to clean, dry skin on upper arm q24-48hr before chemotherapy or radiation

---

- Do not cut in pieces
- Apply immediately after opening pouch

SUBCUT route
- **Preparation:** Extended-release injection is for **SUBCUT** use only
- Remove the extended-release kit from the refrigerator at least 60 min prior to use; all contents should warm to room temperature
- Once at room temperature, activate one of the syringe warming pouches. Wrap the syringe in the warming pouch for 5-6 min
- Do not use if particulate matter or discoloration is observed, the tip cap is missing or has been tampered with, or the Luer fitting is missing or dislodged. The injection is a sterile, clear, colorless to slightly yellow, viscous liquid

Administer: Complete administration instructions with illustrations are in the kit
- A topical anesthetic may be used at the injection site prior to administration. Do not inject anywhere the skin is burned, hardened, inflamed, swollen, or otherwise compromised
- Using aseptic technique, give as a single slow SUBCUT injection in the back of the upper arm or the skin of the abdomen (at least 1 inch away from the umbilicus) over up to 20-30 sec; due to viscosity, pressing the plunger harder will not expel the solution faster

Direct IV route
- May give undiluted over 30 sec via Y-site

Intermittent IV INFUSION route
- Dilute in 0.9% NaCl for inj or D_5W (20-50 mL); give over 5-15 min 30 min before chemotherapy
- Store at room temperature for 24 hr after dilution; do not freeze vials
- Do not admix

Solution compatibilities: D_5W, 0.9% NaCl

Y-site compatibilities: Acetaminophen, alemtuzumab, alfentanil, allopurinol, amifostine, amikacin, aminophylline, amphotericin B cholesteryl, ampicillin, ampicillin/sulbactam, amsacrine, aztreonam, bleomycin, bumetanide, buprenorphine, butorphanol, calcium gluconate, CARBOplatin, carmustine, ceFAZolin, cefepime, cefonicid, cefotaxime, cefoTEtan, cefOXitin, cefTAZidime, ceftizoxime, cefTRIAXone, cefuroxime, chlorproMAZINE, cimetidine, ciprofloxacin, CISplatin, cladribine, clindamycin, cyclophosphamide, cytarabine, dacarbazine, DACTINomycin, DAUNOrubicin, dexamethasone, diphenhydrAMINE, DOBUTamine, DOPamine, DOXOrubicin, DOXOrubicin liposome, doxycycline, droperidol, enalaprilat, etoposide, famotidine, filgrastim, fluconazole, fluorouracil, floxuridine, fludarabine, furosemide, gallium, ganciclovir, gentamicin, haloperidol, heparin hydrocortisone, HYDROmorphone, hydrOXYzine, IDArubicin, ifosfamide, imipenem-cilastatin, leucovorin, LORazepam, magnesium sulfate, melphalan, meperidine, mesna, methotrexate, methylPREDNISolone, metoclopramide, metroNIDAZOLE, mezlocillin, miconazole, minocycline, mitoMYcin, mitoXANtrone, morphine, nalbuphine, netilmicin, ofloxacin, PACLitaxel, piperacillin, piperacillin/tazobactam, plicamycin, potassium chloride, prochlorperazine, promethazine, propofol, ranitidine, sargramostim, sodium bicarbonate, streptozocin, teniposide, thiotepa, ticarcillin, ticarcillin/clavulanate, tobramycin, trimethoprim-sulfamethoxazole, vancomycin, vinBLAStine, vinCRIStine, vinorelbine, voriconazole, zidovudine, zoledronic acid

Transdermal route
- Apply to dry, clean intact skin of upper outer arm 24-48 hr before chemotherapy, firmly press on skin, keep on during chemotherapy; can bathe, avoid swimming, whirlpool; remove ≥24 hr after chemotherapy completion; do not cut patch

SIDE EFFECTS
CNS: *Headache, asthenia,* anxiety, dizziness, stimulation, insomnia, drowsiness
CV: Hypertension, QT prolongation
GI: Diarrhea, *constipation,* increased AST, ALT, *nausea*
MISC: Rash, serotonin syndrome

Side effects: *italics* = common; red = life-threatening

PHARMACOKINETICS

Metabolized in liver to an active metabolite, half-life 10-12 hr, protein binding 65%, distributed to erythrocytes excreted by the kidney

PO: Peak 60 min, duration 24 hr, IV: Peak 30 min, duration up to 24 hr
TD: Peak 24 hr

INTERACTIONS

Increase: QT prolongation—amoxapine, arsenic, β-blockers, chloroquine, class IA, III antidysrhythmics, cloZAPine, dasatinib, dolasetron, dronedarone, droperidol, erythromycin, flecainide, fluconazole, halogenated/local anesthetics, haloperidol, lapatinib, maprotiline, methadone, octreotide, ondansetron, palonosetron, pentamidine, phenothiazines, pimozide, posaconazole, propafenone, ranolazine, risperiDONE, sertindole, SUNItinib, tacrolimus, telithromycin, tricyclics, troleandomycin, vardenafil, voriconazole, vorinostat, ziprasidone

Increase: EPS—anytipsychotics

Increase: Serotonin syndrome—SSRIs, tricyclics, MAOIs, lithium, buspirone, fentanyl

NURSING CONSIDERATIONS

Assess:
• For absence of nausea, vomiting during chemotherapy
• **Hypersensitivity reaction:** rash, bronchospasm
• **Extrapyramidal symptoms:** grimacing, shuffling gait, tremors, involuntary movements, rare
• **QT prolongation:** monitor ECG in those with heart disease or renal disease or in the elderly
• **Serotonin syndrome:** hallucinations, seizures, diaphoresis, dizziness, flushing, hyperthermia, nausea, vomiting, diarrhea, discontinue
• **Pregnancy/breastfeeding:** use only if benefits outweigh fetal risk
Evaluate:
• **Therapeutic response:** absence of nausea, vomiting during cancer chemotherapy

Teach patient/family:
• To report diarrhea, constipation, rash, changes in respirations
• That headache requiring an analgesic is common
• To take second dose of PO 12 hr after first dose
• That allergic reactions can occur up to 7 days after use (ext rel), or later (SUBCUT)
• **Serotonin syndrome:** to report mental changes, including agitation, hallucinations, dizziness, sweating, flushing, tremors, seizures; discontinue immediately and notify prescriber

guaiFENesin (OTC, Rx)

(gwye-fen′e-sin)

Altarussin, Bidex, Buckleys Chest Congestion, Chest Congestion Relief, Diabetic Tussin, Fenesin IR, Geri-Tussin, GoodSense Mucus Relief, Liquibid, Mucinex Fast-Max Chest Congestion MS, Mucinex For Kids, Mucinex Maximum Strength, Mucinex, Mucos, Mucus Relief ER, Mucus Relief Max St, Mucus Relief, Pharbinex, Refenesen 400, Refenesen, Robafen Mucus/Chest Congestion, Robafen, Siltussin, Siltussin SA, Tussin Mucus & Chest Conges, Tussin, Xpect

Func. class.: Expectorant

Do not confuse:
guaiFENesin/guanfacine
Mucinex/Mucomyst

ACTION: Increases the volume and reduces the viscosity of secretions in the trachea and bronchi to facilitate secretion removal

USES: Productive and nonproductive cough

CONTRAINDICATIONS

Hypersensitivity; chronic, persistent cough

Precautions: Pregnancy, breastfeeding, HF, asthma, emphysema, fever

DOSAGE AND ROUTES
• **Adult and adolescent: PO** 200-400 mg q4hr; **EXT REL** 600-1200 mg q12hr, max 2.4 g/day
• **Child 6-11 yr: PO** 100-200 mg q4hr; **EXT REL** 600 mg q12hr, max 1.2 g/day
• **Child 2-5 yr: PO** 50-100 mg q4hr; max 600 mg/day; ext rel 300 mg q12hr, max 600 mg/day
Available forms: Tabs 100, 200, 400 mg; oral sol 100 mg/5 mL; ext rel tabs 600, 1200 mg; syrup 100 mg/5 mL; oral granules 50, 100 mg/packet, caps 200 mg; liquid 100, 200 mg/5 mL
Administer:
Do not break, crush, chew ext rel tabs
• Store at room temperature

SIDE EFFECTS
CNS: Drowsiness, headache, dizziness
GI: Nausea, anorexia, vomiting, diarrhea

PHARMACOKINETICS
Half-life 1 hr, excreted in urine (metabolites)

NURSING CONSIDERATIONS
Assess:
• **Cough:** type, frequency, character, including sputum; fluids should be increased to 2 L/day
• Increased fluids, room humidification to liquefy secretions
• **Pregnancy/breastfeeding:** use only if benefits outweigh fetal risk
Evaluate:
• **Therapeutic response:** productive cough, thinner secretions
Teach patient/family:
• To avoid driving, other hazardous activities if drowsiness occurs (rare)
• To avoid smoking, smoke-filled room, perfumes, dust, environmental pollutants, cleansers
• To consult health care provider if cough lasts >7 days
• To avoid if breastfeeding

• To avoid use in a child <2 yr
• To use as prescribed, not to double or skip doses
• Not to drive or operate machinery until response is known; drowsiness, dizziness may occur
• To notify health care professional of change in heartbeat or if feeling faint
TD: Not to use near heat such as heating pad or expose to sunlight, tanning, not to cut patch, or use in MRI

guanfacine (Rx)
(gwahn´fa-seen)
Intuniv
Func. class.: Alpha$_2$-adrenergic agonist/antihypertensive

USES: Attention-deficit/hyperactivity disorder (extended release only), hypertension (immediate release only)

DOSAGE AND ROUTES
Hypertension (alternative agent)
Adult: PO IR: Initial: 0.5 to 1 mg daily at bedtime; may increase as needed after 3 to 4 wk up to 3 mg daily at bedtime
ADHD
Child ≥6 yr and adolescents ≤45 kg:
PO: Initial: 0.5 mg daily at bedtime; may titrate q3-4days in 0.5-mg/day increments to 0.5 mg bid, then 0.5 mg tid, then 0.5 mg qid; max daily dose: Patient weight 27 to 40.4 kg: 2 mg/day; 40.5 to 45 kg: 3 mg/day; **>45 kg:** Initial: 1 mg daily at bedtime; may titrate q3-4days in 1-mg/day increments to 1 mg bid, then 1 mg tid, then 1 mg qid max daily dose: 4 mg/day
Children and adolescents 6 to 17 yr:
Extended-release product (Intuniv):
PO: Initial: 1 mg daily at the same time of day (in the morning or evening); may titrate by no more than 1 mg/wk based upon response; max 7 mg/day for age 13-17, max 4 mg/day for age 6-12
Available forms: Tabs 1, 2 mg; tabs, ext rel 1, 2, 3, 4 mg

guselkumab (Rx)
(gus-elk′-ue-mab)

Tremfya

Func. class.: Antirheumatic agent (disease modifying), immunomodulator, anti-TNF

Chem. class.: Recombinant human IgG1 monoclonal antibody, DMARD

USES: For the treatment of moderate to severe plaque psoriasis in those who are candidates for phototherapy or systemic therapy, psoriatic arthritis

DOSAGE AND ROUTES
• **Adult:** SUBCUT 100 mg at week 0, week 4, and every 8 wk thereafter

Available forms: Prefilled syringe 100 mg/mL

halcinonide topical
See Appendix B

haloperidol (Rx)
(hal-oh-pehr'ih-dol)
Haldol Decanoate, Haldol
Func. class.: Antipsychotic, neuroleptic
Chem. class.: Butyrophenone

ACTION: Blocks neurotransmission produced by DOPamine at synapse; exhibits strong α-adrenergic, anticholinergic blocking action; mechanism for antipsychotic effects unclear

USES: Tourette's syndrome, prolonged parenteral therapy in chronic schizophrenia, emergency sedation of severely agitated or delirious patients, ADHD, oppositional defiant disorder
Unlabeled uses: Autistic disorder, delirium, mania, hiccups, chemotherapy-induced nausea/vomiting

CONTRAINDICATIONS
Hypersensitivity, coma, Parkinson's disease
Precautions: Pregnancy, breastfeeding, geriatric patients, seizure disorders, hypertension, pulmonary/cardiac/hepatic disease, QT prolongation, torsades de pointes, prostatic hypertrophy, hyperthyroidism, thyrotoxicosis, children, blood dyscrasias, brain damage, bone marrow depression, alcohol and barbiturate withdrawal states, angina, epilepsy, urinary retention, closed-angle glaucoma, CNS depression

Black Box Warning: Increased mortality in elderly patients with dementia-related psychosis

DOSAGE AND ROUTES
Schizophrenia
• **Adult:** PO 0.5-2 mg bid-tid depending on severity
Severe symptoms: 3-5 mg orally 2-3 times a day; **haloperidol lactate IM** 2-5 mg

q4-8hr, max 20 mg/day; **Haloperidol decanoate IM** Max initial dose 100 mg; if greater than 100 mg is needed, the dose should be given in 2 separate injections (100 mg followed by the balance in 3-7 days). **Maintenance** 10-15 times the previous daily PO dose, given IM monthly, titrate to response; max 450 mg/mo
Tourette syndrome
Adult: PO 0.5-5 mg bid or as needed, max 100 mg/day
Child 3-12 yr and 15-40 kg: PO 0.05-0.075 mg/kg/day divided max 15 mg/day
Available forms: Tabs 0.5, 1, 2, 5, 10, 20 mg; **lactate:** oral sol 2 mg/mL; inj 5 mg/mL, **decanoate:** 50 mg/mL, 100 mg/mL
Administer:
• Reduced dose to geriatric patients
• Antiparkinsonian agent if EPS occurs
• Avoid use with CNS depressants
PO route
• Store in tight, light-resistant container
• **Oral liquid:** use calibrated device; do not mix in coffee or tea
• PO with food or milk
• Avoid skin contact with oral suspension or solution—may cause contact dermatitis
IM route (long acting)
• IM inj into large muscle mass, use 21-G, 2-in needle, use Z track method; give no more than 3 mL/inj site; patient should remain recumbent for 30 min, protect from light

SIDE EFFECTS
CNS: *EPS: pseudoparkinsonism, akathisia, dystonia, tardive dyskinesia; drowsiness, headache,* seizures, neuroleptic malignant syndrome, confusion
CV: *Orthostatic hypotension,* ECG changes, tachycardia, QT prolongation, torsades de pointes
EENT: Blurred vision, glaucoma, dry eyes
GI: *Dry mouth, nausea, vomiting, anorexia, constipation,* weight gain, ileus, hepatitis
HEMA: Agranulocytosis, anemia, neutropenia, leukopenia
GU: Urinary retention, urinary frequency, impotence
INTEG: *Rash,* photosensitivity, dermatitis
RESP: Respiratory depression
SYST: Risk for death (dementia)

Side effects: *italics* = common; red = life-threatening

PHARMACOKINETICS

Metabolized by liver; excreted in urine, bile; crosses placenta; enters breast milk; protein binding 92%; half-life 12-36 hr (metabolites)

PO: Onset erratic, peak 2-6 hr, half-life 14-37 hr

IM (Lactate): Onset 15-30 min, peak 15-20 min, half-life 21 hr

IM (Decanoate): Peak 4-11 days, half-life 3 wk

> **Black Box Warning:** Increase: respiratory depression, death opioids

INTERACTIONS

Increase: serotonin syndrome, neuroleptic malignant syndrome—SSRIs, SNRIs

Increase: QT prolongation—class IA, III antidysrhythmics, tricyclics, amoxapine, maprotiline, phenothiazines, pimozide, risperiDONE, sertindole, ziprasidone, β-blockers, chloroquine, cloZAPine, dasatinib, dolasetron, droperidol, dronedarone, flecainide, halogenated/local anesthetics, lapatinib, methadone, erythromycin, telithromycin, troleandomycin, octreotide, ondansetron, palonosetron, pentamidine, propafenone, ranolazine, SUNItinib, tacrolimus, vardenafil, vorinostat, usually with IV use

> **Black Box Warning: Increase:** oversedation—opioids, other CNS depressants, alcohol, barbiturate anesthetics

Increase: toxicity—EPINEPHrine, lithium
Increase: anticholinergic effects—anticholinergics
Drug/Lab Test
Increase: LFTs

NURSING CONSIDERATIONS
Assess:

• **Mental status:** Monitor mood, behavior, orientation, affect, LOC, sleep patterns, presence of delusions, hallucinations; baseline, periodically

• Monitor prolactin, CBC, urinalysis, ophthalmic exam before and during prolonged therapy

> **Black Box Warning:** Assess for dementia, affect, orientation, LOC, reflexes, gait, coordination, sleep pattern disturbances, risk for death in dementia-related psychosis

• **CV:** B/P standing, lying; take pulse, respirations during initial treatment; establish baseline before starting treatment; report drops of 20 mm Hg

• Dizziness, faintness, palpitations, tachycardia on rising

• **Fall risk assessment:** Assess for fall potential baseline and during treatment; supervised ambulation until patient stabilized on medication; do not involve patient in strenuous exercise program, fainting is possible; patient should not stand still for long periods

• **Extrapyramidal symptoms,** including akathisia (inability to sit still, no pattern to movements), tardive dyskinesia (bizarre movements of jaw, mouth, tongue, extremities), pseudoparkinsonism (rigidity, tremors, pill rolling, shuffling gait) after long-term use

• **Neuroleptic malignant syndrome/ serotonin syndrome:** hyperthermia, muscle rigidity, altered mental status, increased CPK, seizures, hypo/hypertension, tachycardia; notify prescriber immediately

• Constipation, urinary retention daily; if these occur, increase bulk, water in diet

• **Abrupt discontinuation:** do not withdraw abruptly, taper

• **QT prolongation:** more common with IV use at high doses; monitor ECG in those with CV disease

• **Esophageal aspiration risk:** assess for aspiration risk in pneumonia, dementia

> **Black Box Warning Beers: avoid use in older adults** except for schizophrenia, bipolar disorder; increased risk of stroke and cognitive decline, mortality

• **Pregnancy/breastfeeding:** no well-controlled studies; use in 3rd trimester results in infant extrapyramidal symptoms; avoid breastfeeding
Evaluate:

• **Therapeutic response:** decrease in emotional excitement, hallucinations, delusions, paranoia; reorganization of patterns of thought, speech; improvement in specific behaviors

Teach patient/family:
• That orthostatic hypotension occurs often; to rise from sitting or lying position gradually; to remain lying down after IM inj for at least 30 min
• To avoid hazardous activities until stabilized on medication and effects are known
• To avoid abrupt withdrawal of this product because EPS may result; to withdraw slowly
• To avoid OTC preparations (cough, hay fever, cold) unless approved by prescriber; serious product interactions may occur; to avoid use with alcohol, as increased drowsiness may occur
• About EPS and the necessity of meticulous oral hygiene because oral candidiasis may occur

Black Box Warning: Opioids: Discuss with patient, family, caregivers to report immediately, dizziness, severe drowsiness, slowed breathing, to obtain emergency services

• To report impaired vision, jaundice, tremors, muscle twitching
• To use sunscreen, protective clothing to minimize photosensitivity, avoid overheating
• To take as prescribed; not to use OTC, herbal products or alcohol unless directed by prescriber
• To use good oral hygiene, frequent sips of water, sugarless gum, candy for dry mouth

TREATMENT OF OVERDOSE: Lavage if recently ingested orally; provide an airway; do not induce vomiting; provide supportive care

⚠ HIGH ALERT

heparin (Rx)
(hep′a-rin)
Hepalean ✤, Heparin Leo ✤, Heparin Sodium Injection, Hep-Lock, Hep-Lock U/P, Monoject Prefill ✤
Func. class.: Anticoagulant, antithrombotic

Do not confuse:
heparin/Hespan

ACTION: Prevents conversion of fibrinogen to fibrin and prothrombin to thrombin by enhancing inhibitory effects of antithrombin III

USES: Prevention treatment of deep venous thrombosis, PE, MI, open heart surgery, disseminated intravascular clotting syndrome, atrial fibrillation with embolization, as an anticoagulant in transfusion and dialysis procedures, to maintain patency of indwelling venipuncture devices; diagnosis, treatment of DIC

CONTRAINDICATIONS
Bleeding, hypersensitivity to this product, corn, porcine protein (pork product)
Precautions: Pregnancy, children, geriatric patients, alcoholism, hyperlipidemia, diabetes, renal disease, heparin-induced thrombocytopenia (HIT), hemophilia, leukemia with bleeding, peptic ulcer disease, severe thrombocytopenic purpura, severe renal/hepatic disease, blood dyscrasias, severe hypertension, subacute bacterial endocarditis, acute nephritis; benzyl alcohol products in neonates/infants/pregnancy/lactation

DOSAGE AND ROUTES
Anticoagulation
• Adult: IV BOLUS (intermittent) 10,000 units, then 5000-10,000 q4-6hr CONTINUOUS IV INFUSION 5000 units, then 20,000-40,000 give over 24 hr; SUBCUT 5000 units, then 10,000-20,000 units, then 8000-10,000 q8hr
• Child >1 yr: IV bolus (intermittent) 50-100 units/kg q4hr; continuous IV infusion 75 units/kg then 20 units/kg/hr, adjust to aPTT by 65-85 sec
• Neonates, infants <1 yr: Continuous IV infusion 75 units/kg, then 28 units/kg/hr, adjust to aPTT 65-85 sec
Thromboembolism prevention
• Adult: SUBCUT 5000 units q8-12hr
CV surgery
• Adult: IV ≥150 units/kg (300 units) for procedure <60 min, 400 units/kg for procedure ≥60 min

Side effects: *italics* = common; red = life-threatening

Line flush
• **Adult/child:** **IV** 10-100 units/mL (10 units: infants) to fill heparin lock
TPN
• **Adult/child IV** 0.5-1 units/mL
Available forms: Sol for inj 10, 100, 1000, 2000, 5000, 7500, 10,000, 20,000 units/mL; premixed 1000 units/500 mL, 2000 units/1000 mL, 12,500 units/250 mL, 25,000 units/250 mL, 25,000 units/500 mL; lock flush preparations 10 units/mL
Administer:
• Cannot be used interchangeably (unit for unit) with LMWHs or heparinoids
• At same time each day to maintain steady blood levels; always check dose with another nurse before use or a change in dose
• Store at room temperature
Heparin lock route
• Do not mistake heparin sodium inj 10,000 units/mL and Hep-Lock U/P 10 units/mL; they have similar blue labeling; deaths in pediatric patients have occurred when heparin sodium inj vials were confused with heparin flush vials
• Inject to prevent clots in heparin lock; inject dilute heparin solution 10-100 units/0.5-1 mL after each injection or q8hr flush lock before and after each use with sterile water or 0.9% NaCl
SUBCUT route
• Give deeply with 25-G ⅜-½-in needle; do not massage area or aspirate when giving SUBCUT inj; give in abdomen between pelvic bones, inject at 45- or 90-degree angle, rotate sites; do not pull back on plunger; apply gentle pressure for 1 min
• Do not give IM
• Avoid all IM inj that may cause bleeding, hematoma
Direct IV route
• Give loading dose undiluted, over ≥1 min; use before continuous infusion
Continuous IV INFUSION route
• Obtain baseline coagulation tests before use

• Use infusion pump; make sure pressure dressings are used after drawing blood
• Draw coagulation studies 30 min before next dose; never draw from tubing or from infused vein; use other arm
• Dilute 25,000 units/250-500 mL 0.9 NaCl or D₅W; 50-100 units/mL solutions are premixed and ready for use
• When product is added to infusion sol for cont IV, invert container at least 6 times to ensure adequate mixing

Y-site compatibilities: Acetaminophen, acetylcysteine, acyclovir, alcohol 10%, dextrose 5%, alemtuzumab, alfentanil, allopurinol, amifostine, aminocaproic acid, aminophylline, amphotericin B lipid complex, amphotericin B liposome, anidulafungin, argatroban, arsenic trioxide, ascorbic acid injection, asparaginase, atenolol, atropine, azaTHIOprine, azithromycin, aztreonam, benztropine, betamethasone, bivalirudin, bleomycin, bretylium, bumetanide, buprenorphine, butorphanol, caffeine, calcium chloride/gluconate, cangrelor, CARBOplatin, carmustine, cefamandole, ceFAZolin, cefotaxime, cefoTEtan, cefotiam, cefOXitin, ceftaroline, cefTAZidime, ceftizoxime, ceftobiprole, cefTRIAXone, cefuroxime, chloramphenicol succinate, chlordiazePOXIDE, chlorothiazide, chlorpheniramine, cimetidine, CISplatin, cladribine, clindamycin, cloxacillin, codeine, colistimethate, cyanocobalamin, cyclophosphamide, cycloSPORINE, cytarabine, DACTINomycin, DAPTOmycin, DAUNOrubicin citrate liposome, dexamethasone, dexmedetomidine, dexrazoxane, digoxin, DOCEtaxel, DOPamine, doripenem, doxacurium, doxapram, DOXOrubicin liposomal, edetate calcium disodium, edrophonium, enalaprilat, ePHEDrine sulfate, EPINEPHrine, epoetin alfa, eptifibatide, ergonovine, ertapenem, esmolol, estrogens conjugated, ethacrynate, etoposide, etoposide phosphate, famotidine, fenoldopam, fentaNYL, flecainide, fluconazole, fludarabine, fluorouracil, folic acid (as sodium salt), foscarnet, gallamine, gallium, ganciclovir, gemcitabine, gemtuzumab, glycopyrrolate, granisetron, hydrocortisone,

HYDROmorphone, ibuprofen lysine, ifosfamide, imipenem-cilastatin, indomethacin, irinotecan, isoproterenol, ketorolac, lactated Ringer's injection, lansoprazole, leucovorin, lidocaine, lincomycin, linezolid, LORazepam, magnesium sulfate, mannitol, mechlorethamine, melphalan, mephentermine, meropenem, mesna, metaraminol, methadone, methohexital, methotrexate, methoxamine, methyldopa, methylergonovine, metoclopramide, metoprolol, metroNIDAZOLE, micafungin, midazolam, milrinone, minocycline, mitoMYcin, mivacurium, morphine, moxifloxacin, multiple vitamins injection, nafcillin, nalbuphine, nalorphine, naloxone, neostigmine, nitroglycerin, nitroprusside, norepinephrine, octreotide, ondansetron, oxacillin, oxaliplatin, oxytocin, PACLitaxel (solvent/surfactant), palonosetron, pamidronate, pancuronium, PEMEtrexed, penicillin G potassium, sodium, PENTobarbital, PHENobarbital, phentolamine, phenylephrine, phytonadione, piperacillin sodium, piperacillin-tazobactam, potassium acetate/chloride, procainamide, prochlorperazine, promazine, propofol, propranolol, pyridostigmine, pyridoxine, raNITIdine, remifentanil, Ringer's injection, riTUXimab, rocuronium, sargramostim, scopolamine, sodium acetate, bicarbonate/fusidate, succinylcholine, SUFentanil, tacrolimus, theophylline, thiamine, thiopental, thiotepa, ticarcillin, ticarcillin-clavulanate, tigecycline, tirofiban, tolazoline, topotecan, TPN (2-in-1), tranexamic acid, trastuzumab, trimetaphan, trimethobenzamide, tubocurarine, urokinase, vasopressin, vecuronium, verapamil, vinBLAStine, vinCRIStine, voriconazole, warfarin, zidovudine, zoledronic acid

SIDE EFFECTS

CNS: *Fever,* chills, headache
GU: Hematuria
HEMA: Hemorrhage, *thrombocytopenia,* anemia, heparin-induced thrombocytopenia (HIT)
INTEG: *Rash,* dermatitis, urticaria, pruritus, alopecia, hematoma, cutaneous necrosis (SUBCUT), inj-site reactions

META: Hyperkalemia, hypoaldosteronism, rebound hyperlipidemia, vitamin D deficiency
GI: Elevated LFTs
MS: Osteoporosis (child)
SYST: Anaphylaxis

PHARMACOKINETICS

Half-life 1-2 hr (dose dependent); excreted in urine; 95% bound to plasma proteins; does not cross placenta or alter breast milk; removed from the system via the lymph and spleen; partially metabolized in kidney, liver; excreted in urine (<50% unchanged)
SUBCUT: Onset 20-60 min, peak 2-4 hr duration 8-12 hr, well absorbed >35,000 IU/24 hr
IV: Peak 5 min, duration 2-6 hr

INTERACTIONS

Increase: heparin action—oral anticoagulants, salicylates, dextran, NSAIDs, platelet inhibitors, cephalosporins, penicillins, ticlopidine, dipyridamole, antineoplastics, clopidogrel, SSRIs, SNRIs, quinidine, valproic acid
Decrease: heparin action—digoxin, tetracyclines, antihistamines, cardiac glycosides, nicotine, nitroglycerin
Drug/Herb
Increase: bleeding risk—arnica, anise, chamomile, clove, dong quai, garlic, ginger, ginkgo, feverfew, green tea, horse chestnut
Drug/Lab Test
Increase: ALT, AST, INR, PT, PTT, potassium
Decrease: platelets

NURSING CONSIDERATIONS
Assess:
• **Bleeding, hemorrhage:** gums, petechiae, ecchymosis, black tarry stools, hematuria, epistaxis, decrease in Hct, B/P; HIT may occur after product discontinuation; check periodically for sign of decreasing clots
• Blood studies (Hct, occult blood in stools) q3mo
• **Thrombosis:** monitor for increased thrombosis daily, in affected areas
• Partial prothrombin time, which should be 1.5-2.5× control; for continuous IV infusion, check aPTT baseline 6 hr after initiation

and 6 hr after any dose change; use aPTT for dosing adjustments; after therapeutic aPTT has been measured 2×, check aPTT daily

• **Heparin-induced thrombocytopenia (HIT):** platelet count q2-3days; thrombocytopenia may occur on 4th day of treatment and resolves even during continued treatment; HIT may occur on the 5th-10th day of treatment, with platelets to 5000 mm³; this may lead to HITT (venous/arterial thrombosis) even after discontinued therapy

• **Hypersensitivity:** rash, chills, fever, itching; report to prescriber

Evaluate:

• **Therapeutic response:** prevention of DVT and pulmonary emboli; adequate anticoagulation based on aPTT, PTT 1.5-2.5× control

Teach patient/family:

• To avoid OTC preparations that may cause serious product interactions unless directed by prescriber; to notify all health care providers of heparin use

• That product may be held during active bleeding (menstruation), depending on condition

• About subcut injection technique if self-administered; to rotate sites, not to inject into irritated or broken skin

• To use soft-bristle toothbrush to avoid bleeding gums; to avoid contact sports; to use an electric razor; to avoid IM inj

• To carry emergency ID identifying product taken

• **Bleeding:** to report to prescriber any signs of bleeding: gums, under skin, urine, stools

• To report to prescriber any signs of hypersensitivity: rash, chills, fever, itching

TREATMENT OF OVERDOSE:

Withdraw product; administer 1 mg protamine/100 units heparin

---

hepatitis B immune globulin (HBIG) (Rx)

HepaGam B, HyperHEP B S/D, Nabi-HB

Func. class.: Immune globulin

USES: Prevention of hepatitis B virus in exposed patients, including passive immunity in neonates born to HBsAg-positive mother, prevention of hepatitis B recurrence after liver transplant in HBsAg-positive patients

DOSAGE AND ROUTES
Hepatitis B exposure in high-risk patients

• **Adult/child:** IM 0.06 mL/kg (usual 3-5 mL) within 7 days of exposure; repeat 28 days after exposure if patient wishes to not receive hepatitis B vaccine

Neonates born to hepatitis B surface-antigen–positive persons

• **Neonate:** IM 0.5 mL within 12 hr of birth

Prevention of hepatitis B infection recurrence after liver transplant

• **Adult:** IV (HepaGam B only) 20,000 international units concurrent with grafting transplanted liver, then 20,000 international units/day on days 1-7, then 20,000 international units q2wk starting on day 14, then 20,000 international units/mo starting with month 4

Available forms: Injection: 1-, 5-mL vials; 0.5-mL neonatal single-dose syringe; 1-mL single-dose syringe

---

homatropine ophthalmic

See Appendix B

---

hydrALAZINE (Rx)

(hye-dral′a-zeen)

Apresoline ✦

Func. class.: Antihypertensive, direct-acting peripheral vasodilator

Chem. class.: Phthalazine

Do not confuse:

hydrALAZINE/hydrOXYzine

ACTION: Vasodilates arteriolar smooth muscle by direct relaxation; reduction in

---

blood pressure with reflex increases in heart rate, stroke volume, cardiac output

USES: Essential hypertension; hypertensive emergency/urgency
Unlabeled uses: HF

CONTRAINDICATIONS
Hypersensitivity to hydrALAZINEs, mitral valvular rheumatic heart disease, CAD
Precautions: Pregnancy, breastfeeding, geriatric patients, CVA, advanced renal disease, hepatic disease, SLE, dissecting aortic aneurysm

DOSAGE AND ROUTES
Hypertension
• **Adult:** PO 10 mg qid 2-4 days, then 25 mg for rest of 1st wk, then 50 mg qid, max 300 mg/day
• **Child ≥1 yr (unlabeled):** PO 0.75-1 mg/kg/day in 2-4 divided doses, max 25 mg/dose, increase over 3-4 wk to max 7.5 mg/kg/day or 200 mg, whichever is less
Hypertensive crisis
• **Adult: IV BOL** 10-20 mg q4-6hr, administer **PO** as soon as possible; **IM** 10-50 mg q4-6hr
• **Child: IM/IV BOL** 0.1-0.2 mg/kg/dose q4hr may increase the dose slowly up to 0.6 mg/kg/dose (Max: 20 mg/dose)
Preeclampsia/eclampsia
Adult female IV 5-10 mg over 2 min
HF (unlabeled)
• **Adult:** PO 10-25 mg tid, max 100 mg tid
Available forms: Inj 20 mg/mL; tabs 10, 25, 50, 100 mg
Administer:
PO route
• Give with meals (PO) to enhance absorption
IM route
• Do not admix, switch to PO as soon as possible, use only in those that cannot use PO
• No dilution needed, inject deeply in large muscle, aspirate
Direct IV route
• IV undiluted; give through Y-tube or 3-way stopcock, give each 10 mg over ≥1 min
• To recumbent patient, keep recumbent for 1 hr after administration

Y-site compatibilities: Alemtuzumab, anidulafungin, argatroban, atenolol, bivalirudin, bleomycin, DACTINomycin, DAPTOmycin, dexrazoxone, diltiazem, DOCEtaxel, etoposide, fludarabine, gatifloxacin, gemcitabine, granisetron, HYDROmorphone, IDArubicin, irinotecan, leucovorin, linezolid, mechlorethamine, metroNIDAZOLE, milrinone, mitoXANtrone, octreotide, oxaliplatin, PACLitaxel, palonosetron, pancuronium, potassium chloride, tacrolimus, teniposide, thiotepa, tirofiban, vecuronium, vinorelbine, vitamin B/C, voriconazole

SIDE EFFECTS
CNS: *Headache, dizziness,* drowsiness, peripheral neuritis
CV: *Palpitations, tachycardia, angina,* orthostatic hypotension, shock
GI: *Nausea, vomiting, anorexia, diarrhea,* hepatotoxicity
EENT: Nasal congestion
RESP: Dyspnea
HEMA: Agranulocytosis
GU: Urinary retention
INTEG: Rash, pruritus, flushing
MISC: *Lupuslike symptoms,* muscle cramps

PHARMACOKINETICS
Half-life 3-7 hr, metabolized by liver, 12%-14% excreted in urine, protein binding 89%; half of Mexicans, blacks, South Indians, and Caucasians are at risk for toxicity
PO: Onset 20-30 min, peak 1-2 hr, duration 2-4 hr
IM: Onset 10-30 min, peak 1 hr, duration 2-6 hr
IV: Onset 5-30 min, peak 10-80 min, duration up to 12 hr

INTERACTIONS
Increase: Severe hypotension risk—MAOIs
Increase: Tachycardia, angina—sympathomimetics (EPINEPHrine, norepinephrine)
Increase: Hypotension—other antihypertensives, alcohol, thiazide diuretics
Increase: Effects of β-blockers (metoprolol, propranolol)

Side effects: *italics* = common; red = life-threatening

Decrease: HydrALAZINE effects—NSAIDs, estrogens

Drug/Lab Test

Decrease: HB, WBC, RBC, platelets, neutrophils

Positive: ANA titer

Drug/Food

Increase: drug absorption; have patient take with food

NURSING CONSIDERATIONS

Assess:

• **Cardiac status:** B/P q15min × 2 hr, then q1hr × 2 hr, then q4hr after IV dose; pulse, jugular venous distention q4hr, after IV administration

• **Electrolytes, blood studies:** potassium; sodium; chloride; carbon dioxide; CBC; serum glucose; LE prep; ANA titer before, during treatment; assess for fever, joint pain, rash, sore throat (lupuslike symptoms); notify prescriber

• Number of refills to determine compliance (PO)

• Weight daily; I&O; edema in feet, legs daily; skin turgor; dryness of mucous membranes for hydration status

• **For renal disease:** dosage and administration are altered in reduced CCr, dialysis

• Crackles, dyspnea, orthopnea

• IV site for extravasation, rate

• **Mental status:** affect, mood, behavior, anxiety; check for personality changes

• **Beers:** use with caution in older adults; may exacerbate syncope in those with a history of syncope

• **Pregnancy/breastfeeding:** use only if benefits outweigh fetal risk; 3rd-trimester toxicity has occurred; use caution in breastfeeding

Evaluate:

• **Therapeutic response:** decreased B/P

Teach patient/family:

• To take with food to increase bioavailability (PO)

• To avoid OTC, herbals, supplements unless directed by prescriber

• To notify prescriber if chest pain, severe fatigue, fever, muscle or joint pain, rash, sore throat; tingling, pain in hands, feet, pyridoxine can be used

• To rise slowly to prevent orthostatic hypotension

• That follow-up will be needed; to comply with other requirements, such as exercise, weight loss, avoidance of smoking

• To notify providers of product use prior to surgery

• To avoid driving or other hazardous activities until response is known; drowsiness, dizziness may occur

• To weigh 2× per wk and check lower extremities for swelling

• To take as prescribed, not to skip or double doses, to take at the same time of the day, if dose is missed, take when remembered, do not discontinue abruptly

• To notify prescriber if pregnancy is suspected or planned or if breastfeeding

TREATMENT OF OVERDOSE:

Administer vasopressors, volume expanders for shock; if PO, lavage if recently ingested, digitalization

---

hydrochlorothiazide (Rx)

(hye-droe-klor-oh-thye′a-zide)

Func. class.: Thiazide diuretic, antihypertensive

Chem. class.: Sulfonamide derivative

ACTION: Acts on distal tubule and ascending limb of loop of Henle by increasing excretion of water, sodium, chloride, potassium

USES: Edema, hypertension, diuresis, HF; idiopathic lower extremity edema therapy

Unlabeled uses: Diabetes insipidus, hypercalciuria, nephrolithiasis, premenstrual syndrome, renal calculus

---

CONTRAINDICATIONS

Hypersensitivity to thiazides or sulfonamides, preeclampsia, anuria, renal decompensation

Precautions: Pregnancy, breastfeeding, hypokalemia, renal/hepatic disease, gout, COPD, LE, diabetes mellitus, hyperlipidemia, CCr <30 mL/min, hypomagnesemia

DOSAGE AND ROUTES
Hypertension

Adult/adolescent: PO 12.5-25 mg/day, may increase to 50 mg/day in 1-2 divided doses, max 100 mg/day

Child 6 mo-12 yr: PO 1-2 mg/kg/day in 1 or 2 divided doses, may increase to max 37.5 mg/day (child 6 mo-2 yr) 100 mg/day (child 2-12 yr)

Child <6 mo: PO 1-3 mg/kg/day in 1 or 2 divided doses, max 37.5 mg/day

Edema

Adult: PO 25-100 mg in 1-2 divided doses
Renal dose:
• **Adult: PO** CCr <30 mL/min, do not use; not effective

Available forms: Tabs 12.5, 25, 50, 100 ✤ mg; caps 12.5 mg
Administer:
PO route

• In AM to avoid interference with sleep if using product as a diuretic; tab may be crushed, mixed with food
• Potassium replacement if potassium <3 mg/dL, replace magnesium if needed
• With food; if nausea occurs, absorption may be decreased slightly

SIDE EFFECTS

CNS: Drowsiness, paresthesia, depression, headache, *dizziness, fatigue, weakness,* fever

CV: Irregular pulse, *orthostatic hypotension,* palpitations, volume depletion, allergic myocarditis

EENT: Blurred vision

ELECT: *Hypokalemia,* hypercalcemia, hyponatremia, hypochloremia, hypomagnesemia

GI: *Nausea, vomiting, anorexia,* constipation, diarrhea, cramps, pancreatitis, GI irritation, hepatitis, jaundice

GU: *Urinary frequency,* polyuria, uremia, glucosuria, hyperuricemia, renal failure, erectile dysfunction

HEMA: Aplastic anemia, hemolytic anemia, leukopenia, agranulocytosis, thrombocytopenia, neutropenia

INTEG: *Rash,* urticaria, purpura, photosensitivity, alopecia, erythema multiforme

META: *Hyperglycemia, hyperuricemia,* increased creatinine, BUN

SYST: Stevens-Johnson syndrome

PHARMACOKINETICS

PO: Onset 2-6 hr, peak 1-5 hr, duration 6-12 hr, half-life 6-15 hr, excreted unchanged by kidneys, crosses placenta, enters breast milk

INTERACTIONS

Increase: hyperglycemia, hyperuricemia, hypotension risk—diazoxide

Increase: hypokalemia risk—corticosteroids, amphotericin B, topiramate

Increase: toxicity—lithium, nondepolarizing skeletal muscle relaxants, cardiac glycosides

Increase: hypersensitivity reaction risk: with allopurinol, monitor level

Decrease: thiazide effect—NSAIDs, monitor renal function

Increase: effects—loop diuretics

Decrease: effects—antidiabetics, monitor glucose

Decrease: thiazides absorption—cholestyramine, colestipol

Drug/Herb

Increase: severe hypokalemia—licorice

Drug/Lab Test

Increase: parathyroid test, uric acid, calcium, glucose, cholesterol, triglycerides

Decrease: potassium, sodium, HB, WBC, platelets

NURSING CONSIDERATIONS
Assess:

• B/P, pulse; weight, I&O, electrolytes baseline and periodically to determine fluid loss; effect of product may be decreased if used daily

• **Hypersensitivity to sulfonamides:** if skin rash occurs, discontinue product; fatal Stevens-Johnson syndrome may occur

---

Side effects: *italics* = common; red = life-threatening

• **Hypertension:** B/P lying, standing; postural hypotension may occur
• **Blood studies:** BUN, blood glucose, CBC, serum creatinine, uric acid
• **Signs of hypokalemia:** postural hypotension, malaise, fatigue, tachycardia, leg cramps, weakness, dehydration; monitor potassium
• **Signs of metabolic alkalosis,** restlessness, drowsiness
• Confusion, especially in geriatric patients; take safety precautions if needed
• **Beers:** use with caution in older adults; may exacerbate or cause syndrome of inappropriate antidiuretic hormone secretion or hyponatremia
• **Pregnancy, breastfeeding:** may affect fetus, crosses placental barrier, if using for hypertension before pregnancy continue; do not breastfeed

Evaluate:
• **Therapeutic response:** improvement in edema of feet, legs, sacral area daily; decreased B/P

Teach patient/family:
• To rise slowly from lying or sitting position to prevent postural hypotension
• To notify prescriber of muscle weakness, cramps, nausea, dizziness; hypokalemia is common; rash
• That product may be taken with food or milk
• To use sunscreen for photosensitivity
• That blood glucose may be increased in diabetics
• To take early in day at same time of day to avoid nocturia
• To avoid alcohol, OTC meds unless approved by prescriber
• To monitor weight and notify prescriber of changes
• To discuss dietary potassium requirements
• That follow-ups and routine lab tests will be required
• How to take B/P, to continue with other medical regimens (weight loss, exercise), that effect in hypertension may take several weeks

TREATMENT OF OVERDOSE: Lavage if recently ingested orally; monitor electrolytes; administer dextrose in saline; monitor hydration, CV, renal status; provide supportive care

---

⚠ HIGH ALERT

HYDROcodone (Rx)
REMS
(hye-droe-koe′done)
Hysingla ER, Zohydro ER
HYDROcodone/ acetaminophen (Rx)
Lorcet, Lortab, Norco
Func. class.: Antitussive opioid analgesic/nonopioid analgesic
Controlled Substance Schedule II

Do not confuse:
HYDROcodone/hydrocortisone/ oxycodone/HYDROmorphone

ACTION: Binds to opiate receptors in CNS to reduce pain

USES: Moderate to severe pain

CONTRAINDICATIONS
Abrupt discontinuation; hypersensitivity to this product, benzyl; GI obstruction; status asthmaticus

Black Box Warning: Respiratory depression

Precautions: Pregnancy, breastfeeding, neonates, addictive personality, increased intracranial pressure, MI (acute), severe heart disease, renal/ hepatic disease, bowel impaction, urinary retention, viral infection, ulcerative colitis, seizures, sulfite hypersensitivity, psychosis, hypertension, hyperthyroidism

---

Black Box Warning: Accidental exposure; neonatal opioid withdrawal syndrome; potential for overdose or poisoning, substance abuse, ethanol ingestion, benzodiazepines

DOSAGE AND ROUTES
Analgesic
• **Adult: PO** 2.5-10 mg q3-6hr as needed; if using with acetaminophen max 4 g/day, total of 5 tablets with ibuprofen combination tablets; **ext rel (Zohydro ER)** 10 mg q12hr, may increase by 10 mg q12hr q3-7days as needed; **ext rel (Hysingla)** 20 mg daily, may increase by 10-20 mg q3-5day
• **Child 1-3 yr: PO** 0.1-0.2 mg/kg q3-4hr
Antitussive
• **Adult: PO** 5 mg q4-6hr as needed
• **Child: PO** 0.6 mg/kg/day divided q6-8hr, max <2 yr, 1.25 mg/dose; 2-12 yr, 5 mg/dose; >12 yr, 10 mg/dose
Renal dose
• **Adult: PO** CCr <45 mL/min-Hysingla decrease dose by 50% initially
Hepatic dose
• **Adult: PO** Hysingla decrease by 50% initially

Available forms: *HYDROcodone:* Extended release (Zohydro ER) 10, 15, 20, 30, 40, 50 mg; **(Hysingla ER)** 20, 30, 40, 60, 80, 100, 120 mg; syrup: 1 mg/mL *HYDROcodone/acetaminophen:* Tablet 2.5 mg HYDROcodone/325 acetaminophen; 5 mg HYDROcodone/325 acetaminophen; 7.5 mg HYDROcodone/325 acetaminophen; 15 mg HYDROcodone/325 acetaminophen; 10 mg HYDROcodone/325 acetaminophen; **oral solution** 7.5 mg HYDROcodone/325 acetaminophen/15 mL, 10 mg HYDROcodone/325 acetaminophen/15 mL
Administer:
• Check product carefully before using; fatalities have occurred using wrong dose, wrong product, given only by those knowledgable in use of opioids
• Do not break, crush, or chew tabs; only scored tabs can be broken
• With antiemetic after meals if nausea or vomiting occurs

Black Box Warning: Do not exceed 4 g acetaminophen with combination product

• Give with food or milk to prevent gastric upset
• Store in light-resistant area at room temperature
Extended-release route
• May need short- or rapid-acting opioid for breakthrough pain
• Swallow caps whole, do not crush or chew

SIDE EFFECTS
CNS: *Drowsiness,* dizziness, lightheadedness, confusion, headache, sedation, euphoria, dysphoria, weakness, hallucinations, mood changes, dependence, seizures
CV: Tachycardia, bradycardia, QT prolongation (Hysingla)
EENT: Blurred vision, miosis, diplopia
GI: *Nausea, vomiting, anorexia, constipation,* esophageal obstruction, choking
GU: Urinary retention
INTEG: Rash, sweating, flushing, pruritus
META: Dehydration
RESP: Respiratory depression, cough, respiratory arrest (child), pulmonary edema

PHARMACOKINETICS
HYDROcodone: Onset unknown, peak 6-30 hr (Hysingla ER), 5 hr (Zohydro ER), duration unknown, half-life 7-9 hr
HYDROcodone/acetaminophen: Onset 10 min, peak 1-1.6 hr (HYDROcodone), 0.5-1 hr (acetaminophen); duration 4-8 hr, half-life 3.3-4.4 hr, metabolized in liver, excreted in urine, crosses placenta

INTERACTIONS
Black Box Warning: **Increase:** anticholinergic effects—anticholinergics

Black Box Warning: **Increase:** CNS depression—alcohol, opioids, sedative/hypnotics, phenothiazines, skeletal muscle relaxants, general anesthetics, tricyclics

Side effects: *italics* = common; red = life-threatening

Black Box Warning: Increase HYDRO-codone effect—CYP3A4 inhibitors

Increase: Serotonin syndrome—SNRIs, SSRIs, TCAs, traZODone, vilazodone, monitor for serotonin syndrome
Increase: Severe reactions—MAOIs, separate by ≥14 days

Black Box Warning: Decrease: HYDRO-codone effect—CYP3A4 inducers

Drug/Herb
Increase: CNS depression—lavender, valerian, chamomile, kava
Decrease: HYDROcodone effect—St. John's wort
Drug/Lab Test
Increase: cholesterol, GGT
Decrease: potassium

NURSING CONSIDERATIONS
Assess:
• **Pain:** intensity, type, location, other characteristics before, 1 hr after giving product; titrate upward by 25% until pain reduced by half; need for pain medication, physical dependence; opioid is more effective before pain is severe
• **CNS changes:** dizziness, drowsiness, hallucinations, euphoria, LOC, pupil reaction

Black Box Warning: Respiratory depression: do not use in those with respiratory depression; monitor for decreased respiratory rate, reduced urge to breathe, sighing breathing pattern; CO_2 retention, respiratory depression may worsen, sedation; an opioid antagonist may be needed

• **Hypersensitivity:** Assess for reactions in those with hypersensitivity to other opiates

Black Box Warning: Accidental exposure: may cause fatal overdose; do not use with ethanol; check all medications for alcohol content

• **Opioid addiction:** identify opioid addiction or use before starting product; if

product has been used by snorting, fatal reactions have occurred
• B/P, pulse, respirations before, periodically; if respirations <10/min, dose may need to be reduced, oversedation may occur
• May decrease sex hormone levels after long-term use
• **Bowel status:** constipation; provide fluids, fiber in diet; may need stimulant laxatives if opioid use exceeds 3 days

Black Box Warning: Neonatal opioid withdrawal syndrome: monitor neonate for withdrawal (irritability, hyperactivity, abnormal sleep patterns, high-pitched crying, tremor, vomiting, diarrhea)

• **Allergic reactions:** rash, urticaria; stop product
• Cough and respiratory dysfunction: respiratory depression, character, rate, rhythm
• **Beers:** avoid in older adults unless safer alternative is unavailable; may cause ataxia, impaired psychomotor function

Black Box Warning: Pregnancy/breast-feeding: use only if benefits outweigh fetal risk; neonatal withdrawal syndrome may occur if used for prolonged periods in pregnancy; do not use in breastfeeding, excretion in breast milk

Evaluate:
• **Therapeutic response:** decrease in pain or cough
Teach patient/family:
• To report any symptoms of CNS changes, allergic reactions
• That physical dependency may result when used for extended periods
• That withdrawal symptoms may occur: nausea, vomiting, cramps, fever, faintness, anorexia
• To avoid driving, other hazardous activities because drowsiness occurs
• To avoid other CNS depressants; they will enhance sedating properties of this product
• To change positions slowly to reduce orthostatic hypotension

- To take as directed, not to double doses or exceed doses, not to discontinue abruptly, taper, there is a high abuse potential
- To notify provider if pain is not adequately controlled
- For dry mouth, use sugarless gum, frequent sips of water, use food, good oral hygiene
- To notify prescriber of relief of pain

Black Box Warning: Not to exceed 4000 mg in combination product with acetaminophen; check all other products that may contain acetaminophen

Black Box Warning: Ethanol ingestion: that a patient's use with ethanol can lead to serious overdose or death; not to use with other medications containing ethanol unless directed by prescriber

Black Box Warning: Neonatal opioid withdrawal syndrome: that this syndrome can be fatal; that it results from prolonged maternal use of long-acting opioids

- To notify prescriber if pregnancy is planned or suspected

TREATMENT OF OVERDOSE: Naloxone HCl (Narcan) 0.2-0.8 mg IV, O_2, IV fluids, vasopressors

hydrocortisone (Rx)
(hy-dro-kor'tih-sone)
Alkindi Sprinkle, Cortef, Cortenema
hydrocortisone acetate (topical/rectal) (Rx)
Anusol HC, Cortaid, Corticaine, Cortifoam
hydrocortisone sodium succinate (Rx)
Solu-Cortef
Func. class.: Corticosteroid
Chem. class.: Short-acting glucocorticoid

Do not confuse:
hydrocortisone/HYDROcodone/hydroxychlorothiazide
Solu-Cortef/Solu-Medrol

ACTION: Decreases inflammation by suppression of migration of polymorphonuclear leukocytes, fibroblasts, reversal of increased capillary permeability, and lysosomal stabilization

USES: Severe inflammation, adrenal insufficiency, ulcerative colitis, collagen disorders, asthma, COPD, SLE, Stevens-Johnson syndrome, ulcerative colitis, TB
Unlabeled uses: Carpal tunnel syndrome, Churg-Strauss syndrome, endophthalmitis, mixed connective-tissue disease, multiple myeloma, polyarteritis nodosa, polychondritis, pulmonary edema, temporal arteritis, Wegener's granulomatosis, septic shock

CONTRAINDICATIONS
Fungal infection, hypersensitivity
Precautions: Pregnancy, breastfeeding, children <2 yr, diabetes mellitus, glaucoma, osteoporosis, seizure disorders, ulcerative colitis, HF, myasthenia gravis, renal disease, esophagitis, peptic ulcer, metastatic carcinoma, psychosis, idiopathic thrombocytopenia (IM), acute glomerulonephritis, amebiasis, nonasthmatic bronchial disease, AIDS, TB, recent MI (associated with left ventricular rupture), Cushing syndrome, hepatic disease, hypothyroidism, coagulopathy, thromboembolism

DOSAGE AND ROUTES
Most disorders
- **Adult: PO** 20-240 mg daily in divided doses; **IM/IV** 100-500 mg (succinate), may repeat q2-6hr
- **Child: PO** 2-8 mg/kg/day (60-240 mg/ m^2/day as a single or divided dose; **IM/IV** 0.666-4 mg/kg (20-120 mg/m^2) q12-24hr
Adrenocortical insufficiency
- **Child: PO** 0.56 mg/kg/day (15-20 mg/m^2/day) as a single dose or divided

dose; **IM/IV** 0.186-0.28 mg/kg/day (10-12 mg/m²/day) in 3 divided doses

Shock prevention

• **Adult: IM/IV** (succinate) 50 mg/kg repeated after 4 hr; repeat q24hr as needed

Colitis

• **Adult: PO** 20-240 mg (base)/day in 2-4 divided doses; **ENEMA** 100 mg nightly for 21 days; **FOAM** 1 applicatorful 1-2×/day × 2-3 wk

• **Child: PO** 2-8 mg (base)/kg/day or 60-240 mg (base)/m²/day in 3-4 divided doses

Available forms: Hydrocortisone: enema: 100 mg/60 mL; tabs 5, 10, 20 mg; oral granules in capsule for opening; **Acetate: rectal suppository:** 25, 30 mg; tabs 5, 10, 20 mg; **Succinate:** injection 100-, 250-, 500-, 1000-mg vial

Administer:

Daily dose in AM for better results

• In one dose in AM to prevent adrenal suppression; avoid SUBCUT administration, may damage tissue

• Do not use acetate or susp for IV; salts are not interchangeable

PO route

• With food or milk for GI symptoms

IM route

• IM inj deep in large muscle mass; rotate sites; avoid deltoid; use 21-G needle

IV route

• **Succinate:** IV in mix-o-vial or reconstitute ≤250 mg/2 mL bacteriostatic water for inj (50 mg/mL); mix gently; give direct IV over ≥1 min; may be further diluted in 100, 250, 500, or 1000 mL of D₅W, D₅ 0.9%, NaCl 0.9% given over ordered rate; for doses ≥500 mg give over 10 min

Sodium succinate

Y-site compatibilities: Acyclovir, acetaminophen, alemtuzumab, alfentanil, allopurinol, amifostine, amphotericin B cholesteryl, ampicillin, amrinone, amsacrine, atracurium, atropine, aztreonam, betamethasone, calcium gluconate, cefepime, cefmetazole, cephalothin, chlordiazePOXIDE, chlorproMAZINE, cisatracurium, cladribine, cyanocobalamin, cytarabine, dexamethasone, digoxin, diphenhydrAMINE, DOPamine, DOXOrubicin liposome, droperidol, edrophonium, enalaprilat, EPINEPHrine, esmolol, estrogens conjugated, ethacrynate, famotidine, fentaNYL, fentaNYL/droperidol, filgrastim, fludarabine, fluorouracil, foscarnet, furosemide, gallium, granisetron, heparin, hydrALAZINE, insulin (regular), isoproterenol, kanamycin, lidocaine, LORazepam, magnesium sulfate, melphalan, menadiol, meperidine, methicillin, methoxamine, methylergonovine, minocycline, morphine, neostigmine, norepinephrine, ondansetron, oxacillin, oxytocin, PACLitaxel, pancuronium, penicillin G potassium, pentazocine, phytonadione, piperacillin/tazobactam, prednisoLONE, procainamide, prochlorperazine, propofol, propranolol, pyridostigmine, remifentanil, scopolamine, sodium bicarbonate, succinylcholine, tacrolimus, teniposide, theophylline, thiotepa, trimethaphan, trimethobenzamide, vecuronium, vinorelbine, zoledronic acid

SIDE EFFECTS

CNS: *Depression, flushing, sweating,* psychosis, headache, mood changes, pseudotumor cerebri, euphoria, insomnia, seizures

CV: *Hypertension,* edema

EENT: Increased intraocular pressure, blurred vision, cataracts, glaucoma

GI: *Diarrhea, nausea,* abdominal distention, GI hemorrhage, pancreatitis, vomiting

HEMA: Thrombophlebitis, thromboembolism

INTEG: Acne, poor wound healing, ecchymosis, petechiae

MISC: Adrenal insufficiency (after stress/withdrawal), pheochromocytoma

MS: Fractures, osteoporosis, weakness

PHARMACOKINETICS

Metabolized by liver, excreted in urine (17-OHCS, 17-KS), crosses placenta

PO: Peak 1-2 hr, duration 1-1½ days

IM/IV: Onset 20 min, peak 4-8 hr, duration 1-1½ days

IV: Peak 1-2 hr

RECT: Onset 3-5 hr

INTERACTIONS
Increase: GI bleeding risk—salicylates, NSAIDs, acetaminophen

Increase: side effects—alcohol, amphotericin B, digoxin, cycloSPORINE, diuretics

Increase: neurologic reactions—live virus vaccines/toxoids

Decrease/Increase: anticoagulation—oral anticoagulants

Decrease: hydrocortisone action—bosentan, cholestyramine, colestipol, barbiturates, rifAMPin, phenytoin, theophylline, carBAMazepine

Decrease: anticoagulant effects, anticonvulsants, antidiabetics, calcium supplements, toxoids, vaccines

Drug/Herb
Decrease: hydrocortisone levels—ephedra

Drug/Lab Test
Increase: cholesterol, sodium, blood glucose, uric acid, calcium, glucose

Decrease: calcium, potassium, T_4, T_3, thyroid ^{131}I uptake test, urine 17-OHCS, 17-KS

False negative: skin allergy tests

NURSING CONSIDERATIONS
Assess:
• **Labs:** Potassium, blood glucose, urine glucose while patient receiving long-term therapy; hypokalemia and hyperglycemia; potassium depletion: paresthesias, fatigue, nausea, vomiting, depression, polyuria, dysrhythmias, weakness

• **Vitals:** B/P, pulse; notify prescriber of chest pain

• I&O ratio; be alert for decreasing urinary output, increasing edema; weight daily, notify prescriber of weekly gain >5 lb

• **Cushingoid symptoms:** weight gain, purple striae, bruising skin, weakness, acne, personality changes, hypertension, unusual hair growth

• **Adrenal insufficiency:** nausea, anorexia, hypotension, weight loss, disorientation, fatigue, dizziness, weakness

• Plasma cortisol levels during long-term therapy (normal level: 138-635 nmol/L SI units when drawn at 8 AM)

• **Infection:** increased temperature, WBC even after withdrawal of medication; product masks infection

• **Mental status:** affect, mood, behavioral changes, aggression

• **GI effects:** nausea, vomiting, anorexia or appetite stimulation, diarrhea, constipation, abdominal pain, hiccups, gastritis, pancreatitis, GI bleeding/perforation with long-term treatment

• **Beers:** avoid in older adults with delirium or at high risk for delirium

• **Pregnancy/breastfeeding:** use only if benefits outweigh fetal risk, avoid use in 1st trimester, usually compatible with breastfeeding

Evaluate:
Therapeutic response: decreased inflammation, GI symptoms

Teach patient/family:
• That emergency ID as corticosteroid user should be carried

• To immediately report abdominal pain, black tarry stools because GI bleeding/perforation can occur; if received by epidural route, to report immediately a change in vision, severe headache, seizures, weakness (emergency response needed)

• To notify prescriber if therapeutic response decreases; that dosage adjustment may be needed; about signs of infection

• Not to discontinue abruptly because adrenal crisis can result; that product should be tapered

• That supplemental calcium/vit D may be needed if patient is receiving long-term therapy

• That product can mask infection and cause hypo/hyperglycemia (diabetic)

• To avoid OTC, herbals, supplements: salicylates, alcohol in cough products, cold preparations unless directed by prescriber

• **About adrenal insufficiency:** nausea, anorexia, fatigue, dizziness, dyspnea, weakness, joint pain, moon face

• To avoid live-virus vaccines if using steroids long term

hydrocortisone nasal
See Appendix B

Side effects: *italics* = common; red = life-threatening

hydrocortisone (topical) (OTC)

(hye-droe-kor′ti-sone)

Ala-Cort, Ala-Scalp, Anusol HC, Cetacort, Cortizone-10 Scalpion, Procort, Texacort

hydrocortisone butyrate (Rx)

Locoid, Locoid Lipocream

hydrocortisone probutate (Rx)

Pandel

hydrocortisone valerate (Rx)

Func. class.: Corticosteroid, topical

ACTION: Crosses cell membrane to attach to receptors to decrease inflammation, itching, inhibits multiple inflammatory cytokines

USES: Inflammation/itching in corticosteroid-responsive dermatoses on the skin, rectal area

CONTRAINDICATIONS

Hyper-sensitivity
Precautions: Pregnancy, breastfeeding, children

DOSAGE AND ROUTES
Corticosteroid-responsive dermatoses, inflammation, pruritus
• **Adult/child: TOP** apply to affected area 1 to 4 times per day
Inflammation from proctitis
• **Adult: RECTAL** 1 applicator full of foam once or twice a day × 2-3 wk, then every other day as needed; suppository: 1 bid × 2 wk
Available forms:
Hydrocortisone: cream 0.5%, 1%, 2.5%; gel 1%, 2%; lotion 0.25%, 1%, 2%, 2.5%; ointment 0.5%, 1%, 2.5%; rectal cream 1%; rectal ointment 1%; spray 1%; solution 1%, 2.5%;

Hydrocortisone acetate: cream 0.5%, 1%, 2%, 2.5%; lotion 0.5%; ointment 0.5%, 1%; rectal foam 90 mg/application; suppositories 25 mg, 30 mg; **Hydrocortisone butyrate:** cream 0.1%; ointment 0.1%; lotion; **Hydrocortisone probutate:** cream 0.1%; **Hydrocortisone valerate:** cream 0.2%, ointment 0.2%
Administer:
Topical route
• May be used with dressings
Cream/ointment/lotion
• Apply sparingly in a thin film and rub gently

SIDE EFFECTS
CNS: Seizures, increased intracranial pressure, headache
CV: Hypertension
EENT: Cataracts, glaucoma
INTEG: Burning, folliculitis, pruritus, dermatitis, maceration
MISC: Hyperglycemia, glycosuria, HPA suppression

PHARMACOKINETICS
Unknown, minimally absorbed

NURSING CONSIDERATIONS
Assess:
• Skin reactions: burning, pruritus, folliculitis, dermatitis
Evaluate:
• Decreasing itching, inflammation on the skin, rectal area
Teach patient/family:
Topical route
• That product may be used with dressings
Cream/ointment/lotion
• To apply sparingly in a thin film and rub gently into the affected area
Gel
• To apply sparingly in a thin film and rub gently
Rectal
• To remove wrapper and insert suppository

⚠ HIGH ALERT

HYDROmorphone (Rx)

REMS

(hye-droe-mor'fone)

Dilaudid, Hydromorph Contin, Jurnista ✦

Func. class.: Opiate analgesic

Chem. class.: Semisynthetic phenanthrene

Controlled Substance Schedule II

Do not confuse:

HYDROmorphone/meperidine/morphine
Dilaudid/Demerol

ACTION: Inhibits ascending pain pathways in CNS, increases pain threshold, alters pain perception

USES: Moderate to severe pain

CONTRAINDICATIONS

Hypersensitivity to this product/sulfite, COPD, cor pulmonale, emphysema, GI obstruction, ileus, increased intracranial pressure, obstetric delivery, status asthmaticus

Black Box Warning: Respiratory depression, opioid-naive patients

Precautions: Pregnancy, breastfeeding, children <18 yr, addictive personality, renal/hepatic disease, abrupt discontinuation, adrenal insufficiency, angina, asthma, biliary tract disease, bladder obstruction, hypothyroidism, hypovolemia, hypoxemia, IBD, IV use, lactase/paraben deficiency, labor, latex hypersensitivity, myxedema, seizure disorders, sleep apnea

Black Box Warning: Substance abuse, accidental exposure, potential for overdose/poisoning, neonatal opioid withdrawal syndrome

DOSAGE AND ROUTES
Analgesic

• **Adult: PO** (oral solution) 2.5-10 mg q3-6hr or (tabs) 2-4 mg q4-6hr; **EXT REL:** convert to **EXT REL** by giving total daily dose of immediate release/day, in 1 daily dose, if needed titrate **EXT REL** q3-4days until adequate pain relief; use 25%-50% increase for each titration step, if more than 2 doses of rescue medication needed in 24 hr consider titration; **IV** 0.2-1 mg q2-3hr given over 2-3 min; **IM/SUBCUT** 1-2 mg q4-6hr prn, may be increased (opioid-naive patients may require lower dose); **RECT** 3 mg q6-8hr prn

• **Geriatric: PO** 1-2 mg q4-6hr

• **Child >50 kg (unlabeled): PO** 2-4 mg q3-4hr in opioid-naive patients, titrate; **IV** 0.2-1 mg q2-4hr or 0.3 mg/kg infusion (opioid-naive will require lower dose)

• **Infant >6 mo/child <50 kg (unlabeled): PO** 0.04-0.08 mg/kg q3-4hr in opioid-naive patients, titrate; **IV** 0.015-0.02 mg/kg q2-4hr or 0.006 mg/kg/hr infusion (opioid-naive)

Renal dose

• **Adult: PO (moderate impairment) ext rel** decrease dose by 50%, **severe impairment** decrease dose by 75%

Hepatic disease

• **Adult: Child-Pugh B, or C (oral liquid, immediate rel tab, supp)** give reduced dose based on response, impairment **(parenteral),** give 25%-50% of dose **(moderate impairment)**

Available forms: Powder for inj 250 mg; inj 1, 2, 4, 10 mg/mL; tabs 2, 4, 8 mg; supp 3 mg; oral sol 5 mg/5 mL; ext rel tab 8, 12, 16, 32 mg

Administer:

PO route

• Give with food or milk for GI irritation

• **Ext rel:** discontinue all other ext rel opioids, give q24hr; do not crush, break, chew

• When pain is beginning to return; determine interval by response

• Store in light-resistant area at room temperature

Black Box Warning: Do not use ext rel products in opioid-naive patients or with other ext rel opioids; do not use with other ext rel hydromorphone products; may be fatal

Extended release

• **Converting from oral opioids:** initiate ext rel tabs at 50% of total daily equivalent dose of ext rel, give q24hr; max increase q3-4days, titrate increases of 25%-50% with each step

• **Converting from transdermal patch (fentaNYL):** initiate ext rel tabs 18 hr after removal of patch; for each 25 mcg/hr dose of transdermal fentaNYL dose is 12 mg q24hr, start dose at 50% of HYDROmorphone ext rel dose q24hr; titrate no more often than q3-4days, may increase dose of 25%-50% with each step; if more than 2 rescue doses are required in 24 hr, consider titration

SUBCUT route

• Use short 30-G needle; make sure not to inject IV

• Rotate inj sites

IM route

• Rotate sites

IV route

• **Direct,** diluted with 5 mL sterile water or NS; give through Y-connector or 3-way stopcock; give ≤2 mg over 3-5 min, very slowly

• **IV INFUSION:** Dilute each 0.1-1 mg/mL NS (0.1-1 mg/mL), deliver by opioid syringe infuser; may be diluted in D_5W, D_5/NaCl, 0.45% NaCl, NS for larger amounts, delivery through infusion pump

Y-site compatibilities: Acyclovir, allopurinol, amifostine, amikacin, amsacrine, aztreonam, cefamandole, cefepime, cefoperazone, cefotaxime, cefOXitin, cefTAZidime, ceftizoxime, cefuroxime, chloramphenicol, cisatracurium, CISplatin, cladribine, clindamycin, cyclophosphamide, cytarabine, dilTIAZem, DOBUTamine, DOPamine, DOXOrubicin, DOXOrubicin liposome, doxycycline, EPINEPHrine, erythromycin lactobionate, famotidine, fentaNYL, filgrastim, fludarabine, foscarnet, furosemide, gentamicin, granisetron, heparin, kanamycin, labetalol, LORazepam, magnesium sulfate, melphalan, methotrexate, metroNIDAZOLE, midazolam, milrinone, morphine, nafcillin, niCARdipine, nitroglycerin, norepinephrine, ondansetron, oxacillin, PACLitaxel, penicillin G potassium, piperacillin, piperacillin/tazobactam, propofol, ranitidine, remifentanil, teniposide, thiotepa, ticarcillin, tobramycin, trimethoprim-sulfamethoxazole, vancomycin, vecuronium, vinorelbine

SIDE EFFECTS

CNS: *Drowsiness, dizziness, confusion, headache, sedation, euphoria,* mood changes, seizures

CV: Palpitations, bradycardia, change in B/P, hypotension, tachycardia, peripheral vasodilation

EENT: Tinnitus, blurred vision, miosis, diplopia

GI: *Nausea, vomiting, anorexia, constipation, cramps,* dry mouth, paralytic ileus

GU: Increased urinary output, dysuria, urinary retention

INTEG: *Rash,* urticaria, bruising, flushing, diaphoresis, pruritus

RESP: Respiratory depression, dyspnea

MISC: Physical/psychologic dependence

PHARMACOKINETICS

IM: Onset 15-30 min, peak ½-1 hr, duration 4-5 hr, metabolized by liver, excreted by kidneys, crosses placenta, excreted in breast milk, half-life 2-3 hr

INTERACTIONS

Increase: effects—other CNS depressants (alcohol, opiates, sedative/hypnotics, antipsychotics, skeletal muscle relaxants)

Increase: CNS, respiratory depression—MAOIs, separate by ≥14 days

Decrease: HYDROmorphone effects—opiate antagonists

Drug/Herb

Increase: action—chamomile, hops, kava, lavender, St. John's wort, valerian

Drug/Lab Test

Increase: amylase

NURSING CONSIDERATIONS

Assess:

• **Pain:** control, sedation by scoring on 0-10 scale, around-the-clock dosing is best for pain control

• I&O ratio; check for decreasing output; may indicate urinary retention
• **CNS changes:** dizziness, drowsiness, hallucinations, euphoria, LOC, pupil reaction
• Bowel function, constipation
• **Allergic reactions:** rash, urticaria
• Need for pain medication, physical dependence
• Assistance with ambulation
• **Safety measures:** side rails, nightlight, call bell within easy reach
• **Beers:** avoid in older adults unless safer alternative is unavailable; may cause ataxia, impaired psychomotor function
• **Pregnancy/breastfeeding:** use only if benefits outweigh fetal risk; neonatal withdrawal syndrome may occur if used in pregnancy for prolonged periods; do not breastfeed
Evaluate:
• **Therapeutic response:** decrease in pain
Teach patient/family:
• To report any symptoms of CNS changes, allergic reactions
• That product is contained in a hard tablet shell that may be seen in a bowel movement, which is normal
• Not to stop taking the product without discussing with provider

• To avoid driving, other hazardous activities because drowsiness occurs; to take with food if nausea occurs

• To notify provider if pain is not controlled adequately
• To use sugarless gum, frequent sips of water for dry mouth, use good oral hygiene

TREATMENT OF OVERDOSE: Naloxone (Narcan) 0.2-0.8 mg IV (nontolerant patients), O_2, IV fluids, vasopressors

hydroxychloroquine (Rx)

(hye-drox-ee-klor'oh-kwin)
Apo-Hydroxyquine ✦, Plaquenil
Func. class.: Antimalarial, antirheumatic (DMARDs)
Chem. class.: 4-Aminoquinoline derivative

ACTION: Impairs complement-dependent antigen–antibody reactions

USES: Malaria caused by susceptible strains of *Plasmodium vivax, P. malariae, P. ovale, P. falciparum* (some strains); SLE, rheumatoid arthritis
Unlabeled uses: Lupus nephritis, polymorphous-light eruptions

CONTRAINDICATIONS
Hypersensitivity to this product or chloroquine; retinal field changes
Precautions: Pregnancy, breastfeeding, blood dyscrasias, severe GI disease, neurologic disease, alcoholism, hepatic disease, G6PD deficiency, psoriasis, eczema, children, ocular disease

DOSAGE AND ROUTES
Malaria
• **Adult: PO Suppression or prevention:** 400 mg/wk, begin 2 wk before travel to endemic area, continue 4 wk after returning; **treatment:** 800 mg, then 400 mg after 6-8 hr, then 400 mg/day on 2nd and 3rd day, total dose 2 g
• **Child: PO Suppression or prevention:** 6.4 mg/kg (5 mg/kg base) weekly,

begin 1-2 wk before travel to endemic area, continue 4 wk after returning; **treatment:** 10 mg/kg, 6.4 mg/kg (5 mg/kg base) at 6, 18, 24 hr after 1st dose

Lupus erythematosus

• **Adult: PO** 200-400 mg (310 mg base) daily or divided twice daily; length depends on patient response; maintenance: 200-400 mg/day

• **Child (unlabeled): PO** 5 mg/kg/day, max 400 mg/day; long-term therapy is contraindicated

Rheumatoid arthritis

• **Adult: PO** 400-600 mg daily or divided twice daily for 4-12 wk, then 200-400 mg/day after good response

Available forms: Tabs 200 mg

Administer:

PO route

• Tabs may be crushed and mixed with food, fluids

• With food or milk; at same time each day to maintain product level

• Store in tight, light-resistant container at room temperature; keep inj in cool environment

SIDE EFFECTS

CNS: Headache, fatigue, irritability, seizures, bad dreams, dizziness, confusion, psychosis, anxiety, suicidal ideation

CV: HF, torsades de pointes, QT prolongation, asystole with syncope

EENT: *Blurred vision, corneal changes,* tinnitus, vertigo, nystagmus, corneal deposits

GI: *Nausea, vomiting, anorexia,* diarrhea, cramps

HEMA: Thrombocytopenia, agranulocytosis, leukopenia, aplastic anemia

INTEG: Pruritus, exfoliative dermatitis, alopecia, Stevens-Johnson syndrome, photosensitivity, DRESS, rash, pruritus

PHARMACOKINETICS

Peak 3 hr; half-life 32-50 days; metabolized in liver; excreted in urine, feces, breast milk; crosses placenta, protein binding 45%

INTERACTIONS

Increase: digoxin, methotrexate levels

Increase: antibody titer—rabies vaccine

Decrease: hydroxychloroquine action—magnesium or aluminum compounds

Decrease: effect of—live virus vaccines, botulinum toxoids

NURSING CONSIDERATIONS

Assess:

• **SLE, malaria symptoms:** before treatment and daily

• **Rheumatoid arthritis:** pain, swelling, ROM, temperature of joints; for decreased reflexes: knee, ankle

• Ophthalmic exam at baseline for retinal toxicity then annually after 5 yr of use, or annually in those with increased risk factors

• Hepatic studies weekly: AST, ALT, bilirubin if patient receiving long-term treatment

• **Blood dyscrasias:** blood studies: CBC, platelets; WBC, RBC, platelets may be decreased; if severe, product should be discontinued; assess for malaise, fever, bruising, bleeding (rare)

• **ECG** during therapy: watch for depression of T waves, widening of QRS complex

• **Allergic reactions:** pruritus, rash, urticaria

• **Ototoxicity** (tinnitus, vertigo, change in hearing); audiometric testing should be done before, after treatment

• **Toxicity:** blurring vision, difficulty focusing, headache, dizziness, knee, ankle reflexes; product should be discontinued immediately

• **Pregnancy/breastfeeding:** increased rate of birth defects in the literature; CDC recommends this product for pregnant women with malaria or may be used in those with lupus; cautious use in breastfeeding

Evaluate:

• **Therapeutic response:** decreased symptoms of malaria, SLE, rheumatoid arthritis

Teach patient/family:

• To use sunglasses in bright sunlight to decrease photophobia; to wear protective clothing (photosensitivity)

• That urine may turn rust or brown; that skin may become blue-black

- To report hearing, visual problems, fever, fatigue, bruising, bleeding, which may indicate blood dyscrasias

RA: To report to provider if there is no change in condition, may need several months for results

Malaria prevention

- Discuss how to prevent mosquitoes in the environment
- Not to use with alcohol

TREATMENT OF OVERDOSE: Induce vomiting; gastric lavage; administer barbiturate (ultrashort acting), vasopressor, ammonium chloride; tracheostomy may be necessary

hydroxyprogesterone caproate (Rx)

(hye-droks-ee-proe-jes′te-rone cap′ro-ate)

Makena

Func. class.: Hormone, progesterone

USES: To reduce the risk of preterm birth

CONTRAINDICATIONS

Hypersensitivity to hydroxyprogesterone caproate or any component; current or history of thrombosis or thromboembolic disorders; breast cancer or other hormone-sensitive cancer; undiagnosed abnormal vaginal bleeding unrelated to pregnancy; cholestatic jaundice of pregnancy; liver tumors (benign or malignant) or active liver disease; missed abortion; uncontrolled hypertension; as a diagnostic test for pregnancy

DOSAGE AND ROUTES

Adult female: IM (vial): 250 mg q7days
SUBCUT 275 mg q7days; treatment may begin between 16 wk, 0 days and 20 wk, 6 days of gestation. Continue weekly administration until 37 wk (through 36 wk, 6 days) gestation or until delivery, whichever comes first

⚠ HIGH ALERT

hydroxyurea (Rx)

(hye-drox′ee-yoo-ree-ah)

Droxia, Hydrea, Siklos

Func. class.: Antineoplastic, antimetabolite

Chem. class.: Synthetic urea analog

Do not confuse:
hydroxyurea/hydrOXYzine
Hydrea/Lyrica

ACTION: Acts by inhibiting DNA synthesis without interfering with RNA or protein synthesis; incorporates thymidine into DNA, thereby causing direct damage to DNA strands; specific for S phase of cell cycle

USES: Melanoma, chronic myelogenous leukemia, recurrent or metastatic ovarian cancer, squamous cell carcinoma of the head and neck, sickle cell anemia
Unlabeled uses: Acute myeloid leukemia, essential thrombocythemia, hypereosinophilic syndrome, meningioma, polycythemia vera

CONTRAINDICATIONS

Pregnancy, breastfeeding, hypersensitivity, leukopenia ($<2500/mm^3$), thrombocytopenia ($<100,000/mm^3$), anemia (severe)
Precautions: Renal disease (severe), anemia, bone marrow suppression, dental disease, geriatric patients, HIV, hyperkalemia, hyperphosphatemia, hyperuricemia, hypocalcemia, infection, infertility, IM injection, tumor lysis syndrome, vaccinations

Black Box Warning: Secondary malignancy, bone marrow suppression

DOSAGE AND ROUTES
Ovarian cancer, malignant melanoma
- **Adult: PO** 80 mg/kg as a single dose q3days or 20-30 mg/kg as a single dose daily

Ovarian cancer in combination with radiation
• **Adult: PO** 80 mg/kg as a single dose q3days

Sickle cell anemia
• **Adult: PO** 15 mg/kg/day, may increase by 5 mg/kg/day q12wk, max 35 mg/kg/day

Chronic myelogenous leukemia (CML)/acute myelogenous leukemia (unlabeled)
• **Adult: PO** WBC >100,000/mm³, 50-75 mg/kg/day; WBC <100,000/mm³, 10-30 mg/kg/day; adjust for WBCs
• **Child: PO** 10-20 mg/kg/day, adjust to hematologic response

Renal disease
• **Adult: PO** CCr <59 mL/min use 50% of dose

Available forms: Caps 200, 300, 400, 500 mg

Administer:
• Gloves should be worn when handling bottles or caps, including by caregivers; wash hands immediately and thoroughly
• Do not crush or chew caps; caps can be opened and contents mixed with water
• Antiemetic 30-60 min before product and prn

SIDE EFFECTS

CNS: Headache, confusion, hallucinations, dizziness, seizures
CV: Angina, ischemia
GI: Nausea, vomiting, anorexia, diarrhea, stomatitis, constipation, hepatotoxicity, pancreatitis
GU: Increased BUN, uric acid, creatinine, temporary renal function impairment
HEMA: Leukopenia, anemia, thrombocytopenia, megaloblastic erythropoiesis
INTEG: *Rash,* urticaria, pruritus, dry skin, facial erythema
META: Hyperphosphatemia, hyperuricemia, hypocalcemia
MISC: Fever, chills, malaise, secondary cancers, tumor lysis syndrome
RESP: Pulmonary fibrosis, diffuse pulmonary infiltrates

PHARMACOKINETICS

Readily absorbed; peak 1-4 hr; degraded in liver; excreted in urine; almost totally eliminated within 24 hr; crosses blood-brain barrier; eliminated as CO_2; half-life 3.5-4.5 hr

INTERACTIONS

Increase: pancreatitis/hepatotoxicity—didanosine, stavudine
Increase: toxicity—radiation or other antineoplastics
Increase: bleeding risk—NSAIDs, anticoagulants, thrombolytics, salicylates, platelet inhibitors
Increase: uric acid levels—probenecid, sulfinpyrazone
• Do not use with live virus vaccines
• Do not use hematopoietic progenitor cells (sargramostim, filgrastim) 24 hr before or after antineoplastic

Drug/Lab Test
Increase: BUN, creatinine, LFTs, uric acid
False increase: urea, uric acid, lactic acid
Decrease: HB, WBC, platelets, phosphate, calcium

NURSING CONSIDERATIONS
Assess:

Black Box Warning: Bone marrow suppression: HB, total leukocyte count, and platelet count at least once a week during entire course; if the WBC is ≤2500/mm³ or platelets are ≤100,000/mm³, interrupt Hydrea until values closer to normal; if severe anemia occurs, manage without interrupting Hydrea; for Droxia, monitor blood counts q2wk and interrupt if neutrophils are <2000/mm³, platelets are <80,000/mm³, hemoglobin is <4.5 g/dL, or reticulocytes are <80,000/mm³ when the HB <9 g/dL; after recovery, Droxia may be resumed at lower dosage; Droxia requires an experienced clinician knowledgeable in the use of this medication for the treatment of sickle cell anemia

- **Renal studies:** BUN; serum uric acid; urine CCr; electrolytes before, during therapy
- **Tumor lysis syndrome;** hyperkalemia, hyperphosphatemia, hyperuricemia, hypocalcemia; uric acid nephropathy, acute renal failure, metabolic acidosis can also occur; alkalinization of urine, allopurinol may help prevent this
- I&O ratio; report fall in urine output to <30 mL/hr
- Monitor temperature; fever may indicate beginning infection
- **Hepatic studies** before, during therapy: bilirubin, alk phos, AST, ALT, LDH; prn or monthly; pancreatitis may also occur
- **Cutaneous vasculitic toxicity and gangrene:** more common in those who are receiving interferon
- **Bleeding:** hematuria, guaiac, bruising or petechiae, mucosa or orifices q8hr
- Buccal cavity for dryness, sores or ulceration, white patches, oral pain, bleeding, dysphagia; rinsing of mouth tid-qid with water, club soda; brushing of teeth bid-tid with soft brush or cotton-tipped applicators for stomatitis; use unwaxed dental floss
- **Pulmonary reactions:** assess for pulmonary fibrosis, fever, dyspnea, diffuse pulmonary infiltrates
- **Symptoms indicating severe allergic reaction:** rash, urticaria, itching, flushing
- **Neurotoxicity:** headaches, hallucinations, seizures, dizziness

Black Box Warning: Secondary malignancy: leukemia may occur after extended use

- **Pregnancy/breastfeeding:** do not use in pregnancy/breastfeeding
Evaluate:
- **Therapeutic response:** decreased tumor size, spread of malignancy
Teach patient/family:
- **To report signs of infection:** elevated temperature, sore throat, flulike symptoms
- **To report signs of anemia:** fatigue, headache, faintness, SOB, irritability

- To report bleeding; to avoid use of razors, commercial mouthwash
- To avoid use of aspirin products, ibuprofen (thrombocytopenia)
- To avoid foods with citric acid, hot or rough texture if stomatitis is present
- **To report stomatitis:** any bleeding, white spots, ulcerations in the mouth; to examine mouth daily, report symptoms
- To inform provider if planning to receive vaccinations
- To wear gloves, wash hands before and after handling capsules
- To notify prescriber if pregnancy is planned or suspected
- To notify prescriber of fever, chills, sore throat, nausea, vomiting, anorexia, diarrhea, bleeding, bruising; may indicate blood dyscrasias; mental status changes, pancreatitis, hepatotoxicity

hydrOXYzine (Rx)
(hye-drox'i-zeen)
Atarax ✦, Vistaril
Func. class.: Antianxiety/antihistamine/sedative/hypnotic, antiemetic
Chem. class.: Piperazine derivative

Do not confuse:
hydrOXYzine/hydrALAZINE

ACTION: Depresses subcortical levels of CNS, including limbic system, reticular formation; competes with H_1-receptor sites

USES: Anxiety preoperatively, prevention of nausea, vomiting postoperatively; to potentiate opioid analgesics; sedation; pruritus

CONTRAINDICATIONS
Pregnancy 1st trimester, breastfeeding; hypersensitivity to this product or cetirizine; acute asthma
Precautions: Pregnancy (2nd/3rd trimester), geriatric patients, debilitated patients, renal/hepatic disease, closed-angle glaucoma, COPD, prostatic hypertrophy, asthma

656   hydrOXYzine

DOSAGE AND ROUTES

Anxiety
- **Adult:** PO 50-100 mg qid, max 400 mg/day; **IM** 50-100 mg q4-6hr
- **Child ≥6 yr:** PO 50-100 mg/day in divided doses, max 100 mg/day or 2 mg/kg/day
- **Child <6 yr:** PO 50 mg/day in divided doses, max 50 mg/day or 2 mg/kg/day

Alcohol withdrawal
- **Adult:** IM 50-100 mg q4-6hr

Preoperatively/postoperatively (nausea/vomiting)
- **Adult:** IM 25-100 mg q4-6hr
- **Child:** IM 1.1 mg/kg as a single dose

Pruritus
- **Adult:** PO 25 mg tid-qid; **IM** 50-100 mg, then q4-6hr prn, switch to **PO** as soon as feasible
- **Child ≥6 yr:** PO 50-100 mg/day in divided doses; **IM** 0.5-1 mg/kg/dose q4-6hr prn, use **PO** when possible
- **Child <6 yr:** PO 50 mg/day in divided doses

Renal dose
- **Adult:** PO CCr <50 mL/min, give 50% of dose

Available forms: Tabs 10, 25, 50 mg; caps 25, 50, 100 mg; syrup 2 mg/mL ✦, 10 mg/5 mL; inj 25, 50 mg/mL; oral susp 25 mg/5 mL

Administer:
PO route
- Without regard to meals
- Crushed if patient is unable to swallow medication whole
- Shake oral susp before giving

IM route
- Does not need to be diluted; give by Z-track inj in large muscle to decrease pain, chance of necrosis; never give IV/SUBCUT (HCl)

SIDE EFFECTS

CNS: *Dizziness, drowsiness,* confusion, headache, tremors, fatigue, depression, seizures
CV: Hypotension
GI: Dry mouth, increased appetite, nausea, diarrhea, weight gain

PHARMACOKINETICS

PO: Onset 15-60 min, duration 4-6 hr, half-life 3 hr, metabolized by liver, excreted by kidneys

INTERACTIONS

Increase: CNS depressant effect—barbiturates, opioids, analgesics, alcohol, sedative/hypnotics, other CNS depressants
Increase: anticholinergic effects—phenothiazines, quiNIDine, disopyramide, antihistamines, antidepressants, atropine, haloperidol, MAOIs

Drug/Lab Test
False negative: skin allergy testing
False increase: 17-hydroxycorticosteroids

NURSING CONSIDERATIONS

Assess:
- **Anticholinergic effects:** dry mouth, dizziness, confusion, hypotension, increased sedation; monitor B/P
- **Fall risk:** assistance with ambulation during beginning therapy, since drowsiness, dizziness occurs
- **Beers:** avoid use in older adults; anticholinergic effects, toxicity may occur
- **Pregnancy/breastfeeding:** do not use in pregnancy/breastfeeding

Evaluate:
- **Therapeutic response:** decreased anxiety

Teach patient/family:
- To avoid OTC preparations (cold, cough, hay fever) unless approved by prescriber
- To avoid driving, activities that require alertness
- To avoid alcohol, psychotropic medications
- Not to discontinue medication quickly after long-term use
- To rise slowly because fainting may occur
- To report urinary retention, constipation, or other serious anticholinergic symptoms to provider, discontinue use

TREATMENT OF OVERDOSE:
VS, supportive care; IV norepinephrine for hypotension

ibalizumab (Rx)

(eye-ba-liz´ue-mab)

Trogarzo

Func. class.: HIV antiviral
Chem. class.: HIV-1 entry inhibitor/
fusion inhibitor

ACTION: Blocks HIV-1 from infecting CD4, T cells by binding to CD4 and interfering with the steps required for the entry of HIV-1 virus into host cells, preventing viral transmission

USES: Human immunodeficiency virus type 1 (HIV-1) infection in heavily treatment-experienced adults with multidrug-resistant HIV-1 infection failing their current antiretroviral regimen

CONTRAINDICATIONS

Hypersensitivity

Precautions: Autoimmune disease, breastfeeding, Graves' disease, Guillain-Barré disease, immune reconstitution syndrome, pregnancy, progressive multifocal leukoencephalopathy, immune reconstitution syndrome

DOSAGE AND ROUTES

• **Adult: IV** 2000 mg once, then 800 mg q2wk as part of combination therapy
Available forms: Sol for infusion 200 mg/1.33 mL
Administer:
IV route
• Visually inspect for particulate matter and discoloration before use
Dilution
• Select the appropriate number of vials necessary for either the loading dose (10 vials) or maintenance dose (4 vials)
• Withdraw 1.33 mL from each vial and transfer into a 250-mL IV bag of 0.9% sodium chloride for injection. Do not use other diluents
• Once diluted, solution should be given immediately

• **Storage:** diluted solution may be stored at room temperature (20° C-25° C or 68° F-77° F) for up to 4 hr or refrigerated (2° C-8° C or 36° F-46° F) for up to 24 hr. If refrigerated, allow to stand at room temperature for at least 30 min, but no more than 4 hr before use

Intermittent IV infusion route:
• Do not administer as an IV push or bolus
• Administer in the cephalic vein of the patient's arm or an appropriate vein located elsewhere
• Infuse the loading dose (2000 mg) over no less than 30 min
• If there are no infusion-associated adverse reactions, the maintenance doses (800 mg) can be decreased to no less than 15 min
• Flush with 30 mL of 0.9% NaCl for injection after the completion
• Observe for 1 hr after completion for at least the first infusion. If there are no adverse reactions, observation time can be reduced to 15 min
Missed doses
• If a maintenance dose (800 mg) is missed by 3 days or longer, a loading dose (2000 mg) should be given as early as possible
• Resume maintenance dosing (800 mg) q14days thereafter

SIDE EFFECTS

CNS: Dizziness
ENDO: Increased serum glucose and uric acid
GI: Nausea, diarrhea
INTEG: Rash
MISC: Thrombocytopenia, dizziness, rash, hyperglycemia, neutropenia

PHARMACOKINETICS

Half-life 64 hr

INTERACTIONS

None known

NURSING CONSIDERATIONS

Assess:

• HIV: monitor CD4+ T-cell count, plasma HIV RNA baseline and periodically

• **Immune reconstitution syndrome:** Monitor beginning treatment when used with combination antiretrovirals; an inflammatory response to opportunistic infections may occur

• Blood studies: blood glucose, CBC with differential, LFTs, pregnancy testing, serum bilirubin (total and direct), serum creatinine/BUN baseline and periodically

• **Pregnancy/breastfeeding:** no adequate human data available. Report cases of antiretroviral drug exposure to the Antiretroviral Pregnancy Registry, 800-258-4263 or http://www.apregistry.com/. Avoid breastfeeding

Evaluate:

• **Therapeutic response:** increased CD4+ counts, plasma HIV-1 RNA levels, decreased viral load, slowing progression of HIV-1 infection

Teach patient/family:

• That lab work will be necessary at the start of treatment and periodically thereafter

• **Pregnancy/breastfeeding:** to notify health care provider if pregnancy is planned or suspected; that pregnancy test will be required before starting treatment; to enroll in Antiretroviral Pregnancy Registry, which monitors fetal outcomes of pregnant women exposed to this product; not to breastfeed, HIV-1 can be passed to the baby in breast milk

• To report nausea, diarrhea if severe

• To read the patient information provided

• **Immune reconstitution syndrome:** to inform health care provider immediately of any symptoms of infection

• That product is given q2wk as recommended by the health care provider; not to change the dosing schedule or any antiretroviral medication without consulting the health care provider

• To notify health care provider immediately if patient stops taking this product or any other drug in his or her antiretroviral regimen

• That product is not a cure for HIV-1 but controls symptoms and that disease still can be passed to others; to use in combination with other antiretrovirals

---

ibandronate (Rx)

(eye-ban′dro-nate)

Boniva

Func. class.: Bone-resorption inhibitor, electrolyte modifier

Chem. class.: Bisphosphonate

ACTION: Inhibits bone resorption, without inhibiting bone formation and mineralization; absorbs calcium phosphate crystals in bone and may directly block dissolution of hydroxyapatite crystals of bone; more potent than other products

USES: Postmenopausal osteoporosis and prophylaxis

Unlabeled uses: Hypercalcemia of malignancy, osteolytic metastases, Paget's disease

CONTRAINDICATIONS

Achalasia, esophageal stricture, hypocalcemia, intraarterial administration, renal failure, hypersensitivity to bisphosphonates, inability to stand or sit upright

Precautions: Pregnancy, breastfeeding, children, geriatric patients, anemia, chemotherapy, coagulopathy, dental disease, diabetes mellitus, dysphagia, GI/renal disease, GERD, hypertension, infection, multiple myeloma, phosphate hypersensitivity, vit D deficiency

DOSAGE AND ROUTES

Postmenopausal osteoporosis/ prophylaxis

• **Adult: PO** 150 mg/mo; **IV BOL** 3 mg q3mo

Hypercalcemia of malignancy (unlabeled)

• **Adult: IV INFUSION** 2 mg infused over 2 hr in moderate hypercalcemia, 4 mg in

---

severe hypercalcemia (>3 mmol/L). The use of 6 mg should be reserved for serum calcium levels >3.5 mmol/L

Renal dose
• **Adult: PO** CCr <30 mL/min, avoid use
Available forms: Tabs 150 mg; sol for inj 1 mg/mL (3 mg/3 mL in prefilled syringes)
Administer:
PO route
• Give early ᴀᴍ with a glass of water; if monthly, give on same day of each month
• Patient to remain upright for ≥1 hr after taking
• Do not suck/chew; throat ulcers may occur
• Store at room temperature
Direct IV route
• Use single-dose prefilled syringe; discard unused portion; give over 15-30 sec; give q3mo; do not use if discolored or contains particulates
• Do not admix
• Store at room temperature

SIDE EFFECTS
CNS: Fever, insomnia, dizziness, headache
CV: Hypertension
EENT: Ocular pain/inflammation, uveitis, esophageal ulceration
GI: Constipation, nausea, vomiting, diarrhea, dyspepsia, esophageal/GI cancer
INTEG: Rash, inj-site reaction
MS: *Bone pain, myalgia,* osteonecrosis of the jaw
SYST: Stevens-Johnson syndrome, erythema multiforme, dermatitis bullosa

PHARMACOKINETICS
Half-life tabs 1.5-6 days, IV 4.5-25.5 hr; 91%-99% protein binding; taken up mainly by bones, primarily in areas of high bone turnover; eliminated primarily by kidneys (60%); **PO:** onset unknown, peak ½-2 hr, duration unknown; **IV:** onset rapid, peak 3 hr

INTERACTIONS
Increase: GI irritation—NSAIDs, salicylates
Increase: QTc prolongation—drugs that prolong QTc
Decrease: ibandronate effect—PPIs

Decrease: ibandronate effect—calcium/vit D/iron/aluminum/magnesium salts; separate by 1 hr
Drug/Food
• Do not take with food, calcium products; give product on empty stomach
Drug/Lab Test
Decrease: Alk phos, magnesium, calcium, phosphate

NURSING CONSIDERATIONS
Assess:
• **Osteoporosis:** before and during treatment; DEXA scan for bone mineral density; correct electrolyte imbalances (calcium, magnesium, phosphate) before starting therapy
• **Anaphylaxis (IV) rare:** swelling of face, lips, mouth, rash, sweating, wheezing, trouble breathing; discontinue immediately, provide supportive treatment
• **Dental health:** before dental extraction, may require drug holiday for up to 2 mo; osteonecrosis of the jaw may occur
• **Labs:** electrolytes, creatinine/BUN, calcium, vit D, alkaline phosphatase; correct deficiencies before treatment
• **For bone pain;** use analgesics; may begin within 24 hr or even years after treatment; pain usually subsides after treatment is discontinued
• **Esophageal irritation/ulceration:** heartburn, painful swallowing; avoid use in those with swallowing difficulties
Evaluate:
• **Therapeutic response:** increased bone mineral density
Teach patient/family:
• **To report hypercalcemic relapse:** nausea, vomiting, bone pain, thirst, unusual muscle twitching, muscle spasms, severe diarrhea, constipation
• To continue with dietary recommendations, including calcium, vit D
• To obtain an analgesic from provider for bone pain, which may occur rapidly or within months
• That if nausea, vomiting occur; small, frequent meals may help
• **To report vision symptoms:** blurred vision, edema, inflammation

• To exercise regularly, stop smoking, decrease alcohol intake

• To notify health care professional of osteonecrosis of the jaw, after dental procedures, pain, draining, swelling, to notify dentist before dental procedures

• To take PO first thing in AM at least 60 min before other medications, food, beverages; to take monthly dose on same day; that if IV dose is missed, to reschedule as soon as able and to reschedule subsequent doses on new time schedule; not to receive IV dose more than once in 3 mo

• To sit upright for ≥60 min after PO to prevent irritation; to swallow tab whole, not to chew or suck

• To report whether pregnancy is planned or suspected or if planning to breastfeed

---

⚠ HIGH ALERT

ibrutinib (Rx)

(eye-broo′ti-nib)

Imbruvica

Func. class.: Antineoplastic-biologic response modifier

Chem. class.: Signal transduction inhibitor (STIs)—kinase inhibitor

---

ACTION: Irreversible inhibitor of Bruton's tyrosine kinases in B cells responsible for tumor growth

USES: Recurrent mantle cell lymphoma in patients who have received at least 1 prior treatment, Waldenström macroglobulinemia, chronic lymphocytic leukemia (CLL) including those with 17 p deletion; dependent or steroid refractory chronic graft-versus-host disease (cGVD)

CONTRAINDICATIONS

Pregnancy, breastfeeding, hypersensitivity, hepatic disease

Precautions: Children, geriatric patients, active infections, anticoagulant therapy (3 × 140-mg caps once daily until disease progression), bleeding, hepatic/renal disease, neutropenia, surgery

DOSAGE AND ROUTES
CLL, WM, cGVHD
• **Adult: PO** 420 mg/day
MCL
• **Adult: PO** 560 mg (4 × 140-mg caps) daily

Dosage adjustment for ≥grade 3 nonhematologic toxicities, ≥grade 3 neutropenia with infection or fever, or grade 4 hematologic toxicities: Interrupt therapy; resume upon recovery to grade 1 or baseline as indicated below:

• **First occurrence:** Resume dosing at original dose (daily dose = 560 mg/day)

• **Second occurrence:** Reduce dose by 1 capsule (daily dose = 420 mg/day)

• **Third occurrence:** Reduce dose by 2 capsules (daily dose = 280 mg/day)

• **Fourth occurrence:** Discontinue

Available forms: Caps 140 mg

Administer:
• At same time of day with water; without regard to food; if dose is missed, take as soon as possible on same day, do not double

• Do not open, break, chew cap, swallow whole

• Use safe handling procedures

• Store at room temperature, avoid moisture

SIDE EFFECTS
CNS: *Fatigue, fever,* headache, insomnia
CV: Hypertension, atrial fibrillation, peripheral edema
EENT: Sinusitis
GI: *Nausea,* vomiting, dyspepsia, anorexia, *abdominal pain,* constipation, stomatitis, *diarrhea,* GI bleeding
GU: Increased serum creatinine, UTI, renal failure
HEMA: *Neutropenia, thrombocytopenia, anemia,* bleeding, epistaxis, transient lymphocytosis, *febrile neutropenia*
INTEG: *Rash,* skin infections, *bruising*
MS: *Pain,* arthralgia, muscle cramps
RESP: Cough, dyspnea
SYST: Secondary malignancy, infection

PHARMACOKINETICS
Protein binding 97.3%; metabolized by CYP3A4/CYP2D6; primarily excreted in feces, small amount in urine; peak 1-2 hr, half-life 4-8 hr

INTERACTIONS
Increase: ibrutinib effect—avoid use with moderate or strong CYP3A4 inhibitors (clarithromycin, indinavir, itraconazole, ketoconazole, nelfinavir, posaconazole, ritonavir, saquinavir, voriconazole)
Decrease: ibrutinib effect—avoid use with moderate or strong CYP3A4 inducers (carBAMazepine, phenytoin, rifAMPin)
Drug/Herb
Decrease: SUNItinib concentration—St. John's wort
Drug/Food Test
Increase: plasma concentrations—grapefruit juice; avoid use
Drug/Lab Test
Increase: lymphocytes, uric acid, creatinine

NURSING CONSIDERATIONS
Assess:
• **Bleeding:** bruising; grade 3 or higher bleeding events may occur, may be fatal; CBC
• **Hypersensitivity:** trouble breathing, fever, itching, wheezing; swelling of face, lips, tongue; stop product immediately, provide supportive treatment
• **Renal failure:** monitor (BUN, creatinine), maintain hydration, monitor for hyperuricemia
• **Infection:** fever, sore throat, malaise; infections may be fatal
• **Cardiac changes/hypertension:** monitor B/P and for cardiac changes
• **Secondary malignancies:** monitor for new malignancies
• Hepatic/renal function; signs and symptoms of infections
• **Surgery:** may interrupt treatment a few days before surgery
• **Pregnancy/breastfeeding:** identify whether pregnancy is planned or suspected or if breastfeeding
Evaluate:
• **Therapeutic response:** decrease in progression of disease
Teach patient/family:

• About reason for treatment, expected result
• **That many adverse reactions may occur:** high B/P, bleeding, mouth swelling, shortness of breath, report immediately
• To avoid persons with known upper respiratory infections; that immunosuppression is common
• To avoid grapefruit juice or medications, herbs; there are many interactions
• To report if pregnancy is planned or suspected, or if breastfeeding
• To report bleeding, severe infections, renal toxicity (maintain hydration), development of second malignancies, diarrhea (contact physician if it persists)
• To take with water at same time each day; do not open, break, or chew

ibuprofen (OTC, Rx)
(eye-byoo-proe'fen)
Addaprin, Advil Junior Strength, Advil Liqui-Gels minis, Advil Migraine, Advil, Childrens Advil, Childrens Ibuprofen, Childrens Motrin, Dyspel, Genpri, GoodSense Ibuprofen Childrens, GoodSense Ibuprofen, IBU, IBU-200, Ibupak, Ibuprofen Childrens, Infants Advil, KS Ibuprofen, Motrin Childrens, Motrin IB, Motrin Infants Drop
ibuprofen (injection) (Rx)
Caldolor; NeoProfen (lysine)
Func. class.: NSAID
Chem. class.: Propionic acid derivative

Do not confuse:
Motrin/neurontin
ibuprofen/acetaminophen

ACTION: Inhibits COX-1, COX-2 by blocking arachidonate; analgesic, antiinflammatory, antipyretic

USES: Inflammatory disorders: Rheumatoid arthritis, osteoarthritis, primary dysmenorrhea, dental pain,

Side effects: *italics* = common; red = life-threatening

musculoskeletal disorders, fever, migraine, patent ductus arteriosus, headache

Unlabeled uses: Ankylosing spondylitis, bone pain, cystic fibrosis, gouty arthritis, psoriatic arthritis

CONTRAINDICATIONS

Pregnancy 3rd trimester; hypersensitivity to this product, NSAIDs, salicylates; asthma; severe renal/hepatic disease; perioperative pain in CABG, severe HF, active GI ulcer, IBD, risk of bleeding

Precautions: Pregnancy 1st and 2nd trimesters, breastfeeding, children, geriatric patients, bleeding disorders, GI disorders, renal disorders, cardiac disorders, hypersensitivity to other antiinflammatory agents, HF, CCr <25 mL/min

Black Box Warning: GI bleeding, MI, stroke

DOSAGE AND ROUTES
Self-treatment of minor aches/pains
• **Adult/adolescent: PO** (OTC product) 200 mg q4-6hr, may increase to 400 mg q4-6hr if needed, max 1200 mg/day
• **Child 11 yr (72-95 lb): PO** 300 mg q6-8hr
• **Child 9-10 yr (60-71 lb): PO** 250 mg q6-8hr
• **Child 6-8 yr (48-59 lb): PO** 200 mg q6-8hr
• **Child 4-5 yr (36-47 lb): PO** 150 mg q6-8hr
• **Child 2-3 yr (24-35 lb): PO** 100 mg q6-8hr
• **Child 12-23 mo (18-23 lb): PO** 75 mg q6-8hr
• **Child 6-11 mo (12-17 lb): PO** 50 mg q6-8hr
Analgesic
• **Adult: PO** 200-400 mg q4-6hr, max 3.2 g/day; OTC use max 1200 mg/day
• **Child: PO** 4-10 mg/kg/dose q6-8hr
Moderate to severe pain (hospitalized patients) (Caldolor)
• **Adult: IV** 400-800 mg q6hr as an adjunct to opiate-agonist therapy

Dysmenorrhea
• **Adult: PO** 400 mg q4-6hr, max 1200 mg/day
Antipyretic
• **Child 6 mo-12 yr: PO** 5 mg/kg (temperature <102.5° F or 39.2° C), 10 mg/kg (temperature >102.5° F), may repeat q6-8hr, max 40 mg/kg/day or 2400 mg/day whichever is less
Antiinflammatory
• **Adult: PO** 400-800 mg tid-qid, max 3.2 g/day
• **Child 6 mo-12 yr: PO** 30-50 mg/kg/day in 3-4 divided doses, max 50 mg/kg/day or 2400 mg/day whichever is less
Juvenile arthritis
• **Child: PO** 30-50 mg/kg/day divided in 3-4 doses, max 2.4 g per day
Patent ductus arteriosus (PDA) (NeoProfen)
• **Premature neonate ≤32 wk gestation who weighs 500-1500 g: IV** 10 mg/kg initially, then, if needed, 2 doses of 5 mg/kg at 24-hr intervals; if oliguria occurs, hold dose
Cystic fibrosis (unlabeled)
• **Child 6 mo-12 yr: PO** 20-30 mg/kg/dose twice daily, max 1600 mg per dose
Available forms: Caps 200 mg; tabs 100, 200, 300 ✿, 400, 600, 800 mg; cap, liq gels 200 mg; oral susp 40 mg/mL, 100 mg/5 mL; liq 100 mg/5 mL; chew tabs 100 mg; oral drops 50 mg/1.25 mL; inj 10 mg/mL (NeoProfen), single-dose IV bag
Administer:
PO route
• With food, milk, or antacid to decrease GI symptoms; if nausea and vomiting occur or persist, notify prescriber
• Shake suspension well before use
• Do not break, crush, chew enteric- or film-coated products
• Do not use in pregnancy after 30 wk gestation
• Store at room temperature

IV route
• Patient must be well hydrated before administration
• Dilute to ≤4 mg/mL with 0.9% NaCl, LR, D_5W; infuse over ≥30 min; do not give IM
• Discard unused portion

✿ Canada only   🙵☜☞ Genetic warning

• Visually inspect for particulate prior to use
• **Ibuprofen lysine:** dilute with dextrose or saline to appropriate volume (10 mg/mL of ibuprofen is recommended); give within 30 min of preparation; give via IV port nearest insertion site; give over 15 min
• Check for extravasation; do not give in same line with TPN; interrupt TPN for 15 min before and after product administration

SIDE EFFECTS

CNS: *Headache,* dizziness, drowsiness, fatigue
CV: Tachycardia, *peripheral edema,* palpitations, dysrhythmias, CV thrombotic events, MI, stroke, HF
EENT: Tinnitus, hearing loss, blurred vision
GI: Nausea, *anorexia,* vomiting, diarrhea, jaundice, constipation, flatulence, cramps, dry mouth, peptic ulcer, GI bleeding, ulceration, necrotizing enterocolitis, GI perforation
GU: Nephrotoxicity, dysuria, hematuria, oliguria, azotemia
HEMA: Blood dyscrasias, increased bleeding time
INTEG: Purpura, *rash,* pruritus, urticaria, necrotizing fasciitis, photosensitivity, photophobia
ENDO: Hyperkalemia, hyperuricemia, hypoglycemia, hyponatremia
SYST: Anaphylaxis, Stevens-Johnson syndrome

PHARMACOKINETICS

PO: Onset ½ hr, peak 1-2 hr, duration 4-6 hr; IV: duration 4-6 hr, half-life 1.8-2 hr (adult), 1-2 hr (child) metabolized in liver (inactive metabolites), excreted in urine (inactive metabolites), 90%-99% protein binding, does not enter breast milk, well absorbed

INTERACTIONS

Increase: renal dysfunction risk—ACEI/ARBs
Increase: bleeding risk—valproic acid, thrombolytics, antiplatelets, anticoagulants, salicylates, SSRIs
Increase: blood dyscrasia risk—antineoplastics, radiation

Increase: toxicity—lithium, oral anticoagulants, cycloSPORINE, methotrexate
Increase: GI reactions—aspirin, corticosteroids, NSAIDs, alcohol, tobacco
Increase: hypoglycemia—oral antidiabetics
Decrease: effect of antihypertensives, thiazides, furosemide
Decrease: ibuprofen action—aspirin

Drug/Herb

Increase: bleeding risk—feverfew, fish oil garlic, ginger, ginkgo, ginseng *(Panax),* horse chestnut, red clover

Drug/Lab Test

Increase: BUN, creatinine, LFTs, potassium
Decrease: HB/Hct, blood glucose, WBC, platelets

NURSING CONSIDERATIONS
Assess:

Black Box Warning: GI bleeding/perforation: chronic use can cause gastritis with or without bleeding; for those with a prior or history of peptic ulcer disease or GI bleeding, initiate treatment at lower dose; geriatric patients are at greater risk and those who consume >3 alcoholic drinks/day

• **Labs:** BUN, creatinine, AST, ALT, HB, stool guaiac, before treatment, periodically thereafter; monitor electrolytes as needed; make sure patient is well hydrated
• **Perioperative pain in CABG:** MI and stroke can result for 10-14 days; can be fatal; those taking NSAIDs are at greater risk of MI and stroke even in first few weeks of therapy
• **Cardiac status:** edema (peripheral), tachycardia, palpitations; monitor B/P, pulse for character, quality, rhythm, especially in patients with cardiac disease, geriatric patients
• **Pain:** note type, duration, location, intensity with ROM 1 hr after administration
• **PDA closure:** monitor for bleeding, oliguria, infection; in preterm neonates, use only doses needed for ductus arteriosus closure, hold dose if renal output <0.6 mL/kg/hr on 2nd/3rd dose
• **Dysmenorrhea:** give at onset of menses

- Audiometric, ophthalmic exam before, during, after long-term treatment; for eye, ear problems: blurred vision, tinnitus; may indicate toxicity
- **Infection:** may mask symptoms; fever: temperature before and 1 hr after administration
- For history of peptic ulcer disorder, asthma, aspirin use, hypersensitivity; check closely for hypersensitivity reactions
- **Serious skin disorders:** for skin rash or swelling of lips, face, tongue; if present, discontinue immediately, provide supportive care
- **Beers:** avoid chronic use in older adults unless other alternatives are ineffective; increased risk of GI bleeding
- **Pregnancy:** identify if pregnancy is planned or suspected, or if breastfeeding; do not use after 30 wk gestation; use only if benefits outweigh fetal risk before 30 wk gestation; do not breastfeed

Evaluate:
- **Therapeutic response:** decreased pain, stiffness in joints; decreased swelling in joints; ability to move more easily; reduction in fever or menstrual cramping

Teach patient/family:
- To use sunscreen, sunglasses, and protective clothing to prevent photosensitivity, photophobia
- To report blurred vision, ringing, roaring in ears (may indicate toxicity); that eye and hearing tests should be done during long-term therapy
- To avoid driving, other hazardous activities if dizziness or drowsiness occurs

Black Box Warning: GI Bleeding: Assess for bleeding, bruising, ulceration, perforation of stomach

- **Nephrotoxicity:** to report change in urinary pattern, increased weight, edema, increased pain in joints, fever, blood in urine
- To avoid alcohol, NSAIDs, salicylates; bleeding may occur
- To report use of this product to all health care providers
- **Pregnancy:** to notify prescriber if pregnancy is planned or suspected; avoid after 30 wk

- To avoid driving or other hazardous activities until effect is known

Black Box Warning: MI/stroke: to report signs/symptoms of MI/stroke immediately; discontinue product, seek emergency medical treatment

- To take with full glass of water; to sit upright for 30 min after use; to take with food to lessen GI effects

ibuprofen/famotidine (Rx)
(eye-byoo-proe′fen/fa-moe′ t-deen)
Duexis
Func. class.: Nonopioid analgesic/ histamine H2 antagonist/NSAID

USES: Osteoarthritis, RA

Black Box Warning: GI bleeding/perforation, CABG

DOSAGE AND ROUTES
- **Adult: PO:** One tablet (ibuprofen 800 mg/famotidine 26.6 mg) TID, avoid in CCr <50 mL/min

Available forms: Tablet: ibuprofen 800 mg/famotidine 26.6 mg

⚠ HIGH ALERT

ibutilide (Rx)
(eye-byoo′tih-lide)
Corvert
Func. class.: Antidysrhythmic (class III)
Chem. class.: Methane sulfonamide

ACTION: Prolongs duration of action potential and effective refractory period

USES: For rapid conversion of atrial fibrillation/flutter, including within 1 wk of coronary artery bypass or valve surgery

CONTRAINDICATIONS
Hypersensitivity breastfeeding, children <18 yr

Precautions: Pregnancy, geriatric patients, sinus node dysfunction, 2nd- or 3rd-degree AV block, electrolyte imbalances, bradycardia, renal/hepatic disease, HF

Black Box Warning: Life threatening dysrrhthmias: QT prolongation, torsades de pointes, ventricular arrhythmias, ventricular tachycardia, cardiac dysrhythmias, atrial fibrillation

DOSAGE AND ROUTES
Atrial fibrillation/flutter
• **Adult ≥60 kg: IV INFUSION** 1 vial (1 mg) given over 10 min, may repeat same dose after 10 min
• **Adult <60 kg: IV INFUSION** 0.01 mg/kg given over 10 min, may repeat same dose after 10 min
Available forms: Inj 0.1 mg/mL in 10-mL vials
Administer:
• Ice compress after stopping infusion for extravasation; tubing should be removed and attempt to aspirate product; elevate affected areas

IV route
• Do not use if discolored or particulate is present
• Undiluted or diluted in 50 mL 0.9% NaCl, or D$_5$W (0.017 mg/mL); give over 10 min
• Solution is stable for 48 hr refrigerated or 24 hr at room temperature
• Do not admix with other sol, products
• Reduce dosage slowly with ECG monitoring
• Stop infusion as soon as arrhythmia is controlled

SIDE EFFECTS
CNS: *Headache,* syncope, stroke
CV: *Hypotension, bradycardia,* sinus arrest, HF, dysrhythmias, torsades de pointes, hypertension, extrasystoles, ventricular tachycardia, bundle branch block, AV block, palpitations, supraventricular extrasystoles, syncope, prolonged QT interval
GI: Nausea

PHARMACOKINETICS
Half-life 6 hr, metabolized by liver, excreted by kidneys

INTERACTIONS
Increase: prodysrhythmia—phenothiazines, tricyclics, tetracyclics, antidepressants, H$_1$-receptor antagonists, antihistamines
Increase: masking of cardiotoxicity—digoxin
• Do not use within 5 hr of ibutilide: class Ia antidysrhythmics (disopyramide, quiNIDine, procainamide), class III agents (amiodarone, sotalol); QT prolongation may occur

NURSING CONSIDERATIONS
Assess:

Black Box Warning: ECG continuously for ≥4 hr to determine product effectiveness; measure PR, QRS, QT intervals, check for PVCs, other dysrhythmias; discontinue if atrial fibrillation/flutter ceases; continue until QT interval corrected for heart rate (QTc) returned to baseline; if atrial fibrillation lasts more than 2 days, anticoagulation must be adequate >2 wk before use

• I&O ratio; electrolytes: potassium, sodium, chlorine
• Hepatic studies: AST, ALT, bilirubin, alk phos
• Dehydration or hypovolemia
• Rebound hypertension after 1-2 hr
• Cardiac rate, respiration: rate, rhythm, character, chest pain
• **Pregnancy/breastfeeding:** use only if benefits outweigh fetal risk; avoid breastfeeding, excretion unknown
Evaluate:
• **Therapeutic response:** decrease in atrial fibrillation/flutter
Teach patient/family:
• To report side effects immediately, pain at injection site
• About reason for medication

---

icatibant (Rx)
Firazyr
Func. class.: Bradykinin receptor antagonists

USES: Hereditary angioedema

DOSAGE AND ROUTES:
• **Adult: SUBCUT** 30 mg at onset of acute attack, may repeat dose every 6 hr as needed for recurring symptoms or inadequate response, max 3 doses (90 mg total)/24 hr
Available forms: Injection (SUBCUT) 10 mg/mL (30 mg)

---

icosapent (Rx)
(eye-koe´sa-pent)
Vascepa
Func. class.: Antilipidemic
Chem. class.: Omega-3 fatty acid ethylester

USES: As adjunct to diet in adults with severe hypertriglyceridemia (≥500 mg/dL); adjunct to statin therapy to reduce risk of MI, stroke

CONTRAINDICATIONS
Hypersensitivity to icosapent ethyl

DOSAGE AND ROUTES
• **Adult: PO** 2 g bid with food
Available forms: Soft gel cap 0.5 g, 1 g

⚠ HIGH ALERT

IDArubicin (Rx)
(eye-dah-roob´ih-sin)
Idamycin PFS
Func. class.: Antineoplastic, antibiotic

USES: Used in combination with other antineoplastics for acute myelocytic leukemia in adults

Black Box Warning: Myelosuppression, bilirubin >5 mg/dL

Black Box Warning: Renal/hepatic disease, heart failure

DOSAGE AND ROUTES
• **Adult: IV** 8-12 mg/m^2/day × 3 days in combination with cytarabine (induction)
• **Adolescent/child (unlabeled): IV** 10-12 mg/m^2/day × 3 days

Black Box Warning: **Renal/hepatic dose: Adult: IV** CCr >2.5 mg/dL, reduce dose; bilirubin 2.5-5 mg/dL, reduce dose by 50%; bilirubin >5 mg/dL, do not use

Available forms: Inj 1 mg/mL in 5-mL, 10-mL, 20-mL single-use vials

---

idarucizumab (Rx)
(eye-da-roo-siz´uh-mab)
Praxbind
Func. class.: Antidote (dabigatran)
Chem. class.: Monoclonal antibody

Do not confuse:
Praxbind/digibind
Idarucizumab/idarubicin

ACTION:
A humanized monoclonal antibody fragment (Fab) that binds specifically to dabigatran and its acylglucuronide metabolites with a higher affinity for dabigatran to thrombin and neutralizes the anticoagulant effect within minutes

USES:
Reversal of dabigatran

CONTRAINDICATIONS
Hypersensitivity, fructose intolerance, sobitol parenterally, children <18 yr
Precautions: Pregnancy, breastfeeding, liver disease

DOSAGE AND ROUTES
Adult IV Bolus: 5 g (given as 2 separate 2.5-g/50 mL doses no more than 15 min apart)
Available forms: Injection 2.5 g/50 mL in single-use vials

Administer:

IV route
- For IV use only
- Do not shake
- Prior to use, flush preexisting IV line with NSS
- Give dose undiluted as an IV bolus by syringe or as an infusion by hanging the vials
- Do not mix with other drugs or give any other infusion in the same IV line
- Give promptly once solution has been removed from vial. Infusion of each vial should take no longer than 5-10 min, with the second vial of 2.5 g administered no later than 15 min after the end of the first 2.5-g vial
- Store intact vials at 2° C - 8° C (36° F-46° F) in original packaging (to protect from light), do not freeze. May store intact vials in the original packaging (to protect from light) at room temperature, 25° C (77° F), for up to 48 hr or up to 6 hr if exposed to light

SIDE EFFECTS
CNS: Headache, delirium
GI: Constipation
MISC: Hypersensitivity (fever, pruritus, rash)
RESP: Bronchospasm, pneumonia
CV: Thrombotic event
GU: UTI

PHARMACOKINETICS
Onset a few minutes, peak unknown, duration 24 hr, half-life 10.3 hr

INTERACTIONS:
None known
Drug/Lab: Increase: aPtt, ecarin clotting time (ECT)
Decrease: Potassium

NURSING CONSIDERATIONS
Assess:
- **Thrombotic risk:** Resume anticoagulant treatment as soon as possible to decrease the risk of thrombosis formation, may restart after 24 hr
- **Hypersensitivity:** Assess for hypersensitivity (bronchospasm, fever, pruritus, dyspnea, rash); hereditary fructose intolerance, product contains sorbitol

- **Pregnancy/breastfeeding:** No well-controlled studies, use only if clearly needed, cautious use in breastfeeding
Evaluate:
- **Therapeutic response:** Dabigatran reversal
Teach patient/family:
- Reason for product and expected result
- **Pregnancy/breastfeeding:** To notify provider if pregnancy is planned or suspected or if breastfeeding

> ### ⚠ HIGH ALERT
>
> ## idelalisib (Rx)
> (eye-del′a-lis′ib)
> Zydelig
> *Func. class.:* Antineoplastic, biologic response modifier
> *Chem. class.:* Signal transduction inhibitor (STI)

ACTION: Selective, small-molecule inhibitor of one kinase (expressed in both normal and malignant B-cells). Induces apoptosis and inhibited proliferation, inhibits several cell signaling pathways

USES: Treatment of relapsed chronic lymphocytic leukemia (CLL), in combination with riTUXimab, in those for whom riTUXimab alone should not be used; non-Hodgkin's lymphoma (NHL), relapsed follicular B-cell non-Hodgkin's lymphoma in those who have received at least 2 prior systemic therapies and are refractory to both riTUXimab/alkylating agent

CONTRAINDICATIONS
Infusion-related reaction, serious rash, pregnancy
Precautions: Serious allergic reactions, grade 3 or 4 neutropenia, breastfeeding, hyperglycemia/hypoglycemia

Black Box Warning: Serious hepatotoxicity, grade 3 or higher diarrhea or colitis, fatal/serious pneumonitis, GI perforation, infection

Side effects: *italics* = common; red = life-threatening

DOSAGE AND ROUTES
Follicular lymphoma
- **Adult: PO** 150 mg bid until disease progression or unacceptable toxicity

Chronic lymphocytic leukemia
- **Adult: PO** 150 mg bid with rituximab 375 mg/m² **IV**, then 500 mg/m² **IV** q2wk for 4 doses, then q4wk for 3 doses, for a total of 8 infusions

Hepatic dose
- **AST/ALT >3-5 × ULN:** No change; monitor AST/ALT at least every week until ≤1 × ULN
- **AST/ALT >5-20 × ULN:** Hold doses, monitor AST/ALT at least every week, when AST/ALT are ≤1 × ULN, resume at 100 mg bid
- **AST/ALT >20 × ULN:** Permanently discontinue
- **Bilirubin >1.5-3 × ULN:** No change; monitor bilirubin at least every week until ≤1 × ULN
- **Bilirubin >3-10 × ULN:** Hold treatment; monitor bilirubin at least every week; when bilirubin is ≤1 × ULN, resume treatment at 100 mg bid
- **Bilirubin >10 × ULN:** Permanently discontinue

Available forms: Tabs 100, 150 mg
Administer:
- Take without regard to food; do not crush or dissolve tabs
- Do not take 2 doses at the same time; if a dose is missed by <6 hr, take the dose, take next dose at usual time

Therapeutic drug monitoring: dosage adjustments due to treatment-related toxicity
- **Moderate diarrhea (4-6 stools/day over baseline):** Continue current dosing; monitor at least every week until diarrhea is resolved
- **Severe diarrhea (≥7 stools/day over baseline) or diarrhea requiring hospitalization:** Hold treatment, and monitor at least every week for resolution. When diarrhea has resolved, resume with 100 mg bid
- **Life-threatening diarrhea:** Permanently discontinue treatment

- **Neutropenia: ANC 1000-1499 cells/mm³:** no change; ANC 500-999 cells/mm³: continue current dosing; monitor ANC at least every week; **ANC <500 cells/mm³:** hold treatment and monitor ANC at least every week, when ANC ≥500 cells/mm³, resume treatment at 100 mg bid
- **Thrombocytopenia: Platelet count 50,000-75,000 cells/mm³:** no change; **platelet count 25,000-49,000 cells/mm³:** continue dose; monitor platelet count at least every week; **platelet count <25,000 cells/mm³:** hold treatment, monitor platelet count at least every week, when platelet count ≥25,000 cells/mm³, resume treatment at 100 mg bid
- **Symptomatic pneumonitis (any severity):** Discontinue treatment
- **Other severe or life-threatening toxicities:** Hold until toxicity is resolved; if resuming treatment, reduce the dose to 100 mg bid; permanently discontinue treatment for any recurrence of severe or life-threatening toxicity after rechallenge

SIDE EFFECTS
CNS: Insomnia, fatigue, *fever, headache, chills, pain*
RESP: Pneumonitis, dyspnea, cough, severe infection
ENDO: Hypoglycemia, hyperglycemia, hyponatremia
INTEG: Rash
EENT: Sinusitis
GI: Nausea, vomiting, hepatic failure, GI perforation, stomatitis, colitis, diarrhea, anorexia, abdominal pain, GERD
HEMA: Thrombocytopenia, neutropenia, anemia
SYST: Serious/fatal rashes, infection, sepsis

PHARMACOKINETICS
84% protein binding, half-life 8.2 hr, peak 1.5 hr

INTERACTIONS
Avoid use with CYP3A4 inhibitors, inducers, substrates
- **Decrease:** Action with strong CYP3A inducers (phenytoin, carBAMazepine, rifAMPin) may need dosage increase

• **Increase toxicity**—CYP3A inhibitors (ketoconazole, verapamil, dilTIAZem)
• **Increase:** CYP3A substrates (cycloSPORINE, fentaNYL, tacrolimus, ergots, warfarin), avoid concurrent use

Drug/Lab Test
Increase: LFTs

NURSING CONSIDERATIONS
Assess:

Black Box Warning: Hepatic failure: increased LFTs within the first 12 wk and were reversible with dose interruption. Monitor LFTs q2wk × 3 mo, then q4wk for 3 mo, and q1-3mo thereafter; monitor weekly if AST or ALT are >3 times the upper limit of normal (ULN) or bilirubin >1.5 × ULN. Hepatotoxicity may require treatment interruption, dose reduction, or discontinuation of therapy

Black Box Warning: Severe diarrhea/GI perforation: The occurrence of ≥7 stools/day over baseline or hospitalization due to diarrhea may require interruption, dose reduction, or permanent discontinuation. Assess for abdominal pain, chills, fever, or nausea/vomiting. If intestinal perforation occurs, permanently discontinue

Black Box Warning: Infections/pneumonitis: monitor for cough, dyspnea, hypoxia, and bilateral interstitial infiltrates, or a decline in O_2 saturation by >5%. If pneumonitis is suspected, hold therapy. Permanently discontinue for pneumonitis and consider corticosteroids

• **Pregnancy/breastfeeding:** do not use in pregnancy/breastfeeding

Evaluate:
• **Therapeutic response:** Decreased disease progression

Teach patient/family:
• **Pregnancy/breastfeeding:** to report planned or suspected pregnancy; to use effective contraception during treatment and for at least 1 mo after the last dose; to avoid breastfeeding
• To report new or worsening side effects

• To take tabs whole, not to crush or chew; to take with food for GI upset

⚠ HIGH ALERT

ifosfamide (Rx)
(i-foss'fa-mide)
Ifex
Func. class.: Antineoplastic alkylating agent
Chem. class.: Nitrogen mustard

USES: Germ cell testicular cancer in combination
Unlabeled uses: Soft tissue sarcoma, ALL, Ewing sarcoma, NHL, NSCLC, osteogenic sarcoma, penile cancer

Black Box Warning: Coma, hemorrhagic cystitis, bone marrow suppression, neurotoxicity, nephrotoxicity, encephalopathy

DOSAGE AND ROUTES
Germ cell testicular cancer
• Give with mesna for uroprotective treatment
• **Adult: IV** 1.2-2 g/m^2/day × 5 days, repeat course q3wk, given with mesna, in combination with 1-2 other antineoplastic agents
Sarcoma of soft tissue (orphan drug designation) (unlabeled)
• **Adult: IV INFUSION MAID regimen:** DOXOrubicin 60 mg/m^2 and dacarbazine 1000 mg/m^2, mixed or administered separately via **CONT IV INFUSION** over 4 days, ifosfamide 6000 mg/m^2 and mesna 10,000 mg/m^2 mixed or infused separately over 3 days (ifosfamide) and 4 days (mesna); repeat q21days if tolerated; OR MAID regimen: DOXOrubicin 60 mg/m^2 and dacarbazine 900 mg/m^2, mixed and administered through central venous access via **CONT IV INFUSION** over 3 days, ifosfamide 7500 mg/m^2 and mesna 10,000 mg/m^2 mixed or infused separately through a peripheral line via a **CONT IV INFUSION** over 3

days (ifosfamide) and 4 days (mesna); repeat q21days if tolerated

Renal dose

• **Adult: IV** CCr 31-60 mL/min, give 75% of dose; CCr 10-30 mL/min, give 50% of dose; CCr <10 mL/min, do not give

Available forms: Powder for Inj 1-, 3-g vials; IV solution 1 g/20 mL

---

iloperidone (Rx)

(eye-loe-pehr'ih-dohn)

Fanapt

Func. class.: 2nd-generation atypical antipsychotic

Chem. class.: Benzisoxazole derivative

Do not confuse:
Fanapt/Xanax

ACTION: Unknown; may be mediated through both DOPamine type 2 (D2) and serotonin type 2 (5-HT2) antagonism, high receptor binding affinity for norepinephrine (alpha 1)

USES: Schizophrenia

CONTRAINDICATIONS

Breastfeeding, hypersensitivity

Precautions: Pregnancy, children, geriatric patients, renal/hepatic disease, breast cancer, Parkinson's disease, dementia with Lewy bodies, seizure disorder, QT prolongation, bundle branch block, acute MI, ambient temperature increase, AV block, stroke, substance abuse, suicidal ideation, tardive dyskinesia, torsades de pointes, blood dyscrasias, dysphagia

Black Box Warning: Increased mortality in elderly patients with dementia-related psychosis; opioids

DOSAGE AND ROUTES

• **Adult: PO** 1 mg bid, may increase to target dose of 6-12 mg bid with daily dose adjustment of max 2 mg bid, titrate slowly; max 24 mg/day in 2 divided doses; reduce dose by 50% 🧬 in patient who is a poor

metabolizer of CYP2D6 or when used with strong CYP2D6/CYP3A4 inhibitors

Available forms: Tabs 1, 2, 4, 6, 8, 10, 12 mg; titration pack

Administer:

• Use without regard to meals
• Reduced dose in geriatric patients
• Anticholinergic agent for EPS
• Avoid use with CNS depressants
• Store in tight, light-resistant container

SIDE EFFECTS

CNS: *EPS, pseudoparkinsonism, akathisia, dystonia, tardive dyskinesia; drowsiness,* seizures, neuroleptic malignant syndrome, dizziness, delirium, depression, paranoia, fatigue, hostility, lethargy, restlessness, vertigo, tremor

CV: Orthostatic hypotension, heart failure, AV block, QT prolongation, tachycardia

EENT: Blurred vision, cataracts, nystagmus, tinnitus, nasal congestion

GI: *Nausea,* vomiting, *anorexia, constipation,* jaundice, weight gain/loss, abdominal pain, stomatitis, xerostomia, dry mouth

GU: Urinary retention/incontinence, priapism

HEMA: Agranulocytosis, leukopenia, neutropenia

MISC: 🧬, Decreased bone density hyperglycemia, dyslipidemia

SYST: Anaphylaxis, angioedema

PHARMACOKINETICS

PO: Extensively metabolized by liver to major active metabolite by 🧬 CYP2D6, CYP3A4; protein binding 95%; peak 2-4 hr; excreted in urine and feces; 🧬 terminal half-life 18 hr in extensive metabolizers; 33 hr in poor metabolizers

INTERACTIONS

Increase: sedation—other CNS depressants, alcohol, opioids

Increase: iloperidone effect, decreased clearance—CYP2D6 (FLUoxetine, paroxetine), CYP3A4 inhibitors (delavirdine, indinavir, isoniazid, itraconazole, dalfopristin, ritonavir, tipranavir); reduce dose

Increase: QT prolongation—class IA/III antidysrhythmics, some phenothiazines, β-agonists, local anesthetics, tricyclics, haloperidol, methadone, chloroquine, clarithromycin, droperidol, erythromycin, pentamidine

Decrease: iloperidone action—CYP2D6, CYP3A4 inducers (carBAMazepine, barbiturates, phenytoins, rifAMPin)

Drug/Lab Test

Increase: prolactin levels, cholesterol, glucose, lipids, triglycerides

Decrease: potassium

NURSING CONSIDERATIONS

Assess:

• AIMS assessment, lipid panel, blood glucose, CBC, glycosylated hemoglobin A1c, LFTs, neurologic function, pregnancy test, serum creatinine, electrolytes, prolactin, thyroid function studies, weight

• Affect, orientation, LOC, reflexes, gait, coordination, sleep-pattern disturbances

• **Vitals:** B/P standing and lying, pulse, respirations q4hr during initial treatment; establish baseline before starting treatment; report drops of 30 mm Hg; watch for ECG changes; QT prolongation may occur; dizziness, faintness, palpitations, tachycardia on rising

• **Extrapyramidal symptoms,** including akathisia, tardive dyskinesia (bizarre movements of the jaw, mouth, tongue, extremities), pseudoparkinsonism (rigidity, tremors, pill rolling, shuffling gait)

• Check to see the patient swallows the medication

Black Box Warning: Dementia-related psychosis: sudden death; not to be used in the elderly with dementia

• **Neuroleptic malignant syndrome:** hyperthermia, increased CPK, altered mental status, muscle rigidity, seizures, diaphoresis; discontinue immediately, notify prescriber

Black Box Warning: Opioids: Use only if alternative agents are not effective

• Constipation, urinary retention daily; if these occur, increase water and fiber in the diet

• Weight gain, BMI, waist circumference, hyperglycemia, metabolic changes in diabetes

• **Fall risk:** Supervised ambulation until patient is stabilized on medication; do not involve patient in strenuous exercise program because fainting is possible; patient should not stand still for long periods

• Sips of water, candy, gum for dry mouth

• **Hyperprolactemia:** sexual dysfunction, galactorrhea, change in menses

• **Beers:** avoid in older adults except for schizophrenia, bipolar disorder, or short-term use as an antiemetic during chemotherapy; increased risk of stroke

• **Pregnancy/breastfeeding:** use only if benefits outweigh fetal risk; infant exposed to product during 3rd trimester may exhibit EPS; do not breastfeed, excretion unknown

Evaluate:

• **Therapeutic response:** decrease in emotional excitement, hallucinations, delusions, paranoia; reorganization of patterns of thought, speech

Teach patient/family:

• That orthostatic hypotension may occur; to rise from sitting or lying position gradually

• To avoid hot tubs, hot showers, tub baths because hypotension may occur; that heat stroke may occur in hot weather; to take extra precautions to stay cool

• To avoid abrupt withdrawal of product because extrapyramidal symptoms may result; that product should be withdrawn slowly; to review symptoms of neuroleptic malignant syndrome

Black Box Warning: Opioids: Teach patient/family/caregiver, to seek medical care immediately if dizziness, drowsiness, trouble breathing occur

• To avoid OTC preparations (cough, hay fever, cold), herbals, supplements unless discussed by prescriber because serious product interactions may occur; to avoid use of alcohol because increased drowsiness may occur

• To use gum, lozenges for dry mouth

• To avoid hazardous activities if drowsy or dizziness occurs

---

Side effects: *italics* = common; red = life-threatening

• To comply with product regimen, to take as prescribed, not to skip or double doses, if medication is missed for >3 days start as initial dose

• To report impaired vision, tremors, muscle twitching

• That follow-up exams will be needed

• **Pregnancy/breastfeeding:** To use contraception; to inform prescriber if pregnancy is planned or suspected; if pregnant, should enroll in the Atypical Antipsychotic National Pregnancy Registry: 866-961-2388

TREATMENT OF OVERDOSE:
Lavage if orally ingested; provide airway; *do not induce vomiting*

---

iloprost (Rx)
[eye′-loe-prost]
Ventavis
Func. class.: Pulmonary vasodilator
Chem. class.: Prostacyclin analog

ACTION: Produces vasodilation and antiproliferative effects; mechanism for vasodilation is unclear. Hemodynamic effects following relaxation of vascular smooth muscle and vasodilation include decreased pulmonary vascular resistance, increased cardiac index, increased oxygen delivery. Also decreases platelet aggregation

USES: PAH in those with NYHA Class III or IV symptoms

CONTRAINDICATIONS
Hypersensitivity
Precautions: Asthma, breastfeeding, children, COPD, driving, geriatrics, hepatic disease, hypotension, pregnancy, pulmonary edema

DOSAGE AND ROUTES
• **Adult:** INH 2.5 mcg using adaptive aerosol delivery (AAD) may increase to 5 mcg 6-9×/day as needed separated by ≥2 hr, max 5 mcg 9×/day
Available forms: INH solution 10, 20 mcg/mL

Administer:
• Use only delivery device provided
• Do not take orally; avoid ocular exposure, contact with skin
• If signs of pulmonary edema occur in those with pulmonary hypertension, treatment should be stopped immediately; this may be a sign of pulmonary venous hypertension

SIDE EFFECTS
CNS: Headache, insomnia, syncope
CV: Hypotension, chest pain, vasodilation, palpitations, heart failure, supraventricular tachycardia, edema
GI: Nausea, vomiting, mouth/tongue discomfort
GU: Renal failure
RESP: Cough, dyspnea, pneumonia, flu-like symptoms

PHARMACOKINETICS
Half-life 30 min, peak 5 min, duration 30-60 min

INTERACTIONS
Increase: bleeding risk—anticoagulants, platelet inhibitors; assess for bleeding
Increase: hypotension—antihypertensives, vasodilators; monitor B/P
Drug/Lab Test:
Increase: alkaline phosphatase

NURSING CONSIDERATIONS
Assess:
• **Pulmonary arterial hypertension (PAH):** dizziness, light-headedness, fainting because of lowered B/P; patients should use caution when driving or operating machinery until effect is known
• **Syncope:** because of risk of syncope, vital signs should be monitored while initiating; in those with low systemic blood pressure, avoid further hypotension; do not use in systolic blood pressure <85 mm Hg; if syncope occurs during physical exertion, dose may need to be adjusted
• **Renal failure:** monitor closely in patients with renal impairment; effect may be extended
• **Bronchospasm:** may occur especially in susceptible patients with hyperreactive

airways; avoid use in COPD, severe asthma, acute respiratory infection

• **Pregnancy/breastfeeding:** use during pregnancy only if benefits to mother clearly outweigh potential risk to fetus; not known whether product crosses placenta

Teach patient/family:

• To take as prescribed; not to double doses; to take 2 hr before physical exertion; not to save leftover product; to always keep enough product and backup inhalation device; not to mix with other medications; not to miss doses or stop abruptly, risk of rebound hypertension

• To keep away from skin and eyes

• To avoid driving or other hazardous activities until reaction is known; dizziness, syncope may occur; to rise slowly to minimize orthostatic hypotension

• To monitor B/P; do not take if systolic B/P <85 mm Hg

⚠ HIGH ALERT

imatinib (Rx)

(im-ah-tin′ib)

Gleevec

Func. class.: Antineoplastic—miscellaneous

Chem. class.: Protein-tyrosine kinase inhibitor

ACTION: Inhibits ⊶ Bcr-Abl tyrosine kinase created in patients with chronic myeloid leukemia (CML), also inhibits tyrosine kinases

USES: Treatment of ⊶ CML; Philadelphia chromosome–positive (Ph+) in blast-cell crisis or in chronic failure; gastrointestinal stromal tumors (GIST) positive for c-Kit; chronic eosinophilic leukemia (CEL), Ph+ acute lymphocytic leukemia, dermatofibrosarcoma protuberans, myelodysplastic syndrome, systemic mastocytosis, HES

CONTRAINDICATIONS

Pregnancy, hypersensitivity

Precautions: Breastfeeding, children, geriatric patients, cardiac/renal/hepatic disease, GI bleeding, bone marrow suppression, infection, thrombocytopenia, neutropenia, immunosuppression

DOSAGE AND ROUTES

For the treatment of Ph+ CML chronic phase as initial therapy

• **Adult:** PO 400 mg/day, continue as long as beneficial; may increase to 600 mg/day in the absence of severe adverse reactions and severe non–leukemia-related neutropenia or thrombocytopenia

• **Adolescent/child >2 yr:** PO 340 mg/m²/day, max 600 mg/day; the daily dose may be given as a single dose or split into 2 doses given once in the morning and once in the evening

Ph+ acute lymphocytic leukemia (ALL)

• **Adult:** PO 600 mg every day, continue as long as beneficial

GIST

• **Adult:** PO 400-600 mg every day, may increase to 400 mg bid

Adjuvant treatment of *Kit* (CD117)-positive GIST after complete gross resection

• **Adult:** PO 400 mg/day

HES/CEL

• **Adult:** PO 400 mg/day in those who are FIP1L1-PDGFR α-fusion kinase negative or unknown; for HES/CEL patients with demonstrated FIP1L1-PDGFR α-fusion kinase, 100 mg/day, may increase to 400 mg

MDS/MPD

• **Adult:** PO 400 mg/day

Aggressive systemic mastocytosis (ASM) without D816V c-Kit mutation or with c-Kit mutation status unknown

• **Adult:** PO 400 mg/day

DFSP

• **Adult:** PO 400 mg twice daily

Renal dose

• **Adult:** PO **CCr 40-59 mL/min,** max 600 mg/day; **CCr 20-39 mL/min,** decrease initial dose by 50%, max 400 mg/day; **CCr <20 mL/min,** use with caution, 100 mg/day

Hepatic dose

Severe hepatic bilirubin 3-10 times ULN and any AST

Adult: PO Decrease recommended dose by 25%

Available forms: Tabs 100, 400 mg

Administer:
• With meal and large glass of water to decrease GI symptoms; doses of 800 mg should be given as 400 mg bid
• Tab may be dispersed in a glass of water or apple juice, use 50 mL of liquid for 100-mg tab, 200-mL liquid for 400-mg tab
• Use low-molecular-weight anticoagulant for anticoagulation if needed, not warfarin
• Continue as long as beneficial
• Store at 77° F (25° C)

SIDE EFFECTS

CNS: Headache, dizziness, insomnia, subdural hematoma, CNS hemorrhage
CV: Hemorrhage, heart failure, cardiac tamponade, cardiac toxicity
EENT: Blurred vision, conjunctivitis
GI: *Nausea,* hepatotoxicity, vomiting, dyspepsia, *anorexia, abdominal pain,* GI perforation, diarrhea
HEMA: Neutropenia, thrombocytopenia, bleeding, hypereosinophilia
INTEG: *Rash, pruritus,* alopecia, photosensitivity, drug rash with eosinophilia and systemic symptoms (DRESS)
META: *Fluid retention, hypokalemia, edema*
MISC: Fatigue, epistaxis, pyrexia, night sweats, increased weight, flulike symptoms, hypothyroidism, tumor lysis syndrome
MS: Cramps, pain, arthralgia, myalgia
RESP: Cough, dyspnea, nasopharyngitis, pneumonia, pleural effusion

PHARMACOKINETICS

Well absorbed (98%); protein binding 95%; metabolized by CYP3A4; excreted in feces, small amount in urine; peak 2-4 hr; duration 24 hr (imatinib), 40 hr (metabolite); half-life 18-40 hr

INTERACTIONS

Increase: imatinib concentrations—CYP3A4 inhibitors (ketoconazole, itraconazole, erythromycin, clarithromycin)
Increase: plasma concentrations of simvastatin, calcium channel blockers, ergots
Increase: plasma concentration of warfarin; avoid use with warfarin; use low-molecular-weight anticoagulants instead

Decrease: imatinib concentrations—CYP3A4 inducers (dexamethasone, phenytoin, carBAMazepine, rifAMPin, PHENobarbital)

Drug/Herb
Decrease: imatinib concentration—St. John's wort

Drug/Food
Increase: effect of grapefruit juice, avoid use

Drug/Lab Test
Increase: bilirubin, amylase, LFTs
Decrease: albumin, calcium, potassium, sodium, phosphate, platelets, neutrophils, leukocytes, lymphocytes

NURSING CONSIDERATIONS

Assess:
• **Bone marrow suppression:** ANC, platelets; during chronic phase, if ANC <1 × 10^9/L and/or platelets <50 × 10^9/L, stop until ANC >1.5 × 10^9/L and platelets >75 × 10^9/L; during accelerated phase/blast crisis, if ANC <0.5 × 10^9/L and/or platelets <10 × 10^9/L, determine whether cytopenia related to biopsy/aspirate; if not, reduce dose by 200 mg; if cytopenia continues, reduce dose by another 100 mg; if cytopenia continues for 4 wk, stop product until ANC ≥1 × 10^9/L
• Monitor CBC weekly for first month, biweekly next month and periodically thereafter; may cause neutropenia (2-3 wk) and thrombocytopenia (3-4 wk) and anemia; may need dosage decrease or discontinuation
• **Renal toxicity:** if bilirubin >3 × UNL, withhold imatinib until bilirubin levels return to <1.5 × UNL
• **DRESS:** swelling of face, fever, rash, later hepatitis, myocarditis may occur, discontinue if present (rare)
• **Hepatotoxicity:** monitor LFTs before and during treatment monthly; if liver transaminases >5 × UNL, withhold imatinib until transaminase levels return to <2.5 × UNL
• Signs of fluid retention, edema: weigh, monitor lung sounds, assess for edema; some fluid retention is dose dependent
• **Pregnancy/breastfeeding:** do not use in pregnancy and for 14 days after last dose, breastfeeding

---

Evaluate:
• **Therapeutic response:** decrease in leukemic cells or size of tumor
Teach patient/family:
• To report adverse reactions immediately: shortness of breath, swelling of extremities, bleeding
• About reason for treatment, expected results
• That effect on male infertility is unknown
• Not to stop or change dose
• To avoid hazardous activities until response is known, dizziness may occur
• To take with food and water; for those unable to swallow tabs, to mix in liquid (30 mL for 100 mg); after dissolved, stir and consume; avoid grapefruit juice
• To avoid OTC products unless approved by prescriber
• To notify prescriber if pregnancy is planned or suspected; not to breastfeed; to use effective contraception

---

imipenem/cilastatin (Rx)

(i-me-pen′em/sye-la-stat′in)

Primaxin IM, Primaxin IV

Func. class.: Antiinfective—miscellaneous

Chem. class.: Carbapenem

ACTION: Interferes with cell-wall replication of susceptible organisms; osmotically unstable cell-wall swells, bursts from osmotic pressure; addition of cilastatin prevents renal inactivation that occurs with high urinary concentrations of imipenem

USES: Serious infections caused by gram-positive *Streptococcus pneumoniae,* group A β-hemolytic streptococci, *Staphylococcus aureus,* enterococcus; gram-negative *Klebsiella, Proteus, Escherichia coli, Acinetobacter, Serratia, Pseudomonas aeruginosa, Salmonella, Shigella, Haemophilus influenzae, Listeria* sp.; lower respiratory tract infections, UTIs, septicemia, endocarditis, bone/joint infections, skin structure infections

CONTRAINDICATIONS
Hypersensitivity to this product, amide local anesthetics, or carbapenems; AV block, shock (IM), breastfeeding
Precautions: Pregnancy, breastfeeding, children, geriatric patients, seizure disorders, renal disease, head trauma; hypersensitivity to cephalosporins, penicillins; CDAD, ulcerative colitis, diabetes mellitus

DOSAGE AND ROUTES
Doses based on imipenem content are to be used IV infusion only
Most infections
• **Adult IV** 500-1000 mg every 6-8 hr depending on indication and organism susceptibility; max 4 g/day
• **Adolescent/child/infant ≥3 mo: IV** 15-25 mg/kg every 6 hr
• **Infant 1-3 mo and ≥1500 g: IV** 25 mg/kg every 6 hr
• **Neonate 1-4 wk and ≥1500 g: IV** 25 mg/kg every 8 hr
• **Neonate <7 days and ≥1500 g: IV** 25 mg/kg every 12 hr
Neutropenic fever (unlabeled) Adult: IV 500 mg q6hr until a febrile for ≥48 hr and ANC 500 cells/mm^3 and increases

Renal dose
• **Adult: CCr 60-89 mL/min:** adjust to 400 mg every 6 hr for starting dose of 500 mg every 6 hr, to 500 mg every 6 hr for starting dose of 1 g every 8 hr, to 750 mg every 8 hr for starting dose of 1 g every 6 hr
CCr 30-59 mL/min: adjust to 300 mg every 6 hr for starting dose of 500 mg every 6 hr, to 500 mg every 8 hr for starting dose of 1 g every 8 hr, to 500 mg every 6 hr for starting dose of 1 g every 6 hr
CCr 15-29 mL/min: adjust to 200 mg every 6 hr for starting dose of 500 mg every 6 hr, to 500 mg every 12 hr for starting dose of 1 g every 6 or 8 hr
CCr <15 mL/min: Do not use unless hemodialysis is instituted within 48 hr
Available forms: Powder for sol inj 250/250, 500/500 mg

Side effects: *italics* = common; red = life-threatening

Administer:
• After C&S is taken, may start treatment before results are received
Intermittent IV infusion route
• After reconstitution of 250 or 500 mg with 10 mL of diluent and shake, add to ≥100 mL of same infusion sol
• 250-500 mg over 20-30 min; ≥750 mg over 40-60 min; give through Y-tube or 3-way stopcock; do not give by IV bolus or if cloudy, do not admix with other antibiotics separate by ≥1 hr (aminoglycosides)
• **Storage:** 4 hr at room temperature, 24 hr refrigerated

Y-site compatibilities: Acyclovir, alfentanil, amifostine, amikacin, aminocaproic acid, anidulafungin, argatroban, ascorbic acid, atenolol, atracurium, atropine, benztropine, bivalirudin, bleomycin, bumetanide, buprenorphine, butorphanol, CARBOplatin, carmustine, caspofungin, ceFAZolin, cefotaxime, cefoTEtan, cefOXitin, cefTAZidime, cefuroxime, chloramphenicol, cimetidine, cisatracurium, CISplatin, clindamycin, codeine, cyanocobalamin, cyclophosphamide, cycloSPORINE, cytarabine, DACTINomycin, dexamethasone, dexrazoxane, digoxin, diltiaZEM, diphenhydrAMINE, DOCEtaxel, dolasetron, DOPamine, doxacurium, DOXOrubicin, DOXOrubicin liposomal, doxycycline, enalaprilat, famotidine, fludarabine, foscarnet, granisetron, IDArubicin, insulin (regular), melphalan, methotrexate, ondansetron, propofol, remifentanil, tacrolimus, teniposide, thiotepa, vinorelbine, zidovudine

SIDE EFFECTS
CNS: *Fever, somnolence, seizures,* confusion, *dizziness,* weakness, myoclonus, drowsiness
CV: Hypotension, palpitations, tachycardia
GI: *Diarrhea, nausea, vomiting,* CDAD, hepatitis, glossitis, gastroenteritis, abdominal pain, jaundice

HEMA: Eosinophilia
INTEG: *Rash, urticaria, pruritus,* pain at inj site, phlebitis, erythema at inj site, erythema multiforme, Stevens-Johnson syndrome, toxic epidermal necrolysis, angioedema
EENT: Hearing loss, tinnitus
SYST: Anaphylaxis, electrolyte abnormalities

PHARMACOKINETICS
IV: Onset immediate, peak 20 min-1 hr; duration 6-8 hr
70%-80% excreted unchanged in urine

INTERACTIONS
Increase: imipenem plasma levels—probenecid
Increase: antagonistic effect—β-lactam antibiotics
Increase: seizure risk—ganciclovir, theophylline, aminophylline, cycloSPORINE
Decrease: effect of valproic acid
Decrease: effect aminoglycosides if admixed
Drug/Lab Test
Increase: AST, ALT, LDH, BUN, alk phos, bilirubin, creatinine, potassium, chloride
Decrease: sodium
False positive: direct Coombs' test

NURSING CONSIDERATIONS
Assess:
• Renal studies: creatinine/BUN, electrolytes
• **Seizures:** product decreases seizure threshold and may decrease effectiveness of seizure medications; monitor closely
• **Infection:** increased temperature, WBC, characteristics of wounds, sputum, urine or stool culture
• Sensitivity to penicillin, other β-lactams—may have sensitivity to this product
• Renal disease: lower dose may be required
• **CDAD:** Bowel pattern daily; if severe diarrhea occurs, product should be discontinued; may indicate CDAD

- **Allergic reactions, anaphylaxis:** rash, urticaria, pruritus, wheezing, laryngeal edema; may occur a few days after therapy begins; have EPINEPHrine, antihistamine, emergency equipment available
- **Overgrowth of infection:** perineal itching, fever, malaise, redness, pain, swelling, drainage, rash, diarrhea, change in cough, sputum
- **Pregnancy/breastfeeding:** use only if benefit outweighs fetal risk; use caution in breastfeeding, excretion unknown

Evaluate:
- **Therapeutic response:** negative C&S; absence of signs and symptoms of infection

Teach patient/family:
- To report severe diarrhea; may indicate CDAD

TREATMENT OF ANAPHYLAXIS: EPINEPHrine, antihistamines; resuscitate if needed

imipenem/cilastatin/relebactam (Rx)

(im'i-pen'em/sye'la-stat'in/rel'e-bak'tam)

Recarbrio

Func. class.: Antiinfective

USES: Intraabdominal infection, complicated; pneumonia, hospital acquired or ventilator associated; urinary tract infection, complicated (including pyelonephritis)

DOSAGE AND ROUTES
Intra-abdominal infection, complicated
Adult: IV: 1.25 g every 6 hr. Total duration of therapy is 4 to 7 days following adequate source control
Pneumonia, hospital acquired or ventilator associated:
Adult: IV: 1.25 g every 6 hr × 7 days as part of an appropriate combination regimen

Urinary tract infection, complicated (including pyelonephritis)
Adult: IV: 1.25 g every 6 hr × 5 to 14 days
Available forms: Powder for injection

imipramine (Rx)

(im-ip'ra-meen)
Func. class.: Antidepressant, tricyclic
Chem. class.: Dibenzazepine, tertiary amine

Do not confuse:
imipramine/desipramine

ACTION: Blocks reuptake of norepinephrine, serotonin into nerve endings, thereby increasing action of norepinephrine, serotonin in nerve cells

USES: Major depression, enuresis
Unlabeled uses: Bulimia, neuropathic pain, panic disorder, ADHD, stress/urge incontinence, social phobia

CONTRAINDICATIONS
Pregnancy, hypersensitivity to this product or carBAMazepine; acute MI, MAOI therapy
Precautions: Breastfeeding, geriatric patients, suicidal patients, severe depression, increased intraocular pressure, closed-angle glaucoma, urinary retention, cardiac/hepatic disease, hyperthyroidism, electroshock therapy, elective surgery, seizure disorders, prostatic hypertrophy, MI, AV block, bundle branch block, ileus, QT prolongation, hypersensitivity to tricyclics

Black Box Warning: Children; suicidal ideation

DOSAGE AND ROUTES
Depression
- **Adult: PO** 75-100 mg/day in divided doses, may increase by 25-50 mg to 200 mg/day (outpatients), 300 mg/day (inpatients); may give daily dose at bedtime

• **Adolescent/geriatric: PO** 30-40 mg at bedtime, may increase to 100 mg/day in divided doses
• **Child ≥6 yr (unlabeled): PO** 1.5 mg/kg/day in divided doses, max 2.5 mg/kg/day

Enuresis
• **Adolescents: PO** 25 mg daily, 1 hr prior to bedtime, max 75 mg/day
• **Child 6-12 yr: PO** 25 mg daily 1 hr prior to bedtime; max 50 mg/day

Available forms: Tabs 10, 25, 50, ✦ mg; caps 75, 100, 125, 150 mg

Administer:

PO route
• Improvement may take 1-2 wk (sleep, energy); 1-4 wk (improved mood) 6-12 wk (optimal mood)
• Not to break, crush, or chew caps
• With food or milk for GI symptoms
• Dosage at bedtime if oversedation occurs during day; may take entire dose at bedtime; geriatric patients may not tolerate once-daily dosing
• Sugarless gum, hard candy, or frequent sips of water for dry mouth
• Do not discontinue abruptly, taper 50% × 3 days, another 50% × 3 days, then stop
• Store in tight container at room temperature; do not freeze

SIDE EFFECTS

CNS: *Dizziness, drowsiness,* confusion, seizures, headache, anxiety, insomnia, suicidal ideation, paresthesia
CV: *Orthostatic hypotension, ECG changes, tachycardia,* dysrhythmias
EENT: Blurred vision, mydriasis, tinnitus
ENDO: Hyperglycemia, hypo/hyperthyroidism, SIADH
GI: *Diarrhea, dry mouth,* nausea, vomiting, paralytic ileus, increased appetite, taste change
GU: *Retention,* decreased libido
HEMA: Agranulocytosis, thrombocytopenia, eosinophilia, leukopenia
INTEG: Rash, urticaria, pruritus, photosensitivity
SYST: serotonin syndrome

PHARMACOKINETICS

Metabolized to desipramine in liver by CYP2D6; excreted in urine, breast milk, feces; crosses placenta; half-life 8-16 hr, protein binding 90%-95%

INTERACTIONS

• **Increase:** Hyperpyretic crisis, seizures, hypertensive episode: MAOIs, cloNIDine
• **Increase:** serotonin syndrome, neuroleptic malignant syndrome—SSRIs, SNRIs, serotonin-receptor agonists, bupropion, cyclobenzapine, trazadone, tramadil, tricyclics; avoid concurrent use, linezolid, methylene blue IV

Increase: QT interval—class IA/III antidysrhythmics, tricyclics, gatifloxacin, levoFLOXacin, moxifloxacin, ziprasidone

Increase: effects of direct-acting sympathomimetics (EPINEPHrine), alcohol, barbiturates, benzodiazepines, CNS depressants

Decrease: effects of guanethidine, cloNIDine, indirect-acting sympathomimetics (ePHEDrine)

Drug/Herb
Increase: serotonin syndrome—SAM-e, St. John's wort
Increase: sedation—chamomile, kava, valerian

Drug/Lab Test
Increase: serum bilirubin, alk phos, blood glucose, LFTs
Mental status: mood, sensorium, affect, **suicidal tendencies** especially in children, young adults; increase in psychiatric symptoms: depression, panic, monitor weekly × 1 mo, then 3 wk give limited amount of product

NURSING CONSIDERATIONS

Assess:

Black Box Warning: Depression: mood, behavior, sleep, lability; mental status, suicidal tendencies especially in children, young adults; increase in psychiatric symptoms, panic, monitor weekly × 1 mo, then q3wk, give limited amount of medication

- **CV:** B/P (lying, standing), pulse; if systolic B/P drops 20 mm Hg, hold product, notify prescriber, monitor HR, rhythm, take ECG baseline in those with CV disease
- **Blood studies:** CBC, leukocytes, differential, cardiac enzymes, serum imipramine levels (125-250 ng/mL) if patient is receiving long-term therapy
- **Hepatic studies:** AST, ALT, bilirubin
- Weight weekly; appetite may increase with product
- **QT prolongation:** monitor ECG for flattening of T wave, bundle branch block, AV block, dysrhythmias in cardiac patients
- EPS primarily in geriatric patients: rigidity, dystonia, akathisia
- Urinary retention, constipation; constipation is more likely to occur in children, geriatric patients; increase fluids, bulk in diet
- **Withdrawal symptoms:** headache, nausea, vomiting, muscle pain, weakness, diarrhea, insomnia, restlessness; not usual unless product is discontinued abruptly
- **Serotonin syndrome, hypertensive episodes, orthostatic hypotension:** identify drug interactions before use of product
- Alcohol consumption; if alcohol is consumed, hold dose until morning
- Assistance with ambulation during beginning therapy because drowsiness, dizziness, orthostatic hypotension may occur
- Safety measures, primarily for geriatric patients
- **Beers:** avoid in older adults; highly anticholinergic, high risk of delirium, orthostatic hypotension

Evaluate:
- **Therapeutic response:** decreased depression, enuresis

Teach patient/family:
- That full therapeutic effects may take 2-3 wk
- That product may be dispensed in small amounts because of suicide potential, especially at beginning of therapy

- To use caution when driving, performing other activities requiring alertness because of drowsiness, dizziness, blurred vision
- To report urinary retention immediately
- To avoid alcohol, other CNS depressants during treatment
- Not to discontinue medication abruptly after long-term use; may cause nausea, headache, malaise
- To wear sunscreen or large hat because photosensitivity occurs
- To rise slowly, orthostatic hypotension may occur

Black Box Warning: To report suicidal thoughts, behaviors immediately; more common in children, young adults

- **Pregnancy/breastfeeding:** Identify if pregnancy is planned or suspected or if breastfeeding

TREATMENT OF OVERDOSE:
ECG monitoring; lavage if recently ingested; sodium bicarbonate (cardiac effects); administer anticonvulsant, antidysrrthmics

immune globulin IM (IMIG/IGIM) (Rx)
GamaSTAN
immune globulin IV (IGIV, IVIG) (Rx)
Flebogamma 10% DIF, Gammagard S/D, Gammagard Liquid 10%, Gammaked, Gammaplex, Gamunex, Octagam, Privigen
immune globulin SC (SCIG/IGSC) (Rx)
Gammagard 10%, Gammaked, Gamunex 10%, Hizentra
Func. class.: Immune serum
Chem. class.: IgG

USES: Replacement for primary and secondary hormonal immunodeficiency syndrome; B-cell chronic lymphocytic leukemia; Kawasaki syndrome; bone marrow transplantation; pediatric HIV infection; agammaglobulinemia; hepatitis A, B exposure; measles exposure; measles vaccine complications; purpura; rubella exposure; chickenpox exposure; chronic inflammatory demyelinating polyneuropathy, multifocal motor neuropathy, MS, RA, myasthenia gravis

CONTRAINDICATIONS

Hypersensitivity, coagulopathy, hemophilia, IgA deficiency, thrombocytopenia, fructose intolerance

DOSAGE AND ROUTES

Immune globulin IM (IMIG, IGIM)
Hepatitis A prophylaxis
• **Adult/geriatric/adolescent/child/infant (unlabeled): IM** 0.02 mL/kg for those who have not received hepatitis A vaccine and have been exposed during the prior 2 wk
Measles prophylaxis (exposed during prior 6 days)
• **Adult: IM** 0.25 mL/kg (immunocompetent)
• **Child (unlabeled): IM** 0.5 mL/kg as a single dose, max 15 mL (immunocompromised)
Varicella prophylaxis
• **Adult: IM** 0.6-1.2 mL/kg as soon as possible and if varicella-zoster immune globulin is not available
Rubella prophylaxis in exposed/susceptible individual who will not consider a therapeutic abortion
• **Adult pregnant women: IM** 0.55 mL/kg
Immunoglobulin deficiency
• **Adult: IM** 1.32 mL/kg, then 0.66 mL/kg (≥100 mg/kg) q3-4wk
Immune globulin IV (IVIG, IGIV)
Primary immunodeficiency
Gammagard S/D
• **Adult/adolescent/child: IV** 300-600 mg/kg q3-4wk
Gamunex
• **Adult/adolescent/child: IV INFUSION** 300-600 mg/kg (3-6 mL/kg) q3-4wk,

initial infusion rate 1 mg/kg/min (max 8 mg/kg/min)
Gammagard Liquid/Flebogamma 5%
• **Adult/adolescent/child: IV** 300-600 mg/kg q3-4wk
Privigen
• **Adult/adolescent/child ≥3 yr: IV** 200-800 mg q3wk

Idiopathic thrombocytopenic purpura (ITP)
Gammagard S/D
• **Adult/adolescent/child: IV** 1000 mg/kg as a single dose; may give on alternate days for up to 3 doses
Gamunex
• **Adult/adolescent/child: IV INFUSION** total dose of 2000 mg/kg on 2 consecutive days; initial rate is 1 mg/kg/min (max 8 mg/kg/min); if after 1st dose, adequate platelets are observed after 24 hr, may withhold 2nd dose
Privigen
• **Adult/adolescent ≥15 yr: IV** 1 g/kg/day × 2 days

Kawasaki disease
Gammagard S/D
• **Infant/child: IV** 1000 mg/kg as a single dose or 400 mg/kg/day × 4 days beginning within 7 days of fever onset, with aspirin 80-100 mg/kg/day × 4 divided doses
Immune globulin SC (SCIG/IGSC)
• **Adult/child >2 yr: SUBCUT INFUSION** 100-200 mg/kg weekly, **Vivaglobin** brand of SCIG 160 mg IgG/mL, **SUBCUT** inj 15 mL/inj site, given at max of 20 mL/hr
Hizentra
• **Adult/child:** multiply the previous IVIG dose by 1.37, then divide into weekly dose based on previous week treatment

---

imiquimod (Rx)
(i-mi-kwi′mod)
Aldara, Vyloma ✦,
Zyclara, Zyclara Pump
Func. class.: Immunosuppressant

USES:

Actinic keratosis, genital and perianal warts, superficial basal cell carcinoma

DOSAGE AND ROUTES
Actinic keratosis
Adult: Topical: 2.5% and 3.75% cream: Apply thin film (using up to 2 packets or 2 full pump actuations) daily before bedtime for 2 wk to the skin of the affected area (either the entire face or balding scalp, but not both concurrently); leave on for ~8 hr, then remove with mild soap and water. After a 2-wk period of no treatment, repeat with a second 2-wk treatment (do not extend treatment cycles because of missed doses or rest periods)
Genital and perianal warts
Adult/child ≥12
Topical: 3.75% cream: Apply a thin layer once daily (using up to 1 packet or 1 full actuation of pump) prior to bedtime; leave on skin for ~8 hr, then remove with mild soap and water. Continue treatment until there is total clearance of the warts or for a maximum duration of therapy of 8 wk
Superficial basal cell carcinoma (Aldara 5% cream)
Adult: Topical: Apply once daily 5 days per week, prior to normal sleeping hours, for 6 wk; leave on skin for ~8 hr, then remove with mild soap and water. Apply enough cream to cover the treatment area, including 1 cm of skin surrounding the tumor. Tumor treatment area should not exceed 3 cm

---

indapamide (Rx)
(in-dap′a-mide)
Func. class.: Diuretic—thiazide-like, antihypertensive
Chem. class.: Indoline

USES: Edema of HF, mild-moderate hypertension may be used alone or in combination
DOSAGE AND ROUTES
Edema
• **Adult: PO** 2.5 mg/day in ᴀᴍ; may be increased to 5 mg/day if needed after 1 wk
Antihypertensive
• **Adult: PO** 1.25 mg/day in ᴀᴍ; may increase to 2.5 mg/day after 4 wk; if not effective after 4 wk, may increase to max dose of 5 mg/day
Available forms: Tabs 1.25, 2.5 mg

---

indomethacin (Rx)
(in-doe-meth′a-sin)
Indocin, Indocin IV
Func. class.: Nonsteroidal antiinflammatory product (NSAID), antirheumatic
Chem. class.: Acetic acid derivative

ACTION: Inhibits prostaglandin synthesis by decreasing enzyme needed for biosynthesis; analgesic, antiinflammatory, antipyretic

USES: RA, ankylosing spondylitis, osteoarthritis, bursitis, tendinitis, acute gouty arthritis; closure of patent ductus arteriosus in premature infants (IV)
CONTRAINDICATIONS
Pregnancy after 30 wk, aortic coarctation, bleeding, salicylate/NSAID hypersensitivity, GI bleeding

Black Box Warning: Perioperative pain in CABG, GI bleeding/perforation

Precautions: Pregnancy before 30 wk, breastfeeding, children, bleeding disorders, GI disorders, cardiac disorders, depression, renal/hepatic disease, asthma, diabetes, acute bronchospasm, ulcerative colitis, seizures, Parkinson's disease, neonates, stroke

Black Box Warning: Stroke, MI, those taking NSAIDs are at greater risk of MI and stroke, even in first few weeks of therapy, thromboembolism

DOSAGE AND ROUTES
Arthritis/antiinflammatory
• **Adult/child ≥15 yr: PO** 25-50 mg bid-tid; max 200 mg/day; **EXT REL** 75 mg/day, may increase to 75 mg bid

---

Gout
• **Adult/child >15 yr: PO** 50 mg tid; use only for acute attack, then reduce dose
Rectal route for all uses
• **Adult: PR** 50 mg bid or 100 mg at bedtime (max 200 mg/day)
Patent ductus arteriosus
• **Neonate >8 days: IV** Initially, 0.2 mg/kg, then, if necessary, 2 more doses of 0.25 mg/kg at 12-hr intervals if urine output is >1 mL/kg/hr after prior dose or at 24-hr intervals if urine output is <1 mL/kg/hr; hold in cases of oliguria (<0.6 mL/kg/hr) or anuria
• **Neonate 2-7 days: IV** Initially, 0.2 mg/kg, then, if necessary, 2 more doses of 0.2 mg/kg at 12-hr intervals if urine output is >1 mL/kg/hr after prior dose or at 24-hr intervals if urine output is <1 mL/kg/hr; hold in cases of oliguria (<0.6 mL/kg/hr) or anuria
• **Neonate <2 days: IV** Initially, 0.2 mg/kg, then, if necessary, 1 or 2 doses of 0.1 mg/kg at 12-hr intervals if urine output is >1 mL/kg/hr after prior dose or at 24-hr intervals if urine output is <1 mL/kg/hr; hold in cases of oliguria (<0.6 mL/kg/hr) or anuria
• **Neonate: PO** Doses of 0.3 mg/kg daily × 2 days have been used
Available forms: Caps 20, 25, 50 mg; ext rel caps 75 mg; powder for inj 1-mg vial; rectal suppository 50, 100 ♣ mg; oral susp 5 mg/mL (25 mg/5 mL)
Administer:
PO route
• Do not break, crush, or chew sus rel cap or reg caps
• With food to decrease GI symptoms and prevent ulcerations
• Shake susp; do not mix with other liquids
• Store at room temperature
Rectal route
• Use suppository that is not soft, may place in refrigerator for 15 min before use
Direct IV route
• After reconstituting 1 mg with 1 or 2 mL NS or sterile water for inj without preservative; to give 1 or 0.5 mg/mL, respectively; do not dilute further
• Infuse over 20-30 min; avoid extravasation
• Do not inject/infuse via umbilical catheter to avoid dramatic shift in cerebral blood flow

SIDE EFFECTS
CNS: Dizziness, drowsiness, fatigue, confusion, insomnia, anxiety, depression, *headache*
CV: Peripheral edema, hypertension, CV thrombotic events, MI, stroke
EENT: Tinnitus, hearing loss, blurred vision
GI: *Nausea,* anorexia, *vomiting,* diarrhea, jaundice, *constipation,* flatulence, cramps, peptic ulcer, ulceration, perforation, GI bleeding
GU: Nephrotoxicity: dysuria, hematuria, oliguria; azotemia (IV)
HEMA: Blood dyscrasias, prolonged bleeding
INTEG: Purpura, rash, pruritus, sweating, phlebitis at IV site

PHARMACOKINETICS
PO: Onset 30 min; peak 2 hr; duration 4-6 hr; metabolized in liver, kidneys; excreted in urine 60%, feces 33%; crosses placenta; excreted in breast milk; 99% protein binding; half-life 1 hr 1st pass, 2.6-11.2 hr 2nd pass

INTERACTIONS
Increase: hyperkalemia—potassium-sparing diuretics
Increase: toxicity—lithium, methotrexate, cycloSPORINE, probenecid, cidofovir
Increase: effect of—digoxin, phenytoin, aminoglycosides
Increase: bleeding risk—anticoagulants, abciximab, clopidogrel, eptifibatide, plicamycin, ticlopidine, tirofiban, thrombolytics, aspirin, SSRIs, SNRIs
Decrease: effect of—antihypertensives, diuretics
Drug/Herb
Increased: bleeding risk—chamomile, clove, dong quai, garlic, ginger, ginkgo
Drug/Lab
Increase: Potassium, LFTs
Decrease: Hb, Hct

NURSING CONSIDERATIONS
Assess:
• **Arthritis symptoms:** ROM, pain, swelling before and 2 hr after treatment

• **Hypersensitivity:** monitor for rash (those with aspirin sensitivity, nasal polyps are at greater risk)

Black Box Warning: Cardiac disease, CV, thrombotic events (MI, stroke) before administration, not to be used in perioperative pain in CABG surgery

• Patent ductus arteriosus: respiratory rate, character, heart sounds
• **Renal, hepatic, blood studies:** BUN, creatinine, AST, ALT, HB before treatment, periodically thereafter; if renal function has decreased, do not give subsequent doses
• **Eye/ear problems:** blurred vision, tinnitus; may indicate toxicity; audiometric, ophthalmic exam before, during, after treatment if patient receiving long-term therapy
• Confusion, mood changes, hallucinations, especially among geriatric patients
• Asthma, nasal polyps, aspirin sensitivity, may develop hypersensitivity to indomethacin

Black Box Warning: GI bleeding/perforation: chronic use can lead to GI bleeding, use cautiously in those with a history of active GI disease

Black Box Warning: MI, stroke: may be greater with longer-term use and in those with CV risk factors

• **Beers:** avoid use in older adults; more likely to cause CNS effects
• **Pregnancy/breastfeeding:** do not use after 30 wk gestation; use only if benefits outweigh fetal risk <30 wk gestation; do not breastfeed, excreted in breast milk
Evaluate:
• **Therapeutic response:** decreased pain, stiffness, swelling in joints; ability to move more easily, PDA closure
Teach patient/family:
• To report blurred vision, ringing, roaring in ears; may indicate toxicity
• To avoid driving, other hazardous activities if dizziness, drowsiness occurs

• To report change in urine pattern, increased weight, edema, increased pain in joints, fever, blood in urine; may indicate nephrotoxicity
• To take with food for GI upset, to use as prescribed, not to skip or double doses, to take with 8 oz of water
• To report signs of GI bleeding: dark stools, hematemesis
• To report mood changes: anxiety, depression
• To use sunscreen, protective clothing, hat to prevent burns
• That therapeutic antiinflammatory effects may take up to 1 mo
• To avoid alcohol, NSAIDs, salicylates because bleeding may occur, discuss all OTC, Rx, herbals, supplements with health care professional
• To report use to all health care providers

Black Box Warning: MI/stroke: to immediately report and seek medical attention for signs/symptoms of MI/stroke; discontinue product

inFLIXimab (Rx)
(in-fliks′ih-mab)
Remicade
infliximab-abda (Rx)
Renflexis
infliximab-dyyb (Rx)
Inflectra
infliximab-qbtx (Rx)
Ixifi
Func. class.: Biologic response modifiers
Chem. class.: Tumor necrosis factor modifiers

Do not confuse:
Remicade/Renacidin
inFLIXimab/riTUXimab

ACTION: Monoclonal antibody that neutralizes the activity of tumor necrosis factor-alpha (TNF-α) found in Crohn's disease; decreased infiltration of inflammatory cells

USES: Ankylosing spondylitis, Crohn's disease (adult/child), plaque psoriasis, psoriatic arthritis, rheumatoid arthritis, ulcerative colitis (adult/child)

Unlabeled uses: Behcet's (uveitis) syndrome, resistant Kawasaki disease, multisystem inflammatory syndrome in children

CONTRAINDICATIONS

Hypersensitivity to murines, moderate to severe HF (NYHA class III/IV)

Precautions: Pregnancy, breastfeeding, children, geriatric patients, COPD, hepatotoxicity, hematologic abnormalities, hepatitis B, Guillain-Barré syndrome, seizures, multiple sclerosis

Black Box Warning: Infection, neoplastic disease, TB

DOSAGE AND ROUTES

Rheumatoid arthritis (in combination with methotrexate therapy)

Adult: IV: 3 mg/kg at 0, 2, and 6 wk, followed by a maintenance regimen of 3 mg/kg every 8 wk thereafter; may adjust dose up to 10 mg/kg every 4-8 wk

Ankylosing spondylitis

Adult: IV: 5 mg/kg at 0, 2, and 6 wk, followed by 5 mg/kg every 6 wk thereafter

Crohn's disease

Adult: IV: 5 mg/kg at 0, 2, and 6 wk, followed by 5 mg/kg every 8 wk thereafter; may increase to 10 mg/kg every 8 wk in patients who respond but then lose their response. If no response by wk 14, consider discontinuing therapy

Inflectra/Renflexis:

Child ≥6 yr/adolescent: IV Initial: 5 mg/kg/dose at 0, 2, and 6 wk, followed by maintenance: 5 mg/kg/dose every 8 wk thereafter

Plaque psoriasis

Adult: IV: 5 mg/kg at 0, 2, and 6 wk, followed by 5 mg/kg every 8 wk thereafter

Psoriatic arthritis (with or without methotrexate)

Adult: IV: 5 mg/kg at 0, 2, and 6 wk, followed by 5 mg/kg every 8 wk thereafter

Ulcerative colitis

Adult

IV: 5 mg/kg at 0, 2, and 6 wk, followed by 5 mg/kg every 8 wk thereafter

Child ≥6 yr/adolescent: IV Initial: 5 mg/kg/dose at 0, 2, and 6 wk, followed by maintenance: 5 mg/kg/dose every 8 wk thereafter

Juvenile idiopathic arthritis; refractory to conventional disease-modifying drugs:

Children ≥4 yr and adolescents: IV: Initial: 3 mg/kg at 0, 2, and 6 wk; then 3 to 6 mg/kg/dose every 8 wk thereafter in combination with methotrexate during induction and maintenance. Alternatively, some studies used 6 mg/kg/dose starting at wk 14 of a methotrexate induction regimen (wk 0 to 13); repeat dose (6 mg/kg/dose) at wk 16 and 20, then every 8 wk thereafter

Available forms: Powder for inj 100 mg

Administer:

Intermittent IV INFUSION route

• Pretreat with diphenhydrAMINE, acetaminophen, predniSONE if a reaction is infusion related

• Give immediately after reconstitution; reconstitute each vial with 10 mL sterile water for inj; further dilute total dose/250 mL of 0.9% NaCl inj to a total concentration of 0.4-4 mg/mL; use 21-G or smaller needle for reconstitution; direct sterile water at glass wall of vial; gently swirl; do not shake; may foam; allow to stand for 5 min, give within 3 hr

• Give over ≥2 hr, use polyethylene-lined infusion with in-line, sterile, low–protein-binding filter

• Do not admix

• Refrigerated storage; do not freeze

SIDE EFFECTS

CNS: *Headache, dizziness, depression, vertigo, fatigue, anxiety, fever,* seizures, *chills, flulike symptoms,* demyelinating disease

CV: Chest pain, hypo/hypertension, tachycardia, HF, acute coronary syndrome

GI: *Nausea, vomiting, abdominal pain, stomatitis, constipation, dyspepsia, flatulence*

GU: Dysuria, urinary frequency

HEMA: Anemia, leukopenia, thrombocytopenia, pancytopenia

INTEG: *Rash, dermatitis, urticaria,* dry skin, sweating, flushing, hematoma, pruritus, keratoderma blenorrhagicum

MS: Myalgia, back pain, arthralgia

RESP: URI, pharyngitis, bronchitis, cough, dyspnea, sinusitis

SYST: Anaphylaxis, fatal infections, sepsis, malignancies, immunogenicity, Stevens-Johnson syndrome, toxic epidermal necrolysis, sarcoidosis

PHARMACOKINETICS
Distributed to vascular compartment, half-life 9.5 days

INTERACTIONS
Increase: infections, neutropenia—TNF blockers (abatacept, anakinra, golimumab, rilonacept); avoid concurrent use
• Do not administer live vaccines concurrently

NURSING CONSIDERATIONS
Assess:
• **RA:** pain, joints involved, ROM, aggravating ameliorating factors baseline and periodically
• **Plaque psoriasis:** lesions, body areas affected baseline and periodically
• **Ulcerative colitis/Crohn's disease:** pain, cramping, diarrhea, change in life style baseline and periodically
• **GI symptoms:** nausea, vomiting, abdominal pain
• **Labs:** Periodic blood counts (CBC with differential), ANA titer, LFTs, baseline and periodically, may cause blood dyscrasia, discontinue if present; obtain TB test before using
• **CV status:** B/P, pulse, chest pain
• **Allergic reaction, anaphylaxis:** rash, dermatitis, urticaria, dyspnea, hypotension, fever, chills; discontinue

if severe, administer EPINEPHrine, corticosteroids, antihistamines; assess for allergies to murine proteins before starting therapy

Black Box Warning: Fatal infections: discontinue if infection occurs, do not administer to patients with active infection; identify TB before beginning treatment; a TB test should be obtained; if present, TB should be treated before patient receives product; exercise caution when switching from 1 DMARD to another

Black Box Warning: For neoplastic disease in those <18 yr, including hepatosplenic T-cell lymphoma; usually occurs in those with inflammatory bowel disease

• **Pregnancy/breastfeeding:** Avoid use in pregnancy, effect unknown, do not breastfeed
Evaluate:
• **Therapeutic response:** absence of fever, mucus in stools
Teach patient/family:
• That infusion reaction should be reported immediately
• To notify prescriber immediately if infection occurs
• To notify prescriber of GI symptoms, hypersensitivity reactions, heart symptoms
• Not to operate machinery or drive if dizziness, vertigo occur
• To avoid live virus vaccinations; bring up-to-date before use
• **Malignancy:** check skin for changes, growths, or color changes
• **Pregnancy/breastfeeding:** identify if pregnancy is planned or suspected

---

inotersen (Rx)
(in-oh-ter′sen)
Tegsedi
Func. class.: Metabolic agent

USES:
Polyneuropathy of hereditary transthyretin mediated amyloidosis

Black Box Warning: Glomerulonephritis, thrombocytopenia

DOSAGE AND ROUTES
Adult: SUBCUT 284 mg once weekly on same day each wk
Available forms: Prefilled syringe solution for injection 284 mg/1.5 mL

⚠ HIGH ALERT

inotuzumab ozogamicin (Rx)
(ih-noh-too′-zoo-mab oh′-zoh-ga-MIH-sin)

Besponsa
Func. class.: Antineoplastic monoclonal antibodies

ACTION: A CD22-directed antibody-drug conjugate; CD22 is expressed on pre–B cells and mature B cells. It consists of a cytotoxic agent; it induces DNA breaks, resulting in cell-cycle arrest and apoptotic cell death

USES: For the treatment of adults with relapsed or refractory B-cell precursor acute lymphoblastic leukemia

CONTRAINDICATIONS
Pregnancy, hypersensitivity

Black Box Warning: Hepatic disease, hepatotoxicity, mortality, sinusoidal obstructive disease, veno-occlusive disease

Precautions: Alcoholism, bleeding, breastfeeding, contraception requirements, diabetes mellitus, electrolyte imbalances, females, geriatric patients, infertility, male-mediated teratogenicity, neutropenia, bone marrow suppression, infection, reproductive risk, thrombocytopenia, thyroid disease, QT prolongation

DOSAGE AND ROUTES
Relapsed or refractory B-cell precursor ALL
• **Adult:** IV 0.8 mg/m^2 day 1 and 0.5 mg/m^2 days 8 and 15 (cycle 1). Length of cycle 1 is 21 days, may increase to 28 days
Management of treatment-related toxicity
• Do not interrupt doses within a treatment cycle (day 8 or day 15 dose) for neutropenia or thrombocytopenia. Dosing interruptions within a cycle are recommended for nonhematologic toxicity. If a dose reduction is necessary, do not re-escalate the dose
Hematologic toxicity
• **Absolute neutrophil count (ANC) of ≥1 × 10^9 cells/L before starting therapy:** if the ANC decreases, hold next cycle until recovery of the ANC to 1 × 10^9 cells/L or greater. Discontinue therapy if low ANC lasts >28 days and is suspected to be due to inotuzumab ozogamicin
• **Platelet count of ≥50 × 10^9 cells/L before starting therapy:** if platelet count decreases, hold next cycle until the platelet count recovers to 50 × 10^9 cells/L or greater. Discontinue therapy if low platelet count lasts >28 days and is suspected to be due to inotuzumab ozogamicin
• **ANC was <1 × 10^9 cells/L and/or platelet count was <50 × 10^9 cells/L before starting therapy:** if the ANC or platelet count decreases, hold the next cycle until at least 1 of the following occurs: the ANC and platelet counts recover to baseline or better for the prior cycle; the ANC recovers to 1 × 10^9 cells/L or greater and the platelet count recovers to 50 × 10^9 cells/L or greater; the patient has stable or improved disease (based on most recent bone marrow assessment) and the ANC and platelet count decrease is considered to be due to the underlying disease and not product-related toxicity

---

Available forms: Powder for injection 0.9 mg
Administer:
IV route
• Visually inspect for particulate matter and discoloration before use
• Follow cytotoxic handling procedures
• Available as a single-dose, preservative-free, 0.9-mg lyophilized powder vial
• Premedication with a corticosteroid, an antipyretic agent (acetaminophen), and an antihistamine before each dose is recommended; observe patients during and for at least 1 hr after the end of the infusion for symptoms of infusion-related reactions

Reconstitution
• After calculating the number of vials needed, add 4 mL of sterile water for injection to each vial for a final vial concentration of 0.25 mg/mL (0.9 mg/3.6 mL); gently swirl the vial to dissolve powder; do not shake
• The reconstitution solution should be clear to opalescent, colorless to slightly yellow, and free of visible foreign matter
• **Storage of reconstituted vials:** if not further diluted immediately, vials may be stored in the refrigerator (at 2° C-8° C or 36° F-46° F) for up to 4 hr after reconstitution; protect from light, do not freeze
Dilution:
• Add required dose/volume from the reconstituted vials to an infusion container made of polyvinyl chloride (PVC) (or non–DEHP-containing), polyolefin (polypropylene and/or polyethylene), or ethylene vinyl acetate (EVA); discard any unused portion
• Add 0.9% sodium chloride injection to the infusion container for a final total volume of 50 mL; gently invert to mix, do not shake
• **Storage of admixture:** if not infused immediately, the diluted solution may be stored at room temperature (20° C-25° C or 68° F-77° F) for up to 4 hr or refriger-

ated (2° C-8° C or 36° F-46° F) for up to 3 hr; protect from light and do not freeze
Intravenous (IV) Infusion:
• Allow refrigerated admixtures to warm to room temperature for 1 hr before use
• Give admixture (protected from light) as an IV infusion over 1 hr through an infusion line made of PVC, polyolefin (polypropylene and/or polyethylene), or polybutadiene
• Complete infusion within 8 hr of reconstitution
• The diluted solution does not need to be filtered; if it is filtered, use polyethersulfone (PES)-, polyvinylidene fluoride (PVDF)-, or hydrophilic polysulfone (HPS)-based filters
• Do not use filters made of nylon or mixed cellulose ester (MCE)
• Do not mix with or administer as an infusion with other drugs

SIDE EFFECTS
CNS: Fatigue, fever, headache, migraine, chills
GI: Nausea, vomiting, diarrhea, stomatitis, constipation, anorexia, abdominal pain, hepatotoxicity
HEMA: Anemia, thrombocytopenia, bleeding, hematoma, hematuria, ecchymosis, veno-occlusive disease
MISC: Infection, asthenia, QT prolongation, tumor lysis syndrome, sinusoidal obstruction syndrome

PHARMACOKINETICS
Protein binding 97%

INTERACTIONS
Increase: QT prolongation—other products that increase QT prolongation
Drug/Lab Test
Increase: LFTs

NURSING CONSIDERATIONS
Assess:
• **Serious infection:** some may be fatal. Monitor patients for signs and symptoms of infection; use prophylactic anti-infectives as appropriate
• **Severe myelosuppression/bone marrow suppression:** thrombocytopenia, neutropenia; obtain a CBC before each

dose; therapy interruption or permanent discontinuation may be necessary in patients who develop severe myelosuppression

• **QT prolongation:** obtain an electrocardiogram (ECG) and monitor serum electrolytes before the start of treatment and periodically as needed. Use with caution in a history of QT prolongation or electrolyte imbalance

Black Box Warning: Severe or life-threatening hepatotoxicity including veno-occlusive disease (VOD)/sinusoidal obstruction syndrome (SOS): monitor liver function tests (LFTs), total bilirubin, alkaline phosphatase levels before and following each dosage change; therapy interruption, dose reduction, or permanent discontinuation may be necessary in those who develop LFT abnormalities. Closely monitor for VOD/SOS (hepatomegaly, rapid weight gain, and ascites). Permanently discontinue in those who develop VOD/SOS; in those who undergo a hematopoietic stem-cell transplant (HSCT), monitor LFTs frequently during the first month post-HSCT; then, continue to monitor LFTs but less often. Time from HSCT to onset of VOD/SOS was 15 days (range, 3-57 days). The risk of VOD/SOS may be greater in patients who receive an HSCT or a conditioning regimen that contains 2 alkylating agents before HSCT and in patients who have an increased total bilirubin level before an HSCT; other risk factors include hepatic disease (e.g., cirrhosis, nodular regenerative hyperplasia, active hepatitis), a prior HSCT, increased age, later salvage lines, and a greater number of treatment cycles

Black Box Warning: Mortality: those who underwent a hematopoietic stem-cell transplant (HSCT) may have a higher 100-day post-HSCT nonrelapse mortality; monitor closely for post-HSCT toxicity. The most common causes of post-HSCT death were veno-occlusive disease/sinusoidal obstruction syndrome and infectious complications

• **Pregnancy/breastfeeding:** product can cause fetal harm; females of reproductive

potential should avoid becoming pregnant during and for 8 mo after final dose; obtain pregnancy test before starting product; do not breastfeed during and for at least 2 mo after last dose; men with female partners of reproductive potential should avoid fathering a child and use effective contraception during and for at least 5 mo after therapy

Evaluate:

• **Therapeutic response:** improving blood counts

Teach patient/familiy:

• **To report adverse reactions immediately:** bleeding; report diarrhea, hepatic, hematologic symptoms/toxicity, flulike symptoms

• About reason for treatment, expected results

• That monitoring for infusion reactions will be needed for at least 1 hr after infusion has ended

• **Pregnancy/breastfeeding:** to notify provider if pregnancy is planned or suspected; to use effective contraception during treatment and for 8 mo after discontinuing treatment; not to breastfeed during treatment or for 2 mo after final dose; that men with female partners of reproductive potential should avoid fathering a child and use effective contraception during and for at least 5 mo after therapy

⚠ HIGH ALERT
INSULINS

Rapid Acting

insulin aspart (Rx)
Fiasp, Kirsty ✦ NovoLOG, NovoLOG Flexpen, NovoLOG Pen Fill, Novo Rapid ✦, Trurapi ✦

insulin glulisine (Rx)
Apidra, Apidra SoloStar

Inhaled insulin
Afreeza

insulin lispro (Rx)
Admelog, HumaLOG

insulin lispro-aabc (Rx)
Lyumjev

Short Acting
insulin, regular (OTC, Rx)
HumuLIN R, NovoLIN R
Intermediate Acting
insulin, isophane suspension (NPH) (OTC, Rx)
HumuLIN N, Hypurin NPH ✤, NovoLIN ge NPH ✤, NovoLIN N, NovoLIN N Prefilled

Long Acting

insulin detemir (Rx)
Levemir, Levemir FlexTouch
insulin glargine (Rx)
Basaglar, Lantus, Rezvoglar, Semglee, Toujeo SoloStar

Ultra Long Lasting
insulin degludec (Rx)
Tresiba

Mixtures
insulin degludec, insulin aspart (Rx)
Ryzodeg 70/30
insulin degludec, liraglutide
Xultophy
regular insulin/NPH mixture
Humulin 70/30, Novolin 70/30, Novolinge 30/70 ✤, Novolin ge 40/60 ✤, Novolin ge 50/50 ✤
insulin lispro mixture (Rx)
HumaLOG Mix 75/25, HumaLOG Mix 50/50
insulin aspart/aspart protein mixture (Rx)
NovoLOG 70/30, NovoLOG Mix Flexpen Prefilled Syringe 70/30, NovoMix 30 ✤

insulin glargine/ lixisenatide (Rx)
Soliqua 100/33
insulin lispro protamine/ insulin lispro (Rx)
Humalog Kwik Pen Mix 75/25, Humalog Mix 75/25
Func. class.: Antidiabetic, pancreatic hormone
Chem. class.: Modified structures of endogenous human insulin

Do not confuse
Humulin N/Humalog/Novolin N/ Humulin/Novolin/Nogolog

ACTION: Decreases blood glucose; by transport of glucose into cells and the conversion of glucose to glycogen, indirectly increases blood pyruvate and lactate, decreases phosphate and potassium; insulin may be human (processed by recombinant DNA technologies)

USES: Type 1 diabetes mellitus, type 2 diabetes mellitus, gestational diabetes; insulin lispro may be used in combination with sulfonylureas in children >3 yr

CONTRAINDICATIONS
Hypersensitivity to protamine; creosol (aspart)
Precautions: Pregnancy

DOSAGE AND ROUTES
Insulin glulisine
• **Adult/adolescent/child ≥4 yr: SUBCUT** dosage individualized, give within 15 min before or 20 min after starting a meal
• **Adult: IV** dilute to 1 unit/mL in infusion systems with 0.9% NaCl, use PVC Viaflex infusion bags and PVC tubing, use dedicated line
Insulin aspart
• **Adult/adolescent/child ≥6 yr: INTERMITTENT SUBCUT** Total daily dose is given as 2-4 inj/day just before beginning of meal; in general, 50%-70% of total daily insulin may be given as insulin aspart, remainder should be intermediate- or long-acting insulin; **CONTINUOUS SUBCUT** used with external insulin

Side effects: *italics* = common; red = life-threatening

pump via cont SUBCUT insulin infusion (CSII), insulin dose should be based on insulin dose from previous regimen

Insulin lispro
• **Adult/adolescent/child ≥3 yr: SUBCUT** 15 min before meals; **CONT SUBCUT INFUSION (external insulin pump):** total daily dose should be based on insulin dose from previous regimen, 50% of total dose can be given as meal-related boluses, remainder as basal infusion; intermittent SUBCUT (Lyumjev)
• **Adult: SUBCUT** 0.4-1 unit/kg/day

Human regular
• **Adult: SUBCUT** ½-1 hr before meals

Insulin, isophane suspension
• **Adult: SUBCUT** dosage individualized by blood, urine glucose; usual dose 7-26 units; may increase by 2-10 units/day if needed

Insulin degludec
• **Adult: SUBCUT** dosage individualized

Insulin detemir
• **Adult/adolescent/child ≥2 yr: SUBCUT** 1-2×/day; if 1×, give with evening meal

Insulin glargine
• **Adult and child ≥6 yr: SUBCUT** 10 units/day, range 2-100 units/day, but may go much higher

Regular insulin (ketoacidosis)
• **Adult:** IV 5-10 units, then 5-10 units/hr until desired response, then switch to **SUBCUT** dose; **IV/INFUSION** 2-12 units (50 units/500 mL of normal saline)
• **Child:** IV 0.1 units/kg

Replacement
• **Adult/child: SUBCUT** 0.5-1 units/kg/day qid given 30 min before meals
• **Adolescent: SUBCUT** 0.8-1.2 units/kg/day; this dosage is used during rapid growth

Available forms: *NPH* Inj 100 units/mL; *regular* inj 100 units/mL, cartridges 100 units/mL; *insulin analog* inj 100 units/mL; *isophane insulin* inj 100 units/mL, cartridges 100 units/mL; **insulin lispro** 100 units/mL, 1.5-mL cartridges, Huma-LOG Pen sol for inj 100 units/mL,

Humalog KwikPen; *insulin glulisine* inj 100 units/mL; *insulin glargine* inj 100, 300 units/mL; 3-mL single prefilled pen; *insulin degludec* solution for inj 100 units/mL (u-100), 200 units/mL (u-200); *insulin detemir* inj 100 units/mL in 10 vials, 3-mL cartridges; *insulin aspart* inj 100 units/mL

Administer:
• Store at room temperature for <1 mo (some insulins); keep away from heat and sunlight; refrigerate all other supply; NPH, premixed insulins are cloudy; regular, rapid-acting analogs, long-acting analogs are clear; do not freeze—IV route, regular only

SUBCUT route
• After warming to room temperature by rotating in palms; use only insulin syringes with markings or syringe matching units/mL; rotate inj sites within one area: abdomen, upper back, thighs, upper arm, buttocks; keep record of sites
• Increased dosages if tolerance occurs
• Premixed insulins, NPH are cloudy suspensions
• Regular human insulin, rapid-acting analogs, long-acting analogs are clear; do not use if cloudy, thick, or discolored

CONT SUBCUT route (insulin infusion CSII)
• Do not mix with other insulins when using a pump
• Insulin lispro 3-mL cartridges to be used in Disetronic H-TRON plus V100 pump using Disetronic rapid infusion sets; infusion set and cartridge adapter should be changed q3days; replace 3-mL cartridge q6days

IV route (insulin glulisine only)
• Dilute to 1 international unit/mL in infusion systems with 0.9% NaCl using PVC viaflex infusion bags and PVC tubing; use dedicated line; do not admix

IV route (regular only)
When regular insulin is administered IV, monitor glucose, potassium often to prevent fatal hypoglycemia, hypokalemia
• IV direct, undiluted via vein, Y-site, 3-way stopcock; give at ≤50 units/min
• By cont infusion after diluting with IV sol and run at prescribed rate; use

IV infusion pump for correct dosing; give reduced dose at serum glucose level of 250 mg/100 mL

Y-site compatibilities: Amiodarone, ampicillin, ampicillin/sulbactam, aztreonam, ceFAZolin, cefoTEtan, DOBUTamine, esmolol, famotidine, gentamicin, heparin, heparin/hydrocortisone, imipenem/cilastatin, indomethacin, magnesium sulfate, meperidine, meropenem, midazolam, morphine, nitroglycerin, oxytocin, PENTobarbital, potassium chloride, propofol, ritodrine, sodium bicarbonate, sodium nitroprusside, tacrolimus, terbutaline, ticarcillin, ticarcillin/clavulanate, tobramycin, vancomycin, vit B/C

SIDE EFFECTS
EENT: Blurred vision, dry mouth
INTEG: Flushing, rash, urticaria, warmth, lipodystrophy, lipohypertrophy, swelling, redness
META: *Hypoglycemia,* rebound hyperglycemia (Somogyi effect 12-72 hr or longer)
MISC: Peripheral edema
SYST: Anaphylaxis

PHARMACOKINETICS
Rapid acting
Insulin glulisine: Onset 15-30 min, peak ½-1½ hr, duration 3-4 hr
Insulin aspart: Onset 10-20 min, peak 1-3 hr, duration 3-5 hr
Insulin lispro: Onset 15-30 min, peak ½-1½ hr, duration 3-5 hr
Short acting
Insulin regular: Onset 30 min, peak 2.5-5 hr, duration up to 7 hr
Intermediate acting
Insulin, isophane suspension (NPH): Onset 1.5-4 hr, peak 4-12 hr, duration ≤24 hr
Insulin degludec: Peak 12 hr, duration 42 hr after 8 doses
Long acting
Insulin detemir: Onset 0.8-2 hr, peak unknown, duration ≤24 hr (concentration dependent)
Insulin glargine: Onset 1.5 hr, no peak identified, duration ≥24 hr

Mixtures
Insulin, isophane suspension and regular insulin (70/30): Onset 10-20 min, peak 2.4 hr, duration ≤24 hr
Insophane insulin suspension (NPH) and insulin mixtures (50/50): Onset ½-1 hr, peak dual, duration 10-16 hr

INTERACTIONS
Increase: hypoglycemia—salicylate, alcohol, β-blockers, anabolic steroids, phenylbutazone, sulfinpyrazone, guanethidine, oral hypoglycemics, MAOIs, tetracycline
Decrease: hypoglycemia—thiazides, thyroid hormones, oral contraceptives, corticosteroids, estrogens, DOBUTamine, EPINEPHrine
Drug/Lab Test
Increase: VMA
Decrease: potassium, calcium
Interference: LFTs, thyroid function studies

NURSING CONSIDERATIONS
Assess:
• Fasting blood glucose; A1c may be drawn to identify treatment effectiveness q3mo
• Urine ketones during illness; insulin requirements may increase during stress, illness, surgery
• Hypoglycemic reaction that can occur during peak time (sweating, weakness, dizziness, chills, confusion, headache, nausea, rapid weak pulse, fatigue, tachycardia, memory lapses, slurred speech, staggering gait, anxiety, tremors, hunger)
• **Hyperglycemia:** acetone breath; polyuria; fatigue; polydipsia; flushed, dry skin; lethargy
• **Beers:** avoid use of short- or rapid-acting insulin in older adults; sliding-scale insulin poses a higher risk of hypoglycemia without improvement in hyperglycemia management
Evaluate:
• **Therapeutic response:** decrease in polyuria, polydipsia, polyphagia; clear sensorium; absence of dizziness; stable gait, blood glucose HBA1c within normal limits
Teach patient/family:

• That blurred vision occurs; not to change corrective lenses until vision is stabilized after 1-2 mo
• To keep insulin, equipment available at all times; to carry a glucagon kit, candy, or oral glucose preparation to treat hypoglycemia
• That product does not cure diabetes but controls symptoms
• To carry emergency ID as diabetic
• **To recognize hypoglycemia reaction:** headache, tremors, fatigue, weakness, tachycardia
• **To recognize hyperglycemia reaction:** frequent urination, thirst, fatigue, hunger
• About the dosage, route, mixing instructions, diet restrictions (if any), disease process
• **About the symptoms of ketoacidosis:** nausea; thirst; polyuria; dry mouth; decreased B/P; dry, flushed skin; acetone breath; drowsiness; Kussmaul respirations
• That a plan is necessary for diet, exercise; that all food on diet should be eaten; that exercise routine should not vary
• About blood glucose testing; how to determine glucose level
• To avoid OTC products unless directed by prescriber

Interferon alfa 2b (Rx)

(In'ter-fear'on al'fa 2b)

Intron A

Func. class.: Antineoplastic, interferon

USES: Hairy cell leukemia, malignant melanoma, follicular lymphoma, Kaposi sarcoma caused by AIDS, some genital warts, and chronic hepatitis B or C in adults and to treat chronic hepatitis B in children ≥1 yr old

DOSAGE AND ROUTES

Hairy cell leukemia: NOTE: Administer interferon alfa-2b subcutaneously as opposed to intramuscularly if the patient's platelet count is <50,000/mm³.

Adults: IM/SUBCUT 2 million international units/m² 3 times a wk for up to 6 mo

Aggressive, follicular non-Hodgkin lymphoma (NHL) with an anthracycline
• **Adults: SUBCUT** 5 million IU 3 times per wk for up to 18 mo in combination with an anthracycline

AIDS-related Kaposi sarcoma
• **Adult: IM/SUBCUT** 30 million international units/m², 3 times/wk, continue for max response after 16 wk

Chronic HBV infection
• **Adult: IM/SUBCUT** 30-35 million IU/wk × 16 weeks either as 5 million IU/day or 10 million IU 3 × per wk
• **Child 1-17 yr: SUBCUT** 3 million IU/m² 3 × per week for the first week, then escalated to 6 million IU/m² (max 10 million IU) 3 × per week × 16 to 24 wk

Available forms: Solution for injection 18, 25 million international units (6 and 10 million international units/mL); powder for injection 10, 18, 50 million international units/vial with diluent

---

interferon beta-1a (Rx)

(in-ter-feer'on)

Avonex, Rebif

interferon beta-1b (Rx)

Betaseron, Extavia

Func. class.: Antiviral

Chem. class.: Interferon, *Escherichia coli* derivative

ACTION: Antiviral, immunoregulatory; action not clearly understood; biologic response-modifying properties mediated through specific receptors on cells, inducing expression of interferon-induced gene products

USES: Ambulatory patients with relapsing or remitting MS

CONTRAINDICATIONS

Hypersensitivity to natural or recombinant interferon-β or human albumin, hamster protein, rotavirus vaccine

Precautions: Pregnancy, breastfeeding, children <18 yr, chronic progressive MS, depression, mental disorders, seizure disorder, latex allergy, autoimmune disorders, bone marrow suppression, hepatotoxicity, cardiac disease, alcoholism, chickenpox, herpes zoster

DOSAGE AND ROUTES
Interferon beta-1a
Multiple sclerosis
• **Adult: IM** (Avonex) 30 mcg/wk
• **Adult: SUBCUT** (Rebif) 22 or 44 mcg 3×/wk with each dose 48 hr apart, titrate to full dose over 4-wk period
Interferon beta-1b
Multiple sclerosis
• **Adult: SUBCUT** 0.0625 mg every other day for wk 1 and 2, then 0.125 mg every other day for wk 3 and 4, then 0.1875 mg every other day for wk 5 and 6, then 0.25 mg every other day thereafter; higher doses should not be used
Available forms: *beta-1a:* (Avonex) 30 mcg (6.6 million international units/vial) (autoinjector pen); (Rebif) 22 mcg, 44 mcg/0.5 mL; *beta-1b:* powder for inj 0.3 mg kit
Administer
Interferon beta-1a
• Visually inspect parenteral products for particulate matter and discoloration before use
• Store in refrigerator; do not freeze
IM route
• Premedicate with acetaminophen or ibuprofen and give at bedtime to lessen flulike symptoms
• Interferon-β1a (Avonex) 30 mcg = 6 million IU
• If a dose is missed, give it as soon as possible; continue regular schedule but do not give 2 injections within 2 days; all products are single-use only; do not reuse needles, syringes, prefilled syringes, or autoinjectors
• Rotate injection sites to minimize injection-site reactions
• Do not inject into an area where skin is irritated, reddened, bruised, infected, or scarred

• Check site after 2 hr for redness, edema, or tenderness
• The manufacturer of Avonex offers free training on IM use for patients and health care partners; contact Above MS for more information (800-456-2255)
Reconstitution and administration of Avonex lyophilized powder for IM route
• Use aseptic technique for preparation of solution
• Sites include the thigh or upper arm
• Slowly add 1.1 mL sterile water for injection, preservative-free (supplied by manufacturer) to the vial; rapid addition of the diluent can cause foaming
• Gently swirl; do not shake; final concentration should be 30 mcg/mL (6 million IU/mL)
• The solution should be clear to slightly yellow without particles; discard if the reconstituted product contains particulate or is discolored
• Withdraw 1 mL of reconstituted solution into a syringe; attach the sterile needle and inject IM
• A 25-G 1-inch needle for IM may be substituted for the 23-G 1¼-inch needle provided
• **Storage:** Use within 6 hr of reconstitution; store reconstituted solution in refrigerator; *do not freeze;* discard any unused solution; both drug and diluent vials are single-use only
Administration of Avonex prefilled syringe
• The first injection should be performed under the supervision of an appropriately qualified person
• If self-injecting, rotate injection site between thighs
• Wash hands before handling the Dose Pack
• Remove prefilled syringe from the refrigerator to warm to room temperature (usually 30 min before use); do not use external heat sources such as hot water to warm the syringe
• Refer to the Patient Medication Guide for detailed instructions for preparing and giving a dose

- **Storage:** Store refrigerated; if refrigeration is unavailable, may store at 77° F or less for up to 7 days; after removing from refrigerator, do not store product above 25° C

Administration of Avonex prefilled auto-injector

- The first injection should be performed under the supervision of provider
- Remove one Administration Dose Pack from the refrigerator to warm to room temperature (about 30 min before use); do not use external heat sources such as hot water to warm the syringe Dose Pack
- Do not use the injection if the liquid is colored, cloudy, or has lumps or particles; air bubbles will not affect the dose
- Avonex Pen should be injected into the upper outer thigh
- Refer to the Patient Medication Guide for detailed instructions for preparing and giving a dose
- **Storage:** Store at 36° F-46° F (2° C-8); if refrigeration is unavailable, may store at 77° F or less for up to 7 days; after removing from refrigerator, do not store product above 25° C; do not expose to high temperatures; do not freeze; protect from light

Subcutaneous administration

- Give at the same time (preferably late in the afternoon or evening) on the same days of the week at least 48 hr apart
- Do not give on 2 consecutive days; if a dose is missed, administer the dose as soon as possible, then skip the following day; return to the regular schedule the following week
- Premedication with acetaminophen or ibuprofen can lessen the severity of flu-like symptoms
- Interferon-β1a (Rebif) 44 mcg is equivalent to 12 million IU
- Rotate injection sites
- A Starter Pack containing a lower dose of Rebif syringes is available for the initial titration period

Injection (Rebif)

- Interferon-β1a (Rebif) is available in a prefilled syringe with a 29-G needle
- Inject subcut into the outer surface of the upper arm, abdomen, thigh, or buttock, do not inject the area near the navel or waistline; take care not to inject intradermally
- Discard any unused solution; prefilled syringes do not contain preservatives and are single-use only

Interferon beta-1b

SUBCUT route

- The manufacturers of Betaseron and of Extavia offer materials to assist with training on subcut use, call 800-788-1467 (Betaseron), 888-669-6682 (Extavia)
- Premedication with acetaminophen or ibuprofen and use of product at bedtime can lessen the severity of flulike symptoms
- Visually inspect parenteral products for particulate matter and discoloration before use; do not use if particulate matter is present

Reconstitution

- Add 1.2 mL of 0.54% sodium chloride injection (supplied by the manufacturer) to the vial by using the vial adapter to attach the prefilled syringe that contains the diluent
- If not used immediately, store in the refrigerator for up to 3 hr; do not freeze; discard any unused portion after 3 hr

Injection

- Withdraw the desired amount of the reconstituted solution into the syringe
- Choose an injection site on the upper back arm, abdomen, buttock, or front thigh; do not inject within 2 inches of the navel or in a site where the skin is red, bruised, infected, broken, painful, uneven, or scabbed; rotate injection sites
- Inject subcut; take care not to inject intradermally

SIDE EFFECTS

CNS: *Headache, fever, pain, chills, mental changes, depression,* hypertonia, suicide attempts, seizures

CV: *Migraine, palpitations, hypertension,* tachycardia, peripheral vascular disorders

EENT: *Conjunctivitis,* blurred vision

GI: *Diarrhea, constipation, vomiting, abdominal pain*
GU: *Dysmenorrhea, irregular menses, metrorrhagia,* cystitis, breast pain
HEMA: Decreased lymphocytes, ANC, WBC, *lymphadenopathy,* anemia
INTEG: *Sweating, inj-site reaction*
MS: *Myalgia,* myasthenia
RESP: *Sinusitis,* dyspnea

PHARMACOKINETICS
β-1a: Onset ≤12 hr, peak 16 hr, duration 4 days, half-life 8.6 hr
β-1b: Onset rapid, peak 2-8 hr, duration unknown, half-life 8 min-4.3 hr

INTERACTIONS
Increase: hepatic damage—antiretrovirals (NNRTIs, NRTIs, protease inhibitors)
Increase: myelosuppression—antineoplastics
Decrease: clearance of zidovudine
Drug/Herb
• Change in immunomodulation: astragalus, echinacea, melatonin
Drug/Lab Test
Interference: vaccines, toxoids; avoid concurrent use
Increase: LFTs

NURSING CONSIDERATIONS
Assess:
• **Blood, hepatic studies:** CBC, differential, platelet counts, BUN, creatinine, ALT, urinalysis; if absolute neutrophil count <750/mm³ or if AST/ALT is 10× normal, discontinue product
• **CNS symptoms:** headache, fatigue, depression
• **GI status:** diarrhea or constipation, vomiting, abdominal pain
• **Cardiac status:** increased B/P, tachycardia
• **Mental status:** depression, depersonalization, suicidal thoughts, insomnia
• Lupus-like symptoms
• Multiple sclerosis symptoms
Evaluate:
• **Therapeutic response:** decreased symptoms of multiple sclerosis

Teach patient/family:
• With written, detailed information about product
• That blurred vision, hearing loss, sweating may occur
• That female patients may experience irregular menses, dysmenorrhea or metrorrhagia, breast pain
• To use sunscreen to prevent photosensitivity
• About injection technique, care of equipment
• To notify prescriber of increased temperature, chills, muscle soreness, fatigue, depression, symptoms of hepatotoxicity
• To notify prescriber if pregnancy is suspected

interferon gamma-1b (Rx)
(in-ter-feer'on)
Actimmune
Func. class.: Biologic response modifier
Chem. class.: Lymphokine, interleukin type

USES: Serious infections associated with chronic granulomatous disease, osteopetrosis

DOSAGE AND ROUTES
• **Adult:** SUBCUT 50 mcg/m² (1.5 million units/m²) for patients with surface area >0.5 m²; 1.5 mcg/kg/dose for patients with surface area <0.5 m²; give Monday, Wednesday, Friday for 3×/wk dosing
Available forms: Injection 100 mcg (2 million Ib/0.5-mL vial

⚠ HIGH ALERT

ipilimumab (Rx)
(ip-i-lim'ue-mab)
Yervoy
Func. class.: Antineoplastic; biologic response modifier
Chem. class.: CTLA-4-directed blocking antibody

ACTION: Human IgGIk monoclonal antibody that binds to the cytotoxic T-lymphocyte–associated antigen 4 (CTLA-4); action is indirect, possibly through T-cell–mediated antitumor immune responses

USES: Colorectal cancer, metastatic (microsatellite instability-high or mismatch repair deficient), hepatocellular carcinoma, adjuvant treatment, melanoma, unresectable or metastatic, non-small cell lung cancer (metastatic), non-small cell lung cancer (metastatic or recurrent), advanced renal cell carcinoma

CONTRAINDICATIONS

Hypersensitivity

Precautions: Pregnancy, breastfeeding, Crohn's disease, hepatitis, immunosuppression, inflammatory bowel disease, iritis, ocular disease, organ transplant, pancreatitis, renal disease, rheumatoid arthritis, sarcoidosis, systemic lupus erythematosus, thyroid disease, ulcerative colitis, uveitis adrenal insufficiency, diarrhea, Guillain-Barré syndrome, hepatic disease, myasthenia gravis, hypo/hyperthyroidism, hypopituitarism, peripheral neuropathy, serious rash, hypophysitis

DOSAGE AND ROUTES

When given in combination with nivolumab, if nivolumab is withheld, ipilimumab should also be withheld, and if ipilimumab is withheld, nivolumab should be withheld

Colorectal cancer, metastatic

Adult IV: 1 mg/kg every 3 wk (in combination with nivolumab) for 4 combination doses, followed by nivolumab monotherapy until disease progression or unacceptable toxicity

Hepatocellular carcinoma

Adult: IV: 3 mg/kg once every 3 wk (in combination with nivolumab) for 4 combination doses, followed by nivolumab monotherapy until disease progression or unacceptable toxicity

Melanoma, unresectable or metastatic

Adult: IV: 3 mg/kg every 3 wk for a maximum of 4 doses

Children ≥12 yr and adolescents: IV:

3 mg/kg every 3 wk for a maximum of 4 doses; doses may be delayed due to toxicity, but all doses must be administered within 16 wk of the initial dose

Non-small cell lung cancer, metastatic, PD-L1 expressing

Adult: IV: 1 mg/kg once every 6 wk (in combination with nivolumab; refer to nivolumab monograph for nivolumab dosing information) until disease progression, unacceptable toxicity, or up to 2 yr in patients without disease progression

Non-small cell lung cancer, metastatic or recurrent

Adult: IV: 1 mg/kg once every 6 wk (in combination with nivolumab and 2 cycles of histology-based platinum-doublet chemotherapy; refer to nivolumab monograph for nivolumab dosing information) until disease progression, unacceptable toxicity, or up to 2 yr in patients without disease progression

Renal cell cancer, advanced, combination therapy

Adult: IV: 1 mg/kg once every 3 wk (in combination with nivolumab) for 4 combination doses, followed by nivolumab monotherapy (refer to nivolumab monograph for nivolumab dosing information) until disease progression or unacceptable toxicity. **Small cell lung cancer, progressive (unlabeled use): IV:** 3 mg/kg every 3 wk (in combination with nivolumab) for 4 combination doses, followed by nivolumab monotherapy

Available forms: Sol for inj 50 mg/10 mL, 200 mg/40 mL
Administer:
Intermittent IV INFUSION route
• Visually inspect parenteral products for particulate matter and discoloration before using; sol may have a pale yellow color and have translucent to white, amorphous particles; discard the vial if sol is cloudy, if there is pronounced discoloration, or if particulate matter is present
• Allow to stand at room temperature for 5 min before infusion preparation; withdraw the required volume and transfer into an IV bag; discard partially used vials or empty vials; dilute with 0.9% sodium chloride injection or 5% dextrose injection to a final concentration (1-2 mg/mL); mix diluted sol by gentle inversion; do not admix
• Give infusion over 90 min (melanoma) 30 min (renal cell or colorectal cancer) through an IV line with a low-protein binding in-line filter, do not give with other products; after each infusion, flush the line with 0.9% sodium chloride injection or 0.5% dextrose injection
• Store once diluted for no more than 24 hr refrigerated or at room temperature

SIDE EFFECTS
CNS: Severe and fatal immune-mediated neuropathies, fatigue, headache, fever
EENT: Uveitis, iritis, episcleritis
ENDO: Severe and fatal immune-mediated endocrinopathies
GI: Severe and fatal immune-mediated enterocolitis, hepatitis, pancreatitis, abdominal pain, nausea, diarrhea, appetite decreased, vomiting, constipation, colitis
INTEG: Severe and fatal immune-mediated dermatitis, pruritus, rash, urticaria
MISC: Cough, dyspnea, anemia, eosinophilia, nephritis
SYST: Antibody formation, Stevens-Johnson syndrome, toxic epidermal necrolysis

PHARMACOKINETICS: Steady-state by 3rd dose; terminal half-life 15.4 days

NURSING CONSIDERATIONS
Assess:
• **Serious skin disorders: Stevens-Johnson syndrome, toxic epidermal necrolysis:** permanently discontinue in these or rash complicated by full-thickness dermal ulceration; give systemic corticosteroids at a dose of 1-2 mg/kg/day of predniSONE or equivalent; when dermatitis is controlled, taper corticosteroids over at least 1 mo, withhold in patients with moderate to severe reactions; for mild to moderate dermatitis (localized rash and pruritus), give topical or systemic corticosteroids
• **Immune-mediated reactions:** before starting treatment, assess for enterocolitis, hepatitis, dermatitis, neuropathy, endocrinopathy; take LFTs, ACTH, and thyroid function tests; permanently discontinue if these conditions occur
• **Hepatotoxicity:** LFTs baseline and before each dose; increase the frequency of liver function test monitoring until resolution; permanently discontinue in grade 3-5 toxicity; give systemic corticosteroids at a dose of 1-2 mg/kg/day of predniSONE or equivalent
• **Neuropathy:** monitor for motor or sensory neuropathy (unilateral or bilateral weakness, sensory alterations, or paresthesias) before each dose; permanently discontinue if severe neuropathy (interfering with daily activities), such as Guillain-Barré–like syndromes, occurs
• **Endocrinopathy:** monitor thyroid function tests at baseline and before each dose; monitor hypophysitis, adrenal insufficiency, adrenal crisis, hypo/hyperthyroidism (fatigue, headache, mental status changes, abdominal pain, unusual bowel habits, hypotension, or nonspecific symptoms that may resemble other causes)
• **Vision changes:** uveitis, iritis, episcleritis; corticosteroids may be used
• **Pregnancy/breastfeeding:** do not use in pregnancy, breastfeeding

Side effects: *italics* = common; red = life-threatening

Evaluate:
• Decreasing spread or recurrence of malignant melanoma

Teach patient/family:
• To immediately report allergic reactions, skin rash, severe abdominal pain, yellowing of skin or eyes, tingling of extremities, change in bowel habits
• About the reason for treatment and expected results; to read medication guide provided
• **Pregnancy/breastfeeding:** to notify prescriber if pregnancy is planned or suspected or if breastfeeding; to use contraception during and for 3 mo after final dose

---

ipratropium (Rx)

(i-pra-troe′pee-um)

Atrovent HFA, Atrovent Nasal Spray, Ipravent ✦

Func. class.: Anticholinergic, bronchodilator

Chem. class.: Synthetic quaternary ammonium compound

ACTION: Inhibits interaction of acetylcholine at receptor sites on the bronchial smooth muscle, thereby resulting in decreased cGMP and bronchodilation

USES: Maintenance treatment of bronchospasm associated with COPD; rhinorrhea (nasal spray)

CONTRAINDICATIONS
Hypersensitivity to this product, atropine, bromide, soybean or peanut products
Precautions: Breastfeeding, children <12 yr, angioedema, heart failure, surgery, acute bronchospasm, bladder obstruction, closed-angle glaucoma, prostatic hypertrophy, urinary retention, pregnancy

DOSAGE AND ROUTES
Bronchospasm in chronic bronchitis/emphysema
• **Adult: INH** 2 sprays (17 mcg/spray) 3-4×/day, max 12 **INH**/24 hr; **SOL** 500

mcg (1 unit dose) given 3-4×/day by nebulizer; nasal spray: 2 sprays (42 mcg/spray) 3-4×/day
• **Child 5-11 yr: INH** 4-8 inhalations q20min as needed for ≤3 hr (asthma, unlabeled); **NEB** 250-500 mcg q20min as needed for ≤3 hr (asthma, unlabeled)

Rhinorrhea perennial rhinitis
• **Adult/child ≥6 yr: INTRANASAL** 2 sprays (43 mcg)/nostril bid or tid
• **Child 5-12 yr: INTRANASAL** 2 sprays (0.03%) in each nostril 3×/day

Available forms: Aerosol 17 mcg/actuation; nasal spray 0.03%, 0.06%; sol for inh ✦, 0.02%

Administer:
• Store at room temperature
Nebulizer route
• Use sol in nebulizer with a mouthpiece rather than a face mask
Intranasal route
• Priming pump initially requires 7 actuations of pump; priming again is not necessary if used regularly, tilt head backward after dose

SIDE EFFECTS
CNS: *Anxiety, dizziness, headache,* nervousness
CV: Palpitation
EENT: Dry mouth, blurred vision, nasal congestion
GI: *Nausea, vomiting, cramps*
INTEG: Rash
RESP: *Cough, worsening of symptoms,* bronchospasms

PHARMACOKINETICS
Half-life 2 hr, does not cross blood-brain barrier

INTERACTIONS
Increase: toxicity—other bronchodilators (INH)
Increase: anticholinergic action—phenothiazines, antihistamines, disopyramide
Drug/Herb
Increase: anticholinergic effect—belladonna
Increase: bronchodilator effect—green tea (large amounts), guarana

NURSING CONSIDERATIONS
Assess:

• **Palpitations:** if severe, product may have to be changed

• Tolerance over long-term therapy; dose may have to be increased or changed

• **Atropine sensitivity:** patient may also be sensitive to this product

• **Respiratory status:** rate, rhythm, auscultate breath sounds before and after administration, vital capacity, FEV, ABGs/VBGs, heart rate, rhythm

• Hard candy, frequent drinks, sugarless gum to relieve dry mouth

• **Pregnancy/breastfeeding:** use only if benefit outweighs fetal risk; use caution in breastfeeding, excretion unknown

Evaluate:

• **Therapeutic response:** ability to breathe adequately

Teach patient/family:

• That compliance is necessary with number of inhalations/24 hr or overdose may occur; about spacer device for geriatric patients; that max therapeutic effects may take 2-3 mo

• How to use equipment properly and take medication as directed; to take missed doses as soon as remembered unless almost time for the next dose; to space remaining doses evenly during the day; not to double doses

• That rinsing mouth after use of the inhaler, good oral hygiene, and sugarless gum or candy may minimize dry mouth; to notify health care professional if stomatitis occurs or if dry mouth persists for more than 2 wk

• **Inhalation:** not to exceed 12 doses within 24 hr; to notify heath care professional if symptoms do not improve within 30 min after administration of medication or if condition worsens

• About the need for pulmonary function tests baseline and periodically during therapy to determine effectiveness

• To avoid spraying in eyes; may cause irritation

• To inform prescriber if cough, nervousness, headache, dizziness, nausea occurs

• **Nasal spray:** instruct patient in proper use of nasal spray. Clear nasal passages before use. Do not inhale during administration. Prime pump initially with 7 actuations. If used regularly, no further priming is needed. If not used in 24 hr, prime with 2 actuations. If not used for >7 days, prime with 7 actuations

---

ipratropium/albuterol (Rx)
(i-pra-troe′pee-um/al-byoo-ter-ole)

Combivent Respimat
Func. class.: Anticholinergic agent, beta$_2$-adrenergic agonist

USES: COPD

DOSAGE AND ROUTES

Adult: Oral inhalation (soft-mist inhaler) 1 INH 4 times daily (max 6 INH/day); NEB: Initial: 1 vial (3 mL) (ipratropium bromide 0.5 mg/albuterol 2.5 mg) every 6 hr (max: 6 vials [18 mL]/day)

Available forms: metered dose inhaler 20 mcg ipratropium/100 mcg albuterol; nebulizer solution 0.5 mg ipratropium and 2.5 mg albuterol

---

irbesartan (Rx)
(er-be-sar′tan)

Avapro
Func. class.: Antihypertensive
Chem. class.: Angiotensin II receptor blocker (Type AT$_1$)

Do not confuse:
Avapro/Anaprox

ACTION: Blocks the vasoconstrictor and aldosterone-secreting effects of angiotensin II; selectively blocks the binding of angiotensin II to the AT$_1$ receptor found in tissues

USES: Hypertension, alone or in combination; nephropathy in type 2 diabetic patients; proteinuria

CONTRAINDICATIONS
Hypersensitivity

Side effects: *italics* = common; red = life-threatening

Black Box Warning: Do not use in pregnancy

Precautions: Breastfeeding, children <6 yr, geriatric patients, hypersensitivity to ACE inhibitors; hepatic/renal disease; renal artery stenosis, ☞ African descent, angioedema

DOSAGES AND ROUTES
Hypertension
• **Adult: PO** 150 mg/day; may be increased to 300 mg/day, volume-depleted patients: start with 75 mg/day
Nephropathy in type 2 diabetic patients
• **Adult: PO** maintenance dose 300 mg/day, start 75 mg/day
Available forms: Tabs 75, 150, 300 mg
Administer:
• Without regard to meals
• May be used with other antihypertensives, diuretic
• Volume depletion should be corrected before use

SIDE EFFECTS
CNS: *Dizziness,* anxiety, *headache, fatigue,* syncope
CV: Hypotension
GI: *Diarrhea, dyspepsia,* hepatitis, cholestasis
HEMA: Thrombocytopenia
MISC: Edema, chest pain, rash, tachycardia, UTI, angioedema, hyperkalemia
RESP: *Cough, upper respiratory tract infection,* sinus disorder, pharyngitis, rhinitis

PHARMACOKINETICS
Peak 1.5-2 hr, extensively metabolized by CYP2C9, half-life 11-15 hr, highly bound to plasma proteins, excreted in urine and feces, protein binding 90%

INTERACTIONS
Increase: hyperkalemia—potassium-sparing diuretics, potassium salt substitutes, ACE inhibitors

Increase: irbesartan level—CYP2C9 inhibitors (amiodarone, delavirdine, fluconazole, FLUoxetine, fluvastatin, fluvoxaMINE, imatinib, sulfonamides, sulfinpyrazone, voriconazole, zafirlukast)
Decrease: antihypertensive effect—NSAIDs
Drug/Herb
Increase: antihypertensive effect—black cohosh, garlic, goldenseal, hawthorn, kelp
Increase or decrease: antihypertensive effect—astragalus, cola tree
Decrease: antihypertensive effect—guarana, khat, licorice, yohimbe

NURSING CONSIDERATIONS
Assess:
• **Hypotension:** for severe hypotension, place in supine position and give IV infusion of NS, drug may be continued after B/P is restored
• B/P, pulse q4hr; note rate, rhythm, quality
• Baselines of renal/hepatic studies before therapy begins; periodically monitor LFTs, total/direct bilirubin
• Skin turgor, dryness of mucous membranes for hydration status; edema in feet, legs daily

Evaluate:
• **Therapeutic response:** decreased B/P
Teach patient/family:
• To comply with dosage schedule, even if feeling better; that max therapeutic effects may take 2-3 mo, to take without regard to food
• That product may cause dizziness, fainting, light-headedness
• To rise slowly to sitting or standing position to minimize orthostatic hypotension
• Not to stop product abruptly

Black Box Warning: To notify prescriber if pregnancy is suspected; discontinue if pregnant

irbesartan/hydrochloro-thiazide (Rx)

(ir-be-sar'tan/hye-droe-klor-oh-thye'a-zide)

Avalide

Func. class.: Angiotensin II receptor blocker, antihypertensive, diuretic, thiazide

USES: Hypertension

CONTRAINDICATIONS

Hypersensitivity to irbesartan, hydrochlorothiazide, sulfonamide-derived drugs; concomitant use with aliskiren in those with diabetes mellitus; anuria

Black Box Warning: Pregnancy

DOSAGE AND ROUTES

Adult PO Initial therapy: Irbesartan 150 mg/hydrochlorothiazide 12.5 mg once daily. If initial response is inadequate, may titrate dose after 1 to 2 wk (max daily dose: irbesartan 300 mg/hydrochlorothiazide 25 mg)

Available forms: Tablets 150 mg irbesartan/12.5 mg hydrochlorothiazide, 300 mg irbesartan/12.5 mg hydrochlorothiazide

---

⚠ HIGH ALERT

irinotecan (Rx)

(eye-ri-noe-tee'kan)

Camptosar

Func. class.: Antineoplastic

Chem. class.: Camptothecin analog

ACTION: Cytotoxic by producing damage to single-strand DNA during DNA synthesis; binds to topoisomerase I

USES: Metastatic carcinoma of the colon or rectum or 1st-line treatment in combination with 5-FU and leucovorin for metastatic colon or rectal carcinomas

Unlabeled uses: Pancreatic cancer

CONTRAINDICATIONS

Pregnancy, hypersensitivity to this product or fructose, use with ketoconazole or St. John's wort

Precautions: Breastfeeding, children, geriatric patients, irradiation, hepatic disease, ⊘ decreased UGT 1A1 action, reproductive potential (women), males with partners of reproductive potential

Black Box Warning: Myelosuppression, diarrhea/dehydration

DOSAGE AND ROUTES

Premedications: atropine 0.25-1 mg IV or SUBCUT in patients with cholinergic symptoms (increased salivation, rhinitis, miosis, diaphoresis, abdominal cramping) or early-onset diarrhea. Antiemetics are recommended

First-line treatment colorectal cancer, metastatic with 5-FU

Adult: IV: 125 mg/m^2 over 90 min followed by leucovorin 20 mg/m^2 IV bolus, then 5-FU 500 mg/m^2 IV bolus on days 1, 8, 15, and 22 of a 6-wk treatment cycle (may adjust upward to 150 mg/m^2 if tolerated)

Non-small cell lung cancer, advanced (unlabeled)

Adult: IV: 60 mg/m^2 days 1, 8, and 15 every 4 wk (in combination with cisplatin)

Pancreatic cancer, advanced or metastatic (unlabeled)

Adult: IV: FOLFIRINOX regimen: 180 mg/m^2 over 90 min every 2 wk (in combination with oxaliplatin, leucovorin, and fluorouracil)

Available forms: Inj 20 mg/mL

Administer:

• Use cytotoxic handling precautions

IV route

• Premedicate with antiemetic dexamethasone plus another antiemetic agent, such as a 5-HT$_3$ blocker, given at least 30 min before use

• Before beginning a course of therapy, the granulocyte count should be ≥1.5 × 10 9/L, the platelet count recovered to ≥100 × 10 9/L, and treatment-related diarrhea should be fully resolved

---

Side effects: *italics* = common; red = life-threatening

Dilution
• Dilute appropriate dose in D₅W (preferred) or NS injection to a final concentration of 0.12-2.8 mg/mL
• Store up to 24 hr at room temperature and room lighting; however, because of possible microbial contamination during preparation, an admixture prepared with D₅W or NS should be used within 6 hr, solutions prepared with D₅W, refrigerated, protected from light must be used within 48 hr; avoid refrigeration if prepared with NS

Intravenous infusion
• Infuse over 90 min

Y-site compatibilities: Alemtuzumab, alfentanil, amifostine, amikacin, aminocaproic acid, aminophylline, amiodarone, ampicillin, ampicillin-sulbactam, anidulafungin, argatroban, atenolol, atracurium, azithromycin, aztreonam, bivalirudin, bleomycin, bretylium, bumetanide, buprenorphine, butorphanol, calcium chloride/gluconate, capreomycin, CARBOplatin, caspofungin, ceFAZolin, cefotetan, cefOXitin, cefTAZidime, cefTAZidime (L-arginine), ceftizoxime, cefuroxime, cimetidine, ciprofloxacin, cisatracurium, CISplatin, clindamycin, cyclophosphamide, cycloSPORINE, cytarabine, dacarbazine, DAPTOmycin, DAUNOrubicin liposome, DAUNOrubicin, dexamethasone, dexrazoxane, digoxin, diltiaZEM, diphenhydrAMINE, DOBUTamine, DOCEtaxel, dolasetron, DOPamine, doxacurium, DOXOrubicin, DOXOrubicin liposomal, doxycycline, enalaprilat, ePHEDrine, EPINEPHrine, ertapenem, erythromycin, esmolol, etoposide, etoposide phosphate, famotidine, fenoldopam, fentaNYL, fluconazole, foscarnet, gallium, garenoxacin, gatifloxacin, gemtuzumab, gentamicin, granisetron, haloperidol, heparin, hydrALAZINE, hydrocortisone, HYDROmorphone, hydrOXYzine, IDArubicin, imipenem-cilastatin, inamrinone, insulin, regular, isoproterenol, ketorolac, labetalol, lepirudin, leucovorin, levoFLOXacin, LEVOleucovorin, levorphanol, lidocaine, linezolid, LORazepam, magnesium sulfate, mannitol, meperidine, meropenem, mesna, metaraminol, methadone, methyldopate, metoclopramide, metoprolol, metroNIDAZOLE, midazolam, milrinone, minocycline, mitoXANTRONE, mivacurium, morphine, moxifloxacin, nalbuphine, naloxone, nesiritide, niCARDipine, nitroglycerin, norepinephrine, octreotide, ondansetron, oxaliplatin, PACLitaxel (solvent/surfactant), palonosetron, pancuronium, pantoprazole, pentamidine, pentazocine, PHENobarbital, phentolamine, phenylephrine, polymyxin B, potassium acetate, chloride/phosphates, procainamide, prochlorperazine, promethazine, propranolol, quiNIDine, quinupristin-dalfopristin, raNITIdine, remifentanil, riTUXimab, rocuronium, sodium acetate, bicarbonate/phosphates, succinylcholine, SUFentanil, sulfamethoxazole-trimethoprim, tacrolimus, teniposide, theophylline, thiotepa, ticarcillin, ticarcillin-clavulanate, tigecycline, tirofiban, tobramycin, tolazoline, trimethobenzamide, vancomycin, vasopressin, vecuronium, verapamil, vinBLAStine, vinorelbine, voriconazole, zidovudine, zoledronic acid

SIDE EFFECTS
CNS: Fever, headache, chills, dizziness
CV: Vasodilation, edema, thromboembolism
GI: Severe diarrhea, *nausea, vomiting,* anorexia, constipation, cramps, flatus, stomatitis, dyspepsia, hepatotoxicity
HEMA: Leukopenia, anemia, neutropenia
INTEG: Irritation at site, rash, sweating, alopecia
MISC: Edema, asthenia, weight loss, back pain
RESP: Dyspnea, increased cough, rhinitis

PHARMACOKINETICS
Rapidly and completely absorbed, excreted in urine and bile as metabolites, half-life 6-12 hr, bound to plasma proteins 30%-68%, increased risk for toxicity in patients homozygous for UGT1A1 28

INTERACTIONS

Increase: toxicity—fluorouracil

Increase: bleeding risk—NSAIDs, anticoagulants

Increase: irinotecan levels—some CYP3A4 inhibitors (ketoconazole)

Increase: myelosuppression, diarrhea—other antineoplastics, radiation

Increase: lymphocytopenia, hyperglycemia—dexamethasone

Increase: akathisia—prochlorperazine

Increase: dehydration—diuretics

Decrease: irinotecan levels—CYP3A4 inducers (phenytoin, carBAMazepine, PHENobarbital)

Drug/Herb

Decrease: product level—St. John's wort; avoid concurrent use

Drug/Lab Test

Increase: alk phos, LFTs, bilirubin

Decrease: platelets, WBC, neutrophils, HB/HcT

NURSING CONSIDERATIONS

Assess:

• CNS symptoms: fever, headache, chills, dizziness

Black Box Warning: Myelosuppression: CBC, differential, platelet count weekly; use colony-stimulating factor if WBC <2000/mm³ or platelet count <100,000/mm³, HB ≤9 g/dL, neutrophil ≤1000/mm³; notify prescriber of results; product should be discontinued

• Buccal cavity for dryness, sores or ulceration, white patches, oral pain, bleeding, dysphagia

Black Box Warning: GI symptoms: frequency of stools; cramping; severe, life-threatening diarrhea may occur with fluid and electrolyte imbalances, treat diarrhea within 24 hr of use with 0.25-1 mg atropine IV; treat diarrhea >24 hr of use with loperamide, diarrhea >24 hr (late diarrhea) can be fatal

• **Signs of dehydration:** rapid respirations, poor skin turgor, decreased urine output, dry skin, restlessness, weakness

• **Bone marrow suppression:** bruising; bleeding; blood in stools, urine, sputum, emesis

• Increased fluid intake to 2-3 L/day to prevent dehydration unless contraindicated

Evaluate:

• **Therapeutic response:** decrease in tumor size, spread of cancer

Teach patient/family:

• To avoid foods with citric acid, hot temperature, or rough texture if stomatitis is present; to drink adequate fluids

• To report stomatitis; any bleeding, white spots, ulcerations in mouth; to examine mouth daily, report symptoms

• To report signs of anemia: fatigue, headache, faintness, SOB, irritability, infection, rash

• To use contraception during therapy

• To avoid salicylates, NSAIDs, alcohol because bleeding may occur; to avoid all products unless approved by prescriber

• About alopecia; that when hair grows back, it may be different in texture, thickness

• To avoid vaccinations while taking this product

Black Box Warning: To report diarrhea that occurs 24 hr after administration; severe dehydration can occur rapidly, may be fatal

• To report immediately injection site pain, irritation

• To report vomiting, dizziness

• That regular lab exams will be needed

• To report if pregnancy is planned or suspected; to use contraception during therapy and for 6 mo after last dose; to avoid breastfeeding during and for 7 days after last dose

irinotecan liposome (Rx)
(eye-rye-no-tee´-kan lye-po-so´m)

Onivyde
Func. class.: Antineoplastic agent,
camptothecin, topoisomerase I
inhibitor

USES: Pancreatic adenocarcinoma,
metastatic

CONTRAINDICATIONS
Severe hypersensitivity to irinotecan liposome, irinotecan hydrochloride, or any
component

Black Box Warning: Diarrhea, GI obstruction, neutropenia

DOSAGE AND ROUTES
**Pancreatic adenocarcinoma,
metastatic**
Adult: IV: 70 mg/m^2 once every 2 wk (in
combination with fluorouracil and leucovorin); reduce initial starting dose to
50 mg/m^2 in patients known to be homozygous for the UGT1A1*28 allele; the
dose may be increased to 70 mg/m^2 as
tolerated in subsequent cycles
Available forms: Injection 43 mg/10 mL

iron dextran, injection (Rx)
Dexiron ♣, INFeD
Func. class.: Hematinic
Chem. class.: Ferric hydroxide
complex with dextran

ACTION: Iron is carried by transferrin
to the bone marrow, where it is incorporated into hemoglobin

USES: Iron-deficiency anemia

CONTRAINDICATIONS
Repeated blood transfusions, vitamin E
deficiency

Black Box Warning: Hypersensitivity

Precautions: Pregnancy, breastfeeding,
neonates, infants <4 mo, children, acute
renal disease, asthma, rheumatoid
arthritis (IV), ankylosing spondylitis,
lupus, hypotension, all anemias excluding iron-deficiency anemia, hepatic/cardiac/renal disease

DOSAGE AND ROUTES
• **Adult/child: IM** 0.5 mL as a test dose
by Z-track, then no more than the following total dose including test dose per day
• **Adult/adolescent/child (>15 kg):** Total
iron dextran dose in mL = [0.0442 ×
(Desired Hb – observed Hb) × LBW] +
(0.26 × LBW), max of undiluted is 100
mg (2 mL)/day
• **Child (10-15 kg):** Total iron dextran
dose in mL = [0.0442 × (Desired Hb –
observed Hb) × LBW] + (0.26 × ABW),
max of undiluted iron dextran is 100 mg
(2 mL)/day
• **Child/Infant >4 mo (5-9.9 kg):** Total
iron dextran dose in mL = [0.0442 ×
(Desired Hb – observed Hb) × LBW] +
(0.26 × ABW)
• **Infants >4 mo (<5 kg):** Total iron
dextran dose in mL = [0.0442 × (Desired Hb – observed Hb) × LBW] +
(0.26 × ABW)
Administer:
• D/C oral iron before parenteral; give
only after test dose of 25 mg by preferred
route; wait at least 1 hr before giving remaining portion
• Store at room temperature in cool environment
• Recumbent position 30 min after IV inj
to prevent orthostatic hypotension
IM route
• IM deeply in large muscle mass; use
Z-track method, 19- to 20-G 2- to 3-in
needle; ensure needle long enough to
place product deep in muscle; change
needles after withdrawing product and
before injecting to prevent skin, tissue
staining
• Only with EPINEPHrine available in case
of anaphylactic reaction during dose

IV route
• IV after flushing with 10 mL 0.9% NaCl; give undiluted; may be diluted in 50-250 mL NS for infusion; give ≤1 mL (50 mg) over ≥1 min; flush line after use with 10 mL 0.9% NaCl; patient should remain recumbent for ½-1 hr
• IV inj requires single-dose vial without preservative; verify on label that IV use approved

SIDE EFFECTS
CNS: Headache, paresthesia, dizziness, shivering, weakness, seizures
CV: Chest pain, shock, hypotension, tachycardia
GI: *Nausea,* vomiting, metallic taste, abdominal pain
HEMA: Leukocytosis
INTEG: Rash, pruritus, urticaria, fever, sweating, chills, brown skin discoloration, pain at inj site, necrosis, sterile abscesses, phlebitis
OTHER: Anaphylaxis
RESP: Dyspnea

PHARMACOKINETICS
IM: Excreted in feces, urine, bile, breast milk; crosses placenta; most absorbed through lymphatics; can be gradually absorbed over weeks/months from fixed locations

INTERACTIONS
Increase: toxicity—oral iron; do not use
Decrease: reticulocyte response—chloramphenicol

Drug/Lab Test
False increase: serum bilirubin
False decrease: serum calcium
False positive: ^{99m}Tc diphosphate bone scan, iron test (large doses >2 mL)

NURSING CONSIDERATIONS
Assess:
• Observe for 1 hr after first dose to monitor for anaphylactic reactions
• Blood studies: Hct, HB, reticulocytes, transferrin, plasma iron concentrations, ferritin, total iron binding, bilirubin before treatment, at least monthly

Black Box Warning: Allergy: anaphylaxis, rash, pruritus, fever, chills, wheezing; notify prescriber immediately, keep emergency equipment available

• **Cardiac status:** anginal pain, hypotension, tachycardia
• **Nutrition:** amount of iron in diet (meat, dark green leafy vegetables, dried beans, dried fruits, eggs)
• Cause of iron loss or anemia, including use of salicylates, sulfonamides
• **Toxicity:** nausea, vomiting, diarrhea, fever, abdominal pain (early symptoms), cyanotic-looking lips, nailbeds, seizures, CV collapse (late symptoms)
• **Pregnancy/breastfeeding:** use only if benefit outweighs fetal risk; use caution in breastfeeding, trace amounts appear in breast milk

Evaluate:
• **Therapeutic response:** increased serum iron level, increased HB, Hct

Teach patient/family:
• That iron poisoning may occur if increased beyond recommended level; not to take oral iron preparation or vitamins containing iron
• That delayed reaction may occur 1-2 days after administration and last 3-4 days (IV), 3-7 days (IM); to report fever, chills, malaise; muscle, joint aches; nausea, vomiting, backache
• To avoid breastfeeding
• That stools may become dark

TREATMENT OF OVERDOSE:
Discontinue product, treat allergic reaction, give diphenhydrAMINE or EPINEPHrine as needed, give iron-chelating product for acute poisoning

---

iron sucrose (Rx)
Velphoro, Venofer
Func. class.: Hematinic
Chem. class.: Ferric hydroxide complex with dextran

ACTION: Iron is carried by transferrin to the bone marrow, where it is incorporated into hemoglobin

USES: Iron-deficiency anemia, hyperphosphatemia in chronic kidney disease on dialysis

Unlabeled uses: Dystrophic epidermolysis bullosa (DEB)

CONTRAINDICATIONS

Hypersensitivity, all anemias excluding iron-deficiency anemia, iron overload

Precautions: Pregnancy, breastfeeding, children, geriatric patients, abdominal pain, anaphylactic shock, arthralgia, chest pain, cough, diarrhea, dizziness, dyspnea, edema, increased LFTs, fever, headache, heart failure, hypo/hypertension, infection, MS pain, nausea/vomiting, seizures, weakness

DOSAGE AND ROUTES

Iron-deficiency anemia (on dialysis)

• **Adult: IV** 5 mL (100 mg of elemental iron) given during dialysis; most will need 1000 mg of elemental iron over 10 sequential dialysis sessions

Available forms: Inj 20 mg/mL (elemental iron), 2.5-mL, 5-mL, 10-mL single-dose vials

Iron-deficiency anemia (not on dialysis)

Adult: IV 200 mg (undiluted) over 2-5 min or as an infusion 200 mg/1000 mL or less in normal saline over 15 min on 5 sessions in 14 days (total 1000 mg)

IV route

• Do not use if particulate is present or if discolored

• Give directly in dialysis line by slow inj or infusion; give by slow inj at 1 mL/min (5 min/vial); for infusion, dilute each vial exclusively in ≤100 mL 0.9% NaCl, give at 100 mg of iron/15 min; discard unused portions

• Do not use with IV products

• Store at room temperature in cool environment; do not freeze

SIDE EFFECTS

CNS: Headache, dizziness

CV: Chest pain, hypo/hypertension, hypervolemia, heart failure

GI: *Nausea, vomiting, abdominal pain*

INTEG: Rash, pruritus, urticaria, fever, sweating, chills

OTHER: Anaphylaxis, hyperglycemia

RESP: Dyspnea, pneumonia, cough

PHARMACOKINETICS

Excreted in urine, half-life 6 hr

INTERACTIONS

Decrease: absorption of oral iron products, avoid using together

NURSING CONSIDERATIONS

Assess:

• **Blood studies:** Hct, HB, reticulocytes, transferrin, plasma iron concentrations, ferritin, total iron binding; bilirubin before treatment, at least monthly

• **Allergy, anaphylaxis:** rash, pruritus, fever, chills, wheezing; notify prescriber immediately, keep emergency equipment available

• **Cardiac status:** hypo/hypertension, hypervolemia

• **Toxicity:** nausea, vomiting, diarrhea, fever, abdominal pain (early symptoms), cyanotic-looking lips, nailbeds, seizures, CV collapse (late symptoms)

• **Pregnancy/breastfeeding:** use only if clearly needed; cautious use in breastfeeding

Evaluate:

• **Therapeutic response:** increased serum iron levels, Hct, HB

Teach patient/family:

• To report itching, rash, chest pain, headache, vertigo, nausea, vomiting, abdominal pain, joint/muscle pain, numbness, tingling

• That iron poisoning may occur if dosage is increased beyond recommended level; not to take oral iron preparation

TREATMENT OF OVERDOSE:

Discontinue product, treat allergic reaction, give diphenhydrAMINE or EPINEPHrine as needed, give iron-chelating product for acute poisoning

---

isavuconazonium (Rx)

(eye-sa-vue-koe-na-zoe'nee-um)

Cresemba

Func. class.: Antifungal, systemic

Chem. class.: Azole

ACTION: Exerts antifungal activity by inhibiting the synthesis of ergosterol, an essential component of the fungal cell membrane. The depletion of ergosterol within the fungal cell membrane results in increased cellular permeability, causing leakage of cellular content

USES: *Aspergillus flavus, Aspergillus fumigatus, Aspergillus niger, Rhizopus oryzae, Mucormycetes* species; do NOT use for infections of *Candida, Blastomyces, Histoplasma*

CONTRAINDICATIONS

Hypersensitivity, short QT syndrome

Precautions: Azole hypersensitivity, pregnancy, breastfeeding, infusion-related reactions, hepatic disease

DOSAGE AND ROUTES

• **Adult: PO/IV** loading dose of (372 mg) q8hr × 6 doses. Then, (372 mg) daily. Start maintenance dosing 12-24 hr after the last loading dose; treatment may last 6-12 wk up to 6 mo

Available forms: Caps 186 mg; powder for injection 382 mg

Administer:

PO route

• Swallow whole; do not chew, crush, dissolve, open the capsules; may be used without regard to food

IV route

• Visually inspect for particulate matter and discoloration; diluted solution may contain translucent to white particulates that will be removed by the in-line filter

Reconstitution

• Reconstitute the dry powder with 5 mL sterile water for injection, gently shake until dissolved

• Storage: the reconstituted solution may be stored below 77° F (25° C) for a maximum of 1 hr before further dilution

Dilution

• Remove 5 mL of the reconstituted solution and add it to 250 mL of either 0.9% NaCl or D₅W (1.5 mg/mL)

• Gently mix the solution or roll the bag. DO NOT shake. Do not place in a pneumatic transport system

• Apply an in-line filter (0.2-1.2 microns), adhere an in-line filter reminder sticker to the infusion bag

• Give within ≤6 hr of dilution

• Storage: may be stored immediately after dilution at 36° F-46° F (2° C-8° C); administration MUST be completed within 24 hr of the time of dilution. Do NOT freeze

• Product only after C&S confirms organism, product needed to treat condition; make sure product is used in life-threatening infections

• Flush IV lines with 0.9% sodium chloride or 5% dextrose in water before and after administration of the infusion

• Must be administered through a 0.2- to 1.2-micron filter; give over ≥1 hr. Do not give by bolus

• Do not admix

SIDE EFFECTS

CNS: *Headache,* paresthesias, peripheral neuropathy, *hallucinations,* depression, insomnia, dizziness, fever, vertigo, tremor, confusion

CV: Tachypnea, supraventricular tachycardia, atrial fibrillation/flutter

EENT: Tinnitus

GI: Nausea, vomiting, anorexia, diarrhea, cramps, hepatitis, stomatitis

GU: *Hypokalemia,* renal failure

HEMA: Anemia, eosinophilia, hypomagnesemia, thrombocytopenia, leukopenia

INTEG: *Burning, irritation,* pain, necrosis at inj site with extravasation, *rash*

MISC: Cough

PHARMACOKINETICS

Metabolized by CYP3A4, CYP3A5, UGT, P-gp, OCT2 enzymes; eliminated in urine/feces; peak 2 hr (PO), Chinese patients (levels 40% lower), protein binding >99%

INTERACTIONS

Increase: effects of benzodiazepines, calcium channel blockers, cycloSPORINE, ergots, HMG-CoA reductase inhibitors, pimozide, quiNIDine, prednisoLONE, sirolimus, sulfonylureas, tacrolimus, vinca alkaloids, warfarin, rifabutin, proton pump inhibitors, NNRTIs, protease inhibitors, phenytoin

Increase: isavuconazonium effect—CYP3A4 substrates

Decrease: isavuconazonium effect—CYP3A4 inhibitors

Decrease: bupropion effect—dose may need to be increased

Drug/Herb

• Do not use with St. John's wort

Drug/Lab Test

Increase: AST/ALT, alk phos, creatinine, bilirubin

Decrease: HB/Hct, platelets, WBC

NURSING CONSIDERATIONS

Assess:

• **Short QT syndrome:** do not use in this condition

• VS q15-30min during first infusion; note changes in pulse, B/P

• Blood studies: CBC, potassium, sodium, calcium, magnesium, q2wk; obtain culture and sensitivity before starting first dose; may start treatment before results are received

• **Hepatotoxicity:** increases in AST, ALT, alk phos, bilirubin, baseline and periodically

• **Allergic reaction:** dermatitis, rash; product should be discontinued, antihistamines (mild reaction) or epinephrine (severe reaction) administered

• **Hypokalemia:** anorexia, drowsiness, weakness, decreased reflexes, dizziness, increased urinary output, increased thirst, paresthesias

• **Ototoxicity:** tinnitus (ringing, roaring in ears), vertigo

• **Infusion-related reactions:** dizziness, chills, fever, hypotension, dyspnea; discontinue if these occur

• **Pregnancy/breastfeeding:** test for pregnancy before starting treatment; do not use in breastfeeding

Evaluate:

• **Therapeutic response:** resolution of fungal infection, negative C&S

Teach patient/family:

• That long-term therapy may be needed to clear infection (2 wk-3 mo, depending on type of infection); not to discontinue unless approved by prescriber

• To notify prescriber of bleeding, bruising, soft-tissue swelling, dark urine, persistent nausea or diarrhea, headache, rash, yellow skin/eyes

• That women of childbearing age should use effective contraceptive during and for 28 days after last dose; not to breastfeed

• To notify provider of all OTC, Rx, herbal products or supplements taken and to avoid new products unless approved by prescriber

• That lab exams will be required

---

isoniazid (Rx)

(eye-soe-nye'a-zid)

Func. class.: Antitubercular

Chem. class.: Isonicotinic acid hydrazide

ACTION: Bactericidal interference with lipid, nucleic acid biosynthesis

USES: Treatment, prevention of TB

CONTRAINDICATIONS
Hypersensitivity

Black Box Warning: Acute hepatic disease

Precautions: Pregnancy, renal disease, diabetic retinopathy, cataracts, ocular defects, IV drug users, >35 yr, postpartum, HIV, neuropathy

Black Box Warning: Alcoholism, females (African descent/Hispanic patients)

DOSAGE AND ROUTES
• **Adult/adolescent: PO/IM** 5 mg/kg/day up to 300 mg/day or 15 mg/kg 2-3×/wk, max 900 mg 2-3×/wk
• **Child/infant: PO/IM** 10-15 mg/kg/day, max 300 mg/day (active TB); 20-40 mg 2 × per wk (latent TB)
Available forms: Tabs 50 🍁, 100, 300 mg; inj 100 mg/mL; oral sol 10 mg/mL
Administer:
PO route
• PO with meals to decrease GI symptoms; better to take on empty stomach 1 hr before or 2 hr after meals
IM route
• IM deep in large muscle mass; massage; rotate injection site; warm inj to room temperature to dissolve crystals

SIDE EFFECTS
CNS: *Peripheral neuropathy, dizziness,* memory impairment, seizures, psychosis
EENT: Blurred vision, optic neuritis
GI: *Nausea, vomiting,* fatal hepatitis
HEMA: Agranulocytosis, hemolytic, aplastic anemia, thrombocytopenia, eosinophilia, methemoglobinemia
Hypersensitivity: DRESS, Stevens-Johnson syndrome, toxic epidermal necrolysis, rash, fever

PHARMACOKINETICS
Metabolized in liver, 🌑 50% of patients may metabolize slowly, increasing toxicity; excreted in urine (metabolites), crosses placenta, excreted in breast milk; half life 1-4 hr (slow acetylators), 0.5-1.5 hr (fast acetylators)
PO: Peak 1-2 hr

IM: Peak 45-60 min

INTERACTIONS
Increase: toxicity—tyramine foods, alcohol, cycloSERINE, ethionamide, rifAMPin, carBAMazepine, phenytoin, benzodiazepines, meperidine
Increase: serotonin syndrome—SSRIs, SNRIs
Decrease: absorption—aluminum antacids
Decrease: effectiveness of BCG vaccine—ketoconazole
Drug/Food
• Do not give with high-tyramine foods, alcohol
Drug/Lab Test
Increase: LFTs, bilirubin, glucose
Decrease: platelets, granulocytes

NURSING CONSIDERATIONS
Assess:

Black Box Warning: Hepatic studies weekly: baseline in all patients, those >35 yr and all women should be monitored periodically; ALT, AST, bilirubin; increased test results may indicate hepatitis; hepatic status: decreased appetite, jaundice, dark urine, fatigue; 🌑 those with fast acetylation may metabolize product more than 5 times faster (black, Asian patients are at greater risk than some Caucasian patients); fatal hepatitis is a greater risk in Black or Hispanic patients after giving birth

• **DRESS:** fever, flulike symptoms, rash, lymphadenopathy, facial swelling, may involve other organ systems
• **Stevens-Johnson syndrome, toxic epidermal necrolysis:** rash, fever, fatigue, blistering, discontinue immediately if these occur
• **Mental status often:** affect, mood, behavioral changes; psychosis may occur
• Paresthesia in hands, feet
• 🌑 **Susceptibility testing:** 🌑 obtain susceptibility tests before treatment and periodically; half of Mexicans, Blacks, Whites, and Native Americans may be

slow acetylators; Asians, Eskimos may be fast acetylators

• **Pregnancy/breastfeeding:** use during pregnancy even 1st trimester for active TB, use only if benefits outweigh fetal risk for other indications; compatible with breastfeeding

Evaluate:

• **Therapeutic response:** decreased symptoms of TB

Teach patient/family:

• That compliance with dosage schedule, duration is necessary; not to skip or double dose

• That scheduled appointments must be kept or relapse may occur

• To avoid alcohol while taking product; may increase risk for hepatic injury

• If diabetic, to use blood glucose monitor to obtain correct result

• To report weakness, fatigue, loss of appetite, nausea, vomiting, jaundice of skin or eyes, tingling/numbness of hands/feet

Black Box Warning: Fatal hepatitis: to notify prescriber immediately of yellow skin/eyes, dark urine, loss of appetite

---

⚠ **HIGH ALERT**

isoproterenol (Rx)
(eye-soe-proe-ter′-e-nole)

Isuprel

Func. class.: Beta$_1$- and beta$_2$-adrenergic agonist agent

USES: Acute bronchospasm, Adam-Stokes syndrome, cardiac arrest, cardiogenic shock, HF, septic shock AV block

CONTRAINDICATIONS

Angina, preexisting ventricular arrhythmias, tachyarrhythmias; cardiac glycoside intoxication

DOSAGE AND ROUTES
Bradyarrhythmias, AV nodal block

Adult: Continuous IV infusion: Usual range: 2 to 10 mcg/min; titrate to patient response

Cardiogenic shock due to bradycardia (unlabeled)

Adult: Continuous IV infusion: N2 to 20 mcg/min

Provocation during tilt table testing for syncope (unlabeled):

Adult: Continuous IV infusion: Initial: 1 mcg/min; increase as necessary based on response; maximum dose: 5 mcg/min

Provocation of ventricular arrhythmias in suspected arrhythmogenic right ventricular cardiomyopathy (unlabeled)

Adult: 45 mcg/min for 3 min (regardless of initial heart rate) followed by evaluation for arrhythmia

---

isosorbide dinitrate (Rx)
(eye-soe-sor′bide)

Isordil

isosorbide mononitrate (Rx)

Imdur ♣

Func. class.: Antianginal, vasodilator
Chem. class.: Nitrate

Do not confuse:
Isordil/Plendil/Isuprel/Inderal

ACTION: Relaxation of vascular smooth muscle, which leads to decreased preload, afterload, which is responsible for decreasing left ventricular end-diastolic pressure, systemic vascular resistance, and reducing cardiac oxygen demand

USES: Treatment, prevention of chronic stable angina pectoris
Unlabeled uses: Heart failure (dinitrate), esophageal spasms without GERD

CONTRAINDICATIONS
Hypersensitivity to this product or nitrates; severe anemia, closed-angle glaucoma
Precautions: Pregnancy, breastfeeding, children, orthostatic hypotension, MI,

---

HF, severe renal/hepatic disease, increased intracranial pressure, cerebral hemorrhage, acute MI, geriatric patients, GI disease, syncope

DOSAGE AND ROUTES
Dinitrate (HF)
• **Adult: PO** 5-20 mg bid-tid initially, maintenance 10-40 mg bid-tid; **EXT REL** 40-80 mg q8-12hr, max 160 mg/day
Mononitrate
• **Adult: PO** (tablets) 10-20 mg bid, 7 hr apart; (extended release) initiate at 30-60 mg/day as a single dose, increase q3days as needed, may increase to 120 mg/day, max 240 mg/day

Available forms: *Dinitrate:* ext rel tabs 40 mg; tabs 5, 10, 20, 30, 40 mg; *mononitrate:* tabs 10, 20 mg; ext rel 30, 60, 120 mg
Administer:
• After checking expiration date
• PO with 8 oz water on empty stomach
• **Extended release capsule/tablet:** allow dosing interval >18 hr
• Do not break, crush, or chew extended release capsules

SIDE EFFECTS
CNS: *Vascular headache, flushing, dizziness,* weakness
CV: *Orthostatic hypotension,* tachycardia, collapse, syncope
GI: Nausea, vomiting
INTEG: Pallor, sweating, rash
MISC: Twitching, hemolytic anemia, methemoglobinemia, tolerance, xerostomia

PHARMACOKINETICS
Dinitrate
Metabolized by liver, excreted in urine as metabolites (80%-100%)
PO: Onset 15-30 min, duration 4-6 hr, half-life 5-6 hr
SUS REL: Onset ≤4 hr, duration 6-8 hr
Mononitrate
SUS REL: Onset 30-60 min, peak 1-4 hr, duration 6-8 hr, half-life 5 hr

INTERACTIONS
• Fatal hypotension: avanafil, sildenafil, tadalafil, vardenafil; do not use together

Increase: hypotension—β-blockers, diuretics, antihypertensives, alcohol, calcium channel blockers, phenothiazines
Increase: heart rate, B/P—sympathomimetics
Increase: myocardial ischemia—rosiglitazone; avoid concurrent use

NURSING CONSIDERATIONS
Assess:
• **Anginal pain:** duration, time started, activity being performed, character
• **Methemoglobinemia (rare):** cyanosis of lips, nausea/vomiting, coma, shock; usually caused by high dose of product but may occur with normal dosing
• **Vitals:** B/P, pulse, respirations during beginning therapy and periodically thereafter
• Tolerance if taken over long period; to prevent, allow intervals of 12-14 hr/day without product
• Headache, light-headedness, decreased B/P; may indicate a need for decreased dosage, treat headache with OTC analgesics
• **Beers:** use with caution in older adults; may exacerbate episodes of syncope
• **Pregnancy/breastfeeding:** use only if benefit outweighs fetal risk; cautious use in breastfeeding, excretion unknown
Evaluate:
• **Therapeutic response:** decrease or prevention of anginal pain
Teach patient/family:
• To leave tabs in original container
• To avoid alcohol, OTC products unless approved by prescriber
• That product may cause headache; that taking with meals may reduce or eliminate headache; to take no later than 7 PM (last dose)
• To avoid hazardous activities if dizziness occurs
• About the importance of complying with complete medical regimen
• To make position changes slowly to prevent orthostatic hypotension
• Not to use with avanafil, sildenafil, tadalafil, vardenafil with nitrates; may cause serious drop in B/P
• Not to discontinue abruptly, may cause heart attack

Side effects: *italics* = common; red = life-threatening

• To use at beginning of angina symptoms, may repeat every 15 min; if no relief, seek medical attention immediately

isosorbide/hydralazine (Rx)
(eye-soe-sor'bide/hye-dral'a-zeen)
BiDil
Func. class.: Antihypertensive, vasodilator

USES: Heart failure with reduced ejection fraction (HFrEF)

CONTRAINDICATIONS
Hypersensitivity to organic nitrates or any component; concomitant use with phosphodiesterase 5 inhibitors (avanafil, sildenafil, tadalafil, vardenafil); concomitant use with riociguat

DOSAGE AND ROUTES
Heart failure with reduced ejection fraction (HFrEF)
Adult: PO Initial: 1 tablet (20 mg isosorbide/37.5 mg hydralazine) 3 times daily; titrate dose in 2 to 4 wk to a max 2 tablets (total of 40 mg isosorbide/75 mg hydralazine) 3 times daily
Available forms: Tablet 20 mg/37.5 mg

ISOtretinoin (Rx)
(eye-soe-tret'i-noyn)
Absorica, Accutane, Amnesteem, Claravis, Clarus, E Puris, Myorisan, Sotret, Zenatane
Func. class.: Antiacne agent, retinoid

USES: Severe recalcitrant nodulocystic acne

CONTRAINDICATIONS
Hypersensitivity to this product, parabens, retinoids, inflamed skin, blood donation

Black Box Warning: Pregnancy

DOSAGE AND ROUTES
• **Adult: PO** 0.5-2 mg/kg/day in 2 divided doses × 15-20 wk; if relapse occurs, repeat after 2 mo off product
Available forms: Capsule 8,10, 20, 25, 30, 35, 40 mg

istradefylline (Rx)
(iz-tra'de-fye'leen)
Nourianz
Func. class.: Anti-Parkinson agent
Chem. class.: Adenosine receptor antagonist

ACTION: Adenosine A_{2A} receptor antagonist that acts through a nondopaminergic mechanism to improve motor function

USES: Adjuvant treatment in patients with Parkinson's disease experiencing "off" episodes

CONTRAINDICATIONS
Hypersensitivity, severe psychosis, pregnancy, severe hepatic disease
Precautions:
Behavioral changes, breastfeeding, children, contraception requirements, dyskinesia, geriatric, hepatic disease, impulse control symptoms, infants, pregnancy, psychosis, reproductive risk, tobacco smoking

DOSAGE AND ROUTES
Adults PO 20 mg daily; adjust dose based on response and tolerability; max: 40 mg daily; 20 or more cigarettes, 40 mg daily
Hepatic dose:
Adult: PO Child-Pugh B max 20 mg/day
Available forms: Tabs 10, 40 mg
Administer: May give without regard to meals

SIDE EFFECTS
CNS: *Dyskinesia,* psychosis, dizziness, hallucinations, insomnia
GI: Nausea, constipation
INTEG: Rash
ENDO: Hyperuricemia, hyperglycemia

PHARMACOKINETICS

• Protein binding 98%, metabolized by CYP1A1, CYP3A4, with a minor contribution from CYP1A2, CYP2B6, CYP2C8, CYP2C9, CYP2C18, and CYP2D6 metabolites 39% and excreted urine (39%), feces (48%); half-life 83 hr; dosage modifications are needed in heavy smoking; peak 4 hr (fasting), increased with high-fat meal

INTERACTIONS

Increased: istradefylline effect—strong CYP3A4 inhibitors (ketoconazole, itraconazole, clarithromycin); max 20 mg daily
Decreased: istradefylline effect—strong CYP3A4 inducers (carBAMazepine, rifAMPin, phenytoin, St. John's wort); avoid using together
Drug: herb
Decreased: istradefylline effect—St. John's wort; avoid using together

NURSING CONSIDERATIONS
Assess:
• **Parkinson's disease:** Assess for decreasing "off" episodes, tremors usually first appearing in hands/foot while at rest, slow movement, rigidity, postural instability, problems with speech and voice, incontinence, difficulty swallowing, inability to start movements or continue repeated movement, excessive sweating, constipation, dry skin, mood changes
• **Dyskinesia:** Assess for grimacing, eye blinking, lip smacking, repetitive movements, these should lessen with treatment
• **Hallucinations/psychosis/impulse control/compulsive behaviors:** Assess for these effects, and if present, decreased dose or discontinuation of treatment may be needed
• Monitor LFTs in hepatic disease
Evaluate:
• **Therapeutic response:** decreasing symptoms of Parkinson's disease, decreased "off" time
Teach patient/family:
• To identify if tobacco is used and, if so, how much per day; dosage change may be needed
• To identify all Rx, OTC, herbals, supplements that are used and discuss with health care provider

• **Pregnancy/breastfeeding:** Identify if pregnancy is planned or suspected or if breastfeeding, use in pregnancy is not recommended; adequate contraception should be used in women of childbearing age

itraconazole (Rx)
(it-ra-con′a-zol)
Onmel ✤, Sporanox, Tolsura
Func. class.: Antifungal, systemic
Chem. class.: Triazole derivative

ACTION: Alters cell membranes; inhibits several fungal enzymes

USES: Histoplasmosis, blastomycosis (pulmonary and extrapulmonary), aspergillosis, onychomycosis of toenail/fingernail
Unlabeled uses: Dermatomycosis, histoplasmosis, chromoblastomycosis, coccidioidomycosis, pityriasis versicolor, seboposoriasis, vaginal candidiasis, cryptococcus, subcutaneous mycoses, dimorphic infections, fungal keratitis, zygomycosis, superficial mycoses (dermatophytosis), chronic mucocutaneous candidiasis

CONTRAINDICATIONS
Hypersensitivity, fungal meningitis; onychomycosis or dermatomycosis with cardiac dysfunction, in pregnant women

Black Box Warning: Heart failure, ventricular dysfunction, coadministration with other products

Precautions: Pregnancy, breastfeeding, children, cardiac/renal/hepatic disease, achlorhydria or hypochlorhydria (product-induced), dialysis, hearing loss, cystic fibrosis neuropathy

DOSAGE AND ROUTES
Capsules and oral solution are not interchangeable, oral solution is used only for oral/esophageal candidiasis
Pulmonary or disseminated extrapulmonary blastomycosis
Adults PO (capsules) 200 mg PO 3 times daily for 3 days followed by 200 mg

PO 1 or 2 times daily for 6-12 mo; **PO (Tolsura)** 130 mg PO once daily with 65-mg increment dose increases to a maximum of 260 mg/day if there is no obvious improvement or there is evidence of progressive fungal disease. Administer doses above 130 mg/day in 2 divided doses

Treatment of serious, life-threatening systemic fungal infections

Adult: PO (Capsules): Loading dosage of 200 mg 3 times daily (600 mg daily) for the first 3 days, then 200-400 mg daily, usually continued for 3 mo and until clinical parameters and laboratory tests indicate that the active fungal infection has subsided

Treatment of pulmonary or extrapulmonary aspergillosis

Adult: PO (Capsules): 200-400 mg daily × at least 3 mo

Treatment of pulmonary or extrapulmonary blastomycosis

Adult: PO (Capsules): 200 mg once daily. If there is evidence of progression or no apparent improvement, increase dosage in 100-mg increments daily up to a max 400 mg daily for 6-12 mo

Treatment of oropharyngeal candidiasis

Adult PO (Oral solution): 200 mg (20 mL) daily for 1-2 wk. Generally resolves within several days; retreatment in patients who failed to respond to or are refractory to oral fluconazole: Manufacturer recommends 100 mg (10 mL) twice daily. A response to itraconazole in these patients generally is evident within 2-4 wk; relapse may be expected shortly after the drug is discontinued

HIV-infected adults PO (oral solution): 200 mg daily × 7-14 days

Treatment of esophageal candidiasis

Adult PO Oral solution: 100 mg (10 mL) daily; depending on patient response, up to 200 mg (20 mL) daily may be given for >3 wk, continue for 2 wk after symptoms resolve

Available forms: Caps 100 mg; oral sol 10 mg/mL; tab 200 mg

Pulmonary or disseminated extrapulmonary blastomycosis

Adults: PO (capsules) 200 mg PO 3 times daily for 3 days followed by 200 mg PO 1 or 2 times daily for 6-12 mo; **PO (Tolsura)** 130 mg PO once daily with 65-mg-increment dose increases to a maximum of 260 mg/day if there is no obvious improvement or there is evidence of progressive fungal disease. Administer doses above 130 mg/day in 2 divided doses

Treatment of serious, life-threatening systemic fungal infections

Adult: PO (capsules) Loading dosage of 200 mg 3 times daily (600 mg daily) for the first 3 days, then 200-400 mg daily, usually continued for 3 mo and until clinical parameters and laboratory tests indicate that the active fungal infection has subsided

Treatment of pulmonary or extrapulmonary aspergillosis

Adult: PO (capsules) 200-400 mg daily for at least 3 mo

Treatment of pulmonary or extrapulmonary blastomycosis

Adult: PO (capsules) 200 mg once daily. If there is evidence of progression or no apparent improvement, increase dosage in 100-mg increments daily up to a max 400 mg daily for 6-12 mo

Treatment of oropharyngeal candidiasis

Adult: PO (oral solution) 200 mg (20 mL) daily for 1-2 wk. Generally resolves within several days; retreatment in patients who failed to respond to or are refractory to oral fluconazole: Manufacturer recommends 100 mg (10 mL) twice daily. A response to itraconazole in these patients generally is evident within 2-4 wk; relapse may be expected shortly after the drug is discontinued

HIV-infected adults PO (oral solution) 200 mg daily × 7-14 days

Treatment of esophageal candidiasis

Adult: PO (oral solution) 100 mg (10 mL) daily; depending on patient response, up to 200 mg (20 mL) daily may be given for ≥3 wk, continue for 2 wk after symptoms resolve

Administer:
- In the presence of acid products only; do not use alkaline products, antacids within 2 hr of product; may give coffee, tea, acidic fruit juices

PO route
- Swallow caps whole; do not break, crush, or chew caps
- Give caps after full meal to ensure absorption
- Oral sol: patient should swish in mouth vigorously, use on empty stomach
- Oral sol and caps are not interchangeable on mg/mg basis
- Store in tight container at room temperature, do not freeze

SIDE EFFECTS
CNS: *Headache, dizziness,* insomnia, somnolence, depression
CV: Hypertension, HF
GI: *Nausea, vomiting, anorexia, diarrhea,* cramps, *abdominal pain,* flatulence, GI bleeding, hepatotoxicity
GU: Gynecomastia, impotence, decreased libido
INTEG: *Pruritus,* fever, *rash,* toxic epidermal necrolysis, Stevens-Johnson syndrome
MISC: *Edema, fatigue,* malaise, hypokalemia, tinnitus, rhabdomyolysis
RESP: Rhinitis, sinusitis, upper respiratory infection, pulmonary edema

PHARMACOKINETICS
PO: Peak 3-4 hr; half-life 21 hr, IV 35.4 hr; metabolized in liver; excreted in bile, feces, urine 40%; requires acid pH for absorption; distributed poorly to CSF; 99.8% protein bound; inhibits CYP3A4

INTERACTIONS
- Life-threatening CV reactions—pimozide, quiNIDine, dofetilide, levomethadyl, dronedarone
Increase: tinnitus, hearing loss—quiNIDine
Increase: hepatotoxicity—other hepatotoxic products
Increase: edema—calcium channel blockers

Increase: severe hypoglycemia—oral hypoglycemics
Increase: sedation—ALPRAZolam, clorazepate, diazePAM, estazolam, flurazepam, triazolam, oral midazolam
Increase: levels, toxicity—busPIRone, busulfan, clarithromycin, cycloSPORINE, diazePAM, digoxin, felodipine, fentaNYL, atorvastatin, carBAMazepine, disopyramide, indinavir, isradipine, niCARdipine, NiFEdipine, niMODipine, phenytoin, quiNIDine, QUEtiapine, ritonavir, saquinavir, tacrolimus, warfarin
Decrease: itraconazole action—antacids, H$_2$-receptor antagonists, rifamycins, didanosine, carBAMazepine, isoniazid, proton pump inhibitors

Drug/Food
- Food increases absorption
- Grapefruit juice decreases itraconazole level

Drug/Lab Test
Increase: LFTs, alk phos, bilirubin, triglyceride, GGT

NURSING CONSIDERATIONS
Assess:
- **HF:** if present, discontinue product
- Type of infection; may begin treatment before obtaining results
- **Infection:** temperature, WBC, sputum at baseline and periodically
- I&O ratio, potassium levels
- Hepatic studies (ALT, AST, bilirubin) if patient receiving long-term therapy
- **Allergic reaction:** rash, photosensitivity, urticaria, dermatitis
- **Hepatotoxicity:** nausea, vomiting, jaundice, clay-colored stools, fatigue
- **Pregnancy/breastfeeding:** do not use in onychomycosis; use for other conditions only if benefits outweigh fetal risk; do not use in breastfeeding
Evaluate:
- **Therapeutic response:** decreased fever, malaise, rash, negative C&S for infecting organism
Teach patient/family:
- That long-term therapy may be needed to clear infection (1 wk-6 mo, depending on infection)

• To avoid hazardous activities if dizziness occurs

• To take 2 hr before administration of other products that increase gastric pH (antacids, H₂-blockers, omeprazole, sucralfate, anticholinergics); to avoid grapefruit juice; to notify health care provider of all medications taken; to take after a full meal (caps) or on empty stomach (oral sol)

• About the importance of compliance with product regimen; to use alternative methods of contraception

• To notify prescriber of GI symptoms; signs of hepatic dysfunction (fatigue, jaundice, nausea, anorexia, vomiting, dark urine, pale stools); heart failure (trouble breathing, unusual weight gain, fatigue, swelling); hearing changes

ivacaftor (Rx)

(eye′va-kaf′tor)

Kalydeco

Func. class.: Respiratory agent

USES: Cystic fibrosis in those with G551D, G1244E, G1349D, G178R, G5515S, S1255P, S549N, S549R mutation in the CFTR gene

DOSAGE AND ROUTES

• **Adult/adolescent/child ≥6 yr: PO** 150 mg q12hr with fat-containing food

Child 4-6 mon, ≥5 kg: PO One 25-mg packet of granules q12 hr with fat-containing food; **6 mo-<6 yr, 5-<7 kg:** One 25-mg packet of granules q12 hr; mix with fat containing food; **6-<6 yr, 7-<14 kg:** One 50-mg packet of granules q12hr; mix with fat containing food; **6 mo-<6 yr, ≥14 kg:** One 75-mg packet of granules q12hr with fat containing food

ivabradine (Rx)

Corlanor

Func. class.: CV agent, misc

DOSAGE AND ROUTES

Stable symptomatic heart failure

• **Adults: PO** 5 mg bid; after 2 wk, adjust to achieve a resting HR between 50 and 60 bpm

• **Child/adolescent ≥40 kg: PO** 2.5 mg bid, adjust by 2.5 mg at 2-wk intervals to a target HR reduction of at least 20% based on tolerability

• **Child/adolescent <40 kg: PO** 0.05 mg/kg/dose bid, adjust by 0.05 mg/kg at 2-wk intervals to a target HR reduction of at least 20% based on tolerability

• **Infants 6-11 mo: PO** 0.05 mg/kg/dose bid, adjust by 0.05 mg/kg at 2-wk intervals to a target HR reduction of at least 20% based on tolerability

Available forms: Tablets 5, 7.5 mg; oral solution 5 mg/5 mL (1 mg/mL)

ivosidenib (Rx)

(I′-voh-sih′-deh-nib)

Tibsovo

Func. class.: Antineoplastic

USES: Relapsed or refractory AML with an isocitrate dehydrogenase-1 (IDH1) mutation

CONTRAINDICATIONS

Hypersensitivity, pregnancy

Black Box Warning: Differentiation syndrome

DOSAGE AND ROUTES

• **Adult: PO** 500 mg daily until disease progression or unacceptable toxicity

⚠ HIGH ALERT

ixabepilone (Rx)

(ix-ab-ep′i-lone)

Ixempra

Func. class.: Antineoplastic—miscellaneous

Chem. class.: Epothilone, B analogue

ACTION: Microtubule stabilizing agent; microtubules are needed for cell division

USES: Breast cancer resistant to taxanes and anthracyclines

CONTRAINDICATIONS

Pregnancy, breastfeeding, hypersensitivity to products with polyoxyethylated castor oil, neutropenia of <1,500/mm^3, thrombocytopenia

Black Box Warning: Hepatic disease (AST or ALT >2.5 times upper limits, bilirubin >1 time upper limit)

Precautions: Children, geriatric patients, alcoholism, bone marrow suppression, cardiac dysrhythmias, cardiac/renal disease, diabetes mellitus, peripheral neuropathy, ventricular dysfunction

DOSAGE AND ROUTES
• **Adult: IV INFUSION** 40 mg/m^2 over 3 hr q3wk
Dosage reduction in those taking a strong CYP3A4 inhibitor
• **Adult: IV INFUSION** 20 mg/m^2 over 3 hr q3wk
Hepatic dose
• **Adult:** IV 20 mg/m^2 q3wk, max 30 mg/m^2
Available forms: Powder for inj 15, 45 mg
Administer:
• Premedicate with histamine antagonists 1 hr before use, prevents hypersensitivity
• Antiemetic 30-60 min before product and prn
IV route
• Let kit stand at room temperature for 30 min; to reconstitute, withdraw supplied diluent (8 mL for 15-mg vials, 23.5 mL for 45-mg vials); slowly inject sol into vial; gently swirl and invert to mix, final concentration 2 mg/mL; further dilute in LR in DEHP-free bags, final concentration should be between 0.2 and 0.6 mg/mL; after added, mix by manual rotation
• Diluted sol stable for 6 hr at room temperature; infusion must be completed within 6 hr
• Use in-line filter, 0.2-1.2 micron
• Give over 3 hr

SIDE EFFECTS
CNS: *Peripheral neuropathy,* impaired cognition, chills, fatigue, fever, flushing, headache, insomnia, *asthenia*

CV: Bradycardia, *hypotension,* abnormal ECG, angina, atrial flutter, cardiomyopathy, chest pain, edema, MI, vasculitis
GI: *Nausea, vomiting, diarrhea,* abdominal pain, anorexia, colitis, constipation, gastritis, jaundice, GERD, hepatic failure, trismus
GU: Renal failure
HEMA: Neutropenia, thrombocytopenia, anemia, infections, coagulopathy
INTEG: *Alopecia,* rash, hot flashes
META: Hypokalemia, metabolic acidosis
MS: *Arthralgia, myalgia*
RESP: Bronchospasm, cough, dyspnea
SYST: *Hypersensitivity reactions,* anaphylaxis, dehydration, radiation recall reaction

PHARMACOKINETICS
Metabolized in liver by CYP3A4; excreted in feces (65%) and urine (21%); terminal half-life 52 hr

INTERACTIONS
Increase: ixabepilone level—CYP3A4 inhibitors (amiodarone, amprenavir, aprepitant, atazanavir, chloramphenicol, clarithromycin, conivaptan, cycloSPORINE, danazol, darunavir, dalfopristin, delavirdine, diltiaZEM, erythromycin, estradiol, fluconazole, fluvoxaMINE, fosamprenavir, imatinib, indinavir, isoniazid, itraconazole, ketoconazole, lopinavir, miconazole, nefazodone, nelfinavir, propoxyphene, ritonavir, RU-486, saquinavir, tamoxifen, telithromycin, troleandomycin, verapamil, voriconazole, zafirlukast), toxicity, avoid using together
Decrease: ixabepilone levels—CYP3A4 inducers (aminoglutethimide, barbiturates, bexarotene, bosentan, carBAMazepine, dexamethasone, efavirenz, griseofulvin, modafinil, nafcillin, nevirapine, OXcarbazepine, phenytoin, rifamycin, topiramate), avoid using together
Drug/Herb
• Avoid use with St. John's wort
Drug/Food
• Avoid use with grapefruit products

Side effects: *italics* = common; red = life-threatening

NURSING CONSIDERATIONS
Assess:
• CBC, differential, platelet count before treatment and weekly; withhold product if WBC is <1,500/mm³ or platelet count is <100,000/mm³, notify prescriber
• Monitor temperature q4hr (may indicate beginning infection)

Black Box Warning: Hepatic disease: liver function tests before, during therapy (bilirubin, AST, ALT, LDH) prn or monthly; check for jaundiced skin and sclera, dark urine, clay-colored stools, itchy skin, abdominal pain, fever, diarrhea; contraindicated in combination with capecitabine if AST or ALT is >2.5 × ULN or bilirubin >1 × ULN due to risk of toxicity and neutropenia-related death

• VS during 1st hr of infusion; check IV site for signs of infiltration
• **Hypersensitivity reactions, anaphylaxis** including hypotension, dyspnea, angioedema, generalized urticaria; discontinue infusion immediately; keep emergency equipment available
• Effects of alopecia on body image; discuss feelings about body changes
• **Pregnancy/breastfeeding:** do not use in pregnancy or breastfeeding
Evaluate:
• **Therapeutic response:** decreased tumor size, spread of malignancy
Teach patient/family:
• **To report signs of infection:** fever, sore throat, flulike symptoms
• **To report signs of anemia:** fatigue, headache, faintness, SOB
• To report any complaints or side effects to nurse or prescriber
• That hair may be lost during treatment; that a wig or hairpiece may make patient feel better; that new hair may be different in color, texture
• That pain in muscles and joints 2-5 days after infusion is common
• To use nonhormonal type of contraception

• To avoid receiving vaccinations while receiving product

---

ixazomib (Rx)
(ix-az′-oh-mib)
Ninlaro
Func. class.: Antineoplastic agent
Chem. class.: Proteasome inhibitor

ACTION: Reversibly inhibits proteasomes, enzyme complexes that regulate protein homeostasis within the cell; reversibly inhibits chymotrypsin-like activity of the beta 5 subunit of the 20S proteasome, leading to activation of signaling cascades, cell-cycle arrest, and apoptosis

USES: Multiple myeloma

CONTRAINDICATIONS
Hypersensitivity
Precautions:
• Bone marrow suppression, dermatologic toxicity, gastrointestinal toxicity, hepatic disease, herpes zoster infection, peripheral edema, peripheral neuropathy, thrombotic microangiopathy, renal disease

SIDE EFFECTS
CV: Peripheral edema
INTEG: Rash
GI: Constipation, diarrhea, nausea, vomiting
HEMA: Thrombocytopenia, neutropenia
CNS: Peripheral neuropathy, peripheral sensory neuropathy
MS: Back pain
EENT: Eye disease
RESP: URI

PHARMACOKINETICS
Onset unknown, peak 1 hr, duration unknown, half-life 9.5 days

INTERACTIONS
Decrease: ixazomib effect—CYP3A4 inducers (carBAMazepine, phenytoins, rifamycins), avoid using together

---

Drug/Herb

Decrease: ixazomib effect—St. John's wort, avoid using together

DOSAGE AND ROUTES
Multiple myeloma
Adult: PO 4 mg once weekly on days 1, 8, and 15 of a 28-day treatment cycle (in combination with lenalidomide and dexamethasone); continue until disease progression or unacceptable toxicity

Available forms:
Capsules 2.3, 3, 4 mg

Administer:
• Use cytotoxic handling procedure, do not touch capsules, use gloves
• Give 1 hr before or 2 hr after food, capsules should be swallowed whole
• If a dose is missed, give only if the next scheduled dose is ≥72 hr, do not take a missed dose within 3 days of the next scheduled dose; do not double doses to make up for the missed dose. If vomiting occurs, do not repeat the dose; resume dosing at the next scheduled dose
• Store at room temperature, do not freeze

NURSING CONSIDERATIONS
Assess:
• **Bone marrow suppression:** Platelet nadirs (14-21 days) of each cycle with a recovery to baseline by the start of the next cycle. Monitor platelet counts at least monthly, more frequent monitoring during the initial 3 cycles. May require therapy interruption, dosage reduction, and/or platelet transfusions. Monitor CBC (with differential) for neutropenia; therapy interruption or dosage modification may be needed; monitor for bleeding, bruising
• **Dermatologic toxicity:** Monitor for dermatologic toxicity and use supportive care or dosage modification of ixazomib and/or lenalidomide (for grade 2 or higher toxicity); SJS may occur (rare)
• **Gastrointestinal toxicity:** Monitor diarrhea, constipation, nausea, and vomiting have been reported, antidiarrheals, antiemetics, and supportive

care, dosage change for grade 3 or 4 symptoms
• **Hepatotoxicity:** Monitor LFTs baseline and regularly; may require dosage adjustment for grade 3 or 4 toxicity
• **Herpes zoster infection:** May use an antiviral prophylaxis to decrease the risk of herpes zoster reactivation
• **Peripheral edema:** Assess for potential underlying causes and provide supportive care
• **Peripheral neuropathy:** Monitor for neuropathy; may require dosage adjustment (of ixazomib and/or lenalidomide) or treatment discontinuation
• **Thrombotic microangiopathy:** Monitor for signs/symptoms. Interrupt therapy if TTP/HUS is suspected
• **Renal disease:** Reduced initial doses for 30 mL/min or end-stage renal disease requiring dialysis
• **Pregnancy/breastfeeding:** Males and females of reproductive potential should use effective contraception during and for 90 days after last dose. Women using hormonal contraception should also use a barrier method

Evaluate:
• **Therapeutic response:** Delayed progression of multiple myeloma with minimum toxicity

Teach patient/family:
• To take at the same time of day on the same day of the week for 3 wk out of 4 wk, do not double or skip doses, take whole
• Not to touch capsule, use gloves
• To notify provider of adverse reactions: bleeding, bruising, severe diarrhea, constipation, burning/tingling of feet or hands, weight gain, rash, yellow skin, eyes, clay-colored stools, pain in right upper area of abdomen
• **Pregnancy/breastfeeding:** To report if pregnancy is planned or suspected or if breastfeeding; not to use during pregnancy, both males and females should use contraception during and for 90 days after last dose, women taking hormonal contraceptive should also use barrier method, not to breastfeed

ixekizumab (Rx)

(ix'e-kiz'ue-mab)

Taltz

Func. class.: Immunosuppressive
Chem. class.: Interleukin antagonist

ACTION: A human IgG4 monoclonal antibody that selectively binds to the interleukin 17A (IL-17A) cytokine, inhibiting its interaction with the IL-17 receptor. Treatment inhibits the release of proinflammatory cytokines and chemokines

USES: The treatment of moderate to severe plaque psoriasis in adults who are candidates for systemic therapy or phototherapy, active psoriatic arthritis, ankylosing spondylitis, no radiographic axial spondyloarthritis

CONTRAINDICATIONS

Risk of serious hypersensitivity reactions or anaphylaxis

Precautions: Breastfeeding, children, Crohn's disease, immunosuppression, infection, inflammatory bowel disease, pregnancy, tuberculosis, ulcerative colitis, vaccination

DOSAGE AND ROUTES

Plaque psoriasis

Child 6-18 yr and >50 kg: SUBCUT 160 mg, then 80 mg q4wk; 25-50 kg: 80 mg then 40 mg q4wk

Acute psoriatic arthritis/ankylosing spondylitis

Adult: SUBCUT 160 mg, then 80 mg q4wk

Active nonradiographic axial spondyloarthritis

Adult: SUBCUT 80 mg q4wk

• **Adult: SUBCUT** 160 mg at week 0 (administered as two 80-mg injections) followed by 80 mg at weeks 2, 4, 6, 8, 10, and 12, then 80 mg q4wk; for active psoriatic arthritis maintenance 80 mg q4wk

• **Available forms:** Solution for injection 80 mg/mL, autoinjector 80 mg/mL

Administer:

SUBCUT route

• Administer by subcutaneous injection only

• Visually inspect for particulate matter and discoloration before use. The solution should be free of visible particles, clear, and colorless to slightly yellow

• Available as a prefilled syringe and as an autoinjector; each device contains 80 mg

• Use upper arms, thighs, and any quadrant of the abdomen for injection sites

• Do not use where skin is tender, bruised, erythematous, indurated, or affected by psoriasis; rotate sites with each dose

• Does not contain preservatives; discard any unused product

• **Missed doses:** If a dose is missed, give as soon as possible. Then, resume dosing at the regular scheduled time

• **Storage of unopened prefilled syringes and autoinjectors:** Protect from light; store refrigerated at 2° C-8° C (36° F-46° F) until time of use. Do not freeze and do not use the injection if it has been frozen. Do not shake

SIDE EFFECTS

SYST: antibody formation, infection, angioedema

INTEG: injection site reaction, urticaria

HEMA: neutropenia

PHARMACOKINETICS

Half-life is 13 days; bioavailability 60% to 81%, injection in the thigh achieved higher bioavailability; peak 4 days

INTERACTIONS

• Do not use concurrently with vaccines; immunizations should be brought up-to-date before treatment

• Avoid use with immunosuppressives

NURSING CONSIDERATIONS

Assess:

• **TB:** TB testing should be done before use c

• For injection-site reactions, redness, swelling, pain

• Bring immunizations up-to-date before use
• **Infection:** monitor for fever, sore throat, cough; do not use in active infections
• **Pregnancy/breastfeeding:** avoid in pregnancy and breastfeeding
Evaluate:
• **Therapeutic response:** decreased lesions and spread, decreased painful joints, inflammation in psoriatic arthritis

Teach Patient/Family:
• That product must be continued for prescribed time to be effective, to use as prescribed
• Not to receive vaccinations during treatment
• **Infection:** to notify prescriber of possible infections, respiratory or other, or of allergic reactions
• Injection techniques and disposal of equipment, not to reuse needles, syringes

ketoconazole (Rx)

(kee-toe-koe′na-zole)

Func. class.: Antifungal
Chem. class.: Imidazole derivative

USES: Chronic mucocandidiasis, oral thrush, candiduria, coccidioidomycosis, histoplasmosis, chromomycosis, paracoccidioidomycosis, blastomycosis; tinea cruris, tinea corporis, tinea versicolor, *Pityrosporum ovale* in patients who are intolerant to other antifungal therapies or for whom other antifungal therapies have failed

CONTRAINDICATIONS

Breastfeeding, hypersensitivity, fungal meningitis

> **Black Box Warning:** Coadministration with other products (ergot derivatives, cisapride, or triazolam) may cause fatal cardiac arrhythmias due to inhibition of CYP3A4 enzyme system

> **Black Box Warning:** Hepatic disease

DOSAGE AND ROUTES

• **Adult:** PO 200-400 mg/day for 1-2 wk (candidiasis), 6 mo (other infections)
• **Child ≥2 yr:** PO 3.3-6.6 mg/kg/day as a single daily dose, max 400 mg/day

Prostate cancer (unlabeled)
• **Adult:** PO 400 mg tid with PO hydrocortisone

Available forms: Tabs 200 mg

ketoconazole (topical) (Rx)

(kee-toe-koe′na-zole)

Extina, Ketoderm ✦, Ketozole ✦, Nizoral, Nizoral A-D, Xolegel
Func. class.: Topical antifungal
Chem. class.: Imidazole derivative

ACTION: Antifungal activity results from altering cell membrane permeability

USES: Seborrheic dermatitis (immunocompromised), tinea corporis, tinea cruris, tinea pedis, tinea versicolor, dandruff

CONTRAINDICATIONS

Hypersensitivity, sulfite allergy
Precautions: Pregnancy, breastfeeding, children

DOSAGE AND ROUTES
Seborrheic dermatitis
• **Adult/child ≥12 yr: TOP FOAM** apply to affected areas bid × 4 wk; **GEL** apply to affected areas daily × 2 wk

Tinea corporis, tinea cruris, tinea pedis, tinea versicolor
• **Adult: TOP** cover areas daily × 2 wk

Dandruff
• **Adult: SHAMPOO** wet hair, lather, massage for 1 min, rinse, repeat 2×/wk spaced by 3 days, for up to 8 wk, then as needed

Available forms: Topical gel, foam, cream 2%; shampoo 1%, 2%

Administer:
Topical route
• For external use only; do not use skin products near the eyes, nose, or mouth; wash hands before and after use
• **Cream/lotion:** Apply to the cleansed affected area, massage gently into affected areas, do not use on skin that is broken or irritated

SIDE EFFECTS
INTEG: Irritation, stinging, pustules, pruritus

NURSING CONSIDERATIONS
Assess allergic reaction:
• Assess for hypersensitivity; product may need to be discontinued
• Assess for sulfite allergy; may be life-threatening

Evaluate:
• Therapeutic response: decreased itching, scaling

Teach patient/family:
Topical route
• These products are not for intravaginal therapy, external use only; do not use skin products near the eyes, nose, or mouth; wash hands before and after use; do not wash affected area for ≥3 hr after application
• **Cream/ointment/lotion:** apply a thin film to the cleansed affected area, massage gently

• **Foam formulations:** do not dispense foam directly onto hands or face; dispense directly into the cap or onto a cool surface; cover the affected area(s); to apply, pick up small amounts of the foam with the fingertips and gently massage into the affected areas

• To continue for prescribed time, tinea corporis/cruris ≥2 wk

ketoprofen (OTC, Rx)
(ke-toe-proe′fen)

Apo-Keto ✦

Func. class.: Nonsteroidal antiinflammatory product (NSAID), antirheumatic, analgesic

Chem. class.: Propionic acid derivative

Do not confuse:
ketoprofen/ketorolac

ACTION: May inhibit prostaglandin synthesis; analgesic, antiinflammatory, antipyretic

USES: Mild to moderate pain, osteoarthritis, rheumatoid arthritis, dysmenorrhea; OTC relief of minor aches, pains

Black Box Warning: CABG, GI bleeding/perforation, thromboembolism

DOSAGE AND ROUTES
Analgesic
• **Adult: PO** 25-50 mg q6-8hr, max 300 mg/day
Rheumatoid arthitis, osteoarthritis
• **Adult: PO** 50 mg qid or 75 mg tid, max 300 mg/day or **EXT REL** up to 200 mg/day
Dysmenorrhea
• **Adult: PO** 25-50 mg q6-8hr (immediate release) up to max 300 mg/day
Ankylosing spondylitis (unlabeled)
• **Adults: PO** 100 bid
Renal/hepatic dose
• **Adult: PO** GFR <25 mL/min/1.73m², albumin <3.5 g/dL, decreased hepatic function, or ESRD, max 100 mg/day

Available forms: Caps 25, 50, 75, 100 mg; ext rel cap 200 mg

ketorolac (ophthalmic) (Rx)
(kee′toe-role-ak)

Acular, Acular LS, Acuvail

Func. class.: Antiinflammatory (ophthalmic)

Chem. class.: Nonsteroidal antiinflammatory drug (NSAID)

ACTION: Inhibits miosis by inhibiting the biosynthesis of ocular prostaglandins; prostaglandins play a role in the miotic response produced during ocular surgery by constricting the iris sphincter

USES: Pain and inflammation after cataract surgery, refractive surgery, seasonal allergic conjunctivitis

CONTRAINDICATIONS
Hypersensitivity to this product, NSAIDs, salicylates

Precautions: Bleeding disorders, complicated ocular surgery, corneal denervation, diabetes mellitus, rheumatoid arthritis, dry eye syndrome, pregnancy, breastfeeding, children, contact lenses

DOSAGE AND ROUTES
Seasonal allergic conjunctivitis (Acular)
• **Adult/child ≥2 yr: OPHTH** Instill 1 drop into affected eye qid
Inflammation after cataract extraction (Acular)
• **Adult: OPHTH** 1 drop in affected eye qid beginning 24 hr after surgery × 2 wk
Corneal refracture surgery, pain, burning (Acular LS)
• **Adult: OPHTH** 1 drop in affected eye qid × ≤4 days
Cataract surgery, pain, inflammation (Acuvail)
• **Adult: OPHTH** 1 drop bid in affected eye, starting 1 day before surgery, on the day of surgery, × 2 wk after surgery

Side effects: *italics* = common; red = life-threatening

Available forms: Ophthalmic solution Acular (0.5%), Acular LS (0.4%), Acuvail (0.45%)

Administer:

• Apply topically to the eye, separate by ≥5 min when using with other ophthalmics
• Remove contact lenses before instillation of solution
• Instruct patient on proper instillation of eye solution
• Do not touch the tip of the dropper to the eye, fingertips, or other surface
• Do not share bottle with other patients

SIDE EFFECTS

CNS: Headache
EENT: Abnormal sensation in eye, conjunctival hyperemia, ocular irritation, ocular pain, ocular pruritus, conjunctival hyperemia, iritis, keratitis, blurred vision, transient burning/stinging

NURSING CONSIDERATIONS

Assess:

• **Eyes:** for pain, inflammation, burning, redness after cataract surgery, visual acuity

Evaluate:

• Therapeutic response: decreased pain and inflammation after cataract surgery, refractive surgery, seasonal allergic conjunctivitis

Teach patient/family:

• To apply topically to the eye
• To remove contact lenses before instillation of solution, wait 10 min before reinserting
• Proper instillation of eye solution
• Not to touch the tip of the dropper to the eye, fingertips, or other surface
• Not to share bottle with other patients

---

ketorolac (systemic, nasal) (Rx)

(kee-toe′role-ak)

Toradol ✦, Sprix

Func. class.: NSAIDs
Chem. class.: Acetic acid

Do not confuse:
ketorolac/Ketalar, ketoprofen

ACTION: Inhibits prostaglandin synthesis; analgesic antiinflammatory antipyretic effects

USES: Mild to moderate pain (short term), including postsurgery

CONTRAINDICATIONS

Pregnancy 3rd trimester, hypersensitivity to this product, salicylates, asthma, hepatic disease, peptic ulcer disease, CV bleeding, C-section, intracranial bleeding

Black Box Warning: Severe renal disease, L&D, before major surgery, epidural/intrathecal administration, GI bleeding/perforation, hypovolemia, NSAID hypersensitivity, peptic ulcer disease, CABG, hematologic disease, intracranial bleeding

Precautions: Pregnancy/breastfeeding, GI/cardiac disorders, hypersensitivity to other antiinflammatory agents, CCr <25 mL/min

Black Box Warning: Bleeding, MI, stroke; limit duration of use; geriatric patients, children, infants/neonates, serious hypersensitivity reactions or anaphylaxis

DOSAGE AND ROUTES

Max 5 combined days of all routes, only use PO as continuation to IV/IM

• **Adult: IM/IV: Single dose:** ≥50 kg 60 mg IM or 30 mg IV once; **<50 kg** 30 mg IM or 15 mg IV once
• **Adult: IM/IV: Multiple dose:** ≥50 kg 30 mg IM/IV q6hr as needed; max 120 mg/day; **Nasal** 31.5 mg q6-8hr (1 spray each nostril); **<50 kg** 15 mg IM/IV q6hr as needed; max 60 mg/day; **Nasal** 15.75 mg q6-8hr (1 spray in 1 nostril). Continuation therapy (should not be given as an initial dose)
• **Adult: PO ≥50 kg** 20 mg once, then 10 mg q4-6hr as needed; **<50 kg:** 10 mg, then 10 mg q4-6hr as needed, max 40 mg/day

Renal dose

• **Adults: PO** 10 mg, then 10 mg q4-6hr, max 40 mg

Available forms: Inj 15, 30 mg/mL (prefilled syringes), 60 mg/2 mL; tab 10 mg; nasal spray 15.75 mg/spray
Administer:
• Store at room temperature
IM route
• IM inj deeply and slowly in large muscle mass, painful
Nasal route
• Prime pump before using for the first time, point away from person/pets, pump activator 5 times, no need to reprime
• For single-use only, discard 24 hr after opening if not used
• Do not share with others
• Have patient blow nose, sit upright to spray
IV route
• Give undiluted over ≥15 sec, protect from light

SIDE EFFECTS
CNS: Dizziness, *drowsiness,* tremors, seizures, headache
CV: Hypertension, pallor, edema, CV thrombotic events, MI, stroke
EENT: Tinnitus, hearing loss, blurred vision
GI: Nausea, anorexia, vomiting, diarrhea, constipation, flatulence, cramps, dry mouth, peptic ulcer, GI bleeding, perforation, taste change, hepatic failure
GU: Nephrotoxicity: dysuria, hematuria, oliguria
HEMA: Blood dyscrasias, prolonged bleeding
INTEG: Purpura, rash, pruritus, sweating, angioedema, Stevens-Johnson syndrome, toxic epidermal necrolysis

PHARMACOKINETICS
Enters breast milk, metabolized by liver, excreted by kidneys
PO: Onset 30-60 min, peak 2-3 hr, duration 4-6 hr, half-life 2-9 hr
IM: Onset 30 min, duration 4-6 hr, half-life 2-9 hr
IV: Onset 30 min, peak 2-3 hr, duration 4-6 hr

INTERACTIONS
Increase: toxicity—methotrexate, lithium, cycloSPORINE, pentoxifylline, probenecid, cidofovir

Increase: bleeding risk—anticoagulants, salicylates, tirofiban, thrombolytics, SSRIs, SNRIs
Increase: renal impairment—ACE inhibitors, ARBs
Increase: GI effects—corticosteroids, alcohol, aspirin, NSAIDs
Decrease: effects—antihypertensives, diuretics
Drug/Lab Test
Increase: AST, ALT, LDH, bleeding time

NURSING CONSIDERATIONS
Assess:

Black Box Warning: Aspirin sensitivity, asthma: patients may be more likely to develop hypersensitivity to NSAIDs; monitor for hypersensitivity

• **Pain:** type, location, intensity, ROM before and 1 hr after treatment, do not use long term or for minor pain

Black Box Warning: Renal, hepatic, blood studies: BUN, creatinine, AST, ALT, HB before treatment, periodically thereafter; check for dehydration

Black Box Warning: Bleeding: check for bruising, bleeding, occult blood in urine, stool guaiac, can prolong bleeding time

Black Box Warning: Do not use epidurally, intrathecally; alcohol is present in the solution

• **Eye/ear problems:** blurred vision, tinnitus (may indicate toxicity)
• **Hepatic dysfunction:** jaundice, yellow sclera and skin, clay-colored stools

Black Box Warning: **CV thrombotic events:** MI, stroke; do not use in perioperative pain in CABG

• Audiometric, ophthalmic exam before, during, after treatment

Side effects: *italics* = common; red = life-threatening

Black Box Warning: **Beers:** avoid in older adults; increased risk of GI bleeding, peptic ulcer disease; those >65 and 50 kg, adjust dose to CCr, risk is increased; max 60 mg/day

Evaluate:
• **Therapeutic response:** decreased pain, stiffness, swelling in joints, ability to move more easily

Teach patient/family:

Black Box Warning: To report blurred vision, ringing/roaring in ears (may indicate toxicity)

• To avoid driving, other hazardous activities if dizziness or drowsiness occurs

Black Box Warning: To report change in urine pattern, weight increase, edema; pain increase in joints, fever, blood in urine **(indicates nephrotoxicity);** bruising, black tarry stools **(indicates bleeding);** pruritus, jaundice, nausea, right upper quadrant pain, abdominal pain **(hepatotoxicity);** to notify prescriber immediately

• To report immediately signs of MI, stroke
• To maintain hydration
• To take with food (PO)
• That pain may occur with IM
• To avoid alcohol, salicylates, other NSAIDs
• To report product use to all health care providers, not to use with other products unless approved by prescriber; use for ≤5 days
• **Nasal:** to discard within 24 hr of opening; may cause irritation, may drink water after dose, to read instructions provided

Black Box Warning: **Pregnancy/breast-feeding:** to notify prescriber if pregnancy is planned or suspected; not to breast-feed; contraindicated during labor and delivery

ketotifen (ophthalmic) (Rx)

(kee-toe-tye′fen)

Alaway, Zaditor, ZyrTEC Itchy Eye, Claritin Eye

Func. class.: Antihistamine (ophthalmic)

Chem. class.: Histamine 1 receptor antagonist/mast cell stabilizer

ACTION: A topically active, direct H_1-receptor antagonist and mast cell stabilizer; by reducing these inflammatory mediators, relieves the ocular pruritus associated with allergic conjunctivitis

USES: For the temporary relief of ocular pruritus due to ragweed, pollen, grass, animal hair, animal dander

CONTRAINDICATIONS
Hyper-sensitivity
Precautions: Pregnancy, breastfeeding, children, contact lenses

DOSAGE AND ROUTES
• **Adult/child ≥3 yr: OPHTH** instill 1 drop in affected eye(s) every 8-12 hr
Available forms: Ophthalmic solution 0.025%
Administer:
Ophthalmic route
• For topical ophthalmic use only
• Wash hands before and after use; squeeze drops into the conjunctival sac
• Do not touch the tip of the dropper to the eye, fingertips, or other surface
• Wait ≥10 min after instilling the ophthalmic solution before inserting contact lenses; contact lenses should not be worn if eye is red

SIDE EFFECTS
CNS: Headache
EENT: Conjunctival hyperemia, rhinitis, allergic reactions, ocular irritation consisting of burning or stinging, conjunctivitis, eyelid disorder, flu syndrome, keratitis, lacrimation disorder, mydriasis, ocular discharge, ocular pain, pharyngitis,

photophobia, pruritus, rash, xerophthalmia (dry eyes)

NURSING CONSIDERATIONS
Assess:
• Eyes: for itching, redness, tearing, use
of soft or hard contact lens
Evaluate:
• Absence of redness, itching in the
eyes
Teach patient/family:
Ophthalmic route
• That product is for topical ophthalmic
use only
• To wash hands before and after use;
tilt the head back slightly and pull the
lower eyelid down with the index finger;
squeeze drops into the conjunctival sac
and gently close eyes for 1-2 min; not to
blink
• Not to touch the tip of the dropper to
the eye, fingertips, or other surface
• To wait ≥10 min after instilling the
ophthalmic solution before inserting
contact lenses; contact lenses should not
be worn if eye is red
• Not to share ophthalmic drops with
others
• To remove contact lenses before use;
the preservative benzalkonium chloride
may be absorbed by soft contact
lenses

K

> ## ⚠ HIGH ALERT

labetalol (Rx)
(la-bet'a-lole)

Trandate ✦

Func. class.: Antihypertensive, antianginal

Chem. class.: α-1/β-Blocker

Do not confuse:
labetalol/Lamictal/lamotrigine

ACTION: Produces decreases in B/P without reflex tachycardia or significant reduction in heart rate through mixture of α-blocking, β-blocking effects; elevated plasma renins are reduced

USES: Mild to moderate hypertension; treatment of severe hypertension (IV)

CONTRAINDICATIONS
Hypersensitivity to β-blockers, cardiogenic shock, heart block (2nd or 3rd degree), sinus bradycardia, HF, bronchial asthma

Precautions: Pregnancy, breastfeeding, geriatric patients, major surgery, diabetes mellitus, thyroid/renal/hepatic disease, COPD, well-compensated heart failure, nonallergic bronchospasm, peripheral vascular disease

> **Black Box Warning:** Abrupt discontinuation

DOSAGE AND ROUTES
Hypertension
• **Adult: PO Outpatient** 100 mg bid; may be given with diuretic; may increase to 200 mg bid after 2 days; may increase q1-3days; max 2400 mg/day in divided doses; **Inpatient** 200 mg then 200-400 mg in 6-12 hr, depends on response; may increase by 200 mg bid at 1-day intervals, max 2400 mg/day
• **Child/adolescent (unlabeled): PO** 1-3 mg/kg/day, titrate to max 10-12 mg/kg/day based on B/P, max 12 mg/kg/day, max 1200 mg/day; **IV** 0.2-1 mg/kg over 2 min; **IV INFUSION** 0.25-3 mg/kg/hr, max 3 mg/kg/hr

Hypertensive crisis
• **Adult: IV Intermittent** 10-20 mg over 2 min; may repeat 20-80 mg over 2 min q10min, max 300 mg; **IV Cont INFUSION** after loading dose give 0.5-2 mg/min until desired response or max 300 mg

Available forms: Tabs 100, 200, 300 mg; inj 5 mg/mL, 20-, 40-mL vials

Administer:
PO route
• PO before meals, or with meals; tab may be crushed or swallowed whole; give with meals to increase absorption
• Take pulse before use; if <50 bpm, hold dose, notify prescriber
• Take apical pulse before use; if <50 bpm, withhold; notify prescriber
• When discontinuing IV and starting PO, begin PO when B/P rises; start at 200 mg, then 200-400 mg in 6-12 hr; adjust as needed
• Do not discontinue before surgery or abruptly
• Store in dry area at room temperature; do not freeze

Direct IV route
• Give undiluted (5 mg/mL) over 2 min
Continuous IV INFUSION route
• Give at a rate of 2 mg/min after diluting in LR, D_5W, D_5 in 0.2%, 0.9%, 0.33% NaCl, Ringer's inj; infusion is titrated to patient response; 200 mg of product/160 mL sol = 1 mg/mL; 300 mg of product/240 mL sol = 1 mg/mL; 200 mg of product/250 mL sol = 2 mg/3 mL; use infusion pump
• Keep patient recumbent during and for 3 hr after administration; monitor VS q5-15min

Y-site compatibilities: Alemtuzumab, alfentanil, amikacin, aminocaproic acid, aminophylline, amiodarone, anidulafungin, argatroban, arsenic trioxide, ascorbic acid injection, atracurium, atropine, azithromycin, aztreonam, benztropine, bivalirudin, bleomycin, bretylium, bumetanide, buprenorphine, butorphanol, calcium chloride/gluconate, CARBOplatin, carmustine, caspofungin, ceFAZolin, cefotaxime, cefoTEtan, cefOXitin, ceftaroline, cefTAZidime, ceftizoxime, chlorproMAZINE, cimetidine, CISplatin, cloNIDine, cyanocobalamin, cyclophosphamide, cycloSPORINE, cytarabine, DACTINomycin, DAPTOmycin, DAUNOrubicin liposome, dexmedetomidine, dexrazoxane, digoxin, diltiazem, diphenhydrAMINE, DOBUTamine, DOCEtaxel, dolasetron, DOPamine, doripenem, doxacurium, DOXOrubicin, DOXOrubicin liposomal, doxycycline, enalaprilat, ePHEDrine, EPINEPHrine, epirubicin, epoetin alfa, eptifibatide, ertapenem, erythromycin lactobionate, esmolol, etoposide, etoposide phosphate, famotidine, fenoldopam, fentaNYL, fluconazole, fludarabine, fluorouracil, folic acid, gallium, ganciclovir, gatifloxacin, gemcitabine, gentamicin, glycopyrrolate, granisetron, HYDROmorphone, hydroxyzine, IDArubicin, ifosfamide, imipenem-cilastatin, inamrinone, irinotecan, isoproterenol, lactated Ringer's injection, lepirudin, leucovorin, levofloxacin, lidocaine, linezolid injection, LORazepam, magnesium sulfate, mannitol, mechlorethamine, meperidine, metaraminol, methyldopate, methylPREDNISolone, metoclopramide, metoprolol, metroNIDAZOLE, midazolam, milrinone, minocycline, mitoXANtrone, morphine, moxifloxacin, multiple vitamins injection, mycophenolate, nalbuphine, naloxone, netilmicin, niCARdipine, nitroglycerin, nitroprusside, norepinephrine, octreotide, ondansetron, oxacillin, oxaliplatin, oxytocin, palonosetron, pamidronate, pancuronium, papaverine, PEMEtrexed, pentamidine, pentazocine, PENTobarbital, PHENobarbital, phentolamine, phenylephrine, phytonadione, polymyxin B, potassium acetate/chloride/phosphates, procainamide, prochlorperazine, promethazine, propofol, propranolol, protamine, pyridoxine, quiNIDine, quinupristin-dalfopristin, ranitidine, Ringer's injection, rocuronium, sodium acetate/bicarbonate, succinylcholine, SUFentanil, tacrolimus, telavancin, teniposide, theophylline, thiamine, thiotepa, ticarcillin-clavulanate, tigecycline, tirofiban, tobramycin, tolazoline, urokinase, vancomycin, vasopressin, vecuronium, verapamil, vinBLAStine, vinCRIStine, vinorelbine, voriconazole, zoledronic acid

SIDE EFFECTS
CNS: *Dizziness,* mental changes, drowsiness, *fatigue,* headache, depression, anxiety, nightmares, paresthesias, lethargy
CV: *Orthostatic hypotension, bradycardia,* HF, chest pain, ventricular dysrhythmias
EENT: Visual changes; double vision; dry, burning eyes; floppy iris syndrome; nasal congestion
ENDO: Hyperkalemia
GI: *Nausea, vomiting, diarrhea,* dyspepsia, taste distortion, hepatotoxicity
GU: Impotence, dysuria, ejaculatory failure
INTEG: Rash, urticaria, pruritus, fever
RESP: Bronchospasm, dyspnea, wheezing

PHARMACOKINETICS
Half-life 2.5-8 hr, metabolized by liver (metabolites inactive), excreted in urine, crosses placenta, excreted in breast milk, protein binding 50%
PO: Onset 30 min, peak 1-4 hr, duration 8-24 hr
IV: Onset 2-5 min, peak 5-15 min, duration 2-4 hr

INTERACTIONS
• Do not use within 2 wk of MAOIs
Increase: myocardial depression—hydantoins, general anesthetics, verapamil, class I antidysrhythmics
Increase: tremor—tricyclic antidepressants
Increase: hypotension—diuretics, other antihypertensives, cimetidine, nitroglycerin, alcohol, nitrates
Decrease: effects of—sympathomimetics, lidocaine, theophylline, β-blockers, bronchodilators, xanthines
Decrease: antihypertensive effect—NSAIDs, salicylates
Increase or decrease: effects of—antidiabetics; monitor blood glucose
Drug/Herb
Increase: antihypertensive effect—hawthorn

Decrease: antihypertensive effect—ephedra (ma huang)

Drug/Lab Test

Increase: ANA titer, blood glucose, alk phos, LDH, AST, ALT, uric acid

False increase: urinary catecholamines

NURSING CONSIDERATIONS
Assess:

• **Hypertension:** monitor B/P before starting treatment, periodically thereafter; note pulse, rate, rhythm, quality; apical/radial pulse before administration; notify prescriber of any significant changes, watch for orthostatic hypotension

• **HF:** I&O, weight daily; fluid overload: weight gain, jugular venous distention, edema, crackles in lungs; report weight gain >5 lb

• **Abrupt discontinuation:** product should be tapered to prevent adverse reactions

• Baselines of renal/hepatic studies before therapy begins

• **Pregnancy/breastfeeding:** use only if benefits outweigh fetal risk; use caution in breastfeeding

Evaluate:

• **Therapeutic response:** decreased B/P after 1-2 wk

Teach patient/family:

• Not to discontinue product abruptly; to taper over 2 wk; may cause precipitate angina

• Not to use OTC products containing α-adrenergic stimulants (nasal decongestants, OTC cold preparations) unless directed by prescriber

• To report bradycardia, dizziness, confusion, depression, fever, difficulty breathing, cold extremities, confusion, rash, sore throat

• To take pulse at home; advise when to notify prescriber

• May mask symptoms of hypoglycemia; monitor blood glucose closely in diabetes

• To avoid alcohol, smoking, increased sodium intake

• **Hypertension:** To comply with weight control, dietary adjustments, modified exercise program

• To carry emergency ID to identify product, allergies

• To avoid hazardous activities if dizziness is present

• To avoid hot baths, showers

• **To report symptoms of HF:** difficulty breathing, especially on exertion or when lying down; night cough; swelling of extremities

• To advise providers of use before surgery

• To avoid driving or other hazardous activities until response is known; dizziness, drowsiness, may occur

TREATMENT OF OVERDOSE:
IV glucagon or atropine for bradycardia, theophylline (nebulizer) for bronchospasm; digoxin, O₂, diuretic for cardiac failure; hemodialysis useful for removal/hypotension; administer vasopressor, cardiac monitor (hypertensive urgency)

lacosamide (Rx)
(la-koe′sa-mide)

Vimpat

Func. class.: Anticonvulsant, miscellaneous

Chem. class.: Functionalized amino acid

Controlled Substance Schedule V

ACTION: May act through action at sodium channels; exact action is unknown

USES: Partial-onset seizures

CONTRAINDICATIONS
Hypersensitivity

Precautions: Pregnancy, breastfeeding, children <18 yr, geriatric patients, allergies, cardiac/renal/hepatic disease, acute MI, atrial fibrillation/flutter, AV block, bradycardia, HF, dehydration, depression, dialysis, hazardous activity, electrolyte imbalance, heart failure, labor, PR prolongation, sick sinus syndrome, substance abuse, suicidal ideation, syncope, torsades de pointes

DOSAGE AND ROUTES
Adjunct therapy
• **Adult and adolescent ≥17 yr: PO** 50 mg bid, may increase weekly by 100 mg bid to 200-400 mg/day; **IV** 50 mg bid, infuse over 30-60 min, may be increased by 100 mg/day weekly up to 200-400 mg/day maintenance
Monotherapy
• **Adult: PO** 100 mg bid; may increase weekly by 100 mg/day in 2 divided doses, increase to 300-400 mg/day in 2 divided doses or 200-mg single loading dose then 12 hr later start 100 mg bid
Renal/hepatic dose
• **Adult: PO/IV** max 300 mg/day for mild to moderate hepatic disease or CCr ≤30 mL/min; do not use in severe hepatic disease; reduce dose in renal/hepatic disease in those who are taking strong CYP3A4, CYP2C9 inhibitors
Available forms: Film-coated tabs 50, 100, 150, 200 mg; solution for injection IV 20-mL single-use vials (200 mg/20 mL); oral sol 10 mg/mL
Administer:
• Store PO products/IV vials at room temperature; sol is stable for 24 hr when mixed with compatible diluents in glass or PVC bags at room temperature
PO route
• **Tablet:** give without regard to meals
• **Oral sol:** measure with calibrated measuring device
IV route
• May give undiluted or mixed in 0.9% NaCl, D_5W, or LR
• Infuse over 30-60 min
• Do not use if discolored or if particulates are present; discard unused portions

SIDE EFFECTS
CNS: Dizziness, syncope, tremor, drowsiness, fever, paresthesias, depression, fatigue, headache, suicidal ideation

CV: Atrial fibrillation/flutter, bradycardia, orthostatic hypotension, palpitations
EENT: Diplopia, blurred vision, tinnitus
GI: Nausea, constipation, vomiting, hepatitis, diarrhea, dyspepsia
HEMA: Anemia, neutropenia, agranulocytosis
INTEG: Rash, erythema, inj-site reaction, pruritus
SYST: Drug reaction with eosinophilia, systemic symptoms (DRESS), Stevens-Johnson syndrome, toxic epidermal necrolysis

PHARMACOKINETICS
Metabolized by liver; excreted by kidneys, 40%; protein binding <15%
PO: Peak 1-4 hr
IV: Peak 30-60 min; half-life 13 hr

INTERACTIONS
• **Increase:** PR prolongation—β-blockers, calcium channel blockers, atazanavir, dronedarone, digoxin, lopinavir, ritonavir
• **Increase:** lacosamide effect—CYP2C19 inhibitors (fluconazole, isoniazid, miconazole)
Drug/Lab Test
Increase: LFTs

NURSING CONSIDERATIONS
Assess:
• **Seizures:** duration, type, intensity, precipitating factors
• **Renal function:** albumin concentration
• **CV status:** orthostatic hypotension, PR prolongation; monitor cardiac status throughout treatment; ECG prior to therapy (IV), AV block may occur
• **Mental status:** mood, sensorium, affect, memory (long, short term), depression, suicidal ideation, psychologic dependence
• **Serious skin reactions:** discontinue product at first sign of rash
• **Pregnancy/breastfeeding:** Pregnant patient should enroll in North American Antiepileptic Drugs Pregnancy Registry, 888-233-2334; use only if benefits outweigh fetal risk; do not breastfeed, excretion unknown

• **Beers:** avoid in older adults unless safer alternatives are unavailable; may cause ataxia, impaired psychomotor function

Evaluate:

• **Therapeutic response:** increased seizure control

Teach patient/family:

• Not to discontinue product abruptly; to taper over 1 wk because seizures may occur

• To report blurred vision, nausea, dizziness, syncope; to avoid hazardous activities until stabilized on product

• To carry emergency ID stating product use

• To notify prescriber of suicidal thoughts/behaviors, syncope, cardiac changes

• To report rash, fever, fatigue, yellowing of skin, eyes, dark urine; may be hypersensitivity reaction

• To notify prescriber immediately if pregnancy is planned or suspected; to enroll in pregnancy registry at 888-233-2334, www.aedpregnancyregistry.org

• That interactions with other medications may occur; to report all OTC, Rx medications, herbals and supplements taken; not to use with alcohol

• To consult MedGuide for proper use, risks, and review with patient

---

lactitol (Rx)

(lac'ti-tol)

Pizensy

Func. class.: Laxative

Chem. class.: Hyperosmolar product

ACTION:
Influx of water into the small intestine by osmosis, provide a laxative effect

USES:
Chronic idiopathic constipation

CONTRAINDICATIONS
GI obstruction/perforation, galactosemia

Precautions: Pregnancy, children, breastfeeding

DOSAGE AND ROUTES

• **Adult: PO** 20 g with meals daily

Available forms: Powder for oral solution 10 g (single dose), 280 g, 560 g

Administer:

• Give with meals, if possible

• Give other oral medications separated by ≥2 hr

• Dilute powder for oral solution before use

• Using lactitol multidose bottle: **20-g dose:** Fill the measuring cap twice to the top of the white section in cap marked by the arrow; **10-g dose:** Fill the measuring cap once to the top of the white section in cap marked by the arrow

• Pour the measured dose into an empty 8-oz glass

• Add 120 mL to 240 mL (4-8 oz) of water, juice, or other common beverage (coffee, tea, soda) and stir to dissolve

• Have the patient drink the entire contents of the glass

• Using lactitol unit-dose packets: pour the contents of 1 or 2 unit-dose packets, as prescribed, into an empty 8-oz glass; add 120 mL to 240 mL (4-8 oz) of water, juice, or other common beverage (coffee, tea, soda) and stir to dissolve; have the patient drink the entire contents of the glass

SIDE EFFECTS

CV: Hypertension

GI: Abdominal pain, diarrhea, distention/flatulence

GU: UTI

PHARMACOKINETICS
Peak 3.6 hr, half-life 2.4 hr

INTERACTIONS

• All medications (PO): separate by 2 hr

NURSING CONSIDERATIONS

Assess:

• **Constipation:** Assess for continuing constipation or relief

• Identify if pregnancy is suspected, not known if there is harm to fetus

Evaluate:

• **Therapeutic response:** Relief of constipation

Teach patient/family:
• To separate all other oral medications by ≥2 hr

lactulose (Rx)
(lak′tyoo-lose)

Constulose, Enulose, Generlac, Kristalose

Func. class.: Laxative; ammonia detoxicant (hyperosmotic)
Chem. class.: Lactose synthetic derivative

Do not confuse:
lactulose/lactose

ACTION: Prevents absorption of ammonia in colon by acidifying stool; increases water, softens stool

USES: Chronic constipation, portal-systemic encephalopathy (PSE) in patients with hepatic disease

CONTRAINDICATIONS
Hypersensitivity, low-galactose diet
Precautions: Pregnancy, breastfeeding, geriatric patients, debilitated patients, diabetes mellitus

DOSAGE AND ROUTES
Chronic constipation
• **Adult: PO** 15-30 mL/day (10-20 g), may increase to 60 mL/day prn
• **Child: PO** 1.5-3 mL/kg/day once or twice daily
Portal systemic (Hepatic) encephalopathy (PSE)
• **Adult: PO** 30-45 mL (20-30 g) tid or qid until stools soft; **RETENTION ENEMA** 300 mL (200 g) diluted with 700 mL water or NS every 4-6 hr as needed
• **Child: PO (unlabeled)** 40-90 mL/day in 3-4 divided doses
• **Infant: PO (unlabeled)** 2.5-10 mL/day in divided doses
Available forms: Oral sol 10 g/15 mL; single-use packets 10, 20 g; rectal sol 10 g/15 mL
Administer:
PO route

• With 8 oz fruit juice, water, milk to increase palatability of oral form; for rapid effect, give on empty stomach
• Increased fluids to 2 L/day; do not give with other laxatives; if diarrhea occurs, reduce dosage
• **Kristalose:** dissolve contents of packet/4 oz water
Rectal route
• **Retention enema (no commercial product)** by diluting 300 mL lactulose/700 mL of water; administer by rectal balloon catheter; retain for >30 min; if retained for <30 min, repeat

SIDE EFFECTS
GI: *Nausea, vomiting, anorexia, abdominal cramps,* diarrhea, flatulence, distention, belching
META: Hypernatremia, hypokalemia; hyperglycemia (diabetes)

PHARMACOKINETICS
Metabolized in colon, excretion kidneys, unchanged, onset 1-2 days, peak unknown, duration unknown

INTERACTIONS
• Do not use with other laxatives (hepatic encephalopathy)
Decrease: lactulose effects—other oral antiinfectives, antacids
Drug/Herb
Increase: laxative action—flax, senna
Drug/Lab Test
Increase: blood glucose (diabetic patients)
Decrease: blood ammonia

NURSING CONSIDERATIONS
Assess:
• **Stool:** amount, color, consistency, frequency, abdominal pain/distention, bowel sounds prior to use and after use
• **Cause of constipation;** determine whether fluids, bulk, or exercise is missing from lifestyle; use of constipating products
• **Hepatic encephalopathy:** blood ammonia level (15-45 mcg/dL or 35-65 umol/L is normal range); may decrease ammonia level by 25%-50%; monitor for clearing of confusion, lethargy, restlessness, irritability if portal-systemic encephalopathy; monitor sodium in higher doses

L

- Monitor sodium in higher levels
- Blood, urine electrolytes if product used often; may cause diarrhea, hypokalemia, hyponatremia
- I&O ratio to identify fluid loss, replace any loss
- Cramping, rectal bleeding, nausea, vomiting; if these symptoms occur, product should be discontinued

Evaluate:
- **Therapeutic response:** decreased constipation, decreased blood ammonia level, clearing of mental state

Teach patient/family:
- Not to use as a laxative long term, to use as prescribed
- To dilute with water or fruit juice to counteract sweet taste
- To store in cool environment; not to freeze
- To take on an empty stomach for rapid action
- To report diarrhea, number, amount, consistency of stools; may indicate overdose

---

lamiVUDine 3TC (Rx)

(lam-i-voo'deen)

Epivir, Epivir HBV, Heptovir ♣

Func. class.: Antiretroviral

Chem. class.: Nucleoside reverse transcriptase inhibitor (NRTI)

Do not confuse:
lamiVUDine/lamoTRIgine
Epivir/Epivir HBV

ACTION: Inhibits replication of HIV virus by incorporating into cellular DNA by viral reverse transcriptase, thereby terminating cellular DNA chain

USES: HIV-1–related infection in combination with at least 2 other antiretrovirals; chronic hepatitis B (Epivir HBV)

Unlabeled uses: HIV-1 nonoccupational postexposure prophylaxis, prevention of perinatal HIV transmission

CONTRAINDICATIONS

Hypersensitivity, other combination products with lamivudine or emtricitubine

Precautions: Pregnancy, breastfeeding, children <3 yr, geriatric patients, granulocyte count <1000/mm³ or HB <9.5 g/dL, renal disease, pancreatitis, peripheral neuropathy, coinfection with hepatitis B

Black Box Warning: Hepatitis B exacerbation

DOSAGE AND ROUTES

HIV in combination with other antiretroviral agents (Epivir)
- **Adult:** PO Tablet/Solution 300 mg once daily or 150 mg twice daily
- **Child/adolescent ≥25 kg:** PO Tablet 150 mg twice daily; solution 5 mg/kg/dose twice daily
- **Child 20-24 kg:** PO Tablet 75 mg once daily in the morning and 150 mg once daily in the evening
- **Child 14-19 kg:** 75 mg twice daily

Chronic hepatitis B infection, with HPV replication/active liver involvement (Epivir HBV)
- **Adult:** PO 100 mg once daily
- **Child/adolescent 2-17 yr:** PO 3 mg/kg/dose once daily (max: 100 mg/dose)

Renal dose
- **Adult/adolescents:** PO CCr 30-49 mL/min: **Epivir** 150 mg/day; **Epivir HBV** 100 mg 1st dose, then 50 mg/day; CCr 15-29 mL/min: **Epivir** 150 mg 1st dose, then 100 mg/day; **Epivir** HBV 100 mg 1st dose, then 25 mg/day; CCr 5-14 mL/min: **Epivir** 150 mg 1st dose, then 50 mg/day; **Epivir** HBV 35 mg 1st dose, then 15 mg/day; CCr <5 mL/min: **Epivir** 50 mg 1st dose, then 25 mg/day; **Epivir HBV** 35 mg 1st dose, then 10 mg/day

Available forms: (Epivir) oral sol 10 mg/mL; tabs 150, 300 mg; (Epivir HBV) oral sol 5 mg/mL; tabs 100 mg

Administer:
- PO daily or bid, without regard to meals
- Epivir and Epivir HBV are not interchangeable
- Use with other antiretrovirals only; do not use triple antiretroviral with abacavir or didanosine; resistance may occur

---

lamiVUDine 3TC 735

- Store in cool environment; protect from light

SIDE EFFECTS

CNS: *Fever, headache, malaise, dizziness, insomnia, depression, fatigue, chills,* seizures, peripheral neuropathy, paresthesias
EENT: Taste change, hearing loss, photophobia
GI: *Nausea, vomiting, diarrhea,* anorexia, cramps, dyspepsia, hepatomegaly with steatosis; pancreatitis (more common in children)
HEMA: Neutropenia, anemia, thrombocytopenia
INTEG: *Rash*
MS: *Myalgia, arthralgia, pain*
RESP: *Cough*
SYST: Lactic acidosis, anaphylaxis, Stevens-Johnson syndrome, immune reconstitution syndrome

PHARMACOKINETICS

Rapidly absorbed, distributed to extravascular space, excreted unchanged in urine, protein binding <36%, half-life 5-7 hr, child 2 hr, peak 3.2 hr

INTERACTIONS

Decrease: both products—zalcitabine; avoid concurrent use
Increase: pancreatitis—other products that cause pancreatitis
Increase: lamotrigine level—sulfamethoxazole-trimethoprim, may need dose decrease
- Do not use with emtricitabine, duplication

Drug/Lab Test
Increase: ALT, bilirubin, CK
Decrease: HB, neutrophil, platelet count

NURSING CONSIDERATIONS
Assess:
- **HIV:** Test for HIV before starting treatment, blood counts q2wk; watch for neutropenia, thrombocytopenia, HB, CD4, viral load; if low, therapy may have to be discontinued and restarted after hematologic recovery; blood transfusions may be required; assess for lessening of symptoms; if HBV is present, a higher dose of Epivir HBV is needed

- **Labs:** Monitor CBC, with differential, platelets, blood glucose, cholesterol/lipids, urinalysis, BUN, creatinine baseline and periodically during treatment; obtain resistance testing before starting treatment

Black Box Warning: Hepatitis B exacerbation: fatigue, anorexia, pruritus, jaundice during and for several months after discontinuation; AST, ALT, bilirubin; amylase, lipase, triglycerides periodically during treatment

- **Children for pancreatitis:** abdominal pain, nausea, vomiting, neuropathy; discontinuing may be required; monitor amylase, lipase; use cautiously in children

- **Lactic acidosis, severe hepatomegaly with steatosis:** obtain baseline LFTs; if elevated, discontinue treatment; discontinue even if LFTs are normal if lactic acidosis, severe hepatomegaly develops; may be fatal, especially in women

- **Pregnancy/breastfeeding:** Epivir is a drug that is used in pregnancy to treat HIV; enroll patient in the Antiretroviral Pregnancy Registry at 800-258-4263; do not breastfeed. Obtain pregnancy test prior to starting therapy
Evaluate:
- **Therapeutic response:** decreasing symptoms of HIV, CD4, viral load
Teach patient/family:
- That GI complaints, insomnia resolve after 3-4 wk of treatment
- That product is not a cure for HIV but will control symptoms; that compliance is necessary; to take as directed; to complete full course of treatment even if feeling better
- To notify prescriber of sore throat, swollen lymph nodes, malaise, fever, peripheral neuropathy; other infections may occur
- To report symptoms of pancreatitis, immune reconstitution syndrome immediately
- That patient is still infective, may pass HIV virus on to others

Side effects: *italics* = common; red = life-threatening

• That follow-up visits must be continued since serious toxicity may occur; that blood counts must be done

• That other products may be necessary to prevent other infections

• That product may cause fainting or dizziness

• **Pregnancy/breastfeeding:** to enroll in the Antiretroviral Pregnancy Registry at 800-258-4263; not to breastfeed, a pregnancy test will be required prior to beginning therapy in those who can become pregnant

---

lamivudine/tenofovir disoproxil (Rx)

(lam-i-voo′deen/ten-oh-foh′veer)

Cimduo, Temixys

Func. class.: Antiretroviral

USES: In combination with other antiretrovirals for human immunodeficiency virus (HIV) infection

CONTRAINDICATIONS

Hypersensitivity

Black Box Warning: Hepatitis B exacerbation

DOSAGE AND ROUTES

• **Adult/adolescent/child ≥35 kg: PO**
1 tablet (lamivudine 300 mg; tenofovir 300 mg) daily

Available forms: Tabs 300 mg/300 mg

---

lamivudine/ zidovudine (Rx)

(la-mi′vyoo-deen/zye-doe′vyoo-deen)

Combivir

Func. class.: Antiretroviral, reverse transcriptase inhibitor, nucleoside

---

USES: Treatment of HIV-1 infection in combination with other antiretrovirals

Black Box Warning: Bone marrow suppression, hepatitis B exacerbation, hepatotoxicity, lactic acidosis, myopathy

DOSAGE AND ROUTES

Adult: PO 1 tablet (lamivudine 150 mg/ zidovudine 300 mg) bid in combination with other antiretrovirals

Children and adolescents ≥30 kg: PO 1 tablet bid, use in combination with at least one other antiretroviral agent

Available forms: Tabs 150 mg/300 mg

---

lamoTRIgine (Rx)

(la-moe′tri-green)

LaMICtal, Lamictal CD, LaMICtal ODT, LaMICtal Starter, LaMICtal XR, Subvenite, Subvenite Starter Kit-Blue, Subvenite Starter Kit-Green, Subvenite Starter Kit-Orange

Func. class.: Anticonvulsant—miscellaneous

Chem. class.: Phenyltriazine

Do not confuse:
lamoTRIgine/lamiVUDine/levothyroxine
LaMICtal/LamISIL

ACTION: Inhibits voltage-sensitive sodium channels, thus decreasing seizures

USES: Adjunct for the treatment of partial, tonic-clonic seizures; children with Lennox-Gastaut syndrome, bipolar disorder

Unlabeled uses: Absence seizures

CONTRAINDICATIONS

Hypersensitivity, mania

Precautions: Pregnancy (cleft lip/palate during 1st trimester), breastfeeding, geriatric patients, cardiac/renal/hepatic disease, severe depression, suicidal thoughts, blood dyscrasias, children <16 yr, risk of hemophagocytic lymphohistiocytosis (HLH), abrupt discontinuation, autoimmune disease, SLE

Black Box Warning: Serious rash (STS, TEN)

DOSAGE AND ROUTES
Seizures: monotherapy
• **Adult/adolescent ≥16 yr: PO** 50 mg/day while receiving 1 enzyme-inducing AED (carBAMazepine, PHENobarbital, phenytoin, primidone but not valproic acid) week 1-2, then increase to 100 mg divided bid week 3-4; maintenance 300-500 mg/day; **EXT REL** 50 mg/day × 1-2 wk, then 100 mg/day week 3-4, then 200 mg/day week 5, then 300 mg/day week 6, then 400 mg/day week 7; after week 7, range is 400-600 mg/day
• **Adolescent <16 yr/child: PO** 0.3 mg/kg/day week 1-2, then 0.6 mg/kg/day week 3-4; depends on use of AED; usual dose 4.5-7.5 mg/kg/day, max 300 mg/day
Monotherapy for patients taking valproate
• **Adult/adolescent ≥16 yr receiving lamoTRIgine and valproate without enzyme-inducing drug: PO** (immediate release) stabilize on valproate, target dose is 200 mg/day lamoTRIgine; if patient is not taking lamoTRIgine 200 mg/day, increase dose by 25-50 mg/day q1-2wk to reach 200 mg/day; while maintaining lamoTRIgine 200 mg/day, decrease valproate to 500 mg/day by ≤500 mg/day/wk, maintain valproate at 500 mg/day × 1 wk, then increase lamoTRIgine to 300 mg/day while decreasing valproate 250 mg/day × 1 wk, then discontinue valproate and increase lamoTRIgine by 100 mg/day/wk to maintenance of 500 mg/day
Seizures: multiple therapy with valproate
• **Adult/adolescent ≥16 yr: PO** 25 mg every other day for weeks 1-2, then 25 mg/day week 3-4, increase by 25-50 mg q1-2wk, maintenance 100-500 mg/day
• **Adolescent <16 yr/child: PO** 0.1-0.2 mg/kg/day initially, then increase q2wk as needed to 1-5 mg/kg/day or 200 mg/day

Hepatic dose
• **Adult: PO** moderate hepatic impairment or severe without ascites: reduce by 25%; severe hepatic impairment with ascites: reduce by 50%

Available forms: Tabs 25, 100, 150, 200 mg; **PO** ext rel 25-50-100, 50-100-200 mg titration kit; **PO** 25-100 mg starter kit; **ext rel** 25, 50, 100, 250, 300 mg; **chew dispersible tabs** 5, 25 mg; **oral disintegrating tab** 25, 50, 100, 200 mg; **oral disintegrating tab** 25-50, 50-100-200 mg, 25-50-100 mg titration kit

Administer:
• Correct starter kit; severe side effects have occurred from incorrect starter kit
• Discontinue all products gradually over ≥2 wk; abrupt discontinuation can increase seizures
• All forms may be given without regard to meals
• Extended-release product is not to be used for conversion to monotherapy for ≥2 antiepileptic products
• **Orange starter kit:** for those **NOT** taking carBAMazepine, phenytoin, PHENobarbital, primidone, rifAMPin, valproate
• **Green starter kit:** for those taking carBAMazepine, phenytoin, PHENobarbital, primidone, rifAMPin but **NOT** valproate
• **Blue starter kit:** for those taking valproate
• If a dose is missed, take as soon as remembered unless next dose is in <4 hr, then skip and take next regularly scheduled dose
• **Chewable dispersible tab:** may be swallowed whole, chewed, mixed in water or fruit juice; to mix, add to small amount of liquid in glass or spoon; tabs will dissolve in 1 min, then mix in more liquid and swirl and swallow immediately; do not cut tabs in half
• **Orally disintegrating tabs:** place on tongue, move around in mouth; when disintegrated, swallow; examine blister pack be-

L

fore use, do not use if blisters are torn or missing

• **Extended-release tabs:** swallow whole; do not cut, break, chew; without regard to food

SIDE EFFECTS

CNS: *Dizziness,* ataxia, *headache,* fever, insomnia, tremor, depression, anxiety, suicidal ideation, seizures, poor concentration

EENT: Nystagmus, diplopia, blurred vision

GI: Nausea, vomiting, anorexia, abdominal pain, hepatotoxicity

GU: *Dysmenorrhea*

HEMA: Anemia, DIC, leukopenia, thrombocytopenia

INTEG: Rash (potentially life-threatening), alopecia, photosensitivity

CV: Chest pain, palpitations

MS: Neck pain, myalgias

SYST: Stevens-Johnson syndrome, angioedema, toxic epidermal necrolysis, DRESS

PHARMACOKINETICS

Half-life varies depending on dose; half-life 24 hr, 15 hr with enzyme inducers; rapidly, completely absorbed; metabolized by glucuronic acid conjunction; protein binding 55%; peak 1.4-2.3 hr, XR 4-10 hr; crosses placenta; excreted in breast milk

INTERACTIONS

Decrease: metabolic clearance of lamoTRIgine—valproic acid, CYP3A4 inhibitors

Decrease: lamoTRIgine concentration—carBAMazepine, acetaminophen, phenytoin, primidone, PHENobarbital, OXcarbazepine

Drug/Herb

Increase: anticonvulsant effect—ginkgo

Decrease: anticonvulsant effect—ginseng

Drug/Lab

False positive: PCP (rapid drug screen)

NURSING CONSIDERATIONS

Assess:

• **Seizure:** duration, type, intensity, halo before seizure baseline and periodically

Black Box Warning: Rash (Stevens-Johnson syndrome, toxic epidermal necrolysis) in pediatric patients: product should be discontinued at first sign of rash; more common in those taking multiple products for seizures; rash usually occurs during 2-8 wk of therapy

• **Bipolar disorder:** suicidal thoughts/behaviors

• **DRESS:** monitor for fever, rash, lymphadenopathy; may occur with hepatitis, nephritis, myocarditis; discontinue immediately, may involve multiple organ systems

• **Risk of hemophagocytic lymphohistiocytosis (HLH):** monitor for persistent fevers, rash, enlarged liver/spleen/lymph nodes, anemia, low platelets

Evaluate:

• **Therapeutic response:** decrease in severity of seizures or of bipolar symptoms

Teach patient/family:

• To take PO doses divided, with or after meals to decrease adverse effects; not to discontinue product abruptly because seizures may occur

• To avoid hazardous activities until stabilized on product

• To carry emergency ID; to notify prescriber of skin rash, increased seizure activity; to use sunscreen, protective clothing if photosensitivity occurs

Black Box Warning: Rash: to notify prescriber immediately if rash, fever, or swollen lymph nodes occur

• To notify prescriber immediately of suicidal thoughts/behaviors, new or worsening depression, anxiety, aggression

• **Pregnancy/breastfeeding:** to notify prescriber if pregnancy is planned or suspected; to use a nonhormonal contraceptive; to enroll with the North American Antiepileptic Drug Pregnancy Registry at 888-233-2334 (www.aedpregnancyregistry.org); that product decreases folate; to avoid breastfeeding

lanadelumab-flyo (Rx)
(lan'a-del'ue-mab)
Takhzyro
Func. class.: Complement inhibitors
Chem. class.: Plasma kallikrein inhibitor

USES
Prophylaxis to prevent attacks of hereditary angioedema (HAE) in those ≥12

DOSAGE AND ROUTES
Adult/child ≥12 yr: SUBCUT 300 mg q2wk; consider using q4wk when attack free for >6 months
Available forms: Injection: 300 mg/2 mL (150 mg/mL) solution in a single-dose vial

lansoprazole (Rx, OTC)
(lan-so-prey'zole)
Prevacid, Prevacid SoluTab
Func. class.: Antiulcer, proton pump inhibitor
Chem. class.: Benzimidazole

ACTION: Suppresses gastric secretion by inhibiting hydrogen/potassium ATPase enzyme system in gastric parietal cell; characterized as gastric acid pump inhibitor because it blocks the final step of acid production

USES: Gastroesophageal reflux disease (GERD), severe erosive esophagitis, poorly responsive systemic GERD, pathologic hypersecretory conditions (Zollinger-Ellison syndrome, systemic mastocytosis, multiple endocrine adenomas); possibly effective for treatment of duodenal, gastric ulcers, maintenance of healed duodenal ulcers

Unlabeled uses: Dyspepsia, stress ulcer prophylaxis in critically-ill patients, GERD (infants/neonates), eosinophilic esophagitis

CONTRAINDICATIONS
Hypersensitivity
Precautions: Pregnancy, breastfeeding, children, hypomagnesemia, osteoporosis

DOSAGE AND ROUTES
Frequent heartburn
• **Adult: PO (OTC)** 15 mg daily up to 14 days
Duodenal ulcer (*H. pylori* eradication)
• **Adult: PO** 15 mg/day before eating for 4 wk, then 15 mg/day to maintain healing of ulcers; associated with *Helicobacter pylori*: 30 mg lansoprazole bid, 1 g amoxicillin bid; clarithromycin 500 mg bid × 10-14 day or lansoprazole tid with 1 g amoxicillin tid × 14 days
Pathologic hypersecretory conditions
• **Adult: PO** 60 mg/day, may give up to 90 mg bid, administer doses of >120 mg/day in divided doses
NSAID-related ulcer (continuing use)
• **Adult: PO** 30 mg daily × 8 wk
GERD/esophagitis
• **Adult/adolescent: PO** 15-30 mg/day × 8 wk
• **Child 1-11 yr (>30 kg): PO** 30 mg/day ≤12 wk
• **Child 1-11 yr (≤30 kg): PO** 15 mg/day ≤12 wk
• **Infant (unlabeled): PO** 1-2 mg/kg/day; limited data available
• **Neonate (unlabeled): PO** 0.5-1 mg/kg/day
Stress gastric prophylaxis
• **Adult: NG** Use 30 mg del rel caps or 30 mg disintegrating tab once daily
Available forms: Del rel caps 15, 30 mg; orally disintegrating tabs 15, 30 mg

Administer:

PO route

• Swallow caps whole 30 min before eating; do not crush or chew caps; caps may be opened and contents sprinkled on food

Delayed-release capsules

• Swallow intact, do not chew or crush, may be opened and contents sprinkled on 1 Tbsp applesauce or other soft food, swallow immediately; or contents may be mixed into a small volume of juice, mixed and swallowed, rinse with 2 or more oz volume of liquid and have patient take

NG route

• **Oral cap:** open cap and pour ¼ of granules into NG feeding syringe with plunger removed, slowly add water and depress plunger, repeat until all granules used; flush tube with 15 mL water

• Place on tongue, allow to dissolve, use without regard to water

• **Oral syringe:** dissolve 15 mg/4 mL or 30 mg/10 mL water, use extra water in syringe to remove all of the product

NG tube

• **Oral disintegrating tab:** mix 30-mg tab in 10 mL water, give via NG tube, flush tube with 10 mL sterile water, clamp for 60 min

SIDE EFFECTS

CNS: *Headache,* dizziness

GI: Diarrhea, abdominal pain, nausea, *constipation,* flatulence, acid regurgitation, anorexia, irritable colon, CDAD

GU: Hematuria, glycosuria, impotence, kidney calculus, breast enlargement

PHARMACOKINETICS

Absorption after granules leave stomach 80%; half-life 1½-2 hr; protein binding 97%; extensively metabolized in liver; excreted in urine, feces; clearance decreased in geriatric patients, renal/hepatic impairment, onset 1-3 hr, peak 1.7 hr, duration 24 hr

INTERACTIONS

Increase: bleeding risk—warfarin

Decrease: lansoprazole absorption—sucralfate

Decrease: absorption of ketoconazole, itraconazole, iron salts, calcium carbonate, atazanavir, ampicillin

Increase: hypomagnesemia—loop/thiazide diuretics

Decrease: lansoprazole effect—antimuscarinics, H₂-blockers

• Avoid use with dasatinib, delavirdine

Drug/Herb

• Avoid use with red yeast rice, St. John's wort

Drug/Food

• Food decreases rate of absorption; use before food

NURSING CONSIDERATIONS

Assess:

• **CDAD:** bowel sounds, abdomen for pain, swelling; anorexia, blood in stool; may occur even after completion of therapy

• **Hepatic studies:** AST, ALT, alk phos during treatment

• INR and prothrombin time when taking warfarin

• **Magnesium:** low magnesium may occur, palpitations, muscle spasm, tremors

• **Beers:** avoid scheduled use for >8 wk unless for high-risk patients (oral corticosteroids/chronic NSAIDs use)

• **Pregnancy/breastfeeding:** use only if clearly needed; do not breastfeed

Evaluate:

• **Therapeutic response:** absence of epigastric pain, swelling, fullness

Teach patient/family:

• To report severe diarrhea, cramping, blood in stools, fever; product may have to be discontinued

• That hypoglycemia may occur if diabetic; to monitor blood glucose

• To avoid hazardous activities; that dizziness may occur

• To avoid alcohol, salicylates, ibuprofen; may cause GI irritation

- That if using OTC for heartburn, it may take 1-4 days to see full benefit
- Teach patient the reason for use and how to take, to take 30-60 min before eating
- Symptoms of low magnesium levels
- **Pregnancy:** to notify provider if pregnancy is planned or suspected or if breastfeeding

lansoprazole/ amoxicillin/ clarithromycin (Rx)
Func. class.: GI-related disorder agent

USES:
Helicobacter pylori eradication

DOSAGE AND ROUTES
H. pylori eradication:
- **Adults:** PO 30 mg lansoprazole, 1000 mg amoxicillin, 500 mg clarithromycin bid × 10 days

Available forms: Triple therapy pack/ daily

lanthanum (Rx)
(lan'-tha-num)
Fosrenol
Func. class.: Phosphate binder

USES: End-stage renal disease to reduce serum phosphate

DOSAGE AND ROUTES
- **Adult:** PO 750-1500 mg/day in divided doses with meals; titrate dose q2-3wk until an acceptable phosphate level is reached; tabs should be chewed completely before swallowing; intact tabs should not be swallowed; maintenance dose 1500-3000 mg/day divided with meals; max 4500 mg/day

Available forms: Tabs, chewable 500, 750, 1000 mg; oral powder 750, 1000 mg

⚠ HIGH ALERT

lapatinib (Rx)
(la-pa'tin-ib)
Tykerb
Func. class.: Antineoplastic—miscellaneous
Chem. class.: Biologic response modifier, signal transduction inhibitor (STIs)

USES: Advanced metastatic breast cancer patients with tumor that overexpresses HER2 protein and who have received previous chemotherapy

Black Box Warning: Hepatotoxicity

DOSAGE AND ROUTES
Advanced/metastatic breast cancer with HER2 overexpression who have received previous therapy
- **Adult:** Lapatinib PO 1250 mg (5 tabs)/ day 1 hr before or after food on days 1-21 plus **capecitabine** 2000 mg/m^2/ day in 2 divided doses on days 1-14 in a repeating 21-day cycle; continue until therapeutic response or toxicity occurs

Lapatinib/letrozole combination
- **Adult:** PO lapatinib 1500 mg (6 tablets) q2days with letrozole PO 2.5 mg daily

Metastatic breast cancer with HER2 overexpression for whom hormonal therapy is indicated
- **Adult:** PO 1500 mg (6 tabs) 1 hr before food with letrozole 2.5 mg/day

Hepatic dose
- **Adult:** PO (Child-Pugh C) 750 mg/day (with capecitabine); 1000 mg/day (with letrozole)

Available forms: Tabs 250 mg

⚠ HIGH ALERT

larotrectinib (Rx)
(layr'oh-trek'tih-nib)
Vitrakvi
Func. class.: Antineoplastic—TRK inhibitor

USES: Metastatic or surgically unresectable neurotrophic receptor tyrosine kinase (NTRK) gene fusion–positive solid tumors with no known acquired resistance mutation, in patients with no satisfactory alternative treatments or in patients who have progressed following treatment

DOSAGE AND ROUTES
• **Adult/adolescent/child/infant: PO** For BSA ≥1 m^2, 100 mg bid; for BSA <1 m^2, 100 mg/m^2 bid; continue therapy until disease progression
Available forms: Oral solution 20 mg/mL; capsules 25, 100 mg

---

lasmiditan (Rx)
(las-mid′i-tan)

Reyvow
Func. class.: Antimigraine

USES: Migraine with or without aura in adults

DOSAGE AND ROUTES
• **Adults: PO** 50, 100, or 200 mg as a single dose; max: 1 dose in 24 hr
Available forms: Tabs 50, 100 mg

---

latanoprost (ophthalmic) (Rx)
(lah-tan′oh-prost)

Xalatan
Func. class.: Antiglaucoma agent
Chem. class.: Prostaglandin agonist

Do not confuse:
latanoprost/bimatoprost

ACTION: Increases aqueous humor outflow

USES: Increased intraocular pressure in those who have open-angle glaucoma/ocular hypertension and who do not respond to other IOP-lowering products

CONTRAINDICATIONS
Hypersensitivity to this product, benzalkonium chloride
Precautions: Eye infections, angleclosure glaucoma, renal/hepatic function impairment, children, contact lenses, uveitis, keratitis

DOSAGE AND ROUTES
• **Adult: OPHTH** Instill 1 drop in each affected eye (conjunctival sac) every night
Available forms: Ophthalmic solution 0.005% (50 mcg/mL)
Administer:
Ophthalmic route
• Wash hands before and after use; contact lenses should be removed before using the product, reinsert 15 min after use; contains benzalkonium chloride, which may be absorbed by soft contact lenses
• The solution may be used concomitantly with other topical ophthalmic drug products to lower IOP; if more than one topical ophthalmic drug is being used, the drugs should be administered at least 5 min apart
• Store unopened bottle refrigerated; once opened, it may be stored at room temperature, protected from light, for up to 6 wk

SIDE EFFECTS
EENT: *Conjunctival hyperemia, iris color change, ocular pruritus,* xerophthalmia, visual disturbance, ocular irritation/burning, foreign body sensation, ocular pain, blepharitis, cataracts, and superficial punctate keratitis
INTEG: Rash, allergic reactions
MISC: Flulike symptoms
CV: Angina

PHARMACOKINETICS
Ophthalmic: Onset 3-4 hr, peak 8-12 hr; half-life 3 hr

NURSING CONSIDERATIONS
Assess:
• **Intraocular pressure:** in those with ongoing increased IOP
Evaluate:
• **Therapeutic response:** decreasing IOP

Teach patient/family:
Ophthalmic route
• To wash hands before and after use; that contact lenses should be removed, reinsert 15 min after use; contains benzalkonium chloride, which may be absorbed by soft contact lenses
• Tilt the head back slightly and pull lower eyelid down to form a pouch; squeeze drops into the pouch and close the eyes for 1-2 min; not to blink; to avoid contamination, do not touch the tip of the dropper to the eye, fingertips, or other surface
• May be used concomitantly with other topical ophthalmic products to lower IOP; if more than one is used, the drugs should be administered at least 5 min apart, do not exceed dose
• To store unopened bottle refrigerated; once opened, it may be stored at room temperature, protected from light, for up to 6 wk

---

⚠ HIGH ALERT

ledipasvir/sofosbuvir (Rx)
(le-dip′as-vir/soe-fos′bue-veer)
Harvoni
Func. class.: Antiviral, antihepatitis agent
Chem. class.: NS5A inhibitor

ACTION: A combination product with an HCV NS5A inhibitor (ledipasvir) and a nucleotide analog HCV NS5B polymerase inhibitor (sofosbuvir)

USES: Chronic hepatitis C virus (HCV) genotype 1 infection in patients with compensated liver disease

CONTRAINDICATIONS
Hypersensitivity
Precautions: Decompensated hepatic disease, decompensated cirrhosis, severe renal impairment (eGFR <30 mL/min/1.73 m^2), end-stage renal failure requiring dialysis, pregnancy, breastfeeding

Black Box Warning: Hepatitis B exacerbation

DOSAGE AND ROUTES
Chronic hepatitis C virus (HCV) genotype 1 infection:
• **Adult (treatment-naïve) without cirrhosis: PO** 1 tablet (90 mg ledipasvir; 400 mg sofosbuvir) daily with or without food; the recommended duration of treatment is 12 wk; however, 8-wk treatment can be considered for patients with a baseline HCV RNA <6 million IU/mL. Recommendation includes patients coinfected with HIV

Genotype 1
• **Adult (treatment-naïve) with compensated (Child-Pugh A) cirrhosis: PO** 1 tablet (90 mg ledipasvir; 400 mg sofosbuvir) daily with or without food; the recommended duration of treatment is 12 wk (recommendation includes patients coinfected with HIV)
• **Adult (treatment-experienced) without cirrhosis: PO** 1 tablet (90 mg ledipasvir; 400 mg sofosbuvir) daily with or without food; the recommended duration of treatment is 12 wk (recommendation includes patients coinfected with HIV)
• **Adult (treatment-experienced) with compensated (Child-Pugh A) cirrhosis: PO** 1 tablet (90 mg ledipasvir; 400 mg sofosbuvir) daily with or without food; for 24 wk
• **Adult (treatment-naïve and experienced) with decompensated (Child-Pugh B or C) cirrhosis: PO** 1 tablet (90 mg ledipasvir; 400 mg sofosbuvir) **PO** daily with ribavirin (600 mg **PO** daily) for 12 wk. Ribavirin must be administered with food
• **Adult (treatment-naïve and experienced) transplantation and is without cirrhosis or has compensated (Child-Pugh A) cirrhosis: PO** 1 tablet (90 mg ledipasvir; 400 mg sofosbuvir) daily with ribavirin for 12 wk. Ribavirin must be administered with food

L

• **Child/adolescent 12-17 yr (treatment-naïve) without cirrhosis or with compensated (Child-Pugh A) cirrhosis:** **PO** 1 tablet (90 mg ledipasvir; 400 mg sofosbuvir) daily with or without food × 12 wk

• **Child/adolescent 12-17 yr (treatment-experienced) without cirrhosis:** **PO** 1 tablet (90 mg ledipasvir; 400 mg sofosbuvir) daily with or without food × 12 wk

• **Child/adolescent 12-17 yr (treatment-experienced) with compensated (Child-Pugh A) cirrhosis: PO** 1 tablet (90 mg ledipasvir; 400 mg sofosbuvir) daily with or without food × 24 wk

For the treatment of chronic hepatitis C virus (HCV) genotype 4, 5, 6 infection

• **Adult (treatment-naïve or experienced) without cirrhosis or who have compensated (Child-Pugh A) cirrhosis:** **PO** 1 tablet (90 mg ledipasvir; 400 mg sofosbuvir) daily with or without food × 12 wk

• **Adult (treatment-naïve or experienced) who has undergone liver transplantation and is without cirrhosis or has compensated (Child-Pugh A) cirrhosis: PO** 1 tablet (90 mg ledipasvir; 400 mg sofosbuvir) daily with ribavirin for 12 wk. Ribavirin must be administered with food in 2 divided doses

• **Child/adolescent 12-17 yr (treatment-naïve or experienced) without cirrhosis or who has compensated (Child-Pugh A) cirrhosis: PO** 1 tablet (90 mg ledipasvir; 400 mg sofosbuvir) daily with or without food × 12 wk

Available forms: Tab 90 mg ledipasvir/400 mg sofosbuvir
Administer:
• Without regard to food

SIDE EFFECTS
CNS: *Fatigue, headache,* insomnia
GI: Nausea, vomiting, diarrhea
INTEG: Rash
MS: Myalgia

PHARMACOKINETICS
Ledipasvir: >99.8% protein binding, elimination biliary excretion, half-life 47 hr, peak 4-5 hr
Sofosbuvir: 61%-65% protein binding, elimination by the kidneys, 80% recovered in the urine, peak 0.8-1 hr, half-life 0.4 hr, metabolite 27 hr

INTERACTIONS
Increase: digoxin level—digoxin
Decrease: ledipasvir level—antacids; separate by ≥4 hr
Decrease: ledipasvir/sofosbuvir level—anticonvulsants, antimycobacterials (rifabutin, rifapentine), P-glycoprotein inducers; avoid using together
Decrease: ledipasvir level—H_2 receptor antagonists (famotidine), separate by ≥12 hr, max dose of H_2 receptor antagonist should not exceed famotidine 40 mg bid equivalent
Drug/Lab Test:
Increase: bilirubin, lipase, CK

NURSING CONSIDERATIONS
Assess:
• **Hepatitis C:** monitor hepatitis C RNA, serum bilirubin, creatinine
• **Pregnancy/breastfeeding:** use only if benefits outweigh fetal risk; cautious use in breastfeeding, excretion unknown

Black Box Warning: Hepatitis B: test prior to initiating therapy; risk of fulminant hepatitis and death

Evaluate:
• **Therapeutic response:** hepatitis C RNA reduction
• CHC is decreased
Teach patient/family:
• To report effects to the prescriber
• To notify all providers of product use
• To take at the same time each day, to use for full course even if feeling better, to take missed doses when remembered on the same day; not to double doses
• That the product will not decrease transmission of infection in others
• If antacids (magnesium, aluminum) are needed, take 4 hr before or after this product

lefamulin (Rx)

(le-FAMue-lin)

Xenleta

Func. class.: Antiifective

Chem. class.: Pleuromutilin antibiotics

ACTION: May be bacteriostatic or bactericidal depending on the organism; inhibits bacterial protein synthesis through interactions (hydrogen bonds, hydrophobic interactions, and Van der Waals forces) in rRNA of the 50S subunit

USES: Treatment of community acquired bacterial pneumonia caused by *Chlamydophila pneumoniae, Haemophilus influenzae (β-lactamase negative), Haemophilus influenzae (β-lactamase positive), Haemophilus parainfluenzae, Legionella pneumophila, Moraxella catarrhalis, Mycoplasma pneumoniae, Staphylococcus aureus* (MRSA), *Staphylococcus aureus* (MSSA), *Streptococcus agalactiae* (group B streptococci), *Streptococcus anginosus, Streptococcus mitis, Streptococcus pneumoniae, Streptococcus pyogenes* (group A β-hemolytic streptococci), *Streptococcus salivarius*

CONTRAINDICATIONS

Hypersensitivity to this product or pleuromutilin antibiotics; use with CYP3A4 substrates

Precautions:

Alcoholism, bradycardia, breastfeeding, cardiac disease, contraception requirements, CAD, diabetes mellitus, dialysis, diarrhea, geriatrics, hepatic disease, hypertension, hypocalcemia, hypokalemia, hypomagnesemia, long QT syndrome, renal failure, reproductive risk, thyroid disease, torsades de pointes, ventricular dysrhythmias

DOSAGE AND ROUTES

• **Adults: PO** 600 mg q12hr × 5 days; IV 150 mg q12hr × 5-7 days

Hepatic dose

• **Adults: IV** Give over 60 min q24hr (Child-Pugh Class C); PO not recommended for patients with moderate (Child-Pugh Class B) or severe (Child-Pugh Class C)

Available forms:

Tablet 600 mg; solution for injection 150 mg/15 mL (10 mg/mL)

Administer:

PO route

• If a dose is missed, give the dose as soon as possible and anytime up to 8 hr before the next scheduled dose; if less than 8 hr remain before the next scheduled dose, do not give the missed dose, and resume dosing at the next scheduled dose

• Administer at least 1 hour before a meal or 2 hr after a meal

• Swallow tablet whole with 6 to 8 ounces of water; do not crush or divide tablets

• **Intermittent IV route** Visually inspect for particulate matter and discoloration prior to use, do not use if present

Dilution: Dilute the entire 15-mL vial into the supplied diluent bag; mix thoroughly; do not use the diluent bag in series connections, do not admix

Storage: Store up to 24 hr at room temperature and up to 48 hr when refrigerated at 2° C-8° C (36° F-46° F)

• Infuse over 60 min

SIDE EFFECTS

GI: Nausea, diarrhea, CDAD, vomiting

CNS: Insomnia, headache

META: Hypokalemia

PHARMACOKINETICS

Protein binding 94.8% to 97.1%, metabolized by CYP3A4; excreted urine 15.5% (9.6%-14.1% unchanged) after IV, 5.3% (unchanged after PO, excreted feces 77.3% (4.2%-9.1% unchanged) after IV and 88.5% (7.8%-24.8% unchanged) after PO; half-life is 3-20 hr; is a CYP3A4 and P-glycoprotein (P-gp) substrate; inhibits CYP2C8, breast cancer resistance protein (BCRP), and MATE1; PO peak 0.88-2 hr

INTERACTIONS

Decreased: Lefamulin effect—strong or moderate CYP3A inducers or P-gp inducers; avoid using together; if used, monitor for reduced effect

Increased: lefamulin effect—strong CYP3A inhibitors or P-gp inhibitors;

L

avoid using together; if used together, monitor for adverse reactions

Increased: QT interval—CYP3A substrates; do not use together

NURSING CONSIDERATIONS
Assess:
• **Pneumonia:** Assess for signs of pneumonia
• QT prolongation: Assess for QT prolongation
Evaluate:
Therapeutic response: decreasing symptoms of pneumonia, culture negative
Teach patient/family:
• Advise patients to take at least 1 hr before a meal or 2 hr after a meal and should be swallowed whole with water (6-8 ounces); do not crush or divide
• That nausea/vomiting is common
• That serious allergic reactions may occur and require immediate attention
• To take exactly as directed, not to skip doses or not complete the full course of therapy
• **CDAD, diarrhea:** Assess for diarrhea that is watery or has mucous, with or without fever, stomach cramps that may occur up to 2 months after final dose
• **Pregnancy/breastfeeding:** Identify if pregnancy is planned or suspect, or if breastfeeding, pregnancy testing will be needed before use; use adequate contraception during use and for 2 days after final dose; not to be used in pregnancy; if used inadvertently during pregnancy or if a patient becomes pregnant while receiving product, report exposure by calling 1-855-5NABRIVA to enroll; if breastfeeding, pump and discard milk for the duration of treatment and for 2 days after the final dose

---

leflunomide (Rx)
(leh-floo'noh-mide)
Arava
Func. class.: Antirheumatic (DMARDs)
Chem. class.: Immune modulator, pyrimidine synthesis inhibitor

ACTION: Inhibits an enzyme involved in pyrimidine synthesis; has antiproliferative, antiinflammatory effect

USES: RA: to reduce disease process and symptoms
Unlabeled uses: Juvenile RA, BK virus (viremia or nephropathy; in kidney transplant), cytomegalovirus disease (in transplant patients resistant to standard antivirals)

CONTRAINDICATIONS
Breastfeeding, hypersensitivity

Black Box Warning: Pregnancy

Precautions: Children, renal disorders, vaccinations, infection, alcoholism, immunosuppression, jaundice, lactase deficiency, hepatic disease

Black Box Warning: Hepatic disease (ALT >2 × ULN)

DOSAGE AND ROUTES
Rheumatoid arthritis
• **Adult: PO** Loading dose 100 mg/day × 3 days, maintenance 20 mg/day; may be decreased to 10 mg/day if not well tolerated
Juvenile rheumatoid arthritis (unlabeled)
• **Adolescent/child >40 kg: PO** 20 mg/day
• **Adolescent/child 20-40 kg: PO** 15 mg/day
• **Adolescent/child 10-19.9 kg: PO** 10 mg/day
Available forms: Tabs 10, 20 mg
Administer:
• With food for GI upset, give same time each day, loading dose is recommended
• **Drug elimination:** give cholestyramine 8 g tid × 11 days; check levels

SIDE EFFECTS
CNS: *Headache,* dizziness, insomnia, depression, paresthesia, anxiety, migraine, neuralgia
CV: Palpitations, hypertension, chest pain, angina pectoris, peripheral edema

EENT: Pharyngitis, oral candidiasis, stomatitis, dry mouth, blurred vision
GI: *Nausea, anorexia, vomiting, constipation, flatulence, diarrhea, elevated LFTs,* hepatotoxicity, weight loss
HEMA: Anemia, ecchymosis, hyperlipidemia
INTEG: Rash, pruritus, alopecia, acne, hematoma, herpes infections
RESP: Pharyngitis, rhinitis, bronchitis, cough, respiratory infection, pneumonia, sinusitis, interstitial lung disease
SYST: Opportunistic/fatal infections, Stevens-Johnson syndrome, toxic epidermal necrolysis, DRESS

PHARMACOKINETICS
Metabolized in liver to active metabolite, half-life of metabolite 2 wk, excreted in urine, protein binding, 99%, crosses placenta, onset 99 min, peak up to 6 min of RA effect

INTERACTIONS
Increase: NSAID effect—NSAIDs
Increase: hepatotoxicity—hepatotoxic agents, methotrexate
Increase: leflunomide levels—rifampin
Increase: bleeding risk—warfarin
Decrease: antibody response—live virus vaccines
Decrease: leflunomide effect—cholestyramine, use for overdose

NURSING CONSIDERATIONS
Assess:
• **Arthritic symptoms:** ROM, mobility, swelling of joints at baseline and during treatment
• Screen for latent TB before starting treatment; if TB is present, pretreat before using product
• **Interstitial lung disease:** increased or worsening cough, SOB, fever; product may need to be discontinued and drug elimination procedure initiated (rare)

Black Box Warning: Hepatic necrosis/failure: monitor LFTs, if ALT elevations are >2 × baseline, reduce dose to 10 mg/day; monitor monthly or more frequently

• **Labs:** CBC with differential monthly × 6 mo, then q6-8wk thereafter; pregnancy test; serum electrolytes
• **Infections:** fatal infections can occur
• **Hypertension:** B/P, weight; edema can occur
• **Stevens-Johnson syndrome, toxic epidermal necrolysis:** monitor for rash during treatment; if rash with fever, fatigue, joint aches, blisters is present, discontinue immediately, initiate drug elimination procedure

Black Box Warning: Pregnancy: determine that patient is not pregnant before treatment; not to be given to women of childbearing potential who are not using reliable contraception, not to use in males who could potentially father a child, use barrier protection during therapy and up to 2 yr after last dose

Evaluate:
• **Therapeutic response:** decreased inflammation, pain in joints
Teach patient/family:
• That continuing monitoring will be needed
• That product must be continued for prescribed time to be effective, that up to a month may be required for improvement, that other treatment may continue corticosteroids, NSAIDs
• To take with food, milk, or antacids to avoid GI upset; to take at same time of day
• To use caution when driving because drowsiness, dizziness may occur
• To take with a full glass of water to enhance absorption, may continue with correct prescribed treatment with other antiinflammatories
• To discuss with health care professional all Rx, OTC, herbals, supplements used
• That hair may be lost; review alternatives
• To avoid live virus vaccinations during treatment
• To notify prescriber of weight loss
• **Overdose treatment:** give cholestyramine 8 g tid × 11 days

Black Box Warning: Pregnancy/breastfeeding: not to become pregnant while taking this product; not to breastfeed while taking this product; men should also discontinue product and begin leflunomide removal protocol if pregnancy is planned

⚠ HIGH ALERT

lemborexant (Rx)
(lem-boe-rex'ant)
Dayvigo
Func. class.: Hypnotic
Chem. class.: Orexin receptor

Controlled Substance Schedule IV

ACTION:
Competitive antagonism of orexin receptors that are responsible for wakefulness

USES:
Insomnia

CONTRAINDICATIONS
Hypersensitivity, narcolepsy
Precautions: Substance abuse, breastfeeding, pregnancy, depression, suicidal ideation, elderly, sleep apnea, COPD

DOSAGE AND ROUTES
Insomnia with sleep onset and/or sleep maintenance difficulties:
• **Adults:** PO 5 mg nightly immediately before going to bed, with at least 7 hr remaining before the planned time of awakening. The dose may be increased to the 10 mg max if needed
Available forms: Tabs 5, 10 mg
Administer:
• Give immediately before going to bed, with at least 7 hr remaining before the planned time of awakening
• Do not use >10 mg per night

SIDE EFFECTS
CNS: Fatigue, headache, nightmares, hallucinations, sleep paralysis, suicidal ideation

PHARMACOKINETICS
Peak 1-3 hr, half-life 17-19 hr, protein binding 94%

INTERACTIONS
Increase: CNS depression—other CNS depressants
Increase: lemborexant level: CYP3A4 inhibitors
Decrease: lemborexant level: CYP3A4 inducers

Decrease: effect of—CYP2B6 substrates

NURSING CONSIDERATIONS
Assess:
• **Mental status:** reason for medication, type of sleep problem, trouble falling asleep, staying asleep, complex sleep-related behaviors, sleep paralysis, suicidal ideation, depression
Evaluate:
• **Therapeutic response:** Ability to sleep throughout the night
Teach patient/family:
• **Suicidal ideation:** have patient report immediately
• To report complex sleep disorders, sleep paralysis, hallucinations, nightmares
• To avoid other CNS depressants
• Not to take others, medication, herbs without discussing with prescriber
• **Pregnancy/breastfeeding:** to notify prescriber if pregnancy is planned or suspected or if breastfeeding

⚠ HIGH ALERT

lenvatinib (Rx)
(len-va'-ti-nib)
Lenvima
Func. class.: Antineoplastic

USES: Locally recurrent or metastatic, progressive, radioactive iodine-refractory differentiated thyroid cancer (DTC)

CONTRAINDICATIONS
Hypersensitivity

DOSAGE AND ROUTES
Thyroid cancer
• **Adult:** PO 24 mg (two 12 mg capsules)
Advanced renal cell carcinoma after 1 prior treatment, used with everolimus
• **Adult:** PO 18 mg/day with everolimus 5 mg/day
Hepatocellular cancer, unrectable
• **Adult ≥60 kg:** PO 12 mg daily; <60 kg: PO 8 mg once daily
Available forms: Capsules 4, 8, 10, 12, 14, 18, 20, 24 mg

letermovir (Rx)

(le-term-oh-vir)

Prevymis

Func. class.: Antiviral

USES: For the prevention of cytomegalovirus following allogenic hematopoietic stem cell transplant

DOSAGE AND ROUTES
Cytomegalovirus (CMV) disease prophylaxis

• **Adult: PO/IV** 480 mg/day started between day 0 and day 28 after transplantation (before or after engraftment) and continued through day 100 after transplantation

Cytomegalovirus (CMV) disease prophylaxis in patients with concurrent cycloSPORINE

• **Adult: PO/IV** 240 mg/day started between day 0 and day 28 after transplantation (before or after engraftment) and continued through day 100 after transplantation. If cycloSPORINE is initiated after starting letermovir, reduce letermovir to 240 mg with the next dose. If cycloSPORINE is discontinued after starting letermovir, increase the dose of letermovir to 480 mg. If cycloSPORINE dosing is interrupted due to high cycloSPORINE concentrations, no dosage adjustment of letermovir is needed

Available forms: Tabs 240, 480 mg; injection 240 mg/12 mL; 480 mg/24 mL single-use vials

⚠ HIGH ALERT

letrozole (Rx)

(let′roe-zole)

Femara

Func. class.: Antineoplastic, non-steroidal aromatase inhibitor

Do not confuse:
Femara/Femhrt

ACTION: Binds to the heme group of aromatase; inhibits conversion of androgens to estrogens to reduce plasma estrogen levels

USES: Early, advanced, or metastatic breast cancer in postmenopausal women who are hormone receptor positive

Unlabeled uses: Infertility, ovarian cancer, idiopathic short stature, constitutional delayed puberty

CONTRAINDICATIONS
Pregnancy, premenopausal females, hypersensitivity

Precautions: Respiratory/hepatic disease, osteoporosis

DOSAGE AND ROUTES
• **Adult: PO** 2.5 mg/day
Infertility (unlabeled)
• **Adult: PO** 2.5, 5, 7.5 mg/day × 5 days, usually days 3-7 of menstrual cycle
Idiopathic short stature, constitutional delayed puberty (unlabeled)
• **Adolescent and child ≥9 (male): PO** 2.5 mg/day; use with testosterone for delayed puberty
Available forms: Tabs 2.5 mg
Administer:
• Without regard to meals; with small glass of water
• May administer bisphosphonates to increase bone density

SIDE EFFECTS
CNS: *Headache, lethargy,* somnolence, dizziness, depression, anxiety
CV: Angina, MI, CVA, thromboembolic events, hypertension, peripheral edema
GI: *Nausea, vomiting, anorexia,* constipation, heartburn, diarrhea
GU: Endometrial cancer, vaginal bleeding, endometrial proliferation disorders
INTEG: *Rash, pruritus,* alopecia, sweating
MISC: Hot flashes, night sweats, second malignancies, anaphylaxis, angioedema, infections
MS: Arthralgia, arthritis, bone fracture, myalgia, osteoporosis
RESP: Dyspnea, cough

PHARMACOKINETICS
Metabolized in liver, excreted in urine, peak 2 days, terminal half-life 48 hr, steady state 2-6 wk

Side effects: *italics* = common; red = life-threatening

INTERACTIONS
Decrease: letrozole effect—estrogens, oral contraceptives

NURSING CONSIDERATIONS
Assess:
• **Pain:** Assess pain baseline and periodically
• Hepatic studies before, during therapy (bilirubin, AST, ALT, LDH) as needed or monthly
• Bone density studies, cholesterol/ lipid levels, pregnancy testing
Evaluate:
• **Therapeutic response:** decrease in size of tumor
Teach patient/family:
• To report allergic reactions (rash; hives; difficulty breathing; tightness in chest; swelling of mouth, face, lips, tongue)
• To report vaginal bleeding, diarrhea, chest/bone pain
• To use adequate contraception in perimenopausal, recently postmenopausal women, fetal risk
• To avoid driving or other hazardous activities until response is known, dizziness may occur

---

leucovorin (Rx)
(loo-koe-vor'in)
Func. class.: Vitamin, folic acid/ methotrexate antagonist antidote
Chem. class.: Tetrahydrofolic acid derivative

Do not confuse:
leucovorin/Leukeran/levoleucovorin

USES: Megaloblastic or macrocytic anemia caused by folic acid deficiency, overdose of folic acid antagonist, methotrexate/pyrimethamine/trimetrexate/ trimethoprim toxicity, pneumocystosis, toxoplasmosis

CONTRAINDICATIONS
Hypersensitivity to this product or folic acid, benzyl alcohol; anemias other than megaloblastic not associated with vit B_{12} deficiency

DOSAGE AND ROUTES
Methotrexate toxicity/leucovorin rescue
• **Adult/child: PO/IM/IV normal elimination** given 6 hr after dose of methotrexate (10 mg/m^2) until methotrexate $<5 \times 10^{-8}$ m, CCr $>50\%$ above prior level, or methotrexate level 5×10^{-8} m at 24 hr or $>9 \times 10^{-8}$ m at 48 hr; give leucovorin 100 mg/m^2 q3hr until level drops to $<10^{-8}$ m
Megaloblastic anemia caused by enzyme deficiency (folate)
• **Adult/child: IV/IM** 1 mg/day
Pyrimethamine/trimethoprim toxicity prevention
• **Adult/child: PO/IV/IM** 5-15 mg/day
Advanced colorectal cancer
• **Adult: IV** 200 mg/m^2, then 5-FU 370 mg/m^2 or leucovorin 20 mg/m^2, then 5-FU 425 mg/m^2; give daily × 5 days q4-5wk

---

⚠ HIGH ALERT

leuprolide (Rx)
(loo-proe'lide)
Camcevi, Eligard, Fensolvi, Lupron Depot, Lupron Depot-Ped, Lupron ✦
Func. class.: Antineoplastic hormone
Chem. class.: Gonadotropin-releasing hormone

ACTION: Causes initial increase in circulating levels of LH, FSH; continuous administration results in decreased LH, FSH; in men, testosterone is reduced to castrate levels; in premenopausal women, estrogen is reduced to menopausal levels

USES: Metastatic prostate cancer (inj implant), management of endometriosis, central precocious puberty, uterine leiomyomata (fibroids)

Unlabeled uses: Breast cancer, hormone therapy for transgender females (male-to-female), paraphilia

CONTRAINDICATIONS
Pregnancy, breastfeeding, hypersensitivity to GnRH or analogs, thromboembolic disorders, undiagnosed vaginal bleeding; Eligard should not be used in women, children

Precautions: Edema, hepatic disease, CVA, MI, seizures, hypertension, diabetes mellitus, HF, depression, osteoporosis, spinal cord compression, urinary tract obstruction

DOSAGE AND ROUTES
Advanced prostate cancer
• **Adult:** SUBCUT 1 mg/day; **IM** 7.5 mg/depot dose monthly; **IM** 22.5 mg depot q3mo; or **IM** 30 mg depot q4mo; or **IM** 45 mg depot q6mo; **SUBCUT** (Eligard) 7.5 mg monthly; **SUBCUT** 22.5 mg (Eligard) q3mo; **SUBCUT** 45 mg (Eligard) qmo every 6 mo

Endometriosis
• **Adult:** IM 3.75 mg depot monthly for 6 mo or 11.25 mg q3mo for 6 mo or 30 mg q4mo

Anemia related to uterine fibroids
• **Adult:** IM 3.75 mg depot monthly × 3 mo or 11.25 mg depot as a single dose

Central precocious puberty
• **Child:** SUBCUT 50 mcg/kg/day; may increase by 10 mcg/kg/day as needed
• **Child >37.5 kg:** IM Lepron Depot-Ped 15 mg q4wk
• **Child 25-37.5 kg:** IM Lepron Depot-Ped 11.25 mg q4wk
• **Child ≤25 kg:** IM Lepron Depot-Ped 7.5 mg q4wk

Benign prostatic hyperplasia (BPH) (unlabeled)
• **Adult:** SUBCUT (sol for inj) 1 mg/day, **IM** (injection susp) 3.75 mg q28day × 24 wk

Available forms: Depot inj: 3.75, 7.5, 11.25, 15, 22.5, 30, 45 mg; Solution for Subcut Inj: 5 mg/mL (2.8-mL multidose vials); emulsion for injection 42 mg injection kit

Administer:
• Never give IV
• Store in tight container at room temperature
• **SUBCUT:** No dilution needed if patient self-administering; make sure patient is using syringes provided by manufacturer
• **SUBCUT Eligard** bring to room temperature, once mixed, give within 30 min, prepare the 2 syringes for mixing, join the 2 syringes together by pushing in and twisting until secure; mix the product by pushing the contents of both syringes back and forth between syringes until uniform; should be light tan to tan, draw entire mixed product into syringe B (short, wide syringe) by depressing the syringe A plunger and slightly withdrawing syringe B plunger, uncouple syringe A, while pushing down on syringe A plunger, small air bubbles will remain, hold syringe B upright, remove pink cap, attach needle cartridge to the end of syringe B, remove needle cover, give by subcut

IM route
• **Monthly:** reconstitute single-use vial with 1 mL of diluent; if multiple vials used, withdraw 0.5 mL, inject into each vial (1 mL); withdraw all, inject at 90-degree angle (3.75 mg)
• **3-mo:** reconstitute microspheres using 1.5 mL of diluent, inject into vial; shake, withdraw, inject

SIDE EFFECTS
CNS: Memory impairment, *depression*, seizures
CV: MI, PE, dysrhythmias, peripheral edema
GI: *Nausea, vomiting, anorexia, diarrhea*, GI bleeding
GU: *Edema, hot flashes, impotence, decreased libido, amenorrhea, vaginal dryness*, gynecomastia, profuse vaginal bleeding
INTEG: Alopecia
MS: Bone pain
RESP: Dyspnea, pulmonary fibrosis, interstitial lung disease

PHARMACOKINETICS

IM/SUBCUT: Peak 1-2 mo, duration 1-3 mo; absorbed rapidly (SUBCUT), slowly (IM depot); half-life 3 hr

INTERACTIONS

Increase: antineoplastic action—flutamide, megestrol

Increase: seizure risk—SSRIs

Drug/Herb

• Do not use with black cohosh or chaste tree fruit; may interfere with treatment

NURSING CONSIDERATIONS

Assess:

• **Prostate cancer:** increased bone pain for first 4 wk of treatment; those with metastases in spinal column may exhibit severe back pain

• **Symptoms of endometriosis** (lower abdominal pain)/**fibroids** (pelvic pain, excessive vaginal bleeding, bloating) before, during, after treatment

• **Central precocious puberty (CPP)** diagnosis should have been confirmed by secondary S_4 characteristics in children <9 yr, estradiol/testosterone levels, GnRH test, tomography of head, adrenal steroids, chorionic gonadotropin, wrist x-ray, height, weight

• Hepatic studies (bilirubin, AST, ALT, LDH) before, during therapy monthly, as needed; PSA, calcium, testosterone with prostate cancer; bone mineral density; blood glucose, HbA1c

• Pituitary gonadotropic and gonadal function during therapy and 4-8 wk after therapy is discontinued

• **QT prolongation (depot):** ECG in CV patients using depot route

• **Tumor flare:** worsening of signs and symptoms; normal during beginning therapy

• Fatigue; increased pulse, pallor, lethargy; edema in feet, joints; stomach pain

• **Severe allergic reaction:** rash, pruritus, urticaria, purpuric skin lesions, itching, flushing

Evaluate:

• **Therapeutic response:** decreased tumor size and spread of malignancy; decrease in lesions, pain with endometriosis,

fibroids, correction of CPP; increased follicle maturation

Teach patient/family:

• To notify prescriber if menstruation continues; menstruation should stop

• That bone pain will disappear after 1 wk

• To report any complaints, side effects to nurse, prescriber; that hot flashes may occur; to record weight, report gain of >2 lb/day

• How to prepare, give; to rotate sites for SUBCUT/IM inj; to use only syringes provided by manufacturer; to store depot at room temperature; to refrigerate unopened vials, to protect all from heat

• To keep accurate records of dose

• **That tumor flare may occur:** increase in size of tumor, increased bone pain, will subside rapidly; may take analgesics for pain, usually in prostate cancer or central precocious puberty

• That ongoing treatment is needed in central precocious puberty

• That voiding problems may increase during beginning of therapy but will decrease in several weeks

• **Pregnancy:** to notify prescriber if pregnancy is planned or suspected; not to breastfeed; to use nonhormonal form of contraception (women of childbearing age)

---

levalbuterol (Rx)

(lev-al-byoo′ter-ole)

Xopenex, Xopenex HFA

Func. class.: Bronchodilator, adrenergic β_2-agonist

ACTION: Causes bronchodilation by action on β_2 (pulmonary) receptors by increasing levels of cAMP, which relaxes smooth muscle; produces bronchodilation, CNS, cardiac stimulation as well as increased diuresis and gastric acid secretion

USES: Treatment or prevention of bronchospasm (reversible obstructive airway disease), asthma

CONTRAINDICATIONS

Hypersensitivity to sympathomimetics, this product, albuterol

Precautions: Pregnancy, breastfeeding, hyperthyroidism, diabetes mellitus, hypertension, prostatic hypertrophy, angle-closure glaucoma, seizures, renal disease, QT prolongation, tachydysrhythmias, severe cardiac disease, hypokalemia, children

DOSAGE AND ROUTES
Prevention of bronchospasm in reversible obstructive airway disease
• **Adult/child ≥12 yr: INH** 0.63 mg tid q6-8hr by nebulization, may increase 1.25 mg q8hr
• **Adult/adolescent/child >4 yr:** (HFA, metered dose) 90 mcg **(2INH)** q4-6hr
• **Child 6-11 yr: INH** 0.31 mg tid by nebulization, max 0.63 mg tid
Available forms: Sol, inh pediatric 0.31 mg/3 mL; 0.63 mg/3 mL; 1.25 mg/3 mL; 1.25 mg/0.5 mL; 45 mcg per actuation (HFA)
Administer:
• Every 6-8 hr; wait ≥1 min between inhalation of aerosols
Inhalation route
• Keep unopened until ready for use; after opening, use within 2 wk; protect from light, heat
• Shake well before use; use a spacer device; prime with 4 test sprays in new canister or when not used for >3 days
Nebulizer route
• Dilute concentrated (1.25 mg/0.5 mL) with normal sterile saline before use

SIDE EFFECTS
CNS: *Tremors, anxiety,* insomnia, *headache,* dizziness
CV: Tachycardia
EENT: Dry nose, irritation of nose and throat, rhinitis
GI: Diarrhea, dyspepsia
INTEG: Rash
META: *Hypokalemia, hyperglycemia*
MS: Muscle cramps
RESP: Cough, dyspnea, bronchospasm
MISC: Flu-like symptoms

PHARMACOKINETICS
Metabolized in the liver and tissues; crosses placenta, breast milk, blood-brain barrier; half-life 3.3-4 hr
INH sol: Onset 10-17 min, peak 1½ hr, duration 5-6 hr; **INH aerosol:** onset 4.5-10.2 min, peak 76-78 min, duration ≤6 hr

INTERACTIONS
Increase: hypokalemia—loop/thiazide diuretics
Increase: action of aerosol bronchodilators
Increase: levalbuterol action—tricyclics, MAOIs, other adrenergics; avoid use within 2 wk of MAOIs
Decrease: levalbuterol action—other β-blockers; severe bronchospasm may occur
Decrease: digoxin effect—digoxin
Drug/Herb
Increase: stimulation—black/green tea, coffee, cola nut, guarana, yerba maté

NURSING CONSIDERATIONS
Assess:
• **Respiratory function:** vital capacity, pulse oximetry, forced expiratory volume, ABGs, lung sounds, heart rate and rhythm (baseline); character of sputum: color, consistency, amount
• Cardiac status: palpitations, increase/decrease in B/P, dysrhythmias
• **For evidence of allergic reactions, paradoxic bronchospasm, anaphylaxis, angioedema;** if these occur, hold dose, notify prescriber at once; bronchospasm may occur with new canister or vial
• **Pregnancy/breastfeeding:** avoid use in pregnancy, do not breastfeed, reaction is unknown
Evaluate:
• **Therapeutic response:** absence of dyspnea, wheezing after 1 hr; improved airway exchange, ABGs/VBGs
Teach patient/family:
• Not to use OTC medications because excess stimulation may occur
• To avoid getting aerosol in eyes because blurring may result

• To avoid smoking, smoke-filled rooms, persons with respiratory infections
• That paradoxic bronchospasm may occur; to stop product immediately, contact prescriber
• To limit caffeine products such as chocolate, coffee, tea, colas, and herbs such as cola nut, guarana, yerba maté
• **Inhaler:** to shake well before using and to breathe normally while using and mist goes into reservoir; to spray 4 times before first use or if not used for 3 days; to wash at least weekly
• To use this product first if using other inhalers; to wait 5 min or more between products; to rinse mouth with water after each dose to prevent dry mouth
• **Diabetes:** that diabetes may be exacerbated; that medications for diabetes may need to be adjusted

TREATMENT OF OVERDOSE:
Administer a β_1-adrenergic blocker

---

levETIRAcetam (Rx)
(lev-eh-teer-ass'eh-tam)
Keppra, Keppra XR, Spritam
Func. class.: Anticonvulsant
Chem. class.: Pyrrolidine derivative

Do not confuse:
Keppra/Kaletra/Keflex
levETIRAcetam/lamotrigine/levocarnitine/levofloxacin

ACTION: Unknown; may inhibit nerve impulses by limiting influx of sodium ions across cell membrane in motor cortex

USES: Adjunctive therapy for partial-onset seizures, primary generalized tonic-clonic seizures, myoclonic seizures in juvenile patients

CONTRAINDICATIONS
Hypersensitivity, breastfeeding
Precautions: Pregnancy, children, geriatric patients, renal/cardiac disease, psychosis

DOSAGE AND ROUTES
Adjunctive treatment of partial-onset seizures
• **Adult/adolescent ≥16 yr: IV** 500 mg bid, may be titrated by 1000 mg/day q2wk, max 3000 mg/day in divided doses; **EXT REL** 1000 mg/day, may increase q2wk, max 3000 mg/day
• **Adolescent <16 yr/child: 1 mo to <6 mo** (immediate-release tablet, injection or oral solution): Initially, 7 mg/kg **IV/PO** bid; increase by 14 mg/kg/day in 2 divided doses q2wk to target dose of 42 mg/kg/day in 2 divided doses. For **PO,** use oral sol with weight of ≤20 kg
6 mo to <4 yr (immediate-release tablet, injection, or oral sol): Initially, 10 mg/kg **IV/PO** bid; increase by 20 mg/kg/day in 2 divided doses q2wk to target dose of 50 mg/kg/day in 2 divided doses as tolerated. For oral administration, use oral sol with weight of ≤20 kg
4 yr to <16 yr and 20-40 kg (immediate-release tablet): Initially, 250 mg **PO** bid; titration, increase by 500 mg/day in 2 divided doses q2wk to max 1500 mg/day in 2 divided doses
4 yr to <16 yr and >40 kg (immediate-release tablet): Initially, 500 mg **PO** bid; increase by 1000 mg/day q2wk in 2 divided doses to max 3000 mg/day in 2 divided doses
4 yr to <16 yr (oral sol): Initially, 10 mg/kg orally bid; increase by 20 mg/kg/day in 2 divided doses q2wk to target dose of 60 mg/kg/day in 2 divided doses as tolerated
Myoclonic seizures/tonic-clonic seizures/partial seizures
• **Adult/adolescent ≥16 yr: PO/IV** 500 mg bid, may increase by 1000 mg/day q2wk, max 3000 mg/day in 2 divided doses
Adjunctive treatment of partial onset seizures in those with epilepsy (Spritam)
• **Adult/child ≥4 yr and >40 kg: PO** 500 mg bid, may increase q2wk by 500 mg bid, max 1500 mg bid

---

Renal dose
• **Adult: PO** CCr 50-80 mL/min, 500-1000 mg q12hr or **EXT REL** 1000-2000 mg q24hr, max 2000 mg/day; CCr 30-49 mL/min, 250-750 mg q12hr or **EXT REL** 500-1500 mg q24hr, max 1500 mg/day; CCr <30 mL/min, 250-500 mg q12hr or **EXT REL** 500-1000 mg q24hr, max 1000 mg/day

Available forms: Tabs 250, 500, 750, 1000 mg; oral sol 100 mg/mL; sol for inj 100 mg/mL; ext rel tab 500, 750 mg; pre-mixed solution 1000 mg/100 mL 0.75% NaCl, 1500 mg/100 mL, 500 mg/100 mL 0.82% NaCl; tabs for oral suspension (Spirtam) 250, 500, 750, 1000 mg

Administer:
PO route
• Extended-release product should not be used in dialysis patients
• Swallow tab whole; do not break, crush, or chew
• With food, milk to decrease GI symptoms (rare) if needed
• Store at room temperature (PO)
Child:
• <20 kg should be given oral solution; use calibrated device
Tabs for oral suspension (Spirtam)
• Give only whole tabs
• Peel foil from blister; do not push through foil
• Place on tongue and swallow with a sip of liquid; do not swallow whole
• Tab can be added to a tablespoon of liquid in a cup; swirl gently, consume
Intermittent IV INFUSION route
• Single-use vials: dilute in 100 mL of 0.9% NaCl, D5W, LR; give over 15 min, discard unused vial contents, do not use product with particulates or discoloration
• **Child:** max concentration of product 15 mg/mL (diluted solution); infuse over 15 min
• Diluted preparation stable for 24 hr at room temperature in polyvinyl bags
• Store vials at room temperature

SIDE EFFECTS
CNS: Dizziness, somnolence, asthenia, psychosis, suicidal ideation, nonpsychotic behavioral symptoms, headache, ataxia
EENT: Diplopia, conjunctivitis
GI: Nausea, vomiting, anorexia, diarrhea, constipation, hepatitis
HEMA: Infection, leukopenia
INTEG: Pruritus, rash
MISC: Infection, abdominal pain, pharyngitis
SYST: Stevens-Johnson syndrome, toxic epidermal necrolysis; dehydration (child <4 yr)

PHARMACOKINETICS
Rapidly absorbed; not protein bound; excreted via kidneys 66% unchanged; half-life 6-8 hr, longer in geriatric patients or with renal disease

INTERACTIONS
Increase: sedation—TCAs, antihistamines, benzodiazepines, other CNS depressants, alcohol
• Possible increased carBAMazepine toxicity: carBAMazepine
Decrease: levETIRAcetam absorption—sevelamer; separate by 1 hr before, 3 hr after sevelamer
Drug/Lab Test
Decrease: Hct/HB, WBC, RBC

NURSING CONSIDERATIONS
Assess:
• **Seizures:** type, location, duration, character, intensity, precipitating factors; provide seizure precautions
• **Renal studies:** urinalysis, BUN, urine creatinine q3mo
• **Blood studies:** CBC, LFTs
• **Mental status:** mood, sensorium, affect, behavioral changes, **suicidal** thoughts/behaviors; if mental status changes, notify prescriber
• Assistance with ambulation during early part of treatment; dizziness occurs
• **Beers:** avoid in older adults unless safer alternative is unavailable; may cause ataxia, impaired psychomotor function

• **Pregnancy:** if used during pregnancy, patient should enroll in the Antiepileptic Drug Pregnancy Registry at 888-233-2334; do not breastfeed

Evaluate:

• **Therapeutic response:** decreased seizure activity; document on patient's chart

Teach patient/family:

• To take with or without food

• Not to crush, break, chew tablets

• To carry emergency ID stating patient's name; products taken; condition; prescriber's name, phone number

• How to use oral sol; if trouble swallowing, measure oral sol in medicine cup or dropper, do not use teaspoon

• To avoid driving, other activities that require alertness until response is known; drowsiness occurs during first month

• Not to discontinue medication quickly after long-term use because withdrawal seizure may occur

• To immediately report suicidal thoughts or behaviors, mood changes, hostility; thoughts of death, dying

• **Pregnancy/breastfeeding:** to notify prescriber if pregnant, intending to become pregnant; not to breastfeed, excreted in breast milk

---

levobetaxolol ophthalmic

See Appendix B

---

levobunolol (ophthalmic) (Rx)

(lee′voe-byoo′no-lahl)

Betagan

Func. class.: Antiglaucoma

Chem. class.: β-Blocker

ACTION: Can decrease aqueous humor and increase outflows

USES: Treatment of chronic open-angle glaucoma and ocular hypertension

CONTRAINDICATIONS

Hypersensitivity, AV block, heart failure, bradycardia, sick sinus syndrome, asthma

Precautions: Abrupt discontinuation, children, pregnancy, breastfeeding, COPD, depression, diabetes mellitus, myasthenia gravis, hyperthyroidism, pulmonary disease, sulfite sensitivity, angle-closure glaucoma

DOSAGE AND ROUTES

• **Adult:** Instill 1-2 drops in the affected eyes once a day (0.5% solution), bid (0.25% solution)

Available forms: Ophthalmic solution 0.25%, 0.5%

Administer:

• For ophthalmic use only

• To prevent contamination, do not touch the tip of the dropper to the eye, fingertips, or other surface

• Wash hands before and after use; tilt head back slightly and pull the lower eyelid down with the index finger to form a pouch; squeeze the prescribed number of drops into the pouch; close eyes to spread drops; to avoid excessive systemic absorption, apply finger pressure on the lacrimal sac for 1-2 min after use

• If more than one topical ophthalmic drug product is being used, the drugs should be administered at least 5 min apart

• To avoid contamination or the spread of infection, do not use dropper for more than one person

• Decreased intraocular pressure can take several weeks; monitor IOP after a month

SIDE EFFECTS

CNS: Insomnia, headache, dizziness

CV: Palpitations

EENT: Eye stinging/burning, tearing, photophobia

RESP: Bronchospasm

PHARMACOKINETICS
Onset 60 min, peak 2-6 hr, duration 24 hr

INTERACTIONS
Increase: β-blocking effect—oral β-blockers

Increase: intraocular pressure reduction—topical miotics, dipivefrin, EPINEPHrine, carbonic anhydrase inhibitors; this may be beneficial

Increase: depression of AV nodal conduction, bradycardia, or hypotension—adenosine, cardiac glycosides, disopyramide, other antiarrhythmics, class 1C antiarrhythmic drugs (flecainide, propafenone, moricizine, encainide, quiNIDine), or drugs that significantly depress AV nodal conduction

Increase: Antihypertensive effect—other antihypertensives

NURSING CONSIDERATIONS
Assess:
• **Systemic absorption:** when used in the eye, systemic absorption is common with the same adverse reactions and interactions
• **Glaucoma:** monitor intraocular pressure
Evaluate:
• **Therapeutic response:** decreasing intraocular pressure
Teach patient/family:
• That product is for ophthalmic use only
• Not to touch the tip of the dropper to the eye, fingertips, or other surface to prevent contamination
• To wash hands before and after use; tilt the head back slightly and pull the lower eyelid down with the index finger to form a pouch; squeeze the prescribed number of drops into the pouch; close eyes to spread drops; to avoid excessive systemic absorption by applying finger pressure on the lacrimal sac for 1-2 min following use
• That if more than one topical ophthalmic drug product is being used, the drugs should be administered at least 5 min apart

• To avoid contamination or the spread of infection by not using dropper for more than one person

---

levocabastine ophthalmic
See Appendix B

---

levocetirizine (Rx)
(lee-voh-se-teer'ah-zeen)
Children's Xyzal Allergy 24 HR, Xyzal Allergy 24 HR
Func. class.: Antihistamine, low sedating
Chem. class.: H₁ histamine blocker

L

ACTION: Acts on blood vessels, GI, respiratory system by competing with histamine for H_1-receptor site; decreases allergic response by blocking pharmacologic effects of histamine; minimal anticholinergic action

USES: Perennial or seasonal rhinitis, allergy symptoms, chronic idiopathic urticaria

CONTRAINDICATIONS
Breastfeeding; children 6-11 yr with renal disease; end-stage renal disease; dialysis; hypersensitivity to this product, cetirizine, hydrOXYzine
Precautions: Pregnancy, driving, renal disease

DOSAGE AND ROUTES
• **Adult and child ≥12 yr:** PO 2.5-5 mg/day in the evening
• **Child 6-11 yr:** PO (oral solution) 2.5 mg/day in the evening
• **Child 2-5 yr:** PO (oral solution) 1.25 mg/day in the evening
• **Geriatric:** PO 2.5-5 mg/day in the evening

Renal dose

• **Adult: PO** CCr 50-80 mL/min, 2.5 mg/day; CCr 30-49 mL/min, 2.5 mg every other day; CCr 10-29 mL/min, 2.5 mg 2×/wk; CCr <10 mL/min, do not use

Available forms: Tabs 5 mg; oral sol 2.5 mg/5 mL

Administer:

• Without regard to meals in the evening; tabs scored, may be broken in half

• Store in tight, light-resistant container

SIDE EFFECTS

CNS: *Drowsiness, fatigue,* asthenia, dizziness

GI: Dry mouth, increased LFTs, hepatitis

MISC: Urinary retention

PHARMACOKINETICS

Rapid absorption; peak 0.9 hr; protein binding 91%-92%; half-life 8 hr; excreted in urine 85.4%, feces 12.9%

INTERACTIONS

Increase: CNS depression—alcohol, other CNS depressants

Increase: anticholinergic/sedative effect—MAOIs, phenothiazines, tricyclics

Decrease: clearance of levocetirizine—ritonavir

Drug/Lab Test

False negative: skin allergy tests

NURSING CONSIDERATIONS

Assess:

• **Allergy symptoms:** pruritus, urticaria, watering eyes at baseline, during treatment

• **Respiratory status:** rate, rhythm, increase in bronchial secretions, wheezing, chest tightness

• Liver function tests, serum creatinine, BUN

• **Pregnancy/breastfeeding:** use only if clearly needed; do not breastfeed, excreted in breast milk

Evaluate:

• **Therapeutic response:** absence of running or congested nose or rashes

Teach patient/family:

• About all aspects of product use; to notify prescriber if confusion, sedation, hypotension occur, not to exceed recommended dose

• To avoid driving, other hazardous activities if drowsiness occurs

• To avoid alcohol, other CNS depressants

• Do not breastfeed

---

levodopa-carbidopa (Rx)

(lee-voe-doe′pa-kar-bi-doe′pa)

Duopa, Sinemet, Rytary

Func. class.: Antiparkinson agent
Chem. class.: Catecholamine

ACTION: Decarboxylation of levodopa in periphery is inhibited by carbidopa; more levodopa is made available for transport to the brain and for conversion to DOPamine in the brain

USES: Parkinson's disease, parkinsonism resulting from carbon monoxide, chronic manganese intoxication, cerebral arteriosclerosis, motor fluctuations in those with advanced Parkinson's disease

Unlabeled uses: Restless legs syndrome

CONTRAINDICATIONS

Hypersensitivity, malignant melanoma, history of malignant melanoma or undiagnosed skin lesions resembling melanoma

Precautions: Pregnancy, breastfeeding, diabetes, closed-angle glaucoma, respiratory/cardiac/renal/hepatic disease, MI with dysrhythmias, seizures, peptic ulcer, depression

DOSAGE AND ROUTES

Parkinson's disease

• **Adult: PO (immediate-release tablets)** 1 carbidopa 25 mg/levodopa 100-mg tablet tid, may increase by 1 tablet daily or every other day, max: 2,000 mg/day levodopa. **Maintenance:** At least 70-100 mg of carbidopa per day should be used

Converting patients from levodopa to carbidopa-levodopa IR to ER

25% of the previous dose of levodopa; usual dosage is 1 carbidopa 50 mg/levodopa 200-mg ext-rel tablet bid

---

For the treatment of restless legs syndrome (RLS) (unlabeled)
• **Adult: PO** A bedtime dose starting at 25 mg/100 mg levodopa

Available forms: Tabs 10 mg carbidopa/100 mg levodopa, 25 mg carbidopa/100 mg levodopa, 25 mg carbidopa/250 mg levodopa; ext rel tab 25 mg carbidopa/100 mg levodopa, 50 mg carbidopa/200 mg levodopa (Sinemet CR); oral disintegrating tab 10 mg carbidopa/100 mg levodopa, 25 mg carbidopa/100 mg levodopa, 25 mg carbidopa/250 mg levodopa; ext rel caps (Rytary) 23.75 mg/95 mg, 36.25 mg/145 mg, 48.75 mg/195 mg, 61.25 mg/245 mg; enteral suspension (Duopa) 20 mg/mL levodopa/4.63 mg/mL carbidopa

Administer:
• Pyridoxine (B$_6$) not effective for reversing Sinemet

PO route
• Do not crush or chew **ext rel tabs;** they may be broken in half; adjust dosage to response
• **Oral disintegrating tab** by gently removing from bottle, placing on tongue and swallowing with saliva; after tab dissolves, liquid is not necessary
• With meals if GI symptoms occur; limit protein taken with product
• Only after nonselective MAOIs have been discontinued for 2 wk; if patient has been previously treated with levodopa, discontinue for at least 12 hr before change to carbidopa-levodopa

Enteral route
• Fully thaw in refrigerator; remove 1 cassette from refrigerator 20 min before use, give through NG tube or a percutaneous endoscopic gastrostomy jejunostomy tube connected to the CADD-Legacy pump; disconnect after use and flush with water; cassettes are single-use only, label in order to be used based on date

SIDE EFFECTS
CNS: *Involuntary choreiform movements, hand tremors, fatigue, headache, anxiety, twitching, numbness, weakness, confusion, agitation, insomnia, nightmares,* psychosis, hallucination, hypomania, severe depression, dizziness, impulsive behaviors, neuroleptic malignant syndrome, suicidal ideation

CV: *Orthostatic hypotension,* tachycardia, hypertension, palpitation, MI

EENT: Blurred vision, diplopia, dilated pupils

GI: *Nausea, vomiting, anorexia, abdominal distress, dry mouth, flatulence, dysphagia,* bitter taste, diarrhea, constipation, GI bleeding

HEMA: Hemolytic anemia, leukopenia, agranulocytosis, thrombocytopenia

INTEG: Rash, sweating, alopecia

MISC: Urinary retention, incontinence, weight change, dark urine, increased libido, hypersensitivity, dark sweat

PHARMACOKINETICS
PO: Onset 30 min, peak 1-3 hr, excreted in urine (metabolites)
EXT REL: Onset 4-6 hr
Enteral: Peak 2.5 hr

INTERACTIONS
Increase: hypertensive crisis—nonselective MAOIs
Increase: risk for sedation—CNS depressants
Increase: hypotension—antihypertensives
Increase: CV reactions—dobutamine, dopamine, epinephrine, isoproterenol, norepinephrine, TCAs
Increase: effects of levodopa—antacids, metoclopramide
Decrease: effects of levodopa—anticholinergics, hydantoins, papaverine, pyridoxine, benzodiazepines, antipsychotics

Drug/Lab Test
Increase: BUN, AST, ALT, bilirubin, alk phos, LDH, serum glucose
Decrease: BUN, creatinine, uric acid
False positive: urine ketones (dipstick), Coombs' test
False negative: urine glucose
False increase: urine protein

Drug/Food
Decrease: absorption of levodopa—protein

NURSING CONSIDERATIONS
Assess:

- **Parkinson's symptoms:** tremors, pill rolling, drooling, akinesia, rigidity; shuffling gait before, during treatment
- B/P, respiration; orthostatic B/P
- **Mental status:** affect, mood, behavioral changes, depression, complete suicide assessment
- **Toxicity:** muscle twitching, blepharospasm
- Renal, hepatic, hematopoietic tests; also for diabetes, acromegaly if on long-term therapy
- End-of-dose akinesia, on/off phenomenon; akinesia paradoxica
- **Pregnancy/breastfeeding:** use only if benefits outweigh fetal risk; product is excreted in breast milk

Evaluate:

- **Therapeutic response:** decrease in akathisia/bradykinesis, tremor, rigidity, improved mood

Teach patient/family:

- To change positions slowly to prevent orthostatic hypotension, especially during beginning of treatment
- That falling asleep when engaged in activities may occur
- To report side effects: twitching, eye spasms because these indicate overdose
- To use product as prescribed; not to double doses; if discontinued abruptly, parkinsonian crisis, neuroleptic malignant syndrome (NMS) may occur; to gradually taper
- To use ODT immediately after removing from container, to dissolve on tongue, swallow with saliva
- That urine, sweat may darken
- To use physical activities to maintain mobility, lessen spasms
- To use with meals to decrease GI upset; do not use high-protein meals
- That improvement may not occur for 2-4 mo; about "on-off phenomenon"
- Not to chew or crush extended-release product
- To immediately report nausea, vomiting, abdominal pain, ongoing constipation if using enteral product

---

levodopa-carbidopa-entacapone (Rx)

(lee-voe-doe′pa-kar-bi-doe′pa-en-ta′ka-pone)

Stalevo

Func. class.: Antiparkinson agent
Chem. class.: COMT inhibitor/decarboxylase inhibitor/dopamine precursor

ACTION

Levodopa: The precursor of dopamine, a chemical depleted in Parkinson disease. Levodopa is able to circulate in the plasma and cross the blood-brain barrier, converted by striatal enzymes to dopamine

Carbidopa: Inhibits the peripheral plasma breakdown of levodopa by inhibiting its decarboxylation; increases available levodopa at the blood–brain barrier

Entacapone: A reversible and selective inhibitor of catechol-O-methyltransferase (COMT). Alters the pharmacokinetics of levodopa, resulting in more sustained levodopa serum levels and increased concentrations available for absorption across the blood-brain barrier

USES: Parkinson disease

CONTRAINDICATIONS

Hypersensitivity, malignant melanoma, history of malignant melanoma or undiagnosed skin lesions resembling melanoma

Precautions: Pregnancy, breastfeeding, diabetes, closed-angle glaucoma, respiratory/cardiac/renal/hepatic disease, MI with dysrhythmias, seizures, peptic ulcer, depression

DOSAGE AND ROUTES

Adult: PO max daily dose: 8 tablets of Stalevo 50, 75, 100, 125, or 150, or 6 tablets of Stalevo 200, those receiving <70 to 100 mg of the carbidopa component may experience nausea and vomiting; **those previously treated with**

---

carbidopa/levodopa immediate-release tablets (ratio of 1:4): with current entacapone therapy: May switch directly to corresponding strength of combination tablet; **without entacapone therapy:** If current levodopa dose is >600 mg daily or history of moderate or severe dyskinesias: levodopa dose reduction may be required when adding entacapone to therapy; titrate dose using individual products, first carbidopa/levodopa immediate release with a ratio of 1:4 plus entacapone 200 mg; then transfer to combination product once stabilized; if current levodopa dose is <600 mg and without a history of dyskinesias: May transfer to corresponding dose of combination product

Available forms: Tablets 50, 75, 100, 125, 150, 200 mg

Administer:
• Administer whole; do not cut, break, or crush
• Avoid giving with a high-fat meal

SIDE EFFECTS

CNS: Involuntary choreiform movements, hand tremors, fatigue, headache, anxiety, twitching, numbness, weakness, confusion, agitation, insomnia, nightmares, psychosis, hallucination, hypomania, severe depression, dizziness, impulsive behaviors, neuroleptic malignant syndrome, suicidal ideation

CV: Orthostatic hypotension, tachycardia, hypertension, palpitation, MI

EENT: Blurred vision, diplopia, dilated pupils

GI: Nausea, vomiting, anorexia, abdominal distress, dry mouth, flatulence, dysphagia, bitter taste, diarrhea, constipation, GI bleeding

HEMA: Hemolytic anemia, leukopenia, agranulocytosis, thrombocytopenia

INTEG: Rash, sweating, alopecia

MISC: Urinary retention, incontinence, weight change, dark urine, increased libido, hypersensitivity, dark sweat

PHARMACOKINETICS

PO: Onset unknown, peak 1-3 hr, duration unknown

Interactions

Increase: hypertensive crisis—nonselective MAOIs

Increase: risk for sedation—CNS depressants

Increase: hypotension—antihypertensives

Increase: CV reactions—dobutamine, dopamine, epinephrine, isoproterenol, norepinephrine, TCAs

Increase: effects of levodopa—antacids, metoclopramide

Decrease: effects of levodopa—anticholinergics, hydantoins, papaverine, pyridoxine, benzodiazepines, antipsychotics

Drug/Lab Test

Increase: BUN, AST, ALT, bilirubin, alk phos, LDH, serum glucose

Decrease: BUN, creatinine, uric acid

False positive: urine ketones (dipstick), Coombs' test

False negative: urine glucose

False increase: urine protein

Drug/Food

Decrease: absorption of levodopa—protein

NURSING CONSIDERATIONS

Assess:
• **Parkinson symptoms:** tremors, pill rolling, drooling, akinesia, rigidity; shuffling gait before, during treatment
• **Vitals:** B/P, respiration; orthostatic B/P
• **Mental status:** affect, mood, behavioral changes, depression, complete suicide assessment
• Toxicity: muscle twitching, blepharospasm
• Renal, hepatic, hematopoietic tests; also for diabetes, acromegaly if on long-term therapy
• End-of-dose akinesia; on/off phenomenon, akinesia paradoxica
• **Pregnancy/breastfeeding:** use only if benefits outweigh fetal risk; product is excreted in breast milk

Evaluate:
• **Therapeutic response:** decrease in akathisia/bradykinesis, tremor, rigidity, improved mood

Teach patient/family:
• To change positions slowly to prevent orthostatic hypotension, especially during beginning of treatment

L

Side effects: *italics* = common; red = life-threatening

- **To report side effects:** twitching, eye spasms because these indicate overdose
- That falling asleep when engaged in activities may occur
- To use product as prescribed; not to double doses; if discontinued abruptly, parkinsonian crisis, neuroleptic malignant syndrome (NMS) may occur; to gradually taper
- That urine, sweat may darken
- To use physical activities to maintain mobility, lessen spasms
- To use with meals to decrease GI upset; do not use high-protein meals, distribute protein throughout the day

---

levofloxacin (Rx)

(lee-voh-floks′a-sin)
Func. class.: Antiinfective
Chem. class.: Fluoroquinolone

Do not confuse:
levofloxacin/levetiracetam

ACTION: Interferes with conversion of intermediate DNA fragments into high-molecular-weight DNA in bacteria; DNA gyrase inhibitor; inhibits topoisomerase IV

USES: Acute sinusitis, acute chronic bronchitis, community-acquired pneumonia, uncomplicated skin infections, UTI, cellulitis, prostatitis, inhalational anthrax (postexposure); acute pyelonephritis caused by *Streptococcus pneumoniae, Streptococcus pyogenes, Haemophilus influenzae, Haemophilus parainfluenzae, Moraxella catarrhalis, Escherichia coli, Serratia marcescens, Klebsiella pneumoniae, Chlamydia pneumoniae, Legionella pneumophila, Mycoplasma pneumoniae, Enterococcus faecalis, Staphylococcus epidermidis, Staphylococcus pyogenes, Staphylococcus aureus, Bacillus anthracis;* inhalation anthrax in children

Unlabeled uses: Adnexitis, Bartholin abscess, bartholinitis, cervicitis,

epididymitis, gastroenteritis, *H. pylori* eradication, mastitis, MAC, nongonococcal urethritis, obstetric infections, PID, plague, SARS, shigellosis, TB, typhoid fever, disseminated; otitis media, otitis externa, tonsillitis, pharyngitis, sialadenitis

CONTRAINDICATIONS

Hypersensitivity to quinolones
Precautions: Pregnancy, breastfeeding, children, photosensitivity, acute MI, atrial fibrillation, colitis, dehydration, diabetes, QT prolongation, myasthenia gravis, renal disease, seizure disorder, syphilis

Black Box Warning: Tendon pain/rupture, tendinitis, myasthenia gravis, neurotoxicity, peripheral neuropathy, psychiatric events

DOSAGE AND ROUTES
Most infections
- **Adult: PO/IV** 250-750 mg q24hr

Inhalational anthrax postexposure
- **Adult: PO/IV** 500 mg daily × 60 days
- **Child >50 kg: PO/IV** 500 mg daily × 60 days
- **Child <50 kg, ≥6 mo: PO/IV** 8 mg/kg q12hr × 60 days, max 250 mg/dose

Plague
- **Adult: PO/IV** 500 mg q24hr × 10-14 days
- **Child >50 kg: PO/IV** 500 mg daily × 10-14 days
- **Child <50 kg ≥6 mo: PO/IV** 8 mg/kg q12hr × 10-14 days, max 250 mg/dose

Renal disease
- **Adult: PO/IV** CCr 20-49 mL/min for 750-mg doses, give 750 mg q48hr; for 500-mg doses, give 500 mg once, then 250 mg q24hr; for 250-mg doses, no adjustment; **CCr 10-19 mL/min** for 750-mg dose, give 750 mg once, then 500 mg q48hr; for 500-mg dose, give 500 mg once, then 250 mg q48hr; for 250-mg dose, give 250 mg q48hr, except when treating complicated UTI, then no dose adjustment; **CCr <10 mL/min** for 750 mg, give 500 mg, then 500 mg q2days, if 500

mg, give 500 mg, then 250 mg q2days, if 250 mg then 250 mg q2days

Available forms: Single-use vials 500, 750 mg; premixed flexible containers 250 mg/50 mL D$_5$W, 500 mg/100 mL D$_5$W, 750 mg/150 mL D$_5$W; tabs 250, 500, 750 mg; oral sol 25 mg/mL; ophthalmic solution 0.5%

Administer:

• Obtain C&S before treatment and periodically to determine resistance to product, treatment can start before results are obtained

• PO 2 hr before or after antacids, iron, calcium, zinc, sucralfate; give fluids

• **Oral solution:** Give 1 hr before or 2 hr after food

Intermittent IV INFUSION route

• Discard any unused sol in single-dose vial

• Visually inspect for particulate matter/discoloration before use

• Do not give by rapid or bolus IV, only slow infusion ≥60 min 250-, 500-mg dose, ≥90 min 750-mg dose

• Do not use flexible containers in series connections, could result in air embolism

• Do not admix with levofloxacin in 5% dextrose injections or infused through the same IV line; if the same line is used for additional infusions of multiple drugs, flush prior to and after use

IV (single-use vial)

• **500-mg/20-mL vials:** To prepare a dose of 500 mg, withdraw 20 mL from a 20-mL vial and dilute with a compatible IV solution (D$_5$W, NS) to a total volume of 50 mL; to prepare a 500-mg dosage, withdraw all 20 mL from the vial and dilute with a compatible intravenous solution to a total volume of 100 mL

• **750-mg/30-mL vials:** To prepare a dose of 750 mg, withdraw 30 mL from a 30-mL vial and dilute with a compatible intravenous solution (D$_5$W, NS) to a total volume of 150 mL

• The concentration of the diluted solution should be 5 mg/mL before administration; solutions contain no preservatives; any unused portions must be discarded

• **Storage:** The diluted solution may be stored for up to 72 hr at room temperature or 14 days refrigerated; solutions may be frozen for up to 6 mo

Premixed IV solution

• No dilution is necessary

Ophthalmic

• Do not share with others

• Do not touch tip to eye

SIDE EFFECTS

CNS: *Headache,* dizziness, *insomnia,* anxiety, seizures, *encephalopathy,* paresthesia, pseudotumor cerebri

CV: Chest pain, palpitations, vasodilation, QT prolongation, hypotension (rapid infusion)

EENT: Dry mouth, visual impairment, tinnitus

GI: *Nausea,* flatulence, *vomiting,* diarrhea, abdominal pain, CDAD, hepatotoxicity, esophagitis, pancreatitis

GU: Vaginitis, crystalluria

HEMA: Eosinophilia, hemolytic anemia, lymphopenia

INTEG: Rash, pruritus, *photosensitivity,* epidermal necrolysis, injection-site reaction, edema

MISC: Hypoglycemia, hypersensitivity, tendinitis, tendon rupture, rhabdomyolysis

RESP: Pneumonitis

SYST: Anaphylaxis, multisystem organ failure, Stevens-Johnson syndrome, angioedema, toxic epidermal necrolysis

PHARMACOKINETICS

Excreted in urine unchanged, half-life 6-8 hr, peak 1-2 hr

INTERACTIONS

Black Box Warning: Increase: tendon rupture—corticosteroids; assess for tendon pain

• Do not use with magnesium in same IV line

Increase: QT prolongation—products causing a QT prolongation; avoid concurrent use

Increase: levofloxacin levels—probenecid

Increase: CNS stimulation, seizures—NSAIDs, foscarnet, cycloSPORINE

Increase: bleeding risk—warfarin; monitor INR/PT

Decrease: levofloxacin absorption—antacids containing aluminum, magnesium; sucralfate, zinc, iron, calcium; give 2 hr before or after products

Decrease: clearance of theophylline; toxicity may result; monitor theophylline level

Drug/Herb

Increase: photosensitivity—St. John's wort

Drug/Lab Test

Increase: PT, INR

Decrease: glucose, lymphocytes

NURSING CONSIDERATIONS

Assess:

• Previous sensitivity reaction to quinolones

• **Signs/symptoms of infection:** characteristics of sputum, WBC >10,000/mm^3, fever; obtain baseline information before, during treatment

• C&S before beginning product therapy to identify if correct treatment initiated

• **Allergic reactions, anaphylaxis:** rash, urticaria, pruritus, chills, fever, joint pain; may occur a few days after therapy begins; EPINEPHrine and resuscitation equipment should be available for anaphylactic reaction

• **CDAD:** bowel pattern daily; if severe diarrhea, fever occur, product should be discontinued; assess for signs/symptoms of CDAD daily, abdominal pain/cramping, blood/pus in stool

• **Overgrowth of infection:** perineal itching, fever, malaise, redness, pain, swelling, drainage, rash, diarrhea, change in cough, sputum

• Renal function (BUN/creatinine) increase fluid to 2 L/day to prevent crystalluria

• **Peripheral neuropathy:** tingling, pain, numbness, burning in extremities, can be permanent

• **Retinal detachment:** may occur up to 1 yr after last dose of oral treatment

Black Box Warning: Tendon rupture: discontinue product at first sign of tendon pain or inflammation, usually the Achilles tendon is affected; can occur up to a few months after treatment and may require surgical repair; risk is increased in elderly patients, transplant patients, or with use of steroids

Black Box Warning: Myasthenia gravis: do not use this product with this disease; may lead to life-threatening weakness of the respiratory muscles

Black Box Warning: Neurotoxicity: may occur within hours to weeks after starting use; may be irreversible; avoid use in those who have experienced peripheral neuropathy (numbness, tingling, burning in extremities); report to prescriber immediately

• Increased fluid intake to 2 L/day to prevent crystalluria

• **Seizures:** use with caution in those with CNS disorder

• **Hepatotoxicity:** acute hepatitis, liver failure has occurred; LFTs baseline and periodically

• **Pregnancy/breastfeeding:** avoid use in pregnancy; do not use in breastfeeding

Evaluate:

• **Therapeutic response:** absence of signs, symptoms of infection (WBC <10,000/mm^3, temperature WNL)

Teach patient/family:

• **Superinfection:** To contact prescriber if vaginal itching; loose, foul-smelling stools; furry tongue occur (may indicate superinfection); to report itching, rash, pruritus, urticaria, change in heartbeat

• **CDAD:** To notify prescriber of diarrhea with blood or purulent discharge in stool

• To take product 2 hr before or after antacids, iron, calcium, zinc products

• To complete full course of therapy, not to skip or double doses

• To avoid driving or other hazardous activities until response is known, dizziness may occur

• To use frequent rinsing of mouth, sugarless candy, or gum for dry mouth

• To avoid other medication unless approved by prescriber

• To prevent sun exposure or to use sunscreen to prevent photosensitivity
• To monitor glucose (diabetes); to notify prescriber of changes
• Not to use contact lenses if using ophthalmic product

Black Box Warning: To notify prescriber of tendon pain, inflammation; to avoid corticosteroids with this product

• **Pregnancy/breastfeeding:** identify if pregnancy is planned or suspected or if breastfeeding

levofloxacin ophthalmic
See Appendix B

levomilnacipran (Rx)
[lee′voe-mil-na′si-pran]
Fetzima, Fetzima Titration

milnacipran (Rx)
(mil-na′si-pran)
Savella, Savella Titration Pack
Func. class.: Antidepressant
Chem. class.: Serotonin-norepinephrine reuptake inhibitor (SNRI)

Do not confuse:
Fetzima/Farxiga

ACTION: May potentiate serotonergic, adrenergic activity in the CNS; is a potent inhibitor of adrenal serotonin and norepinephrine reuptake

USES: Major depressive disorder in adults

CONTRAINDICATIONS
Hypersensitivity, MAOI therapy
Precautions: Pregnancy, breastfeeding, geriatric patients, mania, hypertension, renal/cardiac disease, seizures, increased intraocular pressure, anorexia, bleeding, dehydration, diabetes, hypotension, hypovolemia, orthostatic hypotension, abrupt product withdrawal, alcohol intoxication, alcoholism, closed-angle glaucoma

Black Box Warning: Children, suicidal ideation

DOSAGE AND ROUTES
Major depressive disorder (levomilnacipran)
• **Adult: PO** 20 mg/day × 2 days, then 40 mg/day; may increase in increments of 40 mg at intervals of at least 2 days, max 120 mg/day; max 80 mg/day (strong CYP3A4 inhibitors therapy)
Major depressive disorder (milnacipran)
• **Adult: PO** 12.5-25 mg bid, may titrate to 100 mg bid, max 200 mg/day
Fibromyalgia (levomilnacipran)
• **Adult: PO** 12.5 mg daily, increase to 12.5 mg bid on days 2 and 3, then 25 mg bid on days 4 to 7; increase to 50 mg bid after day 7; may increase to 100 mg bid as needed
Fibromyalgia (milnacipran)
• **Adult/adolescent ≥17 yr: PO** 12.5 mg once on day 1, then 12.5 mg bid on days 2-3, then 25 mg bid on days 4-7, and 50 mg bid thereafter
Renal dose (levomilnacipran)
• **Adult: PO** CCr 15-29 mL/min, max 40 mg/day; CCr 30-59 mL/min, max 80 mg/day; CCr <15 mL/min, do not use
Renal dose (milnacipran)
• **Adult: PO** CCr 5-29 mL/min, reduce maintenance dose by 50% (25-50 mg bid)
Available forms: Ext rel caps 20, 40, 80, 120 mg (levomilnacipran); tabs 12.5, 25, 50, 100 mg (milnacipran)
Administer:
• Swallow cap whole; do not break, crush, or chew; do not sprinkle on food or mix with liquid
• Without regard to food
• Give at the same time each day

SIDE EFFECTS
CNS: Dizziness, agitation, hallucinations, seizures, drowsiness, mania, migraine, paresthesias, suicidal ideation, syncope
CV: Hypertension, palpitations, dysrhythmia, sinus tachycardia
EENT: Teeth grinding, blurred vision
GI: Constipation, diarrhea, nausea, vomiting, anorexia, dry mouth, abdominal pain

Side effects: *italics* = common; red = life-threatening

GU: Urinary retention
SYST: Serotonin syndrome, Stevens-Johnson syndrome

PHARMACOKINETICS

Peak 6-8 hr metabolized (CYP2D6) in the liver; excretion 58% (urine), 22% protein binding, half-life 12 hr (levomilnacipran) 6-10 hr (milnacipran)

INTERACTIONS

• Do not use with linezolid or methylene blue IV, or within 14 days of MAOIs
• **Increase:** levomilnacipran effect—CYP34A inhibitors
Increase: serotonin syndrome—SSRIs, serotonin receptor agonists, SNRIs, lithium
Increase: bleeding risk—anticoagulants, antiplatelets, salicylates, NSAIDs
Increase: risk of neuroleptic malignant syndrome—antipsychotics, DOPamine antagonists; avoid concurrent use
Increase: bleeding risk—alfalfa, feverfew, dong quai, fish oil, ginseng, garlic, ginkgo biloba
Drug/Herb
• **Serotonin syndrome:** St. John's wort
Increase: CNS depression—kava, valerian

NURSING CONSIDERATIONS
Assess:
• **Neuroleptic malignant syndrome:** hyperthermia, rigidity, rapid fluctuations of vital signs, mental status changes; MAOIs: coadministration contraindicated within 14 days of MAOI

> **Black Box Warning: Depression:** mood, sensorium, affect, suicidal tendencies, increase in psychiatric symptoms; panic; monitor children weekly face to face during first 4 wk, or dosage change, then every other week for the next 4 wk, then at 12 wk

• B/P lying, standing; pulse; if systolic B/P drops 20 mm Hg, hold product, notify prescriber; take VS more often in patients with CV disease
• **Hepatic studies:** AST, ALT, bilirubin baseline and periodically
• **Withdrawal symptoms:** headache, nausea, vomiting, muscle pain, weakness; not common unless product is discontinued abruptly
• Avoid alcohol, rapid absorption may occur

> **Black Box Warning: Serotonin syndrome:** nausea, vomiting, dizziness, facial flush, shivering, sweating

• **Beers:** use with caution in older adults; may exacerbate or cause SIADH; monitor for hyponatremia
• **Pregnancy/breastfeeding:** use only if benefits outweigh fetal risk; SSRIs should not be used; do not use in 3rd trimester; do not breastfeed
Evaluate:
• **Therapeutic response:** decreased depression
Teach patient/family:
• About signs and symptoms of bleeding (GI bleeding, nosebleed, ecchymosis, bruising)
• To use with caution when driving and performing other activities requiring alertness because of drowsiness and blurred vision
• To avoid ingestion of alcohol, MAOIs, other CNS depressants; not to use within 14 days of MAOIs; to notify all providers of use of this product
• Not to discontinue medication quickly after long-term use; may cause headache, malaise; taper
• That product may be used with or without food
• To swallow caps whole; do not break, crush, chew

> **Black Box Warning:** That clinical worsening and suicidal risk may occur, usually worse in first few months of treatment; to notify prescriber immediately if suicidal thoughts/behaviors, aggression, hostility, agitation, panic attacks occur

• That improvement may occur in 4-8 wk or up to 12 wk (geriatric patients)
• To report trouble with urination

• **Serotonin syndrome:** to report immediately nausea, vomiting, dizziness, facial flush, shivering, sweating
• **Pregnancy/breastfeeding:** to notify prescriber if pregnancy is planned or suspected or if breastfeeding

---

levothyroxine (T$_4$) (Rx) (NTI)

(lee-voe-thye-rox'een)

Eltroxin ✦, Euthyrox, Levoxyl, Synthroid, Tirosint, Tirosint-SOL, Unithroid

Func. class.: Thyroid hormone
Chem. class.: Levoisomer of thyroxine

Do not confuse:
Synthroid/Symmetrel
levothyroxine/lamotrigine/Lanoxin/liothyronine/Loxitane

ACTION: Increases metabolic rate; controls protein synthesis; increases cardiac output, renal blood flow, O$_2$ consumption, body temperature, blood volume, growth, development at cellular level via action on thyroid hormone receptors

USES: Hypothyroidism, myxedema coma, thyroid hormone replacement, thyrotoxicosis, congenital hypothyroidism, some types of thyroid cancer, pituitary TSH suppression

CONTRAINDICATIONS
Adrenal insufficiency, recent MI, thyrotoxicosis, hypersensitivity to beef, alcohol intolerance (inj only)

Black Box Warning: Obesity treatment

Precautions: Pregnancy, breastfeeding, geriatric patients, angina pectoris, hypertension, ischemia, cardiac disease, diabetes

DOSAGE AND ROUTES
Hypothyroidism
• **Adult ≤50 yr: PO** 1.6 mcg/kg/day, 6-8 wk, average dose 100-200 mcg/day;
IM/IV 50-100 mcg/day as single dose or 50% of usual oral dosage
• **Adult >50 yr without heart disease or <50 yr with heart disease: PO** 25-50 mcg/day, titrate q6-8wk
• **Adult >50 yr with heart disease: PO** 12.5-25 mcg/day, titrate by 12.5-25 mcg q6-8wk
• **Child (puberty complete): PO** 1.7 mcg/kg/day
• **Child >12 yr (incomplete puberty): PO** 2-3 mcg/kg/day as single dose in AM
• **Child 6-12 yr: PO** 4-5 mcg/kg/day as single dose in AM
• **Child 1-5 yr: PO** 5-6 mcg/kg/day as single dose in AM
• **Child 6-12 mo: PO** 6-8 mcg/kg/day as single dose in AM
• **Child 3-6 mo: PO** 8-10 mcg/kg/day as single dose in AM
• **Infant/neonate to age 3 mo: PO** 10-15 mcg/kg/day; use in lower dose in those at risk for cardiac failure; may increase q4-6wk if needed
Myxedema coma
• **Adult: IV** 300-500 mcg initially, may increase by 100-300 mcg after 24 hr; give oral medication as soon as possible
Subclinical hypothyroidism
• **Adult: PO** 1 mcg/kg/day
Available forms: Powder for inj 100, 200, 500 mcg/vial; tabs 25, 50, 88, 100, 112, 125, 137, 150, 175, 200, 300 mcg; cap (liquid filled) 13, 25, 50, 75, 88, 100, 112, 125, 137, 150 mcg
Administer:
• Store in tight, light-resistant container; sol should be discarded if not used immediately
• Withdrawal of medication 4 wk before RAIU test
PO route
• In AM if possible as single dose to decrease sleeplessness; at same time each day to maintain product level; take on empty stomach
• Only for hormone imbalances; not to be used for obesity, male infertility, menstrual conditions, lethargy
• Use 8 oz of water on empty stomach

• Lowest dose that relieves symptoms; lower dose to geriatric patients and for those with cardiac diseases

• Crush and mix with water, nonsoy formula (decreased absorption), or breast milk for infants, children; give by spoon or dropper; may crush and sprinkle over applesauce or other food

• Separate antacids, iron, calcium products by 4 hr

Direct IV route

• IV after reconstituting with 5 mL normal saline injection (500 mcg/5 mL, 200 mcg/2 mL); shake; give through Y-tube or 3-way stopcock; give ≤100 mcg/1 min; do not add to IV infusion

• Considered to be incompatible in syringe with all other products

SIDE EFFECTS

CNS: *Anxiety, insomnia, tremors,* headache, thyroid storm, excitability

CV: *Tachycardia, palpitations, angina, dysrhythmias,* hypertension, cardiac arrest

GI: Nausea, diarrhea, increased or decreased appetite, cramps

MISC: Menstrual irregularities, weight loss, sweating, heat intolerance, fever, alopecia, decreased bone mineral density

PHARMACOKINETICS

Half-life euthyroid 6-7 days, hypothyroid 9-10 days, hyperthyroid 3-4 days, distributed throughout body tissues, protein binding 99%

PO: Onset 24 hr
IV: Onset 6-8 hr

INTERACTIONS

Increase: levothyroxine need—SSRIs, antiepileptics (carBAMazepine, OXcarbazepine, phenobarbital, primidone, phenytoin), antimicrobials (rifAMPin, efavirenz, rifabutin, rifapentine); monitor levels of levothyroxine

Increase or decrease: glucose levels—insulin, antidiabetics; monitor blood glucose, adjust levels

Increase: cardiac insufficiency risk—EPINEPHrine products

Increase: effects of both products—tricyclics, tetracyclics

Increase: effects of anticoagulants, sympathomimetics, tricyclics; monitor PT, INR if using with anticoagulants

Decrease: levothyroxine absorption—bile acid sequestrants, orlistat, ferrous sulfate

Decrease: levothyroxine effect—estrogens, antacids, sucralfate, aluminum, magnesium, calcium, iron, rifampin, rifabutin

Drug/Herb

Decrease: thyroid hormone effect—soy, horseradish

Drug/Lab Test

Increase: blood glucose

Decrease: thyroid function tests

Drug/Food

Decrease: product absorption—fiber, walnuts; avoid concurrent use or adjust dose

NURSING CONSIDERATIONS

Assess:

• B/P, pulse periodically during treatment

• Weight daily in same clothing, using same scale, at same time of day

• Height, growth rate of child

• Patient may require decreased anticoagulant; check for bleeding, bruising

• **Cardiac status:** angina, palpitation, chest pain, change in VS

• **CAD:** monitor for coronary insufficiency; also watch for cardiac changes in those receiving high, rapid dosing

• **Bone density:** test bone density baseline and periodically; bone loss may occur with long-term therapy

• **Pregnancy/breastfeeding:** may be used in pregnancy and breastfeeding

Hypothyroidism:

• T₃, T₄, FTIs, which are decreased; radioimmunoassay of TSH, which is increased; radio uptake, which is increased if patient is receiving too low a dose of medication

• Increased nervousness, excitability, irritability, which may indicate too high a dose of medication, usually after 1-3 wk of treatment

Evaluate:
• **Therapeutic response:** absence of depression; increased weight loss, diuresis, pulse, appetite; absence of constipation, peripheral edema, cold intolerance; pale, cool, dry skin; brittle nails, alopecia, coarse hair, menorrhagia, night blindness, paresthesias, syncope, stupor, coma, rosy cheeks
Teach patient/family:
• That hair loss will occur in child, is temporary; that hypothyroid child will show almost immediate behavior/personality change
• To report excitability, irritability, anxiety, which indicate overdose
• Not to switch brands unless approved by prescriber; to protect from light, moisture

Black Box Warning: That product is not to be taken to reduce weight

• To avoid OTC preparations with iodine; to read labels; to separate antacids, iron, calcium products by 4 hr
• To take in AM on empty stomach, at least 30 min before food
• To avoid iodine-rich food, iodized salt, soybeans, tofu, turnips, high-iodine seafood, some bread products
• That product is not a cure but controls symptoms; that treatment is lifelong, full effect may take up to 6 wk
• That all products are not interchangeable
• **Pregnancy/breastfeeding:** to continue using during pregnancy, breastfeeding
• **Anticoagulants:** to have anticoagulant level monitored, dose adjusted as needed

⚠ HIGH ALERT

lidocaine (parenteral) (Rx)
(lye'doe-kane)
LidoPen Auto-Injector, Xylocaine, Xylocard ✦
Func. class.: Antidysrhythmic (Class Ib)
Chem. class.: Aminoacyl amide

ACTION: Increases electrical stimulation threshold of ventricle, His-Purkinje system, which stabilizes cardiac membrane, decreases automaticity

USES: Ventricular tachycardia, ventricular dysrhythmias during cardiac surgery, digoxin toxicity, cardiac catheterization
Unlabeled uses: Attenuation of intracranial pressure increased during intubation/endotracheal tube suctioning

CONTRAINDICATIONS
Hypersensitivity to amides, severe heart block, supraventricular dysrhythmias, Adams-Stokes syndrome, Wolff-Parkinson-White syndrome
Precautions: Pregnancy, breastfeeding, children, geriatric patients, renal/hepatic disease, HF, respiratory depression, malignant hyperthermia, myasthenia gravis, weight <50 kg

DOSAGE AND ROUTES
Ventricular arrhythmias caused by MI, cardiac manipulation/glycosides
• **Adult:** IV BOL 50-100 mg (1-1.5 mg/kg) 25-50 mg/min, repeat q5min until arrhythmias are controlled, max 300 mg in 1 hr; begin IV INFUSION; IV INFUSION 1-4 mg/min (20-50 mcg/kg/min)
• **Child:** IV/INTRAOSSEUS BOL 1 mg/kg; start infusion at 30 mcg/kg/min
Renal/hepatic dose with heart failure
• **Adult <50 kg:** IV reduce dose
Available forms: IV INFUSION 0.2% (2 mg/mL), 0.4% (4 mg/mL), 0.8% (8 mg/mL); IV 4% (40 mg/mL), 10% (100 mg/mL), 20% (200 mg/mL); IV dir 1% (10 mg/mL), 2% (20 mg/mL); Inj (to IV admix) 20% (200 mg/mL)
Administer:
IV route
• Bolus undiluted (1%, 2% only), give ≤50 mg/1 min or dilute 1 g/250-500 mL D₅W; titrate to patient response; use infusion pump; pediatric infusion 120 mg

lidocaine/100 mL D$_5$W; 1-2.5 mL/kg/hr = 20-50 mcg/kg/min; use only 1%, 2% sol for IV bol
- Use a cardiac monitor
- Additive syringes/single-use vials are for infusions and must be diluted

Y-site compatibilities: Acetaminophen, alemtuzumab, alfentanil, alteplase, amikacin, aminocaproic acid, aminophylline, amiodarone, amphotericin B lipid/liposome, anidulafungin, argatroban, ascorbic acid injection, atenolol, atropine, atracurium, azithromycin, aztreonam, benztropine, bivalirudin, bleomycin, bumetanide, buprenorphine, butorphanol, calcium chloride/gluconate, CARBOplatin, carmustine, ceFAZolin, cefotaxime, cefoTEtan, cefOXitin, ceftaroline, cefTAZidime, ceftizoxime, cefTRIAXone, cefuroxime, chloramphenicol, chlorproMAZINE, cimetidine, ciprofloxacin, cisatracurium, CISplatin, clarithromycin, clindamycin, cyanocobalamin, cyclophosphamide, cycloSPORINE, cytarabine, DACTINomycin, DAPTOmycin, DAUNOrubicin, dexamethasone, dexmedetomidine, dexrazoxane, digoxin, diltiazem, diphenhydrAMINE, DOBUTamine, DOCEtaxel, dolasetron, DOPamine, doxacurium, DOXOrubicin, DOXOrubicin liposomal, doxycycline, enalaprilat, EPINEPHrine, epirubicin, epoetin alfa, eptifibatide, ertapenem, erythromycin, esmolol, etomidate, etoposide, etoposide phosphate, famotidine, fenoldopam, fentaNYL, fluconazole, fludarabine, fluorouracil, folic acid, furosemide, gentamicin, granisetron, haloperidol, heparin, hydrocortisone, imipenem/cilastatin, inamrinone, insulin, isoproterenol, ketorolac, labetalol, levofloxacin, linezolid, LORazepam, magnesium sulfate, meperidine, methylPREDNISolone sodium succinate, metoclopramide, metoprolol, metroNIDAZOLE, micafungin, midazolam, morphine, nafcillin, niCARDipine, nitroglycerin, nitroprusside, norepinephrine, ondansetron, palonosetron, penicillin G potassium, phenylephrine, phytonadione, piperacillin/tazobactam, potassium chloride, procainamide, prochlorperazine, promethazine, propofol, propranolol, protamine, quinupristin/dalfopristin, ranitidine, remifentanil, sodium bicarbonate, streptokinase, tacrolimus, theophylline, ticarcillin/clavulanate, tigecycline, tirofiban, tobramycin, vancomycin, vasopressin, verapamil, vitamin B complex with C, voriconazole, warfarin

SIDE EFFECTS
CNS: *Headache, dizziness,* involuntary movement, confusion, tremor, drowsiness, euphoria, seizures, shivering
CV: *Hypotension, bradycardia,* heart block, CV collapse, arrest
EENT: Tinnitus, blurred vision
GI: Nausea, vomiting, anorexia
HEMA: Methemoglobinemia
INTEG: Rash, urticaria, edema, swelling, petechiae, pruritus
MISC: Febrile response, phlebitis at inj site
RESP: Dyspnea, respiratory depression

PHARMACOKINETICS
Half-life 8 min, 1-2 hr (terminal); metabolized in liver; excreted in urine; crosses placenta
IV: Onset 2 min, duration 20 min

INTERACTIONS
Increase: cardiac depression, toxicity—amiodarone, phenytoin, procainamide, propranolol, quiNIDine
Increase: hypotensive effects—MAOIs, antihypertensives
Increase: neuromuscular blockade—neuromuscular blockers, tubocurarine; monitor for adverse effects
Increase: lidocaine effects, toxicity—cimetidine, β-blockers, protease inhibitors, ritonavir
Increase: hypotension—ergots; avoid concurrent use
Decrease: lidocaine effects—barbiturates, ciprofloxacin, voriconazole
Decrease: effect of—cycloSPORINE

NURSING CONSIDERATIONS
Assess:
- **CV:** B/P continuously for circulatory collapse, decompensation; ECG continuously to determine increased PR or QRS segments; if these develop, discontinue

or reduce rate; watch for increased ventricular ectopic beats, may have to rebolus; B/P

• **Drug levels:** therapeutic level 1.5-5 mcg/mL

• I&O ratio, electrolytes (potassium, sodium, chlorine)

• **Toxicity:** monitor for seizures, confusion, tremors; if these occur, discontinue immediately, notify prescriber; keep emergency equipment nearby

• **Malignant hyperthermia:** tachypnea, tachycardia, changes in B/P, increased temperature

• **Respiratory status:** rate, rhythm, lung fields for crackles, watch for respiratory depression; lung fields, bilateral crackles may occur with HF; increased respiration, pulse; product should be discontinued

• **CNS effects:** dizziness, confusion, psychosis, paresthesias, convulsions; product should be discontinued

• **Pregnancy/breastfeeding:** use only if clearly needed; use caution in breastfeeding, excreted in breast milk
Evaluate:
• **Therapeutic response:** decreased dysrhythmias
Teach patient/family:
• About the use of automatic lidocaine injection device if ordered for personal use
• To report signs of toxicity immediately

TREATMENT OF OVERDOSE: O₂, artificial ventilation, ECG; administer DOPamine for circulatory depression, diazepam or thiopental for seizures; decrease product if needed

lidocaine ophthalmic
See Appendix B

lidocaine topical
See Appendix B

lifitegrast ophthalmic (Rx)
(lif-i-teg'rast)
Xiidra
Func. class.: Lymphocyte function-associated antigen 1 (LFA-1) antagonist

USES: Signs and symptoms of dry eye disease

CONTRAINDICATIONS
Hypersensitivity

DOSAGE AND ROUTES
Adult: Ophthalmic: Instill 1 drop into each eye q12h

Available forms: Opthalmic solution 5%

linaclotide (Rx)
(lin-ak'loe-tide)
Constella ✤, Linzess
Func. class.: Gastrointestinal agent, miscellaneous

USES: Chronic idiopathic constipation, IBS in adults

CONTRAINDICATIONS
Hypersensitivity, child <6 yr; GI obstruction

DOSAGE AND ROUTES
Constipation
Adult PO: 72 or 145 mcg daily
Irritable bowel syndrome
• **Adult PO** 290 mcg daily on an empty stomach at least 30 min prior to first meal of the day
Available forms: Capsules 72, 145, 290 mcg

⚠ HIGH ALERT

linagliptin (Rx)
(lin'a-glip'tin)
Tradjenta, Trajenta ✤
Func. class.: Antidiabetic
Chem. class.: Didipeptidyl peptidase-4 inhibitor

Do not confuse:
Tradjenta/Tanzeum/Tresiba/Trulicity

ACTION: Slows the inactivation of incretin hormones; concentrations of the active, intact hormones are increased, thereby increasing and prolonging the action of these hormones; incretin hormones are released by the intestine throughout the day, and levels are increased in response to a meal

USES: Type 2 diabetes mellitus

CONTRAINDICATIONS

Hypersensitivity to linagliptin, type 1 diabetes mellitus, diabetic ketoacidosis (DKA)
Precautions: Pregnancy, breastfeeding, adolescents or children <18 yr, debilitated physical condition, malnutrition, uncontrolled adrenal insufficiency, pituitary insufficiency, hypo/hyperthyroidism, diarrhea, gastroparesis, GI obstruction, ileus, female hormonal changes, high fever, severe psychologic stress, uncontrolled hypercortisolism, HF

DOSAGE AND ROUTES

• **Adult: PO** 5 mg daily; when used with a sulfonylurea or insulin, a lower dose of the sulfonylurea may be necessary to minimize the risk of hypoglycemia
Available forms: Tab 5 mg
Administer:
• Once daily; may give without regard to food
• May require an increased dose in stress, fever, surgery, trauma
• Store at room temperature

SIDE EFFECTS

CNS: Headache
EENT: Nasopharyngitis
ENDO: Hypoglycemia, hyperuricemia, hypertriglyceridemia
GI: Body weight loss, pancreatitis
INTEG: Serious hypersensitivity reactions, urticaria, angioedema, exfoliative dermatitis
MISC: Arthralgia, back pain
RESP: Bronchial hyperreactivity (with bronchospasm), nasopharyngitis, cough

PHARMACOKINETICS

Extensively distributed to tissues, protein binding is concentration-dependent, weak to moderate inhibitor of CYP3A4, half life of >100 hr; effective half-life 12 hr, 90% excreted unchanged, 85% excreted enterohepatic system urine (5%), rapidly absorbed, peak in 1.5 hr; bioavailability 30%

INTERACTIONS

• Long-term treatment in combination with strong CYP3A4 inducers, may reduce glycemic lowering effect of linagliptin
Increase: hypoglycemia—sulfonylureas, β-blockers, ACE inhibitors, angiotensin II receptor antagonists, disopyramide, guanethidine, cloNIDine, octreotide, fenfluramine, dexfenfluramine, fibric acid derivatives, monoamine oxidase inhibitors (MAOIs), FLUoxetine, salicylates
Increase: masking of the signs and symptoms of hypoglycemia—reserpine, β-blockers
Increase: need for dosing change—cisapride, metoclopramide, tegaserod, androgens, alcohol, lithium, quinolones
Decrease: hypoglycemic effect—dextrothyroxine, bumetanide, furosemide, ethacrynic acid, torsemide, estrogens, progestins, oral contraceptives, thyroid hormones, glucocorticoids, glucagon, carbonic anhydrase inhibitors, phenytoin, fosphenytoin, or ethotoin; atypical antipsychotics (ARIPiprazole, cloZAPine, OLANZapine, QUEtiapine, risperiDONE, and ziprasidone), phenothiazine, niacin (nicotinic acid), triamterene, thiazide diuretics
Decrease: effect of linagliptin—CYP3A4 inducers (topiramate, rifabutin, pioglitazone, OXcarbazepine, carBAMazepine, nevirapine, modafinil, metyrapone, etravirine, efavirenz, bosentan, barbiturates, aprepitant, fosaprepitant)
Drug/Herb
Decrease: linagliptin effect—St. John's wort
Drug/Lab Test
Increase: uric acid
Decrease: HbA1c level, fasting blood glucose

NURSING CONSIDERATIONS
Assess
• **Diabetes:** monitor blood glucose, A1c during treatment to determine diabetes control; monitor for hypoglycemia: confusion, sweating, tachycardia, anxiety; hyperglycemia: polydipsia, polyuria, polyphagia
• CBC baseline and periodically during treatment; report decreased blood counts
• **Pancreatitis (rare):** severe abdominal pain, nausea, vomiting; may be fatal; discontinue product immediately, use supportive therapy; monitor amylase, lipase, electrolytes
• **Arthralgia:** may be severe, but temporary
• **Pregnancy/breastfeeding:** use only if clearly needed; use caution in breastfeeding, excretion is unknown
Evaluate:
• **Therapeutic response:** improving blood glucose level, A1c; decreasing polydipsia, polyphagia, polyuria, clear sensorium, absence of dizziness
Teach patient/family:
• About the symptoms of hypo/hyperglycemia and what to do about each; to have glucagon emergency kit available, to carry sugar packets
• That product must be continued on a daily basis, about the consequences of discontinuing product abruptly; to take only as directed
• To avoid OTC products unless approved by prescriber
• That diabetes is a lifelong illness, that product will not cure diabetes
• To carry emergency ID with prescriber, condition and medications taken
• To immediately report skin disorders, swelling, difficulty breathing, or severe abdominal pain
• **Pregnancy/breastfeeding:** to notify provider if pregnancy is planned or suspected, or if breastfeeding

---

linagliptin/metformin (Rx)
(lin-a-glip′tin/met-for′min)
Jentadueto, Jentadueto XR
Func. class.: Antidiabetic agent, biguanide/dipeptidyl peptidase 4 (DPP-4) inhibitor

USES: An adjunct to diet and exercise to improve glycemic control in adults with type 2 diabetes mellitus

CONTRAINDICATIONS
Hypersensitivity to linagliptin, metformin, or any component; severe renal impairment (eGFR <30 mL/min/1.73 m²); metabolic acidosis, diabetic ketoacidosis

Black Box Warning: Fatal lactic acidosis

DOSAGE AND ROUTES
Adult: PO (Immediate release): to 1 g bid; **(extended release)** linagliptin **those currently on metformin:** Initial: linagliptin 5 mg/day plus current daily dose of metformin; **those not on metformin:** Initial: linagliptin 5 mg/metformin 1 g/day; **conversion from IR to ER:** May switch to extended-release product containing linagliptin 5 mg and current daily dose of metformin once daily
Available forms: Tabs 2.5/500, 2.5/850, 2.5/1000 mg; tabs ext rel 2.5/1000, 5/1000 mg

---

lindane (Rx)
(lin′dane)
Func. class.: Scabicide, pediculicide
Chem. class.: Chlorinated hydrocarbon (synthetic)

ACTION: Stimulates nervous system of arthropods, resulting in seizures, death

USES: Scabies, lice (head/pubic/body), nits in those intolerant to or who do not respond to other agents

CONTRAINDICATIONS
Hypersensitivity, patients with known seizure disorders, Norwegian (crusted) scabies

Black Box Warning: Seizure disorder

Precautions: Pregnancy, breastfeeding, infants, children <10 yr, avoid contact with eyes

---

Black Box Warning: Neurotoxicity

DOSAGE AND ROUTES
Lice
• **Adult/child:** shampoo using 30 mL: work into lather, rub for 5 min, rinse, dry with towel; comb with fine-toothed comb to remove nits; most require 1 oz, max 2 oz
Available forms: shampoo, (1%)
Administer:
• Caregivers should wear gloves less permeable to lindane, thoroughly clean hands after application; avoid natural latex gloves
• **Shampoo:** for lice only; do not use other hair products before use; shake well; hair should be completely dry; use only enough shampoo to lightly coat hair and scalp, work into hair, do not use water; allow to remain only 4 min, rinse, lather away, towel briskly
• To scalp only; do not apply to face, lips, mouth, eyes, any mucous membrane, anus, or meatus
• Topical corticosteroids as ordered to decrease contact dermatitis; antihistamines
• Lotions of menthol or phenol to control itching
• Topical antibiotics for infection

SIDE EFFECTS
CNS: Seizures, CNS toxicity, stimulation, dizziness
INTEG: *Pruritus, rash, irritation, contact dermatitis*

PHARMACOKINETICS
Onset 3 hr, half-life 18-22 hr

INTERACTIONS
• Oils may increase absorption; if oil-based hair dressing used, shampoo, rinse, dry hair before applying lindane shampoo

NURSING CONSIDERATIONS
Assess:

Black Box Warning: Abrasions, skin inflammation, breaks in skin: do not use on these areas, increased risk of neurotoxicity

• **Infestation:** head, hair for lice, nits before and after treatment; if scabies present, check all skin surfaces; identify source of infection: school, family, sexual contacts
• Isolation until areas on skin, scalp have cleared, treatment completed
• Removal of nits with fine-toothed comb rinsed in vinegar after treatment; use gloves

Black Box Warning: Seizures: avoid use in children with uncontrolled seizure disorders

Black Box Warning: Neurotoxicity: when large amounts are used, absorbed systemically, may cause death; use only second line

• **Pregnancy/breastfeeding:** avoid in pregnancy, breastfeeding
Evaluate:
• **Therapeutic response:** decreased crusts, nits, brownish trails on skin, itching papules in skin folds, decreased itching after several weeks
Teach patient/family:
• To wash all inhabitants' clothing using insecticide; that preventive treatment may be required of all persons living in same house, using lotion or shampoo to decrease spread of infection; to use rubber gloves when applying product
• That itching may continue for 4-6 wk
• That product must be reapplied if accidentally washed off or treatment will be ineffective
• Not to apply to face; if accidental contact with eyes occurs, flush with water

Black Box Warning: To remove product after specified time to prevent toxicity

• To treat sexual contacts simultaneously

Black Box Warning: To check for CNS toxicity: dizziness, cramps, anxiety, nausea, vomiting, seizures

linezolid (Rx)

(line-zoe'lide)

Zyvox, Zyvoxam ✤

Func. class.: Broad-spectrum antiinfective

Chem. class.: Oxazolidinone

Do not confuse:

Zyvox/Vioxx/Zovirax

ACTION: Inhibits protein synthesis by interfering with translation; binds to bacterial 23S ribosomal RNA of the 50S subunit, thus preventing formation of the bacterial translation process in primarily gram-positive organisms

USES: Vancomycin-resistant *Enterococcus faecium* infections, hospital-acquired pneumonia caused by *Staphylococcus aureus* or *Streptococcus pneumoniae*, uncomplicated or complicated skin and skin-structure infections, community-acquired pneumonia, *Pasteurella multocida*, viridans streptococci, *E. faecium* infections, *S. aureus, S. pyogenes;* can be used for MSSA/MRSA/MDRSP strains

CONTRAINDICATIONS

Hypersensitivity

Precautions: Pregnancy, breastfeeding, children, thrombocytopenia, bone marrow suppression, hypertension, hyperthyroidism, pheochromocytoma, seizure disorder, ulcerative colitis, MI, PKU, renal/GI disease

DOSAGE AND ROUTES

Vancomycin-resistant *Enterococcus faecium* infections

• **Adult/adolescent/child ≥12 yr: IV/PO** 600 mg q12hr × 14-28 days; max 1200 mg/day

• **Child <12 yr/infant/term neonate: IV/PO** 10 mg/kg q8hr × 14-28 days

Pneumonia/complicated skin infections

• **Adult: IV/PO** 600 mg q12hr × 10-14 days; max 1200 mg/day

• **Child birth-11 yr: PO/IV** 10 mg/kg q8hr × 10-14 days

Uncomplicated skin infections caused by *S. aureus* (MSSA only) or *S. pyogenes*

• **Adult: PO** 600 mg q12hr × 10-14 days; max 1200 mg/day

• **Adolescent: PO** 600 mg q12hr × 10-14 days; max 1200 mg/day

• **Child 5-11 yr: PO** 10 mg/kg q12hr × 10-14 days

• **Neonate ≥7 days old/infant/child <5 yr: PO** 10 mg/kg q8hr × 10-14 days

• **Infant preterm <7 days old: PO** 10 mg/kg q12hr × 10-14 days

Available forms: Tabs 600 mg; oral susp 100 mg/5 mL; premixed infusion 200 mg/100 mL, 400 mg/200 mL, 600 mg/mL (2 mg/mL)

Administer:

• Obtain culture and sensitivity before starting treatment, may give before results are received

PO route

• With/without food

• Store reconstituted oral susp at room temperature; use within 3 wk

Intermittent IV INFUSION route

• Do not use if particulate is present, yellow color is normal

• Premixed sol ready to use (2 mg/mL), give over 30-120 min; do not use IV infusion bag in series connections; do not use with additives in sol; do not use with another product, administer separately, flush line before and after use

• Store at room temperature in original packaging

Y-site compatibilities: Acyclovir, alfentanil, amikacin, aminophylline, ampicillin, aztreonam, buprenorphine, butorphanol, calcium gluconate, CARBOplatin, ceFAZolin, cefoTEtan, cefOXitin, cefTAZidime, ceftizoxime, cefuroxime, cimetidine, ciprofloxacin, cisatracurium, CISplatin, clindamycin, cyclophosphamide, cycloSPORINE, cytarabine, digoxin, furosemide, ganciclovir, gemcitabine, gentamicin, heparin, HYDROmorphone, ifosfamide, labetalol, leucovorin, levofloxacin, lidocaine, LORazepam, magnesium sulfate, mannitol, meperidine, meropenem, mesna, methotrexate, methyl-PREDNISolone, metoclopramide, metro-NIDAZOLE, midazolam, minocycline, mito-XANtrone, morphine, nalbuphine, naloxone, nitroglycerin, ofloxacin, ondansetron, PACLitaxel, PENTobarbital, PHENobarbital, piperacillin, potassium chloride, prochlorperazine, promethazine, propranolol, ranitidine, remifentanil, SUFentanil, theophylline, ticarcillin, tobramycin, vancomycin, vecuronium, verapamil, vinCRIStine, zidovudine

Solution compatibilities: D_5W, 0.9% NaCl, LR

SIDE EFFECTS

CNS: *Headache*, dizziness, insomnia
GI: *Nausea, diarrhea,* CDAD, increased ALT/AST, *vomiting,* taste change, tongue-color change
EENT: Optic neuropathy
HEMA: Myelosuppression
MISC: Vaginal moniliasis, fungal infection, oral moniliasis, lactic acidosis, anaphylaxis, angioedema, Stevens-Johnson syndrome, serotonin syndrome

PHARMACOKINETICS

Peak 1-2 hr, terminal half-life 4-5 hr, rapidly and extensively absorbed, protein binding 31%, metabolized by oxidation of the morpholine ring

INTERACTIONS

Do not use with MAOIs (or within 2 wk) or with products that possess MAOI-like action (furazolidone, isoniazid, INH, procarbazine); hypertensive crisis may occur

Increase: hypertensive crisis, seizures, coma—amoxapine, maprotiline, mirtazapine, traZODone, cyclobenzaprine, tricyclics, methyldopa
Increase: serotonin syndrome—bupropion, cyclobenzaprine, tramadol, trazadone, SSRIs, SNRIs, serotonin receptor agonists; notify prescriber immediately
Increase: effects of adrenergic agents (DOPamine, EPINEPHrine, pseudoephedrine); monitor B/P
Drug/Herb

• Avoid use with green tea, valerian, ginseng, yohimbine, kava, guarana, St. John's wort
Drug/Food
• Tyramine foods: avoid; increased pressor response
Drug/Lab Test
Increase: LFTs, alkaline phosphatase, amylase, lipase, BUN
Decrease: WBC, platelets, blood glucose

NURSING CONSIDERATIONS
Assess:
• **Infection:** VS, characteristics of sputum, wounds, stool, emesis; WBC baseline, periodically
• Vision change, optic neuritis may occur
• CBC with differential weekly, assess for myelosuppression (anemias, leukopenia, pancytopenia, thrombocytopenia)
• **Serotonin syndrome:** at least 2 wk should elapse between discontinuing linezolid and starting serotonergic agents; assess for increased heart rate, shivering, sweating, dilated pupils, tremor, high B/P, hyperthermia, headache, confusion; if these occur, stop linezolid, administer a serotonin antagonist if needed
• **Lactic acidosis:** repeated nausea/vomiting, unexplained acidosis, low bicarbonate level; notify prescriber immediately
• **Anaphylaxis/angioedema/Stevens-Johnson syndrome:** rash, pruritus, difficulty breathing, fever; have emergency equipment nearby
• **CNS symptoms:** headache, dizziness
• **Hepatic studies:** AST, ALT
• **Diabetes mellitus:** monitor those receiving insulin or oral antidiabetics for increased hypoglycemia
• **CDAD:** diarrhea, abdominal pain, fever, fatigue, anorexia, possible anemia, elevated WBC, low serum albumin; stop product, usually either vancomycin or IV metroNIDAZOLE given
• **Pregnancy/breastfeeding:** avoid use in pregnancy and breastfeeding
Evaluate:

• **Therapeutic response:** decreased symptoms of infection, blood cultures negative

Teach patient/family:

• If dizziness occurs, to ambulate, perform activities with assistance

• To complete full course of product therapy, use as directed, not to skip or double dose when remembered, unless close to next dose

• **Serotonin syndrome:** to notify prescriber immediately of fever, sweating, diarrhea, confusion

• To contact prescriber if adverse reaction occurs

• To inform prescriber if SSRIs or cold products, decongestants being used

• To avoid large amounts of high-tyramine foods (aged cheeses, red wine), drinks; provide list

• To report diarrhea, signs/symptoms of superinfection

• To notify health care professional of vision change

• To discuss with health care professional all Rx, OTC, herbals, supplements used

• **Pregnancy/breastfeeding:** Identify if pregnancy is planned or suspected or if breastfeeding

liothyronine (T₃) (Rx) (NTI)

(lye-oh-thye′roe-neen)

Cytomel, Triostat
Func. class.: Thyroid hormone
Chem. class.: Synthetic T₃

Do not confuse:
liothyroxine/levothyroxine

USES: Hypothyroidism, myxedema coma, thyroid hormone replacement, congenital hypothyroidism, nontoxic goiter, T₃ suppression test

CONTRAINDICATIONS

Adrenal insufficiency, MI, thyrotoxicosis, untreated hypertension

Black Box Warning: Obesity treatment

DOSAGE AND ROUTES

• **Adult:** PO 25 mcg/day, increase by 12.5-25 mcg q1-2wk until desired response, maintenance dose 25-75 mcg/day, max 100 mcg/day

• **Geriatric:** PO 5 mcg/day, increase by 5 mcg/day q1-2wk, maintenance 25-75 mcg/day

Congenital hypothyroidism

• **Child >3 yr:** PO 50-100 mcg/day

• **Child <3 yr:** PO 5 mcg/day, increase by 5 mcg q3-4days titrated to response, infant maintenance 20 mcg/day; 1-3 yr 50 mcg/day

Myxedema, severe hypothyroidism

• **Adult:** PO 25-50 mcg, then may increase by 5-10 mcg q1-2wk; maintenance dose 50-100 mcg/day

Myxedema coma/precoma

• **Adult:** IV 25-50 mcg initially, 5 mcg in geriatric patients, 10-20 mcg with cardiac disease; give doses q4-12hr

Nontoxic goiter

• **Adult:** PO 5 mcg/day, increase by 12.5-25 mcg q1-2wk; maintenance dose 75 mcg/day

Suppression test

• **Adult:** PO 75-100 mcg/day × 1 wk; radioactive ¹³¹I given before and after 1-wk dose

Available forms: Tabs 5, 25, 50 mcg; injection 10 mcg/mL/vial

⚠ HIGH ALERT

liraglutide (Rx)

(lir′a-gloo′tide)

Saxenda, Victoza
Func. class.: Antidiabetic agent
Chem. class.: Incretin mimetics

ACTION: Improved glycemic control and potential weight loss via activation of the glucagon-like peptide-1 (GLP-1) receptor

USES: Type 2 diabetes mellitus in combination with diet/exercise (Victoza), obesity (Saxenda)

Side effects: *italics* = common; red = life-threatening

CONTRAINDICATIONS

Hypersensitivity, medullary thyroid carcinoma (MTC), multiple endocrine neoplasia syndrome type 2 (MEN 2), thyroid cancer, pregnancy

Precautions: Breastfeeding, children, geriatric patients, alcoholism, cholelithiasis, ketoacidosis, diarrhea, fever, gastroparesis, hepatic/renal disease, hypoglycemia, infection, surgery, thyroid disease, trauma, vomiting, pancreatitis

Black Box Warning: Thyroid C-cell tumors

DOSAGES AND ROUTES

• **Adult: SUBCUT (Victoza)** 0.6 mg/day × 1 wk, then increase to 1.2 mg/day, max 1.8 mg/day; **Saxenda** (Initial BMI >27 kg/m²): 0.6 mg/day × 1 wk, then 1.2 mg/day × 1 wk then 1.8 mg × 1 wk, then 2.4 mg/day × 1 wk, then 3 mg/day

Available forms: Solution for injection 0.6, 1.2, 1.8, 2.4, 3 mg prefilled pen (Saxenda); solution for injection 0.6, 1.2, 1.8 mg prefilled pen (Victoza)

Administer:

SUBCUT route

• Give subcut only, inspect for particulate matter, discoloration; do not use if unusually viscous, cloudy, discolored, or if particles present; give daily anytime, without regard to meals; pen needles must be purchased separately, use Novo Nordisk needle; before first use, prime, see manual for directions; give in thigh, abdomen, or upper arm; lightly pinch fold of skin, insert needle at 90-degree angle (45-degree angle if thin), release skin; aspiration is not needed, give over 6 sec, rotate injection sites

• If dose is missed, resume once-daily dosing at next scheduled dose; if >3 days have elapsed since last dose, reinitiate at 0.6 mg, titrate

• Storage: do not store pen with needle attached; avoid direct heat and sunlight; discard 30 days after first use; after first use may be stored at room temperature or refrigerated; do not freeze

SIDE EFFECTS

CNS: Dizziness, headache

CV: Hypertension

ENDO: Hypoglycemia

EENT: Sinusitis

GI: Abdominal pain, anorexia, constipation, diarrhea, dyspepsia, nausea, vomiting, pancreatitis

INTEG: erythema, injection site reaction, urticaria

MS: Back pain

SYST: Antibody formation, infection, influenza, secondary thyroid malignancy, anaphylaxis, angioedema

INTERACTIONS

Increase: hypoglycemic reactions—angiotensin II receptor antagonists, ACE inhibitors, other antidiabetics, β-blockers, dexfenfluramine, fenfluramine, disopyramide, FLUoxetine, fibric acid derivatives, mecasermin, MAOIs, octreotide, pegvisomant, salicylates

Decrease: liraglutide effect—protease inhibitors, phenothiazines, baclofen, atypical antipsychotics, corticosteroids, cycloSPORINE, tacrolimus, carbonic anhydrase inhibitors, dextrothyroxine, diazoxide, phenytoin, fosphenytoin, ethotoin, isoniazid, INH, niacin, nicotine, estrogens, progestins, oral contraceptives, growth hormones, sympathomimetics

Increase or decrease: hypoglycemic reactions—androgens, bortezomib, quinolones, cloNIDine, alcohol, lithium, pentamidine

Increase or decrease: effects of—atorvastatin, acetaminophen, griseofulvin

Decrease: levels of digoxin

Drug/Lab Test

Increase: calcitonin, lipase

Decrease: glucose

PHARMACOKINETICS

Protein binding (98%); half-life 12-13 hr; binds to albumin, then released into circulation; peak 8-12 hr; body weight significantly affects pharmacokinetics

NURSING CONSIDERATIONS
Assess:

Black Box Warning: Thyroid C-cell tumors; monitor during treatment; if calcitonin is elevated or if nodules can be felt, referral is needed; do not use in those with a family history of MTC or in those with multiple endocrine neoplasia syndrome type 2

• **Diabetes:** that may occur soon after meals: hunger, sweating, weakness, dizziness, tremors, restlessness, tachycardia; serum glucose, A1c, CBC during treatment
• Hypersensitivity to this product
• **Insulin use with Victoza:** monitor for hypoglycemic reactions often
• **Stress:** those diabetic patients exposed to stress, surgery, fever, infections may require insulin administration temporarily
• **Serious skin reactions:** angioedema, hypersensitivity responses
• **Pancreatitis:** monitor for nausea, vomiting, severe abdominal pain; product should be discontinued; give supportive care; monitor amylase, lipase, electrolytes
Evaluate:
• **Therapeutic response:** stable and improved serum glucose, A1c, weight loss
Teach patient/family:
• **Hypersensitivity:** to report any allergic symptoms
• About symptoms of hypoglycemia/hyperglycemia and what to do for each; to have glucagon emergency kit available; to carry a carbohydrate source at all times
• About adverse reactions associated with therapy, such as nausea and vomiting; that upward dose titration can be delayed or ignored, depending on tolerance
• That diabetes is a lifelong illness; that product does not cure disease and must be continued on a daily basis
• To carry emergency ID with prescriber's phone number and medications taken
• To continue with other recommendations: diet, exercise

• To test blood glucose using a blood glucose meter
• To avoid other medications, herbs, supplements unless approved by prescriber
• To report serious skin effects, abdominal pain with nausea/vomiting immediately
• To consult written instructions if self-administration is ordered; to discard pen after 30 days
• That continuing follow-up exams will be needed
• That secondary malignancy is possible; that routine monitoring may be needed; to report trouble breathing, continuous hoarseness, lump in neck region immediately
• Not to share product with others; infections such as hepatitis may occur
• **Pregnancy/breastfeeding:** that product is not to be used in pregnancy or breastfeeding, that insulin is usually used in pregnancy, to notify health care professional if pregnancy is planned or suspected or if breastfeeding

lisdexamfetamine (Rx)
(lis-dex′am-fet′a-meen)
Vyvanse
Func. class.: CNS stimulant
Chem. class.: Amphetamine

Controlled Substance Schedule II

ACTION: Increases release of norepinephrine, DOPamine in cerebral cortex to reticular activation system

USES: Attention-deficit/hyperactivity disorder (ADHD), binge eating disorder

CONTRAINDICATIONS
Breastfeeding, hyperthyroidism, hypertension, glaucoma, severe arteriosclerosis, hypersensitivity to sympathomimetic amines

Black Box Warning: Substance abuse

Precautions: Pregnancy, children <6 yr, Gilles de la Tourette's disorder, depression, anorexia nervosa, psychosis, seizure disorder, suicidal ideation, MI, heart failure, alcoholism, aortic stenosis, bipolar disorder, CV disease

DOSAGE AND ROUTES
ADHD
• **Adult/child 6-17 yr: PO** 30 mg/day in AM; may increase by 10-20 mg/day at weekly intervals, max 70 mg/day
Moderate to severe binge eating disorder
• **Adult: PO** 30 mg/day in AM, increase by 20 mg weekly to target of 50-70 mg/day
Renal dose
• **Adult: PO** Severe impairment (GFR 15-<30 mL/min/1.73 m^2): max 50 mg/day; ESRD (GFR <15 mL/min/1.73 m^2): max 30 mg/day
Available forms: Caps 10, 20, 30, 40, 50, 60, 70 mg
Administer:
• Give daily in AM
• Without regard to meals
• Caps: may take whole or opened and contents dissolved in water, take immediately

SIDE EFFECTS
CNS: *Hyperactivity, insomnia, restlessness, talkativeness,* dizziness, headache, dysphoria, irritability, CNS tumor, dependence, addiction, mild euphoria, somnolence, lability, psychosis, mania, hallucinations, aggression; movement disorders, psychiatric events (child)
CV: *Palpitations, tachycardia,* hypertension, decrease in heart rate, dysrhythmias, MI, cardiomyopathy
EENT: Blurred vision, mydriasis, diplopia
ENDO: Growth inhibition
GI: *Anorexia,* dry mouth, diarrhea, weight loss
GU: Impotence, change in libido
INTEG: Urticaria, angioedema, Stevens-Johnson syndrome, toxic epidermal necrolysis
MISC: Rhabdomyolysis

PHARMACOKINETICS
Metabolized by liver; urine excretion pH dependent; crosses placenta, breast milk; half-life <1 hr

INTERACTIONS
• **Hypertensive crisis:** MAOIs or within 14 days of MAOIs
Increase: serotonin syndrome, neuroleptic malignant syndrome—SSRIs, SNRIs, serotonin-receptor agonists
Increase: lisdexamfetamine effect—acetaZOLAMIDE, antacids, sodium bicarbonate, urinary alkalinizers
Increase: CNS effect—haloperidol, tricyclics, phenothiazines, modafinil, meperidine, PHENobarbital, phenytoin
Increase: CNS stimulation—melatonin
Decrease: absorption of phenytoin
Decrease: lisdexamfetamine effect—ascorbic acid, ammonium chloride, urinary acidifiers
Decrease: effect of—adrenergic blockers, antidiabetics
Drug/Herb
• **Serotonin syndrome:** St. John's wort
Increase: stimulant effect—khat, melatonin, green tea, guarana
Decrease: stimulant effect—eucalyptus
Drug/Food
Increase: amine effect—caffeine

NURSING CONSIDERATIONS
Assess:
• **ADHD:** obtain history from parents, patient, counselors, as well as testing; confirm diagnosis before use
• **Binge eating disorder:** obtain history of diet bingeing times and food
• VS, B/P; product may reverse antihypertensives; check patients with cardiac disease often
• CBC, urinalysis; in diabetes: blood glucose; insulin changes may be required because eating may decrease
• Height, growth rate in children; growth rate may be decreased; treatment should be discontinued if this is present
• **Mental status:** mood, sensorium, affect, stimulation, insomnia, irritability
• **Serotonin syndrome, neuroleptic malignant syndrome:** increased heart rate, shivering, sweating, dilated pupils, tremors, high B/P, hyperthermia, headache, confusion; if these occur, stop product, administer serotonin antagonist

---

if needed; at least 2 wk should elapse between discontinuation of serotonergic agents and start of product

- **Tolerance or dependency:** increased amount of product may be used to get same effect; will develop after long-term use
- **Overdose:** pain, fever, dehydration, insomnia, hyperactivity

Black Box Warning: Before giving this product, identify presence of substance abuse; high potential for abuse, may be fatal

- **Psychotic manic episodes:** may occur when patients have underlying psychiatric conditions
- Gum, hard candy, frequent sips of water for dry mouth
- **Pregnancy/breastfeeding:** avoid use in pregnancy and breastfeeding

Evaluate:
- **Therapeutic response:** increased CNS stimulation, decreased drowsiness

Teach patient/family:
- **Seizures:** that product may decrease seizure threshold; those with a seizure disorder should notify prescriber if seizure occurs
- To report CNS changes, blurred vision; decrease in dose may be needed
- To decrease caffeine consumption (coffee, tea, cola, chocolate); may increase irritability, stimulation
- To avoid OTC preparations unless approved by prescriber
- To taper product over several weeks; depression, increased sleeping, lethargy may occur
- To avoid alcohol ingestion
- To avoid breastfeeding
- To avoid hazardous activities until stabilized on medication
- To get needed rest; patient will feel more tired at end of day

Black Box Warning: Serious CV effects may occur from increasing dose

- **Pregnancy/breastfeeding:** to avoid use in pregnancy, breastfeeding

TREATMENT OF OVERDOSE: Administer fluids, antihypertensive for increased B/P, ammonium chloride for increased excretion, chlorproMAZINE for antagonizing CNS effects

lisinopril (Rx)

(lyse-in'oh-pril)
Prinivil, Qbrelis
Func. class.: Antihypertensive, angiotensin-converting enzyme 1 (ACE) inhibitor
Chem. class.: Enalaprilat lysine analog

Do not confuse:
lisinopril/RisperDAL/Lipitor
Prinivil/Plendil/Proventil/PriLOSEC

ACTION: Selectively suppresses renin-angiotensin-aldosterone system; inhibits ACE, thereby preventing conversion of angiotensin I to angiotensin II

USES: Mild to moderate hypertension, adjunctive therapy of systolic HF, acute MI
Unlabeled uses: Diabetic retinopathy, proteinuria, post MI

CONTRAINDICATIONS
Hypersensitivity, angioedema

Black Box Warning: Pregnancy

Precautions: Breastfeeding, renal disease, hyperkalemia, renal artery stenosis, HF, aortic stenosis

DOSAGE AND ROUTES
Hypertension
- **Adult: PO** initially 10 mg, 10-40 mg/day; max 80 mg/day
- **Child ≥6 yr: PO** 0.07 mg/kg/day up to 5 mg/day; titrate q1-2wk up to 0.6 mg/kg/day or 40 mg/day
- **Geriatric: PO** 2.5-5 mg/day, increase q7days

Heart failure
- **Adult: PO** 5 mg/day, increase if needed max 40 mg/day in hypernatremia of

<130 mEqL or creatinine >3 mg/dL or CCr <30 mL/min, 2.5 mg/day initially

Acute myocardial infarction
• **Adult: PO** give 5 mg within 24 hr of onset of symptoms, then 5 mg after 24 hr, 10 mg after 48 hr, then 10 mg daily

Renal dose
• **Adult: PO** CCr <30 mL/min, reduce dose by 50%, initially 5 mg/day, max 40 mg/day; CCr <10 mL/min, 2.5 mg/day, max 40 mg/day

Available forms: Tabs 2.5, 5, 10, 20, 30, 40 mg

Administer:
• Severe hypotension may occur after 1st dose of product; may be prevented by reducing or discontinuing diuretic therapy 3 days before beginning lisinopril therapy
• Without regard to food

SIDE EFFECTS

CNS: *Vertigo,* depression, stroke, insomnia, paresthesias, *headache, fatigue,* asthenia, *dizziness*

CV: Chest pain, *hypotension,* sinus tachycardia

EENT: Blurred vision, nasal congestion

GI: Nausea, vomiting, anorexia, constipation, flatulence, GI irritation, diarrhea, hepatic failure, hepatic necrosis, pancreatitis

GU: Proteinuria, renal insufficiency, sexual dysfunction, impotence

HEMA: Neutropenia, agranulocytosis

INTEG: Rash, pruritus

MISC: Muscle cramps, *hyperkalemia*

RESP: Dry cough, dyspnea

SYST: Angioedema, anaphylaxis, toxic epidermal necrolysis

PHARMACOKINETICS
Onset 1 hr, peak 6-8 hr, duration 24 hr, excreted unchanged in urine, half-life 12 hr

INTERACTIONS
Increase: hyperkalemia—potassium salt substitutes, potassium-sparing diuretics, potassium supplements, cycloSPORINE

Increase: possible toxicity—lithium

Increase: hypotensive effect—diuretics, other antihypertensives, probenecid, phenothiazines, nitrates, acute alcohol ingestion

Increase: hypersensitivity—allopurinol

Decrease: lisinopril effects—aspirin, indomethacin, NSAIDs; dose may need adjustment

Drug/Food
• High-potassium diet (bananas, orange juice, avocados, nuts, spinach) should be avoided; hyperkalemia may occur; monitor potassium levels

Drug/Lab Test
Interference: glucose/insulin tolerance tests, LFTs, BUN, creatinine

Drug/Herb
Increase: hypotensive effect—garlic
Increase: hypotensive effect—black licorice

NURSING CONSIDERATIONS
Assess:
• **Heart failure:** edema in feet, legs daily; weight daily; dyspnea, wet crackles
• Skin turgor, dryness of mucous membranes for hydration status
• **Acute MI:** can be used in combination with salicylates, β blockers, thrombolytics
• **Hypertension:** B/P, pulse q4hr during beginning treatment and periodically; black patients should take in combination with diuretics thereafter; note rate, rhythm, quality; apical/pedal pulse before administration; notify prescriber of any significant changes
• Blood studies, platelets; WBC with differential at baseline, periodically q3mo; if neutrophils <1000/mm^3, discontinue treatment (recommended with collagen-vascular disease)
• Baselines of renal, hepatic studies before therapy begins, periodically; LFTs, uric acid, glucose may be increased
• **Angioedema, anaphylaxis, toxic epidermal necrolysis:** facial swelling, dyspnea, tongue swelling (rare); have emergency equipment nearby; may be more common in Black patients
• **Electrolytes:** potassium, sodium, chlorine

Black Box Warning: Pregnancy/breastfeeding: assess pregnancy, breastfeeding status before giving this product; if pregnant, do not use; do not breastfeed

Evaluate:
• **Therapeutic response:** decreased B/P, HF symptoms

Teach patient/family:
• Not to discontinue product abruptly; to taper
• To rise slowly to sitting or standing position to minimize orthostatic hypotension
• To avoid increasing potassium in the diet
• To report dry cough

Black Box Warning: Pregnancy/breastfeeding: to report if pregnancy is planned or suspected; not to breastfeed

TREATMENT OF OVERDOSE:
Lavage, IV atropine for bradycardia, IV theophylline for bronchospasm, digoxin, O_2, diuretic for cardiac failure

lisinopril/hydrochlorothiazide (Rx)

(lyse-in'oh-pril/hye-droe-klor-oh-thye'a-zide)

Zestoretic

Func. class.: Antihypertensive, angiotensin-converting enzyme 1 (ACE) inhibitor/diuretic, thiazide
Chem. class.: Enalaprilat lysine analog

ACTION:
Lisinopril: Competitive inhibitor of ACE; prevents conversion of angiotensin I to angiotensin II, a potent vasoconstrictor; results in lower levels of angiotensin II, which causes an increase in plasma renin activity and a reduction in aldosterone secretion
Hydrochlorothiazide: Inhibits sodium reabsorption in the distal tubules causing increased excretion of sodium, water, potassium

USES: Hypertension not controlled by monotherapy

CONTRAINDICATIONS
Hypersensitivity to lisinopril, hydrochlorothiazide, sulfonamide-derived drugs, or any component, angioedema related to use with an ACE inhibitor; idiopathic/hereditary angioedema; use with aliskiren in patients with diabetes mellitus; coadministration with or within 36 hr of switching to or from a neprilysin inhibitor (sacubitril); anuria

Black Box Warning: Pregnancy

Precautions: Breastfeeding, renal disease, hyperkalemia, renal artery stenosis, HF, aortic stenosis

DOSAGE AND ROUTES
Adult: PO Initial: lisinopril 10 mg/hydrochlorothiazide 12.5 mg or lisinopril 20 mg/hydrochlorothiazide 12.5 mg daily in those not controlled on monotherapy; titrate dosage after 2 to 3 wk; max lisinopril 80 mg/hydrochlorothiazide 50 mg per day
Available forms: Tablets: 10/12.5: Lisinopril 10 mg and hydrochlorothiazide 12.5 mg; 20/12.5: Lisinopril 20 mg and hydrochlorothiazide 12.5 mg; 20/25: Lisinopril 20 mg and hydrochlorothiazide 25 mg
Administer:
• Without regard to food

SIDE EFFECTS
CNS: *Vertigo,* depression, insomnia, paresthesias, *headache, fatigue,* asthenia, *dizziness*
CV: Chest pain, *hypotension,* sinus tachycardia
EENT: Blurred vision, nasal congestion
GI: Nausea, vomiting, anorexia, constipation, flatulence, GI irritation, diarrhea
GU: Sexual dysfunction, impotence
INTEG: Rash, pruritus
MISC: Muscle cramps, *hyperkalemia, hypokalemia*

RESP: Dry cough, dyspnea

PHARMACOKINETICS
Lisinopril: Onset 1 hr, peak 6-8 hr, duration 24 hr, excreted unchanged in urine, half-life 12 hr
Hydrochlorothiazide: Onset 2 hr, peak 4 hr, duration 6-12 hr, half-life 5.6-14.8 hr

INTERACTIONS
Increase: hyperkalemia—potassium salt substitutes, potassium-sparing diuretics, potassium supplements, cycloSPORINE
Increase: possible toxicity—lithium
Increase: hypotensive effect—diuretics, other antihypertensives, probenecid, phenothiazines, nitrates, acute alcohol ingestion
Increase: hypersensitivity—allopurinol
Decrease: lisinopril effects—aspirin, indomethacin, NSAIDs; dose may need adjustment
Drug/Food
• High-potassium diet (bananas, orange juice, avocados, nuts, spinach) should be avoided; hyperkalemia may occur; monitor potassium levels
Drug/Lab Test
Interference: glucose/insulin tolerance tests, LFTs, BUN, creatinine

NURSING CONSIDERATIONS
Assess:
• **Hypertension:** B/P, pulse q4hr during beginning treatment and periodically; Black patients should take in combination with diuretics thereafter; note rate, rhythm, quality; apical/pedal pulse before administration; notify prescriber of any significant changes
• Baselines of renal, hepatic studies before therapy begins, periodically; LFTs, uric acid, glucose may be increased
• **Angioedema, anaphylaxis, toxic epidermal necrolysis:** facial swelling, dyspnea, tongue swelling (rare); have emergency equipment nearby; may be more common in Black patients
• **Electrolytes:** potassium, sodium, chlorine

Black Box Warning: Pregnancy/breastfeeding: assess pregnancy, breastfeeding status before giving this product; if pregnant, do not use; do not breastfeed

Evaluate:
• **Therapeutic response:** decreased B/P
Teach patient/family:
• Not to discontinue product abruptly; to taper
• To rise slowly to sitting or standing position to minimize orthostatic hypotension
• To avoid increasing potassium in the diet
• To report dry cough

Black Box Warning: Pregnancy/breastfeeding: to report if pregnancy is planned or suspected; not to breastfeed

lithium (Rx) (NTI)
(li'thee-um)
Carbolith ♣, Lithane ♣, Lithamax ♣
Func. class.: Psychotropic agent—antimanic
Chem. class.: Alkali metal ion salt

Do not confuse:
lithium/lanthanum/Ultram

ACTION: May alter sodium, potassium ion transport across cell membrane in nerve, muscle cells; may balance biogenic amines of norepinephrine, serotonin in CNS areas involved in emotional responses

USES: Bipolar disorders (manic phase), prevention of bipolar manic-depressive psychosis
Unlabeled uses: Major depression (augmented use)

CONTRAINDICATIONS
Pregnancy, breastfeeding, children <12 yr, hepatic disease, brain trauma, organic brain syndrome, schizophrenia, severe cardiac/renal disease, severe dehydration

Precautions: Geriatric patients, thyroid disease, seizure disorders, diabetes mellitus, systemic infection, urinary retention, QT prolongation

Black Box Warning: Lithium level >1.5 mmol/L

DOSAGE AND ROUTES—NTI
Bipolar disorder (mania)
• **Adult:** PO 300 mg 3 times daily, initially. Adjust by 300 mg every 3 days based on clinical response, tolerability, and serum lithium concentration. Usual dose: 600 mg 2 to 3 times daily; **EXT REL** 900 mg q12hr; dose should be individualized to maintain blood levels at 1-1.5 mEq/L or 0.6-1.2 mEq/L (maintenance)
• **Geriatric:** PO 300 mg bid, increase q7days by 300 mg to desired dose
• **Child:** PO 10-30 mg/kg/day in 3-4 divided doses; increase as needed; do not exceed adult doses; maintain blood levels at 0.4-0.5 mEq/L
Depression (unlabeled use)
Adult PO: PO 600 mg tid or 10 mL oral solution tid
Renal dose
• **Adult:** PO CCr 10-50 mL/min give 50%-75% of normal dose, CCr <10 mL/min give 25%-50% of normal dose
Available forms: Caps 150, 300, 600 mg; tabs 300 mg; ext rel tabs 300, 450 mg; oral solution 300 mg/5 mL (8 mEq/5 mL)
Administer:
• Do not break, crush, chew caps, ext rel tabs
• Reduced dose to geriatric patients
• With meals to avoid GI upset
• Adequate fluids (2-3 L/day) to prevent dehydration during initial treatment, 1-2 L/day during maintenance

SIDE EFFECTS
CNS: *Headache, drowsiness, dizziness,* tremors, twitching, ataxia, seizure, slurred speech, restlessness, confusion, stupor, memory loss, clonic movements, fatigue
CV: *Hypotension,* ECG changes, dysrhythmias, circulatory collapse, edema, Brugada syndrome, QT prolongation

EENT: Tinnitus, blurred vision
ENDO: Hyponatremia, goiter, hyperglycemia, hypo/hyperthyroidism
GI: *Dry mouth, anorexia, nausea, vomiting, diarrhea,* incontinence, abdominal pain, metallic taste
GU: Polyuria, glycosuria, proteinuria, albuminuria, urinary incontinence, polydipsia
HEMA: Leukocytosis
INTEG: Drying of hair, alopecia, rash, pruritus, hyperkeratosis, acneiform lesions, folliculitis
MS: Muscle weakness

PHARMACOKINETICS
PO: Onset rapid, peak ½-3 hr, half-life 18-36 hr depending on age, crosses blood-brain barrier, 80% of filtered lithium reabsorbed by renal tubules, excreted in urine, crosses placenta, enters breast milk, well absorbed by oral method

INTERACTIONS
Increase: hypothyroid effects—antithyroid agents, calcium iodide, potassium iodide, iodinated glycerol
Increase: effects of neuromuscular blocking agents
Increase: renal clearance—sodium bicarbonate, acetaZOLAMIDE, mannitol, aminophylline
Increase: lithium level—ACE inhibitors
Increase: QT interval—antiarrhythmics, other QT prolongation products
Increase: masking of lithium toxicity—β-blockers used for lithium tremor
Increase: toxicity—indomethacin, diuretics, NSAIDs
Increase: lithium effect/toxicity—carBAMazepine, FLUoxetine, methyldopa, thiazide diuretics, probenecid; monitor drug levels
Decrease: lithium effects—calcium channel blockers
Drug/Herb
• Avoid use with kava, St. John's wort, valerian
Decrease: lithium levels—black/green tea, guarana
Drug/Food
• Significant changes in sodium intake will alter lithium excretion

L

Decrease: lithium levels—caffeine; adjust dose as needed

Drug/Lab Test

Increase: potassium excretion, urine glucose, blood glucose, protein, BUN

Decrease: VMA, T_3, T_4, ^{131}I

NURSING CONSIDERATIONS

Assess:

• **Mental status:** manic symptoms; mood; behavior before, during treatment

Black Box Warning: **Lithium toxicity:** diarrhea, vomiting, tremor, twitching, poor coordination, lassitude; **major toxicity,** coarse tremors, severe thirst, tinnitus, dilute urine; serum lithium levels week initially, then q2mo (therapeutic level: 0.5-1.5 mEq/L); toxic level >1.5 mcg/L; the drug has a narrow therapeutic index (NTI), measure level before AM dose

• Weight daily; check for, report edema in legs, ankles, wrists

• **Sodium intake:** decreased sodium intake with decreased fluid intake may lead to lithium retention; increased sodium, fluids may decrease lithium retention

• Skin turgor at least daily

• Urine for albuminuria, glycosuria, uric acid during beginning treatment, q2mo thereafter; specific gravity, any level <1.005 may indicate diabetes insipidus and should be reported to prescriber

• **Thyroid tests (TSH, T4)** baseline and q6mo to 1 yr, hypo/hyperthyroidism may occur

• **Neurologic status:** LOC, gait, motor reflexes, hand tremors

• ECG in those >50 yr with CV disease; cardiology consult is recommended in those with risk factor; QT prolongation may occur

• **Pregnancy/breastfeeding:** do not use in pregnancy, breastfeeding

Evaluate:

• **Therapeutic response:** decrease in excitement, manic phase

Teach patient/family:

• **About the symptoms of minor toxicity:** vomiting, diarrhea, poor coordination, fine motor tremors, weakness, lassitude; major toxicity: coarse tremors, severe thirst, tinnitus, diluted urine; to seek medical care immediately

• To monitor urine specific gravity, emphasize need for follow-up care to determine lithium levels; to monitor lithium levels to ensure effective levels and treatment

• Not to operate machinery until lithium levels are stable

• To use emergency ID with diagnosis, product used

• That beneficial effects may take 1-3 wk

• About products that interact with lithium (provide list); about need for adequate, stable intake of salt and fluids; not to use OTC products unless approved by prescriber

• **Pregnancy/breastfeeding:** that contraception is necessary because lithium may harm fetus; not to breastfeed

TREATMENT OF OVERDOSE:

Induce emesis or lavage, maintain airway, respiratory function; dialysis for severe intoxication

lixisenatide (Rx)

(lix'i-sen'a-tide)

Adlyxin

Func. class.: Antidiabetic agent

Chem. class.: GLP-1 receptor agonist

ACTION: An incretin mimetic; a glucagon-like peptide-1 (GLP-1) receptor agonist; binds and activates the GLP-1 receptor. GLP-1 is an important, gut-derived, glucose homeostasis regulator that is released after the oral ingestion of carbohydrates or fats

USES: Treatment of type 2 diabetes mellitus in combination with diet and exercise

CONTRAINDICATIONS

Angioedema

Precautions: Alcoholism, breastfeeding, children, cholelithiasis, diabetic ketoacidosis, gastroparesis, hypoglycemia, pancreatitis, pregnancy, renal failure, renal impairment, risk of serious hypersensitivity reactions or anaphylaxis, type 1 diabetes mellitus

DOSAGE AND ROUTES
• **Adult: SUBCUT** Initially, 10 mcg/day within 1 hr before the morning meal. If a dose is missed, give within 1 hr before the next meal. Continue 10 mcg/day × 14 days; on day 15, increase the dose to the maintenance dose of 20 mcg/day, max 20 mcg/day

Renal dose
• **Adult:** eGFR 60 to 89 mL/min/1.73 m^2: no dosage adjustment needed; eGFR 30 to 59 mL/min/1.73 m^2: no change; monitor closely for adverse reactions; eGFR <15 mL/min/1.73 m^2: do not use

Available forms: Solution for injection 10 mcg, 20 mcg prefilled pen starter pack, maintenance pack

Administer:

SUBCUT route
• May be used as monotherapy or with other antidiabetic medications. Dose adjustment of metformin or a thiazolidine is not usually required. A reduction in the dose of a sulfonylurea may be needed to reduce the risk of hypoglycemia
• Give subcut injection only. Do not give IV/IM
• Visually inspect for particulate matter and discoloration before use; do not use if unusually viscous, cloudy, discolored, or if particles are present
• Available as a prefilled pen. Each pen must be activated before the first use
• Administer daily within 1 hr before the first meal of the day, preferably the same meal each day. If a dose is missed, give within 1 hr before the next meal
• Inject subcut into the thigh, abdomen, or upper arm
• Rotate sites with each injection to prevent lipodystrophy
• **Storage:** Protect pen from light and keep in its original packaging; discard pen 14 days after its first use

SIDE EFFECTS
GI: Nausea, vomiting, diarrhea, constipation, abdominal pain, dyspepsia, pancreatitis (rare)

CNS: Dizziness, headache

MISC: Antibody formation, hypoglycemia, injection site reactions, hypotension; anaphylactoid reaction, bronchospasm, renal failure, laryngeal edema

PHARMACOKINETICS
Eliminated through glomerular filtration and proteolytic degradation, terminal half-life 1-3 hr; peak 1-3.5 hr; elimination prolonged in renal disease, with mild (CCr 60 to 89 mL/min), moderate (CCr 30 to 59 mL/min), and severe renal impairment (CCr 15 to 29 mL/min) was increased by approximately 34%, 69%, and 124%, respectively; use with caution in renal disease

INTERACTIONS
Increase: hypoglycemia—antidiabetes, sulfonylureas

Decrease: effect of hormonal contraceptives, oral antiinfectives, atorvastatin, to be taken 1 hr before

NURSING CONSIDERATIONS
Assess:
• **Diabetes:** fasting blood glucose, A1c level during treatment to determine diabetic control
• **Pancreatitis:** severe abdominal pain with or without nausea and vomiting, product should be discontinued immediately
• **Renal disease**: monitor BUN, creatinine in mild renal disease; do not use in severe renal disease
• **Hypoglycemia/hyperglycemia:** reaction can occur soon after meals; for severe hypoglycemia, give IV D$_{50}$W, IV dextrose solution

Evaluate:
• **Therapeutic response:** decreasing polydipsia, polyuria, polyphagia, clear sensorium, improving A1c, weight

Teach patient/family:
• How to prepare and use the pen; include a practice injection
• About the signs and symptoms of hypoglycemia/hyperglycemia and what to do about each; to have emergency glucagon kit available at all times, to carry glucose source (sugar, candy)

• That product must be taken on a continuing basis; not to discontinue without prescriber's approval

• That diabetes is a lifelong condition; that product will not cure condition; to carry emergency ID with condition, products taken, prescriber's phone number and name

• To continue weight control, dietary restrictions, exercise, hygiene

• That regular lab testing and A1c will be necessary

• **Pancreatitis:** to seek medical care immediately if severe abdominal pain occurs with or without nausea, vomiting

• **Pregnancy:** to notify prescriber if pregnant or planning to become pregnant; if taking oral contraceptives, to take at least 1 hr before this product

---

Iodoxamide ophthalmic

See Appendix B

Iofexidine (Rx)

(loe-FEX-i-deen)

Lucemyra

Func. class.: Opioid withdrawal agent
Chem. class.: Central alpha-2 agonist

ACTION: A central alpha-2 agonist that binds to adrenergic receptors, resulting in a reduction in the release of norepinephrine and a decrease in sympathetic tone

USES: For the mitigation of opioid withdrawal symptoms to facilitate abrupt opioid discontinuation in adults

CONTRAINDICATIONS

Hypersensitivity

Precautions: Abrupt discontinuation, acute MI, alcoholism, bradycardia, breastfeeding, cardiac dysrhythmias, CV disease, children, coadministration with other CNS depressants, coronary artery disease, dehydration, diabetes mellitus, dialysis, driving or operating machinery, electrolyte imbalance, ethanol ingestion, females, geriatric patients, heart failure, hepatic disease, hypertension, hypocalcemia, hypomagnesemia, hypotension, infertility, long QT syndrome, malnutrition, poor metabolizers, pregnancy, renal disease, syncope, thyroid disease

DOSAGE AND ROUTES

• **Adult: PO** Initially, 0.54 mg (3×0.18-mg tablets) $4\times$ daily during peak withdrawal symptoms (first 5-7 days after last use of opioid), with dosing based on opiate withdrawal symptoms and tolerability; may use up to 14 days. Space dosing 5-6 hr apart; max 0.72 mg (4 tabs) as a single dose; max 2.88 mg (16 tabs) per day. To discontinue, gradually taper dose over 2-4 days to reduce drug withdrawal symptoms (reduce by 1 tab per dose every 1-2 days)

Available forms: Tabs 0.18 mg

Administer:

• May administer orally without regard to meals

PHARMACOKINETICS

Protein binding 55%, 30% of dose is converted to inactive metabolites during first-pass metabolism by CYP2D6, CYP1A2, and CYP2C19, excretion kidney 15%-20%, half-life 17-22 hr after repeated dosing, peak 3-5 hr

INTERACTIONS

• **Increase:** QT prolongation—type IA, IC, III antidysrhythmics, antihistamines, antidepressants; monitor ECG if used concurrently

• **Increase:** CNS effects and sedation—other CNS depressants; if used concurrently, monitor for increased sedation

• **Increase:** hypotension—antihypertensives; avoid concurrent use if possible

• **Increase:** hypotension, bradycardia—CYP2D6 inhibitors

NURSING CONSIDERATIONS

Assess:

• **QT prolongation:** Monitor ECG in heart failure, bradyarrhythmias, liver or kidney impairment, or during concurrent use of other medications that lead to QT prolongation

• **Electrolyte imbalances** (hypokalemia, hypomagnesemia) should be corrected before use; monitor electrolytes for changes

• **Somnolence and sedation** may cause impairment of cognitive and motor skills; may be increased when coadministered with other CNS depressants (benzodiazepines, ethanol, and barbiturates)

• **Abrupt discontinuation:** monitor B/P during tapering; a significant increase in B/P may occur with abrupt discontinuation. May also cause diarrhea, insomnia, anxiety, chills, hyperhidrosis, and extremity pain

• **Hepatic disease:** may reduce drug clearance. Dosage reductions are recommended based on degree of hepatic impairment

• **Renal impairment:** may reduce drug clearance. Dosage reductions may be needed based on degree of renal impairment, including renal failure (end-stage renal disease, patients on dialysis); may be used without regard to timing of dialysis

• **Geriatric patients:** caution is recommended when administering to patients over age 65. Dose adjustments may be needed

• **Fertility:** infertility has been noted in some animal studies

• **Pregnancy/breastfeeding:** safety not established. Consider the benefits of breastfeeding, the risk of potential infant drug exposure, and the risk of an untreated or inadequately treated condition

Teach patient/family

• About self-monitoring for hypotension, bradycardia, and related symptoms; that moving from a supine to upright position may increase the risk for hypotension or orthostatic effects

• To stay hydrated; to recognize symptoms of hypotension; if hypotension occurs, to sit or lie down; to carefully rise from a sitting or lying position

• To withhold doses when experiencing hypotension or bradycardia and to contact health care provider for guidance on dose adjustments

• To use caution or avoid performing activities that require mental alertness, such as driving or operating machinery, until effect of product is known

• Not to discontinue without consulting health care provider, taper

• To inform health care provider of other medications being taken, including ethanol ingestion

• That patients who complete opioid discontinuation are at an increased risk of fatal overdose should they resume opioid use

lomitapide (Rx)

(loe-mi′ta-pide)

Juxtapid

Func. class.: Antilipemic

Chem. class.: Microsomal triglyceride transfer protein (MTP) inhibitor

ACTION: Directly binds to and inhibits MTP, which is located in the lumen of the endoplasmic reticulum. MTP inhibition prevents the assembly of apo-B–containing lipoproteins in enterocytes and hepatocytes resulting in reduced production of chylomicrons and VLDL and subsequently reduces plasma LDL-C concentrations

USES: Homozygous familial hypercholesterolemia

CONTRAINDICATIONS
Hypersensitivity, pregnancy, breastfeeding

Black Box Warning: Hepatotoxicity, requires an experienced clinician

Precautions: Contraception requirements, dialysis, ethanol ingestion, hepatic disease, lactase deficiency, malabsorption syndrome, pancreatic insufficiency, renal impairment, requires an experienced clinician

DOSAGE AND ROUTES

Adult: PO Initial: 5 mg daily; after ≥2 wk, may increase to 10 mg daily; then ≥4-wk intervals, may increase to 20 mg daily, then to 40 mg daily, max 60 mg/day

Available forms: Capsule 5 mg, 10 mg, 20 mg, 30 mg, 40 mg, 60 mg

Administer:

• Give with water only

• Give ≥2 hr after the evening meal to lessen GI adverse effects

• Avoid grapefruit and grapefruit juice

• Swallow capsules whole (do not open, crush, chew)

• To take supplements of vitamin E 400 IU, linoleic acid 200 mg, ALA 210 mg, EPA 110 mg, DHA 80 mg; take ≥2 hr of product

• Store at 20° C-25° C (68° F-77° F); excursions permitted between 15° C and 30° C (59° F and 86° F). Protect from moisture

SIDE EFFECTS

CV: Chest pain, angina pectoris, palpitations

CNS: Fatigue, dizziness, headache

GI: Diarrhea, nausea, dyspepsia, vomiting, abdominal pain, weight loss, abdominal distention, constipation, flatulence, gastroenteritis, liver steatosis, increased LFTs, GERD, tenesmus, bowel urgency, hepatotoxicity

MS: Back pain

RESP: Nasopharyngitis, nasal congestion

MISC: Fever, infection

PHARMACOKINETICS

Onset and duration unknown, peak 6 hr; half-life 40 hr

Interactions

Increase: lomitapide effect—CYP3A4 inhibitors

Increase: myopathy—lovastatin, simvastatin, decrease dose of statin

Increase: substrate level—P-gp substrates, decrease dose of substrate

Increase: hepatotoxicity—acetaminophen, monitor LFTs

Increase: bleeding risk—warfarin, monitor INR

Decrease: lomitapide effect—bile acid sequestrants

Drug/Herb

Increase: lomitapide effect—Ginkgo biloba

Drug/Food

Do not use with grapefruit juice

NURSING CONSIDERATIONS

Assess:

> **Black Box Warning:** Available only through the Juxtapid REMS program at www.Juxtapid.com

> **Black Box Warning: Hepatotoxicity:** Monitor LFTs baseline and periodically, if 3 × ULN, discontinue; contraindicated in **moderate or severe hepatic impairment** (based on Child-Pugh category B or C) or **active hepatic disease**

• Monitor serum alkaline phosphatase, serum bilirubin, serum cholesterol profile baseline and periodically

• **Dialysis:** Do not exceed a dose of lomitapide 40 mg PO

• **Pregnancy/breastfeeding:** Do not use in pregnancy, rule out before starting treatment, if pregnancy occurs, discontinue immediately and enroll in Global Lomitapide Pregnancy Exposure Registry 877-902-4099, do not breastfeed

Evaluate:

• **Therapeutic response:** Reduction in LDL cholesterol

Teach patient/family:

• To notify provider of chest pain, change in heartbeat, flulike symptoms, severe/persistent nausea/vomiting/abdominal pain/diarrhea, dry skin/mouth/eyes, increased thirst, dizziness, confusion

• To notify provider of dark urine, fatigue, lack of appetite, light-colored stools, yellow skin/eyes

• To continue with a low-fat diet and to take product ≥2 hr after evening meal to prevent GI upset

• To not consume more than 1 alcoholic drink per day

• **Allergic reaction:** Rash, itching; red, swollen, blistered, peeling skin; wheezing; tightness in the chest or throat; trouble breathing, swallowing, talking; swelling of the mouth, face, lips, tongue, throat

• Not to double dose if missed, take at next scheduled time

• **Pregnancy/breastfeeding:** To notify provider if pregnancy is planned or suspected, if using hormonal contraceptives or if breastfeeding. Additional contraceptive measures are required

---

⚠ HIGH ALERT

lomustine (Rx)
(loe-mus'teen)
Gleostine
Func. class.: Antineoplastic agent, alkylating agent (Nitrosourea)

USES: Treatment of primary and metastatic brain tumors after appropriate surgical and/or radiotherapeutic treatment (in combination with other chemotherapy agents) of Hodgkin lymphoma that has progressed following initial chemotherapy

CONTRAINDICATIONS
Hypersensitivity to lomustine or any component

Black Box Warning: Severe leukopenia and/or thrombocytopenia, potential for overdose/poisoning

DOSAGE AND ROUTES
Adult/child: PO: 130 mg/m² as a single dose q6wk; reduce dose to 100 mg/m² as a single dose q6wk in patients with compromised bone marrow function

Available forms: Capsules 5, 10, 40, 100 mg

lonapeg-somatropin-tcgd (Rx)
(loe-na-peg-soe-ma-TROE-pin-tcgd)
Skytrofa
Func. class.: Human growth hormone

USES: Pediatric growth hormone deficiency

DOSAGE AND ROUTES
• **Child ≥1 yr and ≥11 kg: SUBCUT** usually 0.24 mg per kg of body weight injected weekly

Available forms: Injection 3 mg, 3.6 mg, 4.3 mg, 5.2 mg, 6.3 mg, 7.6 mg, 9.1 mg, 11 mg, 13.3 mg

loncastuximab tesirine-lpyl (Rx)
Zynlonta
Func. class.: Antineoplastic-alkylating agent

USES: Relapsed or refractory large B-cell lymphoma

DOSAGE AND ROUTES
• **Adult: IV** 0.15 mg/kg over 30 min on day 1 of each cycle (q3wk) × 2 cycles, then 0.075 mg/kg over 30 min q3wk for subsequent cycles

Available forms: Lyophilized powder for injection; for IV use 10 mg

loperamide (OTC, Rx)
(loe-per'a-mide)
Diamode, Imodium ✚,
Imodium A-D
Func. class.: Antidiarrheal
Chem. class.: Piperidine derivative

Do not confuse:
Loperamide/furosemide

L

ACTION: Direct action on intestinal muscles to decrease GI peristalsis; reduces volume, increases bulk; electrolytes not lost

USES: Diarrhea (cause undetermined), travelers' diarrhea, chronic diarrhea, to decrease amount of ileostomy discharge

CONTRAINDICATIONS
Hyper-sensitivity, CDAD, constipation, dysentery, GI bleeding/obstruction/perforation, ileus, vomiting

Black Box Warning: Children, cardiac arrest, torsade de pointes

Precautions: Pregnancy, breastfeeding, children <2 yr, hepatic disease, dehydration, gastroenteritis, toxic megacolon, geriatric patients, severe ulcerative colitis

DOSAGE AND ROUTES
• **Adult: PO** 4 mg, then 2 mg after each loose stool, max 16 mg/day
• **Child 9-12 yr: PO** 2 mg, then 1 mg after each loose stool, max 6 mg/24 hr
• **Child 6-8 yr: PO** 2 mg, then 1 mg after each loose stool, max 4 mg/day
• **Child 2-5 yr: PO** 1 mg, then 1 mg after each loose stool, max 3 mg/24 hr
Available forms: Caps 2 mg; oral solution 1 mg/5 mL; tabs 2 mg
Administer:
• Do not break, crush, or chew caps
• For 48 hr only
• Do not mix oral sol with other sol

SIDE EFFECTS
CNS: Dizziness, drowsiness, fatigue
GI: *Nausea, dry mouth, vomiting, constipation,* abdominal pain, anorexia, toxic megacolon, bacterial enterocolitis, flatulence
INTEG: Rash
MISC: Hyperglycemia
SYST: Anaphylaxis, angioedema, toxic epidermal necrolysis

PHARMACOKINETICS
PO: Duration 24 hr, protein binding 97%, half-life 9-14 hr, metabolized in liver, excreted in feces as unchanged product, small amount in urine

INTERACTIONS
Increase: CNS depression—alcohol, antihistamines, analgesics, opioids, sedative/hypnotics
Drug/Herb
Increase: CNS depression—chamomile, hops, kava, valerian

NURSING CONSIDERATIONS
Assess:
• **Stools:** volume, color, characteristics, frequency; bowel pattern before product; rebound constipation
• Electrolytes (potassium, sodium, chlorine) if receiving long-term therapy
• Response after 48 hr; if no response, product should be discontinued
• Abdominal distention, toxic megacolon in those with ulcerative colitis
• Dehydration, CNS change in children, hepatic disease
• **Pregnancy/breastfeeding:** use only if benefits outweigh fetal risk; breastfeeding is not recommended
Evaluate:
• **Therapeutic response:** decreased diarrhea (48 hr); decreased chronic diarrhea (10 days)
Teach patient/family:
• To avoid OTC products unless directed by prescriber
• That ileostomy patient may take product for extended time
• Not to operate machinery if drowsiness occurs
• To use hard candy, sips of water for dry mouth
• To notify health care professional if diarrhea continues over 48 hr or 10 days if distention, fever, or abdominal pain occurs

lopinavir/ritonavir (Rx)

(low-pin′ah-veer/ri-toe′na-veer)

Kaletra

Func. class.: Antiretroviral

Chem. class.: Protease inhibitor

Do not confuse:

Kaletra/Keppra

ACTION: Inhibits human immunodeficiency virus (HIV-1) protease and prevents maturation of the infectious virus

USES: HIV-1 in combination with or without other antiretrovirals

CONTRAINDICATIONS

Hypersensitivity to this product or polyoxyethylated castor oil (oral solution), CYP3A4 metabolized products

Precautions: Pregnancy, breastfeeding, hepatic disease, pancreatitis, diabetes, hemophilia, AV block, hypercholesterolemia, immune reconstitution syndrome, neonates, cardiomyopathy, congenital long-QT prolongation, hypokalemia, elderly patients, Graves' disease, polymyositis, Guillain-Barré syndrome, children, HBV/HCV coinfection

DOSAGE AND ROUTES

HIV-1 infection, treatment without efavirenz, nelfinavir, or nevirapine Adult: PO Twice-daily dosing: Therapy-naive or therapy-experienced: Lopinavir 400 mg/ritonavir 100 mg bid; **once-daily dosing: Therapy-naive or experienced patients with <3 lopinavir resistance-associated substitutions:** Lopinavir 800 mg/ritonavir 200 mg daily; once-daily dosing is not recommended in those receiving efavirenz, fosamprenavir, nevirapine, nelfinavir, carbamazepine, phenobarbital, or phenytoin.

Pregnant women (with no lopinavir resistance–associated amino acid substitutions): PO Lopinavir 400 mg/ritonavir 100 mg bid; once-daily dosing is not recommended. Tablets are recommended; avoid use of the oral solution

Child >6 mo/adolescents:

PO (solutions) 230 mg/57.5 mg per m²/dose bid

HIV-1 infection with combination therapy with efavirenz, nelfinavir, or nevirapine. Adult: PO Twice-daily dosing: Therapy-naive and therapy-experienced patients: Solution: Lopinavir 520 mg/ritonavir 130 mg (6.5 mL) bid; Tablet: Lopinavir 500 mg/ritonavir 125 mg bid; once-daily dosing: not recommended

Children >6 mo/adolescents: PO (solution) 300 mg/75 mg per m²/dose bid

HIV-1 infection not receiving concomitant efavirenz, nelfinavir, or nevirapine

Available forms: Oral solution 400 mg lopinavir/100 mg ritonavir/5 mL; tablets 100 mg lopinavir/25 mg ritonavir, 200 mg lopinavir/50 mg ritonavir

Administer:

PO route

• **TAB:** take without regard to food; swallow whole; do not crush, break, chew

• **ORAL SOL:** shake well, use calibrated measuring device

• Drug-resistance testing should be done before beginning therapy in antiretroviral-naive patients and before changing therapy for treatment failure

SIDE EFFECTS

CNS: Paresthesia, *headache, seizures, fever, dizziness, insomnia, asthenia,* intracranial bleeding, encephalopathy

CV: QT, PR interval prolongation, deep vein thrombosis

EENT: Blurred vision, otitis media, tinnitus

L

GI: Diarrhea, buccal mucosa ulceration, abdominal pain, nausea, taste perversion, dry mouth, vomiting, anorexia
INTEG: Rash
MISC: Asthenia, angioedema, anaphylaxis, Stevens-Johnson syndrome, increased lipids, lipodystrophy
MS: Pain, rhabdomyolysis, myalgias

PHARMACOKINETICS
Well absorbed, 98% protein binding, hepatic metabolism, peak 4 hr, terminal half-life 6 hr

INTERACTIONS
Increase: toxicity—amiodarone, avanafil, azole antifungals, benzodiazepines, buPROPion, cloZAPine, desipramine, dihydroergotamine, encainide, ergotamine, flecainide, HMG-CoA reductase inhibitors, interleukins, meperidine, midazolam, pimozide, piroxicam, propafenone, quiNIDine, ranolazine, rivaroxaban, saquinavir, triazolam, zolpidem
Increase: QT prolongation—class IA/III antidysrhythmics, some phenothiazines, β-agonists, local anesthetics, tricyclics, haloperidol, chloroquine, droperidol, pentamidine, CYP3A4 inhibitors (amiodarone, clarithromycin, erythromycin, telithromycin, troleandomycin), arsenic trioxide, levomethadyl, CYP3A4 substrates (methadone, pimozide, QUEtiapine, quiNIDine, risperiDONE, ziprasidone)
Increase: ritonavir levels—fluconazole
Increase: level of both products—clarithromycin, ddI
Increase: levels of bosentan
Decrease: ritonavir levels—rifamycins, nevirapine, barbiturates, phenytoin, budesonide, predniSONE
Decrease: levels of anticoagulants, atovaquone, divalproex, ethinyl estradiol, lamoTRIgine, phenytoin, sulfamethoxazole, theophylline, voriconazole, zidovudine

Drug/Lab Test
Increase: AST, ALT, CPK, cholesterol, GGT, triglycerides, uric acid, glucose
Decrease: Hct, HB, RBC, neutrophils, WBC

Drug/Herb
Decrease: ritonavir levels—St. John's wort; avoid concurrent use
• Avoid use with red yeast rice, evening primrose oil

NURSING CONSIDERATIONS
Assess:
• **HIV:** viral load, CD4 at baseline, throughout therapy; blood glucose, plasma HIV RNA, serum cholesterol/lipid profile; resistance testing before starting therapy and after treatment failure
• Signs of infection, anemia
• **Hepatic studies:** ALT, AST baseline and periodically
• Bowel pattern before, during treatment; if severe abdominal pain with bleeding occurs, discontinue product; monitor hydration
• Skin eruptions; rash
• **Rhabdomyolysis:** muscle pain, increased CPK, weakness, swelling of affected muscles, tea-colored dark urine; if these occur and if confirmed by CPK, product should be discontinued
• **QT prolongation:** ECG for QT prolongation, ejection fraction; assess for chest pain, palpitations, dyspnea
• **Serious skin disorders:** Stevens-Johnson syndrome, angioedema, anaphylaxis
• **Pregnancy/breastfeeding:** all pregnant women who experience adverse reactions should have provider report the reactions to Antiretroviral Pregnancy Registry, 800-258-4263; avoid breastfeeding

Evaluate:
• **Therapeutic response:** improvement in HIV symptoms; improving viral load, CD4+ T cells

Teach patient/family:
• To take as prescribed; if dose is missed, to take as soon as remembered up to 1 hr before next dose; not to double dose
• That product is not a cure for HIV; that opportunistic infections can continue to be acquired
• That redistribution of body fat or accumulation of body fat may occur

---

- That others can continue to contract HIV from patient
- To avoid OTC, prescription medications, herbs, supplements unless approved by prescriber; not to use St. John's wort because it decreases product's effect; that taking this product with ED drugs may increase adverse reactions
- That regular follow-up exams and blood work will be required
- To report a change in heart rhythm or abnormal heartbeats
- **Pregnancy/breastfeeding:** to use a nonhormonal contraceptive, to notify provider if pregnancy is planned or suspected, avoid breastfeeding

loratadine (OTC)
(lor-a′ti-deen)

Alavert, Childrens Loratadine, Claritin Allergy Childrens, Claritin Childrens, Claritin Reditabs, Claritin, Clear-Atadine ♣, Dimetapp ♣, Triaminic AllerChews ♣

Func. class.: Antihistamine, 2nd generation
Chem. class.: Selective histamine (H$_1$)-receptor antagonist

Do not confuse:
loratadine/lovastatin/ LORazepam/losartan

ACTION: Binds to peripheral histamine receptors, thereby providing antihistamine action without sedation

USES: Seasonal rhinitis, chronic idiopathic urticaria for those ≥2 yr

CONTRAINDICATIONS
Hypersensitivity, acute asthma attacks, lower respiratory tract disease
Precautions: Pregnancy, breastfeeding, increased intraocular pressure, bronchial asthma, hepatic/renal disease

DOSAGE AND ROUTES
- **Adult and child ≥6 yr: PO** 10 mg/day
- **Child 2-5 yr: PO** 5 mg/day
Renal/hepatic dose
- **Adult: PO** CCr <30 mL/min or hepatic disease, 10 mg every other day
- **Child 2-5 yr: PO** GFR <50 mL/min; 5 mg every other day
Available forms: Tabs 10 mg; rapid-disintegrating tabs 10 mg; orally disintegrating tabs 10 mg; syr 1 mg/mL; susp 5 mg/mL, ext rel tab 10 mg
Administer:
- **Rapid-disintegrating tabs** by placing on tongue, to be swallowed after disintegrated with/without water
- Use within 6 mo of opening pouch and immediately after opening blister pack
- On empty stomach daily
Ext Rel Tab
- Do not break, crush, or chew

SIDE EFFECTS
CNS: Sedation (more common with increased doses), headache, fatigue, restlessness
EENT: Dry mouth

PHARMACOKINETICS
Onset 1-3 hr, peak 8-12 hr, duration 24 hr, metabolized in liver to active metabolites, excreted in urine, active metabolite desloratadine half-life 20 hr

INTERACTIONS
Increase: CNS depressant effects—alcohol, antidepressants, other antihistamines, sedative/hypnotics, MAOIs
Increase: loratadine level—cimetidine, ketoconazole, macrolides (clarithromycin, erythromycin)
Drug/Herb
Increase: CNS depression—chamomile, kava, valerian
Drug/Lab Test
False negative: skin allergy tests (discontinue antihistamine 3 days before testing)

NURSING CONSIDERATIONS
Assess:
- **Allergy:** hives, rash, rhinitis; monitor respiratory status
- **Beers:** avoid in older men; may decrease urinary flow and cause urinary retention
- **Pregnancy/breastfeeding:** use only if clearly needed; cautious use in breastfeeding

Evaluate:
- **Therapeutic response:** absence of running or congested nose, other allergy symptoms

Teach patient/family:
- To avoid driving, other hazardous activities if drowsiness occurs
- To avoid use of other CNS depressants

⚠ HIGH ALERT

loratadine/ pseudoephedrine (OTC)
(lor-at′a-deen/soo-doe-e-fedrin)
Claritin-D, Claritin-D 24 hour
Func. class.: Alpha/beta agonist, decongestant, histamine H1 antagonist

---

USES: Temporary relief of sinus and nasal congestion; runny nose; sneezing; itching of nose or throat and itchy, watery eyes due to common cold, hay fever (allergic rhinitis), or other upper respiratory allergies or sinusitis

CONTRAINDICATIONS
Hypersensitivity to loratadine, pseudoephedrine, or any component; within 14 days of MAOI therapy; severe hypertension, coronary heart disease

DOSAGE AND ROUTES
Adult/child ≥12 yr PO: loratadine 5 mg/pseudoephedrine 120 mg per tablet: 1 tablet q12hr (max: 2 tablets/day); loratadine 10 mg/pseudoephedrine 240 mg per tablet: 1 tablet daily (max: 1 tablet/day)
Available forms: Tabs ext rel 5/120, 10/240 mg

⚠ HIGH ALERT

LORazepam (Rx)
(lor-a′ze-pam)
Ativan
Func. class.: Sedative, hypnotic; antianxiety
Chem. class.: Benzodiazepine, short acting

Controlled Substance Schedule IV

Do not confuse:
LORazepam/ALPRAZolam/clonazePAM

ACTION: Potentiates the actions of GABA, especially in the limbic system and the reticular formation

USES: Anxiety, irritability with psychiatric or organic disorders, preoperatively; insomnia; adjunct for endoscopic procedures, status epilepticus, insomnia
Unlabeled uses: Antiemetic before chemotherapy, rectal use, alcohol withdrawal, seizure prophylaxis, agitation, insomnia, sedation maintenance

CONTRAINDICATIONS
Pregnancy, breastfeeding, hypersensitivity to benzodiazepines, benzyl alcohol; closed-angle glaucoma, psychosis, history of drug abuse, COPD, sleep apnea
Precautions: Children <12 yr, geriatric patients, debilitated patients, renal/hepatic disease, addiction, suicidal ideation, abrupt discontinuation

Black Box Warning: Coadministration with other CNS depressants, abrupt discontinuation, substance abuse

DOSAGE AND ROUTES
Anxiety
- **Adult/adolescent ≥12 yr: PO** 2-3 mg/day in divided doses, max 10 mg/day
- **Geriatric: PO** 1-2 mg/day in divided doses or 0.5-1 mg at bedtime
- **Child <11 yr (unlabeled): PO** 0.025-0.05 mg/kg/dose (max q4hr)

Preoperatively for sedation
• **Adult: IM** 50 mcg/kg 2 hr before surgery, max 4 mg; **IV** 44 mcg/kg 15-20 min before surgery, max 2 mg
• **Child ≥12 yr: IV** 0.05 mg/kg, max 4 mg
Status epilepticus
• **Adult: IM/IV** 0.1 mg/kg/dose (Max: 4 mg/dose) as a single dose; may repeat dose once in 5-15 min
• **Neonate: IV** 0.05-0.1 mg/dose, may repeat every 10-15 min
• **Child: IV** 0.05-0.1, may repeat every 5-15 min, up to 4 mg/dose
Insomnia
• **Adult: PO** 2-4 mg at bedtime; only minimally effective after 2 wk continuous therapy
• **Geriatric: PO** 0.5-1 mg initially
Sedation in mechanically ventilated patients (unlabeled)
• **Adult/adolescent: INTERMITTENT IV** 0.044 mg/kg q2-4hr, prn, max 4-mg single dose
• **Adult/adolescent: IV INFUSION** 0.5-8 mg/hr, titrate, use loading dose of 2-4 mg
Alcohol withdrawal (unlabeled)
• **Adult: PO** 2 mg q6hr × 4 doses, then 1 mg q6hr for 8 doses
Available forms: Tabs 0.5, 1, 2 mg; inj 2, 4 mg/mL; oral sol 2 mg/mL
Administer:
PO route
• With food or milk for GI symptoms; crushed if patient is unable to swallow medication whole
• Sugarless gum, hard candy, frequent sips of water for dry mouth
• Give largest dose before bedtime if giving in divided doses
• **Oral solution:** use calibrated dropper; add to food/drink; consume immediately
IM route
• Deep into large muscle mass
• Use this route when IV is not feasible
Direct IV route
• Prepare immediately before use; short stability time
• IV after diluting in equal vol sterile water, 5% dextrose, or 0.9% NaCl for inj; give through Y-tube or 3-way stopcock; give at ≤2 mg/1 min; do not give rapidly
• To reduce amount of benzyl alcohol to a neonate, dilute with preservative-free sterile water injection (0.4 mg/mL) for IV use

Y-site compatibilities: Acetaminophen, acyclovir, albumin, allopurinol, amifostine, amikacin, amoxicillin, amoxicillin/clavulanate, amphotericin B cholesteryl, amsacrine, atenolol, atracurium, bivalirudin, bleomycin, bumetanide, butorphanol, calcium chloride/gluconate, CARBOplatin, ceFAZolin, cefepime, cefotaxime, cefoTEtan, cefOXitin, cefTAZidime, ceftizoxime, ceftobiprole, cefTRIAXone, cefuroxime, chloramphenicol, chlorproMAZINE, cimetidine, ciprofloxacin, cisatracurium, CISplatin, cladribine, clindamycin, cloNIDine, cyclophosphamide, cycloSPORINE, cytarabine, DACTINomycin, DAPTOmycin, dexamethasone, dexmedetomidine, diltiazem, DOBUTamine, DOCEtaxel, DOPamine, doripenem, DOXOrubicin, DOXOrubicin liposomal, droperidol, enalaprilat, ePHEDrine, EPINEPHrine, epirubicin, eptifibatide, erythromycin, esmolol, etomidate, famotidine, fenoldopam, fentaNYL, filgrastim, fluconazole, fludarabine, fosphenytoin, furosemide, ganciclovir, gatifloxacin, gemcitabine, gentamicin, glycopyrrolate, granisetron, haloperidol, heparin, hydrocortisone, HYDROmorphone, hydrOXYzine, ifosfamide, inamrinone, insulin (regular), irinotecan, isoproterenol, ketorolac, labetalol, lidocaine, linezolid, magnesium sulfate, mannitol, mechlorethamine, melphalan, meropenem, metaraminol, methadone, methotrexate, methyldopa, methylPREDNISolone, metoclopramide, metoprolol, metroNIDAZOLE, micafungin, midazolam, milrinone, minocycline, mitoXANtrone, morphine, mycophenolate, nafcillin, nalbuphine, naloxone, nesiritide, niCARdipine, nitroglycerin, nitroprusside, norepinephrine, octreotide, oxaliplatin, oxytocin, PACLitaxel, palonosetron, pamidronate, pancuronium, PEMEtrexed, pentamidine, PENTobarbital, PHENobarbital, piperacillin, piperacillin-tazobactam, polymyxin B, potassium chloride, propofol, ranitidine,

Side effects: *italics* = common; red = life-threatening

remifentanil, tacrolimus, teniposide, theophylline, thiotepa, ticarcillin, ticarcillinclavulanate, tigecycline, tirofiban, tobramycin, TPN, trastuzumab, trimethobenzamide, trimethoprimsulfamethoxazole, vancomycin, vasopressin, vecuronium, verapamil, vinCRIStine, vinorelbine, voriconazole, zidovudine

SIDE EFFECTS

CNS: *Dizziness, drowsiness,* confusion, headache, anxiety, tremors, stimulation, fatigue, depression, insomnia, hallucinations, weakness, unsteadiness

CV: *Orthostatic hypotension,* ECG changes, tachycardia, hypotension, apnea, cardiac arrest (IV, rapid)

EENT: *Blurred vision,* tinnitus, mydriasis

GI: Constipation, dry mouth, nausea, vomiting, anorexia, diarrhea

INTEG: Rash, dermatitis, itching

MISC: Acidosis

PHARMACOKINETICS

Metabolized by liver; excreted by kidneys; crosses placenta, excreted in breast milk; half-life 42 hr (neonates), 10.5 hr (older child), 12 hr (adult), 91% protein bound

PO: Onset 1 hr, peak 2 hr, duration 12-24 hr

IM: Onset 15-30 min, peak 1-1½ hr, duration 6-8 hr

IV: Onset 5 min, peak 1-1½ hr, duration 6-8 hr

INTERACTIONS

Black Box Warning: Increase: LORazepam effects—CNS depressants, opioids, alcohol, disulfiram

Increase: delirium, sedation—cloZAPine

Increase: LORazepam effect of probenecid, valproate reduce dose by 50%

Decrease: LORazepam effects—oral contraceptives; change dose as needed

Drug/Herb

Increase: CNS depression—chamomile, kava, valerian

Drug/Lab Test

Increase: AST, ALT

NURSING CONSIDERATIONS

Assess:

• **Anxiety:** decrease in anxiety; mental status: mood, sensorium, affect, sleeping pattern, drowsiness, dizziness, suicidal tendencies

Black Box Warning: Coadministration with other CNS depressants (especially opioids) should be avoided; if used together, use lower dose

• Renal/hepatic/blood status if receiving high-dose therapy

• **Physical dependency, withdrawal symptoms:** headache, nausea, vomiting, muscle pain, weakness, tremors, seizures; after long-term, excessive use

• **Beers:** avoid in older adults; may increase cognitive impairment, delirium

• **Pregnancy/breastfeeding:** use only if clearly needed; neonatal withdrawal syndrome may occur; do not breastfeed unless benefits outweigh risk; excreted in breast milk

Evaluate:

• **Therapeutic response:** decreased anxiety, restlessness, insomnia

Teach patient/family:

• That product may be taken with food

• Not to take more than prescribed amount; may be habit forming

• To avoid OTC preparations (cough, cold, hay fever) unless approved by prescriber

• To avoid driving, activities that require alertness since drowsiness may occur

Black Box Warning: To avoid alcohol, other psychotropic medications, opioids unless directed by prescriber; to notify prescriber immediately of trouble breathing, dizziness, coma, or if no response

• Not to discontinue medication abruptly after long-term use, taper

• To rise slowly because fainting may occur, especially among geriatric patients

• That drowsiness may worsen at beginning of treatment

• To report suicidal ideation

• **Pregnancy/breastfeeding:** not to use in pregnancy or breastfeeding; to use contraception while using this product

TREATMENT OF OVERDOSE: Lavage, VS, supportive care, flumazenil

⚠ HIGH ALERT

lorlatinib (Rx)

(lor-la′ti-nib)
Lorbrena
Func. class.: Antineoplastic

USES: Metastatic ALK-positive non–small-cell lung cancer (NSCLC) with disease progression on either alectinib or ceritinib as the first ALK inhibitor for metastatic disease, or disease progression on crizotinib and at least one other ALK inhibitor for metastatic disease

CONTRAINDICATIONS
Hypersensitivity

DOSAGE AND ROUTES
• **Adult: PO** 100 mg daily until disease progression or unacceptable toxicity
Available forms: Tabs 25, 100 mg

losartan (Rx)

(lo-zar′tan)
Cozaar
Func. class.: Antihypertensive
Chem. class.: Angiotensin II receptor (type AT$_1$) antagonist

Do not confuse:
losartan/valsartan
Cozaar/Zocor

ACTION: Blocks the vasoconstrictor and aldosterone-secreting effects of angiotensin II; selectively blocks the binding of angiotensin II to the AT$_1$ receptor found in tissues

USES: Hypertension, alone or in combination; nephropathy in type 2 diabetes; proteinuria; stroke prophylaxis for hypertensive patients with left ventricular hypertrophy
Unlabeled uses: Heart failure

CONTRAINDICATIONS
Hypersensitivity

Black Box Warning: Pregnancy

Precautions: breastfeeding, children, geriatric patients, hypersensitivity to ACE inhibitors, hepatic disease, angioedema, renal artery stenosis, ☞ African descent, hyperkalemia, hypotension

DOSAGE AND ROUTES
Hypertension
• **Adult: PO** 50 mg/day alone or 25 mg/day in combination with diuretic; maintenance 25-100 mg/day
• **Child ≥6 yr: PO** 0.7 mg/kg/day, max 50 mg/day
Hypertension with left ventricular hypertrophy to reduce stroke
• **Adult: PO** 50 mg/day; add hydrochlorothiazide 12.5 mg/day and/or increase losartan to 100 mg/day, then increase hydrochlorothiazide to 25 mg/day
Nephropathy in type 2 diabetic patients/proteinuria
• **Adult: PO** 50 mg/day, may increase to 100 mg/day
Heart failure (unlabeled)
• **Adult: PO** 25-50 mg/day initially, then titrate to max 50-150 mg/day maintenance
Hepatic dose/volume depletion
• **Adult: PO** 25 mg/day as starting dose
• **Child: PO** Don't use in eGFR <30 mL/min/1.73 m^2
Available forms: Tabs 25, 50, 100 mg
Administer:
• Without regard to meals
• If product is compounded into suspension, store in refrigerator and shake well before use
• May use alone or in combination

L

SIDE EFFECTS

CNS: *Dizziness, insomnia,* anxiety, confusion, abnormal dreams, migraine, tremor, vertigo, headache, malaise, depression, fatigue

CV: Angina pectoris, 2nd-degree AV block, cerebrovascular accident, *hypotension,* MI, dysrhythmias

EENT: Blurred vision, burning eyes, conjunctivitis

GI: *Diarrhea, dyspepsia,* anorexia, constipation, dry mouth, flatulence, gastritis, vomiting

GU: Impotence, nocturia, urinary frequency, UTI, renal failure

HEMA: Anemia, thrombocytopenia

INTEG: Alopecia, dermatitis, dry skin, flushing, photosensitivity, rash, pruritus, sweating, angioedema

META: Gout, hyperkalemia, hypoglycemia

MS: Cramps, myalgia, pain, stiffness

RESP: *Cough, upper respiratory infection,* congestion, dyspnea, bronchitis

MISC: Diabetic vascular disease

PHARMACOKINETICS

Peak 1 hr, extensively metabolized, half-life 2 hr, metabolite 6-9 hr, excreted in urine/feces, protein binding 98.7%

INTERACTIONS

Increase: lithium toxicity—lithium; monitor lithium level

Increase: antihypertensive effect—garlic

Increase: hyperkalemia—potassium-sparing diuretics, potassium supplements, ACE inhibitors

Decrease: antihypertensive effect—NSAIDs

Drug/Herb

Decrease: antihypertensive effects—ma huang, black licorice

Drug/Lab Test

Increase: AST, ALT

NURSING CONSIDERATIONS

Assess:

• B/P with position changes, pulse before and periodically during treatment; note rate, rhythm, quality; ✤☞ Black patients should use combination therapy for better control of B/P

• Baselines of renal, hepatic, electrolyte studies before therapy begins and periodically thereafter

• Skin turgor, dryness of mucous membranes for hydration status

• Angioedema: facial swelling, dyspnea, wheezing; may occur rapidly; tongue swelling (rare)

• **HF:** jugular venous distention; edema in feet/legs, weight daily

• **Blood dyscrasias:** thrombocytopenia, anemia (rare)

Black Box Warning: Pregnancy/breast-feeding: assess for pregnancy before starting treatment; do not use in pregnancy; do not breastfeed

Evaluate:

• **Therapeutic response:** decreased B/P, slowing diabetic neuropathy

Teach patient/family:

• To avoid sunlight or to wear sunscreen if in sunlight; that photosensitivity may occur

• To comply with dosage schedule, even if feeling better; not to discontinue abruptly; not to share with others

• To notify prescriber of mouth sores, fever, swelling of hands or feet, irregular heartbeat, chest pain

• That excessive perspiration, dehydration, vomiting, diarrhea may lead to fall in B/P; to consult prescriber if these occur

• That product may cause dizziness, fainting, light-headedness; to avoid hazardous activities until reaction is known

• To rise slowly to sitting or standing position to minimize orthostatic hypotension

Black Box Warning: Pregnancy/breast-feeding: to use contraception while taking this product; not to breastfeed

• To avoid salt substitutes, alcohol, OTC products unless approved by prescriber

---

losartan/
hydrochlorothiazide (Rx)
(loe-SAR-tan/hye-droe-klor-oh-THYE-a-zide)

Hyzaar

Func. class.: Angiotensin II receptor blocker, antihypertensive, diuretic, thiazide

---

USES: Hypertension

CONTRAINDICATIONS
Hypersensitivity to losartan, hydrochlorothiazide, sulfonamide-derived drugs, or any component; use with aliskiren in diabetes mellitus; anuria

Black Box Warning: Pregnancy

DOSAGE AND ROUTES
Adult: PO Losartan 50 mg/hydrochlorothiazide 12.5 mg or losartan 100 mg/hydrochlorothiazide 12.5 mg or losartan 100 mg/hydrochlorothiazide 25 mg once daily; adjust dose base on blood pressure response. Max losartan 100 mg/hydrochlorothiazide 25 mg per day
Available forms: Tabs 50 mg/12.5 mg, 100 mg/12.5 mg, 100 mg/25 mg

---

loteprednol ophthalmic
See Appendix B

---

lovastatin (Rx)
(loh-vah-stat'in)

Altoprev, Mevacor ✦

Func. class.: Antilipemic

Chem. class.: HMG-CoA reductase inhibitor

Do not confuse:
Mevacor/Benicor

ACTION: Inhibits HMG-CoA reductase enzyme, which reduces cholesterol synthesis

USES: As an adjunct for primary hypercholesterolemia (types IIa, IIb), atherosclerosis; heterozygous familial hypercholesterolemia (adolescents)

CONTRAINDICATIONS
Pregnancy, breastfeeding, hypersensitivity, active hepatic disease
Precautions: Children, past hepatic disease, alcoholism, severe acute infections, trauma, hypotension, uncontrolled seizure disorders, severe metabolic disorders, electrolyte imbalances, visual disorder

DOSAGE AND ROUTES
To prevent/treat CAD, hyperlipidemia
• **Adult:** PO 20 mg/day with evening meal; may increase to 20-80 mg/day in single or divided doses at 4-wk intervals, max 80 mg/day; **EXT REL** 20-60 mg/day at bedtime, max 60 mg/day
Heterozygous familial hypercholesterolemia ✦
• **Adolescent 10-17 yr:** PO 10-80 mg with evening meal
Primary prevention of CV disease
• **Adult 40-75 yr with type 1 or 2 diabetes:** PO 40 mg immediate release daily
Secondary prevention of CV disease
• **Adult >75 yr (not candidate for high-intensity use):** PO 40 mg immediate release daily
Renal dose
• **Adult:** PO CCr <30 mg/min, max 20 mg/day unless titrated
Available forms: Tabs 10, 20, 40 mg; ext rel tab 20, 40, 60 mg
Administer:
• In evening with meal; if dose is increased, take with breakfast and evening meal (immediate release); use at bedtime (extended release)
• Altroprev is not equivalent to Mevacor
• Do not crush, chew ext rel tab
• Store in cool environment in airtight, light-resistant container

L

SIDE EFFECTS

CNS: *Dizziness, headache, tremor,* insomnia, paresthesia
EENT: *Blurred vision,* lens opacities
GI: Flatus, nausea, constipation, diarrhea, dyspepsia, abdominal pain, heartburn, hepatic dysfunction, vomiting, acid regurgitation, dry mouth, dysgeusia
HEMA: Thrombocytopenia, hemolytic anemia, leukopenia
INTEG: *Rash, pruritus,* photosensitivity
MS: *Muscle cramps, myalgia,* myositis, rhabdomyolysis; leg, shoulder, or localized pain

PHARMACOKINETICS

PO: Peak 2 hr; peak response 4-6 wk, ext rel peak 14 hr; metabolized in liver (metabolites); highly protein bound; excreted in urine 10%, feces 83%; crosses blood-brain barrier, placenta; excreted in breast milk; half-life 1 hr

INTERACTIONS

Increase: myalgia, myositis, rhabdomyolysis—azole antifungals, clarithromycin, clofibrate, cycloSPORINE, danazol, diltiazem, erythromycin, gemfibrozil, niacin, protease inhibitors, quinupristin-dalfopristin, telithromycin, verapamil; avoid concurrent use
Increase: bleeding—warfarin
Increase: lovastatin effects—diltiazem
Decrease: effects of lovastatin—bile acid sequestrants, exenatide, bosentan
Decrease: lovastatin metabolism, avoid combining with >40 mg/day amiodarone

Drug/Herb
Decrease: effect—pectin, St. John's wort
Increase: adverse reactions—red yeast rice
Drug/Food
• Possible toxicity: grapefruit juice
Increase: levels of lovastatin with food; must be taken with food
Decrease: absorption—oat bran
Drug/Lab Test
Increase: CK, LFTs
Interference: T_3, T_4, T_7, TSH

NURSING CONSIDERATIONS

Assess:
• **Diet:** obtain diet history including fat, cholesterol in diet
• Fasting cholesterol, LDL, HDL, triglycerides periodically during treatment
• Hepatic studies at initiation, 6 wk, 12 wk after initiation or change in dose, periodically thereafter; AST, ALT, LFTs may increase
• Renal function in patients with compromised renal system: BUN, creatinine, I&O ratio
• **Pregnancy/breastfeeding:** not to be used in pregnancy, breastfeeding
Evaluate:
• **Therapeutic response:** decreased triglycerides, sLDL, total cholesterol; increased HDL; slowing CAD
Teach patient/family:
• That blood work, ophthalmic exam will be necessary during treatment
• To report blurred vision, severe GI symptoms, dizziness, headache, muscle pain, weakness
• To use sunscreen or to stay out of the sun to prevent photosensitivity
• That previously prescribed regimen will continue: low-cholesterol diet, exercise program, smoking cessation
• That product should be taken with food; not to crush, chew ext rel product; to take immediate-release product in the AM, PM if used bid; to take ext rel product at bedtime
• Not to use with grapefruit juice, large amounts of alcohol
• To protect product from light and moisture

• **Pregnancy/breastfeeding:** to report suspected pregnancy; not to breastfeed

---

loxapine (Rx)

(lox'a-peen)

Adasuve, Loxapac ✦, Xylac
Func. class.: Antipsychotic, neuroleptic
Chem. class.: Dibenzoxazepine

USES: Schizophrenia, bipolar disorder
Unlabeled uses: Anxiety

CONTRAINDICATIONS
Hypersensitivity, coma

Black Box Warning: Acute bronchospasm, asthma, COPD, emphysema, dementia, requires a specialized care setting

DOSAGE AND ROUTES
• **Adult:** PO 10 mg bid-qid initially, may be rapidly increased depending on severity of condition, maintenance 60-100 mg/day; max 250 mg/day; inhalation powder 10 mg as a single dose in 24 hr
• **Geriatric:** PO 5-10 mg daily-bid, increase q4-7days by 5-10 mg, max 250 mg/day

Available forms: Powder for inhalation 10 mg; capsule 5, 10, 25, 50 mg

---

lubiprostone (Rx)
(loo-bi-pros′tone)
Amitiza
Func. class.: GI agent, miscellaneous

USES: Chronic idiopathic constipation, IBS with constipation, opioid-induced constipation

CONTRAINDICATIONS
Hypersensitivity, known or suspected mechanical GI obstruction

DOSAGE AND ROUTES
Chronic idiopathic constipation
Adult: PO 24 mcg bid
IBS with constipation
Adult: Females ≥18 yr: PO 8 mcg bid
Opioid-induced constipation
Adult: PO 24 mcg bid
Available forms: Capsules 8, 24 mcg

---

luliconazole topical
See Appendix B

---

lumacaftor/ivacaftor (Rx)
(loo-ma-kaf′tor/eye-va-kaf′tor)
Orkambi
Func. class.: Cystic fibrosis agent

USES: Cystic fibrosis

CONTRAINDICATIONS
Hypersensitivity

DOSAGE AND ROUTES
• **Adult/child ≥12 yr:** PO Lumacaftor 400 mg/ivacaftor 250 mg q12h
• **Child ≥2-5 yr <14 kg:** PO Lumacaftor 100 mg/ivacaftor 125-mg granule packet: 1 packet q12h; **≥14 kg:** Lumacaftor 150 mg/ivacaftor 188-mg granule packet: 1 packet q12h
• **Child ≥6-11 yr:** PO Lumacaftor 100 mg/ivacaftor 125-mg tablets: 2 tablets q12h (lumacaftor 200 mg/ivacaftor 250 mg per dose)
Available forms: Tabs 100 mg/125 mg, 200 mg/125 mg; granules 100 mg/125 mg, 150 mg/188 mg

---

lumasiran (Rx)
(loo′ma-sir′an)
Oxlumo
Func. class.: Metabolic disorder agent

USES: Primary hyperoxaluria type 1

CONTRAINDICATIONS
Hypersensitivity, breastfeeding, pregnancy

DOSAGE AND ROUTES
Adults: SUBCUT 3 mg/kg/dose monthly × 3 doses, then 3 mg/kg/dose q3mo
Child/adolescent ≥20 kg: SUBCUT 3 mg/kg/dose monthly × 3 doses, then 3 mg/kg/dose q3mo
Infant/child 10-19 kg: SUBCUT 6 mg/kg/dose monthly × 3 doses, then 6 mg/kg/dose q3mo
Infant/child <10 kg: SUBCUT 6 mg/kg/dose monthly × 3 doses, then 3 mg/kg/dose monthly
Neonates: SUBCUT 6 mg/kg/dose monthly × 3 doses, then 3 mg/kg/dose monthly

---

lumateperone (Rx)
(luma-tep′-erone)
Caplyta
Func. class.: Antipsychotic

USES: Schizophrenia, bipolar depression

CONTRAINDICATIONS
Hypersensitivity

Black Box Warning: Dementia-related psychosis, children, suicidal ideation

DOSAGE AND ROUTES
• **Adult: PO** 42 mg/day
Available forms: Capsules 42 mg

---

lurasidone (Rx)
(loo-ras'i-done)
Latuda
Func. class.: Atypical antipsychotic
Chem. class.: Dopamine-serotonin receptor antagonist derivative

---

ACTION: May modulate central DOPaminergic and serotonergic activity; high affinity for DOPamine-D2 receptors, serotonin 5-HT2A receptors; partial agonist at serotonin 5-HT1A receptor

USES: Schizophrenia, depression associated with bipolar disorder I

CONTRAINDICATIONS
Hypersensitivity
Precautions: Pregnancy, breastfeeding, geriatric patients, abrupt discontinuation, ambient temperature increase, breast cancer, cardiac disease, dehydration, diabetes, ketoacidosis, driving, operating machinery, dysphagia, heart failure, hematologic/hepatic/renal disease, hypotension, hypovolemia, MI, infertility, obesity, Parkinson's disease, seizures, strenuous exercise, stroke, substance abuse, syncope, tardive dyskinesia

Black Box Warning: Dementia: antipsychotics (e.g., lurasidone) not approved for treatment of dementia-related psychosis in geriatric patients; may increase risk of death in this population, children, suicidal ideation

DOSAGE AND ROUTES
Schizophrenia
• **Adult: PO** 40 mg/day, range 40-160 mg/day; for those receiving CYP3A4 inhibitors max 80 mg/day, do not use with strong CYP3A4 inducers/inhibitors
• **Child 13-17 yr: PO** 40 mg daily, may increase to max 80 mg daily
Bipolar Disorder I
• **Adult: PO** 20 mg daily, max 120 mg/day
• Child 10-17 PO 20 mg daily, max 80 mg daily
Hepatic/renal dose
• **Adult: PO** CCr <50 mL/min, hepatic disease CTP A start dose 20 mg/day, max 80 mg/day; hepatic disease CTP B start dose 20 mg/day, max 40 mg/day
Available forms: Tabs 20, 40, 80, 120 mg
Administer:
• Give with meal of ≥350 calories

SIDE EFFECTS
CNS: Agitation, akathisia, anxiety, dizziness, drowsiness, fatigue, hyperthermia, insomnia, dystonic reactions, pseudoparkinsonism, restlessness, seizures, suicidal ideation, syncope, tardive dyskinesia, vertigo
CV: Angina, AV block, bradycardia, hypertension, orthostatic hypotension, sinus tachycardia, stroke
EENT: Blurred vision
ENDO: Diabetes mellitus, ketoacidosis, hyperglycemia, hyperprolactinemia
GI: Abdominal pain, diarrhea, dyspepsia, nausea, vomiting, gastritis, weight gain/loss
GU: Amenorrhea, breast enlargement, dysmenorrhea, impotence, dysuria, renal failure
HEMA: Agranulocytosis, anemia, leukopenia, neutropenia
INTEG: Pruritus, rash
MS: Back pain, dysarthria; rhabdomyolysis (rare)
SYST: Angioedema

PHARMACOKINETICS
99% protein binding; excreted 80% in feces, 9% in urine; elimination half-life

---

18 hr; 9%-19% absorbed; peak 1-3 hr, steady-state 7 days

INTERACTIONS
• Do not use with metoclopramide
Increase: hypertensive risk—antihypertensive
Increase: lurasidone effect—strong CYP3A4 inhibitors; do not use concurrently
Increase: serotonin syndrome, neuroleptic malignant syndrome—SSRIs, SNRIs
Increase: sedation, respiratory depression—other CNS depressants, alcohol, opioids; avoid using together
Decrease: lurasidone effect—CYP3A4 inducers (carbamazepine, rifampin); do not use concurrently

Drug/Herb
Decrease: product effect—St. John's wort; do not use together

Drug/Food
• Do not use with grapefruit, grapefruit juice

NURSING CONSIDERATIONS
Assess:
• **Schizophrenia:** hallucinations, delusions, agitation, social withdrawal; monitor orientation, behavior, mood before and periodically during therapy
• **Temperature regulation:** avoid strenuous activities, excessive heat, dehydration, concomitant anticholinergic medications; risk of hyperthermia
• **Coadministration with other CNS depressants (opioids):** if given together, assess for excessive sedation, slow breathing; avoid concurrent use
• AIMS assessment, thyroid function tests, LFTs, lipid panel, electrolytes
• **EPS:** restlessness, difficulty speaking, loss of balance, pill rolling, masklike face, shuffling gait, rigidity, tremors, muscle spasms; monitor before and periodically during therapy; report tardive dyskinesia immediately

Black Box Warning: Dementia: this product is not approved for geriatric patients with dementia-related psychosis

Black Box Warning: Suicidal ideation/children: avoid use in children; there may be increased risk of suicide in young adults (<24 yr) and children; assess for worsening depression, suicidal thoughts/behaviors; product should be dispensed in small quantities

• Weight gain, hyperglycemia, metabolic changes in diabetes
• **Beers:** avoid in older adults except for schizophrenia, bipolar disorder, or short-term use as an antiemetic for chemotherapy; increased risk of stroke, cognitive decline
• **Pregnancy/breastfeeding:** use only if clearly needed; cautious use in breastfeeding; excretion is unknown

Evaluate:
• **Therapeutic response:** decreasing hallucinations, delusions, agitation, social withdrawal

Teach patient/family:
• About reason for treatment, expected results; not to use grapefruit juice, alcohol
• That lab work will be needed regularly
• To avoid hazardous activities until response is known
• To avoid OTC products unless approved by prescriber; serious reactions may occur
• To report fast heartbeat, extra beats, trouble breathing, sweating, stiffness, thirst, urinating more than usual
• To report EPS symptoms, blood dyscrasias: sore throat, fever, unusual bleeding/bruising

Black Box Warning: Suicidal ideation/children: to be aware of and report immediately any worsening depression, suicidal thoughts/behaviors, hostility, irritability

lurbinectedin (Rx)
(loor'bin-ek'te-din)
Zepzelca
Func. class.: Antineoplastic, alkylating agent

USES: Treatment of metastatic small cell lung cancer with disease progression after platinum-type chemotherapy

CONTRAINDICATIONS
Hypersensitivity

DOSAGE AND ROUTES
Small cell lung cancer, metastatic
• **Adult: IV:** 3.2 mg/m² q21days until disease progression/unacceptable toxicity

luspatercept-aamt (Rx)
(lus-pat'er-sept)
Reblozyl
Func. class.: Hematopoietic

USES:
Anemia in beta thalassemia

DOSAGE AND ROUTES
Anemia in beta thalassemia that requires regular RBC transfusions:
• **Adults: SUBCUT** 1 mg/kg q3wk
Available forms: Injection 25-, 75-mg single-use vials

lusutrombopag (Rx)
(lew-soo-trom'bow-pag)
Mulpleta
Func. class.: Antihemorrhagic

USES: Thrombocytopenia in chronic hepatic disease in patients who are scheduled to undergo a procedure

CONTRAINDICATIONS
Hypersensitivity

DOSAGE AND ROUTES
• **Adult: PO** 3 mg daily × 7 days beginning 8 to 14 days before a scheduled procedure. Schedule the procedure for 2 to 8 days after the last dose
Available forms: Tabs 3 mg

lymphocyte immune globulin (Rx)
Atgam
Func. class.: Immune globulin

USES: Treatment of moderate-to-severe aplastic anemia in those not considered suitable for bone marrow transplantation

CONTRAINDICATIONS
Hypersensitivity to this product or any other equine gamma globulin preparation

Black Box Warning: Anaphylaxis

DOSAGE AND ROUTES
• **Adult/child: IV:** 10 to 20 mg/kg daily for 8 to 14 days, may administer every other day for 7 more doses for a total of 21 doses in 28 days
Available forms: Inj 50 mg/5 mL ampule

---

mafenide topical
See Appendix B

MAGNESIUM SALTS

magnesium chloride (Rx)
(12% mg, 9.8 Eq mg/g)
Chloromag, Slow-Mag
magnesium citrate (OTC)
(16.2% mg, 4.4 mEq mg/g)
Citrate of magnesia, Citroma,
Citromag ✦
magnesium gluconate (OTC)
(5.4% mg, 4.4 mEq mg/g)
Magtrate, Magonate
magnesium oxide (OTC)
(60.3% mg, 49.6 mEq mg/g)
Mag-Ox 400, Uro-Mag
magnesium hydroxide (OTC)
(41.7% mg, 34.3 mEq mg/g)
Dulcolax magnesium tablets,
MOM, Phillips' Milk of Magnesia

⚠ HIGH ALERT

magnesium sulfate (Rx)
(9.9% mg, 8.1 mEq mg/g)
Func. class.: Electrolyte; anticonvulsant; saline laxative, antacid

ACTION: Increases osmotic pressure, draws fluid into colon, neutralizes HCl

USES: Constipation, dyspepsia; bowel preparation before surgery or exam; anticonvulsant for preeclampsia, eclampsia (magnesium sulfate); electrolyte; cardiac glycoside–induced arrhythmias, nutritional supplement

CONTRAINDICATIONS
Hypersensitivity, abdominal pain, nausea/vomiting, obstruction, acute surgical abdomen, rectal bleeding, heart block, myocardial damage

Precautions: Pregnancy (magnesium sulfate), renal/cardiac disease

DOSAGE AND ROUTES
Laxative
• **Adult:** PO (milk of magnesia) 15-60 mL at bedtime
• **Adult/child >12 yr:** PO (magnesium sulfate) 15 g in 8 oz water; PO (concentrated milk of magnesia) 5-30 mL; PO (magnesium citrate) 5-10 oz at bedtime
• **Child 2-12 yr:** PO (Magnesium citrate) 100 mL; (magnesium hydroxide) 15-30 mL
• **Child 2-6 yr:** PO (milk of magnesia) 5-15 mL/day
Prevention of magnesium deficiency (mg of magnesium)
• **Adult/child ≥10 yr:** PO (male) 350-400 mg/day; (female) 280-300 mg/day; (breastfeeding) 335-350 mg/day; (pregnancy) 320 mg/day
• **Child 8-10 yr:** PO 170 mg/day
• **Child 4-7 yr:** PO 120 mg/day
Magnesium sulfate deficiency (mg of magnesium)
• **Adult:** PO 200-400 mg in divided doses tid-qid; IM 1 g q6hr × 4 doses; IV 5 g (severe)
• **Child 6-12 yr:** PO 3-6 mg/kg/day in divided doses tid-qid
Preeclampsia/eclampsia (magnesium sulfate)
• **Adult:** IM/IV 4-5 g IV infusion; with 5 g IM in each gluteus, then 5 g q4hr or 4 g IV INFUSION, then 1-3 g/hr CONT INFUSION, max 30-40 g/24 hr or 20 g/48 hr in severe renal disease
Available forms: Chloride: sus rel tabs 535 mg (64 mg Mg); enteric tabs 833 mg (100 mg Mg); **citrate:** oral sol 240-, 296-, 300-mL bottles (77 mEq/100 mL); **gluconate:** tabs 500 mg; liquid 54 mg/5 mL; **oxide:** tabs 400 mg; caps 140 mg; **hydroxide:** liq 400 mg/5 mL; concentration liq 800 mg/5 mL; chew tabs 300, 600 mg; **sulfate:** 500 mg/mL; premixed infusion 1 g/100 mL, 2 g/100 mL, 4 g/50 mL, 4 g/100 mL, 20 g/500 mL, 40 g/1000 mL

M

Side effects: *italics* = common; red = life-threatening

Administer:

PO route

- With 8 oz water
- Refrigerate magnesium citrate before giving
- Shake susp before using as antacid at least 2 hr after meals
- Tablets should be chewed thoroughly before patient swallows; give 4 oz of water afterward
- **Laxative:** give on empty stomach with full glass of liquid, do not give at bedtime

IM route (magnesium sulfate)

- Give deeply in gluteal site

IV route (magnesium sulfate)

- Only when calcium gluconate is available for magnesium toxicity

Direct IV route

- Dilute 50% sol to ≤20%, give at ≤150 mg/min

Continuous IV INFUSION route

- May dilute to 20% sol, infuse over 3 hr
- IV at less than 125 mg/kg/hr; circulatory collapse may occur; use INFUSION pump

Y-site compatibilities: Acyclovir, aldesleukin, alemtuzumab, alfentanil, amifostine, amikacin, aminocaproic acid, argatroban, arsenic trioxide, ascorbic acid injection, asparaginase, atenolol, atosiban, atracurium, atropine, azithromycin, aztreonam, benztropine, bivalirudin, bleomycin, bumetanide, buprenorphine, butorphanol, calcium gluconate, cangrelor, CARBOplatin, carmustine, caspofungin, cefotaxime, cefoTEtan, cefOXitin, cefTAZidime, ceftizoxime, cephapirin, chloramphenicol, chlorproMAZINE, cimetidine, cisatracurium, CISplatin, clindamycin, cloNIDine, codeine, cyanocobalamin, cyclophosphamide, cytarabine, DACTINomycin, DAPTOmycin, DAUNOrubicin liposome, DAUNOrubicin, dexmedetomidine, dexrazoxane, digoxin, diltiaZEM, dimenhyDRINATE, diphenhydrAMINE, DOBUTamine, DOCEtaxel, dolasetron, DOPamine, doripenem, doxacurium chloride, DOXOrubicin liposomal, doxycycline, enalaprilat, ePHEDrine, EPINEPHrine, epoetin alfa, eptifibatide, ertapenem, esmolol, etoposide, etoposide phosphate, famotidine, fenoldopam, fentaNYL, fluconazole, fludarabine, fluorouracil, folic acid (as sodium salt), foscarnet, gallium, gatifloxacin, gemcitabine, gemtuzumab, gentamicin, glycopyrrolate, granisetron, heparin, HYDROmorphone, hydrOXYzine, IDArubicin, ifosfamide, imipenem-cilastatin, insulin (regular), irinotecan, isoproterenol, kanamycin, ketamine, ketorolac, labetalol, lactated Ringer's injection, lepirudin, leucovorin, lidocaine, linezolid, LORazepam, mannitol, mechlorethamine, mesna, metaraminol, methotrexate, methyldopate, metoclopramide, metoprolol, metroNIDAZOLE, micafungin, midazolam, milrinone, minocycline, mitoMYcin, mitoXANTRONE, mivacurium, morphine, moxifloxacin, multiple vitamins injection, mycophenolate mofetil, nafcillin, nalbuphine, nesiritide, netilmicin, niCARdipine, nitroglycerin, nitroprusside, norepinephrine, octreotide, ondansetron, oxaliplatin, oxytocin, PACLitaxel, palonosetron, pamidronate, pancuronium, papaverine, PEMEtrexed, penicillin G potassium/sodium, pentazocine, PENTobarbital, PHENobarbital, phentolamine, phenylephrine, piperacillin, piperacillin tazobactam, polymyxin B, potassium acetate/chloride, procainamide, prochlorperazine, promethazine, propranolol, protamine, pyridoxine, quiNIDine, quinupristin-dalfopristin, raNITIdine, remifentanil, Ringer's injection, riTUXimab, rocuronium, sargramostim, sodium acetate/bicarbonate, succinylcholine, SUFentanil, tacrolimus, telavancin, teniposide, theophylline, thiamine, thiotepa, ticarcillin, ticarcillin-clavulanate, tigecycline, tirofiban, TNA (3-in-1), tobramycin, tolazoline, topotecan, TPN (2-in-1), trastuzumab, urokinase, vancomycin, vasopressin, vecuronium, verapamil, vinBLAStine, vinCRIStine, vinorelbine, vitamin B complex with C, voriconazole, zoledronic acid

SIDE EFFECTS

CNS: Muscle weakness, flushing, sweating, confusion, sedation, depressed reflexes, flaccid paralysis, hypothermia

CV: Hypotension, heart block, circulatory collapse, vasodilation
GI: *Nausea, vomiting, anorexia, cramps,* diarrhea
HEMA: Prolonged bleeding time
META: Electrolyte, fluid imbalances
RESP: Respiratory depression/paralysis

PHARMACOKINETICS
PO: Onset 1-2 hr
IM: Onset 1 hr, duration 4 hr
IV: Duration ½ hr
Excreted by kidney, effective anticonvulsant serum levels 2.5-7.5 mEq/L

INTERACTIONS
Increase: effect of neuromuscular blockers
Increase: hypotension—antihypertensives, calcium channel blockers
Decrease: absorption of tetracyclines, fluoroquinolones, nitrofurantoin
Decrease: effect of digoxin

NURSING CONSIDERATIONS
Assess:
• **Laxative:** cause of constipation; lack of fluids, bulk, exercise; cramping, rectal bleeding, nausea, vomiting; product should be discontinued
• **Eclampsia:** seizure precautions, B/P, ECG (magnesium sulfate); magnesium toxicity: thirst, confusion, decrease in reflexes; I&O ratio; check for decrease in urinary output
• **Pregnancy/breastfeeding:** use only if clearly needed (chloride), contraindicated in labor, toxemia during 2 hr prior to delivery, appears in breast milk
Evaluate:
• **Therapeutic response:** decreased constipation, absence of seizures (eclampsia), normal serum calcium levels
Teach patient/family:
• Not to use laxatives for long-term therapy because bowel tone will be lost
• That chilling improves taste of magnesium citrate
• To shake suspension well
• Not to give at bedtime as a laxative, may interfere with sleep; that milk of magnesia is usually given at bedtime

• To give citrus fruit after administering to counteract unpleasant taste
• About reason for product, expected results

---

mannitol (Rx)
(man´i-tole)
Osmitrol, Resectisol
Func. class.: Diuretic, osmotic; GU irrigant
Chem. class.: Hexahydric alcohol

ACTION: Acts by increasing osmolarity of glomerular filtrate, which inhibits reabsorption of water and electrolytes and increases urinary output

USES: Edema; promotion of systemic diuresis in cerebral edema; decrease in intraocular/intracranial pressure; improved renal function in acute renal failure, chemical poisoning, urinary bladder irrigation, kidney transplant

CONTRAINDICATIONS
Active intracranial bleeding, hypersensitivity, anuria, severe pulmonary congestion, edema, severe dehydration, progressive heart/renal failure, acute MI, aneurysm, stroke
Precautions: Pregnancy, breastfeeding, geriatric patients, dehydration, severe renal disease, HF, electrolyte imbalances

Black Box Warning: Acute bronchospasm (inhalation test kit), asthma

DOSAGE AND ROUTES
• **Test dose:** Administer a test dose to patients with marked oliguria or suspected inadequate renal function to establish renal response before therapy is initiated.
• A response is considered adequate if at least 30-50 mL of urine per hour is excreted over the next 2-3 hr
• If an adequate response is not attained, a second test dose may be given
• If a satisfactory response is not obtained after the second test dose, reevaluate patient, and mannitol should not be used

---

• **Rate of administration:** Test dose in adults and children >12 yr: Infuse over a period of 3-5 min to produce urine flow of ≥30-50 mL/hr

• Treatment of oliguria in adults: Infuse over 90 min to several hours

• Cerebral or ocular edema in children >12 yr: Usually infuse over 30-60 min

• Reduction of intracranial or IOP in adults: Usually infuse over 30-60 min

• Edema and ascites in adults and children >12 yr: Has been infused over 2-6 hr

• **Transurethral irrigation:** Sorbitol-mannitol irrigation solution is for urologic irrigation only; do *not* use for injection

• Administer only by transurethral instillation using appropriate and disposable urologic instrumentation

• Placing the flexible irrigation container >60 cm above the operating table may increase intravascular absorption of irrigation solution

Oliguric acute renal failure

• **Test dose: Children >12 yr:** IV 0.2 g/kg or 6 g/m² as a single dose

• **Therapeutic purposes: Children >12 yr:** IV 2 g/kg or 60 g/m²

Cerebral or ocular edema

• **Children >12 yr:** IV 2 g/kg or 60 g/m² administered as a 15% or 20% solution

Urinary excretion of toxins

• **Children >12 yr:** IV 2 g/kg or 60 g/m² administered as a 5% or 10% solution as needed

Edema and ascites

• **Children >12 yr:** IV 2 g/kg or 60 g/m² administered as a 15% or 20% solution

General dosage

• **Adult/child ≥12 yr:** IV 20-100 g 25% solution q24h

Test dose: Adult: IV 0.2 g/kg or 12.5 g infused as a 15% or 20% solution (usually 100 or 75 mL of a 15% or 20% solution, respectively)

Oliguric acute renal failure—prevention

• **Adult:** IV 50-100 g as a 5%, 10%, or 15% solution. Usually, a concentrated solution is given and then followed by a 5% or 10% solution

Treatment of oliguria

• **Adult:** IV 100 g infused as a 15% or 20% solution

Management of nephrotoxicity associated with amphotericin B

• **Adult:** IV 12.5 g given immediately prior to and after each dose of amphotericin B

Reduction of intracranial pressure (ICP)

• **Adult:** IV 0.25 g/kg given q6-8h or 1.5-2 g/kg infused as a 15%, 20%, or 25% solution

Reduction of intraocular pressure (IOP)

• **Adult:** IV 1.5-2 g/kg infused as a 15%, 20%, or 25% solution

Urinary excretion of toxins

• **Adult:** IV Maintain a urinary output of >100 mL/hr, but preferably 500 mL/hr, and a positive fluid balance of 1-2 L; initially, 25 g, followed by infusion of a solution at a rate that will maintain a urinary output of ≥100 mL/hr

Transurethral prostatic resection

• **Urogenital irrigation** Administer a sufficient volume of sorbitol-mannitol irrigation solution; volume determined at the discretion of clinician

Hyperuricemia (unlabeled)

• **Adult:** IV 50 g/m² per 24 hr

Available forms: Inj 5%, 10%, 15%, 20%, 25%; GU irrigation: 5%; inhalation capsule challenge kit

Administer:

Intermittent/continuous IV route

• Precipitate may occur with PVC

• Change IV set q24hr

• May warm solution to dissolve crystals

• In 15%-25% sol with filter; rapid infusion may worsen HF; warm in hot water, shake to dissolve, use in-line filter 0.2-0.5 micron; do not give as direct injection; to redissolve, run bottle under hot water and shake vigorously; cool to body temperature before using

• Run at 30-50 mL/hr in oliguria; 30-60 min in ICP; increased over 30 min in intraocular pressure; 60-90 min after surgery

• Give 20 mEq NaCL/L of product solution if blood is given concurrently

• Assess site for pain, redness, inflammation often during infusion

SIDE EFFECTS
CNS: *Dizziness, headache,* confusion

CV: Edema, thrombophlebitis, hypo/hypertension, tachycardia, angina-like chest pains, fever, chills, HF, circulatory overload

ELECT: Fluid, electrolyte imbalances, electrolyte loss, dehydration, hypo/hyperkalemia

GI: *Nausea, vomiting,* dry mouth

GU: Marked diuresis, urinary retention, thirst

INTEG: Injection-site reaction

PHARMACOKINETICS

IV: Onset 1-3 hr for diuresis, ½-1 hr for intraocular pressure, 15 min for cerebrospinal fluid; duration 4-8 hr for intraocular pressure, 3-8 hr for cerebrospinal fluid; excreted in urine; half-life 100 min

INTERACTIONS

Increase: elimination of mannitol—lithium; monitor lithium level

Increase: excretion of imipramine

Increase: hypokalemia—cardiac glycosides

Increase or Decrease: sodium, potassium, magnesium

Drug/Lab Test

Interference: inorganic phosphorus, ethylene glycol

NURSING CONSIDERATIONS
Assess:

• Monitor I&O, B/P, pulse hourly; report decreasing urine output; monitor weight, **electrolytes:** potassium, sodium, chloride daily; BUN, serum creatinine daily, blood pH, PAP, CVP, ABGs, CBC

• Use urinary catheter in those who are comatose; I&O must be precise

• **Metabolic acidosis:** drowsiness, restlessness

• **Hypokalemia:** postural hypotension, malaise, fatigue, tachycardia, leg cramps, weakness, or hyperkalemia

• Rashes, temperature daily

• **CNS toxicity:** Confusion, lethargy, coma; risk factors: hyponatremia, impaired renal function, hyperosmolarity, high mannitol level

• **Fluid shift/dehydration:** Hydration including skin turgor, thirst, dry mucous membranes; provide adequate fluids, mouth care frequently; assess for HF, fluid electrolyte shifts, circulatory overload, (dyspnea, respiratory congestion, dry mouth)

• Blurred vision, pain in eyes before, during treatment **(increased intraocular pressure);** neurologic checks, intracranial pressure during treatment **(increased intracranial pressure)**

• **Pregnancy/breastfeeding:** use only if clearly needed; cautious use in breastfeeding, unknown if excreted in breast milk

Black Box Warning: Bronchospasm/asthma (inhalation test kit): test for bronchial hyperresponsiveness should not be performed in any person with asthma or baseline pulmonary function test FEV1 <1-1.5 liters or <70% of predicted values

• **Beers:** use with caution in older adults; may cause or exacerbate SIADH

Evaluate:

• **Therapeutic response:** improvement in edema of feet, legs, sacral area daily if medication being used with HF; decreased intraocular pressure, prevention of hypokalemia, increased excretion of toxic substances; decreased ICP

Teach patient/family:

• To rise slowly from lying or sitting position

• About the reason for, method of treatment

• To report signs of electrolyte imbalance, confusion, pain at injection site, hearing loss, blurred vision

TREATMENT OF OVERDOSE:
Discontinue infusion; correct fluid, electrolyte imbalances; hemodialysis; monitor hydration, CV status, renal function including output/serum creatinine

⚠ HIGH ALERT

maraviroc (Rx)
(mah-rav′er-rock)

Celsentri ✦, Selzentry
Func. class.: Antiretroviral
Chem. class.: Fusion inhibitor,
CCR5-receptor antagonist

ACTION: Interferes with entry into HIV-1 by inhibiting the fusion of the virus and the cell membrane

USES: CCR5-tropic HIV in combination with other antiretroviral agents for treating experienced patients

CONTRAINDICATIONS
Hypersensitivity, dialysis, renal impairment
Precautions: Pregnancy, ⚲ Asian patients, breastfeeding, renal/hepatic/cardiac disease, electrolyte imbalance, dehydration, immune reconstitution syndrome, infection, MI, orthostatic hypotension, children, geriatric patients, Graves' disease, Guillain-Barré syndrome, polymyositis, fever, serious rash

Black Box Warning: Hepatotoxicity

DOSAGE AND ROUTES
Those not taking CYP3A inhibitors/inducers:
Adult/adolescent: PO 300 mg bid
Those taking CYP3A4 inhibitors with/without a CYP3A inducer
• Adult/adolescent ≥16 yr: **PO** 150 mg bid
Those taking CYP3A4 inducers without a strong CYP3A inhibitor
• Adult/adolescent ≥16 yr: **PO** 600 mg bid
Available forms: Tabs 25, 75, 150, 300 mg; oral solution 20 mg/mL
Administer:
• May give without regard to meals, with 8 oz water; swallow whole; do not crush, chew, break
• Do not double missed dose, take next dose as soon as remembered
• Store at room temperature

SIDE EFFECTS
CV: MI, cardiac ischemia, orthostatic hypotension
CNS: Dizziness, depression, viral meningitis, disturbances in consciousness, peripheral neuropathy, paresthesia, dysesthesia, fever
EENT: Gingival hyperplasia, visual changes
GI: Diarrhea, constipation, dyspepsia, CDAD, hepatotoxicity
INTEG: Rash, urticaria, pruritus, folliculitis
MS: Joint pain, leg pain, muscle cramps
RESP: Cough, upper respiratory tract infection, sinusitis, bronchitis, pneumonia, bronchospasm, obstruction, dyspnea
SYST: Herpes virus, lipodystrophy, malignancy

PHARMACOKINETICS
Metabolized by P450 system; CYP3A metabolism; excreted 20% urine, 76% feces; protein binding 76%; terminal half-life 14-18 hr

INTERACTIONS
Increase: maraviroc levels—CYP3A inhibitors (amiodarone, aprepitant, chloramphenicol, clarithromycin, conivaptan, cycloSPORINE, dalfopristin, danazol, diltiaZEM, erythromycin, estradiol, fluconazole, fluvoxaMINE, imatinib, isoniazid, itraconazole, ketoconazole, miconazole, nefazodone, niCARdipine, propoxyphene, RU-486, tamoxifen, telithromycin, troleandomycin, verapamil, voriconazole, zafirlukast); reduce dose
Decrease: maraviroc levels—CYP3A4 inducers (efavirenz, aminoglutethimide, barbiturates, bexarotene, bosentan, carBAMazepine, dexamethasone, griseofulvin, modafinil, nafcillin, OXcarbazepine, phenytoin, fosphenytoin, rifabutin, rifAMPin, rifapentine, topiramate, tipranavir); increase dose
Drug/Herb
• Decreased maraviroc effect: St. John's wort
Drug/Food
• High-fat meal decreases absorption 33%

Drug/Lab Test
Increase: AST, ALT, bilirubin, amylase, lipase, CK
Decrease: ANC

NURSING CONSIDERATIONS
Assess:
• **HIV:** CD4, T-cell count, plasma HIV RNA, CCR5-tropic HIV-1; assess for changes in symptoms, other infections during treatment
• Severe renal disease (ESRD CCr <30 mL/min): for those taking CYP3A inhibitors/inducers and with severe renal disease, drug is contraindicated
• Bowel pattern before, during treatment
• **Allergies:** skin eruptions, rash, urticaria, itching; discontinue product

Black Box Warning: **Hepatotoxicity:** dark urine, vomiting, abdominal pain; yellowing of skin, eyes; hepatomegaly; discontinue product, monitor LFTs

• **Serious skin rash (Stevens-Johnson syndrome, toxic epidermal necrolysis, DRESS):** assess for serious rash; if symptoms develop, discontinue product immediately, provide supportive treatment
• **Pregnancy/breastfeeding:** provide during pregnancy in those who are HIV positive; avoid breastfeeding to reduce risk of HIV transmission; register pregnant patient with Antiretroviral Pregnancy Registry, 800-258-4263
Evaluate:
• **Therapeutic response:** improvement in CD4, viral load, T-cell count
Teach patient/family:
• To take as prescribed; if dose is missed, to take as soon as remembered up to 1 hr before next dose; not to double dose; that product does not cure condition; should not be shared with others
• Not to stop product without approval of prescriber
• That product does not cure infection, just controls symptoms and does not prevent infecting others
• To report sore throat, fever, fatigue **(may indicate superinfection)**; yellow skin/eyes, abdominal pain, vomiting, dark urine, nausea **(hepatitis)**; itching, SOB **(allergic reaction)**
• That product must be taken in equal intervals around the clock to maintain blood levels for duration of therapy
• To avoid all OTC products unless approved by prescriber
• To avoid driving, other hazardous activities until reaction is known; that dizziness may occur
• To make position changes slowly to prevent postural hypotension
• To notify prescriber if pregnancy is planned or suspected; not to breastfeed

mebendazole (Rx)
(me-ben′da-zole)
Emverm, Vermox ♣
Func. class.: Anthelmintic

USES: Broad spectrum to anthelmintic activity, including Ancylostoma duodenale (hookworm), Ascaris lumbricoides (roundworm), Enterobius vermicularis (pinworm), Necator americanus (hookworm), Trichuris trichiura (large tapeworm)

DOSAGE AND ROUTES
Trichuriasis (whipworm infection) or ascariasis (roundworm infection) or mixed infections with these parasites
• **Adults/child 2-17 yr: PO** 500 mg as a single dose or 100 mg bid × 3 days. If not cured 3 wk after treatment, a second course of therapy is recommended
Enterobiasis (pinworm infection):
• **Adults/child 2-17 yr: PO** 100 mg in a single dose; repeat dose in 2 wk
Hookworm infection: Adults/child 2-17 yr: PO 500 mg as a single dose or 100 mg bid × 3 days. If not cured 3 wk after treatment, a second course of therapy is recommended
Available forms: Chewable tablets 100 mg

maribavir (Rx)
Increlex
Func. class.: Antiviral-kinase inhibitor

Side effects: *italics* = common; red = life-threatening

USES: Posttransplant CMV infection/disease

DOSAGE AND ROUTES
• **Adult/child:** SUBCUT ≥12 yr and older, ≥35 kg: 400 mg (2 tablets) bid
Available forms: Tabs 200 mg

---

mecasermin (Rx)
Increlex
Func. class.: Biologic response modifier; insulin-like growth factor

---

USES: Growth failure in children with severe primary insulin-like growth factor-1 (IGF-1) deficiency (primary IGFD) or with growth hormone (GH) gene deletion who have developed neutralizing antibodies to GH

CONTRAINDICATIONS
Hypersensitivity, benzyl alcohol, closed epiphyses, active/suspected neoplasia, IV use

DOSAGE AND ROUTES
• **Child ≥2 yr:** SUBCUT 0.04-0.08 mg/kg (40-80 mcg/kg) bid; if well tolerated for 1 wk, may increase by 0.04 mg/kg/dose, max 0.12 mg/kg bid

---

meclizine (OTC, Rx)
(mek′li-zeen)
Antivert, Bonine
Func. class.: Antiemetic, antihistamine, anticholinergic
Chem. class.: H$_1$-receptor antagonist, piperazine derivative

---

Do not confuse:
Antivert/Axert

ACTION: Suppresses vestibular end-organ receptors and inhibits activation of cholinergic pathways

USES: Vertigo, motion sickness

CONTRAINDICATIONS:
Hypersensitivity to cyclizines
Precautions: Pregnancy, breastfeeding, children, geriatric patients, closed-angle glaucoma, prostatic hypertrophy, hepatic/renal disease, urinary retention, GI obstruction, contact lenses

DOSAGE AND ROUTES
Vertigo
• **Adult/adolescent:** PO 25-100 mg/day in divided doses
Motion sickness
• **Adult/adolescent:** PO 25-50 mg 1 hr before traveling, repeat dose q24hr prn
Available forms: Tablets 12.5, 25, 50 mg; chewable tablets 25 mg; ODT 25 mg
Administer:
PO route
• May give without regard to food
• **Chew tab:** give without regard to water or may be swallowed whole with water
• Lowest possible dose for geriatric patients; anticholinergic effects

SIDE EFFECTS
CNS: *Drowsiness,* fatigue
EENT: Blurred vision
GI: Dry mouth

PHARMACOKINETICS
PO: Onset 1 hr, duration 8-24 hr, half-life 6 hr

INTERACTIONS
Increase: sedation—CYP2D6, inhibitors
Increase: anticholinergic effects—other antihistamines, atropine, antidepressants, phenothiazines
Increase: effect of alcohol, opioids, other CNS depressants
Drug/Lab Test
False negative: allergy skin testing (allergen extracts)

NURSING CONSIDERATIONS
Assess:
• **Vertigo/motion sickness:** nausea, vomiting after 1 hr; assess vertigo periodically
• **Signs of toxicity:** CNS depression, constipation; consider other causes of symptoms; may mask symptoms of other diseases, such as brain tumor, intestinal obstruction

• For urinary disease obstruction, decreased urinary output; may exacerbate symptoms; monitor urinary output
• Observe for drowsiness, dizziness, level of consciousness
• **Pregnancy/breastfeeding:** use only if needed; occasional doses should not pose a risk in breastfeeding
• **Beers:** use caution in older adults; higher risk of anticholinergic effects

Evaluate:
• **Therapeutic response:** absence of dizziness, vomiting in motion sickness; decreased vertigo

Teach patient/family:
• That a false-negative result may occur with skin testing for allergies; that these procedures should not be scheduled for ≤4 days after discontinuing use
• To avoid hazardous activities, activities requiring alertness because dizziness may occur; to request assistance with ambulation
• To avoid alcohol, other depressants; not to breastfeed; to report severe side effects
• To use sugarless gum, frequent sips of water for dry mouth
• **Motion sickness prophylaxis:** to take ≥1 hr before event that may cause motion sickness

---

medroxyPROGESTER-one (Rx)

(me-drox′ee-proe-jess′te-rone)
Depo-Provera, Depo-SubQ Provera 104, Medroxy ♣, Proclim ♣, Provera
Func. class.: Antineoplastic, hormone, contraceptive
Chem. class.: Progesterone derivative

Do not confuse:
medroxyPROGESTERone/
methylPREDNISolone
Provera/Proscar/Prozac

ACTION: Inhibits secretion of pituitary gonadotropins, which prevents follicular maturation and ovulation; antineoplastic action against endometrial cancer

USES: Uterine bleeding (abnormal); secondary amenorrhea; prevention of endometrial changes associated with estrogen replacement therapy (ERT); contraceptive

CONTRAINDICATIONS

Pregnancy, hypersensitivity, reproductive cancer, genital bleeding (abnormal, undiagnosed), missed abortion, stroke, cerebrovascular disease, cervical cancer, hepatic disease, uterine/vaginal cancer

Black Box Warning: Breast cancer, MI, stroke, thromboembolic disease, thrombophlebitis

Precautions: Breastfeeding, hypertension, asthma, blood dyscrasias, gallbladder disease, HF, diabetes mellitus, bone disease, depression, migraine headache, seizure disorders, renal/hepatic disease, family history of cancer of breast or reproductive tract, bone mineral density loss, ocular disorders, AIDS/HIV, alcoholism, children, hyperlipidemia, cardiac disease

Black Box Warning: Dementia, osteoporosis

DOSAGE AND ROUTES
Secondary amenorrhea
• **Adult: PO** 5-10 mg/day × 5-10 days, start during any time of menstrual cycle
Uterine bleeding
• **Adult: PO** 5-10 mg/day × 5-10 days starting on 16th or 21st day of menstrual cycle
With ERT
• **Adult: PO** 5-10 mg daily × 10-14 or more days/mo (sequential estrogen); 2.5-5 mg daily (continuous estrogen)
Contraceptive
• **Adult (women): IM** (contraceptive inj) 150 mg (Depo-Provera) q13wk; **SUBCUT** (depot SUBCUT; Depo-SubQ Provera 104 inj) 104 mg q12-14 wk, give first dose during the first 5 days of menstrual period, only within the first 5 days postpartum (no breastfeeding), only at 6th postpartum wk (breastfeeding)

Side effects: *italics* = common; red = life-threatening

Endometriosis pain
• **Adult: SUBCUT** 104 mg q12-14wk; begin on day 5 of normal menses; avoid use >2 yr

Hot flashes/symptoms of menopause (unlabeled)
• **Adult (female): PO** 20 mg/day; **IM** 150 mg monthly

Available forms: Tabs 2.5, 5, 10 mg; inj susp, 104 mg/0.65 mL; 150, 400 mg/mL

Administer:
• Store in dark area

PO route
• Give without regard to food
• Take missed dose as soon as possible unless close to next dose

IM route
• Visually inspect for particulate matter or discoloration before use

Depo-Provera contraceptive injection suspension
• IM only, *never* IV; use only 150 mg/mL vial
• Instruct patient on risks and warnings associated with hormonal contraceptives (see Patient Information)
• The possibility of pregnancy should be excluded before giving the first dose of medroxyPROGESTERone or whenever >14 wk has passed since the last dose
• Do not dilute
• Shake vigorously immediately before administration
• Inject deeply into the gluteal or deltoid muscle; aspirate before injection to avoid injection into a blood vessel

Depo-Provera sterile aqueous suspension, preserved
• IM only, *never* IV
• Instruct patient on risks and warnings associated with progestin use (see Patient Information)
• Shake vigorously immediately before use
• When multidose vials are used, take special care to prevent contamination
• Inject deeply into the gluteal or deltoid muscle; aspirate before injection

SUBCUT route
Depo-SubQ Provera 104 contraceptive injection suspension only
• For subcut only, *never* give IM or IV
• Instruct patient on risks and warnings associated with hormonal contraceptives (see Patient Information)
• Shake vigorously for at least 1 min before use
• Inject the entire contents of the pre-filled syringe subcut into the anterior thigh or abdomen, avoiding bony areas and the umbilicus; press lightly on the injection site with a clean cotton pad for a few seconds; do not rub the area

SIDE EFFECTS
CNS: Dizziness, *headache,* migraines, depression, fatigue, nervousness
CV: Thrombophlebitis, edema, thromboembolism, stroke, PE, MI
GI: *Nausea, increased weight, abdominal pain*
GU: *Amenorrhea,* cervical erosion, breakthrough bleeding, dysmenorrhea, vaginal candidiasis, breast changes, vaginitis
INTEG: Acne, hirsutism, alopecia, injection-site reaction
META: Hyperglycemia
MS: Decreased bone density
SYST: Angioedema, anaphylaxis, breast cancer

PHARMACOKINETICS
PO: Duration 3-5 days; **IM** duration 3-4 mo; excreted in urine and feces, breast milk; metabolized in liver, half-life 14.5 hr

INTERACTIONS
Decrease: medroxyPROGESTERone action—strong CYP3A4 inducers (carBAMazepine, phenytoin, rifAMPin, rifabutin, PHENobarbital); avoid concurrent use
Increase: medroxyPROGESTERone level—strong CYP3A4 inhibitors (clarithromycin, ketoconazole, itraconazole, atazanavir, indinavir, ritonavir, voriconazole), avoid using together
Increase or Decrease: medroxyPROGESTERone levels—NNRTIs, protease inhibitors; may diminish progestin level; to provide contraception use nonhormonal method
Decrease: bone mineral density—anticoagulants, corticosteroids
Decrease: contraception—carBAMazepine, phenytoin, rifAMPin, rifabutin;

avoid concurrent use, or use additional nonhormonal method of contraception
Drug/Lab Test
Increase: LFTs, HDL, triglycerides, coagulation tests
Decrease: GTT
Drug/Herb
Decreased levels—St. John's wort; avoid concurrent use

NURSING CONSIDERATIONS
Assess:
• **Menstrual history:** duration of menses, bleeding, spotting, age at menarche, regularity; start on any day in those with amenorrhea, or on day 16 or 21 in dysfunctional bleeding
• Pelvic exam, Pap smear, pregnancy test before treatment, periodically
• **Severe allergic reaction, angioedema;** have EPINEPHrine and resuscitative equipment available
• Weight daily; notify prescriber of weekly weight gain >5 lb; bone mineral density
• B/P at beginning of treatment and periodically
• Hepatic studies: ALT, AST, bilirubin baseline and periodically during long-term therapy; triglycerides, caution if preexisting elevation, product may exacerbate levels
• Mental status: affect, mood, behavioral changes, depression

Black Box Warning: This product should not be given to those with breast cancer, MI, stroke, thromboembolic disorders; assess for these conditions before using

• **Bone mineral density loss:** those taking anticoagulants, corticosteroids with Depo-Provera or Depo-SubQ Provera are at greater risk

Black Box Warning: Use of product shown to increase dementia in women ≥65 yr old; use may increase osteoporosis in long-term treatment; those who smoke also at greater risk; adequate calcium and vit D should be taken

• **Ectopic pregnancy:** severe abdominal pain may indicate ectopic pregnancy if patient is pregnant

Evaluate:
• **Therapeutic response:** decreased abnormal uterine bleeding, absence of amenorrhea
Teach patient/family:
• To take with food if nausea occurs
• To have complete physical exam, including reproductive exam, yearly
• To avoid sunlight or to use sunscreen; photosensitivity can occur
• To report breast lumps, vaginal bleeding, edema, jaundice, dark urine, clay-colored stools, dyspnea, headache, blurred vision, abdominal pain, sudden change in speech/coordination, numbness or stiffness in legs, chest pain; males to report impotence, gynecomastia immediately
• That product doesn't protect against sexually transmitted diseases, including HIV
• That injection (subcut) must be given q3mo for contraception; missing dose may lead to pregnancy

Black Box Warning: Long-term use decreases bone density; exercise, calcium, vitamin D, supplements can help lessen osteoporosis

• Review package insert with patient; patient must understand all possible adverse reactions
• **Pregnancy/breastfeeding:** not to use in pregnancy; to report suspected pregnancy; that fertility returns 6-12 mo after discontinuing; not to breastfeed

mefloquine (Rx)
Func. class.: Antimalarial

USES:
Malaria

DOSAGE AND ROUTES
Malaria:
• **Adults:** PO 1250-mg single dose or 750 mg then 500 mg at 6-12 hours after initial dose
• **Infants, children, and adolescents 6 mo to 17 yr:** PO 20-25 mg/kg/dose (max: 1250 mg/dose) single dose or 15 mg/kg/

dose (max: 750 mg/dose) then 10 mg/kg/dose (max: 500 mg/dose) at 6-12 hours after initial dose
Available forms: Tablet 25 mg

⚠ HIGH ALERT

megestrol (Rx)

(me-jess′trole)
Megace ✦
Func. class.: Antineoplastic hormone
Chem. class.: Progestin

ACTION: Inhibits pituitary and adrenal function

USES: Breast, endometrial cancer; to treat cachexia, anorexia, weight loss with AIDS
Unlabeled uses: Hot flashes, endometriosis

CONTRAINDICATIONS
Pregnancy, hypersensitivity, breastfeeding
Precautions: Diabetes, thrombosis, adrenal insufficiency

DOSAGE AND ROUTES
Endometrial carcinoma (palliative)
• **Adult: PO** 40-320 mg/day in divided doses
Anorexia, cachexia, severe weight loss in AIDS
• **Adult: PO** (oral suspension) 400-800 mg daily; 625 mg (5-mL concentrated oral suspension) daily
Breast carcinoma (palliative)
• **Adult: PO** 40 mg qid or 160 mg/day (tablets)
Hot flashes (unlabeled)
• **Adult: PO** 20 mg bid
Available forms: Tabs 20, 40, 160 ✦ mg; oral susp 40, concentrated oral solution 125 mg/mL
Administer:
• Oral susp for AIDS patients; shake well
• Do not confuse concentrated product with regular
• Without regard to food
• Store in tight container at room temperature

SIDE EFFECTS
CNS: Mood swings, insomnia, fever, lethargy, depression
CV: Thrombophlebitis, thromboembolism, hypertension
ENDO: Adrenal insufficiency
GI: Nausea, vomiting, *diarrhea*, abdominal cramps, *weight gain*, flatus, indigestion
GU: Gynecomastia, fluid retention, vaginal bleeding, discharge, *impotence*, decreased libido, menstruation disorders
INTEG: Alopecia, *rash*, pruritus
MISC: Tumor flare, leukopenia

PHARMACOKINETICS
PO: Half-life 13-105 hr, suspension 20-50 hr, tablets 1-3 hr; metabolized in liver; excreted in feces, urine, breast milk; food increases bioavailability of oral sol, protein binding >90%; peak 5 hr (susp), 1-3 hr (tablets)

INTERACTIONS
• **Increase:** serious arrhythmias—dofetilide; avoid using concurrently
• **Increased INR:** warfarin, monitor often
• **Decrease:** megestrol effect—antidiabetics; may need to increase megestrol dose
• **Decrease:** effect of indinavir; may need to increase indinavir dose
Drug/Lab Test
Increase: glucose

NURSING CONSIDERATIONS
Assess:
• PSA levels in men (prostate cancer); blood glucose, LFTs, serum calcium, weight
• **Psychosocial:** effects of alopecia on body image; feelings about body changes
• Frequency of stools, characteristics: cramping, acidosis, signs of dehydration (poor skin turgor, decreased urine output, dry skin, restlessness, weakness), rapid respirations
• **AIDS:** Anorexia, nausea, vomiting, constipation, weakness, loss of muscle tone
• **Thrombophlebitis:** unilateral increase in leg girth; edema; warm, red skin; pain in extremity; notify prescriber immediately

- **HPA axis suppression:** in chronic users, do not discontinue abruptly; wear medical ID; monitor for hypotension during stress, trauma, acute illness
- **Beers:** avoid in older adults as an appetite stimulant; minimal effect on weight; increased risk of thrombotic events
- **Pregnancy/breastfeeding:** do not use in pregnancy or breastfeeding

Evaluate:
- **Therapeutic response:** decreased tumor size, spread of malignancy; weight gain in AIDS patients; resolved dysfunctional uterine bleeding

Teach patient/family:
- To report vaginal bleeding
- That gynecomastia, alopecia can occur; reversible after discontinuing treatment
- To recognize signs of fluid retention, thromboemboli; to report these immediately
- To monitor blood glucose if diabetic
- That products may be taken without food
- **Pregnancy/breastfeeding:** that nonhormonal contraception should be used during and for 4 mo after treatment

---

meloxicam (Rx)
(mel-oks′i-kam)
Anjeso, Mobic, Mobicox ✤, Qmiiz ODT, Vivlodex
Func. class.: Antirheumatic, NSAIDs

USES: **IV: Pain:** Moderate to severe pain in adults, alone or in combination with nonsteroidal antiinflammatory drug analgesics; **PO** Osteoarthritis, RA (ODT tablet and suspension only)

CONTRAINDICATIONS
Hypersensitivity to meloxicam or any component; history of asthma, urticaria, other allergic-type reactions after taking aspirin or other nonsteroidal antiinflammatory drugs; CABG; phenylketonuria (orally disintegrating tablet only); moderate to severe renal disease who are at risk for renal

failure due to volume depletion (injection only)

Black Box Warning: CABG, GI bleeding/perforation, thromboembolism

DOSAGE AND ROUTES
Osteoarthritis
Adult: Capsule (Vivlodex): PO Initial: 5 mg daily; may increase to max 10 mg daily
Osteoarthritis, rheumatoid arthritis
Adult: tablet/suspension: PO Initial: 7.5 mg once daily; may increase to max 15 mg daily
Pain, moderate to severe
Adult: IV Bolus: 30 mg once daily. Use for the shortest duration consistent with individual patient treatment goals; may be used as monotherapy or in combination with nonsteroidal antiinflammatory drug analgesics
Juvenile idiopathic arthritis (JIA)
Child ≥2 yr/adolescent: Oral suspension, tablets: 0.125 mg/kg daily; max 7.5 mg/day; ODT:
Child/adolescent ≥60 kg: 7.5 mg daily
Available forms: Tabs 7.5, 15 mg; suspension 7.5 mg/5 mL; solution for injection 30 mg/mL; capsules 5, 10 mg

---

⚠ HIGH ALERT

melphalan (Rx)
(mel′fa-lan)
Alkeran ✤, Evomela
Func. class.: Antineoplastic, alkylating agent
Chem. class.: Nitrogen mustard

Do not confuse:
melphalan/Myleran/Leukeran

ACTION: Responsible for cross-linking DNA strands, thereby leading to cell death; activity is not cell-cycle–phase specific

USES: Multiple myeloma, advanced ovarian cancer, stem cell transplant preparation (multiple myeloma)
Unlabeled uses: Neuroblastoma conditioning treatment before stem cell transplantation

Side effects: *italics* = common; red = life-threatening

CONTRAINDICATIONS
Pregnancy, breastfeeding, hypersensitivity
Precautions: Children, radiation therapy, infections, renal disease

> **Black Box Warning:** Bone marrow depression, secondary malignancy, radiation therapy, bleeding, infection, risk of serious hypersensitivity reaction; requires an experienced clinician

DOSAGE AND ROUTES
Multiple myeloma (palliative)
• **Adult:** PO 6 mg daily 2-3 wk, adjust weekly then stop for ≤4 wk or until WBC/platelets begin to rise; maintenance 2 mg/day
• **Adult:** IV INF 16 mg/m² ; give over 15-20 min; give at 2-wk intervals 4 doses, then at 4-wk intervals; adjust to blood counts
Multiple myeloma conditioning treatment before stem cell transplantation (Evomela only)
• **Adult: IV INFUSION** 100 mg/m²/day over 30 min for 2 days before stem cell transplant (day 3, day 2; day 0 [transplant]); >130% of ideal body weight or renal disease BUN >30 mg/day: reduce dose by 50%
Epithelial ovarian carcinoma
• **Adult:** PO 0.2 mg/kg/day × 5 days q4-5wk; repeat q4-5wk depending on blood counts
Neuroblastoma conditioning treatment before stem cell transplantation (unlabeled)
Child: IV INF 140 mg/m² with busulfin before transplantation
Available forms: Tabs 2 mg, powder for inj 50 mg
Administer:
• Antiemetic 30-60 min before product to prevent vomiting
PO route
• Give on empty stomach
• Protect from light; store refrigerated

Intermittent IV INF route
• Use gloves during administration; if skin exposure occurs, wash immediately with soap and water, use cytotoxic handling procedures

Evomela
Reconstitution:
• Add 8.6 mL of 0.9% NaCl injection to the vial for a final vial concentration of 5 mg/mL
• Negative pressure should be present in the vial; discard any vial that does not have a vacuum present during reconstitution
• Storage after reconstitution: Store at room temperature for up to 1 hr or refrigerated up to 24 hr

IV infusion:
• Dilute the appropriate dose with 0.9% NaCl to a final concentration not to exceed 0.45 mg/mL
• The diluted solution may be stored at room temperature for up to 4 hr (in addition to 1 hr after reconstitution)
• Give over 30 min when used as conditioning treatment before stem cell transplant or IV over 15-20 min when used as palliative treatment in multiple myeloma
• Infuse into an injection port or by injecting slowly into a fast-running IV infusion via a central venous line to avoid extravasation

Alkeran/generic melphalan reconstitution:
• Using a 20-gauge or larger needle, rapidly inject 10 mL of the supplied diluent into a 50-mg vial for a final concentration of 5 mg/mL
• Immediately shake the vial until clear and all material is dissolved
• Dilute the reconstituted vial immediately; the solution is unstable
• Do not refrigerate the reconstituted vial; a precipitate will form
IV infusion:
• Dilute the dose in 0.9% NaCl to a final concentration max 0.45 mg/mL
• Give over 15-20 min; and complete the infusion within 60 min from vial reconstitution
• The diluted solution is unstable; about 1% of the labeled dose hydrolyzes every 10 min after dilution with sodium chloride
• Infuse through a central line to avoid extravasation

Y-site compatibilities: Acyclovir, amikacin, aminophylline, ampicillin, aztreonam, bleomycin, bumetanide, buprenorphine, butorphanol, calcium gluconate, CARBOplatin, carmustine, ceFAZolin, cefepime, cefoperazone, cefotaxime, cefoTEtan, cefTAZidime, ceftizoxime, cefTRIAXone, cefuroxime, cimetidine, CISplatin, clindamycin, cyclophosphamide, cytarabine, dacarbazine, DACTINomycin, DAUNOrubicin, dexamethasone, diphenhydrAMINE, DOXOrubicin, doxycycline, droperidol, enalaprilat, etoposide, famotidine, floxuridine, fluconazole, fludarabine, fluorouracil, furosemide, gallium, ganciclovir, gentamicin, granisetron, haloperidol, heparin, hydrocortisone, hydrocortisone sodium phosphate, HYDROmorphone, hydrOXYzine, IDArubicin, ifosfamide, imipenem-cilastatin, LORazepam, mannitol, mechlorethamine, meperidine, mesna, methotrexate, methylPREDNISolone, metoclopramide, metroNIDAZOLE, miconazole, minocycline, mitoMYcin, mitoXANTRONE, morphine, nalbuphine, netilmicin, ondansetron, pentostatin, piperacillin, plicamycin, potassium chloride, prochlorperazine, promethazine, raNITIdine, sodium bicarbonate, streptozocin, teniposide, thiotepa, ticarcillin, ticarcillin/clavulanate, tobramycin, trimethoprim-sulfamethoxazole, vancomycin, vinBLAStine, vinCRIStine, vinorelbine, zidovudine

SIDE EFFECTS
GI: *Nausea, vomiting, stomatitis, diarrhea,* hepatotoxicity, *abdominal pain, anorexia, constipation*
GU: *Amenorrhea,* infertility
HEMA: Thrombocytopenia, neutropenia, leukopenia, anemia
INTEG: Pruritus, necrosis, extravasation, alopecia, rash
RESP: Dyspnea, pneumonitis, bronchospasm
SYST: Anaphylaxis, allergic reactions, new primary malignancies, edema
CNS: *Fatigue, fever,* dizziness
META: *Hypokalemia, hypophosphatemia*
ENDO: Menstrual irregularities

PHARMACOKINETICS
Metabolized in liver, excreted in urine, half-life 2 hr, protein binding ≤30%

INTERACTIONS (IV MELPHALAN)
Increase: toxicity—antineoplastics, radiation
Increase: bleeding risk—NSAIDs, anticoagulants, salicylates, thrombolytics, platelet inhibitors; avoid concurrent use
Decrease: antibody response—live virus vaccines; bring up-to-date before use or postpone 3 mo after conclusion of treatment
Drug/Lab Test
Increase: BUN
Decrease: HB, RBC, WBC, platelets
False-positive: Direct Coombs' test

NURSING CONSIDERATIONS
Assess:

Black Box Warning: Bone marrow depression: full nadir 2-3 wk; CBC, differential, platelet count weekly; notify prescriber, withhold product if WBC is <3000/mm³ or platelet count is <100,000/mm³; recovery usually occurs in 6 wk; IV product causes more myelosuppression

• Renal studies: BUN, serum uric acid before, during therapy
• I&O ratio; report fall in urine output to 30 mL/hr
• **Infection:** fever, cough, temperature, chills, sore throat; notify prescriber

Black Box Warning: New primary malignancy: acute leukemia, myeloproliferative syndrome may occur due to chromosome damage; risk is increased when using long-term treatment

Black Box Warning: Requires an experienced clinician: product should be used only by clinician knowledgeable in use of chemotherapy

• **Hepatotoxicity:** hepatic studies before, during therapy (bilirubin, AST, ALT,

Side effects: *italics* = common; red = life-threatening

LDH) as needed; assess for jaundiced skin and sclera, dark urine, clay-colored stools, itchy skin, abdominal pain, fever, diarrhea

• **Bleeding:** hematuria, guaiac, bruising or petechiae, mucosa or orifices often, no rectal temperature, IM injections if possible, use pressure on IV/IM sites

• Buccal cavity for dryness, sores, ulceration, white patches, oral pain, bleeding, dysphagia

• Local irritation, pain, burning, discoloration at inj site

Black Box Warning: Severe allergic reaction: rash, pruritus, urticaria, purpuric skin lesions, itching, flushing; assess allergy to chlorambucil; cross-sensitivity may occur in 2% of patients; avoid

• Increase fluid intake to 2-3 L/day to prevent urate deposits, calculi formation

• Rinsing of mouth tid-qid with water, club soda; brushing of teeth bid-tid with soft brush or cotton-tipped applicators for stomatitis; use unwaxed dental floss

• **Pregnancy/breastfeeding:** Do not use during pregnancy or breastfeeding; male patients with female partners of childbearing potential and female patients should use adequate contraception during and for 3 mo after last dose; do not breastfeed during and for 1 wk after last dose

Evaluate:

• **Therapeutic response:** decreased tumor size, spread of malignancy

Teach patient/family:

• To avoid foods with citric acid, hot temperature, or rough texture

• To report any bleeding, white spots, or ulcerations in mouth to prescriber; to examine mouth daily

• **To report signs of infection:** fever, sore throat, flulike symptoms

• To report signs of anemia: fatigue, headache, faintness, SOB, irritability, nausea/vomiting, dehydration, decreased urine output

• To avoid use of aspirin products, NSAIDs, alcohol

• **Hepatotoxicity:** to report immediately yellowing of skin or eyes, dark urine, clay-colored stools, itchy skin, abdominal pain, fever, diarrhea

• **Pregnancy/breastfeeding:** to report suspected pregnancy; that usually sterility, amenorrhea occur; reversible after discontinuing treatment

---

memantine (Rx)

(me-man'teen)

Ebixa ♣, Namenda, Namenda XR

Func. class.: Anti-Alzheimer's agent
Chem. class.: N-methyl-D-aspartate receptor antagonist

Do not confuse:
memantine/methadone

ACTION: Antagonist action of CNS NMDA receptors that may contribute to the symptoms of Alzheimer's disease

USES: Moderate to severe dementia in Alzheimer's disease

CONTRAINDICATIONS

Children, hypersensitivity

Precautions: Pregnancy, breastfeeding, renal disease, GU conditions that raise urine pH, seizures, severe hepatic disease, renal failure

DOSAGE AND ROUTES

• **Adult:** PO 5 mg/day, may increase dose in 5-mg increments ≥1-wk intervals over a 3-wk period; recommended target dose is 10 mg bid at wk 4; ext rel 7 mg daily, increased by 7 mg ≥1 wk up to target dose of 28 mg daily

Renal dose

• **Adult:** PO CCr 5-29 mL/min, a target of 5 mg bid **immediate release** or 14 mg/day **extended release**

Available forms: Tabs 5, 10 mg; tab (Namenda Titration Pak) 5, 10 mg; oral sol 2 mg/mL (10 mg/5 mL); cap ext rel 7, 14, 21, 28 mg

Administer:

• Can be taken without regard to meals

• Twice a day if dose >5 mg

• Dosage adjusted to response no more than q1wk

• **Ext rel caps:** do not crush, chew, divide; swallow whole or open and sprinkle on applesauce
• When switching from immediate-release product, begin the ext rel the day after the last dose of immediate-release product. Those on 10 mg bid should be switched to ext rel 28 mg daily
• **Oral sol:** Use device provided; remove dosing syringe, green cap, plastic tube from plastic; attach tube to green cap; open cap by pushing down on cap, turning counterclockwise; remove unscrewed cap; remove seal from bottle, discard; insert plastic tube fully into bottle, screw green cap tightly onto bottle by turning cap clockwise; keeping bottle upright on table, remove lid; with plunger fully depressed, insert tip of syringe into cap; while holding syringe, gently pull up on plunger; remove syringe; invert syringe, slowly press plunger to level that removes large air bubbles; keep plunger in inverted position; few small air bubbles may be present

SIDE EFFECTS

CNS: *Dizziness, confusion,* headache, stroke
CV: Hypertension, HF
GI: Vomiting, *constipation*
INTEG: Rash
MISC: Back pain, fatigue, flulike symptoms

PHARMACOKINETICS

Rapidly absorbed PO, 44% protein binding, very little metabolism, 57%-82% excreted unchanged in urine, half-life 60-80 hr; peak 3-7 hr (tabs), 9-12 hr (caps)

INTERACTIONS

Increase/decrease: both products: hydroCHLOROthiazide, triamterene, cimetidine, quiNIDine, raNITIdine, nicotine; monitor for effect
Increase: effect—levodopa, some ergots
Decrease: clearance of memantine, increased level—products that make urine alkaline (sodium bicarbonate, carbonic anhydrase inhibitors); monitor for effect

• Use cautiously with amantadine, dextromethorphan, ketamine; reaction unknown
Drug/Food
Increase: product level—foods that cause urine alkalinity (fruits, vegetables, nuts, dairy)

NURSING CONSIDERATIONS
Assess:
• **Alzheimer's dementia:** affect, mood, behavioral changes; hallucinations, confusion, attention, orientation, memory; monitor serum creatinine
• Provide assistance with ambulation during beginning therapy; dizziness may occur
• **Adverse reactions:** patient may be unable to verbalize reactions
Evaluate:
• **Therapeutic response:** decrease in agitation, even with no improvement in symptoms
Teach patient/family:
• **To report side effects:** restlessness, psychosis, visual hallucinations, stupor, LOC; may indicate overdose
• To use product exactly as prescribed; to avoid alcohol, nicotine
• To use oral sol dispenser provided
• To avoid OTC, herbal products unless approved by prescriber
• That product doesn't cure Alzheimer's disease but controls symptoms
• Not to smoke or use alcohol
• Not to crush, chew ext rel caps, may be opened and sprinkled on applesauce; do not mix oral sol with other liquids
• That product may cause dizziness

⚠ HIGH ALERT

meperidine (Rx)
(me-per´i-deen)
Demerol
Func. class.: Opioid analgesic
Chem. class.: Phenylpiperidine derivative

Controlled Substance Schedule II

Do not confuse:
meperidine/HYDROmorphone/
meprobamate/morphine
Demerol/Dilaudid

ACTION: Depresses pain impulse transmission at the spinal cord level by interacting with opioid receptors

USES: Moderate to severe pain preoperatively, postoperatively, general anesthesia maintenance, sedation induction
Unlabeled uses: Obstetric/regional analgesic, acute severe headache/migraine, shaking chills induced by IV amphotericin B or postoperative shivering

CONTRAINDICATIONS
Hypersensitivity, GI obstruction, ileus

Black Box Warning: MAOI therapy, respiratory depression

Precautions: Pregnancy, breastfeeding, children, geriatric patients, addictive personality, increased intracranial pressure, renal/hepatic disease, seizure disorder, abrupt discontinuation, chronic pain, cardiac disease, adrenal insufficiency, alcoholism, angina, anticoagulant therapy, asthma, atrial flutter, biliary tract disease, bladder obstruction, cardiac dysrhythmias, COPD, CNS depression, coagulopathy, constipation, cor pulmonale, dehydration, diarrhea, driving, epidural use, geriatric patients, GI obstruction, head trauma, heart failure, hypotension, hypothyroidism, ileus, IBS, IM/intrathecal/IV use, labor, myxedema, thrombocytopenia

Black Box Warning: Coadministration with other CNS depressants, accidental exposure, neonatal opioid withdrawal syndrome, potential for overdose or poisoning, substance abuse

DOSAGE AND ROUTES
Moderate-severe pain
• **Adult:** PO/SUBCUT/IM 50-150 mg q3-4hr prn; **IV CONT INF** 15-35 mg/hr

• **Child:** PO/SUBCUT/IM 1-1.8 mg/kg q3-4hr prn, max single dose 150 mg; IV **CONT INF** 0.5-1 mg/kg loading dose then 0.3 mg/kg/hr
PCA
• **Adult:** IV 10 mg, range 1-5 mg increments, lock out interval 6-10 min
Labor analgesia
• **Adult:** SUBCUT/IM 50-100 mg given when contractions regularly spaced, repeat q1-3hr prn
Preoperative analgesia
• **Adult:** IM/SUBCUT 50-100 mg 30-90 min before surgery
• **Child:** IM/SUBCUT 1-2.2 mg/kg 30-90 min before surgery, max 100 mg

Coadministration with other CNS depressants
• **Adult:** PO/IM/SUBCUT/IV Reduce dose by 25%-50%

Renal dose
• **Adult:** PO/IM/SUBCUT/IV CCr 10-50 mL/min give 75% of dose; CCr <10 mL/min give 50% of dose
Available forms: Inj 10, 25, 50, 75, 100 mg/mL; tabs 50 mg; oral sol 50 mg/5 mL
Administer:
• Doses given regularly before pain returns are more effective
PO route
• May give with food or milk to decrease GI irritation
• Store in light-resistant container at room temperature
• Do not use in severe respiratory insufficiency
• **Oral solution:** dilute in 4 oz water; less effective than IM
IM/SUBCUT route
• Patient should remain recumbent for 1 hr after IM/SUBCUT route
• With antiemetic for nausea, vomiting
• When pain beginning to return; determine dosage interval by patient response
• In gradually decreasing dose after long-term use; withdrawal symptoms may occur
• Inject IM into large muscle mass; IM preferred route for multiple inj

PCA route
• Refer to package insert for instructions and agency protocol
• Have emergency equipment and opiate/antagonist nearby

Direct IV route
• Dilute to concentration of ≤10 mg/mL with sterile water for inj or NS
• Inject slowly ≤25 mg/min over at least 5 min, rapid administration may cause respiratory depression, hypotension, circulatory collapse
• Have emergency equipment and opiate antagonist on hand

Intermittent IV INFUSION route
• Dilute to concentration of 1 mg/mL
• Infuse using infusion pump over 15-30 min, titrate

Continuous intrathecal INFUSION route
• Use controlled infusion device; implantable controlled microinfusion device used for highly concentrated infusion; monitor for several days after implantation
• Filling of infusion reservoir should be done only by those fully qualified
• To prevent pain, depletion of reservoir should be avoided

SIDE EFFECTS
CNS: *Drowsiness, dizziness, confusion, headache, sedation, euphoria,* increased intracranial pressure, seizures, serotonin syndrome
CV: Palpitations, bradycardia, hypotension, change in B/P, tachycardia (IV)
EENT: Tinnitus, blurred vision, miosis, diplopia, depressed corneal reflex
GI: Nausea, vomiting, anorexia, constipation, cramps, biliary spasm, paralytic ileus
GU: Urinary retention, dysuria
INTEG: Rash, urticaria, bruising, flushing, diaphoresis, pruritus
RESP: Respiratory depression
SYST: Anaphylaxis

PHARMACOKINETICS
Metabolized by liver (to active/inactive metabolites), excreted by kidneys; crosses placenta, excreted in breast milk; half-life 3-4 hr; toxic by-product accumulation can result from regular use or renal disease; protein binding 65%-75%
PO: Onset 15 min, peak 1.5 hr, duration 2-4 hr, absorption 50%
SUBCUT/IM: Onset 10 min, peak 30-60 min, duration 2-4 hr, well absorbed
IV: Onset immediate, peak 5-7 min, duration 2 hr

INTERACTIONS

Black Box Warning: May cause fatal reaction: MAOIs, procarbazine within 14 days

Increase: serotonin syndrome, neuroleptic malignant syndrome—SSRIs, SNRIs, serotonin-receptor agonists, tricyclics, 5-HT3 receptor antagonists

Black Box Warning: Increase: effects, severe respiratory depression with other CNS depressants, alcohol, opioids, sedative/hypnotics, antipsychotics, skeletal muscle relaxants

Increase: adverse reactions—protease inhibitor antiretrovirals

Black Box Warning: Increase: opioid toxicity serious respiratory depression—CYP3A4 inhibitors (fluconazole, ketoconazole, itraconazole, clarithromycin, nefazodone, verampamil), assess often if taken together

Decrease: meperidine effect—phenytoin, nalbuphine, pentazocine
Increase: sedation—kava, hawthorn, lavender, valerian
Drug/Herb
Increase: CNS depression, serotonin syndrome—St. John's wort, avoid using together
Drug/Lab Test
Increase: amylase, lipase
Decrease: cortisol, LH

NURSING CONSIDERATIONS
Assess:

M

Side effects: *italics* = common; red = life-threatening

- **Pain:** location, type, character; give product before pain becomes extreme; reassess after 60 min (IM, SUBCUT, PO) and 5-10 min (IV)
- B/P, pulse, respirations baseline and during use
- Renal function prior to initiating therapy; poor renal function can lead to accumulation of toxic metabolite and seizures; monitor BUN, serum creatinine
- I&O ratio; check for decreasing output; may indicate urinary retention

Black Box Warning: Opioids/benzodiazepines: use only if alternative products cannot be used; excessive sedation and death may occur; if used, monitor closely

- **Abrupt discontinuation:** withdraw slowly; if stopped abruptly, assess for withdrawal
- **Sex hormone changes:** assess for libido, changes in menstrual cycle, erectile dysfunction, infertility; if androgen deficiency is suspected, lab tests should be done
- **Adrenal insufficiency:** assess for anorexia, nausea, vomiting, decreased B/P, weakness; if suspected, confirm with cortisol, sodium, potassium levels; if present, do not abruptly discontinue meperidine, but gradually withdraw

Black Box Warning: Serotonin syndrome when given with SSRIs, SNRIs, and serotonin receptor agonists: monitor for hyperthermia, hypertension, rigidity, delirium, coma; do not use within 14 days of MAOIs

- **Bowel function:** for constipation; increase fluids, bulk in diet; give stimulant laxatives if needed
- **CNS changes:** dizziness, drowsiness, hallucinations, euphoria, LOC, pupil reactions with chronic or high-dose use; risk of toxicity increases with >600 mg/day

Black Box Warning: CYP3A4 inhibitors: avoid concomitant use as increased plasma concentrations of meperidine may occur, resulting in serious effects, respiratory depression, or death

- Allergic reactions: rash, urticaria

Black Box Warning: Respiratory dysfunction: depression, character, rate, rhythm; notify prescriber if respirations are <12/min

- CNS stimulation with chronic or high doses
- **Children:** monitor for restlessness; changes in respirations may occur more frequently than in adults
- **Beers:** avoid in older adults, especially those with chronic disease; may cause neurotoxicity; monitor for delirium frequently

Black Box Warning: Pregnancy/breastfeeding: Do not use during pregnancy, risk of neonatal opioid withdrawal syndrome; notify prescriber of intended or suspected pregnancy; do not breastfeed

Evaluate:
- **Therapeutic response:** decrease in pain

Teach patient/family:

Black Box Warning: Avoid CNS depressants (alcohol, sedatives/hypnotizers, benzodiazepines) for at least 24 hr after taking this product

- To report any symptoms of CNS changes, allergic reactions

Black Box Warning: That physical dependency may result from extended use; use should be short-term only

- That drowsiness, dizziness may occur
- That withdrawal symptoms may occur: nausea, vomiting, cramps, fever, faintness, anorexia
- To make position changes slowly; orthostatic hypotension can occur
- To avoid OTC medications, alcohol, herbals unless directed by prescriber
- Not to be used long term
- That nausea may be decreased by lying down

Black Box Warning: Serotonin syndrome: to report symptoms immediately, hypertension, fever, delirium, confusion, diluted pupils, twitching

TREATMENT OF OVERDOSE:
Naloxone (Narcan) 0.2-0.8 mg IV, caution in physically dependent patients, O_2, IV fluids, vasopressors

---

mepolizumab (Rx)
(me-poe-liz-ue-mab)
Nucala
Func. class.: Miscellaneous respiratory agent

USES:
Asthma: Add-on maintenance treatment of severe asthma in adults and pediatric patients ≥6 yr of age with an eosinophilic phenotype

CONTRAINDICATIONS
Hypersensitivity

DOSAGE AND ROUTES
Add-on maintenance treatment for Asthma
Adult/child ≥12 yr: SUBCUT: 100 mg q4wk
Eosinophilic granulomatosis with polyangiitis
Adult: SUBCUT: 300 mg q4wk, given in 3 separate injections
Hypereosinophilic syndrome
Adult: SUBCUT: 300 mg q4wk
Available forms: Powder for SUBCUT injection 100 mg; solution for injection 40 mg/0.4 mL, 100 mg/mL autoinjector, prefilled syringe

---

⚠ HIGH ALERT

mercaptopurine (6-MP) (Rx)
(mer-kap-toe-pyoor′een)
Purinethol 🍁, Purixan
Func. class.: Antineoplastic-antimetabolite
Chem. class.: Purine analog

Do not confuse:
purinethol/propylthiouracil

ACTION: Inhibits purine metabolism at multiple sites, which inhibits DNA and RNA synthesis; specific for S phase of cell cycle

USES: Acute lymphocytic leukemia in combination
Unlabeled uses: Acute promyelocytic leukemia maintenance

CONTRAINDICATIONS
Pregnancy, breastfeeding, patients with prior product resistance, hypersensitivity
Precautions: Renal/hepatic disease, tumor lysis syndrome, dental disease, herpes, radiation therapy, leukopenia, thrombocytopenia, anemia, requires an experienced clinician, secondary malignancy, infection, hypocalcemia, hyperuricemia, hyperphosphatemia, hyperkalemia

DOSAGE AND ROUTES
Acute lymphocytic leukemia
• **Adult/child: PO** 1.5-2.5 mg/kg/day in combination with other agents; start mercaptopurine therapy after a complete hematologic remission
Renal dose
• **Adult: PO** CCr <50 mL/min, give dose q48hr; if used with allopurinol, reduce usual dose by at least 25%
Acute promyelocytic leukemia, maintenance (unlabeled)
Adult PO 60 mg/m²/day × 1 yr or more with methotrexate and tretinoin
Ulcerative colitis (unlabeled)
Adult PO 50 mg q day, initially, then 1.5 mg/kg/day after 2 wk if WBC 4 × 109 or more and has not decreased by more than 50% from baseline and liver function tests and amylase are not rising
Child ≥3 yr PO 1-1.5 mg/kg/day
Available forms: Tabs 50 mg; oral susp 20 mg/mL
Administer:
• Store in tightly closed container in cool environment
• Give product after evening meal, before bedtime, on an empty stomach; risk of relapse is lower with evening dose
• Use cytotoxic handling procedures

• **Suspension:** Shake well; wash syringe with warm, soapy water; rinse; move plunger up and down several times; use only after dry; after opening, use within 6 wk

SIDE EFFECTS

CNS: Fever
EENT: Oral lesions
GI: *Nausea, vomiting, anorexia, diarrhea, stomatitis,* hepatotoxicity (high doses), jaundice, gastritis, pancreatitis
GU: Hyperuricemia
HEMA: Thrombocytopenia, leukopenia, myelosuppression, anemia
INTEG: *Rash,* dry skin, urticaria, alopecia
RESP: Fibrosis
MISC: Secondary malignancy, infection

PHARMACOKINETICS

Incompletely absorbed when taken orally, metabolized in liver, excreted in urine, peak 1-2 hr, terminal half-life 47 min (adult), 21 min (child)

INTERACTIONS

Increase: effects of mercaptopurine—allopurinol; avoid use or decrease dose by at least 25%
Increase: effects—radiation or other antineoplastics, immunosuppressants
Increase: bone marrow suppresion—azaTHIOprine, sulfamethoxazole-trimethoprim; avoid concurrent use or monitor blood counts
Increase: anticoagulant action—anticoagulants, NSAIDs, thrombolytics, platelet inhibitors, salicylates; monitor PT, INR
Decrease: antibodies—live virus vaccines; bring vaccinations up-to-date before use
Decrease: TPMT, rapid bone marrow suppression—balsalazide, olsalazine, mesalamine, sulfaSALAzine; use cautiously

Drug/Lab Test

Increase: alk phos, bilirubin, uric acid
Decrease: platelets, WBC, RBC

NURSING CONSIDERATIONS

Assess:

• **Bone marrow suppression:** CBC, differential, platelet count weekly during induction and monthly during maintenance; withhold product at first sign of abnormally large decrease in blood counts unless bone marrow aplasia is the goal

• **Thiopurine methyltransferase (TPMT) deficiency:** individuals are prone to rapid bone marrow suppression; dosage reduction may be required in homozygous TPMT–deficient persons

• **Tumor lysis syndrome:** monitor for increased potassium, uric acid, phosphate; decreased urine output, calcium

• **Renal studies:** BUN; serum uric acid; urine CCr; electrolytes before, during therapy

• I&O ratio; report fall in urine output to <30 mL/hr; increase fluids to 3 L/day unless contraindicated

• Monitor temperature; fever may indicate beginning infection; no rectal temperature

• **Hepatotoxicity:** hepatic studies before, during therapy: bilirubin, alk phos, AST, ALT weekly during beginning therapy; hepatic encephalopathy, toxic hepatitis, ascites can be fatal; monitor for jaundice, dark urine, clay-colored stools, abdominal pain; reversible after completion of treatment

• **Bleeding:** hematuria, guaiac, bruising, petechiae, mucosa, or orifices; avoid IM inj if platelets are <100,000/mm³; blood transfusions may be needed

• **Stomatitis:** buccal cavity for dryness, sores, ulceration, white patches, oral pain, bleeding, dysphagia

• Increase fluid intake to 2-3 L/day to prevent urate deposits, calculi formation, unless contraindicated

• Rinsing of mouth tid-qid with water, club soda; brushing of teeth bid-tid with soft brush or cotton-tipped applicators for stomatitis; use unwaxed dental floss

• **Pregnancy/breastfeeding:** identify whether pregnancy is planned or suspected, or if breastfeeding

Evaluate:

• **Therapeutic response:** decreased size of tumor, spread of malignancy

Teach patient/family:

• To avoid foods with citric acid, hot temperature, or rough texture for stomatitis; to report stomatitis: any bleeding, white spots, ulcerations in mouth; to examine mouth daily, report symptoms

• To drink 10-12 8-oz glasses of fluid/day
• To notify prescriber of fever, chills, sore throat, nausea, vomiting, anorexia, diarrhea, bleeding, bruising, all of which may indicate blood dyscrasias/infection
• **To report signs of infection:** fever, sore throat, flulike symptoms
• **To report signs of anemia:** fatigue, headache, faintness, SOB, irritability
• To report bleeding; to avoid use of razors, commercial mouthwash
• To avoid use of aspirin products, NSAIDs
• To take entire dose at one time; how to safely handle and dispose of product
• **Pregnancy/breastfeeding:** that contraceptive measures are recommended during therapy and for 6 mo after last dose, not to breastfeed

---

meropenem (Rx)

(mer-oh-pen′em)

Merrem

Func. class.: Antiinfective—miscellaneous

Chem. class.: Carbapenem

ACTION: Bactericidal; interferes with cell-wall replication of susceptible organisms

USES: *Acinetobacter* sp., *Aeromonas hydrophila, Bacteroides distasonis, Bacteroides fragilis, Bacteroides ovatus, Bacteroides thetaiotaomicron, Bacteroides uniformis, Bacteroides ureolyticus, Bacteroides vulgatus, Campylobacter jejuni, Citrobacter diversus, Citrobacter freundii, Clostridium difficile, Clostridium perfringens, Enterobacter cloacae, Enterococcus faecalis, Escherichia coli, Eubacterium lentum, Fusobacterium* sp., *Haemophilus influenzae* (beta-lactamase negative), *Haemophilus influenzae* (beta-lactamase positive), *Hafnia alvei, Klebsiella oxytoca, Klebsiella pneumoniae, Moraxella catarrhalis, Morganella morganii, Neisseria meningitidis, Pasteurella multocida, Peptostreptococcus* sp., *Porphyromonas asaccharolytica, Prevotella bivia, Prevotella intermedia, Prevotella melaninogenica, Propionibacterium acnes, Proteus mirabilis, Proteus vulgaris, Pseudomonas aeruginosa, Salmonella* sp., *Serratia marcescens, Shigella* sp., *Staphylococcus aureus* (MSSA), *Staphylococcus epidermidis, Streptococcus agalactiae* (group B streptococci), *Streptococcus pneumoniae, Streptococcus pyogenes* (group A beta-hemolytic streptococci), viridans streptococci, *Yersinia enterocolitica;* appendicitis, bacteremia, intraabdominal infections, meningitis, peritonitis, skin/skin structure infections

Unlabeled uses: Febrile neutropenia, hospital-acquired pneumonia, sepsis, drug-resistant TB with clavulanic acid, UTI, typhoid fever, anthrax

CONTRAINDICATIONS

Hypersensitivity to this product, carbapenems, hypersensitivity to cephalosporins, penicillins

Precautions: Pregnancy, breastfeeding, geriatric patients, renal disease, seizure disorder, gram-negative infection, hypersensitivity to pneumonia

DOSAGE AND ROUTES
Intraabdominal infections (complicated appendicitis, peritonitis)
• **Adult IV** 1-2 g q8h × 3-7 days
• **Infant child/adolescent: IV** 20 mg/kg q8hr × 3-7 days
Complicated skin and skin structure infections
• **Adult/adolescents/child >50 kg: IV** 500 mg q8hr over 15-30 min, 1 g q8hr for *Pseudomonas aeruginosa*
• **Infants ≥3 mo/children/adolescents ≤50 kg: IV** 10 mg/kg q8hr over 15-30 min; 20 mg/kg q8hr for *Pseudomonas aeruginosa,* max 1 g q8hr for *Pseudomonas aeruginosa*
Bacterial Meningitis
• **Adult/child/adolescent >50 g: IV** 2 g q8hr
• **Infant/child/adolescent ≤50 kg: IV** 40 mg/kg q8hr, max 2 g q8hr

---

Renal disease
• **Adult:** IV CCr 26-50 mL/min, give dose q12hr; CCr 10-25 mL/min, give ½ dose q12hr; CCr <10 mL/min, give ½ dose q24hr

Available forms: Powder for inj 500 mg, 1 g; premixed infusion 500 mg/5 mL in 0.9% NaCl, 1 g/50 mL in 0.9% NaCl

Administer:
• After C&S is taken may start treatment before results are received
• If dose is missed, give as soon as remembered, readjust subsequent doses
• Monitor injection site periodically for redness, inflammation, phlebitis

Direct IV route (bolus)
• Reconstitute 500-mg or 1-g vials with 10, 20 mL of sterile water for inj, respectively; shake to dissolve; let stand until clear (average concentration 50 mg/ mL); reconstituted sol may be stored for 3 hr at room temperature or for 13 hr refrigerated; inject up to 1 g in 5-20 mL over 3-5 min

Intermittent IV INFUSION route
• Vials may be directly reconstituted **and diluted** with compatible infusion fluid (NS, D₅W) to 2.5-50 mg/mL; vials with NS can be stored 2 hr at room temperature or for ≤18 hr refrigerated, D₅W solutions may be stored for up to 1 hr at room temperature or ≤15 hr refrigerated; infuse over 15-30 min

SIDE EFFECTS

CNS: Seizures, dizziness, *headache*
CV: Hypotension, tachycardia
ENDO: Hypoglycemia
GI: Diarrhea, nausea, vomiting, CDAD; thrush (child), hepatitis, glossitis, jaundice
INTEG: *Rash,* urticaria, *pruritus,* pain at inj site, phlebitis, erythema at inj site, DRESS
RESP: Apnea, pneumonia
SYST: Anaphylaxis, Stevens-Johnson syndrome, angioedema

PHARMACOKINETICS

IV: Onset immediate, peak dose dependent, half-life 1 hr, excreted unchanged in urine (70%), duration 8 hr

INTERACTIONS

Increase: meropenem plasma levels— probenecid; avoid concurrent use
Decrease: effect of valproic acid; monitor for seizures

Drug/Lab Test
Increase: AST, ALT, LDH, BUN, alk phos, bilirubin, creatinine
Increase or decrease: INR, platelets, PT, PTT
False positive: direct Coombs' test, urine glucose

NURSING CONSIDERATIONS

Assess:
• Sensitivity to carbapenem antibiotics, penicillins, cephalosporins before starting this product
• **Renal disease:** lower dose may be required; monitor serum creatinine/BUN before, during therapy; monitor weight, fluid balance
• **CDAD:** bowel pattern daily; if severe diarrhea, fever, abdominal pain, fatigue occurs, product should be discontinued
• **Infection:** temperature, sputum, characteristics of wound, WBC, stool; vital signs before, during, and after treatment
• **Allergic reactions, anaphylaxis:** rash, laryngeal edema, wheezing, urticaria, pruritus; may occur immediately or several days after therapy begins; identify if there has been hypersensitivity to penicillins, cephalosporins, beta-lactams; cross-sensitivity may occur; have emergency equipment nearby
• **DRESS:** Rash, fever, swelling of face, lymphadenopathy, may lead to other organ systems
• **Seizures:** may occur in those with brain lesions, seizure disorder, bacterial meningitis, or renal disease; stop product, notify prescriber if seizures occur, seizure threshold is lowered
• **Overgrowth of infection:** perineal itching, fever, malaise, redness, pain, swelling, drainage, rash, diarrhea; change in cough, sputum
• **Pregnancy/breastfeeding:** use only if clearly needed; no well-controlled studies; use cautiously in breastfeeding, excreted in breast milk

Evaluate:
• **Therapeutic response:** negative C&S; absence of symptoms and signs of infection
Teach patient/family:
• **CDAD:** to report severe diarrhea, diarrhea with pus; not to self treat
• To avoid driving or other hazardous activities until response is known, dizziness may occur
• To discuss all OTC, Rx, herbals, supplements with prescriber
• To report sore throat, bruising, bleeding, joint pain; may indicate blood dyscrasias (rare)
• **To report overgrowth of infection:** black, furry tongue; vaginal itching; foul-smelling stools; seizures
• To avoid breastfeeding; product is excreted in breast milk

TREATMENT OF ANAPHYLAXIS: EPINEPHrine, antihistamines; resuscitate if necessary

meropenem/
vaborbactam (Rx)

(mer-oh-pen'em/va-bor-bak'tam)

Vabomere
Func. class.: Antiinfective—miscellaneous
Chem. class.: Carbapenem

ACTION: Bactericidal; interferes with cell-wall replication of susceptible organisms

USES: For the treatment of complicated urinary tract infections caused by *Citrobacter freundii, Citrobacter koseri, Enterobacter aerogenes, Enterobacter cloacae, Escherichia coli, Klebsiella oxytoca, Klebsiella pneumoniae, Morganella morganii, Proteus mirabilis, Providencia* sp., *Pseudomonas aeruginosa, Serratia marcescens*

CONTRAINDICATIONS
Hypersensitivity to this product, carbapenems
Precautions: Pregnancy, breastfeeding, geriatric patients, renal disease, seizure disorder, gram-negative infection, pneumonia; hypersensitivity to cephalosporins, penicillins

DOSAGE AND ROUTES
Complicated urinary tract infection (UTI), including pyelonephritis
• **Adult:** IV 4 g (2 g meropenem and 2 g vaborbactam) q8hr for up to 14 days
Renal dose
• **Adult:** IV eGFR ≥50 mL/min/1.73 m²: no change; **eGFR 30-49 mL/min/1.73 m²:** 2 g (1 g meropenem and 1 g vaborbactam) q8hr; **eGFR 15-29 mL/min/1.73 m²:** 2 g (1 g meropenem and 1 g vaborbactam) q12hr; **eGFR <15 mL/min/1.73 m²:** 1 g (0.5 g meropenem and 0.5 g vaborbactam) q12hr
Intermittent hemodialysis
• Meropenem and vaborbactam are removed by hemodialysis; give drug after hemodialysis
Available forms: Powder for inj 2 g
Administer:
IV route
• Visually inspect for particulate matter and discoloration before use
• **Reconstitution:** Constitute the appropriate number of vials as needed for the dose
• 2 vials are used for 4-g dose (2 g meropenem and 2 g vaborbactam)
• 1 vial is used for 2-g (1 g meropenem and 1 g vaborbactam) or 1-g (0.5 g meropenem and 0.5 g vaborbactam) doses
• **Withdraw** 20 mL of 0.9% sodium chloride injection from an infusion bag, and constitute each vial
• For 4-g (2 g meropenem and 2 g vaborbactam) dose/250 to 1000 mL
• For 2-g (1 g meropenem and 1 g vaborbactam) dose/125 to 500 mL
• For 1-g (0.5 g meropenem and 0.5 g vaborbactam) dose/70 to 250 mL
• Mix gently to dissolve
• The constituted solution is concentrations of 0.05 g/mL meropenem /0.05 g/mL vaborbactam; the final volume is 21.3 mL
• Further dilute before use; do not use by direct injection
• **Dilution:** withdraw the full or partial constituted vial contents from each vial and add back into the 0.9% sodium chloride injection infusion bag

Side effects: *italics* = common; red = life-threatening

• The final concentration of meropenem and vaborbactam will be between 2 and 8 mg/mL
• **Storage:** complete infusion within 4 hr if stored at room temperature or 22 hr if refrigerated at 2° C-8° C (36° F-46 °F)
Intermittent IV Infusion:
• Give over 3 hr

SIDE EFFECTS

GI: Diarrhea, nausea, vomiting, CDAD, hepatitis, glossitis, jaundice
RESP: Dyspnea, hyperventilation, cough, sputum
SYST: Anaphylaxis, Stevens-Johnson syndrome, angioedema
INTEG: Rash, urticaria, pruritus, pain at inj site, phlebitis, erythema at inj site
CNS: Seizures, dizziness, weakness, headache, insomnia, agitation, confusion, drowsiness
CV: Hypotension, tachycardia
ENDO: Hypoglycemia

PHARMACOKINETICS

Protein binding 2% for meropenem, 33% for vaborbactam; excreted by kidneys; half-life 1.22 hr meropenem, 1.68 hr vaborbactam; meropenem is a substrate of OAT1 and OAT3 transporters; use after hemodialysis

INTERACTIONS

Increase: effect of—valproic acid
Drug/Lab Tests
Increase: AST, ALT, LDH, BUN, alk phos, bilirubin, creatinine
Decrease: prothrombin time
False positive: direct Coombs test

NURSING CONSIDERATIONS

Assess:
• Obtain culture and sensitivity before first dose; product can be given while waiting for results
• **Infusion site reactions:** assess for redness, inflammation, pain, and phlebitis at infusion site
• Sensitivity to carbapenem antibiotics, penicillins, cephalosporins
• **Renal disease:** lower dose may be required; monitor serum creatinine/BUN, sodium, before, during therapy

• **CDAD:** bowel pattern daily; if severe diarrhea, abdominal pain, fatigue occurs, product should be discontinued
• **Infection:** temperature; sputum; characteristics of wound before, during, and after treatment
• **Allergic reactions, anaphylaxis:** rash, laryngeal edema, wheezing, urticaria, pruritus; may occur immediately or several days after therapy begins; identify whether there has been hypersensitivity to penicillins, cephalosporins, beta-lactams; cross-sensitivity may occur
• **Seizures:** may occur in those with brain lesions, seizure disorder, bacterial meningitis, or renal disease; stop product, notify prescriber if seizures occur
• **Overgrowth of infection:** perineal itching, fever, malaise, redness, pain, swelling, drainage, rash, diarrhea, change in cough, sputum
Evaluate:
• **Therapeutic response:** negative C&S; absence of symptoms and signs of infection
Teach patient/family:
• **CDAD:** to report severe diarrhea, diarrhea with blood, pus; not to self-treat
• To report sore throat, bruising, bleeding, joint pain; may indicate blood dyscrasias (rare)
• To report overgrowth of infection: black furry tongue, vaginal itching, foul-smelling stools
• To avoid driving, hazardous tasks until response is known, dizziness, drowsiness, seizures may occur

mesalamine, 5-ASA (Rx)
(me-sal'a-meen)
Apriso, Asacol ✤, Ascol DR ✤, Asacol HD, Canasa, Delzicol, Lialda, Mezavant ✤, Pentasa, Rowasa, Salofalk ✤, SfRowasa
Func. class.: GI antiinflammatory
Chem. class.: 5-Aminosalicylic acid

Do not confuse:
Asacol/Os-Cal

ACTION: May diminish inflammation by blocking cyclooxygenase, inhibiting prostaglandin production in colon; local action only

USES: Mild to moderate active distal ulcerative colitis, proctitis, proctosigmoiditis

CONTRAINDICATIONS
Hypersensitivity to this product or salicylates, 5-aminosalicylates

Precautions: Pregnancy, breastfeeding, children, geriatric patients, renal disease, sulfite sensitivity, pyloric stenosis, GI obstruction

DOSAGE AND ROUTES
Treatment of ulcerative colitis
• **Adult:** RECT 60 mL (4 g) at bedtime, retained for 8 hr × 3-6 wk; **DEL REL TAB (Lialda)** 2.4-4.8 g/day × 8 wk; **DEL REL TAB (Asacol HD)** 1.6 g × 6 wk; **DEL REL TAB (Asacol)** 800 mg tid × 6 wk; **CONTROLLED REL CAP (Pentasa)** 1 g qid up to 8 wk; **RECT SUPP** 500 mg bid retained for 1-3 hr × 3-6 wk until remission, may increase tid if needed; **DEL REL CAP (Delzicol)** 800 mg tid × 6 wk
• **Child ≥5 yr and 54-90 kg:** PO (Delzicol) 27-44 mg/kg/day in divided doses × 6 wk, max 2.4 g/day
• **Child ≥5 yr and 33-53 kg:** PO (Delzicol) 37-61 mg/kg/day in 2 divided doses × 6 wk, max 2 g/day
• **Child ≥5 yr and 17-32 kg PO:** (Delzicol) 36-71 mg/kg/day in 2 divided doses × 6 wk, max 1.2 g/day
Maintenance of remission
• **Adult:** DEL REL TAB (Asacol) 800 mg bid or 400 mg qid; **DEL REL TAB (Apriso)** 1500 mg (4 caps) each AM; **DEL REL TAB (Lialda)** 2.4 g (2 tabs) daily with meal; **DEL REL TAB (Delzicol)** 800 mg bid; **(Pentasa) Adult** 1000-mg capsules qid (4 g) × 8 wk
Treatment of ulcerative proctosis-moiditis/proctitis
• **Adult:** (Rectal) (Rowasa) 4 g enema (60 mL) at bedtime retained for 8 hr × 3-6 wk
Available forms: Rectal susp 4 g/60 mL (Rowasa); ext rel tab 500 mg; ext rel cap 250, 500 mg (Pentasa); 0.375 g (Apriso);

del rel tab 400 mg (Asacol), 800 mg (Asacol HD); del rel tab (Lialda) 1.2 g; rectal supp 1000 mg (Canasa); del rel cap (Delzicol) 400 mg; enema suspension 4 g/60 mL (SfRowasa)

Administer:
PO route
• Swallow tabs whole; do not break, crush, or chew tabs; give with a full glass of water
• **Lialda:** take with meal
• **Apriso caps:** take without regard to meals in AM
• **Delzicol caps:** give ≥1 hr before a meal or 2 hr after a meal
Rectal suspension
• Product should be given at bedtime, retained until morning (8 hr); empty bowel before insertion, shake well
Rectal suppository
• Moisten before insertion; suppository should be retained for 1-3 hr

SIDE EFFECTS
CNS: *Headache, fever, dizziness,* insomnia, asthenia, weakness, fatigue
CV: Chest pain, palpitations, pericarditis
EENT: Pharyngitis, rhinitis
GI: *Cramps, gas, nausea, diarrhea,* rectal pain, constipation, vomiting, pancreatitis
GU: Nephrotoxicity, interstitial nephritis
INTEG: *Rash, itching,* acne, Stevens-Johnson syndrome, hair loss
SYST: Anaphylaxis, acute intolerance syndrome, angioedema, DRESS

PHARMACOKINETICS
RECT: Primarily excreted in feces unchanged but some in urine as metabolite; half-life 1 hr, metabolite half-life 12 hr PO, ½-1½ hr rectal

INTERACTIONS
Increase: action, adverse reactions of azaTHIOprine, mercaptopurine
Decrease: mesalamine absorption—lactulose, antacids
Decrease: effect of—warfarin
Drug/Lab Test
Increase: AST, ALT, alk phos, LDH, GGTP, amylase, lipase, BUN, serum creatinine
Decrease: CCr, Hb, Hct

M

NURSING CONSIDERATIONS
Assess:

• **Allergy to salicylates, sulfonamides, sulfites:** if allergic reactions occur, discontinue product

• **Renal studies:** BUN, creatinine before, periodically during treatment; renal toxicity may occur; increase fluids to maintain urine at ≥1200 mL/day to prevent crystalluria; also monitor CBC periodically

• **Bowel disorders:** cramps, gas, nausea, diarrhea, rectal pain, abdominal pain baseline and periodically; if severe, product should be discontinued

• **Pregnancy/breastfeeding:** avoid in pregnancy; excreted in breast milk, avoid use

Evaluate:

• **Therapeutic response:** absence of pain, bleeding from GI tract, decrease in number of diarrhea stools

Teach patient/family:

• To report immediately trouble breathing, rash, hives

• To use rectal suspension dose at bedtime, teach how to use

• That follow-up exams and blood work will be needed, including possible proctoscopy or sigmoidoscopy

• Not to drive or engage in other hazardous activities until response is known, dizziness may occur

• That usual initial course of therapy is 3-6 wk; to notify prescriber if symptoms do not improve after 2 mo of treatment; to continue to take even if feeling better; not to miss doses; if a dose is missed, to take when remembered, if almost time for next dose, skip it; do not double doses; do not use PO with antacids

• To shake bottle well (rectal susp)

• To inform prescriber of GI symptoms

• To report abdominal cramping, pain, diarrhea with blood, headache, fever, rash, chest pain, bruising, bleeding, mouth sores; product should be discontinued

---

mesna (Rx)

(mes′na)

Mesnex, Uromitexan ✦

Func. class.: Antidote, chemoprotective agent

ACTION: Binds to ifosfumide urotoxic metabolism

USES: Prevention of ifosfamide-induced hemorrhagic cystitis

CONTRAINDICATIONS
Hypersensitivity

DOSAGE AND ROUTES
Prevention of ifosfamide-induced hemorrhagic cystitis

Adult standard-dose ifosfamide: **IV:** Each mesna dose is equal to 20% of the daily ifosfamide dose given for 3 doses: With the ifosfamide dose (hour 0), hour 4, and at hour 8 after the ifosfamide dose (total daily mesna dose is 60% of the daily ifosfamide dose); PO mesna (following IV mesna; for ifosfamide doses ≤2 g/m²/day): Mesna dose (IV) is equal to 20% of the daily ifosfamide dose at hour 0, followed by 2 mesna doses (orally), each equal to 40% of the daily ifosfamide dose given 2 and 6 hr after the ifosfamide dose (total daily mesna dose is 100% of the daily ifosfamide dose)

Adult: Short infusion standard-dose ifosfamide (<2.5 g/m²/day): **IV:** Total mesna dose is equal to 60% of the ifosfamide dose, in 3 divided doses (each mesna dose as 20% of daily ifosfamide dose), given 15 min before the ifosfamide dose and 4 and 8 hr after each dose of ifosfamide

Adult: Continuous infusion standard-dose ifosfamide (<2.5 g/m²/day):
IV: Mesna dose (as a bolus) is equal to 20% of the daily ifosfamide dose, followed by a continuous infusion of mesna at 40% of the daily ifosfamide dose; continue mesna infusion for 12 to 24 hr after completion of ifosfamide infusion

Prevention of cyclophosphamide-induced hemorrhagic cystitis Adults <40 yr of age: **IV:** Cycles 1, 2, 3, and 6 (cyclophosphamide-containing regimen): 2.1 g/m²/day continuous infusion (mesna dose is equivalent to the daily cyclophosphamide dose) for 2 days with cyclophosphamide infusion during cycles 1, 2, 3, and 6

> **⚠ HIGH ALERT**

metFORMIN (Rx)

(met-for'min)

Glumetza, Glycon ✦, Riomet ER

Func. class.: Antidiabetic, oral
Chem. class.: Biguanide

Do not confuse:

metformin/metroNIDAZOLE

ACTION: Inhibits hepatic glucose production and increases sensitivity of peripheral tissue to insulin

USES: Type 2 diabetes mellitus

CONTRAINDICATIONS

Diabetic ketoacidosis, metabolic acidosis, renal failure, radiographic contrast use, creatinine ≥1.5 mg/mL (males)

Black Box Warning: Lactic acidosis

Precautions: Pregnancy, breastfeeding, geriatric patients, previous hypersensitivity, thyroid disease, HF, type 1 diabetes mellitus, hepatic disease, alcoholism, cardiopulmonary disease, acidemia, acute MI, cardiogenic shock, renal disease, heart failure

DOSAGE AND ROUTES

Type 2 diabetes mellitus

• **Adult: PO** 500 mg bid or 850 mg/day, **max 2550 mg/day; EXT REL** (Glucophage XR) 500 mg daily with evening meal, may increase by 500 mg per wk, max 2000 mg/day; (Glumetza) 1000 mg daily with food, preferably with PM meal, may increase by 500 mg per wk, max 2000 mg daily; **extended-release suspension (Riomet ER)** 500 mg daily, initially. May increase dose by 500 mg/wk if needed. Max: 2,000 mg/day; may consider 1,000 mg twice daily if needed

Renal dose

• **Adult: PO** eGFR 30-45 mL/min/1.73 m², avoid use; if eGFR >45 mL/min/1.73 m² then falls <45 mL/min/1.73 m², assess benefits/risks of treatment; discontinue if eGFR falls <30 mL/min/1.73 m²

Available forms: Tabs 500, 850, 1000 mg; ext rel tab 500, 750, 1000 mg; oral sol 500 mg/5 mL; extended-release suspension 500 mg/5 mL

Administer:

PO route

• Conversion from other oral hypoglycemic agents; change may be made without gradual dosage change; monitor serum glucose, urine ketones tid during conversion
• Store in tight container in cool environment
• Monitor eGFR at least annually
• Do not use in dialysis
• **Immediate rel product:** bid given with meals to decrease GI upset and provide the best absorption; immediate rel tabs crushed, mixed with meal, fluids for patients with difficulty swallowing
• **Ext rel product** may also be taken as single dose; titrate slowly to therapeutic response, side effect tolerance
• **Ext rel tabs:** do not chew, break, crush; may be given with evening meal
• **Oral solution:** use calibrated spoon, oral syringe or container to measure; give with meals
• **Oral extended-release suspension:** shake well, use dosing cup, give with evening meal

SIDE EFFECTS

ENDO: Lactic acidosis, hypoglycemia
GI: *Nausea, vomiting, diarrhea,* heartburn, anorexia, metallic taste

PHARMACOKINETICS

Excreted by kidneys unchanged 35%-50%, half-life 6 hr, peak 2-3 hr (immediate release); 7 hr (ext release); 2½ hr (solution)

INTERACTIONS

• Do not give with radiologic contrast media; may cause renal failure
• Do not use with dofetilide; may cause lactic acidosis

Increase: digoxin levels—digoxin; monitor digoxin level

Increase: metFORMIN level—cimetidine, digoxin, morphine, procainamide, quiNIDine, raNITIdine, triamterene, vancomycin; monitor blood glucose

Increase: hyperglycemia—calcium channel blockers, corticosteroids, estrogens, oral contraceptives, phenothiazines, sympathomimetics, diuretics,

M

Side effects: *italics* = common; red = life-threatening

phenytoin, β-blockers; monitor blood glucose

Drug/Herb

Increase: hyperglycemia—glucosamine

Increase: hypoglycemia—chromium, coenzyme Q10, garlic, green tea, horse chestnut

Drug/Lab Test

Decrease: vit B_{12}

NURSING CONSIDERATIONS

Assess:

• **Hypoglycemic reactions** (sweating, weakness, dizziness, anxiety, tremors, hunger); hyperglycemic reactions soon after meals; these occur rarely with product, may occur when product combined with sulfonylureas

• **Labs:** CBC (baseline, q3mo) during treatment; check LFTs periodically, AST, LDH, renal studies: BUN, creatinine during treatment; glucose, A1c; folic acid, vit B_{12} q1-2yr

• **Surgery:** product should be discontinued temporarily for surgical procedures when patient is NPO or if contrast medium is used; resume when patient is eating

Black Box Warning: Lactic acidosis: malaise, myalgia, abdominal distress; risk increases with age, poor renal function; monitor electrolytes, lactate, pyruvate, blood pH, ketones, glucose; suspect in any diabetic patient with metabolic acidosis, with ketoacidosis; immediately stop product if hypoxemia or significant renal dysfunction occurs; do not use in those >80 yr unless CCr is normal; alcohol use may increase lactic acidosis risk

• **Renal status:** obtain BUN, creatinine before use; if elevated, a dose reduction is required

• **Pregnancy/breastfeeding:** avoid use in pregnancy, do not use in breastfeeding; if an antidiabetic is needed during pregnancy, use insulin

Evaluate:

• **Therapeutic response:** decrease in polyuria, polydipsia, polyphagia; clear sensorium; absence of dizziness; stable gait; blood glucose, A1c at normal level

Teach patient/family:

Black Box Warning: Lactic acidosis: hyperventilation, fatigue, malaise, chills, myalgia, somnolence; to notify prescriber immediately, stop product; not to use in excessive alcohol intake that is chronic

• To regularly self-monitor blood glucose with blood-glucose meter

• About signs, symptoms of hypoglycemia/hyperglycemia; what to do about each (rare)

• That product must be continued on daily basis; about consequences of discontinuing product abruptly; to take as prescribed; not to double doses

• To avoid OTC medications, alcohol unless approved by prescriber

• That diabetes is a lifelong illness; that product is not a cure, only controls symptoms

• To carry emergency ID and glucagon emergency kit

• That XR tab may appear in stool

• To report adverse reactions; if GI upset occurs, it usually decreases over time

• To take with meals; not to break, crush, chew ext rel product

• **Pregnancy:** that PCOS patients with insulin resistance may be at risk of conception; to use adequate contraception if pregnancy is not desired

---

⚠ HIGH ALERT

methadone (Rx) REMS

(meth′a-done)

Metadol ✦, Metadol-D ✦, Methadose

Func. class.: Opioid analgesic

Chem. class.: Synthetic diphenylheptane derivative

Controlled Substance Schedule II

Do not confuse:

methadone/methylphenidate/morphine

ACTION: Depresses pain impulse transmission at the spinal cord level by interacting with opioid receptors; produces CNS depression

USES: Severe pain, opioid withdrawal
Unlabeled uses: Neonatal abstinence syndrome

CONTRAINDICATIONS
Hypersensitivity, asthma, ileus

Black Box Warning: Respiratory depression

Precautions: Breastfeeding, children <18 yr, geriatric patients, addictive personality, increased intracranial pressure, MI (acute), severe heart disease, respiratory depression, pulmonary/renal/hepatic disease, respiratory insufficiency, torsades de pointes, COPD, seizures

Black Box Warning: QT prolongation, pain, substance abuse, potential for overdose, poisoning, accidental exposure, coadministration with other CNS depressants, IV use, pregnancy, requires an experienced clinician

DOSAGE AND ROUTES
Severe pain
• **Adult: PO** 2.5 mg q8-12hr in opioid-naive, titrate; **IV/IM/SUBCUT** 2.5-10 mg q8-12hr in opioid-naive
Opioid detoxification
• **Adult: PO** 25-30 mg qday, max initial dose 30 mg; maintenance 80-120 mg qday
Available forms: Inj 10 mg/mL; tabs 1 mg ✽, 5, 10, 25 ✽ mg; oral sol 1 mg/mL ✽; 5, 10 mg/5 mL; 10 mg/mL (concentrate); dispersible tabs for maintenance 40 mg
Administer:
PO route
• When using during a methadone maintenance program, use only PO according to NATA guidelines
• PO is half as potent as parenteral
IM route

• Rotating inj sites, give deep in large muscle mass (IM)
• Protect from light
IV route
• Used as PCA
• Protect from light
SUBCUT route
• Pain and induration may occur at site

SIDE EFFECTS
CNS: *Drowsiness, dizziness, confusion, headache, sedation,* euphoria, seizures
CV: Bradycardia, change in B/P, hypotension, torsades de pointes, QT prolongation
EENT: Blurred vision, miosis, diplopia
ENDO: adrenal insufficiency
MISC: Dependence, tolerance
GI: *Nausea, vomiting, anorexia, constipation*
GU: Urinary retention
INTEG: *Rash,* flushing, diaphoresis
RESP: Respiratory depression

PHARMACOKINETICS
Metabolized by liver; excreted by kidneys; crosses placenta; excreted in breast milk; half-life 15-23 hr, extended interval with continued dosing; 90% bound to plasma proteins
PO: Onset 30-60 min, peak 1-1.5 hr, duration 6-8 hr, cumulative 22-48 hr; PO half as active as INJ
SUBCUT/IM: Onset 10-20 min, peak 1½-2 hr, duration 4-6 hr, cumulative 22-48 hr

INTERACTIONS
• **Unpredictable reactions:** MAOIs; do not use together
• Do not use within 2 wk of selegiline
Increase: serotonin syndrome—linezolid, methylene blue, mirtazapine, tramadol, trazodone, SSRIs, SNRIs, MAOIs, tricyclics, 5-HT3 receptor antagonists
Increase: fatal reaction: benzodiazepines
Increase: effects with other CNS depressants—alcohol, opiates, sedative/hypnotics, antipsychotics, skeletal muscle relaxants
Increase: toxicity—CYP2C9 inhibitors, CYP2C19 inhibitors, CYP2D6 inhibitors,

M

Side effects: *italics* = common; red = life-threatening

CYP3A4 inhibitors (aprepitant, antiretroviral protease inhibitors, clarithromycin, danazol, delavirdine, diltiaZEM, erythromycin, fluconazole, FLUoxetine, fluvoxaMINE, imatinib, ketoconazole, mibefradil, nefazodone, telithromycin, voriconazole)
Increase: QT prolongation—class IA antiarrhythmics (disopyramide, procainamide, quiNIDine), class III antiarrhythmics (amiodarone, dofetilide, ibutilide, sotalol), astemizole, arsenic trioxide, cisapride, chloroquine, clarithromycin, levomethadyl, pentamidine, some phenothiazines, pimozide, terfenadine
Decrease: analgesia—rifAMPin, phenytoin, nalbuphine
Decrease: methadone effect—CYP2C9 inducers, CYP2C19 inducers CYP3A4 inducers (barbiturates, bosentan, carBAMazepine, efavirenz, phenytoins, nevirapine, rifabutin, rifAMPin); withdrawal symptoms may occur

Drug/Food
• Avoid use with grapefruit juice
Drug/Herb
• Avoid use with St. John's wort; withdrawal may result
Increase: CNS depression—chamomile, hops, kava, valerian
Drug/Lab Test
Increase: amylase, lipase

NURSING CONSIDERATIONS
Assess:
• **Pain:** type, location, intensity, grimacing before, 1½-2 hr after administration; use pain scoring; monitor for cumulative reactions; use during entire 24-hr period for severe pain
• I&O ratio; check for decreasing output; may indicate urinary retention
• **CNS changes:** dizziness, drowsiness, hallucinations, euphoria, LOC, pupil reaction
• **Allergic reactions:** rash, urticaria

Black Box Warning: Respiratory dysfunction: respiratory depression, character, rate, rhythm; notify prescriber if respirations are <10/min; avoid use with other CNS depressants (benzodiazepines)

Black Box Warning: QT prolongation: may be dose related or use with other products that increase QT; titrate doses carefully, may be fatal

Black Box Warning: Accidental exposure: make sure product is not accessible to children, pets

Black Box Warning: Overdose, poisoning: advise persons involved in correct use

Black Box Warning: Substance abuse: may occur but has less psychologic dependence than other opiate agonists

• **Opioid detoxification:** goal in detoxification is only prevention of withdrawal symptoms, not to provide analgesia or pain relief

Black Box Warning: B/P, pulse, ECG; hypotension, palpitations may occur

• Bowel changes, bulk, fluids, laxatives should be used for constipation
• **Beers:** avoid in older adults unless safer alternatives are unavailable; may cause ataxia, impaired psychomotor function
• **Pregnancy/breastfeeding:** do not use in pregnancy, neonatal opioid withdrawal syndrome may result; do not use in breastfeeding, serious sedation of the infant may occur, with respiratory depression
Evaluate:
• **Therapeutic response:** decrease in pain, successful opioid withdrawal
Teach patient/family:
• To report any symptoms of CNS changes, allergic reactions, extreme sedation, trouble breathing
• That physical dependency may result from extended use
• **That withdrawal symptoms may occur:** nausea, vomiting, cramps, fever, faintness, anorexia
• To maintain proper hydration; to avoid alcohol use
• To avoid use with other products without approval of prescriber; many drug interactions

• To use correctly, exactly as directed; not to increase unless directed by prescriber

• That drowsiness, dizziness may occur; not to perform hazardous tasks until effect is known; to ask for assistance when getting out of bed

• That regular ECGs will be needed

• To change positions slowly to minimize orthostatic hypotension

• To advise all providers of product taken

• **Pregnancy/breastfeeding:** not to use in pregnancy, breastfeeding

TREATMENT OF OVERDOSE:
Naloxone (Narcan) 0.2-0.8 mg IV, O_2, IV fluids, vasopressors

---

methimazole (Rx)

(meth-im′a-zole)

Tapazole

Func. class.: Thyroid hormone antagonist (antithyroid)

Chem. class.: Thioamide

Do not confuse:

methimazole/metoprolol/minoxidil

ACTION: Inhibits synthesis of thyroid hormones by decreasing iodine use in manufacture of thyroglobulin and iodothyronine; does not affect circulatory T_4, T_3

USES: Hyperthyroidism

CONTRAINDICATIONS
Pregnancy, breastfeeding, hypersensitivity

Precautions: Infection, bone marrow suppression, hepatic disease, bleeding disorders

DOSAGE AND ROUTES
Hyperthyroidism
• **Adult:** PO 15 mg/day (mild hyperthyroidism); 30-40 mg/day (moderate to severe); 60 mg/day (severe); maintenance 5-15 mg/day; may be divided

• **Child:** PO 0.4 mg/kg/day in divided doses q8hr; continue until euthyroid; maintenance dose 0.2 mg/kg/day in divided doses q8hr, max 30 mg/24 hr; may be divided

Available forms: Tabs 5, 10, 20 ♣ mg

Administer:

• With meals to decrease GI upset

• At same time each day to maintain product level

• Lowest dose that relieves symptoms

• Use gloves to give tablets, hazardous

SIDE EFFECTS

CNS: *Drowsiness, headache, vertigo, fever,* paresthesias, neuritis

ENDO: *Enlarged thyroid*

GI: *Nausea, diarrhea, vomiting,* jaundice, hepatitis, loss of taste

GU: Nephritis

HEMA: Agranulocytosis, leukopenia, thrombocytopenia, hypothrombinemia, lymphadenopathy, bleeding, vasculitis

INTEG: *Rash, urticaria, pruritus, alopecia, hyperpigmentation,* lupuslike syndrome

MS: Myalgia, arthralgia, nocturnal muscle cramps

PHARMACOKINETICS
Onset rapid; peak 1-2 hr; half-life 4-6 hr; excreted in urine, breast milk; crosses placenta

INTERACTIONS
Increase: bone marrow depression—radiation, antineoplastic agents

Increase: response to digoxin; monitor digoxin level, reduce dose if needed

Decrease: effectiveness—amiodarone, potassium iodide; methIMAzole dose may need to be increased

Decrease: anticoagulant effect—warfarin; monitor PT, INR

Drug/Lab Test

Increase: PT, AST, ALT, alk phos

NURSING CONSIDERATIONS
Assess:

• **Hyperthyroidism:** palpitations, nervousness, loss of hair, insomnia, heat intolerance, weight loss, diarrhea; product adjustment may be needed

M

• **Hypothyroidism:** constipation, dry skin, weakness, fatigue, headache, intolerance to cold, weight gain; adjustment may be needed; check for edema: puffy hands, feet, periorbits; these indicate hypothyroidism

• Pulse, B/P, temperature

• Weight daily; same clothing, scale, time of day; weight increase or decrease is a sign of need to adjust product dose

• Monitor lab work: T_3, T_4, which are increased; serum TSH, which is decreased; free thyroxine index, which is increased if dosage too low; discontinue product 3-4 wk before RAIU

• **Blood dyscrasias:** CBC; monitor leukopenia, thrombocytopenia, agranulocytosis; if these occur, product should be discontinued and other treatment initiated; may occur at doses >40 mg/day

• **Hypersensitivity:** rash, enlarged cervical lymph nodes; product may have to be discontinued

• **Hypoprothrombinemia:** bleeding, petechiae, ecchymosis

• **Clinical response:** after 3 wk should include increased weight; decreased T_4, pulse

• **Bone marrow suppression:** sore throat, fever, fatigue

• **Pregnancy/breastfeeding:** may cause fetal harm; do not use in pregnancy; avoid use in breastfeeding

Evaluate:

• **Therapeutic response:** weight gain, decreased pulse, decreased T_4, B/P

Teach patient/family:

• Not to breastfeed

• To take pulse daily

• To report redness, swelling, sore throat, mouth lesions, fever, which indicate blood dyscrasias

• To keep graph of weight, pulse, mood

• To avoid OTC products, seafood that contain iodine, other iodine products

• Not to discontinue product abruptly because thyroid crisis may occur; stress patient response

• That response may take several months if thyroid is large

• **Symptoms and signs of overdose:** periorbital edema, cold intolerance, mental depression

• **Symptoms of inadequate dose:** tachycardia, diarrhea, fever, irritability

• To take medication as prescribed; not to skip or double dose

• To report yellowing of skin/eyes, dark urine, anorexia, right upper abdominal pain; may indicate hepatic dysfunction

---

⚠ *HIGH ALERT*

methotrexate (Rx)

(meth-oh-trex′ate)

Metoject ✦, Otrexup, Rasuvo, Rheumatrex ✦, Trexall, Xatmep

Func. class.: Antineoplastic-antimetabolite (vesicant)

Chem. class.: Folic acid antagonist

Do not confuse:

methotrexate/metolazone/MTX patch/mitoxantrone

ACTION: Inhibits an enzyme that reduces folic acid, which is needed for nucleic acid synthesis in all cells; specific to S phase of cell cycle; immunosuppressive

USES: Acute lymphocytic leukemia; in combination for breast, lung, head, neck carcinoma; lymphoma, sarcoma, gestational choriocarcinoma, hydatidiform mole, psoriasis, RA, mycosis fungoides, osteosarcoma

Unlabeled uses: Active Crohn's disease, metastatic bladder cancer in combination, SLE, psoriatic arthritis

CONTRAINDICATIONS

Hypersensitivity, leukopenia (<3500/mm^3), thrombocytopenia (<100,000/mm^3), anemia; psoriatic patients with severe renal disease, alcoholism, AIDS, hepatic disease

Black Box Warning: Pregnancy, bone marrow suppression

Precautions: Breastfeeding, children, exfoliative dermatitis

Black Box Warning: Renal disease, ascites, diarrhea, infection, intrathecal administration, lymphoma, pleural effusion, pulmonary toxicity, radiation therapy, stomatitis, tumor lysis syndrome, gastroenteritis, GI bleeding/perforation, hepatotoxicity, intrauterine fetal death, nephrotoxicity, requires an experienced clinician

DOSAGE AND ROUTES
Breast cancer
• **Adult: IV** 40 mg/m² on day 1, 8 of every 21-28 days with other antineoplastics

Acute lymphocytic leukemia (except Otrexup, Rasuvo)
• **Adult/child: IM/IV** 3.3 mg/m²/day × 4-6 wk or until remission, with predniSONE 60 mg/m²/day, then 30 mg/m² **PO/IM** weekly in 2 divided doses or 2.5 mg/kg **IV** × q2wk; **IT adult:** 12 mg/m²
• **Child ≥3 yr:** 12 mg; **2 yr,** 10 mg; **1 yr,** 8 mg; **<1 yr,** 6 mg

Choriocarcinoma/hydatidiform mole
• **Adult/child: PO/IM** 15-30 mg/day × 5 days, then off 1 wk; may repeat, max 5 courses

Meningeal leukemia
• **Adult: Intrathecally** ≤12 mg/m² q2-5days until CSF is normal, then 1 additional dose, max 15 mg
• **Child ≥3-9 yr:** Intrathecally 12 mg q2days or up to twice a wk
• **Child 2-3 yr:** IT 10 mg q2days or up to twice a wk
• **Child 1-2 yr:** IT 8 mg q2days or up to twice a wk

Osteosarcoma
• **Adult/child: IV** 12 g/m² given over 4 hr, then leucovorin rescue

Psoriasis
• **Adult: PO/IM/IV** 10-25 mg/wk or 2.5 mg **PO** q12hr × 3 doses/wk, may increase to 25 mg/wk, max 30 mg/wk

Epidermal head/neck cancer
• **Adult/child: IV** 40 mg/m² on days 1 and 15, q21days alone or in combination with bleomycin, CISplatin
• **Adult: PO** 25-50 mg/m² q7days
• **Child: PO** 7.5-30 mg/m² q7-14days

Rheumatoid arthritis
• **Adult: PO** 7.5 mg/wk or in divided doses of 2.5 mg q12hr × 3 doses once a wk; max 20 mg/wk

Polyarticular-course juvenile RA
• **Child: PO/IM** 10 mg/m²/wk

Burkitt's lymphoma (stages I, II)
• **Adult/adolescent/child: IV** 10-25 mg/day × 4-8 days; give in combination for stage III

Active Crohn's disease (unlabeled)
• **Adult: IM** 25 mg/wk; **SUBCUT** 15 mg/kg/wk × 16 wk

Renal dose
• **Adult: PO/IM/IV** CCr 46-60 mL/min, give 65% of standard dose; CCr 31-45 mL/min, give 50% of standard dose; CCr ≤30 mL/min, not recommended

Available forms: Tabs 2.5, 5, 7.5, 10, 15 mg; inj 10 mg/mL ❧; 25 mg/mL single-use vials; lyophilized powder: 1000 mg preservative-free vials; oral solution 2.5 mg/mL; single-use autoinjector: 7.5, 10, 12.5, 15, 17.5, 20, 22.5, 25, 30 mg

Administer:
Intrathecal route

Black Box Warning: Use preservative-free sol, reconstitute with NS; dose should be drawn into 5- to 10-mL syringe after LP, vol of CSF should be withdrawn equal to vol of methotrexate; allow CSF to flow into syringe and mix, inject over 15-30 sec with bevel of needle upward

• Use safe handling procedures for chemotherapeutic agents
PO route
• This route is preferred for low-dose therapy
• Methotrexate absorption is dose-dependent; absorption of single doses more than 40 mg/m² is significantly less than that of lower doses

• Weekly therapy with Rheumatrex Dose Packs is not intended for doses more than 15 mg PO/wk

• **Oral liquid formulations:** Mistaken daily use of the recommended dose has led to fatal toxicity

• Measure using a calibrated oral measuring device

• **Storage:** store at room temperature (68° F-77° F) for up to 60 days

Injectable route

• Visually inspect parenteral products for particulate matter and discoloration before use

• The preserved solutions contain benzyl alcohol and should not be used for intrathecal, intermediate-, or high-dose therapy

• **Reconstitution of lyophilized powders:** reconstitute each vial with sterile, preservative-free solution (D$_5$W, 0.9% NaCl injection). Reconstitute the 25-mg vial to a concentration ≤25 mg/mL. The 1-g vial should be reconstituted with 19.4 mL to a concentration of 50 mg/mL; prepare immediately before use. Discard unused portions

Intravenous route

• **Direct IV injection:** inject as a slow push via Y-site or 3-way stopcock into a free-flowing IV solution

• **Intermittent/continuous IV infusion:** further dilute in D$_5$W, D$_5$/0.8% NaCl, 0.9% NaCl injection before infusion, check vein patency by flushing with 5 to 10 mL of 5% dextrose injection or 0.9% sodium chloride injection; infuse at prescribed rate. Following infusion, flush IV tubing

IV infusion of intermediate- or high-dose methotrexate (500 mg/m^2 over <4 hr or more than 1 g/m^2 over >4 hr)

• Before use, the following laboratory parameters should be confirmed: WBC >1,500/mm^3, neutrophil count >200/mm^3, platelet count >75,000/mm^3, serum bilirubin <1.2 mg/dL, normal serum creatinine, and SGPT <450 U. Creatinine clearance should be >60 mL/min. If serum creatinine has increased by 50% or more compared to a prior value, creatinine clearance should be measured and documented as more than 60 mL/min even if the serum creatinine is still within normal limits

• Give 1 L/m^2 of IV fluids over 6 hr before initiation of the methotrexate infusion; continue hydration at 125 mL/m^2/hr during the methotrexate infusion and for 2 days after the infusion has been completed

• Alkalinize the urine using sodium bicarbonate to maintain the urine pH more than 7 during the methotrexate infusion and leucovorin therapy

• Repeat serum creatinine and methotrexate serum level determinations 24 hr after starting methotrexate and at least daily until the methotrexate level is below 5×10^{-8} mol/L (0.05 micro-M)

IM route

• Inject deeply into a large muscle

• Aspirate before injection

Subcut route

• Otrexup and Rasuvo are methotrexate formulations for subcutaneous use only

• Both Otrexup and Rasuvo are single-use auto-injectors. Otrexup is available in 5-mg increments for doses between 10 and 25 mg; Rasuvo is available in 2.5-mg increments for doses between 7.5 and 30 mg. Neither formulation should have lumps or particles floating in it

• Administer Otrexup and Rasuvo in the abdomen or thigh; do NOT administer within 2 inches of the navel, on the arms, on any other areas of the body, or on skin that is tender, bruised, red, scaly, hard, or has scars or stretch marks

• If self-injection is deemed appropriate, patients or caregivers should practice injections using a training device with guidance from a health care professional

Use of Otrexup auto-injector

• Immediately before use, twist cap to remove; flip the safety clip

• Place needle end of Otrexup against thigh or stomach (abdomen) at a 90-degree angle and firmly push until you hear a click; hold for 3 sec before removing

Use of Rasuvo auto-injector:

• Pull the yellow cap straight off. Do not twist

• Position the uncapped end of the auto-injector at a 90-degree angle to the skin. Without pressing the button, push firmly onto the skin until the stop point is felt, which will unlock the yellow injection button

• Press the yellow injection button until a click is heard. Hold Rasuvo against the skin until all medication is injected. This can take up to 5 sec

• Visually inspect the transparent control zone to ensure there is no liquid left in the syringe

Intrathecal administration

• Use preservative-free solutions. The preserved solutions contain benzyl alcohol and should NOT be used for intrathecal therapy

• Reconstitute the preservative-free powder for injection with preservative-free 0.9% sodium chloride injection. The desired dose should be drawn into a 5- to 10-mL syringe

• After lumbar puncture is complete, withdraw an amount of CSF equivalent to the volume of methotrexate injection to be administered. If puncture was traumatic, wait 2 days before attempting to administer methotrexate intrathecally

• Allow CSF (approximately 10% of estimated CSF total volume) to flow into the syringe and mix with the product

• Inject intrathecally over 15 to 30 sec with the bevel of the needle directed upward

SIDE EFFECTS

CNS: Dizziness, seizures, leukoencephalopathy, headache, confusion, encephalopathy, hemiparesis, malaise, fatigue, chills, fever; arachnoiditis (intrathecal)

EENT: Blurred vision, optic neuropathy

GI: *Nausea, vomiting, anorexia, diarrhea, ulcerative stomatitis,* hepatotoxicity, cramps, ulcer, gastritis, GI hemorrhage, abdominal pain, hematemesis, hepatic fibrosis, acute toxicity

GU: Urinary retention, renal failure, menstrual irregularities, defective spermatogenesis, hematuria, azotemia, uric acid nephropathy

HEMA: Leukopenia, thrombocytopenia, myelosuppression, anemia

INTEG: *Rash, alopecia,* dry skin, urticaria, photosensitivity, folliculitis, vasculitis, petechiae, ecchymosis, acne, alopecia, severe fatal skin reaction

RESP: Methotrexate-induced lung disease

SYST: Sudden death, *Pneumocystis jiroveci,* tumor lysis syndrome, secondary malignancy

PHARMACOKINETICS

Not metabolized; excreted in urine (unchanged); crosses placenta, blood-brain barrier; 50% plasma protein bound; terminal half-life 10-12 hr

PO: Readily absorbed

PO/IM/IV: Onset, duration unknown

IT: Onset, peak, duration unknown

INTERACTIONS

Do not use with proton pump inhibitors

Increase: toxicity—salicylates, sulfa products, other antineoplastics, radiation, alcohol, probenecid, NSAIDs, phenylbutazone, theophylline, penicillins

Increase: hypoprothrombinemia—oral anticoagulants

Increase: hepatitis—acitretin; avoid concurrent use

Decrease: effect of oral digoxin, vaccines, phenytoin, fosphenytoin

Decrease: antibody response—live virus vaccines

Decrease: effect of methotrexate—folic acid supplements, asparaginase

NURSING CONSIDERATIONS

Assess:

• Make sure product is taken weekly in RA, JRA

Black Box Warning: Infection: those with active infections should be treated for infection before product use; monitor temperature, fever may indicate beginning of infection; more common during neutropenia

• **Rheumatoid arthritis:** ROM; pain; joint swelling before, during treatment

Side effects: *italics* = common; red = life-threatening

• **Psoriasis:** skin lesions before, during treatment

• Make sure drug–drug interacting products are discontinued before therapy, and do not resume until methotrexate level is safe

• **Bone marrow suppression:** CBC, differential, platelet count weekly; avoid use until WBC is >1500/mm^3 or platelet count is >75,000/mm^3, neutrophils >200/mm^3; notify prescriber; WBC, platelet nadirs occur on day 7

Black Box Warning: Nephrotoxicity: avoid use in renal failure; BUN, serum uric acid, urine CCr, electrolytes before, during therapy; I&O ratio; report fall in urine output to <30 mL/hr

• Monitor vital signs during use; report changes if significant

• Monitor for stomatitis, diarrhea, abdominal cramping or pain; if severe, product may need to be discontinued

• **Anemia:** extreme fatigue, increased heart rate, dyspnea, headache, dizziness, pale skin

• **Gout:** joint warmth, pain, edema, increased uric acid level; use of allopurinol and alkalinization of urine will decrease uric acid

• **Bleeding:** bleeding time, coagulation time during treatment; bleeding: hematuria, guaiac, bruising, petechiae, hematemesis, assess in mucosa or orifices; avoid IM injections, rectal temperature when platelets are low

Black Box Warning: Pulmonary toxicity: may start with dry, nonproductive cough; those with ascites or pleural effusion at greater risk for toxicity; fluid should be removed before treatment; monitor plasma methotrexate levels

Black Box Warning: Tumor lysis syndrome: hyperkalemia, hyperphosphatemia, hyperuricemia, hypocalcemia, decreased urine output; use aggressive hydration, allopurinol to correct severe electrolyte imbalances, renal toxicity

Black Box Warning: Hepatotoxicity: jaundiced skin and sclera, dark urine, clay-colored stools, pruritus, abdominal pain, fever, diarrhea, hepatic studies before and during therapy: bilirubin, alk phos, AST, ALT; liver biopsy should be done before start of therapy (psoriasis)

• Monitor methotrexate levels; adjust leucovorin dose based on level

• Buccal cavity for dryness, sores, ulceration, white patches, oral pain, bleeding, dysphagia

Black Box Warning: Serious skin reaction: Stevens-Johnson syndrome, exfoliative dermatitis, skin necrosis, erythema multiforme may occur within days of receiving product by any route; product should be discontinued

• **Stroke-like encephalopathy:** common in high-dose therapy; assess for confusion, hemiparesis, seizures, coma; usually transient

• Increased fluid intake to 2-3 L/day to prevent urate deposits, calculi formation unless contraindicated

• Rinsing of mouth tid-qid with water, club soda; brushing of teeth bid-tid with soft brush or cotton-tipped applicators for stomatitis; use unwaxed dental floss

• **Pregnancy/breastfeeding:** do not use in pregnancy or breastfeeding; females of childbearing potential should use contraception during and for 6 mo after last dose, males with partners of childbearing potential should use adequate contraception during and for 3 mo after last dose

Evaluate:

• **Therapeutic response:** decreased tumor size, spread of malignancy; decreased joint inflammation, pain in RA

Teach patient/family:

• That hair may be lost during treatment; that wig or hairpiece may make patient feel better; that new hair may be different in color, texture (alopecia rare)

• To avoid foods with citric acid, hot temperature, or rough texture if stomatitis is present
• To report stomatitis and any bleeding, white spots, ulcerations in mouth to prescriber; to examine mouth daily; to report symptoms to nurse; to use good oral hygiene
• To drink 10-12 glasses of fluid/day
• To avoid alcohol, salicylates, live vaccines
• To avoid use of razors, commercial mouthwash; to use soft-bristle toothbrush
• To use sunblock to prevent burns
• To use good dental care to prevent overgrowth of infection in the mouth
• How to use this product with leucovorin rescue
• To continue leucovorin until told it is safe to stop
• To report CNS symptoms, vision changes
• To report fever, other symptoms of infection
• To report decreased urine output
• To avoid crowds, persons with known infections
• To advise all health care providers that methotrexate is being taken; not to use Rx, OTC medications, herbs, or supplements unless approved by prescriber
• **Subcut route:** Teach patient self-injection technique and use and disposal of equipment

---

⚠ **HIGH ALERT**

methyldopa (Rx)

(meth-ill-doe′pa)
Func. class.: Antihypertensive
Chem. class.: Centrally acting α-adrenergic inhibitor

Do not confuse:
methyldopa/L-dopa/levodopa

ACTION: Stimulates central inhibitory α-adrenergic receptors or acts as false transmitter, resulting in reduction of arterial pressure

USES: Hypertension

CONTRAINDICATIONS

Active hepatic disease, hypersensitivity, MAOI therapy
Precautions: Pregnancy, geriatric patients, cardiac disease, autoimmune disease, depression, dialysis, hemolytic anemia, Parkinson's disease, pheochromocytoma, sulfite hypersensitivity

DOSAGE AND ROUTES
Hypertension
• **Adult: PO** 250-500 mg bid or tid, then adjusted q2days as needed, 0.5-2 g/day in 2-4 divided doses (maintenance), max 3 g/day
Available forms: Tabs 125 🍁, 250, 500 mg
Administer:
PO route
• Increase in dose should be done in the evening to minimize drowsiness
• Product should not be withdrawn abruptly

SIDE EFFECTS
CNS: *Drowsiness, weakness, dizziness, sedation, headache,* depression, psychosis, paresthesias, parkinsonism, Bell's palsy, nightmares, drug fever
CV: Bradycardia, myocarditis, orthostatic hypotension, angina, edema, weight gain, HF, paradoxic pressor response (IV)
EENT: Nasal congestion
ENDO: Breast enlargement, gynecomastia, amenorrhea
GI: Nausea, vomiting, diarrhea, constipation, hepatic dysfunction, sore or "black" tongue, pancreatitis, colitis, flatulence
GU: Impotence, failure to ejaculate
HEMA: Leukopenia, thrombocytopenia, hemolytic anemia, granulocytopenia, positive Coombs' test
INTEG: Rash, toxic epidermal necrolysis, lupuslike syndrome

PHARMACOKINETICS
PO: Onset 4-6 hr, duration 24-48 hr
Metabolized by liver, excreted in urine, half-life 2 hr

M

Side effects: *italics* = common; red = life-threatening

INTERACTIONS

• **Lithium toxicity:** lithium

Increase: pressor effect—sympathomimetic amines, MAOIs; do not use concurrently with MAOIs

Increase: hypotension, CNS toxicity—levodopa

Increase: hypotension—diuretics, other antihypertensives

Increase: psychosis—haloperidol

Increase: CNS depression—alcohol, antihistamines, antidepressants, analgesics, sedative/hypnotics

Increase: B/P—phenothiazines, β-blockers, amphetamines, NSAIDs, tricyclics, barbiturates

Increase: hypoglycemia—TOLBUTamide

Decrease: methyldopa absorption—iron

Drug/Lab Test

Increase: creatinine, LFTs

Decrease: platelets, WBC, HB/HcT

Interference: urinary uric acid, serum creatinine, AST

False increase: urinary catecholamines

NURSING CONSIDERATIONS

Assess:

• Blood studies: neutrophils, decreased platelets, CBC

• **Hemolytic anemia:** direct Coombs' test before and after 6 and 12 mo of therapy; a positive test may indicate hemolytic anemia; usually reverses within weeks to months after discontinuing treatment; monitor HB/Hct and RBC; do not start therapy in those with hemolytic anemia

• Baselines of renal, hepatic studies before therapy begins

• **Drug-induced hepatitis/drug fever:** usually subsides within 3 mo of discontinuing therapy

• **Hypertension:** B/P when beginning treatment, periodically thereafter; report significant changes

• **Allergic reaction:** rash, fever, pruritus, urticaria; product should be discontinued if antihistamines fail to help

• CNS symptoms, especially in geriatric patients; depression, change in mental status

• **HF:** edema, dyspnea, wet crackles, B/P

• **Renal symptoms:** polyuria, oliguria, urinary frequency; I&O ratio, weight; report weight gain >5 lb

• **Product tolerance:** may occur within 3 mo of starting treatment; a dosage change and other products may be needed

• **Beers:** avoid in older adults; high risk of CNS effects; may cause bradycardia and orthostatic hypotension

• **Pregnancy/breastfeeding:** use cautiously in pregnancy, breastfeeding; has been used for pregnancy-induced hypertension

Evaluate:

• **Therapeutic response:** decrease in B/P

Teach patient/family:

• To avoid hazardous activities

• Not to discontinue product abruptly because withdrawal symptoms may occur: anxiety, increased B/P, headache, insomnia, increased pulse, tremors, nausea, sweating

• To rise slowly to sitting or standing position to minimize orthostatic hypotension

• To notify prescriber of mouth sores, sore throat, fever, swelling of hands or feet, irregular heartbeat, chest pain, signs of angioedema

• That excessive perspiration, dehydration, vomiting, diarrhea may lead to fall in B/P; to consult prescriber

• That dizziness, fainting, light-headedness may occur during first few days of therapy

• Not to use OTC (cough, cold, allergy) products unless directed by prescriber; that compliance is necessary; not to skip or stop product unless directed by prescriber

• That product may cause skin rash

TREATMENT OF OVERDOSE: Gastric evacuation, sympathomimetics may be indicated; if severe, hemodialysis

methylergonovine (Rx)

(meth-ill-er-goe-noe′veen)

Methergine

Func. class.: Oxytocic

Chem. class.: Ergot alkaloid

USES: Prevention, treatment of hemorrhage postpartum or postabortion, uterine contractions

DOSAGE AND ROUTES

• **Adult: PO** 0.2 mg tid-qid × ≤7 days during puerperium; **IM/IV** 0.2 mg after delivery of shoulder, placenta, or puerperium, then q2-4hr × 1-5 doses

Available forms: Inj 0.2 mg/mL; tabs 0.2 mg

---

methylnaltrexone (Rx)

(meth-il-nal-trex'one)

Relistor

Func. class.: GI agent

Chem. class.: Opioid antagonist

ACTION: Peripheral µ-opioid receptor antagonist that reduces constipation associated with opiate agonists

USES: Treatment of opioid-induced constipation in patients with advanced illness who are receiving palliative care when response to laxative therapy has been insufficient; treatment of opioid-induced constipation in chronic noncancer pain

CONTRAINDICATIONS

Hypersensitivity, GI obstruction, IV route, eclampsia, elective induction of labor, hypertension, preeclampsia, pregnancy

Precautions: Pregnancy, breastfeeding, children, geriatric patients, renal disease, diarrhea, driving, operating machinery, neoplastic disease, Crohn's disease, peptic ulcer, ulcerative colitis

DOSAGE AND ROUTES

Opiate-agonist–induced constipation

• **Adult >114 kg: SUBCUT** 0.15 mg/kg every other day prn, max 0.15 mg/kg/24 hr

• **Adult 62-114 kg: SUBCUT** 12 mg every other day prn, max 12 mg/24 hr

• **Adult 38-<62 kg: SUBCUT** 8 mg every other day prn, max 8 mg/24 hr

• **Adult <38 kg: SUBCUT** 0.15 mg/kg every other day prn, max 0.15 mg/kg/24 hr

Opioid-induced constipation with noncancer pain

• **Adult: PO** 450 mg daily in the AM; **SUBCUT** 12 mg daily, discontinue laxative before starting this product

Renal dose

• **Adult: SUBCUT** CCr <60 mL/min, reduce normal adult dose by 50%; **PO** 150 mg/day

Available forms: Sol for inj 12 mg/0.6 mL (single-use vials), 8 mg/0.4 mL (prefilled syringes); tab 150 mg

Administer:

PO route

• Take on empty stomach at least 30 min before first meal of the day

SUBCUT route

Do not give IV; IV dosing for urinary retention investigational

• Store at 59° F-86° F (15° C-30° C); do not freeze

• Store away from light

• Inspect sol before use; should be clear, colorless to pale yellow aqueous sol; do not use if particulate matter or discoloration is present

• Withdraw needed amount of sol into sterile syringe; syringe may be kept at room temperature for ≤24 hr; immediately discard any unused portion in vial; no preservatives are present

• Administer into upper arm, abdomen, or thigh ≤1×/24 hr; rotate inj sites; do not inject in same spot each time; do not inject into areas where skin is tender, bruised, red, or hard; avoid areas with scars or stretch marks

• If using with retractable needle, slowly push down on plunger past resistance point until the syringe is empty and click is heard

PO route

• Give with water on empty stomach 30 min before morning meal

SIDE EFFECTS

CNS: Dizziness

GI: Nausea, vomiting, diarrhea, flatulence, abdominal pain, GI perforation

PHARMACOKINETICS

Half-life 8 hr, protein binding 11%-15.3%; dose adjustment is required for patients with CCr <60 mL/min

SUBCUT: Peak 30 min

Side effects: *italics* = common; red = life-threatening

NURSING CONSIDERATIONS
Assess:
• Serum creatinine, BUN, baseline and periodically
• **Opioid-induced constipation:** stool characteristics, bowel sounds during treatment
• **Pain:** monitor characteristics of pain; this product does not affect analgesics
• **Beers:** avoid in older adults unless safer alternatives are unavailable; may cause ataxia, impaired psychomotor function
Evaluate:
• **Therapeutic response:** decreasing constipation
Teach patient/family:
• That, after 30 min, to remain near toilet facilities because bowel relaxation occurs; not to use more than 1 dose in 24 hr
• To notify prescriber of abdominal pain, continuous or severe diarrhea, nausea, vomiting
• To notify prescriber before taking all other OTC, prescription, or herbal products
• Not to drive or perform other hazardous activities until response is known; dizziness may occur
• To continue other products for constipation unless directed by prescriber not to
• **Opioid withdrawal:** to report severe diarrhea, abdominal pain, chills
• **Pregnancy/breastfeeding:** to avoid use in pregnancy unless absolutely necessary; to avoid in breastfeeding

---

methylphenidate (Rx)
(meth-ill-fen´i-date)
Adhansia XR, Aptensio XR, Biphentin ✦, Concerta, Cotempla XR-ODT, Daytrana, Jornay PM, Quillivant XR, Ritalin, Ritalin LA, QuilliChew ER, Relexxii
Func. class.: Cerebral stimulant
Chem. class.: Piperidine derivative
Controlled Substance Schedule II

Do not confuse:
methylphenidate/methadone
Ritalin/ritodrine/Ritalin LA

ACTION: Increases release of norepinephrine, DOPamine in cerebral cortex to reticular activating system; exact action not known

USES: Attention deficit disorder (ADD), attention-deficit/hyperactivity disorder (ADHD); narcolepsy (except Concerta, Metadate CD, Ritalin LA)

CONTRAINDICATIONS
Hypersensitivity, anxiety, history of Gilles de la Tourette's syndrome; glaucoma, hereditary fructose intolerance
Precautions: Pregnancy, breastfeeding, hypertension, depression, seizures, abrupt discontinuation, acute MI, aortic stenosis, arteriosclerosis, bipolar disorder, cardiac dysrhythmias, cardiomyopathy, chemical leukoderma, child depression, dysphagia, esophageal stricture, growth inhibition, heart failure, hepatic disease, hypertension, hyperthyroidism, ileus, mania, peripheral vascular disease, PKU, psychosis, Raynaud's disease, schizophrenia, stroke, suicidal ideation, visual disturbances

Black Box Warning: Substance abuse, alcoholism

DOSAGE AND ROUTES
Attention-deficit/hyperactivity disorder (ADHD) initial treatment, not currently on methylphenidate

Regular release: Ritalin, Methylin
• **Adult:** PO 20-30 mg/day, range 10-60 mg/day in 2-3 divided doses, 30-45 min before meals
• **Child ≥6 yr:** PO 5 mg bid initially, increase 5-10 mg/day weekly, usual dose 0.3-2 mg/kg/day, max 60 mg/day

Extended-release once-daily tabs: Concerta, Relexxii
• **Adult:** PO 18-36 mg/day initially, then adjust by 18 mg/wk, max 72 mg/day
• **Adolescent:** PO 18 mg/day initially, then adjust by 18 mg/wk, max 72 mg/day
• **Child ≥6 yr:** PO 18 mg/day initially, then adjust by 18 mg/wk, max 54 mg/day

Extended-release once-daily capsules: Ritalin LA

• **Adult/adolescent/child ≥6 yr: PO** 10-20 mg daily in ᴀᴍ initially, adjust by 10 mg/wk, max 60 mg/day

Extended release once-daily ᴘᴍ capsule:

• **Child >6 yr and adolescents: PO** 20 mg in evening; may increase weekly by 20 mg, max 100 mg/day

Transdermal: Daytrana

• **Adolescent/child ≥6 yr: TD** wk 1: 10 mg/day (9-hr patch); wk 2: 15 mg/day (9-hr patch); wk 3: 20 mg/day (9-hr patch); wk 4: 30 mg/day (9-hr patch)

Conversion to once-daily treatment from other forms for ADHD

Extended-release once-daily capsules: Ritalin LA

• **Adult/adolescent/child ≥6 yr: PO** give no more than total daily dose of other forms; may adjust by 10 mg/wk, max 60 mg/day

Extended-release once-daily tablets: Concerta

• **Adult/adolescent/child ≥6 yr (currently on 10-15 mg/day): PO** 18 mg every ᴀᴍ initially, adjust by 18 mg/wk, max 72 mg/day (adult); max 72 mg/day, 2 mg/kg/day (adolescent); 54 mg/day (child)

• **Adult/adolescent/child ≥6 yr (currently receiving 20-30 mg/day): PO** 36 mg every ᴀᴍ, adjust by 18 mg/wk, max 72 mg/day (adult); 72 mg/day, 2 mg/kg/day (adolescent); 54 mg/day (child)

• **Adult/adolescent/child ≥6 yr (currently receiving 30-45 mg/day): PO** 54 mg every ᴀᴍ, adjust by 18 mg/wk, max 72 mg/day (adult); 72 mg/day, 2 mg/kg/day (adolescent); 54 mg/day (child)

• **Adult/adolescent/child ≥6 yr (currently receiving 40-60 mg/day): PO** 72 mg every ᴀᴍ, 72 mg/day

Extended-release once-daily suspension: Quillivant XR

• **Adolescent/child ≥6 yr: PO** give 20 mg in ᴀᴍ, increase in 10-20 mg increments weekly

Narcolepsy

Immediate release: Ritalin

• **Adult: PO** 20-30 mg/day, range 10-60 mg/day in 2-3 divided doses

• **Child ≥6 yr: PO** 5 mg bid, may increase by 5-10 mg/wk, max 60 mg/day

Available forms: Tabs 5, 10, 20 mg; ext rel tabs 10, 20 mg; ext rel tabs (Concerta) 18, 27, 36, 54 mg; ext rel caps 10, 20, 30, 40 mg; ext rel chewable tabs (QuillChew ER) 20, 30, 40 mg; oral sol 5 mg/5 mL, 10 mg/5 mL; chew tabs (Methylin) 2.5, 5, 10 mg; transdermal patch 12.5 cm² (10 mg), 18.75 cm² (15 mg), 25 cm² (20 mg), 37.5 cm² (30 mg); ext rel oral susp 300 mg/60 mL, 600 mg/120 mL; 750 mg/150 mL, 900 mg/180 mL; capsule (Journay ᴘᴍ) 20 mg

Administer:

PO route

• **Chewable tablets:** give with at least 8 oz of fluid to avoid choking

• **Immediate-release dosage forms (Ritalin),** give 30-45 min before meal; twice-daily dosages may be used in ᴀᴍ and noon

• **Ext-rel tablets:** may be given without regard to meals. Give whole; do not cut, crush, or chew. Give the last dose of the day several hours before bedtime. Ext-rel tablets may be used when the determined 8-hr dose of immediate-release methylphenidate tablets equals the 8-hr dosage of the ext-rel tablets

• **Once-daily ext-rel tablets (Concerta Relexxii):** may be given without regard to meals. Give whole; do not cut, crush, or chew; portion of this tablet may appear intact in the stool

• **Once-daily ext-rel capsules (Ritalin LA, Aptensio XR):** may be given without regard to meals; establish a routine pattern with regard to meals. Give with an adequate amount of fluid. Do not cut, crush, or chew. If swallowing is difficult, capsule may be opened and the contents sprinkled on 1 tablespoon of applesauce and swallowed immediately. The capsule contents (beads) should not be crushed or chewed. Instruct patient to drink fluids (water, milk, or juice) after taking sprinkles with applesauce

• **Once-daily ext-rel chewable tablets (QuilliChew ER):** give daily in the ᴀᴍ with

or without food. The tablet may be broken in half for 10-mg and 15-mg doses
• **Immediate-release oral solution (Methylin):** measure dose with oral syringe or calibrated measuring device. Give 30-45 min before meals in divided doses 2 to 3 times/day. Twice-daily dosages may be administered in AM and around noon. Give last dose of day before 6 PM
• **Once-daily ext-rel oral suspension (Quillivant XR):** vigorously shake before use; measure dose with calibrated oral dosing dispenser provided. Give in AM without regard to meals
• **Reconstitution of once-daily ext-rel oral suspension (Quillivant XR):** review manufacturer's instructions; before reconstitution, tap bottle to loosen powder. Add specified amount of water to bottle, fully insert the bottle adapter into the bottle neck, replace the cap, and vigorously shake for at least 10 sec. Store reconstituted suspension at 77° F; dispense in original packaging (bottle in container). Reconstituted suspension is stable for 4 mo from date of reconstitution
Topical route
• **Daytrana transdermal system:** apply patch 2 hr before effect is needed
• Do not cut or trim patch
• Apply patch immediately after opening. Do not use if pouch seal is broken. Do not touch adhesive side of patch during application to avoid absorption. Wash hands immediately if adhesive side of patch is touched. Discard patch if difficulty is encountered in separating patch from the release liner, or if tearing or other damage occurs. Discard patch if adhesive containing medication has transferred to the liner during removal of patch from the liner
• Place on a dry, clean area of the hip, and hold in place for 30 sec with palm of hand. Do not apply to oily, damaged, or irritated skin. Do not apply topical preparations to the application site immediately before patch application. Avoid waistline area where patch could be rubbed by clothing

• Application sites should be alternated from one hip to the next each day
• Adherence of patch may be affected by showering, bathing, or swimming
• Avoid exposing the application site to hair dryers, heating pads, electric blankets, heated water beds, or other direct external heat sources
• Do not apply or reapply the patch with dressings, tape, or adhesives
• Total daily wear time max not exceed 9 hr, regardless of patch replacement
• Peel off slowly. Patch removal may be aided by applying an oil-based product (petroleum jelly, mineral oil, olive oil) to the patch edges
• **For disposal,** instruct patient and/or caregiver to fold used patch so that the adhesive side of the patch adheres to itself, and then flush it down the toilet or dispose of in an appropriate lidded container

SIDE EFFECTS
CNS: *Hyperactivity, insomnia, restlessness, talkativeness,* dizziness, drowsiness, toxic psychosis, headache, akathisia, dyskinesia, masking or worsening of Tourette's syndrome, seizures, hallucinations, malignant neuroleptic syndrome, aggression; cerebral vasculitis, hemorrhage, stroke (rare)
CV: *Palpitations, tachycardia,* B/P changes, angina, dysrhythmias, sudden death
ENDO: Growth retardation
GI: Nausea, anorexia, dry mouth, weight loss, abdominal pain
HEMA: Leukopenia, anemia, thrombocytopenic purpura
INTEG: Exfoliative dermatitis, urticaria, rash, erythema multiforme, hypersensitivity reactions; patch: permanent loss of skin color, anaphylaxis, angioedema
MISC: Fever, arthralgia, scalp hair loss, rhabdomyolysis

PHARMACOKINETICS
PO: Varies with formulation, metabolized by liver, excreted by kidneys, half-life 3-4 hr

INTERACTIONS
Increase: hypertensive crisis—MAOIs or within 14 days of MAOIs, vasopressors
Increase: effects of tricyclics, SSRIs, anticonvulsants, SNRIs, CNS stimulants; monitor for adverse reactions
Decrease: effect of antihypertensives
Drug/Herb
Increase: CNS stimulation—cola nut, guarana, horsetail, yerba maté, yohimbe
Drug/Food
Increase: stimulation—caffeine

NURSING CONSIDERATIONS
Assess:
• **ADHD:** attention span, decreased hyperactivity, impulsivity, socialization

Black Box Warning: Substance abuse: there is a high potential for abuse; use caution in those with history of substance abuse

• VS, B/P; may reverse antihypertensives; check patients with cardiac disease more often for increased B/P
• CBC with differential, platelets, LFTs, urinalysis; in diabetes: blood glucose, urine glucose; insulin changes may have to be made because eating will decrease
• Height, growth rate q3mo in children; growth rate may be decreased, but normal growth will resume when product is discontinued
• **Mental status:** mood, sensorium, affect, stimulation, insomnia, aggressiveness; may produce euphoria, rebound depression after product wears off
• **Withdrawal symptoms:** headache, nausea, vomiting, muscle pain, weakness; usually not associated with drug holidays
• Appetite, sleep, speech patterns
• **Narcolepsy:** identify frequency, length of narcoleptic episodes
• Skin pigmentation when using TD product; may cause loss of pigmentation around site

• **Beers:** avoid use in older adults; CNS stimulant effects
• **Pregnancy/breastfeeding:** use only if benefit outweighs risk to fetus; no well-controlled studies; cautious use in breastfeeding
Evaluate:
• **Therapeutic response:** decreased hyperactivity (ADHD); increased ability to stay awake (narcolepsy)
Teach patient/family:
• To decrease caffeine consumption (coffee, tea, cola, chocolate); may increase irritability, stimulation; not to use guarana, yerba maté, cola nut
• To avoid OTC preparations unless approved by prescriber
• To always use dosing dispenser provided for oral suspension dose
• To taper off product over several weeks because depression, increased sleeping, lethargy will occur
• To avoid driving, hazardous activities if dizziness, blurred vision occur
• To avoid alcohol
• To get needed rest; patients will feel more tired at end of day
• That shell of Concerta tab may appear in stools
• To take regular tab at least 6 hr before sleep, 10 hr for ext rel; to use dosing syringe, not household teaspoon, to measure liquid
• **Seizures:** that those with seizure disorders may have lower seizure threshold
• **Transdermal:** to use in AM; after tray is opened, to use within 2 mo; not to store patches without protective covering; to notify prescriber if skin irritation or rash occurs; that if patch comes off, to use a new one on a different skin site; to tell child not to remove or share with others

TREATMENT OF OVERDOSE:
Administer fluids; hemodialysis or peritoneal dialysis; antihypertensive for increased B/P; administer short-acting barbiturate before lavage

methylPREDNISolone (Rx)

(meth-il-pred-niss'oh-lone)

DEPO-Medrol, Medrol, SOLU-Medrol

Func. class.: Corticosteroid, synthetic
Chem. class.: Glucocorticoid, intermediate acting

Do not confuse:
methylPREDNISolone/predniSONE/
medroxyPROGESTERone/
methylTESTOSTERone

ACTION: Decreases inflammation by suppression of migration of polymorphonuclear leukocytes, fibroblasts; reversal of increased capillary permeability and lysosomal stabilization

USES: Severe inflammation, shock, adrenal insufficiency, collagen disorders, management of acute spinal cord injury, multiple sclerosis, acute lymphocytic leukemia, anaphylaxis, angioedema, asthma, Crohn's disease, eczema, gouty arthritis

CONTRAINDICATIONS

Hypersensitivity, intrathecal use, neonates
Precautions: Pregnancy, breastfeeding, diabetes mellitus, glaucoma, osteoporosis, seizure disorders, ulcerative colitis, HF, myasthenia gravis, renal disease, esophagitis, peptic ulcer, tartrazine, benzyl alcohol, corticosteroid hypersensitivity, viral infection, TB, traumatic brain injury, Cushing syndrome, measles, varicella, fungal infections

DOSAGE AND ROUTES
Severe inflammation/ immunosuppresion

• **Adult/child: PO** 4-48 mg daily (acetate) depending on condition or IM/IV 10-40 mg/day (succinate)
• **Child: PO/IM/IV** 0.11-1.6 mg/kg/day divided (succinate)

Available forms: Tabs 2, 4, 8, 16, 32 mg; inj 20, 40, 80 mg/mL acetate; inj 40, 125, 500, 1000, 2000 mg/vial succinate

Administer:
• Titrated dose; use lowest effective dose

PO route
• With food or milk to decrease GI symptoms (PO)
• Once-a-day dose should be given in AM to coincide with body's normal cortisol secretion

IM route
• IM inj deep in large muscle mass; rotate sites; avoid deltoid; use 21-G needle; after shaking suspension (parenteral); inj-site reaction may occur (induration, pain at site, atrophy)
• In one dose in AM to prevent adrenal suppression; avoid SUBCUT administration; may damage tissue

IV route
• Use only methylprednisolone sodium succinate; never use acetate product

Direct IV route
• After diluting with diluent provided; agitate slowly; give ≤500 mg/≥1 min directly over 3-15 min; doses ≥2 mg/kg or 250 mg should be given by intermittent IV infusion unless potential benefits outweigh risks

Intermittent/continuous INFUSION route
• Dilute further in D₅W, NS, D₅NS; haze may form; give over 15-60 min; large dose (≥500 mg) should be given over 30-60 min

Y-site compatibilities: Acetaminophen, acyclovir, amifostine, amphotericin B cholesteryl, amrinone, aztreonam, cefepime, CISplatin, cladribine, cyclophosphamide, cytarabine, DOPamine, DOXOrubicin, enalaprilat, famotidine, fludarabine, granisetron, heparin, melphalan, meperidine, methotrexate, metroNIDAZOLE, midazolam, morphine, piperacillin/tazobactam, remifentanil, sodium bicarbonate, tacrolimus, teniposide, theophylline, thiotepa

SIDE EFFECTS
CNS: Depression, flushing, sweating, headache, mood changes

CV: Hypertension, circulatory collapse, thrombophlebitis, embolism, tachycardia

EENT: Fungal infections, increased intraocular pressure, blurred vision, cataracts

GI: Diarrhea, nausea, abdominal distention, GI hemorrhage, increased appetite, pancreatitis

HEMA: Thrombocytopenia

INTEG: Acne, poor wound healing, ecchymosis, petechiae

MS: Fractures, osteoporosis, weakness

MISC: Hypernatremia

PHARMACOKINETICS

Half-life >3½ hr (plasma), 18-36 hr (tissue); crosses placenta, enters breast milk in small amounts; metabolized in liver; excreted by kidneys (unchanged)

PO: Peak 1-2 hr, duration 1½ days, well absorbed

IM: Peak 4-8 days, duration 1-4 wk, well absorbed

Intraarticular: Peak 1 wk

INTERACTIONS

Increase: side effects—amphotericin B, diuretics

Increase: GI bleeding—salicylates, NSAIDs; assess for GI bleeding

Increase: methylPREDNISolone action—oral contraceptives, estrogens

Increase: adrenal suppression—CYP3A4 inhibitors (aprepitant, antiretroviral protease inhibitors, clarithromycin, danazol, delavirdine, diltiaZEM, erythromycin, fluconazole, FLUoxetine, fluvoxaMINE, imatinib, ketoconazole, mibefradil, nefazodone, telithromycin, voriconazole); dose may need to be decreased

Decrease: methylPREDNISolone effect—CYP3A4 inducers (barbiturates, bosentan, carBAMazepine, efavirenz, phenytoins, nevirapine, rifabutin, rifAMPin); dose may need to be increased

Decrease: effects of antidiabetics, vaccines, somatrem

Drug/Herb

Avoid use with St. John's wort

Drug/Food

Do not use with grapefruit/grapefruit juice; level of methylPREDNISolone will be increased

Drug/Lab Test

Increase: cholesterol, blood glucose

Decrease: calcium, potassium, T_4, T_3, thyroid ^{131}I uptake test, urine 17-OHCS, 17-KS

False negative: skin allergy tests

NURSING CONSIDERATIONS

Assess:

• **Potassium depletion:** parethesias, fatigue, nausea, vomiting, depression, polyuria, dysrhythmias, weakness

• Edema, hypertension, cardiac symptoms

• **Mental status:** affect, mood, behavioral changes, aggression

• Monitor potassium, blood glucose, urine glucose while receiving long-term therapy; hypokalemia and hyperglycemia

• Assess joint mobility, pain, edema if product given intraarticularly

• B/P q4hr, pulse; notify prescriber of chest pain, crackles

• I&O ratio; be alert for decreasing urinary output, increasing edema; weight daily; notify prescriber of weekly gain >5 lb

• **Adrenal insufficiency:** weight loss, nausea, vomiting, confusion, anxiety, hypotension, weakness; plasma cortisol levels during long-term therapy (normal level: 138-635 nmol/L SI units when drawn at 8 AM)

• Growth in children receiving long-term treatment

• **Infection:** increased temperature, WBC, even after withdrawal of product; product masks infection

• **Beers:** avoid in older adults with delirium or at high risk for delirium; assess for confusion, delirium frequently

• **Pregnancy/breastfeeding:** use only if benefits outweigh risk to fetus, no well-controlled studies; do not breastfeed, excreted in breast milk

Evaluate:

• **Therapeutic response:** ease of respirations, decreased inflammation; decreased symptoms of adrenal insufficiency

M

Teach patient/family:
• To increase intake of potassium, calcium, protein
• To carry emergency ID as corticosteroid user, with product used and prescriber's information
• To notify prescriber if therapeutic response decreases; that dosage adjustment may be needed
• Not to discontinue abruptly because adrenal crisis can result
• To take PO with food, milk to decrease GI symptoms
• To avoid OTC products: salicylates, alcohol in cough products, cold preparations unless directed by prescriber; to avoid vaccinations because immunosuppression occurs
• **Adrenal insufficiency:** nausea, anorexia, fatigue, dizziness, dyspnea, weakness, joint pain
• **Cushingoid symptoms:** buffalo hump, moon face, rapid weight gain, excess sweating, when to notify prescriber
• **Infection:** to avoid persons with known infections; corticosteroids can mask symptoms of infection

---

methyltestosterone (Rx)
(meth-il-tes-tos′te-rone)
Methitest
Func. class.: Androgen

USES: Breast cancer, metastatic (females); advancing inoperable metastatic (skeletal) mammary cancer who are 1-5 yr postmenopausal; delayed puberty (males)

CONTRAINDICATIONS
Hypersensitivity, men with breast cancer/prostate cancer; pregnancy

DOSAGE AND ROUTES
Breast cancer, metastatic (females)
Adult PO: 50-200 mg daily
Delayed puberty (males)
Adolescent PO: 5-25 mg daily; for 4-6 mo
Available forms: Capsules 10 mg; tablets 10 mg

---

metipranolol ophthalmic
See Appendix B

---

metoclopramide (Rx)
(met-oh-kloe-pra′mide)
Gimoti, Maxeran ✤, Metonia ✤, Reglan
Func. class.: Cholinergic, antiemetic, GI stimulant
Chem. class.: Central dopamine receptor antagonist

Do not confuse:
metoclopramide/metOLazone

ACTION: Enhances response to acetylcholine of tissue in upper GI tract, which causes the contraction of gastric muscle; relaxes pyloric, duodenal segments; increases peristalsis without stimulating secretions; blocks DOPamine in chemoreceptor trigger zone of CNS

USES: Prevention of nausea, vomiting induced by chemotherapy, radiation, delayed gastric emptying, gastroesophageal reflux

CONTRAINDICATIONS
Hypersensitivity to this product, procaine, or procainamide; seizure disorder, pheochromocytoma, GI obstruction, hemorrhage/perforation, child <1 yr
Precautions: Pregnancy, breastfeeding, Parkinson's disease, breast cancer (prolactin dependent), abrupt discontinuation, cardiac disease, children, depression, diabetes mellitus, G6PD deficiency, geriatrics, heart failure, hypertension, infertility, malignant hyperthermia, methemoglobinemia, procainamide/paraben hypersensitivity, renal impairment

Black Box Warning: Tardive dyskinesia

DOSAGE AND ROUTES
Nausea/vomiting (chemotherapy)
• **Adult: IV** 1-2 mg/kg 30 min before administration of chemotherapy, then q2hr × 2 doses, then q3hr × 3 doses

---

• **Child (unlabeled): IV** 2 mg/kg/dose IV infusion, 30 min prior to chemotherapy, then repeated at intervals 2 to 4 hr later (Max: 5 doses/day) have been used for highly emetogenic chemotherapy regimens. 1 mg/kg/dose IV infusion regimens have been used clinically for less emetogenic chemotherapy

Facilitate small-bowel intubation for radiologic exams
• **Adult and child >14 yr: IV** 10 mg over 1-2 min
• **Child <6 yr: IV** 0.1 mg/kg
• **Child 6-14 yr: IV** 2.5-5 mg

Diabetic gastroparesis
• **Adult: PO** 10 mg 30 min before meals, at bedtime × 2-8 wk; **Nasal spray:**
Adult <65 yr: 1 spray (15 mg) in 1 nostril, 30 min before meals and bedtime × 2-8 wk (max 4 sprays/day; >65 yr not recommended
• **Geriatric: PO** 5 mg 30 min before meals, at bedtime, increase to 10 mg if needed

Gastroesophageal reflux
• **Adult: PO** 10-15 mg qid 30 min before meals and at bedtime
• **Child: PO** 0.4-0.8 mg/kg/day in 4 divided doses; max: 10 mg/dose

Renal dose
• **Adult: PO** CCr <60 mL/min, 5 mg qid, max 20 mg/day, or CCr 10-15 mL/min give 75% of normal dose; CCr <10 mL/min give 50% of normal dose

Available forms: Tabs 5, 10 mg; syr 1 mg/mL ✿, solution for inj 5 mg/mL, 10 mg/2 mL; oral sol 5 mg/5 mL, 10 mg/10 mL; orally disintegrating tab 5, 10 mg; nasal spray 15 mg/actuation

Administer:
• Total daily dose, max 0.5 mg/kg except in platinum-based chemotherapy

PO route
• ½-1 hr before meals and at bedtime for better absorption
• Gum, hard candy, frequent rinsing of mouth for dry oral cavity
• **Oral disintegrating:** place on tongue, allow to dissolve, swallow; remove from blister immediately before use; give ≥30 min before meals and at bedtime; do not use if tablet breaks

Nasal spray
• Prime before first use, use 10 sprays

• Lean head slightly forward to use, close other nostril with finger, press firmly, while inhaling, wipe tip when done

IM route
• Give for postoperative nausea, vomiting before end of surgery

Direct IV route
• DiphenhydrAMINE IV or benztropine IM for EPS
• Undiluted if dose ≤10 mg; give by slow injection over 2 min

Intermittent IV INFUSION route
• **10-mL and 30-mL vials (50 mg and 150 mg, respectively, in 5 mg/mL) are used for IV infusion with dilution:** Dilute calculated amount in ≥50 mL D₅W, NaCl, given over ≥15 min
• Max 5 mg/min infusion rate
• Infusions are stable at room temperature for 24 hr
• Discard unused portions

Y-site compatibilities: Acetaminophen, alfentanil, amifostine, amikacin, aminophylline, ascorbic acid, atracurium, atropine, azaTHIOprine, aztreonam, bivalirudin, bleomycin, bumetanide, buprenorphine, butorphanol, calcium chloride/gluconate, CARBOplatin, caspofungin, ceFAZolin, cefonicid, cefoperazone, cefotaxime, cefoTEtan, cefOXitin, cefTAZidime, ceftizoxime, cefTRIAXone, cefuroxime, chloramphenicol, chlorproMAZINE, cimetidine, ciprofloxacin, cisatracurium, CISplatin, cladribine, clindamycin, cyanocobalamin, cyclophosphamide, cycloSPORINE, cytarabine, DACTINomycin, DAPTOmycin, dexamethasone, dexmedetomidine, digoxin, diltiaZEM, diphenhydrAMINE, DOBUTamine, DOCEtaxel, DOPamine, doripenem, doxapram, DOXOrubicin hydrochloride, doxycycline, droperidol, enalaprilat, ePHEDrine, EPINEPHrine, epiRUBicin, epoetin alfa, ertapenem, erythromycin, esmolol, etoposide, etoposide phosphate, famotidine, fenoldopam, fentaNYL, filgrastim, fluconazole, fludarabine, folic acid, foscarnet, gallium nitrate, gemcitabine, gentamicin, glycopyrrolate, granisetron, heparin, hydrocortisone, HYDROmorphone, IDArubicin, ifosfamide, imipenem/cilastatin,

Side effects: *italics* = common; red = life-threatening

indomethacin, insulin, isoproterenol, ketorolac, labetalol, leucovorin, levoFLOXacin, lidocaine, linezolid, LORazepam, magnesium sulfate, mannitol, mechlorethamine, melphalan, meperidine, meropenem, metaraminol, methadone, methotrexate, methoxamine, methyldopate, methylPREDNISolone, metoprolol, metroNIDAZOLE, miconazole,midazolam, milrinone, minocycline, mitoMYcin, morphine, moxalactam, multiple vitamins, nafcillin, nalbuphine, naloxone, nesiritide, nitroglycerin, nitroprusside, norepinephrine, octreotide, ondansetron, oxaliplatin, oxytocin, PACLitaxel, palonosetron, pantoprazole, papaverine, PEMEtrexed, penicillin G, pentamidine, pentazocine, PENTobarbital, PHENobarbital, phentolamine, phenylephrine, phytonadione, piperacillin/tazobactam, potassium chloride, procainamide, prochlorperazine, promethazine, propranolol, protamine, pyridoxine, quinupristin/dalfopristin, raNITIdine, remifentanil, riTUXimab, rocuronium, sargramostim, sodium acetate/bicarbonate, succinylcholine, SUFentanil, tacrolimus, teniposide, theophylline, thiamine, thiotepa, ticarcillin/clavulanate, tigecycline, tirofiban, tobramycin, tolazoline, topotecan, trastuzumab, trimethaphan, urokinase, vancomycin, vasopressin, vecuronium, verapamil, vinBLAStine, vinCRIStine, vinorelbine, voriconazole, zidovudine

SIDE EFFECTS

CNS: *Sedation, fatigue, restlessness, headache, sleeplessness, dystonia,* dizziness, drowsiness, suicidal ideation, seizures, EPS, neuroleptic malignant syndrome; tardive dyskinesia (>3 mo, high doses)

CV: Hypotension, supraventricular tachycardia

GI: Dry mouth, constipation, nausea, anorexia, vomiting, diarrhea

GU: Decreased libido, prolactin secretion, amenorrhea, galactorrhea

HEMA: Neutropenia, leukopenia, agranulocytosis

INTEG: Urticaria, rash

PHARMACOKINETICS

Metabolized by liver, excreted in urine, half-life 2½-6 hr

PO: Onset ½-1 hr, duration 1-2 hr

IM: Onset 10-15 min, duration 1-2 hr
IV: Onset 1-3 min, duration 1-2 hr

INTERACTIONS

• Avoid use with MAOIs; may increase hypertension

Increase: sedation—alcohol, other CNS depressants; avoid concurrent use

Increase: risk for EPS—haloperidol, phenothiazines; assess for EPS

Decrease: action—anticholinergics, opiates; avoid using together or assess carefully

Drug/Lab Test

Increase: prolactin, aldosterone, thyrotropin

NURSING CONSIDERATIONS
Assess:

> **Black Box Warning: EPS, tardive dyskinesia;** more likely to occur in treatment >3 mo, geriatric patients and may be irreversible; assess for involuntary movements often; avoid using phenothiazines, haloperidol

• **Neuroleptic malignant syndrome:** hyperthermia, change in B/P, pulse, tachycardia, sweating, rigidity, altered consciousness (rare)

• **Mental status:** depression, anxiety, irritability

• **GI complaints:** nausea, vomiting, anorexia, constipation; assess bowel sounds

• **Pregnancy/breastfeeding:** use only if clearly needed; no studies in pregnancy; do not breastfeed, appears in breast milk

• **Beers:** avoid in older adults unless for gastroparesis; can cause extrapyramidal effects; monitor for EPS frequently

Evaluate:

• **Therapeutic response:** absence of nausea, vomiting, anorexia, fullness; decreased GERD

Teach patient/family:

• To avoid driving, other hazardous activities until stabilized on product

• To avoid alcohol, other CNS depressants that will enhance sedating properties of this product

Black Box Warning: Symptoms of EPS, tardive dyskinesia; to report to prescriber

• How to use oral disintegrating product

metolazone (Rx)

(me-tole'a-zone)
Func. class.: Diuretic, antihypertensive
Chem. class.: Thiazide-like quinazoline derivative

Do not confuse:
metolazone/methotrexate/methadone/metoclopramide

ACTION: Acts on distal tubule by increasing excretion of water, sodium, chloride, potassium, magnesium, bicarbonate; decreases GFR

USES: Edema, hypertension, heart failure, nephrotic syndrome

CONTRAINDICATIONS
Hypersensitivity to thiazides, sulfonamides; anuria, hepatic coma, hepatic encephalopathy
Precautions: Pregnancy, breastfeeding, geriatric patients, hypokalemia, renal/hepatic disease, gout, COPD, lupus erythematosus, diabetes mellitus, hypotension, history of pancreatitis; electrolyte imbalance

DOSAGE AND ROUTES
Edema in heart failure/renal disease
• **Adult: PO** 5-20 mg/day; max 20 mg/day
Hypertension
• **Adult: PO** 2.5-5 mg/day
• **Child: PO** 0.2-0.4 mg/kg/day in divided doses q12-24hr
Available forms: Tabs 2.5, 5, 10 mg
Administer:
• In AM to avoid interference with sleep if using product as diuretic
• Potassium replacement if potassium <3 mg/dL
• With food if nausea occurs; absorption may be decreased slightly

SIDE EFFECTS
CNS: Drowsiness, lethargy
CV: *Orthostatic hypotension,* palpitations, hypotension, chest pain, volume depletion
ELECT: *Hypokalemia,* hypercalcemia, hyponatremia, hyperuricemia, hypomagnesemia, hypophosphatemia, hypovolemia
GI: *Nausea, vomiting, anorexia,* constipation, diarrhea, cramps, pancreatitis, GI irritation, dry mouth, jaundice, hepatitis
GU: *Urinary frequency,* polyuria, uremia, glucosuria, nocturia, impotence, *hyperuricemia*
HEMA: Aplastic anemia, hemolytic anemia, leukopenia, agranulocytosis, neutropenia
EENT: Blurred vision
INTEG: *Rash,* urticaria, purpura, photosensitivity, fever, dry skin, toxic epidermal necrolysis, Stevens-Johnson syndrome
ENDO: *Hyperglycemia,* increased creatinine, BUN
MS: Muscle cramps, joint pain, swelling

PHARMACOKINETICS
Protein binding 33%, peak 8 hr, duration 12-24 hr, excreted unchanged by kidneys, crosses placenta, enters breast milk, half-life 14 hr

INTERACTIONS
Increase: hyperglycemia—antidiabetics
Increase: hypokalemia—mezlocillin, piperacillin, amphotericin B, glucocorticoids, digoxin, stimulant laxatives
Increase: hypotension—alcohol (large amounts), nitrates, antihypertensives, barbiturates, opioids
Increase: toxicity—lithium
Increase: metOLazone effects—loop diuretics
Decrease: action of metOLazone, increase renal failure risk—NSAIDs, salicylates
Drug/Food
Increase: severe hypokalemia—licorice
Drug/Herb
Decrease: antihypertensive effect—ephedra (ma huang)
Increase: antihypertensive effect—hawthorn
Drug/Lab Test

M

Side effects: *italics* = common; red = life-threatening

Increase: calcium, cholesterol, glucose, triglycerides
Decrease: potassium, sodium, chloride, magnesium, WBC, Hb
Interference: parathyroid function tests

NURSING CONSIDERATIONS
Assess:
• **Weight, I&O daily** to determine fluid loss; effect of product may be decreased if used daily
• **HF:** improvement in edema of feet, legs, sacral area daily if product being used
• **Hypertension:** B/P lying, standing; postural hypotension may occur
• **Electrolytes:** potassium, magnesium, sodium, chloride; include BUN, blood glucose, CBC, serum creatinine, blood pH, ABGs, uric acid, calcium
• **Hypokalemia:** postural hypotension, malaise, fatigue, tachycardia, leg cramps, weakness
• Rashes, temperature daily
• Confusion, especially among geriatric patients; take safety precautions if needed
• **Hepatic encephalopathy:** do not use in hepatic coma or precoma; fluctuations in electrolytes can occur rapidly and precipitate hepatic coma; use caution in patients with impaired hepatic function
• **Beers:** use with older adults may exacerbate or cause SIADH; monitor sodium level frequently
• **Pregnancy/breastfeeding:** use in pregnancy only if needed, no well-controlled studies; do not breastfeed, appears in breast milk
Evaluate:
• **Therapeutic response:** decreased edema, B/P
Teach patient/family:
• To rise slowly from lying or sitting position
• To notify prescriber of muscle weakness, cramps, nausea, dizziness
• That product may be taken with food or milk
• To use sunscreen, protective clothing for photosensitivity
• That blood glucose may be increased in diabetics
• To take early in day to avoid nocturia, to take at same time of day, not to skip or double doses, that skipped dose should be taken when remembered if not close to next dose
• To avoid alcohol
• To avoid sodium foods; to increase potassium foods in diet
• Not to stop product abruptly

TREATMENT OF OVERDOSE:
Lavage if taken orally; monitor electrolytes; administer dextrose in saline; monitor hydration, CV, renal status

---

⚠ HIGH ALERT

metoprolol (Rx)
(meh-toe′proe-lole)
Kapspargo Sprinkle, Lopressor, Toprol ✦, Toprol-XL
Func. class.: Antihypertensive, antianginal
Chem. class.: β₁-Blocker

Do not confuse:
Lopressor/Lyrica
Toprol-XL/Topamax

ACTION: Lowers B/P by β-blocking effects; reduces elevated renin plasma levels; blocks β₂-adrenergic receptors in bronchial, vascular smooth muscle only at high doses; negative chronotropic effect

USES: Mild to moderate hypertension, acute MI to reduce cardiovascular mortality, angina pectoris, NYHA class II, III heart failure, cardiomyopathy

CONTRAINDICATIONS
Hypersensitivity to β-blockers, cardiogenic shock, heart block (2nd, 3rd degree), sinus bradycardia, sick sinus syndrome
Precautions: Pregnancy, breastfeeding, geriatric patients, major surgery, diabetes mellitus, thyroid/renal/hepatic disease, COPD, CAD, nonallergic bronchospasm, bronchial asthma, CVA, children, depression, vasospastic angina, pheochromocytoma

Black Box Warning: Abrupt discontinuation

DOSAGE AND ROUTES
Angina
• **Adult: PO** 100 mg/day as a single dose or in 2 divided doses, increase weekly prn or 100 mg **EXTENDED RELEASE** daily, max 400 mg/day extended release and regular release

Hypertension
• **Adult: PO** 50 mg bid or 100 mg/day; may give up to 100-450 mg in divided doses; **EXT REL** 25-100 mg daily, titrate at weekly intervals; max 400 mg/day
• **Geriatric: PO** 25 mg/day initially, increase weekly as needed
• **Child and adolescent 6-16 yr: PO Regular release** 1 to 2 mg/kg/day divided twice daily, initially. May increase dose if needed up to a max of 6 mg/kg/day (Max: 200 mg/day); **PO EXT REL** 1 mg/kg/dose (Max: 50 mg/dose) q day, initially. May increase if further control is needed up to a max of 2 mg/kg/day (Max: 200 mg/day)

Myocardial infarction
• **Adult: IV BOL (early treatment)** 5 mg q2min × 3, then 50 mg **PO** 15 min after last dose and q6hr × 48 hr; **(late treatment) PO** maintenance 50-100 mg bid for 1-3 yr

Available forms: Tabs 25, 50, 100 mg; inj 1 mg/mL; ext rel tab (succinate) (XL) 25, 50, 100, 200 mg; ext rel tabs, tartrate: 100 mg, sprinkle 25, 50, 100, 200 mg
Administer:
PO route
• Take apical pulse before giving; if <50 bpm, hold and notify prescriber
• Do not break, crush, or chew ext rel tabs
• Regular release tab after meals, at bedtime; tab may be crushed or swallowed whole; take at same time each day
Sprinkle capsule: May be swallowed whole or opened and sprinkled on a small amount of soft food
• Store in dry area at room temperature; do not freeze
Direct IV route
• IV, undiluted, give 1 mg/mL over 1 min × 3 doses at 2- to 5-min intervals; start **PO** 15 min after last IV dose
• Check dose with another person to prevent errors that could be fatal

Y-site compatibilities: Abciximab, acyclovir, alemtuzumab, alfentanil, alteplase, amikacin, aminophylline, amiodarone, amphotericin B liposome, anidulafungin, argatroban, ascorbic acid, atracurium, atropine, azaTHIOprine, aztreonam, benztropine, bivalirudin, bleomycin, bumetanide, buprenorphine, butorphanol, calcium chloride/gluconate, CARBOplatin, caspofungin, ceFAZolin, cefonicid, cefoperazone, cefotaxime, cefoTEtan, cefOXitin, cefTAZidime, ceftizoxime, cefTRIAXone, cefuroxime, chloramphenicol, chlorproMAZINE, cimetidine, CISplatin, clindamycin, cyanocobalamin, cyclophosphamide, cycloSPORINE, cytarabine, DACTINomycin, DAPTOmycin, dexamethasone, dexmedetomidine, digoxin, diltiaZEM, diphenhydrAMINE, DOBUTamine, DOCEtaxel, DOPamine, doxacurium, DOXOrubicin, doxycycline, enalaprilat, ePHEDrine, EPINEPHrine, epiRUBicin, epoetin alfa, eptifibatide, esmolol, etoposide, etoposide phosphate, famotidine, fenoldopam, fentaNYL, fluconazole, fludarabine, fluorouracil, folic acid, furosemide, ganciclovir, gemcitabine, gentamicin, glycopyrrolate, granisetron, heparin, hydrocortisone, HYDROmorphone, IDArubicin, ifosfamide, imipenem/cilastatin, indomethacin, insulin, isoproterenol, ketorolac, labetalol, linezolid, LORazepam, magnesium sulfate, mannitol, mechlorethamine, meperidine, metaraminol, methotrexate, methoxamine, methyldopate, methylPREDNISolone, metoclopramide, metroNIDAZOLE, midazolam, milrinone, mitoXANTRONE, morphine, multivitamins, nafcillin, nalbuphine, naloxone, nitroprusside, norepinephrine, octreotide, ondansetron, oxacillin, oxaliplatin, oxytocin, PACLitaxel, palonosetron, pancuronium, papaverine, PEMEtrexed, penicillin G, pentamidine, pentazocine, PENTobarbital, PHENobarbital, phentolamine, phenylephrine, phytonadione, piperacillin/tazobactam, potassium chloride, procainamide, prochlorperazine, promethazine, propranolol, protamine, pyridoxime, quinupristin/dalfopristin, raNITIdine, rocuronium, sodium bicarbonate, succinylcholine, SUFentanil,

M

tacrolimus, teniposide, theophylline, thiamine, thiotepa, ticarcillin/clavulanate, tigecycline, tirofiban, tobramycin, tolazoline, trimetaphan, urokinase, vancomycin, vasopressin, vecuronium, verapamil, vinCRIStine, vinorelbine, voriconazole

SIDE EFFECTS
CNS: *Insomnia, dizziness,* mental changes, hallucinations, depression, anxiety, headaches, nightmares, confusion, fatigue, weakness
CV: *Hypotension,* bradycardia, HF, *palpitations,* dysrhythmias, cardiac arrest, AV block, pulmonary/peripheral edema, chest pain
EENT: Blurred vision
GI: *Nausea, vomiting,* colitis, cramps, *diarrhea,* constipation, flatulence, dry mouth, *hiccups*
GU: Impotence, urinary frequency
HEMA: Agranulocytosis, eosinophilia, thrombocytopenia, purpura
INTEG: Rash, purpura, alopecia, dry skin, urticaria, pruritus
RESP: Bronchospasm, dyspnea, wheezing
ENDO: Hyper/hypoglycemia

PHARMACOKINETICS
Half-life 3-10 hr, metabolized in liver (metabolites) by CYP2D6 ⚠ some may be poor metabolizers, excreted in urine; crosses placenta, enters breast milk
PO: Peak 2-4 hr, duration 13-19 hr
PO-ER: Peak 6-12 hr, duration 24 hr
IV: Onset immediate, peak 20 min, duration 6-8 hr

INTERACTIONS
Increase: hypoglycemic digoxin, diltiazem, bradycardia effects—verapamil, insulin, oral antidiabetics
Increase: metoprolol level—cimetidine
Increase: effects of benzodiazepines
Decrease: antihypertensive effect—salicylates, NSAIDs
Decrease: metoprolol level—barbiturates
Decrease: effects of—xanthines
Decrease: effects of each—dopamine, theophylline
Drug/Food
Increase: absorption with food

Drug/Lab Test
Increase: LDH, AST, ALT

NURSING CONSIDERATIONS
Assess:

Black Box Warning: Abrupt withdrawal: may cause MI, ventricular dysrhythmias, myocardial ischemia; taper dose over 7-14 days

• **Hypertension/angina:** ECG directly when giving IV during initial treatment
• I&O, weight daily; check for heart failure (weight gain, jugular venous distention, crackles, edema, dyspnea)
• Monitor B/P during initial treatment, periodically thereafter; pulse; note rate, rhythm, quality; apical/radial pulse before administration; notify prescriber of any significant changes or pulse <50 bpm; atropine 0.25-0.5 mg IV may be given for heart rate <40 bpm
• Baselines of renal, hepatic studies before therapy begins
• **Pregnancy/breastfeeding:** use only if clearly needed, no well-controlled studies, excreted in breast milk in small quantities; American Academy of Pediatrics considers this product to be compatible with breastfeeding
Evaluate:
• **Therapeutic response:** decreased B/P after 1-2 wk, decreased anginal pain
Teach patient/family:
• To take immediately after meals; to take medication at bedtime to prevent effect of orthostatic hypotension

Black Box Warning: Not to discontinue product abruptly; to taper over 2 wk; may cause angina

• Not to use OTC products containing α-adrenergic stimulants (nasal decongestants, OTC cold preparations) unless directed by prescriber; to avoid alcohol, smoking, sodium intake
• To report bradycardia, dizziness, confusion, depression, fever, sore throat, SOB, decreased vision to prescriber

- To take pulse, B/P at home; when to notify prescriber
- To comply with weight control, dietary adjustments, modified exercise program
- To carry emergency ID to identify product, allergies, prescriber
- To monitor blood glucose closely if diabetic, hypo/hyperglycemia
- To avoid hazardous activities if dizziness is present
- To report symptoms of heart failure: difficult breathing, especially on exertion or when lying down; night cough; swelling of extremities
- To rise slowly to decrease orthostatic hypertension
- To report Raynaud's symptoms
- That product may increase sensitivity to cold

TREATMENT OF OVERDOSE:
Lavage, IV atropine for bradycardia, IV theophylline for bronchospasm, digoxin, O_2, diuretic for cardiac failure, hemodialysis, administer vasopressor

metoprolol/
hydrochlorothiazide (Rx)
Dutoprol, Lopressor
Func. class.: β-blocker/thiazide diuretic

USES: Hypertension

DOSAGE AND ROUTES

Black Box Warning: Abrupt discontinuation

Hypertension in those who do not respond to monotherapy:
- **Adults (regular release): PO** 100-200 mg of metoprolol with 25-50 mg of hydrochlorothiazide, given in 1-2 divided doses; **(extended-release)** 25 mg to 200 mg metoprolol with 12.5 mg to 25 mg hydrochlorothiazide daily

Available forms: Tabs 50 mg/12.5 mg, 100 mg/12.5 mg, 100 mg/50 mg metoprolol/hydrochlorothiazide

metroNIDAZOLE (Rx)
(me-troe-ni′da-zole)
Flagyl
Func. class.: Antiinfective—miscellaneous
Chem. class.: Nitroimidazole derivative

Do not confuse:
metroNIDAZOLE/metFORMIN
Combinations: Helidac: metroNIDAZOLE 250 mg, bismuth 262 mg, tetracycline 500 mg; Pylera: metroNIDAZOLE 125 mg, bismuth 140 mg, tetracycline 125 mg

ACTION: Direct-acting amebicide/trichomonacide binds and disrupts DNA structure, thereby inhibiting bacterial nucleic acid synthesis

USES: Intestinal amebiasis, amebic abscess, trichomoniasis, refractory trichomoniasis, bacterial anaerobic infections, giardiasis, septicemia, endocarditis; bone, joint, lower respiratory tract infections; rosacea
Unlabeled uses: Giardiasis

CONTRAINDICATIONS
Pregnancy 1st trimester, breastfeeding, hypersensitivity to this product
Precautions: Pregnancy/2nd/3rd trimester, geriatric patients, *Candida* infections, heart failure, fungal infection, dental disease, bone marrow suppression, hematologic disease, GI/renal/hepatic disease, contracted visual or color fields, blood dyscrasias, CNS disorders

Black Box Warning: New primary malignancy

DOSAGE AND ROUTES

Black Box Warning: **Carcinogenic:** Use only for specified conditions

Trichomoniasis
- **Adult: PO** 500 mg bid × 7 days or 2 g as single dose; do not repeat treatment for 4-6 wk

- **Child ≥45 kg (unlabeled): PO** 2 g once
- **Child <45 kg (unlabeled): PO** 15 mg/kg/day in 3 divided doses × 7-10 days
- **Infant (unlabeled): PO** 15 mg/kg/day divided in 3 doses × 7 days

Amebic hepatic abscess

- **Adult: PO** 750 mg tid × 7-10 days
- **Child: PO** 35-50 mg/kg/day in 3 divided doses × 7-10 days

Intestinal amebiasis

- **Adult: PO** 750 mg tid × 7-10 days
- **Child: PO** 35-50 mg/kg/day in 3 divided doses × 7-10 days, then oral iodoquinol

Anaerobic bacterial infections

- **Adult: IV INFUSION** 15 mg/kg over 1 hr, then 7.5 mg/kg **IV** or **PO** q6hr, not to exceed 4 g/day; 1st maintenance dose should be administered 6 hr after loading dose

Bacterial vaginosis (nonpregnant)

- **Adult: PO** regular rel 500 mg bid or 250 mg tid × 7 days; ext rel 750 mg/day × 7 days

Giardiasis (unlabeled)

- **Adult: PO** 250-500 mg tid or 500 mg bid × 5-7 days

Available forms: Tabs 250, 500 mg; ext rel tab (ER) 750 mg; caps 375 mg; injection solution 5 mg/mL

Administer:

- Store in light-resistant container; do not refrigerate

PO route

- Do not break, crush, or chew ext rel product, give on empty stomach
- PO with or after meals to avoid GI symptoms, metallic taste; crush tabs if needed

IV route

Intermittent INFUSION (vial 5 mg/mL)

- **Premixed infusion bags:** prediluted, ready to use infusion over 30-60 min
- **Lyophilized vials:** dilute 500 mg with 4.4 mL sterile water, 0.9% NaCl; must be diluted further with ≤8 mg/mL with 0.9% NaCl, D_5W, or LR; must neutralize with 5 mEq $NaCO_3$/500 mg; CO_2 gas will be generated and may require venting; run over 30-60 min; primary IV must be discontinued; may be given as cont infusion; do not use aluminum products; IV may require venting
- Do not use aluminum needles or other equipment to prepare product

Incompatible: aztreonam, some cephalosporins, penicillin G, sodium lactate 5%, dextrose 10% injection and others

SIDE EFFECTS

CNS: *Headache, dizziness,* confusion, irritability, restlessness, ataxia, depression, fatigue, drowsiness, insomnia, paresthesia, peripheral neuropathy, seizures, incoordination, depression, encephalopathy, aseptic meningitis (IV)

CV: Flattening of T waves

EENT: Blurred vision, sore throat, retinal edema, dry mouth, metallic taste, furry tongue, glossitis, stomatitis, photophobia, optic neuritis

GI: *Nausea, vomiting, diarrhea,* epigastric distress, *anorexia,* constipation, *abdominal cramps,* CDAD, xerostomia, metallic taste, abdominal pain, pancreatitis

HEMA: Leukopenia, bone marrow supression, aplasia, thrombocytopenia

GU: Genital candida infection

INTEG: Rash, pruritus, urticaria, flushing, Stevens-Johnson syndrome, phlebitis at injection site, toxic epidermal necrolysis

PHARMACOKINETICS

Crosses placenta, enters breast milk, metabolized by liver 30%-60%, excreted in urine (60%-80%), half-life 6-8 hr

PO: Peak 2 hr, absorbed 80%-85%

IV: Onset immediate, peak end of infusion

INTERACTIONS

- Do not use with aprenavir
- Avoid use with zalcitabine, disulfiram, bortezomib, norfloxacin

Decrease: metroNIDAZOLE level—cholestyramine

Increase: disulfiram reaction—alcohol, oral ritonavir, any product with alcohol

Increase: busulfan toxicity—busulfan; avoid concurrent use

Increase: metroNIDAZOLE level, toxicity—cimetidine

Increase: lithium, CYP3A4 substrates

Increase: action of warfarin, phenytoin, lithium, fosphenytoin

Increase: leukopenia—azaTHIOprine, fluorouracil
Drug/Lab Test
Altered: AST, ALT, LDH, glucose
Decrease: WBC, neutrophils
False decrease: triglycerides

NURSING CONSIDERATIONS
Assess:
• **Infection:** WBC, wound symptoms, fever, skin or vaginal secretions; start treatment after C&S is obtained, waiting for results is not needed; for opportunistic fungal infections; superinfection: fever, monilial growth, fatigue, malaise
• Stools during entire treatment; should be clear at end of therapy; stools should be free of parasites for 1 yr before patient considered cured (amebiasis)
• Vision by ophthalmic exam during, after therapy; vision problems often occur
• **Allergic reaction:** fever, rash, itching, chills; product should be discontinued if these occur, if fever, facial swelling, blisters occur, discontinue immediately
• **Renal, reproductive dysfunction:** dysuria, polyuria, impotence, dyspareunia, decreased libido, I&O; weight daily

Black Box Warning: **New primary malignancy:** use only when indicated; avoid unnecessary use

• **Giardiasis:** stool samples before starting to confirm diagnosis, then 3-4 week after treatment
• **Pregnancy/breastfeeding:** not to be used in breastfeeding or 1st trimester of pregnancy
Evaluate:
• **Therapeutic response:** decreased symptoms of infection
Teach patient/family:
• That urine may turn dark reddish brown; that product may cause metallic taste; that both are normal
• About proper hygiene after bowel movement; handwashing technique
• To notify provider about numbness or tingling of extremities
• To avoid hazardous activities because dizziness can occur

• About need for compliance with dosage schedule, duration of treatment; to take extended-release tabs 1 hr before or 2 hr after meals; to take PO with meals to prevent GI upset
• To discuss all OTC, Rx, herbals, supplements taken with provider
• To notify provider immediately of rash, fever, facial swelling, blisters
• To use condoms if treatment for trichomoniasis or cross-contamination may occur; to notify prescriber if pregnant or planning to become pregnant; that treatment of both partners is necessary for trichomoniasis
• To use frequent sips of water, sugarless gum, candy for dry mouth
• Not parations containing alcohol during use or for 48 hr after use of product; disulfiram-like reaction can occur
• To notify if pregnancy is planned or suspected, or if breastfeeding

metroNIDAZOLE (topical, vaginal) (Rx)
(met-roe-ni′da-zole)
MetroCream, MetroGel, Noritate, Vandazole
Func. class.: Antiprotozoal, antibacterial
Chem. class.: Nitroimidazole

ACTION: Antibacterial and antiprotozoal activity may result from interacting with DNA

USES: Acne rosacea, bacterial vaginosis

CONTRAINDICATIONS
Hypersensitivity to this product or nitroimidazoles, parabens
Precautions: Hepatic disease, blood dyscrasias; CNS conditions (vaginal), children, pregnancy

DOSAGE AND ROUTES
Acne rosacea
• **Adult: TOP** apply to affected areas bid (0.75%) or daily (1%); adjust therapy based on response

Side effects: *italics* = common; red = life-threatening

Bacterial vaginosis
• **Adult: VAG** 1 applicatorful daily × 5 days

Available forms: Topical cream 0.75%, 1%; gel 0.75%, 1%; lotion 0.75%; vaginal gel 0.75%

Administer:
Topical route
• Topical skin products are not for intravaginal therapy and are for external use only; do not use skin products near the eyes, nose, or mouth
• Wash hands before and after use; wash affected area and gently pat dry
• **Cream/gel/lotion:** Apply a thin film to the cleansed affected area; massage gently into affected areas

Intravaginal route
• Only use dosage formulations specified for intravaginal use; intravaginal dosage forms are not for topical therapy; do not ingest
• Avoid vaginal intercourse during treatment
• **Cream:** Use applicator(s) supplied by the manufacturer

SIDE EFFECTS
GU: Vaginitis, cervicitis
GI: Nausea, vomiting, cramping
INTEG: Redness, burning, dermatitis, rash, pruritus

INTERACTIONS
• Possible lithium toxicity (vaginal gel)

NURSING CONSIDERATIONS
Assess:
• **Allergic reaction:** assess for hypersensitivity; product may need to be discontinued
• **Infection:** assess for number of lesions and severity of acne rosacea, itching in vaginosis
• **Pregnancy/breastfeeding:** not to be used in breastfeeding, systemic absorption; use in pregnancy only if clearly needed, no adequate studies

Evaluate:
• Decreased severity of acne rosacea, infection in vaginosis

Teach patient/family:
• That topical skin products are not for intravaginal therapy and are for external use only; not to use skin products near the eyes, nose, or mouth
• To wash hands before and after use; to wash affected area and gently pat dry
• **Cream/gel/lotion:** to apply a thin film to the cleansed affected area and massage gently into affected areas
• **Intravaginal route:** to use only dosage formulations specified for intravaginal use; not to ingest intravaginal dosage forms because these are not for topical therapy; to avoid vaginal intercourse during treatment
• **Cream:** to use applicator(s) supplied by the manufacturer

---

micafungin (Rx)
(my-ca-fun′gin)

Mycamine
Func. class.: Antifungal, systemic
Chem. class.: Echinocandin

ACTION: Inhibits an essential component of fungal cell walls; causes direct damage to fungal cell wall

USES: Treatment of esophageal candidiasis; prophylaxis for *Candida* infections in patients undergoing hematopoietic stem-cell transplantation (HSCT); susceptible *Candida* sp.: *C. albicans, C. glabrata, C. krusei, C. parapsilosis, C. tropicalis*

CONTRAINDICATIONS
Hypersensitivity to this product or other echinocandins

Precautions: Pregnancy, breastfeeding, children, geriatric patients, severe hepatic disease, renal impairment, hemolytic anemia

DOSAGE AND ROUTES
Esophageal candidiasis
• **Adult: IV INFUSION** 150 mg/day given over 1 hr × 15 days × 14-21 days
• **Child ≥4 mo, >30 kg: IV INFUSION** 2.5 mg/kg/day, max 150 mg/day × 14-21 days
• **Child ≥4 mo, ≤30 kg: IV INFUSION** 3 mg/kg/day × 14-21 days

Candidemia/acute disseminated candidiasis, abscess/peritonitis

• **Adult:** IV 100 mg/day over 1 hr × 15 days; treat for 2 wk after clearance from the bloodstream and resolution of signs and symptoms

• **Child ≥4 mo and >30 kg:** IV 2 mg/kg/day, max 100 mg/day; **≥4 mo and ≤30 kg:** 2 mg/kg/day; treat for 2 wk after clearance from the bloodstream and resolution of signs and symptoms

Prophylaxis for *Candida* infections in hemapoietic stem-cell transplant patients

• **Adult:** IV INFUSION 50 mg/day given over 1 hr

• **Adolescent/child/infant ≥4 mo:** IV INFUSION 1 mg/kg/day, max 50 mg/day

Administer:

Available forms: Powder for inj 50 mg, in single-dose vials 50-, 100-mg vial

IV route

Intermittent IV infusion

• Visually inspect for particulate matter and discoloration prior to use

• *Reconstitution:* Reconstitute each 50-mg vial or 100-mg vial with 5 mL of either 0.9% sodium chloride injection (without bacteriostatic agent) or 5% dextrose injection for a resultant concentration of 10 mg/mL or 20 mg/mL, respectively

• Gently dissolve by swirling the vial. In order to minimize excessive foaming, do not vigorously shake the vial

• *Storage:* Reconstituted product may be stored in the original vial protected from light for up to 24 hr at room temperature (77° F [25° C])

• *Dilution*

• **Adults:** Transfer the needed amount of reconstituted micafungin to an IV bag containing 100 mL of 0.9% sodium chloride injection or 5% dextrose injection

• **Pediatrics:** Withdraw the calculated volume of reconstituted micafungin and add to an IV bag or syringe containing 0.9% sodium chloride injection or 5% dextrose injection (final concentration 0.5-4 mg/mL); label infusion bags or syringes containing micafungin concentrations more than 1.5 mg/mL for administration through a central catheter only

• Discard partially used vials; micafungin is preservative-free.

• *Storage:* The final diluted solution may be stored protected from light for up to 24 hr at room temperature (77° F [25° C])

• To minimize the risk of infusion-related reactions, infuse solutions with concentrations more than 1.5 mg/mL via a central catheter

• If an existing IV line will be used, flush the line with 0.9% sodium chloride injection prior to and after infusion

• **Run** as a slow IV infusion over 1 hr. If administered more rapidly, more frequent histamine-mediated reactions may occur. Do not give as a bolus

• Do not mix or coinfuse micafungin with other medications. Micafungin has been shown to precipitate when mixed directly with several commonly used medications

• Protect diluted micafungin from light; not necessary to cover the drip chamber or the tubing during use

SIDE EFFECTS

GI: Abdominal pain, *nausea, anorexia, vomiting, diarrhea, hyperbilirubinemia,* hepatitis

GU: Renal failure

HEMA: Hemolytic anemia

INTEG: *Rash, pruritus, inj-site pain*

MISC: Allergic reactions

PHARMACOKINETICS

Metabolized in liver; excreted in feces, urine; terminal half-life 14-17.2 hr; protein binding 99%

INTERACTIONS

Increase: plasma concentrations—CYP3A4 substrates (aripiprazole, dofetilide, pimozide); itraconazole, sirolimus, NIFEdipine; may need dosage reduction

Drug/Lab Test

Increase: ALT/AST, alk phos, bilirubin, potassium, sodium, LDH, BUN, creatinine

Decrease: blood glucose platelets, HB, WBCs

NURSING CONSIDERATIONS
Assess:
• **Infection,** clearing of cultures during treatment; obtain culture at baseline and during treatment; product may be started as soon as culture is taken (esophageal candidiasis); monitor cultures during HSCT for prevention of *Candida* infections
• CBC (RBC, Hct, HB), differential, platelet count baseline, periodically; notify prescriber of results
• Renal studies: BUN, urine CCr, electrolytes before and during therapy
• Hepatic studies before and during treatment: bilirubin, AST, ALT, alk phos as needed
• **Bleeding:** hematuria, heme-positive stools, bruising, petechiae, mucosa or orifices; blood dyscrasias can occur
• **For hypersensitivity:** rash, pruritus, facial swelling, phlebitis
• For hemolytic anemia
• **GI symptoms:** frequency of stools, cramping; if severe diarrhea occurs, electrolytes may need to be given
• **Pregnancy/breastfeeding:** use cautiously in breastfeeding; use in pregnancy if benefit outweighs risk to fetus, no adequate studies
Evaluate:
• **Therapeutic response:** prevention of *Candida* infection with HSCT or decreased symptoms of *Candida* infection, negative culture
Teach patient/family:
• To avoid breastfeeding while taking this product, to notify prescriber if pregnancy is planned or suspected
• To report bleeding, facial swelling, wheezing, difficulty breathing, itching, rash, hives, increasing warmth, flushing
• To report signs of infection: increased temperature, sore throat, flulike symptoms: nausea, vomiting, clay-colored stools, anorexia, yellowing skin/eyes, dark urine, hepatotoxicity may occur

miconazole (Rx)
(mi-kon′a-zole)
Oravig
miconazole nitrate (OTC)
Baza, Desenex, Fungoid, Lotrimin AF, Micaderm, Micatin, Micozole ♣, Monistat-1, Monistat-3, Monistat-7, M-Zole 3, Vagistat-3, Zeasorb-AF
Func. class.: Antifungal
Chem. class.: Imidazole

Do not confuse:
miconazole/clotrimazole/metroNIDAZOLE

ACTION: Antifungal activity results from disruption of cell membrane permeability

USES: Treatment of topical fungal infection, vulvovaginal candidiasis; athlete's foot (tinea pedis), jock itch (tinea cruris), and ringworm (tinea corporis)

CONTRAINDICATIONS
Hypersensitivity to this product or imidazoles; pregnancy first trimester (vaginal)
Precautions: Breastfeeding, children

DOSAGE AND ROUTES
Oropharyngeal candidiasis (thrush)
• **Adult/adolescent ≥16 yr: BUCCAL** apply 1 tab (50 mg) to upper gum region, just above incisor daily × 14 days
Tinea corporis, cruris, pedis; cutaneous candidiasis
• **Adult/child >2 yr: TOP** apply bid × 2-4 wk
Tinea versicolor
• **Adult/child >2 yr: TOP** use bid × 2 wk, apply sparingly every day
Vulvovaginal candidiasis
• **Adult/child ≥12 yr: VAG** 1 applicatorful of Monistat-7 (100 mg) or 1 supp (100 mg) at bedtime × 7 days, repeat if needed, or Monistat-3 (200 mg) × 3 days or a 1200 mg supp × 1 day

Available forms: Topical cream, ointment, lotion, powder, aerosol, powder 2%; aerosol spray 2%; vag cream 2, 4%; vag supp 100, 200, 1200 mg; buccal tab 50 mg
Administer:
• Type of product is based on area involved
Transmucosal use (adhesive buccal tablet)
• Place the rounded surface of the tab against the upper gum just above the incisor tooth, hold in place with slight pressure over the upper lip for 30 sec to assure adhesion
• The tab will gradually dissolve
• Administration of subsequent tab should be made to alternate sides of the mouth
• Before applying the next tab, clear away any remaining tab material
• Do not crush, chew, or swallow; food and drink can be taken normally; avoid chewing gum
• If tab does not adhere or falls off within the first 6 hr, the same tab should be repositioned; if the tab still does not adhere, a new tab should be used
• If the tab falls off or is swallowed after it was in place for 6 hr or more, a new tab should not be applied until the next regularly scheduled dose
Topical route
• Topical skin products are not for intravaginal therapy and are for external use only; do not use skin products near the eyes, nose, or mouth
• Wash hands before and after use; was affected area and gently pat dry
• **Cream/ointment/lotion/solution:** apply a thin film to the cleansed affected area; massage gently into affected areas
• **Intravaginal route:** only use dosage formulations specified for intravaginal use
• **Suppository:** unwrap, use applicator(s) supplied by the manufacturer
• **Cream:** use applicator(s) supplied by the manufacturer

SIDE EFFECTS
CNS: Headache
GI: Diarrhea, nausea

GU: Pruritus, irritation, vaginal burning
INTEG: Burning, dermatitis, rash

DRUG INTERACTIONS
Increase: anticoagulant   effect—(buccal) monitor PT, INR
Decrease: effect (vaginal)—progesterone
Drug/Lab
Decrease: WBC, RBC (buccal)

NURSING CONSIDERATIONS
Assess:
• **Allergic reaction:** assess for hypersensitivity; product may need to be discontinued
• **Infection:** assess for severity of infection
• **Pregnancy/breastfeeding:** use cautiously in breastfeeding; use PO form in pregnancy only if benefits outweigh risk to fetus, no adequate studies
Evaluate:
• Decreasing severity of infection

Teach patient/family:
Topical route
• That topical skin products are not for intravaginal therapy and are for external use only; not to use skin products near the eyes, nose, or mouth
• To wash hands before and after use; wash affected area and gently pat dry
• **Cream/ointment/lotion/solution:**   to apply a thin film to the cleansed affected area and massage gently into affected areas
Intravaginal route
• To only use dosage formulations specified for intravaginal use; not to ingest intravaginal dosage forms; not to use tampons, douches, spermicides; not to engage in sexual activity; product may damage condoms, diaphragms, cervical caps
• **Suppository:** to unwrap vaginal ovule (suppository) before inserting; to use applicator(s) supplied by the manufacturer
• **Cream:** to use applicator(s) supplied by the manufacturer

M

> ### ⚠ HIGH ALERT

midazolam (Rx)
(mid′ay-zoe-lam)

Nayzilam (nasal spray)

Func. class.: Anxiolytic

Chem. class.: Benzodiazepine, short-acting

Controlled Substance Schedule IV

ACTION: Depresses subcortical levels in CNS; may act on limbic system, reticular formation; may potentiate γ-aminobutyric acid (GABA) by binding to specific benzodiazepine receptors

USES: Preoperative sedation, general anesthesia induction, sedation for diagnostic endoscopic procedures, intubation, anxiety

Unlabeled uses: Acute agitation, cocaine, methamphetamine intoxication, palliative/end-of-life sedation, rapid sequence intubation, status epilepticus

CONTRAINDICATIONS
Pregnancy, hypersensitivity to benzodiazepines, acute closed-angle glaucoma, epidural/intrathecal use

Precautions: Breastfeeding, children, geriatric patients, COPD, HF, chronic renal failure, chills, debilitated patients, hepatic disease, shock, coma, alcohol intoxication, status asthmaticus

Black Box Warning: Neonates (contains benzyl alcohol), IV administration, respiratory depression/insufficiency, specialized care setting, experienced clinician, coadministration with other CNS depressants, abrupt discontinuation, hypotension

DOSAGE AND ROUTES
• Use lean body weight for obese patient

Preoperative sedation/amnesia induction

• **Adult/child ≥12 yr: IM** 0.07-0.08 mg/kg ½-1 hr before general anesthesia

• **Child 6 yr-12 yr: IV** 0.025-0.05 mg/kg; total dose of 0.4 mg/kg may be necessary

• **Child 6 mo-5 yr: IV** 0.05-0.1 mg/kg; total dose of 0.6 mg/kg may be necessary

Induction of general anesthesia

• **Adult >55 yr:** (ASA I/II) **IV** 150-300 mcg/kg over 30 sec; (ASA III) **IV** limit dose to 250 mcg/kg (nonpremedicated) or 150 mcg/kg (premedicated)

• **Adult <55 yr: IV** 200-350 mcg/kg over 20-30 sec; if patient has not received premedication, may repeat by giving 20% of original dose; if patient has received premedication, reduce dose by 50 mcg/kg

• **Child:** no safe and effective dose established; however, doses of 50-200 mcg/kg **IV** have been used

Continuous infusion for mechanical ventilation (critical care)

• **Adult: IV** 0.01-0.05 mg/kg over several min; repeat at 10- to 15-min intervals until adequate sedation, then 0.02-0.10 mg/kg/hr maintenance; adjust as needed

• **Child: IV** 0.05-0.2 mg/kg over 2-3 min then 0.06-0.12 mg/kg/hr by cont infusion; adjust as needed

• **Neonate: IV** 0.03 mg/kg/hr, titrate using lowest dose

Status epilepticus (unlabeled)

• **Child and infant >2 mo: IV** 0.15 mg/kg then **CONT IV** 1 mcg/kg/min, titrate upward q5min until seizures controlled

Available forms: Inj 1, 5 mg/mL (preservative free); injection 1 mg/mL, 5 mg/mL; syr 2 mg/mL; nasal spray 5 mg

Administer:

• Store at room temperature; protect from light

PO route (syrup)

• **Press-in-bottle adaptor (PIBA)** Remove cap of press-in bottle adapter, push adapter into neck of bottle; close with cap; remove cap, insert tip of dispenser, insert into adapter; turn upside-down, withdraw correct dose; place in mouth

IM route

• IM deep into large muscle mass

IV route

• May be given diluted or undiluted 1 mg/mL or 5 mg/mL (undiluted) or 0.03-3 mL (diluted)

• After diluting with D₅W or 0.9% NaCl, give over 2-5 min (conscious sedation) or over 30 sec (anesthesia induction)

Continuous IV infusion route

• Dilute in 0.9% NaCl or D₅W to 0.5-1 mg/mL, dose is calculated on patient's weight and use

Black Box Warning: Do not use rapid injection in neonates

Y-site compatibilities: Abciximab, acetaminophen, alemtuzumab, alfentanil, amikacin, amiodarone, anidulafungin, argatroban, atracurium, atropine, aztreonam, benzotropine, calcium gluconate, ceFAZolin, cefotaxime, cefOXitine, cefTRIAXone, cimetidine, ciprofloxacin, CISplatin, clindamycin, cloNIDine, cyanocobalamin, cycloSPORINE, DACTINomycin, digoxin, diltiaZEM, diphenhydrAMINE, DOCEtaxel, DOPamine, doxycycline, enalaprilat, EPINEPHrine, erythromycin, esmolol, etomidate, etoposide, famotidine, fentaNYL, fluconazole, folic acid, gatifloxacin, gemcitabine, gentamicin, glycopyrrolate, granisetron, heparin, hetastarch, HYDROmorphone, hydrOXYzine, inamrinone, isoproterenol, labetalol, lactated Ringer's, levoFLOXacin, lidocaine, linezolid, LORazepam, magnesium, mannitol, meperidine, methadone, methyldopa, methylPREDNISolone, metoclopramide, metoprolol, metroNIDAZOLE, milrinone, morphine, nalbuphine, naloxone, niCARdipine, nitroglycerin, nitroprusside, norepinephrine, ondansetron, oxacillin, oxytocin, PACLitaxel, palonosetron, pancuronium, papaverine, phytonadione, piperacillin, potassium chloride, propranolol, protamine, pyridoxine, raNITIdine, remifentanil, sodium nitroprusside, succinylcholine, SUFentanil, teniposide, theophylline, thiotepa, ticarcillin, tobramycin,

vancomycin, vasopressin, vecuronium, verapamil, voriconazole, zoledronic acid

SIDE EFFECTS

CNS: Retrograde amnesia, headache, paresthesia, chills, paradoxic reactions

CV: Hypotension, PVCs, nodal rhythm, cardiac arrest

EENT: Nystagmus, blurred vision

GI: *Nausea, vomiting,* hiccups

INTEG: Urticaria; pain, swelling, pruritus at inj site; rash

RESP: Coughing, apnea, respiratory depression

PHARMACOKINETICS

Protein binding 97%; half-life 1-5 hr, metabolized in liver; by CYP3A4 to metabolites excreted in urine; crosses placenta, blood-brain barrier

PO: Onset 10-30 min

IM: Onset 15 min, peak ½-1 hr, duration 2-3 hr

IV: Onset 1.5-5 min, onset of anesthesia 1½-2½ min, duration 2 hr

INTERACTIONS

Increase: hypotension—antihypertensives, opiates, alcohol, nitrates

Increase: extended half-life—CYP3A4 inhibitors (cimetidine, erythromycin, raNITIdine), adjust dose if needed

Increase: respiratory depression—other CNS depressants, alcohol, barbiturates, opiate analgesics, verapamil, ritonavir, indinavir, fluvoxaMINE, protease inhibitors

Decrease: midazolam metabolism—CYP3A4 inducers (azole antifungals, theophylline), adjust dose if needed

Drug/Herb

Increase: sedation—kava, valerian

Decrease: midazolam effect—St. John's wort

Drug/Food

Increase: (PO) midazolam effect—grapefruit juice, do not use together

NURSING CONSIDERATIONS

Assess:

• B/P, pulse, respirations during IV; emergency equipment should be nearby

M

Side effects: *italics* = common; red = life-threatening

- Inj site for redness, pain, swelling

Black Box Warning: Should be used only in a specialized care setting by those trained in use

Black Box Warning: Respiratory depression/insufficiency: apnea, respiratory depression may be increased in geriatric patients

- Assistance with ambulation until drowsy period ends
- Immediate availability of resuscitation equipment, O_2 to support airway; do not give by rapid bolus
- **Beers:** avoid in older adults with delirium or at high risk for delirium; assess frequently for confusion, delirium; degree of amnesia in geriatric patients may be increased
- **Pregnancy/breastfeeding:** do not use in pregnancy; avoid use in breastfeeding, excreted in breast milk

Evaluate:
- **Therapeutic response:** induction of sedation, general anesthesia

Teach patient/family:
- That amnesia occurs; that events may not be remembered; to give with instructions
- To avoid driving, other hazardous activities until effects are known
- Reason for product, expected results

TREATMENT OF OVERDOSE: Flumazenil, O_2

⚠ HIGH ALERT

midostaurin (Rx)
(mye-doe-staw´-rin)
Rydapt
Func. class.: Antineoplastic

USES: Newly diagnosed FLT3 mutation–positive AML in combination with standard cytarabine and DAUNOrubicin induction and consolidation therapy and for the treatment of aggressive systemic mastocytosis, systemic mastocytosis with associated hematologic neoplasm, or mast cell leukemia

DOSAGE AND ROUTES
Newly diagnosed FLT3 mutation–positive AML
- **Adult: PO** 50 mg bid on days 8 to 21 of each cycle of induction therapy with cytarabine and DAUNOrubicin; additionally, give midostaurin 50 mg bid on days 8 to 21 of each cycle of consolidation with high-dose cytarabine therapy

Aggressive systemic mastocytosis, systemic mastocytosis
- **Adult: PO** 100 mg bid until disease progression

Available forms: Capsule 25 mg

---

migalastat (Rx)
(mi-gal´a-stat)
Galafold
Func. class.: Metabolic agent
Chem. class.: Pharmacologic chaperone

USES Treatment of a confirmed diagnosis of Fabry disease and an amenable galactosidase alpha gene (GLA) variant

DOSAGE AND ROUTES
Adult: PO 123 mg every other day
Available forms: Capsules 123 mg

---

miglitol (Rx)
(mig´lih-tol)
Glyset
Func. class.: Oral hypoglycemic
Chem. class.: α-Glucosidase inhibitor

ACTION: Delays digestion and absorption of ingested carbohydrates, which results in a smaller rise in blood glucose after meals; does not increase insulin production

USES: Type 2 diabetes mellitus, alone or in combination

CONTRAINDICATIONS

Hypersensitivity, diabetic ketoacidosis, cirrhosis, inflammatory bowel disease, colonic ulceration, partial intestinal obstruction, chronic intestinal disease, ileus

Precautions: Pregnancy, breastfeeding, children, diarrhea, hiatal hernia, hypoglycemia, renal disease, type 1 diabetes, vomiting

DOSAGE AND ROUTES
Type 2 diabetes
• **Adult:** PO 25 mg tid initially, with 1st bite of meal; maintenance dose may be increased to 50 mg tid; may be increased to 100 mg tid if needed with dosage adjustment at 4- to 8-wk intervals

Available forms: Tabs 25, 50, 100 mg
Administer:
• Tid with first bite of each meal
• Store in tight container at room temperature

SIDE EFFECTS
GI: *Abdominal pain, diarrhea, flatulence,* hepatotoxicity
INTEG: Rash

PHARMACOKINETICS
Peak 2-3 hr, not metabolized, excreted in urine as unchanged product, half-life 2 hr

INTERACTIONS
Increase: hypoglycemia risk—insulin, other antidiabetics
Decrease: levels of digoxin, propranolol, raNITIdine; adjust dose as needed
Decrease: miglitol levels—digestive enzymes, intestinal adsorbents; do not use together
Drug/Food
Increase: diarrhea—carbohydrates

NURSING CONSIDERATIONS
Assess:
• **Hypo/hyperglycemia;** even though product does not cause hypoglycemia, if patient receiving sulfonylureas or insulin, hypoglycemia may be additive (rare)
• Blood glucose levels, hemoglobin, A1c, LFTs; if hypoglycemia occurs with monotherapy, treat with glucose

• Identify medical regimen prescribed—diet, exercise, lab work
• Monitor blood glucose testing more often in stress, trauma, surgery
• **Pregnancy/breastfeeding:** use of insulin during pregnancy is recommended, don't use this product unless clearly needed; excreted in breast milk, avoid use
Evaluate:
• **Therapeutic response:** decreased signs, symptoms of diabetes mellitus (polyuria, polydipsia, polyphagia; clear sensorium, absence of dizziness; stable gait); improved blood glucose, A1c
Teach patient/family:
• About the symptoms of hypo/hyperglycemia; what to do about each; that during periods of stress, infection, or surgery, insulin may be required
• To carry oral glucose or glucagon to treat low glucose, do not use simple sugar in fruit juices, candy, table sugar
• How to use a glucose monitor and when to monitor; how to identify low blood glucose levels
• That medication must be taken as prescribed, tid with first bite of each meal; about consequences of discontinuing medication abruptly
• To avoid OTC medications unless approved by health care provider
• That diabetes is lifelong; that product is not a cure; to continue with medical regimen of diet, exercise, lab work
• To carry ID for emergency purposes
• About GI side effects that are common during several weeks of treatment, that they improve with continued treatment

> **⚠ HIGH ALERT**
>
> ## milrinone (Rx)
> (mill′rih-nohn)
> *Func. class.:* Inotropic/vasodilator agent
> *Chem. class.:* Bipyridine phosphodiesterase inhibitor

ACTION: Positive inotropic agent; increases contractility of cardiac muscle with vasodilator properties; reduces preload and afterload by direct relaxation on vascular smooth muscle

USES: Short-term management of advanced heart failure that has not responded to other medication

CONTRAINDICATIONS
Hypersensitivity to this product, severe aortic disease, severe pulmonic valvular disease, acute MI
Precautions: Pregnancy, breastfeeding, children, geriatric patients, renal/hepatic disease, atrial flutter/fibrillation

DOSAGE AND ROUTES
Short-term treatment of acutely decompensated heart failure
• **Adult: IV BOL** 50 mcg/kg given over 10 min (loading dose); start infusion of 0.375-0.75 mcg/kg/min, titrate based on response
Renal dose
• **Adult: IV** CCr 41-50 mL/min, 0.43 mcg/kg/min, titrate up; CCr 31-40 mL/min, 0.38 mcg/kg/min, titrate up; CCr 21-30 mL/min, 0.33 mcg/kg/min, titrate up; CCr 11-20 mL/min, 0.28 mcg/kg/min; CCr 6-10 mL/min, 0.23 mcg/kg/min; CCr ≤5 mL/min, 0.20 mcg/kg/min; max for all doses 0.75 mcg/kg/min
Available forms: Inj 1 mg/mL; premixed inj 200 mcg/mL in D_5W
Administer:
• Potassium supplements if ordered for potassium levels <3 mg/dL
Direct IV route
• Give IV loading dose undiluted over 10 min, use infusion device
Continuous IV route
• Dilute 20-mg vial with 80, 113, 180 mL of 0.45% NaCl, 0.9% NaCl, or D_5W to a concentration of 200, 150, 100 mcg/mL, respectively
• Titrate rate based on hemodynamic and clinical response, use infusion device
• Diluted solution must be kept at room temperature and used within 24 hr
• Precipitation will form when furosemide is injected into line with milrinone

Y-site compatibilities: Acyclovir, alfentanil, allopurinol, amifostine, amikacin, aminocaproic acid, aminophylline, amiodarone, amphotericin B liposome, ampicillin, ampicillin-sulbactam, anidulafungin, argatroban, atenolol, atracurium, aztreonam, bivalirudin, bleomycin, bumetanide, buprenorphine, busulfan, butorphanol, calcium chloride/gluconate, CARBOplatin, caspofungin, ceFAZolin, cefepime, cefotaxime, cefoTEtan, cefOXitin, cefTAZidime, ceftizoxime, cefTRIAXone, cefuroxime, chloramphenicol, chlorproMAZINE, cimetidine, ciprofloxacin, cisatracurium, CISplatin, clindamycin, cyclophosphamide, cycloSPORINE, cytarabine, DACTINomycin, DAPTOmycin, dexamethasone, digoxin, diltiaZEM, DOBUTamine, DOCEtaxel, DOPamine, doripenem, doxacurium, DOXOrubicin, doxycycline, droperidol, enalaprilat, ePHEDrine, EPINEPHrine, epiRUBicin, eptifibatide, ertapenem, erythromycin, etoposide, famotidine, fenoldopam, fentaNYL, fluconazole, fludarabine, fluorouracil, gallium, ganciclovir, gatifloxacin, gemcitabine, gentamicin, glycopyrrolate, granisetron, haloperidol, heparin, hydrALAZINE, hydrocortisone, HYDROmorphone, IDArubicin, ifosfamide, insulin (regular), irinotecan, isoproterenol, ketorolac, labetalol, levoFLOXacin, linezolid, LORazepam, magnesium sulfate, mannitol, mechlorethamine, melphalan, meperidine, meropenem, methohexital, methotrexate, methyldopate, methylPREDNISolone, metoclopramide, metoprolol, metroNIDAZOLE, micafungin, midazolam, mitoXANTRONE, morphine, mycophenolate, nafcillin, nalbuphine, naloxone, nesiritide, niCARdipine, nitroglycerin, nitroprusside, norepinephrine, octreotide, oxacillin, oxaliplatin, oxytocin, PACLitaxel, palonosetron, pamidronate, pancuronium, PEMEtrexed, pentamidine, pentazocine, PENTobarbital, PHENobarbital, phenylephrine, piperacillin, piperacillin-tazobactam, polymyxin B, potassium chloride/phosphates, prochlorperazine, promethazine, propofol, propranolol, quiNIDine, quinupristin-dalfopristin, raNITIdine, remifentanil, rocuronium, sodium acetate/bicarbonate/phosphates, streptozocin, succinylcholine, SUFentanil, sulfamethoxazole-trimethoprim, tacrolimus, teniposide, theophylline, thiopental, thiotepa, ticarcillin, ticarcillin-clavulanate, tigecycline, tirofiban, tobramycin, torsemide, vancomycin, vasopressin, vecuronium, verapamil, vinCRIStine, vinorelbine, voriconazole, zidovudine, zoledronic acid

SIDE EFFECTS
CNS: Headache
CV: Ventricular dysrhythmias, hypotension, chest pain, *PVCs, palpitations, angina,* ventricular tachycardia
HEMA: Thrombocytopenia
MISC: Inj site reactions

PHARMACOKINETICS
IV: Onset 2-5 min, peak 10 min, duration variable; half-life 2.3 hr; metabolized in liver; excreted in urine as product (83%), metabolites (12%)

INTERACTIONS
None significant

NURSING CONSIDERATIONS
Assess:
• Monitor ECG continuously during IV; ventricular dysrhythmia can occur, PEWP, CVP index often during infusion; B/P, pulse q5min during infusion; if B/P drops 30 mm Hg, stop infusion, call prescriber
• **Electrolytes:** potassium, sodium, chloride, calcium, correct as needed; **renal studies:** BUN, creatinine; **blood studies:** platelet count
• ALT, AST, bilirubin daily
• I&O ratio, weight daily; diuresis should increase with continuing therapy
• **Pregnancy/breastfeeding:** use in pregnancy if benefit outweighs risk to fetus; no well-controlled studies; cautious use in breastfeeding, not known if excreted in breast milk

Evaluate:
• **Therapeutic response:** increased cardiac output, decreased PCWP, adequate CVP; decreased dyspnea, fatigue, edema, ECG
Teach patient/family:
• To report angina, palpitations immediately during infusion
• To report headache, which can be treated with analgesics

TREATMENT OF OVERDOSE:
Discontinue product, support circulation

miltefosine (Rx)
(mil′-te-foe′-seen)
Impavido
Func. class.: Antiprotozoal/antileishmanial

USES: Treatment of visceral leishmaniasis caused by *L. donovani,* mucosal leishmaniasis caused by *L. braziliensis,* and cutaneous leishmaniasis caused by *L. braziliensis, L. guyanensis,* and *L. panamensis*

CONTRAINDICATIONS
Hypersensitivity, pregnancy

DOSAGE AND ROUTES
• **Adult/adolescent/child ≥12 yr and ≥45 kg: PO** 50 mg tid × 28 days
• **Adult/adolescent/child ≥12 yr and 30-44 kg: PO** 50 mg bid × 28 days; HIV guidelines suggest 100 mg daily × 4 wk in adults and adolescents regardless of weight
Available forms: capsule 50 mg

minocycline (Rx)
(min-oh-sye′kleen)
Arestin ✦, Minocin, Minolira, Solodyn, Ximino
Func. class.: Broad-spectrum antiinfective
Chem. class.: Tetracycline

ACTION: Inhibits protein synthesis, phosphorylation in microorganisms by binding to ribosomal subunits, reversibly binding to ribosomal subunits; bacteriostatic

USES: *Acinetobacter* sp., *Actinomyces israelii, Actinomyces* sp., *Bacillus anthracis, Bartonella bacilliformis, Bordetella pertussis, Borrelia burgdorferi, Borrelia recurrentis, Brucella* sp., *Burkholderia mallei, Burkholderia pseudomallei, Campylobacter fetus, Chlamydia trachomatis, Chlamydophila psittaci, Clostridium perfringens, Clostridium* sp., *Clostridium tetani, Coxiella burnetii, Eikenella corrodens, Entamoeba* sp., *Enterobacter aerogenes, Escherichia coli, Francisella tularensis, Fusobacterium fusiforme, Fusobacterium nucleatum, Haemophilus ducreyi, Haemophilus influenzae (beta-lactamase negative), Haemophilus influenzae (beta-lactamase positive), Klebsiella granulomatis, Klebsiella* sp., *Legionella mophila, Leptospira* sp., *Leptotrichia buccalis, Listeria monocytogenes, Mycobacterium marinum, Mycoplasma hominis, Mycoplasma pneumoniae, Neisseria gonorrhoeae, Neisseria meningitidis, Nocardia* sp., *Pasteurella multocida, Porphyromonas gingivalis, Prevotella intermedia, Propionibacterium acnes, Propionibacterium propionicum, Rickettsia akari, Rickettsia prowazekii, Rickettsia rickettsii, Rickettsia tsutsugamushi, Shigella* sp., *Spirillum minus, Staphylococcus aureus* (MRSA), *Staphylococcus aureus* (MSSA), *Streptobacillus moniliformis, Streptococcus pneumoniae, Treponema pallidum, Treponema pertenue, Ureaplasma urealyticum, Vibrio cholerae, Vibrio parahaemolyticus, Yersinia enterocolitica, Yersinia pestis*

CONTRAINDICATIONS
Pregnancy, children <8 yr, hypersensitivity to tetracyclines

Precautions: Hepatic disease, breastfeeding

DOSAGE AND ROUTES
Most infections
• Adult: PO/IV 200 mg, then 100 mg q12hr, max 400 mg/24 hr IV
• Child/adolescents 9-17 yr: PO/IV 4 mg/kg, max 200 mg, then 2 mg/kg/dose (max 100 mg/dose) q12hr
Rickettsial infections
• Adult: PO/IV 200 mg, then 100 mg q12hr
• Child ≥9 yr/adolescent: PO/IV 4 mg/kg, then 2 mg/kg q12hr, max adult dose
Gonorrhea (allergic to penicillin)
• Adult: PO 200 mg, then 100 mg q12hr × ≥4 days, cultures 2-3 days after use
Syphilis (allergic to penicillin)
• Adult: PO 200 mg, then 100 mg q12hr × 10-15 days
Meningococcal carrier state
• Adult: PO 100 mg q12hr × 5 days
Uncomplicated gonococcal urethritis in men
• Adult: PO 100 mg q12hr × 5 days
Acne vulgaris (Solodyn only)
• Adult/adolescent/child ≥12 yr: PO ext rel 1 mg/kg/day × 12 wk or those weighing 126-136 kg—135 mg/day; 111-125 kg—115 mg/day; 97-110 kg—105 mg/day; 85-96 kg—90 mg/day; 72-84 kg—80 mg/day; 60-71 kg—65 mg/day; 50-59 kg—55 mg/day; 45-49 kg—45 mg/day
Acne vulgaris (all except Solodyn)
• Adult/adolescent/child ≥12 yr: PO ext rel 1 mg/kg/day × 12 wk or those weighing 91-136 kg—135 mg/day; 60-90 kg—90 mg/day; 45-59 kg—45 mg/day
Available forms: Caps 50, 75, 100 mg; inj 100 mg; tabs 50, 75, 100 mg; ext rel tabs 45, 55, 65, 80, 90, 105, 115, 135 mg
Administer:
• After C&S obtained before first dose; begin treatment as soon as drawn
• Store in airtight, light-resistant container at room temperature; do not expose to light
• **Fanconi's syndrome:** do not use outdated products; may cause nephrotoxicity

PO route
• With full glass of water; with food for GI symptoms
• Use extended-release tabs at same time each day, without regard to food
• Swallow caps, extended-release tabs whole; do not crush, chew
• 2 hr before or after laxative or ferrous products; 3 hr after antacid

IV route
• After reconstituting 100 mg/5 mL sterile water for inj; further dilute in 100-1000 mL of NaCl, dextrose sol; give over 1-6 hr, do not give rapidly or 250-1000 mL with Ringer's or LR, do not admix
• Change to PO dose as soon as possible to reduce thrombophlebitis risk

Y-site compatibilities: Alfentanil, amikacin, atracurium, benztropine, buprenorphine, butorphanol, calcium chloride, CARBOplatin, caspofungin, cefonicid, chlorproMAZINE, cimetidine, cisatracurium, codeine, cyclophosphamide, cycloSPORINE, cytarabine, DACTINomycin, dexmedetomidine, diltiaZEM, diphenhydrAMINE, DOBUTamine, DOCEtaxel, doxacurium, doxycycline, enalaprilat, ePHEDrine, EPINEPHrine, eptifibatide, etoposide, fenoldopam, fentaNYL, filgrastim, fludarabine, gatifloxacin, gemcitabine, gentamicin, glycopyrrolate, granisetron, heparin, hetastarch, IDArubicin, ifosfamide, inamrinone, isoproterenol, labetalol, levoFLOXacin, lidocaine, linezolid, LORazepam, magnesium sulfate, mannitol, melphalan, metaraminol, methotrexate, methyldopa, metoclopramide, metoprolol, midazolam, mitoXANTRONE, nalbuphine, naloxone, perphenazine, potassium chloride, remifentanil, sargramostim, teniposide, vinorelbine, vit B/C

SIDE EFFECTS
CNS: *Dizziness,* fever, light-headedness, vertigo, seizures, increased intracranial pressure, headache
CV: Pericarditis, thrombophlebitis
EENT: Permanent discoloration of teeth, oral candidiasis, tinnitus
GI: *Nausea, vomiting, diarrhea,* anorexia, hepatotoxicity, CDAD
GU: Renal failure
HEMA: Eosinophilia, neutropenia, thrombocytopenia, hemolytic anemia, pancytopenia
RESP: Bronchospasm, cough, dyspnea
INTEG: *Rash, urticaria, photosensitivity, increased pigmentation,* exfoliative dermatitis, pruritus, blue-gray color of skin, mucous membranes
MS: Myalgia, arthritis; bone growth retardation (<8 yr)
SYST: Angioedema, Stevens-Johnson syndrome, DRESS

PHARMACOKINETICS
PO: Peak 1-4 hr, half-life 11-22 hr; excreted in urine, feces, breast milk; crosses placenta

INTERACTIONS
Increase: effect of warfarin, digoxin, insulin, oral anticoagulants, theophylline, neuromuscular blockers
Increase: chance of pseudomotor cerebri—retinoids; do not use concurrently
Decrease: effect of hormonal contraceptives, use another form of contraception
Decrease: effect of live virus vaccines, bring up to date before use
Decrease: minocycline absorption, give 2 hr before or 3 hr after iron products; laxatives (calcium, aluminum, magnesium) antidiarrhea
Decrease: effect of penicillins, avoid using together
Drug/Lab Test
False negative: urine glucose with Clinistix or Tes-Tape
Increase: BUN, FTs, eosinophils
Decrease: HB, platelets, neutrophils

NURSING CONSIDERATIONS
Assess:
• **CDAD:** diarrhea, abdominal cramps, fever; may start up to 2 mo after treatment ends; if diarrhea occurs, evaluate
• I&O ratio
• Age and tooth development
• **Blood tests:** PT, CBC, AST, ALT, BUN, creatinine
• **Signs of anemia:** Hct, HB, fatigue
• **Serious allergic reactions (anaphylaxis, Stevens-Johnson syndrome, DRESS):**

M

assess for rash, fever, fatigue, fluid-filled blisters, abnormal LFTs; product should be discontinued immediately

• Nausea, vomiting, diarrhea; administer antiemetic, antacids as ordered

• **Overgrowth of infection:** fever, malaise, redness, pain, swelling, drainage, perineal itching, diarrhea; changes in cough or sputum; black, furry tongue in long-term therapy

• **Beers:** Avoid in older adults, may exacerbate syncope, monitor frequently

• **Pregnancy/breastfeeding:** do not use in pregnancy, can cause fetal harm; if pregnancy occurs, stop immediately; do not breastfeed, excreted in breast milk

Evaluate:

• **Therapeutic response:** decreased temperature, absence of lesions, negative C&S

Teach patient/family:

• To avoid sunlight, wear protective clothing; that sunscreen does not seem to decrease photosensitivity

• That all prescribed medication must be taken to prevent superinfection; not to use outdated product because Fanconi's syndrome may occur

• To report diarrhea that can occur several months after discontinuing product

• To avoid taking antacids, iron, cimetidine; to use 2 hr before, 6 hr after this product, absorption may be decreased; to take with a full glass of water; to take with food; not to take at bedtime, esophageal irritation may occur

• That teeth discoloration, joint or muscle pain may occur

• To use backup contraception; effectiveness may be decreased

• Not to use during pregnancy, breastfeeding; not to use for acne if trying to conceive

• To avoid driving, other hazardous activities until reaction is known

• To swallow extended-release product whole, do not crush, chew, split; not to increase, double doses, take at same time of day

---

minoxidil (Rx, OTC)

(mi-nox′i-dill)

Hair Regrowth Treatment Men, Minoxidil for Men, Rogaine Mens Extra Strength, Rogaine Mens, Rogaine Womens (topical)

Func. class.: Antihypertensive
Chem. class.: Vasodilator, peripheral

USES: Topically to treat alopecia

DOSAGE AND ROUTES
Alopecia

• **Adult: TOP** 1 mL bid, rub into scalp daily, max 2 mL/day

Available forms: Topical 2%, 5% sol; topical foam 5%

---

mirabegron (Rx)

(mir′a-beg′ron)

Myrbetriq

Func. class.: Bladder antispasmodic
Chem. class.: β_3-Adrenergic receptor agonist

ACTION: Relaxes smooth muscles in urinary tract, increase bladder capacity

USES: Overactive bladder (urinary frequency, urgency), urinary incontinence, neurogenic detrusor overactivity

CONTRAINDICATIONS
Hypersensitivity

Precautions: Pregnancy, breastfeeding, children, kidney/liver disease, bladder obstruction, dialysis, hypertension

DOSAGE AND ROUTES
Overactive bladder

• **Adult: PO** 25 mg/day, may increase to 50 mg/day if needed, may be given with solifenacin

---

Hepatic/renal dose
• **Adult: PO** Child-Pugh B or CCr 15-29 mL/min, max 25 mg/day; Child-Pugh C or CCr <15 mL/min, not recommended

Neurogenic detrusor overactivity
• **Child ≥3 yr and ≥35 kg:** Ext Rel tab 25 mg qday, may increase to 50 mg/day after 4-8 wk; **Ext Rel Suspension** 48 mg qday, may increase to 80 mg qday after 4-8 wk
• **Child ≥3 yr and 22 to <35 kg:** Ext **Rel suspension** 32 mg qday, may increase to 64 mg qday after 4-8 wk
• **Child ≥3 yr and 11 to <22 kg:** Ext **Rel suspension** 24 mg qday may increase to 48 mg qday after 4-8 wk

Available forms: Tabs ext rel 25, 50 mg; granules for ext rel suspension 8 mg/mL after reconstitution

Administer:
• Give whole; take with liquids; do not crush, chew, or break ext rel product; use without regard to meals
• Missed dose should not be taken; take at next selected time
• **Suspension:** Use 100 mL of water and add granules, shake well for 1 min, let stand 10-30 min, shake again for 1-2 min until dissolved; use dosing device; store reconstituted at room temperature for up to 28 days

SIDE EFFECTS

CNS: Fatigue, *dizziness, headache*
CV: *Hypertension,* tachycardia
EENT: Xerophthalmia, blurred vision
GI: Anorexia, abdominal pain, constipation, diarrhea, nausea, vomiting
GU: Urinary retention, frequency, UTI, bladder discomfort
INTEG: Stevens-Johnson syndrome, rash, pruritis
MS: Arthralgia, back pain

PHARMACOKINETICS

71% protein binding, excretion 25% unchanged in urine, half-life 50 hr, peak 3.5 hr

INTERACTIONS

Increase: effect of CYP2D6 substrates
Increase: effect of digoxin, warfarin, desipramine
Increase: mirabegron effect—CYP3A4 inhibitors
Increase: urinary retention risk—antimuscarinic agents (atropine, scopolamine)

Drug/Lab Test
Increase: LFTs, digoxin, INR, LDH

NURSING CONSIDERATIONS
Assess:
• **Urinary patterns:** distention, nocturia, frequency, urgency, incontinence
• **Angioedema (rare):** swelling of face, lips, tongue, dyspnea; discontinue immediately, have emergency equipment nearby
• LFTs at baseline, periodically
• Monitor B/P, pulse often
• **Pregnancy/breastfeeding:** use only if benefits outweigh risks to fetus; no well-controlled studies, discontinue product, not known if excreted in breast milk
Evaluate:
• Decreasing dysuria, frequency, nocturia, incontinence
Teach patient/family:
• **Hypertension:** to report fast heartbeat; monitor B/P, P at home
• **Angioedema (rare):** to report immediately swelling of face, lips, tongue
• To avoid hazardous activities; dizziness can occur; may take up to 8 wk for full effect
• Not to drink liquids before bedtime
• About the importance of bladder maintenance
• Not to breastfeed; to report if pregnancy is planned or suspected
• Not to crush, chew, split; to take without regard to food, not to skip, double doses, if missed take at regularly scheduled next day, provide "Patient Information Materials"
• To discuss all OTC, Rx, herbals, supplements with provider

mirtazapine (Rx)
(mer-ta′za-peen)
Remeron, Remeron SolTab
Func. class.: Antidepressant
Chem. class.: Tetracyclic

ACTION: Blocks reuptake of norepinephrine and serotonin into nerve endings, antagonist of central α_2-receptors; blocks histamine receptors

USES: Depression; dysthymic disorder; bipolar disorder: depressed, agitated depression

CONTRAINDICATIONS

Hypersensitivity to tricyclics, recovery phase of MI, agranulocytosis, jaundice, MAOIs

Precautions: Pregnancy, geriatric patients, suicidal patients, severe depression, increased intraocular pressure, closed-angle glaucoma, urinary retention, cardiac/renal/hepatic disease, hypo/hyperthyroidism, electroshock therapy, elective surgery, seizure disorder, bone marrow suppression, thrombocytopenia

> **Black Box Warning:** Suicidal ideation, children, young adults

DOSAGE AND ROUTES
Major depressive disorder
• **Adult:** PO 15 mg/day at bedtime, maintenance to continue for 6 mo, titrate up to 45 mg/day at intervals of ≥1 wk
• **Geriatric:** PO 7.5 mg at bedtime, increase by 7.5 mg q1-2wk to desired dose, max 45 mg/day
Available forms: Tabs 7.5, 15, 30, 45 mg; orally disintegrating tab (SolTab) 15, 30, 45 mg
Administer:
• Increased fluids, bulk in diet for constipation, especially for geriatric patients
• Without regard to meals
• Dosage at bedtime if oversedation occurs during day; may take entire dose at bedtime; geriatric patients may not tolerate once-daily dosing
• Gum, hard candy, or frequent sips of water for dry mouth
• Store in tight container at room temperature; do not freeze
• **Orally disintegrating tab:** no water needed; allow to dissolve on tongue, do not split; contains phenylalanine

SIDE EFFECTS

CNS: *Dizziness, drowsiness,* confusion, nightmares, abnormal dreams, neuroleptic malignant syndrome, suicidal thoughts
CV: *Orthostatic hypotension, ECG changes,* tachycardia, twitching
EENT: *Blurred vision,* tinnitus, mydriasis
GI: *Dry mouth,* nausea, vomiting, increased appetite, cramps, epigastric distress, constipation, weight gain
GU: Urinary frequency
HEMA: Agranulocytosis, thrombocytopenia, eosinophilia, leukopenia
META: Hyponatremia, hypercholesterolemia
INTEG: Rash, urticaria, sweating, pruritus, photosensitivity
MS: Back pain, myalgia
RESP: Cough, dyspnea
SYST: Flulike symptoms, serotonin syndrome

PHARMACOKINETICS
PO: Peak 2 hr, metabolized by CYP1A2, 2D6, 3A4 in liver; excreted in urine, feces; crosses placenta; half-life 20-40 hr, protein binding 85%

INTERACTIONS
Increase: hyperpyretic crisis, seizures, hypertensive episode—MAOIs; avoid within 14 days
Increase: CNS depression—alcohol, barbiturates, benzodiazepines, other CNS depressants
Increase: serotonin syndrome, risk—SSRIs, buspropion, SNRIs, serotonin-receptor agonists, fentanyl, triptans, tricyclics, linezolid, methylene blue; monitor for symptoms
Decrease: effects of cloNIDine, indirect-acting sympathomimetics (ePHEDrine)
Drug/Herb
• **Serotonin syndrome:** St. John's wort; monitor for symptoms
Increase: CNS depression—kava
Drug/Lab Test
Increase: cholesterol, triglycerides

NURSING CONSIDERATIONS
Assess:

• B/P (lying, standing), pulse often; if systolic B/P drops 20 mm Hg, hold product, notify prescriber; vital signs more frequently in patients with CV disease

• **Seizures:** in those with seizure disorder, may be increased, provide seizure precautions

• **Neuroleptic malignant syndrome:** fever, dyspnea, sweating, change in B/P, discontinue immediately

• **Blood studies:** ECG, lipid profile, blood glucose, LFTs, serum creatinine/BUN if patient is receiving long-term therapy

• Weight weekly; appetite may increase with product

Black Box Warning: Mental status: mood, sensorium, affect, suicidal tendencies (especially among adolescents, young adults), increase in psychiatric symptoms: depression, panic; product should be discontinued in those who exhibit worsening depression, emergent suicidality; EPS primarily in geriatric patients: rigidity, dystonia, akathisia

• **Serotonin syndrome:** hyperthermia, hypertension, myoclonus, rigidity, delirium, coma (if using other serotonergic products)

• Alcohol consumption; if alcohol consumed, hold dose until morning

• Assistance with ambulation during beginning therapy because drowsiness, dizziness occurs

• **Pregnancy/breastfeeding:** use only if clearly needed; excreted in breast milk, discontinue product or breastfeeding

Evaluate:

• **Therapeutic response:** decreased depression

Teach patient/family:

• That therapeutic effects may take 2-3 wk; to take at bedtime; that there is decreased sedation with increased doses; not to discontinue abruptly

• To use caution when driving, performing other activities requiring alertness because of drowsiness, dizziness, blurred vision

• To avoid alcohol, other CNS depressants without prescriber approval

• **Infection:** to report flulike symptoms, other signs of infection

• **Serotonin syndrome:** to report immediately symptoms that include fever, delirium, rigidity; may occur in combination with other products

• About how to take orally disintegrating tabs; dissolve on tongue, swallow

• Not to crush, break, chew ODT product

• To notify prescriber immediately if pregnancy is suspected, or if breastfeeding

• Not to use within 14 days of MAOIs

• That follow-up exams will be needed

Black Box Warning: To notify prescriber immediately of suicidal thoughts, behavior

TREATMENT OF OVERDOSE:
ECG monitoring, lavage; administer anticonvulsant, IV fluids

mirvetuximab (Rx)
(mir-ve-tux-i-mab)
Elahere
Func. class.: Antineoplastic

USES: Adults with FRα-positive, platinum-resistant epithelial ovarian, fallopian tube, or primary peritoneal cancer who have received 1-3 prior systemic regimens

DOSAGE AND ROUTES
Adult: IV INF 6 mg/kg q3wk until disease progression or unacceptable toxicity; premedicate with a corticosteroid, antihistamine, and antipyretic; antiemetic; ophthalmic topical steroids; and lubricating eye drops
Available forms: Injection: 100 mg/20 mL (5 mg/mL) in a single-dose vial

misoprostol (Rx)
(mye-soe-prost'ole)
Cytotec
Func. class.: Gastric mucosa protectant, antiulcer
Chem. class.: Prostaglandin E_1 analog

Do not confuse:
miSOPROStol/metoprolol/mifepristone

USES: Prevention of NSAID-induced gastric ulcers, pregnancy termination

CONTRAINDICATIONS
Hypersensitivity to this product or prostaglandins

Black Box Warning: Pregnancy, females

DOSAGE AND ROUTES
NSAID-induced gastroduodenal ulcers and treatment of duodenal ulcers caused by peptic ulcer disease
• Adult: PO 200 mcg qid with food for duration of NSAID therapy, with last dose given at bedtime; if 200 mcg is not tolerated, 100 mcg may be given
Active duodenal/gastric ulcer (unlabeled)
• Adult: PO 100-200 mcg qid with meals at bedtime × 4-8 wk
Pregnancy termination before 70th day (unlabeled)
• Adult: INTRAVAGINALLY 800 mcg 5-7 days after methotrexate IM
Cervical ripening induction for term pregnancy (unlabeled)
• Adult: INTRAVAGINALLY 25 mcg q3-6hr

⚠ HIGH ALERT

mitoMYcin (Rx)
(mye-toe-mye'sin)
Jelmyto
Func. class.: Antineoplastic, antibiotic

Do not confuse:
mitoMYcin/mitoXANTRONE

ACTION: Inhibits DNA synthesis, primarily; derived from *Streptomyces caespitosus;* appears to cause cross-linking of DNA; vesicant

USES: Pancreatic, stomach, colorectal, bladder cancer
Unlabeled uses: Palliative treatment of anal, bladder, head, neck, colon, biliary, cervical, lung malignancies

CONTRAINDICATIONS
Pregnancy, breastfeeding, hypersensitivity, as single agent, coagulation disorders, thrombocytopenia
Precautions: Accidental exposure, acute bronchospasm, anemia, children, dental disease/work, extravasation, females, infection, radiation therapy, surgery, vaccines, renal/respiratory disease, leukopenia

Black Box Warning: Bone marrow suppression, hemolytic uremic syndrome, requires an experienced clinician and specialized care setting

DOSAGE AND ROUTES
Disseminated adenocarcinoma of stomach/pancreas in combination
• Adult: IV 20 mg/m² q6-8wk
Anal cancer (unlabeled)
• Adult: IV 10 mg/m² on days 1 and 29, max 20 mg, use with 5-FU and radiation therapy or 10 mg/m² on day 1 with capecitabine and radiation therapy
Bladder cancer (unlabeled)
• Adult: IV 12 mg/m² on day 1 with 5-FU and radiation therapy
Upper Tract Urothelial Cancer
• Adult: Instill Jelmyto 4 mg per mL via ureteral catheter or a nephrostomy tube, with total instillation volume based on pyelography, max 15 mL (60 mg of mitomycin). Instill weekly × 6 wk, those with a complete response after 3 mo may be used monthly for a max of 11 additional doses
Available forms: Inj 5, 20, 40 mg/vial; powder for pyelocalyceal solution

Administer:
- **Cytotoxic:** use safe handling and disposal procedures
- **Vesicant:** check for extravasation; do not give IM/subcut, may result in extreme tissue damage

Direct IV route
- Use port or central line if possible
- Antiemetic 30-60 min before product to prevent vomiting
- IV after reconstituting 5 mg/10 mL, 20 mg/40 mL, 40 mg/80 mL (0.5 mg/mL) sterile water for inj; shake, allow to stand, protect from light, give slow IV push or infuse over 15-30 min; color of reconstituted sol is gray
- Avoid excessive heat; store unreconstituted product at room temperature

Y-site compatibilities: Amifostine, amphotericin B lipid complex, amphotericin B liposome, anidulafungin, argatroban, atenolol, bivalirudin, bleomycin, caspofungin, CISplatin, cyclophosphamide, DACTINomycin, dolasetron, DOXOrubicin, droperidol, epiRUBicin, ertapenem, fluorouracil, furosemide, granisetron, heparin, leucovorin, melphalan, methotrexate, metoclopramide, nesiritide, octreotide, ondansetron, oxaliplatin, PACLitaxel, palonosetron, PEMEtrexed, riTUXimab, teniposide, thiotepa, tigecycline, tirofiban, trastuzumab, vinBLAStine, vinCRIStine, voriconazole, zoledronic acid

SIDE EFFECTS
CNS: Fever, headache, confusion, drowsiness, syncope, fatigue
CV: Edema
EENT: Blurred vision
GI: *Nausea, vomiting, anorexia, stomatitis,* hepatotoxicity, diarrhea
GU: Urinary retention, renal failure, infertility
HEMA: Thrombocytopenia, leukopenia, anemia
INTEG: *Rash,* alopecia, extravasation, nail discoloration
MISC: Hemolytic uremic syndrome
RESP: Fibrosis, pulmonary infiltrate

PHARMACOKINETICS
Half-life 1 hr, metabolized in liver, 10% excreted in urine (unchanged)

INTERACTIONS
Increase: toxicity—other antineoplastics, radiation
Increase: bleeding risk—NSAIDs, anticoagulants
- Avoid use with vaccines

Drug/Lab Test
Increase: BUN, creatinine
Decrease: platelets, WBCs

NURSING CONSIDERATIONS
Assess:

Black Box Warning: Bone marrow suppression: monitor CBC, differential, platelet count weekly; withhold product if WBC is <4000/mm^3, serum creatinine >1.7 mg/dL, or platelet count is <100,000/mm^3, nadir of leukopenia, thrombocytopenia is 4-8 wk, recovering within 10 wk; notify prescriber; bleeding: hematuria, guaiac, bruising, petechiae, mucosa, or orifices, avoid IM injections when platelets are low

Black Box Warning: Fatal hemolytic uremic syndrome: assess for hypertension, thrombocytopenia, microangiopathic hemolytic anemia; occurs in those receiving long-term therapy; most cases are caused by doses ≥60 mg; transfusion may worsen syndrome

- **Nephrotoxicity:** Renal studies: BUN, uric acid, urine CCr, before, during therapy; adjust dose based on renal function; I&O ratio; report fall in urine output to <30 mL/hr
- Monitor temperature; fever may indicate beginning infection
- **Hepatotoxicity:** hepatic studies before, during therapy: bilirubin, AST, ALT, alk phos as needed or monthly; check for jaundiced skin and sclera, dark urine, clay-colored stools, itchy skin, abdominal pain, fever, diarrhea

---

Side effects: *italics* = common; red = life-threatening

• **Pulmonary fibrosis:** bronchospasm, dyspnea, crackles, unproductive cough; chest pain, tachypnea, fatigue, increased pulse, pallor, lethargy; pulmonary function tests; chest x-ray before, during therapy; chest x-ray should be obtained q2wk during treatment

• Effects of alopecia on body image; discuss feelings about body changes

• Buccal cavity q8hr for dryness, sores, ulceration, white patches, oral pain, bleeding, dysphagia

• Local irritation, pain, burning at inj site

• GI symptoms: frequency of stools, cramping

• Adequate fluids (2-3 L/day) unless contraindicated

• Rinsing of mouth tid-qid with water; brushing of teeth with baking soda bid-tid with soft brush or cotton-tipped applicators for stomatitis; use unwaxed dental floss

• **Cardiac toxicity (rare):** HF may be treated with diuretics, cardiac glycosides; most with this condition received doxorubicin

• **Pregnancy/breastfeeding:** do not use in pregnancy or breastfeeding

Evaluate:

• **Therapeutic response:** decreased tumor size, spread of malignancy

Teach patient/family:

• That hair may be lost during treatment; that wig or hairpiece may make patient feel better; that new hair may be different in color, texture

• To avoid foods with citric acid, hot temperature, or rough texture

• To report any bleeding, white spots, ulcerations in mouth; to examine mouth daily

• To report sign of IV site reaction: redness, inflammation, burning, pain

• To avoid crowds, persons with infections if granulocyte count is low

• **Infection:** to report fever, flulike symptoms, sore throat

• To immediately report urine retention, absence of urine, dyspnea, bleeding, jaundice, signs of pulmonary toxicity

• **Pregnancy/breastfeeding:** to report if pregnancy is planned or suspected; not to breastfeed, use adequate contraception during for and 6 mo after last dose

⚠ HIGH ALERT

mitoXANTRONE (Rx)

(mye-toe-zan′trone)
Func. class.: Antineoplastic, antiinfective, immunomodulator
Chem. class.: Synthetic anthraquinone

Do not confuse:
mitoXANTRONE/mitoMYcin/mitotane/MTX patch

ACTION: DNA reactive agent; cytocidal effect on both proliferating and nonproliferating cells; topoisomerase II inhibitor (vesicant)

USES: Acute myelogenous leukemia (adult), relapsed leukemia; used with steroids to treat bone pain (advanced prostate cancer), multiple sclerosis (MS)

CONTRAINDICATIONS
Pregnancy, hypersensitivity
Precautions: Breastfeeding, children; myelosuppression, renal/cardiac/hepatic disease; gout

Black Box Warning: Bone marrow suppression, cardiotoxicity, SUBCUT/IM/intraarterial/intrathecal, requires an experienced clinician, new primary malignancy

DOSAGE AND ROUTES
Acute myelogenous leukemia/induction
• **Adult: IV INFUSION** 12 mg/m^2/day on days 1-3 and 100 mg/m^2 cytarabine × 7 days as continuous 24-hr infusion may use 2nd induction
Consolidation
• **Adult: IV** 12 mg/m^2 given as short 5- to 15-min infusion for 2 days with cytarabine × 5 days, use 6 wk after induction, and another course after 4 wk
Advanced prostate cancer
• **Adult: IV** 12-14 mg/m^2 as single dose or short infusion q21days

Multiple sclerosis, relapsing
• **Adult: IV INFUSION** 12 mg/m^2 as 5- to 15-min infusion q3mo, cumulative lifetime dose 140 mg/m^2

Available forms: Solution for inj 2 mg/mL

Administer:
• Antiemetic 30-60 min before product to prevent vomiting
• **Cytotoxic:** use precautions for handling, preparing, and disposal of this product; use goggles, gloves, gown during preparation and administration; rinse accidentally exposed skin with warm water
• Undiluted solution may be stored for 7 days (room temperature), 14 days (refrigerated); do not freeze

Direct IV route
• IV after **diluting** with ≥50 mL NS or D$_5$W; discard unused portion immediately; do not mix in same infusion with heparin; **give** over 3-5 min into running IV of D$_5$W or NS; check for extravasation; do not give IM, SUBCUT, or intraarterially

Intermittent IV INFUSION route
• May be diluted further in D$_5$W, NS (0.02-0.5 mg/mL), run over 15-30 min

Continuous IV INFUSION route
• Give over 24 hr

Y-site compatibilities: Acyclovir, alemtuzumab, alfentanil, allopurinol, amikacin, aminocaproic acid, aminophylline, amiodarone, anidulafungin, argatroban, arsenic trioxide, atracurium, bivalirudin, bleomycin, bretylium, bumetanide, buprenorphine, butorphanol, calcium chloride, calcium gluconate, CARBOplatin, carmustine, caspofungin, cefoTEtan, ceftizoxime, chloramphenicol, chlorproMAZINE, cimetidine, ciprofloxacin, cisatracurium, CISplatin, cladribine, codeine, cyclophosphamide, cycloSPORINE, cytarabine, DACTINomycin, DAPTOmycin, DAUNOrubicin citrate liposome, dexmedetomidine, dexrazoxane, diltiaZEM, diphenhydrAMINE, DOBUTamine, DOCEtaxel, dolasetron, DOPamine, doxacurium, doxycycline, droperidol, enalaprilat, ePHEDrine, EPINEPHrine, erythromycin, esmolol, etoposide, etoposide phosphate, famotidine, fenoldopam, fentaNYL, filgrastim, fluconazole, fludarabine, fluorouracil, ganciclovir, gatifloxacin, gemcitabine, gentamicin, glycopyrrolate, granisetron, haloperidol, hydrALAZINE, hydrocortisone sodium succinate, HYDROmorphone, hydrOXYzine, ifosfamide, imipenem-cilastatin, inamrinone, insulin (regular), irinotecan, isoproterenol, ketorolac, labetalol, leucovorin, levoFLOXacin, levorphanol, lidocaine, linezolid, LORazepam, magnesium sulfate, mannitol, melphalan, meperidine, meropenem, mesna, metaraminol, methohexital, methotrexate, methyldopate, metoclopramide, metoprolol, metroNIDAZOLE, midazolam, milrinone, minocycline, mivacurium, morphine sulfate, nalbuphine, naloxone, nesiritide, niCARdipine, nitroglycerin, norepinephrine, octreotide, ondansetron, oxaliplatin, palonosetron, pamidronate, pancuronium, pentamidine, pentazocine, PENTObarbital, PHENObarbital, phentolamine, phenylephrine, polymyxin B, potassium acetate, potassium chloride, procainamide, prochlorperazine, promethazine hydrochloride, propranolol, quiNIDine gluconate, quinupristin-dalfopristin, raNITIdine, remifentanil, riTUXimab, rocuronium, sargramostim, sodium acetate, sodium bicarbonate, succinylcholine, SUFentanil, sulfamethoxazole-trimethoprim, tacrolimus, teniposide, theophylline, thiopental, thiotepa, tigecycline, tirofiban, tobramycin, tolazoline, trastuzumab, trimethobenzamide, vancomycin, vasopressin, vecuronium, verapamil, vinCRIStine, vinorelbine, zidovudine, zoledronic acid

SIDE EFFECTS
CNS: Headache, seizures, fatigue
CV: Cardiotoxicity, dysrhythmias, HF
EENT: Conjunctivitis, blue/green sclera, blurred vision
GI: *Nausea, vomiting, diarrhea, anorexia, stomatitis,* hepatotoxicity, abdominal pain, constipation
GU: Amenorrhea, menstrual disorders, blue-green urine, renal failure

Side effects: *italics* = common; red = life-threatening

HEMA: Thrombocytopenia, leukopenia, myelosuppression, anemia, secondary leukemia

INTEG: *Rash, necrosis at inj site,* dermatitis, thrombophlebitis at inj site, alopecia

MISC: Fever, hyperuricemia, infections

RESP: Cough, dyspnea

SYST: Tumor lysis syndrome, sepsis

PHARMACOKINETICS

Protein binding 78%; excreted via renal, hepatobiliary systems; half-life 23-215 hr

INTERACTIONS

Increase: bone marrow depression toxicity—radiation, other antineoplastics

Increase: adverse reactions—live virus vaccines, trastuzumab

Increase: oral mucositis—palifermin, do not use within 24 hr of mitoxantrone

Increase: immunosuppression—tofacitinib, avoid using together

Increase: infection risk—natalizumab

Increase: bleeding risk—NSAIDs, anticoagulants

Increase: mitoXANTRONE, effects of—cyclosporine

Decrease: digoxin, hydration level—monitor levels, adjust dose

Drug/Lab Test

Increase: LFTs, uric acid, bilirubin

Decrease: HcT/HB, platelets, WBC, calcium, sodium, granulocytes

NURSING CONSIDERATIONS
Assess:

Black Box Warning: Bone marrow depression: CBC, differential, platelet count weekly; withhold product if WBC is <1500/mm³; leukopenia, neutropenia, thrombocytopenia are expected, leukocyte nadir 10-14 days, recovers in 2-3 wk

Black Box Warning: Extravasation: avoid extravasation; not traditionally considered a vesicant; serious skin necrosis requiring debridement, skin graft has occurred; if extravasation occurs, stop product, place ice packs on area

• **Hepatotoxicity:** hepatic studies before, during therapy: bilirubin, AST, ALT, alk phos

prn or monthly; dose reduction needed with hepatic disease; jaundiced skin and sclera, dark urine, clay-colored stools, itchy skin, abdominal pain, fever, diarrhea

• Renal studies: BUN; serum uric acid; urine CCr; electrolytes before, during therapy

• Bleeding, hematuria, guaiac, bruising or petechiae, mucosa or orifices q8hr

Black Box Warning: **Cardiotoxicity:** ECG, ECHO, chest x-ray, MUGA, RAI angiography; assess ejection fraction before and during treatment; cardiotoxicity may develop during treatment or months to years after treatment; use vigilant cardiac monitoring in MS; risk is greater in cumulative dose >140 mg/m²

Black Box Warning: **New primary malignancy** can develop after taking this product

• **Multiple sclerosis:** obtain MUGA, LVEF baselines; repeat LVEF if symptoms of HF occur or if cumulative dose is >100 mg/m²; do not administer to patients who have received lifetime dose of ≥140 mg/m² or if LVEF <50% or significant LVEF or if neutrophils <1500/mm³

• Rinsing of mouth tid-qid with water, club soda; brushing of teeth bid-qid with soft brush or cotton-tipped applicators for stomatitis; use unwaxed dental floss

• Provide increased fluids to 2-3 L/day unless contraindicated

Black Box Warning: Requires a specialized care setting with an experienced clinician: use only in a setting with emergency equipment, those trained in administration of cytotoxic products

• **Pregnancy/breastfeeding:** do not use in pregnancy, breastfeeding; obtain pregnancy test for all women of childbearing age, even if birth control is used

Evaluate:

• **Therapeutic response:** decreased tumor size, spread of malignancy, prevention of relapse in MS

Teach patient/family:
• To immediately report bleeding, dyspnea, possible infections, seizure, jaundice, fever, cough, or dyspnea
• To avoid hot foods or those with citric acid, rough texture
• To report any bleeding, white spots, ulcerations in mouth; to examine mouth daily
• To avoid crowds, persons with infections
• To provide package insert and review with patient
• To report immediately yellow eyes, skin, clay-colored stools, dark urine, diarrhea
• That follow-up exams and blood work will be needed
• That sclera, urine may turn blue or green; that hair loss may occur
• To notify prescriber if pregnancy is suspected or planned; to use effective contraception, do not breastfeed

---

mobocertinib (Rx)
(moe-boe-SER-ti-nib)
Exkivity
Func. class.: Antineoplastic, kinase inhibitor

USES: Epidermal growth factor receptor (EGFR) exon 20 insertion mutation–positive metastatic non–small cell lung cancer

DOSAGE AND ROUTES
• **Adult:** PO 160 mg daily until disease progression or unacceptable toxicity

Available forms: Capsules 40 mg

---

modafinil (Rx)
(mo-daf'i-nil)
Alertec ✦, Provigil
Func. class.: CNS stimulant
Chem. class.: Racemic compound

Controlled Substance Schedule IV

ACTION: Similar action as that of sympathomimetics; does not alter release of DOPamine, norepinephrine

USES: Narcolepsy, shift-work sleep disturbance, obstructive sleep apnea
Unlabeled uses: ADHD, fatigue in MS, Parkinson's disease

CONTRAINDICATIONS
Hypersensitivity, ischemic heart disease, left ventricular hypertrophy, chest pain, dysrhythmias
Precautions: Pregnancy, breastfeeding, child <16 yr, geriatric patients, unstable angina, history of MI, severe hepatic disease

DOSAGE AND ROUTES
To improve wakefulness with daytime sleepiness
• **Adult/adolescent ≥17 yr:** PO 200 mg daily
Hepatic dose (severe hepatic disease)
• **Adult:** PO 100 mg daily
Available forms: Tabs 100, 200 mg
Administer:
• Give 1 hr before start of shift work or in AM for those with narcolepsy or sleep apnea
• Store at room temperature
• Give without regard to food

SIDE EFFECTS
CNS: *Headache,* anxiety, cataplexy, depression, dizziness, insomnia, amnesia, confusion, ataxia, tremors, paresthesia, dyskinesia, suicidal ideation
CV: Dysrhythmias, hypo/hypertension, chest pain, vasodilation
EENT: Change in vision, *rhinitis,* pharyngitis, epistaxis
GI: Nausea, vomiting, changes in LFTs, anorexia, diarrhea, thirst, mouth ulcers
GU: Ejaculation disorder, urinary retention, albuminuria
HEMA: Eosinophilia
INTEG: Rash, dry skin, herpes simplex, Stevens-Johnson syndrome
MISC: Infection, hyperglycemia, neck pain
RESP: *Dyspnea,* lung changes

PHARMACOKINETICS
Absorbed rapidly, 60% protein binding, metabolized by the liver (90%), half-life 15 hr, peak 2-4 hr

---

INTERACTIONS

Increase: altered levels of CYP3A4 inhibitors (azole antibiotics, some SSRIs); reaction difficult to predict; monitor for reaction

Increase: levels of CYP2C19 substrates (diazePAM, phenytoin, some tricyclics), adjust dose if needed

Decrease: effects of—cycloSPORINE, hormonal contraceptives, theophylline, estrogens

Delayed effect modafinil by 1 hr: methylphenidate

Altered: levels of CYP3A4 inducers (carBAMazepine, phenytoin, rifAMPin, cycloSPORINE, theophylline)

Drug/Herb

Increase: stimulation—cola nut, guarana, yerba maté, coffee, tea

Drug/Lab Test

Increase: LFTs, glucose, eosinophils

NURSING CONSIDERATIONS

Assess:

• Narcolepsy, shift work, history of sleep apnea

• **Stevens-Johnson syndrome:** rash, fever, fatigue, blisters; discontinue immediately if these occur; provide supportive therapy

• Depression, suicidal ideation

• Monitor B/P in those with hypertension

• **Pregnancy/breastfeeding:** pregnant patients should enroll in the pregnancy registry, 866-404-4106; use only when benefits outweigh risk to the fetus; avoid use in breastfeeding

• **Beers:** avoid in older adults; CNS stimulant effects

Evaluate:

• Ability to stay awake

Teach patient/family:

• To take only as directed; that product may be taken with/without food

• **Pregnancy/breastfeeding:** To use other form of contraception during and for ≥30 days after discontinuing medication if using hormonal birth control; to notify prescriber if pregnancy is planned or suspected or if breastfeeding

• To notify prescriber of allergic reaction, tremors, confusion, trouble breathing

• To avoid all OTC medications unless approved by prescriber; not to use alcohol

• To avoid hazardous activities until drug effect is known

---

moexipril (Rx)

(moe-ex'ih-prill)

Func. class.: Antihypertensive

Chem. class.: Angiotensin-converting enzyme inhibitor

USES: Hypertension, alone or in combination with thiazide diuretics

CONTRAINDICATIONS

Breastfeeding, children, hypersensitivity, heart block, bilateral renal stenosis, history of angioedema

Black Box Warning: Pregnancy

DOSAGE AND ROUTES

• **Adult:** PO 7.5 mg 1 hr before meals initially; may be increased or divided depending on B/P response; maintenance dosage 7.5-30 mg/day in 1-2 divided doses 1 hr before meals

Renal dose

• **Adult:** PO CCr <40 mL/min, 3.75 mg/day; titrate to desired dose; max 15 mg/day

Available forms: Tablet 7.5, 15 mg

---

mogamulizumab-kpkc (Rx)

(moh-gam'-yoo-lih'-zoo-mab)

Poteligeo

Func. class.: Antineoplastic

USES: Cutaneous T-cell lymphoma (CTCL) (mycosis fungoides or Sézary syndrome) in those who have received at least 1 prior systemic therapy

CONTRAINDICATIONS

Hypersensitivity, pregnancy

DOSAGE AND ROUTES

• **Adult:** IV 1 mg/kg on days 1, 8, 15, and 22 in cycle 1, then 1 mg/kg on days 1 and 15 in subsequent cycles until dis-

---

ease progression; therapy cycles are repeated q28days

Available forms: Solution for injection 20 mg/5 mL

---

mometasone (Rx)

(moe-met′a-sone)

Asmanex, Asmanex HFA, Propel, Sinuva

Func. class.: Antiinflammatory
Chem. class.: Corticosteroid

ACTION: May depress the formation, release, and activity of endogenous chemical mediators of inflammation (kinins, histamine, liposomal enzymes, prostaglandins)

USES: Inhalation: Maintenance treatment of asthma as prophylactic therapy in those ≥4 yr of age; allergic rhinitis, nasal congestion

DOSAGE AND ROUTES
Asthma
Adult/child ≥12 yr: Oral inhalation:
Asmanex HFA: Metered-dose inhaler: *Patients with no prior treatment with inhaled corticosteroid:* Mometasone 100 mcg: Initial: 200 mcg twice daily; max 400 mcg twice daily (800 mcg/day); those *who previously received oral corticosteroids:* Mometasone 200 mcg: Initial: 400 mcg twice daily; max 400 mcg twice daily (800 mcg/day); **Asmanex Twisthaler:** Dry powder inhaler: *Those who previously received bronchodilators alone:* Initial: 220 mcg once daily in the evening; max 440 mcg/day; *those who previously received inhaled corticosteroids:* Initial: 220 mcg once daily in the evening; maximum dose: 440 mcg/day; *those who previously received oral corticosteroids:* Initial: 440 mcg twice daily; max 880 mcg/day
Allergic rhinitis (seasonal and perennial)
Adult: Intranasal: 2 sprays (100 mcg) in each nostril once daily (total daily dose: 200 mcg)

Nasal congestion associated with seasonal rhinitis
Adult/child ≥12 yr: Intranasal: 2 sprays (100 mcg) in each nostril once daily (total daily dose: 200 mcg)
Nasal polyps
Adult: Intranasal: 2 sprays (100 mcg) in each nostril twice daily (total daily dose: 400 mcg); 2 sprays (100 mcg) in each nostril once daily may be effective in some patients
Seasonal allergic rhinitis (prophylaxis)
Adult/child ≥12 yr: Intranasal: 2 sprays (100 mcg) in each nostril once daily (total daily dose: 200 mcg); treatment should begin 2-4 wk before the anticipated start of pollen season

Available forms: Inhalation aerosol 100 mcg, 200 mcg/actuation; inhalation powder 110 mcg, 220 mcg/actuation, cream 0.1%, lotion 0.1%, ointment 0.1%, nasal spray 50 mcg/spray

Administer:
Nasal route:
• Spray: For intranasal administration only
• Prime pump (press 10 times or until fine spray appears) before first use
• If 7 or more days have elapsed since last use, reprime pump with 2 sprays or until a fine mist appears
• Shake before using. Blow nose
• Insert applicator into nostril, tilt head slightly forward keeping bottle upright, and close off the other nostril. Breathe in through nose
• While inhaling, press pump, exhale through mouth
• After each use, wipe tip with a tissue and replace cap
• Avoid spraying directly into nasal septum, eyes, mouth, face
• Discard after 120 medicated sprays have been used, even if not completely empty

SIDE EFFECTS
CNS: Headache, fatigue, depression
GI: Oral candidiasis, abdominal pain, dyspepsia, nausea, vomiting, anorexia, gastroenteritis

---

Side effects: *italics* = common; red = life-threatening

MS: MS pain, arthralgia
RESP: Sinusitis, allergic rhinitis, URI, pharyngitis
GU: Dysmenorrhea, UTI

PHARMACOKINETICS
Nasal: Onset, peak, duration unknown
Inhalation: Onset, duration unknown, peak 1-2½ hr

INTERACTIONS
Increase: adverse reactions—CYP3A4 inhibitors, use cautiously

NURSING CONSIDERATIONS
Assess:
• **Asthma:** Monitor signs, symptoms of asthma, not to be used for acute asthma attacks, wean from corticosteroids (systemic)
• **Cushing symptoms:** Assess for excess sweating, excessive hairiness, excessive hunger, fatigue, flushing, high blood pressure, osteoporosis, abnormal pad of fat between the shoulder blades, acne, darkening of the skin, stretch marks, or thinning, muscle weakness or loss of muscle, anxiety, depression, easy bruising, hair loss, headache, infertility, insomnia, irritability, pot belly, round face from gradual swelling, swelling in extremities, or weight gain
Evaluate:
• **Therapeutic response:** decrease symptoms of asthma or seasonal/perennial rhinitis
Teach patient/family:
• Teach patient how to use inhalation or nasal spray
• If only using once/day use before bedtime
• Not to be used for acute asthma attack

**mometasone/
formoterol (Rx)**
(moe-met′sone/formoh′te-rol)
Dulera
Func. class.: Corticosteroid, inhalant/beta₂ agonist, long-acting

---

USES: Asthma

CONTRAINDICATIONS
Hypersensitivity

DOSAGE AND ROUTES
Adult/child ≥12 yr: INH 2 INH of mometasone furoate 100 mcg/formoterol fumarate 5 mcg/inhalation or mometasone furoate 200 mcg/formoterol fumarate 5 mcg/INH bid, if no response after 2 wk, may increase to mometasone furoate 200 mcg/formoterol fumarate 5 mcg/INH bid; max, 2 INH bid of mometasone furoate 200 mcg/formoterol fumarate 5 mcg (800 mcg/20 mcg/day)
Available forms: 50, 100, 200 mcg/5 mcg actuation

---

montelukast (Rx)
(mon-teh-loo′kast)
Singulair
Func. class.: Bronchodilator
Chem. class.: Leukotriene receptor antagonist, cysteinyl

Do not confuse:
Singulair/SINEquan

ACTION: Inhibits leukotriene (LTD₄) formation; leukotrienes exert their effects by increasing neutrophil, eosinophil migration; aggregation of neutrophils, monocytes; smooth muscle contraction, capillary permeability; these actions further lead to bronchoconstriction, inflammation, edema

USES: Chronic asthma in adults and children, seasonal allergic rhinitis, bronchospasm prophylaxis

CONTRAINDICATIONS
Hypersensitivity
Precautions: Pregnancy, breastfeeding, children <6 yr, acute attacks of asthma, alcohol consumption, severe hepatic disease, corticosteroid withdrawal, phenylketonuria, suicidal ideation, depression

---

Black Box Warning: Neurologic/psychiatric events

DOSAGE AND ROUTES
Asthma, seasonal/perennial allergic rhinitis
- **Adult/child ≥15 yr: PO** 10 mg/day in PM
- **Child 6-14 yr: PO** 5-mg chew tab/day in PM
- **Child 2-5 yr: PO** (chew tab/granules) 4 mg/day
- **Child 12-23 mo: PO** 1 packet (4 mg) qday in PM

Exercise-induced bronchoconstriction prevention
- **Adult/child ≥15 yr: PO** 10 mg 2 hr before exercise; do not take another dose within 24 hr
- **Child 6 yr-15 yr: PO** 5 mg once given 2 hr before exercise, max 1 dose/24 hr

Available forms: Tabs 10 mg; chew tabs 4, 5 mg; oral granules 4 mg/packet

Administer:
PO route
- In PM daily for all uses except exercise-induced bronchoconstriction; then take 2 hr before exercise
- Granules directly in mouth or mixed with spoonful of soft food (carrots, applesauce, ice cream, rice)
- Do not open granules packet until ready to use; mix whole dose; give within 15 min

SIDE EFFECTS
CNS: *Dizziness, fatigue, headache,* behavior changes, hallucinations, seizures, agitation, anxiety, depression, fever, drowsiness, suicidal ideation, memory impairment, hostility, somnambulism

GI: *Abdominal pain,* dyspepsia, nausea, vomiting, diarrhea, pancreatitis

HEMA: Thrombocytopenia

INTEG: Rash, pruritus, erythema

MS: Asthenia, myalgia, muscle cramps

RESP: *Influenza, cough,* nasal congestion

SYST: Churg-Strauss syndrome, Stevens-Johnson syndrome, toxic epidermal necrolysis

PHARMACOKINETICS
Rapidly absorbed; peak 3-4 hr, chew tab (5 mg) 2-2.5 hr; half-life 2.7-5.5 hr, extended in hepatic disease; protein binding 99%; metabolized by liver; excreted via bile

INTERACTIONS
Increase: adverse reactions of CYP2C8 substrates

Decrease: montelukast levels—barbiturates, rifabutin, rifapentine, carBAMazepine, fosphenytoin, phenytoin, rifAMPin

Drug/Herb
Increase: stimulation—black, green tea, guarana

Drug/Lab Test
Increase: ALT, AST

NURSING CONSIDERATIONS
Assess:
- **Respiratory symptoms:** wheezing, decrease in asthma exacerbations, rhinitis, urticaria
- **Churg-Strauss syndrome (rare):** assess adult patients carefully for symptoms: eosinophilia, vasculitic rash, worsening pulmonary symptoms, cardiac complications, neuropathy
- For behavioral changes, suicidal ideation, other neuropsychiatric reactions
- **Severe hepatic disease:** use cautiously
- **Stevens-Johnson syndrome:** rash, fever, blisters, fatigue, muscle/joint aches; if these occur, discontinue, provide supportive therapy
- **Pregnancy/breastfeeding:** use in pregnancy only if clearly needed, no well-controlled studies; use cautiously in breastfeeding, unknown if excreted in breast milk

Evaluate:
- **Therapeutic response:** ability to breathe more easily

Teach patient/family:
- To check OTC medications, stimulation; to avoid alcohol
- To avoid hazardous activities; dizziness may occur
- If aspirin sensitivity is known, not to take NSAIDs while taking this product

- To report mood, behavioral changes to prescriber
- Not to use for acute asthma/acute exercise-induced bronchospasm; not effective
- To take even if no symptoms are present
- To continue to use inhaled β-agonists if exercise-induced asthma occurs
- **Granules:** to give directly in mouth or mixed in a spoonful of room temperature soft food (use only applesauce, carrots, rice, or ice cream); use within 15 min of opening packets; discard unused portions

---

⚠ HIGH ALERT

morphine (Rx)

(mor'feen)

Arymo ER, Astramorph PF, Doloral ✦, Duramorph PF, Infumorph, M-Eslon ✦, Mitigo ✦, MS IR ✦, MS Contin, Statex ✦

Func. class.: Opioid analgesic
Chem. class.: Alkaloid

Controlled Substance Schedule II

Do not confuse:
morphine/HYDROmorphone
MS Contin/OxyCONTIN

ACTION: Depresses pain impulse transmission at the spinal cord level by interacting with opioid receptors

USES: Moderate to severe pain
Unlabeled uses: Agitation, bone/dental pain, dyspnea in end-stage cancer or pulmonary disease, sedation induction, rapid-sequence intubation

CONTRAINDICATIONS

Hypersensitivity, addiction (opioid/alcohol), hemorrhage, bronchial asthma, increased intracranial pressure, paralytic ileus, hypovolemia, shock, MAOI therapy

Black Box Warning: Respiratory depression

Precautions: Pregnancy, breastfeeding, children <18 yr, geriatric patients, addictive personality, acute MI, severe heart disease, renal/hepatic disease, bowel impaction, abrupt discontinuation, seizures

Black Box Warning: Accidental exposure, epidural/intrathecal/IM/subcut administration, opioid-naïve patients, substance abuse, coadministration with other CNS depressants, ethanol ingestion, neonatal opioid withdrawal syndrome, potential for overdose or poisoning, requires a specialized care setting

DOSAGE AND ROUTES

Acute and chronic moderate pain or severe pain
PO Route IR
Adults: Initially, 10-30 mg q4hr as needed in opioid-naive patients. Titrate to pain relief. Only use the concentrated oral morphine solution (20 mg/mL) in opioid-tolerant patients
Infants, children, and adolescents 6 mo to 17 yr (unlabeled): Initially, 0.2-0.3 mg/kg/dose q3-6 hr as needed
Intermittent IV, IM, or SUBCUT
Adults: Initially, 2-10 mg q3-4hr as needed, titrated to pain relief
Infants >6 mo and older, children, and adolescents: 0.05-0.2 mg/kg/dose q2-4hr as needed; begin at the lower end of dosage range and titrate to effect (usual max dose: 4 mg for children or 8 mg for adolescents)
Neonates (unlabeled) and infants <6 mo: Initially, 0.03-0.1 mg/kg/dose q3-4hr as needed. Titrate upward as needed for adequate pain relief

IV dosage (patient-controlled analgesia [PCA])
Adults: Starting dose should be based on the patient's recent exposure to opioids. Titrate to patient response. Larger doses may be needed in opioid-tolerant

---

patients. For OPIOID-NAIVE patients, start with a demand dose of 1 mg (range: 0.5-2.5 mg) and lockout interval of 6 min (range: 5-10 min), with a maximal dosing rate of 10 mg/hr. For OPIOID TOLERANT patients, start with a demand dose of 2-5 mg IV and lockout interval of 6 min (range: 5-10 min), with a maximal dosing rate of 30 mg/hr

Children >7 yr and adolescents
Demand dose: 0.01-0.025 mg/kg IV (max: 1 mg/dose)
Lockout interval: 5-10 min
Doses per hour: 5

Epidural dosage (morphine sulfate injection, but not DepoDur)
Adults: Initially, inject 5 mg epidurally in the lumbar region and assess the patient in 1 hr; if pain relief is not adequate, give incremental doses of 1-2 mg, with sufficient time between injections to appropriately assess for efficacy. Max: 10 mg per 24 hr. For continuous epidural infusion, initiate at 2-4 mg per 24 hr, with additional doses of 1-2 mg given if pain relief is not achieved

Intrathecal dosage (morphine sulfate injection, but not DepoDur)
Adults: 0.2-1 mg in the lumbar area as a single dose or to establish dosage for continuous intrathecal infusion

Rectal dosage
Adults: 10-20 mg q4hr, as needed

PO route
PO [extended-release tablets (Arymo ER, MS Contin) or capsules] in opioid nontolerant adult patients
Adults: 15 mg q8hr or q12hr **(Arymo ER, MS Contin)** Capsules. For opioid nontolerant patients, initiate with 15 mg q12hr (MS Contin), adjust the dose every 1-2 days based upon the total daily morphine requirements (ER dose plus breakthrough doses)

PO dosage [ER tablets (Arymo ER, MS Contin) or capsules] in adult patients receiving other opioid agonist therapy
Adults: Discontinue all other around-the-clock opioids. To convert from other morphine formulations, calcu-

late the morphine 24-hr oral requirement; the 24-hr oral dose is 3 times the 24-hr parenteral requirement. Initiate dosing, using the 24-hr oral requirement (round down to the closest available tablet/capsule strength), for: **Arymo ER, MS Contin** at one-half of the requirement every 12 hr or one-third q8hr; Avinza at the total requirement once q24hr; and ER capsule at one-half q12hr or the total once q24hr. Initiate dosing for: **Arymo ER, or MS Contin** at 15 mg q8hr or q12hr; and ER Caps at 30 mg q24hr

Available forms: IR tablets 15, 30 mg; ER tablets (Arymo ER) 15, 30, 60 mg; ER tablets (MS Contin) 15, 30, 60, 100, 200 mg; ER tablets 15, 30, 60, 100 mg; ER capsules 10, 20, 30, 40, 50, 60, 75, 80, 100, 130, 150, 200 mg; oral solution 1 mg/mL ✿, 2 mg/mL, 4 mg/mL, 5 mg/mL ✿, 20 mg/mL; rectal suppositories 5, 10, 20, 30 mg; solution for injection (IM, IV, SUBCUT) 1 mg/mL, 2 mg/mL, 4 mg/mL, 5 mg/mL, 8 mg/mL, 10 mg/mL, 15 mg/mL, 25 mg/mL, 50 mg/mL; solution for epidural, IV (no preservative) 0.5 mg/mL, 1 mg/mL; solution for IT or epidural, continuous microinfusion device; no preservative 10 mg/mL, 25 mg/mL; solution for IV (PCA device) 1 mg/mL, 2 mg/mL, 3 mg/mL, 5 mg/mL

Administer:
PO route
• Give with food or milk to minimize GI effects
• Begin with immediate-release products and titrate to correct dose and convert to a sustained-release product
• **Immediate-release cap:** may swallow whole, or cap may be opened and contents sprinkled on cool food (pudding or applesauce) or added to juice; give immediately or delivered via gastric or NG tube by either adding to or following with liquid
• **Extended-release and controlled-release tabs:** swallow whole; do not crush, break, dissolve, or chew

• The use of MS Contin 100-mg or 200-mg tabs should be limited to opioid-tolerant patients requiring oral doses equivalent to ≥200 mg/day; use of the 100-mg or 200-mg tablet is only recommended for patients who have already been titrated to a stable analgesic regimen using lower strengths of MS Contin or other opioids

• **Sustained-release caps:** swallow; do not chew, crush, or dissolve; caps may be opened and contents sprinkled on applesauce (at room temperature or cooler) immediately before ingestion; do not chew, crush, or dissolve the pellets/beads inside the cap; the applesauce should be swallowed without chewing; if the pellets/beads are chewed, an immediate release of a potentially fatal morphine dose may be delivered; rinse mouth

Oral liquid

• Check dose before use because many concentrations of oral solution are available; may be diluted in fruit juice; protect from light

Injectable administration

• Visually inspect for particulate matter, discoloration before use; do not use if a precipitate is present after shaking; do not use the Duramorph solution if a precipitate is present or if the color is darker than pale yellow

Intrathecal/epidural route

• Morphine sulfate injection is not interchangeable with morphine sulfate extended-release liposome injection (DepoDur); DepoDur is only for epidural administration

• Do not use Infumorph (10 mg/mL or 25 mg/mL) for single-dose neuraxial injection because lower doses can be more reliably administered with Duramorph (0.5 mg/mL or 1 mg/mL)

Rectal route

• Moisten the suppository with water before insertion; if suppository is too soft, chill in the refrigerator for 30 min or run cold water over it before removing the wrapper

IV route

• Before use, an opiate antagonist and emergency facilities should be available

• Do not use the highly concentrated morphine injections (10-25 mg/mL) for IV, IM, or SC administration of single doses; these injection solutions are intended for use via continuous, controlled microinfusion devices

• **Direct IV route:** dilute dose with ≥5 mL of sterile water for injection or NS injection; inject 2.5-15 mg directly into a vein or into the tubing of a freely flowing IV solution over 4-5 min; do not give rapidly

• **Continuous IV infusion:** dilute in D$_5$W to (0.1-1 mg/mL) use a controlled-infusion device; adjust dosage and rate based on patient response

• **Patient-controlled analgesia (PCA):** a compatible patient-controlled infusion device must be used; dilute solutions to a concentration of 1 or 10 mg/mL for ease in calculations and programming of PCA pumps; adjust dosage and rate based on patient response; consult the patient-controlled infusion device manual for directions on rate of infusion

Y-site compatibilities: Acetaminophen, aldesleukin, allopurinol, amifostine, amikacin, aminophylline, amiodarone, amsacrine, atenolol, atracurium, aztreonam, bumetanide, calcium chloride, cefamandole, ceFAZolin, cefotaxime, cefoTEtan, cefOXitin, cefTAZidime, ceftizoxime, cefTRIAXone, cefuroxime, cephalothin, chloramphenicol, cisatracurium, cladribine, clindamycin, cyclophosphamide, cytarabine, dexamethasone, digoxin, diltiaZEM, DOBUTamine, DOPamine, doxycycline, enalaprilat, EPINEPHrine, erythromycin, esmolol, etomidate, famotidine, fentaNYL, filgrastim, fluconazole, fludarabine, foscarnet, gentamicin, granisetron, heparin, hydrocortisone, HYDROmorphone, kanamycin, labetalol, lidocaine, LORazepam, magnesium sulfate, melphalan, meropenem, methotrexate, methyldopa, methylPREDNISolone, metoclopramide, metoprolol, metroNIDAZOLE, midazolam, milrinone, nafcillin, niCARdipine, nitroglycerin, norepinephrine, ondansetron, oxacillin, oxytocin, PACLitaxel, pancuronium, penicillin G potassium, piperacillin, piperacillin/tazobactam, potassium chloride, propranolol, raNITIdine, remifentanil, sodium bicarbonate, teniposide, thiotepa, ticarcillin, ticarcillin/clavulanate, tigecycline, tobramycin, vancomycin, vecuronium, vinorelbine, vit B/C, warfarin, zidovudine, zoledronic acid

SIDE EFFECTS
CNS: Drowsiness, dizziness, confusion, headache, sedation, euphoria, insomnia, seizures
CV: Palpitations, bradycardia, change in B/P, shock, cardiac arrest, chest pain, hypo/hypertension, edema, tachycardia
EENT: Blurred vision, miosis, diplopia
ENDO: Gynecomastia
GI: Nausea, vomiting, anorexia, constipation, cramps, biliary tract pressure
GU: Urinary retention, impotence, gonadal suppression
HEMA: Thrombocytopenia
INTEG: Rash, urticaria, bruising, flushing, diaphoresis, pruritus
RESP: Respiratory depression, respiratory arrest, apnea

PHARMACOKINETICS
PO: Onset variable, peak 60 min, duration 4-5 hr
IM: Onset ½ hr, peak 30-60 min, duration 4-5 hr
SUBCUT: Onset 15-20 min, peak 50-90 min, duration 4-5 hr
IV: Peak 20 min, duration 4-5 hr
RECT: Peak ½-1 hr, duration 3-7 hr
Intrathecal: Onset rapid, duration ≤24 hr. Metabolized by liver, crosses placenta; excreted in urine, breast milk; half-life IM 3-4 hr; Kadian 11-13 hr

INTERACTIONS
• **Unpredictable reaction, avoid use: MAOIs**
• **Greater risk of cross-sensitivity with organic and semiorganic opioids**

Increase: serotonin syndrome risk—SSRIs, SNRIs, tricyclics, MAOIs, amoxapine, dolasetron, palonosetron, antimigraine agents, linezolid, lithium, methylene blue, traZODone; monitor for serotonin syndrome
Increase: effects with other CNS depressants—alcohol, opiates, sedative/hypnotics, antipsychotics, skeletal muscle relaxants, general anesthetics, benzodiazepine; avoid using together; increased respiratory depression
Decrease: morphine effect—butorphanol, nalbuphine, pentazocine; consider using another product; withdrawal symptoms may occur
Decrease: morphine action—rifAMPin
Drug/Herb
Increase: CNS depression—chamomile, hops, kava, St. John's wort, valerian
Drug/Lab Test
Increase: amylase, lipase

NURSING CONSIDERATIONS
Assess:
• **Pain:** location, intensity, type, character; check for pain relief 20 min following IV, 1 hr following PO/IM/Subcut; titrate to relieve pain; give dose before pain becomes severe
• **Bowel status:** constipation common, use stimulant laxative if needed; provide increased bulk, fluids in diet
• I&O ratio; check for decreasing output; may indicate urinary retention; monitor serum sodium
• B/P, pulse, respirations (character, depth, rate)
• **CNS changes:** dizziness, drowsiness, hallucinations, euphoria, LOC, pupil reaction
• **Abrupt discontinuation:** gradually taper to prevent withdrawal symptoms; decrease by 50% q1-2days; avoid use of narcotic antagonists
• Allergic reactions: rash, urticaria

Black Box Warning: Accidental exposure: if Duramorph or Infumorph gets on skin, remove contaminated clothing, rinse affected area with water

Black Box Warning: Requires a specialized care setting: patient should be observed for ≥24 hr; have emergency equipment nearby

Black Box Warning: Respiratory dysfunction: depression, character, rate, rhythm; notify prescriber if respirations are <12/min; accidental overdose has occurred with high-potency oral sols

• Gradual withdrawal after long-term use

Black Box Warning: Pregnancy/breastfeeding: use only if benefits outweigh risk to fetus; longer use can result in neonatal opioid withdrawal syndrome; do not breastfeed

Evaluate:
• **Therapeutic response:** decrease in pain intensity
Teach patient/family:

Black Box Warning: To keep out of the reach of children, pets

Black Box Warning: To notify health care professional if pregnancy is planned or suspected

• To avoid driving, hazardous activities until response is known
• To turn, cough, and deep breathe if on bed rest
• To report constipation, as other products will need to be used
• To change position slowly; orthostatic hypotension may occur
• To report any symptoms of CNS changes, allergic reactions
• That physical dependency may result from long-term use
• To avoid use of alcohol, CNS depressants
• That withdrawal symptoms may occur: nausea, vomiting, cramps, fever, faintness, anorexia
• To take exactly as directed; do not crush, break, chew, or dissolve caps or tabs

TREATMENT OF OVERDOSE:
Naloxone (Narcan) 0.2-0.8 mg IV

(caution with opioid-tolerant individuals), O_2, IV fluids, vasopressors

⚠ HIGH ALERT

moxetumomab pasudo-tox-tdfk (Rx)
(mox-e-toom'oh-mab pa-soo'doe-tox)
Lumoxiti
Func. class.: Antineoplastic

USES: Relapsed or refractory hairy-cell leukemia in patients who have received at least 2 prior systemic therapies, including treatment with a purine nucleoside analog

CONTRAINDICATIONS
Hypersensitivity

Black Box Warning: Capillary leak syndrome, hemolytic-uremic syndrome

DOSAGE AND ROUTES
• **Adult: IV** 0.04 mg/kg (actual body weight) over 30 min on days 1, 3, and 5 repeated q28days until disease progression or a maximum of 6 cycles
Available forms: Powder for injection 1 mg

moxifloxacin (Rx)
(mocks-ah-flox'a-sin)
Avelox
Func. class.: Antiinfective
Chem. class.: Fluoroquinolone

ACTION: Interferes with conversion of intermediate DNA fragments into high-molecular-weight DNA in bacteria; DNA gyrase inhibitor

USES: Acute bacterial sinusitis: *Streptococcus pneumoniae, Haemophilus influenzae, Moraxella catarrhalis;* acute bacterial exacerbation of chronic bronchitis: *S. pneumoniae, H. influenzae, Haemophilus parainfluenzae, Klebsiella pneumoniae, Staphylococcus aureus, M. catarrhalis;* community-acquired pneumonia: *S. pneumoniae, H. influenzae, Mycoplasma pneumoniae, Chlamydia pneumoniae, M. catarrhalis;* uncomplicated skin/skin-structure infections: *S. aureus, Streptococcus pyogenes;* complicated intraabdominal infections including polymicrobial infections: *E. coli, Bacteroides fragilis, S. anginosus, S. constellatus, Enterococcus faecalis, Proteus mirabilis, Clostridium perfringens, Bacteroides thetaiotaomicron, Peptostreptococcus* sp.; complicated skin, skin-structure infections caused by methicillin-susceptible bacteria: *S. aureus, E. coli, K. pneumoniae, Enterobacter cloacae;* prophylaxis and treatment of plague caused by *Yersinia pestis,* including pneumonic and septicemic plague

Unlabeled uses: Anthrax treatment/prophylaxis, gastroenteritis, MAC, nongonococcal urethritis, shigellosis, surgical infection prophylaxis, TB

CONTRAINDICATIONS
Hypersensitivity to quinolones
Precautions: Pregnancy, breastfeeding, children, hepatic/cardiac/renal/GI disease, epilepsy, uncorrected hypokalemia, prolonged QT interval; patients receiving class IA, III antidysrhythmics; seizure disorder, CDAD, diabetes mellitus

Black Box Warning: Tendon pain, rupture; tendinitis, myasthenia gravis, neurotoxicity, peripheral neuropathy, psychiatric events

DOSAGE AND ROUTES
Acute bacterial sinusitis
• **Adult: PO/IV** 400 mg q24hr × 10 days
Acute bacterial exacerbation of chronic bronchitis
• **Adult: PO/IV** 400 mg q24hr × 5 days
Community-acquired pneumonia
• **Adult: PO/IV** 400 mg q24hr × 7-14 days

Uncomplicated skin/skin-structure infections
• **Adult: PO/IV** 400 mg q24hr × 7 days
Complicated intraabdominal infections
• **Adult: IV** 400 mg/day × 7-21 days
Complicated skin, skin-structure infections
• **Adult: PO/IV** 400 mg/day × 7-21 days
Plague
• **Adult: PO/IV** 400 mg q24hr × 10-14 days

Available forms: Tabs 400 mg; inj premix 400 mg/250 mL
Administer:
PO route
• 4 hr before or 8 hr after antacids, zinc, iron, calcium, sucralfate, multivitamins
• Without regard to food
• Store at room temperature; do not refrigerate, do not use if particulate is present
IV route
• Do not use if particulate matter is present
• Give PO 4 hr before or 8 hr after antacids, sucralsulfate, multivitamins
• Do not give SUBCUT, IM
• Available as premixed sol; may be diluted at ratios from 1:10 to 10:1; do not refrigerate; give by direct infusion or through Y-type infusion set; do not add other medications to sol or infusion through same IV line at same time
• Flush line with compatible sol before and after use
• Do not admix

Solution compatibilities: 0.9% NaCl, D$_5$, D$_{10}$, LR, sterile water for inj

SIDE EFFECTS
CNS: *Headache,* dizziness, fatigue, insomnia, depression, *restlessness,* seizures, confusion, increased intracranial pressure, peripheral neuropathy, pseudotumor cerebri, fever
CV: Prolonged QT interval, dysrhythmias, torsades de pointes, tachycardia
EENT: Blurred vision, tinnitus, taste changes
GI: *Nausea, diarrhea,* increased ALT, AST, flatulence, heartburn, *vomiting,* oral candidiasis, dysphagia, CDAD,

abdominal pain, dyspepsia, constipation, gastroenteritis, xerostomia

GU: Renal failure

INTEG: *Rash*, pruritus, urticaria, photosensitivity, flushing, fever, chills, injection-site reactions

MISC: Candidiasis vaginitis

MS: Tremor, arthralgia, tendinitis, tendon rupture, myalgia

SYST: Anaphylaxis, Stevens-Johnson syndrome, angioedema, toxic epidermal necrolysis

PHARMACOKINETICS

Excreted in urine as active product, metabolites; parent product excreted in urine (20%), feces (25%); half-life PO 12-16 hr, IV 8-15 hr, peak 1 hr (PO), 1-3 hr (IV)

INTERACTIONS

Increase: QT prolongation—drugs that increase QT interval; avoid using concurrently

Increase: moxifloxacin serum levels—probenecid

Increase: warfarin, cycloSPORINE effect

Increase: seizure risk—NSAIDs; monitor, adjust or use different product

> **Black Box Warning: Increase:** tendon rupture—corticosteroids

Increase: anticoagulant level—warfarin; monitor PT/INR

Decrease: moxifloxacin absorption—magnesium antacids, aluminum hydroxide, zinc, iron, sucralfate, calcium, enteral feeding, didanosine

Drug/Lab Test

Increase: glucose, lipids, triglycerides, uric acid, LDH ALT, ionized calcium, chloride, globulin, albumin, PT, INR, WBC

Decrease: potassium, glucose, amylase, RBC, eosinophils, Hb, Hct

NURSING CONSIDERATIONS

Assess:

• **CNS symptoms:** headache, dizziness, fatigue, insomnia, depression, seizures

• **Renal, hepatic studies:** BUN, creatinine, AST, ALT, electrolytes

• I&O ratio, urine pH <5.5 is ideal

• **Allergic reactions, Stevens-Johnson syndrome, toxic epidermal necrolysis, anaphylaxis:** fever, flushing, rash, urticaria, pruritus, sore throat, fatigue, ulcers, other lesions; keep EPINEPHrine, emergency equipment nearby for anaphylaxis

> **Black Box Warning:** Tendon pain, rupture, tendinitis; if tendon becomes inflamed, product should be discontinued; more common in Achilles tendon

• **Cardiac status:** prolonged QT or use of products that increase QT prolongation

• **CDAD:** assess for diarrhea, abdominal pain, fever, fatigue, anorexia; possible anemia, elevated WBC, low serum albumin; stop product; usually either vancomycin or IV metroNIDAZOLE given

• Increased fluids to 3 L/day to avoid crystallization in kidneys

> **Black Box Warning: Myasthenia gravis:** assess for increased weakness when using this product; avoid using in this condition

> **Black Box Warning: Peripheral neuropathy:** assess for pain, numbness, tingling in extremities; report

• **Pregnancy/breastfeeding:** risks to fetus are unknown; adverse events observed in some animal studies; discuss risks, benefits of treatment

Evaluate:

• **Therapeutic response:** decreased pain, C&S; absence of infection

Teach patient/family:

> **Black Box Warning:** To notify prescriber of tendon pain, inflammation, or burning, tingling, weakness; stop drug

• Not to take any products containing magnesium or calcium (such as antacids), iron, or aluminum with this product or 4 hr before or 8 hr after

• That photosensitivity may occur; to avoid sunlight or use sunscreen to prevent burns

- To use frequent rinsing of mouth, sugarless candy or gum for dry mouth
- To take as prescribed; not to double or miss doses; to take without regard to meals
- To report immediately rash, diarrhea, rapid heartbeat
- If dizziness occurs, to ambulate, perform activities with assistance
- To complete full course of product therapy
- To contact prescriber if abnormal heart rhythm or seizures occur

moxifloxacin (ophthalmic) (Rx)

(mocks-ih-floks′a-sin)

Vigamox, Moxeza

Func. class.: Ophthalmic antiinfective
Chem. class.: Fluoroquinolone

Do not confuse:
moxifloxacin/ciprofloxacin/gatifloxacin/levoFLOXacin

ACTION: Inhibits DNA gyrase, thereby decreasing bacterial replication

USES: Bacterial conjunctivitis (aerobic gram-positive/negative organisms), *Chlamydia trachomatis*

CONTRAINDICATIONS
Hypersensitivity to this product or fluoroquinolones
Precautions: Pregnancy, breastfeeding

DOSAGE AND ROUTES
Bacterial conjunctivitis
- **Adult/adolescent/child ≥1 yr: ophthalmic SOL** 1 drop in affected eye(s) bid (Moxeza) or tid (Vigamox) × 7 days
Available forms: Ophthalmic solution 0.5%
Administer:
Ophthalmic route
- Commercially available ophthalmic solutions are not for injection subconjunctivally or into the anterior chamber of the eye

- Apply topically to the eye, taking care to avoid contamination
- Do not touch the tip of the dropper to the eye, fingertips, or other surface
- Apply pressure to lacrimal sac for 1 min after instillation
- Avoid wearing contact lenses during treatment

SIDE EFFECTS
EENT: Hypersensitivity, pruritus, blurred vision, tearing

PHARMACOKINETICS
Half-life 13 hr

NURSING CONSIDERATIONS
Assess:
- **Allergic reaction:** assess for hypersensitivity; discontinue product
Evaluate:
- Decreased ophthalmic infection
Teach patient/family:
Ophthalmic route
- To apply topically to the eye, taking care to avoid contamination
- That product is for ophthalmic use only
- Not to touch the tip of the dropper to the eye, fingertips, or other surface
- To apply pressure to lacrimal sac for 1 min after instillation
- To avoid wearing contact lenses during treatment

mupirocin (topical, nasal) (Rx)

(myoo-pihr′oh-sin)

Bactroban ✦, Centany, Centany AT
Func. class.: Topical antiinfective

ACTION: Antibacterial activity results from inhibition of protein synthesis; bacteriostatic at low concentration, bactericidal at high concentration

USES: Impetigo, skin lesions *(Staphylococcus aureus/Streptococcus pyogenes);* nasal: methicillin-resistant *S. aureus*

CONTRAINDICATIONS
Hypersensitivity to this product
Precautions: Open wounds, burns, severe kidney disease, children, pregnancy, breastfeeding

DOSAGE AND ROUTES
Impetigo
• **Adult/child: TOP** apply to affected area tid × 1-2 wk
Skin lesions
• **Adult/child: TOP** apply to affected area tid × 10 days
Methicillin-resistant *S. aureus* in the nose
• **Adult/child ≥12 yr: NASAL** divide ointment in single use tube in half; use in each nostril bid × 5 days
Available forms: Topical cream, ointment 2%; intranasal ointment 2%
Administer:
Topical route
• Do not use skin products near the eyes, nose, or mouth
• Wash hands before and after use; wash affected area and gently pat dry
• May cover treated areas with gauze dressing
Cream/ointment
• Apply a thin film to the cleansed affected area; massage gently into affected areas; do not use near eyes, mouth
• **Nasal:** Close nostrils by squeezing and releasing and gently massaging over 1 min

SIDE EFFECTS
CNS: Headache
EENT: Burning, pharyngitis, rhinitis (nasal)
GI: Taste change, nausea
INTEG: Burning, rash, pruritus

INTERACTIONS
Decrease: Effect of other nasal products

NURSING CONSIDERATIONS
Assess:
• **Allergic reaction:** assess for hypersensitivity; product may need to be discontinued
• **Infection:** assess for number of lesions, severity in impetigo, other skin disorders

Evaluate:
• Decreased lesions in impetigo, other skin disorders
Teach patient/family:
Topical route
• Not to use skin products near the eyes, nose, or mouth
• To wash hands before and after use and to wash affected area and gently pat dry
• **Cream/ointment:** to apply a thin film to the cleansed affected area; to cover treated areas with gauze dressing if desired
• **Nasal:** to close nostrils by squeezing and releasing and gently massaging over 1 min

---

mycophenolate mofetil (Rx)
(mye-koe-phen'oh-late)
CellCept
mycophenolate acid
Myfortic
Func. class.: Immunosuppressant

ACTION: Inhibits inflammatory responses that are mediated by the immune system

USES: Prophylaxis for organ rejection in allogenic cardiac, hepatic, renal transplants
Unlabeled uses: Nephrotic syndrome

CONTRAINDICATIONS
Hypersensitivity to this product or mycophenolic acid

Black Box Warning: Pregnancy

Precautions: Breastfeeding, lymphomas, neutropenia, renal disease, accidental exposure, anemia

Black Box Warning: Infection, neoplastic disease; requires an experienced clinician and a specialized care setting

DOSAGE AND ROUTES
For kidney transplant rejection prophylaxis with or without antithymocyte induction
• **Adult: IV** 1 g over at least 2 hr bid in combination with corticosteroids and

---

cycloSPORINE; initial dose should be given within 24 hr of transplantation

Oral dosage

The delayed-release tablets (mycophenolate sodium) and the capsules, oral suspension, and tablets (mycophenolate mofetil) are not interchangeable on an mg basis

• **Adult: PO** (regular release) 1 g mycophenolate mofetil or **PO** (extended release) 720-mg mycophenolate sodium bid in combination with corticosteroids and cyclosporine

• **Child: PO** (oral suspension) 600 mg/m^2 bid, max 2 g/day. Mycophenolate mofetil capsules may be given at dose of 750 mg bid for those with a body surface area (BSA) of 1.25-1.5 m^2 or 1 g bid for those with a BSA >1.5 m^2; mycophenolate sodium delayed-release tablets 400 mg/m^2 bid, max 720 mg bid

• **Infant ≥3 mo: PO** (oral suspension) 600 mg/m^2 bid, max 2 g/day

For heart transplant rejection prophylaxis

• **Adult: IV** 1.5 g over at least 2 hr bid in combination with corticosteroids and cycloSPORINE. The first dose may be administered within 24 hr after transplantation

• **Adult: PO** (regular release) (mycophenolate mofetil) 1.5 g bid in combination with corticosteroids and cycloSPORINE. Initial oral dose should be administered as soon as possible after transplantation

For liver transplant rejection prophylaxis

• **Adult: IV** 1 g over at least 2 hr bid in combination with corticosteroids and cycloSPORINE; the first dose may be administered within 24 hr after transplantation

• **Adult: PO** (mycophenolate mofetil) 1.5 g bid in combination with corticosteroids and cycloSPORINE; give initial dose as soon as possible after transplantation

Available forms: Caps 250 mg; tabs 500 mg; inj (powder) 500 mg/20-mL vial; powder for oral susp 200 mg/mL; delayed rel tab (Myfortic) 180, 360 mg

Administer:

• May be given in combination with corticosteroids, cycloSPORINE

• **Cytotoxic:** Use safe handling procedures; avoid inhalation or direct contact with skin, mucous membranes; teratogenic in animals; wash skin if product comes in contact with skin

PO route

• Do not break, crush, or chew tabs; do not open caps

• Give at same time each day

• **Oral susp:** tap closed bottle several times to loosen powder; use 94 mL of water in graduated cylinder; add ½ total amount of water for reconstitution and shake the closed bottle; add remaining water and shake again; remove child-resistant cap; push adapter into neck of bottle; close tightly, may give by NG tube ≥8 French catheter

• Give alone for better absorption

Intermittent IV INFUSION route

• Reconstitute each vial with 14 mL D$_5$W; shake gently; further dilute to 6 mg/mL; dilute 1 g/140 mL D$_5$W, 1.5 g/210 mL D$_5$W; give by slow IV infusion ≥2 hr; never give by bolus or rapid IV inj

• Do not give with other medications or sol, do not use if particulates are present

Y-site compatibilities: Alemtuzumab, alfentanil, amikacin, anidulafungin, argatroban, bivalirudin, caspofungin, cefepime, DAPTOmycin, DOPamine, norepinephrine, octreotide, oxytocin, tacrolimus, tigecycline, tirofiban, vancomycin, zoledronic acid

SIDE EFFECTS

CNS: *Tremor, dizziness, insomnia, headache, fever,* anxiety, pain, progressive multifocal leukoencephalopathy, asthenia, paresthesia

CV: *Hypertension, chest pain,* hypotension, edema

GI: *Diarrhea, constipation, nausea, vomiting,* stomatitis, GI bleeding, abdominal pain, anorexia, dyspepsia

GU: *UTI, hematuria,* renal tubular necrosis, polyomavirus-associated nephropathy
HEMA: Leukopenia, thrombocytopenia, anemia, pancytopenia, pure red cell aplasia, neutropenia
INTEG: *Rash*
META: *Peripheral edema, hypercholesterolemia, hypophosphatemia, edema, hyperkalemia, hypokalemia, hyperglycemia,* hypocalcemia, hypomagnesemia
MS: Arthralgia, muscle wasting, back pain, weakness
RESP: *Dyspnea, respiratory infection, increased cough, pharyngitis, bronchitis, pneumonia,* plural effusion, pulmonary fibrosis
SYST: Lymphoma, *nonmelanoma skin carcinoma,* sepsis

PHARMACOKINETICS
Rapidly and completely absorbed; metabolized to active metabolite (MPA); excreted in urine, feces; protein binding (MPA) 97%; half-life (MPA) 17.9 hr

INTERACTIONS
Increase: bone marrow suppression—azaTHIOprine; do not use concurrently
Increase: bleeding risk—anticoagulants, NSAIDs, thrombolytics, salicylates
Increase: toxicity—acyclovir, ganciclovir, valACYclovir; monitor if used together
Increase: effects of both products—phenytoin, theophylline
Increase: mycophenolate levels—probenecid, immunosuppressives, salicylates; monitor for adverse reactions
Decrease: mycophenolate levels—antacids (magnesium, aluminum), cholestyramine, cycloSPORINE, rifamycin; separate dosing times by several hours
Decrease: protein binding of phenytoin, theophylline
Decrease: effect of live attenuated vaccines, oral contraceptives
Drug/Herb
Interference with immunosuppression: astragalus, cat's claw, echinacea, melatonin

Drug/Food
Decrease: absorption if taken with food
Drug/Lab Test
Increase: serum creatinine, BUN, cholesterol, potassium, WBC

NURSING CONSIDERATIONS
Assess:
• **Progressive multifocal leukoencephalopathy:** may be fatal; ataxia, confusion, apathy, hemiparesis, visual problems, weakness; side effects should be reported to FDA
• **Pure red cell aplasia (PRCA):** occurs when used in combination with other immunosuppressants; assess for fatigue, pulmonary tachycardia; may cause graft rejection
• Blood studies: CBC during treatment monthly, may monitor mycophenolate levels in those at high risk for organ rejection
• Hepatic studies: alk phos, AST, ALT, bilirubin
• Renal studies: BUN, CCr, electrolytes

Black Box Warning: **Pregnancy/breastfeeding:** pregnancy test within 1 wk before initiation of treatment; confirm negative pregnancy test; if patient becomes pregnant, enroll in Mycophenolate Pregnancy Registry 800-617-8191; do not breastfeed during treatment and for 6 wk after final dose

Black Box Warning: **Requires a specialized setting and experienced clinician:** should be used by those experienced in the use of immunosuppressive therapy in a facility equipped for transplants

Evaluate:
• **Therapeutic response:** absence of graft rejection
Teach patient/family:
• About the need for repeated lab tests and follow-up exams

Black Box Warning: Pregnancy/breast-feeding: to use 2 forms of contraception before, during, and for 6 wk after therapy; not to breastfeed during and for 6 wk after final dose; that pregnancy test is required the week before start of therapy and 8-10 days later

• To take at same time each day; not to crush, chew caps, or ext rel tab; swallow whole, take on empty stomach

Black Box Warning: Infection: to report fever, chills, sorze throat, fatigue; serious infections may occur; avoid crowds, persons with known infections

Black Box Warning: Neoplastic disease: lymphoma and other neoplastic diseases may occur, particularly skin cancer; limit UV exposure by wearing protective clothing, sunscreen

M

> ⚠️ **HIGH ALERT**

nadolol (Rx)
(nay-doe′lole)

Corgard

Func. class.: Antihypertensive, antianginal

Chem. class.: β-Adrenergic receptor blocker

ACTION: Long-acting, nonselective β-adrenergic receptor blocking agent, blocks β_1 in the heart and β_2 in the lungs, uterus, and circulatory system; mechanism is similar to that of propranolol

USES: Chronic stable angina pectoris, mild to moderate hypertension

CONTRAINDICATIONS
Hypersensitivity to this product, cardiac failure, cardiogenic shock, 2nd-/3rd-degree heart block, bronchospastic disease, sinus bradycardia, HF, COPD, asthma
Precautions: Pregnancy, breastfeeding, diabetes mellitus, renal disease, hyperthyroidism, peripheral vascular disease, myasthenia gravis, major surgery, nonallergic bronchospasm

Black Box Warning: Abrupt discontinuation, ischemic heart disease may be more severe

DOSAGE AND ROUTES
Angina pectoris
• **Adult:** PO 40 mg/day, increase by 40-80 mg q3-7days; **maintenance** 40-240 mg/day
Hypertension
• **Adult PO** 40 mg daily, increase by 40-80 mg every 2 to 14 days until therapeutic response; maintenance, 40-320 mg/day

Renal dose
• **Adult:** PO CCr 31-50 mL/min, give q24-36hr; CCr 10-30 mL/min, give q24-48hr; CCr <10 mL/min, give q40-60hr
Available forms: Tabs 20, 40, 80, 160
🍁 mg

Administer:
• With 8 oz water, check apical pulse before use; if <60 bpm, withhold; notify prescriber
• Give without regard to food
• Tabs may be crushed and mixed with food

Black Box Warning: Taper over 1-2 wk to discontinue product; do not stop abruptly, may worsen angina pectoris

SIDE EFFECTS
CNS: Depression, *dizziness, fatigue,* drowsiness
CV: *Bradycardia, hypotension,* HF, palpitations, chest pain, peripheral ischemia, flushing, edema, vasodilation

PHARMACOKINETICS
PO: Onset variable, peak 3-4 hr, duration 17-24 hr; half-life 20-24 hr; not metabolized; excreted in urine 70% (unchanged), bile, breast milk; protein binding 30%

INTERACTIONS
Increase: orthostatic hypertension—MAOIs; monitor B/P
Increase: peripheral ischemia—ergots, avoid if possible
Increase: bradycardia—digoxin; monitor for bradycardia
Increase: hypotension, bradycardia—cloNIDine, EPINEPHrine
Increase: lack of stability of dose in diabetes—antidiabetics, insulin, dose may need to be changed
Increase: hypotensive effects—amphetamines, methylphenidate, other antihypertensives, antipsychotics (2nd generation), barbiturates, calcium channel blockers, PDE5 inhibitors, prostacyclin analogues, other hypotensive agents, phenothiazines, general anesthetics, monitor B/P, consider stopping nadolol before surgery
Decrease: β-blocking effect—thyroid hormones
Decrease: antihypertensive effect—NSAIDs, monitor B/P

🍁 Canada only   ⚕️Ⓖⓔⓧ Genetic warning

Drug/Herb

Increase: orthostatic hypertension—dong quai, garlic, ginseng, yohimbe; avoid concurrent use

NURSING CONSIDERATIONS
Assess:
• **Hypertension:** check that prescriptions have been filled; B/P, pulse, respirations during beginning therapy and periodically thereafter
• Monitor for orthostatic hypotension
• **Angina:** monitor frequency of angina, alleviating factors; duration, time started, activity being performed, character
• Headache, light-headedness, decreased B/P; may indicate a need for decreased dosage
• **HF:** daily weight, report gain of 2-3 lb/wk or unexpected weight gain
• **Dyspnea:** shortness of breath, wheezing, allergic rhinitis
• I&O ratio, serum creatinine/BUN

Black Box Warning: Abrupt discontinuation: can result in MI, myocardial ischemia, ventricular dysrhythmias, severe hypertension; withdraw slowly by tapering over 1-2 wk; if symptoms return, restart

• **Pregnancy/breastfeeding:** use only if benefits outweigh risk to fetus; discontinue product or breastfeeding, excreted in breast milk
Evaluate:
• **Therapeutic response:** decreased B/P, heart rate, symptoms of angina
Teach patient/family:
• That product may mask signs of hypoglycemia or alter blood glucose in patients with diabetes
• To avoid OTC products unless prescriber approves; to take as prescribed, at same time each day, do not double; to take missed dose as soon as remembered if less than 8 hr before next dose
• To avoid hazardous activities if dizziness occurs
• **Hypertension:** to comply with complete medical regimen; to report weight gain of >5 lb, swelling, unusual bruising, bleeding
• To rise slowly to prevent orthostatic hypotension

• About how and when to check B/P, pulse; to hold dose, contact prescriber if pulse ≤60 bpm, systolic B/P <90 mm Hg

Black Box Warning: Not to discontinue abruptly; may cause life-threatening cardiac changes

nafarelin (Rx)
Nah-far'eh-lin
Synarel
Func. class.: Gonadotropin-releasing hormone analogue

USES: Central precocious puberty, endometriosis
CONTRAINDICATIONS
Hypersensitivity to gonadotropin-releasing hormone (GnRH), GnRH-agonist analogs, or any component; undiagnosed abnormal vaginal bleeding; pregnant women or those who may become pregnant; breastfeeding

DOSAGE AND ROUTES
Endometriosis: Adult female:
Intranasal: 1 spray (200 mcg) into 1 nostril each morning and 1 spray (200 mcg) into the other nostril each evening starting between days 2 and 4 of menstrual cycle (total: 2 sprays [400 mcg] daily). If regular menstruation persists after 2 mo of therapy, may increase dose to 2 sprays (400 mcg; 1 spray in each nostril) in the morning and evening (total: 4 sprays [800 mcg] daily), max 6 mo
Central precocious puberty
Child males (≤9 yr)/females (≤8 yr): Intranasal: 2 sprays (400 mcg) into each nostril in the morning and 2 sprays (400 mcg) into each nostril in the evening
Available forms: Nasal spray 2 mg/mL/200 mcg/spray

nafcillin (Rx)
(naf-sill'in)
Func. class.: Antibiotic, broad-spectrum
Chem. class.: Penicillinase-resistant penicillin

ACTION: Bacteriocidal, interferes with cell-wall replication of susceptible organisms

USES: Effective for gram-positive cocci (*Staphylococcus aureus, Streptococcus viridans, Streptococcus pneumoniae*), infections caused by penicillinase-producing *Staphylococcus*

CONTRAINDICATIONS

Hypersensitivity to penicillins

Precautions: Pregnancy, breastfeeding, neonates; hypersensitivity to cephalosporins or carbapenems; GI disease, asthma, electrolyte imbalances, hepatic/renal disease, CDAD

DOSAGE AND ROUTES

• **Adult: IV** 1-2 g q4hr for severe infections
• **Child and infant >1 mo: IV** 100-200 mg/kg/day in divided doses, Max: 2 g/dose, max 12 g/day
• **Neonate** 25 mg/kg/dose q6h × 14 days
Available forms: Powder for inj 1 g/vial, 2 g/vial, 10 g/vial; premixed infusion 1 g/50 mL D_5W, 2 g/100 mL
Administer:
• Product after C&S has been drawn, begin therapy while waiting for results
• Check for allergy to penicillins, cephalosporins
IM route
• Reconstitute vials: Add 3.4 mL to 1-g vial, 6.6 mL to 2-g vial (250 mg/mL)
• After reconstitution, inject in deep muscle mass
• Use sterile water for injection or 0.9% NaCl to prevent using benzyl alcohol (neonate)
• **Store:** Stable for 3 days at room temperature, 7 days refrigerated, 90 days frozen
• Do not use benzyl alcohol preparations for reconstitution
• Give deep in gluteal, rotate sites
IV route
• Reconstitute vials: Add 3.4 mL to 1-g vial, 6.6 mL to 2-g vial (250 mg/mL)
Direct IV route
• Give over 5-10 min
Intermittent IV route
• Vials, further dilute reconstituted sol to 10-40 mg/mL infuse ≥ 30-60 min
• Change IV site q48hr to prevent irritation, check for extravasation often

Y-site compatibilities: Acyclovir, alfentanil, amikacin, aminophylline, amphotericin B lipid complex (Abelcet), anidulafungin, argatroban, ascorbic acid injection, atenolol, atracurium, atropine, aztreonam, benztropine, bivalirudin, bleomycin, bretylium, bumetanide, buprenorphine, butorphanol, calcium chloride/gluconate, CARBOplatin, carmustine, cefamandole, ceFAZolin, cefoperazone, cefotaxime, cefoTEtan, cefOXitin, cefTAZidime, ceftizoxime, cefTRIAXone, cefuroxime, chlorproMAZINE, cimetidine, CISplatin, clindamycin, cyanocobalamin, cyclophosphamide, cycloSPORINE, DACTINomycin, DAPTOmycin, DAUNOrubicin liposome, dexamethasone, digoxin, DOBUTamine, DOCEtaxel, DOPamine, DOXOrubicin liposomal, enalaprilat, EPHEDrine, EPINEPHrine, epoetin alfa, erythromycin, etoposide, etoposide phosphate, famotidine, fenoldopam, fentaNYL, fluconazole, fludarabine, foscarnet, furosemide, gallium, ganciclovir, gatifloxacin, gemtuzumab, gentamicin, glycopyrrolate, granisetron, heparin, hydrocortisone, HYDROmorphone, imipenem-cilastatin, indomethacin, isoproterenol, ketorolac, lactated Ringer's, lepirudin, leucovorin, lidocaine, linezolid injection, LORazepam, magnesium sulfate, mannitol, methyldopa, methylPREDNISolone, metoclopramide, metoprolol, metroNIDAZOLE, milrinone, morphine, multiple vitamins injection, naloxone, niCARdipine, nitroglycerin, nitroprusside, norepinephrine, octreotide, ondansetron, oxacillin, oxaliplatin, oxytocin, PACLitaxel (solvent/surfactant), pamidronate, pancuronium, pantoprazole, PEMEtrexed, penicillin G potassium/sodium, PENTobarbital, perphenazine, PHENobarbital, phentolamine, phenylephrine, phytonadione, piperacillin, polymyxin B, potassium acetate/chloride, procainamide, prochlorperazine, propofol, propranolol, ranitidine, Ringer's injection, sodium bicarbonate, SUFentanil, tacrolimus, teniposide, theophylline, thiamine, thiotepa, ticarcillin, ticarcillin-clavulanate, tigecycline, tirofiban, TNA (3-in-1), tobramycin, tolazoline, TPN (2-in-1),

urokinase, vasopressin, vinBLAStine, voriconazole, zidovudine, zoledronic acid

SIDE EFFECTS
CNS: Neurotoxicity, seizures
GI: *Nausea, vomiting, diarrhea,* CDAD
GU: Proteinuria, glomerulonephritis, interstitial nephritis
HEMA: Neutropenia, thrombocytopenia, leukopenia, agranulocytosis, anemia
INTEG: Tissue necrosis, extravasation at inj site, rash, pruritus, exfoliative dermatitis
SYST: Anaphylaxis, serum sickness, Stevens-Johnson syndrome

PHARMACOKINETICS
Half-life 30-60 min; metabolized by liver; excreted in bile, urine; 70%-90% protein bound; peak rapid (IV) peak 30-60 min (IM)

INTERACTIONS
Increase: nafcillin concentrations—probenecid, used to increase nafcillin action
Decrease: effect of cycloSPORINE—warfarin, monitor closely
Decrease: nafcillin effect—tetracyclines, aminoglycosides
Decrease: effect of live virus vaccines, do not use together
Decrease: effects of CYP3A4 substrates, bedaquiline, clarithromycin, cloZAPine, fentaNYL, lurasidone, zolpidem, monitor closely
Decrease: effect of hormonal contraceptives, use additional contraceptives
Drug/Lab Test
Increase: LFTs
Decrease: HB/HcT, neutrophils
False positive: urine glucose, urine protein, Coombs test

NURSING CONSIDERATIONS
Assess:
• **Infection:** signs, symptoms of infection, including characteristics of wounds, sputum, urine, stool, WBC >10,000/mm³, earache, fever, obtain information baseline, during treatment
• I&O ratio; report hematuria, oliguria; high doses are nephrotoxic

• **CDAD:** diarrhea, abdominal pain, fever, fatigue, anorexia; possible anemia, elevated WBC, low serum albumin; stop product; usually either vancomycin or IV metroNIDAZOLE given
• **Renal studies:** urinalysis, BUN, creatinine; abnormal urinalysis may indicate nephrotoxicity
• C&S before product therapy; product may be given as soon as culture is taken
• **Allergies before initiation of treatment;** monitor for anaphylaxis, dyspnea, rash, laryngeal edema; stop product; keep emergency equipment nearby; skin eruptions after administration of penicillin to 1 wk after discontinuing product
• **IV site:** for redness, swelling, pain at site
• **Pregnancy/breastfeeding:** use only if clearly needed; use caution in breastfeeding, excreted in breast milk
Evaluate:
• **Therapeutic response:** absence of signs/symptoms of infection
Teach patient/family:
• To report vaginal itching; loose, foul-smelling stools; furry tongue; sore throat; fever; fatigue (may indicate superinfection); CNS reactions; CDAD (diarrhea, fever, abdominal pain, fatigue)
• Inform patient that product must be taken as prescribed
• Advise patient to report pain, burning, redness at IV site
• To wear or carry emergency ID if allergic to penicillins

TREATMENT OF ANAPHYLAXIS: Withdraw product; maintain airway; administer EPINEPHrine, aminophylline, O₂, IV corticosteroids

⚠ **HIGH ALERT**

nalbuphine (Rx)
(nal′byoo-feen)
Nubain ✦
Func. class.: Opioid analgesic
Chem. class.: Synthetic opioid agonist, antagonist

Do not confuse:

nalbuphine/naloxone

ACTION: Depresses pain impulse transmission by interacting with opioid receptors

USES: Moderate to severe pain, supplement to anesthesia, sedation prior to surgery

CONTRAINDICATIONS

Hypersensitivity to this product or parabens, bisulfites, addiction (opiate)

Precautions: Pregnancy, breastfeeding, addictive personality, increased intracranial pressure, MI (acute), severe heart disease, respiratory depression, renal/hepatic disease, bowel impaction, abrupt discontinuation

Black Box Warning: Coadministration with other CNS depressants, respiratory depression

DOSAGE AND ROUTES
Analgesic (nonopioid tolerant)

• **Adult: SUBCUT/IM/IV** 10 mg q3-6hr prn (based on 70-kg body weight), max 160 mg/day; max 20 mg/dose if opiate naïve

• **Child: SUBCUT/IM/IV** 0.1-0.15 mg/kg q3-6hr, max 20 mg/dose, 160 mg/day

Balanced anesthesia adjunct

• **Adult: IV** 0.3-3 mg/kg given over 10-15 min; may give 0.25-0.5 mg/kg as needed for maintenance

Available forms: solution for inj 10, 20 mg/mL

Administer:

• With antiemetic if nausea, vomiting occur

• When pain beginning to return; determine dosage interval by response

• Store in light-resistant area at room temperature

IM route

• IM deep in large muscle mass, rotate inj sites, protect from light

Direct IV route

• Undiluted ≤10 mg over 2-3 min into free-flowing IV line of D_5W, NS, or LR

SUBCUT route

• Rotate injection sites, protect from light

SIDE EFFECTS

CNS: *Drowsiness, dizziness, confusion, headache, sedation*

CV: Bradycardia, change in B/P

EENT: Blurred vision

GI: *Nausea, vomiting, constipation,* xerostomia, bitter taste

INTEG: Diaphoresis, pruritus

RESP: Respiratory depression

PHARMACOKINETICS

IV: Onset rapid, peak 2-3 min, duration 3-6 hr; **IM/SUBCUT:** Onset up to 15 min, peak 10-15 min, duration 3-6 hr metabolized by liver, excreted by kidneys, half-life 5 hr

INTERACTIONS

Black Box Warning: Increase: effects with other CNS depressants—alcohol, opiates, sedative/hypnotics, antipsychotics, skeletal muscle relaxants, avoid using together

Increase: severe reactions—MAOIs; decrease dose to 25%

Black Box Warning: Increase: serotonin syndrome risk SSRIs, SNRIs, TCAs, some antiemetics, antimigraine agents, MAOIs, monitor for serotonin syndrome

Drug/Herb

Increase: CNS depression—kava, valerian, hops, chamomile

Increase: serotonin syndrome risk St. John's wort, monitor closely

NURSING CONSIDERATIONS
Assess:

• **Pain:** type, location, intensity before and 30 min after administration; titrate upward with 25%-50% until 50% of pain reduced; need for pain medication by pain sedation scoring, can repeat if initial

dose is not adequately effective, not for long-term use
• Bowel status; constipation is common; may need laxative or stool softener

Black Box Warning: Withdrawal reactions in opiate-dependent individuals: PE, vascular occlusion; abscesses, ulcerations, nausea, vomiting, seizures

• **CNS changes:** dizziness, drowsiness, hallucinations, euphoria, LOC, pupil reaction
• Allergic reactions: rash, urticaria
• Monitor for serotonin syndrome in those taking serotonergic drugs
• Monitor for adrenal insufficiency (rare): nausea, vomiting, weakness, hypotension, dizziness; if confirmed, treat with corticosteroids and slowly withdraw opiates

Black Box Warning: Avoid coadministration with other CNS depressants: coadministration increases the risk for respiratory depression, low B/P, and death

Black Box Warning: Respiratory dysfunction: respiratory depression, character, rate, rhythm; notify prescriber if respirations are <10/min, respiratory depression may be fatal

• **Pregnancy/breastfeeding:** use only if clearly needed, labor use can result in fatal bradycardia, monitor closely; if used in long-term pregnancy, neonatal withdrawal syndrome may occur; cautious use in breastfeeding
Evaluate:
• **Therapeutic response:** decrease in pain without respiratory depression
Teach patient/family:
• That physical dependency may result from long-term use
• **That withdrawal symptoms may occur:** nausea, vomiting, cramps, fever, faintness, anorexia, profuse sweating,

twitching; without treatment symptoms resolve in 5-14 days, chronic abstinence syndrome may last 2-6 mo
• To report all OTC/Rx/herbals/supplements taken
• To increase bulk water in diet, or add stool softeners for constipation
• That naloxone may be used in overdose
• To report troubled, slowed breathing; symptoms of serotonin syndrome; allergic reactions

Black Box Warning: To avoid use with CNS depressants, alcohol, benzodiazepines, and notify prescriber of unresponsiveness, trouble breathing

• To avoid driving, operating machinery if drowsiness occurs, to have help with activities to prevent falls at home if dizzy, drowsy
• To use sugarless gum or candy and good oral hygiene for dry mouth

TREATMENT OF OVERDOSE: Naloxone (Narcan) 0.2-0.8 mg IV, O_2, IV fluids, vasopressors

naloxegol (Rx)
(Nal-ox′ee-gol)
Movantik
Func. class.: Antidote, opioid antagonist

USES: Treatment of opioid-induced constipation with chronic noncancer pain, including patients with chronic pain related to prior cancer or its treatment who do not require frequent (weekly) opioid dosage escalation

DOSAGE AND ROUTES
Adult: PO 25 mg daily, 1 hr before or 2 hr after morning meal if not tolerated, reduce to 12.5 mg daily; moderate CYP3A4 inhibitor use: 12.5 mg daily

Renal dose

• **Adult: PO** CCr <60 mL/min 12.5 mg daily, may increase to 25 mg daily if needed

Available forms: Tablet 12.5, 25 mg

---

naloxone (Rx)

(nal-oks′one)

Evzio, Kloxxado, Narcan, S.O.S., Zimhi

Func. class.: Opioid antagonist, antidote
Chem. class.: Thebaine derivative

Do not confuse:
naloxone/naltrexone/nalbuphine/
Naloxegol

ACTION: Competes with opioids at opiate receptor sites

USES: Respiratory depression induced by opioids, opiate agonist overdose
Unlabeled uses: Pruritus (opiate induced)

CONTRAINDICATIONS

Hypersensitivity

Precautions: Pregnancy, breastfeeding, children, neonates, CV disease, opioid dependency, seizure disorder, drug dependency, hepatic disease

DOSAGE AND ROUTES

• Duration of some opioids may exceed duration of naloxone, additional doses may be needed
Opioid-induced respiratory/CNS depression (known or suspected opiate agonist overdose)
• **Adult: IV/SUBCUT/IM** 0.4-2 mg, repeat q2-3min if needed, max 10 mg; **IV INFUSION** loading dose 0.005 mg/kg, then 0.0025 mg/kg/hr; **IM/SUBCUT (Zimhi autoinjector only)** 5 mg, may repeat q2-3min if needed
• **Child/adolescent 5-17 yr or ≥20 kg: IV** 2 mg, may repeat
• **Child/infant <5 yr or ≤20 kg: IV** 0.01 mg/kg slowly followed by 0.1 mg/kg if

needed, may give IM/SUBCUT if IV not possible
• **Neonates: IM/IV/SUBCUT** 0.01 mg/kg, repeat q2-3min until adequate response
• **Adult/adolescent/child: NASAL** 1 spray, may repeat q2-3min if needed
Postoperative opioid-induced respiratory depression
• **Adult: IV** 0.1-0.2 mg q2-3min prn
• **Infant/child/adolescent: IV** 0.005-0.01 mg/kg q2-3min prn
Available forms: Inj 0.4 mg/mL, 1 mg/mL; auto injector 2 mg/0.4 mL, 5/0.5 mL; nasal spray 4 mg/0.1 mL; 8 mg (equal to 7.2 naloxone)/0.1 mL unit dose device; solution for injection (Zimhi 5 mg/5 mL)
Administer:
• Only with resuscitative equipment, O_2 nearby
• Store in dark area at room temperature
• Double-check dose; those taking opioids >1 wk are sensitive to this product
• Solution should be clear
Direct IV route
• Undiluted (suspected opioid overdose) or diluted with sterile water for inj; give ≤0.4 mg over 15 sec
Continuous IV INFUSION route
• Dilute 2 mg/500 mL 0.9% NaCl or D_5W (4 mcg/mL); titrate to response
• Do not admix with bisulfite, sulfites

IM route with standard syringe
• Inject deeply into a large muscle mass; aspirate
• Use prepared solution within 24 hr
IM route with autoinjector (Evzio)
• Remove red safety guard; Evzio must be used immediately or disposed of properly. Give quickly into the anterolateral aspect of the thigh, through clothing if necessary. Press firmly and hold in place 5 sec
• Upon activation, the needle is automatically inserted, delivers the injection, and then retracts fully
• After initial injection, seek immediate medical attention. Keep patient under

continued surveillance because the duration of action of most opioids is longer than that of naloxone. Repeat doses q2-3min as needed

• Do NOT attempt to reuse Evzio; each device contains a single dose of naloxone

Subcut

• Inject undiluted or diluted solution, taking care not to inject intradermally

Nasal route

• Give as quickly as possible if a patient is unresponsive and an opioid overdose is suspected

• Place the patient in the supine position. Assure that the device nozzle is inserted into one of the patient's nostrils and provide support to the back of the neck to allow the head to tilt back. Do NOT prime or test the device before administration

• Press firmly on the device plunger

• Turn the patient on his or her side (recovery position) and seek immediate medical assistance after the first dose of naloxone

• Do NOT attempt to reuse; each device contains a single dose

• Using a new nasal spray device, re-administer naloxone q2-3min if the patient does not respond or responds and then relapses into respiratory depression

• Administer the nasal spray in alternate nostrils with each dose

Y-site compatibilities: Acyclovir, alfentanil, amikacin, aminocaproic acid, aminophylline, anidulafungin, ascorbic acid, atenolol, atracurium, atropine, azaTHIOprine, aztreonam, benztropine, bivalirudin, bleomycin, bumetanide, buprenorphine, butorphanol, calcium chloride/gluconate, CARBOplatin, caspofungin, cefamandole, ceFAZolin, cefmetazole, cefonicid, cefoperazone, cefotaxime, cefoTEtan, cefOXitin, cefTAZidime, ceftizoxime, cefTRIAXone, cefuroxime, cephalothin, cephapirin, chloramphenicol, chlorproMAZINE, cimetidine, CISplatin, clindamycin, cyanocobalamin, cyclophosphamide, cycloSPORINE, cytarabine, DACTINomycin, DAPTOmycin, dexamethasone, digoxin, diltiazem, diphenhydrAMINE, DOBUTamine, DOCEtaxel, DOPamine, doxacurium, DOXOrubicin, doxycycline, enalaprilat, ePHEDrine, EPINEPHrine, epirubicin, epoetin alfa, eptifibatide, ertapenem, erythromycin, esmolol, etoposide, etoposide phosphate, famotidine, fenoldopam, fentaNYL, fluconazole, fludarabine, fluorouracil, folic acid, furosemide, ganciclovir, gatifloxacin, gemcitabine, gentamicin, glycopyrrolate, granisetron, heparin, hydrocortisone, hydrOXYzine, IDArubicin, ifosfamide, imipenem-cilastatin, inamrinone, indomethacin, insulin (regular), irinotecan, isoproterenol, ketorolac, labetalol, levofloxacin, lidocaine, linezolid, LORazepam, mannitol, mechlorethamine, meperidine, metaraminol, methicillin, methotrexate, methoxamine, methyldopate, methylPREDNISolone, metoclopramide, metoprolol, metroNIDAZOLE, mezlocillin, miconazole, midazolam, milrinone, minocycline, mitoXANtrone, morphine, moxalactam, multiple vitamins, mycophenolate, nafcillin, nalbuphine, nesiritide, netilmicin, nitroglycerin, nitroprusside, norepinephrine, octreotide, ondansetron, oxacillin, oxaliplatin, oxytocin, PACLitaxel, palonosetron, pamidronate, pancuronium, papaverine, PEMEtrexed, penicillin G potassium/sodium, pentamidine, pentazocine, PENTobarbital, PHENobarbital, phentolamine, phenylephrine, phytonadione, piperacillin, piperacillin-tazobactam, polymyxin B, potassium chloride, procainamide, prochlorperazine, promethazine, propofol, propranolol, protamine, pyridoxine, quiNIDine, quinupristin-dalfopristin, ranitidine, ritodrine, rocuronium, sodium acetate/bicarbonate, succinylcholine, SUFentanil, tacrolimus, teniposide, theophylline, thiamine, ticarcillin, ticarcillin-clavulanate, tigecycline, tirofiban, tobramycin, tolazoline, trimetaphan, urokinase, vancomycin, vasopressin, vecuronium, verapamil, vinCRIStine, vinorelbine, voriconazole, zoledronic acid

N

SIDE EFFECTS

CV: Rapid pulse, ventricular tachycardia, fibrillation, hypo/hypertension
GI: Nausea, vomiting
CNS: Headache, seizures
MS: Pain
INTEG: Injection site reactions
MISC: Withdrawal symptoms in those dependent
EENT: Nasal dryness

PHARMACOKINETICS

Well absorbed IM, SUBCUT; metabolized by liver, crosses placenta; excreted in urine, breast milk; half-life 30-81 min
IM/SUBCUT: Onset 2-5 min, peak 5-15 min, duration 45-60 min
IV: Onset 1 min, peak 5 min, duration 45 min
Nasal: Peak 20 min

INTERACTIONS

Increase: seizure risk—traMADol overdose
Increased withdrawal risk: methylnatrexone, naldemedine, naloxegel; avoid using together
Decreased reversal risk: partial mixed opioid agonists, antagonists; monitor closely
Decrease: effect of opioid analgesics

NURSING CONSIDERATIONS

Assess:
• **Withdrawal:** cramping, hypertension, anxiety, vomiting tachypnea; signs of withdrawal in drug-dependent individuals may occur ≤2 hr after administration; severity depends on length of time opioids were taken, naloxone dose; **infant withdrawal:** seizures, hyperreflexia, can be life-threatening
• **Respiratory dysfunction:** respiratory depression, character, rate, rhythm; if respirations are <10/min, administer naloxone; probably due to opioid overdose; monitor LOC, ECG, B/P
• Vital signs q3-5min
• Arterial blood gases, including PO_2, PCO_2
• **Cardiac status:** tachycardia, hypertension, monitor ECG
• **Pain:** duration, intensity, location before and after administration; analgesia will be decreased; may be used for respiratory depression

• **Acute opioid reversal:** patients may become very agitated and violent after use
• **Pregnancy/breastfeeding:** use only if clearly needed, cautious use in breastfeeding
Evaluate:
• **Therapeutic response:** reversal of respiratory depression; LOC—alert
Teach patient/family:
• When patient is lucid, about the reasons for, expected results of product; for nasal administration, teach family, caregivers correct use, use of autoinjector
Opioid emergency:
• Teach patient and family increased sleepiness, coma, trouble breathing are a sign of overdose; discuss family's use of this product for overdose

---

naltrexone (Rx)

(nal-trex'one)
ReVia ✤, Vivitrol
Func. class.: Opioid antagonist, antidote
Chem. class.: Thebaine derivative

Do not confuse:
naltrexone/naloxone/naloxegol

ACTION: Competes with opioids at opioid-receptor sites

USES: Blockage of opioid analgesics; used for treatment of opiate addiction, alcoholism, opiate agonist overdose

CONTRAINDICATIONS

Hypersensitivity, opioid dependence
Precautions: Pregnancy, breastfeeding, children, renal disease, depression, suicidal ideation, coagulopathy, respiratory depression, IV use, hepatic impairment

DOSAGE AND ROUTES

Treatment should not be attempted until the patient has remained opioid free for 7-10 days
Narcan challenge (to identify opioid-free state)
• Should not be performed in a patient showing clinical signs of opioid withdrawal or urine positive for opioids

---

• Positive signs: nausea, vomiting, dysphoria, yawning, sweating, tearing, rhinorrhea, stuffy nose, craving for opioids, poor appetite, abdominal cramps, uneasiness, poor ability to focus, mental lapses, muscle aches or cramps, pupillary dilation, piloerection, fever, changes in B/P, pulse, or temperature; anxiety, depression, irritability, backache, bone or joint pains, tremors, sensations of skin crawling

• If signs or symptoms of withdrawal appear, the test is positive and no additional Narcan (naloxone hydrochloride injection) should be administered

• **Adult: IV** 0.5 mL (0.2 mg) Narcan (naloxone injection) (0.4 mg/mL); observe for 20 min for withdrawal; if no evidence of withdrawal, give another 1.5 mL (0.6 mg) of Narcan and observe for an additional 20 min

• **Adult: SUBCUT** 2 mL (0.8 mg) Narcan (naloxone hydrochloride injection) (0.4 mg/mL); observe patient for 20 min for signs or symptoms of withdrawal

Treatment of opioid dependence

• Treatment should not be started until opioid free for 7-10 days

• Negative Narcan challenge; negative urine test

• **Adult: PO** 25 mg naltrexone; if no withdrawal symptoms in 1 hr, then 25 mg naltrexone; if no withdrawal symptoms, then 50 mg naltrexone daily, or 100 mg q2days or 150 mg q3days; IM 380 mg q4wk

Treatment of alcoholism (within a comprehensive psychosocial program)

• **Adult: PO** 50 mg naltrexone daily × 12 wk; IM 380 mg q4wk

Available forms: Tabs 25, 50, 100 mg; inj 380 mg kit

Administer:

PO route

• Give with food or after meals, to prevent nausea, vomiting

• Store in tight container

IM route

• Do not give until opioid-free for 7-10 days to prevent opioid withdrawal (relapse only)

• Allow to come to room temperature

• IM deep in gluteal, alternate inj sites; use supplied needle to prevent inj-site reaction; aspirate before inj

• Do not use IV or SUBCUT

• Store refrigerated up to 1 wk, do not freeze

SIDE EFFECTS

CNS: *Stimulation, drowsiness,* dizziness, confusion, seizures, headache, flushing, hallucinations, nervousness, irritability, suicidal ideation, syncope, anxiety

CV: Rapid pulse, pulmonary edema, hypertension, DVT

EENT: Tinnitus, hearing loss, blurred vision

GI: *Nausea, vomiting, diarrhea, heartburn,* hepatotoxicity, constipation, abdominal pain

GU: Delayed ejaculation, impotence

INTEG: *Rash,* urticaria, bruising, oily skin, acne, pruritus, inj-site reactions

MISC: Increased thirst, chills, fever

MS: Joint and muscle pain

RESP: Wheezing, hyperpnea, nasal congestion, rhinorrhea, sneezing, sore throat, pneumonia

PHARMACOKINETICS

Metabolized by liver, excreted by kidneys; crosses placenta, excreted in breast milk; half-life 4 hr; IM half-life 5-10 days; extensive first-pass metabolism; protein binding 21%-28%

PO: Onset 15-30 min, peak 1 hr

IM: Peak 2-3 days, duration >1 month

INTERACTIONS

Increase: lethargy—phenothiazines

Increase: bleeding risk—anticoagulants

Increase: hepatotoxicity—disulfiram

NURSING CONSIDERATIONS

Assess:

• **Hepatic status:** LFTs, jaundice, hepatitis, hepatic failure, discontinue if hepatitis is diagnosed

• ABGs including PO_2, PCO_2, LFTs, VS q3-5min

• Signs of withdrawal in drug-dependent individuals; use naltrexone challenge to test opioid dependence; must be free of opioids for 7-10 days before using this product, or withdrawal symptoms can occur

• **Respiratory dysfunction:** respiratory depression, character, rate, rhythm; if respirations <10/min, respiratory stimulant should be administered

• Mental status: depression, suicidal ideation

• **Beers:** avoid in older adults unless safer alternatives are unavailable; may cause ataxia, impaired psychomotor function

• **Pregnancy/breastfeeding:** use only if clearly needed; use cautiously in breastfeeding

Evaluate:

• **Therapeutic response:** blocking opiate ingestion; successful nicotine, alcohol withdrawal

Teach patient/family:

• That patient must be drug-free to start treatment

• That using opioid while taking this product could prove fatal because high dose is needed to overcome this antagonist; not to self-dose with OTC products unless approved by prescriber

• To carry emergency ID stating product used

• That, if surgery is needed, all involved should be aware of this product

• To use caution while driving or performing other hazardous tasks until effect is known

• That suicidal thoughts/behaviors may occur; to report these immediately

---

naphazoline (ophthalmic)

(na-faz'oh-leen)

Clear Eyes Redness Relief

Func. class.: Ophthalmic vasoconstrictor

Chem. class.: Sympathomimetic

USES: Ocular congestion, irritation, itching of the eye

DOSAGE AND ROUTES

• **Adult: OPHTH** instill 1-2 drops in affected eye in the conjunctival sac every 3-4 hr, up to qid

Available forms: ophthalmic solution 0.0125%, 0.03%

---

naproxen (Rx, OTC)

Aleve, Anaprox DS, EC-Naprosyn, Mediproxen, Motrimax ❦, Naprelan, Naprosyn

Func. class.: Nonsteroidal antiinflammatory, nonopioid analgesic

Chem. class.: Propionic acid derivative

ACTION: Inhibits COX-1, COX-2 by blocking arachidonate; synthesis analgesic, antiinflammatory, antipyretic

USES: Osteoarthritis; rheumatoid, gouty arthritis; primary dysmenorrhea; ankylosing spondylitis, bursitis, tendinitis, myalgia, dental pain, juvenile rheumatoid arthritis

CONTRAINDICATIONS

Pregnancy ≥20 wk; hypersensitivity to NSAIDs, salicylates; perioperative pain in CABG surgery; MI; stroke

Precautions: Breastfeeding, children <2 yr, geriatric patients, bleeding disorders, GI disorders, cardiac disorders, hypersensitivity to other antiinflammatory agents, CCr <30 mL/min, asthma, renal failure, hepatic disease; corticosteroid, anticoagulant therapy, pregnancy <20 wk

Black Box Warning: GI bleeding, thromboembolism

DOSAGE AND ROUTES

200 mg base = 220 mg naproxen sodium

Ankylosing spondylitis, osteoarthritis, RA:

• **Adult: PO** Naproxen Sodium: 275-550 mg bid or 250-500 mg (tablet or suspension) bid or Naproxen DEL REL Tablet 375-500 mg bid or Naproxen EXT REL Tablet 750-1000 mg qday

Acute gout

• **Adult: Naproxen:** 750 mg once, then 250 mg q8h until attack has subsided; naproxen sodium 825 mg, then 275 mg q8hr

---

Pain (mild to moderate), dysmenorrhea, acute tendinopathy, bursitis:
• **Adult: PO Naproxen:** 500 mg, then 250 mg q6-8hr; max: 1250 mg/day; **Naproxen sodium:** 550 mg, then 550 mg q12hr, or 275 mg q6-8hr, Max: 1,375 mg on day 1, then 1,100 mg/day.

Juvenile idiopathic arthritis
Child ≥2 yr: PO Naproxen sodium: 5 mg/kg/dose (Max: 500 mg/dose) twice daily, max 1000 mg/day.

Available forms: Naproxen: tabs 250, 375, 500 mg; del rel tabs (EC-Naprosyn) 250 ♣, 375, 500, 750 mg; oral susp 125 mg/5 mL; **naproxen sodium:** tabs 220, 275, 550 mg; capsules 200, 220 mg ♣; ext rel tabs 375, 500, 750 mg

Administer:
• Store at room temperature
• With food to decrease GI symptoms; take on empty stomach to facilitate absorption; give with full glass of liquid
• Do not crush, break, or chew ext rel tabs
• OTC for ≤10 days unless approved by prescriber
• Adequately hydrate in those taking angiotensin receptor blockers/angiotensin-converting enzyme inhibitors
• **Oral susp:** shake well; use measuring cup provided or other calibrated device

SIDE EFFECTS

CNS: Dizziness, drowsiness, fatigue, tremors, confusion, insomnia, anxiety, depression
CV: Tachycardia, peripheral edema, palpitations, dysrhythmias, MI, stroke
EENT: Tinnitus, hearing loss, blurred vision
GI: Nausea, anorexia, vomiting, diarrhea, jaundice, hepatitis, constipation, flatulence, cramps, peptic ulcer, GI perforation, bleeding
GU: Nephrotoxicity: dysuria, hematuria, oliguria, azotemia
HEMA: Blood dyscrasias, prolonged bleeding time
INTEG: Purpura, rash, pruritus, sweating
SYST: Anaphylaxis, Stevens-Johnson syndrome

PHARMACOKINETICS
PO: Peak 2-4 hr, half-life 10-20 hr (adult), 8-10 hr (child), metabolized in liver; excreted in urine (metabolites), breast milk; 99% protein binding

INTERACTIONS
• Avoid use with adefovir, cidofovir, nephrotoxicity is increased
Decrease: effect of these drugs—ACE inhibitors, angiotensin II antagonists, monitor B/P closely
Increase: toxicity risk—methotrexate, lithium, antineoplastics, probenecid, radiation treatment

Black Box Warning: Increase: bleeding risk—oral anticoagulants, thrombolytic agents, eptifibatide, tirofiban, clopidogrel, ticlopidine, plicamycin, SSRIs, SNRIs, tricyclics, avoid using together

Increase: GI side effects risk—aspirin, corticosteroids, alcohol, NSAIDs
Decrease: effect of antihypertensives, loop/thiazide diuretics, monitor B/P closely
Decrease: absorption of naproxen—antacids, sucralfate, cholestyramine
Drug/Herb
• Bleeding risk: feverfew, garlic, ginger, ginkgo, ginseng *(Panax)*
Drug/Lab Test
Increase: BUN, alk phos, LFTs, potassium, glucose, cholesterol
Decrease: potassium, sodium
False increase: 5-HIAA, 17KS

NURSING CONSIDERATIONS
Assess:
• **Pain:** frequency, characteristics, intensity; relief before and 1-2 hr after product
• **Arthritis:** range of motion, pain, swelling before and 1-2 hr after use
• **Fever:** before, 1 hr after use
• **Cardiac status:** CV thrombotic events, MI, stroke; may be fatal; not to be used with CABG

Black Box Warning: GI status: ulceration, bleeding, perforation; may be fatal; obtain stool guaiac

• Asthma, aspirin hypersensitivity or nasal polyps; increased risk of hypersensitivity

Side effects: *italics* = common; red = life-threatening

• **Renal, hepatic blood studies:** BUN, creatinine, AST, ALT, HB, LDH, blood glucose, Hct, WBC, platelets, CCr before treatment, periodically thereafter during long-term therapy
• Monitor B/P baseline and periodically
• **Beers:** avoid chronic use in older adults unless other alternatives are unavailable; increased GI bleeding risk, peptic ulcer disease
• **Pregnancy/breastfeeding:** use only if benefits outweigh fetal risk; avoid in ≥20 wk gestation; avoid use in breastfeeding

Evaluate:
• **Therapeutic response:** decreased pain, stiffness, swelling in joints; ability to move more easily

Teach patient/family:
• To report ringing, roaring in ears
• To avoid driving, other hazardous activities if dizziness or drowsiness occurs
• To report change in urine pattern, weight increase, edema (face, lower extremities), pain increase in joints, fever, blood in urine (indicates nephrotoxicity); black stools, flulike symptoms, signs of MI, stroke
• That therapeutic effects may take up to 1 mo in arthritis

Black Box Warning: To avoid aspirin, alcohol, steroids, or other OTC medications without prescriber approval; increased risk of GI bleeding

• To take with food or milk to prevent GI upset
• To report use to all health care providers
• To notify prescriber if pregnancy is planned or suspected; to avoid breastfeeding

---

naproxen/esomeprazole (Rx)

(na-proks′en/es-oh-me′pray-zol)
Vimovo
Func. class.: NSAID/proton pump inhibitor

USES: Reduction of the risk of NSAID-associated gastric ulcers in those who require an NSAID for the relief of signs and symptoms of osteoarthritis, rheumatoid arthritis, and ankylosing spondylitis in adults; juvenile idiopathic arthritis ≥12 yr and >38 kg

Black Box Warning: CABG surgery

DOSAGE AND ROUTES
Osteoarthritis, rheumatoid arthritis, ankylosing spondylitis
Adult: PO 1 tablet bid
Juvenile idiopathic arthritis
Child/adolescents ≥12 yr; weight ≥38 kg to <50 kg: PO 1 tablet bid
Available forms: Tabs 375 mg naproxen/20 mg esomeprazole, 500 mg naproxen/20 mg esomeprazole

---

naratriptan (Rx)

(nair′ah-trip-tan)
Amerge
Func. class.: Antimigraine agent
Chem. class.: 5-HT₁ receptor agonist

ACTION: Binds selectively to the vascular 5-HT₁ B/D receptor subtype; exerts antimigraine effect; causes vasoconstriction in cranial arteries

USES: Acute treatment of migraine with/without aura

CONTRAINDICATIONS
Hypersensitivity, angina pectoris, history of MI, documented silent ischemia, ischemic heart disease, concurrent ergotamine-containing preparations, uncontrolled hypertension, CV syndromes, hemiplegic or basilar migraines, severe renal disease (CCr <15 mL/min); severe hepatic disease (Child-Pugh grade C)
Precautions: Pregnancy, breastfeeding, children, geriatric patients, postmenopausal women, men >40 yr, CAD risk, hypercholesterolemia, obesity, diabetes, impaired renal/hepatic function, peripheral vascular disease overuse

---

DOSAGE AND ROUTES
Acute migraine
• **Adult:** PO 1 or 2.5 mg with fluids; if headache returns, repeat 1× after 4 hr; max 5 mg/24 hr
Hepatic/renal dose
• **Adult: PO CCr 15-39 mL/min or mild to moderate hepatic disease** max 2.5 mg/24 hr
Available forms: Tabs 1, 2.5 mg
Administer:
• With fluids as soon as symptoms appear; may take another dose after 4 hr; do not take >5 mg during any 24-hr period
• Swallow whole; use without regard to food
• Use for >4 headaches/30 days has not been established

SIDE EFFECTS
CNS: Dizziness, sedation, fatigue, drowsiness, paresthesia
CV: Increased B/P, palpitations, tachydysrhythmias, PR, QTc prolongation, ST/T wave changes, PVCs, atrial flutter/fibrillation, coronary vasospasm in those with cardiac disease
EENT: EENT infections, photophobia
GI: *Nausea, vomiting,* dry mouth
MISC: Temperature change sensations; tightness, pressure sensations
MS: *Weakness, neck stiffness,* myalgia

PHARMACOKINETICS
Onset 2-3 hr; peak 2-3 hr; 28%-31% protein binding; half-life 6 hr; metabolized in liver (metabolite); excreted in urine, feces; may be excreted in breast milk

INTERACTIONS
Increase: serotonin syndrome, neuroleptic malignant syndrome—SSRIs (FLUoxetine, fluvoxaMINE, PARoxetine, sertraline), SNRIs, serotonin receptor agonists, sibutramine, tramadol
Increase: QT prolongation—antidysrhythmics, some phenothiazines, dolasetron, mefloquine, ziprasidone; monitor QT closely in cardiac patients
Increase: vasospastic effects—ergot, ergot derivatives, other 5-HT$_1$ agonists
Increase: adverse reactions risk—MAOIs; do not use together

Drug/Herb
• **Serotonin syndrome:** SAM-e, St. John's wort

NURSING CONSIDERATIONS
Assess:
• **Migraine symptoms:** aura, duration, effect on lifestyle, aggravating/alleviating factors
• **Serotonin syndrome, neuroleptic malignant syndrome:** increased heart rate, shivering, sweating, dilated pupils, tremors, high B/P, hyperthermia, headache, confusion; if these occur, stop product, administer serotonin antagonist if needed; at least 2 wk should elapse between discontinuation of serotonergic agents and start of product
• **Cardiac status:** ECG, increased B/P, dysrhythmias, monitor for PR, QT prolongation, ST-T wave changes, PVCs in those with cardiac disease
• Stress level, activity, recreation, coping mechanisms
• Neurologic status: LOC, blurred vision, nausea, vomiting, tingling in extremities preceding headache
• Quiet, calm environment with decreased stimulation (noise, bright light, excessive talking)
• **Pregnancy/breastfeeding:** use only if benefits outweigh fetal risk; cautious use in breastfeeding
Evaluate:
• **Therapeutic response:** decrease in frequency, severity of headache
Teach patient/family:
• To report pain, tightness in chest, neck, throat, or jaw; seek emergency services if sudden, severe abdominal pain, difficulty breathing occurs
• Not to use if another 5-HT$_1$ agonist or ergot preparation has been used during past 24 hr; to avoid using >2 days/wk because rebound headache may occur
• To notify prescriber if pregnancy is planned or suspected; to avoid breastfeeding
• To discuss all OTC, Rx, herbals, supplements with health care professional
• To take as soon as headache is starting, only use to treat, not prevent, migraine
• That drowsiness, dizziness may occur, not to drive or perform other hazardous tasks until response is known

N

Side effects: *italics* = common; red = life-threatening

• To maintain adequate hydration while using

natalizumab (Rx)

(na-ta-liz'u-mab)

Tysabri

Func. class.: Immunomodulator, immunoglobulins, monoclonal antibody

ACTION: Biologic-response-modifying properties mediated through specific receptors on cells; may be secondary to blockade of the interaction of inflammatory cells with vascular endothelial cells

USES: Ambulatory patients with relapsing/remitting MS who have not responded to other treatment; those with moderate to severe Crohn's disease

CONTRAINDICATIONS

Hypersensitivity, immunocompromised individuals (HIV, AIDS, leukemia, lymphoma, transplants), PML, murine (mouse) protein allergy

> **Black Box Warning:** Progressive multifocal leukoencephalopathy

Precautions: Pregnancy, breastfeeding, geriatric patients, chronic progressive MS, depression, mental disorders, diabetes, TB, active infections, hepatotoxicity

DOSAGE AND ROUTES
Relapsing/remitting MS

• **Adult: IV INFUSION** 300 mg; give over 1 hr q4wk

Available forms: Single-use vial, 300 mg/15 mL

Administer:

• Acetaminophen for fever, headache

Intermittent IV INFUSION route

• Use only clear, colorless solution, without particulates

• **Withdraw** 15 mL from the vial inj concentration into 100 mL 0.9% NaCl; do not use other diluents; mix completely; do not shake; **infuse** immediately or refrigerate for ≤8 hr; flush with 0.9% NaCl before, after infusion; do not admix or use in same line with other agents

• Store sol in refrigerator; do not freeze or shake; protect from light

> **Black Box Warning:** Withhold product at first sign of PML. Prescribers must be registered in the TOUCH Prescribing Program (800-456-2255)

SIDE EFFECTS

CNS: *Headache, fatigue,* rigors, syncope, tremors, *depression,* progressive multifocal leukoencephalopathy (PML), suicidal ideation, anxiety

CV: Chest discomfort, hypo/hypertension, tachycardia

GI: *Abdominal discomfort,* abnormal LFT, gastroenteritis, severe hepatic injury, weight change

GU: Amenorrhea, *UTI, irregular menses,* vaginitis, urinary frequency

INTEG: *Rash,* dermatitis, pruritus, skin melanoma, infusion-related reactions

HEMA: Thrombocytopenia

MS: *Arthralgia,* myalgia

RESP: *Lower respiratory tract infection,* dyspnea

SYST: Anaphylaxis, angioedema

PHARMACOKINETICS

Half-life approximately 11 days

INTERACTIONS

• Do not use with vaccines

Increase: infection—immunosuppressants, antineoplastics, immunomodulators, tumor necrosis factors

NURSING CONSIDERATIONS
Assess:

• **MS symptoms;** product should be used only by patients who have not responded to other treatments and for relapsing forms of MS and Crohn's disease; restricted prescribing program; discuss risks, benefits; obtain baseline MRI

> **Black Box Warning: Progressive multifocal leukoencephalopathy** (weakness, paralysis, vision loss, impaired

speech, cognitive deterioration; obtain gadolinium-enhanced MRI scan of the brain, possibly cerebrospinal fluid for JC viral DNA); incidence of PML increases with number of doses, over 2 yr immunosuppressants and anti-JC virus antibody, withhold drug

• **Infection:** report serious opportunistic infections to the manufacturer; those with Crohn's disease and chronic oral corticosteroids may be at greater risk of infection

• **Labs:** CBC, differential, platelet counts, BUN, creatinine, ALT, urinalysis, antibody testing

• **CNS symptoms:** headache, fatigue, depression, rigors, tremors

• **GI status:** abdominal discomfort, gastroenteritis, severe hepatic injury, abnormal LFTs

• **Mental status:** depression, depersonalization, suicidal thoughts, insomnia

• **Anaphylaxis:** SOB, hives; swelling, tightness in throat, chest pain; usually within 2 hr of infusion

• **Pregnancy/breastfeeding:** use only if benefits outweigh fetal risk; avoid breastfeeding

Evaluate:

• **Therapeutic response:** decreased symptoms of MS, Crohn's disease

Teach patient/family:

• Purpose of medication, regimen

• That dizziness may occur, to be aware falls may occur and protect patient from injury

• To discuss with prescriber all OTC, Rx, herbals, and supplements taken

• Provide patient or family member with written, detailed information about product (med guide)

• To discuss possible liver injury, change in weight

• That enrollment in TOUCH program is required

• **To notify prescriber of possible infection:** sore throat, cough, increased temperature, infusion-site reactions

• That continuing follow-up will be needed at 3, 6 mo after first dose, then every 6 mo

• To inform all prescribers of product use

• **Pregnancy/breastfeeding:** That female patients may experience irregular menses, amenorrhea; may worsen over several days; to notify prescriber if pregnancy is suspected; to avoid breastfeeding while taking this product; if pregnant, call the Tysabri Pregnancy Exposure Registry (800-456-2255)

---

natamycin ophthalmic
See Appendix B

---

nateglinide (Rx)
(na-te-glye′nide)
Starlix
Func. class.: Antidiabetic-meglitinide derivatives

USES: Type 2 diabetes as an adjunct to diet and exercise

CONTRAINDICATIONS
Hypersensitivity

DOSAGE AND ROUTES
Adult: PO 120 mg tid before meals
Available forms: Tabs 60, 120 mg

⚠ HIGH ALERT

necitumumab (Rx)
(ne-si-toom′oo-mab)
Portrazza
Func. class.: Antineoplastic agent, epidermal growth factor receptor (EGFR) inhibitor

USES: First-line treatment of metastatic squamous non-small cell lung cancer (NSCLC) in combination with gemcitabine and cisplatin

---

CONTRAINDICATIONS
Hypersensitivity, pregnancy

Black Box Warning: Cardiopulmonary arrest, hypomagnesemia

DOSAGE AND ROUTES
Non-small cell lung cancer (squamous), metastatic
Adult: IV: 800 mg on days 1 and 8 of each 3-wk treatment cycle (in combination with gemcitabine and cisplatin); continue until disease progression or unacceptable toxicity
Available forms: 800 mg/50 mL solution for injection

---

nefazodone
(nef-ay′zoe-done)
Func. class.: Antidepressant, SSRI

USES: Depression

DOSAGE AND ROUTES

Black Box Warning: Suicidal thoughts, behaviors, children, young adults, hepatic failure

Adult: PO Initial: 100 mg bid or 50-100 mg/day, then gradually increase by 100-200 mg/day (in 2 divided doses) and intervals ≥1 wk to a usual dose of 150-600 mg/day in 2 divided doses.
Geriatric/debilitated: PO 50 mg bid initially
Available forms: Tabs 50, 100, 150, 200, 250 mg

⚠ HIGH ALERT

nelarabine (Rx)
(nel-ay′re-been)
Arranon, Atriance ✦
Func. class.: Antineoplastic, antimetabolite (purine analog)

USES: Relapsed/refractory T-cell acute lymphoblastic leukemia/lymphoma

CONTRAINDICATIONS
Hypersensitivity, pregnancy

Black Box Warning: Neurotoxicity (seizures)

DOSAGE AND ROUTES
T-cell acute lymphoblastic leukemia/lymphoma
Adult: IV: 1500 mg/m²/dose on days 1, 3, and 5; repeat q21days until a transplant candidate, disease progression, unacceptable toxicity
• **Child >1 yr:** IV 650 mg/m²/dose × 5 days, repeat q21days
Available forms: Injection 5 mg/mL (50-mL vial)

---

nelfinavir (Rx)
(nell-fin′a-ver)
Viracept
Func. class.: Antiretroviral
Chem. class.: Protease inhibitor

Do not confuse:
Viracept/Viramune

ACTION: Inhibits human immunodeficiency virus (HIV-1) protease, which prevents maturation of the infectious virus
Uses: HIV-1 in combination with other antiretrovirals

CONTRAINDICATIONS
Hypersensitivity to protease inhibitors
Precautions: Pregnancy, breastfeeding, renal/hepatic disease, hemophilia, PKU, pancreatitis, diabetes, infection, immune reconstitution syndrome

DOSAGE AND ROUTES
HIV infection
• **Adult/child >13 yr: PO** 750 mg tid or 1250 mg bid, max 2500 mg/day in combination
• **Child 2-12 yr: PO** 25-35 mg/kg tid or 45-55 mg/kg bid, max 2500 mg/day bid or 2250 mg/day tid in combination
Available forms: Tabs 250, 625 mg

Administer:
PO route
- Give with food
- Do not mix with juice or acidic fluids
- **Tabs** may be crushed and dispersed in water or mixed with food; consume immediately, rinse and have patient consume all liquid

SIDE EFFECTS
CNS: Headache, asthenia, poor concentration, seizures, suicidal ideation
CV: Bleeding, QTc prolongation, torsades de pointes
ENDO: Hyperglycemia, hyperlipidemia
GI: *Diarrhea,* anorexia, dyspepsia, *nausea, flatulence,* hepatitis, pancreatitis
GU: Sexual dysfunction
HEMA: Anemia, leukopenia, thrombocytopenia, HB abnormalities
INTEG: *Rash,* dermatitis, anaphylaxis
MISC: Hypoglycemia, redistribution/accumulation of body fat, immune reconstitution syndrome
MS: Pain, arthralgia, myalgia, myopathy

PHARMACOKINETICS
Half-life 3½-5 hr, excreted in feces (87%), peak 2-4 hr, 98% protein binding; metabolized by CYP3A4 enzyme system; potent inhibitor of CYP3A4

INTERACTIONS
- Many drug interactions
Increase: serious dysrhythmias—amiodarone, ergots, lovastatin, midazolam, pimozide, quiNIDine, simvastatin, triazolam, salmeterol, monitor cardiac status
Increase: effect of—atorvastatin, azithromycin, rifabutin, indinavir, saquinavir, cycloSPORINE, tacrolimus, sirolimus, sildenafil, alfentanil, alosetron, buprenorphine, busPIRone, bortezomib, calcium channel blockers, cilostazol, disopyramide, dofetilide, DOCEtaxel, donepezil, ethosuximide, fentaNYL, galantamine, gefitinib, levomethadyl, systemic lidocaine, PACLitaxel, sibutramine, SUFentanil, vinca alkaloids, ziprasidone,

zonisamide, traZODone, tricyclic antidepressants, sildenafil
Increase: adverse reactions of sildenafil, taudalafil, vardenafil; dosage reduction will be needed
Increase: nelfinavir levels—ketoconazole, indinavir, ritonavir; delavirdine, other HIV protease inhibitors
Decrease: nelfinavir levels—rifamycins, nevirapine, PHENobarbital, phenytoin, carBAMazepine
Decrease: effect of—didanosine, methadone, oral contraceptives, phenytoin
Drug/Herb
Decrease: antiretroviral effect—St. John's wort; do not use concurrently
Drug/Lab Test
Increase: AST, ALT, alk phos, total bilirubin, CPK, LDH, lipids, uric acid
Decrease: WBC, platelets

NURSING CONSIDERATIONS
Assess:
- **HIV:** serum lipid profile, plasma HIV RNA, LFTs, blood glucose, viral load, CD4 cell counts at baseline and throughout treatment
- Resistance testing at initiation, or with failure of treatment
- Signs of infection, anemia
- Hepatic studies: ALT, AST
- Bowel pattern before, during treatment; if severe abdominal pain with bleeding occurs, product should be discontinued; monitor hydration
- **Infection:** assess for opportunistic infections (fever, flulike symptoms; increased white count)
- **Immune reconstitution syndrome:** occurs with combination therapy, including MAC, CMV, PCP, TB, requiring treatment
- **Anaphylaxis, hypersensitivity reaction:** wheezing, flushing; swelling of lips, tongue, throat, skin eruptions, rash, urticaria, itching
- **Pregnancy/breastfeeding:** enroll pregnant patients in Antiretroviral Pregnancy Registry (800-258-4263); use only if potential benefit is greater than risk; do not breastfeed; alternate (nonhormonal contraception) should be used

Evaluate

• **Therapeutic response:** decreased viral load, improved CD4+ cell count, reduced opportunistic infections

Teach patient/family:

• To avoid taking with other medications unless directed by prescriber

• **Diarrhea** is most common side effect; may use loperamide to control

• That product does not cure but does manage symptoms; that product does not prevent transmission of HIV to others

• **Sexual dysfunction:** If using with sildenafil report change in vision, pain with erection, decreased B/P, do not use ≥25 mg/48 hr

• If dose is missed, to take as soon as remembered up to 1 hr before next dose; not to double dose; to take with food

• To report symptoms of hyperglycemia, bleeding, abdominal pain; yellowing of skin, eyes

• **Phenylketonuria:** that powder contains phenylalanine

• To advise all providers of this product; to advise prescriber of all OTC products, prescription products, or herbal products taken

• **Pregnancy:** To report if pregnancy is planned or suspected; to use a nonhormonal form of birth control while taking this product if using contraceptives, do not breastfeed

---

neomycin (Rx)

(nee-oh-mye'sin)

Func. class.: Antiinfective—aminoglycoside

USES: Severe systemic infections of CNS, respiratory, GI, urinary tract, eye, bone, skin, soft tissues; hepatic coma, preoperatively to sterilize bowel, infectious diarrhea caused by enteropathogenic *E. coli, Enterobacter* sp., *Escherichia coli, Klebsiella* sp. May be effective for *Acinetobacter* sp., *Bacillus anthracis,* *Citrobacter* sp., *Haemophilus influenzae* (beta-lactamase negative), *Haemophilus influenzae* (beta-lactamase positive), *Neisseria* sp., *Proteus mirabilis, Proteus vulgaris, Providencia* sp., *Salmonella* sp., *Serratia* sp., *Shigella* sp., *Staphylococcus aureus* (MSSA), *Staphylococcus epidermidis*

CONTRAINDICATIONS

Infants, children, bowel obstruction (oral use), severe renal disease, hypersensitivity, GI disease

Precautions: Dehydration, geriatric patients, respiratory insufficiency

Black Box Warning: Hearing impairment, neuromuscular disease, renal disease

DOSAGE AND ROUTES

Hepatic encephalopathy

• **Adult:** PO 4-12 g/day in divided doses q6hr × 5-6 days

• **Child:** PO 50-100 mg/kg/day in divided doses q6hr × 5-6 days

Preoperative intestinal antisepsis

• **Adult:** PO 1 g neomycin, and 1 g erythromycin dose at 1 PM, 2 PM, 11 PM on day before morning surgery, give after saline laxative

Available forms: Tablet 500

⚠ *HIGH ALERT*

nepafenac ophthalmic

See Appendix B

⚠ *HIGH ALERT*

neratinib (Rx)

(ne-ra′-ti-nib)

Nerlynx

Func. class.: Antineoplastic

Chem. class.: Tyrosine kinase inhibitors

ACTION: It is an irreversible inhibitor of the epidermal growth factor receptor (EGFR) and the human epidermal receptor type 2 (HER2) and HER4.

USES: For the extended adjuvant treatment of early-stage ♥♥ HER2-positive breast cancer after completion of adjuvant trastuzumab; advanced metastatic HER-2-positive breast cancer with capecitabine in those who have received ≥2 regimens

CONTRAINDICATIONS
Hypersensitivity

Precautions: Breastfeeding, contraception requirements, geriatric patients, hepatic disease, hepatotoxicity, infertility, pregnancy, pregnancy testing, reproductive risk

DOSAGE AND ROUTES
Extended adjuvant treatment of early-stage HER2-positive breast cancer
• **Adult: PO** 240 mg/day with food, × ≤1 yr, or escalation 120 mg/day × 7 days then 160 mg/day × 7 days, then 240 mg/day for up to 1 yr

Advanced metastatic HER2-positive breast cancer with capecitabine
• **Adult: PO** 240 mg/day with food for 21 days each cycle with capecitabine 750 mg/mL bid for 14 days of a 21-day cycle or escalation 120 mg/day wk 1, day 1-7, 160 mg/day wk 2 day 8-14, then 240 mg/day day 15 and thereafter

Hepatic dose
• **Adult: PO Child-Pugh C:** reduce starting dose to 80 mg/day

Available forms: Tabs 40 mg

Administer:
• With food at the same time every day
• Swallow tablets whole; do not chew, crush, or split
• If a dose is missed, do not replace the missed dose. Resume with the next scheduled daily dose
• **Antidiarrheal prophylaxis** is recommended during the first 2 cycles (56 days) of treatment during nondose escalation, and should be initiated with the first dose of neratinib; loperamide should be taken as directed below, titrating to 1-2 bowel movements/day; additional antidiarrheal

agents may be required to manage patients with loperamide-refractory diarrhea
• Weeks 1-2 (days 1-14): take loperamide 4 mg tid
• Weeks 3-8 (days 15-56): take loperamide 4 mg bid
• Weeks 9-52 (days 57-365): take loperamide 4 mg as needed (max 16 mg/day)
• Store at room temperature

SIDE EFFECTS
GI: *Diarrhea, abdominal pain, anorexia, nausea, vomiting*
MS: Muscle cramps
INTEG: Rash, dry skin, nail changes, fissures
GU: UTI
MISC: Infection

PHARMACOKINETICS
Protein binding >99%; half-life 7-17 hr; fecal excretion 97.1%; metabolized in the liver by CYP3A4; avoid with strong and moderate CYP3A4 inhibitors and inducers

INTERACTIONS
Decrease: neratinib effect—gastric acid–reducing agents; avoid concomitant use with proton pump inhibitors (PPI) and H₂-receptor antagonists; separate by 3 hr after antacid dosing
Increase: neratinib effect—strong or moderate CYP3A4 inhibitors; avoid concomitant use
Decrease: neratinib effect—strong or moderate CYP3A4 inducers; avoid concomitant use
Increase: CNS and CV adverse reactions—P-glycoprotein (P-gp) substrates; monitor for adverse reactions of narrow therapeutic agents that are P-gp substrates

NURSING CONSIDERATIONS
Assess
• **Hepatotoxicity:** use with caution in those with preexisting hepatic disease; a dose reduction is required for patients with severe (Child-Pugh C) hepatic disease at baseline. Monitor LFTs (total bilirubin, AST, ALT, alkaline phosphatase) baseline, monthly × 3 mo and then q3mo thereafter and as needed. Monitor LFTs (including fractionated bilirubin and pro-

thrombin time) in those experiencing grade 3 diarrhea or any signs of hepatotoxicity (fatigue, nausea, vomiting, right upper quadrant tenderness, fever, rash, eosinophilia)

• **Geriatric patients >65 yr:** monitor geriatric patients more closely for toxicities (vomiting, diarrhea, renal failure, dehydration) during treatment

• **Infection:** may occur after completion of adjuvant trastuzumab-based therapy; assess for urinary tract infection, cellulitis and erysipelas

• **Pregnancy/breastfeeding:** avoid drug in females of reproductive potential; use contraception during treatment and for at least 1 mo after the last dose; can cause fetal harm or death; discontinue breastfeeding during treatment and for 1 mo after the final dose. Presence in breast milk unknown. Obtain a pregnancy test before starting treatment. Males with female partners of reproductive potential should avoid pregnancy and use effective contraception during treatment and ≥3 mo after last dose

Evaluate:

• **Therapeutic outcome:** decrease in size of cancerous tumor

Teach patient/family

• That infection may occur; to report urinary pain, hesitancy; skin redness, pain, heat; fever, shaking, chills

• **Diarrhea:** to report number of loose stools per day or change in stools to provider and complete prophylaxis with loperamide

• That follow-ups and lab work will be needed

• **Pregnancy/breastfeeding:** not to use in pregnancy, breastfeeding; to use contraception during treatment and for at least 1 mo after last dose; men with a partner who may become pregnant should use contraception during treatment and for at least 3 mo after last dose

---

netarsudil (Rx)
(ne-tar′soo-dil)

Rhopressa
Func. class.: Antiglaucoma agent, Rho kinase inhibitor

USES: Reduction of elevated IOP in patients with open-angle glaucoma or ocular hypertension

DOSAGE AND ROUTES
Adult: Ophthalmic: Instill 1 drop into affected eye(s) daily in the evening
Available forms: Ophthalmic solution 0.02%

---

netarsudil/latanoprost (Rx)
(ne-tar′soo-dil/la-ta′noe-prost)

Rocklatan
Func. class.: Antiglaucoma agent, Rho kinase inhibitor/prostaglandin F2 alpha analogue

---

USES: Reduction of elevated intraocular pressure (IOP) in open-angle glaucoma or ocular hypertension

DOSAGE AND ROUTES
Adult: Ophthalmic: One drop in the affected eye(s) daily in the evening
Available forms: Ophthalmic solution netarsudil 0.2 mg/mL, latanoprost 0.05 mg/mL

---

nevirapine (Rx)
(ne-veer′a-peen)

Viramune, Viramune XR
Func. class.: Antiretroviral
Chem. class.: Nonnucleoside reverse transcriptase inhibitor (NNRTI)

Do not confuse:
nevirapine/nelfinavir
Viramune/Viracept

ACTION: Binds directly to reverse transcriptase and blocks RNA, DNA, thus causing a disruption of the enzyme's site

USES: HIV-1 in combination with other highly active antiretroviral therapy (HAART)

CONTRAINDICATIONS
Hypersensitivity
Precautions: Pregnancy, breastfeeding, children, renal disease, ⌖ Hispanic patients, hepatitis

---

Black Box Warning: serious rash, hepatotoxicity

DOSAGE AND ROUTES
HIV infection
• **Adult/adolescent: PO** 200 mg/day × 2 wk, then 200 mg bid in combination; **EXT REL** 200 mg/day × 14 days with other antiretrovirals; if no consistent rash present, then 400 mg/day ER tab with other antiretrovirals
• **Child/adolescent ≥6 yr and BSA ≥1.17 m^2 PO** 150 mg/m^2 daily (max 200 mg/day) × 14 days, then **ext rel** 400 mg/day, max 400 mg/day
• **Child/infant/neonate ≥15 days old: PO** 150 mg/m^2/dose × 14 days, then 150 mg/m^2 bid, max 200 mg/dose
Hepatic dose
• **Adult: PO** do not use with Child-Pugh grade B or C
Available forms: Tabs 200 mg; oral susp 50 mg/5 mL; ext rel 100, 400 mg
Administer:
• Do not initiate treatment in females when CD4 counts >250 cells/mm^3 or in males when >400 cells/mm^3 unless benefits outweigh risks
• Use for 2 wk at lower dose (200 mg) to prevent skin reactions
• Use safe handling procedures as per agency policy
• Without regard to meals
• Use in combination with at least 1 other antiretroviral, missed doses of >1 wk: restart at lower dose
• **Ext rel:** swallow whole; do not crush, chew
• **Oral susp** should be shaken before giving, use oral syringe, dosing cup if possible

SIDE EFFECTS
CNS: *Paresthesia, headache, fever, peripheral neuropathy*
GI: *Diarrhea,* abdominal pain, *nausea, stomatitis,* hepatotoxicity, hepatic failure
HEMA: Neutropenia
INTEG: *Rash,* toxic epidermal necrolysis
MISC: Stevens-Johnson syndrome, anaphylaxis
MS: Pain, myalgia

PHARMACOKINETICS
Rapidly absorbed, peak 4 hr, 60% bound to plasma proteins, metabolized by liver; metabolized by hepatic P450 enzyme system, excreted 91% in urine, terminal half-life 25-30 hr, 50% removed by peritoneal dialysis; with hepatic disease and in ✎ Hispanic patients, African-American patients, slower rate of clearance

INTERACTIONS
Increase: nevirapine levels—cimetidine, macrolide antiinfectives, fluconazole, voriconazole
Increase: effect of warfarin
Decrease: effects of protease inhibitors, oral contraceptives, ketoconazole, methadone, itraconazole, boceprevir, telaprevir, clarithromycin, efavirenz, fosamprenavir, saquinavir rifamycins, anticonvulsants, clonazePAM, diazepam
Drug/Herb
Decrease: action of antiretroviral—St. John's wort; do not use concurrently
Drug/Lab Test
Increase: ALT, AST, GGT, bilirubin, HB
Decrease: neutrophil count

NURSING CONSIDERATIONS
Assess:
• **HIV:** blood studies during treatment: ALT, AST, viral load, CD4, plasma HIV RNA, renal studies; if LFTs elevated significantly, product should be withheld; glucose levels in patients with diabetes; if treatment is interrupted by >1 wk, restart at initial dose
• Resistance testing before therapy and when therapy fails
• Signs of infection, anemia, hepatotoxicity, immune reconstitution syndrome; hepatitis B or C, liver toxicity may occur

Black Box Warning: Hepatotoxicity: may be fatal; usually occurs within the first 18 wk of treatment, may have rash, fever; assess for anorexia, jaundice, clay-colored stools, nausea, fatigue, hepatic pain; higher risk in females with higher CD4+ counts, if AST/ALT is elevated, stop treatment; do not restart

N

- Do not start therapy in females, including pregnant women, with CD4+ cell counts >250 cell/mm^3 or adult males with CD4+ >400 cells/mm^3
- **Rhabdomyolysis:** pain, tenderness, weakness, edema; product should be discontinued
- Bowel pattern before, during treatment; if severe abdominal pain with bleeding occurs, product should be discontinued; monitor hydration

Black Box Warning: Stevens-Johnson syndrome, toxic epidermal necrolysis: allergies before treatment, reaction to each medication; assess for skin eruptions; rash, urticaria, itching; if rash is severe or systemic symptoms occur, discontinue immediately, usually occurs within first 6 wk of treatment

- **Hypersensitivity reaction:** usually within first 18 wk of treatment; rash, fever, fatigue, muscle/joint pain, oral lesions
- **Pregnancy/breastfeeding:** use only if benefits outweigh fetal risk, those who are pregnant should enroll in the Antiretroviral Pregnancy Registry (800-258-4263), may cause infertility, do not breastfeed if HIV is present

Evaluate:
- **Therapeutic response:** absence of AIDS-defining symptoms, improvement in quality of life; decreased viral load, increase in CD4 count

Teach patient/family:

Black Box Warning: To stop drug and report immediately any right quadrant pain, yellowing of eyes or skin, dark urine, nausea, anorexia, muscle pain or tenderness, rash

- That follow-up exams and blood work will be needed
- That product may be taken with food, antacids
- To take as prescribed; if dose is missed, to take as soon as remembered up to 1 hr before next dose; not to double dose

- To notify health care provider immediately if infection/fever, flulike symptoms occur, hypersensitive reactions (blistering, swelling on facial, tongue, rash) occur
- That product is not a cure, does not prevent transmission; controls symptoms of HIV
- To avoid all agents unless approved by prescriber
- That body fat redistribution may occur
- **Pregnancy/breastfeeding:** To use a nonhormonal form of contraception during treatment in those using contraceptives, not to breastfeed

niacin (OTC, Rx)
(nye'a-sin)

Niacor, Niaspan, Niodan ♣, Slo-Niacin
niacinamide (OTC, Rx)
Func. class.: Vit B$_3$, antihyperlipidemic
Chem. class.: Water-soluble vitamin

USES: Pellagra, hyperlipidemias (types 4, 5), peripheral vascular disease that presents a risk for pancreatitis

CONTRAINDICATIONS
Breastfeeding, hypersensitivity, peptic ulcer, hepatic disease, hemorrhage, severe hypotension, history of gouty arthritis, uncontrolled hyperglycemia

DOSAGE AND ROUTES
Niacin deficiency
- **Adult:** PO 100-500 mg/day in divided doses
- **Child:** PO ≤300 mg/day in divided doses

Adjunct in hyperlipidemia
- **Adult:** PO 250 mg after evening meal; may increase dose at 1-4 wk intervals to 1-2 g tid, max 6 g/day; **EXT REL** 500 mg at bedtime × 4 wk, then 1000 mg at bedtime for wk 5-8; do not increase by >500 mg q4wk, max 2000 mg/day

Available forms: Extended-release capsule 250 mg; tablet 50, 100, 250, 500; extended-release tablet 250, 500, 750, 1000 mg

niCARdipine (Rx)
(nye-card'i-peen)

Cardene IV

Func. class.: Calcium channel blocker, antianginal, antihypertensive
Chem. class.: Dihydropyridine

Do not confuse:
niCARdipine/NIFEdipine/nimodipine
Cardene/Cardizem

ACTION: Inhibits calcium ion influx across cell membrane during cardiac depolarization; produces relaxation of coronary vascular smooth muscle, peripheral vascular smooth muscle; dilates coronary vascular arteries; increases myocardial oxygen delivery in patients with vasospastic angina

USES: Chronic stable angina pectoris, hypertension

CONTRAINDICATIONS
Sick sinus syndrome, 2nd-/3rd-degree heart block; hypersensitivity to this product or dihydropyridine; advanced aortic stenosis
Precautions: Pregnancy, breastfeeding, children, geriatric patients, HF, hypotension, hepatic injury, renal disease

DOSAGE AND ROUTES
Angina
• **Adult: PO** 20 mg tid; may be adjusted q3days; may use 20-40 mg tid
Hypertension
• **Adult: PO IR** 20 mg tid initially; may increase after 3 days (range 20-40 mg tid) may increase to 60 mg bid or **IV** 5 mg/hr; may increase by 2.5 mg/hr q15min; max 15 mg/hr; **extended-release** 30 mg bid, titrate
Renal dose
• **Adult: PO** 20 mg tid
Hepatic dose
• **Adult: PO** 20 mg bid

Available forms: Capsules 20, 30 mg; injection 2.5 mg/mL, premixed 20 mg/200 mL, 40 mg/200 mL
Administer:
PO route
• Without regard to meals
• To start PO, give 1 hr prior to discontinuing IV nicardipine
• Avoid use with grapefruit, grapefruit juice
IV route
• To convert from PO to IV for adults: if PO 20 mg q8hr, start infusion at 0.5 mg/hr; if PO 30 mg q8hr, start infusion at 1.2 mg/hr; if PO 40 mg q8hr, start infusion at 2.2 mg/hr
Continuous IV INFUSION
• Dilute each 25 mg/240 mL of compatible sol (0.1 mg/mL), give slowly, titrate to patient response, change IV site q12hr
• Stable at room temperature for 24 hr
Solution compatibilities: D₅W, D₅/0.45% NaCl, D₅/0.9% NaCl

Y-site compatibilities: Alemtuzumab, amikacin, aminophylline, aztreonam, bivalirudin, butorphanol, calcium gluconate, CARBOplatin, caspofungin, ceFAZolin, ceftizoxime, chloramphenicol, cimetidine, CISplatin, clindamycin, cytarabine, DAPTOmycin, dexmedetomidine, diltiazem, DOBUTamine, DOCEtaxel, DOPamine, DOXOrubicin hydrochloride, enalaprilat, EPINEPHrine, epirubicin, erythromycin, esmolol, famotidine, fenoldopam, fentaNYL, gentamicin, hydrocortisone, HYDROmorphone, labetalol, lidocaine, linezolid, LORazepam, magnesium sulfate, mechlorethamine, methylPREDNISolone, metroNIDAZOLE, midazolam, milrinone, morphine, nafcillin, nesiritide, nitroglycerin, nitroprusside, norepinephrine, octreotide, oxaliplatin, oxytocin, palonosetron, penicillin G potassium, potassium chloride/phosphate, quinupristin/dalfopristin, ranitidine, rocuronium, tacrolimus, tirofiban, tobramycin, trimethoprim/sulfamethoxazole, vancomycin, vasopressin, vecuronium, vinCRIStine, voriconazole, zoledronic acid

SIDE EFFECTS

CNS: *Headache, dizziness,* anxiety, depression, confusion, paresthesia

CV: Edema, hypotension, palpitations, tachycardia, angina

GI: Nausea, vomiting, abdominal cramps, dry mouth

INTEG: Rash, infusion-site discomfort, Stevens-Johnson syndrome

OTHER: Myalgia (IV)

PHARMACOKINETICS

Metabolized by liver, excreted in urine 60%, feces 35%, half-life 2-5 hr

PO: Onset ½-2 hr, peak 1-2 hr, duration 8 hr

IV: Onset 1 min, peak 45 min, duration ≤8 hr

INTERACTIONS

Increase: effects of digoxin, neuromuscular blocking agents, theophylline, other antihypertensives, nitrates, alcohol, quiNIDine

Increase: hypotension—antihypertensives, neuromuscular blockers, nitrates, protease inhibitors, fentanyl

Increase: toxicity—cycloSPORINE, prazosin, carBAMazepine, quiNIDine, propranolol, cimetidine

Decrease: antihypertensive effect—NSAIDs, rifampin, protease inhibitors

Drug/Herb

Increase: effect—ginkgo, ginseng, hawthorn

Decrease: effect—ephedra, melatonin, St. John's wort, yohimbe

Drug/Food

Increase: hypotensive effect—grapefruit, grapefruit juice, avoid use

Decreased: absorption of high-fat foods

NURSING CONSIDERATIONS

Assess:

• **Anginal pain:** intensity, location, duration; alleviating, precipitating factors

• **HF:** weight gain, crackles, peripheral edema, jugular venous distention, dyspnea, I&O

• **Cardiac status:** B/P baseline and frequent intervals, pulse, respiration, ECG during long-term treatment

• Potassium, renal, hepatic studies periodically if on long-term treatment

• **Allergic reactions (Stevens-Johnson syndrome):** if rash is severe, with joint aches, mouth lesions, discontinue immediately

• **Hypertension:** decreasing B/P; assess salt in diet, smoking, exercise, weight, monitor B/P often

• **Pregnancy/breastfeeding:** use only if benefits outweigh fetal risk; cautious use in breastfeeding

Evaluate:

• **Therapeutic response:** decreased anginal pain, decreased B/P

Teach patient/family:

• How to take pulse and what to report

• To avoid hazardous activities until stabilized on product, dizziness is no longer a problem

• To limit caffeine consumption; to avoid alcohol products; to take without regard to food, avoid high-fat foods, to avoid grapefruit, grapefruit juice

• **Hypertension:** to comply in all areas of medical regimen: diet, exercise, stress reduction, product therapy

• To notify prescriber of irregular heartbeat, SOB, swelling of feet and hands, pronounced dizziness, constipation, nausea, hypotension, change in severity/pattern/incidence of angina

• To rise slowly from sitting or lying down to prevent orthostatic hypotension

TREATMENT OF OVERDOSE:

Defibrillation, β-agonists, IV calcium, diuretics, atropine for AV block, vasopressor for hypotension

---

nicotine

(nik′o-teen)

nicotine chewing gum (OTC)

Nicorette

nicotine inhaler (OTC, Rx)

Nicotrol Inhaler

---

nicotine lozenge (OTC)
Nicorette
nicotine nasal spray (Rx)
Nicotrol NS
nicotine transdermal (OTC, Rx)
Nicoderm CQ, Habitrol ✦
Func. class.: Smoking deterrent
Chem. class.: Ganglionic cholinergic agonist

ACTION: Agonist at nicotinic receptors in peripheral, central nervous systems; acts at sympathetic ganglia, on chemoreceptors of aorta, carotid bodies; also affects adrenalin-releasing catecholamines

USES: Deter cigarette smoking

CONTRAINDICATIONS
Pregnancy (transdermal, inhaler); hypersensitivity, immediate post-MI recovery period, severe angina pectoris
Precautions: Pregnancy (gum); breastfeeding, vasospastic disease, dysrhythmias, diabetes mellitus, hyperthyroidism, pheochromocytoma, esophagitis, peptic ulcer, coronary/renal/hepatic disease; MRI (patch); soy hypersensitivity (mint lozenge)

DOSAGE AND ROUTES
Nicotine chewing gum
• **Adult:** chew 1 piece of gum (2 mg nicotine) whenever urge to smoke occurs; dose varies; usually 20 mg/day during first mo, max 24 pieces/day, max 3 mo
Nicotine inhaler
• **Adult: INH** 6 cartridges/day (24-64 mg) for up to 12 wk, then gradual reduction over 12 wk
Nicotine lozenge
• **Adult:** if cigarette is desired >30 min after awakening, start with 2-mg lozenge; if <30 min after awakening, start with 4-mg lozenge, then again q1-2hr,

max 20 lozenges/day or 5 lozenges/6 hr × 6 wk, then 1 lozenge q2-4hr × 2 wk, then 1 lozenge q4-8hr × 2 wk, then discontinue
Nicotine nasal spray
• **Adult:** 1 spray in each nostril 1-2×/hr, max 5×/hr or 40×/day, max 3 mo
Nicotine transdermal/inhaler system
• **Nicoderm:** 21 mg/day × 4-8 wk; 14 mg/day × 2-4 wk; 7 mg/day × 2-4 wk
• **Nicotrol:** 15 mg/day × 12 wk; 10 mg/day × 2 wk; 5 mg/day × 2 wk
• **Nicotrol inhaler:** delivers 30% of nicotine that smoker receives from an actual cigarette
Available forms: Transdermal patch delivering 7, 14, 21 mg/day; **nicotine inhaler** 4 mg delivered; **nasal spray** 0.5 mg nicotine/actuation; **gum** 2, 4 mg/piece; **lozenge** 2 mg, 4 mg
Administer:
• **Gum:** chew gum slowly for 30 min to promote buccal absorption of product; do not chew >45 min
• Do not expose to light; gum will turn color
• Begin product withdrawal after 3 mo of use; do not exceed 6 mo
• **Transdermal patch:** 1× day to non-hairy, clean, dry area of skin on upper body or upper outer arm; rotate sites to prevent skin irritation; can remove before bed if patient has strange dreams
• **Nasal spray/inhaler:** puffing on mouthpiece delivers nicotine through mouth
• **Lozenge:** allow to dissolve slowly

SIDE EFFECTS
CNS: Dizziness, vertigo, insomnia, headache, confusion, seizures, numbness, tinnitus, strange dreams
CV: Dysrhythmias, tachycardia, palpitations, edema, flushing, hypertension
EENT: Jaw ache, irritation in buccal cavity
GI: *Nausea, vomiting, anorexia, indigestion,* diarrhea, abdominal pain, constipation, eructation, irritation

N

RESP: Breathing difficulty, cough, hoarseness, sneezing, wheezing, bronchial spasm

PHARMACOKINETICS
Onset 15-30 min, metabolized in liver, excreted in urine, half-life 2-3 hr, 30-120 hr (terminal)

INTERACTIONS
Increase: vasoconstriction—ergots, bromocriptine, cabergoline
Increase: effect after smoking cessation—adrenergic antagonists, β blockers
Increase: effect of—adenosine
Increase: B/P—buPROPion
Decrease: effect of—α-blockers, insulin
Decrease: nicotine clearance—cimetidine
Drug/Food
• Avoid use of gum with acidic foods (colas, coffee) and for 15 min after

NURSING CONSIDERATIONS
Assess:
• **Smoking:** number of cigarettes smoked, years used, brand; **withdrawal:** headache, cravings, restlessness, irritation, drowsiness, insomnia, sore throat, periodic increase in appetite
• **Adverse reaction:** irritation of buccal cavity, dislike of taste, jaw ache, gum should not be used if temporomandibular condition exists
• **Toxicity:** nausea, vomiting, diarrhea, headache, dizziness, dyspnea, hypertension
• **Pregnancy/breastfeeding:** whenever possible, avoid in pregnancy; cautious use in breastfeeding
Evaluate:
• **Therapeutic response:** decrease in urge to smoke, decreased need for gum after 3-6 mo
Teach patient/family:
• To discontinue if patient is unable to stop smoking after 4th wk of therapy
• **Gum:** about all aspects of product use; give package insert to patient and explain
• That gum will not stick to dentures, dental appliances
• That gum is as toxic as cigarettes; that it is to be used only to deter smoking; to call prescriber immediately, stop use if difficulty breathing or rash occurs
• To avoid use during pregnancy

• **Transdermal patch:** that patch is as toxic as cigarettes; to be used only to deter smoking
• Not to use during pregnancy because birth defects may occur; not to breast-feed
• To keep used and unused system out of reach of children and pets
• To stop smoking immediately when beginning patch treatment
• To apply promptly after removing from protective patch because system may lose strength
• **Nasal spray:** to tilt head back; not to swallow or inhale during administration; after smoking is stopped, to use spray up to 8 wk, then discontinue over 6 wk by tapering
• **Lozenges:** to allow to dissolve; to avoid swallowing; not to chew
• **Inhalation:** to use by inhaler for 20 min by frequent puffs
• **Pregnancy/breastfeeding:** Identify if pregnancy is planned or suspected or if breastfeeding

---

NIFEdipine (Rx)
(nye-fed′i-peen)
Adalat CC, Adalat OROS ✤, Procardia XL
Func. class.: Calcium channel blocker, antianginal, antihypertensive
Chem. class.: Dihydropyridine

Do not confuse:
NIFEdipine/niCARdipine/niMODipine

ACTION: Inhibits calcium ion influx across cell membrane during cardiac depolarization; relaxes coronary vascular smooth muscle; dilates coronary arteries; increases myocardial oxygen delivery in patients with vasospastic angina; dilates peripheral arteries

USES: Chronic stable angina pectoris, variant angina, hypertension

CONTRAINDICATIONS
Hypersensitivity to this product or dihydropyridine; cardiogenic shock
Precautions: Pregnancy, breastfeeding, children, hypotension, sick sinus

syndrome, 2nd-/3rd-degree heart block, hypotension <90 mm Hg systolic, hepatic injury, renal disease, acute MI, aortic stenosis, GERD, heart failure

DOSAGE AND ROUTES
Angina
• **Adult: PO** Immediate release 10 mg tid, increase in 10-mg increments q7-14days, max 180 mg/24 hr or single dose of 30 mg; **EXTENDED RELEASE** 30-60 mg/day, may increase q7-14days, max 120 mg/day

Hypertension
• **Adult: PO EXTENDED RELEASE** 30-60 mg daily, titrate upward as needed, max 90 mg/day (Adalat CC), 120 mg/day (Procardia XL)

• **Child/adolescent (unlabeled): PO EXT REL** 0.25-0.5 mg/kg/day in 1-2 divided doses, max 3 mg/kg/day or 120 mg, whichever is less

Available forms: Caps 10, 20 mg; ext rel tabs (XL) 20 ✿, 30, 60, 90 mg

Administer:
• Do not break, crush, or chew ext rel tabs, do not use immediate-release caps within 7 days of MI, coronary syndrome; do not use caps (SL) to reduce severe hypertension, may cause death
• Without regard to meals; avoid grapefruit juice
• Give ext rel (Adalat CC) on empty stomach
• Protect caps from direct light, keep in dry area, do not freeze

SIDE EFFECTS
CNS: *Headache,* fatigue, drowsiness, *dizziness,* anxiety, depression, weakness, insomnia, light-headedness, paresthesia, tinnitus, blurred vision, nervousness, tremor, *flushing*
CV: Dysrhythmias, edema, hypotension, palpitations, tachycardia
GI: Nausea, vomiting, diarrhea, gastric upset, constipation, increased LFTs, dry mouth, flatulence, gingival hyperplasia
GU: *Nocturia, polyuria*
HEMA: Bruising, bleeding, petechiae

INTEG: Rash, pruritus, flushing, hair loss, Stevens-Johnson syndrome, toxic epidermal necrolysis, exfoliative dermatitis
MISC: Sexual difficulties, cough, fever, chills

PHARMACOKINETICS
Metabolized by liver; excreted in urine 60%-80% (metabolites), feces 15%; protein binding 92%-98%, half-life 2-7 hr, well absorbed
PO: Onset 20 min, duration 6-8 hr
PO-ER: Onset 20 min, duration 24 hr

INTERACTIONS
• Contraindicated with strong CYP3A4 inducers
Increase: level of digoxin, phenytoin, cycloSPORINE, prazosin, carBAMazepine β-blockers, antihypertensives, vincristine, warfarin, diuretics
Increase: NIFEdipine effect—ACE inhibitors, alpha blockers, cimetidine, antiretrovirals, verapamil, CYP3A4 inhibitors azole antifungals, dilTIAZem
Increase: hypotension: PDE5 inhibitors, monitor B/P
Increase: NIFEdipine, toxicity—cimetidine, raNITIdine

Drug/Food
Increase: NIFEdipine level—grapefruit juice
Drug/Herb
Decreased: hypotensive effect—St. John's wort, avoid using together
Drug/Lab Test
Increase: CPK, LDH, AST
Positive: ANA, direct Coombs' test

NURSING CONSIDERATIONS
Assess:
• **Anginal pain:** location, intensity, duration, character, alleviating, aggravating factors
• **HTN:** Monitor B/P, pulse, respirations especially those using other cardiac products (ACE inhibitors, diuretics, β-blockers and any other antihypertensives)
• Potassium, renal, hepatic studies periodically during treatment
• For bruising, petechiae, bleeding

N

• **GI obstruction:** ext rel products have been associated with rare reports of obstruction in those with strictures and no known GI disease

• **Serious skin disorders:** rash that starts suddenly, fever, cutaneous lesions that may have pustules present; discontinue product if fever present or if rash is severe

• **Beers:** avoid in older adults; potential for hypotension, myocardial ischemia

• **Pregnancy/breastfeeding:** often used in pregnancy for hypertension; avoid breastfeeding

Evaluate:

• **Therapeutic response:** decreased anginal pain, B/P; activity tolerance

Teach patient/family:

• To avoid hazardous activities until stabilized on product, dizziness is no longer a problem

• To limit caffeine consumption; to avoid alcohol products

• To avoid OTC products unless directed by prescriber; give without regard to meals, not to use with grapefruit juice

• That empty tab shells may appear in stools and are not significant

• To prevent direct light on ext rel product

• To swallow ext rel product whole

• **Hypertension:** to comply with all areas of medical regimen: diet, exercise, stress reduction, product therapy

• To change position slowly because orthostatic hypotension is common

• To notify prescriber of dyspnea, edema of extremities, nausea, vomiting, severe ataxia, severe rash; changes in pattern, frequency, severity of angina

• To check for gingival hyperplasia and report promptly

• Not to discontinue abruptly; to gradually taper, may cause increased angina

• About fall risk for older adults

TREATMENT OF OVERDOSE:

Defibrillation, atropine for AV block, vasopressor for hypotension

⚠ HIGH ALERT

nilotinib (Rx)

(nye-loe′ti-nib)

Tasigna

Func. class.: Antineoplastic—miscellaneous

Chem. class.: Protein-tyrosine kinase inhibitor

ACTION: Inhibits BCR-ABL tyrosine kinase created in patients with chronic myeloid leukemia (CML)

USES: ✎ Chronic phase/accelerated phase Philadelphia chromosome–positive CML that is resistant or intolerant to imatinib

CONTRAINDICATIONS

Pregnancy, breastfeeding, hypersensitivity

Black Box Warning: Hypokalemia, hypomagnesemia, QT prolongation

Precautions: Children, females, geriatric patients, active infections, anemia, cardiac disease, bone marrow suppression, cholestasis, diabetes, gelatin hypersensitivity, infertility, galactose-free diet, lactase deficiency, neutropenia, pancreatitis, thrombocytopenia, hepatic disease, alcoholism, angina, ascites, tumor lysis syndrome

DOSAGE AND ROUTES

• **Adult:** PO 300 mg q12hr, continue until disease progression (chronic phase, newly diagnosed); 400 mg q12hr, continue until disease progression or unacceptable toxicity (accelerated phase). Use with a strong CYP3A4 inducer 200-300 mg daily, depending on the indication

• **Child/adolescent:** PO 230 mg/m² q12hr until disease progression or unacceptable toxicity. Round the dose to the nearest 50 mg to a max single dose of 400 mg

Adjustment after discontinuation of a strong CYP3A4 inhibitor

• **Adult:** PO reduce to 400 mg bid

Use with a strong CYP3A4 inhibitor
• **Adult: PO** reduce dose to 200-300 mg/day depending on indication

QT prolongation
• QTcF >480 msec: withhold dose

Myelosuppression
• ANC 1 × 10⁹/L or platelets <50 × 10⁹/L: withhold dose

Hepatic dose
• **Adult: PO** (Child-Pugh A/B/C) newly diagnosed CML 200 mg bid, then escalation to 300 mg bid initially

Available forms: Caps 50, 150, 200 mg

Administer:
• Do not break, crush, or chew caps; if whole capsule cannot be swallowed, disperse capsule contents in 1 tsp applesauce
• On empty stomach; separate doses by 12 hr; make-up dose should not be taken if dose is missed
• Store at 59° F-86° F (15° C-30° C)

SIDE EFFECTS

CNS: Headache, dizziness, fatigue, fever, flushing, paresthesia

CV: QT prolongation, palpitations, torsades de pointes, AV block

GI: *Nausea,* hepatotoxicity, vomiting, dyspepsia, *anorexia, abdominal pain,* constipation, pancreatitis, diarrhea, xerostomia

HEMA: Neutropenia, thrombocytopenia, anemia, pancytopenia

INTEG: *Rash,* alopecia, erythema

META: Hyperamylasemia, hyperbilirubinemia, hyperglycemia, hyperkalemia, hypocalcemia, hyponatremia, hypomagnesemia

MISC: Diaphoresis, anxiety

MS: Arthralgia, myalgia, back or bone pain, muscle cramps

RESP: Cough, dyspnea

SYST: Bleeding, tumor lysis syndrome

PHARMACOKINETICS

Protein binding 98%, metabolized by CYP3A4, plasma levels 3 hr, elimination half-life 17 hr

INTERACTIONS

• Product interactions are numerous
• Do not use with phenothiazines, pimozide, ziprasidone

Increase: QT prolongation—class IA/III antidysrhythmics, some phenothiazines, β agonists, local anesthetics, tricyclics, haloperidol, chloroquine, droperidol, pentamidine; CYP3A4 inhibitors (amiodarone, clarithromycin, erythromycin, telithromycin, troleandomycin), arsenic trioxide, levomethadyl; CYP3A4 substrates (methadone, pimozide, QUEtiapine, quiNIDine, risperiDONE, ziprasidone)

Increase: hepatotoxicity—acetaminophen

Increase: concentrations—ketoconazole, itraconazole, erythromycin, clarithromycin

Increase: plasma concentrations of simvastatin, calcium channel blockers

Increase: plasma concentration of warfarin; avoid use with warfarin, use low-molecular-weight anticoagulants instead

Decrease: concentrations—dexamethasone, phenytoin, carBAMazepine, rifampin, PHENobarbital

Drug/Herb
Decrease: concentration—St. John's wort

Drug/Food
Increase: plasma concentrations—grapefruit juice

NURSING CONSIDERATIONS
Assess:
• **Tumor lysis syndrome:** maintain hydration, correct uric acid before use with this product

Black Box Warning: QT prolongation can occur; monitor ECG, left ventricular ejection fraction (LVEF) at baseline, periodically; hypertension, assess for chest pain, palpitations, dyspnea

Black Box Warning: Hepatotoxicity: monitor LFTs before treatment and monthly; if liver transaminases >5 × IULN, withhold until transaminase levels return to <2.5 × IULN

• **Myelosuppression:** Monitor CBC ×2 mo, then monthly, differential, platelet count; for bleeding: epistaxis, rectal, gingival, upper GI, genital and wound bleeding; tumor-related hemorrhage may occur rapidly

---

Side effects: *italics* = common; red = life-threatening

• ANC and platelets: if ANC $<1 \times 10^9$/L and/or platelets $<50 \times 10^9$/L, stop until ANC $>1.5 \times 10^9$/L and platelets $>75 \times 10^9$/L

• **Electrolytes:** calcium, potassium, magnesium, sodium; lipase, phosphate; hypokalemia, hypomagnesemia should be corrected before use

• **AST/ALT/bilirubin/lipase/amylase:** if increased to grade 3, withhold product; resume at 400 mg daily when levels return to grade 1 or below

• **Pregnancy/breastfeeding:** do not use in pregnancy, breastfeeding

Evaluate:

• **Therapeutic response:** decrease in progression of disease

Teach patient/family:

• **Infection:** to report immediately cough, fever, chills

• To report bleeding gums; blood in stools, urine, emesis

• About reason for treatment, expected results

• That many adverse reactions may occur

• To avoid persons with known upper respiratory tract infections; immunosuppression is common

• To watch for signs, symptoms of low potassium or magnesium

• To notify prescriber of all OTC, prescription, and herbal products used; not to receive vaccinations without prescriber's approval

• **Pregnancy/breastfeeding:** to use contraception during treatment; not to breastfeed

---

nimodipine (Rx)

(nye-moe'di-peen)

Nymalize

Func. class.: Subarachnoid hemorrhage agent, calcium channel blocker

---

USES: For the improvement of neurologic outcome by reducing the incidence and severity of ischemic deficits in those with subarachnoid hemorrhage

CONTRAINDICATIONS

Use with strong CYP3A4 inhibitors (clarithromycin, telithromycin, delavirdine, indinavir, nelfinavir, ritonavir, saquinavir, ketoconazole, itraconazole, voriconazole, nefazodone)

DOSAGE AND ROUTES
Subarachnoid hemorrhage

Adult: PO 60 mg q4h × 21 days, start therapy within 96 hr of the onset of subarachnoid hemorrhage

Hepatic dose

• **Adult: PO** 30 mg q4h × 21 days

Available forms: Capsules 30 mg; oral solution 6 mg/mL (30 mg/5 mL), prefilled syringe 60 mg/10 mL

---

nintedanib (Rx)

(nin-ted'a-nib)

Ofev

Func. class.: Interstitial lung disease agent

Chem. class.: Idiopathic pulmonary fibrosis agent

USES: Idiopathic pulmonary fibrosis (IPF)

DOSAGE AND ROUTES

• **Adults PO** 150 mg q12hr

Available forms: Capsule 100, 150 mg

⚠ HIGH ALERT

niraparib (Rx)

(nye-rap'-a-rib)

Zejula

Func. class.: Antineoplastic

USES: Recurrent epithelial ovarian, fallopian tube, or primary peritoneal cancer

DOSAGE AND ROUTES

• **Adult: PO** 200 mg/day until disease progression or unacceptable toxicity. Begin therapy no later than 12 wk after last platinum-containing regimen

Available forms: Capsule 100 mg

---

nisoldipine (Rx)

(nye-sole′dih-peen)

Sular

Func. class.: Calcium channel blocker, antihypertensive

Chem. class.: Dihydropyridine

USES: Essential hypertension, alone or in combination with other antihypertensives, ischemic heart disease

CONTRAINDICATIONS

Hypersensitivity to this product or dihydropyridines; sick sinus syndrome; 2nd-/3rd-degree heart block; aortic stenosis

DOSAGE AND ROUTES
Hypertension

• **Adult: PO EXTENDED RELEASE** 17 mg/day initially, may increase by 8.5 mg/wk, usual dose 17-34 mg/day, max 34 mg/day

• **Geriatric/hepatic dose: PO EXTENDED RELEASE** 8.5 mg/day, increase based on patient response up to 34 mg/day

Hepatic dose

• **Adult: PO EXTENDED RELEASE** 8.5 mg/day

Available forms: Tabs ext rel 8.5, 17, 20, 25.5, 30, 34, 40 mg

nitazoxanide (Rx)

(nye-ta-zox′a-nide)

Alinia

Func. class.: Antiprotozoal

USES: Treatment of diarrhea caused by Cryptosporidium parvum or Giardia lamblia

CONTRAINDICATIONS

Hypersensitivity to nitazoxanide or any component

DOSAGE AND ROUTES
Infectious diarrhea caused by *C. parvum* or *G. lamblia*

Oral suspension or tablets. Adult/child ≥12 yr: PO 500 mg q12h for 3 days

Child 4-11 yr: PO 200 mg q12h for 3 days

Child 1-3 yr: PO 100 mg q12h for 3 days

Available forms: Tabs 500 mg; oral suspension 100 mg/5 mL

nitrofurantoin (Rx)

(nye-troe-fyoor′an-toyn)

Furadantin, Macrobid, Macrodantin

Func. class.: Urinary tract antiinfective

Chem. class.: Synthetic nitrofuran derivative

ACTION: Inhibits bacterial acetyl-CoA interference with carbohydrate metabolism

USES: Urinary tract infections caused by *Escherichia coli, Klebsiella, Pseudomonas, Proteus vulgaris, Proteus morganii, Serratia, Citrobacter, Staphylococcus aureus, Staphylococcus epidermidis, Enterococcus, Salmonella, Shigella*

CONTRAINDICATIONS

Infants <1 mo, hypersensitivity, anuria, severe renal disease CCr <60 mL/min, at term pregnancy (38-42 wk), labor, delivery, cholestatic jaundice due to nitrofurantoin therapy

Precautions: Pregnancy, breastfeeding, geriatric patients, ✺ G6PD deficiency, GI disease, diabetes

DOSAGE AND ROUTES
Active UTI

• **Adult/child >12 yr: PO** 50-100 mg qid after meals or 100 mg (Macrobid) q12hr × 7 days

• **Child 1 mo-12 yr: PO** 5-7 mg/kg/day in 4 divided doses, Max: 100 mg/dose

UTI prevention

• **Adult: PO** 50-100 mg q PM

• **Child: PO** 1-2 mg/kg/day in PM or 0.5-1 mg/kg q12hr if dose not well tolerated

Available forms: oral suspension (microcrystals) 25 mg/5 mL; capsules 25, 50, 100 mg macrocrystalline

N

Administer:
PO route

• Give with meals, food, or milk
• Do not break, crush, chew, or open tabs, caps, store in original container
• Two daily doses if urine output is high or if patient has diabetes
• Oral suspension: Shake, use calibrated device to measure liquid product; may mix water, fruit juice; rinse mouth after liquid product; staining of teeth may occur, protect from light

SIDE EFFECTS

CNS: *Dizziness, headache,* drowsiness, peripheral neuropathy, chills, confusion, vertigo, polyneuropathy (high dose)
CV: Bundle chest pain
GI: *Nausea, vomiting, abdominal pain, diarrhea,* cholestatic jaundice, loss of appetite, CDAD, hepatitis, pancreatitis
HEMA: Anemia, agranulocytosis, hemolytic anemia, leukopenia, thrombocytopenia
INTEG: Pruritus, rash, urticaria, angioedema, alopecia, tooth staining, exfoliative dermatitis, Stevens-Johnson syndrome
MS: Arthralgia, myalgia, numbness, peripheral neuropathy
RESP: Cough, dyspnea, pneumonitis, pulmonary fibrosis or infiltrate
SYST:
Superinfection, SLE-like syndrome

PHARMACOKINETICS

PO: Half-life 20-60 min; crosses blood-brain barrier, placenta; enters breast milk; excreted as inactive metabolites in liver, unchanged in urine; protein binding 60%-90%

INTERACTIONS

Increase: nitrofurantoin toxicity—topical dapsone/tetracaine, prilocaine, sodium nitrate, monitor closely
Increase: levels of nitrofurantoin—probenecid, sulfinpyrazone, avoid using together
Decrease: absorption of magnesium antacid, separate by ≥1 hr
Decrease: effect of live virus vaccines, avoid using together

Drug/Food
Food: Increased absorption
Drug/Lab Test
Increase: BUN, alk phos, bilirubin, creatinine, blood glucose
Decrease: WBC, platelets, HB

NURSING CONSIDERATIONS
Assess:

• **Urinary tract infection:** burning, pain on urination; fever; cloudy, foul-smelling urine; I&O ratio: C&S before treatment, after completion; serum creatinine, BUN
• Blood count during chronic therapy, LFTs, pulmonary function tests
• **CDAD:** diarrhea with mucus, abdominal pain, fever, fatigue, anorexia; may be treated with vancomycin or metroNIDAZOLE
• **CNS symptoms:** insomnia, vertigo, headache, drowsiness, seizures
• **Hepatotoxicity:** yellowing of skin or eyes, dark urine, clay-colored stools; monitor AST, ALT, stop drug immediately in hepatitis
• **Pulmonary fibrosis, pneumonitis:** dyspnea, tachypnea, persistent cough
• **Serious skin disorders:** fever, flushing, rash, urticaria, pruritus
• **Peripheral neuropathy:** paresthesias (more common in diabetes mellitus, electrolyte imbalances, vit B deficiency, debilitated patients)
• **Beers:** avoid in older adults; potential for pulmonary, hepatic toxicity, peripheral neuropathy
• **Pregnancy/breastfeeding:** do not use in gestation of 38-42 wk or in labor/delivery; cautious use in breastfeeding, excreted in breast milk

Evaluate:
• **Therapeutic response:** decreased dysuria, fever; negative C&S

Teach patient/family:
• To notify prescriber of continued symptoms of UTI, fever, myalgias, arthralgias, numbness or tingling of extremities
• To take as prescribed even if better
• To take with food or milk; to avoid alcohol
• To protect susp from freezing; shake well before taking
• That product may cause drowsiness; to seek aid with walking, other activities;

not to drive or operate machinery while taking medication
• That patients with diabetes should monitor blood glucose levels
• That product may turn urine rust-yellow to brown
• **CDAD:** to report immediately symptoms of fever; diarrhea with mucus, pus, or blood

---

nitroglycerin IV (Rx)
extended release caps (Rx)

Nitro-Time

topical ointment (Rx)

Nitro-Bid, Nitrol ✦

rectal ointment

Rectiv

SL (Rx)

Nitrostat

SL Powder (Rx)

GoNitro

translingual spray (Rx)

Nitrolingual, NitroMist

transdermal (Rx)

Transderm ✦, Minitran, Nitro-Dur, Trinipatch ✦

Func. class.: Coronary vasodilator, antianginal
Chem. class.: Nitrate

ACTION: Decreases preload and afterload, which are responsible for decreasing left ventricular end-diastolic pressure, systemic vascular resistance; dilates coronary arteries, improves blood flow through coronary vasculature, dilates arterial and venous beds systemically

USES: Chronic stable angina pectoris, prophylaxis of angina pain, HF, acute MI, controlled hypotension for surgical procedures, anal fissures

CONTRAINDICATIONS

Hypersensitivity to this product or nitrites; severe anemia, increased intracranial pressure, cerebral hemorrhage, closed-angle glaucoma, cardiac tamponade, cardiomyopathy, constrictive pericarditis

Precautions: Pregnancy, breastfeeding, children, postural hypotension, severe renal/hepatic disease, acute MI, abrupt discontinuation, hyperthyroidism

DOSAGE AND ROUTES

• **Adult: IV:** Run at 5 mcg/min, may increase by 5 mcg/min q3-5min, up to 100 mcg/min, may be used (hypertension in HF, MI, surgery); **SL** Dissolve tab under tongue when pain begins; may repeat q5min until relief occurs; take ≤3 tabs/15 min; use 1 tab prophylactically 5-10 min before activities; **TOP** 1-2 inches q8hr, increase to 4 inches q4hr as needed; **TRANS PATCH** apply a patch daily to a site free of hair; remove patch at bedtime to provide 10-12 hr nitrate-free interval to avoid tolerance

Anal fissures (Rectiv)
• **Adult: Rectal** Apply 1 inch of 0.4% ointment q12hr × 3 wk

Available forms: SL tabs 0.3, 0.4, 0.6 mg; **topical oint** 2%; **trans syst** 0.1, 0.2, 0.3, 0.4, 0.6, 0.8 mg/hr; **inj sol** 5 mg/mL; **rectal ointment** 0.4% (Rectiv); SL powder 400 mcg; **SL/translingual spray** 400 mcg/spray

Administer:
• **Topical ointment** should be measured on papers supplied; use paper to spread on nonhairy area of chest, abdomen, thigh skin; thin layer spread over 2-3 inches; do not rub

PO route
• Swallow sus rel products whole; do not break, crush, or chew
• With 8 oz water on empty stomach (oral tablet) 1 hr before or 2 hr after meals
• **SL:** should be dissolved under tongue, or between gum and cheek, not swallowed
• **Aerosol** sprayed under tongue (**nitrolingual**), not inhaled; prime before 1st-time use or if product has not been used in >6 wk; press valve head with forefinger

N

Side effects: *italics* = common; red = life-threatening

Transdermal route
• Apply new TD patch daily; remove after 12-14 hr to prevent tolerance

Rectal route
• Cover finger with plastic wrap, disposable glove, or finger cot; lay finger alongside 1-inch dosing line on carton; squeeze tube until equal to 1-inch dosing line; insert covered finger gently into anal canal no further than 1st finger joint and apply to sides; wash hands thoroughly; if too painful, apply directly to outside of anus

Continuous IV INFUSION route
• Diluted in D_5, D_5W, 0.9% NaCl for infusion to 200-400 mcg/mL, depending on patient's fluid status; common dilution 50 mg/250 mL, use controlled infusion device; titrate to patient response; do not use filters

Y-site compatibilities: Acyclovir, alfentanil, amikacin, aminocaproic acid, aminophylline, amiodarone, amphotericin B cholesteryl, amphotericin B lipid complex, amphotericin B liposome, anidulafungin, argatroban, ascorbic acid, atenolol, atracurium, atropine, azaTHIOprine, aztreonam, benztropine, bivalirudin, bleomycin, bumetanide, buprenorphine, butorphanol, calcium chloride/gluconate, CARBOplatin, caspofungin, cefamandole, ceFAZolin, cefmetazole, cefonicid, cefoperazone, cefotaxime, cefoTEtan, cefOXitin, cefTAZidime, ceftizoxime, cefTRIAXone, cefuroxime, cephalothin, cephapirin, chloramphenicol, chlorproMAZINE, cimetidine, cisatracurium, CISplatin, clindamycin, cloNIDine, cyanocobalamin, cyclophosphamide, cycloSPORINE, cytarabine, DACTINomycin, dexamethasone, digoxin, diltiazem, diphenhydrAMINE, DOBUTamine, DOCEtaxel, DOPamine, doxacurium, DOXOrubicin, doxycycline, drotrecogin alfa, enalaprilat, ePHEDrine, EPINEPHrine, epirubicin, epoetin alfa, eptifibatide, ertapenem, erythromycin, esmolol, etoposide, famotidine, fenoldopam, fentaNYL, fluconazole, fludarabine, fluorouracil, folic acid, ganciclovir, gatifloxacin, gemcitabine, gemtuzumab, gentamicin, glycopyrrolate, granisetron, heparin, hydrocortisone, HYDROmorphone, hydrOXYzine, IDArubicin, ifosfamide, imipenem-cilastatin, indomethacin, insulin (regular), irinotecan, isoproterenol, ketorolac, labetalol, lidocaine, linezolid, LORazepam, magnesium sulfate, mannitol, mechlorethamine, meperidine, metaraminol, methicillin, methotrexate, methoxamine, methyldopate, methylPREDNISolone, metoclopramide, metroNIDAZOLE, mezlocillin, micafungin, miconazole, midazolam, milrinone, minocycline, mitoXANtrone, morphine, moxalactam, mycophenolate, nafcillin, nalbuphine, naloxone, nesiritide, netilmicin, niCARdipine, nitroprusside, norepinephrine, octreotide, ondansetron, oxacillin, oxaliplatin, oxytocin, PACLitaxel, palonosetron, pamidronate, pancuronium, pantoprazole, papaverine, PEMEtrexed, penicillin G potassium/sodium, pentamidine, pentazocine, PENTobarbital, PHENobarbital, phentolamine, phenylephrine, phytonadione, piperacillin, piperacillin-tazobactam, polymyxin B, potassium chloride, procainamide, prochlorperazine, promethazine, propofol, propranolol, protamine, pyridoxine, quiNIDine, quinupristin-dalfopristin, ranitidine, remifentanil, ritodrine, rocuronium, sodium bicarbonate, succinylcholine, SUFentanil, tacrolimus, teniposide, theophylline, thiamine, thiopental, thiotepa, ticarcillin, ticarcillin-clavulanate, tigecycline, tirofiban, tobramycin, tolazoline, trimetaphan, urokinase, vancomycin, vasopressin, vecuronium, verapamil, vinCRIStine, vinorelbine, voriconazole, warfarin, zoledronic acid

SIDE EFFECTS
CNS: *Headache, flushing, dizziness*
CV: *Postural hypotension,* tachycardia, collapse, syncope, palpitations
GI: Nausea, vomiting
INTEG: Pallor, sweating, rash

PHARMACOKINETICS
Metabolized by liver, excreted in urine, half-life 1-4 min

SL: Onset 1-3 min, duration 30 min
TRANSDERMAL: Onset 30 min-1 hr, duration 12-24 hr
AEROSOL: Onset 2 min, duration 30-60 min
TOPICAL OINT: Onset 30-60 min, duration 2-12 hr
IV: Onset 1-2 min, duration 3-5 min

INTERACTIONS
• **Severe hypotension, CV collapse:** alcohol
Increase: effects of β-blockers, diuretics, antihypertensives, calcium channel blockers
Increase: fatal hypotension—avanafil, sildenafil, tadalafil, vardenafil; do not use together
Increase: nitrate level—aspirin
Decrease: heparin—IV nitroglycerin
Drug/Lab Test
Increase: urine catecholamine, urine VMA
False increase: cholesterol

NURSING CONSIDERATIONS
Assess:
• **Chest pain/angina:** duration, time started, activity being performed, character
• **Hypotensive episodes:** Orthostatic B/P, pulse before and after administration
• Tolerance if taken over long period
• Headache, light-headedness, decreased B/P; may indicate a need for decreased dosage
• **Pregnancy/breastfeeding:** use only if clearly needed; cautious use in breastfeeding
Evaluate:
• **Therapeutic response:** decrease, prevention of anginal pain
Teach patient/family:
• To place SL tab under tongue and wait to dissolve, or spray on or under tongue
• To keep tabs in original container; to replace q6mo because effectiveness is lost; to keep away from heat, moisture, light
• That if 3 SL tabs in 15 min do not relieve pain, to seek immediate medical attention
• To avoid alcohol

• That product may cause headache; that tolerance usually develops; to use nonopioid analgesic
• That product may be taken before stressful activity: exercise, sexual activity
• That SL may sting when product comes in contact with mucous membranes
• To avoid hazardous activities if dizziness occurs
• To comply with complete medical regimen
• To make position changes slowly to prevent fainting
• Never to use erectile dysfunction products (sildenafil, tadalafil, vardenafil); may cause severe hypotension, death

---

⚠ HIGH ALERT

nitroprusside (Rx)
(nye-troe-pruss´ide)
Nipride, Nipride RTU
Func. class.: Antihypertensive, vasodilator

ACTION: Directly relaxes arteriolar, venous smooth muscle, thereby resulting in reduction in cardiac preload and afterload

USES: Hypertensive crisis/urgency/induction; to decrease bleeding by creating hypotension during surgery; acute HF

CONTRAINDICATIONS
Hypersensitivity, hypertension (compensatory) due to aortic coarctation or AV shunting, acute HF associated with reduced peripheral vascular resistance, toxic amblyopia, hypothyroidism
Precautions: Anemia, increased intracranial pressure, pregnancy, breastfeeding, children, geriatric patients, hypovolemia, electrolyte imbalances, renal/hepatic disease, hypothyroidism

Black Box Warning: Hypotension, cyanide toxicity

Side effects: *italics* = common; red = life-threatening

DOSAGE AND ROUTES
• **Adult/child:** IV INFUSION 0.25-10 mcg/kg/min; max 10 mcg/kg/min × 10 min

Renal dose
• **Adult:** IV INFUSION CCr <60 mL/min, maintain doses <3 mcg/kg/min to reduce thiocyanate accumulation

Available forms: Inj 50 mg/2 mL

Administer:
• Antidote is sodium thiosulfate

Continuous IV INFUSION route

• **Black Box Warning:** Reconstitute 50 mg/2-3 mL of D_5W, further dilute in 250, 500, or 1000 mL of D_5W to 200, 100, 50 mcg/mL, respectively; use infusion pump only; wrap bottle with aluminum foil to protect from light; observe for color change in infusion; discard if highly discolored (blue, green, dark red); titrate to patient response

• **Black Box Warning:** Stop infusion if B/P is not lowered sufficiently within 10 min

• **Black Box Warning:** Monitor continuously

• Do not exceed max dose as cyanide may accumulate

Y-site compatibilities: Alfentanil, alprostadil, amikacin, aminocaproic acid, aminophylline, amphotericin B lipid complex, amphotericin B liposome, anidulafungin, argatroban, atenolol, atropine, aztreonam, benztropine, bivalirudin, bleomycin, bumetanide, buprenorphine, butorphanol, calcium chloride/gluconate, CARBOplatin, cefamandole, ceFAZolin, cefmetazole, cefonicid, cefoperazone, cefotaxime, cefoTEtan, cefOXitin, cefTAZidime, ceftizoxime, cefTRIAXone, cefuroxime, cephalothin, chloramphenicol, cimetidine, CISplatin, clindamycin, cyanocobalamin, cyclophosphamide, cycloSPORINE, cytarabine, DACTINomycin, DAPTOmycin, dexamethasone, digoxin, diltiazem, DOCEtaxel, DOPamine, doxacurium, DOXOrubicin, doxycycline, enalaprilat, ePHEDrine, EPINEPHrine, epirubicin, epoetin alfa, eptifibatide, ertapenem, esmolol, etoposide, famotidine, fenoldopam, fentaNYL, fluconazole, fludarabine, fluorouracil, folic acid, furosemide, ganciclovir, gatifloxacin, gemcitabine, gemtuzumab, gentamicin, glycopyrrolate, granisetron, heparin, hydrocortisone, HYDROmorphone, IDArubicin, ifosfamide, inamrinone, indomethacin, insulin (regular), isoproterenol, ketorolac, labetalol, lidocaine, linezolid, LORazepam, magnesium sulfate, mannitol, mechlorethamine, meperidine, metaraminol, methicillin, methoxamine, methyldopate, methylPREDNISolone, metoclopramide, metoprolol, metroNIDAZOLE, mezlocillin, micafungin, miconazole, midazolam, milrinone, minocycline, morphine, moxalactam, multiple vitamins injection, nafcillin, nalbuphine, naloxone, nesiritide, netilmicin, niCARdipine, nitroglycerin, norepinephrine, octreotide, ondansetron, oxacillin, oxaliplatin, oxytocin, PACLitaxel, palonosetron, pamidronate, pancuronium, pantoprazole, penicillin G potassium/sodium, pentamidine, PENTobarbital, PHENobarbital, phentolamine, phenylephrine, phytonadione, piperacillin, piperacillin-tazobactam, polymyxin B, potassium chloride/phosphates, procainamide, propofol, propranolol, protamine, pyridoxine, ranitidine, ritodrine, rocuronium, sodium acetate/bicarbonate, succinylcholine, SUFentanil, tacrolimus, teniposide, theophylline, thiamine, ticarcillin, ticarcillin-clavulanate, tigecycline, tirofiban, tobramycin, tolazoline, trimetaphan, urokinase, vancomycin, vasopressin, vecuronium, verapamil, vinCRIStine, zoledronic acid

SIDE EFFECTS
CNS: *Dizziness, headache,* agitation, twitching, decreased reflexes, *restlessness*

CV: *Bradycardia,* ECG changes, tachycardia, *hypotension*

GI: Nausea, vomiting, abdominal pain

INTEG: Pain, irritation at inj site, sweating

MISC: Cyanide, thiocyanate toxicity, flushing, hypothyroidism

PHARMACOKINETICS
IV: Onset 1-2 min, duration 1-10 min, half-life 2 min; metabolized in liver, excreted in urine

INTERACTIONS
Increase: severe hypotension—ganglionic blockers, volatile liquid anesthetics, halothane, enflurane, circulatory depressants
Drug/Herb
Increase: antihypertensive effect—hawthorn

NURSING CONSIDERATIONS
Assess:
• **Electrolytes:** potassium, sodium, chloride, CO_2, CBC, serum glucose, serum methemoglobin if pulmonary O_2 levels are decreased; use IV 1-2 mg/kg methylene blue given over several min for methemoglobinemia, ABGs
• **Renal studies:** catecholamines, BUN, creatinine
• **Hepatic studies:** AST, ALT, alk phos

Black Box Warning: **Hypotension:** B/P by direct means if possible; check ECG continuously; pulse, jugular venous distention; PCWP; rebound hypertension may occur after nitroprusside is discontinued, give only with emergency equipment nearby, rapid decrease in B/P may occur; check weight, I&O daily

Black Box Warning: **Thiocyanate, lactate, cyanide toxicity:** obtain levels daily if infusion >3 mcg/kg/min; thiocyanate toxicity occurs at plasma levels of 50-100 mcg/mL; thiocyanate toxicity includes confusion, weakness, seizures, hyperreflexia, psychosis, tinnitus, coma

• Nausea, vomiting, diarrhea
• Edema in feet, legs daily; skin turgor, dryness of mucous membranes for hydration status
• Crackles, dyspnea, orthopnea q30min
• For decrease in bicarbonate, $PaCO_2$, blood pH, acidosis

• **Pregnancy/breastfeeding:** prolonged use may result in death of the fetus (cyanide toxicity); do not breastfeed
Evaluate:
• **Therapeutic response:** decreased B/P, decreasing symptoms of cardiogenic shock or cardiac pump failure
Teach patient/family:
• To report headache, dizziness, loss of hearing, blurred vision, dyspnea, faintness, pain at IV site
• About the reason for giving product and expected results

nivolumab (Rx)
(nye-vol'ue-mab)
Opdivo
Func. class.: Antineoplastic, monoclonal antibody

USES: Treatment of BRAF V600 mutation-positive unresectable/metastatic melanoma, Hodgkin's disease, non–small-cell lung cancer (NSCLC), renal cell cancer, mesothelioma

CONTRAINDICATIONS
Hypersensitivity

DOSAGE AND ROUTES
• **Adult: IV INFUSION** 240 mg over 30 min q2wk OR 480 mg over 30 min q4wk, until disease progression or unacceptable toxicity
Available forms: Injection 10 mg/mL

⚠ HIGH ALERT

nivolumab/relatlimab (Rx)
(nye-vol'-ue-mab/rel-at-li-mab)
Opdualag
Func. class.: Antineoplastic
Chem. class.: Human IgG4 monoclonal antibody

ACTIONS: A combination product with a programmed death receptor-1 (PD-1) blocking antibody and a lymphocyte

N

activation gene-3 (LAG-3) blocking antibody. When combined leads to additive inhibitory effects on T-cell function and results in improved tumor response in melanoma

USES: Unresectable or metastatic melanoma in adults and those over 12 yr

CONTRAINDICATIONS
Hypersensitivity

Precautions: Pregnancy, breastfeeding, Crohn disease, hepatitis, immunosuppression, inflammatory bowel disease, iritis, ocular disease, organ transplant, pancreatitis, renal disease, rheumatoid arthritis, sarcoidosis, systemic lupus erythematosus, thyroid disease, ulcerative colitis, uveitis, adrenal insufficiency, diarrhea, Guillain-Barré syndrome, hepatic disease, myasthenia gravis, hypo/hyperthyroidism, hypopituitarism, peripheral neuropathy, serious rash, hypophysitis

DOSAGE AND ROUTES
• **Adult/child >12 yr and >40 kg: IV** 480 mg nivolumab and 160 mg relatlimab q4wk; max volume 160 mL (nivolumab: 3 mg/mL to 12 mg/mL; relatlimab: 1 mg/mL to 4 mg/mL)

Available forms: Injection: 240 mg nivolumab and 80 mg relatlimab per 20 mL (12 mg and 4 mg per mL) in a single-dose vial

Administer:

Intermittent IV INFUSION route

• May be administered diluted or undiluted and administered at a final concentration as ordered

• Withdraw the required volume of and transfer into an IV container made of PVC, EVA, PO

• If diluting, dilute solution with 0.9% NaCl injection, USP or 5% dextrose injection, USP to final concentration and maximum infusion volume, mix by inversion, do not shake

• Discard any unused solution

• Run over 30 min, do not give with other products; after each infusion, flush the line with 0.9% sodium chloride injection

• Store once diluted for no more than 24 hr refrigerated, 8 hr at room temperature

SIDE EFFECTS
CNS: Severe and fatal immune-mediated neuropathies, fatigue, headache, fever

EENT: Uveitis, iritis, episcleritis

ENDO: Severe and fatal immune-mediated endocrinopathies

GI: Severe and fatal immune-mediated enterocolitis, hepatitis, pancreatitis, abdominal pain, nausea, diarrhea, appetite decreased, vomiting, constipation, colitis

INTEG: Severe and fatal immune-mediated dermatitis, pruritus, rash, urticaria

MISC: Cough, dyspnea, anemia, eosinophilia, nephritis

SYST: Antibody formation, Stevens-Johnson syndrome, toxic epidermal necrolysis

PHARMACOKINETICS:
Terminal half-life 26.5 days

NURSING CONSIDERATIONS
Assess:

• Serious skin disorders: Stevens-Johnson syndrome, toxic epidermal necrolysis: permanently discontinue in these or rash complicated by full-thickness dermal ulceration; give systemic corticosteroids at a dose of 1-2 mg/kg/day of predniSONE or equivalent; when dermatitis is controlled, taper corticosteroids over at least 1 mo, withhold in patients with moderate to severe reactions; for mild to moderate dermatitis (localized rash and pruritus), give topical or systemic corticosteroids

• Immune-mediated reactions: prior to starting treatment, assess for enterocolitis, hepatitis, dermatitis, neuropathy, endocrinopathy; take LFTs, ACTH, and thyroid function tests; permanently discontinue if these conditions occur

• Hepatotoxicity: LFTs baseline and prior to each dose; increase the frequency of liver function test monitoring until resolution; permanently discontinue in grade 3-5 toxicity; give systemic corticosteroids at a dose of 1-2 mg/kg/day of predniSONE or equivalent

• Neuropathy: monitor for motor or sensory neuropathy (unilateral or bilateral weakness, sensory alterations, or paresthesias) prior to each dose; permanently discontinue if severe neuropathy (interfering with daily activities), such as Guillain-Barré–like syndromes, occurs

• Endocrinopathy: monitor thyroid function tests at baseline and prior to each dose; monitor hypophysitis, adrenal insufficiency, adrenal crisis, hypo/hyperthyroidism (fatigue, headache, mental status changes, abdominal pain, unusual bowel habits, hypotension, or nonspecific symptoms that may resemble other causes)

• Vision changes: uveitis, iritis; corticosteroids may be used

• Pregnancy/breastfeeding: do not use in pregnancy, breastfeeding, pregnancy testing prior to first dose

Evaluate:

• Decreasing spread or recurrence of malignant melanoma

Teach patient/family:

• To immediately report allergic reactions, skin rash, severe abdominal pain, yellowing of skin or eyes, tingling of extremities, change in bowel habits, diarrhea, cough, chest pain, decreased urine

• About the reason for treatment and expected results; to read medication guide provided

• Pregnancy/breastfeeding: to notify prescriber if pregnancy is planned or suspected or if breastfeeding; to use contraception during and for 5 mo after final dose, not to breastfeed

---

nizatidine (Rx)

(ni-za'ti-deen)
Func. class.: H$_2$-receptor antagonist
Chem. class.: Substituted thiazole

USES: Benign gastric and duodenal ulceration, prevention of duodenal ulcer recurrence, symptomatic relief of gastroesophageal reflux, heartburn prevention

CONTRAINDICATIONS
Hypersensitivity

DOSAGE AND ROUTES
Gastric and duodenal ulcer

• **Adult: PO** 300 mg at night or 150 mg bid for 4-8 wk; maintenance 150 mg at night

Prophylaxis of duodenal ulcer

• **Adult: PO** 150 mg/day at bedtime

Gastroesophageal reflux

• **Adult and child ≥12 yr: PO** 150 mg bid × ≤12 wk, max 300 mg/day

Heartburn prevention

• **Adult: PO** 75 mg before eating up to bid, max 150 mg/day

Renal dose

• **Adult: PO** CCr 20-50 mL/min, give 150 mg every other day; CCr <20 mL/min, give 150 mg q72hr

---

⚠ HIGH ALERT

norepinephrine (Rx)

(nor-ep-i-nef'rin)
Levophed
Func. class.: Vasopressor
Chem. class.: α/β-agonist

Do not confuse:
norepinephrine/EPINEPHrine

ACTION: Causes increased contractility and heart rate by acting on β-receptors in heart; also acts on α-receptors, thereby causing vasoconstriction in blood vessels; B/P is elevated, coronary blood flow improves, and cardiac output increases

USES: Acute hypotension, shock

CONTRAINDICATIONS
Hypersensitivity to this product or cyclopropane/halothane anesthesia, hypovolemia, mesenteric thrombosis

Precautions: Pregnancy, breastfeeding, geriatric patients, arterial embolism, peripheral vascular disease, hypertension, hyperthyroidism, cardiac disease, ventricular fibrillation, tachydysrhythmias, pheochromocytoma, hypotension, sulfite hypersensitivity, extravasation

N

DOSAGE AND ROUTES
• **Adult: IV INFUSION** 0.5-1 mcg/min titrated to B/P; maintenance 2-4 mcg/min; max 30 mcg/min
• **Child: IV INFUSION** 0.1 mcg/kg/min titrated to B/P; max 2 mcg/kg/min
Available forms: Inj 1 mg/mL
Administer:
Plasma expanders for hypovolemia; correct volume depletion before starting treatment
Continuous IV INFUSION route
• Premixed infusion bags do not require dilution
• Monitor at all times while infusing
• Dilute with 500-1000 mL D₅W or D₅/0.9% NaCl; average dilution 4 mg/1000 mL diluent (4 mcg base/mL); give as infusion 2-3 mL/min; titrate to response; discontinue gradually
• Store reconstituted sol in refrigerator ≤24 hr, protect from light, store unopened product at room temperature, do not use discolored sol

Y-site compatibilities: Alemtuzumab, alfentanil, amikacin, amiodarone, anidulafungin, argatroban, ascorbic acid, atenolol, atracurium, atropine, aztreonam, benztropine, bivalirudin, bleomycin, bumetanide, buprenorphine, butorphanol, calcium chloride/gluconate, CARBOplatin, caspofungin, cefamandole, ceFAZolin, cefmetazole, cefonicid, cefoperazone, cefotaxime, cefoTEtan, cefOXitin, cefTAZidime, ceftizoxime, ceftobiprole, cefTRIAXone, cefuroxime, cephalothin, chloramphenicol, chlorproMAZINE, cimetidine, cisatracurium, CISplatin, clindamycin, cloNIDine, cyanocobalamin, cyclophosphamide, cycloSPORINE, cytarabine, DAPTOmycin, dexamethasone, digoxin, diltiazem, diphenhydrAMINE, DOBUTamine, DOCEtaxel, DOPamine, doripenem, doxycycline, enalaprilat, ePHEDrine, EPINEPHrine, epirubicin, epoetin alfa, ertapenem, erythromycin, esmolol, etoposide, famotidine, fenoldopam, fentaNYL, fluconazole, fludarabine, gatifloxacin, gemcitabine, gentamicin, glycopyrrolate, granisetron, heparin, hydrocortisone, HYDROmorphone, hydrOXYzine, IDArubicin, ifosfamide, imipenem-cilastatin, irinotecan, isoproterenol, ketorolac, labetalol, lidocaine, linezolid, LORazepam, magnesium sulfate, mannitol, mechlorethamine, meperidine, meropenem, metaraminol, methicillin, methotrexate, methoxamine, methyldopate, methylPREDNISolone, metoclopramide, metoprolol, metroNIDAZOLE, mezlocillin, micafungin, miconazole, midazolam, milrinone, minocycline, mitoXANtrone, morphine, moxalactam, multiple vitamins injection, mycophenolate, nafcillin, nalbuphine, naloxone, netilmicin, niCARdipine, nitroglycerin, nitroprusside, octreotide, ondansetron, oxacillin, oxaliplatin, oxytocin, PACLitaxel, palonosetron, pamidronate, pancuronium, papaverine, PEMEtrexed, penicillin G potassium/sodium, pentamidine, pentazocine, phenylephrine, phytonadione, piperacillin, piperacillin-tazobactam, polymyxin B, potassium chloride, procainamide, prochlorperazine, promethazine, propofol, propranolol, protamine, pyridoxine, quiNIDine, ranitidine, remifentanil, ritodrine, succinylcholine, SUFentanil, tacrolimus, teniposide, theophylline, thiamine, thiotepa, ticarcillin, ticarcillin-clavulanate, tigecycline, tirofiban, tobramycin, tolazoline, trimetaphan, urokinase, vancomycin, vasopressin, vecuronium, verapamil, vinCRIStine, vinorelbine, vitamin B complex with C, voriconazole, zoledronic acid

SIDE EFFECTS
CNS: *Headache,* anxiety, dizziness, insomnia, restlessness, tremor, cerebral hemorrhage
CV: *Palpitations, tachycardia, hypertension, ectopic beats, angina*
GI: *Nausea, vomiting*
GU: Decreased urine output
INTEG: Necrosis, tissue sloughing with extravasation, gangrene
RESP: Dyspnea
SYST: Anaphylaxis

PHARMACOKINETICS
IV: Onset 1-2 min; metabolized in liver; excreted in urine (inactive metabolites); crosses placenta

INTERACTIONS
• Do not use within 2 wk of MAOIs, antihistamines, ergots, methyldopa, oxytocics, tricyclics because hypertensive crisis may result

Increase: B/P—oxytocics

Increase: pressor effect—tricyclics, MAOIs

Decrease: norepinephrine action—α-blockers

NURSING CONSIDERATIONS
Assess:
• I&O ratio; notify prescriber if output <30 mL/hr
• B/P, pulse q2-3min after parenteral route, ECG during administration continuously; if B/P increases, product is decreased, CVP or PWP during infusion if possible
• Paresthesias and coldness of extremities; peripheral blood flow may decrease
• **Extravasation:** inj site: tissue sloughing; change injection sites if blanching or vasoconstriction occurs
• Sulfite sensitivity, which may be life-threatening
• **Pregnancy/breastfeeding:** use only if clearly needed; cautious use in breastfeeding

Evaluate:
• **Therapeutic response:** increased B/P with stabilization, adequate tissue perfusion

Teach patient/family:
• About the reason for product administration; to report dyspnea, dizziness, chest pain

TREATMENT OF OVERDOSE:
Administer fluids, electrolyte replacement

---

norethindrone (Rx)
(nor-eth-in′drone)
Camila, Errin, Heather, Incassia, Jencycla, Movisse ✦, Nor-QD
Func. class.: Progestogen

ACTION: Inhibits the secretion of pituitary gonadotropins, which prevents follicular maturation and ovulation; stimulates growth of mammary tissue; antineoplastic action against endometrial cancer

USES: Uterine bleeding (abnormal), amenorrhea, endometriosis, contraception

CONTRAINDICATIONS
Pregnancy, breast cancer, hypersensitivity, thromboembolic disorders, reproductive cancer, genital bleeding (abnormal, undiagnosed), liver tumors, hepatic disease

Precautions: Breastfeeding, hypertension, asthma, blood dyscrasias, HF, diabetes mellitus, depression, migraine headache, seizure disorders, bone/gallbladder/renal/hepatic disease, family history of breast or reproductive tract cancer, smoking, HIV

DOSAGE AND ROUTES
Amenorrhea, abnormal uterine bleeding (acetate)
• **Adult: PO** 2.5 to 10 mg daily for 5 to 10 days during the second half of the theoretical menstrual cycle

Endometriosis (acetate)
• **Adult: PO** 5 mg/day × 2 wk, then increased by 2.5 mg/day × 2 wk up to 15 mg/day, may continue for 6-9 mo

Contraception
• **Adult: PO** 0.35 mg on 1st day of menses, then 0.35 mg/day

Available forms: Tabs 5 mg; tabs 0.35 mg
Administer:
• Use safe handling procedures
• Titrated dose; use lowest effective dose
• One dose in AM; do not interrupt between pill packs; give at roughly same time of day
• Without regard to meals
• Store in dark area

SIDE EFFECTS
CNS: *Dizziness, headache,* migraines, depression, fatigue
CV: Hypotension, thrombophlebitis, edema, thromboembolism, CVA, stroke, PE, MI
EENT: Diplopia
GI: *Nausea,* vomiting, anorexia, cramps, increased weight, cholestatic jaundice
GU: Amenorrhea, cervical erosion, breakthrough bleeding, dysmenorrhea,

Side effects: *italics* = common; red = life-threatening

vaginal candidiasis, breast changes, (gynecomastia, testicular atrophy, impotence), endometriosis, spontaneous abortion, *breast tenderness*

INTEG: Rash, urticaria, acne, hirsutism, alopecia, oily skin, seborrhea, purpura, melasma

META: Hyperglycemia

PHARMACOKINETICS
Excreted in urine, feces; metabolized in liver, half-life 5-14 hr

INTERACTIONS
Decrease: progestin effect—barbiturates, carBAMazepine, fosphenytoin, phenytoin, rifampin

Drug/Herb
Decrease: contraception—St. John's wort

Drug/Food
Increase: caffeine level—caffeine

Drug/Lab Test
Increase: LDL
Decrease: GTT, HDL, alk phos

NURSING CONSIDERATIONS
Assess:
• **Weight daily:** notify prescriber of weekly weight gain >5 lb
• B/P at beginning of treatment and periodically
• I&O ratio; be alert for decreasing urinary output, increasing edema
• **Hepatic studies:** ALT, AST, bilirubin periodically during long-term therapy
• Edema, hypertension, cardiac symptoms, jaundice, thromboembolism
• **Mental status:** affect, mood, behavioral changes, depression
• Monitor for hypercalcemia
• Monitor Pap smear

Evaluate:
• **Therapeutic response:** decreased abnormal uterine bleeding, absence of amenorrhea

Teach patient/family:
• About cushingoid symptoms (fatigue, weakness, increased thirst/urination, anxiety, weight gain, facial puffiness)
• To report vaginal bleeding, amenorrhea, edema, jaundice, dark urine, clay-colored stools, dyspnea, headache, blurred vision, abdominal pain, numbness or stiffness in legs, chest pain; impotence or gynecomastia (men)
• To take at same time of day; not to interrupt between pill packs
• **Pregnancy:** to report suspected pregnancy immediately; to wait ≥3 mo after stopping product to become pregnant; to use backup contraception methods for 48 hr if treatment is not begun on the first day of menstruation
• To avoid smoking; CV reactions may occur
• That product does not protect against HIV, STDs
• That product may mask onset of menopause

---

nortriptyline (Rx)
(nor-trip′ti-leen)
Aventyl ♣, Pamelor
Func. class.: Antidepressant, tricyclic
Chem. class.: Dibenzocycloheptene—secondary amine

Do not confuse:
nortriptyline/amitriptyline

ACTION: Blocks reuptake of norepinephrine and serotonin into nerve endings, thereby increasing action of norepinephrine and serotonin in nerve cells

USES: Major depression

CONTRAINDICATIONS
Hypersensitivity to tricyclics, carBAMazepine; recovery phase of MI
Precautions: Breastfeeding, suicidal patients, severe depression, increased intraocular pressure, closed-angle glaucoma, urinary retention, cardiac/hepatic disease, hyperthyroidism, electroshock therapy, elective surgery, pregnancy, seizure disorders, prostatic hypertrophy

Black Box Warning: Children, suicidal ideation

DOSAGE AND ROUTES
• **Adult:** PO 25 mg tid or qid; may increase to 150 mg/day; may give daily dose at bedtime
• **Adolescent/elderly:** PO 30-50 mg in 1 or 2 divided doses
Available forms: Caps 10, 25, 50, 75 mg; oral sol 10 mg/5 mL
Administer:
• Store in tight, light-resistant container at room temperature
• Increased fluids, bulk in diet if constipation occurs
• Without regard to meals
• Dosage at bedtime to avoid oversedation during day; may take entire dose at bedtime; geriatric patients may not tolerate once-daily dosing
• Gum, hard candy, frequent sips of water for dry mouth
• **Oral solution:** with fruit juice, water, or milk to disguise taste

SIDE EFFECTS
CNS: *Dizziness, drowsiness,* confusion, headache, anxiety, tremors, stimulation, weakness, insomnia, nightmares, EPS (geriatric patients), increased psychiatric symptoms, seizures
CV: *Orthostatic hypotension,* ECG changes, *tachycardia,* hypertension, palpitations, dysrhythmias
EENT: *Blurred vision,* tinnitus, mydriasis, dry eyes
ENDO: SIADH, hyponatremia, hypothyroidism
GI: *Constipation, dry mouth,* nausea, vomiting, paralytic ileus, increased appetite, cramps, epigastric distress, jaundice, hepatitis, stomatitis, weight gain
GU: *Urinary retention,* acute renal failure, sexual dysfunction
HEMA: Agranulocytosis, thrombocytopenia, eosinophilia, leukopenia
INTEG: Rash, urticaria, sweating, pruritus, photosensitivity
SYST: Serotonin syndrome

PHARMACOKINETICS
PO: Steady-state 4-19 days; metabolized by liver; excreted by kidneys; crosses placenta; excreted in breast milk; half-life 18-28 hr, protein binding 93%-95%

INTERACTIONS
Increase: QT prolongation—class IA/III antidysrhythmics, some phenothiazines, β agonists, local anesthetics, tricyclics, haloperidol, chloroquine, droperidol, pentamidine; CYP3A4 inhibitors (amiodarone, clarithromycin, erythromycin, telithromycin, troleandomycin), arsenic trioxide, levomethadyl; CYP3A4 substrates (methadone, pimozide, QUEtiapine, quiNIDine, risperiDONE, ziprasidone)
• Heavy smoking: decreased product effect
• **Hyperpyretic crisis, seizures, hypertensive episode:** MAOI
Increase: effects of direct-acting sympathomimetics (EPINEPHrine), alcohol, barbiturates, benzodiazepines, CNS depressants, products increasing QT interval, other anticholinergics
Increase: serotonin syndrome, neuroleptic malignant syndrome—SSRIs, SNRIs, serotonin receptor agonists, linezolid; methylene blue (IV)
Decrease: effects of guanethidine, cloNIDine, indirect-acting sympathomimetics (ePHEDrine)
Drug/Herb
Increase: CNS effect—evening primrose oil, kava, valerian
Decrease: nortriptyline level—St. John's wort, SAM-e, yohimbe
Drug/Lab Test
Increase: serum bilirubin, blood glucose, alk phos
Decrease: VMA, 5-HIAA
False increase: urinary catecholamines

NURSING CONSIDERATIONS
Assess:

Black Box Warning: Suicidal thoughts/behaviors in children/young adults: not approved for children; monitor for suicidal ideation in depression, adolescents, young adults

• Monitor for glaucoma exacerbation and paralytic ileus

N

Side effects: *italics* = common; red = life-threatening

- B/P (lying, standing), pulse q4hr; if systolic B/P drops 20 mm Hg, hold product, notify prescriber; VS q4hr in patients with CV disease
- **Blood studies:** thyroid function tests, LFTs, serum nortriptyline level/target 50-150 mg/mL if patient is receiving long-term therapy
- Weight weekly; appetite may increase with product
- **PR, QT prolongation:** dysrhythmias in cardiac patients; assess for chest pain, palpitations, dyspnea
- **EPS primarily in geriatric patients:** rigidity, dystonia, akathisia, preferred tricyclic in geriatric patients
- **Mental status changes:** mood, sensorium, affect, suicidal tendencies, increase in psychiatric symptoms, depression, panic
- Urinary retention, constipation; constipation is more likely to occur in children
- **Withdrawal symptoms:** headache, nausea, vomiting, muscle pain, weakness; do not usually occur unless product was discontinued abruptly
- Alcohol intake; if alcohol is consumed, hold dose until AM
- **Serotonin syndrome, neuroleptic malignant syndrome:** assess for increased heart rate, shivering, sweating, dilated pupils, tremors, high B/P, hyperthermia, headache, confusion; if these occur, stop product, administer serotonin antagonist if needed (rare)
- Assistance with ambulation during beginning therapy because drowsiness/dizziness occurs; safety measures including side rails, primarily for geriatric patients
- **Beers:** avoid in older adults; highly anticholinergic, sedating, and may cause orthostatic hypotension
- **Pregnancy/breastfeeding:** use only if benefits outweigh fetal risk; cautious use in breastfeeding

Evaluate:
- **Therapeutic response:** decreased depression

Teach patient/family:
- That therapeutic effects may take 2-3 wk; only small quantities may be dispersed
- To use caution when driving, during other activities requiring alertness because of drowsiness, dizziness, blurred vision
- To avoid alcohol ingestion, other CNS depressants; to avoid MAOIs within 14 days
- Not to discontinue medication quickly after long-term use; may cause nausea, headache, malaise
- To wear sunscreen or large hat because photosensitivity occurs
- To immediately report urinary retention, worsening depression, suicidal thoughts/behaviors

TREATMENT OF OVERDOSE: ECG monitoring; lavage; administer anticonvulsant

---

nusinersen (Rx)

(neu-si-ner′sen)

Spinraza
Func. class.: Miscellaneous CNS agent for muscular dystrophy
Chem. class.: Antisense oligonucleotide

Do not confuse:
Nusinersen/Neurontin
Nucynta, Sprinraza/Spriva

USES: Spinal muscular atrophy

DOSAGE AND ROUTES
Adult/child: Intrathecal 12 mg q14days 3 doses, then 12 mg q30days after third dose; maintenance 12 mg q4mo thereafter
Available forms: Injection 12 mg/5 mL single-use vials

---

nystatin, systemic (Rx)

(nye-stat′in)

Nystop, Nyaderm ✦
Func. class.: Antifungal
Chem. class.: Amphoteric polyene

ACTION: Interferes with fungal DNA replication; binds sterols in fungal cell

---

membrane, which increases permeability, leaking of cell nutrients

USES: *Candida* species causing oral, intestinal infections

CONTRAINDICATIONS
Hypersensitivity
Precautions: Pregnancy, breastfeeding, systemic infection

DOSAGE AND ROUTES
Oral infection
• **Adult/adolescent/child: SUSP** 400,000-600,000 units qid; use ½ dose in each side of mouth; swish and swallow; use for at least 48 hr after symptoms resolved
• **Infant: SUSP** 200,000 units qid (100,000 units in each side of mouth)
• **Newborn and premature infant: SUSP** 100,000 units qid
• **Adult/child: TROCHES** 200,000-400,000 units qid × ≤2 wk
GI infection
• **Adult: PO** 500,000-1,000,000 units tid
Cutaneous candidiasis
• **Adult/child: Top cream/ointment** apply to affected area bid; **powder** apply to affected area bid-tid
Available forms: Tabs 500,000 units; suspension 100,000 mg/mL
Administer:
Store at room temperature for oral susp; tabs in tight, light-resistant containers at room temperature
PO route
• Oral susp dose by placing ½ in each cheek, then swallow; do not mix with food
• Topical dose after cleansing area; mouth may be swabbed; very moist lesions best treated with topical powder

SIDE EFFECTS
GI: Nausea, vomiting, anorexia, diarrhea, cramps

PHARMACOKINETICS
PO: Little absorption, excreted in feces

NURSING CONSIDERATIONS
Assess:
• **Allergic reaction:** rash, urticaria, irritated oral mucous membranes; product may have to be discontinued
• Obtain culture, histologic tests to confirm organism
• Predisposing factors: antibiotic therapy, pregnancy, diabetes mellitus, sexual partner infection (vaginal infections)
• **Pregnancy/breastfeeding:** use only if clearly needed; may breastfeed
Evaluate:
• **Therapeutic response:** culture negative for *Candida*
Teach patient/family:
• That long-term therapy may be needed to clear infection; to complete entire course of medication
• To avoid commercial mouthwashes for mouth infection
• To shake susp before measuring each dose, to swish and swallow
• To notify prescriber of irritation; product may have to be discontinued

---

nystatin topical
See Appendix B

---

obeticholic acid (Rx)
(oh-bet-i-koe′lik as′id)

Ocaliva

Func. class.: Farnesoid X receptor agonist

USES: Treatment of primary biliary cholangitis (PBC) in combination with ursodiol (ursodeoxycholic acid) with an inadequate response to ursodiol, or in those unable to tolerate ursodiol

Black Box Warning: Hepatic decompensation/failure

DOSAGE AND ROUTES
Adult: PO Noncirrhotic or compensated Child-Pugh class A: Initial: 5 mg daily; if an adequate reduction in alkaline phosphatase and/or total bilirubin has not been achieved after 3 mo, increase to 10 mg daily, max 10 mg/day
Hepatic dose
• **Adult: PO** Child-Pugh B-C 5 mg weekly ×3 mo then increase as needed
Available forms: Tabs 5, 10 mg

⚠ HIGH ALERT

obinutuzumab (Rx)
(oh′bi-nue-tooz′ue-mab)

Gazyva

Func. class.: Antineoplastic; biologic response modifier; monoclonal antibody

ACTION: A recombinant, human monoclonal antibody that binds to the gastric B-lymphocyte–associated antibody; action is indirect, possible through T-cell–mediated anti-tumor responses

USES: Chronic lymphocytic leukemia, previously untreated in combination with chlorambucil; non-Hodgkin's lymphoma (follicular lymphoma) in relapse or refractory to rituximab-containing regimen, used in combination; previously untreated stage II bulky, III, or IV follicular lymphoma in combination, then monotherapy

CONTRAINDICATIONS
Hypersensitivity
Precautions: Pregnancy, breastfeeding, cardiac disease, children, human antichimeric antibody (HACA), human antimurine antibody (HAMA), infection, infusion-related reactions, neutropenia, pulmonary disease, thrombocytopenia, tumor lysis syndrome, vaccination

Black Box Warning: Hepatitis B exacerbation, progressive multifocal leukoencephalopathy

DOSAGE AND ROUTES
Chronic lymphocytic leukemia (previously untreated); in combination with chlorambucil
• **Adult: IV: Cycle 1:** 100 mg on day 1, followed by 900 mg on day 2, followed by 1000 mg weekly for 2 doses (days 8 and 15); treatment cycle is 28 days; **cycles 2-6:** 1000 mg on day 1 every 28 days for 5 doses
Follicular lymphoma (relapsed/refractory)
• **Adult: IV: Cycle 1 (in combination with bendamustine):** 1000 mg weekly on days 1, 8, and 15; treatment cycle is 28 days; **cycles 2-6 (in combination with bendamustine):** 1000 mg on day 1 every 28 days for 5 doses; **obinutuzumab monotherapy:** 1000 mg every 2 mo for up to 2 yr
Available forms: Sol for inj 1000 mg/40 mL (25 mg/mL)
Administer:
IV intermittent INFUSION route
• Due to the risk of hypotension, consider withholding antihypertensive medications for 12 hr before, during, and for the 1st hr after use until blood pressure is stable
• Single-use vials do not contain preservatives
• Do not mix with other products
• Give antimicrobial prophylaxis to neutropenic patients throughout treatment; consider antiviral and antifungal prophylaxis as needed

- **Premedication for cycle 1, days 1 and 2:** acetaminophen 650-1000 mg, and diphenhydrAMINE 50 mg at least 30 min before infusion, dexamethasone 20 mg IV or methylPREDNISolone 80 mg IV at least 1 hr before infusion
- **Premedication for cycle 1, days 8 and 15, and cycles 2-6, day 1:** acetaminophen 650-1000 mg at least 30 min before infusion; those with any infusion-related reaction with the previous infusion should also receive diphenhydrAMINE 50 mg at least 30 min before the infusion; if the patient had a grade 3 infusion-related reaction with the previous dose or has a lymphocyte count >25 × 10⁹/L, additionally administer dexamethasone 20 mg IV or methylPREDNISolone 80 mg IV at least 1 hr before infusion
- Use in a facility to adequately monitor and treat infusion reactions
- Visually inspect parenteral products for particulate matter and discoloration before use
- Prepare all doses in 0.9% NaCl; do not admix; use a final concentration of 0.4-4 mg/mL; give as an IV infusion only

Reconstitution: Cycle 1, days 1 and 2:
- Withdraw 4 mL (100 mg) from the vial and dilute into 100 mL 0.9% NaCl for use on day 1; mix by gentle inversion; do not shake, use immediately
- Withdraw the remaining 36 mL (900 mg) and dilute into 250 mL 0.9% NaCl for use on day 2; mix by gentle inversion; do not shake

Cycle 1, days 8 and 15; cycles 2-6:
- Withdraw 40 mL (1000 mg) from the vial and dilute into 250 mL 0.9% NaCl; mix by gentle inversion; do not shake
- Store following reconstitution: store at 2° C-8° C (36° F-46° F) for up to 24 hr; do not freeze; allow to come to room temperature before administration; use a dedicated line, protect from light
- **Day 1 (100-mg dose):** give at initial rate of 25 mg/hr over 4 hr; do not increase the infusion rate

- **Day 2 (900-mg dose):** give at 50 mg/hr × 30 min; if no hypersensitivity or infusion-related events occur, increase the rate by 50 mg/hr q30min to a max rate of 400 mg/hr
- **Subsequent infusions (1000-mg dose):** give at rate of 100 mg/hr for 30 min; if no hypersensitivity or infusion-related events occur, increase the infusion rate by 100 mg/hr q30min, max rate of 400 mg/hr

SIDE EFFECTS
CNS: Headache, *fever,* chills, flushing
CV: Cardiac arrest, MI, sinus tachycardia, hypertension
GI: *Constipation,* decreased appetite, diarrhea, hepatitis/hepatic failure, nausea, vomiting
HEMA: Neutropenia, thrombocytopenia, lymphopenia, leukopenia, *anemia*
META: Lower potassium/*sodium*/calcium, aluminum, higher *potassium*/uric acid
RESP: Wheezing, dyspnea, *cough*
SYST: Tumor lysis syndrome, *infection*
MISC: *Arthralgia*

PHARMACOKINETICS
Terminal half-life 29 days

INTERACTIONS
Increase: adverse reactions—abciximab, belimumab, cloZAPine, pimecrolimus; avoid concurrent use
Increase: infection—denosumab, natalizumab, live virus vaccines
Increase: hypotension—antihypertensives
Increase: thrombocytopenia—chlorambucil
Increase: hematologic toxicity—leflunomide
Increase: immunosuppression—tofacitinib; avoid concurrent use
Drug/Herb
Decrease: obinutuzumab—echinacea
Drug/Lab

NURSING CONSIDERATIONS
Assess:

Black Box Warning: Hepatitis B: reactivation of HBV in those who are HBsAg positive, HBsAg negative, and core antibody anti-HBc positive; may result in fulminant hepatitis, hepatic failure, or death, screen high-risk patients before use, monitor carriers for active HBV infection during and for several months after therapy completion, discontinue treatment of any other antineoplastics if infection is reactivated

Black Box Warning: Progressive multifocal leukoencephalopathy (PML): notify prescriber of any new, worsening neurologic signs/symptoms (ataxia, visual changes, confusion)

• **Tumor lysis syndrome:** can occur within 24 hr of 1st infusion; those with high tumor burden or lymphocyte count $>25 \times 10^9$/L are at increased risk; monitor serum creatinine, potassium, calcium, uric acid, phosphate closely
• **Severe/life-threatening infusion reactions:** ⅔ have a reaction to 1st dose; consider withholding antihypertensives for 12 hr before, during, and for 1 hour after infusion
• **Bone marrow suppression:** CBC with differential before infusion and regularly, platelets
• **Infection:** signs of infection; provide neutropenia precautions
• **Pregnancy/breastfeeding:** use only if benefits outweigh fetal risk; do not breastfeed, excretion unknown
Evaluate:
• **Therapeutic response:** decreased disease progression
Teach patient/family:
• About the reason for treatment and expected results
• To avoid live virus vaccines, that vaccinations should be brought up-to-date before treatment

Black Box Warning: Hepatitis B: to report yellow skin, eyes, fatigue, dark urine; that continuing follow-up will be needed

Black Box Warning: Progressive multifocal leukoencephalopathy (PML): to report confusion, visual changes, dizziness, difficulty walking or talking

---

ocrelizumab (Rx)
(oc′-re-liz′-ue-mab)
Ocrevus, Mycapssa
Func. class.: Multiple sclerosis agent

USES: For the treatment of multiple sclerosis

CONTRAINDICATIONS
Hypersensitivity

DOSAGE AND ROUTES
Relapsing or primary progressive forms of multiple sclerosis
• **Adult: IV INFUSION** 300 mg then a second 300 mg 2 wk later; subsequent infusions of 600 mg are given q6mo
Available forms: Solution for injection 300 mg (30 mg/mL)

---

octreotide (Rx)
(ok-tree′oh-tide)
Bynfezia, Mycapssa, SandoSTATIN, SandoSTATIN LAR Depot
Func. class.: Growth hormone, antidiarrheal
Chem. class.: Synthetic analog of somatostatin

Do not confuse:
SandoSTATIN/SandIMMUNE

ACTION: A potent growth hormone similar to somatostatin

USES: SandoSTATIN: acromegaly, improves symptoms of carcinoid tumors, vasoactive intestinal peptide tumors (VIPomas); **LAR Depot:** long-term maintenance of acromegaly, carcinoid tumors, VIPomas
Unlabeled uses: GI fistula, variceal bleeding, diarrheal conditions, pancreatic fistula, irritable bowel syndrome, dumping syndrome, short bowel syndrome, insulinoma, hepatorenal syndrome

CONTRAINDICATIONS
Hypersensitivity

Precautions: Pregnancy, breastfeeding, children, geriatric patients, diabetes mellitus, hypothyroidism, renal disease

DOSAGE AND ROUTES
Acromegaly
• **Adult: SUBCUT/IV (SandoSTATIN)** 50-100 mcg bid-tid, adjust q2wk based on growth hormone levels or **IM (SandoSTATIN LAR)** 20 mg q4wk × 3 mo, adjust based on growth hormone levels; **PO** 20 mg bid. Monitor IGF-1 levels and patient's signs and symptoms every 2 wk to guide titration. Increase dosage in increments of 20 mg daily. For dosages of 60 mg/day, administer 40 mg PO in the morning and 20 mg PO in the evening. For dosages of 80 mg/day, administer 40 mg PO twice daily. Max: 80 mg/day PO.

Hepatic/renal dose
• **Adult:** LAR Depot IM 10 mg q4wk (cirrhosis); 20-mg capsules qday (renal failure)

VIPomas (watery diarrhea)
• **Adult: SUBCUT (SandoSTATIN)** 200-300 mcg/day in 2-4 doses for 2 wk, or **IM(SandoSTATIN LAR)** 20 mg q4wk × 2 mo, adjust dose

Flushing/diarrhea in carcinoid tumors
• **Adult: SUBCUT (SandoSTATIN)** 100-600 mcg/day in 2-4 doses for 2 wk, titrated to patient response or **IM (SandoSTATIN LAR)** 20 mg q4wk × 2 mo, adjust dose

Gastroentero-pancreatic fistula
• **Adult: SUBCUT (SandoSTATIN)** 100 mcg tid

Variceal bleeding (unlabeled)
• **Adult: IV bolus** 50 mcg; then 50 mcg/ hr continuous IV infusion for 2-5 days

Available forms: Inj (SandoSTATIN) 0.05, 0.1, 0.2, 0.5, 1 mg/mL; inj powder for susp (LAR depot) 10, 20, 30 mg/5 mL; delayed-release capsule 20 mg

Administer:
• Store in refrigerator for unopened amps, vials, or at room temperature for 2 wk; protect from light; do not use discolored or cloudy sol
• Do not use if discolored or if particulates are present

• Do not confuse products

PO route
• Give with water on empty stomach ≥1 hr before or >2 hr after a meal
• Swallow capsules whole; do not cut, break, chew

IM route
• Reconstitute with diluent provided; give in gluteal region, immediately after reconstitution, rotate injection sites

SUBCUT route
• Rotate inj site; use hip, thigh, abdomen
• Avoid using medication that is cold; allow to reach room temperature; do not use LAR depot, do not use if discolored or if particulates are present
• SUBCUT dose should be given with IM depot dose for 2 wk before discontinuing SUBCUT dose (carcinoid tumors, VIPomas)

IV route
• **IV direct:** give over 3 min; may give undiluted
• **Intermittent IV infusion:** dilute in 50-200 mL D₅W, 0.9% NaCl; give over 15-30 min
• Solution is stable for 24 hr, protect from light

Y-site compatibilities: Acyclovir, alfentanil, allopurinol, amifostine, amikacin, aminocaproic acid, aminophylline, amiodarone, amphotericin B colloidal, amphotericin B lipid complex, amphotericin B liposome, ampicillin, ampicillin-sulbactam, anidulafungin, argatroban, arsenic trioxide, atenolol, atracurium, azithromycin, aztreonam, bivalirudin, bleomycin, bumetanide, buprenorphine, busulfan, butorphanol, calcium chloride/gluconate, capreomycin, CARBOplatin, carmustine, caspofungin, ceFAZolin, cefepime, cefotaxime, cefoTEtan, cefOXitin, cefTAZidime, ceftizoxime, cefTRIAXone, cefuroxime, chloramphenicol, chlorproMAZINE, cimetidine, ciprofloxacin, cisatracurium, CISplatin, clindamycin, cyclophosphamide, cycloSPORINE, cytarabine, dacarbazine, DACTINomycin, DAPTOmycin, DAUNOrubicin, DAUNOrubicin liposome, dexamethasone, digoxin, diltiaZEM, diphenhydrAMINE, DOBUTamine, DOCEtaxel, dolasetron, DOPamine, DOXOrubicin, DOXOrubicin liposomal, doxycycline, droperidol, enalaprilat, ePHEDrine, EPINEPHrine, epiRUBicin, eptifibatide, ertapenem, erythromycin, esmolol, etoposide, famotidine, fenoldopam, fentaNYL, fluconazole, fludarabine, fluorouracil, foscarnet, fosphenytoin, furosemide, gallium nitrate, ganciclovir, gatifloxacin, gemcitabine, gentamicin, glycopyrrolate, granisetron, haloperidol, heparin, hydrALAZINE, hydrocortisone, HYDROmorphone, hydrOXYzine, IDArubicin, ifosfamide, imipenem-cilastatin, insulin (regular), irinotecan, isoproterenol, ketorolac, labetalol, lansoprazole, leucovorin, levoFLOXacin, lidocaine, linezolid, LORazepam, magnesium sulfate, mannitol, mechlorethamine, melphalan, meperidine, meropenem, mesna, methohexital, methotrexate, methyldopate, methylPREDNISolone, metoclopramide, metoprolol, metroNIDAZOLE, midazolam, milrinone, minocycline, mitoMYcin, mitoXANTRONE, mivacurium, morphine, moxifloxacin, mycophenolate, nafcillin, nalbuphine, naloxone, nesiritide, niCARdipine, nitroglycerin, nitroprusside, norepinephrine, ondansetron, oxaliplatin, PACLitaxel, palonosetron, pamidronate, pancuronium, PEMEtrexed, pentamidine, pentazocine, PENTobarbital, PHENobarbital, phenylephrine, piperacillin, piperacillin-tazobactam, polymyxin B, potassium acetate/chloride/phosphates, procainamide, prochlorperazine, promethazine, propranolol, quiNIDine, quinupristin-dalfopristin, raNITIdine, remifentanil, rocuronium, sodium acetate/bicarbonate/phosphates, streptozocin, succinylcholine, SUFentanil, sulfamethoxazole-trimethoprim, tacrolimus, teniposide, thiopental, thiotepa, ticarcillin, ticarcillin-clavulanate, tigecycline, tirofiban, tobramycin, topotecan, vancomycin, vasopressin, vecuronium, verapamil, vinBLAStine, vinCRIStine, vinorelbine, voriconazole, zidovudine, zoledronic acid

SIDE EFFECTS

CNS: *Headache, dizziness, fatigue, weakness,* depression, anxiety, tremors, seizure, paranoia
CV: *Sinus bradycardia, conduction abnormalities,* dysrhythmias, chest pain, SOB, thrombophlebitis, ischemia, HF, hypertension, palpitations, QT prolongation
ENDO: *Hypo/hyperglycemia, ketosis, hypothyroidism,* galactorrhea, diabetes insipidus
GI: *Diarrhea, nausea, abdominal pain, vomiting, flatulence, distention, constipation,* increased LFTs, cholelithiasis, ileus
GU: UTI
HEMA: Hematoma of inj site, bruise
INTEG: Rash, urticaria, pain; inflammation at inj site

PHARMACOKINETICS

Absorbed rapidly, completely; peak ½ hr (subcut/IV), 2-3 wk (IM); half-life 1.7 hr, duration 12 hr, excreted unchanged in urine 32%, protein binding 65%

INTERACTIONS

Increase: QT prolongation—class IA/III antidysrhythmics, some phenothiazines, β agonists, local anesthetics, tricyclics, haloperidol, chloroquine, droperidol, pentamidine; CYP3A4 inhibitors (amiodarone, clarithromycin, erythromycin, telithromycin, troleandomycin); arsenic trioxide; CYP3A4 substrates (methadone, pimozide, QUEtiapine, quiNIDine, risperiDONE, ziprasidone)
Increase: effect of β-blockers, quiNIDine, rifAMPin, reduction of dose may be required
Increase: hypoglycemia: MAOIs, salicylates, SSRIs, assess for hypoglycemia
Decrease: effect of insulin, oral antidiabetics, monitor blood glucose
Decrease: effect of—bromocriptine
Decrease: effect of—cycloSPORINE, dose may need to be modified
Drug/Food
Decrease: absorption of dietary fat, vit B_{12} levels
Drug/Lab Test
Increase: glucose
Decrease: T_4, thyroid function tests, vit B_{12}, glucose

NURSING CONSIDERATIONS
Assess:
• Growth hormone antibodies, IGF-1 at 1- to 4-hr intervals for 8-12 hr after dose (**acromegaly**); 5-HIAA, plasma serotonin;

blood glucose, serotonin levels **(carcinoid tumors),** plasma substance P, plasma vasoactive intestinal peptide (VIP) **(VIPoma)**
• Thyroid function tests: T_3, T_4, T_7, TSH to identify hypothyroidism
• Vital signs B/P, pulse, hydration status
• Fecal fat, serum carotene, somatomedin-C q14days, glucose; plasma serotonin levels (carcinoid tumors); plasma vasoactive intestinal peptide levels (VIPoma); serum growth hormone, serum IGF-1 baseline and periodically, diabetes to monitor blood glucose
• Chronic therapy may cause B_{12} absorption issues; monitor B_{12} and replace if necessary
• **Allergic reaction:** rash, itching, fever, nausea, wheezing
• **Cardiac status:** bradycardia, conduction abnormalities, dysrhythmias; monitor ECG for QT prolongation, low voltage, axis shifts, early repolarization, R/S transition, early wave progression
• Gallbladder disease, monitor for abdominal pain, ultrasound of gallbladder baseline, periodically
• **Ileus:** assess character of stools, bowel sounds, baseline and throughout treatment
• **Pregnancy/breastfeeding:** use only if benefits outweigh fetal risk; cautious use in breastfeeding, excreted in breast milk
Evaluate:
• **Therapeutic response:** relief of diarrhea in patients with AIDS; improved symptoms of carcinoid or VIP tumors; decreasing symptoms of acromegaly
Teach patient/family:
• That regular assessments are required; that diabetics need to monitor blood glucose
• To use as prescribed, not to miss, double doses; if a dose is missed, take when remembered unless close to next dose
• About SUBCUT inj if patient or other persons will be giving inj, provide instructions for use
• That product may cause dizziness, drowsiness, weakness; to avoid hazardous activities if these occur; to report abdominal pain immediately
• That patients with diabetes need to monitor glucose regularly
• **Pregnancy/breastfeeding:** Teach patient to report if pregnancy is planned or suspected or if breastfeeding; teach patient pregnancy may occur in acromegaly since fertility may be restored; to use contraceptive if pregnancy is unwanted

odevixibat (Rx)
(OH-de-VIX-i-bat)
Bylvay
Func. class.: Bile acid transport (IBAT) inhibitor

USES: Progressive familial intrahepatic cholestasis for the treatment of pruritus in patients 3 mo of age and older

DOSAGE AND ROUTES
• **Child: PO** Initial dose: 40 mcg/kg daily in the morning; maintenance 40-120 mcg/kg daily in the morning; max 6 mg/day
Available forms: Capsules 400, 1200 mcg; Oral pellets, capsules 200 mcg, 600 mcg

ofloxacin (Rx)
(o-flox´a-sin)
Func. class.: Antiinfective
Chem. class.: Fluoroquinolone

ACTION: Interferes with conversion of intermediate DNA fragments into high-molecular-weight DNA in bacteria; inhibits DNA gyrase

USES: Treatment of lower respiratory tract infections (pneumonia, bronchitis), genitourinary infections (prostatitis, UTIs) caused by *Escherichia coli, Klebsiella pneumoniae, Chlamydia trachomatis,* skin and skin-structure infections; otitis media, PID
Unlabeled uses: Spontaneous bacterial peritonitis

CONTRAINDICATIONS
Hypersensitivity to quinolones
Precautions: Pregnancy, breastfeeding, children, geriatric patients, renal disease, seizure disorders, excessive sunlight, hypokalemia, colitis, QT prolongation

Side effects: *italics* = common; red = life-threatening

Black Box Warning: Tendon pain/rupture, tendinitis, myasthenia gravis, psychiatric event, peripheral neuropathy, neurotoxicity, acute bacterial exacerbations of UTIs/bronchitis

DOSAGE AND ROUTES
Cervicitis/urethritis (acute)
• **Adult:** PO Nongonococcal (due to *Chlamydia trachomatis*): 300 mg q12hr × 7 days; 400 mg as a single dose (gonorrhea)
Chronic bronchitis (acute exacerbation), community-acquired pneumonia, skin and skin structure infections (uncomplicated)
• **Adult:** PO 400 mg q12hr × 10 days
Pelvic inflammatory disease (acute)
• **Adult:** PO: 400 mg q12hr × 10-14 days, use with metronidazole
Prostatitis
• **Adult:** PO 300 mg q12hr × 6 wk
UTI
• **Adult:** PO **Uncomplicated:** 200 mg q12hr × 3-7 days; **complicated:** 200 mg q12hr × 10 days
Spontaneous bacterial peritonitis (unlabeled)
• **Adult:** PO 400 mg q12h × 5-7 days
Renal dose
• **Adult: PO** CCr 20-50 mL/min, give q24hr; CCr <20 mL/min, give 50% of dose q24hr
Hepatic dose
• **Adult (Child-Pugh class C): PO** max 400 mg/day
Available forms: Tabs 200, 300, 400 mg
Administer:
PO route
• 2 hr before or 2 hr after antacids, calcium, iron, zinc products, without regard to food, maintain hydration
• Store at room temperature, protect from light

SIDE EFFECTS
CNS: *Dizziness, headache, fatigue, somnolence,* depression, insomnia, lethargy, malaise, seizures, vertigo
CV: QT prolongation, dysrhythmias, chest pain
EENT: Visual disturbances, pharyngitis

GI: *Diarrhea, nausea, vomiting,* anorexia, flatulence, heartburn, dry mouth, increased AST, ALT, abdominal pain, constipation, CDAD, abnormal taste, xerostomia
HEMA: Blood dyscrasias
INTEG: Rash, pruritus, photosensitivity
MS: Tendinitis, tendon rupture, rhabdomyolysis
SYST: Anaphylaxis, Stevens-Johnson syndrome, toxic epidermal necrolysis

PHARMACOKINETICS
PO: Peak 1-2 hr; half-life 4-8 hr; steady-state 2 days; excreted in urine as active product, metabolites; 90%-95% bioavailability

INTERACTIONS

Black Box Warning: Increase: tendon rupture/tendinitis—corticosteroids

• May alter blood glucose levels: antidiabetics
Possible theophylline toxicity: theophylline
Increase: QT prolongation—class IA/III antidysrhythmics, some phenothiazines, β-agonists, local anesthetics, tricyclics, haloperidol, methadone, chloroquine, clarithromycin, droperidol, erythromycin, pentamidine
Increase: CNS stimulation, seizures—NSAIDs
Increase: anticoagulation—warfarin
Decrease: ofloxacin—sevelamer
Decrease: absorption—antacids with aluminum, magnesium, iron products, sucralfate, zinc products; separate by 2 hr
Drug/Lab Test
Increase: INR

NURSING CONSIDERATIONS
Assess:

Black Box Warning: Tendon rupture/tendinitis: more common in lung, heart, kidney transplants or geriatric patients; assess for pain or inflammation; product should be discontinued; steroids may increase risk

• **Blood studies:** BUN, creatinine, AST, ALT, CBC, blood glucose, INR (warfarin

use); hypoglycemia is more common in diabetes in those >60 yr
• **CNS symptoms:** insomnia, vertigo, headache, agitation, confusion; **seizures, pseudotumor cerebri; if serious CNS reactions occur, stop drug**

Black Box Warning: Myasthenia gravis: product may increase weakness; avoid use in patients with myasthenia gravis

Black Box Warning: Peripheral neuropathy: stop drug immediately if this occurs, may be more common with fluoroquinolones

Black Box Warning: CDAD: assess for diarrhea during and for a few months after discontinuing drug, if CDAD is suspected, discontinue

• For overgrowth of infection in long-term treatment
• **Anaphylaxis, Stevens-Johnson syndrome, toxic epidermal necrolysis:** rash, flushing, urticaria, pruritus, peripheral neuropathy; may be fatal; may occur even after first dose; have emergency equipment nearby
Evaluate:
• **Therapeutic response:** culture negative, absence of symptoms of infection
Teach patient/family:
• To ambulate, perform activities using assistance if dizziness or light-headedness occurs
• To complete full course of therapy; to take with plenty of fluids
• That those with diabetes are more prone to hypoglycemia
• To avoid iron- or mineral-containing supplements within 2 hr before or after dose; to take without regard to meals
• **Anaphylaxis, Stevens-Johnson syndrome, toxic epidermal necrolysis:** that allergic reactions usually occur after first dose but may occur later; to stop product; to report to prescriber rash, fever
• To report bloody diarrhea immediately
• To avoid sun exposure; photosensitivity can occur

• To avoid use with other products unless approved by prescriber
• To notify prescriber immediately if tingling, pain in extremities occurs; muscle/tendon pain, numbness in extremities

ofloxacin ophthalmic
See Appendix B

OLANZapine (Rx) REMS
(oh-lanz′a-peen)
ZyPREXA, ZyPREXA Relprevv, ZyPREXA Zydis
Func. class.: Antipsychotic (1st generation), neuroleptic
Chem. class.: Thienobenzodiazepine

Do not confuse:
OLANZapine/olsalazine
ZyPREXA/CeleXA/ZyrTEC /Zestril/Zolpidem

ACTION: May mediate antipsychotic activity by both DOPamine and serotonin type 2 (5-HT2) antagonists; may antagonize muscarinic receptors, histaminic (H_1)- and α-adrenergic receptors

USES: Schizophrenia, acute manic episodes with bipolar disorder, acute agitation
Unlabeled uses: Chemotherapy-related breakthrough or prevention of nausea, vomiting

CONTRAINDICATIONS
Hypersensitivity
Precautions: Pregnancy, breastfeeding, geriatric patients, hypertension, cardiac/renal/hepatic disease, diabetes, agranulocytosis, abrupt discontinuation, Asian patients, closed-angle glaucoma, coma, leukopenia, QT prolongation, tardive dyskinesia, torsades de pointes, suicidal ideation, stroke history, TIA

Black Box Warning: Increased mortality in elderly patients with dementia-related psychosis, postinjection delirium/sedation syndrome

Side effects: *italics* = common; red = life-threatening

DOSAGE AND ROUTES

Schizophrenia
• **Adult: PO** 5-10 mg/day initially, may increase dosage by 5 mg at ≥1 wk intervals, max 20 mg/day; **ORALLY DISINTEGRATING** tabs: daily, open blister pack, place tab on tongue, let disintegrate, swallow; **ext rel inj** (Zyprexa Relprevv) IM 150-300 mg q2wk or 405 mg q4wk
• **Geriatric/debilitated: PO** 5 mg/day, may increase cautiously at 1-wk intervals, max 20 mg/day
• **Adolescent: PO** 2.5 or 5 mg/day, target 10 mg/day, max 20 mg

Acute mania or associated with bipolar I disorder
• **Adult: PO** 10-15 mg/day, may increase dose after >24 hr by 5 mg, max 20 mg/day, usually for 2 wk
• **Adolescent ≥13 yr: PO** 2.5 or 5 mg/day, target 10 mg/day, max 20 mg/day

Acute agitation associated with schizophrenia, bipolar I mania
• **Adult: IM** (reg rel) 2.5-10, usual dose 10 mg once
• **Geriatrc: IM** (reg rel) 2.5-5 mg once

Short-term treatment of acute mixed/manic episodes of bipolar I disorder with lithium or valproate
• **Adult: PO** 10 mg/day for 6 wk (range 5-20 mg/day)

Bipolar I disorder maintenance
• **Adult: PO** 5-20 mg/day
• **Adolescent ≥13 yr: PO** 2.5 or 5 mg qday, may increase by 1.5 mg or 5 mg, max 20 mg/day, Maintenance: 10 mg/day

Depression associated with bipolar I disorder
• **Adult: PO** 5 mg with fluoxetine 20 mg qday

Treatment-resistant depression
• **Adult: PO** 5 mg with fluoxetine 20 mg/day given in evening, may increase fluoxetine to 50 mg/day and to 20 mg/day OLANZapine

Chemotherapy nausea/vomiting prophylaxis (unlabeled)
• **Adult:** 10 mg on day of chemotherapy, then 10 mg on day 2, 3, 4 with dexamethasone and palonosetron day 1;

breakthrough nausea/vomiting 10 mg daily × 3 days

Available forms: Tab 2.5, 5, 7.5, 10, 15, 20 mg; **orally disintegrating tabs** 5, 10, 15, 20 mg (ZyPREXA Zydis); **powder for inj** 10 mg; **ext rel powder for susp for inj** 210, 300, 405 mg base/vial (ZyPREXA Relprevv)

Administer:
• Decreased dose in geriatric patients
PO route
• With full glass of water, milk, food to decrease GI upset, may give without regard to food
• Store in tight, light-resistant container
• **Orally disintegrating tabs:** open blister pack; place tab on tongue until dissolved; swallow; no water needed; do not break, crush, chew
• Keep recumbent if dizziness occurs
IM route (ZyPREXA intramuscular)
• Inspect for particulate, discoloration before use; if present, do not use
• Dissolve contents of vials with 2.1 mL sterile water for inj (5 mg/mL); use immediately
• Do not use IV or subcut
• Inject slowly, deep into muscle mass
• Keep recumbent if dizziness occurs
IM route (ZyPREXA Relprevv)

Black Box Warning: Available only through restricted distribution program (Zyprexa Relprevv Patient Care Program, 877-772-9390) due to postinjection delirium/sedation syndrome; given at a facility with emergency services; continuous observation; monitor for 3 hr after injection

• Use gloves to prepare; irritating to skin
• Use deep IM gluteal inj only
• Use only diluent provided in kit; give q2-4wk using 19-G, 1.5-inch needle in kit; for obese patients, use 19-G, 2-inch or larger needle

SIDE EFFECTS
CNS: EPS (pseudoparkinsonism, akathisia, dystonia, tardive dyskinesia), seizures, headache, neuroleptic malignant syndrome (rare), agitation, nervousness,

hostility, *dizziness,* hypertonia, *tremor,* euphoria, confusion, *drowsiness,* fatigue, abnormal gait, insomnia, fever, suicidal thoughts

CV: Hypotension, tachycardia, chest pain, heart failure, sudden death (geriatric patients, IM), orthostatic hypotension, peripheral edema

ENDO: Increased prolactin levels (dose related), hypo/hyperglycemia

GI: *Dry mouth, nausea, vomiting, appetite, dyspepsia,* anorexia, *constipation,* abdominal pain, *weight gain,* jaundice, hepatitis

GU: Urinary retention, urinary frequency, enuresis, impotence, amenorrhea, gynecomastia, breast engorgement, premenstrual syndrome

HEMA: Neutropenia, agranulocytosis, leukopenia

INTEG: Rash

MISC: Peripheral edema, accidental injury, hypertonia, hyperlipidemia

MS: *Joint pain,* twitching

RESP: *Cough, pharyngitis;* fatal pneumonia (geriatric patients, IM)

PHARMACOKINETICS

Well absorbed (60%), metabolized by liver, glucuronidation/oxidation by CYP1A2 and CYP2D6; excreted in urine (57%), feces (30%); 93% bound to plasma proteins; half-life 21-54 hr, extended in geriatric patients; clearance decreased in women, increased in smokers, peak PO 6 hr, IM 15-45 min, IM ext rel 7 days

INTERACTIONS

Increase: sedation—other CNS depressants, alcohol, barbiturate anesthetics, antihistamines, sedatives/hypnotics, antidepressants

Increase: OLANZapine levels—CYP1A2 inhibitors (fluvoxaMINE)

Increase: hypotension—antihypertensives, alcohol, diazePAM

Increase: anticholinergic effects—anticholinergics

Black Box Warning: Increase: respiratory depression—opioids

Decrease: OLANZapine levels—CYP1A2 inducers: carBAMazepine, omeprazole, rifAMPin

Decrease: antiparkinson activity—levodopa, bromocriptine, other DOPamine agonists

Drug/Lab Test

Increase: LFTs, prolactin, CPK, glucose, uric acid, eosinophils

Drug/Herb

Increase: toxicity—kava

Decrease: olanzapine effect—St. John's wort; avoid concurrent use

NURSING CONSIDERATIONS
Assess:

Black Box Warning: Postinjection delirium/sedation syndrome (ZyPREXA Relprevv): monitor continuously for ≥3 hr after injection; patient must be accompanied when leaving: assess for sedation, coma, delirium, EPS, slurred speech, altered gait, aggression, dizziness, weakness, hypertension, seizures; before leaving, confirm that patient is alert, oriented, and free of any other symptoms

• **Mental status:** assess orientation, affect, LOC, reflexes, coordination, sleep pattern disturbances, mood, behavior, presence of hallucinations and type before initial administration, monthly; EPS, including akathisia (inability to sit still, no pattern to movements), tardive dyskinesia (bizarre movements of jaw, mouth, tongue, extremities), pseudoparkinsonism (rigidity, tremors, pill rolling, shuffling gait), suicidal thoughts, behaviors

• **Renal status:** I&O ratio; palpate bladder if low urinary output occurs; urinary retention may be cause, especially in geriatric patients; urinalysis recommended before, during prolonged therapy

• Bilirubin, CBC, LFTs

• Vitals: B/P sitting, standing, lying: take pulse, respirations during initial treatment; establish baseline before starting treatment; report drops of 30 mm Hg; obtain baseline ECG

• Dizziness, faintness, palpitations, tachycardia on rising

O

Black Box Warning: Geriatric patients for serious reactions: fatal pneumonia, heart failure, stroke leading to death (IM); do not use in dementia-related psychosis

• **Neuroleptic malignant syndrome:** hyperpyrexia, muscle rigidity, increased CPK, altered mental status, acute dystonia (cheek chewing, swallowing, eyes, pill rolling), stop drug immediately
• **EPS:** May occur after long-term use
• **Hyperthermia:** Monitor for excessive heat, worse with exercising
• Constipation, urinary retention daily; increase bulk, water in diet
• Weight gain, hyperglycemia, metabolic changes in diabetic patients
• Supervised ambulation until patient stabilized on medication; do not involve patient in strenuous exercise program because fainting is possible; patient should not stand still for long periods
• **Hyperglycemia:** increased in diabetic patient, monitor FBS baseline and periodically
• **Metabolic syndrome:** large weight gain, increased B/P, FBS, cholesterol, and triglycerides, BMI
• **DRESS:** may be fatal; fever, hepatitis, cutaneous reactions, eosinophilia, nephritis, pneumonia, myocarditis, discontinue immediately
• **Beers:** avoid in older adults except for schizophrenia, bipolar disorder, or short-term use as an antiemetic during chemotherapy; increased risk of stroke
• **Pregnancy/breastfeeding:** use only if benefits outweigh fetal risk, may cause EPS in infant if used in 3rd trimester; those pregnant should enroll women in the National Pregnancy Registry for Atypical Antipsychotics, 1-866-961-2388; fertility is increased in acromegaly; pregnancy test before LAR; excreted in breast milk, avoid breastfeeding
Evaluate:
• **Therapeutic response:** decrease in emotional excitement, hallucinations, de-

lusion, paranoia, reorganization of patterns of thought, speech
Teach patient/family:

Black Box Warning: About postinjection delirium/sedation syndrome: all symptoms, not to drive or engage in hazardous activities after injection on that day

• To use good oral hygiene; frequent rinsing of mouth; sugarless gum, hard candy, ice chips for dry mouth
• To avoid hazardous activities until product response is determined
• That orthostatic hypotension occurs often; to rise from sitting or lying position gradually
• To avoid hot tubs, hot showers, tub baths because hypotension may occur
• To avoid abrupt withdrawal of this product because EPS may result; product should be withdrawn slowly
• To avoid OTC preparations (cough, hay fever, cold) unless approved by prescriber because serious product interactions may occur; to avoid use with alcohol, CNS depressants, opioids because increased drowsiness may occur
• **Suicidal thoughts, behaviors:** report immediately suicidal thoughts/behaviors
• That in hot weather, heat stroke may occur; to take extra precautions to stay cool
• To take PO without regard to food, how to use ODT
• To notify prescriber if pregnancy is planned or suspected; not to breastfeed

TREATMENT OF OVERDOSE:
Lavage if orally ingested; provide airway; do not induce vomiting or use EPINEPHrine

---

⚠ HIGH ALERT

olaparib (Rx)
(oh-lap′a-rib)
Lynparza
Func. class.: Antineoplastic-PARP

USES: Treatment of deleterious or suspected deleterious germline BRCA-mutated advanced ovarian cancer, fallopian tube, primary peritoneal cancer in patients who have not responded successfully to ≥3 prior courses of chemotherapy, as monotherapy, castration-resistant prostate cancer

DOSAGE AND ROUTES
• **Adult female: PO** 300 mg bid, until disease progression or unacceptable toxicity. Avoid use of concomitant strong and moderate CYP3A4 inhibitors if possible

Available forms: Tablets 100, 150 mg

> ## ⚠ HIGH ALERT
> ## oliceridine (Rx)
> (oh'li-ser'i-deen)
> Olinvyk
> *Func. class.:* Opioid analgesic
> **Controlled Substance Schedule II**

ACTION: Binds to the opioid *mu* receptor to produce analgesia

USES:
Acute pain

CONTRAINDICATIONS
Hypersensitivity, severe respiratory depression, GI obstruction, asthma

Black Box Warning: Respiratory depression

Precautions: Pregnancy, breastfeeding, abuse, neonatal opioid withdrawal syndrome, use with benzodiazepine or other CNS depressants, QT prolongation, chronic pulmonary disease, adrenal insufficiency, hypotension, GI disease, seizures

Black Box Warning: Use with other CNS depressants, neonatal opioid withdrawal syndrome, potential overdose or poisoning, substance abuse

DOSAGE AND ROUTES
Acute pain
• **Adult IV bolus** 1.5 mg; may give another 0.75 mg after 1 hr; doses may be repeated ≥1 hr and titrated based on tolerability and response; max single supplemental dose: 3 mg; max total daily dose: 27 mg
• **Adult: PCA:** 1.5 mg (given by provider); demand dose: range: 0.35-0.5 mg; lockout interval: 6 min; supplemental dose (administered by health care provider): 0.75 mg; may be administered beginning 1 hr after the initial dose and repeated hourly as needed; may be used in addition to the demand dose if needed for adequate response

Max cumulative daily dose: 27 mg; an initial dose of oliceridine 1 mg = morphine 5 mg

Available forms: IV solution (preservative free): 1 mg/mL (1 mL); 2 mg/2 mL (2 mL); 30 mg/30 mL (30 mL)
Administer:
IV direct route
• No dilution needed
• Use the 1 mg/mL and 2 mg/2 mL single-dose vials for direct use only
• **PCA:** Withdraw directly into a PCA syringe or IV bag; no dilution needed; 30-mg/30-mL vial is for PCA only
• Store at room temperature, do not freeze, protect from light

SIDE EFFECTS
CNS: Dizziness, somnolence, sedation, headache, flushing
GI: Nausea, vomiting, constipation
INTEG: Pruritus
RESP: Respiratory depression, decreased O_2 saturation
MS: Back pain

PHARMACOKINETICS
Onset <5 min, half-life 1.3-3 hr, metabolite 44 hr, protein binding 77%

INTERACTIONS
Increase: oliceridine effect—moderate-strong inhibitors of CYP3A4

(macrolides, azoles, protease inhibitors); moderate-strong CYP2D6 inhibitors (fluoxetine, quinidine, bupropion); benzodiazepines, other CNS depressants; monitor for respiratory depression/sedation

Increase: serotonin effects—SSRIs, SNRIs, tricyclic antidepressants, triptans, 5-HT3 receptor antagonists, mirtazapine, trazodone, tramadol, cyclobenzaprine, metaxalone, MAOIs, linezolid, IV methylene blue; observe for serotonin symptoms

Increase: respiratory depression—muscle relaxants; monitor for respiratory depression

Increase: urinary retention, paralytic ileus—anticholinergics; monitor for urinary retention, paralytic ileus

Decrease: oliceridine effect—CYP3A4 inducers (rifAMPin, carBAMzepine, phenytoin), mixed agonist/antagonists, partial agonist opioids; monitor for signs of opioid withdrawal

Decrease: diuretic effect—diuretics, monitor B/P, urinary output

NURSING CONSIDERATIONS
Assess
• **Pain:** Location, intensity, type, character; check for pain relief 20 min following
• **IV,** to relieve pain; give dose before pain becomes severe
• **Bowel status;** constipation is common, use stimulant laxative if needed; provide increased bulk, fluids in diet
• **Vitals:** B/P, pulse, respirations (character, depth, rate)

Black Box Warning: CNS changes: Dizziness, drowsiness, euphoria, LOC, pupil reaction

• **Abrupt discontinuation:** Gradually taper to prevent withdrawal symptoms

• **BBW: Respiratory dysfunction:** Depression, character, rate, rhythm; notify prescriber if respirations are <12/min

• **Pregnancy/breastfeeding:** Use only if benefits outweigh risk to fetus; longer use can result in neonatal opioid withdrawal syndrome; do not breastfeed

Evaluate
• **Therapeutic response:** Control of pain without adverse reactions

Teach patient/family
• To report change in pain control
• To report constipation, as other products will need to be used
• To change position slowly; orthostatic hypotension may occur
• To report any symptoms of CNS changes, allergic reactions
• That physical dependency may result from long-term use
• That withdrawal symptoms may occur: nausea, vomiting, cramps, fever, faintness, anorexia
• To report serotonin syndrome

Treatment of overdose
• Naloxone (Narcan), O_2, IV fluids, vasopressors

---

olmesartan (Rx)
(ol-meh-sar´tan)
Benicar, Olmetec ✦
Func. class.: Antihypertensive
Chem. class.: Angiotensin II receptor (type AT_1) antagonist

Do not confuse:
Benicar/Mevacor

ACTION: Blocks the vasoconstrictor and aldosterone-secreting effects of angiotensin II; selectively blocks the binding of angiotensin II to the AT_1 receptor found in tissues

USES: Hypertension, alone or in combination with other antihypertensives

CONTRAINDICATIONS
Hypersensitivity

Black Box Warning: Pregnancy (fetal/ neonatal morbidity/death)

Precautions: Breastfeeding, children, geriatric patients, hepatic disease, HF, renal artery stenosis, ◑ African descent, hyperkalemia

DOSAGE AND ROUTES
HTN
• **Adult: PO** single agent 20 mg/day initially in patients who are not volume depleted; may be increased to 40 mg/day if needed after 2 wk; **in volume depletion:** start with lower dose
• **Child ≥6 yr/adolescent ≤16 yr weighing ≥35 kg: PO** 20 mg/day; may increase to max 40 mg/day after 2 wk
• **Child ≥6 yr/adolescent ≤16 yr weighing 20-<35 kg: PO** 10 mg daily; may increase to max 20 mg/day after 2 wk
Available forms: Tabs 5, 10 ✦, 20, 40 mg
Administer:
• Without regard to meals
• Compounded suspension may be made in the pharmacy; refrigerate up to 1 mo, shake well before use

SIDE EFFECTS
CNS: *Dizziness,* fatigue, *headache,* insomnia, syncope
CV: Chest pain, peripheral edema, tachycardia, *hypotension*
EENT: Sinusitis, rhinitis, pharyngitis
GI: *Diarrhea,* abdominal pain
META: Hyperkalemia
MS: Arthralgia, pain, rhabdomyolysis
RESP: *Upper respiratory infection,* bronchitis
SYST: Angioedema

PHARMACOKINETICS
Peak 1-2 hr; excreted in urine, (50% unchanged) feces; half-life 13 hr; protein binding 99%

INTERACTIONS
Increase: antihypertensive effects— other antihypertensives, diuretics
Increase: hyperkalemia—potassium supplements, potassium-sparing diuretics, ACE inhibitors

Increase: effect of lithium, antioxidants
Decrease: antihypertensive effect— NSAIDs, colesevelam, COX-2 inhibitors
Drug/Herb
Increase: antihypertensive effect— hawthorn, garlic
Decrease: antihypertensive effect— ephedra, black licorice

NURSING CONSIDERATIONS
Assess:
• **Volume depletion:** correct volume depletion before starting therapy
• **Hypertension:** B/P, pulse; note rate, rhythm, quality; electrolytes: sodium, potassium, chloride; baselines for renal, hepatic studies before therapy begins; may use antihypertensives to control B/P if needed
• **Hypotension:** place supine; may occur with hyponatremia or in those with volume depletion; more common in those taking a diuretic also
• **Heart failure:** monitor for edema, jugular vein distention, dyspnea; monitor weight daily
• ◑ ACE inhibitors should be avoided in black patients

Black Box Warning: Pregnancy/breastfeeding: product can cause fetal death when given during pregnancy; assess for pregnancy before starting therapy; do not breastfeed

Evaluate:
• **Therapeutic response:** decreased B/P
Teach patient/family:
• To comply with dosage schedule, not to double or skip dose, to take missed dose when remembered if not close to next dose
• To notify prescriber of mouth sores, fever, swelling of hands or feet, irregular heartbeat, chest pain, severe chronic diarrhea, severe weight loss
• That excessive perspiration, dehydration, vomiting, diarrhea may lead to fall in B/P; to consult prescriber if these occur; to maintain adequate hydration

Side effects: *italics* = common; red = life-threatening

• That product may cause dizziness, fainting, light-headedness; to avoid hazardous activities

• To rise slowly to sitting or standing position to minimize orthostatic hypotension

• To notify provider immediately of swelling of the face, lips, tongue; trouble breathing

• That follow-up exams will be needed

• To avoid all OTC medications unless approved by prescriber

• That blood glucose may increase and antidiabetic product may need dosage change

• To inform all health care providers of medication use

• To use proper technique for obtaining B/P, and discuss acceptable parameters

Black Box Warning: To notify prescriber immediately if pregnant; not to use during breastfeeding

olodaterol (Rx)
(oh-loe-da'ter-ol)
Striverdi Respimat
Func. class.: β$_2$-adrenergic agonist, long-acting

USES: Long-term maintenance treatment of airflow obstruction in COPD, including chronic bronchitis and/or emphysema

CONTRAINDICATIONS
Hypersensitivity; monotherapy (asthma)

DOSAGE AND ROUTES
COPD
• **Adult:** **PO** Oral inhalation: 2 inhalations daily, max 2 inhalations/day
Available forms: Inhalation aerosol: 2.5 mcg/actuation

olopatadine nasal agent
See Appendix B

olopatadine ophthalmic
See Appendix B

olsalazine (Rx)
(ohl-sal'ah-zeen)
Dipentum
Func. class.: GI antiinflammatory
Chem. class.: Salicylate derivative

Do not confuse:
olsalazine/OLANZapine

ACTION: Bioconverted to 5-aminosalicylic acid, which decreases inflammation

USES: Maintenance of remission of ulcerative colitis in patients intolerant to sulfasalazine

CONTRAINDICATIONS
Hypersensitivity to this product or salicylates
Precautions: Pregnancy, breastfeeding, children <14 yr; impaired renal/hepatic function; severe allergy; bronchial asthma

DOSAGE AND ROUTES
• **Adult:** **PO** 500 mg bid, max 3 g/day
Available forms: Caps 250 mg
Administer:
• Total daily dose evenly spaced to minimize GI intolerance; give with food
• Store in tight, light-resistant container at room temperature

SIDE EFFECTS
CNS: Headache, hallucinations, depression, vertigo, fatigue, dizziness
GI: Nausea, vomiting, abdominal pain, diarrhea, bloating
INTEG: Rash, dermatitis, urticaria

PHARMACOKINETICS
Partially absorbed, peak 1½ hr, half-life 30-90 min (rectal), 2-15 hr (PO), excreted in urine as 5-aminosalicylic acid and metabolites, crosses placenta

INTERACTIONS
Increase: azaTHIOprine toxicity—azaTHIOprine
Increase: myelosuppression—mercaptopurine, thioguanine

Increase: bleeding risk—low-molecular-weight heparins; discontinue before using this product

Increase: Reye's syndrome development—varicella vaccine; do not use within 6 wk of olsalazine

Increase: PT, INR—warfarin

Drug/Lab Test

Increase: AST, ALT

NURSING CONSIDERATIONS
Assess:
• **Colitis:** bowel pattern, number of stools, consistency, frequency, pain, mucus, abdominal pain before treatment and periodically
• **Allergic reaction:** rash, dermatitis, urticaria, pruritus, dyspnea, bronchospasm; allergy to salicylates, sulfonamides
• **Renal disease:** BUN, creatinine in those with renal disease; LFTs (liver disease); monitor I&O, output of 1500 mL/day is needed to prevent crystals in urine
• **Liver disease:** Monitor LFTs baseline and periodically
• **Pregnancy/breastfeeding:** use only if benefits outweigh fetal risk; avoid breastfeeding, excreted in breast milk

Evaluate:
• **Therapeutic response:** absence of fever, mucus in stools, decreased diarrhea, abdominal pain

Teach patient/family:
• To report diarrhea, rash, bleeding, bruising, fever, hallucinations, or if symptoms do not improve after 2 mo of therapy
• That product may cause dizziness; to avoid hazardous activities until reaction is known
• To take even if feeling better; to take as directed; to take missed dose when remembered, but not to double
• That lab work and exams will be needed during treatment

omadacycline (Rx)
(oh-mad'a-sye'kleen)
Nuzyra
Func. class.: Antiinfective

USES: Pneumonia, community acquired; skin/skin structure infections

DOSAGE AND ROUTES
Pneumonia, community acquired
• **Adult:** IV loading dose 200 mg as a single dose on day 1 or 100 mg bid on day 1; PO 300 mg daily × 7-14 days

Skin/skin structure infections
• **Adult:** IV loading dose 200 mg as a single dose on day 1 or 100 mg bid on day 1; **PO** 450 mg daily days 1 and 2; maintenance **IV** 100 mg day; PO 300 mg daily × 7-14 days

Available forms: Tabs 150 mg, IV solution 100 mg

omalizumab (Rx)
(oh-mah-lye-zoo'mab)
Xolair
Func. class.: Antiasthmatic
Chem. class.: Monoclonal antibody

ACTION: Recombinant DNA-derived humanized IgG murine monoclonal antibody that selectively binds to IgE to limit the release of mediators in the allergic response

USES: Moderate to severe persistent asthma, chronic idiopathic urticaria, nasal polyps

CONTRAINDICATIONS
Hypersensitivity to hamster protein

Black Box Warning: Hypersensitivity to this product

Precautions: Pregnancy, breastfeeding, children <12 yr, acute attacks of asthma, lymphoma, nephrotic disease, bronchospasm, neoplastic disease, status asthmaticus

DOSAGE AND ROUTES
Moderate to severe asthma
• **Adult/child ≥6 yr: SUBCUT** 75-375 mg × 2-4 wk; divide inj into 2 sites if dose

>150 mg; dose is adjusted based on IgE levels, significant changes in body weight

Chronic idiopathic urticaria

• **Adult/adolescent >12 yr: SUBCUT** 150-300 mg q4wk, dose is adjusted based on IgE levels, significant changes in body weight

Nasal polyps

• **Adult: SUBCUT** 75-600 mg q2wk or q4wk

Available forms: Powder for inj, lyophilized 202.5 mg (150 mg/1.2 mL after reconstitution); 75 mg/0.5 mL, 150 mg/mL; prefilled syringe

Administer:

SUBCUT route

• Reconstitute using 1.4 mL sterile water for inj (150 mg/1.2 mL or 125 mg/mL); gently swirl to dissolve; allow vial to stand and q5min gently swirl for 5-10 sec to dissolve; some vials may take ≥20 min; do not use if contents do not dissolve within 40 min; should be clear or slightly opalescent; use large-bore needle to withdraw medication; replace needle with small-bore needle

• Given q2-4wk; product is viscous; if >150 mg is given, divide into 2 sites; inj may take 5-10 sec to administer

SIDE EFFECTS

CV: Heart failure, cardiomyopathy, hypotension, MI, PE, thrombosis

HEMA: Serious systemic eosinophilia

INTEG: Pruritus, dermatitis, inj-site reactions, rash

MISC: Earache, dizziness, fatigue, pain, malignancies, viral infections, anaphylaxis, thrombocytopenia, headache

MS: Arthralgia, fracture, leg, arm pain

RESP: Sinusitis, upper respiratory infections, pharyngitis, pulmonary hypertension, bronchospasm

PHARMACOKINETICS

Slowly absorbed, peak 7-8 days, half-life 26 days, degradation by liver, excretion in bile

INTERACTIONS

Increase: toxicity—belimumab, loxapine (inhalation), avoid using together

• Use cautiously with live virus vaccines

Drug/Lab Test

Increase: IgE

NURSING CONSIDERATIONS

Assess:

• **Asthma:** respiratory rate, rhythm, depth; auscultate lung fields bilaterally; notify prescriber of abnormalities; monitor pulmonary function tests; serum IgE (may increase and continue for 1 yr)

• **Inj-site reactions:** inflammation, edema, redness, warmth at site; may occur within 60 min of inj; may decrease with repeated dosing

Black Box Warning: Anaphylaxis, allergic reactions: rash, urticaria, inability to breathe, edema of throat; product should be discontinued; have emergency equipment available; observe for 2 hr; reaction can occur ≤24 hr

• **Pregnancy/breastfeeding:** use only if clearly needed; pregnant patients should enroll in the EXPECT Pregnancy Registry, 866-496-5247; cautious use in breastfeeding, excretion unknown

Evaluate:

• **Therapeutic response:** ability to breathe more easily

Teach patient/family:

• That improvement will not be immediate

• Not to stop taking or decrease current asthma medications unless instructed by prescriber

• To avoid live virus vaccines while taking this product

Black Box Warning: To report signs of allergic reaction immediately, can be life-threatening

<hr>

ombitasvir/paritaprevir/ ritonavir and dasabuvir (Rx)

(om-bit′as-vir/par-i-ta′pre-vir/ri-toe′na-vir da-sa′bue-vir)

Viekira Pak, Viekira XR

Func. class.: Antihepaciviral, NS3/4A protease inhibitor (anti-HCV)

USES: Treatment of adults with chronic hepatitis C virus (HCV) infection genotype 1a without cirrhosis, in combination with ribavirin, and genotype 1b without cirrhosis or with compensated cirrhosis

DOSAGE AND ROUTES

Black Box Warning: Hepatitis B exacerbation

Chronic HCV genotype 1 infection (compensated cirrhosis with or without ribavirin)
• **Adult: PO Immediate release (Viekira Pak):** 2 tablets (ombitasvir 12.5 mg/paritaprevir 75 mg/ritonavir 50 mg per tablet) every morning × 12 wk, dasabuvir tablet: 1 tablet (dasabuvir 250 mg) bid × 12 wk; **extended release (Viekira XR):** 3 tablets (ombitasvir 8.33 mg/paritaprevir 50 mg/ritonavir 33.33 mg/dasabuvir 200 mg per tablet) daily × 12 wk
Available forms: Tablet dasabuvir 250 mg; tablet ombitasvir 12.5 mg/paritaprevir 75 mg/ ritonavir 50 mg packaged together

---

omega-3-fatty acids (Rx)
Lovaza, Vascepa, many brands available
Func. class.: Antilipemic, fatty acid

USES: To reduce triglyceride levels ≥500 mg/dL as adjunct to diet

CONTRAINDICATIONS
Hypersensitivity

DOSAGE AND ROUTES
Adjunct to diet to reduce triglycerides ≥500 mg/dL
• **Adult: PO** 4 g/day (Lovaza) or divided bid
Adjunct to statin therapy to prevent MI, stroke
• **Adult: PO** 2 or 4 g daily
Available forms: Capsules 0.5, 1 g

---

omeprazole (OTC, Rx)
(oh-mep′ray-zole)
Losec ✚, Olex ✚, PriLOSEC, PriLOSEC OTC
Func. class.: Antiulcer, proton pump inhibitor
Chem. class.: Benzimidazole

Do not confuse:
PriLOSEC/Prinivil/PROzac/predniSONE/ Pristiq
omeprazole/fomepizole aripiprazole

ACTION: Suppresses gastric secretion by inhibiting hydrogen/potassium ATPase enzyme system in gastric parietal cells; characterized as gastric acid pump inhibitor because it blocks the final step of acid production

USES: Gastroesophageal reflux disease (GERD), severe erosive esophagitis, poorly responsive systemic GERD, pathologic hypersecretory conditions (Zollinger-Ellison syndrome, systemic mastocytosis, multiple endocrine adenomas); treatment of active duodenal ulcers with/without antiinfectives for *Helicobacter pylori*
Unlabeled uses: Dyspepsia

CONTRAINDICATIONS
Hypersensitivity to this product or benzimidazoles
Precautions: Pregnancy; breastfeeding; children; ✹ Asian, black patients, hepatic disease

DOSAGE AND ROUTES
Active duodenal ulcers
• **Adult: PO** 20 mg/day × 4-8 wk
GERD without esophageal lesions
• **Adult: PO** (del rel cap/del rel susp) 20 mg/day × 4-8 wk
• **Child 1-16 yr, ≥20 kg: PO** 20 mg daily × 4 wk
Child 1-16 yr, 10-20 kg: PO 10 mg daily × 4 wk

Side effects: *italics* = common; red = life-threatening

Pathologic hypersecretory conditions (Zollinger-Ellison syndrome)
• **Adult: PO** 60 mg/day; may increase to 120 mg tid; daily doses >80 mg should be divided

Gastric ulcer
• **Adult: PO** 40 mg/day 4-8 wk

Heartburn (OTC)
• **Adult: PO** 1 del rel tab (20 mg)/day before AM meal with glass of water × 14 days

***H. pylori* infection, duodenal ulcer disease**
• **Adult: PO** 40 mg every AM with clarithromycin 500 mg tid × 14 days

Available forms: Del rel caps 10, 20, 40 mg; del rel tabs 20 mg; granules for oral susp 2.5, 10 mg/packet (del rel); suspension 2 mg/mL

Administer:
• Capsules and tablets are not bioequivalent
• Swallow caps whole; do not crush or chew; caps may be opened and sprinkled over applesauce
• Before eating, usually in the AM, separate with other medications
• **Oral susp powder:** give on empty stomach ≥1 hr before food; if there is NG or enteral feeding tube, do not feed 3 hr before or 1 hr after giving product: contents of packet should be mixed with 1-2 tbsp water; add 20 mL water for NG tube; for oral, stir well, drink, add more water, and drink

SIDE EFFECTS
CNS: *Headache, dizziness, asthenia*
GI: *Diarrhea, abdominal pain, vomiting, nausea, constipation, flatulence, acid regurgitation,* abdominal swelling, anorexia, irritable colon, esophageal candidiasis, dry mouth, hepatic failure, *Clostridium difficile*–associated diarrhea (CDAD)
INTEG: *Rash,* dry skin, urticaria, pruritus, alopecia
MISC: *Back pain,* fever, fatigue, malaise
RESP: *Upper respiratory infections, cough,* epistaxis, pneumonia

PHARMACOKINETICS
Bioavailability 30%-40%; peak ½-3½ hr; half-life ½-1 hr; protein binding 95%; eliminated in urine as metabolites and in feces; in geriatric patients, elimination rate decreased, bioavailability increased; metabolized by CYP2C19 enzyme system; ⟠ some Asian, Black, and Caucasian patients are poor metabolizers

INTERACTIONS
Increase: bleeding—warfarin
Increase: serum levels of diazePAM, phenytoin, flurazepam, triazolam, cycloSPORINE, disulfiram, digoxin, benzodiazepines, methotrexate; saquinavir, tacrolimus, voriconazole
Decrease: effect of iron salts, ketoconazole, cyanocobalamin, calcium carbonate, ampicillin, indinavir, gefitinib, ampicillin, azoles, biphosphates

Drug/Herb
Decrease: omeprazole level— St. John's wort
Drug/Food
Decrease: vitamin B_{12} absorption if omeprazole is used long term
Drug/Lab Test
Increase: alk phos, AST, ALT, bilirubin, gastrin
Decrease: vitamin B_{12}, sodium, glucose

NURSING CONSIDERATIONS
Assess:
• **GI system:** bowel sounds, abdomen for pain, swelling, anorexia, blood in stools, diarrhea, emesis
• ***Clostridium difficile*–associated diarrhea (CDAD):** assess for fever, abdominal pain, bloody stool; may occur up to several weeks after conclusion of therapy; report to the prescriber immediately
• **Electrolyte imbalances:** hyponatremia; hypomagnesemia in patients using product 3 mo-1 yr; if hypomagnesemia occurs, use of magnesium supplements may be sufficient; if severe, discontinue product
• **Vitamin B_{12}:** Assess vitamin B_{12} level if on long-term treatment; dyspnea, weakness, anorexia, palpitations may occur if vitamin B_{12} is low
• **Hepatic enzymes:** AST, ALT, alkaline phosphatase during treatment; **blood studies:** CBC, differential during treatment, blood dyscrasias may occur; vitamin B_{12} in long-term treatment, serum magnesium

• **Fractures:** use over 1 yr has been associated with fractures
• **Beers:** avoid scheduled use >8 wk in patients with hypersecretory condition, esophagitis, risk of *Clostridium difficile,* and fractures
• **Pregnancy/breastfeeding:** use only if benefits outweigh fetal risk; cautious use in breastfeeding, excreted in breast milk
Evaluate:
• **Therapeutic response:** absence of epigastric pain, swelling, fullness, bleeding; decreased GERD, esophagitis symptoms
Teach patient/family:
• To report severe diarrhea; black, tarry stools; abdominal cramps/pain; or continuing headache; product may have to be discontinued
• That if diabetic, hypoglycemia may occur
• To avoid hazardous activities because dizziness may occur
• To avoid alcohol, salicylates, NSAIDs; may cause GI irritation
• To take as directed, even if feeling better; to take missed dose as soon as remembered; not to double; PriLOSEC OTC takes up to 4 days for full effect
• Not to use OTC, prescription, or herbal products without prescriber's consent
• To take as directed at lowest dose possible for shortest time needed
• To report if pregnancy is planned or suspected or if breastfeeding

---

ondansetron (Rx)
(on-dan-seh′tron)
Zuplenz
Func. class.: Antiemetic
Chem. class.: 5-HT$_3$ antagonist

Do not confuse:
Zofran/Zantac

ACTION: Prevents nausea, vomiting by blocking serotonin peripherally, centrally, and in the small intestine

USES: Prevention of nausea, vomiting associated with cancer chemotherapy, radiotherapy; prevention of postoperative nausea, vomiting

CONTRAINDICATIONS
Hypersensitivity; phenylketonuric hypersensitivity (oral disintegrating tab), torsades de pointes
Precautions: Pregnancy, breastfeeding, children, geriatric patients, granisetron hypersensitivity, QT prolongation, torsades de pointes

DOSAGE AND ROUTES
Chemotherapy-induced nausea and vomiting, prevention; highly emetogenic chemotherapy:
• *Day of chemotherapy:* Give before chemotherapy with a neurokinin 1 (NK$_1$) receptor antagonist, dexamethasone, with/without olanzapine
• **Adult: IV** 8 mg or 0.15 mg/kg, max 16 mg/dose; **PO (not film)** 8 mg bid × 2 doses with the first dose given before chemotherapy; **oral soluble film:** 24 mg (three 8-mg doses given together) as a single dose
• **Infants ≥6 mo, children, and adolescents: IV** 0.15 mg/kg/dose; max dose: 16 mg/dose; give first dose 30 min before chemotherapy, then doses given 4 and 8 hr after the first dose (3 total doses)
Moderately emetogenic with carboplatin-based doses
• *Day of chemotherapy:* Give before chemotherapy with an NK$_1$ receptor antagonist and dexamethasone
• **Adult: IV** 8 mg or 0.15 mg/kg, max 16 mg/dose, as a single dose; **PO** 8 mg bid × 2 doses with the first dose given before chemotherapy
Moderately emetogenic chemotherapy with non-carboplatin-based doses
• *Day of chemotherapy:* Give before and with dexamethasone
• **Adult: IV** 8 mg or 0.15 mg/kg, max 16 mg/dose, as a single dose; **PO** 8 mg bid × 2 doses with the first dose given before chemotherapy
• **Children 4-11 yr: PO** 4 mg 30 min before chemotherapy; repeat 4 and 8 hours after initial dose, then 4 mg q8hr × 1-2 days after chemotherapy

O

Side effects: *italics* = common; red = life-threatening

• **Children ≥12 yr and adolescents:**
PO 8 mg 30 min before chemotherapy;
then 8 hr after initial dose, then 8 mg
q12hr × 1-2 days after chemotherapy
Highly emetogenic chemotherapy
• **Adult: PO** 24 mg given 30 min prior to
use of single-dose highly emetogenic che-
motherapy, including 50 mg/m² or more
**Radiation therapy–associated nau-
sea and vomiting, prevention**
• **Adult: PO** 8 mg daily to bid given 1-2
hr before each fraction of radiation; give
with dexamethasone
Hepatic dose
• **Adult: PO/IM/IV** max dose 8 mg/day
Available forms: Inj 2 mg/mL, 4-mg/2
mL; tabs 4, 8, 24 mg; oral sol 4 mg/5 mL;
oral disintegrating tabs 4, 8 mg; oral dissolving film 4, 8 mg
Administer:
PO route
• **Regular tab:** protect from light (4-mg tab)
• **Oral disintegrating tab:** do not push
through foil; gently remove; immediately
place on tongue to dissolve; swallow with
saliva
• **Oral dissolving film:** fold pouch along
dotted line to expose tear notch; tear and
remove film; place film on tongue until
dissolved; swallow after dissolved; to
reach desired dose, administer successive films, allowing each to dissolve before using another
• **Oral solution:** protect from light; measure in calibrated oral syringe or other
calibrated device
IM route
• Visually inspect for particulate or discoloration
• May give 4 mg undiluted IM; inject
deeply in large muscle mass; aspirate
Direct IV route
• Give undiluted, max 16 mg
Intermittent IV infusion
• Check for discoloration or particulate;
if particulate is present, shake to dissolve
• After diluting single dose in 50 mL NS or
D₅W, 0.45% NaCl or NS; give over 15 min
• Do not use IV 32 mg/dose in chemo-
therapy nausea/vomiting due to QT pro-
longation, max 16 mg/dose (adult)

• Store at room temperature for up to
48 hr after dilution

Y-site compatibilities: Aldesleukin, amifostine, amikacin, aztreonam, bleomycin,
CARBOplatin, carmustine, ceFAZolin,
cefmetazole, cefotaxime, cefOXitin, cefTAZidime, ceftizoxime, cefuroxime, chlorpro-
MAZINE, cimetidine, cisatracurium, CISplatin, cladribine, clindamycin,
cyclophosphamide, cytarabine, dacarbazine, DACTINomycin, DAUNOrubicin, dexamethasone, diphenhydrAMINE, DOPamine,
DOXOrubicin, DOXOrubicin liposome,
doxycycline, droperidol, etoposide, famotidine, filgrastim, floxuridine, fluconazole,
fludarabine, gallium, gentamicin, haloperidol, heparin, hydrocortisone, HYDROmorphone, hydrOXYzine, ifosfamide, imipenem-cilastatin, magnesium sulfate,
mannitol, mechlorethamine, melphalan,
meperidine, mesna, methotrexate, metoclopramide, miconazole, mitoMYcin, mito-
XANTRONE, morphine, PACLitaxel, pentostatin, piperacillin/tazobactam, potassium
chloride, prochlorperazine, promethazine,
raNITIdine, remifentanil, streptozocin, teniposide, thiotepa, ticarcillin, ticarcillin-
clavulanate, vancomycin, vinBLAStine, vin-
CRIStine, vinorelbine, zidovudine

SIDE EFFECTS

CNS: *Headache, dizziness, drowsiness,
fatigue*
GI: *Diarrhea, constipation,* abdominal
pain, dry mouth
MISC: Rash, bronchospasm (rare), musculoskeletal pain, wound problems, shivering, fever, hypoxia, urinary retention

PHARMACOKINETICS

IV: Mean elimination half-life 3.5-4.7 hr,
plasma protein binding 70%-76%, extensively metabolized in the liver, excreted
45%-60% in urine

INTERACTIONS

Increase: unconsciousness, hypoten-
sion—apomorphine, do not use together
Increase: QT prolongation—other prod-
ucts that prolong QT
Increase: serotonin syndrome—SSRIs,
SSNRIs, MAOIs, tricyclics, monitor closely
Drug/Herb

Decrease: ondansetron effect—St. John's wort

Decrease: ondansetron effect—rifAMPin, carBAMazepine, phenytoin

Drug/Lab Test

Increase: LFTs

NURSING CONSIDERATIONS

Assess:

• Absence of nausea, vomiting during chemotherapy

• Hypersensitivity reaction: rash, bronchospasm (rare)

• **EPS:** shuffling gait, tremors, grimacing, rigidity periodically

• **QT prolongation:** monitor ECG in those with hypokalemia, hypomagnesemia, cardiac disease or in those receiving other products that increase QT

• **Serotonin syndrome:** occurs when other products are given that increase CNS or peripheral serotonin levels; assess for agitation, confusion, dizziness, diaphoresis, flushing, tremor, seizures, nausea, vomiting, diarrhea; product should be discontinued

• **Pregnancy/breastfeeding:** identify whether pregnancy is planned or suspected; avoid use in pregnancy, cardiac malformations, oral clefts may occur if used in 1st trimester; cautious use in breastfeeding

Evaluate:

• **Therapeutic response:** absence of nausea, vomiting due to chemotherapy, surgery

Teach patient/family:

• To report diarrhea, constipation, rash, changes in respirations, discomfort at insertion site, serotonin symptoms, EPS symptoms

• That headache requiring analgesic is common

• Drink with whole glass of water (PO)

• **Oral disintegrating tabs:** remove strip from pouch, place on tongue, and allow to dissolve; drink water

---

opicapone (Rx)

(oh-pik′a-pone)

Ongentys

Func. class.: Anti-Parkinson agent, COMT inhibitor

USES: Adjunct with levodopa/carbidopa in Parkinson disease "off" episodes

CONTRAINDICATIONS

Hypersensitivity, MAOIs, pheochromocytoma, paraganglioma

DOSAGE AND ROUTES

• **Adult: PO** 50 mg daily at bedtime

Available forms: Capsule 25, 50 mg

---

oritavancin (Rx)

(or-it′a-van′sin)

Orbactiv, Kimyrsa

Func. class.: Antibiotic agents

Chem. class.: Glycopeptide

ACTION: Inhibits bacterial cell wall biosynthesis, disrupts bacterial cell membrane

USES: *Enterococcus faecalis, Enterococcus faecium, Staphylococcus aureus* (MRSA), *Staphylococcus aureus* (MSSA), *Streptococcus agalactiae* (group B streptococci), *Streptococcus anginosus, Streptococcus constellatus, Streptococcus dysgalactiae, Streptococcus intermedius, Streptococcus pyogenes* (group A β-hemolytic streptococci); treatment of acute bacterial skin and skin structure infections due to gram-positive organisms, including cellulitis/erysipelas, major cutaneous abscesses, and wound infections

CONTRAINDICATIONS

Hypersensitivity

Precautions: Anticoagulant therapy, antimicrobial resistance, breastfeeding, colitis, diarrhea, inflammatory bowel disease, infusion reactions, pregnancy, CDAD, vancomycin hypersensitivity, viral infection

DOSAGE AND ROUTES

• **Adult: IV** 1200 mg as a single dose

Available forms: Powder for injection: 400-mg vial

Administer:

IV route

• Draw C&S prior to using

O

• Visually inspect for particulate matter and discoloration beforehand; the reconstituted solution is clear, colorless to pale yellow
• **Reconstitution:** Reconstitute each 400-mg vial with 40 mL sterile water for injection. Three vials are necessary for a single dose; gently swirl until dissolved
• **Dilution:** Withdraw and discard 120 mL from a 1000-mL intravenous bag of D_5W; transfer 40 mL solution from each of the 3 reconstituted vials to the D_5W IV bag (1.2 mg/mL)
• **Storage:** Refrigerate or store at room temperature. The combined storage time (from reconstitution to dilution) and 3-hour infusion time should not exceed 6 hr at room temperature or 12 hr if refrigerated

Intermittent IV INFUSION

• Infuse over 3 hr; do not infuse with other medications or electrolytes; do not use with saline-based solutions

• Avoid heparin for 5 days after use of this product; false elevated aPTT and coagulation studies may occur

SIDE EFFECTS
CNS: Dizziness, flushing, headache
CV: Sinus tachycardia, phlebitis
GI: Nausea, vomiting, diarrhea, CDAD
HEMA: Anemia, eosinophilia
MS: Myalgia, osteomyelitis
INTEG: Rash, vasculitis, pruritus, angioedema, infusion-related reaction
MISC: Wheezing, bronchospasm

PHARMACOKINETICS
85% protein binding, half-life 245 hr, excretion urine, unchanged, peak infusion's end

INTERACTIONS
Increase: toxicity—products metabolized by CYP2D6, CYP3A4
Increase: bleeding risk—warfarin; avoid concurrent use
Drug/Lab Test
Increase: LFTs, uric acid, INR, aPTT

NURSING CONSIDERATIONS
Assess:
• **Infection:** wounds, fever, sputum, urine, monitor WBC baseline and periodically report changes

• CBC and differential
• **Infusion-related reactions:** symptoms of red man syndrome (flushing, urticaria, pruritus); slow or stop infusion
• **Bowel function:** for diarrhea, bloody stools, cramping; assess for fever; report to health care professional, may be *Clostridium difficile*–associated diarrhea (CDAD), may start up to 8 wk after completion of treatment
• **Anticoagulant use:** may increase effects of warfarin; monitor closely, avoid use with heparin; heparin effects may be reduced and lab results altered
• **Pregnancy/breastfeeding:** use only if benefits outweigh fetal risk; cautious use in breastfeeding, excreted in breast milk
Evaluate:
• **Therapeutic response:** resolution of infection
Teach patient/family:
• Reason for product, expected result
• Used only once to resolve infection
• **Hypersensitivity reactions:** to notify prescriber of rash, facial swelling, dyspnea
• To avoid use of other prescription products, OTC products, or herbal products unless approved by prescriber
• **Bowel function:** to notify health care professional of diarrhea, bloody stools, cramping, fever; do not self-treat
• To notify prescriber if pregnancy is planned or suspected

---

orlistat (Rx, OTC)
(or'lih-stat)
Alli, Xenical
Func. class.: Weight-control agent
Chem. class.: Lipase inhibitor

ACTION: Inhibits the absorption of dietary fats

USES: Obesity management

DOSAGE AND ROUTES
• **Adult/children ≥12 yr: PO** (Alli) 60 mg, (Xenical) 120 mg tid with each main meal containing fat, max 360 mg/day
Available forms: Capsules 60, 120 mg

oseltamivir (Rx)

(oss-el-tam´ih-veer)

Tamiflu

Func. class.: Antiviral

Chem. class.: Neuraminidase inhibitor

Do not confuse:

Tamiflu/Thera-Flu

ACTION: Inhibits influenza virus neuraminidase with possible alteration of virus particle aggregation and release

USES: Prevention and treatment of influenza type A or B

Unlabeled uses: Avian flu (H5N1)

CONTRAINDICATIONS

Hypersensitivity

Precautions: Pregnancy, neonates, breastfeeding, infants, children, geriatric patients, renal/hepatic/pulmonary/cardiac disease, psychosis, viral infection

DOSAGE AND ROUTES

• Treatment should begin ≤2 days after onset of symptoms

Treatment of influenza

• **Adult/child >40 kg: PO** 75 mg bid × 5 days

• **Child 23-40 kg and ≥1 yr: PO** 60 mg bid × 5 days

• **Child 15-23 kg and ≥1 yr: PO** 45 mg bid × 5 days

• **Child ≤15 kg and ≥1 yr: PO** 30 mg bid × 5 days

• **Neonate ≥14 days/infant: PO** 3 mg/kg/dose bid × 5 days

Prevention of influenza

• **Adult/child ≥13 yr: PO** 75 mg/day (capsule) or 12.5 mL (suspension) daily × 1 wk after exposure (vaccinated) or 2 wk (unvaccinated)

• **Child/adolescent ≤15 kg: PO** 30 mg daily; **>15 kg to 23 kg: PO** 45 mg daily; **>23 kg to 40 kg: PO** 60 mg daily; **>40 kg: PO** 75 mg daily

Renal dose

• **Adult: PO** Treatment: CCr 10-30 mL/min, 30 mg/day × 5 days; CCr 30-60 mL/min, 30 mg bid × 5 days; Prophylaxis: CCr 10-30 mL/min, 30 mg every other day; CCr 30-60 mL/min, 30 mg daily

H1N1 influenza A virus (unlabeled)

• **Adult/adolescent/child >40 kg: PO** 75 mg bid × 5 days

• **Adolescent/child 24-40 kg: PO** 60 mg bid × 5 days

• **Child >1 yr and 15-23 kg: PO** 45 mg bid × 5 days

• **Child >1 yr and ≤15 kg: PO** 30 mg bid × 5 days

Available forms: Caps 30, 45, 75 mg; powder for oral susp 6 mg/mL

Administer:

• Within 2 days of symptoms of influenza; continue for 5 days

• At least 4 hr before bedtime to prevent insomnia

• Without regard to food; give with food for GI upset

• Take with full glass of water

• Store in tight, dry container

• **Oral susp:** 6 mg/mL concentration, take care to use correct dose; loosen powder from side of bottle, add 55 mL, shake well (6 mg/mL), remove push bottle adapter into neck of bottle, close tightly to ensure sealing, use within 17 days of preparation when refrigerated or within 10 days at room temperature, write expiration date on bottle, shake well before use, use oral syringe provided but only with markings for 30, 45, 60 mg, confirm that dosing instructions are in same units as syringe provided

SIDE EFFECTS

CNS: *Headache, dizziness,* fatigue, *insomnia,* seizures, delirium, self-injury (children)

GI: *Nausea, vomiting*

INTEG: Toxic epidermal necrolysis, Stevens-Johnson syndrome, erythema multiforme

RESP: Cough

PHARMACOKINETICS

Rapidly absorbed, protein binding 3%, converted to oseltamivir carboxylate (active form), active forms half-life 1-3 hr, metabolite 6-10 hr, excreted in urine (99%)

INTERACTIONS

• **Decrease:** effect, live, attenuated influenza virus vaccine, avoid prior to use (2 days before or after 14 days)

NURSING CONSIDERATIONS
Assess:

• Bowel pattern before, during treatment
• **Influenza:** fever, fatigue, sore throat, headache, muscle soreness, aches

Evaluate:

• **Therapeutic response:** absence of fever, malaise, cough, dyspnea in infection

Teach patient/family:

• About all aspects of product therapy
• To avoid hazardous activities if dizziness occurs
• To take as soon as symptoms appear; to take full course even if feeling better
• To take missed dose as soon as remembered if within 2 hr of next dose
• To stop immediately; to report to prescriber skin rash, delirium, psychosis, hallucinations (child)
• That this product should not be substituted for flu shot
• That this product will not treat the common cold
• To avoid other products unless approved by prescriber

---

oteseconazole (Rx)

(o-tes-a-KAA-nuh-zowl)

Vivjoa

Func. class.: Antifungal, systemic
Chem. class.: Azole

ACTIONS: An azole inhibitor targeting the fungal sterol, which is required for fungal cell membrane formation and integrity

USES: Reduces the incidence of recurrent vulvovaginal candidiasis (RVVC) in females with a history of RVVC who are NOT of reproductive potential

CONTRAINDICATIONS

Pregnancy, breastfeeding, hypersensitivity
Precautions: Renal/hepatic disease

DOSAGE AND ROUTES
Esophageal candidiasis

• **Adult: PO Oteseconazole-only dosage regimen: On day 1:** Give 600 mg (as a single dose). **On day 2:** Give 450 mg (as a single dose). **Beginning on day 14:** Give 150 mg once a week (q7days) × 11 wk (wk 2 through 12). **Fluconazole/oteseconazole dosage regimen: On day 1, day 4, day 7.** Give **fluconazole 150 mg PO; on days 14-20.** Give oteseconazole 150 mg once daily × 7 days. **Beginning on day 28:** Give oteseconazole 150 mg once a week (every 7 days) × 11 wk (wk 4-14)

Available forms: Capsule 150 mg
Administer:

• Protect from light when removed from packaging, store at room temperature

SIDE EFFECTS
CNS: Headache
GI: Nausea

PHARMACOKINETICS
Peak 5-10 hr, half-life 139 days

INTERACTIONS
Increased: Breast cancer resistance protein (BCRP) substrate effect, increases the risk of adverse reactions, a lower dose may be needed

NURSING CONSIDERATIONS
Assess:

• Pregnancy/breastfeeding: do not use in pregnancy, may cause fetal harm; do not breastfeed

Evaluate:

• **Therapeutic response:** decreased candidiasis

Teach patient/family:

• Women of childbearing age should use effective contraceptive

---

⚠ HIGH ALERT

oxaliplatin (Rx)

(ox-al-i´plat-in)

Func. class.: Antineoplastic

Chem. class.: 3rd-generation platinum analog, alkylating agent

ACTION: Forms crosslinks, thereby inhibiting DNA replication and transcription; not specific to cell cycle

USES: Metastatic carcinoma of the colon or rectum in combination with 5-FU/leucovorin

CONTRAINDICATIONS

Pregnancy, breastfeeding, radiation therapy or chemotherapy within 1 mo, thrombocytopenia, smallpox vaccination

Black Box Warning: Hypersensitivity to this product or other platinum products

Precautions: Children, geriatric patients, pneumococcus vaccination, renal disease

DOSAGE AND ROUTES

Dosage protocols may vary

Colorectal cancer

• **Adult:** IV 85 mg/m^2 concurrently via Y-site with leucovorin (500 mg/m^2 IV) over 2 hr, followed 1 hr later by fluorouracil (500 mg/m^2 IV bolus) on days 1, 15, and 29. On days 8, 22, and 36, administer leucovorin (500 mg/m^2 IV over 2 hr) without oxaliplatin, followed 1 hr later by fluorouracil (500 mg/m^2 IV bolus). Repeat every 8 wk (56 days) for a total of 3 cycles (24 wk)

Renal dose

• **Adult:** IV CCr <30 mL/min, reduce starting dose to 65 mg/m^2

Available forms: Powder for inj 50, 100-mg single-use vials (5 mg/mL); solution for inj 50 mg/10 mL, 100 mg/20 mL, 200 mg/40 mL

Administer:

Intermittent IV INFUSION route

• Use oxaliplatin first if using 5-FU also

• Do not use ice during infusion, may make reactions worse

• Premedicate with antiemetics including 5HT$_3$ blockers, with or without dexamethasone; prehydration not needed

• Do not reconstitute or dilute with sodium chloride or any chloride-containing sol; do not use aluminum equipment during any preparation or administration; will degrade platinum; do not refrigerate unopened powder or sol; do not freeze; protect from light

• Use cytotoxic handling procedures; prepare in biologic cabinet using gown, gloves, mask; do not allow product to come in contact with skin; use soap and water if contact occurs

• EPINEPHrine, antihistamines, corticosteroids for hypersensitivity reaction

• **Lyophilized powder:** reconstitute vial 50 mg/10 mL or 100 mg/20 mL sterile water for inj or D$_5$W; after reconstitution, sol may be stored for ≤24 hr in refrigerator; after dilution in 250-500 mL D$_5$W, may store ≤24 hr in refrigerator or 6 hr at room temperature; infuse over 2 hr

Y-site compatibilities: Alfentanil, amifostine, amikacin, aminocaproic acid, amiodarone, amphotericin B colloidal, amphotericin B lipid complex, amphotericin B liposome, ampicillin, ampicillin-sulbactam, anidulafungin, atenolol, atracurium, azithromycin, aztreonam, bivalirudin, bleomycin, bumetanide, buprenorphine, butorphanol, calcium chloride/gluconate, CARBOplatin, caspofungin, ceFAZolin, cefotaxime, cefoTEtan, cefOXitin, cefTAZidime, ceftizoxime, cefTRIAXone, cefuroxime, chloramphenicol, chlorproMAZINE, cimetidine, ciprofloxacin, cisatracurium, CISplatin, clindamycin, cyclophosphamide, cycloSPORINE, cytarabine, dacarbazine, DACTINomycin, DAPTOmycin, DAUNOrubicin, dexamethasone, digoxin, diltiaZEM, diphenhydrAMINE, DOBUTamine, DOCEtaxel, dolasetron, DOPamine, doxacurium, DOXOrubicin, doxycycline, droperidol, enalaprilat, ePHEDrine, EPINEPHrine, epiRUBicin, ertapenem, erythromycin, esmolol, etoposide, famotidine, fenoldopam, fentaNYL, fluconazole, fludarabine, foscarnet, fosphenytoin, furosemide, gatifloxacin, gemcitabine, gemtuzumab, gentamicin, glycopyrrolate, granisetron, haloperidol, heparin, hydrALAZINE, hydrocortisone, HYDROmorphone, hydrOXYzine, IDArubicin, ifosfamide, imipenem-cilastatin, inamrinone, insulin (regular), irinotecan, isoproterenol, ketorolac, labetalol, leucovorin, levoFLOXacin, levorphanol, lidocaine, linezolid, LORazepam, magnesium sulfate, mannitol, meperidine, meropenem, mesna, metaraminol, methyldopate, methylPREDNISolone, metoclopramide, metoprolol, metroNIDAZOLE, midazolam, milrinone, minocycline, mitoMYcin, mitoXANTRONE, mivacurium, morphine, nafcillin, nalbuphine, naloxone, nesiritide, niCARdipine, nitroglycerin, nitroprusside, norepinephrine, octreotide, ondansetron, PACLitaxel, palonosetron, pancuronium, PEMEtrexed, pentamidine, pentazocine, phenylephrine, piperacillin, polymyxin B, potassium chloride/phosphates, procainamide, prochlorperazine, promethazine, propranolol, quiNIDine, quinupristindalfopristin, raNITIdine, rocuronium, sodium acetate/phosphates, succinylcholine, SUFentanil, sulfamethoxazole-trimethoprim, tacrolimus, teniposide, theophylline, thiotepa, ticarcillin, ticarcillin-clavulanate, tigecycline, tirofiban, tobramycin, tolazoline, topotecan, trimethobenzamide, vancomycin, vasopressin, vecuronium, verapamil, vinBLAStine, vinCRIStine, vinorelbine, voriconazole, zidovudine, zoledronic acid

SIDE EFFECTS

CNS: Peripheral neuropathy, fatigue, headache, dizziness, insomnia, reversible posterior leukoencephalopathy syndrome
CV: Cardiac abnormalities, thromboembolism
EENT: *Decreased visual acuity, tinnitus, hearing loss*
GI: *Severe nausea, vomiting, diarrhea, weight loss,* stomatitis, anorexia, gastroesophageal reflux, constipation, dyspepsia, mucositis, flatulence
GU: Hematuria, dysuria, creatinine
HEMA: Thrombocytopenia, leukopenia, pancytopenia, neutropenia, anemia, hemolytic uremic syndrome
INTEG: Rash, flushing, extravasation, redness, swelling, pain at inj site
META: Hypokalemia
RESP: Fibrosis, dyspnea, cough, rhinitis, URI, pharyngitis
SYST: Anaphylaxis, angioedema

PHARMACOKINETICS

Metabolized in liver, excreted in urine; after administration, 15% of platinum in systemic circulation, 85% either in tissues or being eliminated in urine; half-life 390 hr; protein binding >90%

INTERACTIONS

Increase: QT prolongation: class Ia/III antidysrhythmias, monitor ECG
Increase: bleeding risk—NSAIDs, alcohol, anticoagulants, platelet inhibitors, thrombolytics, salicylates
Increase: oxaliplatin toxicity—tannins
Increase: myelosuppression—myelosuppressive agents, radiation, taxanes, tofacitinib
Increase: nephrotoxicity—aminoglycosides, loop diuretics
Decrease: antibody response—inactivated vaccines
Drug/Lab Test
Increase: ALT, AST, bilirubin, creatinine
Decrease: potassium, neutrophils, WBC, platelets

NURSING CONSIDERATIONS
Assess:
• **Bone marrow depression:** CBC, differential, platelet count each cycle; withhold product if WBC is <4000/mm³ or platelet count is <100,000/mm³; notify prescriber of results
• **Renal/hepatic studies:** BUN, creatinine, serum uric acid, urine CCr before, electrolytes during therapy; dose should not be given if BUN >19 mg/dL; creatinine <1.5 mg/dL; I&O ratio; report fall in urine output of <30 mL/hr; LFTs

Black Box Warning: **Anaphylaxis:** wheezing, tachycardia, facial swelling, fainting, rash, dyspnea, hives; discontinue product, report to prescriber; resuscitation equipment should be nearby with epinephrine, corticosteroids

• **Pulmonary fibrosis:** cough, crackles, dyspnea, pulmonary infiltrate; discontinue immediately; death may occur
• **Reversible posterior leukoencephalopathy syndrome:** assess for headache, seizures, diarrhea, infection, abnormal vision, change in mental functioning; discontinue immediately
• Monitor temperature; may indicate beginning infection
• Hepatic studies before each cycle (bilirubin, AST, ALT, LDH) as needed or monthly
• **Bleeding:** hematuria, guaiac, bruising or petechiae, mucosa or orifices; obtain prescription for viscous lidocaine (Xylocaine)
• All medications PO if possible; avoid IM inj when platelets <100,000/mm³
• **Pregnancy/breastfeeding:** do not use in pregnancy, breastfeeding, use contraception
Evaluate:
• **Therapeutic response:** decreased tumor size, spread of malignancy
Teach patient/family:
• **To report signs of infection:** increased temperature, sore throat, flulike symptoms
• To report signs of **anemia:** fatigue, headache, faintness, SOB, irritability
• To report **bleeding;** to avoid use of razors, commercial mouthwash
• To avoid aspirin, ibuprofen, NSAIDs, alcohol; may cause GI bleeding
• To report any changes in breathing, coughing
• To report numbness, tingling in face or extremities, poor hearing, or joint pain or swelling
• Not to receive live virus vaccines during treatment
• **Dysesthesias:** to avoid contact with cold (air, ice, liquid)

• To use contraception during treatment and for 4 mo after; that product may cause infertility

⚠ HIGH ALERT

oxazepam (Rx)
(ox-ay´ze-pam)
Func. class.: Sedative/hypnotic; anxiolytic
Chem. class.: Benzodiazepine, short acting

Controlled Substance Schedule IV

ACTION: Potentiates the actions of GABA, especially in the limbic system and the reticular formation

USES: Anxiety, alcohol withdrawal
Unlabeled uses: Insomnia

CONTRAINDICATIONS
Pregnancy, breastfeeding, children <6 yr, hypersensitivity to benzodiazepines, closed-angle glaucoma, psychosis
Precautions: Geriatric patients, debilitated patients, renal/hepatic disease, depression, suicidal ideation, dementia, sleep apnea, seizure disorder

Black Box Warning: Depressants, respiratory depression

DOSAGE AND ROUTES
Anxiety (mild/moderate)
• **Adult /child ≥12 yr: PO** 10-15 mg tid-qid, max 120 mg/day
• **Geriatric: PO** 10 mg daily-bid, max 60 mg/day tid
Alcohol withdrawal, severe anxiety
• **Adult: PO** 15-30 mg tid-qid
Severe anxiety syndrome, agitation, anxiety with depression
• **Adult/child >12 yr: PO** 15-30 mg tid-qid
Available forms: Caps 10, 15, 30 mg
Administer:
• Without regard to food

• Taper product (0.5 mg q3days) before discontinuing

SIDE EFFECTS

CNS: *Dizziness, drowsiness,* confusion, headache, anxiety, tremors, fatigue, depression, insomnia, hallucinations, paradoxical excitement, transient amnesia
CV: *Orthostatic hypotension,* ECG changes, tachycardia, hypotension
EENT: *Blurred vision,* tinnitus, mydriasis
GI: Nausea, vomiting, anorexia, drug-induced hepatitis
HEMA: Leukopenia
INTEG: Rash, dermatitis, itching
SYST: Dependence

PHARMACOKINETICS

Peak 2-4 hr; metabolized by liver; excreted by kidneys; half-life 5-15 hr; crosses placenta, breast milk; protein binding 97%

INTERACTIONS

Black Box Warning: **Increase:** oxazepam effects, respiratory depression—CNS depressants, alcohol, disulfiram, opioids

Decrease: oxazepam effects—oral contraceptives, phenytoin, theophylline, valproic acid
Decrease: effects of levodopa
Drug/Herb
Increase: CNS depression—kava, melatonin, valerian
Drug/Lab Test
Increase: AST, ALT, serum bilirubin
Decrease: WBC

NURSING CONSIDERATIONS
Assess:
• CBC and LFTs periodically in longer-term therapy

Black Box Warning: **Respiratory depression:** not to be used in preexisting respiratory depression; use cautiously in severe pulmonary disease; monitor respirations, avoid use with opioids or other CNS depressants

• **Mental status:** mood, sensorium, affect, sleeping pattern, drowsiness, dizziness, sedation, suicidal thoughts/behaviors
• **Physical dependency, withdrawal symptoms:** headache, nausea, vomiting, muscle pain, weakness, tremors, seizures (long-term use)
• **Beers:** avoid in older adults; delirium, cognitive impairment may occur
• **Pregnancy/breastfeeding:** assess for pregnancy before use; do not use in pregnancy; do not breastfeed
Evaluate:
• **Therapeutic response:** decreased anxiety, restlessness, insomnia
Teach patient/family:
• That product may be taken without regard to food
• That medication is not to be used for everyday stress or used >4 mo unless directed by prescriber; not to take more than prescribed dose because product may be habit forming
• To avoid OTC preparations (cough, cold, hay fever) unless approved by prescriber
• To avoid driving, activities that require alertness because drowsiness may occur
• To avoid alcohol, other psychotropic products unless directed by prescriber
• Not to discontinue product abruptly after long-term use
• To rise slowly because fainting may occur, especially among geriatric patients
• That drowsiness may worsen at beginning of treatment
• To notify prescriber if pregnancy is planned or suspected

OXcarbazepine (Rx)
(ox′kar-baz′uh-peen)
Trileptal, Oxtellar XR
Func. class.: Anticonvulsant, miscellaneous
Chem. class.: CarBAMazepine analog

Do not confuse:

OXcarbazepine/carBAMazepine

ACTION: May inhibit nerve impulses by limiting influx of sodium ions across cell membrane in motor cortex

USES: Partial seizures

CONTRAINDICATIONS

Hypersensitivity

Precautions: Pregnancy, breastfeeding, children <4 yr, hypersensitivity to carBAMazepine, renal disease, fluid restriction, hyponatremia, abrupt discontinuation, suicidal ideation, ☜ positive for HLA-B 1502 allele

DOSAGE AND ROUTES

Partial seizures, adjunctive therapy

• **Adult: PO IR** 300 mg bid, may be increased by 600 mg/day in divided doses bid at weekly intervals; maintenance 1200 mg/day; **ext rel:** 600 mg daily × 1 wk, increase weekly in 600 mg/day increments to 1200-2400 mg daily

Child/adolescent 2 to 16 yr, >39 kg: PO 8 to 10 mg/kg/day (Max: 600 mg/day) divided twice daily, initially. Increase over 2 wk to 1800 mg/day

Child/adolescent 2 to 16 yr, 29.1 to 39 kg: PO 8 to 10 mg/kg/day divided twice daily, initially. Increase the over 2 es to 1200 mg/day

Child/adolescent 2 to 16 yr, 20 to 29 kg: PO 8 to 10 mg/kg/day divided twice daily, initially. Increase over 2 wk to 900 mg/day.

Child 2 to 3 years, <20 kg: PO 8 to 10 mg/kg/day divided twice daily or may consider 16 to 20 mg/kg/day divided twice daily, initially. Increase the dose over 2 to 4 wk to a dose of 60 mg/kg/day

Conversion to monotherapy for partial seizures

• **Adult: PO** 300 mg bid with reduction in other anticonvulsants; increase OXcarbazepine by 600 mg/day each week over 2-4 wk; withdraw other anticonvulsants over 3-6 wk; max 2400 mg/day

Initiation of monotherapy for partial seizures

• **Adult: PO** 300 mg bid, increase by 300 mg/day q3days to 1200 mg in divided doses bid, max 1200 mg/day

Renal dose

• **Adult: PO CCr <30 mL/min,** 150 mg bid, increase slowly

Available forms: Film-coated tabs 150, 300, 600 mg; oral susp 300 mg/5 mL; ext rel tab 150, 300, 600 mg

Administer:

PO route

• Without regard to meals

• Test for HLA-B* 1502 allele in Asian/South Asian patient, if positive consider another treatment

• **Oral susp:** shake well, use calibrated oral syringe provided, use or discard within 7 days of opening

• **Ext rel:** do not crush, break, or chew

• Store at room temperature

SIDE EFFECTS

CNS: *Headache, dizziness, confusion, fatigue,* feeling abnormal, ataxia, abnormal gait, tremors, anxiety, agitation, worsening of seizures, suicidal thoughts/behaviors

CV: *Hypotension,* chest pain, edema, bradycardia, syncope

EENT: *Blurred vision, diplopia, nystagmus,* rhinitis, sinusitis

ENDO: Hypothyroidism, hot flashes

GI: *Nausea, constipation, diarrhea,* anorexia, vomiting, abdominal pain, gastritis

GU: Urinary frequency, hematuria, menses change

INTEG: Purpura, rash, acne

META: Hyponatremia

RESP: Flulike symptoms

SYST: Angioedema, anaphylaxis, Stevens-Johnson syndrome, toxic epidermal necrolysis, drug reaction with eosinophilia and systemic symptoms (DRESS)

PHARMACOKINETICS

PO: Onset unknown; peak 4-6 hr; metabolized by liver to active metabolite; terminal half-life 7-9 hr metabolite; inhibits P450 CYP2C19, induces CYP3A4/5, 95% renal extraction

INTERACTIONS

Increase: CNS depression—alcohol

Decrease: effects—felodipine, oral contraceptive, carBAMazepine

---

Side effects: *italics* = common; red = life-threatening

Decrease: OXcarbazepine levels—car-BAMazepine, PHENobarbital, phenytoin, valproic acid, verapamil

Decrease: effect of substrates—CYP3A4 substrates (cycloSPORINE, itraconazole, rivaroxaban)

Drug/Herb

Increase: anticonvulsant effect—ginkgo

Decrease: anticonvulsant effect—ginseng, santonica

Drug/Lab Test

Decrease: sodium

NURSING CONSIDERATIONS
Assess:

• **Description of seizures:** frequency, duration, aura

• **Hyponatremia:** headache, nausea, confusion, usually within the first 3 mo of treatment, but may occur ≤1 yr, if this product is being used with other products that decrease sodium, monitor sodium levels

• **Serious reactions:** angioedema, anaphylaxis, Stevens-Johnson syndrome

• **CNS/mental status:** mood, sensorium, affect, behavioral changes, confusion, suicidal thoughts/behaviors; if mental status changes, notify prescriber

• **Beers:** avoid in older adults unless safer alternatives are unavailable; ataxia, impaired psychomotor function may occur

• **Pregnancy/breastfeeding:** use only if benefits outweigh fetal risk; may cause lack of seizure control due to a metabolite of OXcarbazepine; monitor seizure control; enroll in the North American Antiepileptic Drug (NAAED) Pregnancy Registry, 888-233-2334; do not breastfeed

Evaluate:

• **Therapeutic response:** decreased seizure activity

Teach patient/family:

• To avoid driving, other activities that require alertness

• Not to discontinue medication quickly after long-term use; seizures may increase

• To inform prescriber if hypersensitive to carBAMazepine; multisystem hypersensitivity may occur; to report fever, other allergic symptoms

• To avoid use of alcohol while taking product

• To use alternative contraception if using hormonal method; to report if pregnancy is planned or suspected

• To report skin rashes immediately; serious skin reactions can occur

• To report suicidal thoughts/behavior immediately

• **Pregnancy/breastfeeding:** if pregnant, to enroll in North American Antiepileptic Drug Pregnancy Registry, 888-233-2334; not to breastfeed, excreted in breast milk

TREATMENT OF OVERDOSE:
Give 0.9% NaCl (hypotensive state), atropine (bradycardia); use benzodiazepines, barbiturates for seizures

---

oxybutynin (Rx)
(ox-i-byoo'ti-nin)

Ditropan XL, Gelnique, Oxytrol

Func. class.: Anticholinergic, urinary antispasmodic

Chem. class.: Synthetic tertiary amine

Do not confuse:
Ditropan/diazePAM/Diprivan

ACTION: Relaxes smooth muscles in urinary tract by inhibiting acetylcholine at postganglionic sites

USES: Antispasmodic for neurogenic bladder, overactive bladder in females (OTC)

CONTRAINDICATIONS
Hypersensitivity, GI obstruction, urinary retention, glaucoma, severe colitis, myasthenia gravis, unstable CV disease

Precautions: Pregnancy, breastfeeding, children <12 yr, geriatric patients, suspected glaucoma, cardiac disease, dementia

DOSAGE AND ROUTES
Overactive bladder

- **Adults: PO IR** 5 mg bid-tid, max: 5 mg qid
- **Geriatric: PO IR** 2.5 mg bid-tid, max: 5 mg qid
- **Child 5-12 yr: PO IR** 5 mg bid, max: 5 mg tid
- **Adults: PO EXT REL** 5-10 mg daily, adjust weekly by 5-mg increments max: 30 mg/day
- **Child/adolescent 6-17 yr: PO EXT REL** 5 mg daily, adjust weekly by 5-mg increments, max: 20 mg/day; symptoms of detrusor overactivity associated with a neurologic condition (spina bifida)
- **Adults: TD** apply 1 patch (3.9 mg/day) twice weekly to the abdomen, hip, or buttock; rotate patch site at each application
- **Adults: TOP** Apply the contents of 1 sachet/actuation of the metered-dose pump daily; apply to the abdomen, upper arms/shoulders, or thighs; rotate sites of application; the same site should not be used on consecutive days

Available forms: Syr 5 mg/5 mL; tabs 5 mg; ext rel tabs 5, 10, 15 mg; TD 3.9 mg/day; top gel 10% (Gelnique)

Administer:

PO route
- Do not crush, break, or chew ext rel tabs
- Without regard to meals
- Use measuring device for syrup

Topical route (gel)
- Wash hands; apply to clean, dry intact skin on abdomen, upper arms/shoulders, thighs; avoid navel, rotate sites
- Squeeze contents into palm of hand or directly on site, rub gently
- Do not bathe, exercise, swim for 1 hr after application
- Allow to dry before putting on clothing
- Do not be near flame, fire, or smoke until gel has dried
- Delivers 100 mg

Transdermal route
- Apply to clean, dry intact skin on abdomen, hip, buttock; use firm pressure; not affected by showering/bathing; rotate sites
- Do not expose to sun
- Do not cut
- Delivers 3.9 mg/day

SIDE EFFECTS

CNS: *Anxiety, restlessness, dizziness, somnolence, insomnia, nervousness,* seizures, headache, *drowsiness,* confusion

CV: *Palpitations, sinus tachycardia,* hypertension, peripheral edema, QT prolongation

EENT: *Blurred vision, dry eyes,* increased intraocular tension, *dry mouth,* dry throat

GI: *Nausea, vomiting, anorexia,* abdominal pain, *constipation, dyspepsia,* diarrhea, taste perversion, GERD

GU: Dysuria, impotence, *urinary retention, hesitancy*

MISC: Hyperthermia, anaphylaxis, angioedema

PHARMACOKINETICS

Onset ½-1 hr, peak 3-6 hr, duration 6-10 hr; metabolized by liver, excreted in urine; terminal half-life 2-3 hr

INTERACTIONS

- Altered pharmacokinetic parameters: CYP3A4 inhibitors

Increase: CNS depression—benzodiazepines, sedatives, hypnotics, opioids

Increase: levels of atenolol, digoxin, nitrofurantoin

Increase: anticholinergic effects—antihistamines, amantadine, other anticholinergics

Increase or decrease: levels of phenothiazines

Decrease: levels of acetaminophen, haloperidol, levodopa

Decrease: effects of oxybutynin—CYP3A4 inducers

NURSING CONSIDERATIONS

Assess:
- **Urinary patterns:** distention, nocturia, frequency, urgency, incontinence, I&O ratios; cystometry to diagnose dysfunction, urinary tract infections should be treated
- **Allergic reactions:** rash, urticaria; if these occur, product should be discontinued; **angio-oedema:** swelling of face, tongue, throat
- **QT prolongation:** ECG for QT prolongation, ejection fraction; assess for chest pain, palpitations, dyspnea

• **CNS effects:** confusion, anxiety; anticholinergic effects in geriatric patients
• **Pregnancy/breastfeeding:** use only if benefit outweighs risks; cautious use in breastfeeding, excretion unknown
• **Beers:** avoid in older adults; delirium risk is increased

Evaluate:
• Absence of dysuria, frequency, nocturia, incontinence

Teach patient/family:
• To avoid hazardous activities because dizziness, blurred vision may occur
• To avoid OTC medications with alcohol, other CNS depressants
• To avoid hot weather, strenuous activity because product decreases perspiration
• About the correct application of each product form
• **Transdermal:** change patch 2×/wk; do not use same site within 7 days; dispose of and use container not accessible to pets/children
• To open patch immediately before using
• Do not use during MRI, remove

Topical gel:
• Rotate sites
• Apply to clean, dry skin on abdomen, upper arm/shoulders/thighs
• Gel is flammable

⚠ HIGH ALERT

oxyCODONE (Rx)
(ox-i-koe′done)
Oxaydo, OxyCONTIN, Oxy IR ✦, OxyNEO ✦ Roxicodone, Supeudol ✦, Xtampza ER, RoxyBond

oxyCODONE/acetaminophen (Rx)
Endocet, Percocet, Nalocet, Prolate, Primlev

oxyCODONE/aspirin (Rx)
Endodan

Func. class.: Opiate analgesic
Chem. class.: Semisynthetic derivative

Controlled Substance Schedule II

Do not confuse:
oxyCODONE/HYDROcodone

ACTION: Inhibits ascending pain pathways in CNS, increases pain threshold, alters pain perception

USES: Moderate to severe pain
Unlabeled uses: Postherpetic neuralgic (cont rel)

CONTRAINDICATIONS
Hypersensitivity, addiction (opiate), asthma, ileus

Black Box Warning: Respiratory depression

Precautions: Pregnancy, breastfeeding, child <18 yr, addictive personality, increased intracranial pressure, MI (acute), severe heart disease, renal/hepatic disease, bowel impaction

Black Box Warning: Opioid-naïve patients, substance abuse, accidental exposure, potential for overdose/poisoning, status asthmaticus

DOSAGE AND ROUTES
OxyCODONE severe pain
• **Adult:** PO 10-30 mg q4hr (5-15 mg q4-6hr for opiate-naïve patients). Concentrated sol is extremely concentrated; do not use interchangeably; **CONT REL** 10 mg q12hr for opiate-naïve patients
• **Child >5 yr/adolescent: PO (unlabeled)** 0.2 mg/kg given 30 min preprocedural

OxyCODONE/acetaminophen moderate to moderately severe pain
• **Adult:** PO IR 2.5-10 mg oxyCODONE and 325 mg acetaminophen q6hr, max 60 mg oxyCODONE or 4 g acetaminophen per day

Acute pain
• **Adult:** PO ext rel 2 tabs q12hr, max acetaminophen 4 g

OxyCODONE/aspirin moderate to moderately severe pain
• **Adult:** PO 1 tab q6hr as needed, max 12 tabs/24 hr

Available forms: OxyCODONE: *cont rel tabs* (OxyCONTIN) 10, 15, 20, 30, 40, 80, 160 mg; *immediate rel tabs* 5, 7.5, 10, 15, 20, 30 mg; *immediate rel caps* 5 mg; *oral sol* 5 mg/5 mL, 20 mg/mL; **oxyCODONE with acetaminophen:** 2.5 mg/325 mg, 5 mg/325 mg, 7.5 mg/325 mg, 7.5 mg/300 mg, 10 mg/325 mg, *oral sol* 5 mg/325 mg/5 mL; *ext rel caps* 9, 13.5, 18, 27, 36 mg; **oxyCODONE with aspirin:** 4.835 mg/325 mg

Administer:
• Clarify all orders; fatalities have occurred
• Regular administration is more effective than PRN; give before pain becomes severe
• Discontinue gradually after long-term use
• Store in light-resistant area at room temperature
• OxyCODONE should be titrated from the initial recommended dosage to the dosage required to relieve pain
• There is no maximum dosage of oxyCODONE; however, careful titration is required until tolerance develops to some of the side effects (drowsiness, respiratory depression)

Oral solid formulations
Immediate-release tablets route
• May be administered with food or milk to minimize GI irritation
Extended-release caps route
• **Xtampza ER brand capsules:** take with food and the same amount of food
• Capsule contents may be sprinkled onto soft foods (applesauce, pudding, yogurt, ice cream, or jam) or into a cup and then given directly into the mouth; swallow immediately and rinse mouth
• Capsule contents may be given through an NG or gastrostomy tube. Flush tube with water. Open a capsule and pour the contents directly into the tube. Do not premix capsule contents with the liquid that will be used to flush the tube. Draw up 15 mL of water into a syringe, insert the syringe into the tube, and flush the contents through the tube. Repeat flushing twice using 10 mL of water with each flush. Extended-release 36-mg capsules are for use ONLY in opioid-tolerant patients
• Monitor patients closely for respiratory depression, particularly within the first 24-72 hr after initiation or dose escalation

Controlled-release tablets route (OxyCONTIN):
• Administer whole; do not crush, chew, or break in half; taking chewed, broken, or crushed controlled-release tablets could lead to the rapid release and absorption of a potentially toxic dose of oxyCODONE
• **OxyCONTIN brand tablets:** do not presoak, lick, or otherwise wet tablet before administering dose; administer 1 tablet at a time; allow patient to swallow each tablet separately with sufficient liquid
• **OxyCODONE controlled-release (OxyCONTIN)** 60-mg and 80-mg tablets are for use only in opioid-tolerant patients
• May be administered without food
Oral liquid formulations
Oral concentrate solution route
• Is a highly concentrated sol (20 mg oxyCODONE/mL), and care should be taken in dispensing and administering this medication; the sol may be added to 30 mL of a liquid or semisolid food; if the medication is placed in liquid or food, consume immediately; do not store diluted oxyCODONE for future use

SIDE EFFECTS
CNS: *Drowsiness, dizziness, confusion, headache, sedation, euphoria,* fatigue, abnormal dreams/thoughts, hallucinations
CV: Palpitations, bradycardia, change in B/P
EENT: Tinnitus, blurred vision, miosis, diplopia
GI: *Nausea, vomiting, anorexia, constipation, cramps,* gastritis, dyspepsia, biliary spasms
GU: Increased urinary output, dysuria, urinary retention
INTEG: *Rash,* urticaria, bruising, flushing, diaphoresis, pruritus
RESP: Respiratory depression

PHARMACOKINETICS
PO: Onset 15-30 min, peak 1 hr, duration reg rel 2-6 hr, cont rel 12 hr, metabolized by liver, excreted in urine, crosses placenta, excreted in breast milk, half-life 3-5 hr, protein binding 45%

INTERACTIONS

Black Box Warning: Increase: effects with other CNS depressants—alcohol, opioids, sedative/hypnotics, antipsychotics, skeletal muscle relaxants

Increase: oxyCODONE level—CYP3A4 inhibitors
Increase: toxicity—cimetidine, MAOIs
Drug/Herb
Increase: sedative effect—kava, St. John's wort, valerian
Drug/Lab Test
Increase: amylase, lipase

NURSING CONSIDERATIONS
Assess:
• **Pain:** intensity, location, type, characteristics; need for pain medication by pain/sedation scoring; physical dependence
• I&O ratio; check for decreasing output; may indicate urinary retention
• **CNS changes:** dizziness, drowsiness, hallucinations, euphoria, LOC, pupil reaction
• **Allergic reactions:** rash, urticaria

Black Box Warning: Respiratory dysfunction: respiratory depression, character, rate, rhythm; notify prescriber if respirations are <10/min; monitor B/P, pulse baseline and periodically

• **Bowel status:** constipation; stimulant laxative may be needed with fluids, fiber

Black Box Warning: Substance abuse: assess for substance abuse in patient/family/friends before prescribing; monitor for abuse; may crush, chew, snort, or inject ext rel product; may be fatal

Black Box Warning: Accidental exposure: dispose of properly away from pets, children

Black Box Warning: Pregnancy/breastfeeding: use only if benefits outweigh fetal risk; neonatal opioid withdrawal syndrome may occur with extended use; avoid breastfeeding, excreted in breast milk

• **Beers:** avoid in older adults; ataxia, impaired psychomotor function may occur
• Assistance with ambulation
• Safety measures: night-light, call bell within easy reach
Evaluate:
• **Therapeutic response:** decrease in pain without dependence
Teach patient/family:
• To report any symptoms of CNS changes, allergic reactions
• That physical dependency may result from extended use
• That withdrawal symptoms may occur after long-term use: nausea, vomiting, cramps, fever, faintness, anorexia
• To avoid CNS depressants, alcohol
• To avoid driving, operating machinery if drowsiness occurs

TREATMENT OF OVERDOSE: Naloxone (Narcan) 0.2-0.8 mg IV, O_2, IV fluids, vasopressors, caution with patients physically dependent on opioids

---

oxymetazoline nasal agent
See Appendix B

---

oxymetazoline ophthalmic
See Appendix B

⚠ HIGH ALERT

oxyMORphone (Rx)
(ox-i-mor′fone)
Func. class.: Opiate analgesic
Chem. class.: Semisynthetic phenanthrene derivative
Controlled Substance Schedule II

Do not confuse:
oxyMORphone/oxyCODONE

ACTION: Inhibits ascending pain pathways in CNS, increases pain threshold, alters pain perception

USES: Moderate to severe pain

CONTRAINDICATIONS
Hypersensitivity, addiction (opiate), asthma, hepatic disease, ileus, intrathecal use, surgery

Black Box Warning: Respiratory depression

Precautions: Pregnancy (short-term), breastfeeding, children <18 yr, addictive personality, increased intracranial pressure, MI (acute), severe heart disease, respiratory depression, renal/hepatic disease, bowel impaction

Black Box Warning: Alcoholism, opioid-naive patients, substance abuse

DOSAGE AND ROUTES
Acute pain
• **Adult: PO IR** 5-10 mg q4-6hr prn (opioid naive)
Chronic pain
• **Adult: PO ext rel** 5 mg q12hr
Available forms: Tabs 5, 10 mg; tabs ext rel 5, 7.5, 10, 15, 20, 30, 40 mg
Administer:
• 1 hr before or 2 hr after food (PO)
• With antiemetic for nausea, vomiting
• When pain is beginning to return; determine interval by response
• Store in light-resistant area at room temperature

SIDE EFFECTS
CNS: *Drowsiness, dizziness, confusion, headache,* hallucinations, increased intracranial pressure, *sedation,* seizures, *euphoria (geriatric patients)*
CV: Palpitations, bradycardia, change in B/P, hypotension
EENT: Tinnitus, blurred vision, miosis, diplopia

GI: *Nausea, vomiting, anorexia, constipation, cramps*
GU: Dysuria, urinary retention
INTEG: *Rash,* urticaria, bruising, flushing, diaphoresis, pruritus
RESP: Respiratory depression

PHARMACOKINETICS
Metabolized by liver, excreted in urine, crosses placenta, half-life: PO: 7-9 hr, ext rel: 9-11 hr
PO: Peak 1 hr (fasting)

INTERACTIONS

Black Box Warning: **Increase:** effects with other CNS depressants—alcohol, opiates, sedative/hypnotics, antipsychotics, skeletal muscle relaxants

• **Increase:** unpredictable effects/reactions—MAOIs
• **Increase:** serotonin syndrome SNRIs, SSRIs, tricyclics, MAOIs
Drug/Herb
Increase: sedative effect—kava, St. John's wort, valerian
Drug/Lab Test
Increase: amylase
Drug/Herb
Increase: Serotonin syndrome—St. John's wort

NURSING CONSIDERATIONS
Assess:
• **Pain:** location, intensity, type, other characteristics before and after need for pain medication, physical dependence, give 25%-50% until pain reduction of 50% on pain rating scale, repeat dose may be given at time of peak if previous dose does not control pain and respiratory depression has not occurred
• I&O ratio for decreasing output; may indicate urinary retention
• **Bowel status:** constipation; may need stimulative laxative if use ≥3 days; increased fluids, fiber for prevention
• **CNS changes:** dizziness, drowsiness, hallucinations, euphoria, LOC, pupil reaction
• **Allergic reactions:** rash, urticaria

Black Box Warning: **Respiratory dysfunction:** respiratory depression, character, rate, rhythm; notify prescriber if respirations are <10/min; dose may need to be decreased by 25%-50%; monitor B/P, pulse also

Black Box Warning: **Accidental exposure:** dispose of properly, away from children/pets

Black Box Warning: **Overdose/poisoning:** avoid alcohol ingestion; do not crush, chew, snort, or inject tabs; high abuse potential, assess for abuse

Black Box Warning: **Opioid-naive patients:** ext rel tabs are not to be used immediately postop (12-24 hr after surgery) in these patients

• **Abrupt discontinuation:** Taper after long-term use, assess for withdrawal: anxiety, restlessness, cramps, nausea/vomiting
• **Pregnancy/breastfeeding:** use only if benefits outweigh fetal risk; neonatal opioid withdrawal syndrome may occur with extended use; avoid breastfeeding
• **Beers:** avoid use in older adults; ataxia, impaired psychomotor function may occur
Evaluate:
• **Therapeutic response:** decrease in pain
Teach patient/family:
• To report any symptoms of CNS changes, allergic reactions, serotonin syndrome
• That physical dependency may result from extended use
• That withdrawal symptoms may occur: nausea, vomiting, cramps, fever, faintness, anorexia
• Not to drive or operate machinery if drowsiness occurs
• Not to use other CNS depressants, alcohol
• To make position changes slowly to prevent orthostatic hypotension
• To notify prescriber of all OTC, Rx, herbs, supplements being taken; not to take new products unless approved by prescriber
• To notify health care professional if pregnancy is planned or suspected; avoid breastfeeding

TREATMENT OF OVERDOSE: Naloxone (Narcan) 0.2-0.8 mg IV (caution with patients physically dependent on opioids), O_2, IV fluids, vasopressors

⚠ HIGH ALERT

oxytocin (Rx)
(ox-i-toe´sin)
Pitocin
Func. class.: Hormone
Chem. class.: Oxytocic, uterine-active agent

ACTION: Acts directly on myofibrils, thereby producing uterine contraction; stimulates milk ejection by the breast; vasoactive antidiuretic effect

USES: Stimulation, induction of labor; missed or incomplete abortion; postpartum bleeding

CONTRAINDICATIONS
Hypersensitivity, serum toxemia, cephalopelvic disproportion, fetal distress, hypertonic uterus, prolapsed umbilical cord, active genital herpes
Precautions: Cervical/uterine surgery, uterine sepsis, primipara >35 yr, 1st/2nd stage of labor

Black Box Warning: Elective induction of labor

DOSAGE AND ROUTES
Postpartum hemorrhage
• **Adult:** IV 10-40 units in 1000 mL nonhydrating diluent infused at 20-40 mU/min
Stimulation of labor
• **Adult:** IV 0.5-1 mU/min, increase by 1-2 mU q15-60min until contractions occur, then decrease dose
Incomplete/elective abortion
• **Adult:** IV INFUSION 10 units/500 mL D_5W or 0.9% NaCl at 10-20 mU/min, max 30 units/12 hr
Available forms: Inj 10 units/mL

Administer:
- Give by IV infusion or IM, not used routinely IM
- Before use, an IV infusion of NS should be already running for use in case of adverse reactions. Magnesium sulfate should be readily available if relaxation of the myometrium is needed
- Visually inspect parenteral product for particulate matter and discoloration before use

IV infusion route
- Administer using an infusion pump to ensure accurate dosing

Induction of labor
- Dilute 1 mL (10 units) in 1000 mL of a compatible IV infusion solution. Rotate infusion bottle for thorough mixing. The resultant infusion should contain 10 milliunits/mL

Control of postpartum uterine bleeding
- Dilute 10-40 units in a compatible IV solution or to an already infusing solution. The maximum concentration is 40 units in 1000 mL of solution

Incomplete, inevitable, or elective abortion
- Dilute 10 units in 500 mL of a compatible IV solution

IM route
- Not used routinely IM
- Inject into a large muscle mass; aspirate before injection to avoid injection into a blood vessel

Y-site compatibilities: Acyclovir, alfentanil, allopurinol, amikacin, aminocaproic acid, aminophylline, amphotericin B liposome (ambisome), anidulafungin, argatroban, ascorbic acid injection, atenolol, atracurium, atropine, azaTHIOprine, azithromycin, aztreonam, benztropine, bivalirudin, bumetanide, buprenorphine, butorphanol, calcium chloride/gluconate, capreomycin, caspofungin, cefamandole, ceFAZolin, cefepime, cefoperazone, cefotaxime, cefoTEtan, cefOXitin, cefTAZidime, ceftizoxime, cefTRIAXone, cefuroxime, chloramphenicol, chlorothiazide, chlorpheniramine, cimetidine, ciprofloxacin, cisatracurium, clindamycin, cloxacillin,

colistimethate, cyanocobalamin, cyclophosphamide, cycloSPORINE, DAPTOmycin, dexamethasone, dexmedetomidine, digoxin, dilTIAZEM, diphenhydrAMINE, DOBUTamine, dolasetron, DOPamine, doxycycline, droperidol, edetate calcium disodium, enalaprilat, ePHEDrine, EPINEPHrine, epoetin alfa, eptifibatide, ergonovine, ertapenem, erythromycin, esmolol, famotidine, fenoldopam, fentaNYL, fluconazole, folic acid (as sodium salt), foscarnet, fosphenytoin, furosemide, gallamine, ganciclovir, gatifloxacin, gentamicin, glycopyrrolate, granisetron, heparin, hydrocortisone sodium succinate, HYDROmorphone, hydrOXYzine, imipenem-cilastatin, isoproterenol, kanamycin, ketamine, ketorolac, labetalol, lactated Ringer's injection, lansoprazole, lepirudin, leucovorin, levoFLOXacin, lidocaine, lincomycin, linezolid, LORazepam, magnesium sulfate, mannitol, mechlorethamine, meperidine, mephentermine, meropenem, metaraminol, methyldopate, methylPREDNISolone, metoclopramide, metoprolol, metroNIDAZOLE, midazolam, milrinone, minocycline, morphine, moxifloxacin, multiple vitamins injection, mycophenolate mofetil, nafcillin, nalbuphine, nalorphine, naloxone, nesiritide, netilmicin, niCARdipine, nitroglycerin, nitroprusside, norepinephrine, ondansetron, oxacillin, palonosetron, pamidronate, papaverine, penicillin G potassium/sodium, pentamidine, pentazocine, PENTobarbital, PHENobarbital, phentolamine, phenylephrine, phytonadione, piperacillin sodium, piperacillin-tazobactam, polymyxin B, potassium acetate/chloride/phosphates, procainamide, prochlorperazine, promazine, promethazine, propranolol, protamine, pyridoxine, quinupristin-dalfopristin, raNITIdine, Ringer's injection, sodium acetate/bicarbonate/phosphates, streptomycin, succinylcholine, SUFentanil, tacrolimus, theophylline, thiamine hydrochloride, ticarcillin disodium, ticarcillin disodium-clavulanate potassium, tigecycline, tirofiban hydrochloride, tobramycin sulfate, tolazoline, trimetaphan, tubocurarine, urokinase, vancomycin, vasopressin, verapamil, vitamin B complex with B, voriconazole, warfarin, zidovudine, zoledronic acid

SIDE EFFECTS
CNS: Seizures, tetanic contractions
CV: Hypo/hypertension, dysrhythmias, increased pulse, bradycardia, tachycardia, PVC
FETUS: Dysrhythmias, jaundice, hypoxia, intracranial hemorrhage
GI: Anorexia, nausea, vomiting, constipation
GU: Abruptio placentae, decreased uterine blood flow
HEMA: Increased hyperbilirubinemia
INTEG: Rash
RESP: Asphyxia
SYST: Water intoxication of mother

PHARMACOKINETICS
IM: Onset 3-7 min, duration 1 hr, half-life 12-17 min
IV: Onset 1 min, duration 30 min, half-life 12-17 min

INTERACTIONS
Increase: oxytocin effects—dinoprostone
Increase: QT prolongation—other drugs that increase QT interval
Increase: hypertension—vasopressors, avoid using together
Drug/Herb
• **Increase:** hypertension—ephedra

NURSING CONSIDERATIONS
Assess:

• Assess for fetal presentation, pelvic dimensions before use
• B/P, pulse; watch for changes that may indicate hemorrhage
• Respiratory rate, rhythm, depth; notify prescriber of abnormalities
• Monitor continuously, discontinue immediately if fetal distress occurs or uterine hyperactivity occurs
• Length, intensity, duration of contraction; notify prescriber of contractions lasting >1 min or absence of contractions; turn patient on her left side; discontinue oxytocin
• **FHTs, fetal distress;** watch for acceleration, deceleration; notify prescriber if problems occur; fetal presentation, pelvic dimensions; turn patient on left side if FHT change in rate, give O2
• **Water intoxication:** confusion, anuria, drowsiness, headache; monitor I&O

Black Box Warning: Elective induction of labor: use for induction only when medically necessary

Evaluate:
• **Therapeutic response:** stimulation of labor, control of postpartum bleeding
Teach patient/family:
• To report increased blood loss, abdominal cramps, fever, foul-smelling lochia, nausea, blurred vision, itching, swelling
• That contractions will be similar to menstrual cramps, gradually increasing in intensity

▲ HIGH ALERT

PACLitaxel (Rx)
(pa-kli-tax'el)
PACLitaxel protein bound particle (Rx)
Abraxane
Func. class.: Antineoplastic—miscellaneous
Chem. class.: Taxane

Do not confuse:
PACLitaxel/PARoxetine/Paxil

ACTION: Inhibits reorganization of microtubule network needed for interphase and mitotic cellular functions; causes abnormal bundles of microtubules during cell cycle and multiple esters of microtubules during mitosis

USES: **PACLitaxel:** metastatic carcinoma of the ovary, breast; AIDS-related Kaposi's sarcoma (2nd-line), non–small-cell lung cancer (1st-line), adjuvant treatment for node-positive breast cancer, prostate cancer, esophageal cancer, melanoma
PACLitaxel Protein Bound Particles: metastatic breast cancer after failure or relapse, metastatic pancreatic adenocarcinoma refractory prostate cancer, bladder cancer
Unlabeled uses: (Paclitaxel) endometrial, penile cancer

CONTRAINDICATIONS
Pregnancy; hypersensitivity to PACLitaxel or other products with polyoxyethylated castor oil, albumin

Black Box Warning: Neutropenia <1500/mm³

Precautions: Breastfeeding, children, females, geriatric patients, cardiovascular/hepatic/renal disease, CNS disorder, bone marrow suppression, dental disease, dental work, extravasation, herpes, infection, infertility, jaundice, ocular exposure, radiation therapy, thrombocytopenia, vaccination

Black Box Warning: Anaphylaxis, bone marrow suppression, requires a specialized care setting, requires an experienced clinician

DOSAGE AND ROUTES
PACLitaxel
Ovarian carcinoma
• **Adult: IV INFUSION** 135 mg/m² given over 24 hr or 175 mg/m² over 3 hr q3wk, then CISplatin 75 mg/m²
Breast carcinoma node positive
• **Adult: IV INFUSION** 175 mg/m² over 3 hr q3wk × 4 courses
AIDS-related Kaposi's sarcoma
• **Adult: IV INFUSION** 135 mg/m² over 3 hr q3wk or 100 mg/m² over 3 hr q2wk
First-line non–small-cell lung cancer
• **Adult: IV INFUSION** 135 mg/m²/24 hr infusion with CISplatin 75 mg/m² × 3 wk
Hepatic dose
• **Adult:** Dose reduction for 135 mg/m² 24-hr **IV INFUSION**—AST/ALT 2-10 × ULN, total bilirubin ≤1.5 mg/dL: give 100 mg/m²; AST/ALT <10 × ULN, total bilirubin 1.6-7.5 mg/dL: 50 mg/m²; AST/ALT ≥10 × ULN or total bilirubin >7.5 mg/dL: avoid use
• **Adult:** Dose reduction for 175 mg/m² 3-hr **IV INFUSION**—AST/ALT <10 × ULN, total bilirubin 1.26-2 × ULN: give 135 mg/m²; AST/ALT <10 × ULN, total bilirubin 2.01-5 × ULN: 90 mg/m²; AST/ALT ≥10 × ULN or total bilirubin >5 × ULN: avoid use

PACLitaxel Protein-Bound Particles
Metastatic pancreatic cancer
• **Adult:** IV infusion 125 mg/m² over 30-40 min on days 1, 8, 15 of each 28-day cycle followed by gemcitabine 1000 mg/m² IV over 30-40 min, on days 1, 8, 15, and 28
Available forms: Inj 6 mg/5 mL, powder for inj, lyophilized 100 mg in single-use vials (Abraxane)

P

Administer:
- If CISplatin is given, use after taxane
- Use cytotoxic handling procedures
- Store prepared sol up to 27 hr in refrigerator

Intermittent IV INFUSION route

> **Black Box Warning:** After premedicating with dexamethasone 20 mg PO 12 hr and 6 hr before PACLitaxel, diphenhydrAMINE 50 mg IV ½-1 hr before PACLitaxel and cimetidine 300 mg or ranitidine 50 mg IV ½-1 hr before PACLitaxel

- Assess for extravasation if given by regular IV, not port

PACLitaxel
Continuous IV INFUSION
- **Dilute** 30-mg vial/5 mL
- After diluting in 0.9% NaCl, D₅W, D₅ and 0.9% NaCl, D₅LR (0.3-1.2 mg/mL), chemo dispensing pin or similar devices with spikes should not be used in vials of PACLitaxel; use in-line filter ≤0.22 micron
- Using only glass bottles, polypropylene, polyolefin bags, and administration sets; do not use PVC infusion bags or sets

PACLitaxel Protein Bound Particles
Intermittent IV INFUSION route
- No premedication for allergic reaction is needed
- **Reconstitute** vial by injecting 20 mL of 0.9% NaCl; slowly inject 20 mL of 0.9% NaCl over at least 1 min to direct sol flow on wall of vial (5 mg/mL); do not inject 0.9% NaCl directly onto lyophilized cake (foaming will occur); allow vial to sit for at least 15 min to ensure proper wetting of lyophilized cake; gently **swirl** or invert vial slowly for ≥2 min until completely dissolved, should look milky
- Calculate dose by dosing vol/mL = total dose (mg) ÷ 5 (mg/mL)
- Use PVC IV bag, do not use filter
- Solution is stable for 8 hr refrigerated
- **Give** over 30 min, monitor for extravasation and hypersensitivity
- Do not admix

SIDE EFFECTS

CNS: *Peripheral neuropathy, dizziness, headache, seizures*

CV: Bradycardia, *hypotension,* abnormal ECG, supraventricular tachycardia (SVT)

GI: *Nausea, vomiting, diarrhea, mucositis, stomatitis, pancreatitis*

HEMA: Neutropenia, leukopenia, thrombocytopenia, anemia

INTEG: *Alopecia,* tissue necrosis, generalized urticaria, *flushing*

MS: *Arthralgia, myalgia*

RESP: Pulmonary embolism, dyspnea, cough

SYST: *Hypersensitivity reactions,* anaphylaxis, Stevens-Johnson syndrome, toxic epidermal necrolysis, angioedema

GU: Renal failure

PHARMACOKINETICS
89%-98% of product serum protein bound, metabolized in liver, excreted in bile and urine; terminal half-life 5.3-17.4 hr

INTERACTIONS
Increase: myelosuppression—other antineoplastics, radiation

Increase: DOXOrubicin levels—DOXOrubicin

Increase: bleeding risk—NSAIDs, anticoagulants, platelet inhibitors, thrombolytics

Decrease: PACLitaxel levels-CYP2C8, CYP 2C9 inducers: phenobarbitol, phenytoin

Decrease: PACLitaxel metabolism—verapampil, cyclosporine, diazePAM, teniposide, etoposide, quinidine, vincristine, testosterone, ketoconazole, estradiol

Decrease: immune response—live virus vaccines

Drug/Lab Test
Increase: AST/ALT, alk phos, triglycerides
Decrease: neutrophils, platelets, WBC, HB

NURSING CONSIDERATIONS
Assess:

> **Black Box Warning:** Requires a specialized care setting such as a hospital or facility with management of complications; should be used by a clinician experienced in cytotoxic agents

---

Black Box Warning: Bone marrow suppression: CBC, differential, platelet count before treatment and weekly; withhold product if WBC is <1500/mm³ or platelet count is <100,000/mm³; notify prescriber

• **Cardiovascular status:** ECG continuously in CV conditions; monitor for hypotension, sinus bradycardia/tachycardia
• **Peripheral neuropathy:** paresthesias, numbness; during infusion, use ice packs on extremities to lessen continued neuropathy; may use acupuncture for some relief; use of ice on extremities when infusing
• **Arthralgia, myalgia:** may begin 2-3 days after infusion and continue for 4-5 days; may use analgesics
• **Nausea, vomiting:** premedicate with antiemetics; nausea and vomiting occur often
• **PACLitaxel:** CBC and differential baseline and periodically, leukocytes <1500/mm, platelets 100,000/mm³ hold, nadir is 11 days (leukopenia) recovery 15-21 days
• **PACLitaxel Protein Bound Particles:** CBC and differential on days 1, 8, 15; hold if neutrophils <1500/mm³ × 1 wk, reduce all doses
• Hepatic studies before, during therapy (bilirubin, AST, ALT, LDH) prn or monthly, check for jaundiced skin and sclera, dark urine, clay-colored stool, itchy skin, abdominal pain, fever, diarrhea
• VS during 1st hr of infusion, check IV site for signs of infiltration

Black Box Warning: Hypersensitivity reactions, anaphylaxis: hypotension, dyspnea, angioedema, generalized urticaria, **Stevens-Johnson syndrome;** discontinue infusion immediately; keep emergency equipment available, monitor continuously during first 30-60 min, then periodically, usually occurs in first few minutes, pretreat with dexamethasone, diphenhydrAMINE

• **Flushing:** for mild to moderate flush, may continue diphenhydrAMINE for ≤48 hr

• Effects of alopecia on body image; discuss feelings about body changes
• **Pregnancy/breastfeeding:** do not use in pregnancy, breastfeeding
Evaluate:
• **Therapeutic response:** decreased tumor size, spread of malignancy
Teach patient/family:
• To report signs of infection: fever, sore throat, flulike symptoms
• To report signs of anemia: fatigue, headache, faintness, SOB, irritability
• To report bleeding; to avoid use of razors, commercial mouthwash; to use soft-bristle toothbrush; to use viscous xylocaine or compounded formula for stomatitis
• To avoid use of aspirin, ibuprofen
• To avoid crowds, persons with known infections
• That hair may be lost during treatment; that a wig or hairpiece may make patient feel better; that new hair may be different in color, texture
• That pain in muscles and joints 2-5 days after infusion is common
• **Pregnancy/breastfeeding:** To notify prescriber if pregnancy is planned or suspected; do not breastfeed, to use contraception during and for 3 wk after last dose
• To avoid receiving vaccinations while taking product

pacritinib (Rx)

(pak-RI-ti-nib)
Vonjo
Func. class.: Antineoplastic/
immunomodulating agent

USES: Myelofibrosis, intermediate- or high-risk primary or secondary (post–polycythemia vera or post–essential thrombocythemia) myelofibrosis in patients with a platelet count below 50×109 cells/L

DOSAGE AND ROUTES
• **Adults: PO** 200 mg bid
Available forms: Capsule 100 mg

> ⚠ **HIGH ALERT**

palbociclib (Rx)

(pal-boe-sye′klib)

Ibrance

Func. class.: Antineoplastic

Chem. class.: Signal transduction inhibitor, kinase inhibitor

ACTION: Inhibits progression of the cell cycle from G_1 into S phase, decreased proliferation of ER-positive breast cancer cell lines. When combined with antiestrogen therapy (letrozole), decreases retinoblastoma protein (Rb) phosphorylation, reducing E2F expression and signaling and increasing growth arrest

USES: Treatment of estrogen receptor (ER)–positive, HER2-negative advanced breast cancer in postmenopausal women, in combination with letrozole as initial endocrine-based therapy

CONTRAINDICATIONS

Hypersensitivity, pregnancy, lactation

Precautions: children, fungal/viral infection, infants, infertility, neutropenia, testicular failure, thromboembolic disease

DOSAGE AND ROUTES

Hormone receptor (HR)-positive, HER2-negative advanced or metastatic breast cancer

• **Adult females:** PO 125 mg daily with food × 21 days, followed by 7 days off, repeat q28days, given with letrozole 2.5 mg/day; give continuously through each cycle

Available forms: Caps 75, 100, 125 mg

Administer:

• Give at the same time of the day with food and letrozole, capsules should be swallowed whole; do not cut, open, chew, do not use if capsule is not intact

SIDE EFFECTS

CNS: Weakness, fever, *fatigue*

EENT: *Stomatitis, oral ulceration,* glossitis, pharyngitis, sinusitis, epistaxis

GI: Vomiting, *nausea, anorexia, diarrhea*

INTEG: Alopecia, rash

HEMA: Thrombocytopenia, *neutropenia, leukopenia,* lymphopenia, anemia

MISC: Peripheral neuropathy, infection, pulmonary embolism, thromboembolism

PHARMACOKINETICS

85% protein bound, elimination half-life was 24-34 hr, metabolized by CYP3A, peak 6-12 hr

INTERACTIONS

Avoid use with CYP3A inhibitors and inducers

Drug/Herb

• Avoid use with St. John's wort

Drug/Food

• Avoid use with grapefruit juice

NURSING CONSIDERATIONS

Assess:

• **Pulmonary embolism/thromboembolic events:** dyspnea/shortness of breath, chest pain, arm or leg swelling, sudden numbness or weakness, severe headache or confusion; or problems with vision, speech, or balance

• **Blood dyscrasias:** CBC/differential prior to and q2wk first 2 cycles, then before each cycle or if change in symptoms

• **GI status:** nausea, diarrhea, anorexia, weight loss

• **Body image:** hair loss, loss of weight

• **Pregnancy:** product can cause fetal harm; identify if the patient is pregnant or if pregnancy is planned

Evaluate: Therapeutic response: decreased progression of disease

Teach patient/family:

• That laboratory testing will be needed during treatment

• Do not take with grapefruit juice

• **Pulmonary/thromboembolic events:** to seek medical attention if dyspnea/shortness of breath, chest pain, arm or leg swelling, sudden numbness or weakness, severe headache or confusion; or problems with vision, speech, or balance develop

---

- To take as prescribed, not to double or skip dose, review "Patient Information Sheet"
- To notify provider of infection
- To discuss all OTC, Rx, herbals, supplements taken
- Identify if pregnancy is planned or suspected. Discuss the need for contraception due to possible fetal harm; avoid breastfeeding

paliperidone (Rx)

(pal-ee-per′i-done)

Invega, Invega Hafyera, Invega Sustenna, Invega Trinza

Func. class.: Antipsychotic, atypical, 2nd generation

Chem. class.: Benzisoxazole derivative

Do not confuse:
Invega/Iveegam
paliperidone/risperiDONE

ACTION: Mediated through both DOPamine type 2 (D_2) and serotonin type 2 (5-HT_2) antagonism

USES: Schizophrenia, schizoaffective disorder

CONTRAINDICATIONS
Breastfeeding, geriatric patients, seizure disorders, AV block, QT prolongation, torsades de pointes; hypersensitivity to this product, risperidone

Precautions: Pregnancy, children, renal/hepatic disease, obesity, Parkinson's disease, suicidal ideation, diabetes mellitus, hematologic disease

Black Box Warning: Dementia-related psychosis (mortality)

DOSAGE AND ROUTES
- **Adult: PO** 6 mg/day, max 12 mg/day; **IM (Invega Sustenna)** 234 mg on day 1, then 156 mg 1 wk later; after 2nd dose, give 117 mg each mo; range 39-234 mg; **(Invega Trinza)** dose based on previous 1-mo injection dose of Invega Sustenna; if last dose of Invega Sustenna was 78 mg, give 273 mg of Invega Trinza; if last dose of Invega Sustenna was 117 mg, give 410

mg of Invega Trinza; if last dose of Invega Sustenna was 156 mg, give 546 mg of Invega Trinza; if last dose of Invega Sustenna was 234 mg, give 819 mg of Invega Trinza; give dose q3mo, adjust as needed
- **Child/adolescent ≥12 yr and ≥51 kg: PO** 3 mg daily, may increase if needed by 3 mg/day in intervals of >5 days, up to max 12 mg/day; <51 kg max 6 mg/day

Invega Hafyera (6-month extended-release injection)
- **Adult:** Initial, only after adequate treatment with once-a month extended-release injection for at least 4 months or an every-3-month extended-release injection (PP3M) for at least one 3-month cycle, 1092 mg or 1560 mg (based upon the previous dose of PP1M or PP3M) IM into the gluteal muscle q6mo maintenance, adjust every 6 months between 1092 and 1560 mg

Renal dose
- **Adult: PO** CCr 50-79 mL/min, 3 mg/day, max 6 mg/day; **EXT REL/IM** 156 mg on day 1, 117 mg 1 wk later, then 78 mg each mo; CCr 10-49 mL/min, 1.5 mg/day, max 3 mg/day; **IM** not recommended

Available forms: Ext rel tabs 1.5, 3, 6, 9 mg; ext rel susp for inj 39 mg/0.25 mL, 78 mg/0.5 mL, 117 mg/0.75 mL, 156 mg/mL, 234 mg/1.5 mL; **Invega Trinza** extended-release suspension 273, 410, 546, 819 mg; **Invega Hafyera:** 1092 mg/3.4 mL, 1560 mg/5 mL extended release suspension

Administer:
- Avoid use with CNS depressants

PO route
- Do not break, crush, or chew ext rel tabs; use plenty of water
- Without regard for food
- Reduced dose for geriatric patients

IM route
- Use for IM only; do not use IV or subcut; inj kits contain prefilled syringe and 2 safety needles; for single use only; **shake** for 10 sec; **deltoid inj:** ≥90 kg, use 1.5-inch, 22-G needle; <90 kg, use 1-inch, 23-G needle; alternate injections between deltoid muscles; **gluteal inj:** use 1.5-inch, 22-G needle; attach needle to Luer connection in clockwise motion; pull needle sheath away using straight pull; bring syringe with at-

P

tached needle upright to de-aerate, de-aerate, inject; after inj, use finger, thumb, or flat surface to activate needle protection system until click heard; use deltoid × 2 doses

SIDE EFFECTS

CNS: *EPS, pseudoparkinsonism, akathisia, dystonia, tardive dyskinesia; drowsiness, insomnia, agitation, anxiety, headache,* seizures, neuroleptic malignant syndrome, dizziness, suicidal thoughts/behaviors

CV: Orthostatic hypotension, tachycardia; heart failure, QT prolongation, dysrhythmias, heart block

EENT: Blurred vision, cough

ENDO: Hyperinsulinemia, weight gain, hyperglycemia, dyslipidemia

GI: *Nausea,* vomiting, *anorexia, constipation,* weight gain in adolescents, xerostomia

GU: Priapism, menstrual irregularities, impotence, priapism

MS: Back pain

MISC: Angioedema, anaphylaxis

HEMA: Agranulocytosis, leukopenia, neutropenia

PHARMACOKINETICS

Peak 24 hr; elimination half-life 23 hr; excreted 80% urine, 11% feces, protein binding >74%

INTERACTIONS

Increase: sedation—other CNS depressants, alcohol, sedative/hypnotics, opiates

Increase: QT prolongation—class IA, III antidysrhythmics, azole antifungals, tricyclics (high doses), some phenothiazines, β-blockers, chloroquine, pimozide, droperidol, some antipsychotics, abarelix, alfuzosin, amoxapine, apomorphine, dasatinib, dolasetron, flecainide, halogenated anesthetics

Increase: neurotoxicity—lithium

Increase: serotonin syndrome, neuroleptic malignant syndrome—SSRIs, SNRIs

Increase: EPS—other antipsychotics

Decrease: levels of carBAMazepine, increased dose of paliperidone may be needed

Decrease: effect of paliperidone—carBAMazepine, other CYP3A4 inducers

Decrease: levodopa effect—levodopa

Drug/Lab Test

Increase: prolactin levels

NURSING CONSIDERATIONS

Assess:

> **Black Box Warning: Mental status:** mood, behavior, confusion, orientation, suicidal thoughts/behaviors; dementia, especially in geriatric patients before initial administration and periodically

• **QT prolongation:** ECG for QT prolongation, ejection fraction; chest pain, palpitations, dyspnea

• AIMS assessment, blood glucose, CBC, glycosylated hemoglobin A1c (HbA1c), LFTs, neurologic function, pregnancy testing, serum creatinine/electrolytes/lipid profile/prolactin, thyroid function tests, weight

• Swallowing of PO medication; check for hoarding, giving of medication to others

• Affect, orientation, LOC, reflexes, gait, coordination, sleep pattern disturbances

• **VS:** B/P (standing, lying), pulse, respirations; often during initial treatment; establish baseline before starting treatment; report drops of 30 mm Hg; watch for ECG changes

• **Hyperprolactinemia:** sexual dysfunction, decreased menstruation, breast pain

• Dizziness, faintness, palpitations, tachycardia on rising

• **EPS:** akathisia, tardive dyskinesia (bizarre movements of jaw, mouth, tongue, extremities), pseudoparkinsonism (rigidity, tremors, pill rolling, shuffling gait)

• **Serotonin syndrome, neuroleptic malignant syndrome:** monitor for hyperthermia, increased CPK, altered mental status, muscle rigidity, fever, seizures; discontinue

• Constipation, urinary retention daily; if these occur, increase bulk and water in diet; monitor for weight gain, especially among adolescents

• **Safety:** Supervised ambulation until patient is stabilized on medication; do not involve patient in strenuous exercise program because fainting is possible; patient should not stand still for a long time

- Increased fluids to prevent constipation
- Sips of water, candy, gum for dry mouth
- **Beers:** avoid in older adults except for schizophrenia, bipolar disorder, or short-term use as an antiemetic in chemotherapy; increase in stroke risk
- **Pregnancy/breastfeeding:** use only if benefits outweigh fetal risk; EPS may result; pregnant patients should enroll in the National Pregnancy Registry for Atypical Antipsychotics, 866-961-2388; do not breastfeed

Evaluate:
- **Therapeutic response:** decrease in emotional excitement, hallucinations, delusions, paranoia; reorganization of patterns of thought, speech

Teach patient/family:
- That orthostatic hypotension may occur; to rise gradually from sitting or lying position
- To avoid abrupt withdrawal of this product, EPS may result; that product should be withdrawn slowly
- To avoid OTC preparations (cough, hay fever, cold) unless approved by prescriber because serious product interactions may occur; to avoid alcohol because increased drowsiness may occur
- To avoid hazardous activities if drowsy or dizzy
- About compliance with product regimen; that nonabsorbable tab shell is expelled in stool
- To report impaired vision, tremors, muscle twitching
- To avoid hot tubs, hot showers, tub baths because hypotension may occur
- That heat stroke may occur in hot weather; to take extra precautions to stay cool
- To use contraception; to inform prescriber if pregnancy is planned or suspected; not to breastfeed

Black Box Warning: Suicidal thoughts/behaviors: to notify prescriber of suicidal thoughts/behaviors, other changes in behavior; identify dementia in the elderly

TREATMENT OF OVERDOSE: Lavage if orally ingested; provide airway; *do not induce vomiting*

palivizumab (Rx)
(pah-li-VIZ-u-mab)
Synagis
Func. class.: Antiviral

USES: Prevention of serious lower respiratory tract disease caused by respiratory syncytial virus (RSV) in pediatric patients at high risk of RSV; pediatric patients with bronchopulmonary dysplasia (BPD); or pediatric patients with hemodynamically significant congenital heart disease (CHD)

CONTRAINDICATIONS
Hypersensitivity, child >24 mo, adolescents/adults

DOSAGE AND ROUTES
Respiratory syncytial virus (RSV), prevention
- **Infant/child <24 mo: IM** 15 mg/kg monthly during RSV season; first dose administered before commencement of RSV season

Available forms: Injection 50-, 100-mg vials

palonosetron (Rx)
(pa-lone-o'se-tron)
Aloxi ✦
Func. class.: Antiemetic
Chem. class.: 5-HT$_3$ receptor antagonist

Combination: palonosetron 0.5 mg/netupitant 300 mg (Akynzeo)

ACTION: Prevents nausea, vomiting by blocking serotonin peripherally, centrally, and in the small intestine at the 5-HT$_3$ receptor

USES: Prevention of nausea, vomiting associated with cancer chemotherapy, postoperative nausea/vomiting

CONTRAINDICATIONS
Hypersensitivity
Precautions: Pregnancy, breastfeeding, children, geriatric patients, hypokalemia, hypomagnesemia, patients taking diuretics

DOSAGE AND ROUTES
Prevention of chemotherapy-induced nausea/vomiting
• **Adult:** IV 0.25 mg as single dose over 30 sec ½ hr before chemotherapy
• **Child 1 mo to <17 yr:** IV 20 mcg/kg, max 1.5 mg given 30 min before chemotherapy
Postoperative nausea/vomiting prophylaxis for ≤24 hr after surgery
• **Adult:** IV 0.075 mg given over 10 sec immediately before induction
Available forms: Inj 0.075 mg/1.5 mL, 0.25 mg/5 mL single use
Administer:
Direct IV route
• Inspect for particulate, discoloration
• Give 30 min before chemotherapy or immediately before anesthesia
• Do not admix with other products, flush IV line with 0.9% NaCL before and after use
• No dilution needed
• **Chemotherapy nausea/vomiting:** give as single dose over 30 sec
• **Postoperative nausea/vomiting:** give over 10 sec immediately before anesthesia induction

SIDE EFFECTS
CNS: *Headache, dizziness, drowsiness, fatigue, insomnia,* fever, anxiety
GI: *Diarrhea, constipation*
MISC: Serotonin syndrome
INTEG: Rash
RESP: Bronchospasm
CV: Hyperkalemia
GU: *Urinary retention*

PHARMACOKINETICS
62% protein bound; metabolized by liver; unchanged product and metabolites excreted by kidney; terminal elimination half-life 40 hr

INTERACTIONS
• **Increase: QT prolongation:** class IA antidysrhythmics (disopyramide, procainamide, quiNIDine), class III antidysrhythmics (amiodarone, dofetilide, ibutilide, sotalol), chloroquine, clarithromycin, dro-peridol, erythromycin, haloperidol, methadone, pentamidine, some phenothiazines, diuretics (except potassium sparing)
Increase: hypotension, severe—apomorphine
Increase: serotonin syndrome: buspirone, fentanyl, lithium, methylene blue, Tramadol, SSRIs, SNRIs, MAOIs, tricyclics, triptans
Drug/Lab
Increase: potassium

NURSING CONSIDERATIONS
Assess:
• For agents that cause QT prolongation, even if manufacturer has removed QT prolongation from warnings
• Absence of nausea, vomiting during chemotherapy
• **Hypersensitivity reaction:** rash, bronchospasm (rare)
• **CV disease:** ECG prior to use
• **Hyperkalemia:** potassium baseline and periodically
• **Pregnancy/breastfeeding:** use only if clearly needed; do not breastfeed
Evaluate:
• **Therapeutic response:** absence of nausea, vomiting during cancer chemotherapy, postoperatively
Teach patient/family:
• To report diarrhea, constipation, rash, changes in respirations, or discomfort at insertion site
• To avoid alcohol, barbiturates
• Use other antiemetics if nausea occurs
• Reason for product, expected results

---

pamidronate (Rx)
(pam-i-drone′ate)
Func. class.: Bone-resorption inhibitor, electrolyte modifier
Chem. class.: Bisphosphonate

ACTION: Inhibits bone resorption, apparently without inhibiting bone formation and mineralization; adsorbs calcium phosphate crystals in bone and may directly block the dissolution of hydroxyapatite crystals of bone

USES: Moderate to severe Paget's disease, hypercalcemia, osteolytic bone metastases in breast cancer, patients with multiple myeloma

CONTRAINDICATIONS
Pregnancy, hypersensitivity to bisphosphonates
Precautions: Children, nursing mothers, renal dysfunction, poor dentition

DOSAGE AND ROUTES
Hypercalcemia of malignancy
• **Adult:** IV INFUSION 60-90 mg as single dose for **moderate hypercalcemia**; 90 mg for **severe hypercalcemia** over 2-24 hr; dose should be diluted in 1000 mL 0.45% NaCl, 0.9% NaCl, or D_5W; wait 7 days before 2nd course
Osteolytic lesions
• **Adult:** IV 90 mg/500 mL of D_5W, 0.45% NaCl, or 0.9% NaCl given over 4 hr each mo **(multiple myeloma)** or over 2 hr q3-4wk **(breast carcinoma)**
Paget's disease
• **Adult:** IV INFUSION 30 mg/day given over 4 hr × 3 days
Available forms: Powder for inj 30, 90 mg/vial; inj 3, 6, 9 mg/mL
Administer:
IV route
• Use saline hydration to produce 2000 mL/24 hr of urine output
• Avoid diuretics before treatment
• After reconstituting by adding 10 mL sterile water for inj to each vial (30 mg/10 mL or 90 mg/10 mL, depending on vial used); add to 1000 mL of sterile 0.45%, 0.9% NaCl, D_5W, run over 2-24 hr **(hypercalcemia)**; dilute reconstituted sol in 500 mL of 0.9% NaCl, 0.45% NaCl, or D_5W, give over 4 hr **(multiple myeloma, Paget's disease)**; dilute reconstituted sol in 250 mL of 0.9% NaCl, 0.45% NaCl, or D_5W; give over 2 hr **(osteolytic bone metastases of breast cancer)**
• Do not mix with calcium-containing infusion sol such as Ringer's sol
• Monitor IV site for pain, redness
• Store infusion sol up to 24 hr at room temperature
• Reconstituted sol with sterile water may be refrigerated for ≤24 hr

Y-site compatibilities: Acyclovir, alfentanil, allopurinol, amifostine, amikacin, aminocaproic acid, aminophylline, amphotericin B lipid complex, amphotericin B liposome, ampicillin, anidulafungin, atenolol, atracurium, azithromycin, aztreonam, bivalirudin, bleomycin, bumetanide, buprenorphine, butorphanol, CARBOplatin, carmustine, ceFAZolin, cefepime, cefoperazone, cefotaxime, cefoTEtan, cefOXitin, cefTAZidime, ceftizoxime, cefTRIAXone, cefuroxime, chloramphenicol, chlorproMAZINE, cimetidine, ciprofloxacin, cisatracurium, CISplatin, clindamycin, cyclophosphamide, cycloSPORINE, cytarabine, dacarbazine, DAPTOmycin, dexamethasone, dexmedetomidine, dexrazoxane, digoxin, diltiaZEM, diphenhydrAMINE, DOBUTamine, DOCEtaxel, dolasetron, DOPamine, doxacurium, DOXOrubicin, doxycycline, droperidol, enalaprilat, ePHEDrine, EPINEPHrine, epirubicin, ertapenem, erythromycin, esmolol, etoposide, famotidine, fenoldopam, fentaNYL, fluconazole, fludarabine, fluorouracil, foscarnet, fosphenytoin, furosemide, gallium, ganciclovir, gatifloxacin, gemcitabine, gentamicin, glycopyrrolate, granisetron, haloperidol, heparin, hetastarch 6%, hydrALAZINE, hydrocortisone, HYDROmorphone, hydrOXYzine, ifosfamide, imipenem-cilastatin, inamrinone, insulin (regular), isoproterenol, ketorolac, labetalol, levoFLOXacin, levorphanol, lidocaine, linezolid, LORazepam, magnesium sulfate, mannitol, mechlorethamine, melphalan, meperidine, meropenem, mesna, metaraminol, methotrexate, methyldopate, methylPREDNISolone, metoclopramide, metoprolol, metroNIDAZOLE, midazolam, milrinone, minocycline, mitoXANTRONE, mivacurium, morphine, mycophenolate, nafcillin, nalbuphine, naloxone, nesiritide, niCARdipine, nitroglycerin, nitroprusside, norepinephrine, octreotide, ondansetron, oxytocin, PACLitaxel, palonosetron, pancuronium, PEMEtrexed, pentamidine, pentazocine, PENTobarbital, PHENobarbital, phenylephrine, piperacillin, polymyxin B, potassium chloride/phosphates, procainamide, prochlorperazine, promethazine, propranolol, quiNIDine, quinupristin-dalfopristin, raNITIdine, remifentanil, rocuronium, sodium acetate/bicarbonate/phosphates, succinylcholine, SUFentanil, sulfamethoxazole-trimethoprim, teniposide, theophylline, thiopental, thiotepa, ticarcillin, ticarcillin-clavulanate, tigecycline, tirofiban, tobramycin, tolazoline, topotecan, trimethobenzamide, vancomycin, vasopressin, vecuronium, verapamil, vinBLAStine, vinCRIStine, vinorelbine, voriconazole, zidovudine

SIDE EFFECTS

CNS: *Fever,* fatigue
CV: Hypertension, atrial fibrillation
EENT: Ocular pain, inflammation, vision impairment
GI: Abdominal pain, anorexia, constipation, nausea, vomiting, dyspepsia
GU: Renal failure
HEMA: Thrombocytopenia, anemia, leukopenia
INTEG: Redness, swelling, induration, pain on palpation at site of catheter insertion
META: *Hypokalemia, hypomagnesemia, hypophosphatemia, hypocalcemia,* hypothyroidism
MS: Severe bone pain, myalgia, osteonecrosis of the jaw
RESP: Coughing, dyspnea, upper respiratory tract infection
SYST: Angioedema, anaphylaxis

PHARMACOKINETICS

Rapidly cleared from circulation and taken up mainly by bones, primarily in areas of high bone turnover; eliminated primarily by kidneys; half-life 21-35 hr, terminal half-life in bone is 300 days

INTERACTIONS

None known
Drug/Lab Test
Increase: creatinine
Decrease: potassium, magnesium, phosphate, calcium, WBC, platelets

NURSING CONSIDERATIONS
Assess:

• **Hypocalcemia:** nausea, vomiting, constipation, thirst, dysrhythmias, hypocalcemia, paresthesia, twitching, laryngospasm, Chvostek's sign, Trousseau's sign;

hypercalcemia: thirst, nausea, vomiting, dysrhythmias

• **Dehydration/hypovolemia:** should be corrected during treatment of hypercalcemia, before therapy, maintain adequate urine output
• **Labs:** Monitor WBCs, platelets, electrolytes, creatinine, BUN, HB/Hct before beginning treatment
• **Dental health:** optimal dental health should be obtained before treatment with this product; cover with antiinfectives for dental extractions
• Temperature may be elevated during the first 3 days after a dose; risk of fever increases as dose increases
• **Renal disease:** max 90-mg single dose, longer infusions >2 hr may increase risk for renal toxicity
• **Bone pain:** use analgesics
• I&O, check for fluid overload, edema, crackles, increased B/P; BUN, creatinine, electrolytes (calcium, potassium, magnesium)
• **Pregnancy/breastfeeding:** do not use in pregnancy/breastfeeding; use contraception

Evaluate:
• **Therapeutic response:** decreased calcium levels

Teach patient/family
• To notify prescriber if pregnancy is planned or suspected; to use contraception while taking this product
• To report hypercalcemic relapse: nausea, vomiting, bone pain, thirst; unusual muscle twitching, muscle spasms; severe diarrhea, constipation
• To continue with dietary recommendations, including calcium and vit D
• To obtain analgesic from provider for bone pain
• That small, frequent meals may help if nausea, vomiting occur
• To report ocular symptoms to prescriber: blurred vision, edema, inflammation
• To maintain good oral hygiene; to get regular dental checkups
• To report dental or jaw pain to prescriber

pancrelipase (Rx)

(pan-kre-li′pase)

Cotazym ✦ Creon, Pancrease MT ✦, Pancreaze, Pertzye, Viokase, Zenpep

Func. class.: Digestant
Chem. class.: Pancreatic enzyme—bovine/porcine

ACTION: Pancreatic enzyme needed for the breakdown of substances released from the pancreas

USES: Exocrine pancreatic secretion insufficiency due to cystic fibrosis (digestive aid), pancreatic enzyme deficiency

CONTRAINDICATIONS

Allergy to pork, acute pancreatitis
Precautions: Pregnancy, ileus, chronic pancreatitis, Crohn's disease, diabetes mellitus, breastfeeding

DOSAGE AND ROUTES
Pancreatic insufficiency due to pancreatectomy
• **Adult/adolescent/child ≥4 yr (del rel caps) Creon Caps, Zenpep Caps, Pancreaze Caps:** PO 500 lipase units/kg/meal, titrate based on patient response, max 2500 lipase units/kg/meal
Cystic fibrosis
• **Adult/adolescent/child >4 yr:** PO 500 lipase units/kg/meal, titrate based on response
• **Child 1-3 yr:** PO 1000 lipase units/kg/meal, titrate based on patient response, max 2500 lipase units/kg/meal
• **Neonates/infants:** PO 2600 lipase units/120 mL of formula or breastfeeding **(Pancreaze)** or 3000 lipase units/120 mL of formula or breastfeeding **(Creon, Zenpep)**
Available forms: Delayed-release capsule lipase 2600, 3000, 4000, 4200, 5000, 6000, 8000, 10,000, 10,500, 12,000, 15,000, 16,000, 16,800, 20,000, 20,800, 21,000, 24,000, 25,000, 36,000, 37,000, 40,000; Tablet lipase/amylase 10, 20 mg (VioKase)

Administer:
• After antacid or cimetidine; decreased pH inactivates product
• Low-fat diet for GI symptoms
• Have patient sit up during administration; give with meals
• Do not crush, chew del rel products, caps, those with spheres, microspheres, or microtablets may be opened and sprinkled on soft food
• Follow PO dose with glass of water or juice, formula or breast milk for infants
Delayed-release route
• Given with meals, snacks, or sufficient fluid
• Do not mix directly in formula
• Viokase is not interchangeable with other products
• Store in tight container at room temperature

SIDE EFFECTS
ENDO: Hypo/hyperglycemia
GI: Anorexia, nausea, vomiting, diarrhea, cramping, bloating
GU: Hyperuricuria, hyperuricemia

INTERACTIONS
Decrease: absorption—cimetidine, antacids, oral iron
Decrease: effect of acarbose, miglitol

NURSING CONSIDERATIONS
Assess:
• Appropriate height, weight development before and periodically; may be delayed
• I&O ratio; watch for increasing urinary output
• Fecal fat, nitrogen, PT during treatment
• **Diabetes mellitus:** for polyuria, polydipsia, polyphagia; monitor glucose level more frequently
• Pork sensitivity; cross-sensitivity may occur
• Adequate hydration
• **Pregnancy/breastfeeding:** use only if clearly needed; do not breastfeed
Evaluate:
• **Therapeutic response:** improved digestion of carbohydrates, protein, fat; absence of steatorrhea

Teach patient/family:

• To notify prescriber of allergic reactions, abdominal pain, cramping, or blood in urine

• To always take with food; not to crush, chew del rel product, caps

• To store at room temperature, away from moisture

• Not to sprinkle capsule contents onto alkaline foods

⚠ HIGH ALERT

pancuronium (Rx)

(pan-kyoo-roe′nee-um)

Func. class.: Neuromuscular blocker (nondepolarizing)

Chem. class.: Synthetic curariform

ACTION: Inhibits transmission of nerve impulses by binding with cholinergic receptor sites, antagonizing action of acetylcholine

USES: Facilitation of endotracheal intubation, skeletal muscle relaxation during mechanical ventilation, surgery, or general anesthesia

CONTRAINDICATIONS

Hypersensitivity to bromide ion

Precautions: Pregnancy, breastfeeding, children <2 yr, neuromuscular/cardiac/renal/hepatic disease, electrolyte imbalances, dehydration, previous anaphylactic reactions (other neuromuscular blockers), respiratory insufficiency

Black Box Warning: Requires an experienced clinician

DOSAGE AND ROUTES

Neuromuscular blockade during surgery

• **Adult/child/infant >1 mo: IV** 0.04-0.1 mg/kg initially or 0.05 mg/kg after initial dose of succinylcholine; maintenance 0.01 mg/kg 60-100 min after initial dose, then 0.01 mg/kg q25-60min as needed

Endotracheal intubation

• **Adult/adolescent/infant: IV** 0.06-0.1 mg/kg/dose, onset of intubating 2-3 min

Neuromuscular blockade during mechanical ventilation

• **Adult: IV** 0.05-0.1 mg/kg/dose as needed based on twitch response

Child/adolescent: IV 0.05-0.15 mg/kg/dose q4-6hr as needed

Available forms: Inj 1, 2 mg/mL

Administer:

Direct IV route

• May be given undiluted over 1-2 min (1 mg/mL [10-mL vial], 2 mg/mL [2-, 5-mL vial])

Intermittent IV INFUSION route

• Add 100 mg of product to 250 mL D₅W, NS, LR (0.4 mg/mL)

• Store in refrigerator; do not store in plastic; use only fresh sol

• Reassurance if communication is difficult during recovery from neuromuscular blockade

• Frequent (q2hr) instillation of artificial tears, covering of eyes to prevent drying of cornea

Y-site compatibilities: Aminophylline, ceFAZolin, cefuroxime, cimetidine, DOBUTamine, DOPamine, EPINEPHrine, esmolol, fenoldopam, fentaNYL, fluconazole, gentamicin, heparin, hydrocortisone, isoproterenol, levoFLOXacin, LORazepam, midazolam, morphine, nitroglycerin, raNITIdine, trimethoprim-sulfamethoxazole, vancomycin

SIDE EFFECTS

CNS: Prolonged neuromuscular blockade

CV: Bradycardia; tachycardia; increased, decreased B/P; ventricular extrasystoles, edema, hypertension

EENT: Increased secretions

INTEG: Rash, flushing, pruritus, urticaria, sweating, salivation

MS: Weakness to prolonged skeletal muscle relaxation
RESP: Prolonged apnea, bronchospasm, cyanosis, respiratory depression, dyspnea
SYST: Anaphylaxis

PHARMACOKINETICS
IV: Onset 3-5 min, dose dependent, peak 3-5 min; metabolized (small amounts), excreted in urine (unchanged), crosses placenta

INTERACTIONS
Increase: dysrhythmias—theophylline
Increase: neuromuscular blockade—aminoglycosides, clindamycin, enflurane, isoflurane, lincomycin, lithium, local anesthetics, opioid analgesics, polymyxin antiinfectives, quiNIDine, thiazides
Drug/Lab Test
Decrease: cholinesterase

NURSING CONSIDERATIONS
Assess:
• **Respiratory recovery:** decreased paralysis of face, diaphragm, leg, arm, rest of body; allow to recover fully before neurologic assessment
• Electrolyte imbalances (K, Mg); may lead to increased action of product
• VS (B/P, pulse, respirations, airway) until fully recovered; rate, depth, pattern of respirations, strength of hand grip
• I&O ratio; check for urinary retention, frequency, hesitancy
• **Allergic reactions, anaphylaxis:** rash, fever, respiratory distress, pruritus; product should be discontinued
• **Pregnancy/breastfeeding:** use only if benefits outweigh fetal risk; breast milk excretion is unknown
Evaluate:
• **Therapeutic response:** paralysis of jaw, eyelid, head, neck, rest of body

TREATMENT OF OVERDOSE:
Neostigmine, atropine, monitor VS; may require mechanical ventilation

---

⚠ HIGH ALERT

panitumumab (Rx)
(pan-i-tue′moo-mab)
Vectibix
Func. class.: Antineoplastic—miscellaneous
Chem. class.: Multikinase inhibitor, signal transduction inhibitor

---

ACTION: Decreases growth and survival of cancer cells by competitive inhibition of EGF receptor

USES: ⌖ EGFR expressing metastatic colorectal cancer; not beneficial with KRAS mutations in codon 12 or 13

CONTRAINDICATIONS
Hypersensitivity, ⌖ RAS (KRAS and NRAS) mutant mCRC or if unknown, child <18 yr
Precautions: Pregnancy, breastfeeding, children, hepatic disease, acute bronchospasm, diarrhea, hamster protein allergy, hypomagnesemia, hypotension, pulmonary fibrosis, sepsis, soft tissue toxicities, infusion-related reactions

Black Box Warning: Exfoliative dermatitis

DOSAGE AND ROUTES
• **Adult: IV INFUSION** 6 mg/kg over 60 min every 2 wk; doses >1000 mg over 90 min
Available forms: Sol for inj 20 mg/mL (100 mg/5 mL, 400 mg/20 mL)
Administer:
Proactive skin treatment
• Skin moisturizer, sunscreen (SPF >15 UVA and UVB, topical steroid cream (1% hydrocortisone), and an oral antibiotic (doxycycline) for possible skin toxicities; patients need to apply moisturizer and sunscreen to face, hands, feet, neck, back, and chest every AM during treatment; and apply topical steroid to face, hands, feet, neck, back, and chest every PM

Intermittent IV INFUSION route
- Assess for KRAS before use
- Give in hospital or clinic setting with full resuscitation equipment
- **Only as IV infusion** using controlled IV infusion pump; do not give IV push or bolus; use low–protein binding 0.2- or 0.22-micron in-line filter; flush line with 0.9% NaCl before and after administration
- Give over 60 min through a peripheral line or indwelling catheter; infuse doses of >1000 mg over 90 min
- **Dilute** in 100 mL of 0.9% NaCl; dilute doses >1000 mg in 150 mL of 0.9% NaCl; mix by inverting; do not exceed 10 mg/mL; use within 6 hr if stored at room temperature; can be stored between 2° C and 8° C for up to 24 hr
- **Dosage adjustment for infusion/dermatologic reaction:** Grade 1 or 2: reduce infusion by 50%; Grade 3 or 4: terminate, permanently discontinue depending on severity/resistance
- Store unopened vials in refrigerator; do not shake; protect from direct sunlight; do not freeze

SIDE EFFECTS
CNS: Fatigue
CV: Peripheral edema
EENT: Ocular irritation, ocular toxicity
GI: *Nausea, diarrhea, vomiting,* anorexia, mouth ulceration, abdominal pain, constipation
HEMA: Thrombophlebitis
INTEG: *Rash,* pruritus, exfoliative dermatitis, skin fissure, angioedema, severe/fatal infusion reactions
META: Hypocalcemia, hypomagnesemia, antibody formation
RESP: Bronchospasm, cough, dyspnea, hypoxia, pulmonary fibrosis/embolism, pneumonitis, wheezing, interstitial lung disease

PHARMACOKINETICS
Bioavailability 38%-49%; elimination half-life 7.5 days; peak 3 hr; high-fat meal decreases bioavailability; plasma protein binding 99.5%; metabolized in liver; oxidative metabolism by CYP3A4, glucuronidation by UGT1A9; 77% excreted in feces

INTERACTIONS
- Do not use in combination with other antineoplastics

NURSING CONSIDERATIONS
Assess:

Black Box Warning: Serious skin disorders: fever, sore throat, fatigue, then lesions in mouth, lips; withhold product, notify prescriber

- Serum electrolytes periodically (calcium, magnesium)
- **Infection:** increased temperature
- Assess for diarrhea

Black Box Warning: Infusion reactions: bronchospasm, fever, chills, hypotension; may require discontinuation, have emergency equipment available

- **Ocular toxicity:** ocular irritation, hyperemia
- **Pulmonary fibrosis:** dyspnea, cough, wheezing; may require discontinuation
- **Pregnancy/breastfeeding:** do not use in pregnancy/breastfeeding
Evaluate:
- **Therapeutic response:** decrease in colon carcinoma progression
Teach patient/family:
- **To report adverse reactions immediately:** difficulty breathing, mouth sores, skin rash, ocular toxicity
- About reason for treatment, expected results, adverse reactions
- To use contraception while taking product, for 6 mo after treatment; not to breastfeed for ≥2 mo after stopping treatment; to enroll in Amgen Pregnancy Surveillance Program, 800-772-6436
- To avoid the sun, use sunscreen while taking product

---

pantoprazole (Rx)

(pan-toe-pray'zole)

Pantoloc ✤, Protonix, Tecta ✤

Func. class.: Proton pump inhibitor
Chem. class.: Benzimidazole

Do not confuse:
Protonix/Lotronex/protamine

ACTION: Suppresses gastric secretion by inhibiting hydrogen/potassium ATPase enzyme system in gastric parietal cell; characterized as gastric acid pump inhibitor because it blocks the final step of acid production

USES: Severe erosive esophagitis; maintenance of long-term pathologic hypersecretory conditions, including Zollinger-Ellison syndrome
Unlabeled uses: Duodenal/gastric ulcer, NSAID ulcer prophylaxis, *Helicobacter pylori*–associated ulcer, dyspepsia, gastroesophageal reflux disease (GERD)

CONTRAINDICATIONS

Hypersensitivity to this product or benzimidazole
Precautions: Pregnancy, breastfeeding, children, proton pump hypersensitivity

DOSAGE AND ROUTES
GERD (unlabeled)
• **Adult: PO** 40 mg/day × 4-8 wk, may repeat course
Erosive esophagitis
• **Adult: IV** 40 mg/day × 7-10 days; **PO** 40 mg/day × 8 wk; may repeat **PO** course.
Child ≥5 yr and >40 kg: PO 40 mg daily for up to 8 wk; **15-39 kg:** 20 mg daily for up to 8 wk
Pathologic hypersecretory conditions
• **Adult: PO** 40 mg bid; **IV** 80 mg q12hr, max 240 mg/day
Peptic ulcer/GI bleed (unlabeled)
• **Adult: IV** 80 mg bolus then 40 mg IV bid × 72 hr
Duodenal ulcer/gastric ulcer/NSAID ulcer prophylaxis (unlabeled)
• **Adult: PO** 40 mg/day

H. pylori–associated ulcers (unlabeled)
• **Adult: PO** 40 or 80 mg bid; may be used with other products
Available forms: Del rel tabs 20, 40 mg; powder for inj 40 mg/vial; del rel granules for susp 40 mg
Administer:
PO route
• Swallow del rel tabs whole; do not break, crush, or chew; take del rel tabs at same time of day
• May take with/without food
• **Suspension:** give in apple juice 30 min before a meal or sprinkled on 1 tbsp of applesauce
IV route
• Use of Protonix IV vials with spiked IV system adapters is not recommended
• Visually inspect for particulate matter and discoloration before use
• When using a Y-site, immediately stop use if a precipitation or discoloration occurs
• **Reconstitution of vial:** use 40-mg vial/10 mL NS; do not freeze
• **Two-minute slow IV infusion injection:** dilute one or two 40-mg vials with 10 mL NS per vial to 4 mg/mL; store ≤24 hr at room temperature before use; infuse slowly over ≥2 min; do not give with other IV fluids or medications; flush line with D$_5$W, NS, or LR before and after each dose
• **Fifteen-minute IV infusion:** dilute each 40-mg dose with 10 mL NS; the reconstituted vial should be further admixed with 100 mL (for 1 vial) or 80 mL (for 2 vials) of D$_5$W, NS, or LR (to 0.4 mg/mL or 0.8 mg/mL, respectively); store ≤6 hr at room temperature before further dilution; the admixed solution (0.4 mg/mL or 0.8 mg/mL) may be stored at room temperature and must be used within 24 hr from the time of initial reconstitution; infuse over 15 min at 7 mL/min; do not administer with other IV fluids or medications; flush IV line with D$_5$W, NS, or LR before and after each dose

Y-site compatibilities: Acyclovir, allopurinol, amifostine, amikacin, aminocaproic acid, aminophylline, amoxicillin-clavulanate, amphotericin B liposome, ampicillin, ampicillin-sulbactam, anidulafungin, azithromycin, bleomycin, bumetanide, calcium gluconate, CARBOplatin, carmustine, ceFAZolin, cefOXitin, cefTAZidime, ceftizoxime, cefTRIAXone, cefuroxime, clindamycin, cyclophosphamide, cycloSPORINE, cytarabine, dextrose 3.3% in sodium chloride 0.3%, digoxin, dimenhyDRINATE, DOCEtaxel, DOPamine, doripenem, doxycycline, enalaprilat, EPINEPHrine, ertapenem, fluorouracil, foscarnet, fosphenytoin, furosemide, ganciclovir, gentamicin, granisetron, heparin, hydrocortisone, HYDROmorphone, imipenem-cilastatin, inamrinone, insulin (regular), irinotecan, isoproterenol, magnesium, mannitol, mesna, methohexital, methyldopate, metoclopramide, nafcillin, nitroglycerin, nitroprusside, ofloxacin, oxytocin, PACLitaxel, pentazocine, PENTobarbital, phenylephrine, piperacillin-tazobactam, potassium chloride, procainamide, rifAMPin, sodium bicarbonate, succinylcholine, SUFentanil, sulfamethoxazole-trimethoprim, teniposide, theophylline, thiopental, ticarcillin, ticarcillin-clavulanate, tigecycline, tirofiban, tobramycin, traMADol, vasopressin, zidovudine

SIDE EFFECTS

CNS: *Headache,* insomnia, asthenia, fatigue, malaise, insomnia, somnolence
GI: *Diarrhea, abdominal pain,* flatulence, pancreatitis, weight changes, CDAD
INTEG: *Rash*
META: Hyperglycemia, weight gain/loss, hyponatremia, hypomagnesemia, vitamin B_{12} deficiency
MS: Myalgia, rhabdomyolysis
SYST: Stevens-Johnson syndrome, toxic epidermal necrolysis, anaphylaxis, angioedema

PHARMACOKINETICS

Peak 2.4 hr, duration >24 hr, half-life 1.5 hr, protein binding 97%, eliminated in urine as metabolites and in feces; in geriatric patients, elimination rate decreased; ✸ some Asian patients (15%-20%) may be poor metabolizers

INTERACTIONS

Increase: pantoprazole levels—clarithromycin, diazePAM, phenytoins, flurazepam, triazolam
Increase: bleeding—warfarin
Decrease: effect of each of these drugs: protease inhibitors (atazanavir, indinavir, nelfinavir)
Decrease: absorption of these products—sucralfate, calcium carbonate, vit B_{12}, ketoconazole, itraconazole, atazanavir, ampicillin, iron salts, separate doses
Decrease: clopidogrel effect
Drug/Herb
Decrease: effect of pantoprazole—St. John's wort

NURSING CONSIDERATIONS
Assess:
• **CDAD:** bowel sounds; abdomen for pain, swelling; anorexia; diarrhea with blood, mucus
• **Hepatic studies:** AST, ALT, alk phos during treatment
• For vit B_{12} deficiency in patients receiving long-term therapy
• **Serious skin reactions:** toxic epidermal necrolysis, Stevens-Johnson syndrome, exfoliative dermatitis: fever, sore throat, fatigue, thin ulcers; lesions in the mouth, lips
• **Electrolyte imbalances:** hyponatremia; hypomagnesemia in patients using product 3 mo to 1 year; if hypomagnesemia occurs, use of magnesium supplements may be sufficient; if severe, discontinuation of product may be required
• **Rhabdomyolysis, myalgia:** muscle pain, increased CPK; weakness, swelling of affected muscles
• **Beers:** avoid in older adults for >8 wk unless for high-risk patients; risk of *Clostridium difficile,* fractures
• **Pregnancy/breastfeeding:** use only if clearly needed; do not breastfeed
Evaluate:
• **Therapeutic response:** absence of epigastric pain, swelling, fullness

Teach patient/family:
• To report severe diarrhea; black, tarry stools; abdominal pain; product may have to be discontinued; do not treat diarrhea with OTC products without approval of provider (CDAD)
• That hyperglycemia may occur in diabetic patients
• To take as directed, not to skip or double dose
• To avoid alcohol, salicylates, NSAIDs; may cause GI irritation
• To continue taking even if feeling better
• **Pregnancy/breastfeeding:** To notify prescriber if pregnant or planning to become pregnant; not to breastfeed

parathyroid hormone (Rx)
(par-a-thye′roid hor′mone)
Natpara
Func. class.: Parathyroid hormone analog

USES: Adjunct to calcium and vitamin D to control hypocalcemia in those with hypoparathyroidism, who are not well controlled on calcium/Vitamin D alone

CONTRAINDICATIONS
Hypersensitivity

Black Box Warning: New primary malignancy

DOSAGE AND ROUTES
Hypoparathyroidism
• **Adult:** SUBCUT *Initial:* 50 mcg daily
Before use, serum calcium concentration should be >7.5 mg/dL and the 25-hydroxyvitamin D is adequate
Available forms: Injection 25, 50, 75, 100 mcg multidose cartridges

paricalcitol (Rx)
(pah-ri-kal′si-tole)
Zemplar
Func. class.: Vitamin D analog

USES: IV: Prevention/treatment of secondary hyperparathyroidism with chronic kidney disease on dialysis; PO: prevention/treatment with secondary hyperparathyroidism with stage 3/4 chronic kidney disease and stage 5 chronic kidney disease hemodialysis/peritoneal dialysis

CONTRAINDICATIONS
Hypersensitivity to paricalcitol or any component; vitamin D toxicity; hypercalcemia

DOSAGE AND ROUTES
Secondary hyperparathyroidism in chronic kidney disease on dialysis
• **Adult: IV:** Initial: 0.04-0.1 mcg/kg (2.8-7 mcg) given no more frequently than every other day at any time during dialysis; adjust dose based on serum intact PTH (iPTH), as follows: iPTH above target and increased: Increase by 2-4 mcg every 2-4 wk; maximum dose: 0.24 mcg/kg/day; iPTH above target and decreased by <30%: Increase by 2-4 mcg every 2-4 wk; maximum dose: 0.24 mcg/kg/day; iPTH above target and decreased by 30%-60%: Maintain paricalcitol dose; iPTH above target, decreased dose
Available forms: Capsule 1, 2, 4 mcg; injection 2, 5 mcg/mL

PARoxetine (Rx)
(par-ox′e-teen)
Paxil, Paxil CR
PARoxetine mesylate (Rx)
Pexeva, Brisdelle
Func. class.: Antidepressant, SSRI
Chem. class.: Phenylpiperidine derivative

Do not confuse:
PARoxetine/FLUoxetine/Piroxicam/PACLitaxel
Paxil/PACLitaxel/Taxol/doxil

ACTION: Inhibits CNS neuron uptake of serotonin but not of norepinephrine or DOPamine

Side effects: *italics* = common; red = life-threatening

USES: Major depressive disorder, obsessive-compulsive disorder, panic disorder, generalized anxiety disorder, posttraumatic stress disorder, premenstrual disorders, social anxiety disorder, hot flashes, menopause

Unlabeled uses: Premature ejaculation (IR only)

CONTRAINDICATIONS

Pregnancy, hypersensitivity, MAOI use, alcohol use

Precautions: Breastfeeding, geriatric patients, seizure history; patients with history of mania, renal/hepatic disease

Black Box Warning: Children, suicidal ideation

DOSAGE AND ROUTES

Generalized anxiety disorder
• **Adult: PO** 20 mg/day in AM, range 20-50 mg/day

Posttraumatic stress disorder (PTSD)
• **Adult: PO** 20 mg/day, range 20-50 mg/day; max 50 mg/day

Depression
• **Adult: PO** 20 mg/day in AM; after 4 wk, if no clinical improvement is noted, dose may be increased by 10 mg/day each wk to desired response, max 50 mg/day or **CONT REL** 25 mg/day, may increase by 12.5 mg/day/wk up to 62.5 mg/day
• **Geriatric: PO** 10 mg/day, increase by 10 mg to desired dose, max 40 mg/day

Obsessive-compulsive disorder
• **Adult: PO** 40 mg/day in AM, start with 20 mg/day, increase in 10-mg/day increments, max 60 mg/day

Panic disorder
• **Adult: PO** start with 10 mg/day, increase in 10-mg/day increments to 40 mg/day, max 60 mg/day or **CONT REL** 12.5 mg/day, max 75 mg/day

Premenstrual dysphoric disorders
• **Adult: CONT REL** 12.5 mg/day in AM

Menopause symptoms/hot flashes
• **Adult: PO (CONT REL)** 12.5 mg/day, may increase to 25 mg/day after 1 wk

Premature ejaculation (unlabeled)
• **Adult: PO** 20 mg/day

Renal dose
• **Adult: PO** CCr 30-60 mL/min, lower doses may be needed; CCr <30 mL/min, 10 mg/day initially, **REGULAR RELEASE:** max 40 mg/day; **CONTINUOUS RELEASE** 12.5 mg/day initially, max 50 mg/day

Hepatic dose
• **Adult: PO** 10 mg/day initially, max 40 mg (REGULAR RELEASE); 12.5 mg/day initially, max 50 mg/day (CONTINUOUS RELEASE)

Available forms: Tabs 10, 20, 30, 40 mg; oral susp 10 mg/5 mL; cont rel tab 12.5, 25, 37.5 mg; cap 7.5 mg

Administer:
• Do not substitute Pexeva with Paxil, Paxil CR, or generic PARoxetine
• Store at room temperature; do not freeze
• Increased fluids, bulk in diet for constipation, urinary retention
• With food, milk for GI symptoms
• Crushed if patient is unable to swallow medication whole (regular rel only)
• Gum, hard candy, frequent sips of water for dry mouth
• Avoid use with other CNS depressants
• **Oral susp:** shake, measure with oral syringe or calibrated measuring device
• **Cont rel tab:** do not cut, chew, crush; do not give concurrently with antacids

SIDE EFFECTS

CNS: *Headache,* nervousness, insomnia, *drowsiness, anxiety, tremors, dizziness,* fatigue, *sedation,* abnormal dreams, agitation, apathy, euphoria, hallucinations, delusions, psychosis, seizures

CV: Vasodilation, postural hypotension, palpitations, bleeding, chest pain

EENT: Visual changes

GI: *Nausea, diarrhea, dry mouth,* anorexia, dyspepsia, *constipation,* cramps, vomiting, taste changes, flatulence, decreased appetite, weight gain

GU: Dysmenorrhea, decreased libido, urinary frequency, UTI, amenorrhea, cystitis, impotence; decreased sperm

quality, decreased fertility, *abnormal ejaculation (male)*
INTEG: *Sweating,* rash, photosensitivity
MS: Pain, arthritis, myalgia, myopathy
RESP: Infection, pharyngitis, nasal congestion, sinus headache, sinusitis, cough, dyspnea, yawning
SYST: Fever, abrupt withdrawal syndrome, Stevens-Johnson syndrome, neuroleptic malignant syndrome, suicidal thoughts/behaviors

PHARMACOKINETICS

PO: Peak 5.2 hr, ext rel peak 6-10 hr; metabolized in liver by CYP2D6 enzyme system, 7% may be poor metabolizers; unchanged products and metabolites excreted in feces and urine; half-life 21 hr (reg rel); 15-20 hr (cont rel); protein binding 95%

INTERACTIONS

Increase: serotonin syndrome—SSRIs, SNRIs, atypical psychotics, serotonin-receptor agonists, tricyclics, amphetamines, bupropion, cyclobenzaprine, linezolid, traMADol
Decrease: level of digoxin
• Do not use with MAOIs, pimozide, thioridazine; potentially fatal reactions can occur
Increase: bleeding—NSAIDs, thrombolytics, salicylates, platelet inhibitors, anticoagulants
Increase: PARoxetine plasma levels—cimetidine
Increase: agitation—L-tryptophan
Increase: side effects—highly protein-bound products
Increase: theophylline levels—theophylline
Increase: toxicity—CYP2D6 inhibitors (aprepitant, delavirdine, imatinib, nefazodone)
Decrease: PARoxetine levels—PHENobarbital and phenytoin
Drug/Herb
• SAMe
• Possible serotonin syndrome: St. John's wort, tryptophan
• **Hypertensive crisis:** ephedra

NURSING CONSIDERATIONS
Assess:

Black Box Warning: Depression/OCD/anxiety/panic attacks: mental status: mood, sensorium, affect, suicidal tendencies (especially in child/young adult), increase in psychiatric symptoms, decreasing obsessive thoughts, compulsive behaviors, restrict amount available

• **Postural hypotension:** B/P (lying/standing), pulse q4hr; if systolic B/P drops 20 mm Hg, hold product, notify prescriber; take vital signs q4hr for patients with CV disease
• Hepatic/renal studies: AST, ALT, bilirubin, creatinine
• Weight weekly; appetite may decrease with product, but weight gain may occur; constipation
• EPS, primarily in geriatric patients: rigidity, dystonia, akathisia
• **Renal status:** BUN, creatinine, urinary retention
• **Withdrawal symptoms:** headache, nausea, vomiting, muscle pain, weakness; not usual unless product discontinued abruptly, taper over 1-2 wk
• Alcohol intake; if alcohol is consumed, hold dose until morning
• **Serotonin, neuroleptic malignant syndrome:** hallucinations, coma, headache, agitation, shivering, sweating, tachycardia, diarrhea, tremors, hypertension, hyperthermia, rigidity, delirium, coma, myoclonus, agitation, nausea, vomiting
• **Beers:** Avoid in geriatrics, highly anticholinergic, sedating
• **Pregnancy/breastfeeding:** use only if clearly needed; do not breastfeed
Evaluate:
• **Therapeutic response:** decreased depression
Teach patient/family:
• That therapeutic effect may take 1-4 wk
• To use caution when driving, performing other activities requiring alertness because of drowsiness, dizziness, blurred vision

P

• Not to discontinue medication quickly after long-term use; may cause nausea, headache, malaise (abrupt withdrawal syndrome)

Black Box Warning: That depression, suicidal thoughts/behaviors in children/adolescents or young adults may worsen, to notify prescriber immediately

• To avoid alcohol ingestion, OTC products unless approved by prescriber
• To report bleeding, headache, nausea, anxiety, or if depression continues
• To discuss sexual side effects: impotence, possible male infertility while taking product

TREATMENT OF OVERDOSE: Gastric lavage, airway; for seizures, give diazepam, symptomatic treatment

patiromer (Rx)
(pa-tir'oh-mer)
Veltassa
Func. class.: Antidote, potassium binder

USES: Treatment of hyperkalemia

CONTRAINDICATIONS
Hypersensitivity

DOSAGE AND ROUTES
• **Adult: PO** Initial: 8.4 g daily; adjust dose at ≥1-wk intervals in increments of 8.4 g (max dose: 25.2 g/day), monitor potassium
Available forms: oral powder 8.4-, 16.8-, 25.2-g packets

patisiran (Rx)
(pat-i-sir'an)
Onpattro
Func. class.: Metabolic agent, anti-transthyretin small interfering ribonucleic acid (siRNA) agent

USES: Treatment of the polyneuropathy of hereditary transthyretin-mediated amyloidosis in adults

CONTRAINDICATIONS
Hypersensitivity

DOSAGE AND ROUTES
At least 1 hr before use, premedicate with a corticosteroid, acetaminophen, an H_1 blocker, and an H_2 blocker to reduce the risk of infusion-related reactions (IRR)
• **Adult:** IV: Base dose on actual body weight; <100 kg: 0.3 mg/kg once q3wk; ≥100 kg: 30 mg once q3wk
Available forms: Injection 2 mg/mL in 5-mL single-dose vials

⚠ HIGH ALERT
pazopanib (Rx)
(paz-oh'pa-nib)
Votrient
Func. class.: Antineoplastic biologic response modifiers/multikinase angiogenesis inhibitor
Chem. class.: Kinase inhibitor

ACTION: Targets vascular endothelial growth factor receptors; a multikinase angiogenesis inhibitor

USES: Advanced renal cell carcinoma; soft-tissue sarcoma patients who have received prior chemotherapy
Unlabeled uses: GI stromal tumors (GISTs)

CONTRAINDICATIONS
Pregnancy, hypothyroidism, QT prolongation, MI, wound dehiscence, hypertension
Precautions: Breastfeeding, children, cardiac/renal/hepatic/dental disease, GI bleeding

Black Box Warning: Hepatic disease (fatalities)

DOSAGE AND ROUTES
• **Adult: PO** 800 mg/day without food (1 hr before, 2 hr after a meal), may decrease to 400 mg/day if not tolerated (renal cell cancer); or adjust in 200-mg increments based

on toxicity (soft-tissue sarcoma); **use with strong CYP3A4 inhibitors** 400 mg daily
Hepatic dose
• **Adult: PO** 200 mg daily (moderate hepatic disease)
Available forms: Tabs 200 mg
Administer:
• Give on an empty stomach (1 hr before or 2 hr after a meal); separate doses by ~24 hr
• Do not crush tablets; may affect rate of absorption and systemic exposure; only intact, whole tablets should be used
• If a dose is missed, it should not be taken if it is <12 hr until the next dose
• Store at room temperature 77° F (25° C)

SIDE EFFECTS

CNS: Intracranial bleeding, headache
CV: Heart failure, hypertension, hypertensive crisis, chest pain, MI, QT prolongation, torsades de pointes
GI: Nausea, hepatotoxicity, vomiting, dyspepsia, GI hemorrhage, anorexia, abdominal pain, GI perforation, pancreatitis, diarrhea; hepatotoxicity (geriatric)
HEMA: Neutropenia, thrombocytopenia, bleeding
INTEG: Rash, alopecia
MISC: Fatigue, epistaxis, pyrexia, hot sweats, increased weight, flulike symptoms, hypothyroidism, hand-foot syndrome, retinal tear/detachment

PHARMACOKINETICS

Protein binding 99%, peak 2-4 hr, duration 24 hr, half-life 31 hr

INTERACTIONS

Increase: QT prolongation—class IA/III antidysrhythmics, some phenothiazines, β-agonists, local anesthetics, tricyclics, haloperidol, chloroquine, droperidol, pentamidine; CYP3A4 inhibitors (amiodarone, clarithromycin, erythromycin, telithromycin, troleandomycin), arsenic trioxide; CYP3A4 substrates (methadone, pimozide, QUEtiapine, quiNIDine, risperiDONE, ziprasidone)
Increase: pazopanib concentrations—CYP3A4 inhibitors (ketoconazole, itraconazole, erythromycin, clarithromycin)

Increase: plasma concentrations of simvastatin, calcium-channel blockers, ergots
Increase: plasma concentration of warfarin; avoid use with warfarin; use low-molecular-weight anticoagulants instead
Decrease: PAZOPanib concentrations—CYP3A4 inducers (dexamethasone, phenytoin, carBAMazepine, rifampin, PHENobarbital)
Drug/Food
Increase: PAZOPanib effect—grapefruit juice; avoid use while taking product
Drug/Herb
Decrease: PAZOPanib concentration—St. John's wort

NURSING CONSIDERATIONS
Assess:

Black Box Warning: Hepatic disease: fatal hepatotoxicity can occur; obtain LFTs baseline and at least every 2 wk × 2 mo, then monthly

• **Fatal bleeding:** from GI, respiratory, GU tracts, permanently discontinue in those with severe bleeding
• **Palmar-plantar erythrodysesthesia (hand-foot syndrome):** more common in those previously treated; reddening, swelling, numbness, desquamation on palms and soles
• **GI perforation/fistula:** discontinue if this occurs, assess for pain in epigastric area, dyspepsia, flatulence, fever, chills
• **Hypertension/hypertensive crisis:** hypertension usually occurs in the first cycle; in those with preexisting hypertension, do not start treatment until B/P is controlled; monitor B/P every wk × 6 wk, then at start of each cycle or more often if needed, temporarily or permanently discontinue for severe uncontrolled hypertension
• **Pregnancy/breastfeeding:** do not use in pregnancy, breastfeeding
Evaluate:
• **Therapeutic response:** decrease in size, spread of tumor
Teach patient/family:
• To report adverse reactions immediately: heart attack, stroke

• About reason for treatment, expected results
• That effect on male fertility is unknown
• Not to crush or chew tabs; to take on an empty stomach 1 hr before or 2 hr after meals; to avoid grapefruit juice
• **Blood clots:** Pain in legs; chest pain; swelling in legs, arms; notify provider immediately
• **Hepatotoxicity:** To notify provider immediately of yellow skin, eyes, clay-colored stools, dark urine; monitor LFTs before and at 3, 5, 7, 9 wk; then 3 mo, 4 mo if symptoms are present

---

⚠ HIGH ALERT

pegaspargase (Rx)
(peg-as′par-jase)
Oncaspar
Func. class.: Antineoplastic agent, miscellaneous

USES: Treatment of acute lymphoblastic leukemia (ALL) with hypersensitivity to L-asparaginase (multiagent chemotherapy); first-line treatment of ALL (combination chemotherapy)

CONTRAINDICATIONS
Hypersensitivity, serious thrombosis with prior L-asparaginase therapy; pancreatitis; serious hemorrhagic events with prior L-asparaginase therapy; severe hepatic disease

DOSAGE AND ROUTES
Acute lymphoblastic leukemia (ALL), as first-line treatment or in patients with hypersensitivity to native asparaginase
• **Adult: IM, IV:** ≤21 yr: 2500 units/m² (as part of a multiagent combination chemotherapy regimen); do not administer more frequently than every 14 days; >21 yr: 2000 units/m² (as part of a multiagent combination chemotherapy regimen); do not administer more frequently than every 14 days

Acute lymphoblastic leukemia (ALL)
• **Infant/child/adolescent: IM, IV:** 2500 units/m²/dose (combination chemotherapy); do not use more frequently than q14days
Available forms: Injection 3750 IU/5 mL in single-use vials

⚠ HIGH ALERT

pegfilgrastim (Rx)
(peg-fill-grass′stim)
Neulasta, Neulasta Onpro Kit
pegfilgrastim apgf
Nyvepria
pegfilgrastim-bmez
Ziextenzo
pegfilgrastim-cbqv
Udenyca (biosimilar)
pegfilgrastim-jmdb
Fulphila (biosimilar)
Func. class.: Hematopoietic agent
Chem. class.: Granulocyte colony-stimulating factor

Do not confuse:
Neulasta/Lunesta/Neumega/Nuedexta

ACTION: Stimulates proliferation and differentiation of neutrophils

USES: To decrease infection in patients receiving antineoplastics that are myelosuppressive; to increase WBC count in patients with product-induced neutropenia

CONTRAINDICATIONS
Hypersensitivity to proteins of *Escherichia coli,* filgrastim
Precautions: Pregnancy, breastfeeding, children <45 kg, adolescents, myeloid malignancies, sickle cell disease, leukocytosis, splenic rupture, ARDS, allergic-type reactions, peripheral blood stem cell (PBSC) mobilization

DOSAGE AND ROUTES
• **Adult/child >45 kg: SUBCUT** 6 mg per chemotherapy cycle, give ≥24 hr after cytotoxic chemotherapy

---

Available forms: Sol for inj 6 mg/0.6 mL

Administer:

SUBCUT route

• Using single-use vials; after dose is withdrawn, do not reenter vial

• Do not use 6-mg fixed dose in infants, children, or others <45 kg

• Inspect sol for discoloration, particulates; if present, do not use

• Do not administer during the period 14 days before and 24 hr after cytotoxic chemotherapy

• Store in refrigerator; do not freeze; may store at room temperature up to 6 hr; avoid shaking, protect from light

SIDE EFFECTS

CNS: Fever, fatigue, headache, dizziness, insomnia, peripheral edema

GI: Splenic rupture

HEMA: Leukocytosis

INTEG: Alopecia

MISC: Chest pain, hyperuricemia, anaphylaxis, capillary leak syndrome

GU: Glomerulonephritis

MS: Skeletal pain

RESP: Respiratory distress syndrome

PHARMACOKINETICS

Half-life: 15-80 hr; 20-38 hr (children)

INTERACTIONS

• Do not use product concomitantly, 2 wk before, or 24 hr after administration of cytotoxic chemotherapy

Increase: release of neutrophils—lithium

Drug/Lab Test

Increase: uric acid, LDH, alk phos

NURSING CONSIDERATIONS

Assess:

• **Allergic reactions, anaphylaxis:** rash, urticaria; discontinue product, have emergency equipment nearby

• **ARDS:** dyspnea, fever, tachypnea, occasionally confusion; obtain ABGs, chest x-ray; product may need to be discontinued

• **Splenic rupture:** upper left quadrant abdominal pain, dizziness, confusion, drop in B/P, pallor

• **Sickle cell crisis** in those with sickle cell disease (may be fatal)

• **Capillary leak syndrome:** edema, hemoconcentration, hypotension, hypoalbuminemia, treatment in ICU may be required

• **Bone pain:** give mild analgesics

• Blood studies: CBC with differential, platelet count before treatment, 2× weekly; neutrophil counts may be increased for 2 days after therapy

• **Vitals:** B/P, respirations, pulse before and during therapy

• **Pregnancy/breastfeeding:** use only if benefits outweigh fetal risk; pregnant women should enroll in Amgen's Pregnancy Surveillance Program, 800-772-6436; cautious use in breastfeeding, excretion unknown

Evaluate:

• **Therapeutic response:** absence of infection

Teach patient/family:

• How to perform the technique for self-administration if product to be given at home: dose, side effects, disposal of containers and needles; provide instruction sheet

• To notify prescriber immediately of allergic reaction, trouble breathing, abdominal pain

---

> **⚠ HIGH ALERT**

P

peginterferon alfa-2a (Rx)

(peg-in-ter-feer'on)

Pegasys, Pegasys ProClick

peginterferon alfa-2b (Rx)

PegIntron, Pegintron Redipen, Sylatron

Func. class.: Immunomodulator

ACTION: Stimulates genes to modulate many biologic effects, including the inhibition of viral replication; inhibits ion cell proliferation, immunomodulation; stimulates effector proteins; decreases leukocyte, platelet counts

USES: Chronic hepatitis C infections in adults with compensated liver disease; chronic hepatitis B in adults who are HBe AG positive, HBe AG negative; HCV

Side effects: *italics* = common; red = life-threatening

patients coinfected with HIV; nonresponders or relapsers with chronic hepatitis C, malignant melanoma

Unlabeled uses: Adenovirus, coronavirus, encephalomyocarditis virus, herpes simplex types 1 and 2, hepatitis D, acute hepatitis C, HIV, HPV, polio virus, rhinovirus, varicella zoster, variola, vesicular stomatitis

CONTRAINDICATIONS

Neonates, infants, sepsis; hypersensitivity to interferons, benzyl alcohol, *Escherichia coli* protein

Precautions: Pregnancy, breastfeeding, children <18 yr, geriatric patients, thyroid disorders, myelosuppression, renal/hepatic disease, suicidal/homicidal ideation, preexisting ophthalmologic disorders, pancreatitis, hemodialysis

Black Box Warning: Cardiac disease, depression, autoimmune disease, infection, use with ribavirin

DOSAGE AND ROUTES
Pegasys
• **Adult: SUBCUT** 180 mcg weekly × 48 wk; if poorly tolerated, reduce dose to 135 mcg weekly; in some cases, reduction to 90 mcg may be needed

Peg-Intron
(chronic hepatitis C with compensated liver disease)
• **Adult >105 kg: SUBCUT** 1.5 mcg/kg/wk plus ribavirin 600 mg in AM and 800 mg in PM plus a HCV NS3/4A protease inhibitor; **86-105 kg:** 150 mcg/0.5 mL (0.5 mL of 150-mcg vial or Redipen) per wk plus ribavirin 1200 mg/day in 2 divided doses plus a HCV NS3/4A protease inhibitor; **81-85 kg:** 120 mcg/0.5 mL (0.5 mL of 120-mcg vial or Redipen) per wk plus ribavirin 1200 mg/day in 2 divided doses plus a HCV NS3/4A protease inhibitor; **76-80 kg:** 120 mcg/0.5 mL (0.5 mL of 120-mcg vial or Redipen) per wk plus ribavirin 400 mg in AM and 600 mg in PM plus a HCV NS3/4A protease inhibitor; **66-75 kg:** 96 mcg/0.4 mL (0.4 mL of 120-mcg vial or Redipen) per wk plus ribavirin 400 mg in AM and 600 mg in PM plus a HCV NS3/4A protease inhibitor; **61-65 kg:** 96 mcg/0.4 mL (0.4 mL of 120-mcg vial or

Redipen) per wk plus ribavirin 800 mg/day in 2 divided doses plus a HCV NS3/4A protease inhibitor; **51-60 kg:** 80 mcg/0.5 mL (0.5 mL of 80-mcg vial or Redipen) per wk plus ribavirin 800 mg/day in 2 divided doses plus a HCV NS3/4A protease inhibitor; **40-50 kg:** 64 mcg/0.4 mL (0.4 mL of 80-mcg vial or Redipen) per wk plus ribavirin 800 mg/day in 2 divided doses plus a HCV NS3/4A protease inhibitor; **<40 kg:** 50 mcg/0.5 mL (0.5 mL of 50-mcg vial or Redipen) per wk plus ribavirin 800 mg/day in 2 divided doses plus a HCV NS3/4A protease inhibitor

Malignant melanoma (Sylatron only)
• **Adult: SUBCUT** 6 mcg/kg/wk × 8 wk then 3 mcg/kg/wk × ≤5 yr, premedicate with acetaminophen 500-1000 mg 30 min before first dose, prn for subsequent doses

Available forms: Pegasys: inj 135, 180 mcg/0.5 mL; **Pegintron:** 50, 80, 120, 150 mcg/0.5 mL; **Sylatron** 200, 300, 600 mcg powder for inj

Administer:
• In evening to reduce discomfort, to allow patient to sleep through some side effects
• Continue pediatric dose in those who turn 18 yr

Interferon alfa-2a
• Use prefilled syringes; store in refrigerator

Interferon alfa-2b
SUBCUT/IM route
• Reconstitute with 1 mL of provided diluent/10-, 18-, or 50-million unit vials, swirl; sol for inj vials do not need reconstitution

SIDE EFFECTS
CNS: *Headache, insomnia, dizziness,* anxiety, hostility, lability, nervousness, depression, fatigue, poor concentration, pyrexia, suicidal ideation, homicidal ideation, relapse of drug addiction, emotional lability, mania, psychosis
CV: Ischemic CV events
ENDO: Hypothyroidism, diabetes
GI: *Abdominal pain, nausea, diarrhea, anorexia, vomiting,* dry mouth, fatal colitis, fatal pancreatitis
HEMA: Thrombocytopenia, neutropenia, anemia, lymphopenia
INTEG: *Alopecia, pruritus, rash,* dermatitis

MISC: Blurred vision, inj-site reaction, rigors
MS: *Back pain,* myalgia, arthralgia
RESP: Cough, dyspnea

PHARMACOKINETICS
Half-life 15-80 hr, large variability in other pharmacokinetics

INTERACTIONS
• Use caution when giving with theophylline, myelosuppressive agents
Increase: hepatic damage—NNRTIs, NRTIs, protein inhibitors
Drug/Lab Test
Increase: triglycerides, ALT
Decrease: HB, platelets, WBCs, neutrophils
Abnormal: thyroid function test

NURSING CONSIDERATIONS
Assess:
• **Neuropsychiatric symptoms:** severe depression with suicidal ideation; monitor q3wk then 8 wk, then q6mo
• B/P, blood glucose, ophthalmic exam, pulmonary function
• ALT, HCV viral load; patients who show no reduction in ALT, HCV unlikely to show benefit of treatment after 6 mo
• Platelet counts, heme concentration, ANC, serum creatinine concentration, albumin, bilirubin, TSH, T₄, AFP
• **Myelosuppression:** hold dose if neutrophil count is <500 × 10⁶/L or if platelets are <50 × 10⁹/L
• **Hypersensitivity:** discontinue immediately if hypersensitivity occurs
• **Infection:** vital signs, increased WBCs, fever; product may need to be discontinued
• **Colitis/pancreatitis:** may be fatal; diarrhea, fever, nausea, vomiting, severe abdominal pain; if these occur, product should be discontinued
• **Pregnancy/breastfeeding:** may cause birth defects if alfa-2b is used with ribavirin; do not use in pregnancy, contraception is needed; do not breastfeed
Evaluate:
• **Therapeutic response:** decreased chronic hepatitis C signs, symptoms; undetectable viral load

Teach patient/family:
• Provide patient or family member with written, detailed information about product
• Use 2 forms of effective contraception throughout treatment and for 6 mo after treatment (men and women) (combination therapy with ribavirin)
• To avoid driving, other hazardous activity if dizziness, confusion, fatigue, somnolence occur
• To use puncture-resistant container for disposal of needles/syringes if using at home
• To report suicidal/homicidal ideation, visual changes, bleeding/bruising, pulmonary symptoms

peginterferon beta-1a (Rx)
(peg-inter-feer′on bay′ta-wun-ay)
Plegridy
Func. class.: Biologic response modulator, interferon

USES: Treatment of relapsing forms of multiple sclerosis, including clinically isolated syndrome, relapsing-remitting disease, and active secondary progressive disease

CONTRAINDICATIONS
Hypersensitivity

DOSAGE AND ROUTES
Multiple sclerosis, relapsing
• **Adult:** SUBCUT Initial: 63 mcg on day 1; 94 mcg on day 15; maintenance: 125 mcg q14days beginning on day 29
Available forms: Injection 125 mcg/0.5-mL syringe; 63, 94 mcg/0.5 mL pen injector

pegloticase (Rx)
(peg-loe′ti-kase)
Krystexxa
Func. class.: Antigout agent
Chem. class.: Pegylated, recombinant, mammalian urate oxidase enzyme

ACTION: Lowers plasma uric acid concentration by converting uric acid to allantoin, which is readily excreted by the kidneys

Side effects: *italics* = common; red = life-threatening

USES: Chronic gout in patients experiencing treatment failure

CONTRAINDICATIONS

Black Box Warning: Hypersensitivity, ⁂ G6PD deficiency

Precautions: Pregnancy, breastfeeding, children/infants/neonates, ⁂ African-American patients, heart failure

Black Box Warning: Requires specialized setting, experienced clinician; serious hypersensitivity; methemoglobinemia

DOSAGE AND ROUTES
• **Adult: IV INFUSION** 8 mg over 2 hr q2wk
Available forms: Sol for inj 8 mg/mL
Administer:
Intermittent IV INFUSION route
• **Reconstitute:** visually inspect for particulate matter, discoloration whenever sol/container permits; use aseptic technique; withdraw 8 mg (1 mL) of product/250 mL 0.9% NaCl or 0.45% NaCl; invert several times to mix, do not shake; discard remaining product in vial
• **Premedicate:** with antihistamines and corticosteroids in all patients and acetaminophen if deemed necessary to prevent anaphylaxis, infusion site reactions
• **Infusion:** if refrigerated, allow to come to room temperature; do not warm artificially; give over 120 min; do not give IV push or bolus; use infusion by gravity feed, syringe-type pump, or infusion pump; given in a specialized setting by those who can manage anaphylaxis or inj-site reactions; monitor during and for 1 hr after infusion; if reaction occurs, slow or stop infusion, may be restarted at a slower rate; do not admix
• Store diluted product in refrigerator or at room temperature for up to 4 hr; refrigerator is preferred; protect from light; do not freeze; use within 4 hr of preparation

SIDE EFFECTS
CNS: Dizziness, fatigue, fever
CV: *Chest pain*, heart failure, hypotension
GI: *Nausea*, vomiting, diarrhea, constipation
GU: Nephrolithiasis
HEMA: Anemia
INTEG: Ecchymosis, *erythema, pruritus, urticaria*
MS: Back pain, arthralgia, muscle spasm
SYST: Antibody formation, infection, anaphylaxis, infusion-related reactions
RESP: *Dyspnea*, upper respiratory infection

PHARMACOKINETICS
Remains primarily in intravascular space after administration, elimination half-life 2 wk, mean nadir uric acid concentration 24-72 hr

INTERACTIONS
Do not use with urate-lowering agents (allopurinol, probenecid, febuxostat, sulfinpyrazone)

NURSING CONSIDERATIONS
Assess:
• **Gout:** pain in big toe, feet, knees, redness, swelling, tenderness lasting a few days to weeks; intake of alcohol, purines, if patient is overweight or taking diuretics
• Obtain uric acid levels at baseline, before administration; 2 consecutive uric acid levels of >6 mg/dL may indicate therapy failure; greater chance of anaphylaxis; infection-related reactions

Black Box Warning: Specialized care setting: use only in facility where emergency equipment is available, anaphylaxis may occur

Black Box Warning: Infusion reactions: monitor for reactions for ≥1 hr after use

Black Box Warning: Assess for G6PD deficiency, methemoglobinemia

---

• **Pregnancy/breastfeeding:** use only if benefits outweigh fetal risk; avoid breastfeeding, excretion unknown

Evaluate:

• **Therapeutic response:** decrease uric acid levels; relief of pain, swelling, redness in toes, feet, knees

Teach patient/family:

• About reason for infusion, expected results

• To notify prescriber during infusion of allergic reactions or redness, swelling, pain at infusion site

• That continuing follow-up exams and uric acid levels will be needed

---

pegvaliase-pqpz (Rx)

(peg-val′i-ase)

Palynziq

Func. class.: Phenylalanine ammonia lyase enzyme

USES: To reduce blood phenylalanine concentrations in phenylketonuria (PKU) patients who have uncontrolled blood phenylalanine concentrations >600 micromol/L on existing management

CONTRAINDICATIONS

Black Box Warning: Serious hypersensitivity or anaphylaxis

DOSAGE AND ROUTES
Phenylketonuria (PKU)

• **Adult: SUBCUT Induction:** 2.5 mg weekly × 4 wk

• **Titration (after 4-wk induction):** 2.5 mg twice weekly × 1 wk, then 10 mg weekly for 1 wk, then 10 mg twice weekly for 1 wk, then 10 mg 4 times/wk for 1 wk, then 10 mg day × 1 wk. Additional time may be required before each dosage escalation based on patient tolerability; maintenance: 20 mg daily × ≥24 wk. Individualize dose to achieve blood phenylalanine concentration ≤600 micromol/L; may increase to 40

mg daily if a response (blood phenylalanine concentration 600 micromol/L or less) has not been achieved after using 20 mg daily × 24 wk, max 60 mg/day

Available forms: Injection 2.5, 10, 20 mg/0.5-mL single-dose syringe

---

⚠ HIGH ALERT

pembrolizumab (Rx)

(pem′broe-liz′ue-mab)

Keytruda

Func. class.: Antineoplastics

Chem. class.: Monoclonal antibodies

ACTION: A human monoclonal antibody that binds to the programmed death receptor-1 (PD-1) found on T-cells and blocks the interaction of PD-1 with its ligands, PD-L1 and PD-L2, on the tumor cell

USES: Unresectable or metastatic malignant melanoma in those who have disease progression after ipilimumab or in ⚹ BRAF V600 mutation–positive patients who have disease progression after ipilimumab and a BRAF inhibitor, metastatic non–small-cell lung cancer with high PD-L1 expression, lacking EGFR or ALK, recurrent head and neck squamous cell carcinoma, Hodgkin lymphoma, MSI-H or dMMR colorectal cancer

CONTRAINDICATIONS

Hypersensitivity, pregnancy, breastfeeding

Precautions: Immune-mediated colitis, immune-mediated hepatitis, immune-mediated hyperthyroidism/hypothyroidism; immune-mediated nephritis, acute interstitial nephritis, and renal failure; immune-mediated pneumonitis, adrenocortical insufficiency, arthritis, exfoliative dermatitis, hemolytic anemia, hypophysitis, myasthenia syndrome, myositis, optic neuritis, pancreatitis, partial seizures after inflammatory foci identified in brain parenchyma, rhabdomyolysis, uveitis, incidence of abortion/stillbirths

P

DOSAGE AND ROUTES
• **Adult:** IV 200 mg over 30 min q3wk or 400 mg over 30 min q6wk until disease progression up to 24 mo
Available forms: Powder for injection 50 mg/vial; solution for injection 25 mg/mL
Administer:
Intermittent IV INFUSION route
• Add 2.3 mL of sterile water for injection, 50-mg vial (25 mg/mL); inject sterile water along the walls of the vial and not directly on the powder
• Gently swirl and allow up to 5 min for bubbles to clear, do not shake, solution will be clear to slightly opalescent, colorless to slightly yellow
• Add the required amount of product to a bag of normal saline (0.9% sodium chloride injection) to a final diluted concentration between 1 and 10 mg/mL; mix by gentle inversion
• Discard any unused solution left in the vial
• **Storage after reconstitution and dilution:** Store at room temperature up to 4 hr or refrigerate up to 24 hr (includes reconstitution, dilution, and administration time). If refrigerated, allow the diluted solution to warm to room temperature before use, give over 30 min
• Use a sterile, nonpyrogenic, low–protein binding 0.2- to 5-micron in-line or add-on filter
• Do not use with other drugs through the same infusion line
• **Grade 2 or 3 toxicity:** Withhold and give corticosteroids; resume when the adverse event recovers to grade ≤1. Permanently discontinue if there is no recovery within 12 wk, if the corticosteroid dose cannot be reduced to ≤10 mg/day of predniSONE (or equivalent) within 12 wk, or for recurrent severe or grade 3 colitis
• **Grade 4 toxicity:** Permanently discontinue, give corticosteroids
Hepatitis:
• **Grade 2 toxicity (AST or ALT >3-5 × upper limit of normal [ULN] or total bilirubin >1.5-3 × ULN):** Withhold and give corticosteroids; resume when adverse event recovers to grade 1 or less.

Permanently discontinue if there is no recovery within 12 wk or if the corticosteroid dose cannot be reduced to ≤10 mg/day of predniSONE (or equivalent) within 12 wk
• **Grade 3 or 4 toxicity (AST or ALT >5 × ULN or total bilirubin >3 × ULN):** Permanently discontinue; give corticosteroids
• **Liver metastases and grade 2 elevated transaminase levels at baseline:** Permanently discontinue if AST/ALT levels increase by ≥50% over baseline and transaminase level elevations persist for at least 1 wk

SIDE EFFECTS
CNS: Seizures, myasthenia, headache, fever, insomnia, chills, dizziness, fatigue
ENDO: Hyponatremia, hypothyroidism/hyperthyroidism, hyperglycemia, hypocalcemia, immune-mediated hypophysitis
EENT: Optic neuritis
GI: Nausea, vomiting, abdominal pain, pancreatitis, colitis, diarrhea, hepatitis, constipation
GU: Interstitial nephritis, renal failure
RESP: Cough, dyspnea, immune-mediated pneumonitis
INTEG: Rash, pruritus, skin discoloration
MS: Myalgia, immune-mediated rhabdomyolysis
SYST: Exfoliative dermatitis

INTERACTIONS
None known
Drug/Lab Test
Increase: LFTs, renal function studies

NURSING CONSIDERATIONS
Assess:
• For hyperthyroidism/hypothyroidism, renal function studies baseline, periodically during therapy, CCr, BUN; monitor for nephritis
• For pneumonitis (new or worsening cough, chest pain, shortness of breath); confirm with radiographic imaging, give corticosteroids ≥ grade 2, withhold in grade 2, resume grade 0-1
• **Immune-mediated hepatitis:** liver function tests and hepatitis, jaundice, severe nausea/vomiting, easy bleeding

or bruising; withhold and give cortico-steroids if grade 2 hepatitis (AST or ALT >3-5 × ULN or total bilirubin >1.5-3 × ULN)
• **Pregnancy:** assess whether pregnancy is planned or suspected or if breastfeeding; do not use in pregnancy, breastfeeding
• **Immune-mediated hypophysitis:** headache, weakness, fainting, dizziness, blurred vision; use corticosteroids if >grade 2, discontinue >grade 3
• **Hyperglycemia:** may cause diabetes mellitus 1 or diabetic ketoacidosis
Evaluate:
• **Therapeutic response:** decreased progression of multiple myeloma
Teach patient/family:
• To notify prescriber immediately of signs of colitis, pneumonitis, hepatitis, hypophysitis
• **Hyperglycemia:** about signs and symptoms of hyperglycemia, diabetes; how to ensure tight glucose control; to report hyperglycemia immediately
• **Pregnancy:** to use highly effective contraceptive methods during and for 4 mo after treatment; to contact health care provider if pregnancy is suspected or confirmed; not to breastfeed

---

⚠ HIGH ALERT

PEMEtrexed (Rx)
(pem-ah-trex′ed)
Alimta, Pemfexy
Func. class.: Antineoplastic-antimetabolite
Chem. class.: Folic acid antagonist

Do not confuse:
PEMEtrexed/PRALAtrexate

ACTION: Inhibits multiple enzymes that reduce folic acid, which is needed for cell replication

USES: Malignant pleural mesothelioma in combination with CISplatin; non–small-cell lung cancer as single agent; nonsquamous non–small-cell lung cancer (1st-line treatment)

CONTRAINDICATIONS
Pregnancy, hypersensitivity, ANC <1500 cells/mm^3, CCr <45 mL/min, thrombocytopenia (<100,000/mm^3), anemia
Precautions: Breastfeeding, children, renal/hepatic disease

DOSAGE AND ROUTES
• **Adult: IV INFUSION** 500-600 mg/m^2 given over 10 min on day 1 of 21-day cycle with CISplatin 75 mg/m^2 infused over 2 hr beginning ½ hr after end of PEMEtrexed infusion
Renal dose
• **Adult: IV INFUSION** CCr <45 mL/min, not recommended
Available forms: Inj, single-use vials, 100, 500 mg; solution for injection 100 mg/4 mL, 50 mg/20 mL, 1 g/40 mL
Administer:
• Store at 77° F, excursions permitted at 59° F to 86° F, not light sensitive, discard unused portions
• Vit B$_{12}$ and low-dose folic acid as prophylactic measure to treat related hematologic, GI toxicity; 400-1000 mcg/day × 7 days before 1st dose and × 21 days after last dose, vit B$_{12}$ 1 mg IM 1 wk before 1st dose and q 3 cycles (9 wk) thereafter
• Premedicate with corticosteroid (dexamethasone) given PO bid day before, day of, and day after administration of PEMEtrexed
Intermittent IV INFUSION route
• Use cytotoxic handling procedures
• Reconstitute 500-mg vial/20 mL 0.9% NaCl inj (preservative free) = 25 mg/mL, swirl until dissolved, further dilute with 100 mL 0.9% NaCl inj (preservative free), give as IV infusion over 10 min
• Use only 0.9% NaCl inj (preservative free) for reconstitution, dilution
• Do not begin a new cycle unless neutrophils (ANC) are ≥1500 cells/mm^3, platelets are ≥100,000 cells/mm^3, CCr is ≥45 mL/min

---

• **Platelet nadir <50,000/mm³ regardless of the ANC:** if necessary, delay until platelet count recovery, reduce PEMEtrexed and CISplatin by 50%; if grade 3/4 toxicity occurs after 2 reductions, discontinue both products

• **ANC nadir <500/mm³ when platelet nadir is ≥50,000/mm³:** if necessary, delay until ANC recovery, reduce PEMEtrexed and CISplatin by 75%; if grade 3/4 toxicity occurs after 2 reductions, discontinue both products

• **CTC Grade 3/4 nonhematologic toxicity including diarrhea requiring hospitalization and excluding neurotoxicity, mucositis, and grade 3 transaminase elevations:** withhold therapy until pretherapy value or condition, reduce by 75% both products; if grade 3 or 4 toxicity occurs after 2 reductions, discontinue both products

• **CTC grade 3/4 mucositis:** withhold therapy until pretherapy condition, reduce 50% of PEMEtrexed; if grade 3 or 4 mucositis occurs after 2 dosage reductions, discontinue both products

• **CTC grade 2 neurotoxicity:** withhold therapy until pretherapy value or condition, reduce dose of CISplatin by 50%

• **CTC grade 3/4 neurotoxicity:** discontinue both products

SIDE EFFECTS

CNS: *Fatigue, fever, mood alteration, neuropathy*
CV: Thrombosis, embolism, *chest pain,* arrhythmia exacerbation
GI: *Nausea, vomiting, anorexia, diarrhea, ulcerative stomatitis, constipation, dehydration*
GU: Renal failure, creatinine elevation
HEMA: Neutropenia, leukopenia, thrombocytopenia, myelosuppression, anemia
INTEG: *Rash, desquamation*
RESP: *Dyspnea*
SYST: Infection with/without neutropenia, radiation recall reaction, toxic epidermal necrolysis, Stevens-Johnson syndrome, anaphylaxis

PHARMACOKINETICS

Not metabolized; excreted in urine (unchanged 70%-90%); not known if excreted in breast milk; half-life 3.5 hr, 81% protein binding

INTERACTIONS

Decrease: clearance of PEMEtrexed—nephrotoxic products, avoid NSAIDs for 2-8 days before use

NURSING CONSIDERATIONS
Assess:

• Previous radiation treatments; radiation recall reactions have occurred (erythema, exfoliative dermatitis, pain, burning)

• **Bone marrow depression:** CBC, differential, platelet count; monitor for nadir, recovery on days 8, 15 of the cycle; new cycle should not begin if ANC <1500 cells/mm³, platelets <100,000 cells/mm³, CCr <45 mL/min

• **Nephrotoxicity:** Renal studies: BUN; serum uric acid; urine CCr; electrolytes before, during therapy; I&O ratio; report fall in urine output to <30 mL/hr

• Monitor temperature; fever may indicate beginning infection; no rectal temperature

• **Neurotoxicity:** CTC grade 2: withhold until resolution to at least pretherapy value/condition, reduce CISplatin by 50%; CTC grade 3-4: immediately discontinue product and CISplatin if given in combination

• **Mucositis:** CTC 3/4: withhold until resolution to at least pretherapy value/condition, reduce dose by 50%; if grade 3/4 occurs after 2 dosage reductions, discontinue product and CISplatin

• **Bleeding:** bleeding time, coagulation time during treatment; bleeding: hematuria, guaiac, bruising or petechiae, mucosa or orifices

• Buccal cavity for dryness, sores, ulceration, white patches, oral pain, bleeding, dysphagia

• **Severe allergic reaction, toxic epidermal necrolysis:** rash, urticaria, itching, flushing

• Rinsing of mouth tid-qid with water, club soda; brushing of teeth bid-tid with soft brush or cotton-tipped applicators for stomatitis; use unwaxed dental floss

• **Pregnancy/breastfeeding:** do not use in pregnancy, breastfeeding

Evaluate:

• Therapeutic response: decreased spread of malignancy

Teach patient/family:

• To report any complaints, side effects to nurse or prescriber: black, tarry stools; chills, fever, sore throat, bleeding, bruising, cough, SOB, dark or bloody urine

• To discuss with provider all OTC, Rx, herbals, supplements taken, to avoid alcohol

• To avoid foods with citric acid, hot temperature, or rough texture if stomatitis is present

• To report stomatitis: any bleeding, white spots, ulcerations in mouth to prescriber; to examine mouth daily; to report symptoms to nurse; to use good oral hygiene

• That prophylactic folic acid and B_{12} injections may be necessary 1 wk before therapy to prevent bone marrow suppression and GI symptoms

• To avoid use of razors, commercial mouthwash

• To eat foods high in folic acid; to take supplements as prescribed

• That contraceptive measures are recommended during therapy, for ≥8 wk after cessation of therapy; to discontinue breastfeeding because toxicity to infant may occur

---

penciclovir topical
See Appendix B

PENICILLINS

penicillin G benzathine (Rx)
(pen-i-sill'in)

Bicillin L-A

Penicillin G potassium (Rx)
penicillin G procaine (Rx)
penicillin G sodium (Rx)
penicillin V potassium (Rx)
Penicillin VR

Func. class.: Broad-spectrum antiinfective
Chem. class.: Natural penicillin

ACTION: Interferes with cell-wall replication of susceptible organisms; lysis is mediated by cell-wall autolytic enzymes, results in cell death

USES: Respiratory infections, scarlet fever, erysipelas, otitis media, pneumonia, skin and soft-tissue infections, gonorrhea; effective for gram-positive cocci *(Staphylococcus, Streptococcus pyogenes, S. viridans, S. faecalis, S. bovis, S. pneumoniae)*, gram-negative cocci *(Neisseria gonorrhoeae)*, gram-positive bacilli *(Actinomyces, Bacillus anthracis, Clostridium perfringens, C. tetani, Corynebacterium diphtheriae, Listeria monocytogenes)*, gram-negative bacilli *(Escherichia coli, Proteus mirabilis, Salmonella, Shigella, Enterobacter, Streptobacillus moniliformis)*, spirochetes *(Treponema pallidum)*

CONTRAINDICATIONS
Hypersensitivity to penicillins
Precautions: Pregnancy, breastfeeding; hypersensitivity to cephalosporins, carbapenem, sulfites; severe renal disease, GI disease, asthma, CDAD, electrolyte imbalance, geriatrics, infants, neonates

Black Box Warning: Penicillin G benzathine: IV use, may be fatal

DOSAGE AND ROUTES
Penicillin G benzathine
Early syphilis
• Adult: IM 2.4 million units in single dose
Congenital syphilis
• Child <2 yr: IM 50,000 units/kg in single dose, max 2.4 million units as single inj
Prophylaxis of rheumatic fever, glomerulonephritis
• Adult/child >27 kg: IM 1.2 million units as single dose
• Child ≤27 kg: IM 600,000 units as single dose
Most infections
• Adult/child >27 kg: IM 1.2 million units as single dose

P

Side effects: *italics* = common; red = life-threatening

• **Child ≤27 kg: IM** 600,000 units as single dose
Available forms: Inj 600,000 units/mL
Penicillin G Potassium
Pneumococcal/streptococcal infections (serious)
• **Adult: IM/IV** 5-24 million units in divided doses q4-6hr
• **Child <12 yr: IV** 150,000-300,000 units/kg/day in 4-6 divided doses; max 24 million units/day
Most infections
• **Adult: IM/IV** 1-5 million units q4-6hr
• **Child: IM/IV** 8333-16,667 units/kg q4hr; 12,550-25,000 units/kg q6hr; up to 250,000 units/kg daily in divided doses, if more serious 300,000 units/kg daily
• **Infant >7 days: IV** 25,000 units/kg q8hr; meningitis up to 75,000 units/kg q6hr
• **Infant <7 days: IV** 25,000 units/kg q12hr, meningitis 100,000-150,000 units/kg daily in divided doses
Renal dose
• CCr <10 mL/min, give full loading dose then ½ of loading dose q8-10hr
Available forms: Powder for inj 1, 5, 20 million units/vial; inj 1, 2, 3 million units/50 mL
Penicillin G procaine
Moderate to severe pneumococcal infections
• **Adult: IM** 600,000-1 million units as single dose or divided bid doses/day for 10 days to 2 wk
• **Child: IM** 50,000 units/kg daily × 10-14 days (congenital syphilis)
Available forms: Inj 600,000, units/mL

Penicillin V
Most infections
• **Adult/adolescent/child >12 yr: PO** 1-4 g in 3-4 divided doses
• **Child <12 yr: PO** 25-100 mg/kg/day in 3-4 divided doses, max 3 g/day
Group A beta-hemolytic streptococcal infections
• **Adult/child >12 yr: PO** 1-4 g/day in divided doses
Available forms: Tabs 250, 500 mg; powder for oral sol 125, 250 mg/5 mL

Administer:
• Store in dry, tight container; oral susp refrigerated 2 wk
Penicillin G benzathine
• No dilution needed, shake well, give slowly deep IM inj in large muscle mass; avoid intravascular inj; aspirate; do not give IV
Penicillin G
• Aspirate before use
• Penicillin G sodium or potassium can be given IM or IV, vials containing 10 or 20 million units not for IM use
Intermittent IV INFUSION route
• Vials/bulk packages: dilute according to manufacturer's directions
• Frozen bags: thaw at room temperature, do not force thaw, no reconstitution needed
• Final concentration (100,000-500,000 units/mL—adults; 50,000 units/mL—neonate/infant)
• Total daily dose divided q4-6hr and given over 1-2 hr (adult), 15 min (infant/neonate)

Penicillin G procaine
• No dilution needed; give deep IM inj; avoid intravascular inj; aspirate; do not give IV

Penicillin V
• Orally on empty stomach for best absorption
• **Oral susp:** tap bottle to loosen, add ½ total amount of water, shake, add remaining water, shake; final concentration 125 or 250 mg/mL, store in refrigerator after reconstitution, discard after 14 days

SIDE EFFECTS
CNS: Lethargy, hallucinations, anxiety, depression, twitching, coma, seizures, hyperreflexia
GI: *Nausea, vomiting, diarrhea,* increased AST, ALT, abdominal pain, glossitis, colitis, CDAD
GU: Oliguria, proteinuria, hematuria, *vaginitis, moniliasis,* glomerulonephritis, renal tubular damage
HEMA: Anemia, increased bleeding time, bone marrow depression, granulocytopenia, hemolytic anemia

META: Hypo/hyperkalemia, alkalosis, hypernatremia
MISC: Anaphylaxis, serum sickness, Stevens-Johnson syndrome, *local pain*, tenderness and fever with IM inj

PHARMACOKINETICS

Penicillin G benzathine: IM: Very slow absorption; time to peak 12-24 hr; duration 21-28 days; excreted in urine, feces, breast milk; crosses placenta
Penicillin G: IV: Peak immediate
IM: Peak ¼-½ hr
PO: Peak 1 hr, duration 6 hr
Excreted in urine unchanged, excreted in breast milk, crosses placenta, half-life 30-60 min
Penicillin G procaine: IM: Peak 1-4 hr, duration 15 hr, excreted in urine
Penicillin V: PO: Peak 30-60 min, half-life 30 min, excreted in urine, breast milk

INTERACTIONS

Increase: penicillin effect—aspirin, probenecid
Increase: effect of heparin, methotrexate
Decrease: effect of oral contraceptives, typhoid vaccine
Decrease: antimicrobial effect of penicillin—tetracyclines
Drug/Lab Test
False positive: urine glucose, urine protein

NURSING CONSIDERATIONS
Assess:
• **Infection:** temperature; characteristics of sputum, wounds, urine; stools before, during, after treatment; C&S before therapy; product may be given as soon as culture is taken
• **GU status:** I&O ratio; report hematuria, oliguria because penicillin in high doses is nephrotoxic; renal tests: urinalysis, protein, blood
• **Renal disease:** any patient with compromised renal system because product is excreted slowly with poor renal system function; toxicity may occur rapidly
• Hepatic studies: AST, ALT

• Blood studies: WBC, RBC, Hct, HB, bleeding time
• **CDAD:** diarrhea, mucus, pus; bowel pattern before, during treatment
• Respiratory status: rate, character, wheezing, tightness in chest
• Allergies before initiation of treatment, reaction to each medication; because of prolonged action, allergic reaction may be prolonged and severe; watch for anaphylaxis: rash, dyspnea, pruritus, laryngeal edema; skin eruptions after administration of penicillin to 1 wk after discontinuing product
• EPINEPHrine, suction, tracheostomy set, endotracheal intubation equipment
• Scratch test to assess allergy after securing order from prescriber; usually done when penicillin is only product of choice
Evaluate:
• **Therapeutic response:** resolution of infection
Teach patient/family:
• To report sore throat, fever, fatigue; may indicate superinfection; CNS effects: depression, hallucinations, seizures
• To wear or carry emergency ID if allergic to penicillins
• **CDAD:** To report diarrhea with blood, pus, mucus to prevent dehydration
• To shake susp well before each dose; to store in refrigerator for up to 2 wk
• To use all medication prescribed

TREATMENT OF ANAPHYLAXIS: Withdraw product; maintain airway; administer EPINEPHrine, aminophylline, O$_2$, IV corticosteroids

---

pentamidine (Rx)
(pen-tam′i-deen)
NebuPent, Pentam
Func. class.: Antiprotozoal
Chem. class.: Aromatic diamide derivative

ACTION: Interferes with DNA/RNA synthesis in protozoa

P

USES: Treatment/prevention of *Pneumocystis jiroveci* infections

Unlabeled uses: PJP (inhalation)

CONTRAINDICATIONS

Hypersensitivity

Precautions: Pregnancy, breastfeeding, children, blood dyscrasias, cardiac/renal/hepatic disease, diabetes mellitus, hypocalcemia, hypo/hypertension, anemia

DOSAGE AND ROUTES

• **Adult and child ≥4 mo: IV/IM** 4 mg/kg/day × 2-3 wk; **NEB** 300 mg via Respirgard II Jet (Nebupent) every 4 weeks; or 150 mg q2wk

Available forms: Inj, aerosol 300 mg/vial; sol for aerosol 300 mg ✤

Administer:

• Store in refrigerator protected from light

Inhalation route

• Through nebulizer, using Respirgard II jet nebulizer; mix contents in 6 mL of sterile water; do not use low pressure (<20 psi); flow rate should be 5-7 L/min (40-50 psi) air or O_2 source over 30-45 min until chamber is empty

IM route

• **Reconstitute** 300 mg in 3 mL sterile water (100 mg/mL), give deep IM by Z-track; if painful by this route, rotate inj site

Intermittent IV INFUSION route

• Check IV site frequently (vesicant properties)

• **Reconstitute** 300 mg/3-5 mL of sterile water for inj, D_5W, withdraw dose and **further dilute** in 50-250 mL D_5W, give over 1-2 hr with patient lying down; check B/P often

Y-site compatibilities: alemtuzumab, alfentanil, aminocaproic acid, anidulafungin, argatroban, atracurium, atropine, benztropine, buprenorphine, calcium gluconate, CARBOplatin, caspofungin, chlorproMAZINE, cimetidine, CISplatin, cyclophosphamide, cycloSPORINE, cytarabine, DACTINomycin, diltiaZEM, gatifloxacin, zidovudine

SIDE EFFECTS

CNS: Disorientation, hallucinations

CV: Severe hypotension, chest pain, ventricular tachycardia, QT prolongation, dysrhythmias

GI: *Nausea, anorexia;* metallic taste, pancreatitis

HEMA: Anemia, leukopenia, thrombocytopenia

INTEG: Sterile abscess, pain at inj site, pruritus, urticaria, *rash*, Stevens-Johnson syndrome

MISC: Night sweats, anaphylaxis

RESP: Cough, SOB, bronchospasm (with aerosol), sore throat

PHARMACOKINETICS

IV: Peak 1 hr

IM: Peak 30 min

Excreted unchanged in urine (66%); half-life 9-12 hr (IM), 6 hr (IV)

INTERACTIONS

• **Nephrotoxicity:** aminoglycosides, amphotericin B, CISplatin, NSAIDs, vancomycin

• **Fatal dysrhythmias:** erythromycin IV

Increase: QT prolongation—class IA/III antidysrhythmics, some phenothiazines, β-agonists, local anesthetics, tricyclics, haloperidol, chloroquine, droperidol, pentamidine; CYP3A4 inhibitors (amiodarone, clarithromycin, erythromycin, telithromycin, troleandomycin, arsenic trioxide); CYP3A4 substrates (methadone, pimozide, QUEtiapine, quiNIDine, risperiDONE, ziprasidone)

Increase: myelosuppression—antineoplastics, radiation

Drug/Lab Test

Decrease: WBC, platelets, HB, Hct, calcium, magnesium

Increase: BUN, creatinine, potassium, LFTs, bilirubin, alkaline phosphatase

NURSING CONSIDERATIONS

Assess:

• Blood tests, blood glucose, CBC, platelets, calcium, magnesium

• **GU:** I&O ratio; report hematuria, oliguria

- **CV:** ECG for cardiac dysrhythmias in cardiac patients; patient should be lying down when receiving product; severe hypotension may develop; monitor B/P during administration and until B/P stable
- **Hepatic studies:** AST, ALT
- **Renal studies:** urinalysis, BUN, creatinine; nephrotoxicity may occur; any patient with compromised renal system; product is excreted slowly with poor renal system function; toxicity may occur rapidly
- Signs of infection, anemia
- **GI:** Bowel pattern before, during treatment
- **Respiratory status:** rate, character, wheezing, dyspnea
- Dizziness, confusion, hallucination
- **Serious skin reactions, allergic reactions:** rash, fever, fatigue, muscle or joint aches, oral lesions, blisters; discontinue product immediately if these occur
- **Pancreatitis:** nausea, vomiting, severe abdominal pain; monitor lab values of lipase and amylase (elevated in pancreatitis); if these signs or symptoms occur, product may need to be discontinued
- Diabetic patients, hypoglycemia may occur, then hyperglycemia with prolonged therapy
- **Pregnancy/breastfeeding:** use only if benefits outweigh fetal risk; cautious use in breastfeeding

Evaluate:

- **Therapeutic response:** resolution of AIDS-related PCP

Teach patient/family:

- To report sore throat, fever, fatigue (may indicate superinfection)
- To maintain adequate fluid intake
- That IM injection is painful
- To complete entire course of medication
- **Pancreatitis:** To report to provider immediately nausea, vomiting, severe abdominal pain
- To report immediately rash, bleeding, fever, sore throat, or flulike symptoms, to avoid crowds, persons with known infections

⚠ HIGH ALERT

pentazocine/naloxone (Rx)

(pen-taz′oh-seen/nal-oks′one)
Func. class.: Analgesic, opioid partial agonist

Controlled Substance Schedule IV

USES: Moderate to severe pain

CONTRAINDICATIONS
Hypersensitivity

Black Box Warning: Addiction, abuse, misuse; opioid analgesic REMS; life-threatening respiratory depression; accidental ingestion; neonatal opioid withdrawal syndrome; use with benzodiazepines, other CNS depressants

DOSAGE AND ROUTES
Pain management

- **Adult:** PO: 1 tablet (pentazocine 50 mg/naloxone 0.5 mg) q3-4 hr; may increase to 2 tablets (pentazocine 100 mg/naloxone 1 mg) if needed, max 12 tablets (pentazocine 600 mg/naloxone 6 mg)/day; max 600 mg/6 mg/day

Available forms: Tabs 50 mg/0.5 mg

⚠ HIGH ALERT

pentoxifylline (Rx)

(pen-toks-if′i-lin)
Func. class.: Hemorrheologic agent, blood viscosity reducer

USES: Treatment of intermittent claudication from chronic occlusive arterial disease of the limbs

CONTRAINDICATIONS
Hypersensitivity to pentoxifylline, xanthines, or any component; recent cerebral/retinal hemorrhage

P

DOSAGE AND ROUTES
Intermittent claudication
• **Adult: PO** 400 mg tid; benefit may take up to 4 wk to develop, take for ≥ 8 wk
Available forms: Ext rel tabs 400 mg

---

peramivir (Rx)
(per-am′i-vir)
Rapivab
Func. class.: Antiviral

ACTION: Competitively binds to the active site of the influenza virus, inhibits the activity of strains of influenza A and B viruses

USES: Treatment of uncomplicated acute influenza (seasonal influenza A virus infection or seasonal influenza B virus infection)
Unlabeled uses: Treatment of H1N1 influenza A virus (swine influenza) infection

CONTRAINDICATIONS
Serious hypersensitivity
Precautions: Breastfeeding, children, dialysis, infants, infection, pregnancy, psychosis, renal impairment

DOSAGE AND ROUTES
Influenza
• **Adult: IV** 600 mg as a single dose infused over 15-30 min, give within 48 hr of onset of influenza symptoms
Renal Dose
• **Adult/adolescent:** CCr ≥50 mL/min, no change; CCr 30-40 mL/min, 200 mg as a single dose; CCr 10-29 mL/min, 100 mg as a single dose
Available forms: Solution for injection 200 mg/20 mL
Administer:
• For IV use only, do not give IM, visually inspect parenteral products for particulate matter and discoloration
• **Dilute** the 10 mg/mL to a max volume of 100 mL, use only 0.9% or 0.45% NaCl, 5% dextrose, or LR
• **Storage of diluted solution:** Use immediately or refrigerate up to 24 hr. Refrigerated

solution should be allowed to reach room temperature before administration. Discard any unused diluted solution after 24 hr
• Give over 15-30 min, do not mix or coadminister with other IV products

SIDE EFFECTS
CNS: Delirium, psychosis, hallucinations, insomnia
GI: Constipation, diarrhea, vomiting
MISC: Rash, Stevens-Johnson syndrome, anaphylaxis

PHARMACOKINETICS
Protein binding <30%

INTERACTIONS
Avoid use with intranasal influenza vaccines, H1N1 vaccines

NURSING CONSIDERATIONS
Assess:
• Hypersensitivity reactions/Stevens-Johnson syndrome
• **Neuropsychiatric reactions:** delirium, psychosis, hallucinations
Evaluate:
• **Therapeutic response:** absence of developing influenza A or B
Teach patient/family:
• That product is for use only within 48 hr of symptoms

---

perampanel (Rx)
(per-am′pa-nel)
Fycompa
Func. class.: Anticonvulsant, AMPA glutamate receptor antagonist

Controlled Substance Schedule III

USES: Treatment of partial-onset seizures with or without secondarily generalized seizures as adjunct or monotherapy in epilepsy (≥4); treatment of primary generalized tonic-clonic seizures as adjunct therapy in epilepsy (≥12)

CONTRAINDICATIONS
Hypersensitivity

Black Box Warning: Serious, life-threatening psychiatric events

DOSAGE AND ROUTES
Partial-onset seizures:
• **Adult:** Initial: 2 mg daily at bedtime; may increase by 2 mg daily ≥ weekly; maintenance 4-12 mg daily at bedtime
Available forms: Tablets 2, 4, 6, 8, 10, 12 mg; oral suspension 0.5 mg/mL

perindopril (Rx)
(per-in'doe-pril)
Coversyl ✦, Coversyl Plus ✦
Func. class.: Antihypertensive, ACE inhibitor

USES: Management of hypertension, MI prophylaxis
Unlabeled uses: HF

CONTRAINDICATIONS
Hypersensitivity

Black Box Warning: Pregnancy second/third trimester

DOSAGE AND ROUTES
Hypertension
• **Adult PO:** Initial: 4 mg daily; titrate dose as needed up to 16 mg daily
Available forms: Tabs 2, 4, 8 mg

permethrin (Rx, OTC)
(per-METH-rin)
Elimite, Kwellada-P ✦, Nix
Func. class.: Pediculocide/scabicidal

USES: Treatment of head lice *(Pediculus humanus capitis)* and its nits (eggs); treatment of scabies *(Sarcoptes scabiei)* infestation

CONTRAINDICATIONS
Hypersensitivity

DOSAGE AND ROUTES
Head lice
• **Adult/child ≥2 mo: Topical: Cream rinse/lotion 1%:** Before application, wash hair with conditioner-free shampoo; rinse with water and towel dry. Apply a sufficient amount of lotion or cream rinse to saturate the hair and scalp (especially behind the ears and nape of neck). Leave on hair for 10 min then rinse with warm water; remove remaining nits with nit comb, may repeat in 7 days if needed
Scabies
• **Adult/child ≥2 mo: Topical: Cream 5%:** Thoroughly massage cream (30 g for adult) from head to soles of feet; leave on for 8-14 hr before removing (shower or bath); for infants and the elderly, also apply on the hairline, neck, scalp, temple, and forehead; may repeat if living mites are observed 14 days after first treatment
Available forms: Cream 5%; lotion 1%✦

perphenazine (Rx)
(per-fen'a-zeen)
Func. class.: Antipsychotic, phenothiazine

P

USES: Schizophrenia, control of severe nausea and vomiting

CONTRAINDICATIONS
Hypersensitivity, opioids, bone marrow suppresion, CNS depression, coma

Black Box Warning: Dementia-related psychosis

DOSAGE AND ROUTES
Schizophrenia
• **Adult/child ≥12:** PO Initial: 8-16 mg/day in divided doses; titrate based on response; max 64 mg/day
Nausea/vomiting
• **Adult:** PO 8-16 mg/day in divided doses; max 24mg/day
Available forms: Tablet 2, 6, 8, 16 mg

perphenazine/ amitriptyline (Rx)

per-fen'a-zeen/am-i-trip'ti-leen
Func. class.: Tricyclic antidepressant/
phenothiazine

USES: Treatment of moderate-to-severe anxiety and/or agitation and depression; schizophrenia with depressive symptoms

CONTRAINDICATIONS

Hypersensitivity to amitriptyline, perphenazine, or any component, other phenothiazines, bone marrow depression; within 14 days of MAOIs; CNS depression (barbiturates, alcohol, opioids, analgesics, antihistamines); during the acute recovery of MI

Black Box Warning: Dementia-related psychosis, children

DOSAGE AND ROUTES
Depression/anxiety
• **Adult:** PO 1 tablet (amitriptyline 25 mg/perphenazine 2 mg or amitriptyline 25 mg/perphenazine 4 mg) tid-qid or 1 tablet (amitriptyline 50 mg/perphenazine 4 mg) bid; max amitriptyline 200 mg/ perphenazine 16 mg; maintenance: usually 1 tablet (amitriptyline 25 mg/perphenazine 2 mg or amitriptyline 25 mg/ perphenazine 4 mg) bid-qid or 1 tablet (amitriptyline 50 mg/perphenazine 4 mg) bid
Schizophrenia with depressive symptoms
• **Adult:** PO 2 tablets (amitriptyline 25 mg/perphenazine 4 mg) tid; may give a fourth dose at bedtime; max amitriptyline 200 mg/perphenazine 16 mg; maintenance: usually 1 tablet (amitriptyline 25 mg/perphenazine 2 mg or amitriptyline 25 mg/perphenazine 4 mg) bid-qid or 1 tablet (amitriptyline 50 mg/perphenazine 4 mg) bid
Available forms: Tabs 2/10, 2/25, 4/10, 4/25, 4/50 mg

⚠ HIGH ALERT

pertuzumab (Rx)

(per-too'zoo-mab)
Perjeta
Func. class.: Antineoplastic
Chem. class.: HER-2/new antagonist

ACTION: Blocks liquid-dependent action of human epidermal growth factor-2 (HER2), inhibiting signal pathways

USES: First-line treatment of 🔖 HER2-positive metastatic breast cancer with trastuzumab and DOCEtaxel

CONTRAINDICATIONS
Hypersensitivity:

Black Box Warning: Pregnancy

Precautions: Breastfeeding, children, infants, neonates, cardiac arrhythmias, MI, cardiac disease, heart failure, hypertension, infusion-related reactions

Black Box Warning: Heart failure, ventricular dysfunction

DOSAGE AND ROUTES
• **Adult:** IV 840 mg over 60 min, then after 3 wk 420 mg over 30-60 min every 3 wk; give with trastuzumab 8 mg/kg IV over 90 min, then after 3 wk 6 mg/kg over 30-90 min every 3 wk and DOCEtaxel 75 mg/m² IV every 3 wk; dosage may be escalated to 100 mg/m²
Available forms: Solution for inj 420 mg/14 mL (single-use vials) (30 mg/mL)
Administer:
• Visually inspect for particulate matter and discoloration
Dilution and preparation
• **Withdraw** the calculated dose from the vial and add to a 250 mL 0.9% sodium chloride PVC or non-PVC polyolefin infusion bag; do not dilute with dextrose 5% solution
• **Dilute** in normal saline only; do not mix or dilute with other drugs or dextrose solutions

---

• Mix the diluted solution by gentle inversion; do not shake

IV infusion

• Administer the diluted solution immediately

• Do not administer as an IV push or bolus

• Give the first dose of 840 mg over 60 min and subsequent 420-mg doses over 30-60 min

• If the diluted solution is not used immediately, store at 2° C-8° C for up to 24 hr

Delayed or missed doses

• If time since previous dose is <6 wk, give 420 mg IV (do not wait for next scheduled dose)

• If time since previous dose is ≥6 wk, give 840 mg IV over 60 min, followed 3 wk later by 420 mg IV over 30-60 min repeated every 3 wk

• If DOCEtaxel is discontinued, this product and trastuzumab may continue

SIDE EFFECTS

CNS: *Headache,* fever, *peripheral neuropathy, chills, fatigue,* asthenia

CV: Heart failure

EENT: Lacrimation, *stomatitis*

GI: *Nausea, vomiting,* diarrhea, dysgeusia, *stomatitis, constipation, anorexia*

HEMA: *Anemia,* neutropenia

MS: *Arthralgia*

RESP: Upper respiratory infection, cough

SYST: Anaphylaxis, antibody formation

INTEG: *Alopecia*

PHARMACOKINETICS

Median half-life 18 days

NURSING CONSIDERATIONS

Assess:

• **HER2 overexpression:** testing should be done to identify HER2 overexpression before using this product

• **Decreased left ventricular ejection fraction (LVEF):** can occur and is increased in those with a history of prior anthracycline use or radiotherapy to the chest; evaluate LVEF at baseline and every 3 mo; withhold therapy ×3 wk if LVEF is <40% or LVEF is 40%-45% with a 10% or greater absolute decrease from baseline; resume therapy if the LVEF is recovered to >45% or to 40%-45% with <10% absolute decrease at reassessment; if the LVEF has not improved or has declined further, consider permanently discontinuing pertuzumab and trastuzumab after a risk/benefit assessment

• **Infusion-related reactions/hypersensitivity:** assess anaphylactoid reaction, acute infusion reaction, cytokine-release syndrome 60 min after the first infusion, 30 min after other infusions; monitor for pyrexia, chills, fatigue, headache, asthenia, hypersensitivity, and vomiting; if a significant reaction occurs, slow or interrupt the infusion; permanent discontinuation may be needed in severe reactions

• **Neutropenia:** can occur, but occurs more commonly when trastuzumab is also used and in ⬥ Asian patients, monitor CBC with differential baseline and periodically

• **Upper respiratory infection:** monitor for dyspnea, shortness of breath, fever

Black Box Warning: Pregnancy: determine whether pregnancy is planned or suspected; patients who become pregnant during therapy should report exposure to the Genentech Adverse Event line at 888-835-2555 and enroll in the MotHER Pregnancy Registry at 800-690-6720, women of childbearing age and men with partners of childbearing age must use contraception during and for 7 mo after last dose

Evaluate:

• Decreased size, spread of tumor

Teach patient/family:

• To notify prescriber immediately of **infection** (cough, fever, chills, sore throat); **bleeding** (gums, bruising, blood in urine/stools/sputum); to avoid persons with known infections

• To avoid all OTC, prescription, herbal, and supplement products unless approved by prescriber; not to use aspirin, NSAIDs, alcohol

• To notify prescriber of peripheral neuropathy

• That hair loss is common

Black Box Warning: Pregnancy/breast-feeding: counsel women of childbearing age and men with partners of childbearing age on the need for contraception during and for 7 mo after therapy; advise patients who suspect pregnancy to contact their health care provider immediately; discontinue breastfeeding

> ## ⚠ HIGH ALERT
>
> ### pexidartinib (Rx)
> (pex′-i-dar′-ti-nib)
> Turalio
> *Func. class.:* Antineoplastic-orphan drug
> *Chem. class.:* Colony stimulating factor-1 receptor (CSF-1R) inhibitor

USES: Symptomatic tenosynovial giant cell tumor

CONTRAINDICATIONS
Hypersensitivity, pregnancy, breastfeeding

Black Box Warning: Hepatotoxicity

DOSAGE AND ROUTES
• **Adults: PO** 250 mg bid, taken with low fat meal until disease progression
Available forms: Capsule 125 mg

> ### phentermine/ topiramate (Rx)
> (fen′ter-meen/toe-pyre′a-mate)
> Qsymia
> *Func. class.:* Anorexiant/anticonvulsant
> **Controlled Substance: Schedule IV**

USES: Adjunct to a reduced-calorie diet and increased physical activity, in patients with either an initial body mass index (BMI) of ≥30 kg/m² or an initial BMI of ≥27 kg/m² and at least one weight-related comorbid condition (HTN, dyslipidemia, type 2 diabetes)

CONTRAINDICATIONS
Hypersensitivity to phentermine, other sympathomimetic amines, CV (arrhythmias, HF, CAD, uncontrolled HTN); hyperthyroidism; glaucoma; agitation; use within 14 days of MAOIs; pregnancy; breastfeeding

Black Box Warning: Substance abuse

DOSAGE AND ROUTES
Weight management
• **Adult: PO** Initial: Phentermine 3.75 mg/topiramate 23 mg daily × 14 days; increase to phentermine 7.5 mg/topiramate 46 mg daily × 12 wk then evaluate, if 3% of body weight has not been lost, discontinue use or increase dose to phentermine 11.25 mg/topiramate 69 mg daily × 14 days, then to phentermine 15 mg/topiramate 92 mg daily, evaluate weight loss after 12 wk on phentermine 15 mg/topiramate 92 mg; if 5% of body weight has not been lost at phentermine 15 mg/topiramate 92 mg gradually discontinue therapy 1 dose every other day for ≥ 1 wk
Available forms: Capsule 3.75/23, 7.5/46, 11.25/69, 15 mg/92 mg

> ## ⚠ HIGH ALERT
>
> ### phentermine (Rx)
> (fen′ter-meen)
> Adipex-P, Lomaira
> *Func. class.:* Anorexiant
> **Controlled Substance: Schedule IV**

USES: Short-term adjunct in a regimen of weight reduction based on exercise, behavioral modification, and caloric restriction in the management of exogenous obesity with an initial body mass index (BMI) ≥30 kg/m² or ≥27 kg/m² in the presence of other risk factors (diabetes, hyperlipidemia, controlled hypertension)

CONTRAINDICATIONS
Hypersensitivity or idiosyncrasy to phentermine, other sympathomimetic amines, or any component; CV (arrhythmias, HF, CAD, uncontrolled HTN); hyperthyroidism; glaucoma; agitation; drug abuse; use within 14 days of MAOIs; pregnancy; breastfeeding

DOSAGE AND ROUTES
Obesity (short-term adjunct)
• **Adult: PO** Capsule/tablet **(excluding Lomaira):** 15-37.5 mg/day in 1-2 divided doses; tablet **(Lomaira only):** 8 mg tid
Available forms: Capsule 15, 18.75, 30, 37.5 mg; tabs 8, 37.5 mg

---

⚠ HIGH ALERT

phentolamine (Rx)
(fen-tole′a-meen)
OraVerse
Func. class.: Antidote (extravasation), alpha₁ blocker

Uses: Diagnosis of pheochromocytoma via phentolamine blocking; prevention/treatment of hypertensive episodes associated with pheochromocytoma; prevention/treatment of dermal necrosis/sloughing after extravasation of norepinephrine; reversal of soft tissue anesthesia

CONTRAINDICATIONS
Hypersensitivity to phentolamine, any component; MI, coronary insufficiency, angina, CAD (excluding OraVerse)

DOSAGE AND ROUTES
Extravasation of norepinephrine, management
• **Adult:** Local infiltration: Inject 5-10 mg (diluted in 10 mL normal saline) into extravasation area
Diagnosis of pheochromocytoma (phentolamine-blocking test)
• **Adult: IM, IV:** 5 mg
Perioperative hypertensive episodes associated with pheochromocytoma, prevention and management
• **Adult:** *Preoperative:* IM, IV: 5 mg 1-2 hr before surgery and repeat if needed; *intraoperative:* IV: 5 mg as needed
Available forms: Powder for injection 5 mg

phenylephrine nasal agent
See Appendix B

phenylephrine ophthalmic
See Appendix B

---

phenytoin (Rx) (NTI)
(fen′i-toh-in)
Dilantin, Dilantin 125, Phenytek, Tremytoine ✦
Func. class.: Anticonvulsant; antidysrhythmic (IB)
Chem. class.: Hydantoin

ACTION: Inhibits spread of seizure activity in motor cortex by altering ion transport; increases AV conduction

USES: Generalized tonic-clonic seizures; status epilepticus; nonepileptic seizures associated with Reye's syndrome or after head trauma; complex partial seizures
Unlabeled uses: Digoxin toxicity; seizures, prophylaxis in head trauma, subarachnoid hemorrhage

CONTRAINDICATIONS
Pregnancy, hypersensitivity, bradycardia, SA and AV block, AV block, Adams-Stokes syndrome
Precautions: Hypersensitivity to carBAMazepine, barbituates, succinimide, geriatric patients, renal/hepatic disease, petit mal seizures, hypotension, myocardial insufficiency, Asian patients positive for HLA-B1502, hepatic failure, acute intermittent porphyria, psychiatric condition, abrupt discontinuation, agranulocytosis, alcoholism, bone fractures

Black Box Warning: IV use (infusion-related reactions)

DOSAGE AND ROUTES—NTI
Seizures
• **Adult: PO** 100 mg 3 times daily, initially. Adjust q 7 to 10 days as needed based on clinical status and/or serum concentrations. Usual dose: 100 mg 3 to 4 times daily. Max: 200 mg 3 times daily **IV** 10 to 15 mg/kg/dose loading dose, then 100 mg 3 to 4 times daily, initially.

Side effects: *italics* = common; red = life-threatening

Adjust q 7 to 10 days as needed based on clinical status and/or serum concentrations. Usual dose: 100 mg 3 to 4 times daily. Max: 200 mg 3 times daily
• **Child: IV/PO** 5 mg/kg/day in 2-3 divided doses, maintenance 4-8 mg/kg/day in 2-3 divided doses, max 300 mg/day

Status epilepticus
• **Adult: IV** 20 mg/kg/dose (Max: 1500 mg/dose) as a single dose; may administer additional 5 to 10 mg/kg/dose as single dose after 10 min if needed
• **Child: IV** 15 to 20 mg/kg/dose (Max: 1500 mg/dose) as a single dose; may administer additional 5 to 10 mg/kg/dose as a single dose after 10 min if needed

Available forms: Susp 25 mg/5 mL; chewable tabs 50 mg; inj 50 mg/mL; ext rel caps 100, 200, 300 mg

Administer:

PO route
• Do not interchange chewable product with caps, not equivalent; only ext rel caps to be used for once-a-day dosing
• **Oral suspension:** shake well before each dose given via G tube/NG tube; dilute susp before administration; flush tube with 20 mL water after dose; hold tube feedings 1 hr before and 1 hr after dose
• Allow 7-10 days between dosage changes
• Divided PO doses with or after meals to decrease adverse effects
• Give 2 hr before or after antacid, enteral feeding

Direct IV route

> **Black Box Warning:** Give undiluted at ≤50 mg/min (adult) 1-3 mg/kg/min (child); 0.5-1 mg/kg/min (neonates), monitor for CV reactions and respiratory depression

Intermittent IV INFUSION route

> **Black Box Warning:** Dilute dose in NS to ≤6.7 mg/mL; complete infusion within 1 hr of preparation; use 0.22- or 0.55-micron in-line particulate final filter between IV catheter and tubing; flush IV line or catheter with NS before and after use; give at ≤50 mg/min (adult), 0.5-1 mg/kg/min (child, infant, neonate)

Additive compatibilities: Do not admix

SIDE EFFECTS

CNS: Dizziness, insomnia, paresthesias, depression, suicidal tendencies, aggression, headache, confusion, slurred speech, peripheral neuropathy
CV: Hypotension, ventricular fibrillation, bradycardia, cardiac arrest
EENT: Nystagmus, diplopia, blurred vision
ENDO: Diabetes insipidus
GI: Nausea, vomiting, constipation, anorexia, weight loss, hepatitis, jaundice, gingival hyperplasia, abdominal pain
GU: Nephritis, urine discoloration, sexual dysfunction
HEMA: Agranulocytosis, leukopenia, aplastic anemia, thrombocytopenia, megaloblastic anemia
INTEG: Rash, lupus erythematosus, Stevens-Johnson syndrome, hirsutism, toxic epidermal necrolysis
SYST: Hypocalcemia, purple glove syndrome (IV), DRESS, anaphylaxis, exacerbates myasthenia gravis

PHARMACOKINETICS

Metabolized by liver, excreted by kidneys, protein binding 90%-95%, half-life 7-42 hr, dose dependent
PO: Onset 2-24 hr, peak 1 ½-2 ½ hr, duration 6-12 hr
PO-ER: Onset 2-24 hr, peak 4-12 hr, duration 12-36 hr
IV: Onset 1-2 hr, duration 12-24 hr

INTERACTIONS

• Do not use with delavirdine; decreased response, resistance
Increase: phenytoin effect—benzodiazepines, cimetidine, tricyclics, salicylates, valproate, cycloSERINE, diazePAM, chloramphenicol, disulfiram, alcohol, amiodarone, sulfonamides, FLUoxetine, gabapentin, H_2 antagonists, azole antifungals, estrogens, succinimides, phenothiazines, methylphenidate, felbamate, traZODone
Decrease: phenytoin effects—alcohol carBAMazepine, rifAMPin, calcium (high dose), folic acid

Drug/Food
Enteral tube feeding: may decrease absorption of oral product; do not use enteral feedings 2 hr before or 2 hr after dose

Drug/Lab Test
Increase: glucose, alk phos, GGT

Decrease: dexamethasone, metyraPONE test serum, PBI, urinary steroids

NURSING CONSIDERATIONS
Assess:
• **Phenytoin hypersensitivity syndrome 3-12 wk after start of treatment:** rash, temperature, lymphadenopathy; may cause hepatotoxicity, renal failure, rhabdomyolysis

• **Serious skin disorders:** for beginning rash that may lead to Stevens-Johnson syndrome or toxic epidermal necrolysis; phenytoin should not be used again; may occur more often among Asian patients with HLA-B 1502

• **Purple glove syndrome** with IV use

• **Phenytoin level:** toxic level 30-50 mcg/mL; therapeutic level 7.5-20 mcg/mL

• **Seizures:** duration, type, intensity, precipitating factors; obtain EEG periodically; monitor therapeutic level

• **Blood studies:** CBC, platelets q2wk until stabilized, then monthly × 12, then q3mo; discontinue product if neutrophils <1600/mm³; renal function: albumin concentration; folic acid levels, LFTs

• **Mental status:** mood, sensorium, affect, memory (long, short), suicidal thoughts/behaviors

• Monitor EKG, B/P, respiratory function during IV loading dose; verify potency of IV access port before IV infusion

• Monitor EEG function and serum levels periodically

• **Renal function:** monitor for serum albumin, dosage adjustment may be needed

• **Blood dyscrasias:** fever, sore throat, bruising, rash, jaundice

• **Beers:** avoid use in older adults unless safer alternatives are unavailable; ataxia, impaired psychomotor function may occur

• **Pregnancy/breastfeeding:** pregnant women should enroll in the Antiepileptic Drug Pregnancy Registry, 888-233-2334; may cause fetal malformations; use other options when possible; breastfeeding is not recommended

Evaluate:
• **Therapeutic response:** decrease in severity of seizures

Teach patient/family:
• That, if diabetic, blood glucose should be monitored

• That urine may turn pink

• Not to discontinue product abruptly because seizures may occur

• **Oral hygiene:** about the proper brushing of teeth using a soft toothbrush, flossing to prevent gingival hyperplasia; about the need to see dentist frequently

• To avoid hazardous activities until stabilized on product

• To carry emergency ID stating product use

• That heavy use of alcohol may diminish effect of product; to avoid OTC medications

• Not to change brands or forms once stabilized on therapy because brands may vary

• Not to use antacids within 2 hr of product

• To notify prescriber of unusual bleeding, bruising, petechiae (bleeding), clay-colored stools, abdominal pain, dark urine, yellowing of skin or eyes (hepatotoxicity); slurred speech, headache, drowsiness

• To report suicidal thoughts/behaviors immediately

• **Pregnancy/breastfeeding:** to use nonhormonal contraception; to notify prescriber if pregnancy is planned or suspected

---

phosphate/biphosphate (OTC)
Func. class.: Laxative, saline

ACTION: Increases water absorption in the small intestine by osmotic action; laxative effect occurs by increased peristalsis and water retention

USES: Constipation, bowel or rectal preparation for surgery, exam

---

Side effects: *italics* = common; red = life-threatening

CONTRAINDICATIONS

Hypersensitivity, rectal fissures, abdominal pain, nausea, vomiting, appendicitis, acute surgical abdomen, ulcerated hemorrhoids, sodium-restricted diet, renal failure, hyperphosphatemia, hypocalcemia, hypokalemia, hypernatremia, Addison's disease, HF, ascites, bowel perforation, megacolon, imperforate anus

Black Box Warning: GI obstruction, renal failure

Precautions: Pregnancy

Black Box Warning: Colitis, geriatric hypovolemia, renal disease

DOSAGE AND ROUTES

• **Adult: PO** 20-30 mL (Phospho-Soda)
• **Child: PO** 5-15 mL (Phospho-Soda)
• **Adult/child >12 yr: RECT** 1 enema (118 mL)
• **Child 2-12 yr: RECT** ½ enema (59 mL)
Available forms: Enema 7 g phosphate/19 g biphosphate/118 mL; oral sol 18 g phosphate/48 g biphosphate/100 mL
Administer:
• Alone for better absorption; do not take within 1-2 hr of other products

SIDE EFFECTS

CV: Dysrhythmias, cardiac arrest, hypotension, widening QRS complex
GI: *Nausea, cramps,* diarrhea
META: Electrolyte, fluid imbalances

PHARMACOKINETICS

Onset 30 min-3 hr, excreted in feces

NURSING CONSIDERATIONS
Assess:
• **Stools:** color, amount, consistency; bowel pattern, bowel sounds, flatulence, distention, fever, dietary patterns, exercise; cramping, rectal bleeding, nausea, vomiting; if these occur, product should be discontinued
• Blood, urine electrolytes if product used often
Evaluate:
• **Therapeutic response:** decrease in constipation

Teach patient/family:
• Not to use laxatives for long-term therapy because bowel tone will be lost
• That normal bowel movements do not always occur daily
• Not to use in presence of abdominal pain, nausea, vomiting
• To notify prescriber if constipation unrelieved or if symptoms of electrolyte imbalance occur: muscle cramps, pain, weakness, dizziness, excessive thirst
• To maintain fluid consumption

physostigmine ophthalmic
See Appendix B

phytonadione (Vitamin K₁) (Rx)
(fye-toe-na-dye′one)
Mephyton, Vitamin K
Func. class.: Vitamin K₁, fat-soluble vitamin

Do not confuse:
Mephyton/methadone

ACTION: Needed for adequate blood clotting (factors II, VII, IX, X)

USES: Vit K malabsorption, hypoprothrombinemia, prevention of hypoprothrombinemia caused by oral anticoagulants, prevention of hemorrhagic disease of the newborn

CONTRAINDICATIONS

Hypersensitivity, severe hepatic disease, last few weeks of pregnancy
Precautions: Pregnancy, neonates, hepatic disease, IV use

Black Box Warning: Risk of anaphylaxis (IV/IM)

DOSAGE AND ROUTES
Hypoprothrombinemia from other causes
• **Adult: PO/IM** 2.5-25 mg, may repeat or increase to 50 mg

---

- **Child: PO** 2.5-5 mg
- **Infant: PO/IM** 2 mg

Prevention of hemorrhagic disease of the newborn

- **Neonate: IM** 0.5-1 mg within 1 hr after birth

Hypoprothrombinemia from other cause

- **Adult/child: PO/SUBCUT/IM** 2.5-10 mg, may repeat 12-48 hr

Warfarin-induced hypoprothrombinemia

- **Adults with INR <4.5 with no significant bleeding:** Lower/omit warfarin dose and monitor INR more frequently; reinitiate therapy at a lower dose when therapeutic INR is reached

INR 4.5-10 with no evidence of bleeding: do not use vitamin K, omit the next 1-2 doses of warfarin, monitor the INR more frequently, reinitiate therapy at a lower dose when therapeutic INR is reached

Serious bleeding at any elevation of INR: 5-10 mg IV by slow infusion in addition to 4-factor prothrombin complex concentrate. Hold warfarin therapy

- **Adults with INR >10 with no significant bleeding PO** 2.5-5 mg with the expectation that the INR would be reduced substantially in 24-48 hr. Hold warfarin, monitor INR more frequently

Infants, children, and adolescents (unlabeled): IV 30 mcg/kg/dose, with excessively prolonged INR (typically more than 8) with no bleeding; **significant bleeding,** immediate reversal using fresh-frozen plasma (FFP), prothrombin complex concentrates, or recombinant factor VIIa

Available forms: Tabs 5 mg; inj 10 mg/mL, 1 mg/0.5 mL

Administer:

- Store in tight, light-resistant container (PO)

IM route

- Use this route only when other routes cannot be used (deaths may occur due to allergic reactions)

Intermittent IV INFUSION route

- After diluting with ≥10 mL D₅W, NS, D₅NS; give by slow infusion over 30-60 min, route/mg/min
- VS q15min, check for hypersensitivity
- INR effect in 4-6 hr
- Do not use direct or bolus

Y-site compatibilities: Alfentanil, amikacin, aminophylline, ascorbic acid, atracurium, atropine, azaTHIOprine, aztreonam, bumetanide, buprenorphine, butorphanol, calcium chloride/gluconate, ceFAZolin, cefonicid, cefoperazone, cefotaxime, cefoTEtan, cefOXitin, cefTAZidime, ceftizoxime, cefTRIAXone, cefuroxime, chloramphenicol, chlorproMAZINE, cimetidine, clindamycin, cyanocobalamin, cycloSPORINE, dexamethasone, digoxin, diphenhydrAMINE, DOPamine, doxycycline, enalaprilat, ePHEDrine, EPINEPHrine, epoetin alfa, erythromycin, esmolol, famotidine, fentaNYL, fluconazole, folic acid, furosemide, ganciclovir, gentamicin, glycopyrrolate, heparin, hydrocortisone, imipenem/cilastatin, indomethacin, insulin, isoproterenol, ketorolac, labetalol, lidocaine, mannitol, meperidine, metaraminol, methoxamine, methyldopate, metoclopramide, metoprolol, metroNIDAZOLE, midazolam, morphine, multivitamins, nafcillin, nalbuphine, naloxone, nitroglycerin, nitroprusside, norepinephrine, ondansetron, oxacillin, oxytocin, papaverine, penicillin G potassium, pentamidine, pentazocine, PENTobarbital, PHENobarbital, phentolamine, phenylephrine, potassium chloride, procainamide, prochlorperazine, propranolol, pyridoxine, raNITIdine, sodium bicarbonate, succinylcholine, SUFentanil, theophylline, thiamine, ticarcillin/clavulanate, tobramycin, tolazoline, trimetaphan, urokinase, vancomycin, vasopressin, verapamil, vit B with C

SIDE EFFECTS

CNS: Headache, brain damage (large doses)

GI: Nausea, decreased LFTs

P

HEMA: Hemolytic anemia, hemoglobinuria, hyperbilirubinemia
INTEG: Rash, urticaria
RESP: Bronchospasm, dyspnea, feeling of chest constriction, respiratory arrest

PHARMACOKINETICS
PO: Onset 6-10 hr; peak 24-48 hr
SUBCUT: Erratic
Crosses placenta, metabolized in the liver, excreted in urine/feces

INTERACTIONS
Decrease: action of phytonadione—bile acid sequestrants, sucralfate, antiinfectives, salicylates, mineral oil
Decrease: action of warfarin—large dose of product

NURSING CONSIDERATIONS
Assess:
• **Increased bleeding risk:** emesis, stools, urine; pressure on all venipuncture sites; avoid all inj if possible
• PT, INR during treatment (2-sec deviation from control time, bleeding time, clotting time, INR); monitor for bleeding, pulse, and B/P
• **Hypersensitivity:** monitor closely
• **Pregnancy/breastfeeding:** usually not needed in pregnancy; may breastfeed
Evaluate:
• **Therapeutic response:** prevention of hemorrhagic disease of the newborn, resolution of hypoprothrombinemia
Teach patient/family:
• Not to take other supplements, OTC products, prescription products unless directed by prescriber
• About the necessary foods for associated diet
• To avoid IM inj; to use soft toothbrush; not to floss; to use electric razor until coagulation defect corrected
• To report symptoms of bleeding
• About the importance of frequent lab tests to monitor coagulation factors
• To notify all health care providers of use of this product
• To carry emergency ID describing condition and products used

---

pilocarpine ophthalmic
See Appendix B

---

pimavanserin (Rx)
(pim-a-van′ser-in)
Nuplazid
Func. class.: Atypical antipsychotic

ACTION: The exact mechanism of action is unknown; may be mediated through inverse agonist and antagonist activity at serotonin 5-HT2A receptors and to a lesser extent at 5-HT2C receptors

USES: The treatment of hallucinations and delusions associated with Parkinson's disease psychosis

CONTRAINDICATIONS
Hypersensitivity
Precautions: Alcoholism, bradycardia, breastfeeding, cardiac arrhythmias, cardiac disease, children, coronary artery disease, diabetes mellitus, females, geriatric patients, heart failure, hepatic disease, hypertension, hypocalcemia, hypokalemia, hypomagnesemia, long QT syndrome, malnutrition, myocardial infarction, pregnancy, QT prolongation, renal failure, renal impairment, stroke, thyroid disease

Black Box Warning: Dementia-related psychosis

DOSAGE AND ROUTES
• **Adult: PO** 34 mg daily
Available forms: Capsule 34 mg; tablet 10, 17 mg
Administer:
• Give without regard to food
• Do not split, chew capsules
• Capsules may be opened and sprinkled on soft food

SIDE EFFECTS
CNS: Confusion, hallucinations, fatigue, stroke, dizziness

GI: Nausea, constipation
MISC: Peripheral edema, infection, QT prolongation

PHARMACOKINETICS

Protein binding 95%, hepatic metabolism occurs through CYP3A4 and CYP3A5 and to a lesser extent CYP2J2, CYP2D6 with a major active metabolite; peak 6 hr, plasma half-lives of drug and metabolite are 57 hr and 200 hr, 0.55% eliminated unchanged in the urine and 1.53% was eliminated in feces after 10 days

INTERACTIONS

Increase: effects of pimavanserin—CYP3A4 inhibitors (ketoconazole, erythromycin), CYP2D6 inhibitors (quiNIDine, FLUoxetine, PARoxetine); reduce dose of pimavanserin
Increase: sedation—other CNS depressants
Increase: QT prolongation—products that cause QT prolongation
Decrease: pimavanserin effects—famotidine, valproate, CYP3A4 inducers (carbamazepine)
Decrease: pimavanserin effect—St. John's wort

NURSING CONSIDERATIONS
Assess:

Black Box Warning: Dementia-related psychosis: at increased risk of death, avoid using

• Swallowing of medication; check for hoarding, giving product to other patients
• AIMS assessment, neurologic function, LFTs, serum electrolytes, creatinine monthly
• Constipation daily; if this occurs, increase fiber, water in diet; stool softeners, laxatives may be needed
• **QT prolongation:** avoid in those with cardiac disease or other risk factors for QT prolongation, torsades de pointes (TdP), and/or sudden death such as cardiac arrhythmias, congenital long QT syndrome, heart failure, bradycardia, myocardial infarction, hypertension, coronary artery disease, hypomagnesemia, hypokalemia, hypocalcemia, or in patients receiving medications known to prolong the QT interval. Females, elderly patients, patients with diabetes mellitus, thyroid disease, malnutrition, alcoholism, or hepatic impairment may also be at increased risk for QT prolongation
• **Stroke:** avoid antipsychotics to treat delirium- or dementia-related behavioral problems unless nonpharmacologic options have failed and the patient is a substantial threat to self or others; avoid use in those with a history of falls or fractures
• **Hyponatremia:** product can cause hyponatremia and SIADH and elderly patients are at increased risk; sodium levels should be closely monitored when starting or changing dosages of antipsychotics in older adults

Evaluate:
• **Therapeutic response:** decrease in hallucinations, delusions, paranoia; reorganization of patterns of thought and speech

Teach Patient/Family:
• To avoid hazardous activities until response is known, dizziness may occur
• That compliance with dose is needed
• To avoid OTC products unless approved by prescriber

---

pimecrolimus topical
See Appendix B

P

---

pimecrolimus (Rx)
(pim-e-kroe′li-mus)
Elidel
Func. class.: Topical skin agent, immunosuppressant

USES: Short-term and noncontinuous long-term treatment of mild to moderate atopic dermatitis in nonimmunocompromised, those ≥2 yr who have failed to respond to other topical prescription treatments

CONTRAINDICATIONS
Hypersensitivity to pimecrolimus or any component

Black Box Warning: Neonates/Infants/children, new primary malignancy

---

DOSAGE AND ROUTES
Atopic dermatitis (mild to moderate)
• **Adult/child 2-17 yr: Topical:** Apply thin layer to affected area bid
Available forms: Cream 1%

⚠ HIGH ALERT

pioglitazone (Rx)
(pie-oh-glye'ta-zone)

Actos
Func. class.: Antidiabetic, oral
Chem. class.: Thiazolidinedione

Do not confuse:
Actos/Actonel

ACTION: Specifically targets insulin resistance; an insulin sensitizer; regulates the transcription of a number of insulin-responsive genes

USES: Type 2 diabetes mellitus

CONTRAINDICATIONS
Breastfeeding, children, hypersensitivity to thiazolidinedione, diabetic ketoacidosis, diabetes mellitus type 1, serious hepatic disease

> **Black Box Warning:** NYHA Class III/IV heart failure

Precautions: Pregnancy, geriatric patients, geriatric patients with CV disease, renal/hepatic/thyroid disease, edema, polycystic ovary syndrome, bladder cancer, osteoporosis, pulmonary disease, secondary malignancy

DOSAGE AND ROUTES
Monotherapy
• **Adult: PO** 15 or 30 mg/day, may increase to 45 mg/day; **with strong CYP2C8,** max 15 mg/day; **with NYHA class I/II heart failure,** max 15 mg/day
Combination therapy
• **Adult: PO** 15 or 30 mg/day with a sulfonylurea, metFORMIN, or insulin; decrease sulfonylurea dose if hypoglycemia occurs; decrease insulin dose by 10%-25% if hypoglycemia occurs or if plasma glucose is <100 mg/dL, max 45 mg/day
Hepatic dose
• Do not use in active hepatic disease or if ALT >2.5 times ULN
Available forms: Tabs 15, 30, 45 mg
Administer:
• Once a day; without regard to meals
• Tabs crushed and mixed with food or fluids for patients with difficulty swallowing

SIDE EFFECTS
CNS: *Headache*
CV: MI, heart failure, death (geriatric patients)
ENDO: Hypo/hyperglycemia
MISC: *Sinusitis, upper respiratory tract infection, pharyngitis,* hepatotoxicity, edema, weight gain, anemia, macular edema; risk of bladder cancer (use >1 yr), peripheral/pulmonary edema
MS: Rhabdomyolysis, fractures (females), myalgia

PHARMACOKINETICS
Maximal reduction in FBS after 12 wk; half-life 3-7 hr, terminal 16-24 hr; protein binding >99%

INTERACTIONS
Decrease: effect of atorvastatin
Decrease: effect of oral contraceptives; use alternative contraceptive method
Decrease: pioglitazone effect—CYP2C8 inducers (ketoconazole, fluconazole, itraconazole, miconazole, voriconazole)
Drug/Herb
Increase: hypoglycemia—garlic, green tea, horse chestnut
Drug/Lab Test
Increase: CPK, LFTs, HDL, cholesterol
Decrease: glucose, Hct/HB

NURSING CONSIDERATIONS
Assess:

> **Black Box Warning: Heart failure:** do not use in NYHA Class III/IV; excessive/rapid weight gain >5 lb, dyspnea, edema; may need to be reduced or discontinued; monitor daily weights

---

- **Bladder cancer:** avoid use in a history of bladder cancer; use of pioglitazone >1 yr has shown an increase in bladder cancer
- **Hypoglycemic reactions:** sweating, weakness, dizziness, anxiety, tremors, hunger; hyperglycemic reactions soon after meals (rare); may occur more often with insulin or other antidiabetics
- **Hepatic disease:** check LFTs periodically: AST, LDH; do not start treatment in active heart disease or if ALT >2.5× upper limit of normal; if treatment has already begun, follow closely with continuing ALT levels; if ALT increases to >3× upper limit of normal, recheck ALT as soon as possible; if ALT remains >3× upper limit of normal, discontinue
- FBS, glycosylated HbA1c, plasma lipids/lipoproteins, B/P, body weight during treatment
- **Fracture:** Assess fall risk, fracture risk, diet, activity level
- CBC with differential before and during therapy; more necessary in those with anemia; Hct/HB (may be decreased in first few months of treatment)
- **Beers:** avoid use in older adults; may promote fluid retention and/or exacerbate heart failure
- **Pregnancy/breastfeeding:** use only if benefits outweigh fetal risk; usually insulin is used in pregnancy; do not breastfeed, excretion unknown

Evaluate:
- **Therapeutic response:** decrease in polyuria, polydipsia, polyphagia; clear sensorium; absence of dizziness; stable gait; blood glucose A1c improvement

Teach patient/family:
- To self-monitor using a blood glucose meter
- About the symptoms of hypo/hyperglycemia; what to do about each
- That product must be continued on daily basis; about the consequences of discontinuing product abruptly
- To avoid OTC medications or herbal preparations unless approved by prescriber
- That diabetes is a lifelong illness; that product is not a cure, it only controls symptoms

- **To report symptoms of hepatic dysfunction:** nausea, vomiting, abdominal pain, fatigue, anorexia, dark urine, jaundice
- To report weight gain, edema, chest pain, palpitations, dyspnea
- That lab work, eye exams will be needed periodically
- To notify prescriber if oral contraceptives are used, effect may be decreased; not to use product if breastfeeding

pioglitazone/metformin (Rx)

(pye-oh-gli'ta-zone/met-for'min)

Actoplus Met
Func. class.: Antidiabetic

USES: As an adjunct to diet and exercise to improve glycemic control in adults with type 2 diabetes mellitus when treatment with both pioglitazone and metformin is needed

CONTRAINDICATIONS
Hypersensitivity to pioglitazone, metformin, or any component; established NYHA class III or IV HF, severe renal disease (eGFR <30 mL/min/1.73 m^2); metabolic acidosis, diabetic ketoacidosis

DOSAGE AND ROUTES
Diabetes mellitus, type 2
- **Adult: PO** *Initial:* Pioglitazone 15 mg/metformin 500 mg bid or pioglitazone 15 mg/metformin 850 mg daily
Available forms: Tabs 15/500, 15/850 mg

piperacillin/tazobactam (Rx)

(pip'er-ah-sill'in/ta-zoe-bak'tam)

Zosyn
Func. class.: Antiinfective, broad spectrum
Chem. class.: Extended-spectrum penicillin, β-lactamase inhibitor

ACTION: Interferes with cell-wall replication of susceptible organisms; tazobactam is a β-lactamase inhibitor that protects piperacillin from enzymatic degradation

USES:

Moderate to severe infections caused by piperacillin-resistant, piperacillin-tazobactam–susceptible, beta-lactamase–producing strains of the following: *Acinetobacter baumannii, Bacteroides fragilis, Bacteroides ovatus, Bacteroides thetaiotaomicron, Bacteroides vulgatus, Citrobacter koseri, Clostridium perfringens, Enterococcus faecalis, Escherichia coli, Haemophilus influenzae (beta-lactamase negative), Haemophilus influenzae (beta-lactamase positive), Klebsiella pneumoniae, Moraxella catarrhalis, Morganella morganii, Neisseria gonorrhoeae, Parabacteroides distasonis, Prevotella melaninogenica, Proteus mirabilis, Proteus vulgaris, Providencia rettgeri, Providencia stuartii, Pseudomonas aeruginosa, Salmonella enteritidis, Serratia marcescens, Staphylococcus aureus (MSSA), Staphylococcus epidermidis, Streptococcus agalactiae (group B streptococci), Streptococcus pneumoniae, Streptococcus pyogenes (group A beta-hemolytic streptococci),* and *Viridans streptococci*
This drug may also be effective against the following: *Bacillus anthracis, Enterobacter* sp., *Fusobacterium nucleatum, Klebsiella oxytoca,* and *Neisseria meningitidis*
Unlabeled uses: Endocarditis, bacteremia, cystic fibrosis, febrile neutropenia, peritoneal dialysis–related peritonitis, pleural empyema, pyelonephritis, sepsis, UTI

CONTRAINDICATIONS

Hypersensitivity to penicillins; neonates; carbapenem allergy
Precautions: Pregnancy, breastfeeding, renal insufficiency in neonates, hypersensitivity to cephalosporins, seizures, GI disease, electrolyte imbalances, biliary obstruction

DOSAGE AND ROUTES
Hospital-acquired pneumonia
• **Adult: IV** 4.5 g q6hr or 3.375 g q4hr with an aminoglycoside or antipseudomonal fluoroquinolone × 1-2 wk
Most infections
• **Adult: IV** 3.375 g (3 g pipercillin/0.375 g tazobactam) q6hr × 7-10 days
Renal dose
• **Adult: IV** CCr 20-40 mL/min, give 3.375 g q6hr (nosocomial pneumonia); give 2.25 g q6hr (all other indications); CCr <20 mL/min, give 2.25 g q6hr (nosocomial pneumonia); give 2.25 g q8hr (all other indications)
Available forms: Powder for inj 2 g piperacillin/0.25 g tazobactam, 3 g piperacillin/0.375 g tazobactam, 4 g piperacillin/0.5 g tazobactam, 36 g piperacillin/4.5 g tazobactam
Administer:
• Separate aminoglycoside from piperacillin to avoid inactivation
• Product after C&S is complete
Intermittent IV INFUSION route
• **Reconstitute** each 1 g of product/5 mL 0.9% NaCl for inj or sterile water for inj, dextrose 5%; shake well; **further dilute** in ≥50 mL compatible IV sol, run as int infusion over ≥30 min
• Store: diluted solution may be stored for ≤24 hr at room temperature

Y-site compatibilities: Alfentanil, allopurinol, amifostine, amikacin, aminocaproic acid, aminophylline, amphotericin B lipid complex, amphotericin B liposome, anidulafungin, argatroban, atenolol, aztreonam, bivalirudin, bleomycin, bumetanide, buprenorphine, busulfan, butorphanol, calcium acetate/chloride/gluconate, CARBOplatin, carmustine, cefepime, chloramphenicol, cimetidine, clindamycin, cyclophosphamide, cycloSPORINE, cytarabine, DACTINomycin, DAPTOmycin, dexamethasone, dexrazoxane, diazePAM, digoxin, diphenhydrAMINE, DOCEtaxel, DOPamine, doxacurium, enalaprilat, ePHEDrine, EPINEPHrine, eptifibatide, erythromycin, esmolol, etoposide, fenoldopam, fentaNYL, floxuridine, fluconazole, fludarabine, fluorouracil, foscarnet, fosphenytoin, furosemide, gallium, granisetron, heparin, hydrocortisone, HYDROmorphone, ifosfamide, isoproterenol, ketorolac, lansoprazole, lepirudin, leucovorin, lidocaine, linezolid, LORazepam, magnesium sulfate, mannitol, mechlorethamine, melphalan, meperidine, mesna, metaraminol, methotrexate, methylPREDNISolone, metoclopramide, metoprolol, metroNIDAZOLE, milrinone, morphine, naloxone, nitroglycerin, nitroprusside, norepinephrine, octreotide, ondansetron, oxytocin, PACLitaxel, palonosetron, pamidronate, pancuronium, PEMEtrexed, PENTobarbital, PHENobarbital, phentolamine, phenylephrine, plicamycin, potassium chloride/phosphates, procainamide, raNITIdine, remifentanil, riTUXimab, sargramostim, sodium acetate/bicarbonate/phosphate, succinylcholine, SUFentanil, sulfamethoxazole-trimethoprim, tacrolimus, telavancin, teniposide, theophylline, thiotepa, tigecycline, tirofiban, trimethobenzamide, vasopressin, vinBLAStine, vinCRIStine, voriconazole, zidovudine, zoledronic acid

SIDE EFFECTS
CNS: Lethargy, hallucinations, anxiety, depression, twitching, insomnia, headache, fever, dizziness, seizures, vertigo
CV: Cardiac toxicity, edema
GI: *Nausea, vomiting, diarrhea;* increased AST, ALT; abdominal pain, glossitis, CDAD, constipation, pancreatitis
GU: Oliguria, proteinuria, hematuria, *vaginitis, moniliasis,* glomerulonephritis, renal failure
HEMA: Anemia, increased bleeding time, bone marrow depression, agranulocytosis, hemolytic anemia
INTEG: Rash, pruritus, exfoliative dermatitis
META: Hypokalemia, hypernatremia
SYST: Serum sickness, anaphylaxis, Stevens-Johnson syndrome

PHARMACOKINETICS
Half-life 0.7-1.2 hr; excreted in urine, bile, breast milk; crosses placenta; 33% bound to plasma proteins

IV: Peak completion of IV

INTERACTIONS
Increase: effect of neuromuscular blockers, oral anticoagulants, methotrexate
Increase: piperacillin concentrations—aspirin, probenecid
Decrease: antimicrobial effect of piperacillin—tetracyclines, aminoglycosides IV

Drug/Lab Test
Increase: eosinophilia, neutropenia, leukopenia, serum creatinine, PTT, AST, ALT, alk phos, bilirubin, BUN, electrolytes
Decrease: Hct, HB, electrolytes
False positive: urine glucose, urine protein, Coombs' test

NURSING CONSIDERATIONS
Assess:
• **Infection:** temperature, stools, urine, sputum, wounds
• **GU status:** I&O ratio; report hematuria, oliguria because penicillin in high doses is nephrotoxic; maintain hydration unless contraindicated
• **Hepatic studies:** AST, ALT before treatment and periodically thereafter
• **Blood studies:** WBC, RBC, Hct, HB, bleeding time before treatment and periodically thereafter; serum potassium
• **Renal studies:** urinalysis, protein, blood, BUN, creatinine before treatment and periodically thereafter
• C&S before product therapy; product may be given as soon as culture is taken
• **CDAD:** diarrhea, bloody stools, fever, abdominal cramps; may occur ≤2 mo after treatment; bowel pattern before and during treatment
• **Skin** eruptions after administration of penicillin to 1 wk after discontinuing product
• **Respiratory status:** rate, character, wheezing, tightness in chest
• **Anaphylaxis:** wheezing, laryngeal edema, rash, itching; discontinue product, have emergency equipment nearby

P

• **Pregnancy/breastfeeding:** use only if clearly needed; cautious use in breastfeeding
Evaluate:
• **Therapeutic response:** absence of fever, purulent drainage, redness, inflammation; culture shows decreased organisms
Teach patient/family:
• That culture may be taken after completed course of medication
• To report sore throat, fever, fatigue (superinfection); CNS effects (anxiety, depression, hallucinations, seizures); pseudomembranous colitis (fever, diarrhea with blood, pus, mucus)
• To wear or carry emergency ID if allergic to penicillins
• CDAD: to notify nurse of diarrhea with blood, pus

TREATMENT OF OVERDOSE:
Withdraw product, maintain airway, administer EPINEPHrine, aminophylline, O_2, IV corticosteroids for anaphylaxis

---

pirfenidone (Rx)
(pir-fen'i-done)
Esbriet
Func. class.: Respiratory agent

USES: Pulmonary fibrosis

CONTRAINDICATIONS
Hypersensitivity

DOSAGE AND ROUTES
• **Adult: PO** 267 mg tid on days 1-7, 534 mg tid on days 8-14, and 801 mg tid from day 15 onward
Available forms: Capsule 267 mg; tabs 267, 801 mg

---

pitavastatin (Rx)
(pit'a-va-stat'-in)
Livalo, Zypitamag
Func. class.: Antilipidemic
Chem. class.: HMG-CoA reductase inhibitor

Do not confuse:
pitavastatin/pravastatin

ACTION: Inhibits HMG-CoA reductase enzyme, which reduces cholesterol synthesis; high doses lead to plaque regression

USES: As an adjunct for primary hypercholesterolemia (types Ia, Ib), dysbetalipoproteinemia, elevated triglyceride levels, prevention of CV disease by reduction of heart risk in those with mildly elevated cholesterol
Unlabeled uses: Atherosclerosis

CONTRAINDICATIONS
Pregnancy, breastfeeding, hypersensitivity, active hepatic disease, cholestasis
Precautions: Past hepatic disease, alcoholism, severe acute infections, trauma, severe metabolic disorders, electrolyte imbalance, seizures, surgery, organ transplant, endocrine disease, females, hypotension, renal disease

DOSAGE AND ROUTES
• **Adult: PO** 2 mg/day, usual range 1-4, max 4 mg/day
Renal dose
• **Adult: PO** CCr 30-<60 mL/min, 1 mg daily, max 2 mg daily; CCr <30 mL/min on hemodialysis, 1 mg daily, max 2 mg daily; CCr <30 mL/min, not recommended
Atherosclerosis (unlabeled)
• **Adult: PO** 4 mg/day
Available forms: Calcium tablets 1, 2, 4 mg; magnesium tablet 1, 2, 4 mg
Administer:
• Total daily dose any time of day without regard to meals
• Store in cool environment in tight container protected from light

SIDE EFFECTS
CNS: Headache
GI: Constipation, diarrhea
INTEG: Rash, pruritus, alopecia
MS: Arthralgia, myalgia, rhabdomyolysis
RESP: Pharyngitis

PHARMACOKINETICS
Peak 1 hr; metabolized in liver, excreted in urine, feces; half-life 12 hr; protein binding 99%; ✹✹ concentrations lower in healthy African Americans

INTERACTIONS
Increase: risk for possible rhabdomyolysis—azole antifungals, cycloSPORINE, erythromycin, niacin, gemfibrozil, clofibrate
Increase: levels of pitavastatin—erythromycin
Drug/Herb
Increase: pitavastatin—red yeast rice
Drug/Lab Test
Increase: bilirubin, alk phos, ALT, AST
Interference: thyroid function tests

NURSING CONSIDERATIONS
Assess:
• **Diet:** obtain diet history including fat, cholesterol in diet
• Cholesterol, triglyceride levels periodically during treatment; check lipid panel 6 wk after changing dose
• Hepatic studies baseline and when clinically indicated; if AST >3× normal, reduce or discontinue; AST, ALT, LFTs may be increased
• Renal studies in patients with compromised renal system: BUN, I&O ratio, creatinine
• **Rhabdomyolysis:** muscle pain, tenderness; obtain CPK if clinically indicated; if markedly increased, product may need to be discontinued
• **Pregnancy/breastfeeding:** do not use in pregnancy, breastfeeding
Evaluate:
• **Therapeutic response:** decrease in cholesterol to desired level after 6 wk
Teach patient/family:
• That blood work will be necessary during treatment
• To report blurred vision, severe GI symptoms, headache, muscle pain, weakness, tenderness
• That previously prescribed regimen will continue: low-cholesterol diet, exercise program, smoking cessation
• That product may increase blood glucose level
• Not to take product if pregnant or if pregnancy is planned or suspected (notify prescriber); to avoid breastfeeding

---

pitolisant (Rx)
(pi-tol'i-sant)
Wakix
Func. class.: Narcolepsy agent
Chem. class.: Histamine receptor modulator

ACTION: Selective antagonist/inverse agonist of the histamine-3 (H3) receptor; activation of histaminergic neurons increases histamine release, which promotes wakefulness, attention, and memory; regulates the release of other neurotransmitters involved in wake promotion, including dopamine, noradrenaline, and acetylcholine

USES: Excessive daytime sleepiness in adults with narcolepsy

CONTRAINDICATIONS
Hypersensitivity, severe hepatic disease

PRECAUTIONS
Alcoholism, bradycardia, CAD, cardiac disease, children, breastfeeding, contraception requirement, diabetes mellitus, females, geriatrics, heart failure, hepatic disease, hypertension, hypocalcemia, hypokalemia, hypomagnesemia, long QT syndrome, MI, malnutrition, poor metabolizers, pregnancy, QT prolongation, renal disease, thyroid disease

DOSAGE AND ROUTES
• **Adults PO** Initially, 8.9 mg daily in the morning on awakening for 1 wk; then increase to 17.8 mg daily for 1 wk; after that, the dose may be adjusted based on efficacy response and tolerability; max: 35.6 mg/day; limit to 17.8 mg/day in CYP2D6 poor metabolizers; up to 8 wk may be necessary
Available forms: Tablets 4.45, 17.8 mg

Administer:
• Give each dose in the morning on patient wakening

SIDE EFFECTS
CNS: *Headache, insomnia, anxiety,* hallucinations, irritability, cataplexy
GI: *Nausea,* abdominal pain, anorexia, dry mouth
INTEG: Rash
RESP: URI
MS: MS pain
CV: Increased heart rate

PHARMACOKINETICS
Protein binding is 91%-96%, metabolized by CYP2D6 and to a lesser extent by CYP3A4; inactive metabolites are further metabolized or conjugated with glycine or glucuronic acid, excreted 90% urine (<2% unchanged), 2.3% feces; half-life 7.5-24.2 hours, absorption 90%; peak 2-5 hr; increased in hepatic/renal disease

INTERACTIONS
Increased: cardiac dysrhythmia risk—drugs that prolong the QT interval (class Ia, III antidysrhythmics); avoid using together
Increased: pitolisant effect—CYP2D6 inhibitors (buPROPion, PARoxetine, FLUoxetine); reduce dose by half
Decreased: pitolisant effect—CYP3A4 inducers (carBAMazepine, phenytoin, rifAMPin); increase dose to double
Decreased: pitolisant effect—histamine-1 receptor antagonists (diphenhydrAMINE, imipramine, clomiPRAMINE); avoid using together
Decreased: CYP3A4 substrates (midazolam, hormonal contraceptives, cycloSPORINE)—use alternative contraception

NURSING CONSIDERATIONS
Assess:
• **Narcolepsy:** assess for trouble staying awake baseline and after 1 wk, 2 wk
• **Hepatic/renal disease:** monitor LFTs, serum bilirubin, BUN, creatinine baseline and periodically
Evaluate:
• **Therapeutic response:** ability to stay awake
Teach patient/family:

• If a dose is missed, skip the missed dose and administer the next dose the following day in the morning on wakening
• Report to health care provider if inability to stay awake continues
• **Pregnancy/breastfeeding:** identify if pregnancy is planned or suspected; if using hormonal contraceptives, an alternative method should be used during and for 21 days after last dose; do not use in pregnancy; encourage to enroll in the WAKIX pregnancy registry if patient becomes pregnant; to enroll or obtain information from the registry, call 800-833-7460; present in breast milk

plasma protein fraction (Rx)
Plasmanate
Func. class.: Plasma volume expander

USES: Shock

CONTRAINDICATIONS
Cardiopulmonary bypass procedures, severe anemia, CHF, increased blood volume

DOSAGE AND ROUTES
• **Adult:** IV: Usual minimum effective dosage: 250-500 mL (12.5-25 g of protein); varies widely based on condition
Available forms: Injection 5% (50 mg/mL) in 50-, 250-mL vials

plazomicin (Rx)
(pla-zoe-mye′sin)
Zemdri
Func. class.: Antiinfective—aminoglycoside

ACTION: Bactericidal; inhibits bacterial protein synthesis through irreversible binding to the 30S ribosomal subunit of susceptible bacteria

USES: Complicated urinary tract infection (UTI), including pyelonephritis

CONTRAINDICATIONS

Aminoglycoside hypersensitivity, pregnancy
Precautions: Breastfeeding, colitis, diarrhea, geriatrics, GI disease, hearing impairment, myasthenia gravis, pseudomembranous colitis, renal disease

Black Box Warning: Nephrotoxicity, neuromuscular blockade, ototoxicity, pregnancy

DOSAGE AND ROUTES

• **Adult: IV** 15 mg/kg q24hr for 4-7 days
Available forms: Solution for injection 500 mg/10 mL

SIDE EFFECTS

CNS: Headache
CV: Hypo/hypertension
GI: Nausea, vomiting, diarrhea
GU: Decreased renal function, nephrotoxicity
MISC: Ototoxicity

PHARMACOKINETICS

Plasma protein binding 20%, not metabolized, excreted by kidneys

INTERACTIONS

Black Box Warning: **Increase:** nephrotoxicity—cephalosporins, acyclovir, vancomycin, amphotericin B, cyclosporine, loop diuretics, cidofovir

Black Box Warning: **Increase:** ototoxicity—IV loop diuretics

Black Box Warning: **Increase:** neuromuscular blockade, respiratory depression—anesthetics, nondepolarizing neuromuscular blockers

NURSING CONSIDERATIONS

Assess:
• Weight before treatment; calculation of dosage is usually based on ideal body weight but may be calculated on actual body weight
• Vital signs during infusion; watch for hypotension, change in pulse

• IV site for thrombophlebitis (pain, swelling, redness); change site if needed; apply warm compress to discontinued site

Black Box Warning: **Nephrotoxicity** is greater in those with impaired renal function, the elderly, and in those receiving other nephrotoxic medications; monitor creatinine clearance in all patients before starting therapy and daily; therapeutic drug monitoring (TDM) is recommended for complicated urinary tract infection patients with CCr <90 mL/min to avoid potentially toxic levels; I&O ratio, urinalysis daily for casts, protein; report sudden drop in urinary output

Black Box Warning: **Ototoxicity:** hearing loss, tinnitus, and/or vertigo; assess hearing baseline and throughout treatment; may be irreversible and may not become evident until after completion of therapy; usually in patients with a family history of hearing loss, with renal impairment, or in those receiving higher doses and/or longer durations of therapy than recommended

Black Box Warning: **Neuromuscular blockade** in those with neuromuscular disorders (myasthenia gravis) or in those receiving neuromuscular blocking agents; respiratory paralysis may occur

• **Pregnancy/breastfeeding:** can cause fetal harm when administered to a pregnant woman; do not use in pregnancy; considered compatible with breastfeeding
• For dehydration; provide adequate hydration of 1500-2000 mL/day
Teach patient/family:

Black Box Warning: **Ototoxicity:** to report hearing loss, ringing, roaring in ears; feeling of fullness in the head

• To report headache, dizziness, symptoms of overgrowth of infection, renal impairment, symptoms of nephrotoxicity

P

Side effects: *italics* = common; red = life-threatening

• To report redness, swelling at infusion site
• To drink plenty of fluids each day
• **Pregnancy/breastfeeding:** to notify health care provider if pregnancy is planned or suspected, or if breastfeeding

---

plecanatide (Rx)
(ple-kan′-a-tide)

Trulance
Func. class.: Laxative
Chem. class.: Guanylate cyclase-C agonist

ACTION: Binds to GC-C and acts locally on the luminal surface of the intestinal epithelium. Activation of GC-C results in an increase in both intracellular and extracellular concentrations of cyclic guanosine monophosphate (cGMP); this action results in increased intestinal fluid and accelerated gastrointestinal (GI) transit

USES: Chronic idiopathic constipation, IBS-C

CONTRAINDICATIONS
Hypersensitivity, GI obstruction

Black Box Warning: Child <6 yr

Precautions: Pregnancy, breastfeeding

DOSAGE AND ROUTES
• **Adult: PO** 3 mg daily
Available forms: Tabs 3 mg
Administer:
• Give without regard to food
• Swallow whole; tablets may be crushed and given with applesauce or in water, may be given orally or via NG tube

SIDE EFFECTS
CNS: Dizziness
GI: Diarrhea, flatulence, abdominal distention, abdominal tenderness, nausea
GU: UTI
RESP: Sinusitis, upper respiratory tract infection

PHARMACOKINETICS
Unknown

INTERACTIONS
Drug/Lab Test
Increase: AST/ALT

NURSING CONSIDERATIONS
Assess:
Bowel pattern: frequency, consistency, baseline and periodically; provide adequate hydration if diarrhea occurs
Evaluate:
• **Therapeutic response:** complete bowel movements
Teach patient/family:
• **Pregnancy/breastfeeding:** to notify health care professional if pregnancy is planned or suspected or if breastfeeding
• To notify all health care professionals of all OTC, Rx, herbals or supplements taken
• To take as directed, not to double or skip doses; that if dose is missed, to take next regularly scheduled dose when due

---

plerixafor (Rx)
(pler-ix′a-fore)

Mozobil
Func. class.: Biologic modifier

USES: Mobilization of hematopoietic stem cells for collection and transplantation (in combination with filgrastim) in non-Hodgkin lymphoma and multiple myeloma

CONTRAINDICATIONS
Hypersensitivity

DOSAGE AND ROUTES
Hematopoietic stem cell mobilization (in non-Hodgkin lymphoma and multiple myeloma)
• **Adult: SUBCUT** Give 11 hr before apheresis: ≤83 kg: 20-mg fixed dose or 0.24 mg/kg daily for up to 4 consecutive days; >83 kg: 0.24 mg/kg daily for up to 4 consecutive days; max 40 mg/day
Available forms: Injection 24 mg/1.2-mL single-use vial

---

pomalidomide (Rx)
(pom–a-lid'oh-mide)

Pomalyst

Func. class.: Antineoplastic, biologic response modifier, hormone

Chem. class.: TNF modifier

USES: Multiple myeloma in those who have received ≥2 treatments including lenalidomide and bortezomib and disease has progressed within 60 days of completion of the treatment or in BRAF V600 mutation-positive patients who have disease progression following ipilimumab and a BRAF inhibitor

CONTRAINDICATIONS
Breastfeeding, hypersensitivity

Black Box Warning: Pregnancy, thrombocytopenia

DOSAGE AND ROUTES
• **Adult: PO** 4 mg on days 1-21, repeat in 28-day cycles

Hepatic/renal dose
• **Adult: PO** bilirubin >2 mg/dL and AST/ALT >3 × ULN or CCr >3 mg/dL, do not use

Available forms: Capsule 1, 2, 3, 4 mg

polatuzumab vedotin-piiq (Rx)
(pol'a-tooz'ue-mab ve-doe'tin)

Polivy

Func. class.: Antineoplastic, antibody drug conjugate

USES: Treatment of relapsed/refractory diffuse large B-cell lymphoma (in combination with bendamustine and rituximab), after at least 2 prior therapies

CONTRAINDICATIONS
Hypersensitivity

DOSAGE AND ROUTES
Diffuse large B-cell lymphoma, relapsed or refractory
• **Adult: IV:** 1.8 mg/kg q21days × 6 cycles (in combination with bendamustine and rituximab)

Available forms: Injection 30-, 140-mg single-use vials

polyethylene glycol (PEG) (Rx)
(pol-i-eth'i-leen gly'kol)

GaviLAX, Gialax, GlycoLAX, HealthyLax, MiraLAX

Func. class.: Laxative

USES: Constipation

CONTRAINDICATIONS
Hypersensitivity, known or suspected bowel obstruction

DOSAGE AND ROUTES
Constipation
• **Adult: PO** 17 g (1 heaping tablespoon) dissolved in 120-240 mL (4-8 oz) of beverage, daily as needed; do not use for >1-2 wk

Available forms: Powder for solution

posaconazole (Rx)
(poe'sa-kon'a-zole)

Noxafil, Posanol ✦

Func. class.: Antifungal—systemic

Chem. class.: Triazole derivative

ACTION: Inhibits a portion of cell-wall synthesis; alters cell membranes and inhibits several fungal enzymes

USES: Prevention of aspergillus, candida infection, oropharyngeal candidiasis in immunocompromised patients, chemotherapy-induced neutropenia, mucocutaneous candidiasis

Unlabeled uses: Aspergillosis, cellulitis, coccidioidomycosis, endocarditis, endophthalmitis, esophageal candidiasis, febrile neutropenia, fungal keratitis, fusariosis, histoplasmosis, infectious arthritis, myocarditis, osteomyelitis, pericarditis, sinusitis, tracheobronchitis

CONTRAINDICATIONS

Hypersensitivity to this product or other systemic antifungals or azoles; fungal meningitis, onychomycosis or dermatomycosis in cardiac dysfunction; use with ergots, sirolimus, CYP3A4 substrates

Precautions: Pregnancy, breastfeeding, children, cardiac/hepatic/renal disease

DOSAGE AND ROUTES

Tablets and oral suspension are not interchangeable for dosing

Invasive aspergillosis

• **Adult/adolescent: PO DELAYED RELEASE /IV** 300 mg twice daily for 1 day, then 300 mg once daily × at least 6 to 12 wk

Oropharyngeal candidiasis

• **Adult: PO** (oral suspension) 100 mg bid × 1 day, then 100 mg/day × 13 days

Available forms: Oral susp 200 mg/5 mL; del rel tab 100 mg; sol for inj 300 mg/16.7 mL

Administer:

Delayed-release tab: do not divide, chew, crush; give with food

IV route

Intermittent IV INFUSION route

• **Dilution:** bring to room temperature; transfer 16.7 mL of posaconazole to IV solution that is sufficient for final concentration of 1-2 mg/mL; use immediately

• Store divided solution up to 24 hr refrigerated

• Use 0.22-micron PES or PVDF filter; **give slowly over 90 min through central line;** if central line is unavailable, may give a single dose through a peripheral line over 30 min; do not give multiple doses by this method

PO route

Oral susp: shake well; use calibrated measuring device; take only with full meal or liquid nutritional supplements such as Ensure; rinse measuring device after each use

• Store in tight container in refrigerator; do not freeze

SIDE EFFECTS

CNS: *Headache, dizziness,* insomnia, fever, rigors, weakness, anxiety

CV: Hypo/hypertension, tachycardia, anemia, QT prolongation, torsades de pointes

GI: *Nausea, vomiting, anorexia, diarrhea,* cramps, abdominal pain, flatulence, GI bleeding, hepatotoxicity

GU: Gynecomastia, impotence, decreased libido

INTEG: *Pruritus,* fever, *rash,* toxic epidermal necrolysis

MISC: *Edema, fatigue,* malaise, hypokalemia, tinnitus, rhabdomyolysis, hypokalemia

PHARMACOKINETICS

Well absorbed, enhanced by food, protein binding 98%-99%, peak 3-5 hr, half-life 35 hr, metabolized in liver, excreted in feces (77% unchanged)

INTERACTIONS

• Do not use with lovastatin, atorvastatin

• **Increase:** QT prolongation—class IA/III antidysrhythmics, some phenothiazines, β agonists, local anesthetics, tricyclics, haloperidol, chloroquine, droperidol, pentamidine; CYP3A4 inhibitors (amiodarone, clarithromycin, erythromycin, telithromycin, troleandomycin); arsenic trioxide; CYP3A4 substrates (methadone, pimozide, QUEtiapine, quiNIDine, risperiDONE, ziprasidone)

Increase: tinnitus, hearing loss—quiNIDine

Increase: hepatotoxicity—other hepatotoxic products

Increase: severe hypoglycemia—oral hypoglycemics

Increase: sedation—triazolam, oral midazolam

Increase: levels, toxicity—busPIRone, busulfan, calcium-channel blockers, clarithromycin, cycloSPORINE, diazePAM, digoxin, felodipine, HMG-CoA reductase inhibitors, indinavir, isradipine, midazolam, niCARdipine, NIFEdipine, niMODipine, phenytoin, quiNIDine, ritonavir, saquinavir, sirolimus, tacrolimus, vinca alkaloids, warfarin

Decrease: posaconazole level—cimetidine, phenytoin

Decrease: posaconazole action—antacids, H₂-receptor antagonists, rifamycin, didanosine

Drug/Food
• Food increases absorption

NURSING CONSIDERATIONS
Assess:

• **Infection:** type of, may begin treatment before obtaining results; temperature, WBC, sputum at baseline and periodically, breakthrough infections may occur when used with fosamprenavir

• **Fluid balance:** I&O ratio, electrolytes; correct electrolyte imbalances before starting treatment

• For **allergic reaction:** rash, photosensitivity, urticaria, dermatitis

• **Rhabdomyolysis:** muscle pain, increased CPK; weakness, swelling of affected muscles; if these occur and if confirmed by CPK, product should be discontinued

• **Hepatotoxicity:** nausea, vomiting, jaundice, clay-colored stools, fatigue; hepatic studies (ALT, AST, bilirubin) if patient receiving long-term therapy

• **QT prolongation:** ECG for QT prolongation, ejection fraction; assess for chest pain, palpitations, dyspnea

• **Pregnancy/breastfeeding:** use only if benefits outweigh fetal risk, may cause malformations; use in breastfeeding is not recommended

Evaluate:

• **Therapeutic response:** decreased symptoms of fungal infection, negative C&S for infecting organism

Teach patient/family:

• That long-term therapy may be needed to clear infection (1 wk-6 mo, depending on infection)

• To avoid hazardous activities if dizziness occurs

• To take 2 hr before administration of other products that increase gastric pH (antacids, H₂ blockers, omeprazole, sucralfate, anticholinergics); to notify health care provider of all medications taken (many interactions)

• About the importance of compliance with product regimen; to use alternative method of contraception

• To notify prescriber of GI symptoms, signs of hepatic dysfunction (fatigue, nausea, anorexia, vomiting, dark urine, pale stools)

• To take during or within 20 min of eating

---

potassium acetate (Rx)
potassium bicarbonate (Rx)
Klor-Con EF, K Effervescent ✤, K-vescent ✤
potassium bicarbonate and potassium chloride (Rx)
Neo-K ✤, K-Lyte ✤
potassium bicarbonate and potassium citrate (Rx)

⚠ HIGH ALERT

potassium chloride (Rx)
Klor-Con, K-Tab
Func. class.: Electrolyte, mineral replacement
Chem. class.: Potassium

ACTION: Needed for the adequate transmission of nerve impulses and cardiac contraction, renal function, intracellular ion maintenance

USES: Prevention and treatment of hypokalemia

CONTRAINDICATIONS
Renal disease (severe), severe hemolytic disease, Addison's disease, hyperkalemia, acute dehydration, extensive tissue breakdown

Precautions: Pregnancy, cardiac disease, potassium-sparing diuretic therapy, systemic acidosis

DOSAGE AND ROUTES
Hypokalemia (prevention)
(bicarbonate, chloride)
• **Adult: PO** 20 mEq/day in 1-2 divided doses
• **Child: PO** 1-2 mEq/kg/day in 1-2 divided doses
Hypokalemia (treatment)
• **Adult: PO** initial 40 mmol/day, titrate to 60 mmol/day, max: 100 mmol/day
Hypokalemia, digoxin toxicity
(acetate, chloride)
• **Adult:** serum potassium concentration >2.5 mEq/L: **IV** max 10 mEq/1 hr with 24-hr max dose 200 mEq, initial dose of 20-40 mEq has been recommended; **PO** 40-100 mEq/day in 2-4 divided doses
• **Child: IV** 0.25-0.5 mEq/kg/dose at 0.25-0.5 mEq/kg/hr; **PO** 2-5 mEq/day in divided doses
Available forms: acetate: Solution for injection 4 mEq/mL; **chloride:** oral capsule, extended release 8 mEq, 10 mEq, oral solution 10%, 20%, 40%, extended-release tablet 10 mEq, 20 mEq; **citrate:** tablet, extended release 5, 10, 15 mE
Administer:
PO route
• Do not break, crush, or chew ext rel tabs, caps, or enteric products
• With or after meals; dissolve effervescent tabs, powder in 8 oz cold water or juice; do not give IM, SUBCUT
• Caps with full glass of liquid
IV route
• Through large-bore needle to decrease vein inflammation; check for extravasation; in large vein, avoid scalp vein in child (IV); never give IV bolus

Potassium acetate
Y-site compatibilities: Ciprofloxacin
Potassium chloride
• Must be diluted; concentrated potassium injections fatal
Continuous IV INFUSION route
• Concentration max 100 mcg/L for peripheral line; 200 mEq/L for central line
• Dehydrated patients should receive 1 L of potassium-free hydrating solution,

then infuse 10 mEq/hr; in severe hypokalemia, rate may be 40 mEq/hr with infusion pump and ECG monitoring, draw potassium levels frequently
• Do not ever use IV push or bolus, cardiac arrest may occur
• Monitor I&O, urine should be >0.5 mL kg/hr to prevent hyperkalemia

Y-site compatibilities: Acyclovir, aldesleukin, allopurinol, amifostine, aminophylline, amiodarone, ampicillin, amrinone, atropine, aztreonam, betamethasone, calcium gluconate, cephalothin, cephapirin, chlordiazePOXIDE, chlorproMAZINE, ciprofloxacin, cladribine, cyanocobalamin, dexamethasone, digoxin, diltiaZEM, diphenhydrAMINE, DOBUTamine, DOPamine, droperidol, edrophonium, enalaprilat, EPINEPHrine, esmolol, estrogens, ethacrynate, famotidine, fentaNYL, filgrastim, fludarabine, fluorouracil, furosemide, gallium, granisetron, heparin, hydrALAZINE, IDArubicin, indomethacin, insulin (regular), isoproterenol, kanamycin, labetalol, lidocaine, LORazepam, magnesium sulfate, melphalan, meperidine, methicillin, methoxamine, methylergonovine, midazolam, minocycline, morphine, neostigmine, norepinephrine, ondansetron, oxacillin, oxytocin, PACLitaxel, penicillin G potassium, pentazocine, phytonadione, piperacillin/tazobactam, prednisoLONE, procainamide, prochlorperazine, propofol, propranolol, pyridostigmine, remifentanil, sargramostim, scopolamine, sodium bicarbonate, succinylcholine, tacrolimus, teniposide, theophylline, thiotepa, trimethaphan, trimethobenzamide, vinorelbine, warfarin, zidovudine

SIDE EFFECTS
CNS: Confusion
CV: Bradycardia, cardiac depression, dysrhythmias, arrest; peaking T waves, lowered R, depressed RST, prolonged P-R interval, widened QRS complex
GI: *Nausea, vomiting, cramps,* pain, *diarrhea,* ulceration of small bowel
GU: Oliguria
INTEG: Cold extremities, rash

PHARMACOKINETICS
PO: Excreted by kidneys and in feces; onset of action ≈30 min
IV: Immediate onset of action

INTERACTIONS
Increase: hyperkalemia—potassium phosphate IV; products containing calcium or magnesium; potassium-sparing diuretic or other potassium products; ACE inhibitors

NURSING CONSIDERATIONS
Assess:
• **Hyperkalemia:** indicates toxicity; fatigue, muscle weakness, confusion, dyspnea, palpitation; ECG for peaking T waves, lowered R, depressed RST, prolonged P-R interval, widening QRS complex, hyperkalemia; product should be reduced or discontinued, administer sodium bicarbonate (metabolic acidosis); potassium level during treatment (3.5-5 mg/dL is normal level)
• Determine hydration status, I&O ratio; watch for decreased urinary output; notify prescriber immediately
• **Cardiac status:** rate, rhythm, CVP, PWP, PAWP if being monitored directly, if infused rate is higher, use cardiac monitoring
• IV site for irritation; decrease rate if irritation occurs
• **Pregnancy/breastfeeding:** use only if clearly needed; cautious use in breastfeeding
Evaluate:
• **Therapeutic response:** absence of fatigue, muscle weakness; decreased thirst, urinary output; cardiac changes
Teach patient/family:
• To add potassium-rich foods to diet: bananas, orange juice, avocados, whole grains, broccoli, carrots, prunes, cocoa after product is discontinued
• To avoid OTC products: antacids, salt substitutes, analgesics, vitamin preparations unless specifically directed by prescriber; to avoid licorice in large amounts because it may cause hypokalemia, sodium retention
• To report hyperkalemia symptoms (lethargy, confusion, diarrhea, nausea, vomiting, fainting, decreased output) or continued hypokalemia symptoms (fatigue, weakness, polyuria, polydipsia, cardiac changes)
• To dissolve powder or tablet completely in ≥120 mL water or juice
• About the importance of regular follow-up visits
• That potassium levels will need to be monitored periodically

potassium iodide (Rx)
SSKI, Lugol's ✤
Func. class.: Thyroid hormone antagonist, antidote
Chem. class.: Iodine product

ACTION: Inhibits secretion of thyroid hormone, fosters colloid accumulation in thyroid follicles, decreases vascularity of gland

USES: Preparation for thyroidectomy, thyrotoxic crisis, neonatal thyrotoxicosis, radiation protectant, thyroid storm
Unlabeled uses: Sporotrichosis, thyroid involution induction, thyrotoxicosis, Grave's disease

CONTRAINDICATIONS
Pregnancy, pulmonary edema, pulmonary TB, bronchitis, hypersensitivity to iodine
Precautions: Breastfeeding, children

DOSAGE AND ROUTES
Hyperthyroidism/thyrotoxicosis
• **Adult/child: PO** (SSKI) 250 mg tid × 10-14 days preoperatively
Preparation for thyroidectomy
• **Adult/child: PO** 3-5 drops strong iodine sol tid or 1-5 drops SSKI in water tid after meals for 10 days before surgery
Radiation exposure (radioactive iodine)
• **Adult: PO** 130 mg/day (distribution by government/public health officials or OTC purchase)
• **Child ≥3 yr: PO** 65 mg daily
• **Child/infant >1 mo-3 yr: PO** 32 mg/day

Side effects: *italics* = common; red = life-threatening

• **Neonate: PO** 16 mg/day

Available forms: Oral sol (Lugol's solution) iodine 5%/potassium iodide 10%; oral sol (SSKI) 1 g/mL 65 mg/mL

Administer:
• Products are not interchangeable
• Strong iodine solution after diluting with water or juice to improve taste
• Through straw to prevent tooth discoloration
• With meals to decrease GI upset
• At same time each day to maintain product level
• At lowest dose that relieves symptoms; discontinue before RAIU

SIDE EFFECTS

CNS: Headache, confusion, paresthesias

CV: Tachycardia, cardiac arrest, dysrrthmias

EENT: Metallic taste, stomatitis, salivation, periorbital edema, sore teeth and gums, cold symptoms

ENDO: Hypothyroidism, hyperthyroid adenoma, hyperkalemia

GI: *Nausea, diarrhea, vomiting,* small-bowel lesions, upper gastric pain, metallic taste

INTEG: Rash, urticaria, angioneurotic edema, acne, mucosal hemorrhage, fever

MS: Myalgia, arthralgia, weakness

PHARMACOKINETICS

PO: Onset 24-48 hr, peak 10-15 days after continuous therapy, uptake by thyroid gland or excreted in urine, crosses placenta

INTERACTIONS

Increase: hypothyroidism—lithium, other antithyroid agents

Increase: hyperkalemia—angiotensin II receptor antagonist, ACE inhibitors, potassium salts, potassium-sparing diuretics

NURSING CONSIDERATIONS

Assess:
• Pulse, B/P, temperature; serum potassium
• I&O ratio; check for edema: puffy hands, feet, periorbit; indicate hypothyroidism

• Weight daily; same clothing, scale, time of day
• T_3, T_4, which is increased; serum TSH, which is decreased; free thyroxine index, which is increased if dosage is too low; discontinue product 3-4 wk before RAIU
• **Overdose:** peripheral edema, heat intolerance, diaphoresis, palpitations, dysrhythmias, severe tachycardia, fever, delirium, CNS irritability
• **Hypersensitivity:** rash; enlarged cervical lymph nodes may indicate product should be discontinued
• **Hypoprothrombinemia:** bleeding, petechiae, ecchymosis
• Clinical response: after 3 wk should include increased weight, pulse; decreased T_4
• Fluids to 3-4 L/day unless contraindicated
• **Pregnancy/breastfeeding:** do not use in pregnancy, breastfeeding

Evaluate:
• **Therapeutic response:** weight gain; decreased pulse, T_4, size of thyroid gland

Teach patient/family:
• To abstain from breastfeeding after delivery
• To keep graph of weight, pulse, mood
• To avoid OTC products that contain iodine
• That seafood, other iodine products may be restricted
• Not to discontinue product abruptly; that thyroid crisis may occur as part of stress response
• That response may take several mo if thyroid is large
• To discontinue product, notify prescriber of fever, rash, metallic taste, swelling of throat; burning of mouth, throat; sore gums, teeth; severe GI distress, enlargement of thyroid, cold symptoms

---

prabotulinumtoxin A (Rx)

Jeuveau

Dermatologic agent

USES:
Facial wrinkles or vertical lines between the eyebrows

DOSAGE AND ROUTE

Black Box Warning: Distant spread of toxin effects

Moderate-severe glabellar lines (facial wrinkles or vertical lines between the eyebrows):
• **Adults:** IM 20 units (0.5 mL) given in 5 equal aliquots of 4 units (0.1 mL) each: 2 injections in each corrugator muscle (1 inferomedial and 1 superior middle) and 1 injection in the midline of the procerus muscle. If needed, repeat doses may be given ≥3 mo
Available forms: Injection 100 units/single-dose vial

pralidoxime (Rx)
(pra-li-doks′eem)
Protopam Chloride
Func. class.: Antidote

USES:
Treatment of muscle weakness and/or respiratory depression secondary to poisoning due to organophosphate anticholinesterase pesticides and terrorism nerve agents; control of overdose of anticholinesterase medications used to treat myasthenia gravis (ambenonium, neostigmine, pyridostigmine)

CONTRAINDICATIONS
Hypersensitivity

DOSAGE AND ROUTES
Organophosphate poisoning (pesticides and nerve agents)
• **Adult/adolescents ≥17 yr: IV** 1-2 g as a 15- to 30-min infusion in 100 mL NS after reconstitution with 1000 mg/20 mL sterile water
• **Neonate/infant/child ≤16 yr: IV** loading dose 20-50 mg/kg (max 2 g) infused

over 15-30 min, then 10-20 mg/kg/hr continuous IV infusion
Anticholinesterase overdose (neostigmine, pyridostigmine)
• **Adult: IV** 1-2 g mg; then increments of 250 mg q5min as needed
Available forms: Powder for solution for injection 1 g

pralsetinib (Rx)
(pral′se′ti′nib)
Gavreto
Func. class.: Antineoplastic
Chem class.: RET kinase inhibitor

ACTION: Inhibits wild-type RET, oncogenic RET fusions, and RET mutations; antitumor activity occurs in cells harboring oncogenic RET fusions or mutations

USES: Treatment of non-small cell lung cancer (NSCLC), thyroid cancer

CONTRAINDICATIONS
Hypersensitivity
Precautions:
Breastfeeding, children, chronic lung disease, contraception requirements, growth inhibition, hepatic disease, hypertension, impaired wound healing, infertility, interstitial lung disease, male-mediated teratogenicity, pneumonitis, pregnancy, renal impairment, surgery, tumor lysis syndrome

DOSAGE AND ROUTES
NSCLC/thyroid cancer
• **Adult: PO** 400 mg daily until disease progression/unacceptable toxicity
Available forms: Capsule 100 mg
Administer:
• On empty stomach ≥1 hr before or ≥2 hr after food
• Store at room temperature

SIDE EFFECTS
CNS: Fatigue
GI: Constipation, diarrhea, xerostomia, increased LFTs, hepatotoxicity
CV: Edema, hypertension

META: Hypocalcaemia, hyponatremia, hyper-hypophosphatemia
HEMA: Decreased HB, neutropenia, lymphocytopenia, thrombocytopenia, hemorrhage
MS: MS pain
GU: Increased serum creatinine, UTI
RESP: Cough, pneumonia, pneumonitis
MISC: Fever, sepsis

PHARMACOKINETICS
Onset unknown, peak 2-4 hr, duration unknown, half-life 22 hr, protein binding 97%

INTERACTIONS
Decrease: Pralsetinib effect—CYP3A4 inducers, depending if moderate or strong, monitor or alter dose
Increase: Pralsetinib effect—Strong CYP3A4 Inhibitors, avoid using together

NURSING CONSIDERATIONS
Assess:
• **Lung cancer:** Obtain RET gene fusion status, hepatitis B surface antigen (HBsAg), hepatitis B core antibody (anti-HBc), total Ig or IgG before starting treatment, treatment may start before results
• **Bone marrow suppression:** Monitor CBC with differential, platelets; anemia, lymphocytopenia, neutropenia, thrombocytopenia may occur
• **Bleeding/hemorrhage:** Monitor for bleeding/hemorrhage, permanently discontinue if severe
• **Hepatotoxicity:** Monitor LFTs baseline, q2wk × 3 months, then monthly; if elevated dosage modification or discontinuation may be needed, evaluate RET gene status
• **Hypertension:** Monitor B/P baseline, after 1 wk and monthly thereafter; do not use in uncontrolled hypertension
• **Interstitial lung disease/pulmonary toxicity:** Monitor for dyspnea, cough, fever, fatigue; withhold pralsetinib, evaluate for interstitial lung disease
• **Poor wound healing:** Withhold ≥5 days before elective surgery; do not use ≥2 wk after major surgery and until after adequate wound healing
• Identify if propylene glycol is present in product used: monitor for toxicity if large amounts are present in the product (lactic acidosis, respiratory changes, seizures)
• **Pregnancy/breastfeeding:** Obtain pregnancy testing before use in females of reproductive potential, do not use in pregnancy or breastfeeding; nonhormonal contraceptive should be used during and for ≥2 wk after last dose; males should use contraception during and for ≥1 wk after last dose in those with partners of reproductive potential
Evaluate:
• Therapeutic response: decreasing tumor growth in lung cancer
Teach patient/family:
• To report immediately poor wound healing after surgery, increased trouble breathing, bloody sputum, other bleeding, cough, fever
• Take 1 hr before or 2 hr after food; do not crush, chew, open capsule; take whole
• Liver dysfunction: To report yellow skin/sclera, clay-colored stools, dark urine
• If a dose is missed, take on the same day; resume the regular dosing next day; do not take another dose if vomiting occurs
• Identify if pregnancy is planned or suspected, not to breastfeed, discuss needed contraception

---

pramipexole (Rx)
(pra-mi-pex′ol)
Mirapex, Mirapex ER
Func. class.: Antiparkinson agent
Chem. class.: DOPamine-receptor agonist, non-ergot

Do not confuse:
Mirapex/Miralax

ACTION: Selective agonist for D_2 receptors (presynaptic/postsynaptic sites); binding at D_3 receptor contributes to antiparkinson effects

USES: Idiopathic Parkinson's disease, restless legs syndrome

CONTRAINDICATIONS
Hypersensitivity

Precautions: Pregnancy, cardiac/renal disease, MI with dysrhythmias, affective disorders, psychosis, preexisting dyskinesias, history of falling asleep during daily activities, rapid dose reduction

DOSAGE AND ROUTES
Parkinson's disease
• **Adult: PO** 0.125 mg tid; increase gradually by 0.125 mg/dose at 5- to 7-day intervals until total daily dose of 4.5 mg/day reached; **ER** 0.375 mg daily initially, then up to 0.75 mg/day; may increase by 0.75 mg/day no more than q5-7days as needed, max 4.5 mg/day

Restless legs syndrome
• **Adult: PO** 0.125 mg 2-3 hr before bedtime, increase gradually, max 0.5 mg/day

Renal dose
• **Adult: PO** CCr 35-59 mL/min, 0.125 mg bid, may increase q5-7days to 1.5 mg bid if required; CCr 15-34 mL/min, 0.125 mg/day, increase q5-7days to 1.5 mg/day

Available forms: Tabs 0.125, 0.25, 0.5, 0.75, 1, 1.5 mg; ER tab 0.375, 0.75, 1.5, 2.25, 3.0, 3.75, 4.5 mg

Administer:
• Adjust dosage to patient response, titrate slowly, taper when discontinuing
• With meals to minimize GI symptoms
• Do not crush, chew, or break ext rel product

SIDE EFFECTS
CNS: *Agitation, insomnia,* psychosis, hallucinations, depression, dizziness, headache, confusion, amnesia, dream disorder, asthenia, dyskinesia, hypersomnolence, sudden sleep onset, impulse control disorders

CV: *Orthostatic hypotension,* edema, syncope, tachycardia, increased B/P, heart rate, heart failure

EENT: Blurred vision, retinal/vision deterioration

ENDO: Antidiuretic hormone secretion (SIADH)

GI: *Nausea, anorexia,* constipation, dysphagia, dry mouth

GU: Impotence, urinary frequency

HEMA: Hemolytic anemia, leukopenia, agranulocytosis

INTEG: Pruritus

PHARMACOKINETICS
Minimally metabolized, peak 2 hr, half-life 8 hr, 8.5-12 hr in geriatric patients

INTERACTIONS
Increase: pramipexole levels—levodopa, cimetidine, raNITIdine, diltiaZEM, triamterene, verapamil, quiNIDine

Decrease: pramipexole levels—DOPamine antagonists, phenothiazines, metoclopramide, butyrophenones

NURSING CONSIDERATIONS
Assess:
• **Parkinson's disease:** involuntary movements: bradykinesia, tremors, staggering gait, muscle rigidity, drooling
• B/P, ECG, respiration during initial treatment; hypo/hypertension should be reported
• **Mental status:** affect, mood, behavioral changes, depression; complete suicide assessment, worsening of symptoms of restless legs syndrome, impulse control disorders
• **Somnolence:** may fall asleep during activities without warning; may need to discontinue medication
• Assistance with ambulation during beginning therapy
• Testing for diabetes mellitus, acromegaly if receiving long-term therapy
• **Pregnancy/breastfeeding:** use only if benefits outweigh fetal risk, may cause fetal harm; do not breastfeed

Evaluate:
• **Therapeutic response:** movement disorder improves

Teach patient/family:
• That therapeutic effects may take several weeks to a few months
• To change positions slowly to prevent orthostatic hypotension

Side effects: *italics* = common; red = life-threatening

• To use product exactly as prescribed; if product is discontinued abruptly, parkinsonian crisis may occur; to avoid alcohol, OTC sleeping products

• To notify prescriber if pregnancy is planned or suspected

• To notify prescriber of impulse control disorders: shopping

---

⚠ HIGH ALERT

pramlintide (Rx)
(pram'lin-tide)

SymlinPen

Func. class.: Antidiabetic

Chem. class.: Synthetic human amylin analog

ACTION: Modulates and slows stomach emptying, prevents postprandial rise in plasma glucagon, decreases appetite, leads to decreased caloric intake and weight loss

USES: As an adjunct prandial to insulin therapy for uncontrolled type 1 or type 2 diabetes

CONTRAINDICATIONS
Hypersensitivity to this product or cresol; gastroparesis

Black Box Warning: Hypoglycemia unawareness

Precautions: Pregnancy, breastfeeding, osteoporosis, thyroid disease, trauma, vomiting, renal failure, fever, diarrhea

DOSAGE AND ROUTES
Type 1 diabetes

• **Adult: SUBCUT** 15 mcg before each meal (≥30 g carbohydrate), titrate up in 15-mcg increments to target dose of 60 mcg/dose; each dose titration should occur after no nausea for 3 days

Type 2 diabetes

• **Adult: SUBCUT** 60 mcg before each meal (≥30 g carbohydrate), titrate up to 120 mcg; **SUBCUT** with each meal after no nausea for 3-7 days

Available forms: PEN 60, 120 (1000 mcg/mL solution for injection)

Administer:

• Store at room temperature for ≤30 days; keep away from heat and sunlight; refrigerate all other supply

• Premeal insulin should be decreased by 50% when starting and adjusted to therapeutic dose to prevent hypoglycemia

SUBCUT route

• Rotate injection sites, allow solution to warm to room temperature before use

• Take immediately before mealtime or if 30 g of carbohydrates will be consumed

• Do not use if a meal is skipped

• Do not use if discolored; do not give in arm; absorption is variable

SIDE EFFECTS
CNS: *Headache,* fatigue, dizziness, confusion

EENT: Blurred vision

GI: *Nausea, vomiting, anorexia,* abdominal pain

INTEG: Inj-site reactions, diaphoresis

META: Hypoglycemia

MS: Arthralgia

RESP: *Cough,* pharyngitis

SYST: *Systemic allergy*

PHARMACOKINETICS
Bioavailability 30%-40%, not extensively bound to blood cells or albumin, 40% bound in plasma, half-life 48 min, metabolized by kidneys, peak 20 min, duration 3 hr

INTERACTIONS
• Do not use with erythromycin, metoclopramide

Increase: effect of acetaminophen

Increase: pramlintide action—antimuscarinics, α-glucosidase inhibitors, diphenoxylate, loperamide, octreotide, opiate agonist, tricyclics

Increase: hypoglycemia—ACE inhibitors, disopyramide, anabolic steroids, androgens, fibric acid derivatives, alcohol, corticosteroids, insulin

Increase: hyperglycemia—phenothiazines

Decrease: hypoglycemia—niacin, dextrothyroxine, thiazide diuretics,

---

triamterene, estrogens, progestins, oral contraceptives, MAOIs

NURSING CONSIDERATIONS
Assess:

Black Box Warning: Fasting blood glucose, 2 hr postprandial (80-150 mg/dL, normal fasting level; 70-130 mg/dL, normal 2 hr level); A1c may also be drawn to identify treatment effectiveness; also monitor weight, appetite

• **Hypoglycemic reaction:** sweating; weakness; dizziness; chills; confusion; headache; nausea; rapid, weak pulse; fatigue; tachycardia; memory lapses; slurred speech; staggering gait; anxiety; tremors; hunger
• **Hyperglycemia:** acetone breath; polyuria; fatigue; polydipsia; flushed, dry skin; lethargy
• **Pregnancy/breastfeeding:** use only if benefits outweigh fetal risk, usually insulin is used in pregnancy; avoid breastfeeding
Evaluate:
• **Therapeutic response:** decrease in polyuria, polydipsia, polyphagia; clear sensorium; absence of dizziness; stable gait; improving blood glucose, A1c
Teach patient/family:
• That product does not cure diabetes but rather controls symptoms
• To carry emergency ID as diabetic
• To recognize hypoglycemia reaction: headache, fatigue, weakness, fast pulse
• About the dosage, route, mixing instructions, diet restrictions, disease process

Black Box Warning: To carry a glucose source (candy or lump sugar, glucose tabs) to treat hypoglycemia

• About the symptoms of ketoacidosis: nausea; thirst; polyuria; dry mouth; decreased B/P; dry, flushed skin; acetone breath; drowsiness; Kussmaul respirations
• That a plan is necessary for diet, exercise; that all food on diet should be eaten; that exercise routine should not vary
• About blood glucose testing; how to determine glucose level

• To avoid OTC products, alcohol unless directed by prescriber
• Not to operate machinery or drive until effect is known
• About how to use pen

TREATMENT OF OVERDOSE:
Glucose 25 g IV or 50 mL dextrose 50% sol or 1 mg glucagon SUBCUT

---

pramoxine topical
See Appendix B

---

prasterone (Rx)
(pras′ter-one)
Intrarosa
Func. class.: Hormone, steroid, synthetic

USES: Treatment of moderate to severe dyspareunia

CONTRAINDICATIONS
Undiagnosed abnormal genital bleeding

DOSAGE AND ROUTES
Dyspareunia
Adult females: Intravaginal: 6.5 mg daily at bedtime
Available forms: Vaginal insert 6.5 mg

⚠ HIGH ALERT

prasugrel (Rx)
(pra′soo-grel)
Effient
Func. class.: Platelet aggregation inhibitor
Chem. class.: ADP receptor antagonist

ACTION: Inhibits ADP-induced platelet aggregation

USES: Reducing the risk of stroke, MI, vascular death, peripheral arterial disease in high-risk patients

---

Side effects: *italics* = common; red = life-threatening

CONTRAINDICATIONS

Hypersensitivity, stroke, TIA, active bleeding, hepatic disease (Child-Pugh C)

> **Black Box Warning:** Active bleeding

Precautions: Pregnancy, breastfeeding, children, geriatric patients, hepatic disease, increased bleeding risk, neutropenia, agranulocytosis, renal disease, surgery, trauma, thrombotic thrombocytopenic purpura, ✱☜ Asian patients, weight <60 kg, CABG, abrupt discontinuation

DOSAGE AND ROUTES

• **Adult/geriatric <75 yr and ≥60 kg: PO** 60 mg, then 10 mg daily with aspirin (75-325 mg/day)
• **Adult/geriatric <75 yr and <60 kg: PO** 60 mg, then 5 mg daily
• **Geriatric ≥75 yr:** not recommended
Available forms: Tabs 5, 10 mg
Administer:
• With food to decrease gastric symptoms
• Do not break tablets, tablet may be crushed and mixed in food, fluids
• Do not discontinue therapy abruptly

SIDE EFFECTS

CNS: Headache, dizziness, intracranial hemorrhage
CV: Edema, atrial fibrillation, bradycardia, chest pain, hypo/hypertension, angina
GI: Nausea, vomiting, diarrhea
HEMA: Epistaxis, leukopenia, thrombocytopenia, neutropenia, anaphylaxis, angioedema, anemia
INTEG: Rash, hypercholesterolemia
MISC: Fatigue, intracranial hemorrhage, secondary malignancy, angioedema anaphylaxis
MS: Back pain

PHARMACOKINETICS

Rapidly absorbed; peak 30 min; metabolized by liver (CYP3A4; CYP2B6); excreted in urine, feces; half-life 7 hr

INTERACTIONS

Increase: bleeding risk—anticoagulants, aspirin, NSAIDs, abciximab, eptifibatide, tirofiban, thrombolytics, ticlopidine, SSRIs, treprostinil, rifAMPin

NURSING CONSIDERATIONS
Assess:
• **Thrombotic/thrombocytic purpura:** fever, thrombocytopenia, neurolytic anemia
• **Hepatic studies:** AST, ALT, bilirubin, creatinine with long-term therapy
• **Blood studies:** CBC, differential, Hct, HB, PT, cholesterol with long-term therapy

> **Black Box Warning: Bleeding:** may be fatal, decreased B/P in those who have had CABG may be the first indication; bleeding should be controlled while continuing product; may use transfusion; do not use within 1 wk of CABG; may use lower doses in those <60 kg

• **Pregnancy/breastfeeding:** use only if benefits outweigh fetal risk
• **Beers:** avoid use in those age ≥75 yr; increased bleeding risk
Evaluate:
• **Therapeutic response:** absence of stroke, MI
Teach patient/family:
• That blood work will be necessary during treatment

> **Black Box Warning:** To report any unusual bruising, bleeding to prescriber; that it may take longer to stop bleeding

• To take with food or just after eating to minimize GI discomfort
• To report diarrhea, skin rashes, subcutaneous bleeding, chills, fever, sore throat
• To tell all health care providers that prasugrel is being used; that product may be held before surgery

---

pravastatin (Rx)
(pra´va-sta-tin)
Func. class.: Antilipemic
Chem. class.: HMG-CoA reductase enzyme

ACTION: Inhibits HMG-CoA reductase enzyme, which reduces cholesterol synthesis

USES: As an adjunct for primary hypercholesterolemia (types IIa, IIb, III, IV), to reduce the risk for recurrent MI, atherosclerosis, primary/secondary CV events, stroke, TIAs

CONTRAINDICATIONS

Pregnancy, breastfeeding, hypersensitivity, active hepatic disease

Precautions: Past hepatic disease, alcoholism, severe acute infections, trauma, severe metabolic disorders, electrolyte imbalances, renal disease

DOSAGE AND ROUTES

• **Adult: PO** 40 mg/day at bedtime (range 10-80 mg/day); start at 10 mg/day if patient also taking immunosuppressants or has significant renal/hepatic disease
• **Adolescent 14-18 yr: PO** 40 mg/day
• **Child 8-13 yr: PO** 20 mg/day
Renal dose
• **Adult: PO** 10-20 mg daily at bedtime, increase at 4-wk intervals
Available forms: Tabs 10, 20, 40, 80 mg
Administer:
• Without regard to meals, at bedtime
• Give 4 hr after bile acid sequestrants
• Store in cool environment in tight container protected from light

SIDE EFFECTS

CNS: Headache, dizziness, fatigue, confusion
CV: Chest pain
EENT: Lens opacities
GI: Nausea, constipation, diarrhea, flatus, abdominal pain, heartburn, hepatic dysfunction, pancreatitis, hepatitis
GU: Renal failure (myoglobinuria)
INTEG: Rash, pruritus
MS: Muscle cramps, myalgia, myositis, rhabdomyolysis
RESP: *Common cold, rhinitis, cough, URI*

PHARMACOKINETICS

Peak 1-1 ½ hr; metabolized by liver; protein binding 50%; excreted in urine 20%, feces 70%, breast milk; crosses placenta; half-life 1.25-2.25 hr

INTERACTIONS

Increase: myopathy, rhabdomyolysis risk—erythromycin, niacin, cycloSPORINE, gemfibrozil, clofibrate, clarithromycin, itraconazole, protease inhibitors
Decrease: bioavailability of pravastatin—bile acid sequestrants
Drug/Herb
Increase: adverse reactions—red yeast rice
Increase: hepatotoxicity—eucalyptus
Decrease: effect—St. John's wort
Drug/Lab Test
Increase: CK, LFTs
Altered: thyroid function tests

NURSING CONSIDERATIONS
Assess:
• **Fasting lipid profile:** LDL, HDL, triglycerides, cholesterol at baseline, q12wk, then q6mo when stable; obtain diet history
• **Hepatic studies:** baseline, then when clinically indicated; LFTs may increase
• **Renal studies:** BUN, creatinine, I&O in those with compromised renal system
• **Rhabdomyolysis:** muscle tenderness, pain; obtain CPK if clinically indicated; therapy should be discontinued
• **Pregnancy/breastfeeding:** do not use in pregnancy, breastfeeding
Evaluate:
• **Therapeutic response:** decrease in LDL total cholesterol, triglycerides; increase in HDL
Teach patient/family:
• That blood work will be necessary during treatment
• To report blurred vision, severe GI symptoms, dizziness, headache, muscle pain, weakness, fever
• That regimen will continue: low-cholesterol diet, exercise program; that if taking a product like cholestyramine, to take this product at least 1 hr prior to or 4 hr after the bile acid resin
• To report suspected, planned pregnancy; not to use product during pregnancy; not to breastfeed

P

• **Hepatic disease:** to notify prescriber of lack of appetite, yellow sclera/skin, dark urine, abdominal pain, weakness

prazosin (Rx)

(pray´zoe-sin)

Minipress

Func. class.: Antihypertensive
Chem. class.: α₁-Adrenergic blocker, peripheral

Do not confuse:
prazosin/predniSONE

ACTION: Blocks α-mediated vasoconstriction of adrenergic receptors, thereby inducing peripheral vasodilation

USES: Hypertension, benign prostatic hypertrophy to decrease urine outflow obstruction
Unlabeled uses: Hypertensive urgency, Raynaud's phenomenon, posttraumatic stress disorder (PTSD), BPH

CONTRAINDICATIONS
Hypersensitivity to this product or other quinazoline products, history of tamsulosin-induced angioedema
Precautions: Pregnancy, breastfeeding, children, geriatric patients, prostate cancer, ocular surgery, orthostatic hypotension, angina, priapism, syncope

DOSAGE AND ROUTES
Hypertension
• **Adult: PO** 1 mg bid or tid increasing to 20 mg/day in divided doses, if required; usual range 2-20 mg/day, max 40 mg/day
• **Child (unlabeled): PO** 5 mcg/kg q6hr; may increase slowly to 25 mcg/kg q6hr; max 400 mcg/kg/day or 15 mg/day
Benign prostatic hyperplasia (unlabeled)
• **Adult: PO** 2 mg bid, maintenance range is 1-9 mg/day
Posttraumatic stress disorder (unlabeled)
• **Adult: PO** 1 mg at bedtime, then titrated to max 15 mg/day
Available forms: Caps 1, 2, 5 mg

Administer:
• 1st dose at bedtime to avoid fainting
• Without regard to meals
• Store at room temperature

SIDE EFFECTS
CNS: *Dizziness, headache, drowsiness,* anxiety, depression, vertigo, *weakness,* fatigue, syncope
CV: *Palpitations, orthostatic hypotension,* tachycardia, edema, rebound hypertension
EENT: Blurred vision, epistaxis, tinnitus, dry mouth, red sclera
GI: *Nausea,* vomiting, diarrhea, constipation, abdominal pain, pancreatitis
GU: Urinary frequency, incontinence, impotence, priapism; water, sodium retention

PHARMACOKINETICS
Onset 2 hr, peak 2-4 hr, duration 6-12 hr, half-life 2-4 hr; metabolized in liver, excreted via bile, feces (>90%), urine (<10%); protein binding 97%

INTERACTIONS
Increase: hypotensive effects—β-blockers, nitroglycerin, alcohol, phosphodiesterase inhibitors (vardenafil, tadalafil, sildenafil); diuretics, other antihypertensives, MAOIs
Decrease: antihypertensive effect—NSAIDs
Increase: antihypertensive effect—hawthorn
Drug/Lab Test
Increase: urinary norepinephrine, VMA, BUN, uric acid, LFTs
Positive: ANA titer

NURSING CONSIDERATIONS
Assess:
• **Hypertension/HF:** B/P (sitting, standing) during initial treatment, periodically thereafter; pulse, jugular venous distention, orthostatic hypotension usually occurs on first dose
• **Labs:** BUN, uric acid if patient receiving long-term therapy
• Weight daily, I&O; edema in feet, legs daily
• **Benign prostatic hypertrophy (unlabeled):** urinary patterns, frequency,

stream, dribbling; flow before, during, and after therapy
• **Beers:** avoid use as an antihypertensive in older adults; high risk of orthostatic hypotension
• **Pregnancy/breastfeeding:** use only if benefits outweigh fetal risk; cautious use in breastfeeding, excreted in breast milk
Evaluate:
• **Therapeutic response:** decreased B/P
Teach patient/family:
• That fainting occasionally occurs after 1st dose; to take 1st dose at bedtime; not to drive or operate machinery for 4 hr after 1st dose; that full effect may take 4-6 wk
• To change positions slowly to prevent orthostatic hypotension
• To avoid OTC medications, alcohol unless approved by prescriber; not to crush, chew caps
• Not to discontinue abruptly

TREATMENT OF OVERDOSE:
Administer volume expanders or vasopressors, discontinue product, place patient in supine position

---

prednisoLONE (Rx)
(pred-niss'oh-lone)
Millipred, Orapred, Orapred ODT, Pediapred, Veripred
Func. class.: Corticosteroid, synthetic
Chem. class.: Glucocorticoid, immediate acting

Do not confuse:
prednisoLONE/predniSONE

ACTION: Decreases inflammation by the suppression of migration of polymorphonuclear leukocytes, fibroblasts; reversal to increase capillary permeability and lysosomal stabilization

USES: Severe inflammation, immunosuppression, neoplasms, asthma

CONTRAINDICATIONS
Hypersensitivity, fungal infections, viral infection, varicella

Precautions: Pregnancy, breastfeeding, children, diabetes mellitus, glaucoma, osteoporosis, seizure disorders, ulcerative colitis, HF, myasthenia gravis, abrupt discontinuation, children, acute MI, GI ulcers, hypertension, hepatitis, psychosis, thromboembolism, peptic ulcer disease, renal disease, Cushing syndrome

DOSAGE AND ROUTES
Most conditions
• **Adult: PO** 5-60 mg per day as a single dose or divided doses
• **Infant/child/adolescent: PO** 0.14-2 mg/kg or 4-60 mg/m^2 per day in 3-4 divided doses
Multiple sclerosis
• **Adult: PO** 200 mg/day × 7 day, then 80 mg every other day × 1 mo
Antiinflammatory
• **Adult: PO** 5-60 mg/day as a single dose or in divided doses
• **Infant/child/adolescent: PO** 0.14-2 mg/kg or 4-60 mg/m^2 per day in 3-4 divided doses
Acute asthma exacerbation
• **Adult/adolescent: PO** 40-60 mg per day as a single dose or in 2 divided doses for 3-10 days
• **Child 5-12 yr: PO** 1-2 mg/kg (up to 60 mg) per day in 2 divided doses for 3-10 days
• **Infant/child ≤4 yr: PO** 1-2 mg/kg (up to 30 mg) per day in 2 divided doses for 3-10 days
Available forms: Tabs 5 mg; oral disintegrating tab 10, 15, 30 mg; oral sol 5 mg/5 mL, 10 mg/5 mL, 15 mg/5 mL, 25 mg/5 mL; oral suspension 15 mg/mL
Administer:
• **Oral sol:** use calibrated measuring device
• **Orally disintegrating tabs:** place on tongue; allow to dissolve, swallow or swallow whole; do not cut, split

SIDE EFFECTS
CNS: *Depression,* headache, mood changes
CV: *Hypertension,* circulatory collapse, thrombophlebitis, embolism, tachycardia

---

Side effects: *italics* = common; red = life-threatening

EENT: Fungal infections, increased intra-ocular pressure, blurred vision

GI: *Diarrhea, nausea, abdominal distention,* GI hemorrhage, increased appetite, pancreatitis

INTEG: Acne, poor wound healing, ecchymosis, petechiae, sweating

MS: Fractures, osteoporosis, weakness, arthralgia, myopathy, tendon rupture

MISC: Hyperglycemia

PHARMACOKINETICS
PO: Peak 1-2 hr, duration 2 days

INTERACTIONS
Increase: tendon rupture—quinolones

Increase: side effects—alcohol, salicylates, indomethacin, amphotericin B, digitalis, cycloSPORINE, diuretics

Increase: prednisoLONE action—salicylates, estrogens, indomethacin, oral contraceptives, ketoconazole, macrolide antibiotics

Increase: prednisoLONE effect—CYP3A4 inhibitors

Increase: toxicity—azole antifungals, cycloSPORINE, NSAIDs

Decrease: prednisoLONE action—cholestyramine, colestipol, barbiturates, rifAMPin, ePHEDrine, phenytoin, theophylline

Decrease: effects of anticoagulants, anticonvulsants, antidiabetics, ambenonium, neostigmine, isoniazid, toxoids, vaccines, anticholinesterases, salicylates, somatrem

Decrease: prednisoLONE effect—CYP3A4 inducers

Drug/Lab Test

Increase: cholesterol, sodium, blood glucose, uric acid, calcium, urine glucose

Decrease: calcium, potassium, T_4, T_3, thyroid ^{131}I uptake test, urine 17-OHCS, 17-KS, PBI

False negative: skin allergy tests

NURSING CONSIDERATIONS
Assess:

• Potassium, blood glucose, urine glucose while patient receiving long-term therapy; hypokalemia, hyperglycemia

• Weight daily; notify prescriber if weekly gain of >5 lb

• B/P q4hr, pulse; notify prescriber if chest pain occurs

• I&O ratio; be alert for decreasing urinary output, increasing edema

• Plasma cortisol levels with long-term therapy; normal level: 138-635 nmol/L SI units when drawn at 8 AM

• **Infection:** increased temperature, WBC, even after withdrawal of medication; product masks infection

• **Potassium depletion:** paresthesias, fatigue, nausea, vomiting, depression, polyuria, dysrhythmias, weakness

• Edema, hypertension, cardiac symptoms

• Mental status: affect, mood, behavioral changes, aggression

• **Adrenal insufficiency:** nausea, vomiting, lethargy, restlessness, confusion, weight loss; hypotension before, during treatment baseline and periodically; HPA suppression may be precipitated by abrupt withdrawal

• **Beers:** avoid in older adults with delirium or at high risk of delirium

• **Pregnancy/breastfeeding:** not recommended in pregnancy; cautious use in breastfeeding

Evaluate:

• **Therapeutic response:** ease of respirations, decreased inflammation

Teach patient/family:

• That emergency ID as steroid user should be carried

• To notify prescriber if therapeutic response decreases; that dosage adjustment may be needed

• Not to discontinue abruptly; that adrenal crisis can result; to take product exactly as prescribed

• To avoid OTC products: salicylates, cough products with alcohol, cold preparations unless directed by prescriber

• About cushingoid symptoms: moon face, buffalo hump, rapid weight gain, excessive sweating, stretch marks

• **About the symptoms of adrenal insufficiency:** nausea, anorexia, fatigue, dizziness, dyspnea, weakness, joint pain

prednisoLONE ophthalmic (Rx)

See Appendix B

predniSONE (Rx)

(pred'ni-sone)

Rayos

Func. class.: Corticosteroid
Chem. class.: Intermediate-acting glucocorticoid

Do not confuse:

predniSONE/methylPREDNISolone/ prednisoLONE/PriLOSEC

ACTION: Decreases inflammation by increasing capillary permeability and lysosomal stabilization, minimal mineralocorticoid activity

USES: Severe inflammation, neoplasms, multiple sclerosis, collagen disorders, dermatologic disorders, pulmonary fibrosis, asthma

CONTRAINDICATIONS

Fungal infections, hypersensitivity
Precautions: Pregnancy, diabetes mellitus, glaucoma, osteoporosis, seizure disorders, ulcerative colitis, HF, myasthenia gravis, renal disease, esophagitis, peptic ulcer, cataracts, coagulopathy, abrupt discontinuation, children, corticosteroid hypersensitivity, Cushing syndrome, diabetes mellitus, ulcerative colitis, thromboembolism, geriatric patients, acute MI

DOSAGE AND ROUTES
Most uses
• **Adult:** PO 5-60 mg/day or divided bid-qid
• **Child:** PO 0.05-2 mg/kg/day divided 1-4×/day
Nephrotic syndrome
• **Child:** PO 2 mg/kg/day in divided doses, until urine is protein-free for 3 consecutive days, then 1-1.5 mg/kg/day every other day × 4 wk
Multiple sclerosis
• **Adult:** PO 200 mg/day × 1 wk, then 80 mg every other day × 1 mo
Asthma
• **Adult/adolescent:** PO 40-80 mg/day in 1-2 divided doses until PEF is 70% of predicted or personal best
• **Child:** PO 1 mg/kg (max 60 mg)/day in 2 divided doses until PEF is 70% of predicted or personal best

Available forms: Tabs 1, 2.5, 5, 10, 20, 50 mg; oral sol 5 mg/5 mL; del rel tab 1, 2, 5 mg
Administer:
• Regular tabs may be crushed and given with foods or fluids
• For long-term use, alternate-day therapy recommended to decrease adverse reactions; give in AM to coincide with normal cortisol secretion
• Titrated dose; use lowest effective dose
• With food or milk to decrease GI symptoms
• **Oral sol:** use calibrated measuring device
• **Del rel tab:** swallow whole; do not break, crush, chew; give once a day

SIDE EFFECTS
CNS: Depression, *flushing, sweating, headache, mood changes*
CV: Hypertension, thrombophlebitis, embolism, tachycardia, fluid retention
EENT: Fungal infections, increased intraocular pressure, blurred vision
GI: *Diarrhea, nausea, abdominal distention,* GI hemorrhage, *increased appetite,* pancreatitis
INTEG: Acne, poor wound healing, ecchymosis, petechiae
META: Hyperglycemia
MS: Fractures, osteoporosis, weakness
MISC: Decreased immune response

PHARMACOKINETICS
PO: Well absorbed PO, peak 1-2 hr; del rel peak 6-6 ½ hr; half-life 3 ½-4 hr, crosses

P

placenta, enters breast milk, metabolized by liver after conversion, excreted in urine

INTERACTIONS

Increase: tendon rupture—quinolones

Increase: side effects—alcohol, salicylates, NSAIDs, amphotericin B, digoxin, cycloSPORINE, diuretics

Increase: predniSONE action—salicylates, estrogens, NSAIDs, oral contraceptives, ketoconazole, macrolide antiinfectives

Increase: predniSONE effect—CYP3A4 inhibitors

Decrease: predniSONE effect—CYP3A4 inducers

Decrease: predniSONE action—cholestyramine, colestipol, barbiturates, rifAMPin, phenytoin, theophylline

Decrease: effects of anticoagulants, anticonvulsants, antidiabetics, neostigmine, isoniazid, toxoids, vaccines, anticholinesterases, salicylates, somatrem

Drug/Herb

Decrease: predniSONE effect—ephedra (ma huang)

Drug/Lab Test

Increase: cholesterol, sodium, blood glucose, uric acid, calcium, urine glucose

Decrease: calcium, potassium, T_4, T_3, thyroid ^{131}I uptake test, urine 17-OHCS, 17-KS, PBI

False negative: skin allergy tests

NURSING CONSIDERATIONS
Assess:

• **Adrenal insufficiency:** nausea, vomiting, anorexia, confusion, hypotension, weight loss before or during treatment; HPA suppression may be precipitated by abrupt withdrawal

• Potassium, blood glucose, urine glucose while patient receiving long-term therapy; hypokalemia and hyperglycemia; plasma cortisol with long-term therapy, normal: 138-635 nmol/L SI units drawn at 8 AM

• Weight daily; notify prescriber of weekly gain of >5 lb

• B/P, pulse; notify prescriber of chest pain; monitor for crackles, dyspnea if edema is present; hypertension, cardiac symptoms

• I&O ratio; be alert for decreasing urinary output, increasing edema, rales, crackles; notify provider if present

• **Infection:** increased temperature, WBC, even after withdrawal of medication; product masks infection

• Potassium depletion: paresthesias, fatigue, nausea, vomiting, depression, polyuria, dysrhythmias, weakness

• Mental status: affect, mood, behavioral changes, aggression

• **Pregnancy/breastfeeding:** use only if benefits outweigh fetal risk; do not breastfeed

• **Beers:** avoid in older adults with a high risk of delirium

Evaluate:

• **Therapeutic response:** ease of respirations, decreased inflammation

Teach patient/family:

• That emergency ID as corticosteroid user should be carried; provide information about product being taken and condition

• To notify prescriber if therapeutic response decreases; that dosage adjustment may be needed

• To avoid vaccinations

• Not to discontinue abruptly; adrenal crisis can result

• To avoid OTC products: salicylates, cough products with alcohol, cold preparations unless directed by prescriber

• **Cushingoid symptoms:** moon face, weight gain; symptoms of adrenal insufficiency: nausea, anorexia, fatigue, dizziness, dyspnea, weakness, joint pain

• That product causes immunosuppression; to report any symptoms of infection (fever, sore throat, cough)

• To notify provider before surgery

• That continuing follow-up and blood work will be needed

• That antidiabetic agents may need adjustment in diabetic patients

• **Pregnancy:** to notify prescriber if pregnancy is planned or suspected; cleft palate, stillbirth, abortion reported

pregabalin (Rx)

(pre-gab′a-lin)
Lyrica, Lyrica CR
Func. class.: Anticonvulsant
Chem. class.: γ-Aminobutyric acid (GABA) analog

Controlled Substance Schedule V

Do not confuse:
Lyrica/Lopressor

ACTION: Binds to high-voltage–gated calcium channels in CNS tissues; this may lead to anticonvulsant action similar to the inhibitory neurotransmitter GABA; anxiolytic, analgesic, and antiepileptic properties

USES: Neuropathic pain associated with spinal cord injury/diabetic peripheral neuropathy, partial-onset seizures, postherpetic neuralgia, fibromyalgia

CONTRAINDICATIONS

Hypersensitivity to this product or gabapentin, abrupt discontinuation
Precautions: Pregnancy, breastfeeding, children <12 yr, geriatric patients, renal disease, PR interval prolongation, creatine kinase elevations, HF (class III, IV), decreased platelets, substance abuse, dependence, glaucoma, myopathy, angioedema history, suicidal behavior

DOSAGE AND ROUTES
Diabetic peripheral neuropathic pain/postherpetic neuralgia
• **Adult: PO/ORAL SOL** 50 mg tid, may increase to 300 mg/day (max) within 1 wk, adjust in patients with renal disease; **EXT REL** 165 mg/day, may increase to 330 mg/day (treatment-naive patients)
Partial-onset seizures
• **Adult: PO/ORAL SOL** 75 mg bid or 50 mg tid; may increase to 600 mg/day (max)

Fibromyalgia, spinal cord injury pain
• **Adult: PO/ORAL SOL** 75 mg bid, may increase to 150 mg bid within 1 wk and 225 mg bid after 1 wk
Renal dose
• **Adult: PO** CCr 30-60 mL/min, 75-300 mg/day in 2-3 divided doses; CCr 15-30 mL/min, 25-150 mg/day in 1-2 divided doses; CCr <15 mL/min, 25-75 mg/day as a single dose

Available forms: Caps 25, 50, 75, 100, 150, 200, 225, 300 mg; oral sol 20 mg/mL; ext rel tabs 82.5, 165, 330 mg
Administer:
• Do not crush or chew caps; caps may be opened and contents put in applesauce or dissolved in juice
• Give without regard to meals
• Gradually withdraw over 7 days; abrupt withdrawal may precipitate seizures
• **Ext rel tablets:** do not split, crush, chew; to be taken after evening meal
• **Oral sol:** should be written in mg and calculated to mL

SIDE EFFECTS
CNS: *Dizziness,* drowsiness abnormal thinking, suicidal ideation
EENT: *Dry mouth,* blurred vision, sinusitis
GI: Constipation, abdominal pain, weight gain, nausea, vomiting, increased appetite
GU: Gynecomastia
HEMA: Thrombocytopenia
MS: Back pain, rhabdomyolysis, myopathy
OTHER: Pruritus, *peripheral edema,* angioedema

PHARMACOKINETICS
Well absorbed, peak 1.5 hr; 90% recovered in urine unchanged; negligible metabolism; not bound to plasma proteins; half-life 6 hr

INTERACTIONS
Increase: weight gain/fluid retention—pioglitazone, rosiglitazone; avoid use if possible

Increase: CNS depression—anxiolytics, sedatives, hypnotics, barbiturates, general anesthetics, opiate agonists, phenothiazines, sedating H_1 blockers, thiazolidinediones, tricyclics, alcohol
Increase: angioedema—ACE inhibitors
Drug/Lab Test
Increase: creatine kinase
Decrease: platelets

NURSING CONSIDERATIONS
Assess:
• **Seizures:** aura, location, duration, activity at onset, use seizure precautions
• **Pain:** location, duration, characteristics if using for diabetic neuropathy, spinal cord injury, neuralgia
• **Renal studies:** urinalysis, BUN, urine creatinine q3mo, creatine kinase; if markedly increased, discontinue product
• **Vision:** monitor for blurred vision, nystagmus, amblyopia
• **CV/respiratory status:** monitor B/P, HR, rhythm, breathing for dyspnea, crackles, wheezing
• Mental status: mood, sensorium, affect, behavioral changes, suicidal thoughts/behaviors; if mental status changes, notify prescriber
• **Angioedema/hypersensitivity:** (rare) monitor for blisters, hives, rash, dyspnea, wheezing; angioedema; if these occur, discontinue; cross-hypersensitivity with this product and gabapentin may occur
• **Rhabdomyolysis and creatinine kinase elevations (rare):** monitor for muscle pain, tenderness, weakness accompanied by malaise or fever; product should be discontinued
• **Beers:** avoid in older adults unless safer alternative is unavailable; may cause ataxia, impaired psychomotor function
• **Pregnancy/breastfeeding:** use only if benefits outweigh fetal risk, may cause fetal toxicity; pregnant patients should enroll in the Antiepileptic Drug Pregnancy Registry, 888-233-2334; do not breastfeed
Evaluate:
• **Therapeutic response:** decreased seizure activity; decrease in neuropathic pain

Teach patient/family:
• To carry emergency ID stating patient's name, products taken, condition, prescriber's name and phone number
• To avoid driving, other activities that require alertness because dizziness, drowsiness may occur, to obtain clearance from provider if driving is acceptable
• Not to discontinue medication quickly after long-term use; to taper over ≥1 wk; that withdrawal-precipitated seizures may occur; not to double doses if dose is missed, to take if 2 hr or more before next dose
• To notify prescriber if pregnancy is planned or suspected; to avoid breastfeeding
• To report muscle pain, tenderness, weakness when accompanied by fever, malaise, suicidal thoughts/behaviors
• To avoid alcohol, live virus vaccines

TREATMENT OF OVERDOSE: Lavage, VS, hemodialysis

pretomanid (Rx)
(pree-toh′mah-nid)
Pretomanid*
*Both trade and generic the same name
Func. class.: Antimycobacterial
Chem. class.: Nitroimidazooxazine

ACTION: Kills actively replicating *Mycobacterium tuberculosis* by inhibiting mycolic acid biosynthesis, thereby blocking cell wall production

USES: Drug-resistant TB

CONTRAINDICATIONS
Hypersensitivity to this product, bedaquiline; linezolid (used in combination)
PRECAUTIONS
Breastfeeding, hepatic disease, myelosuppression, pregnancy, QT prolongation, infertility

DOSAGE AND ROUTES
• **Adult PO Pretomanid** Tablet 200 mg daily × 26 wk; **bedaquiline** 400 mg PO daily × 2 wk, then 200 mg 3 times per wk,

with at least 48 hr between doses, × 24 weeks (total of 26 wk); **linezolid** 1,200 mg PO daily × 26 wk, with adjustments to 600 mg daily and further reduction to 300 mg daily or interruption of dosing for known linezolid adverse reactions of myelosuppression, peripheral neuropathy, and optic neuropathy

Available forms: Tablets 200 mg
Administer:
• Take the combination with food, swallow whole with water
• If the combination is interrupted for safety reasons, missed doses can be made up at the end of the treatment; doses of linezolid alone missed because of linezolid adverse reactions should not be made up
• Combination may be extended beyond 26 wk if needed

SIDE EFFECTS

CNS: Peripheral neuropathy, headache, insomnia
CV: QT prolongation, hypertension
GI: Nausea, vomiting, anorexia, abdominal pain, weight loss, diarrhea, constipation, gastritis, dyspepsia
INTEG: Acne, rash, pruritus, dry skin
RESP: Lower respiratory tract infection, cough, pleuritic pain
HEMA: Thrombocytopenia, neutropenia, anemia
META: Hypoglycemia
MS: MS pain
EENT: Visual impairment, increased hyperamylasemia hemoptysis, hyperlipasemia

PHARMACOKINETICS

Protein binding 86.4%, metabolized by multiple reductive and oxidative pathways; 53% excreted in urine, 38% in feces, as metabolites; half-life 16.9-17.4 hr; CYP3A4 is responsible for 20% of the metabolism; pretomanid significantly inhibits organic anion transporter-3 (OAT3) transporter

INTERACTIONS

Decreased: pretomanid effect—strong or moderate CYP3A4 inducers (rifAMPin, efavirenz); avoid using together

Increased: effect of OAT3 substrates— monitor for adverse reactions; dosage reduction for OAT3 substrate drugs may be needed
Drug/Lab
Increased: AST/ALT, bilirubin, γ-glutamyltransferase

NURSING CONSIDERATIONS
Assess:
• **Hepatotoxicity:** assess for fatigue, anorexia, nausea, jaundice, clay-colored stools, dark urine, liver tenderness, and hepatomegaly; obtain LFTs baseline, at 2 wk, monthly; if new or worsening hepatic dysfunction occurs, test for viral hepatitis and discontinue other hepatotoxic medications; interrupt treatment with the entire regimen if ALT/AST are accompanied by total bilirubin elevation >2× ULN or ALT/AST >8× ULN or ALT/AST >5× ULN and continue >2 wk
• **Myelosuppression:** assess for anemia (may be fatal), leukopenia, thrombocytopenia, pancytopenia; monitor CBC baseline, 2 wk, monthly; decreasing or interrupting dosing may be needed in worsening myelosuppression
• **Peripheral/optic neuropathy, peripheral neuropathy:** monitor visual function; if an impairment occurs, interrupt dosing and obtain ophthalmologic testing
• **QT prolongation:** obtain an ECG baseline, and ≤2, 12, 24 wk; obtain serum potassium, calcium, and magnesium at baseline and correct if abnormal; continue to monitor if QT prolongation occurs; may occur more often in a history of torsades de pointes, congenital long QT syndrome, hypothyroidism, bradydysrhythmia, uncompensated HF or serum calcium, magnesium, or potassium levels less than lower limits of normal
• **Lactic acidosis:** assess for recurrent nausea or vomiting; if this occurs, evaluate immediately bicarbonate and lactic acid levels and possible interruption of combination
Evaluate:
Therapeutic response: TB cultures negative

Teach patient/family:

- To report fatigue, vomiting, anorexia, nausea, jaundice, clay-colored stools, dark urine, liver tenderness, and visual impairment immediately
- To swallow whole with water; that all products must be taken as a combination regimen
- **Pregnancy/breastfeeding:** to report if pregnancy is planned or suspected: not to be used in pregnancy or breastfeeding

---

primaquine (Rx)

(prim′a-kween)

Func. class.: Antimalarial

Chem. class.: Synthetic 8-aminoquinolone

ACTION: Unknown; thought to destroy exoerythrocytic forms by gametocidal action

USES: Malaria caused by *Plasmodium vivax;* in combination with clindamycin for *Pneumocystis jiroveci* pneumonia

CONTRAINDICATIONS

Lupus erythematosus, rheumatoid arthritis; hypersensitivity to this product or iodoquinol

Precautions: Pregnancy, breastfeeding, methemoglobin reductase deficiency, bone marrow suppression, 🖐 hemolytic anemia, 🖐 G6PD deficiency

DOSAGE AND ROUTES

- **Adult:** PO 15-30 mg (base)/day × 2 wk or 45 mg (base)/wk × 8 wk; 26.3-mg tab is 15-mg base
- **Child:** PO 0.8 mg/kg (0.5 mg/base/day) daily × 2 wk

Available forms: Tabs 26.3 mg (15 mg base)

Administer:

PO route

- Before or after meals at same time each day to maintain product level; take with food to decrease GI upset

SIDE EFFECTS

CNS: Headache, dizziness

CV: Hypertension, dysrhythmias

EENT: *Blurred vision, difficulty focusing*

GI: *Nausea, vomiting, anorexia,* cramps

HEMA: Agranulocytosis, granulocytopenia, leukopenia, hemolytic anemia, leukocytosis, mild anemia, methemoglobinemia

INTEG: Pruritus, skin eruptions, pallor, weakness

PHARMACOKINETICS

PO: Metabolized by liver (metabolites), half-life 3.7-9.6 hr

INTERACTIONS

Increase: toxicity: quinacrine

Decrease: effect of carBAMazepine, PHENobarbital, phenytoins, rifamycins, nafcillin

Drug/Food

Increase: primaquine effect—food

Decrease: primaquine effect—grapefruit juice

Drug/Lab Test

Increase: WBC (can be increased or decreased)

Decrease: WBC, RBC, HB

NURSING CONSIDERATIONS

Assess:

- **Hepatic studies weekly:** AST, ALT, bilirubin if patient receiving long-term therapy
- **Blood studies:** CBC; blood dyscrasias occur
- **Allergic reactions:** pruritus, rash, urticaria
- **Blood dyscrasias:** malaise, fever, bruising, bleeding (rare)
- **Renal status:** dark urine, hematuria, decreased output
- **Hemolytic reaction:** chills, fever, chest pain, cyanosis; product should be discontinued immediately; 🖐 hemolytic anemia, G6PD deficiency may be severe in patients of Asian, Mediterranean descent
- **Pregnancy/breastfeeding:** do not use in pregnancy/breastfeeding; pregnancy testing should be completed in sexually active females of childbearing age; adequate contraception should be used while taking this product

---

Evaluate:
• **Therapeutic response:** decreased symptoms of malaria
Teach patient/family:
• To report visual problems, fever, fatigue, dark urine, bruising, bleeding; may indicate blood dyscrasias
• To complete full course of therapy; to take with food to decrease GI upset; if vomiting occurs within 30 min of taking dose, to repeat the dose

---

primidone (Rx)
(pri′mi-done)
Mysoline, Sertan ✦
Func. class.: Anticonvulsant, barbiturate

USES: Management of grand mal, psychomotor, focal seizures

CONTRAINDICATIONS
Hypersensitivity to phenobarbital, porphyria

DOSAGE AND ROUTES
Seizure disorders (grand mal, psychomotor, and focal)
• **Adult/child ≥8 yr: PO Days 1-3:** 100-125 mg/day at bedtime; **days 4-6:** 100-125 mg bid; **days 7-9:** 100-125 mg tid; usual dose 750-1500 mg/day in divided doses 3-4 times/day, max 2 g/day
• **Children <8 yr: PO Days 1-3:** 50 mg at bedtime; **days 4-6:** 50 mg bid; **days 7-9:** 100 mg bid; **maintenance (starting day 10):** 125-250 mg tid
Available forms: Tabs 50, 250 mg

---

probenecid (Rx)
(proe-ben′e-sid)
Func. class.: Uricosuric, antigout agent
Chem. class.: Sulfonamide derivative

ACTION: Inhibits tubular reabsorption of urates, with increased excretion of uric acids

USES: Hyperuricemia in gout, gouty arthritis, adjunct to penicillin treatment

CONTRAINDICATIONS
Hypersensitivity, severe renal/hepatic disease, CCr <50 mg/min, history of uric acid calculus
Precautions: Pregnancy, children <2 yr, sulfonamide hypersensitivity, peptic ulcer

DOSAGE AND ROUTES
Gout/gouty arthritis
• **Adult: PO** 250 mg bid for 1 wk, then 500 mg bid, max 2 g/day; maintenance 500 mg/day × 6 mo
Adjunct in penicillin treatment
• **Adult and adolescent >50 kg: PO** 500 mg qid
• **Child <50 kg: PO** 25 mg/kg, then 40 mg/kg in divided doses qid
Renal dose
• Avoid use if CCr <50 mL/min
Available forms: Tabs 500 mg
Administer:
• After meals or with milk if GI symptoms occur
• Increase fluid intake to 2-3 L/day to prevent urinary calculi

SIDE EFFECTS
CNS: Drowsiness, headache, flushing
CV: Bradycardia
GI: *Gastric irritation, nausea, vomiting, anorexia,* hepatic necrosis
GU: Glycosuria, thirst, frequency, nephrotic syndrome
INTEG: Rash, dermatitis, pruritus, fever
META: *Acidosis, hypokalemia, hyperchloremia,* hyperglycemia
RESP: Apnea, irregular respirations

PHARMACOKINETICS
Peak 2-4 hr, duration 8 hr, half-life 5-8 hr; metabolized by liver; excreted in urine

INTERACTIONS
Increase: effect of acyclovir, barbiturates, allopurinol, benzodiazepines, dyphylline,

P

zidovudine, cephalosporins, penicillins, sulfonamides

Increase: toxicity—sulfa products, dapsone, clofibrate, indomethacin, rifAMPin, naproxen, methotrexate

Decrease: action of probenecid—salicylates

Drug/Lab Test

Increase: theophylline levels

NURSING CONSIDERATIONS

Assess:

• Uric acid levels (3-7 mg/dL); mobility, joint pain, swelling, maintain fluid intake at 2-3 L/day

• Respiratory rate, rhythm, depth; notify prescriber of abnormalities

• Electrolytes; CO_2 before, during treatment

• Urine pH, output, glucose during beginning treatment, poor effect in GFR <30 mL/min

• **For CNS symptoms:** confusion, twitching, hyperreflexia, stimulation, headache; may indicate overdose

• **Beers:** avoid in older adults with creatinine clearance <30 mL/min

Evaluate:

• **Therapeutic response:** absence of pain, stiffness in joints

Teach patient/family:

• To avoid OTC preparations (aspirin) unless directed by prescriber; to increase water intake, avoid alcohol, caffeine

---

probenecid/colchicine (Rx)

(proe-ben'e-sid/kol'chi-seen)
Func. class.: Antiinflammatory agent, antigout, uricosuric

USES: Treatment of chronic gouty arthritis with frequent, recurrent acute attacks of gout

CONTRAINDICATIONS

Hypersensitivity to colchicine, probenecid, or any component; child <2 yr; aspirin usage; blood dyscrasias; uric acid kidney stones; initiation during an acute gout attack; concomitant use of a P-glycoprotein (P-gp) or strong CYP3A4 inhibitor in renal/hepatic disease

DOSAGE AND ROUTES

Gouty arthritis

• **Adult:** PO Colchicine 0.5 mg/probenecid 0.5 g: 1 tablet daily × 1 week, then 1 tablet bid, max 4 tablets/day

Available forms: Tabs 500 mg/0.5 mg

> ### ⚠ HIGH ALERT
>
> ## procainamide (Rx) NTI
> (proe-kane-ah'mide)
> *Func. class.:* Antidysrhythmic (class IA)
> *Chem. class.:* Procaine HCl amide analog

ACTION: Depresses excitability of cardiac muscle to electrical stimulation and slows conduction velocity in atrium, bundle of His, and ventricle; increases refractory period

USES: Life-threatening ventricular dysrhythmias

Unlabeled uses: Atrial fibrillation/flutter, paroxysmal atrial tachycardia, PSVT, Wolff-Parkinson-White (WPW) syndrome

CONTRAINDICATIONS

Hypersensitivity, severe heart block, torsades de pointes

Black Box Warning: Lupus erythematosus

Precautions: Pregnancy, breastfeeding, children, renal/hepatic disease, HF, respiratory depression, cytopenia, dysrhythmia associated with digoxin toxicity, myasthenia gravis, digoxin toxicity

Black Box Warning: Bone marrow failure, cardiac arrhythmias

DOSAGE AND ROUTES—NTI
Ventricular tachycardia during CPR
• **Adult:** IV loading dose 20 mg/min; either ventricular tachycardia resolves or patient becomes hypotensive; QRS complex is widened by 50% of original width or total is 17 mg/kg (1.2 g for a 70-kg patient); may give up to 50 mg/min in urgent situations; maintenance: 1-4 mg/min **CONT IV INFUSION; IM** 50 mg/kg/day in divided doses q3-6hr
• **Child:** IV PALS 15 mg/kg over 30-60 min

Renal dose
• **Adult:** IV CCr 35-59 mL/min, give 70% maintenance dose; CCr 15-34 mL/min, give 40%-60% maintenance dose; CCr <15 mL/min, individualize dose

Available forms: Inj 100, 500 mg/mL
Administer:
IM route
• IM inj in deltoid; aspirate to avoid intravascular administration; use only when unable to use IV
Direct IV route
• Dilute each 100 mg/10 mL of 0.9% NaCl; give at max 50 mg/min
Intermittent IV INFUSION route
• Dilute 0.2-1 g/50-500 mL of D₅W (2-4 mg/mL); give over 30-60 min at max 25-50 mg/min; use infusion pump

Y-site compatibilities: Alfentanil, amikacin, aminocaproic acid, aminophylline, amiodarone, amphotericin B lipid complex, amphotericin B liposome, anidulafungin, ascorbic acid, atenolol, atracurium, atropine, aztreonam, benztropine, bivalirudin, bleomycin, bumetanide, buprenorphine, butorphanol, calcium chloride/gluconate, caspofungin, ceFAZolin, cefmetazole, cefonicid, cefoperazone, cefotaxime, cefoTEtan, cefOXitin, cefTAZidime, cefTRIAXone, cefuroxime, cephalothin, chlorproMAZINE, cimetidine, cisatracurium, CISplatin, clindamycin, cyanocobalamin, cyclophosphamide, cycloSPORINE, cytarabine, DACTINomycin, DAPTOmycin, dexamethasone, digoxin, diphenhydrAMINE, DOBUTamine, DOCEtaxel, DOPamine, doxacurium, DOXOrubicin, doxycycline, enalaprilat, ePHEDrine, EPINEPHrine, epiRUBicin, epoetin alfa, eptifibatide, ertapenem, erythromycin, esmolol, etoposide, etoposide phosphate, famotidine, fenoldopam, fentaNYL, fluconazole, fludarabine, fluorouracil, folic acid, furosemide, gatifloxacin, gemcitabine, gentamicin, glycopyrrolate, granisetron, heparin, hydrocortisone, HYDROmorphone, IDArubicin, ifosfamide, indomethacin, insulin (regular), irinotecan, isoproterenol, ketorolac, labetalol, lidocaine, linezolid, LORazepam, magnesium sulfate, mannitol, mechlorethamine, meperidine, metaraminol, methicillin, methotrexate, methoxamine, methyldopate, methylPREDNISolone, metoclopramide, metoprolol, mezlocillin, miconazole, midazolam, mitoXANTRONE, morphine, moxalactam, multivitamins, mycophenolate, nafcillin, nalbuphine, naloxone, netilmicin, nitroglycerin, nitroprusside, norepinephrine, octreotide, ondansetron, oxacillin, oxaliplatin, oxytocin, PACLitaxel, palonosetron, pamidronate, pancuronium, pantoprazole, papaverine, PEMEtrexed, penicillin G potassium/sodium, pentamidine, pentazocine, PENTobarbital, PHENobarbital, phenylephrine, phytonadione, piperacillin, piperacillin-tazobactam, polymyxin B, potassium chloride, prochlorperazine, promethazine, propranolol, protamine, pyridoxine, quiNIDine, quinupristin-dalfopristin, raNITIdine, remifentanil, ritodrine, rocuronium, sodium bicarbonate, succinylcholine, SUFentanil, tacrolimus, teniposide, theophylline, thiamine, thiotepa, ticarcillin, ticarcillin-clavulanate, tigecycline, tirofiban, tobramycin, tolazoline, trimetaphan, urokinase, vancomycin, vasopressin, vecuronium, verapamil, vinCRIStine, vinorelbine, vitamin B complex/C, voriconazole, zoledronic acid

SIDE EFFECTS
CNS: *Headache, dizziness,* confusion, psychosis, restlessness, irritability, weakness, depression
CV: *Hypotension,* heart block, cardiovascular collapse, arrest, torsades de pointes
GI: Nausea, vomiting, anorexia, diarrhea, hepatomegaly, pain, bitter taste

HEMA: SLE syndrome, agranulocytosis, thrombocytopenia, neutropenia, hemolytic anemia
INTEG: Rash, urticaria, edema, swelling (rare), pruritus, flushing, angioedema
SYST: SLE

PHARMACOKINETICS
Metabolized in liver to active metabolites, excreted unchanged by kidneys (60%), protein binding 15%
IM: Peak 10-60 min, half-life 3 hr

INTERACTIONS
Increase: effects of neuromuscular blockers
Increase: procainamide effects—cimetidine, quiNIDine, trimethoprim, β-blockers, raNITIdine
Increase: toxicity—other antidysrhythmics, thioridazine, quinolones
Drug/Lab Test
Increase: ALT, AST, alk phos, LDH, bilirubin

NURSING CONSIDERATIONS
Assess:

Black Box Warning: Cardiac dysrhythmias: ECG continuously if using IV to determine increased PR or QRS segments; discontinue immediately; watch for increased ventricular ectopic beats, maximum need to rebolus

• Therapeutic blood levels, 4-10 mcg/mL or NAPA levels 10-20 mcg/mL

Black Box Warning: Bone marrow suppression: CBC q2wk × 3 mo; leukocyte, neutrophil, platelet counts may be decreased, treatment may need to be discontinued

• I&O ratio; electrolytes (K, Na, Cl), weight weekly, report gain of >2 lb
• **Toxicity:** confusion, drowsiness, nausea, vomiting, tachydysrhythmias, oliguria
• ANA titer; during long-term treatment, watch for lupuslike symptoms

• Respiratory status: rate, rhythm, character, lung fields; bilateral crackles may occur in HF patient; watch for respiratory depression
• **CNS effects:** dizziness, confusion, psychosis, paresthesias, seizures; product should be discontinued
• **Pregnancy/breastfeeding:** use only if clearly needed; do not breastfeed
Evaluate:
• **Therapeutic response:** decreased dysrhythmias
Teach patient/family:
• That wax matrix may appear in stools
• Not to discontinue without provider's approval

Black Box Warning: To notify prescriber immediately if lupuslike symptoms appear (joint pain, butterfly rash, fever, chills, dyspnea)

Black Box Warning: To notify prescriber of leukopenia (sore mouth, gums, throat) or thrombocytopenia (bleeding, bruising)

• How to take pulse and when to report to prescriber
• To avoid driving, other hazardous activities until product effect is known

TREATMENT OF OVERDOSE:
O₂, artificial ventilation, ECG, administer DOPamine for circulatory depression, diazePAM or thiopental for seizures, isoproterenol

---

⚠ HIGH ALERT

procarbazine (Rx)
(proe-kar′ba-zeen)
Matulane
Func. class.: Antineoplastic, alkylating agent
Chem. class.: Hydrazine derivative

Do not confuse:
Matulane/Materna

ACTION: Inhibits DNA, RNA, protein synthesis; has multiple sites of action; nonvesicant

USES: Lymphoma, Hodgkin's disease, cancers resistant to other therapy

CONTRAINDICATIONS
Pregnancy, breastfeeding, hypersensitivity, thrombocytopenia, bone marrow depression
Precautions: Cardiac/renal/hepatic disease, radiation therapy, seizure disorder, anemia, bipolar disorder, Parkinson's disease

> **Black Box Warning:** Requires a specialized care setting and an experienced clinician

DOSAGE AND ROUTES
• **Adult:** PO 2-4 mg/kg/day for 1st wk; maintain dosage of 4-6 mg/kg/day until platelets, WBC fall; after recovery, 1-2 mg/kg/day, may use as single agent or in combination
• **Child:** PO 50 mg/m^2/day for 7 days, then 100 mg/m^2 until desired response, leukopenia, or thrombocytopenia occurs; 50 mg/m^2/day maintenance after bone marrow recovery
Available forms: Caps 50 mg
Administer:
• In divided doses and at bedtime to minimize nausea and vomiting
• Nonphenothiazine antiemetic 30-60 min before product and 4-10 hr after treatment to prevent vomiting

SIDE EFFECTS
CNS: Headache, dizziness, insomnia, hallucinations, confusion, coma, pain, chills, fever, sweating, paresthesias, seizures, peripheral neuropathy
EENT: Retinal hemorrhage, nystagmus, photophobia, diplopia, dry eyes
GI: *Nausea, vomiting,* anorexia, diarrhea, constipation, dry mouth, stomatitis, elevated hepatic enzymes
GU: Azoospermia, cessation of menses
HEMA: Thrombocytopenia, anemia, leukopenia, myelosuppression, bleeding tendencies, purpura, petechiae, epistaxis, hemolysis
INTEG: *Rash,* pruritus, dermatitis, alopecia, herpes, hyperpigmentation
MS: Arthralgias, myalgias
RESP: Cough, pneumonitis, hemoptysis
SYST: Secondary malignancy

PHARMACOKINETICS
Half-life 1 hr; concentrates in liver, kidney, skin; metabolized in liver, excreted in urine

INTERACTIONS
Increase: hypotension—meperidine; do not use together
Increase: neuroleptic malignant syndrome, seizures, hyperpyrexia—alcohol, MAOIs, tricyclics, sympathomimetic products, SSRIs, SNRIs
Increase: hypertension—guanethidine, levodopa, methyldopa, reserpine, caffeine
Life-threatening hypertension: sympathomimetics
Increase: bleeding risk—NSAIDs, anticoagulants, platelet inhibitors, thrombolytics
Increase: CNS depression—barbiturates, antihistamines, opioids, hypotensive agents, phenothiazines
Drug/Food
• **Hypertensive crisis:** tyramine foods

NURSING CONSIDERATIONS
Assess:
• **Bone marrow suppression:** CBC, differential, platelet count weekly; withhold product if WBC is <4000/mm^3 or platelet count is <100,000/mm^3; notify prescriber
• **Hepatic/renal disease:** can cause accumulation of drug, increased toxicity; renal studies: BUN; serum uric acid; urine CCr; electrolytes before, during therapy; I&O ratio, report fall in urine output to <30 mL/hr; hepatic studies before, during therapy: bilirubin, AST, ALT, alk phos, LDH prn or monthly
• Monitor temperature; fever may indicate beginning of infection

> **Black Box Warning:** To be used only in a specialized care setting with emergency equipment

---

Black Box Warning: To be given only by an experienced clinician knowledgeable in cytotoxic products

• CNS changes: confusion, paresthesias, neuropathies; product should be discontinued
• Tyramine foods in diet; hypertensive crisis can occur
• **Toxicity:** facial flushing, epistaxis, increased PT, thrombocytopenia; product should be discontinued
• **Bleeding:** hematuria, guaiac stools, bruising or petechiae, mucosa or orifices q8hr
• Effects of alopecia on body image; discuss feelings about body changes
• Jaundiced skin, sclera; dark urine, clay-colored stools, itchy skin, abdominal pain, fever, diarrhea
• Buccal cavity for dryness, sores or ulceration, white patches, oral pain, bleeding, dysphagia
• GI symptoms: frequency of stools, cramping
• **Acidosis, signs of dehydration:** rapid respirations, poor skin turgor, decreased urine output, dry skin, restlessness, weakness
• **Pregnancy/breastfeeding:** do not use in pregnancy, breastfeeding
Evaluate:
• **Therapeutic response:** decreasing malignancy
Teach patient/family:
• **To report any complaints, side effects to nurse or prescriber:** CNS changes, diarrhea, cough, SOB, fever, chills, sore throat, bleeding, bruising, vomiting blood; black, tarry stools
• That hair may be lost during treatment and wig or hairpiece may make patient feel better; that new hair may be different in color, texture
• To avoid sunlight or UV exposure; to wear sunscreen or protective clothing
• To avoid foods with citric acid, hot temperature, or rough texture
• To report any bleeding, white spots, ulcerations in mouth to prescriber; to examine mouth daily
• To avoid driving, activities requiring alertness because dizziness may occur

• **Pregnancy/breastfeeding:** to use effective contraception; to avoid breastfeeding; that product may cause infertility
• To avoid the ingestion of alcohol, caffeine, tyramine-containing foods; that cold, hay fever, and weight-reducing products may cause serious product interactions; to avoid smoking
• To avoid crowds, persons with infections if granulocytes are low
• To avoid vaccines

---

prochlorperazine (Rx)
(proe-klor-pair´a-zeen)

Compro
Func. class.: Antiemetic, antipsychotic
Chem. class.: Phenothiazine, piperazine derivative

Do not confuse:
prochlorperazine/chlorproMAZINE

ACTION: Decreases DOPamine neurotransmission by increasing DOPamine turnover through the blockade of the D_2 somatodendritic autoreceptor in the mesolimbic system

USES: Nausea, vomiting, psychotic disorders
Unlabeled uses: Migraine

CONTRAINDICATIONS
Hypersensitivity to phenothiazines, coma; infants, neonates, children <2 yr or <20 lb; surgery
Precautions: Pregnancy, breastfeeding, geriatric patients, seizure, encephalopathy, glaucoma, hepatic disease, Parkinson's disease, BPH

Black Box Warning: Increased mortality in elderly patients with dementia-related psychosis

DOSAGE AND ROUTES
Postoperative nausea/vomiting
• **Adult: IM** 5-10 mg 1-2 hr before anesthesia; may repeat after 30 min; **IV**

5-10 mg 15-30 min before anesthesia;
IV INFUSION 20 mg/L D$_5$W or NS 15-
30 min before anesthesia, max 40 mg/
day

Severe nausea/vomiting
• **Adult: PO** 5-10 mg tid-qid; **SUS REL**
15 mg/day in AM or 10 mg q12hr; **RECT**
25 mg/bid; **IM** 5-10 mg q3-4hr prn, max
40 mg/day

• **Child 18-39 kg: PO** 2.5 mg tid or 5 mg
bid; **IM** 0.132 mg/kg q3-4hr prn, max 15
mg/day

• **Child 14-17 kg: PO/RECT** 2.5 mg bid-
tid; **IM** 0.132 mg/kg q3-4hr prn, max 10
mg/day

• **Child 9-13 kg: PO/RECT** 2.5 mg/day-
bid; **IM** 0.132 mg/kg q3-4hr prn, max
7.5 mg/day

Antipsychotic
• **Adult/child ≥12 yr: PO** 5-10 mg tid-
qid; may increase q2-3days, max 150
mg/day; **IM** 10-20 mg q2-4hr up to 4
doses, then 10-20 mg q4-6hr

• **Child 2-12 yr: PO** 2.5 mg bid-tid;
IM 0.132 mg/kg change to oral ASAP

Antianxiety
• **Adult/child ≥12 yr: PO** 5 mg tid-qid,
max 20 mg/day

• **Child 2-12 yr: IM** 0.132 mg/kg change
to oral ASAP

Available forms: Tabs 5, 10 mg; supp
10 ♣, 25 mg; sol for inj 5 mg/mL
Administer:
• Avoid other CNS depressants
IM route
• IM inj in large muscle mass; aspirate
to avoid IV administration
• Keep patient recumbent for ½ hr
Direct IV route
• May give diluted or undiluted; inject
directly in a vein ≤5 mg/min; do not give
as bolus
Intermittent IV INFUSION route
• May dilute 20 mg/L NaCl and give as
infusion 15-30 min before anesthesia
induction

SIDE EFFECTS
CNS: Neuroleptic malignant syndrome,
*extrapyramidal reactions, tardive dyski-
nesia, euphoria,* depression, *drowsiness,*
restlessness, tremor, dizziness, headache

CV: tachycardia, hypotension, ECG
changes
EENT: Blurred vision
GI: Nausea, vomiting, anorexia, dry
mouth, diarrhea, constipation, weight
loss, metallic taste, cramps
HEMA: Agranulocytosis
MISC: Impotence; urine color change
RESP: Respiratory depression

PHARMACOKINETICS
Metabolized by liver; excreted in urine,
breast milk; crosses placenta; 91%-99%
protein binding
IM: Onset 10-20 min, duration 4-6 hr;
children: 12 hr
PO: Onset 30-40 min, duration 3-4 hr
RECT: Onset 60 min, duration 3-4 hr

INTERACTIONS
Increase: anticholinergic action—anti-
cholinergics, antiparkinson products,
antidepressants
Increase: CNS depression—CNS
depressants
Increase: serotonin syndrome, neurolep-
tic malignant syndrome—SSRIs, SNRIs
Decrease: prochlorperazine effect—bar-
biturates, antacids, lithium
Drug/Herb
Increase: CNS depression—chamomile,
hops, kava, St. John's wort, valerian
Increase: EPS—kava
Drug/Lab Test
Increase: LFTs, cardiac enzymes, choles-
terol, blood glucose, prolactin, bilirubin,
PBI, ^{131}I, alk phos, leukocytes, granulo-
cytes, platelets
Decrease: hormones (blood and urine)
False positive: pregnancy tests, urine
bilirubin
False negative: urinary steroids,
17-OHCS, pregnancy tests

NURSING CONSIDERATIONS
Assess:
• **EPS:** abnormal movement, tardive
dyskinesia, akathisia
• VS, B/P; check patients with cardiac
disease more often
• **Neuroleptic malignant syndrome:**
seizures, hypo/hypertension, fever, tachy-

P

cardia, dyspnea, fatigue, muscle stiffness, loss of bladder control; notify prescriber immediately

• CBC, LFTs during course of treatment; blood dyscrasias, hepatotoxicity may occur

• **Respiratory status** before, during, after administration of emetic; check rate, rhythm, character; respiratory depression can occur rapidly among geriatric or debilitated patients

• **Beers:** avoid in older adults with a high risk of delirium

• **Pregnancy/breastfeeding:** use only if benefits outweigh fetal risk; EPS may result; cautious use in breastfeeding, excreted in breast milk

Evaluate:

• **Therapeutic response:** absence of nausea, vomiting; reduced anxiety, agitation, excitability

Teach patient/family:

• To avoid hazardous activities, activities requiring alertness because dizziness may occur

• To avoid alcohol

• Not to double or skip doses

• That urine may be pink to reddish brown

• That suppositories may contain coconut/palm oil

• To report dark urine, clay-colored stools, bleeding, bruising, rash, blurred vision

• To avoid sun; wear sunscreen, protective clothing

---

progesterone (Rx)

(proe-jess′ter-one)

Crinone, Endometrin, Prometrium

Func. class.: Hormone, Progestogen

Chem. class.: Progesterone derivative

ACTION: Inhibits secretion of pituitary gonadotropins, which prevents follicular maturation, ovulation; stimulates growth of mammary tissue; antineoplastic action against endometrial cancer

USES: Contraception, amenorrhea, premenstrual syndrome, abnormal uterine bleeding, endometrial hyperplasia prevention, assisted reproductive technology (ART) gel

Unlabeled uses: PMS, preterm delivery prophylaxis

CONTRAINDICATIONS

Pregnancy, ectopic pregnancy; hypersensitivity to this product, peanuts, or peanut oil; thromboembolic disorders, reproductive cancer, genital bleeding (abnormal, undiagnosed), cerebral hemorrhage, PID, STDs, thrombophlebitis

Black Box Warning: Breast cancer

Precautions: Breastfeeding, hypertension, asthma, blood dyscrasias, HF, diabetes mellitus, bone disease, depression, migraine headache, seizure disorders, gallbladder/renal/hepatic disease, family history of breast/reproductive tract cancer

Black Box Warning: Cardiac disease, dementia

DOSAGE AND ROUTES

Infertility

• **Adult: VAG** 90 mg/day (micronized gel); 100 mg 2-3 times/day starting day after oocyte retrieval and for ≤10 wk total

Amenorrhea/functional uterine bleeding

• **Adult: IM** 5-10 mg/day × 6-8 doses

Endometrial hyperplasia prevention

• **Adult: PO** 200 mg as a single dose in the evening for 12 sequential days of every 28-day cycle of daily estrogen therapy

Assisted reproductive therapy

• **Adult: GEL** 90 mg (8%) vaginally daily for supplementation; 90 mg (8%) vaginally bid for replacement; if pregnancy occurs, continue × 10-12 wk

Corpus luteum insufficiency (assisted reproductive technology [ART])

• **Adult: VAG INSERT** 90-100 mg bid-tid starting at oocyte retrieval and continuing up to 10-12 wk gestation

---

Available forms: Inj 50 mg/mL; vag gel 4%, 8%; caps 100, 200 mg; vag insert 100 mg; vag supp 25, 100, 200, 500 mg; compounding kit 25, 50, 100, 200, 400 mg; oil for IM injection 50 mg/mL

Administer:

PO route

• Do not break, crush, or chew caps
• Titrated dose; use lowest effective dose
• In 1 dose in AM
• With food or milk to decrease GI symptoms
• Start progesterone 14 days after estrogen dose if given concomitantly

Vaginal route

• Wait at least 6 hr after any vaginal treatment before using vaginal gel, use applicator provided

IM route

• Shake vial, inject deeply into large muscle, aspirate
• Check for particulate matter and discoloration before injecting

SIDE EFFECTS

CNS: *Dizziness, headache,* depression, *fatigue,* mood swings
CV: Hypotension, thrombophlebitis, edema, thromboembolism, stroke, pulmonary embolism, MI
EENT: Diplopia, retinal thrombosis
GI: *Nausea,* vomiting, anorexia, cramps, increased weight, cholestatic jaundice, *constipation,* abdominal pain
GU: Amenorrhea, cervical erosion, breakthrough bleeding, dysmenorrhea, nocturia, breast changes, *gynecomastia,* endometriosis, spontaneous abortion, breast pain, ectopic pregnancy
INTEG: Rash, urticaria, acne, hirsutism, alopecia, photosensitivity
META: Hyperglycemia
SYST: Angioedema, anaphylaxis

PHARMACOKINETICS

Excreted in urine, feces; metabolized in liver
IM/RECT/VAG: Duration 24 hr

INTERACTIONS

Increase: progesterone effect—CYP3A4 inhibitors (ketoconazole, clarithromycin, erythroycin, verapamil)
Decrease: progesterone effect—phenytoin, barbiturates

Drug/Lab Test

Increase: alk phos; nitrogen (urine); pregnanediol; amino acids; factors VII, VIII, IX, X
Decrease: GTT, HDL

NURSING CONSIDERATIONS

Assess:

• **Abnormal uterine bleeding:** vaginal bleeding; obtain pad count, patient menstrual history, breast exam, cervical cytology
• Weight daily; notify prescriber of weekly weight gain of >5 lb
• B/P at beginning of treatment and periodically
• I&O ratio; be alert for decreasing urinary output, increasing edema
• **Hepatic studies:** ALT, AST, bilirubin periodically during long-term therapy
• Edema, hypertension, cardiac symptoms, jaundice, thromboembolism
• **Mental status:** affect, mood, behavioral changes, depression
• **Pregnancy/breastfeeding:** do not use in pregnancy, breastfeeding

Evaluate:

• **Therapeutic response:** decreased abnormal uterine bleeding, absence of amenorrhea

Teach patient/family:

• To report breast lumps, vaginal bleeding, edema, jaundice, dark urine, clay-colored stools, dyspnea, headache, blurred vision, abdominal pain, numbness or stiffness in legs, chest pain
• To avoid gel with other vaginal products; if to be used together, to separate by ≥6 hr; for vaginal route, on proper insertion technique
• To report suspected pregnancy
• To monitor blood glucose if diabetic
• To avoid activities requiring mental alertness until effects are realized; can cause dizziness

P

> ⚠ **HIGH ALERT**

promethazine (Rx)

(proe-meth′a-zeen)

Phenergan, Promethegan

Func. class.: Antihistamine, H_1-receptor antagonist, antiemetic

Chem. class.: Phenothiazine derivative

ACTION: Acts on blood vessels, GI, respiratory system by competing with histamine for H_1-receptor sites; decreases allergic response by blocking histamine

USES: Motion sickness, rhinitis, allergy symptoms, sedation, nausea, preoperative and postoperative sedation

CONTRAINDICATIONS

Hypersensitivity, breastfeeding, agranulocytosis, bone marrow suppression, coma, jaundice, Reye's syndrome

Black Box Warning: Infants, neonates, children, intraarterial/SUBCUT administration, extravasation

Precautions: Pregnancy, cardiac/renal/hepatic disease, asthma, seizure disorder, prostatic hypertrophy, bladder obstruction, glaucoma, COPD, GI obstruction, ileus, CNS depression, diabetes, sleep apnea, urinary retention, IV use

Black Box Warning: Tissue necrosis (IV use)

DOSAGE AND ROUTES

Nausea/vomiting

• **Adult:** PO/IM/IV/RECT 12.5-25 mg; q4-6hr prn

• **Child >2 yr:** PO/IM/IV/RECT 0.25-1 mg/kg q4-6hr prn, max 25 mg/dose

Motion sickness

• **Adult:** PO 25 mg bid, give ½-1 hr before departure, then q8-12hr prn

• **Child ≥2 yr:** PO/IM/RECT 0.25 to 0.5 mg/kg/dose (Max: 25 mg/dose) given 30 min to 2 hr prior to travel and q6-12hr as needed

Sedation

• **Adult:** PO/IM 25-50 mg at bedtime

• **Child ≥2 yr:** PO/IM/RECT 12.5-25 mg at bedtime

Sedation (preoperative/postoperative)

• **Adult:** PO/IM/IV 25-50 mg

• **Child >2 yr:** PO/IM/IV 0.5-1.1 mg/kg, max 25 mg/dose

Allergy/rhinitis (unlabeled)

• **Adult:** PO 12.5 mg qid or 25 mg at bedtime

• **Child ≥2 yr:** PO 6.25-12.5 mg tid or 25 mg at bedtime

Hyperemesis gravidarum (unlabeled)

• **Pregnant female:** PO/RECT/IM/IV 12.5-25 mg q4hr

Available forms: Tabs 12.5, 25, 50 mg; supp 12.5, 25, 50 mg; inj 25, 50 mg/mL

Administer:

Avoid use with other CNS depressants

PO route

• With meals for GI symptoms; absorption may slightly decrease

• When used for motion sickness, 30 min-1 hr before travel

IM route

• IM inj deep in large muscle; rotate site, necrosis may occur from subcut injection, give only IM

Direct IV route

Black Box Warning: Check for extravasation: burning, pain, swelling at IV site; can cause tissue necrosis

• Do not use if precipitate is present

• Rapid administration may cause transient decrease in B/P

• After diluting each 25-50 mg/9 mL of NaCl for inj; give ≤25 mg/2 min

Y-site compatibilities: Alfentanil, amifostine, amikacin, aminocaproic acid, amsacrine, anidulafungin, ascorbic acid, atenolol, atracurium, atropine, aztreonam, benztropine, bivalirudin, bleomycin, bumetanide, buprenorphine, butorphanol, calcium chloride/gluconate, CARBOplatin, caspofungin, chlorproMAZINE, cimetidine, ciprofloxacin, cisatracurium, CISplatin, cladribine, codeine, cyanocobalamin, cyclophosphamide, cycloSPORINE, cytarabine, DACTINomycin, DAPTOmycin, dexmedetomidine, digoxin, diltiaZEM, diphenhydrAMINE, DOBUTamine, DOCEtaxel, DOPamine, doxacurium, DOXOrubicin, doxycycline, enalaprilat, ePHEDrine, EPINEPHrine, epirubicin, epoetin, eptifibatide, erythromycin, esmolol, etoposide, famotidine, fenoldopam, fentaNYL, filgrastim, fluconazole, fludarabine, gemcitabine, gentamicin, glycopyrrolate, granisetron, HYDROmorphone, hydrOXYzine, IDArubicin, ifosfamide, insulin (regular), irinotecan, isoproterenol, labetalol, levoFLOXacin, lidocaine, linezolid, LORazepam, magnesium sulfate, mannitol, mechlorethamine, melphalan, meperidine, metaraminol, methoxamine, methyldopate, metoclopramide, metoprolol, metroNIDAZOLE, miconazole, midazolam, milrinone, mitoXANTRONE, morphine, mycophenolate, nalbuphine, naloxone, netilmicin, nitroglycerin, norepinephrine, octreotide, ondansetron, oxaliplatin, oxytocin, PACLitaxel, palonosetron, pamidronate, pancuronium, PEMEtrexed, pentamidine, pentazocine, phenylephrine, polymyxin B, procainamide, prochlorperazine, propranolol, protamine, pyridoxine, quiNIDine, quinupristin-dalfopristin, raNITIdine, remifentanil, Ringer's, ritodrine, riTUXimab, rocuronium, sargramostim, sodium acetate, succinylcholine, SUFentanil, tacrolimus, teniposide, theophylline, thiamine, thiotepa, tigecycline, tirofiban, TNA, tobramycin, tolazoline, trastuzumab, trimetaphan, vancomycin, vasopressin, vecuronium, verapamil, vinCRIStine, vinorelbine, voriconazole

SIDE EFFECTS

CNS: *Dizziness, drowsiness,* poor coordination, fatigue, anxiety, euphoria, confusion, paresthesia, neuritis, EPS, neuroleptic malignant syndrome

CV: Hypo/hypertension, palpitations, tachycardia, orthostatic hypotension
EENT: Blurred vision, dilated pupils, tinnitus, nasal stuffiness; dry nose, throat, mouth; photosensitivity
GI: *Constipation,* dry mouth, nausea, vomiting, anorexia, diarrhea
GU: *Urinary retention,* dysuria, frequency
INTEG: Rash, urticaria, photosensitivity, tissue necrosis (infiltration IV site)
RESP: Increased thick secretions, wheezing, chest tightness; apnea in neonates, infants, young children

PHARMACOKINETICS
Metabolized in liver; excreted by kidneys, GI tract (inactive metabolites)
PO: Onset 20 min, duration 4-12 hr
IV: Onset 3-5 min

INTERACTIONS
Increase: CNS depression—barbiturates, opioids, hypnotics, tricyclics, alcohol
Increase: promethazine effect—MAOIs
Decrease: oral anticoagulants effect—heparin
Drug/Lab Test
Increase: glucose
False negative: skin allergy test, urine pregnancy test
False positive: urine pregnancy test
Interference: blood grouping (ABO), GTT

NURSING CONSIDERATIONS
Assess:

Black Box Warning: Child: not to be used in children <2 yr, fatal respiratory depression may occur; use cautiously in children >2 yr, seizures, paradoxical CNS stimulation may occur

• **Antiemetic/motion sickness:** nausea, vomiting before, after dose
• I&O ratio; be alert for urinary retention, frequency, dysuria; product should be discontinued
• **Respiratory depression/sedation:** degree of sedation, respiratory risk, CNS depressants may cause increased sedation

- **EPS:** pseudoparkinsonism, dystonia, akathisia, may be worse in geriatric patients
- **Anticholinergic effects:** dry mouth, confusion, urinary retention, more common in geriatric patients
- CBC with differential, LFTs during long-term therapy; blood dyscrasias, jaundice may occur
- Respiratory status: rate, rhythm, increase in bronchial secretions, wheezing, chest tightness
- Cardiac status: palpitations, increased pulse, hypo/hypertension, B/P in those receiving IV doses
- **Neuroleptic malignant syndrome:** fever, confusion, diaphoresis, rigid muscles, elevated CPK, encephalopathy; discontinue product, notify prescriber
- Hard candy, gum, frequent rinsing of mouth for dryness

Evaluate:
- **Therapeutic response:** absence of running, congested nose; rashes; absence of motion sickness, nausea; sedation

Teach patient/family:
- That product may cause photosensitivity; to avoid prolonged exposure to sunlight
- To notify prescriber of confusion, sedation, hypotension, jaundice, fever
- To avoid driving, other hazardous activity if drowsy
- To avoid concurrent use of alcohol or other CNS depressants
- That product may reduce sweating; that there is a risk of heat stroke
- How to use frequent sips of water, gum to decrease dry mouth

---

⚠ HIGH ALERT

propafenone (Rx)
(pro-paff'e-nown)

Rythmol ✦, Rythmol SR

Func. class.: Antidysrhythmic (class IC)

ACTION: Slows conduction velocity; reduces membrane responsiveness; inhibits automaticity; increases ratio of effective refractory period to action potential duration; β-blocking activity

USES: Sustained ventricular tachycardia, atrial fibrillation (single dose), paroxysmal supraventricular tachycardia (PSVT) prophylaxis, supraventricular dysrhythmias
Unlabeled uses: Wolff-Parkinson-White (WPW) syndrome

CONTRAINDICATIONS
2nd/3rd-degree AV block, right bundle branch block, cardiogenic shock, hypersensitivity, bradycardia, uncontrolled HF, sick-sinus syndrome, marked hypotension, bronchospastic disorders, electrolyte imbalance, Brugada syndrome
Precautions: Pregnancy, breastfeeding, children, geriatric patients, HF, hypo/hyperkalemia, nonallergic bronchospasm, renal/hepatic disease, hematologic disorders, myasthenia gravis, COPD

> **Black Box Warning:** Recent MI, cardiac arrhythmias, QT prolongation, torsades de pointes

DOSAGE AND ROUTES
PSVT
- **Adult: PO** 150 mg q8hr; allow 3-4 day interval before increasing dose, max 900 mg/day

Atrial fibrillation
- **Adult: PO** IR: 150 mg q8hr, initially. May increase to 225 mg q8hr, up to 300 mg q8hr after intervals of 3-4 days if needed; SR 225 mg q12hr, may increase to 325 q12hr, max 425 mg q12hr

Available forms: Tabs 150, 225, 300 mg; SR cap 225, 325, 425 mg
Administer:
- Do not break, crush, or chew tabs; swallow whole
- To hospitalized patients because heart monitoring is required
- After hypo/hyperkalemia is corrected
- With dosage adjustment q3-4days
- Without regard to meals

SIDE EFFECTS
CNS: Headache, dizziness, abnormal dreams, syncope, confusion, seizures, insomnia, tremor, anxiety, fatigue
CV: Supraventricular dysrhythmia, ventricular dysrhythmia, bradycardia, prodysrhythmia, palpitations, AV block, intraventricular conduction delay, AV dissociation, hypotension, chest pain, asystole
EENT: Blurred vision, altered taste, tinnitus
GI: *Nausea, vomiting,* constipation, dyspepsia, cholestasis, abnormal hepatic studies, dry mouth, diarrhea, anorexia
HEMA: Leukopenia, agranulocytosis, granulocytopenia, thrombocytopenia, anemia, bruising
INTEG: Rash
RESP: Dyspnea

PHARMACOKINETICS
Peak 3-8 hr, half-life 2-10 hr; poor metabolizers 10-32 hr; metabolized in liver; excreted in urine (metabolite)

INTERACTIONS
Increase: propafenone effects—CYP1A2, CYP2D6, CYP3A4 inhibitors (protease inhibitors, quiNINE, PARoxetine, saquinavir, erythromycin, azole antifungals, sertraline, tricyclics)
Increase: QT prolongation—other class IA/IC antidysrhythmics, arsenic trioxide, chloroquine, clarithromycin, droperidol, erythromycin, haloperidol, methadone, pentamidine, chlorproMAZINE, mesoridazine, thioridazine
Increase: anticoagulation—warfarin
Increase: CNS effects—local anesthetics
Increase: digoxin level—digoxin
Increase: β-blocker effect—propranolol, metoprolol
Increase: cycloSPORINE levels—cycloSPORINE
Decrease: propafenone effect—rifAMPin, cimetidine, quiNIDine
Drug/Food
Increase: propafenone effect—grapefruit juice

Drug/Herb
Decrease: propafenone effect—St. John's wort
Drug/Lab Test
Increase: CPK, Hct, HB
Decrease: WBC, platelets

NURSING CONSIDERATIONS
Assess:
• GI status: bowel pattern, number of stools

Black Box Warning: QT/PR prolongation: ECG or Holter monitor before and during therapy

Black Box Warning: HF: dyspnea, jugular venous distention, crackles, edema in extremities, I&O ratio; check for decreasing output; daily weight

• CBC, ANA titer, LFTs
• Chest x-ray, pulmonary function test during treatment
• Lung fields; bilateral crackles, dyspnea, peripheral edema, weight gain; jugular venous distention may occur in patient with HF
• **Toxicity:** fine tremors, dizziness, hypotension, drowsiness, abnormal heart rate
• **Pregnancy/breastfeeding:** use only if benefits outweigh fetal risk; do not breastfeed, excreted in breast milk
Evaluate:
• **Therapeutic response:** absence of ventricular dysrhythmias; decreasing recurrence of PAF, PSVT
Teach patient/family:
• To avoid hazardous activities until response is known
• To report fever, chills, sore throat, bleeding, SOB, chest pain, palpitations, blurred vision
• To take tab with food; alterations in taste sensation may occur; not to use with grapefruit juice or St. John's wort
• To carry emergency ID identifying medication and prescriber
• To avoid abrupt discontinuation of product; to take as prescribed; not to miss, double doses
• **Pregnancy/breastfeeding:** to notify prescriber if pregnancy is planned or suspected; not to breastfeed

Side effects: *italics* = common; red = life-threatening

TREATMENT OF OVERDOSE:
O₂, artificial ventilation, defibrillation ECG; administer DOPamine for circulatory depression, diazePAM or thiopental for seizures, isoproterenol

---

proparacaine ophthalmic
See Appendix B

> ### ⚠ HIGH ALERT

propofol (Rx)
(pro′poh-fole)
Diprivan
Func. class.: General anesthesia
Chem. class.: Phenol derivative

Do not confuse:
Diprivan/Diflucan/Ditropan

ACTION: Produces dose-dependent CNS depression by activation of GABA receptor, hypnotic

USES: Induction or maintenance of anesthesia as part of balanced anesthetic technique; sedation in mechanically ventilated patients

CONTRAINDICATIONS
Hypersensitivity to this product or soybean oil, egg, benzyl alcohol (some products)
Precautions: Pregnancy, breastfeeding, children, geriatric patients, respiratory depression, severe respiratory disorders, cardiac dysrhythmias, labor and delivery, renal disease, hyperlipidemia

DOSAGE AND ROUTES
Anesthesia
• **Adult <55 yr and ASA-PSI or II: IV** 40 mg q10sec until induction onset, maintenance 100-200 mcg/kg/min or **IV BOL** 20-50 mg prn, allow 3-5 min between adjustments
• **Child ≥3 yr: IV induction** 2.5-3.5 mg/kg over 20-30 sec when not premedicated or lightly premedicated

• **Child 2 mo-16 yr maintenance: IV** 125-300 mcg/kg/min, lower dose for ASA III or IV
Monitored anesthesia care (MAC) sedation
• **Adult <55 yr: IV** 100-150 mcg/kg infusion or 0.5 mg/kg by slow infusion; maintenance 25-75 mcg/kg/min infusion or boluses of 10-20 mg
• **Geriatric debilitated, ASA III/IV:** IV initial, use slower rates; maintenance use 20% less than adult dose
ICU sedation
• **Adult: IV** 5 mcg/kg/min over 5 min; may increase by 5-10 mcg/kg/min over 5-10 min until desired response (Diprivan or generic)
Available forms: Inj 10 mg/mL in 20-mL ampule, vials, syringes
Administer:
IV route
• Shake well before use; dilution is not necessary, but if diluted, use only D₅W to ≥2 mg/mL; give over 3-5 min, titrate to needed level of sedation; use only glass containers when mixing, not stable in plastic; use aseptic technique when transferring from original container
• Only with resuscitative equipment available; only by qualified persons trained in anesthesia
• Store in light-resistant area at room temperature, use within 6 hr of opening
• If transferred from original container to another container, complete infusion within 12 hr (Diprivan), 6 hr (generic propofol)

Y-site compatibilities: Acyclovir, alfentanil, aminophylline, ampicillin, aztreonam, bumetanide, buprenorphine, butorphanol, calcium gluconate, CARBOplatin, ceFAZolin, cefoperazone, cefotaxime, cefoTEtan, cefOXitin, ceftizoxime, cefTRIAXone, cefuroxime, chlorproMAZINE, cimetidine, CISplatin, clindamycin, cyclophosphamide, cycloSPORINE, cytarabine, dexamethasone, diphenhydrAMINE, DOBUTamine, DOPamine, doxycycline, droperidol, enalaprilat, ePHEDrine, EPINEPHrine, esmolol, famotidine, fentaNYL, fluconazole, fluorouracil, furosemide, ganciclovir, glycopyrrolate, granisetron, haloperidol, heparin, hydrocortisone,

HYDROmorphone, hydrOXYzine, ifosfamide, imipenem/cilastatin, inamrinone, insulin (regular), isoproterenol, ketamine, labetalol, levorphanol, lidocaine, LORazepam, magnesium sulfate, mannitol, meperidine, mezlocillin, miconazole, morphine, nafcillin, nalbuphine, naloxone, nitroglycerin, norepinephrine, ofloxacin, PACLitaxel, PENTobarbital, PHENobarbital, piperacillin, potassium chloride, prochlorperazine, propranolol, raNITIdine, scopolamine, sodium bicarbonate, sodium nitroprusside, succinylcholine, SUFentanil, thiopental ticarcillin, ticarcillin/clavulanate, vecuronium, verapamil

Solution compatibilities: if given together via Y-site: D₅W, D₅LR, LR, D₅/0.45% NaCl, D₅/0.2% NaCl

SIDE EFFECTS

CNS: Involuntary movement, headache, fever, dizziness, shivering, abnormal dreams, euphoria, fatigue

CV: *Bradycardia, hypotension,* hypertension

GI: *Nausea, vomiting, abdominal cramping,* dry mouth

GU: Urine retention, green urine, *phlebitis, hives, burning/stinging at inj site,* rash

RESP: Apnea, *cough, hiccups*

SYST: Propofol infusion syndrome

PHARMACOKINETICS

Onset 15-30 sec, rapid distribution, half-life 1-8 min, half-life 3-12 hr; 70% excreted in urine; metabolized in liver by conjugation to inactive metabolites, 95%-99% protein binding, crosses placenta, enters breast milk, crosses blood brain barrier

INTERACTIONS

• Do not use within 10 days of MAOIs

Increase: CNS depression—alcohol, opioids, sedative/hypnotics, antipsychotics, skeletal muscle relaxants, inhalational anesthetics

Drug/Herb

Increase: propofol effect—St. John's wort

NURSING CONSIDERATIONS

Assess:

• Inj site: phlebitis, burning, stinging

• **ECG** for changes: PVC, PAC, ST segment changes; monitor VS, B/P, pulse, respirations

• **Neurologic excitatory symptoms:** movement, tremors, dizziness, LOC, pupil reaction

• Avoid general anesthetic use in child <3 yr; may negatively affect the brain

• Allergic reactions: hives

• **Respiratory dysfunction:** respiratory depression, character, rate, rhythm; notify prescriber if respirations are <10/min, apnea may occur ≥1 min, check airway, ventilation, determine level of sedation

• **Propofol infusion syndrome:** rhabdomyolysis, renal failure, hyperkalemia, metabolic acidosis, cardiac dysrhythmias, heart failure usually between 35 and 93 hr after infusion begun at >5 mg/kg/hr for >48 hr

• **ICU sedation:** test wake up on a daily basis to determine needed dose for sedation, do not discontinue abruptly during test

• **For lipids:** adjust enteral nutrition if receiving; monitor for signs and symptoms of pancreatitis (elevated lipids); propofol contains 1.1 Kcal/mL

• **Pregnancy/breastfeeding:** use only if clearly needed; avoid breastfeeding, excreted in breast milk

Evaluate:

• **Therapeutic response:** induction of anesthesia

Teach patient/family:

• That product will cause dizziness, drowsiness, sedation; to avoid hazardous activities until drug effect wears off

• That drug may cause burning sensation during administration

TREATMENT OF OVERDOSE:

Discontinue product; administer vasopressor agents or anticholinergics, artificial ventilation

---

⚠ HIGH ALERT

propranolol (Rx)

(proe-pran′oh-lole)

Inderal LA, Inderal XL, InnoPran XL, Hemangeol

Func. class.: Antihypertensive, antianginal, antidysrhythmic (class II)

Chem. class.: β-Adrenergic blocker

Side effects: *italics* = common; red = life-threatening

Do not confuse:
Inderal/Adderall

ACTION: Nonselective β-blocker with negative inotropic, chronotropic, dromotropic properties

USES: Chronic stable angina pectoris, hypertension, supraventricular dysrhythmias, migraine prophylaxis, pheochromocytoma, cyanotic spells related to hypertrophic subaortic stenosis, essential tremor, acute MI, vascular headache prophylaxis
Unlabeled uses: Anxiety, prevention of variceal bleeding caused by portal hypertension, akathisia induced by antipsychotics, portal hypertension, sclerodermal renal crisis, unstable angina

CONTRAINDICATIONS
Hypersensitivity to this product; cardiogenic shock, AV heart block; bronchospastic disease; sinus bradycardia; bronchospasm; asthma
Precautions: Pregnancy, breastfeeding, children, diabetes mellitus, hyperthyroidism, COPD, renal/hepatic disease, myasthenia gravis, peripheral vascular disease, hypotension, cardiac failure, Raynaud's disease, sick sinus syndrome, vasospastic angina, smoking, Wolff-Parkinson-White syndrome, thyrotoxicosis

> **Black Box Warning:** Abrupt discontinuation

DOSAGE AND ROUTES
Dysrhythmias
• **Adult: PO** 10-30 mg tid-qid; **IV BOL** 1-3 mg give 1 mg/min; may repeat after 2 min, may repeat q4hr thereafter
• **Child: PO** 0.5 to 1 mg/kg/day divided q6-8hr, initially. Increase by 1 mg/kg/day q3-5 days as needed for clinical effect. Usual dose: 2-4 mg/kg/day. Max: 16 mg/kg/day or 60 mg/day, whichever is less; **IV** 0.01-0.1 mg/kg over 5 min; 0.01 mg/kg/dose q6-8hr as needed. May titrate dosage gradually as needed for clinical effect. Max: 0.15 mg/kg/dose or 3 mg/dose, whichever is less

Hypertension
• **Adult: PO** 40 mg bid or 80 mg/day (ext rel) initially; usual dose 120-240 mg/day bid-tid or 120-160 mg/day (ext rel)
• **Child: PO** 0.5 to 2 mg/kg/day in 2-4 divided doses. Titrate gradually q3-7days as needed for clinical effect; HR rate may be dose-limiting. Usual effective dosage is 1-6 mg/kg/day. Max: 8 mg/kg/day or 640 mg/day, whichever is less

Angina
• **Adult: PO** 10-20 mg bid-qid, increase at 3-7 day intervals up to 160-320 mg/day or **EXT REL** 80 mg daily

MI prophylaxis
• **Adult: PO** 180-240 mg/day divided tid-qid starting 5 days to 2 wk after MI

Pheochromocytoma
• **Adult: PO** 60 mg/day × 3 days preoperatively in divided doses or 30 mg/day in divided doses (inoperable tumor)

Migraine
• **Adult: PO** 80 mg/day (ext rel) or in divided doses; may increase to 160-240 mg/day in divided doses
• **Child >35 kg (unlabeled): PO** 0.6 to 3 mg/kg/day in 2 to 3 divided doses. Max: 120 mg/day
• **Child ≤35 kg (unlabeled): PO** 0.6 to 3 mg/kg/day in 2 to 3 divided doses. Max: 60 mg/day

Essential tremor
• **Adult: PO** 40 mg bid; usual dose 120-320 mg/day

Acute MI
• **Adult: PO** 180-320 mg/day in 3-4 divided doses; **IV** 0.1 mg/kg in 3 divided doses at 2-3 min intervals

Anxiety (unlabeled)
• **Adult: PO** 10-80 mg given 1 hr before anxiety-producing event

Scleroderma renal crisis (unlabeled)
• **Adult: PO** 40 mg bid, may increase q3-7days, max 160-480 mg/day

Esophageal varices (portal hypertension) (unlabeled)
• **Adult: PO** 40 mg bid, titrate to heart rate reduction of 25%
Available forms: Ext rel caps 60, 80, 120, 160 mg; tabs 10, 20, 40, 60, 80, 90 mg; inj

1 mg/mL; oral sol 20 mg, 40 mg/mL; oral sol (Hemangeol) 4.28 mg/mL

Administer:

PO route

• Do not break, crush, chew, or open ext rel cap

• Do not use ext rel cap for essential tremor, MI, cardiac dysrhythmias; do not use InnoPran XL in hypertropic subaortic stenosis, migraine, angina pectoris

• Ext rel caps should be taken daily; InnoPran XL should be taken at bedtime

• May mix oral sol with liquid or semisolid food; rinse container to get entire dose

• With 8 oz water with food; food enhances bioavailability

• Do not give with aluminum-containing antacid; may decrease GI absorption

Direct IV route

IV undiluted or diluted 10 mL D_5W for inj; give 0.5 mg/min (adult), over 10 min (child)

Intermittent IV INFUSION route

• May be diluted in 50 mL NaCl and run over 10-15 min

Y-site compatibilities: Acyclovir, alfentanil, alteplase, amikacin, aminocaproic acid, aminophylline, anidulafungin, ascorbic acid, atracurium, atropine, azaTHIOprine, aztreonam, benztropine, bivalirudin, bleomycin, bumetanide, buprenorphine, butorphanol, calcium chloride/gluconate, CARBOplatin, carmustine, caspofungin, cefamandole, ceFAZolin, cefmetazole, cefonicid, cefoperazone, cefotaxime, cefoTEtan, cefOXitin, cefTAZidime, ceftizoxime, cefTRIAXone, cefuroxime, cephalothin, cephapirin, chloramphenicol, chlorproMAZINE, cimetidine, CISplatin, clindamycin, cyanocobalamin, cyclophosphamide, cycloSPORINE, cytarabine, DACTINomycin, DAPTOmycin, dexamethasone, digoxin, diltiaZEM, diphenhydrAMINE, DOBUTamine, DOCEtaxel, DOPamine, doxacurium, DOXOrubicin, doxycycline, enalaprilat, ePHEDrine, EPINEPHrine, epirubicin, epoetin alfa, eptifibatide, ertapenem, erythromycin, esmolol, etoposide, etoposide phosphate, famotidine, fenoldopam, fentaNYL, fluconazole, fludarabine, fluorouracil, folic acid, furosemide, ganciclovir, gatifloxacin, gemcitabine, gemtuzumab, gentamicin, glycopyrrolate, granisetron, heparin, hydrocortisone, HYDROmorphone, hydrOXYzine, IDArubicin, ifosfamide, imipenem-cilastatin, inamrinone, irinotecan, isoproterenol, ketorolac, labetalol, levoFLOXacin, lidocaine, linezolid, LORazepam, magnesium, mannitol, mechlorethamine, meperidine, metaraminol, methicillin, methotrexate, methoxamine, methyldopa, methylPREDNISolone, metoclopramide, metoprolol, metroNIDAZOLE, mezlocillin, miconazole, midazolam, milrinone, minocycline, mitoXANTRONE, morphine, moxalactam, multiple vitamins, mycophenolate, nafcillin, nalbuphine, naloxone, nesiritide, netilmicin, nitroglycerin, nitroprusside, norepinephrine, octreotide, ondansetron, oxacillin, oxaliplatin, oxytocin, palonosetron, pamidronate, pancuronium, papaverine, PEMEtrexed, penicillin G potassium/sodium, pentamidine, pentazocine, PENTobarbital, PHENobarbital, phenylephrine, phytonadione, piperacillin, polymyxin B, potassium chloride, procainamide, prochlorperazine, promethazine, propofol, protamine, pyridoxine, quiNIDine, quinupristin-dalfopristin, raNITIdine, ritodrine, rocuronium, sodium acetate/bicarbonate, succinylcholine, SUFentanil, tacrolimus, teniposide, theophylline, thiamine, thiotepa, ticarcillin, ticarcillin-clavulanate, tigecycline, tirofiban, tobramycin, tolazoline, trimetaphan, urokinase, vancomycin, vasopressin, vecuronium, verapamil, vinCRIStine, vinorelbine, vitamin B complex/C, voriconazole, zoledronic acid

SIDE EFFECTS

CNS: Depression, hallucinations, *dizziness, fatigue,* lethargy, paresthesias, bizarre dreams, disorientation

CV: Bradycardia, hypotension, HF, palpitations, AV block, peripheral vascular insufficiency, vasodilation, cold extremities, pulmonary edema, dysrhythmias

EENT: Sore throat, laryngospasm, blurred vision, dry eyes

Side effects: *italics* = common; red = life-threatening

GI: Nausea, vomiting, diarrhea, colitis, constipation, cramps, dry mouth, hepatomegaly, gastric pain, acute pancreatitis
GU: Impotence, decreased libido, UTIs
HEMA: Agranulocytosis, thrombocytopenia
INTEG: Rash, pruritus, fever, Stevens-Johnson syndrome, toxic epidermal necrolysis
META: Hyperglycemia, hypoglycemia
MISC: Facial swelling, weight change, Raynaud's phenomenon
MS: Joint pain, arthralgia, muscle cramps, pain
RESP: Dyspnea, respiratory dysfunction, *bronchospasm*, cough

PHARMACOKINETICS
Metabolized by liver; crosses placenta, blood-brain barrier; excreted in breast milk; protein binding 90%; ✡ CYP2D6 enzyme system causes 7% of population to be poor metabolizers
PO: Onset 30 min, peak 1-1½ hr, duration 12 hr, half-life 3-8 hr
PO-ER: Peak 6 hr, duration 24 hr, half-life 8-11 hr
IV: Onset 2 min, peak 1 min, duration 2-4 hr

INTERACTIONS
Increase: toxicity—phenothiazines
Increase: propranolol level—propafenone
Increase: effect of calcium channel blockers, neuromuscular blocker
Increase: negative inotropic effects—disopyramide
Increase: β-blocking effect—cimetidine
Increase: hypotension—quiNIDine, haloperidol, prazosin
Decrease: β-blocking effects—barbiturates
Decrease: propranolol levels—smoking
Drug/Herb
• Avoid use with feverfew
Increase: antihypertensive effect—hawthorn
Decrease: antihypertensive effect—ma huang

Drug/Lab Test
Increase: serum potassium, serum uric acid, ALT, AST, alk phos, LDH
Decrease: blood glucose
Interference: glaucoma testing

NURSING CONSIDERATIONS
Assess:

Black Box Warning: **Abrupt withdrawal:** taper over 1-2 wk, do not discontinue abruptly; dysrhythmias, angina, myocardial ischemia, or MI may recur

• B/P, pulse, respirations during beginning therapy; notify prescriber if pulse <50 bpm or systolic B/P <90 mm Hg
• **ECG** continuously if using as antidysrhythmic IV, PCWP (pulmonary capillary wedge pressure), CVP (central venous pressure)
• Hepatic enzymes: AST, ALT, bilirubin; blood glucose (diabetes mellitus)
• Angina pain: duration, time started, activity being performed, character
• Tolerance with long-term use
• Headache, light-headedness, decreased B/P; may indicate need for decreased dosage; may aggravate symptoms of arterial insufficiency
• **Fluid overload:** weight daily; report gain of >5 lb
• I&O ratio, CCr if kidney damage is diagnosed; fatigue, weight gain, jugular distention, dyspnea, peripheral edema, crackles
• **Pregnancy/breastfeeding:** use only if benefits outweigh fetal risk, cautious use in breastfeeding
Evaluate:
• **Therapeutic response:** decreased B/P, dysrhythmias
Teach patient/family:
• Not to discontinue abruptly; may precipitate life-threatening dysrhythmias, exacerbation of angina, MI; to take product at same time each day, either with or without food consistently; to decrease dosage over 2 wk
• To avoid OTC products unless approved by prescriber; to avoid alcohol
• To avoid hazardous activities if dizzy

• About the importance of compliance with complete medical regimen; to monitor blood glucose, may mask symptoms of hypoglycemia
• To make position changes slowly to prevent fainting
• That sensitivity to cold may occur
• How to take pulse, B/P; to withhold product if <50 bpm or systolic B/P <90 mm Hg

---

propranolol/hydrochlorothiazide (Rx)

(proe-pran'oh-lole/hye-droe-klor-oh-thye'a-zide)
Func. class.: Antihypertensive, nonselective beta-blocker, thiazide diuretic

---

USES: Management of hypertension

CONTRAINDICATIONS
Hypersensitivity to propranolol, hydrochlorothiazide, other beta-blockers, other sulfonamide-derived drugs, or any component; HF; cardiogenic shock; sinus bradycardia; heart block >1st-degree; asthma; anuria

Black Box Warning: Abrupt withdrawal

DOSAGE AND ROUTES
Hypertension
• **Adult:** PO Propranolol 40 mg/hydrochlorothiazide 25 mg bid; may titrate gradually based on B/P; max propranolol 160 mg/hydrochlorothiazide 50 mg/day
Available forms: Tabs 40/25, 80/25 mg

⚠ HIGH ALERT

propylthiouracil (Rx)

(proe-pill-thye-oh-yoor'a-sill)
Func. class.: Thyroid hormone antagonist (antithyroid)
Chem. class.: Thioamide

ACTION: Blocks synthesis peripherally of T_3, T_4 (triiodothyronine, thyroxine), inhibits organification of iodine

USES: Preparation for thyroidectomy, thyrotoxic crisis, hyperthyroidism, thyroid storm

CONTRAINDICATIONS
Pregnancy, breastfeeding, hypersensitivity
Precautions: Infants, bone marrow depression, fever, agranulocytosis, hepatitis, jaundice

Black Box Warning: Hepatic disease, pregnancy

DOSAGE AND ROUTES
Thyrotoxic crisis
• **Adult/child:** PO 200-400 mg q4hr for 1st 24 hr
Preparation for thyroidectomy
• **Adult:** PO 600-1200 mg/day
• **Child:** PO 10 mg/kg/day in divided doses
Hyperthyroidism
• **Adult:** PO 50-150 mg tid increasing to 300 mg q8hr if condition is severe; continue to euthyroid state, then 100 mg daily tid
• **Child >6 yr:** PO 50 mg/day divided q8hr, titrate based on TSH/free T_4 levels
• **Neonate (unlabeled):** PO 5-10 mg/kg/day in divided doses q8hr
Available forms: Tabs 50, 100 ✦ mg
Administer:
• With meals to decrease GI upset
• At same time each day to maintain product level
• At lowest dose that relieves symptoms

SIDE EFFECTS
CNS: *Drowsiness, headache, vertigo, fever,* paresthesias, neuritis
GI: *Nausea, diarrhea, vomiting,* jaundice, hepatitis, loss of taste, liver failure, death
GU: Nephritis
HEMA: Agranulocytosis, leukopenia, thrombocytopenia, hypothrombinemia,

---

lymphadenopathy, bleeding, vasculitis, periarteritis

INTEG: *Rash, urticaria, pruritus, alopecia, hyperpigmentation,* lupuslike syndrome

MS: Myalgia, arthralgia, nocturnal muscle cramps, osteoporosis

PHARMACOKINETICS

Onset up to 3 wk, peak 6-10 wk, duration 1 wk to 1 mo, half-life 1-2 hr; excreted in urine, bile, breast milk; crosses placenta; concentration in thyroid gland

INTERACTIONS

• Bone marrow suppression: radiation, antineoplastics

• Agranulocytosis: phenothiazines

Increase: effects—potassium/sodium iodide, lithium

Decrease: anticoagulant effect—heparin, oral anticoagulants

Drug/Lab Test

Increase: PT, AST, ALT, alk phos

NURSING CONSIDERATIONS

Assess:

• **Hyperthyroidism:** weight loss, nervousness, insomnia, fever, diaphoresis, tremors; **hypothyroidism:** constipation, dry skin, weakness, headache; monitor T_3, T_4, which are increased; serum TSH, which is decreased; free thyroxine index, which is increased if dosage is too low; discontinue product 3-4 wk before RAIU

• Pulse, B/P, temperature

• I&O ratio; check for edema: puffy hands, feet, periorbits; indicates hypothyroidism

• Weight daily; same clothing, scale, time of day

• **Blood dyscrasias:** CBC with differential; leukopenia, thrombocytopenia, agranulocytosis; monitor periodically; agranulocytosis may develop in first 2 mo of treatment; discontinue treatment

• **Overdose:** peripheral edema, heat intolerance, diaphoresis, palpitations, dysrhythmias, severe tachycardia, increased temperature, delirium, CNS irritability

• **Hypersensitivity:** rash, enlarged cervical lymph nodes; product may have to be discontinued

• **Hypoprothrombinemia:** bleeding, petechiae, ecchymosis

• Clinical response: after 3 wk should include increased weight, pulse; decreased T_4

• **Bone marrow suppression:** sore throat, fever, fatigue

> **Black Box Warning: Hepatotoxicity:** LFTs before, during treatment; jaundice, nausea, vomiting, abdominal pain, anorexia, diarrhea, fatigue

• Fluids to 3-4 L/day unless contraindicated

> **Black Box Warning: Pregnancy/breastfeeding:** do not use in pregnancy, breastfeeding

Evaluate:

• **Therapeutic response:** weight gain, decreased pulse, decreased T_4, decreased B/P

Teach patient/family:

• To take pulse daily

• To report redness, swelling, sore throat, mouth lesions, which indicate blood dyscrasias; to report symptoms of hepatic dysfunction (yellow skin or eyes, clay-colored stools, dark urine)

• To keep graph of weight, pulse, mood

• To avoid OTC products that contain iodine

• That seafood, other iodine products may be restricted

• Not to discontinue product abruptly because thyroid crisis may occur; about stress response

• That response may take several months if thyroid is large

• About the symptoms/signs of overdose: periorbital edema, cold intolerance, mental depression

• About the symptoms of an inadequate dose: tachycardia, diarrhea, fever, irritability

• To take medication as prescribed; not to skip or double dose; that missed doses should be taken when remembered up to 1 hr before next dose

• To carry emergency ID listing condition, medication

> **Black Box Warning: Pregnancy:** to notify prescriber immediately if pregnancy is planned or suspected; not to breastfeed

protamine (Rx)

(proe´ta-meen)

Func. class.: Heparin antagonist

Chem. class.: Low-molecular-weight protein

Do not confuse:

protamine/Protonix

ACTION: Binds heparin, thereby making it ineffective

USES: Heparin, LMWH toxicity, hemorrhage

CONTRAINDICATIONS

Black Box Warning: Hypersensitivity

Precautions: Pregnancy, breastfeeding, fish allergy, diabetes, previous exposure to protamine, insulins, heparin rebound or bleeding

Black Box Warning: Requires a specialized care setting

DOSAGE AND ROUTES
Heparin overdose

• **Adult/child:** IV 1 mg of protamine/100 units heparin given; administer slowly over 1-3 min; max 50 mg/10 min

Enoxaparin overdose

• **Adult:** IV 1 mg protamine/1 mg enoxaparin

Dalteparin overdose

• **Adult:** IV 1 mg protamine/100 anti-Xa unit

Available forms: Inj 10 mg/mL

Administer:

• Store at 36° F-46° F (2° C-8° C)

Direct IV route

• May give diluted or undiluted

• After reconstituting 50 mg/5 mL sterile bacteriostatic water for inj; shake, give ≤20 mg over 1-3 min, do not give rapidly

Y-site compatibilities: Alfentanil, amikacin, aminophylline, ascorbic acid, atracurium, atropine, azaTHIOprine, aztreonam, benztropine, bumetanide, buprenorphine, butorphanol, calcium chloride/gluconate, cefTAZidime, chlorproMAZINE, cimetidine, clindamycin, cyanocobalamin, cycloSPORINE, digoxin, diphenhydrAMINE, DOBUTamine, DOPamine, doxycycline, enalaprilat, ePHEDrine, EPINEPHrine, epoetin alfa, erythromycin, esmolol, famotidine, fentaNYL, fluconazole, ganciclovir, gentamicin, glycopyrrolate, hydrOXYzine, imipenem-cilastatin, inamrinone, iohexol, iopamidol, iothalamate, isoproterenol, labetalol, lidocaine, magnesium, mannitol, meperidine, metaraminol, methoxamine, methyldopate, metoclopramide, metoprolol, miconazole, midazolam, minocycline, morphine, multiple vitamins, nalbuphine, naloxone, netilmicin, nitroglycerin, nitroprusside, norepinephrine, ondansetron, oxytocin, papaverine, pentazocine, phenylephrine, polymyxin B, potassium chloride, procainamide, prochlorperazine, promethazine, propranolol, pyridoxine, quiNIDine, raNITIdine, Ringer's, ritodrine, sodium bicarbonate, succinylcholine, SUFentanil, theophylline, thiamine, tobramycin, tolazoline, trimetaphan, urokinase, vancomycin, vasopressin, verapamil

SIDE EFFECTS

CV: Hypotension, bradycardia, circulatory collapse, capillary leak

GI: Nausea, vomiting

HEMA: Bleeding, heparin rebound (cardiac surgery)

INTEG: *Rash,* dermatitis, urticaria

RESP: Dyspnea, pulmonary edema, severe respiratory distress, bronchospasm

SYST: Anaphylaxis, angioedema

PHARMACOKINETICS

IV: Onset 5 min, duration 2 hr, half-life unknown

NURSING CONSIDERATIONS
Assess:

• **Bleeding:** 30 min to 18 hr after dose in cardiac surgery

Black Box Warning: Hypersensitivity: urticaria, cough, wheezing, have emergency equipment nearby; allergy to fish; use with caution; men who have had vasectomies may be more prone to hypersensitivity, also high doses

P

Side effects: *italics* = common; red = life-threatening

- Blood studies (Hct, platelets, occult blood in stools)
- Coagulation tests (aPTT, ACT) 15 min after dose, then again after several hours
- VS, B/P, pulse after 30 min, then 3 hr after dose
- Skin rash, urticaria, dermatitis
- **Pregnancy/breastfeeding:** use only if clearly needed; cautious use in breastfeeding

Evaluate:
- **Therapeutic response:** reversal of heparin overdose

Teach patient/family:
- Not to take if allergic to fish
- The purpose of product, expected result
- To avoid activities in which bleeding may occur—shaving, use of hard-bristle toothbrush, injections, rectal temperature—until risk for bleeding has passed

---

protein C concentrate (Rx)

(proe'teen cee kon'suhn-trate)

Ceprotin

Func. class.: Blood product derivative

USES: Prevention/treatment of venous thrombosis and purpura fulminans in severe congenital protein C deficiency

CONTRAINDICATIONS
None known

DOSAGE AND ROUTES
Severe congenital protein C deficiency
- **Adult/child:** IV: Acute episode/short-term prophylaxis: Initial dose: 100-120 units/kg; subsequent 3 doses: 60-80 units/kg q6hr (adjust to maintain peak protein C activity of 100%); maintenance dose: 45-60 units/kg q6h or 12h (adjust to maintain recommended maintenance trough protein C activity levels >25%); long-term prophylaxis: maintenance dose: 45-60 units/kg q12h (recommended maintenance trough protein C activity levels >25%)

Available forms: Injection 500, 1000 IU/vial

---

prucalopride (Rx)

(proo-kal'oh-pride)

Motegrity, Resotran ♦

Func. class.: GI prokinetic, serotonin 5-HT$_4$ receptor agonist

USES: Treatment of chronic idiopathic constipation

CONTRAINDICATIONS
Hypersensitivity to prucalopride or any component, intestinal perforation/obstruction, Crohn disease, ulcerative colitis, toxic megacolon

DOSAGE AND ROUTES
Chronic idiopathic constipation
- **Adult:** PO 2 mg daily; used as added laxative if no bowel movement within ≥3 days

Available forms: Tabs 1, 2 mg

---

pseudoephedrine (OTC, Rx)

(soo-doh-eh-fed'rin)

Eltor ♦, Sudafed, Sudafed 24 Hour, Sudogest (many products)

Func. class.: Adrenergic

Chem. class.: Substituted phenylethylamine

Controlled Substance Schedule V

Do not confuse:
Sudafed/sotalol

ACTION: Primary activity through α-effects on respiratory mucosal membranes reducing congestion, hyperemia, edema; minimal bronchodilation secondary to β-effects

USES: Nasal decongestant, adjunct for otitis media; with antihistamines

---

CONTRAINDICATIONS

Hypersensitivity to sympathomimetics, closed-angle glaucoma

Precautions: Pregnancy, breastfeeding, cardiac disorders, hyperthyroidism, diabetes mellitus, prostatic hypertrophy, hypertension, child <4 yr

DOSAGE AND ROUTES

• **Adult and child >12 yr: PO** 60 mg q6hr; **EXT REL** 120 mg q12hr or 240 mg q24hr
• **Geriatric: PO** 30-60 mg q6hr prn
• **Child 6-12 yr: PO** 30 mg q6hr, max 120 mg/day
• **Child 4-6 yr: PO** 15 mg q6hr, max 60 mg/day

Available forms: Ext rel caps 120, 240 mg; oral sol 15 mg, 30 mg/5 mL; tabs 30, 60 mg; ext rel tabs 120, 240 mg

Administer:
• Avoid taking at or near bedtime; stimulation can occur
• OTC preparations require an ID for sale; tracked, Schedule V

SIDE EFFECTS

CNS: *Tremors, anxiety,* stimulation, insomnia, headache, dizziness, hallucinations, seizures (geriatric patients)
CV: Palpitations, tachycardia, hypertension, chest pain, dysrhythmias, CV collapse
EENT: Dry nose; irritation of nose and throat
GI: *Anorexia, nausea, vomiting,* dry mouth, ischemic colitis
GU: Dysuria

PHARMACOKINETICS

PO: Onset 15-30 min; duration 4-6 hr, 8-12 hr (ext rel); metabolized in liver; excreted in feces and breast milk; half-life 7 hr (adult), 3 hr (child)

INTERACTIONS

• Do not use with MAOIs or tricyclics; hypertensive crisis may occur
Increase: effect of this product—urinary alkalizers, adrenergics, β-blockers, phenothiazines, tricyclics
Decrease: effect of this product—urinary acidifiers

NURSING CONSIDERATIONS

Assess:
• **Nasal congestion:** auscultate lung sounds; check for tenacious bronchial secretions
• B/P, pulse throughout treatment
• **Beers:** avoid in older adults; CNS stimulant effects, seizures, hallucinations, excitation
• **Pregnancy/breastfeeding:** avoid in pregnancy; cautious use in breastfeeding
Evaluate:
• **Therapeutic response:** decreased nasal, eustachian tube, congestion
Teach patient/family:
• About the reason for product administration
• Ext rel: do not divide, crush, chew, or dissolve
• Do not use within 14 days of MAOIs
• Not to use continuously or to take more than recommended dose because rebound congestion may occur
• To notify prescriber immediately of anxiety, slow or fast heart rate, dyspnea, seizures
• To check with prescriber before using other products because product interactions may occur
• To avoid taking near bedtime because stimulation can occur
• Not to use if stimulation, restlessness, tremors occur
• That use in children may cause excessive agitation
• To notify provider if symptoms do not improve within 7 days or if having a fever

---

psyllium (OTC, Rx)
(sill'ee-um)
Hydrocil, Leader Fiber Laxative, Metamucil, Natural Fiber, Natural Vegetable Fiber, Reguloid, Wal-Mucil, Konsyl
Func. class.: Bulk laxative
Chem. class.: Psyllium colloid

ACTION: Bulk-forming laxative

USES: Chronic constipation, ulcerative colitis

Unlabeled uses: Diarrhea, diverticulosis, irritable bowel syndrome, hypercholesterolemia

CONTRAINDICATIONS

Hypersensitivity, intestinal obstruction, abdominal pain, nausea, vomiting, fecal impaction

Precautions: Pregnancy

DOSAGE AND ROUTES

• **Adult: PO** 1-2 tsp in 8 oz water bid or tid, then 8 oz water or 1 premeasured packet in 8 oz water bid or tid, then 8 oz water

• **Child >6 yr: PO** 1 tsp in 4 oz water at bedtime

Available forms: Chew pieces 1.7, 3.4 g/piece; effervescent powder 3.4, 3.7 g/packet; powder 3.3, 3.4, 3.5, 4.94 g/tsp; wafers 3.4 g/wafer

Administer:

PO route

• Alone for better absorption, separate from other products by 1-2 hr

• In morning or evening (oral dose)

• Immediately after mixing with water or will congeal

• With 8 oz water or juice followed by another 8 oz of fluid

SIDE EFFECTS

GI: *Nausea, vomiting, anorexia, diarrhea,* cramps, intestinal or esophageal blockage

PHARMACOKINETICS

Onset 12-72 hr, excreted in feces, not absorbed in GI tract

INTERACTIONS

Decrease: absorption of cardiac glycosides, oral anticoagulants, salicylates

Drug/Herb

Increase: laxative effect—flax, senna

NURSING CONSIDERATIONS

Assess:

• Blood, urine electrolytes if used often

• I&O ratio to identify fluid loss

• **Constipation:** cause of constipation; fluids, bulk, exercise missing; bowel sounds, distention, usual bowel function; color, consistency, amount, cramping, rectal bleeding, nausea, vomiting; product should be discontinued

• **Pregnancy/breastfeeding:** generally considered safe in pregnancy, breastfeeding

Evaluate:

• **Therapeutic response:** decrease in constipation, decreased diarrhea with colitis

Teach patient/family:

• To maintain adequate fluid consumption

• That normal bowel movements do not always occur daily

• Not to use in presence of abdominal pain, nausea, vomiting

• To notify prescriber if constipation unrelieved or if symptoms of electrolyte imbalance occur: muscle cramps, pain, weakness, dizziness, excessive thirst

---

pyrazinamide (Rx)

(peer-a-zin'a-mide)

Func. class.: Antitububerculotic

USES:

Mycobacterium tuberculosis, drug-susceptible TB as part of combination therapy (without HIV)

DOSAGE AND ROUTES

• **Adults > 90 kg (lean body weight): PO** 15-30 mg/kg/dose once daily (max: 3 g/day) or 50-75 mg/kg/dose twice weekly

• **Adults weighing 76 to 90 kg (lean body weight): PO** 2 g once daily or 5 days/wk, or alternatively, 3 g 3 days/wk or 4 g twice weekly

• **Adults weighing 56 to 75 kg (lean body weight): PO** 1.5 g once daily or 5 days/wk, or alternatively, 2.5 g 3 days/wk or 3 g twice weekly

• **Infants, children, and adolescents 30-40 mg/kg/dose (lean body weight) (max: 2 g/dose): PO** once daily or 5 days/wk, or alternatively, 50 mg/kg/dose (lean body weight) 3 days/wk (max: 3 g/dose) or twice weekly (max: 4 g/dose)

Available forms: Tabs 500 mg

---

pyrethrins/piperonyl (Rx, OTC)

(pi-reth′rinz/pye-per′oh-nil)

Lice Shampoo ♣, RID

Func. class.: Pediculicide, pyrethrin

USES: Treatment of *Pediculus humanus* infestations

CONTRAINDICATIONS
Hypersensitivity

DOSAGE AND ROUTES
Pediculosis capitis (head lice infestation)/pediculosis corporis (body lice infestation)
• **Child:** Topical: Apply to *dry* scalp hair or other affected areas in an amount sufficient to thoroughly wet the area, if treating head lice, first apply behind ears and to back of neck, after 10 min, add warm water to form a good lather, wash, and thoroughly rinse with water until all lather is gone, dry hair with a clean towel and comb with a fine-tooth comb to remove any remaining nits, repeat after 7-10 days

Available forms: Shampoo 0.33%/4%

---

pyridostigmine (Rx)

(peer-id-oh-stig′meen)

Mestinon, Regonol

Func. class.: Cholinergic; anticholinesterase

Chem. class.: Tertiary amine carbamate

ACTION: Inhibits destruction of acetylcholine, which increases concentration at sites where acetylcholine is released; this facilitates the transmission of impulses across the myoneural junction

USES: Nondepolarizing muscle relaxant antagonist, myasthenia gravis, pretreatment for nerve gas exposure (military only)

CONTRAINDICATIONS
Bradycardia; hypotension; obstruction of intestine, renal system; bromide, benzyl alcohol sensitivity; adrenal insufficiency; cholinesterase inhibitor toxicity

Precautions: Pregnancy, seizure disorders, bronchial asthma, coronary occlusion, hyperthyroidism, dysrhythmias, peptic ulcer, megacolon, poor GI motility

DOSAGE AND ROUTES
Myasthenia gravis
• **Adult:** **PO** 600 mg/day in 5-6 divided doses, max 1.5 g/day; **IM/IV** 2 mg; **SUS REL** 180-540 mg/day or bid at intervals of ≥6 hr
• **Child:** **PO** 7 mg/kg/day in 5-6 divided doses; **IM/IV** 0.05-0.15 mg/kg/dose
Nondepolarizing neuromuscular blocker antagonist
• **Adult:** 0.6-1.2 mg **IV** atropine, then 0.1-0.25 mg/kg/dose
• **Child:** **IV** 0.1-0.25 mg/kg/dose
Nerve gas exposure prophylaxis (military)
• **Adult:** **PO** 30 mg q8hr if threat of exposure to Soman gas is anticipated; start several hours before exposure and discontinue upon exposure; after product is discontinued, give antidotes (atropine, pralidoxime)

Available forms: Tabs 60 mg; ext rel tabs 180 mg; syr 60 mg/5 mL; inj 5 mg/mL

Administer:
• Only with atropine sulfate available for cholinergic crisis
• Only after all other cholinergics have been discontinued
• Increased doses for tolerance as ordered
• Larger doses after exercise or fatigue as ordered
• Do not break, crush, or chew sus rel tabs
PO route
• On empty stomach for better absorption

Side effects: *italics* = common; red = life-threatening

Direct IV route

• Undiluted (5 mg/mL), give through Y-tube or 3-way stopcock, give ≤0.5 mg/min (myasthenia gravis); 5 mg/min (reversal of nondepolarizing neuromuscular blockers)

Y-site compatibilities: Heparin, hydrocortisone, potassium chloride, vit B/C

SIDE EFFECTS

CNS: Dizziness, headache, sweating, weakness, seizures, incoordination, paralysis, drowsiness, LOC

CV: Tachycardia, dysrhythmias, bradycardia, AV block, hypotension, ECG changes, cardiac arrest, syncope

EENT: Miosis, blurred vision, lacrimation, visual changes

GI: *Nausea, diarrhea, vomiting, cramps, increased salivary and gastric secretions, peristalsis*

GU: Urinary frequency, incontinence, urgency

INTEG: Rash, urticaria, flushing

RESP: Respiratory depression, bronchospasm, constriction, laryngospasm, respiratory arrest

SYST: Cholinergic crisis

PHARMACOKINETICS

Metabolized in liver, excreted in urine (unchanged)

PO: Onset 20-30 min, duration 3-6 hr

PO-EXT REL: Onset 30-60 min, duration 6-12 hr

IM/IV/SUBCUT: Onset 2-15 min, duration 2 ½-4 hr

INTERACTIONS

Increase: action—succinylcholine

Decrease: action—gallamine, metocurine, pancuronium, tubocurarine, atropine

Decrease: pyridostigmine action—aminoglycosides, anesthetics, procainamide, quiNIDine, mecamylamine, polymyxin, magnesium, corticosteroids, antidysrhythmics, quinolones

NURSING CONSIDERATIONS

Assess:

• **Myasthenia gravis:** fatigue, ptosis, diplopia, difficulty swallowing, SOB, hand/gait before, after product; improvement should be seen after 1 hr

• VS, respiration q8hr

• I&O ratio; check for urinary retention or incontinence

• **Toxicity:** bradycardia, hypotension, bronchospasm, headache, dizziness, seizures, respiratory depression; product should be discontinued if toxicity occurs

• **Pregnancy/breastfeeding:** use only if benefits outweigh fetal risk; cautious use in breastfeeding

Evaluate:

• **Therapeutic response:** increased muscle strength, hand grasp, improved gait, absence of labored breathing (if severe), negative inspiratory force, and vital capacity; reversal of nondepolarizing neuromuscular blockers; prevention of nerve gas toxicity

Teach patient/family:

• **Myasthenia gravis:** that product is not a cure, only relieves symptoms

• To wear emergency ID specifying myasthenia gravis, products taken

• To avoid driving, other hazardous activities until effect is known

• To report muscle weakness (cholinergic crisis or underdosage), bradycardia

• Not to drink alcohol

• To take with food to decrease gastric side effects

• That doses are highly individualized, often 5-6 times per day, and will be based on response to the product

TREATMENT OF OVERDOSE: Discontinue product, atropine 1-4 mg IV

pyridoxine (vit B$_6$) (Rx, OTC)

(peer-i-dox′een)

Cataplex ✦, Pyri 500, Neuro-K

Func. class.: Vit B$_6$, water soluble

Do not confuse:

pyridoxine/Pyridium

ACTION: Needed for fat, protein, carbohydrate metabolism; enhances glycogen release from liver and muscle tissue; needed as coenzyme for metabolic transformations of a variety of amino acids

USES: Vit B$_6$ deficiency of inborn errors of metabolism, seizures, isoniazid therapy, oral contraceptives, alcoholic polyneuritis

CONTRAINDICATIONS
Hypersensitivity
Precautions: Pregnancy, breastfeeding, children, Parkinson's disease; patients taking levodopa should avoid supplemental vitamins with >5 mg pyridoxine

DOSAGE AND ROUTES
RDA
• **Adult: PO** (male) 1.7-2 mg; (female) 1.4-1.6 mg
• **Child 9-13 yr: PO** 1 mg/day
• **Child 4-8 yr: PO** 0.6 mg/day
• **Child 1-3 yr: PO** 0.5 mg/day
• **Infant 7-12 mo: PO** 0.3 mg/day
Vit B$_6$ deficiency
• **Adult: PO** 5-25 mg/day × 3 wk
• **Child: PO** 10 mg until desired response
Pyridoxine deficiency neuritis/seizure (not drug induced)
• **Adult: PO** *without neuritis* 2.5-10 mg/day, after corrected 2-5 mg/day; *with neuritis* 100-200 mg/day × 3wk, then 2-5 mg/day
• **Child: PO** *without neuritis* 5-25 mg/day × 3wk, then 1.5-2.5 mg/day in a multivitamin; *with neuritis:* 10-50 mg/day × 3wk, then 1-2 mg/day
• **Neonate with seizures: IM/IV** 50-100 mg as single dose
Deficiency caused by isoniazid, cycloSERINE, hydrALAZINE, penicillAMINE
• **Adult: PO** 100-300 mg/day
• **Child: PO** 10-50 mg/day
Prevention of deficiency caused by isoniazid, cycloSERINE, hydrALAZINE, penicillAMINE
• **Adult: PO** 25-100 mg/day
• **Child: PO** 1-2 mg/kg/day
Available forms: Tabs 25, 50, 100, 250, 500 mg; ext rel tabs 200, 500 mg; inj 100 mg/mL; ext rel caps 200, 500 mg; capsules 250 mg

Administer:
PO route
• Do not break, crush, or chew ext rel tabs/caps
IM route
• Rotate sites; burning or stinging at site may occur
• Z-track to minimize pain
IV route
• Undiluted or added to most IV sol; give ≤50 mg/1 min if undiluted
Syringe compatibilities: Doxapram

SIDE EFFECTS
CNS: *Paresthesia*, flushing, warmth, lethargy (rare with normal renal function)
INTEG: Pain at inj site

PHARMACOKINETICS
PO/INJ: Half-life 2-3 wk, metabolized in liver, excreted in urine

INTERACTIONS
Decrease: effects of levodopa
Decrease: effects of pyridoxine—oral contraceptives, isoniazid, cycloSERINE, hydrALAZINE, penicillamine, chloramphenicol, immunosuppressants

NURSING CONSIDERATIONS
Assess:
• **Pyridoxine deficiency:** seizures, irritability, cheilitis, conjunctivitis, anemia, confusion, red tongue, weakness, fatigue before and during treatment; monitor pyridoxine levels
• Nutritional status: yeast, liver, legumes, bananas, green vegetables, whole grains
• Blood studies: Hct, HB
• **Malabsorption:** may require injection if abdominal resection has occurred or in malabsorption syndromes
• **Pregnancy/breastfeeding:** safe in pregnancy, breastfeeding
Evaluate:
• **Therapeutic response:** absence of nausea, vomiting, anorexia, skin lesions, glossitis, stomatitis, edema, seizures, restlessness, paresthesia
Teach patient/family:
• To avoid vitamin supplements unless directed by prescriber

Side effects: *italics* = common; red = life-threatening

• To increase meat, bananas, potatoes, lima beans, whole-grain cereals in diet
• To take as directed; to continue with follow-up exams, blood work

---

pyrimethamine (Rx)
(peer-i-meth′a-meen)

Daraprim
Func. class.: Antimalarial

USES: Treatment of toxoplasmosis (in combination with a sulfonamide)

CONTRAINDICATIONS
Hypersensitivity to pyrimethamine or any component, megaloblastic anemia due to folate deficiency

DOSAGE AND ROUTES
Toxoplasmosis treatment
• **Adult: PO** 50-75 mg/day × 1-3 wk depending then reduce dose by 50% and continue for 4-5 wk; use with a sulfonamide in combination with leucovorin
Available forms: Tabs 25 mg

QUEtiapine (Rx)

(kwe-tie'a-peen)

SEROquel, SEROquel XR

Func. class.: Antipsychotic, atypical
Chem. class.: Dibenzothiazepine

DO NOT CONFUSE: Seroquel/
Desyrel//Serzone/Sinequan Quetiapine/
Olanzapine

ACTION: Functions as an antagonist at
multiple neurotransmitter receptors in the
brain, including $5HT_{1A}$, $5HT_2$, dopamine D_1,
D_2, H_1, and adrenergic α_1, α_2 receptors

USES: Bipolar disorder, bipolar I disorder, depression, mania, schizophrenia

CONTRAINDICATIONS
Hypersensitivity, breastfeeding
Precautions: Pregnancy, geriatric patients,
hepatic/cardiac disease, breast cancer,
long-term use, seizures, QT prolongation,
brain tumor, hematologic disease, torsades
de pointes, cataracts, dehydration, abrupt
discontinuation

Black Box Warning: Children, suicidal
ideation, increased mortality in elderly
patients with dementia-related psychosis

DOSAGE AND ROUTES
Bipolar mania
• **Adult: PO** 50 mg bid, initially. Increase
by 100 mg/day every day up to 400 mg/
day. May further increase by 200 mg/day
every day based on clinical response and
tolerability. Usual dose: 400 to 800 mg/
day. Max: 800 mg/day in 2 divided doses:
XL: 300 mg daily for 1 day, then 600 mg
daily for 1 day, then 400 to 800 mg daily.
Adjust dose based on clinical response
and tolerability. Usual dose: 400 to 800
mg/day. Max: 800 mg/day
Schizophrenia
• **Adult: PO** (not at risk for hypotension)
25 mg bid on day 1, increase by 25-50 mg
divided 2 to 3× on day 2 and day 3 to a
target of 300-400 mg/day in divided doses
by day 4, further dosage adjustment can
be made in 25-50 mg bid increments, max

800 mg/day; **(XR)** 300 mg/day in PM,
range 400-800 mg/day, max 800 mg/day
• **Adolescent 13-17 yr: PO** 25 mg bid on
day 1, 50 mg bid on day 2, 100 mg bid on
day 3, 150 mg bid on day 4, 200 mg bid
on day 5. Thereafter, adjustments may be
made within 400 mg/day to 800 mg/day,
given in two or three divided doses based
upon response and tolerability; **ext rel**
50 mg on day 1, then 100 mg on day 2,
200 mg on day 3, 300 mg on day 4, 400
mg on day 5. Adjust based upon response
and tolerability within 400 mg/day to 800
mg/day; max: 800 mg/day
• **Geriatric: PO EXT REL** 50 mg/day
may increase in 50 mg/day increments,
max: 800 mg/day
Major depression
• **Adult: PO EXT REL** 50 mg daily in the
evening on Day 1 and Day 2. On Day 3, 150
mg daily in the evening. Usual range: 150-
300 mg/day
• **Geriatric, debilitated or at risk for hypotension: PO EXT REL** 50 mg on day 1 and
2, may increase by 50 mg/day based on
response, usual range 150-300 mg/day
Available forms: Tabs 25, 50, 100,
200, 300, 400 mg; ext rel tab 50, 150,
200, 300, 400 mg
Administer:
• Reduced dose to geriatric patients
• Avoid use of CNS depressants
• Store in tight, light-resistant container
• If there is a week or more absence of
therapy, initiate at beginning dose
• **Immediate release:** without regard to meals
• **Ext rel:** without food or with light meal
≤300 calories; swallow whole; do not
split, crush, chew; can switch from immediate release to extended release by
giving total daily dose daily

SIDE EFFECTS
CNS: EPS, pseudoparkinsonism, akathisia,
dystonia, tardive dyskinesia; *drowsiness,*
insomnia, agitation, anxiety, *headache,*
seizures, neuroleptic malignant syndrome,
dizziness, dystonia, restless legs
CV: Orthostatic hypotension, tachycardia,
QT prolongation, CV disease, Parkinson's
disease, cardiomyopathy, myocarditis
ENDO: SIADH, hyperglycemia

Side effects: *italics* = common; red = life-threatening

GI: *Pancreatitis, nausea, anorexia, constipation,* abdominal pain, dry mouth
HEMA: Leukopenia, agranulocytosis
INTEG: Rash, DRESS
META: Hyponatremia
MISC: Asthenia, back pain, fever, ear pain
MS: Rhabdomyolysis
RESP: Rhinitis
SYST: Stevens-Johnson syndrome, anaphylaxis

PHARMACOKINETICS

Extensively metabolized by liver, half-life ≥6 hr, peak 1½ hr, ext rel 6 hr, inhibits P450 CYP3A4 enzyme system, 83% protein binding, excretion: <1% unchanged urine

INTERACTIONS

Increase: QT prolongation—class IA/III antidysrhythmics, some phenothiazines, β-agonists, local anesthetics, tricyclics, haloperidol, methadone, chloroquine, clarithromycin, droperidol, erythromycin, pentamidine, macrolides (clarithromycin)
Increase: CNS depression—alcohol, opioid analgesics, sedative/hypnotics, antihistamines
Increase: hypotension—alcohol, antihypertensives
Increase: QUEtiapine clearance, decrease QUEtiapine effect—phenytoin, thioridazine, barbiturates, glucocorticoids, carBAMazepine, rifampin
Increase: QUEtiapine action—fluconazole, itraconazole, ketoconazole (CYP3A4 inhibitors), increase CYP3A4 inhibitor after discontinuation of inhibitor
Decrease: quetiapine action—CYP3A4 inducers (carbamazepine, barbiturates, phenytoins, rifAMPin); reduce CYP3A4 inducer after discontinuation
Decrease: effect of voriconazole, consider dosage change
Decrease: effects of DOPamine agonists, levodopa, LORazepam

Drug/Lab Test
Increase: cholesterol, triglycerides, LFTs, glucose, prolactin
Decrease: thyroid tests, WBC
False positive: methadose/TCAs urine immunoassays

NURSING CONSIDERATIONS
Assess:
• **CV status:** QT prolongation, tachycardia, orthostatic B/P

Black Box Warning: Assess **mental status** before initial administration, AIMS assessment; affect, orientation, LOC, reflexes, gait, coordination, sleep pattern disturbances; suicidal thoughts/behaviors (child/young adult); dementia (geriatric patients), complete a full assessment in all new patients

Black Box Warning: Not to be used in child <10 yr (imm rel) or <18 yr (ext rel)

Black Box Warning: Suicide: restrict amount of product given; usually suicidal thoughts/behaviors occur early during treatment and among children/adolescents/young adults

• Baseline blood glucose, LFTs, neurologic function, ophthalmologic exam, weight, monitor glucose often in diabetes mellitus, thyroid function tests, serum electrolytes/creatinine/lipid profile/prolactin
• **B/P** standing, lying; pulse, respirations; determine q4hr during initial treatment; establish baseline before starting treatment; report drops of 30 mm Hg; watch for ECG changes
• Dizziness, faintness, palpitations, tachycardia on rising
• **EPS:** including akathisia (inability to sit still, no pattern to movements), tardive dyskinesia (bizarre movements of jaw, mouth, tongue, extremities), pseudoparkinsonism (rigidity, tremors, pill rolling, shuffling gait)
• **Serious rash:** assess for Stevens-Johnson syndrome, discontinue product; may cause rash, fever, joint pain, lesions
• **Pancreatitis:** assess for nausea, vomiting, severe abdominal pain
• **Metabolic syndrome:** weight gain, increased cholesterol/triglycerides, increased BMI, hypertension
• **Neuroleptic malignant syndrome:** hyperthermia, increased CPK, altered mental status, muscle rigidity, seizures,

tachycardia, diaphoresis, hypo/hypertension, fatigue; notify prescriber immediately if symptoms occur
• Constipation, urinary retention daily; if these occur, increase bulk, water in diet
• Supervised ambulation until patient stabilized on medication; do not involve patient in strenuous exercise program because fainting possible; patient should not stand still for long period of time
• **DRESS:** fever, hepatitis, swelling of face, myositis, monitor eosinophils that may be elevated, discontinue
• **Hyperprolactinemia:** sexual dysfunction, menstrual changes
• **Beers:** avoid in older adults except for schizophrenia, bipolar disorder, or short-term use as an antiemetic for chemotherapy; increased risk for stroke, dementia-related psychosis
• **Pregnancy/breastfeeding:** use only if benefits outweigh fetal risk; pregnant women taking product should enroll in the National Pregnancy Registry for Atypical Antipsychotics, 866-961-2388; EPS may develop in the infant; breastfeeding isn't recommended, excreted in breast milk
Evaluate:
• **Therapeutic response:** decrease in emotional excitement, hallucinations, delusions, paranoia; reorganization of patterns of thought, speech
Teach patient/family:
• Not to become overheated, to drink plenty of fluids
• To rise slowly to prevent orthostatic hypotension
• To take medication only as prescribed; not to crush, chew ext rel product; not to use with alcohol; to take regular tabs without regard to food or only a light meal <300 calories, ext rel without food; not to use other products unless approved by prescriber
• Not to stop abruptly
• That follow-up is necessary, including LFTs, blood glucose, neurologic, cholesterol profile, weight, to report hypoglycemic symptoms
• If drowsiness occurs, to avoid hazardous activities such as driving

• To avoid use of OTC, herbals, supplements, alcohol meds unless directed by prescriber
• To notify prescriber if pregnancy is planned, suspected; not to breastfeed
• To notify prescriber immediately of fever, difficulty breathing, fatigue, sore throat, rash, bleeding, agitation, panic attacks

Black Box Warning: Suicide: to notify prescriber of suicidal thoughts/behaviors, primarily among children/adolescents/young adults, or worsening depression, severe anxiety, panic attacks, insomnia

• To have eye exam before treatment and yearly q6mo; cataracts may occur
• To notify providers before surgery

quinapril (Rx)
(kwin′a-pril)
Accupril
Func. class.: Antihypertensive
Chem. class.: (ACE) inhibitor

Do not confuse:
Accupril/Aciphex

ACTION: Selectively suppresses renin-angiotensin-aldosterone system; inhibits ACE, prevents conversion of angiotensin I to angiotensin II; results in dilation of arterial, venous vessels

USES: Hypertension, alone or in combination with thiazide diuretics; systolic HF

CONTRAINDICATIONS
Children, hypersensitivity to ACE inhibitors, ACE inhibitor induced angioedema

Black Box Warning: Pregnancy 2nd/3rd trimester

Precautions: Breastfeeding, geriatric patients, impaired renal/hepatic function, dialysis patients, hypovolemia, bilateral renal stenosis, hyperkalemia, aortic stenosis, ⬥ African descent, hypotension, hyponatremia, SLE, bone marrow suppression, CV disease, angioedema

Side effects: *italics* = common; red = life-threatening

DOSAGE AND ROUTES
Hypertension
- **Adult:** PO 10-20 mg/day initially, then 20-80 mg/day divided bid or daily **(monotherapy)**; start at 5 mg/day **(with diuretics)**, titrate ≥2 wk up to 80 mg/day
- **Geriatric:** PO 10 mg/day, titrate to desired response **(monotherapy)**; start at 2.5 mg/day **(with diuretics)**

Heart failure
- **Adult:** PO 5 mg bid, may increase weekly until 20-40 mg/day in 2 divided doses

Renal dose
- **Adult:** PO CCr 61-89 mL/min 10 mg daily (hypertension), 5 mg bid (heart failure); CCr 30-60 mL/min, 5 mg/day initially; CCr 10-29 mL/min, 2.5 mg/day initially

Available forms: Tabs 5, 10, 20, 40 mg
Administer:
- Tabs may be crushed if necessary
- Store in airtight container at room temperature
- Do not use with high-fat meal, decreases absorption

SIDE EFFECTS
CNS: *Headache, dizziness, fatigue,* somnolence, depression, malaise, nervousness, vertigo, syncope
CV: *Hypotension,* postural hypotension, syncope, palpitations, *angina pectoris,* MI, tachycardia, vasodilation, chest pain
GI: *Nausea,* diarrhea, constipation, *vomiting,* gastritis, GI hemorrhage, dry mouth
GU: Increased BUN, creatinine; decreased libido, impotence
INTEG: Angioedema, rash, sweating, photosensitivity, pruritus
META: Hyperkalemia
MISC: Back pain, amblyopia
MS: Myalgia
RESP: *Dry cough,* pharyngitis, dyspnea

PHARMACOKINETICS
Bioavailability ≥60%, onset <1 hr, peak 1-2 hr, duration 24 hr, protein binding 97%, half-life 2 hr, metabolized by liver (active metabolite quinaprilat), metabolites excreted in urine (60%)/feces (37%)

INTERACTIONS
Increase: hyperkalemia—vasodilators, hydrALAZINE, prazosin, potassium-sparing diuretics, sympathomimetics, potassium supplements, ACE/angiotensin II receptor antagonists; aliskiren (diabetic patients)
Increase: hypotension—diuretics, other antihypertensives, ganglionic blockers, adrenergic blockers, phenothiazines, nitrates, acute alcohol ingestion
Increase: toxicity of lithium
Decrease: absorption of tetracycline, quinolone antibiotics
Decrease: hypotensive effect of quinapril—NSAIDs

Drug/Herb
Decrease: antihypertensive effect—black licorice, ma huang, yohimbe

Drug/Food
Hyperkalemia: do not use with potassium-containing salt substitutes; read label carefully

Drug/Lab Test
Increase: potassium, creatinine, BUN, LFTs
False negative: aldosterone/renin ratio

NURSING CONSIDERATIONS
Assess:
- **Hypertension:** B/P, orthostatic hypotension, syncope; monitor B/P before giving dose and after 2 hr; African-American patients are more resistant to antihypertension effect
- **Heart failure:** edema in feet, legs daily; weight daily
- **Collagen-vascular disease:** blood studies: neutrophils, decreased platelets; WBC with differential at baseline, periodically, q3mo; if neutrophils <1000/mm³, discontinue treatment
- Renal studies: protein, BUN, creatinine; watch for increased levels; may indicate nephrotic syndrome
- Baselines of hepatic studies before therapy, periodically; increased LFTs; uric acid, glucose may be increased
- Potassium levels; hyperkalemia is rare, those with diabetes, renal disease are more at risk for hyperkalemia

• **Allergic reactions:** angioedema, rash, fever, pruritus, urticaria, swelling of eyes/face/throat/neck, SOB, difficulty breathing; product should be discontinued; angioedema is more common in ℞ African-American patients

Black Box Warning: Do not use in pregnancy, breastfeeding, stop drug if pregnancy is determined

Evaluate:
• **Therapeutic response:** decrease in B/P
Teach patient/family:
• Not to discontinue product abruptly
• Not to use OTC products (cough, cold, allergy); not to use salt substitutes containing potassium unless directed by prescriber, to avoid high-fat meal at same time as product
• To comply with dosage schedule, even if feeling better
• To rise slowly to sitting or standing position to minimize orthostatic hypotension, to report excessive perspiration, dehydration, vomiting, diarrhea; may lead to fall in B/P; maintain adequate hydration, assess fall risk
• To notify prescriber of mouth sores, sore throat, fever, swelling of hands/feet, irregular heartbeat, chest pain, persistent dry cough
• To report signs of infection (fever, sore throat)
• That product may cause dizziness, fainting, light-headedness; may occur during first few days of therapy
• That product may cause skin rash, impaired taste perception
• How to take B/P, normal readings for age group or individual baseline B/P and HR

Black Box Warning: Pregnancy: to report if pregnancy is planned or suspected; not to breastfeed

TREATMENT OF OVERDOSE:
0.9% NaCl IV infusion

quinapril/hydrochlorothiazide (Rx)

(kwin′a-pril/hye-droe-klor-oh-thye′a-zide)

Accuretic, Quinaretic
Func. class.: Antihypertensive, thiazide diuretic, ACE inhibitor

USES: Hypertension

DOSAGE AND ROUTES
Adult: PO: 1 tablet daily, adjust dose after 2-3 wk; maintenance quinapril 5-40 mg/hydrochlorothiazide 6.25-25 mg daily
Available forms: 10 mg quinapril/12.5 mg hydrochlorothiazide, 20 mg quinapril/12.5 mg hydrochlorothiazide, 20 mg quinapril/20 mg hydrochlorothiazide

⚠ HIGH ALERT

quiNIDine gluconate (Rx)

(kwin′i-deen)

quiNIDine sulfate (Rx)
Func. class.: Antidysrhythmic (Class IA)
Chem. class.: QuiNINE dextroisomer

Do not confuse:
quiNIDine/quiNINE

ACTION: Prolongs duration of action potential and effective refractory period, thus decreasing myocardial excitability; anticholinergic properties

USES: Atrial fibrillation, PAT, ventricular tachycardia, atrial flutter, Wolff-Parkinson-White syndrome; PVST

CONTRAINDICATIONS
Hypersensitivity, idiosyncratic response, digoxin toxicity, blood dyscrasias, myasthenia gravis, AV block

Q

Precautions: Pregnancy, breastfeeding, children, geriatric patients, electrolyte imbalance, renal/hepatic disease, HF, respiratory depression, bradycardia, hypotension, syncope

Black Box Warning: Cardiac arrhythmias, MI

DOSAGE AND ROUTES
QuiNIDine gluconate
• **Adult: PO** (ext rel) 324-648 mg q8-12hr; **IV Initially, up to 0.25 mg/kg per minute (up to 1 mL/kg per hr) of 16-mg/mL dilution. Discontinue IV infusion as soon as sinus rhythm is restored**
QuiNIDine sulfate
PVST/WPW/atrial fibrillation/flutter
• **Adult: PO** 200-300 mg q6-8hr × 5-8 doses; may increase daily until sinus rhythm restored; max 4 g/day given only after digitalization; maintenance 200-300 mg tid-qid or **EXT REL** 300-600 mg q8-12hr
Available forms: *gluconate* ext rel tabs 324 mg; *sulfate:* tabs 200, 300 mg
Administer:
• AV node blocker (digoxin) before starting quinidine to avoid increased ventricular rate
• Do not break, crush, chew ext rel products
• With full glass of water or with food; GI upset occurs
• Do not use with grapefruit juice

SIDE EFFECTS
CV: Hypotension, *bradycardia,* PVCs, heart block, CV collapse, arrest, torsades de pointes, widening QRS complex, ventricular tachycardia
EENT: Cinchonism: tinnitus, blurred vision, hearing loss, mydriasis, disturbed color vision
GI: Nausea, vomiting, anorexia, abdominal pain, *diarrhea,* hepatotoxicity
HEMA: Thrombocytopenia, hemolytic anemia, agranulocytosis, hypoprothrombinemia

INTEG: Rash, urticaria, angioedema, swelling, photosensitivity, flushing with severe pruritus
RESP: Dyspnea, respiratory depression

PHARMACOKINETICS
PO: (sulfate) peak 1-6 hr, duration 6-8 hr, (sulfate ER) peak 4 hr, duration 8-12 hr; (gluconate PO) peak 3-4 hr, duration 6-8 hr, half-life 6-7 hr (prolonged in geriatric patients, cirrhosis, HF), metabolized in liver, excreted unchanged (10%-50%) by kidneys, protein bound (80%-90%)

INTERACTIONS
• Additive vagolytic effect: anticholinergic blockers
Increase: cardiac depression: other antidysrhythmics, phenothiazines, reserpine
Increase: effects of neuromuscular blockers, digoxin, warfarin, tricyclics, propranolol
Increase: QT prolongation—macrolides, quinolones, tricyclics, procainamide, antipsychotics
Increase: quiNIDine effects—cimetidine, sodium bicarbonate, carbonic anhydrase inhibitors, antacids, hydroxide suspensions, amiodarone, verapamil, NIFEdipine, protease inhibitors
Decrease: quiNIDine effects—barbiturates, phenytoin, rifampin, sucralfate, cholinergics
Drug/Herb
Increase: quiNIDine effect—hawthorn, licorice
Drug/Food
• Delayed absorption, decreased metabolism: grapefruit juice, avoid use
Drug/Lab Test
Decrease: platelets, HB, granulocytes

NURSING CONSIDERATIONS
Assess:
• Blood levels (therapeutic level 2-5 mcg/mL), CBC, LFTs
• **For cinchonism:** tinnitus, headache, nausea, dizziness, fever, vertigo, tremors; may lead to hearing loss

Black Box Warning: Cardiac toxicity: asystole, ventricular dysrhythmias, widening QRS, torsades de pointes

• CNS effects: dizziness, confusion, psychosis, paresthesias, seizures; product should be discontinued
• **Hepatotoxicity:** monitor LFTs for first 1-2 mo of treatment
• **Pregnancy/breastfeeding:** use only if clearly needed; avoid use in breastfeeding, excreted in breast milk
Evaluate:
• **Therapeutic response:** decreased dysrhythmias
Teach patient/family:
• That if dizziness, drowsiness occurs, to avoid driving or hazardous activities
• To use sunglasses; product may cause sensitivity to light
• To carry emergency ID stating disease, medication use
• How to take pulse; when to notify prescriber
• To avoid all products unless approved by prescriber

• Not to crush, chew ext rel product
• Not to use grapefruit juice with this product
• **QuiNIDine toxicity (cinchonism):** to report immediately visual changes, nausea, headache, ringing in the ears
• To report diarrhea, anorexia, decreased B/P

quinupristin/dalfopristin (Rx)
(kwi-nyoo′pris-tin/dal-foe′pris-tin)
Synercid
Func. class.: Antiinfective, streptogramin

USES: Treatment of complicated skin/skin structure infections caused by methicillin-susceptible *Staphylococcus aureus* or *Streptococcus pyogenes*

DOSAGE AND ROUTES
Adult/child ≥12 yr: IV: 7.5 mg/kg q12hr for ≥7 days
Available forms: Injection 500-mg vial (150 mg quinupristin/350 mg dalfopristin)

RABEprazole (Rx)

(rah-bep′rah-zole)

Aciphex, Aciphex Sprinkle, Pariet ✤

Func. class.: Antiulcer, proton pump inhibitor

Chem. class.: Benzimidazole

Do not confuse:

Aciphex/Aricept/Accupril

RABEprazole/ARIPiprazole

ACTION: Suppresses gastric secretion by inhibiting hydrogen/potassium ATPase enzyme system in the gastric parietal cells; characterized as a gastric acid pump inhibitor because it blocks the final step of acid production

USES: Gastroesophageal reflux disease (GERD), severe erosive esophagitis, poorly responsive systemic GERD, pathologic hypersecretory conditions (Zollinger-Ellison syndrome, systemic mastocytosis, multiple endocrine adenomas); treatment of active duodenal ulcers with/without antiinfectives for *Helicobacter pylori;* daytime, nighttime heartburn

Unlabeled uses: Gastric ulcer, heartburn, *H. pylori* eradication in children

CONTRAINDICATIONS

Hypersensitivity to this product or proton pump inhibitors (PPIs)

Precautions: Pregnancy, breastfeeding, children, ✖✪✪ Asian patients, diarrhea, geriatric patients, gastric cancer, hepatic/GI disease, IBS, osteoporosis, CDAD, ulcerative colitis, vit B_{12} deficiency

DOSAGE AND ROUTES

Healing of duodenal ulcers

• **Adult:** PO 20 mg/day × ≤4 wk; to be taken after breakfast

Healing of erosive esophagitis or ulcerative GERD

• **Adult:** PO 20 mg/day × 4-8 wk; may use an additional course

• **Adolescent and child ≥12 yr: PO** 20 mg/day up to 8 wk

• **Child 1-11 yr (≥15 kg): PO** (sprinkle) 10 mg daily up to 12 wk

• **Child 1-11 yr (<15 kg): PO** 5 mg daily up to 12 wk; may increase to 10 mg daily if needed

H. pylori eradication

• **Adult:** PO 20 mg bid × 14 days with amoxicillin 1 g bid × 14 days with clarithromycin 500 mg bid × 14 days

Pathologic hypersecretory conditions

• **Adult:** PO 60 mg/day; may increase to 120 mg in 2 divided doses

Gastric ulcer (unlabeled)

• **Adult:** PO 20 mg/day after AM meal × 3-6 wk

Dyspepsia/heartburn (unlabeled)

• **Adult:** PO 20 mg/day × ≤14 days

Available forms: Del rel tabs 10 ✤, 20 mg; del rel sprinkle caps 5, 10 mg

Administer:

PO route

• Do not break, crush, chew del-rel tab; after breakfast daily with full glass of water, without regard to food

• **Delayed-release capsule:** open, use on spoonful of applesauce or liquid, give dose immediately (within 15 min), ½ hr before a meal; do not crush, chew delayed-release product, may be mixed in formula for young children

SIDE EFFECTS

CNS: *Headache, dizziness*

EENT: Tinnitus, taste perversion

GI: *Diarrhea, abdominal pain, vomiting, nausea, constipation, flatulence, acid regurgitation,* abdominal swelling, anorexia, hepatitis, hepatic encephalopathy, *Clostridium difficile*–associated diarrhea

GU: UTI, proteinuria, hematuria

MS: Back pain, arthralgia, myalgia, osteoporosis, fractures

MISC: Infection, Stevens-Johnson syndrome

PHARMACOKINETICS

Eliminated in urine as metabolites and in feces, half-life 1-2 hr, metabolized by

CYP2C19 🕸 enzyme system, protein binding 96.3%

INTERACTIONS

Increase: bleeding risk—warfarin, clopidogrel

Increase: serum levels of RABEprazole—benzodiazepines, phenytoin, clarithromycin, antacids, other proton pump inhibitors, H₂ blockers

Increase: levels of—digoxin, nelfinavir/omeprazole, methotrexate

Decrease: levels of RABEprazole—sucralfate, calcium carbonate, vit B₁₂

Decrease: levels of ketoconazole, itraconazole, iron salts, atazanavir/ritonavir, ampicillin, cycloSPORINE, protease inhibitors

Drug/Herb

Decrease: RABEprazole—St. John's wort

Drug/Lab Test

Decrease: magnesium

NURSING CONSIDERATIONS

Assess:

• GI system: bowel sounds; abdomen for pain, swelling, anorexia, emesis/stool for occult blood

• *Clostridium difficile–associated diarrhea:* may occur with most antibiotic therapy; watery diarrhea, abdominal pain, fever; may occur several weeks after treatment concludes

• **Vit B₁₂/cyanocobalamin deficiency/hypomagnesemia:** may occur several weeks after treatment concludes; use magnesium, vit B₁₂, cyanocobalamin supplement; if severe, discontinuation of product may be needed. Assess for low magnesium level: tremors, muscle soreness, spasms, anxiety, change in heart rate, palpitations

• Hepatic studies: AST, ALT, alk phos during treatment; CBC with differential periodically

• CBC with differential before, periodically during treatment; blood dyscrasias may occur (rare)

• Obtain susceptibility testing if *H. pylori* treatment is ineffective; another anti-infective may be needed

• **Osteoporosis/fractures:** may occur with prolonged use (1 yr or longer) of high dose, usually in those ≥50 yr; make sure adequate vitamin D, calcium are taken

• **Beers:** avoid scheduled use >8 wk in older adults unless for high-risk patients

Evaluate:

• **Therapeutic response:** absence of epigastric pain, swelling, fullness; decreased symptoms of GERD after 4-8 wk

Teach patient/family:

• CDAD to report severe diarrhea or black, tarry stools, abdominal pain, fever; avoid using antidiarrheals; product may have to be discontinued

• To avoid hazardous activities because dizziness, drowsiness may occur

• To avoid alcohol, salicylates, NSAIDs because they may cause GI irritation; to avoid other OTC, herbal products unless approved by prescriber

• That osteoporosis and fractures are more common in those who take the product >1 yr

• To use as directed for length of time prescribed; to take missed dose when remembered; not to double dose; to take del-rel tab whole, do not cut, break; that cap should be opened and sprinkled on food (applesauce) to take within 15 min of being sprinkled and 30 min before meal; to take the tablet form for ulcers after meal, for *H. pylori* with morning/evening meals

• To notify prescriber if pregnancy is planned, suspected

---

rabies immune globulin (Rx)

(ray′beez)

HyperRAB, HyperRAB S/D, Imogam Rabies-HT, Kedrab

Func. class.: Antibody-Immune Globulin

USES: Rabies exposure

CONTRAINDICATIONS

Hypersensitivity, Imogam Rabies-HT (do not give repeated doses)

DOSAGE AND ROUTES
Rabies, postexposure prophylaxis
• **Adult/child: IM** 20 units/kg in a single dose, give as part of rabies vaccine regimen. If anatomically feasible, the full rabies immune globulin dose should be infiltrated around and into the wound(s); remaining volume should be administered IM at a site distant from the vaccine site

---

radioactive iodine (sodium iodide) ^{131}I (Rx)
Func. class.: Antithyroid
Chem. class.: Radiopharmaceutical

USES: *High dose:* Thyroid cancer, hyperthyroidism
Low dose: Visualization to determine thyroid cancer, diagnostic aid for thyroid function studies

CONTRAINDICATIONS
Pregnancy, breastfeeding, age <30 yr, recent MI, large nodular goiter, vomiting/diarrhea, acute hyperthyroidism, use of thyroid products

DOSAGE AND ROUTES
Thyroid cancer
• **Adult: PO** 50-150 mCi; may repeat, depending on clinical status
Hyperthyroidism
• **Adult: PO** 4-10 mCi, depending on serum thyroxine level
Available forms: Capsule 0.75-100 mCi; oral solution 5-150 mCi/vial; concentrated oral solution 1000 mCi/mL; all are set at calibration

---

raloxifene (Rx)
(ral-ox'ih-feen)
Evista
Func. class.: Bone resorption inhibitor
Chem. class.: Hormone modifier, selective estrogen receptor modulator (SERM)

ACTION: Tissue-selective estrogen agonist/antagonist; agonist activity in bone and on lipid metabolism; antagonist activity on breast and uterus; reduces resorption of bone and decreases bone turnover

USES: Prevention, treatment of osteoporosis in postmenopausal women; breast cancer prophylaxis in postmenopausal women with osteoporosis or in postmenopausal women at high risk for developing the disease; invasive breast cancer risk reduction
Unlabeled uses: Uterine leiomyomata in postmenopausal women with osteoporosis or in postmenopausal women who are at high risk for developing the disease

CONTRAINDICATIONS
Pregnancy, breastfeeding, hypersensitivity, children

Black Box Warning: Women with active or history of venous thromboembolic events

Precautions: CV/hepatic disease, cervical/uterine cancer, elevated triglycerides, pulmonary embolism, atrial fibrillation

Black Box Warning: Stroke

DOSAGE AND ROUTES
• **Adult postmenopausal women: PO** 60 mg/day, max 60 mg/day
Available forms: Tabs 60 mg
Administer:
• PO: without regard to meals, give with vit D
• Add calcium supplement if inadequate
• Do not use during immobilization or prolonged bedrest

SIDE EFFECTS
CNS: Insomnia, depression, migraines
CV: Hot flashes, peripheral edema, thromboembolism, stroke, fever, chest pain
EENT: Pharyngitis, sinusitis, laryngitis

GI: *Nausea,* vomiting, diarrhea, dyspepsia, abdominal pain, gastroenteritis
GU: Vaginitis, leukorrhea, cystitis, UTI, vaginal bleeding
INTEG: Rash, sweating
META: Weight gain, peripheral edema
MS: Arthralgia, myalgia, *leg cramps,* arthritis
RESP: Increased cough

PHARMACOKINETICS
Duration 24 hr, elimination half-life 28-32 hr; excreted in feces, breast milk; highly bound to plasma proteins

INTERACTIONS
• Administer cautiously with other highly protein-bound products, (ibuprofen, diazePAM, naproxen, systemic estrogens)
Decrease: action of anticoagulants, desiccated thyroid, levothyroxine, liotrix
Decrease: action of raloxifene—ampicillin, bile acid sequestrants
Drug/Food
Decrease: raloxifene, effect of—soy
Drug/Lab Test
Increase: triglycerides

NURSING CONSIDERATIONS
Assess:

Black Box Warning: History of stroke, TIA, thrombosis, atrial fibrillation, hypertension, smoking; venous thrombosis may occur; avoid prolonged sitting; discontinue 3 days before surgery, other immobilization; mortality is increased after stroke

• Bone density test at baseline, throughout treatment, bone-specific alk phos, osteocalcin
Pregnancy/breastfeeding: do not use in pregnancy/breastfeeding
Evaluate:
• **Therapeutic response:** prevention, treatment of osteoporosis in postmenopausal women; prevention of breast cancer in postmenopausal women with osteoporosis or in those who are at high risk for developing the disease
Teach patient/family:

Black Box Warning: To discontinue product 72 hr before prolonged bedrest; to avoid staying in one position for long periods, to report possible blood clots immediately, usually during first few months of therapy

• To take calcium supplements, vit D if intake is inadequate
• To increase exercise using weights
• To stop smoking; to decrease alcohol consumption
• That product does not help to control hot flashes; hot flashes may be increased, as these are a common side effect
• To report fever, acute migraine, insomnia, emotional distress; urinary tract infection, vaginal burning/itching; swelling, warmth, pain in calves; uterine bleeding, abnormal breast changes
• To notify prescriber if pregnancy is planned or suspected; not to use in pregnancy, breastfeeding
• Provide product package insert and discuss with patient

raltegravir (Rx)
(ral-teg′ra-vir)
Isentress, Isentress HD
Func. class.: Antiretroviral
Chem. class.: HIV integrase strand transfer inhibitor (ISTIs)

ACTION: Inhibits catalytic activity of HIV-1 integrase, which is an HIV-encoded enzyme needed for replication

USES: HIV in combination with other antiretrovirals

CONTRAINDICATIONS
Breastfeeding, hypersensitivity
Precautions: Pregnancy (used often in pregnancy), children, geriatric patients, hepatic disease, immune reconstitution syndrome, hepatitis, antimicrobial resistance, lactase deficiency, rhabdomyolysis; PKU (chew tab)

DOSAGE AND ROUTES

Do not interchange chewable tablets, film-coated 400-mg and high-dose 600-mg tablets

HIV with other antiretroviral agents

- **Adult: PO** (400-mg film-coated tablet) 400 mg bid. During coadministration with rifampin, recommended dosage is 800 mg bid
- **Adolescent/child ≥25 kg: PO** (400-mg film-coated tablet) 400 mg bid
- **Adolescent/child** (weight-based dosage): **PO** (chewable tablets) **≥40 kg,** 300 mg bid; **28-39 kg,** 200 mg bid; **20-27 kg,** 150 mg bid; **14-19 kg,** 100 mg bid; **11-13 kg,** 75 mg bid
- **Child: PO** (powder for suspension) **14-19 kg,** 100 mg (5 mL) bid; **11-13 kg,** 80 mg (4 mL) bid; **≥4 wk of age and 8-10 kg,** 60 mg (3 mL) bid; **≥4 wk and 6-7 kg,** 40 mg (2 mL) bid; **≥4 wk and 4-5 kg,** 30 mg (1.5 mL) bid; **≥4 wk and 3 kg,** 25 mg (1 mL) bid

High-dose regimen

- **Adult: PO** (600-mg film-coated tablet) 1200 mg (2 × 600 mg)/day. Coadministration with rifAMPin is not recommended
- **Adolescent/child ≥40 mg: PO** (600 mg film-coated tablet) 1200 mg (2 × 600 mg)/day. Coadministration with rifampin is not recommended

Available forms: Tabs 400, 600 mg; chew tabs 25, 100 mg; granules for oral suspension 100 mg/packet

Administer:

PO route

- Tablets and chew tablets are not interchangeable
- Chew tabs should be chewed or swallowed whole, for a child may be mixed with 5 mL water then crush, use immediately
- Do not break, crush, chew regular tabs
- May give without regard to meals, with 8 oz of water
- Store at room temperature
- **Oral suspension:** Open foil, use 10 mL of water in provided measuring cup, close, add whole packet (10 mg/mL), swirl, do not turn upside down, use oral syringe to administer, use within 30 min, discard any remaining suspension

SIDE EFFECTS

CNS: *Fatigue,* fever, *dizziness, headache,* asthenia, suicidal ideation, insomnia
CV: MI
GI: *Nausea,* vomiting, diarrhea, abdominal pain, asthenia, gastritis, hepatitis, weight gain
GU: Acute renal failure
HEMA: Anemia, neutropenia
INTEG: Rash, urticaria, pruritus, pain or phlebitis at IV site, unusual sweating, alopecia, Stevens-Johnson syndrome, toxic epidermal necrolysis
META: Hyperamylasemia, hyperglycemia, lipodystrophy
MS: Myopathy, rhabdomyolysis
SYST: Immune reconstitution syndrome

PHARMACOKINETICS

Max absorption 3 hr if taken on an empty stomach; half-life 9 hr; metabolized in the liver by uridine diphosphate glucuronosyltransferase (UGT1A1 enzyme system); excreted in feces 51%, urine 23%

INTERACTIONS

Increase: raltegravir effect—proton pump inhibitors, H$_2$ blockers; UGT1A1 inhibitors (atazanavir)
Increase: rhabdomyolysis, myopathy, elevated CPK—fibric acid derivatives, HMG-CoA reductase inhibitors
Decrease: raltegravir levels—rifAMPin, efavirenz, tenofovir, tipranavir/ritonavir, antacids (magnesium, aluminum)
Decreased effect: strong UGT 1A1 inducers

Drug/Lab Test

Increase: AST, ALT, GGT, total bilirubin, alk phos, amylase/lipase, CK, serum glucose, total/HDL/LDL cholesterol
Decrease: HB, platelets, ANC

NURSING CONSIDERATIONS

Assess:

- **HIV infection:** CD4, T-cell count, plasma HIV RNA, viral load; resistance testing before therapy, at treatment failure

- **Rhabdomyolysis:** assess for muscle pain, darkening of urine, increased CPK; product should be discontinued
- Skin eruptions: rash, urticaria, itching
- **Suicidal thoughts/behaviors:** monitor for depression; more common in those with mental illness
- **Immune reconstitution syndrome,** usually during initial phase of treatment; may give antiinfective before starting; opportunistic infections or autoimmune disorders may occur
- **Stevens-Johnson syndrome:** skin eruptions: rash, urticaria, itching
- **Labs:** Monitor total/HDL/LDL cholesterol, blood glucose, LFTs, serum bilirubin (total and direct), baseline and periodically (all may be elevated); pregnancy test, CBC with differential, hepatitis serology, plasma hepatitis C, RNA, urinalysis, baseline and periodically
- Monitor for increased weight, especially in females, Hispanics, Black women
- **Pregnancy/breastfeeding:** use only if benefits outweigh fetal risk, pregnant women taking this product should enroll in the Antiretroviral Pregnancy Registry, 800-258-4263; do not breastfeed

Evaluate:
- **Therapeutic response:** improvement in CD4 counts, T-cell counts, viral load
- Decreased progression of AIDs, HIV

Teach patient/family:
- To take as prescribed; if dose missed, to take as soon as remembered up to 1 hr before next dose; not to double dose; not to share with others, provide patient with "Patient Information" sheet before use and dosage change
- That sexual partners need to be told that patient has HIV; that product does not cure infection, just controls symptoms; that it does not prevent infecting others
- To report sore throat, fever, fatigue (may indicate immune reconstitution syndrome)
- That product must be taken in equal intervals 2×/day to maintain blood levels for duration of therapy

- To notify prescriber immediately of suicidal thoughts/behaviors
- **Pregnancy/breastfeeding:** to notify prescriber if pregnancy is planned or suspected; not to breastfeed
- To continue with follow-up exams, blood work
- Advise patient to discuss with health care provider all Rx, OTC, herbals, supplements taken; not to use any new products without approval
- To report rash, muscle pain immediately

> **⚠ HIGH ALERT**

ramelteon (Rx)
(rah-mel'tee-on)
Rozerem
Func. class.: Sedative/hypnotic, antianxiety
Chem. class.: Melatonin receptor agonist

Do not confuse:
Rozerem/Razadine

ACTION: Binds selectively to melatonin receptors (MT_1, MT_2); thought to be involved in circadian rhythms and in the normal sleep/wake cycle

USES: Insomnia (difficulty with sleep onset)

CONTRAINDICATIONS Breastfeeding, children, infants, hypersensitivity
Precautions: Pregnancy, hepatic disease, alcoholism, COPD, seizure disorder, sleep apnea, suicidal ideation, angioedema, depression, sleep-related behaviors (sleepwalking), schizophrenia, bipolar disorder; alcohol intoxication, hepatic encephalopathy

DOSAGE AND ROUTES
- **Adult: PO** 8 mg within 30 min of bedtime, max 8 mg/day
Hepatic dose
- Do not use with severe hepatic disease; use with caution for mild to moderate hepatic disease

---

Available forms: Tabs 8 mg
Administer:

• Within 30 min of bedtime for sleeplessness; on empty stomach for fast onset, do not give within 1 hr of high-fat foods

• Do not break, crush, chew tabs; swallow whole

• Store in tight container in cool environment

SIDE EFFECTS

CNS: Dizziness, somnolence, fatigue, headache, worsening insomnia, depression, complex sleep-related reactions (sleep driving, sleep eating), suicidal thoughts/behaviors

GI: Nausea, diarrhea, dysgeusia, vomiting

SYST: Severe allergic reactions, angioedema

PHARMACOKINETICS

Absorbed rapidly; peak ½-1½ hr; protein binding 82%; rapid first-pass metabolism via liver by CYP1A2; 84% excreted in urine, 4% in feces; half-life 2-5 hr metabolite

INTERACTIONS

• **Possible toxicity:** antiretroviral protease inhibitors

Increase: ramelteon effect, toxicity—alcohol; CYP1A2 inhibitors, azole antifungals (ketoconazole, fluconazole), fluvoxaMINE, anxiolytics, sedatives, hypnotics, barbiturates, ciprofloxacin, strong CYP2C9 inhibitors, strong CYP3A4 inhibitors, opioids

Decrease: effect of ramelteon—strong CYP inducer (rifAMPin)

Drug/Food

Prolonged absorption, sleep onset reduced: high-fat/heavy meal

Drug/Lab

Increase: protein level
Decrease: testosterone level

NURSING CONSIDERATIONS

Assess:

• **Severe hypersensitive reactions:** assess for angioedema (facial swelling); product should be discontinued

• **Sleep characteristics:** type of sleep problem: falling asleep, staying asleep; complex sleep disorders (sleep walking/driving/eating) after taking product

• Mental status: mood, sensorium, affect, memory (long, short term), suicidal ideation

• LFTs: before treatment, periodically

• **Beers:** avoid use in older adults with a high risk of delirium; delirium might be induced or worsened

• **Pregnancy/breastfeeding:** use only if benefits outweigh fetal risk, may be fetal toxic; cautious use in breastfeeding, excretion is unknown

Evaluate:

• **Therapeutic response:** ability to sleep at night, decreased amount of early morning awakening

Teach patient/family:

• To avoid driving, other activities requiring alertness until product stabilized; drowsiness may continue the next day

• To avoid alcohol ingestion, CNS depressants

• About alternative measures to improve sleep: reading, exercise several hr before bedtime, warm bath, warm milk, TV, self-hypnosis, deep breathing

• To report if pregnancy is planned or suspected; to avoid breastfeeding

• To take product within 30 min before going to bed

• Not to ingest a high-fat/heavy meal before taking product

• To report cessation of menses, galactorrhea (women), decreased libido, infertility, worsening of insomnia, behavioral changes, severe allergic reactions, suicidal thoughts/behaviors; if insomnia gets worse, swelling of face, tongue, trouble breathing

• Med guide should be given to patient and reviewed

---

ramipril (Rx)

(ra-mi′pril)

Altace

Func. class.: Antihypertensive
Chem. class.: Angiotensin-converting enzyme inhibitor (ACE)

Do not confuse:
ramipril/enalapril
Altace/alteplase

ACTION: Selectively suppresses renin-angiotensin-aldosterone system; inhibits ACE, prevents conversion of angiotensin I to angiotensin II; results in dilation of arterial, venous vessels

USES: Hypertension, alone or in combination with thiazide diuretics; HF (post-MI), reduction in risk for MI, stroke, death from CV disorders

CONTRAINDICATIONS
Breastfeeding, children, hypersensitivity to ACE inhibitors, history of ACE inhibitor–induced angioedema

Black Box Warning: Pregnancy

Precautions: Geriatric patients, impaired renal/hepatic function, dialysis patients, hypovolemia, blood dyscrasias, HF, renal artery stenosis, cough, ⚘ African descent, aortic stenosis, SLE, scleroderma, bone marrow suppression

DOSAGE AND ROUTES
Hypertension
• **Adult: PO** 2.5 mg/day initially, then 2.5-20 mg/day divided bid or daily
HF post-MI
• **Adult: PO** 2.5 mg twice daily, initially. May reduce dose to 1.25 mg twice daily if hypotension occurs. Increase the dose as tolerated after 3 wk up to 5 mg twice daily
Reduction in risk for MI, stroke, death
• **Adult: PO** 2.5 mg/day × 7 days, then 5 mg/day × 21 days, then may increase to 10 mg/day
Renal dose
• **Adult: PO** CCr <40 mL/min, reduce by 25%, titrate upward to max 5 mg/day
Available forms: Caps 1.25, 2.5, 5, 10, 15 ⚘ mg
Administer:
• Without regard to meals
• Swallow cap or tablet whole
• Caps can be opened, added to food; mixture is stable for 24 hr at room temperature, 48 hr refrigerated

• Store in tight container at ≤86° F (30° C)

SIDE EFFECTS
CNS: *Headache, dizziness,* anxiety, insomnia, paresthesia, *fatigue,* depression, malaise, vertigo, syncope
CV: *Hypotension,* chest pain, palpitations, angina, syncope, dysrhythmia, heart failure, MI
GI: *Nausea,* constipation, vomiting, anorexia, diarrhea, abdominal pain
GU: Proteinuria, increased BUN, creatinine, impotence
INTEG: Rash, sweating, photosensitivity, pruritus
META: *Hyperkalemia*
MS: Arthralgia, arthritis, myalgia
RESP: *Dry cough,* dyspnea

PHARMACOKINETICS
Bioavailability >50%-60%, onset 1-2 hr, peak 1-3 hr, duration 24 hr, protein binding 73%, half-life 13-17 hr, metabolized by liver (metabolites excreted in urine, feces)

INTERACTIONS
• Do not use with aliskiren in moderate-severe renal disease
Increase: hyperkalemia—potassium-sparing diuretics, potassium supplement, angiotensin II receptor agonists
Increase: hypotension—diuretics, other antihypertensives, ganglionic blockers, adrenergic blockers, nitrates, acute alcohol ingestion
Increase: toxicity—vasodilators, hydrALAZINE, prazosin, potassium-sparing diuretics, sympathomimetics, potassium supplements
Increase: serum levels of lithium
Decrease: absorption—antacids
Decrease: antihypertensive effect—indomethacin, NSAIDs, salicylates
Drug/Herb
Increase: antihypertensive effect—garlic hawthorn
Decrease: antihypertensive effect—black licorice, ephedra
Drug/Food
Increase: hyperkalemia—potassium salt substitutes; avoid use

Drug/Lab Test
Increase: LFTs, BUN, creatinine, glucose, potassium
Decrease: RBC, HB, platelets

NURSING CONSIDERATIONS
Assess:
• **Hypertension:** monitor B/P baseline and regularly, orthostatic hypotension, syncope
• **Heart failure:** edema in feet, legs daily; weight daily
• **Collagen-vascular disease (SLE, scleroderma):** neutrophils, decreased platelets; WBC with differential at baseline, periodically; if neutrophils <1 × 10⁹/L, discontinue treatment
• **Renal disease:** protein, BUN, creatinine, potassium, sodium at baseline, periodically; increased levels may indicate nephrotic syndrome; renal symptoms: polyuria, oliguria, urinary frequency, dysuria
• **Serious allergic reactions:** angioedema, Stevens-Johnson syndrome, rash, fever, pruritus, urticaria; product should be discontinued if antihistamines fail to help
• Monitor electrolytes baseline and periodically; potassium may be increased

Black Box Warning: **Pregnancy:** identify if pregnant or if pregnancy is planned or suspected; if pregnant, discontinue product; do not use in pregnancy/breastfeeding; can cause injury or death to developing fetus

• For dry cough; notify prescriber as product may need to be discontinued
Evaluate:
• **Therapeutic response:** decrease in B/P, HF, prevention of death from stroke, MI
Teach patient/family:
• Not to discontinue product abruptly; to comply with dosage schedule, even if feeling better
• Not to use OTC products (cough, cold, allergy), herbals, supplements unless directed by prescriber; not to use salt substitutes containing potassium without consulting prescriber

• To rise slowly to sitting or standing position to minimize orthostatic hypotension
• To notify prescriber of mouth sores, sore throat, fever, swelling of hands or feet, irregular heartbeat, chest pain
• To report excessive perspiration, dehydration, vomiting, diarrhea; may lead to fall in B/P; to maintain hydration
• That product may cause dizziness, fainting, light-headedness; that these may occur during first few days of therapy; to avoid hazardous activities until response is known
• That product may cause skin rash, impaired perspiration
• How to take B/P, normal readings for age group
• To report dry cough to provider

Black Box Warning: To inform prescriber if pregnancy is planned or suspected; not to breastfeed

TREATMENT OF OVERDOSE:
0.9% NaCl IV infusion, hemodialysis

ramucirumab (Rx)
(ra-mue-sir′ue-mab)
Cyramza
Func. class.: Antineoplastic
Chem. class.: Vascular endothelial growth factor antagonist

Do not confuse:
Cyramza/Cimzia

ACTION: Binds to vascular endothelial growth factor receptor 2 (VEGFR2; kinase insert domain-containing receptor; KDR), preventing the binding of ligands; as a result, ramucirumab inhibits ligand-induced proliferation and migration of human endothelial cells

USES: As a single agent or in combination with PACLitaxel for advanced or metastatic gastric or gastroesophageal junction adenocarcinoma with disease progression on or after fluoropyrimidine

CONTRAINDICATIONS
Hypersensitivity, pregnancy, breastfeeding
Precautions: Anticoagulant therapy, bleeding, cirrhosis, MI, contraception requirements, GI perforation, hepatic disease, human antihuman antibody (HAHA), hypertension, hypothyroidism, infusion related reactions, renal disease, stroke, surgery

DOSAGE AND ROUTES
Gastric cancer or gastroesophageal junction adenocarcinoma and hepatocellular cancer (single agent)
• **Adults:** IV infusion 8 mg/kg over 60 min q2wk until disease progression or unacceptable toxicity; if first infusion is tolerated, all subsequent infusions may be administered over 30 min
Combination with PACLitaxel
• **Adults:** IV infusion 8 mg/kg over 60 min q2wk with PACLitaxel 80 mg/m² on days 1, 8, and 15 of a 28-day cycle
NSCLC
• **Adults:** IV infusion 10 mg/kg over 60 min with docetaxel (75 mg/m² IV) on day 1, give q21days until disease progression or unacceptable toxicity
mCRC
• **Adults** IV 8 mg/kg over 60 min on day 1 before FOLFIRI use, q2wk until disease progression or unacceptable toxicity; FOLFIRI consists of irinotecan 180 mg/m² IV over 90 min and folinic acid (leucovorin) 400 mg/m² given over 120 min on day 1, followed by fluorouracil 400 mg/m² IV bolus over 2-4 min on day 1, followed by fluorouracil 2400 mg/m² by continuous IV infusion over 46-48 hr; if first infusion is tolerated, all subsequent infusions may be given over 30 min
Hepatic dose
• **Adults:** IV Mild to moderate hepatic impairment (Child-Pugh A; total bilirubin 1.1-3 times ULN and any AST, OR or total bilirubin within ULN and AST greater than ULN):** no change; **severe hepatic impairment (Child-Pugh B or C):** Use only if the potential benefits outweigh the risks
Available forms: Injection 10 mg/mL single-dose vial, requires dilution
Administer:
Intermittent IV infusion route
Intermittent IV infusion route
• Use cytotoxic handling precautions
• Premedicate with an IV histamine-1 (H1) receptor antagonist (diphenhydramine); for patients who have had a prior grade 1 or 2 infusion-related reaction, premedicate with an H1-receptor antagonist, dexamethasone (or equivalent), and acetaminophen before each infusion
• Dilute with normal saline to a final volume of 250 mL; invert to mix; do not shake; stable for 4 hr at room temperature
• Inspect for particles and discoloration before using
• Use a protein-sparing 0.22-micron filter; use separate line; flush with normal saline after use
• Do not admix with other solutions or medications
• Store vials in refrigerator; protect from light, do not freeze

SIDE EFFECTS
CNS: Headache, fatigue, RPLS, stroke
CV: Hypertension, arterial thromboembolic events, hemorrhage, MI, cardiac arrest
EENT: Epistaxis
GI: Intestinal obstruction/perforation, diarrhea
GU: Proteinuria
HEMA: Neutropenia, anemia, bleeding
RESP: Lower respiratory tract infection, cough, pleuritic pain
INTEG: Rash
MISC: Hypothyroidism, hyponatremia, IRR, antibody formation, infusion site reactions, poor wound healing

PHARMACOKINETICS
Onset 2 wk, half-life 15 days

INTERACTIONS
Drug/Lab Test
Increased: urine protein, T5H, RBC, platelets, neutrophils

Decreased: RBCs, serum sodium

NURSING CONSIDERATIONS
Assess
• **Bleeding/hemorrhage:** assess for GI bleeding; perforation (severe abdominal pain, nausea, vomiting, fever) may be fatal; discontinue and do not restart if this occurs

• **Poor wound healing:** assess all wounds for changes, avoid use if present

• **Hypertension:** monitor B/P frequently, at least q2wk; if hypertension occurs, withhold until controlled

• **GI status:** diarrhea, bowel sounds; obstruction/perforation has occurred

• **Infusion-related reactions:** chills, fever, chest discomfort, tachycardia, wheezing

• **CNS, RPLS:** assess for hypertension, blurred vision, impaired consciousness, seizures, headache; may be confirmed with MRI; discontinue and do not restart if confirmed

• **Cardiac status:** assess for serious cardiac events, including MI, stroke; discontinue permanently if these occur

• **Pregnancy/breastfeeding:** do not use in pregnancy; women should use adequate contraception during and for ≥3 months after last dose; if childbearing potential, do not breastfeed

Evaluate:
• **Therapeutic response:** decreased progression of cancer

Teach patient/family:
• **Bleeding:** teach patient that bleeding may occur, to contact provider for bleeding

• **Poor wound healing:** teach patient to report wound changes, to discuss with all providers use of product

• Advise patient to report severe abdominal pain, diarrhea, vomiting, lightheadedness

• **Hypertension:** teach patient to monitor B/P frequently, at least q2wk; if high or if headache is present, notify provider

• **RPLS:** assess for hypertension, blurred vision, impaired consciousness, seizures, headache; may be confirmed with MRI; discontinue and do not restart if confirmed

• **Pregnancy/breastfeeding:** identify if pregnancy is planned or suspected; teach not to use in pregnancy, to use adequate contraception during and for ≥3 months after last dose; if childbearing potential, do not breastfeed; product may impair fertility

---

ranibizumab (Rx)
(ran-ih-biz′oo-mab)

Byooviz, Lucentis, Susvimo

Func. class.: Ophthalmic

Chem. class.: Selective vascular endothelial growth factor antagonist

---

ACTION: Binds to receptor-binding site of active forms of vascular endothelial growth factor A (VEGF-A), which causes angiogenesis and cell proliferation

USES: Age-related macular degeneration (neovascular) (wet), macular edema after retinal vein occlusion (RVO), diabetic macular edema

CONTRAINDICATIONS
Hypersensitivity, ocular infections

Precautions: Pregnancy, breastfeeding, children, retinal detachment, increased intraocular pressure

Black Box Warning: Endophthalmitis

DOSAGE AND ROUTES
Neovascular (wet) age-related macular degeneration (Susvime)
• **Adult: Occular implant (continuous)** 2 mg (0.2 mL of 100 mg/m/solution) refilled every 24 wk

Neovascular (wet) age-related macular degeneration (AMD)/or macular edema after retinal vein occlusion (RVO) (Lucentis, Byuoviz)
• **Adult: INTRAVITREAL** 0.5 mg (0.05 mL) of 10 mg/mL product monthly or 0.5 mg monthly × 4 mo, then 0.5 mg q3mo;

(Susvimo) 2 mg continuously delivered via ocular implant

Diabetic macular edema (Except Byooviz)
• **Adult: INTRAVITREAL** 0.3 mg of 6 mg/mL q28day

Available forms: Sol for inj 6 mg/mL, 10 mg/mL; prefilled syringe 0.3-mg dose; 0.5 mg/0.05 mL solution for injection; 100 mg/mL solution for injection

Administer:
• By ophthalmologist via intravitreal injection using adequate anesthesia; use 19-gauge filter
• Store in refrigerator; do not freeze
• Protect from light

SIDE EFFECTS
CNS: Dizziness, headache, peripheral neuropathy
EENT: Blepharitis, cataract, conjunctival hemorrhage/hyperemia, detachment of retinal pigment epithelium, dry eye, irritation/pain in eye, visual impairment, vitreous floaters, ocular infection
GI: Constipation, nausea
MISC: Hypertension, UTI, thromboembolism, nonocular bleeding, anemia, arthralgia
RESP: Bronchitis, cough, sinusitis, URI, pulmonary embolism
INTEG: Impaired wound healing
CV: Hypertension, thromboembolism, nonocular bleeding, anemia, angina, CAD

PHARMACOKINETICS
Elimination half-life 9 days, peak 1 day

INTERACTIONS
Increase: severe inflammation—verteporfin photodynamic therapy (PDT)

NURSING CONSIDERATIONS
Assess:
• **Eye changes:** redness; sensitivity to light, vision change; increased intraocular pressure change; report infection to ophthalmologist immediately, complete procedure with anesthesia and antibiotic before use, check perfusion of optic nerve after use
• **Hypersensitivity:** monitor for inflammation
• **Infection:** UTI, URI, wound/skin

Evaluate:
• **Therapeutic response:** prevention of increasing macular degeneration
Teach patient/family:
• If eye becomes red, sensitive to light, painful, or if there is a change in vision, to seek immediate care from ophthalmologist
• About reason for treatment, expected results; that product is injected into the eye, an anesthetic will be used

ranolazine (Rx)
(ruh-no'luh-zeen)
Aspruzyo Sprinkle, Ranexa
Func. class.: Antianginal
Chem. class.: Piperazine derivative

ACTION: Antianginal, antiischemic; unknown, may work by inhibiting portal fatty-acid oxidation

USES: Chronic stable angina pectoris; use in patients who have not responded to other treatment options; should be used in combination with other antianginals such as amLODIPine, β-blockers, nitrates
Unlabeled uses: Unstable angina

CONTRAINDICATIONS
Preexisting QT prolongation, hepatic disease (Child-Pugh class A, B, C), hypersensitivity, hypokalemia, renal failure, torsades de pointes, ventricular dysrhythmia, ventricular tachycardia, hepatic cirrhosis
Precautions: Pregnancy, breastfeeding, children, geriatric patients, hypotension, renal disease, females at risk for torsades de pointes

DOSAGE AND ROUTES
Chronic angina
• **Adult: PO** 500 mg bid, increased to 1000 mg bid based on response; max 1000 mg bid; limit to 500 mg bid in those taking **moderate CYP3A4 inhibitors**

Available forms: Ext rel tabs 500, 1000 mg; granules, extended release 500, 1000 mg

Administer:

• Use in combination with H$_2$ blocker, metroNIDAZOLE, proton pump inhibitor, and clarithromycin for *H. pylori*

• Without regard to meals, bid; do not use with grapefruit juice or grapefruit

• **Ext rel tabs:** do not break, crush, chew tabs; take product as prescribed; do not double or skip dose

• **Granules:** Sprinkle on 1 Tbs of soft food, use immediately

SIDE EFFECTS

CNS: *Headache, dizziness,* hallucinations

CV: Palpitations, QT prolongation, orthostatic hypotension

EENT: Tinnitus

GI: Nausea, vomiting, constipation, dry mouth

MISC: Peripheral edema

RESP: Dyspnea

PHARMACOKINETICS

Absorption varied; peak 2-5 hr; half-life 7 hr; extensively metabolized by the liver (CYP3A and less by CYP2D6); excreted in urine (75%), feces (25%); protein binding 62%

INTERACTIONS

Increase: ranolazine action—diltiaZEM, ketoconazole, macrolide antibiotics, dofetilide, PARoxetine, protease inhibitors, quiNIDine, sotalol, thioridazine, verapamil, ziprasidone, avoid using together

Increase: action of digoxin, simvastatin

Increase: ranolazine absorption, toxicity—antiretroviral protease inhibitors

Increase: QT prolongation and torsades de pointes—class IA/III antidysrhythmics, arsenic trioxide, chloroquine, droperidol, haloperidol, methadone, pentamidine, chlorproMAZINE, mesoridazine, thioridazine, pimozide; CYP3A4 inhibitors (ketoconazole, fluconazole, itraconazole, IV miconazole, voriconazole, diltiaZEM, verapamil)

Drug/Food

Do not use with grapefruit, grapefruit juice

Drug/Herb

Decrease: ranolazine level—St. John's wort, don't use together

NURSING CONSIDERATIONS

Assess:

• **Angina:** characteristics of pain (intensity, location, duration, alleviating/precipitating factors)

• **QT prolongation:** ECG for QT prolongation, ejection fraction; assess for chest pain, palpitations, dyspnea; torsades de pointes may occur

• Cardiac status: B/P, pulse, respirations

• LFTs, serum creatinine/BUN (in those with CCr <60 mL/min), magnesium, potassium before treatment, periodically; if BUN and creatinine increase significantly, discontinue product

• **Pregnancy/breastfeeding:** use only if benefits outweigh fetal risk; do not breastfeed, excretion unknown

Evaluate:

• **Therapeutic response:** decreased anginal pain, attacks

Teach patient/family:

• To avoid hazardous activities until stabilized on product, dizziness no longer a problem

• To avoid OTC drugs, grapefruit juice, products prolonging QTc (quiNIDine, dofetilide, sotalol, erythromycin, thioridazine, ziprasidone or protease inhibitors, diltiaZEM, ketoconazole, macrolide antibiotics, verapamil) unless directed by prescriber; to notify prescriber of palpitations, fainting

• To comply with all areas of medical regimen

• To take as directed; not to skip dose, double doses

• Not to chew or crush; not to use with grapefruit juice

• To notify all health care providers of product use

• To notify prescriber of dizziness, edema, dyspnea

• For acute angina, to take other products prescribed; this product does not decrease acute attack

rasagiline (Rx)

(ra-sa′ji-leen)

Azilect

Func. class.: Antiparkinson agent
Chem. class.: MAOI, type B

Do not confuse:
Azilect/Aricept

ACTION: Inhibits MAOI type B at recommended doses; may increase DOPamine levels

USES: Idiopathic Parkinson's disease monotherapy or with levodopa

CONTRAINDICATIONS

Breastfeeding; hypersensitivity to this product, MAOIs; pheochromocytoma
Precautions: Pregnancy, children, psychiatric disorders, moderate to severe hepatic disorders

DOSAGE AND ROUTES
Parkinson's disease
Monotherapy
• **Adult: PO** 1 mg/day
Adjunctive therapy
• **Adult: PO** 0.5 mg/day, may increase 1 mg/day; change of levodopa dose for adjunct therapy; reduced levodopa dose may be needed
Hepatic dose
• **Adult: PO** 0.5 mg for mild hepatic disease
Concomitant ciprofloxacin, other CYP1A2 inhibitors
• **Adult: PO** 0.5 mg; plasma concentrations of rasagiline may double
Available forms: Tabs 0.5, 1 mg
Administer:
• With meals to prevent nausea; continuing therapy usually reduces or eliminates nausea; do not give with foods/liquids containing large amounts of tyramine
• Reduce dose of carbidopa/levodopa cautiously
• Renal failure: in dialysis, increase dose slowly

SIDE EFFECTS
Monotherapy
CNS: Drowsiness, hallucinations, depression, headache, malaise, paresthesia, vertigo, syncope
CV: Angina, orthostatic hypotension
GI: *Nausea,* diarrhea, dry mouth, dyspepsia
GU: Impotence, decreased libido
HEMA: Leukopenia
INTEG: Alopecia, skin cancers
MISC: Conjunctivitis, fever, flu syndrome, neck pain, allergic reaction, alopecia
MS: Arthralgia, arthritis, dyskinesia
RESP: Rhinitis

PHARMACOKINETICS

Onset, peak, duration unknown; 35%-40% absorbed; protein binding >88%-94%; metabolized by CYP1A2 in liver; excreted by kidneys <1%, half-life 1.3 hr

INTERACTIONS

Do not give with meperidine, other analgesics because serious reactions (including coma and death) may occur; do not give with sympathomimetics
Increase: levels of rasagiline up to 2-fold—ciprofloxacin, CYP1A2 inhibitors (atazanavir, mexiletine, taurine)
Increased: dopaminergic adverse reaction risk—levodopa, dopamine agonists
Increase: severe CNS toxicity with antidepressants (tricyclics, SSRIs, SNRIs, mirtazapine, cyclobenzaprine)
Increase: hypertensive crisis—MAOIs
Drug/Herb
Do not give with St. John's wort, yohimbe
Drug/Food
Do not give with foods/liquids that have large amounts of tyramine (cured meats, aged cheese)
Drug/Lab Test
Increase: LFTs
Decrease: WBCs

NURSING CONSIDERATIONS
Assess:
• **Parkinson's symptoms:** tremors, ataxia, muscle weakness and rigidity at baseline, periodically; increased dyskinesia, pos-

tural hypotension if used in combination with levodopa

• Mental status: hallucinations, confusion; notify prescriber

• **Hypertensive crisis:** severe headache, blurred vision, seizures, chest pain, difficulty thinking, nausea, vomiting, signs of stroke; any unexplained severe headache should be considered to be hypertensive crisis

• **Melanoma:** periodic skin exams by a dermatologist for possible skin cancer

• Cardiac status: B/P, ECG periodically, orthostatic hypotension during 2 months of treatment during beginning treatment

• **Tyramine products:** foods, other medications may lead to hypertensive crisis (tachycardia, bradycardia, chest pain, nausea, vomiting, sweating, dilated pupils)

• Drowsiness, daytime sleepiness or falling asleep, may need to be discontinued

• **Serotonin syndrome:** agitation, coma, tachycardia, hyperreflexia, nausea, vomiting, diarrhea; may be precipitated in those taking SSRIs, SNRIs

• **Pregnancy/breastfeeding:** use only if benefits outweigh fetal risk; cautious use in breastfeeding, excretion unknown

Evaluate:

• **Therapeutic response:** improved symptoms in patients with Parkinson's disease

Teach patient/family:

• To change positions slowly to prevent orthostatic hypotension

• To avoid hazardous activities until stabilized on product; that dizziness can occur

• To rinse mouth frequently; to use sugarless gum to alleviate dry mouth

• To take as prescribed; not to miss dose or double doses; to take missed dose as soon as remembered if several hours before next dose

• To prevent hypertensive crisis by avoiding high-tyramine foods (>150 mg), give list to patient, to report signs/symptoms of hypertensive crisis (headache, chest pain, nausea, palpitations, racing heart)

• To avoid CNS depressants, alcohol

• To notify all providers of product use; to avoid elective surgery, other procedures involving CNS depressants

• Check skin periodically for possible skin cancer, higher evidence in Parkinson's disease

---

⚠ HIGH ALERT

rasburicase (Rx)

(rass-burr'i-case)

Elitek, Fasturtec ✦

Func. class.: Enzyme

Chem. class.: Recombinant urate-oxidase enzyme

ACTION: Catalyzes enzymatic oxidation of uric acid into an inactive and soluble metabolite (allantoin)

USES: To reduce uric acid levels in patients with leukemia, lymphoma, or solid tumor malignancies who are receiving chemotherapy

CONTRAINDICATIONS

Hypersensitivity

Black Box Warning: ⚠ G6PD deficiency (Mediterranean, African descent), hemolytic reactions, methemoglobinemia reactions to product

Precautions: Pregnancy, breastfeeding, children <2 yr, anemia, acute bronchospasm, angina, atony, African-American and Mediterranean patients, hypotension

Black Box Warning: Anaphylaxis, interference with uric acid measurements

DOSAGE AND ROUTES

• **Adult/adolescent/infant: IV INFUSION** 0.2 mg/kg as single daily dose × 5 days

Available forms: Powder for inj 1.5, 7.5 mg/vial

Administer:
Intermittent IV INFUSION route

• Determine number of vials that are needed based on weight, concentration required

• **Reconstitute** with diluent provided, add 1 mL of diluent/each vial, swirl, withdraw amount needed, mix with NS to final volume of 50 mL, use within 24 hr, give over 30 min, **do not use filter,** use different line; if not possible, flush with ≥15 mL of saline before, after use

• Chemotherapy started 4-24 hr after 1st dose

SIDE EFFECTS

CNS: *Headache,* fever
CV: Chest pain, hypotension
GI: *Nausea, vomiting, anorexia, diarrhea, abdominal pain, constipation, dyspepsia, mucositis*
HEMA: Neutropenia with fever, hemolysis, methemoglobinemia
INTEG: *Rash*
MISC: Edema
SYST: Anaphylaxis, hemolysis, sepsis

PHARMACOKINETICS
Half-life 16-21 hr, duration up to 12 hr

INTERACTIONS
Increase: methemoglobinemia risk—local anesthetics
Drug/Lab Test

Black Box Warning: **Interference:** uric acid

NURSING CONSIDERATIONS
Assess:

• Blood studies: BUN, serum uric acid, urine creatinine clearance, electrolytes; CBC with differential before, during therapy

• Monitor temperature; fever may indicate beginning infection; no rectal temperatures

Black Box Warning: **Anaphylaxis:** dyspnea, urticaria, flushing, wheezing; swelling of lips, tongue, throat; have emergency equipment nearby

Black Box Warning: **G6PD deficiency, hemolytic reactions, methemoglobinemia;** these patients should not be given this product; screen patients who are at higher risk for these disorders

Black Box Warning: **Altered uric acid measurements:** for accurate results, collect blood in prechilled tubes with heparin, place tubes on ice, test within 4 hr

• GI symptoms: frequency of stools, cramping; if severe diarrhea occurs, fluid, electrolytes may need to be given
Evaluate:
• **Therapeutic response:** decreased uric acid levels in children when antineoplastics causing high uric acid levels used
Teach patient/family:
• About the reason for therapy, expected results
• **Pregnancy/breastfeeding:** identify if pregnancy is planned or suspected or if breastfeeding

ravulizumab (Rx)
(rav′-yoo-liz′-yoo-mab)
Ultomiris
Func. class.: Monoclonal antibody

USES: Atypical hemolytic uremic syndrome in adults and pediatrics, paroxysmal nocturnal hemoglobinuria

CONTRAINDICATIONS
Hypersensitivity

Black Box Warning: Meningococcal infection

DOSAGE AND ROUTES
Treat for at least 6 months
• **Adults ≥100 kg: IV** 3000 mg load, then 3600 mg q8wk starting 2 wk after loading dose

- **Adults 60 to 99 kg: IV** 2700 mg load, then 3300 mg q8wk starting 2 wk after loading dose
- **Adults 40 to 59 kg: IV** 2400 mg load, then 3000 mg q8wk starting 2 wk after loading dose
- **Adolescents ≥100 kg: IV** 3000 mg load, then 3600 mg q8wk starting 2 wk after the loading dose
- **Children and adolescents 60 to 99 kg: IV** 2700 mg load, then 3300 mg q8wk starting 2 wk after loading dose
- **Children and adolescents 40 to 59 kg: IV** 2400 mg load, then 3000 mg q8wk starting 2 wk after loading dose
- **Children and adolescents 30 to 39 kg: IV** 1200 mg load, then 2700 mg q8wk starting 2 wk after loading dose
- **Children 20 to 29 kg: IV** 900 mg load, then 2100 mg q8wk starting 2 wk after the loading dose
- **Infants and children 10 to 19 kg: IV** 600 mg load, then 600 mg q4wk starting 2 wk after loading dose
- **Infants and children 5 to 9 kg: IV** 600 mg load, then 300 mg q4wk starting 2 wk after loading dose

Available forms: Injection 300 mg/30-mL single-dose vial

> ### ⚠ HIGH ALERT
>
> ### regorafenib (Rx)
> (re′goe-raf′e-nib)
> Stivarga
> *Func. class.:* Antineoplastic; multikinase inhibitor
> *Chem. class.:* Signal transduction inhibitor (STI)

ACTION: Inhibits tyrosine kinase in patients with colorectal cancer

USES: Metastatic colorectal cancer in those who have received fluoropyrimidine, oxaliplatin, irinotecan-based chemotherapy, an anti-VEGF therapy; and an anti-EGFR therapy if *KRAS* wild type

CONTRAINDICATIONS
Pregnancy

Precautions: Breastfeeding, children, geriatric patients, cardiac/renal/hepatic/dental disease, fistula, GI bleeding or perforation, bone marrow suppression, infection, wound dehiscence, thrombocytopenia, neutropenia, immunosuppression

Black Box Warning: Hepatic disease

DOSAGE AND ROUTES
- **Adult: PO** 160 mg/day with a low-fat breakfast × 21 days of a 28-day cycle, cycles may be repeated

Available forms: Tabs 40 mg

Administer:
- Store at 77° F (25° C)
- Give at the same time each day with a low-fat breakfast that contains less than 30% fat such as 2 slices of white toast with 1 tbsp of low-fat margarine and 1 tbsp of jelly, and 8 oz of skim milk; or 1 cup of cereal, 8 oz of skim milk, 1 slice of toast with jam, apple juice, and 1 cup of coffee or tea
- Swallow tablets whole
- If a dose is missed, take as soon as possible that day; do not take 2 doses on the same day
- **Hand-foot skin reaction:** Reduce to 120 mg (grade 2 palmar-plantar erythrodysesthesia); hold if grade 2 toxicity does not improve in ≤7 days or recurs; hold for ≥7 days in grade 3 toxicity; reduce to 80 mg for recurrent grade 2 toxicity; discontinue if 80 mg is not tolerated
- **Hypertension:** Hold in grade 2 hypertension

Other severe toxicity (except hepatotoxicity)
- Hold until toxicity resolves in grade 3 or 4 toxicity; consider the risk/benefits of continuing therapy in grade 4 toxicity, reduce dosage to 120 mg; if grade 3 or 4 toxicity recurs, hold until toxicity resolves, then reduce to 80 mg; discontinue in those who do not tolerate 80-mg dose
- **Hepatic dose:** Baseline mild (Child-Pugh class A) or moderate (Child-Pugh

class B): no change; baseline severe hepatic impairment (Child-Pugh class C): use not recommended; AST/ALT elevations during therapy: For grade 3 AST/ALT level elevations, hold dose; if therapy is continued, reduce to 120 mg after levels recover; discontinue in those with AST/ALT >20 × ULN; AST/ALT >3 × ULN and bilirubin >2 × ULN; recurrence of AST/ALT >5 × ULN despite a reduction to 120 mg

SIDE EFFECTS

CNS: Headache, tremor
CV: Hypertensive crisis, MI
EENT: Blurred vision, conjunctivitis
GI: Hepatotoxicity, GI hemorrhage, diarrhea, GI perforation, xerostomia
HEMA: Neutropenia, thrombocytopenia, bleeding
INTEG: Rash, alopecia
META: Hypokalemia
MISC: Fatigue, decreased weight, hand-foot syndrome, hypothyroidism

PHARMACOKINETICS

Protein binding 99%, metabolized by CYP3A4, UGT1A0, half-life 14-58 hr

INTERACTIONS

Increase: regorafenib concentrations—CYP3A4 inhibitors (ketoconazole, itraconazole, erythromycin, clarithromycin), avoid using together
Increase: plasma concentrations of simvastatin, calcium channel blockers, ergots
Increase: plasma concentration of warfarin; avoid use with warfarin; use low-molecular-weight anticoagulants instead
Decrease: regorafenib concentrations—CYP3A4 inducers (dexamethasone, phenytoin, carBAMazepine, rifAMPin, PHENobarbital), avoid using together
Drug/Food
Increase: regorafenib effect—grapefruit juice; avoid use while taking product
Drug/Herb
Decrease: imatinib concentration—St. John's wort

NURSING CONSIDERATIONS
Assess:

Black Box Warning: Hepatic disease: fatal hepatotoxicity can occur; obtain LFTs baseline and at least every 2 wk × 2 mo, then monthly

• Assess any wounds for wound healing; report wound dehiscence, stop medication, notify prescriber
• **Fatal bleeding:** from GI, respiratory, GU tracts; permanently discontinue in those with severe bleeding
• **Palmar-plantar erythrodysesthesia (hand-foot syndrome):** more common in those previously treated; reddening, swelling, numbness, desquamation on palms, soles
• **GI perforation/fistula:** discontinue if this occurs; assess for pain in epigastric area, dyspepsia, flatulence, fever, chills
• **Hypertension/hypertensive crisis:** hypertension usually occurs in the first cycle in those with preexisting hypertension; do not start treatment until B/P is controlled; monitor B/P every week × 6 wk, then at start of each cycle or more often if needed; temporarily or permanently discontinue for severe uncontrolled hypertension
• **Pregnancy/breastfeeding:** identify whether patient is pregnant or if pregnancy is planned; identify contraception type in both men and women; do not use in pregnancy and for 2 mo after last dose, breastfeeding
Evaluate:
• **Therapeutic response:** decrease in spread or size of tumor
Teach patient/family:
• To report adverse reactions immediately: bleeding, rash
• About reason for treatment, expected results
• That effect on male fertility is unknown
• To take at the same time of day with low-fat food; not to use grapefruit juice; to take missed dose on same day; not to take multiple doses on the same day; to keep original container
• To report immediately **hepatic effect** (yellowing skin, eyes, nausea, vomiting, dark urine), **increased B/P** (severe head-

ache), **GI perforation/fistula** (dyspepsia, flatulence, fever, chills, epigastric pain)

• **Pregnancy/breastfeeding:** not to use in pregnancy; to report if pregnancy is suspected or if breastfeeding; for men and women to use contraception during and for 2 mo after termination of treatment

---

remdesivir (Rx)

(rem-de′si-vir)

Veklury

Func. class.: Antiviral
Chem. class.: RNA-polymerase inhibitor

ACTION: Inhibits SARS-CoV-2 RNA–dependent RNA polymerase needed for viral replication

USES: COVID-19

DOSAGE AND ROUTES

• **Adult/child ≥12 yr and 40 kg:** IV: 200 mg (single dose) on day 1, then 100 mg daily × 4 days or until hospital discharge, whichever is first; may continue up to 10 days in those without improvement at day 5; **Child ≥28 days and 3 to <40 kg: IV infusion; Ventilated or ECMO:** 5 mg/kg on day 1, then 2.5 mg/kg qday on day 2 for 5 days **Not ventilated or ECMO:** if no improvement, give for 5 more days; if no improvement, give for 10 more days

Available forms: IV solution (preservative free) 100 mg/20 mL; powder for injection 1000 mg

Administer:

Intermittent IV infusion route

• **Injection solution:** Warm to room temperature before dilution, further dilute in 250 mL NS; withdraw and discard the required volume of NS from the infusion bag (40 mL/200 mg; 20 mL/100 mg) before addition of remdesivir, transfer required volume of remdesivir to the infusion bag and invert to mix; do not shake. Discard unused portion of the injection solution vial

• **Lyophilized powder:** Reconstitute vial/19 mL SWFI; shake for 30 sec, allow to sit for 2-3 min, repeat until contents are dissolved (5 mg/mL); further dilute

in 100-250 mL NS; withdraw and discard the required volume of NS from the infusion bag (40 mL/200 mg; 20 mL/100 mg) before adding remdesivir; transfer needed volume of remdesivir to the infusion bag and invert to mix. Discard unused portion

• Give over 30-120 min

CONTRAINDICATIONS

Hypersensitivity

Precautions: Breastfeeding, child <12 yr, dialysis, hepatic disease, infusion-related reactions, pregnancy, renal disease

> **Black Box Warning:** Remdesivir is not an approved treatment for COVID-19 caused by SARS-CoV-2, but is investigational and is available under an FDA emergency use authorization (EUA) for the treatment of COVID-19 in hospitalized patients only

SIDE EFFECTS

GI: Diarrhea, constipation, increased LFTs, nausea

RESP: Dyspnea, hypoxia, **respiratory arrest,** wheezing

CNS: Fever, headache, delirium, **seizures,** shivering

INTEG: Anaphylaxis, angioedema, infusion-related reactions, phlebitis, rash, ecchymosis

HEMA: Anemia

CV: Atrial fibrillation, bradycardia, hypo-hypertension, **sinus tachycardia**

ENDO: Hyperbilirubinemia, hyperglycemia, hypernatremia, hypokalemia

GU: Hematuria

PHARMACOKINETICS

Protein binding 88%-93%, half-life <1 hr, metabolites up to 27 hr

INTERACTIONS

Decrease: Remdesivir effect—hydroxychloroquine, chloroquine, strong CYP3A4 inducers, avoid using together

NURSING CONSIDERATIONS

Assess:

• **COVID-19:** Confirm presence of CO-VID-19 before starting treatment; obtain

---

CBC with differential, PT, and serum electrolytes before and during treatment

• **Hepatic effects:** Obtain LFTs before and during treatment; discontinue in ALT >10 × ULN; discontinue if ALT elevation with signs/symptoms of liver inflammation occur

• **Hypersensitivity:** Monitor for infusion-related reactions, anaphylaxis, angioedema, diaphoresis, dyspnea, hypo-hypertension, hypoxia, fever, rash, shivering, tachycardia, wheezing; slow infusion rate to max infusion time: 120 min; discontinue and provide treatment if severe

• **Renal disease:** Obtain BUN/creatinine baseline and during treatment; monitor for hematuria; avoid use in eGFR <30 mL/min, significant toxicity with a short duration of therapy 5-10 days is unlikely

• **CV reactions:** Monitor for atrial fibrillation, hyper-hypotension, sinus tachycardia, bradycardia

• **Pregnancy/breastfeeding:** Identify if pregnant or if breastfeeding

Evaluate:

• **Therapeutic response:** Resolution of COVID-19 without serious adverse reactions

Teach patient/family:

• Reason for product and expected results

• To report immediately to provider rash, itching, injection site reactions, trouble breathing, shivering, wheezing, rapid heartbeat

• Provide "fact sheet" to patient/caregiver and review

• That this product has not been approved by the FDA and has been granted for emergency use only

---

⚠ HIGH ALERT

remifentanil (Rx)

(rem-ih-fin′ta-nill)

Ultiva

Func. class.: Opiate agonist analgesic
Chem. class.: μ-Opioid agonist

Controlled Substance Schedule II

ACTION: Inhibits ascending pain pathways in limbic system, thalamus, midbrain, hypothalamus

USES: In combination with other products for general anesthesia to provide analgesia

CONTRAINDICATIONS

Hypersensitivity

Precautions: Pregnancy, breastfeeding, children <12 yr, geriatric patients, increased intracranial pressure, acute MI, severe heart disease, GI/renal/hepatic disease, asthma, respiratory conditions, seizure disorders, bradyarrhythmias

> **Black Box Warning:** Potential for overdose or poisoning, substance abuse

DOSAGE AND ROUTES

• **Adult:** IV induction 0.5-1 mcg/kg/min with hypnotic or volatile agent; **maintenance with isoflurane or propofol** 0.25 mcg/kg/min (range 0.05-2 mcg/kg/min); **CONT INFUSION** 0.025-0.2 mcg/kg/min

• **Child 1-12 yr:** CONT IV INFUSION 0.25 mcg/kg/min with isoflurane

• **Full-term neonate and infant up to 2 mo:** CONT IV INFUSION 0.4 mcg/kg/min with nitrous oxide

Available forms: Powder for inj lyophilized 1, 2, 5 mg

Administer:

• Add 1 mL diluent per mg remifentanil

• Shake well; further dilute to a final concentration of 20, 25, 50, or 250 mcg/mL

• Store in light-resistant area at room temperature

• Interruption of infusion results in rapid reversal (no residual opioid effect within 5-10 min)

Direct IV route

• To be used only during maintenance of general anesthesia; inject into tubing close to venous cannula; give to nonintubated patients over 30-60 sec

Continuous IV INFUSION route

• Use infusion device, max 16 hr; do not use same tubing as blood, do not admix

R

Y-site compatibilities: Acyclovir, alfentanil, amikacin, aminophylline, ampicillin, ampicillin/sulbactam, aztreonam, bumetanide, buprenorphine, butorphanol, calcium gluconate, ceFAZolin, cefepime, cefotaxime, cefoTEtan, cefOXitin, cefTAZidime, ceftizoxime, cefTRIAXone, cefuroxime, cimetidine, ciprofloxacin, cisatracurium, clindamycin, dexamethasone, digoxin, diltiazem, diphenhydrAMINE, DOBUTamine, DOPamine, doxacurium, doxycycline, droperidol, enalaprilat, EPINEPHrine, esmolol, famotidine, fentaNYL, fluconazole, furosemide, ganciclovir, gatifloxacin, gentamicin, haloperidol, heparin, hydrocortisone sodium succinate, HYDROmorphone, hydrOXYzine, imipenem-cilastatin, inamrinone, isoproterenol, ketorolac, lidocaine, LORazepam, magnesium sulfate, mannitol, meperidine, methylPREDNISolone sodium succinate, metoclopramide, metroNIDAZOLE, midazolam, morphine, nalbuphine, nitroglycerin, norepinephrine, ondansetron, phenylephrine, piperacillin, potassium chloride, procainamide, prochlorperazine, promethazine, raNITIdine, SUFentanil, theophylline, thiopental, ticarcillin/clavulanate, tobramycin, vancomycin, zidovudine

Solution compatibilities: D$_5$W, 0.45% NaCl, LR, D$_5$LR, 0.9% NaCl

SIDE EFFECTS

CNS: Drowsiness, *dizziness,* confusion, *headache,* sedation, euphoria, delirium, agitation, anxiety
CV: Palpitations, *bradycardia,* change in B/P, facial flushing, syncope, asystole
EENT: Tinnitus, blurred vision, miosis, diplopia
GI: *Nausea, vomiting,* anorexia, constipation, cramps, dry mouth
GU: Urinary retention, dysuria
INTEG: Rash, urticaria, bruising, flushing, diaphoresis, pruritus
MS: Rigidity
RESP: Respiratory depression, apnea

PHARMACOKINETICS

70% protein binding, terminal half-life 3-10 min, excreted in urine; onset: 1-3 min

INTERACTIONS

Increase: respiratory depression, hypotension, profound sedation: alcohol, sedatives, hypnotics, other CNS depressants; antihistamines, phenothiazines, MAOIs
Drug/Herb
Increase: CNS depression—kava

NURSING CONSIDERATIONS
Assess:
• I&O ratio; check for decreasing output; may indicate urinary retention, especially in geriatric patients
• CNS changes; dizziness, drowsiness, hallucinations, euphoria, LOC, pupil reaction
• GI status: nausea, vomiting, anorexia, constipation
• Allergic reactions: rash, urticaria

Black Box Warning: Substance abuse: assess for risks of addiction, abuse, or misuse before drug initiation, and monitor those who receive opioids; assess for depression or other mental illness in the patient or family members

Black Box Warning: Potential for overdose or poisoning: there is a significant potential; proper patient selection and counseling are needed; keep out of reach of children, pets; accidental overdose and death may occur

• **Respiratory dysfunction:** respiratory depression, character, rate, rhythm; notify prescriber if respirations <12/min; CV status; bradycardia, syncope
• **Pregnancy/breastfeeding:** use only if benefits outweigh fetal risk; avoid use in breastfeeding, excretion unknown
Evaluate:
• **Therapeutic response:** maintenance of anesthesia
Teach patient/family:
• Reason for product, expected results

⚠ HIGH ALERT

repaglinide (Rx)

(re-pag'lih'nide)

Gluconorm ✤

Func. class.: Antidiabetic
Chem. class.: Meglitinide

ACTION: Causes functioning β-cells in pancreas to release insulin, thereby leading to a drop in blood glucose levels; closes ATP-dependent potassium channels in the β-cell membrane; this leads to the opening of calcium channels; increased calcium influx induces insulin secretion

USES: Type 2 diabetes mellitus

CONTRAINDICATIONS

Hypersensitivity to meglitinides; diabetic ketoacidosis, type 1 diabetes

Precautions: Pregnancy, breastfeeding, children, geriatric patients, thyroid/cardiac disease, severe renal/hepatic disease, severe hypoglycemic reactions

DOSAGE AND ROUTES

• **Adult: PO** 0.5-4 mg with each meal, max 16 mg/day; adjust at weekly intervals; oral hypoglycemic–naïve patients or patients with A1c <8% should start with 0.5 mg with each meal

Renal/hepatic dose

• **Adult: PO** CCr 20-39 mL/min, 0.5 mg/day; titrate upward cautiously

Available forms: Tabs 0.5, 1, 2 mg

Administer:

• Up to 15-30 min before meals; 2, 3, or 4×/day preprandially

• Skip dose if meal skipped; add dose if meal added

• Store in tight container at room temperature

• May be added to metFORMIN for better control

SIDE EFFECTS

CNS: *Headache, weakness,* paresthesia
CV: Angina
EENT: Tinnitus, sinusitis

ENDO: Hypoglycemia
GI: Nausea, vomiting, diarrhea, constipation, dyspepsia, pancreatitis
INTEG: Rash, allergic reactions
MISC: Chest pain, UTI, allergy
MS: Back pains, arthralgia
RESP: URI, sinusitis, rhinitis, bronchitis

PHARMACOKINETICS

Completely absorbed by GI route; onset 30 min; peak 1 hr; duration <4 hr; half-life 1 hr; metabolized in liver by CYP3A4; excreted in urine, feces (metabolites); crosses placenta; 98% protein bound

INTERACTIONS

• Do not use with gemfibrozil, isophane insulin (NPH)

Increase: repaglinide effect—CYP3A4, OATP101, CYP2C9 inhibitors

Increase: in both—levonorgestrel/ethinyl estradiol

Increase: repaglinide metabolism—CYP3A4 inducers: rifAMPin, barbiturates, carBAMazepine

Increase: repaglinide effect—NSAIDs, salicylates, sulfonamides, chloramphenicol, MAOIs, coumarins, β-blockers, probenecid, gemfibrozil, simvastatin, fenofibrate, deferasirox

Decrease: repaglinide metabolism—CYP3A4 inhibitors: antifungals (ketoconazole, miconazole), erythromycin, macrolides

Decrease: repaglinide action—calcium channel blockers, corticosteroids, oral contraceptives, thiazide diuretics, thyroid preparations, estrogens, phenothiazines, phenytoin, rifAMPin, isoniazid, PHENobarbital, sympathomimetics

Drug/Herb

Increase: antidiabetic effect—garlic, chromium, horse chestnut

Drug/Food

Decrease: repaglinide level; give before meals

Decrease: repaglinide metabolism—grapefruit juice

Drug/Lab Test

Increase/decrease: glucose

R

NURSING CONSIDERATIONS
Assess:
• **Hypo/hyperglycemic reaction,** which can occur soon after meals: dizziness, weakness, headache, tremors, anxiety, tachycardia, hunger, sweating, abdominal pain, A1c, fasting, postprandial glucose during treatment

• **Pregnancy/breastfeeding:** use only if benefits outweigh fetal risk, usually insulin is used in pregnancy; do not breastfeed, excretion unknown

Evaluate:
• **Therapeutic response:** decrease in polyuria, polydipsia, polyphagia; clear sensorium; absence of dizziness; stable gait; blood glucose, A1c improvement

Teach family/patient:
• About technique for blood glucose monitoring; how to use blood glucose meter
• About the symptoms of hypo/hyperglycemia, what to do about each
• That product must be continued on daily basis; about the consequences of discontinuing product abruptly
• To avoid OTC medications unless ordered by prescriber; not to use alcohol
• That diabetes is a lifelong illness; that product will not cure disease
• That all food included in diet plan must be eaten to prevent hypoglycemia; that if a meal is omitted, dose should be omitted; to have glucagon emergency kit available; to take repaglinide 15-30 min before meals 2, 3, or 4×/day; to carry emergency ID

TREATMENT OF OVERDOSE:
Glucose 25 g IV via dextrose 50% solution, 50 mL or 1 mg glucagon

reslizumab (Rx)
(res-liz'ue-mab)
Cinqair
Func. class.: Respiratory antiinflammatory agent

USES: For add-on maintenance treatment of severe asthma of eosinophilic phenotype

CONTRAINDICATIONS
Hypersensitivity

Black Box Warning: Anaphylaxis

DOSAGE AND ROUTES
• **Adult: IV INFUSION** 3 mg/kg q4wk; discontinue the infusion immediately if a severe systemic reaction, including anaphylaxis, occurs

Available forms: Injection 100-mg/10-mL single-use vial

retapamulin (topical) (Rx)
(re-te-pam'you-lin)
Altabax
Func. class.: Topical antiinfective
Chem. class.: Pleuromutilin

ACTION: Antibacterial activity results from inhibition of protein synthesis

USES: For the treatment of impetigo

CONTRAINDICATIONS
Hypersensitivity to this product
Precautions: Children

DOSAGE AND ROUTES
• **Adult/child ≥9 mo: TOP** apply to affected area bid × 5 days

Available forms: Topical ointment 1%

Administer:
Topical route
• Do not use skin products near the eyes, nose, or mouth
• Wash hands before and after use
• **Ointment:** Apply a thin film to the cleansed affected area and massage gently into affected areas

SIDE EFFECTS
INTEG: Pruritus, irritation, headache, diarrhea, nausea

NURSING CONSIDERATIONS
Assess:
• **Allergic reaction:** hypersensitivity, product may need to be discontinued
• **Infection:** number of lesions, severity of impetigo
Evaluate:
• **Therapeutic response:** decreased lesions, infection in impetigo
Teach patient/family:
Topical route
• Not to use skin products near the eyes, nose, or mouth
• To wash hands before and after use
• **Ointment:** to apply a thin film to the cleansed affected area

---

reteplase (Rx)
(re′ta-plase)
Retavase, Retavase Half-Kit
Func. class.: Thrombolytic, tissue plasminogen

USES: Acute ST-elevation MI to reduce death/HF

CONTRAINDICATIONS
Hypersensitivity, active internal bleeding; recent stroke; intracranial/intraspinal surgery, serious head trauma, neoplasm, AV malformations, aneurysm severe uncontrolled hypertension, suspected aortic dissection, brain injury

DOSAGE AND ROUTES
Acute ST-elevation MI
• **Adult:** IV 10 units over 2 min, then a second dose after 30 min
Available forms: Injection 10.4 units/vial

---

revefenacin (Rx)
(rev′e-fen′a-sin)
Yupelri
Func. class.: Respiratory muscarinic antagonists—long-acting

ACTION: In airways, it exhibits pharmacologic effects through inhibition of the M3 receptor at the smooth muscle, leading to bronchodilation

USES: Maintenance treatment of those with COPD

CONTRAINDICATIONS
Hypersensitivity
Precautions: Acute/paradoxical bronchospasm, acutely deteriorating COPD, acute symptoms, other anticholinergics, breastfeeding, cardiac disease, children, closed-angle glaucoma, dementia, driving or hazardous tasks, geriatric patients, hepatic disease, ocular exposure, pregnancy, prostatic hypertrophy, urinary retention/obstruction

DOSAGE AND ROUTES
• **Adult:** INH 1 175-mcg vial (3 mL) once daily, by oral inhalation only
Available forms: 175 mcg/3 mL sol for inhalation
Administer
Oral inhalation route
• Give by oral inhalation via nebulizer only; do not swallow, no dilution necessary, single-dose vials are ready-to-use
• Remove the unit-dose vial from the foil pouch only immediately before use; product should be colorless; discard if the solution is not colorless
• Do not mix with other drugs
• Give the inhalation solution via a standard jet nebulizer connected to an air compressor; give over 8 min
• Discard the vial and any residual solution after use

SIDE EFFECTS
CNS: Headache
RESP: Cough, nasopharyngitis, upper respiratory tract infection, bronchospasm
MS: Back pain
EENT: Ocular hypertension
INTEG: Angioedema, anaphylaxis

PHARMACOKINETICS
Extensively distributed to tissues, primarily metabolized via hydrolysis to a metabolite, half-life of active metabolite 22-70 hr, excreted 54% feces, 27% urine

INTERACTIONS
Increase: anticholinergic effect—other anticholinergics; avoid coadministration

---

Side effects: *italics* = common; red = life-threatening

Increase: revefenacin effect—OATP1B1, OATP1B3 inhibitors (rifampicin, cyclosporine); avoid coadministration

NURSING CONSIDERATIONS
Assess
• **Respiratory status:** lung sounds, pulse, B/P before and after product is given; note wheezing, shortness of breath, cough; monitor pulmonary function tests baseline and periodically

• **Hypersensitivity:** Monitor for rash, pruritus, difficulty breathing, swelling of face, tongue; if these occur, discontinue immediately and provide supportive care

• **Bronchospasm:** Monitor for trouble breathing, wheezing, tightness in the chest, notify health care provider immediately

• **Pregnancy/breastfeeding:** no well-controlled studies; animal studies showed no evidence of fetal harm; anticholinergics suppress lactation
Evaluate:
• **Therapeutic response:** prevention or relief of the symptoms of COPD
Teach patient/family
• To contact health care provider if symptoms are not relieved or if shortness of breath continues or if bronchospasm occurs

• Advise patient to report immediately if trouble breathing, wheezing, swelling of face, tongue, rash or itching occur

• To notify health care provider of all OTC preparations, other medications, herbs, and supplements taken; not to start or stop products without approval of provider

• Not to swallow during nebulization

• That pulmonary function tests will be monitored periodically

• **Pregnancy/breastfeeding:** to inform health care provider if pregnancy is planned or suspected, or if breastfeeding

---

Rh$_o$(D) immune globulin standard dose IM (Rx)
HyperRHO S/D Full Dose, RhoGAM

Rh$_o$(D) immune globulin microdose IM (Rx)
HyperRHO S/D mini-Dose, Rho(D) immune globulin microdose (IM, IV), Rhophylac
Rh$_o$(D) immune globulin IV (Rx)
WinRho SDF

Func. class.: Immune globulins

ACTION: Suppresses immune response of nonsensitized Rh$_o$(D or D^u)-negative patients who are exposed to Rh$_o$(D or D^u)-positive blood

USES: Prevention of isoimmunization in Rh-negative women given Rh-positive blood after abortions, miscarriages, amniocentesis; chronic idiopathic thrombocytopenia purpura (Rhophylac)

CONTRAINDICATIONS
Previous immunization with this product, Rh$_o$(O)-positive/D^u-positive patient

Black Box Warning: Intravascular hemolysis

Precautions: Pregnancy

Black Box Warning: Requires a specialized setting

DOSAGE AND ROUTES
Rho (D) Immune globulin (for IM Only)
• **Adult:** IM before delivery. Hyper-RHO S/D Full Dose, RhoGam 1 vial standard dose (300 mcg) at 26-28 wk; **after delivery** 1 vial standard dose (300 mcg) within 72 hr of delivery
Pregnancy termination (<13 wk gestation)
• **Adult:** IM HyperRho Minidose, MicroRhoGam 1 vial microdose (50 mcg) within 72 hr of termination
Pregnancy termination (>13 wk gestation)
• **Adult:** IM HyperRHO S/D Full Dose, RhoGam 1 vial standard dose (300 mcg) within 72 hr of termination

---

Massive fetomaternal hemorrhage (>15 mL)
• **Adult:** IM RhoGam 20 mcg/mL of Rho(D) positive fetal RBCs
Transfusion accident
• **Adult: IM Hyper Rho Full Dose, RhoGam** (Rh+ blood given [volume] × Hct of donor blood)/15 will be the number of vials needed (standard dose), round to next whole vial
Rho(D) Immune Globulin IV (for IV/IM use)
• **Adult: IM/IV WinRho SDF,** 1500 IU (300 mcg) at 28 wk; **after delivery** 1 vial; **after delivery** 600 IU (120 mcg) within 72 hr of delivery
Termination of pregnancy, amniocentesis
• **Adult: IM/IV WinRho SDF** 600 IU (120 mcg) with 72 hr
Amniocentesis, chorionic villus sampling
• **Adult: IM/IV WinRho SDF (<34 wk gestation)** 1500 IU (300 mcg) repeat q12wk during pregnancy
Massive fetomaternal hemorrhage (>15 mL)/transfusion accident
• **Adult: IM WinRho SDF** 6000 IU (1200 mcg) repeat q12hr until total dose given by amount of blood loss; **IM WinRho SDF** 3000 IU (600 mcg) repeat q8hr until total dose is given by amount of blood loss
Immune thrombocytopenic purpura (ITP)
• **Adult and child: IV WinRho SDF** 250 IU (50 mcg)/kg, **if HB <10g/dL** use 25-40 mcg (125-200 IU), dosing determined by clinical response
Available forms: IM MICRhoGAM, HyperRho S/D: Minidose 50 mcg/vial; 300 mcg/vial **standard dose; IM/IV** 600 IU (120 mcg)/vial, 1500 IU (300 mcg)/vial 2500 IU (500 mcg)/vial, 5000 IU (1000 mcg)/vial, 15,000 IU (3000 mcg)/vial; prefilled syringe 1500 IU (300 mcg/2 mL)
Administer:
• Store in refrigerator
• HyperRHO S/D, MICRhoGAM, RhoGAM given by IM only; do not give IV

• Do not confuse different types
• Inspect for particulate matter; do not use if particulate matter present
• Reconstitute/dilution: no reconstitution or dilution needed for HyperRHO SD; MICRhoGAM, RhoGAM, or liquid formulation of WinRho SDF
IM route
• Use aseptic technique, observe for 20 min after administration
• Bring Rhophylac to room temperature before use
• Inject into deltoid muscle of upper arm or anterolateral portion of upper thigh; do not inject into gluteal muscle
• If dose calculated requires multiple vials or syringes, use different sites at same time
IV route
• Use aseptic technique
• WinRho SDF: remove entire contents of vial to obtain calculated dose; if partial vial required for dosage calculation, withdraw entire vial contents to ensure correct calculation; infuse correct calculated dose over 3-5 min; do not infuse with other fluids, products
• Rhophylac: bring to room temperature; infuse by slow IV; observe for 20 min

SIDE EFFECTS
CNS: Lethargy, dizziness, headache
CV: Hypo/hypertension
INTEG: Irritation at inj site, fever
MISC: Infection, ARDS, anaphylaxis, pulmonary edema, DIC
MS: Myalgia, arthralgia
HEMA: Anemia, DIC, intravascular hemolysis

INTERACTIONS
Decrease: antibody response—live virus vaccines (measles, mumps, rubella)

NURSING CONSIDERATIONS
Assess:
• Allergies, reactions to immunizations; previous immunization with product
• **Intravascular hemolysis:** back pain, chills, hemoglobinuria, renal insufficiency; usually when WinRho SDF is given

R

in those with immune thrombocytopenia purpura

• Type, crossmatch mother and newborn's cord blood; if mother Rh₀ (D)-negative, Dᵁ-negative and newborn Rh₀ (D)-positive, product should be given

Evaluate:

• Rh₀(D) sensitivity in transfusion error, prevention of erythroblastosis fetalis for normal vision

Teach patient/family:

• How product works; that product must be given after subsequent deliveries if subsequent babies are Rh-positive

• To report immediately: shaking, fever, chills, dark urine, swelling of hands or feet, back pain, SOB (intravascular hemolysis)

---

ribavirin (Rx)

(rye-ba-vye′rin)

Ibavyr ✦, Moderiba ✦, Rebetol, Ribasphere, Ribasphere, RibaPak, Virazole

Func. class.: Antiviral, nucleoside/nucleotides

USES: Treatment of chronic HCV infection when used in combination; RSV infection in hospitalized children

CONTRAINDICATIONS

Hypersensitivity, breastfeeding, pregnancy, sickle cell disease, thalassemia, pancreatitis, CCr 50 mL/min

Black Box Warning: Monotherapy (RCV infection)

DOSAGE AND ROUTES

Respiratory syncytial virus (RSV) infection

• **Infant/child/adolescent: INH** ribavirin 20 mg/mL solution in the drug reservoir of the SPAG-2 unit, continuous aerosol administration for 12-18 hr/day × 3-7 days

Chronic hepatitis C infection with compensated hepatic disease (Child-Pugh A) used in combination with a peginterferon alfa-2b

• **Adults >105 kg: PO (capsules/oral solution):** 600 mg ᴀᴍ and 800 mg ᴘᴍ (1400 mg/day) plus peginterferon alfa-2b; **81-105 kg:** 600 mg bid (1200 mg/day) plus peginterferon alfa-2b; **66-80 kg** (1000 mg/day) 400 mg ᴀᴍ and 600 mg ᴘᴍ plus peginterferon alfa-2b; **<66 kg** 400 mg ᴀᴍ, 400 mg ᴘᴍ plus peginterferon-alpha-2b; duration genotype 1 is 48 wk; genotype 2 or 3 is 24 wk, any failure 48 wk

• **Adolescent >73 kg: PO (capsules)** 15 mg/kg/day or 1200 mg/day given in 2 divided doses (3 capsules in the morning and evening) plus interferon alfa-2b. Duration for genotype 1 is 48 wk; genotype 2 or 3 is 24 wk

• **Child/adolescent 60-73 kg: PO (capsules)** 15 mg/kg/day or 1000 mg/day given in 2 divided doses (2 capsules in the morning and 3 capsules in the evening) plus interferon alfa-2b. Duration for genotype 1 is 48 wk; genotype 2 or 3 is 24 wk

• **Child/adolescent 47-59 kg: PO (capsules)** 15 mg/kg/day or 800 mg/day given in 2 divided doses (2 capsules in the morning and evening) plus interferon alfa-2b. Duration for genotype 1 is 48 wk; genotype 2 or 3 is 24 wk

• **Child/adolescent 3-17 yr, <47 kg: PO (oral solution)** 15 mg/kg/day given in 2 divided doses as the oral solution (in the morning and evening) plus interferon alfa-2b. Duration for genotype 1 is 48 wk; genotype 2 or 3 is 24 wk

Chronic hepatitis C infection in compensated hepatic disease (Child-Pugh A) with interferon alfa-2b alone

• **Adults >75 kg: PO (capsules/oral solution)** 600 mg bid (in the morning and evening) plus interferon alfa-2b. For interferon-alfa-naive patients, treat for 24-48 wk; ≤75 kg: PO (capsules/oral solution) 400 mg ᴀᴍ and 600 mg ᴘᴍ plus interferon-alfa-naive patients, treat for 24-48 wk

• **Adolescent >73 kg: PO** 15 mg/kg/day or 1200 mg/day in 2 divided doses (ᴀᴍ and ᴘᴍ) plus interferon alfa-2b. Duration for

genotype 1 is 48 wk; duration for genotype 2 or 3 is 24 wk
• **Child/adolescent 60-73 kg: PO** 15 mg/kg/day or 1000 mg/day given in 2 divided doses (AM and PM) plus interferon alfa-2b. Duration for genotype 1 is 48 wk. Duration for genotype 2 or 3 is 24 wk
• **Child/adolescent 47-59 kg: PO** 15 mg/kg/day or 800 mg/day given in 2 divided doses AM and PM) plus interferon alfa-2b. Duration for genotype 1 is 48 wk; duration for genotype 2 or 3 is 24 wk
• **Child/adolescent 3-17 yr, <47 kg: PO** 15 mg/kg/day given in 2 divided doses (AM and PM) plus interferon alfa-2b. Duration for genotype 1 is 48 wk; duration for genotype 2 or 3 is 24 wk
Available forms: Capsules 200 mg; tablets 200, 400 ✿ mg, powder for nebulizer solution 6 g

ribociclib (Rx)

(rye-boe-sye′-klib)
Kisqali
Func. class.: Antineoplastic
Chem. class.: Protein kinase inhibitors

ACTION: A cyclin-dependent kinase (CDK) 4 and 6 inhibitor. Regulates cell-cycle progression through phosphorylation of the retinoblastoma protein. The combination of ribociclib and an antiestrogen such as letrozole inhibited tumor growth more than either agent alone

USES: For the initial endocrine-based treatment of hormone receptor (HR)-positive, HER2-negative advanced or metastatic breast cancer in combination with an aromatase inhibitor in postmenopausal women

CONTRAINDICATIONS
Hypersensitivity
Precautions: Breastfeeding, contraception requirements, hepatic disease, hepatotoxicity, infertility, neutropenia, pregnancy, pregnancy testing, reproductive risk, thromboembolic disease

DOSAGE AND ROUTES
Hormone receptor (HR)-positive, HER2-negative advanced or metastatic breast cancer in combination with an aromatase inhibitor in postmenopausal women
• **Adult:** 600 mg/day on days 1 to 21, followed by 7 days of rest, in combination with letrozole (2.5 mg daily) or another aromatase inhibitor on days 1 to 28; repeat cycle q28days

Therapeutic drug monitoring
Neutropenia
• **ANC ≥1000 cells/mm³ (grade ≤2):** no change
• **ANC 500 cells/mm³ to 999 cells/mm³ (grade 3):** hold. For the first occurrence of grade 3 neutropenia, resume at original dose level when the ANC returns to ≥1000 cells/mm³ (grade ≤2); for recurrent grade 3 neutropenia, resume at next lower dose level (reduce 600 mg to 400 mg; reduce 400 mg to 200 mg). If further dose reduction below 200 mg per day is required, discontinue
• **ANC 500 cells/mm³ to 999 cells/mm³ (grade 3 neutropenia) with single episode of fever >38.3° C or >38° C for >1 hr and/or concurrent infection:** hold; resume at the next lower dose level when ANC returns to ≥1000 cells/mm³ (grade 2 or less) (reduce 600 mg to 400 mg; reduce 400 mg to 200 mg). If further dose reduction below 200 mg per day is required, discontinue
QT prolongation
• **QTcF 481-500 msec and no serious arrhythmia:** hold; monitor ECG frequently. For the first occurrence, resume at the same dose when QTcF prolongation resolves to ≤480 msec; for a recurrence of QTcF >480 msec, resume at the next lower dose level (reduce 600 mg to 400 mg; reduce 400 mg to 200 mg). If further dose reduction below 200 mg/day is required, discontinue
• **QTcF >500 msec and no serious arrhythmia:** repeat ECG. If the QTcF >500

R

msec on at least 2 separate ECGs at the same visit, hold; monitor ECG more frequently. Resume at the next lower dose level (reduce 600 mg to 400 mg; reduce 400 mg to 200 mg) when QTcF prolongation resolves to ≤480 msec. If further dose reduction below 200 mg/day is required, discontinue

Hepatic dose
• **Adult: Mild hepatic impairment (Child-Pugh A):** no change; **moderate to severe hepatic impairment (Child-Pugh B or C):** reduce starting dose to 400 mg/day

Renal Dose
• **Adult:** CCr<30 mL/min: use only if benefits outweigh risk

Administer:
• Take ribociclib and letrozole at the same time every day, preferably in the morning
• Swallow tablets whole; do not chew, crush, or split. Do not take if broken, cracked
• If a dose is missed, or if the patient vomits, do not replace the missed dose. Resume with the next scheduled daily dose

SIDE EFFECTS

CV: QT prolongation, peripheral edema
GI: Diarrhea, abdominal pain, anorexia, nausea, vomiting, constipation, stomatitis, weight loss
CNS: Fatigue, headache, insomnia
MS: Back pain
INTEG: Rash, alopecia
HEMA: Leukemia, neutropenia, lymphopenia
MISC: Infection

PHARMACOKINETICS

Protein binding 70%; half-life 29.7-54.7 hr; fecal excretion 97.1%; extensively metabolized (CYP3A4); unchanged drug 17% and 12% in feces and urine, respectively; peak 1-4 hr

INTERACTIONS

Increase: QT prolongation—drugs known to prolong QT interval; avoid concomitant use

Increase: ribociclib effect—strong or moderate CYP3A4 inhibitors; avoid concomitant use; if cannot be avoided, reduce dose
Decrease: ribociclib effect—strong or moderate CYP3A4 inducers; avoid concomitant use

Drug/Lab Test
Increase: LFTs

Drug/Food
Avoid use with pomegranates, pomegranate juice, grapefruit, and grapefruit juice

NURSING CONSIDERATIONS

Assess:
• **Hepatotoxicity,** grade ≥3 was 57 days. Monitor LFTs baseline, q2wk for the first 2 cycles, before the next 4 cycles, and then as needed. A dose interruption, reduction, or discontinuation of therapy may be necessary.
• **Bone marrow suppression:** onset of grade ≥2 neutropenia was 16 days. Monitor CBC baseline, q2wk for the first 2 cycles, before the next 4 cycles, and then as needed. A dose interruption, reduction, or discontinuation of therapy may be needed in those with an absolute neutrophil count (ANC) <1000 cells/mm^3
• **Long QT syndrome:** avoid use in long QT syndrome, uncontrolled or significant cardiac disease (cardiac arrhythmias, recent MI, heart failure, unstable angina, bradycardia or bradyarrhythmias), electrolyte imbalance (hypomagnesemia, hypokalemia, hypocalcemia), with products causing prolonged QT interval or that strongly inhibit CYP3A4. Females, geriatric patients, and patients with diabetes, thyroid disease, malnutrition, alcoholism, or hepatic disease may also be at increased risk for QT prolongation. Assess ECG before starting therapy; do not start product if QTcF >450 msec. Repeat ECG at day 14 of first cycle, at the beginning of second cycle, and then as needed; prolongation of the QTcF interval may require interruption of therapy, dose reduction, or discontinuation of

therapy. Monitor serum electrolytes (potassium, calcium, phosphorous, and magnesium) baseline, at the beginning of the first 6 cycles, and as needed; correct electrolyte imbalances before starting product

• **Pregnancy/breastfeeding:** avoid use by females of reproductive potential during treatment and for at least 3 wk after last dose; can cause fetal harm or death; discontinue breastfeeding during treatment and for 3 wk after final dose; presence in breast milk unknown. Obtain pregnancy test before starting treatment

Evaluate

• Therapeutic outcome: decrease in size of cancerous tumor

Teach patient/family:

• **Hepatotoxicity:** patient should report immediately yellowing of skin or eyes, dark urine

• **QT prolongation:** signs and symptoms of QT prolongation (irregular or rapid heartbeat, fainting). To notify health care provider immediately if any of these occur

• **Neutropenia:** to immediately notify health care provider if a fever occurs; usually may occur with an infection

• **Drug interactions:** to avoid pomegranates, pomegranate juice, grapefruit, and grapefruit juice; that all OTC or prescription medications, herbals, and supplements should be approved by provider

• **Alopecia:** that hair is often lost; make suggestions for wigs, scarves to make patient feel more comfortable about hair loss

• Pregnancy/breastfeeding: not to use drug in pregnancy, breastfeeding; contraception should be used during treatment and for at least 3 wk after last dose

riboflavin (vit B₂) (otc)
(rye′boh-flay-vin)
Func. class.: Vit B₂, water soluble

ACTION: Needed for respiratory reactions by catalyzing proteins

USES: Vit B₂ deficiency or polyneuritis; cheilosis adjunct with thiamine
Unlabeled uses: Migraine prophylaxis

CONTRAINDICATIONS
None known
Precautions: Pregnancy

DOSAGE AND ROUTES
Deficiency
• **Adult: PO** 5-30 mg/day
• **Child ≥12 yr: PO** 3-10 mg/day, then 0.6 mg/1000 calories ingested
RDA
• **Adult: PO** (males) 1.3 mg, (females) 1.1 mg
Available forms: Tabs 5, 10, 25, 50, 100, 250 mg
Administer:
• With food for better absorption
• Store in airtight, light-resistant container

SIDE EFFECTS
GU: Yellow discoloration of urine

PHARMACOKINETICS
Half-life 65-85 min, 60% protein bound, unused amounts excreted in urine (unchanged)

INTERACTIONS
Increase: riboflavin need—alcohol, probenecid, tricyclics, phenothiazines
Decrease: action of tetracyclines
Drug/Lab Test
May cause false elevations of urinary catecholamines

NURSING CONSIDERATIONS
Assess:
• Nutritional status: liver, eggs, dairy products, yeast, whole grains, green vegetables
Evaluate:
• **Therapeutic response:** absence of headache, GI problems, cheilosis, skin lesions, depression; burning, itchy eyes; anemia
Teach patient/family:
• That urine may turn bright yellow

- About the addition of needed foods rich in riboflavin
- To avoid alcohol

---

rifabutin (Rx)

(riff'a-byoo-ten)

Mycobutin

Func. class.: Antimycobacterial agent
Chem. class.: Rifamycin S derivative

Do not confuse:
rifabutin/rifAMPin/rifapentine

ACTION: Inhibits DNA-dependent RNA polymerase in susceptible strains of *Escherichia coli* and *Bacillus subtilis;* mechanism of action against *Mycobacterium avium* unknown

USES: Prevention of *M. avium* complex (MAC) in patients with advanced HIV infection
Unlabeled uses: *Helicobacter pylori* that has not responded to other treatment, TB, MAC

CONTRAINDICATIONS

Hypersensitivity, active TB, WBC <1000/ mm^3 or platelet count <50,000/mm^3
Precautions: Pregnancy, breastfeeding, children, hepatic disease, blood dyscrasias

DOSAGE AND ROUTES

- **Adult: PO** 300 mg/day (may take as 150 mg bid); max 600 mg/day
Renal dose
- **Adult: PO** CCr <30 mL/min, reduce by 50%
Available forms: Caps 150 mg
Administer:
- With food if GI upset occurs; better to take on empty stomach 1 hr before or 2 hr after meals; high-fat foods slow absorption; may take in 2 divided doses, may open capsule, mix with applesauce if unable to swallow whole cap
- Antiemetic if vomiting occurs
- After C&S completed; monthly to detect resistance

SIDE EFFECTS

CNS: *Headache,* fatigue, anxiety, confusion, insomnia
GI: *Nausea, vomiting, anorexia, diarrhea,* heartburn, hepatitis, discolored saliva, CDAD
GU: *Discolored urine*
HEMA: Hemolytic anemia, eosinophilia, thrombocytopenia, leukopenia
INTEG: *Rash*
MISC: Flulike symptoms, shortness of breath, chest pressure
MS: Asthenia, arthralgia, myalgia

PHARMACOKINETICS

53% absorbed, peak 2-3 hr, duration >24 hr, half-life 45 hr, metabolized in liver (active/inactive metabolites), excreted in urine primarily as metabolites

INTERACTIONS

Increase: levels of rifabutin—ritonavir
Decrease: action of amprenavir, anticoagulants, β-blockers, barbiturates, busPIRone, clofibrate, corticosteroids, cycloSPORINE, dapsone, delavirdine, disopyramide, doxycycline, efavirenz, estrogens, fluconazole, indinavir, ketoconazole, losartan, nelfinavir, nevirapine, oral contraceptives, phenytoin, quiNIDine, saquinavir, sulfonylureas, theophylline, tricyclic antidepressants, zidovudine, zolpidem
Drug/Food
High-fat diet decreases absorption
Drug/Lab Test
Interference: folate level, vit B$_{12}$, BSP, gallbladder studies

NURSING CONSIDERATIONS
Assess:
- **Acute TB:** chest x-ray, sputum culture, blood culture, biopsy of lymph nodes, PPD; Do not use in MAC prophylaxis in those with active TB
- CBC for neutropenia, thrombocytopenia, eosinophilia
- **CDAD:** diarrhea, abdominal pain/ cramping, fever, bloody stools; report immediately; may occur several weeks after discontinuing treatment
- Signs of anemia: Hct, HB, fatigue

• **Hepatotoxicity:** ALT, AST, bilirubin; assess weekly for decreased appetite, jaundice, dark urine, fatigue
• Renal status before, each mo: BUN, creatinine, output, specific gravity, urinalysis

Evaluate:
• **Therapeutic response:** not used for active TB because of risk for development of resistance to rifAMPin; culture negative

Teach patient/family:
• That patients using oral contraceptives should consider using nonhormonal methods of birth control, may decrease effect; to notify prescriber if pregnancy planned, suspected
• That compliance with dosage schedule, duration necessary
• That scheduled appointments must be kept because relapse may occur
• That urine, feces, saliva, sputum, sweat, tears may be colored red-orange; that soft contact lenses may be permanently stained
• **To report flulike symptoms:** excessive fatigue, anorexia, vomiting, sore throat; unusual bleeding; yellowish discoloration of skin, eyes; myositis: muscle or bone pain; diarrhea, fever, abdominal cramping, bloody stools

---

rifAMPin (Rx)

(rif'am-pin)

Rifadin, Rifampicin ✥, Rofact ✥

Func. class.: Antitubercular
Chem. class.: Rifamycin B derivative

Do not confuse:
rifAMPin/rifabutin/rifAXIMin

ACTION: Inhibits DNA-dependent polymerase, decreases tubercle bacilli replication

USES: Pulmonary TB, meningococcal carriers (prevention)
Unlabeled uses: Endocarditis, *Haemophilus influenzae type B prophylaxis*, Hansen's disease, *Mycobacterium avium* complex (MAC), orthopedic device–related infection, pruritus, CNS infections

CONTRAINDICATIONS
Hypersensitivity to this product, rifamycins; active *Neisseria meningitidis* infection
Precautions: Pregnancy, breastfeeding, children <5 yr, hepatic disease, blood dyscrasias

DOSAGE AND ROUTES
Tuberculosis
• **Adult: PO/IV** Max 600 mg/day as single dose 1 hr before meals or 2 hr after meals or 10 mg/kg/day 5 days/wk or 2-3×/wk
• **Child >5 yr: PO/IV** 10-20 mg/kg/day as single dose 1 hr before meals or 2 hr after meals, max 600 mg/day with other antituberculars
• **6-mo regimen:** 2 mo treatment of isoniazid, rifAMPin, pyrazinamide, and possibly streptomycin or ethambutol, then rifAMPin and isoniazid 3-4 mo
• **9-mo regimen:** rifAMPin and isoniazid supplemented with pyrazinamide, streptomycin, or ethambutol
Meningococcal carriers
• **Adult: PO/IV** 600 mg bid × 2 days, max 600 mg/dose
• **Child >5 yr: PO/IV** 10-20 mg/kg × 2 days, max 600 mg/dose
• **Infant 3 mo-1 yr: PO** 5 mg/kg bid × 2 days
Prevention of *H. influenzae* type B infection (unlabeled)
• **Adult: PO** 600 mg/day × 4 days
• **Child: PO** 20 mg/kg/day × 4 days
• **Neonates: PO** 10 mg/kg/day × 4 days
MAC (unlabeled)
• **Adult: PO/IV** 600 mg/day used with ≥3 other active microbials
• **Child: PO/IV** 10-20 mg/kg/day used with ≥3 other active microbials
Endocarditis with prosthetic valves (unlabeled)
• **Adult: PO** 300 mg q8hr with gentamicin and vancomycin
• **Child: PO** 20 mg/kg/day in 2 divided doses with gentamicin and vancomycin, max 900 mg/day

R

Available forms: Caps 150, 300 mg; powder for inj 600 mg/vial

Administer:

• After C&S completed; monthly to detect resistance

• Do not give IM, SUBCUT

PO route

• On empty stomach, 1 hr before or 2 hr after meals with full glass of water; give with other products for TB

• Antiemetic if vomiting occurs

• Capsules may be opened, mixed with applesauce or jelly

Intermittent IV INFUSION route

• After diluting each 600 mg/10 mL of sterile water for inj (60 mg/mL), swirl, withdraw dose, and dilute in 100 mL or 500 mL of D₅W given as infusion over 3 hr; if diluted in 100 mL, give over ½ hr; do not admix with other sol or products

Y-site compatibilities: amiodarone, bumetanide, midazolam, pantoprazole, vancomycin

SIDE EFFECTS

CNS: Headache, fatigue, anxiety, drowsiness, confusion

EENT: Visual disturbances

GI: *Nausea, vomiting, anorexia, diarrhea,* CDAD, *heartburn,* sore mouth and tongue, pancreatitis, increased LFTs

GU: Hematuria, acute renal failure, hemoglobinuria

HEMA: Hemolytic anemia, eosinophilia, thrombocytopenia, leukopenia

INTEG: Rash, pruritus, urticaria

MISC: Flulike symptoms, menstrual disturbances, edema, SOB, Stevens-Johnson syndrome, toxic epidermal necrolysis, angioedema, anaphylaxis, DRESS

MS: Ataxia, weakness

MISC: Staining of teeth, contact lens; coloring of urine, sweat, tears

PHARMACOKINETICS

PO: Peak 1-4 hr, half-life 1-5 hr, metabolized in liver (active/inactive metabolites), excreted in urine as free product (30% crosses placenta) and in breast milk

INTERACTIONS

Do not use with protease inhibitors

Increase: hepatotoxicity—isoniazid, alcohol, ketoconazole, pyrazinamide

Decrease: action of acetaminophen, alcohol, anticoagulants, antidiabetics, β-blockers, barbiturates, benzodiazepines, chloramphenicol, clofibrate, corticosteroids, cycloSPORINE, dapsone, digoxin, doxycycline, haloperidol, hormones, imidazole antifungals, NIFEdipine, oral contraceptives, phenytoin, protease inhibitors, theophylline, verapamil, zidovudine

Increase: LFTs

Decrease: HB

Drug/Lab Test

Increase: alk phosphatase, ALT, AST, uric acid, bilirubin, eosinophils

Interference: folate level, vit B₁₂

NURSING CONSIDERATIONS

Assess:

• **Infection:** sputum culture, lung sounds, characteristics of sputum, susceptibility tests baseline and periodically to determine effectiveness and resistance

• Signs of anemia: Hct, HB, fatigue

• Hepatic function monthly: ALT, AST, bilirubin, decreased appetite, jaundice, dark urine, fatigue

• Renal status before, each mo: BUN, creatinine, output, specific gravity, urinalysis

• **Serious skin reactions:** fever, sore throat, fatigue, ulcers; lesions in mouth, lips, rash; can be fatal

• **CDAD:** diarrhea, fever, abdominal pain/cramping, bloody stools; product should be discontinued, prescriber notified

• **DRESS:** Rash, fever, large lymph nodes, discontinue product if these occur

• To take on an empty stomach 1 hr before or 2 hr after food

Evaluate:

• **Therapeutic response:** decreased symptoms of TB, culture negative

Teach patient/family:

• That compliance with dosage schedule, duration necessary

• That scheduled appointments must be kept because relapse may occur

- To avoid alcohol because hepatotoxicity may occur
- That urine, feces, saliva, sputum, sweat, tears may be colored red-orange; that soft contact lenses may be permanently stained
- **To report flulike symptoms:** excessive fatigue, anorexia, vomiting, sore throat; unusual bleeding; yellowish discoloration of skin, eyes; diarrhea with pus, mucus, blood
- To use nonhormonal form of birth control; to notify prescriber if pregnancy is planned, suspected; not to breastfeed

rifamycin (Rx)

(rif′a-mye′sin)

Aemcolo

Func. class.: Antibiotic

USES: Treatment of travelers' diarrhea caused by *Escherichia coli*

CONTRAINDICATIONS
Hypersensitivity

DOSAGE AND ROUTES
- **Adult:** PO 388 bid × 3 days

Available forms: Tablet del rel 194 mg

rifapentine (Rx)

(riff′ah-pen-teen′)

Priftin

Func. class.: Antitubercular
Chem. class.: Rifamycin derivative

Do not confuse:
rifapentine/rifAMPin/rifabutin

ACTION: Inhibits DNA-dependent polymerase, decreases tubercle bacilli replication

USES: Pulmonary TB; must be used with at least one other antitubercular agent

CONTRAINDICATIONS
Hypersensitivity to rifamycins, porphyria

Precautions: Pregnancy, breastfeeding, children <12 yr, geriatric patients, hepatic disease, blood dyscrasias, HIV

DOSAGE AND ROUTES
Intensive phase
- **Adult/adolescent >12 yr:** PO 600 mg (four 150-mg tabs) 2×/wk with an interval of 72 hr between doses × 2 mo; must be given with at least 1 other antitubercular agent

Continuation phase
- **Adult/adolescent >12 yr:** PO 600 mg weekly × 4 mo in combination with isoniazid or other appropriate antitubercular product

Available forms: Tabs 150 mg
Administer:
- May give with food for GI upset; use other products for TB
- Antiemetic if vomiting occurs
- After C&S completed; monthly to detect resistance

SIDE EFFECTS
CNS: Headache, fatigue, anxiety, dizziness
EENT: Visual disturbances
GI: *Nausea, vomiting, anorexia, diarrhea,* bilirubinemia, hepatitis, increased ALT, AST, *heartburn,* pancreatitis, CDAD
GU: Hematuria, pyuria, proteinuria, urinary casts, urine discoloration
HEMA: Thrombocytopenia, leukopenia, neutropenia, lymphopenia, anemia, leukocytosis, purpura, hematoma
INTEG: Rash, pruritus, urticaria, acne
MISC: Increased B/P
MS: Gout, arthrosis

PHARMACOKINETICS
Peak 5-6 hr; half-life 13 hr; metabolized in liver (active/inactive metabolites); excreted in urine, feces, breast milk; protein binding 97%; steady-state 10 days; CYP450 3A4, 2C8/9 inducer

INTERACTIONS
- Do not use with protease inhibitors

Decrease: action of amitriptyline, anticoagulants, antidiabetics, barbiturates, β-blockers, chloramphenicol, clarithromycin, clofibrate, corticosteroids, cycloSPORINE, dapsone, delavirdine, diazePAM, digoxin, diltiaZEM, disopyramide, doxycycline, fentaNYL, fluconazole, haloperidol, indinavir, itraconazole, ketoconazole, methadone, mexiletine, nelfinavir, NIFEdipine, nortriptyline, oral contraceptives, phenothiazines, phenytoin, progestins, quiNIDine, quiNINE, ritonavir, saquinavir, sildenafil, tacrolimus, theophylline, thyroid preparations, tocainide, verapamil, warfarin, zidovudine

Drug/Food
Increase: absorption with food
Drug/Lab Test
Increase: LFTs, platelets
Decrease: HB, WBC
Interference: folate level, vit B_{12}

NURSING CONSIDERATIONS
Assess:
• Baselines of CBC, AST, ALT, bilirubin, platelets
• **Infection:** sputum culture, lung sounds
• Signs of anemia: Hct, HB, fatigue
• Hepatic studies monthly: ALT, AST, bilirubin; decreased appetite, jaundice, dark urine, fatigue
• Renal status monthly: BUN, creatinine, output, specific gravity, urinalysis
• **CDAD:** diarrhea, fever, abdominal pain/cramping, bloody diarrhea; discontinue if present, notify prescriber
Evaluate:
• **Therapeutic response:** decreased symptoms of TB, culture negative
Teach patient/family:
• That compliance with dosage schedule, duration necessary
• That scheduled appointments must be kept because relapse may occur
• That urine, feces, saliva, sputum, sweat, tears may be colored red-orange; that soft contact lenses, dentures may be permanently stained
• **To report flulike symptoms:** excessive fatigue, anorexia, vomiting, sore throat; unusual bleeding, yellowish discoloration of skin, eyes; diarrhea with pus, mucus, blood

• **Pregnancy/breastfeeding:** to use alternative method of contraception; that oral contraceptive action may be decreased; to notify prescriber if pregnancy is planned, suspected; to avoid breastfeeding

---

rifAXIMin (Rx)
(rif-ax'i-min)
Xifaxan, Zaxine ✦
Func. class.: Antiinfective—miscellaneous
Chem. class.: Analog of rifAMPin

Do not confuse:
rifAXIMin/rifAMPin

ACTION: Binds to bacterial-DNA–dependent RNA polymerase, thereby inhibiting bacterial RNA synthesis

USES: Traveler's diarrhea in those ≥12 yr caused by *E. coli*, hepatic encephalopathy, irritable bowel syndrome
Unlabeled uses: Crohn's disease, CDAD, traveler's diarrhea prophylaxis

CONTRAINDICATIONS
Hypersensitivity to product, rifamycins; diarrhea with fever, systemic infections
Precautions: Pregnancy, breastfeeding, children, geriatric patients, CDAD

DOSAGE AND ROUTES
Hepatic encephalopathy
• **Adult: PO** 550 mg bid
Traveler's diarrhea
• **Adult/child ≥12 yr: PO** 200 mg tid × 3 days without regard to meals
Irritable bowel syndrome
• **Adult: PO** 550 mg tid × 14 days, may give another 2 courses if recurrence
Crohn's disease (unlabeled)
• **Adult: PO** 200 mg tid × 16 wk
CDAD (unlabeled)
• **Adult: PO** 400 mg tid × 20 days after 10 days of vancomycin PO for second/third recurrence
Available forms: Tabs 200, 550 mg
Administer:
• Without regard to food

SIDE EFFECTS

CNS: Abnormal dreams, dizziness, insomnia, *headache,* fatigue, depression
CV: Hypotension, chest pain, peripheral edema, ascites
GI: *Abdominal pain, constipation, defecation urgency, flatulence, nausea, rectal tenesmus,* vomiting, ascites, CDAD
GU: Proteinuria, polyuria, increased urinary frequency
MISC: *Pyrexia,* motion sickness, tinnitus, rash, photosensitivity, exfoliative dermatitis
MS: Arthralgia, muscle pain, myalgia
RESP: Dyspnea, cough, pharyngitis

PHARMACOKINETICS

Low systemic absorption, distribution to GI tract, half-life 1.8-4.5 hr, excreted in feces, peak 1-4 hr

INTERACTIONS

Increase: effect of—afatinib
Increase: levels—P-glycoprotein inhibitors
Drug/Lab Test
Increase: LFTs, potassium
Decrease: blood glucose, sodium

NURSING CONSIDERATIONS
Assess:
• **Hepatic encephalopathy:** lethargy, confusion, coma, difficulty thinking, personality changes, poor concentration, sweet breath odor, inverted sleep/wake cycles
• **GI symptoms:** amount, character of diarrhea; abdominal pain, nausea, vomiting, blood in stool; do not use in those with blood in stool, increased temperature with diarrhea
• Overgrowth of infection, CDAD
• **Pregnancy/breastfeeding:** do not use in 1st trimester; use only if benefits outweigh fetal risk; do not breastfeed, excretion unknown
Evaluate:
• **Therapeutic response:** absence of infection
Teach patient/family:
• To discontinue rifAXIMin, notify prescriber if diarrhea persists >24-48 hr, if diarrhea worsens, or if blood in stools and fever present

• To avoid hazardous activities if dizziness occurs
• To notify prescriber if pregnancy is planned, suspected
• That headache, rash, insomnia, abnormal dreams, tinnitus may occur
• To take without regard to food
• To take as directed, consume all of the product prescribed

---

rilpivirine (Rx)
Edurant
Func. class.: Antiretroviral
Chem. class.: Nonnucleoside transcriptase inhibitors (NNTIs)

ACTION: Inhibits HIV-1 reverse transcriptase; binds directly to a site on reverse transcriptase, causing disruption of the enzyme's active site and blocking RNA-dependent and DNA-dependent DNA polymerase

USES: HIV in combination with other antiretrovirals

CONTRAINDICATIONS
Hypersensitivity
Precautions: Pregnancy, breastfeeding, neonates, infants, children, adolescents <18 yr, immune reconstitution syndrome, antimicrobial resistance, pancreatitis, coinfection hepatitis B or C and HIV, hepatic disease, depression, suicidal ideation, QT prolongation, torsades de pointes, hyperlipidemia, hypertriglyceridemia, hypercholesterolemia, immune reconstitution syndrome

DOSAGE AND ROUTES
Antiretroviral treatment-naive adults (HIV) in combination
• **Adult/child ≥12 yr and ≥35 kg: PO** 25 mg/day with a meal; if used with rifabutin, increase rilpivirine dose to 50 mg/day
Available forms: Tab 25 mg
Administer:
• Give with other antiretroviral agents; in antiretroviral treatment-naive adults, rilpivirine is used as an alternative to efavirenz in NNRTI-based treatment regimens;

R

potential rilpivirine-based treatment regimens combine rilpivirine with either tenofovir plus emtricitabine or lamiVUDine; or abacavir plus emtricitabine or lamiVUDine; or zidovudine plus emtricitabine or lamiVUDine

• Give with a meal

• Store at room temperature away from heat and moisture

SIDE EFFECTS

CNS: Depressed mood, dizziness, drowsiness, suicide attempts

GI: Hepatotoxicity, nausea, vomiting, diarrhea

INTEG: Drug reaction with eosinophilia and systemic symptoms (DRESS)

GU: membranous glomerulonephritis/messangio-proliferative glomerulonephritis

MISC: Immune reconstitution syndrome

PHARMACOKINETICS:

Protein binding (99.7%) to albumin; metabolism via oxidation CYP3A; half-life 50 hr, excretion feces (85%), 25% excreted unchanged; urine (6.1%); peak 4-5 hr; increased effect 40% (food), decreased effect 50% (high protein drink)

INTERACTIONS

Increase: rilpivirine effect—CYP3A4 inhibitors (delavirdine, efavirenz, darunavir, tipranavir, atazanavir, fosamprenavir, indinavir, nelfinavir, aldesleukin IL-2, amiodarone aprepitant, basiliximab, boceprevir, bromocriptine, chloramphenicol, clarithromycin, conivaptan, danazol, dalfopristin, dasatinib, diltiaZEM, dronedarone, erythromycin, ethinyl estradiol, fluconazole, FLUoxetine, fluvoxaMINE, fosaprepitant, imatinib, isoniazid, itraconazole, ketoconazole, lanreotide, lapatinib, miconazole, nefazodone, niCARdipine, octreotide, posaconazole, quiNINE, ranolazine, rifaximin, tamoxifen, telaprevir, telithromycin, troleandomycin, verapamil, voriconazole, zafirlukast)

Increase: QT prolongation—class IA/III antidysrhythmics, some phenothiazines, β-agonists, local anesthetics, tricyclics, chloroquine, droperidol, haloperidol, pentamidine; CYP3A4 inhibitors (amiodarone,

clarithromycin, erythromycin, telithromycin, troleandomycin, arsenic trioxide); CYP3A4 substrates (methadone, pimozide, QUEtiapine, quiNIDine, risperiDONE, ziprasidone, lopinavir, saquinavir, fluconazole, posaconazole, dasatinib, dronedarone, lapatinib, octreotide, ranolazine, citalopram, abarelix, alfuzosin, amoxapine, apomorphine, artemether, lumefantrine, asenapine, ofloxacin, ciprofloxacin, cloZAPine, cyclobenzaprine, dolasetron, eriBULin, flecainide, gatifloxacin, gemifloxacin, halogenated anesthetics, iloperidone, levoFLOXacin, maprotiline, mefloquine, moxifloxacin, nilotinib, norfloxacin, OLANZapine, ondansetron, paliperidone, palonosetron, QUEtiapine)

Increase: rilpivirine adverse reactions, fungal infections—fluconazole, voriconazole

Decrease: rilpivirine effect, treatment failure—CYP3A4 inducers (phenytoin, fosphenytoin, barbiturates, OXcarbazepine, carBAMazepine, rifabutin, rifAMPin, rifapentine, dexamethasone), efavirenz, nevirapine, ritonavir; aminoglutethimide, bexarotene, bosentan, griseofulvin, metyraPONE, modafinil, flutamide, nafcillin, pioglitazone, primidone, topiramate; proton pump inhibitors (PPIs)

Decrease: rilpivirine effect, treatment failure—H₂ receptor antagonists (cimetidine, famotidine, nizatidine, raNITIdine), give 12 hr before or 4 hr after rilpivirine

Decrease: rilpivirine effect—antacids, use >2 hr before or 4 hr after rilpivirine

Drug/Herb

Decreased effect—St. John's wort, do not use together

Drug/Food

Increase: adverse reactions—grapefruit juice

NURSING CONSIDERATIONS

Assess:

• **HIV:** Assess symptoms of HIV including opportunistic infections before and during treatment; some may be life-threatening; monitor plasma HIV RNA, CD4+, CD8+ cell counts, serum β-2 microglobulin, serum ICD+24 antigen levels; treatment failures occur more frequently in

those with baseline HIV-1 RNA concentrations >100,000 copies/mL than in patients with concentrations <100,000 copies/mL; monitor serum cholesterol, lipid panel; assess for redistribution of body fat
• Antiretroviral drug resistance testing before initiation of therapy in antiretroviral treatment-naive patients
• For adults and adolescents, initiation of antiretroviral therapy is recommended in any patient with a history of an AIDS-defining infection; with a CD4 ≤500/mm³; who is pregnant; who has HIV-associated nephropathy; or who is being treated for hepatitis B (HBV) infection. Only delay treatment for resistance testing
• **Hepatic disease:** monitor for elevated hepatic enzymes (>2.5 × ULN); grade 3 and 4 may be higher in patients coinfected with hepatitis B or C
• **Suicidal thoughts/actions:** assess for suicidal ideation often, report increase in depressive symptoms
• **DRESS:** may occur in 2-8 wk, skin eruptions, eosinophilia, lymphadenopathy, fever, inflammation of internal organs; if these occur, stop product, report immediately; systemic steroids are usually given
• **Pregnancy/breastfeeding:** use only if benefits outweigh fetal risk; enroll pregnant women taking this product in the Antiretroviral Pregnancy Registry, 800-258-4263; do not breastfeed, excretion unknown

Teach patient/family:
• That product is not a cure but controls symptoms; that continuing use is required
• That product must be taken in combination with other prescribed products; that if dose is missed, not to take if next dose is within 12 hr
• To discuss all products taken, including OTC, Rx, herbals, supplements, as there are many interactions
• To report immediately mood changes and depression
• To report hypersensitivity reactions
• That dizziness may occur, not to drive until response is known

• To immediately report if pregnancy is suspected; not to breastfeed

riluzole (Rx)
(rill′you-zole)
Rilutek, Tiglutik
Func. class.: ALS agent
Chem. class.: Benzothiazole

USES: Amyotrophic lateral sclerosis (ALS)

CONTRAINDICATIONS
Hypersensitivity

DOSAGE AND ROUTES
• **Adult: PO** 50 mg q12hr; take 1 hr before or 2 hr after meals
Available forms: Tabs 50 mg

rimegepant (Rx)
(ri-me′je-pant)
Nurtec ODT
Func. class.: Antimigraine agent
Chem. class.: Calcitonin gene–related peptide receptor antagonist

ACTION: Involved in transmission through second- and third-order neurons and pain modulation in the brainstem

USES: Acute treatment of migraine with or without aura, migraine prophylaxis

CONTRAINDICATIONS
Hypersensitivity
Precautions: Pregnancy, breastfeeding, hepatic/renal disease

DOSAGE AND ROUTES
Migraine
• **Adult: PO** 75 mg as a single dose; max 75 mg/24 hr
Migraine prophylaxis
• **Adult: PO** 75 mg every other day
Available forms: Tablet ODT 75 mg

Administer:
• Peel foil covering blister to remove table with dry hands. Do not push tablet through the foil.
• Place tablet on or under tongue, allow to dissolve
• Can be swallowed without additional fluids
• Store at 20° C to 25° C (68° F to 77° F)

SIDE EFFECTS
GI: Nausea
INTEG: Rash, hypersensitivity
RESP: Dyspnea

PHARMACOKINETICS
Onset ≤2 hr, peak 1.5 hr, duration 48 hr, half-life 11 hr, protein binding 96%

INTERACTIONS
Increase: Effect of CYP3A4 substrates
Increase: Rimegepant effect—CYP3A4 inhibitors
Decrease: Rimegepant effect—CY3A4 inducers

NURSING CONSIDERATIONS
Assess:
• **Migraine:** Baseline and periodically, presence of aura, nausea/vomiting
• Assess for hypersensitivity, rash, dyspnea; reaction may be delayed, discontinue if these occur
• Avoid use in hepatic/renal disease
Evaluate:
• **Therapeutic response:** Resolution of migraine
Teach patient/family:
• Reason for product and expected result
• Identify if pregnancy is planned or suspected

---

rimexolone ophthalmic
See Appendix B

---

riociguat (Rx)
(rye-oh-sig′ue-at)
Adempas
Func. class.: Vasodilator

USES: Treatment of persistent/recurrent chronic thromboembolic pulmonary hypertension (WHO group 4) after surgery or inoperable to improve exercise capacity; treatment of PAH (WHO group 1) to improve exercise capacity

CONTRAINDICATIONS
Hypersensitivity, use with nitrates, amyl nitrite, phosphodiesterase (PDE) inhibitors (sildenafil, tadalafil, vardenafil), nonspecific PDE inhibitors (dipyridamole, theophylline), pulmonary hypertension

Black Box Warning: Pregnancy

DOSAGE AND ROUTES
Chronic thromboembolic pulmonary hypertension/PAH
• **Adult: PO**: 1 mg tid; may start with 0.5 mg tid in those at higher risk of hypotension. If systolic BP remains >95 mm Hg and the patient has no signs or symptoms of hypotension, increase the dose by 0.5 mg tid at intervals of ≥2 wk to a max dose of 2.5 mg tid; if treatment is interrupted for ≥3 days, retitration is needed
Available forms: Tabs 0.5, 1, 1.5, 2, 2.5 mg

⚠ HIGH ALERT

ripretinib (Rx)
(rip-re′ti-nib)
Qinlock
Func. class.: Antineoplastic, tyrosine kinase inhibitor

USES: Treatment of advanced gastrointestinal stromal tumor (GIST) in those who have received ≥3 kinase inhibitors, including imatinib

CONTRAINDICATIONS
Hypersensitivity, pregnancy, breastfeeding

DOSAGE AND ROUTES
• **Adult:** PO 150 mg daily until disease progression or unacceptable toxicity
Available forms: Tablet 50 mg

---

risankizumab (Rx)

(ris'an-kiz'ue-mab)

Skyrizi

Func. class.: Systemic antipsoriasis agents

ACTION: A humanized immunoglobulin G1 (IgG1) monoclonal antibody that selectively binds to the p19 subunit of human interleukin-23 (IL-23), thereby inhibiting its interaction with the IL-23 receptor; human IL-23 is a naturally occurring cytokine involved in inflammatory and immune responses; by blocking IL-23 from binding to its receptor, prevents the release of proinflammatory cytokines and chemokines

USES: Moderate to severe plaque psoriasis, Crohn's disease, psoriatic arthritis

CONTRAINDICATIONS

Hypersensitivity

Precautions: Pregnancy, breastfeeding, TB, infection, immunosuppression

DOSAGE AND ROUTES

Plaque psoriasis
• **Adult: SUBCUT** 150 mg (two 75-mg injections) at wk 0, 4, and q12wk thereafter

Crohn's disease
• **Adult: IV** 600 mg over 1 hr at wk 0, 4, 8; **maintenance: SUBCUT** 180 or 360 mg at wk 12 and q8wk thereafter

Psoriatic arthritis
• **Adult: SUBCUT** 150 mg at wk 0, 4, then 150 mg q12wk

Available forms: Prefilled syringe solution for injection 75 mg/0.83 mL 2-pack, 150 mg/mL, 360 mg/2.4 mL, 600 mg/10 mL

Administer:

Subcut route
• Keep in the original carton to protect from light until time of use
• Do not shake the carton or prefilled syringe
• Before use, allow to reach room temperature out of direct sunlight (15-30 min); do not use other methods to speed warming process
• Visually inspect parenteral products for particulate matter and discoloration; solution should be clear to slightly opalescent, colorless to slightly yellow; solution may contain a few translucent white particles
• Do not use if solution contains large particles or is cloudy or discolored; solution has been frozen; syringe has been dropped or damaged; syringe tray seal is broken or missing
• Only an individual trained in subcut drug delivery should administer the injection
• Wash and dry hands
• Select an injection site (right or left thigh, abdomen at least 2 inches from the navel) and wipe with an alcohol swab; do not inject into skin that is tender, bruised, red, hard, or affected by psoriasis; do not inject into a scar or stretch mark; administer injections at different sites at least 1 inch apart
• Remove needle cover from the 1st prefilled syringe
• With 1 hand, gently pinch cleaned injection site; use the other hand to insert needle at a 45-degree angle using a quick, short movement
• Slowly push plunger until all the solution is injected
• Pull needle out of skin; release plunger and allow prefilled syringe to move up until the entire needle is covered by needle guard
• Apply cotton ball or gauze pad over injection site for 10 sec; do not rub injection site
• To obtain the full dose, repeat the injection process using 2nd prefilled syringe; select and cleanse an alternative injection site that is at least 1 inch away from first site; do not inject into the same site as the 1st syringe
• If a dose is missed, administer as soon as possible; then resume dosing at the regularly scheduled time

SIDE EFFECTS

CNS: *Headache,* fatigue, asthenia
EENT: *Sinusitis, nasal congestion, pharyngitis*
INTEG: *Inj site reaction*

MISC: Flulike symptoms, antibody development to this drug; *risk of infection* (TB, invasive fungal infections, other opportunistic infections)

PHARMACOKINETICS
Bioavailability 89%, peak 3-14 days

INTERACTIONS
Avoid use with live virus vaccines

NURSING CONSIDERATIONS
Assess:
• **Plaque psoriasis:** red, raised, inflamed patches of skin; whitish-silver scales or plaques on the red patches; dry skin that may crack and bleed; soreness around patches; itching and burning sensations around patches; thick, pitted nails; painful, swollen joints
• For inj site pain, swelling, redness—usually occur after 2 inj (4-5 days); use cold compress to relieve pain/swelling
• **Infections** (fever, flulike symptoms, dyspnea, change in urination, redness/swelling around any wounds): stop treatment if present; some serious infections including sepsis may occur; patients with active infections should not be started on this product
• **Latent TB before therapy;** treat before starting this product; TB test before use
• **Labs:** Monitor hepatitis B serology, LFTs, plasma hepatitis CRNA, plasma HIV RNA baseline, periodically
• **Pregnancy/breastfeeding:** use only if clearly needed; no well-controlled studies; cautious use in breastfeeding, no data
Evaluate
• **Therapeutic response:** decreasing plaques; painful, swollen joints
Teach patient/family:
• About self-administration if appropriate: inj should be made in thigh, abdomen, upper arm; rotate sites at least 1 inch from old site; do not inject in areas that are bruised, red, hard
• To refrigerate in container that product was received in; to dispose of needles and equipment as instructed
• That if medication is not taken when due, inject dose as soon as remembered and inject next dose as scheduled

• Not to take any live virus vaccines during treatment
• To report signs of infection, allergic reaction, or TB, immediately

---

risdiplam (Rx)
(ris-dip′lam)
Evrysdi
Func. class.: Spinal muscular atrophy agent

USES: Treatment of spinal muscular atrophy in children ≥2 mo

CONTRAINDICATIONS
Hypersensitivity

DOSAGE AND ROUTES
Spinal muscular atrophy
• **Adult: PO** 5 mg daily
• **Child (<2 mo):** 0.15 mg/kg orally once daily after a meal at approximately the same time each day
• **Child (2 mo to <2 yr):** 0.2 mg/kg orally once daily after a meal at approximately the same time each day
• **Child (≥2 yr, <20 kg):** 0.25 mg/kg orally once daily after a meal at approximately the same time each day
• **Child (≥2 yr, ≥20 kg):** 5 mg orally once daily after a meal at approximately the same time each day

---

risedronate (Rx)
(rih-sed′roh-nate)
Actonel, Atelvia
Func. class.: Bone resorption inhibitor
Chem. class.: Bisphosphonate

Do not confuse:
Actonel/Actos

ACTION: Inhibits bone resorption, absorbs calcium phosphate crystal in bone, and may directly block dissolution of hydroxyapatite crystals of bone

USES: Paget's disease; prevention, treatment of osteoporosis in

---

postmenopausal women; glucocorticoid-induced osteoporosis; osteoporosis in men
Unlabeled uses: Osteolytic metastases

CONTRAINDICATIONS

Hypersensitivity to bisphosphonates, inability to stand or sit upright for ≥30 min, esophageal stricture, achalasia, hypocalcemia
Precautions: Pregnancy, breastfeeding, children, renal disease, active upper GI disorders, dental disease, hyperparathyroidism, infection, vit D deficiency, coagulopathy, chemotherapy, asthma

DOSAGE AND ROUTES
Paget's disease (Actonel)
• **Adult: PO** 30 mg/day × 2 mo; patients with Paget's disease should receive calcium and vit D if dietary intake lacking; if relapse occurs, retreatment advised
Treatment/prevention of postmenopausal osteoporosis
• **Adult: PO** 5 mg/day or 35 mg/wk or 75 mg/day × 2 consecutive days monthly or 150 mg/mo
Glucocorticoid osteoporosis
• **Adult: PO** 5 mg/day
Osteoporosis in men
• **Adult: PO** 35 mg/wk
Bone metastases (unlabeled)
• **Adult: PO** 35 mg weekly
Renal dose
• **Adult: PO** CCr <30 mL/min, avoid use
Available forms: Tabs 5, 30, 150 mg; tab, weekly 35 mg
Administer:
• For 2 mo to be effective for Paget's disease
• With a full glass of water; patient should be in upright position for ½ hr; swallow whole; do not crush, break, chew; give del rel tablet in AM after breakfast, only use with food (del rel)
• Supplemental calcium and vit D for Paget's disease if instructed by prescriber
• Give daily ≥30 min before meals or give weekly
• Store in cool environment, out of direct sunlight

SIDE EFFECTS
CNS: Dizziness, headache, depression, asthenia, dizziness, insomnia, *weakness*

CV: *Chest pain,* hypertension, atrial fibrillation
GI: *Abdominal pain, diarrhea, nausea,* constipation, esophagitis
GU: UTI, renal toxicity, acute renal failure
MISC: Rash, UTI, pharyngitis, hypocalcemia, hypophosphatemia, increase PTH
MS: Osteonecrosis of the jaw, severe muscle/joint/bone pain, femoral fractures
SYST: Angioedema, flulike symptoms

PHARMACOKINETICS
Rapidly cleared from circulation, taken up mainly by bones (50%), eliminated primarily through kidneys, absorption decreased by food, terminal half-life 23 hr, delayed release 560 hr

INTERACTIONS
Increase: hypocalcemic effect—loop diuretics
Increase: GI irritation—NSAIDs, salicylates
Increase: osteonecrosis of the jaw—sunitinib
Decrease: absorption of risedronate—aluminum, calcium, iron, magnesium salts, antacids
Decrease: absorption of del rel risedronate H₂ antagonists, proton pump inhibitors, do not use together
Decrease: proton pump inhibitors, avoid concurrent use with delayed-release tablet
Drug/Food
Decrease: bioavailability—take ½ hr before food or drinks other than water
Drug/Lab Test
Decrease: calcium, phosphorus

NURSING CONSIDERATIONS
Assess:
• **Paget's disease:** headache, bone pain, increased head circumference
• **Osteoporosis:** in men or postmenopausal women; bone density study before and periodically during treatment
• **GI adverse effects:** nausea, diarrhea, gastric reflux, dyspnea
• **CV adverse reactions:** monitor B/P, dysrrhythmias, (tachycardia, bradycardia, atrial fibrillation)

• Phosphate, alkaline phosphatase, calcium; creatinine, BUN (renal disease)
• **Hypocalcemia:** paresthesia, twitching, laryngospasm, Chvostek's/Trousseau's signs
• **Serious skin reactions:** angioedema
• **Dental health:** provide antiinfectives for dental extraction; cover with antiinfectives before dental extraction
• **Pregnancy/breastfeeding:** use only if benefits outweigh fetal risk; do not breastfeed, excretion unknown
Evaluate:
• **Therapeutic response:** increased bone mass, absence of fractures
Teach patient/family:
• To sit upright for ½ hr after dose to prevent irritation
• To notify prescriber immediately if difficulty swallowing, severe heartburn, or pain in chest
• To comply with diet, vitamin/mineral supplements
• To maintain good oral hygiene
• To notify all health care providers of use
• That musculoskeletal pain may occur within a few days/mo after starting but usually resolves; use acetaminophen
• To exercise regularly; to avoid alcohol, tobacco
• To notify prescriber if pregnancy is suspected or if breastfeeding

---

risperiDONE (Rx)

(ris-pehr'ih-dohn)
Perseris, RisperDAL, RisperDAL
Consta
Func. class.: Antipsychotic
Chem. class.: Benzisoxazole
derivative

Do not confuse:
RisperDAL/reserpine

ACTION: Unknown; may be mediated through both dopamine type 2 (D_2) and serotonin type 2 (5-HT$_2$) antagonism

USES: Irritability associated with autism, bipolar disorder, mania, schizophrenia

Unlabeled uses: Acute psychosis, agitation, ADHD, dementia, psychotic depression, Tourette's syndrome

CONTRAINDICATIONS
Hypersensitivity, breastfeeding
Precautions: Pregnancy, children, geriatric patients, cardiac/renal/hepatic disease, breast cancer, Parkinson's disease, CNS depression, brain tumor, dehydration, diabetes, hematologic disease, seizure disorders, abrupt discontinuation, suicidal ideation, phenylketonuria

> **Black Box Warning:** Increased mortality in elderly patients with dementia-related psychosis

DOSAGE AND ROUTES
• **Adult:** PO 2 mg/day as single dose or in 2 divided doses, adjust dose at intervals of ≥24 hr and 1-2 mg/day as tolerated to 4-8 mg/day; **IM** establish dosing with **PO** before **IM** 25 mg q2wk, may increase to max 50 mg q2wk
• **Adolescent:** PO 0.5 mg/day in AM or PM, adjust dose at intervals of ≥24 hr and 0.5-1 mg/day as tolerated to 3 mg/day
• **Geriatric:** PO 0.5 mg daily-bid, increase by 1 mg/wk; **IM** 25 mg q2wk
Hepatic/renal dose
• **Adult:** PO 0.5 mg bid, increase by 0.5 mg bid, increase to 1.5 mg bid at intervals ≥1 wk
Available forms: Tabs 0.25, 0.5, 1, 2, 3, 4 mg; oral sol 1 mg/mL; orally disintegrating tabs 0.25, 0.5, 1, 2, 3, 4 mg; long-acting inj kit (Risperdal Consta) 12.5, 25, 37.5, 50 mg
Administer:
• Reduced dose in geriatric patients
• Anticholinergic agent on order from prescriber, to be used for EPS
• Avoid use with CNS depressants
• Conventional tabs: give without regard to meals
• **Oral disintegrating tab:** do not open blister pack until ready to use; tear at perforation; bend; peel back foil; do not push tab through foil; remove from pack and place product on patient's tongue; tab disintegrates in seconds and can be swal-

lowed with/without liquids, do not split or chew

• **Oral sol:** May dilute 3-4 oz of beverage, measure dose using calibrated pipette; not compatible with tea, cola; compatible with water, coffee, orange juice, low-fat milk

IM route

• Only use diluent and needle provided

• Allow to come to room temperature for 30 min

• Remove colored cap from the vial without removing the gray rubber stopper; wipe top of stopper with an alcohol wipe

• Peel back the blister pouch and remove the Vial Access Device by holding between the white Luer cap and the skirt; do not touch the spike tip at any time

• Place the vial on a hard surface and hold the base; orient the Vial Access Device vertically over the vial so that the spike tip is at the center of the vial's rubber stopper

• While holding the white collar of the syringe, insert and press the syringe tip into the blue circle of the Vial Access Device and twist clockwise

• Inject the entire contents of the syringe containing the diluent into the vial

• Shake the vial vigorously

• Invert completely and slowly withdraw the contents of the suspension from the vial into the syringe; tear the section of the vial label at the perforation and apply the detached label to the syringe

• While holding the white collar of the syringe, unscrew the syringe from the Vial Access Device, then discard both the vial and the Vial Access Device appropriately

• Select the appropriate color-coded needle provided with the kit; they are not interchangeable; do not use the needle intended for gluteal injection for deltoid injection, and vice versa

• Peel the blister pouch of the Needle-Pro safety device open halfway; grasp the transparent needle using the pouch, attach the Luer connection of the orange Needle-Pro to the syringe with an easy clockwise twisting motion

• While holding the white collar of the syringe, grasp the transparent needle

sheath and seat the needle firmly on the orange Needle-Pro device with a push and a clockwise twist

• Pull the transparent needle sheath straight away from the needle

• Resuspension is necessary before administration

• Only for IM; do not give IV

• Remove air bubbles

• Inject the entire contents of the syringe into the upper outer quadrant of the gluteal or deltoid muscle; gluteal injections should be alternated between the two buttocks

• After the injection is complete, press the needle into the orange Needle-Pro safety device

• Do not store the vial after reconstitution or the suspension will settle

• Do not combine 2 different dosage strengths of RisperDAL Consta in a single administration

• The dose pack device is for single use only

• **Stability after reconstitution:** Once in suspension, the product may remain at room temperature; use within 6 hr

SIDE EFFECTS

CNS: *EPS, pseudoparkinsonism, akathisia, dystonia, tardive dyskinesia; drowsiness, insomnia, agitation, anxiety, headache,* seizures, neuroleptic malignant syndrome, dizziness, suicidal ideation, head titubation (shaking)

CV: Orthostatic hypotension, tachycardia, heart failure, sudden death (geriatric patients), AV block

EENT: Blurred vision, tinnitus

GI: *Nausea,* vomiting, *anorexia, constipation,* jaundice, weight gain

GU: Hyperprolactinemia, gynecomastia, dysuria

HEMA: Neutropenia, granulocytopenia

MISC: Renal artery occlusion; hyperprolactinemia (child)

MS: Rhabdomyolysis

RESP: Rhinitis, sinusitis, upper respiratory infection, cough

PHARMACOKINETICS

PO: Extensively metabolized by liver to major active metabolite, ◐ determined by poor metabolizer or average metabolizers; plasma protein binding 90%, peak 1-2 hr, excreted 90% in urine, terminal half-life 3-24 hr

INTERACTIONS

Increase: seizures—traMADol

Increase: possible death in dementia-related psychosis: furosemide

Increase: sedation—other CNS depressants, alcohol

Increase: serotonin syndrome, neuroleptic malignant syndrome—CYP2D6 inhibitors (SSRIs, SNRIs)

Increase: EPS—other antipsychotics

Increase: risperiDONE excretion—carBAMazepine

Increase: QT prolongation—class IA/III antidysrhythmics, some phenothiazines, β-agonists, local anesthetics, tricyclics, haloperidol, methadone, chloroquine, clarithromycin, droperidol, erythromycin, pentamidine, thioridazine, ziprasidone

Increase: risperiDONE levels—acetylcholinesterase inhibitors, CYP2D6 inhibitors, SSRIs, valproic acid, verapamil

Decrease: risperiDONE action—CYP2D6 inducers (carBAMazepine, barbiturates, phenytoins, rifAMPin)

Decrease: levodopa effect—levodopa

Drug/Herb

Decrease: risperiDONE effect—echinacea

Drug/Lab Test

Increase: prolactin levels, blood, glucose, lipids

NURSING CONSIDERATIONS
Assess:

• **Suicidal thoughts/behaviors:** often when depression is lessened; mental status before initial administration

• Thyroid function test, blood glucose, serum electrolytes/prolactin/lipid profile, bilirubin, creatinine, weight, pregnancy test, CBC, LFTs, AIMS assessment, baseline and periodically

• Affect, orientation, LOC, reflexes, gait, coordination, sleep pattern disturbances

• **QT prolongation:** B/P standing, lying; pulse, respirations; take these q4hr during initial treatment; establish baseline

before starting treatment; report drops of 30 mm Hg; watch for ECG changes

• Dizziness, faintness, palpitations, tachycardia on rising

• **EPS:** akathisia, tardive dyskinesia (bizarre movements of the jaw, mouth, tongue, extremities), pseudoparkinsonism (rigidity, tremors, pill rolling, shuffling gait)

• **Serious reactions in geriatric patient:** fatal pneumonia, heart failure, sudden death, dementia

• **Neuroleptic malignant syndrome:** hyperthermia, increased CPK, altered mental status, muscle rigidity, seizures, change in B/P, fatigue, tachycardia

• Constipation, urinary retention daily; if these occur, increase bulk, water in diet

• Decreased stimuli by dimming lights, avoiding loud noises

• Supervised ambulation until patient stabilized on medication; do not involve patient in strenuous exercise program because fainting is possible; patient should not stand still for a long time

• Increased fluids to prevent constipation

• Store in tight, light-resistant container (PO); unopened vials in refrigerator, protect from light; do not freeze

• **Beers:** avoid use in older adults except for schizophrenia, bipolar disorder, or as a short-term antiemetic in chemotherapy

• **Pregnancy/breastfeeding:** use only if benefits outweigh fetal risk; EPS may occur in neonate; enroll pregnant women in the National Pregnancy Registry for Atypical Antipsychotics, 866-961-2388; do not breastfeed, excreted in breast milk

Evaluate:

• **Therapeutic response:** decrease in emotional excitement, hallucinations, delusions, paranoia; reorganization of patterns of thought, speech

Teach patient/family:

• That orthostatic hypotension may occur; to rise from sitting or lying position gradually

• To avoid abrupt withdrawal of product because EPS may result; product should be withdrawn slowly

• To avoid OTC preparations (cough, hay fever, cold) unless approved by pre-

scriber; that serious product interactions may occur; to avoid use of alcohol because increased drowsiness may occur
• To avoid hazardous activities if drowsy or dizzy
• To comply with product regimen
• To report impaired vision, tremors, muscle twitching
• **Heat intolerance:** That heat stroke may occur in hot weather; to take extra precautions to stay cool; to avoid hot tubs, hot showers, tub baths
• **Pregnancy/breastfeeding:** To use contraception; to inform prescriber if pregnancy is planned or suspected; not to breastfeed
• To notify provider of suicidal thoughts/ behaviors

TREATMENT OF OVERDOSE:
Lavage if orally ingested; provide airway; *do not induce vomiting*

ritonavir (Rx)
(ri-toe′na-veer)

Norvir

Func. class.: Antiretroviral
Chem. class.: Protease inhibitor

Do not confuse:
ritonavir/Retrovir

ACTION: Inhibits human immunodeficiency virus (HIV-1) protease and prevents maturation of the infectious virus

USES: HIV-1 in combination with at least 2 other antiretrovirals

CONTRAINDICATIONS
Hypersensitivity

Black Box Warning: Coadministration with other drugs

Precautions: Pregnancy, breastfeeding, hepatic disease, pancreatitis, diabetes, hemophilia, AV block, hypercholesterolemia, immune reconstitution syndrome, neonates, cardiomyopathy, immune reconstitution syndrome, infants 1-6 mo (overdose)

DOSAGE AND ROUTES
HIV in combination

• **Adult/adolescent >16 yr: PO** 600 mg bid; if nausea occurs, begin at ½ dose and gradually increase, max 1200 mg/ day in divided doses
• **Adolescent ≤16 yr: PO** 350-400 mg/ m^2 bid; increase by 50 mg/m^2 bid q2-3days, max 600 mg bid
• **Child: PO** Initial 250 mg/m^2 twice daily, then increase by 50 mg/m^2 every 2-3 days to maintenance of 350-400 mg/ m^2 twice daily, max 600 mg twice daily
Available forms: Oral sol 80 mg/mL; tab 100 mg; oral powder 100 mg
Administer:
Tablet
• Take with food, swallow whole; do not crush, break, chew
• When switching from cap to tab, more GI symptoms may occur, will lessen over time
• Use dosage titration to minimize side effects
• Store caps in refrigerator
• **Oral sol:** shake well, use calibrated measuring device
• Mix liquid formulation with chocolate milk or liquid nutritional supplement to improve taste
• **Oral powder:** Prepare using number of packets needed, pour and mix entire contents over soft food or mix in 4 ounces of liquid
• **Overdose:** infants, children, 43.2% alcohol, 26.57% propylene glycol oral sol, calculate total amount of alcohol, propylene glycol from all products given

SIDE EFFECTS
CNS: *Paresthesia, headache,* seizures, fever, dizziness, insomnia, asthenia, intracranial bleeding
CV: QT, PR interval prolongation
GI: *Diarrhea,* buccal mucosa ulceration, *abdominal pain, nausea, taste perversion,* dry mouth, *vomiting, anorexia,* pancreatitis, CDAD, hepatitis
INTEG: Rash
MISC: Asthenia, angioedema, anaphylaxis, Stevens-Johnson syndrome, increase lipids, lipodystrophy, toxic epidermal necrolysis, immune reconstitution syndrome

R

MS: Pain, rhabdomyolysis, myalgia
HEMA: Leukopenia, thrombocytopenia

PHARMACOKINETICS

Well absorbed, 98% protein binding, hepatic metabolism, peak 2-4 hr, terminal half-life 3-5 hr

INTERACTIONS

Black Box Warning: **Increase:** toxicity—amiodarone, astemizole, azole antifungals, benzodiazepines, buPROPion, CISapride, cloZAPine, desipramine, dihydroergotamine, encainide, ergotamine, flecainide, HMG-CoA reductase inhibitors, interleukins, meperidine, midazolam, pimozide, piroxicam, propafenone, propoxyphene, quiNIDine, ranolazine, saquinavir, terfenadine, triazolam, zolpidem; CYP2D6 inhibitors

Black Box Warning: **Increase:** QT prolongation—class IA/III antidysrhythmics, some phenothiazines, β-agonists, local anesthetics, tricyclics, haloperidol, chloroquine, droperidol, pentamidine, CYP3A4 inhibitors (amiodarone, clarithromycin, dasatinib, erythromycin, telithromycin, troleandomycin), arsenic trioxide, CYP3A4 substrates (methadone, pimozide, QUEtiapine, quiNIDine, risperiDONE, ziprasidone)

Increase: ritonavir levels—fluconazole
Increase: level of both products—clarithromycin, ddI
Increase: levels of—bosentan
Decrease: ritonavir levels—rifamycins, nevirapine, barbiturates, phenytoin
Decrease: levels of anticoagulants, atovaquone, divalproex, ethinyl estradiol, lamoTRIgine, phenytoin, sulfamethoxazole, theophylline, voriconazole, zidovudine

Drug/Herb

Decrease: ritonavir levels—St. John's wort; avoid concurrent use
Avoid use with red yeast rice

Drug/Lab Test

Increase: AST, ALT, K, CK, cholesterol, GGT, triglycerides, uric acid
Decrease: Hct, HB, RBC, neutrophils, WBC

NURSING CONSIDERATIONS

Assess:

• **HIV:** viral load, CD4 at baseline, throughout therapy; blood glucose, plasma HIV RNA, serum cholesterol/lipid profile; resistance testing before starting therapy and after treatment failure
• **Immune reconstitution syndrome:** may occur with combination therapy; may develop inflammatory response with opportunistic infection (MAC, Graves' disease, Guillain-Barré syndrome, TB, PCP); may occur during initial treatment or months after
• Signs of infection, anemia
• Hepatic studies: ALT, AST in those with hepatic disease, monitor q3mo
• Bowel pattern before, during treatment; if severe abdominal pain with bleeding occurs, discontinue product; monitor hydration
• Skin eruptions; rash
• **Rhabdomyolysis:** muscle pain, increased CPK, weakness, swelling of affected muscles, dark urine; if these occur and if confirmed by CPK, product should be discontinued
• **QT prolongation:** ECG for QT prolongation, ejection fraction; assess for chest pain, palpitations, dyspnea
• **Serious skin disorders:** Stevens-Johnson syndrome, angioedema, anaphylaxis, toxic epidermal necrolysis
• **Pregnancy/breastfeeding:** use only if benefits outweigh fetal risk; enroll pregnant women in the Antiretroviral Pregnancy Registry, 800-258-4263; do not breastfeed

Evaluate:

• **Therapeutic response:** improvement in HIV symptoms; improving viral load, CD4+ T cells

Teach patient/family:

• To take as prescribed; if dose is missed, to take as soon as remembered up to 1 hr before next dose; not to double dose
• That product not a cure for HIV; that opportunistic infections may continue to be acquired
• That redistribution of body fat or accumulation of body fat may occur
• That others may continue to contract HIV from patient

Black Box Warning: To avoid OTC, prescription medications, herbs, supplements unless approved by prescriber; not to use St. John's wort because it decreases product's effect

• That regular follow-up exams and blood work will be required

⚠ HIGH ALERT

riTUXimab (Rx)
(rih-tuks'ih-mab)
Rituxan, Rituxan SC 🍁
rituximab-abbs (Rx)
Truxima
rituximab-pvvr (Rx)
Ruxience
Func. class.: Antineoplastic—miscellaneous; DMARDs
Chem. class.: Murine/human monoclonal antibody

ACTION: Directed against the CD20 antigen that is found on malignant B lymphocytes; CD20 regulates a portion of cell-cycle initiation/differentiation

USES: ✒ Non-Hodgkin's lymphoma (CD20+, B-cell), bulky disease (tumors >10 cm), rheumatoid arthritis, Wegener's granulomatosis, microscopic polyangiitis
Unlabeled uses: Antibody-mediated rejection in cardiac transplantation autoimmune hemolytic anemia, Burkitt lymphoma, graft-versus-host disease, Hodgkin lymphoma, lupus nephritis

CONTRAINDICATIONS
Hypersensitivity, murine proteins
Precautions: Pregnancy, breastfeeding, children, geriatric patients, pulmonary/cardiac/renal conditions

Black Box Warning: Exfoliative dermatitis, infusion-related reactions, progressive multifocal leukoencephalopathy, hepatitis B exacerbation

DOSAGE AND ROUTES
Non-Hodgkin's lymphoma (NHL)
• **Adult: IV** 375 mg/m²/wk × 4 doses, may re-treat with 4 more doses of 375 mg/m²/wk
CLL
• **Adult: IV** 375 mg/m² on cycle 1; cycle 2 through 6 500 mg/m², treatment cycles are q28days; given with cyclophosphamide and fludarabine
GPA/MPA
• **Adult: IV** 375 mg/m² weekly × 4 wk (induction) give methylPREDNISolone 100 mg/day 1-3 days, then predniSONE; maintenance 500 mg q2 wkfor 2 doses, then by 500 mg q6mo thereafter based on clinical evaluation. Begin maintenance treatment within 24 wk of, and no sooner than 16 wk after, the last induction infusion based on clinical evaluation
Rheumatoid arthritis
• **Adult: IV** infusion 1000 mg days 1, 15; then repeat the 2-dose course,(two 1,000 mg doses separated by 2 wk) q24wk or based on clinical evaluation, but no sooner than q16wk give methylPREDNISolone 100 mg or similar product 30 min before infusion to decrease reactions
Available forms: Inj 10 mg/mL (100 mg/10 mL, 500 mg/50 mL)
Administer:
Intermittent IV INFUSION route
• Hold antihypertensives 12 hr before administration
• After diluting to final concentration of 1-4 mg/mL; use 0.9% NaCl, D₅W, gently invert bag to mix; do not mix with other products; give 50 mg/hr initially; if no reaction, increase rate by 50 mg/hr to max 400 mg/hr
• Monitor closely during infusion, severe reactions usually occur within 30-120 min
• Store vials at 36° F-40° F; protect vials from direct sunlight; infusion sol is stable at 36° F-46° F × 24 hr and at room temperature for another 12 hr

SIDE EFFECTS
CNS: Life-threatening brain infection (progressive multifocal leukoencephalopathy)
CV: Cardiac dysrhythmias, heart failure, hypertension, MI, supraventricular tachycardia, angina

GI: *Nausea, vomiting, anorexia,* GI obstruction/perforation
GU: Renal failure
HEMA: Leukopenia, neutropenia, thrombocytopenia, anemia
INTEG: *Irritation at site, rash,* fatal mucocutaneous infections (rare)
MISC: *Fever,* chills, asthenia, *headache,* angioedema, hypotension, myalgia, bronchospasm, ARDs
SYST: Toxic epidermal necrolysis, tumor lysis syndrome, Stevens-Johnson syndrome, exfoliative dermatitis
META: Hyperkalemia, hypocalcemia, hyperphosphatemia

PHARMACOKINETICS
Half-life varies, binds to CD20 sites or lymphoma cells

INTERACTIONS
Increase: hypotension—antihypertensives, separate by 12 hr
Increase: nephrotoxicity—CISplatin, avoid concurrent use; if used, monitor renal status
Increase: bleeding—anticoagulant
• Avoid with vaccines, toxoids

NURSING CONSIDERATIONS
Assess:

Black Box Warning: **Fatal infusion reaction:** hypoxia, pulmonary infiltrates, ARDS, MI, ventricular fibrillation, cardiogenic shock; most fatal reactions occur with 1st infusion; potentially fatal

Black Box Warning: **Severe mucocutaneous reactions:** Stevens-Johnson syndrome, lichenoid dermatitis, toxic epidermal lysis; occur 1-13 wk after product given, discontinue treatment immediately

Black Box Warning: **Tumor lysis syndrome:** acute renal failure requiring hemodialysis, hyperkalemia, hypocalcemia, hyperuricemia, hyperphosphatemia; allopurinol and adequate hydration may be needed

Black Box Warning: **Multifocal leukoencephalopathy:** confusion, dizziness, lethargy, hemiparesis; monitor periodically

• **Bone marrow suppression:** CBC, differential, platelet count weekly; withhold product if WBC is <3500/mm^3 or platelet count <100,000/mm^3; notify prescriber of results; product should be discontinued
• **Labs:** CBC with differential, hepatitis B serology, pregnancy test if applicable, ECG, serum creatinine/BUN, electrolytes, uric acid; correct electrolyte imbalances before use; hyperkalemia, hypocalcemia, hyperphosphatemia often occur
• **GI symptoms:** frequency of stools, abdominal pain, perforation/obstruction may occur
• **Infection:** fever, increased temperature, flulike symptoms in those with Wegener's granulomatosis and microscopic polyangiitis in those using DMARDs

Black Box Warning: **Hepatitis B exacerbation:** fulminant hepatitis, hepatic failure, death may occur during or following treatment; screen all patients for HBV infection (HBV/HBsAg and anti-HB$_c$ titers) before use; monitor those with current or prior HBV for signs of hepatitis or for HBV reactivation for several months after therapy; if reactivation occurs, discontinue product

• **Pregnancy/breastfeeding:** use only if benefits outweigh fetal risk; contraception should be used during and for 12 mo after last dose; enroll pregnant women in the Mother To Baby Autoimmune Diseases in Pregnancy Study, 877-311-8972 (patients with RA); do not breastfeed, excretion unknown
Evaluate:
• **Therapeutic response:** prevention of increasing cancer progression
Teach patient/family:
• That scheduled appointment must be kept, as relapse may occur
• To avoid use with vaccines, toxoids
• To report to prescriber possible infection (cough, fever, chills, sore throat), re-

nal issues (painful urination, back/side pain), bleeding (gums, stools, urine, bruising, emesis, fatigue)
• To avoid OTC products, alcohol
• To avoid crowds, those with known infections
• To maintain fluid intake
• To use contraception during and for 12 mo after therapy, not to breastfeed

rivaroxaban (Rx)
Xarelto
Func. class.: Anticoagulant
Chem. class.: Factor Xa inhibitor

ACTION: A novel oral anticoagulant that selectively and potently inhibits coagulation factor Xa

USES: For deep venous thrombosis (DVT) prophylaxis/treatment, pulmonary embolism (PE), in patients undergoing knee or hip replacement surgery; for stroke prophylaxis and systemic embolism prophylaxis in patients with nonvalvular atrial fibrillation

CONTRAINDICATIONS
Severe hypersensitivity

Black Box Warning: Active bleeding

Precautions: Pregnancy, breastfeeding, neonates, infants, children, adolescents, geriatric patients, moderate or severe hepatic disease (Child-Pugh Class B or C), hepatic disease associated with coagulopathy, creatinine clearance <30 mL/min for use as DVT prophylaxis and <15 mL/min for stroke and systemic embolism prophylaxis in nonvalvular atrial fibrillation, dental procedures, aneurysm, diabetes retinopathy, diverticulitis, endocarditis, GI bleeding, hypertension, obstetric delivery, peptic ulcer disease, stroke, surgery

Black Box Warning: Abrupt discontinuation, epidermal/spinal anesthesia

Patients, especially those with dental disease, should be instructed in proper oral hygiene, including caution in use of regular toothbrushes, dental floss, toothpicks

DOSAGE AND ROUTES
DVT prophylaxis (knee or hip replacement)
• **Adult: PO** 10 mg/day × 12 days after knee replacement surgery or × 35 days after hip replacement; administer the initial dose ≥6-10 hr after surgery once hemostasis has been established
DVT/PE treatment/reduction of risk
• **Adult: PO** 15 mg bid with food × 21 days, then 20 mg daily for a total of 6 mo, may continue after 6 mo to reduce risk
Stroke prophylaxis and systemic embolism prophylaxis (with nonvalvular atrial fibrillation)
• **Adult: PO** 20 mg/day with evening meal (CrCl >50 mL/min)
Converting from warfarin to rivaroxaban
• Discontinue warfarin and start rivaroxaban when INR is <3
Converting from another anticoagulant other than warfarin to rivaroxaban
• Start rivaroxaban 0-2 hr before the next scheduled evening administration of anticoagulant (omit that dose of anticoagulant); for continuous infusion of unfractionated heparin, stop the infusion and initiate rivaroxaban simultaneously
Converting from rivaroxaban to another anticoagulant with rapid onset (not warfarin)
• Discontinue rivaroxaban and give the first dose of the other anticoagulant (oral or parenteral) at the time that the next dose of rivaroxaban would have been administered
Hepatic dose
• **Adult: PO** Child-Pugh class B or C: avoid use
Renal dose
• **Adult: PO** (nonvalvular atrial fibrillation) CCr 15-50 mL/min 15 mg daily; CCr <15 mL/min avoid use; (treatment/prophylaxis of DVT/pulmonary embolism) CCr <30 mL/min avoid use

Available forms: Tabs 2.5, 10, 15, 20 mg; granules for oral suspension 1 mg/mL; tablet starter pack 15-20 mg

Administer:

• **For DVT prophylaxis:** give daily without regard to food; give initial dose ≥6-10 hr after surgery when hemostasis has been established

• **For stroke/systemic embolism prophylaxis:** give daily with evening meal

• If dose is not given at correct time, give as soon as possible on the same day

• 15-, 20-mg tabs should be taken with food; for those unable to swallow whole, tabs may be crushed, mixed with applesauce; immediately following administration, instruct to eat; crushed tabs are stable in applesauce for up to 4 hr

• 10-mg tab can be taken without regard to food; all doses ≥15 mg should be given with food

Nasogastric (NG) tube or gastric feeding tube:

• Confirm gastric placement of tube

• Crush 15- or 20-mg tab, suspend in 50 mL of water, and administer via NG or gastric feeding tube

• Enteral feeding should immediately follow administration of a crushed dose

• Crushed tabs are stable in water for up to 4 hr

Missed doses

• Patients receiving 15 mg BID should take their missed dose immediately to ensure intake of 30 mg per day; two 15-mg tabs may be taken at once followed by the regular 15 mg BID dose the next day

• For patients receiving once-daily dosing, take the missed dose as soon as it is remembered

• Store at room temperature

SIDE EFFECTS

GI: Increased hepatic enzymes, hyperbilirubinemia, jaundice, nausea, cholestasis, cytolytic hepatitis

HEMA: Bleeding, intracranial bleeding, epidural hematoma, GI bleeding, retinal hemorrhage, adrenal bleeding, retroperitoneal hemorrhage, cerebral hemorrhage, subdural hematoma, epidural hematoma, hemiparesis, thrombocytopenia

INTEG: Pruritus, blister, hypersensitivity, anaphylactic reaction, anaphylactic shock

SYST: Stevens-Johnson syndrome

PHARMACOKINETICS

Bioavailability 80%-100%, protein binding (92%-95%) albumin, excreted in urine 66% (36% unchanged, 30% metabolites), 28% in feces (7% unchanged, 21% metabolites), unchanged drug excreted in urine (via active tubular secretion, glomerular filtration); terminal elimination half-life 5-9 hr, peak 2-4 hr; increased effect in hepatic/renal disease, Japanese patients, increased terminal half-life in geriatric patients

INTERACTIONS

Increase: rivaroxaban effect, possible bleeding—ketoconazole itraconazole, ritonavir, lopinavir/ritonavir; conivaptan, clarithromycin, erythromycin, salicylates, NSAIDs, other anticoagulants, thrombolytics, platelet inhibitors, niCARdipine, fluconazole

Decrease: rivaroxaban effect—carBAMazepine, phenytoin, rifAMPin

Increase: rivaroxaban effect in renal impairment—telithromycin, darunavir, miFEPRIStone, nelfinavir, pantoprazole, posaconazole, saquinavir, tamoxifen, lapatinib, azithromycin, diltiaZEM, verapamil, quiNIDine, ranolazine, dronedarone, amiodarone, felodipine

Drug/Herb

Decrease: rivaroxaban effect—St. John's wort

Drug/Food

Increase: rivaroxaban effect in renal disease—grapefruit juice

NURSING CONSIDERATIONS

Assess:

Black Box Warning: Bleeding: monitor for bleeding, including bleeding during dental procedures (easy bruising, blood in urine, stools, emesis, sputum, epistaxis); there is no specific antidote

---

Black Box Warning: Abrupt discontinuation: avoid abrupt discontinuation unless an alternative anticoagulant in those with atrial fibrillation; discontinuing puts patients at an increased risk of thrombotic events; if product must be discontinued for reasons other than pathologic bleeding, consider administering another anticoagulant

Black Box Warning: Epidural/spinal anesthesia: epidural or spinal hematomas that result in long-term or permanent paralysis may occur in patients who have received anticoagulants and are receiving neuraxial anesthesia or undergoing spinal puncture; epidural catheter should not be removed <18 hr after the last dose of rivaroxaban; do not administer the next rivaroxaban dose <6 hr after the catheter removal; delay rivaroxaban administration for 24 hr if traumatic puncture occurs; monitor for neuro changes

• **Hepatic/renal disease:** increase in effect of product in hepatic disease (Child-Pugh class B or C), hepatic disease with coagulopathy; renal failure/severe renal impairment (creatinine clearance <30 mL/min in DVT prophylaxis and <15 mL/min for stroke or systemic embolism prophylaxis in nonvalvular atrial fibrillation); product should be discontinued in acute renal failure; reduce dose in those with atrial fibrillation and CrCl 15-50 mL/min; monitor renal function periodically (creatinine clearance, BUN)
• **Beers:** avoid use in older adults with CCr <30 mL/min; reduce dose in CCr 30-50 mL/min
• **Pregnancy/breastfeeding:** use only if benefits outweigh fetal risk; do not breastfeed, excretion unknown; pregnancy-related hemorrhage may occur
Evaluate:
• Prevention of DVT, stroke, and systemic embolism
Teach patient/family:
• To report if pregnancy is planned or suspected; not to breastfeed

Black Box Warning: To report bleeding (bruising, blood in urine, stools, sputum, emesis, heavy menstrual flow); use soft toothbrush, electric shaver

• To inform all health care providers of use; to report to prescriber all products used; to take all medication for the duration, exactly as prescribed to prevent clots; to notify prescriber if unable to take so that a different anticoagulant may be used

Black Box Warning: To avoid abrupt discontinuation without another blood thinner

• To report numbness of extremities, weakness, tingling, contact prescriber immediately (neuraxial anesthesia, spinal puncture)

rivastigmine (Rx)
(riv-as-tig´meen)
Exelon, Exelon Patch
Func. class.: Anti-Alzheimer agent
Chem. class.: Cholinesterase inhibitor

ACTION: Potent, selective inhibitor of brain acetylcholinesterase (AChE) and butyrylcholinesterase (BChE)

USES: Mild to severe Alzheimer's dementia, mild to moderate Parkinson's disease dementia (PDD)
Unlabeled uses: Vascular dementia, dementia with Lewy bodies, Pick's disease

CONTRAINDICATIONS
Hypersensitivity to this product, other carbamates
Precautions: Pregnancy, breastfeeding, children, respiratory/cardiac/renal/hepatic disease, seizure disorder, peptic ulcer, urinary obstruction, asthma, increased intracranial pressure, surgery, GI bleeding, jaundice

DOSAGE AND ROUTES
Dementia of Alzheimer's type
• **Adult: PO** 1.5 mg bid with food; after ≥4 wk, may increase to 3 mg bid; may increase to 4.5 mg bid and thereafter 6 mg bid, max 12 mg/day; **TRANSDERMAL** apply 4.6 mg/24 hr/day, after ≥4 wk may increase to 9.5 mg/24 hr/day; max 13.3 mg/24 hr

Parkinson's disease dementia
• **Adult: PO** 1.5 mg bid, after 4 wk may increase to 3 mg bid, increase dose by 1.5 mg bid at intervals of 4 wk or more to the highest tolerated dose (max 12 mg/day); TD 4.6 mg/24-hr patch daily, after 4 wk, may increase to 9.5 mg/ 24 hr, can then be increased to max 13.3 mg/24 hr

Available forms: Caps 1.5, 3, 4.5, 6 mg; transdermal patch 4.6, 9.5, 13.3 mg/24 hr

Administer:
• With meals; take with morning and evening meal even though absorption may be decreased
• If adverse reactions cause intolerance, discontinue treatment for several doses; restart at same or next lower dosage level
• If treatment is interrupted for more than several days, treatment should be initiated with lowest daily dose and titrated as indicated previously

Transdermal route
• Once a day to hairless, clean, dry skin, not in an area that clothing will rub; rotate sites daily; do not apply to same site more than once q14days; remove liner; apply firmly; may be used during bathing, swimming; avoid excess sunlight or external heat such as saunas; each 5-cm² patch contains 9 mg base, rate of 4.6 mg/24 hr, each 10-cm² patch 18 mg base, rate of 9.5 mg/24 hr

SIDE EFFECTS
CV: QT prolongation, AV block, cardiac arrest, angina, MI, palpitations, bradycardia
CNS: *Tremors, confusion, insomnia,* psychosis, hallucination, depression, dizziness, headache, anxiety, somnolence, fatigue, syncope, EPS, exacerbation of Parkinson's disease
GI: *Nausea, vomiting, anorexia, abdominal distress, flatulence,* diarrhea, constipation, dyspepsia, colitis, eructation, fecal incontinence, GI bleeding/obstruction, GERD, gastritis, pancreatitis
MISC: Urinary tract infection, asthenia, increased sweating, hypertension, flulike symptoms, weight change

PHARMACOKINETICS
Rapidly and completely absorbed; peak 1 hr, metabolized to decarbamylated metabolite; half-life 1.5 hr; excreted via kidneys (metabolites); clearance lowered in geriatric patients, hepatic disease and increased with nicotine use; 40% protein binding

INTERACTIONS
Increase: synergistic effect—cholinergic agonists, other cholinesterase inhibitors
Increase: metabolism—nicotine
Increase: GI effects—NSAIDs
Decrease: rivastigmine effect—anticholinergics, sedating H$_1$ blockers, tricyclics, phenothiazines

NURSING CONSIDERATIONS
Assess:
• Hepatic studies: AST, ALT, alk phos, LDH, bilirubin, CBC
• **Severe GI effects:** nausea, vomiting, anorexia, weight loss, diarrhea, GI bleeding
• **CV status:** B/P, heart rate, respiration during initial treatment; hypo/hypertension should be reported
• **Cognitive/mental status:** affect, mood, behavioral changes, depression, insomnia; complete suicide assessment
• **Gout/mobility:** Assistance with ambulation during beginning therapy; dizziness may occur
• **Skin:** assess for hypersensitivity-related dermatitis
• **TD:** overdoses have occurred and may be fatal
• **Beers:** avoid use in older adults; increased risk of orthostatic hypotension or bradycardia
• **Pregnancy/breastfeeding:** use only if clearly needed; do not breastfeed, excretion unknown

Evaluate:
• **Therapeutic response:** improved mood/cognition

Teach patient/family:
• How to apply **transdermal** product, to fold in half and throw away, not to get in eyes, to wash hands after application; not to use heating pad, sauna, tanning bed
• To notify prescriber of severe GI effects
• That product may cause dizziness, anorexia, weight loss
• That effect may take weeks or months; not to discontinue abruptly
• To notify prescriber if pregnancy is planned or suspected
• To give with food in AM, PM if using oral tablet
• To notify prescriber of history of low heart rate, sick sinus syndrome, risk of bradycardia
• How to take B/P, pulse at home
• To report nausea, vomiting, diarrhea
• To inform prescriber of all products taken

---

rizatriptan (Rx)

(rye-zah-trip′tan)

Maxalt, Maxalt-MLT

Func. class.: Migraine agent
Chem. class.: 5-HT$_{1D}$ receptor agonist, abortive agent-triptan

---

ACTION: Binds selectively to the vascular 5-HT$_{1B/1D}$ receptor subtype; exerts antimigraine effect; causes vasoconstriction of the cranial arteries

USES: Acute treatment of migraine

CONTRAINDICATIONS

Angina pectoris, history of MI, documented silent ischemia, Prinzmetal's angina, ischemic heart disease, concurrent ergotamine-containing preparations, uncontrolled hypertension, hypersensitivity, basilar or hemiplegic migraine
Precautions: Pregnancy, breastfeeding, children, geriatric patients, postmenopausal women, men >40 yr, risk factors for CAD, hypercholesterolemia, obesity, diabetes, impaired renal/hepatic function

DOSAGE AND ROUTES
Acute migraine
• **Adult:** PO 5-10-mg single dose, redosing separated by ≥2 hr, max 30 mg/24 hr

Acute migraine in those using propranolol
• **Adult:** PO 5 mg daily, max 10 mg/day given in 2 doses separated by ≥2 hr; use of rizatriptan oral film and propranolol is contraindicated, and a dosage reduction may be needed for rizatriptan tablets, limit to 5 mg/dose and 15 mg/24 hr for those receiving rizatriptan tablets
Available forms: Tabs (Maxalt) 5, 10 mg; orally disintegrating tabs (Maxalt-MLT) 5, 10 mg
Administer:
• **Orally disintegrating tab:** do not open blister until use; peel blister open with dry hands; place tab on patient's tongue, where it will dissolve, and have patient swallow with saliva (contains phenylalanine)
• Not to be used for more than 3-4 times per month

SIDE EFFECTS
CNS: *Dizziness, drowsiness, headache, fatigue,* warm/cold sensations, flushing
CV: MI, ventricular fibrillation, ventricular tachycardia, coronary artery vasospasm, palpitations, hypertension, peripheral vascular ischemia, ECG changes
ENDO: Hot flashes, mild increase in growth hormone
GI: *Nausea,* dry mouth, diarrhea, abdominal pain, ischemic colitis
RESP: Chest tightness, pressure, dyspnea

PHARMACOKINETICS
Onset of pain relief 10 min-2 hr; peak 1-1½ hr; duration 14-16 hr; 14% plasma protein binding; metabolized in liver (metabolite); excreted in urine (82%), feces (12%); half-life 2-3 hr

INTERACTIONS
Weakness, hyperreflexia, incoordination: SSRIs
Increase: levels of sibutramine
Increase: rizatriptan action—cimetidine, oral contraceptives, MAOIs, nonselective MAOI (type A and B), isocarboxazid, pargyline, phenelzine, propranolol, tranylcypromine
Increase: vasospastic effects—ergot, ergot derivatives, other 5-HT receptor agonists
Drug/Herb
Serotonin syndrome: St. John's wort

Side effects: *italics* = common; red = life-threatening

NURSING CONSIDERATIONS
Assess:
- **Migraine symptoms:** visual disturbances, aura, intensity, nausea, vomiting, photophobia
- Stress level, activity, recreation, coping mechanisms
- Neurologic status: LOC, blurring vision, nausea, vomiting, tingling in extremities preceding headache
- **Ingestion of tyramine foods** (pickled products, beer, wine, aged cheese), food additives, preservatives, colorings, artificial sweeteners, chocolate, caffeine, which may precipitate these types of headaches
- Renal status: urine output
- Quiet, calm environment with decreased stimulation: noise, bright light, excessive talking
- **Pregnancy/breastfeeding:** use only if benefits outweigh fetal risk; enroll in the registry, 800-986-8999; cautious use in breastfeeding, excretion unknown

Evaluate:
- **Therapeutic response:** decrease in frequency, severity of headache

Teach patient/family:
- **About use of orally disintegrating tab:** instruct patient not to open blister until use, to peel blister open with dry hands, to place tab on tongue, where it will dissolve, and to swallow with saliva (contains phenylalanine)
- To report any side effects to prescriber
- To use alternative contraception while taking product if oral contraceptives are being used
- That product does not prevent or reduce number of migraines; if 1st dose does not relieve pain, do not use more, notify prescriber; to avoid use in acute headache, use of agent >10 days a month due to the risk of medication overuse headaches

---

roflumilast (Rx)

Daliresp, Daxas ✦

Func. class.: Respiratory antiinflammatory agent
Chem. class.: Phosphodiesterase-4 (PDE4) inhibitor

ACTION: Roflumilast (and the active metabolite roflumilast N-oxide) selectively inhibit phosphodiesterase-4 (PDE4); not a bronchodilator; decreases inflammatory activity, PDE4 inhibition may affect migration and actions of proinflammatory cells

USES: Add-on treatment to bronchodilator use; for the prevention of COPD exacerbations in patients with severe COPD associated with chronic bronchitis and a history of exacerbations

CONTRAINDICATIONS
Moderate to severe hepatic disease (Child-Pugh B or C)
Precautions: Pregnancy, breastfeeding, neonates, infants, children, adolescents, acute bronchospasm, anxiety, insomnia, depression, suicidal ideation or behavior

DOSAGE AND ROUTES
COPD exacerbation
- **Adult: PO** 250 mcg/day × 4 wk, then increase to 500 mcg/day

Available forms: Tabs 250, 500 mcg
Administer:
PO route
- Give without regard to meals
- Store at room temperature

SIDE EFFECTS
CNS: Insomnia, anxiety, depression, headache, dizziness, tremors, suicidal ideation
EENT: Rhinitis, sinusitis
GI: *Weight loss, diarrhea, nausea,* anorexia, abdominal pain, dyspepsia, gastritis, vomiting
GU: Urinary tract infection
MS: Back pain, muscle cramps/spasm
SYST: Infections, influenza

PHARMACOKINETICS
80% bioavailability; protein binding 99% (roflumilast); 97% (N-oxide metabolite); extensively metabolized (liver); metabolism by CYP3A4 and CYP1A2 produces active metabolite N-oxide; half-life parent drug 17 hr, metabolite 30; 70% excreted in urine; parent drug peak 1 hr (range,

---

0.5-2 hr), metabolite peak 8 hr (range, 4-13 hr)

INTERACTIONS

Increase: roflumilast effect—CYP3A4/CYP1A2 inhibitors (enoxacin, cimetidine, delavirdine, indinavir, isoniazid, itraconazole, dalfopristin, quinupristin, tipranavir)

Increase: roflumilast effect—oral contraceptives (gestodene and ethinyl estradiol)

Decrease: roflumilast effect—CYP3A4 inducers (rifAMPin, barbiturates, carBA-Mazepine, phenytoin, erythromycin, ketoconazole, fluvoxaMINE, alcohol, etravirine, ritonavir, bexarotene, rifabutin, OXcarbazepine, nevirapine, modafinil, metyraPONE, PHENobarbital, bosentan, dexamethasone)

Altered effect of: fosamprenavir

Drug/Herb

Decrease: roflumilast effect—St. John's wort

NURSING CONSIDERATIONS
Assess:
• Lung sounds and respiratory function baseline and periodically thereafter
• Behavioral changes including mood, depression, suicidal thoughts/behaviors
• Liver function tests baseline and periodically thereafter; if increases in liver function studies occur, product should be discontinued
• **CV status:** rate, rhythm, chest pain, dyspnea, palpitations, supraventricular dysrrthmias are common
• **GI symptoms:** Weight; weight loss is common, diarrhea
• **Pregnancy/breastfeeding:** use only if benefits outweigh fetal risk; do not breastfeed, excreted in breast milk

Evaluate:
• Decreasing exacerbations in COPD

Teach patient/family:
• To take product as directed; not to skip or double doses; to take missed doses as soon as remembered unless almost time for next dose
• Not to use OTC or other products without prescriber approval; not to dis-

continue other respiratory products unless approved by prescriber
• Not to be used for acute bronchospasm but may be continued during acute asthma attacks
• **Suicidal thoughts/behaviors:** to notify prescriber of worsening depression or suicidal thoughts/behaviors

rolapitant (Rx)
(roe-la′pi-tant)
Varubi
Func. class.: Antiemetic

USES: Prevention of delayed nausea and vomiting associated with emetogenic cancer chemotherapy, including but not limited to highly emetogenic chemotherapy (in combination with other antiemetic agents)

CONTRAINDICATIONS
Hypersensitivity, use with CYP2D6 substrates (thioridazine, pimozide); child <2 yr

DOSAGE AND ROUTES
Chemotherapy-induced nausea and vomiting (prevention)
• **Adult: PO** 180 mg give within 2 hr before chemotherapy on day 1 only (in combination with dexamethasone given on days 1, 2, 3, and 4 and a 5-HT$_3$ receptor antagonist given on day 1); **IV** 166.5 mg over 30 min on day 1, 1-2 hr prior to chemotherapy, and 30 min prior to chemotherapy

Available forms: Emulsion for injection 166.5 mg/92.5 mL; tablet 90 mg

⚠ HIGH ALERT

romidepsin (Rx)
(roe-mi-dep′sin)
Istodax
Func. class.: Antineoplastics

USES: Treatment of cutaneous T-cell lymphoma (CTC)L or treatment of peripheral T-cell lymphoma (PTCL) in

R

Side effects: *italics* = common; red = life-threatening

those who have received at least one prior therapy

CONTRAINDICATIONS
Hypersensitivity

DOSAGE AND ROUTES
• **Adult:** IV 14 mg/m^2 on days 1, 8, and 15 of a 28-day cycle; repeat cycle as long as beneficial

Available forms: Powder for injection 10-mg vials; solution for injection 27.5 mg/5.5 mL

---

romiPLOStim (Rx)
(roe-mi-ploe′stim)
Nplate
Func. class.: Hematopoietin
Chem. class.: Thrombopoietin receptor agonist

USES: Chronic idiopathic thrombocytopenic purpura in patients who have had an insufficient response to corticosteroids, immunoglobulins, or splenectomy; hematopoietic syndrome of acute radiation syndrome

CONTRAINDICATIONS
Hypersensitivity to this product or mannitol

DOSAGE AND ROUTES
Thrombocytopenia in chronic idiopathic thrombocytopenic purpura (ITP)
• **Adult:** SUBCUT 1 mcg/kg/wk (based on actual body weight); increase the weekly dosage by 1 mcg/kg until platelet count ≥50,000/mm^3; 10 mcg/kg/wk max

Available forms: Injection 125-, 250-, 500-mcg single-use vials

---

romosozumab-aqqg (Rx)
(roe′moe-soz′ue-mab)
Evenity
Func. class.: Osteoporosis agent, sclerostin inhibitor

USES: Treatment of osteoporosis in postmenopausal females at high risk for fracture or those who have failed or are intolerant to other available osteoporosis therapy

CONTRAINDICATIONS
Hypersensitivity, uncorrected hypocalcemia

Black Box Warning: MI, stroke

DOSAGE AND ROUTES
Osteoporosis in postmenopausal women at high risk for fracture
• **Adult female** SUBCUT 210 mg monthly × 12 mo

Available forms: Injection 105 mg/1.17 mL, 210 mg/ 2.34 mL single-use prefilled syringe

---

ropeginterferon alfa-2b (Rx)
(ro-peg-in-ter-feer′on alfa)
Besremi
Func. class.: Immunostimulating agent

ACTION:
Binds to interferon alfa receptor (IFNAR) in the bone marrow

USES:
Polycythemia vera

CONTRAINDICATIONS
Hypersensitivity to interferon, severe psychiatric disorders, severe depression, suicidal ideation/attempt, hepatic disease Child-Pugh B or C, active serious/untreated autoimmune disease, immunosuppressed transplant patients

Precautions: Endocrine/CV/pulmonary/ophthalmologic toxicity, pancreatitis, colitis, hyperlipidemia

DOSAGE AND ROUTES
• **Adult:** SUBCUT 100 mcg q2wk, increase by 50 mcg q2wk to a max 500 mcg until hematocrit <45%, platelets <400 × 10^9

---

cells/L, leukocytes $<10 \times 10^9$ cells/L, continue for at least 1 yr at the dosage that achieves hematologic stability, then the dosing interval may be extended to q4wk **(not receiving a hydroxyurea); SUBCUT** 50 mcg q2wk with hydroxyurea, gradually taper hydroxyurea by reducing the total biweekly dose by 20%-40% q2wk during wk 3-12; discontinue hydroxyurea by wk 13; increase ropeginterferon alfa-2b dose by 50 mcg q2wk to a max dose of 500 mcg until hematocrit <45%, platelets $<400 \times 10^9$ cells/L, leukocytes $<10 \times 10^9$ cells/L; continue for at least 1 yr at the dosage that achieves hematologic stability, then the dosing interval may be extended to q4wk **(with hydroxyurea)**

Available forms: Solution for injection 500 mcg/mL prefilled syringe

Administer

SUBCUT route:

• Visually inspect for particulate matter/discoloration before use

• Allow the refrigerated product to warm to room temperature for 15-30 min; keep the syringe in the carton, attach the covered needle, move air bubbles to the top

• Discard some of the medication to achieve the prescribed dose; push the syringe plunger to align the top of the gray stopper to the correct syringe dose line/numbered markings

• Use the lower stomach/abdomen (at least 2 inches away from the belly button) or the top of thighs as injection sites; rotate sites; do not inject into skin that is irritated, red, bruised, infected, or scarred

• Do not recap the needle; dispose of the used prefilled syringe with the needle still attached into a sharps disposal container

• Store in a refrigerator at 36° F-46° F (2° C-8° C) in the original carton to protect from light, do not freeze

INTERACTIONS

Increased: myelosuppression—myelosuppressive agents, monitor for increased myelosuppression

Increased: CNS toxicity—narcotics, opioids, hypnotic sedatives, avoid use

Increased: adverse reactions—CYP 450 substrates (NTI), dose adjustment may be needed

PHARMACOKINETICS

Half-life 7 days, onset, peak, duration unknown

NURSING CONSIDERATIONS

Assess:

• Assess for history of severe psychiatric disorders, in particular severe depression, suicidal ideation, or suicide attempt; monitor closely for symptoms, change in mood, and need for treatment

• Assess for hypersensitivity reactions; if occurs, stop treatment and manage as needed

• Identify hepatic impairment (Child-Pugh B or C), monitor LFTs and hepatic function baseline and during treatment; reduce dose or discontinue depending on severity

• Monitor blood counts baseline, q2wk during titration, ≥q3-6mo during maintenance

• **Pancreatitis:** Assess for signs/symptoms of pancreatitis, including nausea/vomiting, right upper abdominal pain, may need to be discontinued

• **Pulmonary toxicity:** Discontinue if pulmonary infiltrates or pulmonary function impairment occurs

• **Ophthalmologic toxicity:** Advise patients to have eye examinations before and during treatment. Evaluate eye symptoms promptly and discontinue if needed

Teach patient/family:

• **Dental and periodontal toxicity:** Advise patients to use good oral hygiene and to have regular dental exams

• **Driving/operating machinery:** Advise patients to avoid driving or using machinery if they experience dizziness, hallucinations

• **Depression/suicide:** Inform patients, caregivers, family that suicidal ideation/behavior, new onset/worsening

R

depression may occur. Advise them to be aware of any unusual changes in mood or behavior, new onset or worsening of depression, or the emergence of suicidal thoughts or behavior. Instruct them to report signs or symptoms of depression to their health care provider right away, to discontinue product immediately, and seek immediate medical attention if suicidal ideation or attempts occur

• To notify the health care provider of signs/symptoms of diabetes or thyroid dysfunction, CV adverse reactions, weakness, fever, bruising, nosebleeds, itching, alopecia or rash, trouble breathing, severe diarrhea

• **Hyperlipidemia:** Advise patients that product may increase blood triglycerides and that they will need blood testing to monitor for this toxicity

• **Hepatotoxicity:** Advise patients to report signs or symptoms of hepatic toxicity to their health care provider: yellowing of skin, eyes, abdominal pain, clay-colored stools

• **Renal toxicity:** Advise patients to report signs or symptoms of kidney disease, change in urinary patterns

• **Pregnancy/breastfeeding:** Advise women to use an effective method of contraception and not to breastfeed during and ≥8 wk after the final dose

• Teach patient, caregiver storage, preparation, and administration techniques

---

rOPINIRole (Rx)

(roh-pin′ih-role)

Requip, Requip XL

Func. class.: Antiparkinson agent
Chem. class.: DOPamine-receptor agonist, nonergot

Do not confuse:
rOPINIRole/risperiDONE

ACTION: Selective agonist for D_2 receptors (presynaptic/postsynaptic sites); binding at D_3 receptor contributes to antiparkinson effects

USES: Parkinson's disease, restless legs syndrome (RLS)

CONTRAINDICATIONS
Hypersensitivity
Precautions: Pregnancy, dysrhythmias, affective disorder, psychosis, cardiac/renal/hepatic disease

DOSAGE AND ROUTES
Parkinson's disease
• **Adult:** PO **(regular release)** 0.25 mg tid × 1 wk; gradually titrate at weekly intervals: **Week 2,** 0.5 mg tid; **Week 3,** 0.75 mg tid; **Week 4,** 1 mg tid; **After week 4,** may increase by 1.5 mg/day each week, max 9 mg/day total dosage, and then by 3 mg/day each week, max 24 mg/day

• **PO (ext rel)** 2 mg/day × 1-2 wk, may increase by mg/day at intervals ≥1 wk based upon response; max 24 mg/day; if significant interruption of therapy occurs, retitration may be necessary
Restless legs syndrome
• **Adult:** PO **(reg rel)** 0.25 mg daily 1-3 hr before bedtime; days 3-7, may increase to 0.5 mg daily; at the beginning of week 2 (day 8), the dosage may be increased to 1 mg daily × 1 wk; weeks 3-6, dosage may be titrated up by 0.5 mg each week (from 1.5-3 mg over the 5-wk period) as needed to achieve desired effect, max: 4 mg/day
Available forms: Tabs 0.25, 0.5, 1, 2, 3, 4, 5 mg; ext rel tab 2, 4, 6, 8, 12 mg
Administer:
• Product until NPO before surgery
• Adjust dosage to patient response; taper when discontinuing
• With meals to reduce nausea
• **Extended release:** do not chew, crush, or divide
• Testing for diabetes mellitus, acromegaly if patient receiving long-term therapy

SIDE EFFECTS
CNS: *Agitation, insomnia,* psychosis, hallucination, dystonia, depression, dizziness, somnolence, sleep attacks, impulse control disorders

---

CV: *Orthostatic hypotension,* tachycardia, hypo/hypertension, syncope, palpitations
EENT: Blurred vision
GI: *Nausea, vomiting, anorexia, dry mouth,* constipation, dyspepsia, flatulence
GU: Impotence, urinary frequency
HEMA: Hemolytic anemia, leukopenia, agranulocytosis
INTEG: Rash, sweating
RESP: Pharyngitis, rhinitis, sinusitis, bronchitis, dyspnea

PHARMACOKINETICS
Peak 1-2 hr, half-life 6 hr, extensively metabolized by liver by P450 CYP1A2 enzyme system, protein binding 40%

INTERACTIONS
Increase: rOPINIRole effect—cimetidine, ciprofloxacin, diltiaZEM, enoxacin, erythromycin, fluvoxaMINE, mexiletine, norfloxacin, tacrine, digoxin, theophylline, L-dopa
Decrease: rOPINIRole effects—butyrophenones, metoclopramide, phenothiazines, thioxanthenes

NURSING CONSIDERATIONS
Assess:
• **Parkinsonism:** akinesia, tremors, staggering gait, muscle rigidity, drooling
• B/P, respirations during initial treatment; hypo/hypertension should be reported
• **Sleep attacks:** drowsiness, falling asleep without warning even during hazardous activities
• Mental status: affect, mood, behavioral changes, depression; complete suicide assessment; worsening of symptoms in restless legs syndrome
• **Pregnancy/breastfeeding:** use only if benefits outweigh fetal risk; avoid breastfeeding, excretion unknown
Evaluate:
• **Therapeutic response:** improvement in movement disorder
Teach patient/family:
• To notify prescriber if pregnancy is planned or suspected, or if breastfeeding
• To take with food to prevent nausea

• To report hallucinations, confusion (usually in geriatric patients)
• That therapeutic effects may take several weeks to a few months
• To change positions slowly to prevent orthostatic hypotension
• To report any suspicious skin lesions; that dermatologic or skin examinations should be performed regularly due to risk of melanoma in Parkinson's patients
• To use product exactly as prescribed; that if product is discontinued abruptly, parkinsonian crisis may occur; that product will be titrated weekly
• That drowsiness, sleep attacks may occur; to avoid driving, other hazardous activities until response known
• To avoid alcohol, CNS depressants, cough and cold products
• To notify prescriber if unusual urges occur

⚠ HIGH ALERT

rosiglitazone (Rx)
(ros-ih-glit'ah-zone)
Avandia
Func. class.: Antidiabetic, oral
Chem. class.: Thiazolidinedione

Do not confuse:
rosiglitazone/pioglitazone
Avandia/Prandia

ACTION: Improves insulin resistance by hepatic glucose metabolism, insulin receptor kinase activity, insulin receptor phosphorylation

USES: Type 2 diabetes mellitus, alone or in combination with sulfonylureas, metformin, insulin

CONTRAINDICATIONS
Breastfeeding, children, hypersensitivity to thiazolidinediones, diabetic ketoacidosis, jaundice

Black Box Warning: NYHA III, IV acute heart failure, heart failure

Precautions: Pregnancy, geriatric patients, thyroid disease, renal/hepatic disease, MI, heart failure class I, II NYHA

DOSAGE AND ROUTES
• **Adult: PO** 4 mg/day or in 2 divided doses, may increase to 8 mg/day or in 2 divided doses after 12 wk; may be added to metFORMIN, sulfonylurea for adult dose
Available forms: Tabs 2, 4, 8 mg
Administer:
• Conversion from other oral hypoglycemic agents if needed; change may be made without gradual dosage change; monitor blood glucose during conversion
• Store in tight container in cool environment
PO route
• Once or in 2 divided doses, without regard to food
• Tabs crushed and mixed with food or fluids for patients with difficulty swallowing

SIDE EFFECTS
CNS: Fatigue, *headache*
CV: MI, HF, death (geriatric patients), edema
ENDO: Hypo/hyperglycemia
GI: Weight gain, hepatotoxicity, increase total LDL, HDL cholesterol; decrease free fatty acids, diarrhea
MISC: Accidental injury, URI, sinusitis, anemia, back pain, diarrhea, edema, bone fractures (female), pulmonary/macular/peripheral edema
SYST: Anaphylaxis, Stevens-Johnson syndrome

PHARMACOKINETICS
Maximal reductions in fasting blood sugar after 6-12 wk; protein binding 99.8%; excreted in urine, feces; elimination half-life 3-4 hr; may be excreted in breast milk

INTERACTIONS
Increase: hypoglycemia—gemfibrozil, fluvoxaMINE, ketoconazole, trimethoprim; monitor glucose
• Avoid concurrent use with insulin, nitrates

• May increase or decrease level: CYP2C5 inducer/inhibitors
Drug/Herb
Increase: antidiabetic effect—garlic, horse chestnut
Drug/Lab Test
Increase: ALT, HDL, LDL, total cholesterol, blood glucose
Decrease: HB/Hct

NURSING CONSIDERATIONS
Assess:

Black Box Warning: **HF/MI:** dyspnea, crackles, edema, weight gain ≥5 lb, jugular venous distention; may need to change dose or discontinue product; do not use in acute coronary syndrome, NYHA Class III/IV heart failure

• **Hypoglycemic reactions** (sweating, weakness, dizziness, anxiety, tremors, hunger), hyperglycemic reactions soon after meals
• **Systemic reactions:** anaphylaxis, Stevens-Johnson syndrome
• **Hepatotoxicity:** LFTs periodically, AST, ALT (if ALT >2.5 × ULN, do not use product)
• **Diabetes:** Fasting blood sugar, A1c, plasma lipids/lipoproteins, B/P, body weight during treatment
• To use product provider/patient must be enrolled in the Avandia-Rosiglitazone Medicines Access Program
• **Beers:** avoid in older adults; may promote fluid retention or exacerbate heart failure
• **Pregnancy/breastfeeding:** use only if benefits outweigh fetal risk, usually insulin is used in pregnancy; do not breastfeed, excretion unknown
Evaluate:
• **Therapeutic response:** decrease in polyuria, polydipsia, polyphagia; clear sensorium; absence of dizziness; stable gait; blood glucose, A1c improvement
Teach patient/family:
• To monitor blood glucose; that periodic liver function tests mandatory; to report edema, weight gain

- About the symptoms of hypo/hyperglycemia, what to do about each; that these symptoms are more likely to occur in those using insulin
- That product must be continued on daily basis; about the consequences of discontinuing the product abruptly
- To avoid OTC medications, herbal preparations, nitrates, or insulin unless approved by prescriber
- That diabetes is lifelong; that product is not a cure, only controls symptoms
- That all food included in diet plan must be eaten to prevent hypoglycemia
- To carry emergency ID and glucagon emergency kit
- To report symptoms of hepatic dysfunction (nausea, vomiting, abdominal pain, fatigue, anorexia, dark urine, jaundice) immediately; to report macular edema (change in vision)
- That 2 wk is needed to see reduction in blood glucose level and 2-3 mo needed to see full effect of product
- To notify prescriber if oral contraceptives are used
- That a medication guide should be dispensed with each prescription/refill
- Not to use if breastfeeding; may be secreted in breast milk

rosuvastatin (Rx)

(roe-soo′va-sta-tin)

Crestor, Ezallor Sprinkle

Func. class.: Antilipemic

Chem. class.: HMG-CoA reductase inhibitor

ACTION: Inhibits HMG-CoA reductase enzyme, which reduces cholesterol synthesis

USES: As an adjunct for primary hypercholesterolemia (types IIa, IIb) and mixed dyslipidemia, elevated serum triglycerides, homozygous/heterozygous familial hypercholesterolemia (FH), slowing of atherosclerosis, CV disease prophylaxis, MI, stroke prophylaxis (normal LDL)

CONTRAINDICATIONS

Pregnancy, breastfeeding, hypersensitivity, active hepatic disease

Precautions: Children <10 yr, geriatric patients, past hepatic disease, alcoholism, severe acute infections, trauma, hypotension, uncontrolled seizure disorders, severe metabolic disorders, electrolyte imbalances, severe renal impairment, hypothyroidism, Asian patients

DOSAGE AND ROUTES

Hypercholesterolemia, hyperlipoproteinemia, and/or hypertriglyceridemia

- **Adult: PO** 10 mg/day as usual starting dose; 5 mg/day in those requiring less aggressive LDL cholesterol reductions, in patients with CrCl <30 mL/min, or in patients at higher risk for myopathy; range 5-40 mg/day

For slowing the progression of atherosclerosis

- **Adult: PO** 10 mg/day as usual starting dose; initially 5 mg/day in those requiring less aggressive LDL cholesterol reductions, in patients with CCr <30 mL/min, or in patients at higher risk for myopathy; range 5-40 mg/day

Primary prevention of cardiovascular disease

- **Adult: PO** 10-20 mg/day as usual starting dose; range 5-40 mg/day

Renal dose

- **Adult: PO** CCr <30 mL/min, initially, 5 mg/day in those not receiving dialysis; **max** 10 mg/day

Available forms: Sprinkle capsule 5, 10, 20, 40 mg; tablet 40 mg

Administer

- May be taken at any time of day, with/without food
- Store in cool environment in airtight, light-resistant container

SIDE EFFECTS

CNS: *Headache, dizziness,* insomnia, paresthesia, confusion

GI: *Nausea, constipation, abdominal pain, flatus, diarrhea, dyspepsia, heartburn,* kidney failure, liver dysfunction, vomiting

HEMA: Thrombocytopenia, hemolytic anemia, leukopenia

INTEG: *Rash, pruritus*

MS: *Asthenia, muscle cramps, arthritis, arthralgia, myalgia,* myositis, rhabdomyolysis; leg, shoulder, or localized pain

PHARMACOKINETICS

Peak 3-5 hr, minimal live metabolism (about 10%), 88% protein bound, excreted primarily in feces (90%), crosses placenta, half-life 19 hr, not dialyzable

INTERACTIONS

Increase: toxicity—cycloSPORINE, do not use together

• Do not exceed 20 mg/day when used with clopidogrel, eltrombopag, dronedarone, itraconazole

Increase: hepatotoxicity—alcohol

Increase: myalgia, myositis, rhabdomyolysis—cycloSPORINE, gemfibrozil, niacin, clofibrate, azole antifungals, antiretroviral protease inhibitors, fibric acid derivatives

Increase: bleeding risk—warfarin

Drug/Lab Test

Increase: LFTs

NURSING CONSIDERATIONS

Assess:

• Diet; obtain diet history including fat, cholesterol in diet

• Fasting cholesterol, LDL, HDL, triglycerides at baseline and q4-6wk, then periodically

• Liver function: LFTs at baseline, then if clinically indicated; AST, ALT, LFTs may increase

• Renal function in patients with compromised renal system: BUN, creatinine, I&O ratio

• **Rhabdomyolysis:** muscle pain, tenderness, obtain CPK; if these occur,

product may need to be discontinued; for patients with Asian ancestry: increased blood levels, rhabdomyolysis

• **Pregnancy/breastfeeding:** do not use in pregnancy, breastfeeding

Evaluate:

• **Therapeutic response:** decreased LDL, cholesterol, triglycerides, increased HDL, slowing CAD

Teach patient/family:

• To report suspected pregnancy; to use contraception while taking product; not to breastfeed

• To report weakness, muscle tenderness, pain, fever, liver injury (jaundice, anorexia, abdominal pain)

• That blood work and follow-up exams will be necessary during treatment

• To report severe GI symptoms, dizziness, headache, muscle pain, weakness

• That previously prescribed regimen will continue: low-cholesterol diet, exercise program, smoking cessation

---

⚠ HIGH ALERT

rucaparib (Rx)

(roo-kap′a-rib)

Rubraca

Func. class.: Antineoplastic

Chem. class.: Poly (ADP-ribose) polymerase (PARP) inhibitor

ACTION: Inhibits poly (ADP-ribose) polymerase (PARP) enzymes; inhibition of PARP enzyme activity results in increased PARP-DNA complexes, causing DNA damage, apoptosis, and cell death

USES: BRCA mutation–positive (germline and/or somatic), prostate cancer in patients who have received 2 or more prior chemotherapy regimens, as monotherapy, BRCA 1/2 castration-resistant prostate cancer (mCRPc)

CONTRAINDICATIONS

Hypersensitivity

Precautions: Breastfeeding, contraceptive requirements, leukemia, myelodysplastic syndrome (MDS), pregnancy, pregnancy testing, reproductive risk

DOSAGE AND ROUTES
BRCA mutation–positive prostate cancer
• **Adult: PO** 600 mg bid; continue until disease progression or severe toxicity

Available forms: Tabs 200 mg, 250 mg, 300 mg

SIDE EFFECTS
CNS: Fatigue, dizziness, fever, asthenia
GI: Nausea, vomiting, constipation, anorexia, abdominal pain, diarrhea, dysgeusia
HEMA: Anemia, thrombocytopenia, neutropenia, febrile neutropenia, myelodysplastic syndrome (MDS)/acute myeloid leukemia
INTEG: Pruritus, rash, photosensitivity, hand-foot syndrome
RESP: Dyspnea

PHARMACOKINETICS
70% protein binding, peak 1.9 hr, half-life 17-19 hr, metabolized by CYP2D6 (major) and CYP3A4, CYP1A2 (minor)

INTERACTIONS
None known

Drug/Lab:
Increase: AST, ALT, cholesterol
Decrease: ANC, Hb, platelets

NURSING CONSIDERATIONS
Assess:
• **Myelodysplastic syndrome (MDS)/ acute myeloid leukemia (AML):** monitor for signs and symptoms of MDS/AML; monitor CBC baseline and monthly; do not start until prior hematologic toxicity resolves to grade ≤1. For prolonged hematologic toxicity (>4 wk), hold therapy or reduce dose and check a CBC weekly until recovery; discontinue if a diagnosis of MDS or AML occurs

• **Pregnancy/breastfeeding (rarely used in women):** assess use of effective contraception during treatment and for 6 mo after last dose; pregnancy testing should be done before use; can cause fetal harm or death; do not breastfeed during treatment and for 2 wk after the final dose, obtain pregnancy test in those of reproductive potential; male patients with partners who may become pregnant use contraception during and for 3 mo after last dose

• Monitor AST/ALT, cholesterol, creatinine; all may be elevated

Evaluate:
• **Therapeutic response:** decrease in growth, spread of ovarian cancer

Teach patient/family:
• To notify prescriber of all OTC, Rx, and herbal products taken; not to start new products without prescriber approval
• **Myelodysplastic syndrome (MDS)/ acute myeloid leukemia (AML):** to report weakness, fatigue, bruising, bleeding, trouble breathing, blood in urine, stool, emesis; that continuing blood work will be needed
• **Photosensitivity:** to wear protective clothing, sunscreen or to stay out of sun to prevent burns
• **Pregnancy/breastfeeding:** that product can cause fetal harm or death; that pregnancy testing should be done before use; to use effective contraception during treatment and for 6 mo after final dose; not to breastfeed during treatment or for 2 wk after final dose

R

rufinamide (Rx)
(roo-fin′a-mide)
Banzel
Func. class.: Anticonvulsant
Chem. class.: Triazole derivative

USES: Lennox-Gastaut syndrome
Unlabeled uses: Partial seizures

CONTRAINDICATIONS
Hypersensitivity, familial short QT syndrome

DOSAGE AND ROUTES
Lennox-Gastaut syndrome
• **Adult: PO** 400-800 mg/day divided bid; increase by 400-800 mg/day q2days to 3200 mg/day

• **Child 1 to <17 yr: PO** 10 mg/kg/day divided equally bid; increase by 10 mg/kg/day every other day to 45 mg/kg/day or 3200 mg/day, whichever is less

Available forms: Suspension 40 mg/mL; tabs 200, 400 mg

⚠ HIGH ALERT

ruxolitinib (Rx)
(rux-oh-li'ti-nib)

Jakafi

Func. class.: Antineoplastic agent, Janus-associated kinase inhibitor

---

USES: Treatment of steroid-refractory acute graft-versus-host disease (GVHD); treatment of intermediate or high-risk myelofibrosis including primary myelofibrosis, post-polycythemia vera myelofibrosis, and post-essential thrombocythemia myelofibrosis; treatment of polycythemia vera in those with an inadequate response/hydroxyurea

CONTRAINDICATIONS
Hypersensitivity

Black Box Warning: Fungal infection, lymphoma, MI, new primary malignancy

DOSAGE AND ROUTES
Graft-versus-host disease (acute; treatment), steroid-refractory
• **Adult: PO** 5 mg bid may increase to 10 mg bid after ≥3 days of treatment (if ANC and platelets are not decreased by ≥50% compared to baseline)

Myelofibrosis
• **Adult: PO** Initial dose (based on platelet count, titrate dose thereafter based on efficacy and safety): Platelets >200,000/mm^3: 20 mg bid; platelets 100,000-200,000/mm^3: 15 mg bid; platelets 50,000 to <100,000/mm^3 5 mg bid

Available forms: Tablet 5,10,15, 20, 25 mg; topical cream 1.5%

sacituzumab govitecan-hziy (Rx)

(sak′i-tooz′ue-mab goe′vi-tee′kan)

Trodelvy

Func. class.: Antineoplastic, anti-Trop-2

USES: Treatment of metastatic triple-negative breast cancer who have received ≥2 other therapies

CONTRAINDICATIONS
Hypersensitivity, pregnancy, breastfeeding
DOSAGE AND ROUTES
• **Adult: IV:** 10 mg/kg on days 1 and 8 of a 21-day cycle; continue until disease progression or unacceptable toxicity
Available forms: Powder for injection 180 mg

sacubitril/valsartan (Rx)

(sak-ue′bi-tril/val-sar′tan)

Entresto

Func. class.: Antihypertensive, angiotensin II receptor blocker, neprilysin inhibitor

USES: Reduce the risk of cardiovascular death and hospitalization for heart failure (HF) in patients with chronic HF (New York Heart Association Class II-IV) and reduced ejection fraction; symptomatic HF with systemic left ventricular systolic dysfunction in child ≥1 yr

CONTRAINDICATIONS
Hypersensitivity to sacubitril, valsartan, or any component; use within 36 hr of ACE inhibitors; use with aliskiren in diabetes, angioedema

DOSAGE AND ROUTES
Heart failure
• **Adult: Patients previously taking a moderate- to high-dose ACE inhibitor** (>10 mg/day of enalapril or equivalent) or angiotensin II receptor blocker (>160 mg/day of valsartan or equivalent): PO Sacubitril 49 mg/valsartan 51 mg bid, double the dose after 2-4 wk to the target of sacubitril 97 mg/valsartan 103 mg bid
• **Adult: Patients previously taking low doses of an ACE inhibitor (≤10 mg/day of enalapril or equivalent) or ARB (≤160 mg/day of valsartan or equivalent): PO** Sacubitril 24 mg/valsartan 26 mg bid double the dose q2-4wk to the target of sacubitril 97 mg/valsartan 103 mg bid
• **Adult: Patients not currently taking an ACE inhibitor or an ARB: PO** Sacubitril 24 mg/valsartan 26 mg bid, double the dose q2-4wk to the target of sacubitril 97 mg/valsartan 103 mg bid
Symptomatic HF with systemic left ventricular systolic dysfunction in child ≥1 yr
• **Child/adolescent <40 kg: PO solution (extemporaneously prepared):** Initial: 1.6 mg/kg/dose bid; titrate dose in 2 wk to 2.3 mg/kg/dose bid, then 2 wk later to 3.1 mg/kg/dose bid
• **Child/adolescent 40 to <50 kg: PO Tablets:** Sacubitril 24 mg/valsartan 26 mg bid; titrate dose in 2 wk to sacubitril 49 mg/valsartan 51 mg bid, then 2 wk later to sacubitril 72 mg/valsartan 78 mg (three 24-/26-mg tablets) bid; **≥50 kg:** sacubitril 49 mg/valsartan 51 mg bid; titrate dose in 2 wk to sacubitril 72 mg/valsartan 78 mg (three 24-/26-mg tablets) bid, then 2 wk later to sacubitril 97 mg/valsartan 103 mg bid
Available forms: Tabs 24/26, 49/51, 97/103 mg

safinamide (Rx)

(sa-fin′-a-mide)

Xadago

Func. class.: Antiparkinson agent
Chem. class.: MAO type B inhibitor

ACTION: The precise mechanism of action is unknown; one mechanism may be related to its MAO-B inhibitory activity, which causes an increase in DOPamine levels centrally

USES: For adjunctive treatment to levodopa-carbidopa therapy in patients with Parkinson's disease experiencing "off" episodes

CONTRAINDICATIONS
Hypersensitivity, MAOI therapy

Precautions: Abrupt discontinuation, alcoholism, breastfeeding, pregnancy, cataracts, use with CNS depressants, dental work, diabetic retinopathy, hypertension, hepatic disease, impulse control problems, psychosis, schizophrenia, surgery, uveitis

DOSAGE AND ROUTES
• **Adult: PO** Initially, 50 mg/day. May increase after 2 wk to 100 mg/day based on need and tolerability. Max 100 mg/day

Available forms: Tabs 50, 100 mg

Administer:

• Give at same time each day; may be given with or without food

• If a dose is missed, take the next dose at the usual time on the following day

• Food and drug interactions with safinamide can be serious. Patients should avoid foods/beverages containing large amounts of tyramine

SIDE EFFECTS
CNS: Drowsiness, dyskinesia, insomnia, impulse control symptoms, neuroleptic malignant syndrome, psychosis, serotonin syndrome

CV: Orthostatic hypotension

MISC: Cough, dyspepsia, cataracts

PHARMACOKINETICS
Not highly protein bound, excreted via kidneys 5% (unchanged), 76% recovered in the urine; half-life 20-26 hr, peak 2-3 hr; inhibits intestinal breast cancer resistance protein (BCRP)

INTERACTIONS
• **Increase:** severe somnolence—anxiolytics, sedatives, hypnotics, barbiturates, ALPRAZolam, clonazePAM, zolpidem, zaleplon; avoid using together

• **Increase:** hypertension, hypertensive crisis—MAOIs, linezolid; do not use within 14 days of these products

• **Increase:** serotonin syndrome—meperidine, some other opioids; SNRIs; tricyclic antidepressants and other cyclic antidepressants; triazolopyridine antidepressants; cyclobenzaprine; stimulants (methylphenidate, amphetamines), dextromethorphan; use the lowest dose of safinamide

• **Decrease:** safinamide effects—atypical antipsychotics

NURSING CONSIDERATIONS
Assess:

• **Parkinson's disease:** assess for changes before and during treatment; tremors, pin-rolling, movement, balance, anxiety, drooling, depression, delusions, hallucinations, insomnia, shuffling gait; decreasing of "off" periods

• **Mental status:** affect, depression, mood, complete suicide assessment

• **Hypertension:** Monitor for new-onset hypertension or hypertension not adequately controlled after starting product; adjust dose if needed; monitor for hypertension if used with sympathomimetics

• **Drug interactions:** review before use; there are many serious reactions

• **Impulse control:** Assess for new or worsening impulse control symptoms (gambling, increased sexual urges, binge eating, intense urges to spend money, or other intense urges); if these occur, dose reduction or discontinuation may be needed

• **Hepatic disease:** monitor LFTs baseline and periodically in those with hepatic disease

• **Neuroleptic malignant syndrome-like symptoms:** elevated temperature, muscular rigidity, altered consciousness, and autonomic instability; may occur with rapid dose reduction

• **Serotonin syndrome:** nausea, vomiting, sedation, dizziness, diaphoresis (sweating), facial flushing, mental status changes, myoclonus, restlessness, shivering, and hypertension. If serotonin syndrome occurs, any serotonergic agents should be discontinued

• **Pregnancy/breastfeeding:** may cause fetal harm; use in pregnancy only if the potential benefit outweighs fetal risk; do not use in breastfeeding, serious adverse reactions may occur

Teach patient/family:
• **Impulse control:** that symptoms (gambling, increased sexual urges, binge eating, intense urges to spend money, or other intense urges) may occur; to report to provider
• Not to drive or engage in hazardous activities until effect of product is known; drowsiness may occur
• To take B/P regularly
• To change position slowly to prevent orthostatic hypotension
• To use product as prescribed; if discontinued abruptly, neuroleptic malignant syndrome–like symptoms may occur; to taper gradually; to take at same time of day; to take with levodopa-carbidopa
• To use physical activity to maintain mobility, lessen spasms
• **Serotonin syndrome:** to report dry, hot skin; fever, agitation, delirium, diarrhea; to avoid use with other serotonergic products
• To avoid use of tyramine-containing products; give list to patient
• Pregnancy/breastfeeding: to report if pregnancy is planned or suspected or if breastfeeding

---

salicylic acid topical
See Appendix B

---

salmeterol (Rx)
(sal-met′er-ole)
Serevent Diskus
Func. class.: β₂-Adrenergic agonist (long acting), bronchodilator

ACTION: Causes bronchodilation by action on β₂ (pulmonary) receptors by increasing levels of cAMP, which relaxes smooth muscle with little effect on heart rate; maintains improvement in FEV from 3 to 12 hr; prevents nocturnal asthma symptoms

USES: Prevention of exercise-induced bronchospasm, COPD, asthma

CONTRAINDICATIONS
Hypersensitivity to sympathomimetics, tachydysrhythmias, severe cardiac disease, monotherapy treatment of asthma
Precautions: Pregnancy, breastfeeding, cardiac disorders, hyperthyroidism, diabetes mellitus, hypertension, closed-angle glaucoma, seizures, acute asthma, as a substitute to corticosteroids, QT prolongation

Black Box Warning: Asthma-related death, children <4 yr

DOSAGE AND ROUTES
• **Adult/child ≥4 yr: Asthma INH** 50 mcg (1 inhalation as dry powder) q12hr; **exercise-induced bronchospasm prophylaxis** 50 mcg (1 inhalation) ½-1 hr before exercise
Available forms: Inhalation powder 50 mcg/blister
Administer:
• Gum, sips of water for dry mouth
• Use only as add-on therapy
• Use ½ hr before exercise for exercise-induced bronchospasm prevention, do not use additional doses if using bid
• Use this medication before other medications, allow at least 1 min between other inhaled products
• Do not use spacer with this product
• Store in foil pouch; do not expose to temperature >86° F (30° C); discard 6 wk after removal from foil pouch

SIDE EFFECTS
CNS: *Tremors, anxiety,* insomnia, headache, dizziness, fever
CV: Palpitations, tachycardia, hypo/hypertension, angina
EENT: Dry nose, irritation of nose and throat
GI: Nausea, vomiting, abdominal pain, heartburn
MS: Muscle cramps
RESP: Bronchospasm, cough, asthma-related death

Side effects: *italics* = common; red = life-threatening

PHARMACOKINETICS

INH: Onset 30-50 min; peak 4 hr; duration 12 hr; metabolized in liver; excreted in urine, breast milk; crosses placenta, blood-brain barrier; protein binding 94%-98%; terminal half-life 3-5 hr

INTERACTIONS

Increase: CV effect—CYP3A4 inhibitors (itraconazole, ketoconazole, nelfinavir, nefazodone, saquinavir), avoid using together

Increase: action of aerosol bronchodilators

Increase: action of salmeterol—tricyclics, MAOIs

Decrease: salmeterol action—other β-blockers

NURSING CONSIDERATIONS
Assess:

• **Respiratory function:** vital capacity, forced expiratory volume, ABGs, lung sounds, heart rate and rhythm baseline and periodically

• Product should not be used as monotherapy for asthma; product should not be used for rescue breathing treatment

• **Paradoxical bronchospasm:** dyspnea, wheezing, chest tightness; do not use in bronchospasm

Black Box Warning: Children should not use this product as monotherapy for asthma; use only with persistent asthma in those whose symptoms are not controlled with a long-term asthma agent; after product controls asthma, use another bronchodilator

• **Hypersensitivity:** assess for rash, urticaria; rarely leads to anaphylaxis, angioedema

Black Box Warning: Asthma-related death: long-acting beta agonists have been associated with severe asthma and asthma-related death. If wheezing worsens and cannot be relieved during an acute asthma attack, patients should be instructed to seek immediate medical attention. Avoid use of single-ingredient long-acting beta agonists for asthma. Do not use in those with significantly worsening asthma, which may be life-threatening

• **Pregnancy/breastfeeding:** use only if benefits outweigh fetal risk; cautious use in breastfeeding, excretion unknown

Evaluate:

• **Therapeutic response:** absence of dyspnea, wheezing

Teach patient/family:

Black Box Warning: Asthma-related deaths: to seek medical attention immediately for serious asthma attack; death may be greater in black patients

• Not to use for acute bronchospasm; never to exhale into Diskus; to hold level, keep mouthpiece dry

• Not to use OTC medications, extra stimulation may occur

• If using to prevent exercise-induced bronchospasm, to use ½-1 hr before exercise

• Review package insert with patient

• To avoid getting powder in eyes

• To avoid smoking, smoke-filled rooms, persons with respiratory infections

• Not for treatment of acute exacerbation; a fast-acting β-blocker should be used instead

• To immediately report dyspnea after use if ≥1 canister is used in 2 mo time

• To notify prescriber if >4 inhalations are needed or if product is no longer working

• To take other products as prescribed

• To notify prescriber if pregnancy is suspected or if breastfeeding

TREATMENT OF OVERDOSE:
β_2-Adrenergic blocker

---

saquinavir (Rx)
(sa-kwin′a-veer)
Invirase
Func. class.: Antiretroviral-protease inhibitor

USES: Treatment of HIV-1 infection in adults (>16 yr) in combination with other antiretrovirals. Saquinavir is not recommended as a component of initial therapy for the treatment of HIV

CONTRAINDICATIONS

Hypersensitivity or any component, congenital QT prolongation, refractory hypokalemia/hypomagnesemia, complete AV block, use of saquinavir/ritonavir with CYP3A substrates

DOSAGE AND ROUTES

• **Adult: PO** 1 g bid with ritonavir 100 mg bid; for those already taking ritonavir 100 mg bid, no additional ritonavir is needed

Treatment-naive patients or patients switching from a regimen containing delavirdine

• **Adult: PO Initial:** Saquinavir 500 mg bid with ritonavir 100 mg bid × 7 days
Adult: PO Maintenance: Saquinavir 1 g bid with ritonavir 100 mg bid
Available forms: Tabs 500 mg; capsules 200 mg

---

sarecycline (Rx)
(sar-e-sye′kleen)
Seysara
Func. class.: Antibiotic, tetracycline

USES: Treatment of inflammatory lesions of non-nodular moderate-severe acne vulgaris in those ≥9 yr

CONTRAINDICATIONS

Hypersensitivity to sarecycline, tetracyclines, or any component

DOSAGE AND ROUTES
Acne vulgaris, non-nodular, moderate to severe
Adult/child ≥9 yr PO 33-54 kg: 60 mg daily; **55-84 kg:** 100 mg daily; **85-136 kg:** 150 mg daily
Available forms: Tabs 60, 100, 150 mg

> **⚠ HIGH ALERT**

sargramostim, GM-CSF (Rx)
(sar-gram′oh-stim)
Leukine
Func. class.: Biologic modifier, hematopoietic agent
Chem. class.: Granulocyte macrophage colony-stimulating factor (GM-CSF)

ACTION: Stimulates proliferation and differentiation of hematopoietic progenitor cells (granulocytes, macrophages)

USES: Acceleration of myeloid recovery in patients with non–Hodgkin's lymphoma, acute lymphoblastic leukemia, acute myelogenous leukemia, autologous bone marrow transplantation in Hodgkin's disease; bone marrow transplantation failure or engraftment delay, mobilization and transplant of peripheral blood progenitor cells (PBPCs)
Unlabeled uses: Aplastic anemia, Crohn's disease, ganciclovir- or zidovudine-induced neutropenia, malignant melanoma, myelodysplastic syndrome (MDS)

CONTRAINDICATIONS

Neonates; hypersensitivity to GM-CSF, benzyl alcohol, yeast products; excessive leukemic myeloid blast in bone marrow, peripheral blood
Precautions: Pregnancy, breastfeeding, children; lung/cardiac/renal/hepatic disease; pleural, pericardial effusions, peripheral edema, leukocytosis, mannitol hypersensitivity, hepatic/renal disease

DOSAGE AND ROUTES
Myeloid recovery in Hodgkin's disease, non-Hodgkin's lymphoma, acute lymphocytic leukemia
• **Adult/adolescent/child ≥2 yr:** IV 250 mcg/m²/day over a 2-hr period beginning 2-4 hr after infusion of bone marrow and not <24 hr after last dose of chemotherapy or radiotherapy

S

Following engraftment failure
• **Adult/adolescent/child ≥2 yr:** IV 250 mcg/m²/day × 14 days; give over 2 hr; may repeat in 7 days; may repeat 500 mcg/m²/day × 14 days after another 7 days if no improvement

Mobilization of PBPCs
• **Adult:** CONT IV 250 mcg/m²/24 hr or SUBCUT daily; continue through collection

After PBPC transplantation
• **Adult:** CONT IV 250 mcg/m²/day until ANC >1500 cells/mm³

Aplastic anemia (unlabeled)
• **Adult:** SUBCUT 250-500 mcg/day or 5 mcg/kg/day × 14-90 days, used with erythropoietin or immunosuppressive therapy

Available forms: Powder for inj lyophilized 250 mcg; sol for inj 500 mcg/mL

Administer:
• Store in refrigerator; do not freeze

SUBCUT route
• No further dilution of reconstituted sol is needed; take care not to inject intradermally

Intermittent IV INFUSION route
• After reconstituting with 1 mL sterile water for inj without preservative; do not reenter vial; discard unused portion; direct reconstitution sol at side of vial; rotate contents; do not shake
• Dilute in 0.9% NaCl inj to prepare IV infusion; if final concentration is <10 mcg/mL, add human albumin to make final concentration of 0.1% to NaCl before adding sargramostim to prevent adsorption; for a final concentration of 0.1% albumin, add 1 mg human albumin/1 mL 0.9% NaCl inj run over 2 hr **(bone marrow transplant or failure of graft)**; over 4 hr **(chemotherapy for AML)**; over 24 hr as cont infusion **(PBPCs)**; give within 6 hr after reconstitution

Y-site compatibilities: Amikacin, aminophylline, aztreonam, bleomycin, butorphanol, calcium gluconate, CARBOplatin, carmustine, ceFAZolin, cefepime, cefotaxime, cefoTEtan, ceftizoxime, cefTRIAXone, cefuroxime, cimetidine, CISplatin, clindamycin, cyclophosphamide, cycloSPORINE, cytarabine, dacarbazine, DACTINomycin,

dexamethasone, diphenhydrAMINE, DOPamine, DOXOrubicin, doxycycline, droperidol, etoposide, famotidine, fentaNYL, floxuridine, fluconazole, fluorouracil, furosemide, gentamicin, granisetron, heparin, IDArubicin, ifosfamide, immune globulin, magnesium sulfate, mannitol, mechlorethamine, meperidine, mesna, methotrexate, metoclopramide, metroNIDAZOLE, minocycline, mitoXANTRONE, netilmicin, pentostatin, piperacillin/tazobactam, potassium chloride, prochlorperazine, promethazine, ranitidine, teniposide, ticarcillin, ticarcillin-clavulanate, trimethoprim-sulfamethoxazole, vinBLAStine, vinCRIStine, zidovudine

SIDE EFFECTS
CNS: Fever, malaise, CNS disorder, weakness, chills, dizziness, syncope, headache
CV: Transient supraventricular tachycardia, peripheral edema, pericardial effusion, hypotension, tachycardia
GI: Nausea, vomiting, diarrhea, anorexia, GI hemorrhage, stomatitis, liver damage, hyperbilirubinemia
GU: Urinary tract disorder, abnormal kidney function
HEMA: Blood dyscrasias, hemorrhage
INTEG: Alopecia, rash, peripheral edema
MS: Bone pain, myalgia
RESP: Dyspnea

PHARMACOKINETICS
Half-life elimination: IV 60 min, SUBCUT 2-3 hr; detected within 5 min after administration, peak 2 hr

INTERACTIONS
Increase: myeloproliferation—lithium, corticosteroids
Drug/Lab Test
Increase: bilirubin, BUN, creatinine, eosinophils, LFTs, leukocytes

NURSING CONSIDERATIONS
Assess:
• **Blood studies:** CBC, differential count before treatment, 2× weekly; leukocytosis may occur (WBC >50,000 cells/mm³, ANC >20,000 cells/mm³), platelets; if ANC

>20,000/mm³ or 10,000/mm³ after nadir has occurred or platelets >500,000/mm³, reduce dose by ½ or discontinue; if blast cells occur, discontinue
• Renal, hepatic studies before treatment: BUN, creatinine, urinalysis; AST, ALT, alk phos; 2× weekly monitoring is needed in renal/hepatic disease
• **Hypersensitivity, anaphylaxis** rashes, local inj-site reactions; usually transient
• Body weight, hydration status; increased fluid retention in cardiac disease; pulmonary function
• **Constitutional symptoms:** asthenia, chills, fever, headache, malaise
• Myalgia, arthralgia in legs, feet; use analgesics, antipyretics
• **Gasping syndrome in neonates:** due to benzyl alcohol hypersensitivity, do not use
• **Pregnancy/breastfeeding:** use only if clearly needed; cautious use in breastfeeding, excretion unknown

Evaluate:
• **Therapeutic response:** WBC and differential recovery

Teach patient/family:
• That bone pain may occur with use of the product and is normal
• To report excessive diarrhea, B/P increase, or respiratory symptoms to health care provider immediately
• To review all aspects of product use

---

sarilumab (Rx)

(sar-il′ue-mab)

Kevzara

Func. class.: Antirheumatic, immunosuppressive

Chem. class.: Interleukin antagonist, monoclonal antibody

ACTION: Inhibits interleukin-6 (IL-6) receptors by binding to both forms of IL-6 receptors, antiinflammatory action and a reduction in C-reactive protein

USES: Treatment of adults with moderately to severely active rheumatoid arthritis in patients who have had an inadequate response or intolerance to one or more disease-modifying antirheumatic drugs (DMARDs); used as monotherapy or in combination with methotrexate or DMARDs

CONTRAINDICATIONS

Hypersensitivity, active infections, active severe hepatic disease, ANC <2000/mm³, platelets <150,000/mm³, TB

Precautions: Chronic/recurrent infections, corticosteroid therapy, diabetes mellitus, diverticulitis, risk of GI perforation, hepatic disease (Child-Pugh B), severe renal disease, pregnancy, lactation, children, geriatric patients, HIV, neoplastic disease

Black Box Warning: Infection

DOSAGE AND ROUTES
• **Adult: SUBCUT** 200 mg q2wk

Dosage modifications

Lab Value	Recommendation
ANC 0.5-1 × 10⁹/L	Hold until ANC 1 × 10⁹/L
ANC <0.5 × 10⁹/L	Discontinue
Platelets 50-100 × 10³/ mcl	Hold until >100 × 10³/mcl
Platelets <50 × 10³/mcl	Discontinue
ALT >1 to ≤3 × ULN	Consider dose modification
ALT >3 to ≤5 × ULN	Hold until ALT <3 × ULN
ALT >5 × ULN	Discontinue

Available forms: Sol for SUBCUT inj 150 mg/1.14 mL, 200 mg/1.14 mL single-use prefilled syringes or prefilled pen

Administer:

SUBCUT route
• A TB test before use; do not start therapy if patient has latent TB, treat first

S

• Visually inspect for particulate matter and discoloration before use; product is clear and colorless to pale yellow
• Allow to sit at room temperature for 30 min, do not warm any other way
• Inject full amount of the syringe
• Do not rub the injection site
• Dispose of used syringe or pen properly. Do not recap after use. Do not reuse the pen or syringe
• Rotate injection sites with each injection
• **Missed dose:** Give as soon as possible if it has been ≤3 days; if longer, discuss with health care provider
• **Storage:** Use within 14 days after being taken out of the refrigerator

SIDE EFFECTS

GI: GI perforation, abscess, gastroenteritis
GU: UTI
HEMA: Thrombocytopenia, neutropenia, leukopenia, anemia
INTEG: Injection site reactions, rash, pruritus
MISC: Infections (TB), hypersensitivity, immunosuppression, malignancy
RESP: *URI,* dyspnea, nasopharyngitis

PHARMACOKINETICS

Peak 2-4 days, duration 28-43 days depending on dose, half-life 150-mg dose is 8 days, 200-mg dose 10 days

INTERACTIONS

Increase: immunosuppression, infections—DMARDs, TNF antagonists, corticosteroids, live virus vaccines
Altered effect: CYP450 substrates (cyclosporine, atorvastatin, lovastatin, theophylline, warfarin, hormonal contraceptives); monitor substrate levels

NURSING CONSIDERATIONS

Assess
• **Infection:** flulike symptoms, fever, dyspnea, inflammation of wounds; perform TB test before starting treatment
• **Reactivation of viral herpes zoster:** blisters, rash, hepatitis B, dark urine, jaundice, clay-colored stools, weakness, fatigue, anorexia, nausea, vomiting, abdominal pain; immediately report symptoms

• **GI reactions:** assess for ulceration, abscess, perforation; monitor bowel habits, bowel sounds
• **Blood studies: AST, ALT** at baseline, 4 wk and 8 wk after starting therapy, and q3mo thereafter; **lipid levels:** at baseline, 4 wk and 8 wk after starting treatment, and q6mo thereafter; **platelets** at baseline, 4 wk and 8 wk after starting therapy, and q3mo thereafter; **neutrophils:** at baseline, 4 wk and 8 wk after starting therapy, and q3mo thereafter

Evaluate:
• **Therapeutic response:** slowing progression of rheumatoid arthritis

Teach patient/family:
• The reason for therapy and expected result
• The correct technique for subcut injection and proper disposal of syringes; to review the Medication Guide
• **Infection:** to report immediately fever, flulike symptoms, cough, blood in emesis, urine, stools; hypersensitivity: rash, itching
• To avoid live virus vaccines while taking this product; that vaccinations should be brought up-to-date before treatment
• To avoid OTC, herbal products or supplements without consent of prescriber; to discuss with all prescribers all medications and products taken
• **Pregnancy/breastfeeding:** to notify prescriber if pregnancy is planned or suspected or if breastfeeding; that pregnant women should enroll in the pregnancy registry at 877-311-8972

⚠ HIGH ALERT

SAXagliptin (Rx)

(sax-a-glip′tin)

Onglyza
Func. class.: Antidiabetic, oral
Chem. class.: Dipeptidyl-peptidase-4 inhibitor (DPP-4 inhibitor)

Do not confuse:
SAXagliptin/SITaGLIPtin

ACTION: Slows the inactivation of incretin hormones; improves glucose homeostasis, improves glucose-dependent insulin synthesis, lowers glucagon secretions, and slows gastric emptying time

USES: In adults, type 2 diabetes mellitus as monotherapy or in combination with other antidiabetic agents

CONTRAINDICATIONS
Hypersensitivity, angioedema, serious rash, type 1 diabetes, ketoacidosis
Precautions: Pregnancy, geriatric patients, GI obstruction, surgery, thyroid/renal/hepatic disease, trauma, diabetic, heart failure

DOSAGE AND ROUTES
• **Adult:** PO 2.5-5 mg; may use with other antidiabetic agents other than insulin; if used with insulin, a lower dose may be needed; max 2.5 mg with strong 3A4-5 inhibitors
Renal dose
• **Adult:** PO CCr ≤50 mL/min, 2.5 mg daily; **hemodialysis:** 2.5 mg/day after hemodialysis
Available forms: Tabs 2.5, 5 mg
Administer:
PO route
• May be taken with/without food
• Do not break or cut tabs
• Conversion from other antidiabetic agents; change may be made with gradual dosage change
• Store in tight containers at room temperature

SIDE EFFECTS
CNS: *Headache*
ENDO: Hypoglycemia (renal impairment)
GI: *Nausea, vomiting,* abdominal pain, pancreatitis
INTEG: Urticaria, angioedema, anaphylaxis
CV: Edema, HF
EENT: Sinusitis

PHARMACOKINETICS
Rapidly absorbed, metabolized by liver—CYP3A4, excreted by the kidneys (unchanged 24%), half-life 2.5 hr, 3.1 hr metabolite, peak 2 hr, duration 24 hr

INTERACTIONS
Increase: hypoglycemia—androgens, insulins, β-blockers, cimetidine, corticosteroids, salicylates, MAOIs, fibric acid derivatives, FLUoxetine, insulin, sulfonylureas, ACE inhibitors; strong CYP3A4/5 inhibitors; dosage reduction may be needed

Drug/Herb
Increase: antidiabetic effect—garlic, horse chestnut

Drug/Lab Test
Decrease: lymphocytes, glucose

NURSING CONSIDERATIONS
Assess:
• **Hypoglycemic reactions** (sweating, weakness, dizziness, anxiety, tremors, hunger); monitor blood glucose, HbA1c
• **Renal studies:** BUN, creatinine during treatment
• **Heart failure:** history of risk factors for heart failure; use cautiously in these patients; assess daily weight, edema, dyspnea, crackles, tachycardia/bradycardia
• **Pancreatitis:** abdominal pain, nausea; discontinue product immediately; previous pancreatitis may be a contributing factor
• **Pregnancy/breastfeeding:** use only if clearly needed, usually insulin is used in pregnancy; cautious use in breastfeeding, excretion unknown
Evaluate:
• **Therapeutic response:** decrease in polyuria, polydipsia, polyphagia; clear sensorium; absence of dizziness; stable gait, blood glucose at normal level
Teach patient/family:
• To perform regular self-monitoring of blood glucose using blood-glucose meter
• About the symptoms of hypo/hyperglycemia; what to do about each
• That product must be continued on daily basis; about consequences of discontinuing product abruptly

S

• To avoid OTC medications, alcohol, digoxin, exenatide, insulins, nateglinide, repaglinide, and other products that lower blood glucose unless approved by prescriber
• That diabetes is lifelong; that this product is not a cure, only controls symptoms
• That all food included in diet plan must be eaten to prevent hypo/hyperglycemia
• To carry emergency ID
• To take product without regard to food
• To notify prescriber when surgery, trauma, stress occurs because dose may need to be adjusted or insulin used
• **Pancreatitis:** to immediately report and stop product if severe abdominal pain with vomiting occurs
• **Hypersensitivity:** to immediately get medical assistance and stop product if itching; rash; swelling of face, tongue occurs

---

scopolamine (Rx)
(skoe-pol′a-meen)
Transderm Scop
Func. class.: Cholinergic blocker
Chem. class.: Belladonna alkaloid

USES: Preoperatively to produce amnesia, sedation and to decrease secretions; motion sickness, parkinsonian symptoms

CONTRAINDICATIONS
Hypersensitivity, closed-angle glaucoma, myasthenia gravis, GI/GU obstruction, hypersensitivity to belladonna, barbiturates

DOSAGE AND ROUTES
Motion sickness
• **Adult:** TD 1 patch 4 hr before travel and q3days
Preoperatively
• **Adult: IM/IV/SUBCUT** 0.32-0.65 mg; **TD** apply 1 patch PM before surgery or 1 hr before C-section

Nausea and vomiting
• **Adult: SUBCUT** 0.6-1 mg
• **Child: SUBCUT** 0.006 mg/kg; max 0.3 mg/dose
Available forms: TD patch 1 mg/72 hr (1.5 mg/2.5 m^2)

---

secnidazole (Rx)
Solosec
Func. class.: Antiinfective

USES: Bacterial vaginosis

DOSAGE AND ROUTES
• **Adult: PO** 2 g as a single dose
Available forms: Oral granules 2 g

---

secukinumab (Rx)
(sek′-ue-kin′-ue-mab)
Cosentyx, Cosentyx Sensoready, Cosentyx Sensoready Pen
Func. class.: Immune response modifier
Chem. class.: Monoclonal antibody

ACTION: Interleukin (IL)-12, IL-23 antagonist, decreases inflammatory response

USES: Plaque psoriasis, ankylosing spondylitis, psoriatic arthritis, axial spondyloarthritis

CONTRAINDICATIONS
Hypersensitivity, active TB
Precautions: Pregnancy, breastfeeding, Crohn's disease, infection, latex hypersensitivity, vaccination

DOSAGE AND ROUTES
Ankylosing spondylitis
• **Adult: SUBCUT** 150 mg at weeks 0, 1, 2, 3, and 4 and q4wk thereafter, or 150 mg **SUBCUT** q4wk; consider increasing the dose to 300 mg q4wk if active disease persists
Psoriatic arthritis
• **Adult: SUBCUT** 150 mg at weeks 0, 1, 2, 3, and 4 and q4wk thereafter; may give with or without methotrexate; may consider a dose of 300 mg if active disease persists

---

Psoriatic arthritis with plaque psoriasis:
• **Adult: SUBCUT** Initially, 300 mg (2 injections of 150 mg) at weeks 0, 1, 2, 3, and 4; **Maintenance:** 300 mg (2 injections of 150 mg) q4wk
Available forms: Solution for injection 150 mg/mL (pen, prefilled syringe), 2-pack and single
Administer:
• Visually inspect for particulate matter or discoloration; solution should be slightly yellow and may contain a few small translucent or white particles; do not use if discolored, cloudy, or if foreign particulate matter is present; do not shake
• Use a 27-G, 0.5-inch needle
• May be administered SUBCUT into upper arm, abdomen, or thigh; rotate injection sites
• Use by SUBCUT injection only
• Those with latex hypersensitivity should not handle cap
SUBCUT injection:
• Patients may use the prefilled syringe or Sensoready pen after proper training; the lyophilized powder is for health care provider use only
• Each 300-mg dose is used as 2 SUBCUT injections of 150 mg
• Do not administer where skin is tender, bruised, erythematous, indurated, or affected by psoriasis
• **Reconstitution of lyophilized powder:** allow to warm to room temperature for 15-30 min, use 1 mL sterile water for injection to reconstitute, rotate, do not shake or invert vial, allow to stand for 10 min, again rotate vial, allow to stand for another 5 min (150 mg/mL)
• Storage: use immediately or refrigerate for up to 24 hr. Do not freeze. If refrigerated, allow reconstituted solution to reach room temperature (15-30 min) before administration
• **Preparation for use of prefilled syringe or Sensoready pen:** remove prefilled syringe or Sensoready pen from refrigerator and allow 15-30 min to reach room temperature
• Storage: the prefilled syringe or Sensoready should be used within 1 hr

SIDE EFFECTS
EENT: Ocular infections, sinusitis, oral ulceration, rhinitis
GI: Diarrhea
HEMA: Bleeding
INTEG: *Injection-site reaction*, urticaria
SYST: Serious infections, anaphylaxis, antibody formation, candidiasis
RESP: URI

PHARMACOKINETICS
Maximum serum concentration: 13.5 days after a single 45-mg SUBCUT dose, 7 days after a single 90-mg SUBCUT dose; half-life 14.9-45.6 days

INTERACTIONS
• Do not give concurrently with vaccines; immunizations should be brought up-to-date before treatment
• Avoid use with immunosuppressives
Drug/Lab tests
Increase: LFTs

NURSING CONSIDERATIONS
Assess:
• **TB:** TB testing should be done before starting treatment
• For injection-site pain, swelling
• Bring immunizations up-to-date before starting treatment
• **Infection:** monitor for fever, sore throat, cough; do not use during active infections
• **Malignancy:** skin cancer may occur, especially in older patients who have used ultraviolet treatments with immunosuppressants
• **Pregnancy/breastfeeding:** use only if benefits outweigh fetal risk; cautious use in breastfeeding, excretion unknown
Evaluate:
• **Therapeutic response:** decreased plaque psoriasis
Teach patient/family:
• That product must be continued for prescribed time to be effective; to use as prescribed
• Not to receive live vaccinations during treatment; that vaccinations should be brought up-to-date before use of this product

S

• To notify prescriber of possible infection (upper respiratory or other) or allergic reactions
• To report to provider the presence of inflammatory bowel disease, persistent diarrhea; product can cause inflammatory bowel disease
• To report latex allergy; prefilled injection device (Sensoready) may contain latex
• Not to use pen if fluid contains particulate; to use within 1 hr of removing from refrigerator
• Injection techniques and disposal of equipment; not to reuse needles, syringes; to rotate injection sites with each dose; not to inject into bruised or damaged skin

segesterone/ethinyl estradiol (Rx)

(se-jes′ter-one/eth′in-il es-tra-dye′ole)

Annovera

Func. class.: Contraceptive, estrogen/progestin combination

USES: To prevent pregnancy in females of reproductive potential

CONTRAINDICATIONS

Hypersensitivity to segesterone, ethinyl estradiol, or any component; breast cancer, estrogen/progestin-sensitive cancers, liver tumors, acute hepatitis, severe (decompensated) cirrhosis, undiagnosed abnormal uterine bleeding; use of ombitasvir/paritaprevir/ritonavir, with or without dasabuvir, high risk of arterial/venous thrombotic diseases, migraine headaches if >35 yr of age, hypertension (uncontrolled), subacute bacterial endocarditis, females >35 yr who smoke

Black Box Warning: Tobacco smoking

DOSAGE AND ROUTES
Contraception
• **Adult:** Females: Vaginal: Insert 1 ring vaginally, ring should remain in place for 21 days, then removed for 7 days.

One ring provides contraception for 13 cycles (1 yr)
Available forms: Vaginal ring 103 mg/17.4 mg

selegiline (Rx)

(se-le′ji-leen)

Eldepryl, Emsam, Zelapar

Func. class.: Antiparkinson agent, antidepressant

Chem. class.: MAOI, type B

Do not confuse:
selegiline/Salagen
Zelapar/ZyPREXA

ACTION: Increased dopaminergic activity by inhibition of MAO type B activity; not fully understood

USES: Adjunct management of Parkinson's disease for patients being treated with levodopa/carbidopa who had poor response to therapy; depression (transdermal)

CONTRAINDICATIONS
Children/adolescents (suicide/hypertensive crisis), hypersensitivity, breastfeeding, MAOIs

Black Box Warning: Suicidal ideation

Precautions: Pregnancy, abrupt discontinuation, alcoholism, ambient temperature increase, behavioral changes, bipolar disorders, driving or operating machinery, geriatrics, heating pad, hepatic disease, hypertension, hypotension, melanoma, phenylketonuria, psychosis, renal disease, sunlight exposure

DOSAGE AND ROUTES
• **Adult:** PO 5 mg bid given with levodopa/carbidopa in divided doses, after 2-3 days, begin to reduce dose of levodopa/carbidopa 10%-30%; **ORAL DISINTEGRATING** 1.25 mg (1 tab) × 6 wk or more initially, then 2.5 mg (2 tabs) dissolved on tongue daily before breakfast; max 2.5 mg/day

Major depression

Adult: TD 6 mg/24 hr daily, may increase by 3 mg/24 hr q2wK, up to 12 mg/24 hr if needed

Available forms: Tabs 5 mg; caps 5 mg; oral disintegrating tabs 1.25 mg; transdermal 6 mg/24 hr (20 mg/20 cm²), 9 mg/24 hr (30 mg/30 cm²), 12 mg/24 hr (40 mg/40 cm²)

Administer:

PO route

• Do not use in children due to risk for hypertensive crisis

• Product until NPO before surgery

• Adjust dosage to response

• With meals; limit protein taken with product

• Dosing bid in ᴀᴍ and afternoon; avoid ᴘᴍ or bedtime dosing

• At doses of <10 mg/day because of risks associated with nonselective inhibition of MAO

• **Oral disintegrating tab:** peel back foil; remove tab; do not push through foil; place tab on tongue; allow to dissolve; swallow with saliva; no fluids 5 min before or after use; avoid using >2.5 mg/day, hypertensive crisis is more common

Transdermal route (depression)

• Apply to dry intact skin on upper torso, upper thigh, or outer surface of upper arm q24hr

Black Box Warning: Do not use in children <12 yr

• When using 9 mg/24 hr or 12 mg/24 hr, specific manufacturer's recommendation for tyramine intake must be followed to prevent hypertensive crisis

SIDE EFFECTS

CNS: Increased tremors, tardive dyskinesia, dystonic symptoms, hallucinations, *dizziness,* mood changes, nightmares, delusions, serotonin syndrome, headache, migraine, confusion, anxiety, suicide in child/adolescent, suicidal ideation in adults

CV: Orthostatic hypotension, angina pectoris, hypertensive crisis (children)

EENT: Tinnitus

GI: Nausea, weight loss, vomiting, flatulence

GU: Slow urination, nocturia, prostatic hypertrophy, urinary hesitation, retention, frequency, sexual dysfunction

INTEG: Increased sweating, melanoma, acne, pruritus; site reactions (transdermal)

RESP: Asthma, SOB

PHARMACOKINETICS

PO peak ½-2 hr, orally disintegrating tab 10-15 min, TD 2 wk; rapidly metabolized (active metabolites: *N*-desmethyldeprenyl, amphetamine, methamphetamine); metabolites excreted in urine; half-life 10 hr, orally disintegrating tab 1.3 hr, transdermal 18-25 hr; protein binding up to 85%

INTERACTIONS

• **Fatal interaction:** opioids (especially meperidine); do not administer together

• **Serotonin syndrome (confusion, seizures, fever, hypertension, agitation; death):** FLUoxetine, PARoxetine, sertraline, fluvoxaMINE (discontinue 5 wk before selegiline treatment); do not use together

Increase: side effects of levodopa/carbidopa

Increase: unusual behavior, psychosis—dextromethorphan

Increase: hypotension—antihypertensives

Drug/Lab Test

Decrease: VMA

False positive: urine ketones, urine glucose

False negative: urine glucose (glucose oxidase)

False increase: uric acid, urine protein

NURSING CONSIDERATIONS

Assess:

• **Parkinson's symptoms:** decreased rigidity, unsteady gait, weakness, tremors

• Cardiac status: tachycardia/bradycardia; B/P, respiration throughout treatment

Black Box Warning: Depression: affect, mood, behavioral changes, depression; perform suicide assessment on all patients; suicidal ideation may occur

• **Opioids:** if patient has received, do not administer selegiline; fatal reactions have occurred

• **Orthostatic hypotension:** may occur during first few months of treatment, usually in patients >60 yr

Evaluate:

• **Therapeutic response:** decrease in akathisia, improved mood

Teach patient/family:

• To change positions slowly to prevent orthostatic hypotension

• **Hypertensive crisis:** to notify prescriber immediately of nausea, vomiting, sweating, agitation, change in mental status, headache, chest pain

• **Serotonin syndrome:** to report twitching, sweating, shivering, diarrhea to prescriber immediately

• To use product exactly as prescribed; that if discontinued abruptly, parkinsonian crisis may occur

• To use during the day to prevent insomnia

• To avoid heating pads, hot tubs when using transdermal products

• To avoid hazardous activities until response is known

• To avoid foods high in tyramine: cheese, pickled products, wine, beer, large amounts of caffeine as per manufacturer

Black Box Warning: Suicidal ideation: to report change in symptoms, worsening depression, or suicidal thoughts, behaviors; treatment may need to be changed

• Not to exceed recommended dose of 10 mg (PO) because this might precipitate hypertensive crisis; to report severe headache, other unusual symptoms

• **Pregnancy:** to report if pregnancy is planned or suspected; not to breastfeed

TREATMENT OF OVERDOSE: IV fluids for hypertension, IV dilute pressure agent for B/P titration

selenium topical
See Appendix B

---

selexipag (Rx)
(se-lex′-i-pag)
Uptravi
Func. class.: Vasodilator, prostacyclin

USES: Treatment of PAH (WHO Group I)

CONTRAINDICATIONS
Hypersensitivity, use with strong CYP2C8 inhibitors

DOSAGE AND ROUTES
PAH
• **Adult:** PO 200 mcg bid; increase by 200 mcg bid, usually at weekly intervals, max 1600 mcg bid

Available forms: Tabs ext rel 200, 400, 600, 800, 1000, 1200, 1400, 1600 mcg

---

⚠ HIGH ALERT

selinexor (Rx)
(sel-ih-nex′-or)
Xpovio
Func. class.: Antineoplastic
Chem class.: Small molecule antineoplastic nuclear export inhibitor

USES: Multiple myeloma in those who have received at least 4 prior therapies and who are refractory to at least 2 proteasome inhibitors, at least 2 immunomodulatory agents, and an anti-CD38 monoclonal antibody, in combination with dexamethasone

CONTRAINDICATIONS
Hypersensitivity, pregnancy, breastfeeding

DOSAGE AND ROUTES
• **Adult:** PO 80 mg in combination with dexamethasone 20 mg orally on days 1 and 3 of each week; repeat weekly until disease progression or unacceptable toxicity

---

Available forms: Tablets twice-weekly blister pack 40, 60, 80 mg; once-weekly blister pack 40, 60, 80, 100 mg

---

> **⚠ HIGH ALERT**

selpercatinib (Rx)

Retevmo
Func. class.: Antineoplastic

USES:
Metastatic RET fusion–positive non-small cell lung cancer (NSCLC), advanced or metastatic RET-mutant medullary thyroid cancer who require systemic therapy, or advanced or metastatic RET fusion-positive thyroid cancer who require systemic therapy and who are radioactive iodine-refractory

DOSAGE AND ROUTES
Non-small cell lung cancer/thyroid cancer:
• **Adult: <50 kg: PO** 120 mg bid until disease progression or unacceptable toxicity; **≥50 kg 160 mg** bid until disease progression or unacceptable toxicity
Available forms: Capsules 40, 80 mg

> **⚠ HIGH ALERT**

selumetinib (Rx)

(sel'ue-me'ti-nib)
Koselugo
Func. class.: Antineoplastic

USES: Treatment of neurofibromatosis type 1 in children ≥2 yr

CONTRAINDICATIONS
Hypersensitivity, pregnancy, breastfeeding

DOSAGE AND ROUTES
Child ≥2 yr: body surface area 0.55 m(2) or greater and able to swallow capsule whole: **PO** 25 mg/m(2) twice daily (approximately every 12 hours) until disease progression or unacceptable toxicity;

body surface area 1.9 m(2) or greater, give 50 mg twice daily
Available forms: Capsule 10, 25 mg

---

semaglutide (Rx)

Ozempic, Rybelsus, Wegovy
Func. class.: Antidiabetic

USES: For the treatment of type II diabetes, obesity

DOSAGE AND ROUTES

Black Box Warning: Thyroid-cell tumor, multiple endocrine neoplasm

Type 2 diabetes mellitus with diet and exercise
• **Adult: SUBCUT** 0.25 mg q wk X 4 wk, then 0.5 mg q wk, initially. May increase to 1 mg q wk after 4 wk on 0.5 mg/week and 2 mg q wk after 4 wk on 1 mg/wk if additional glycemic control is needed; **PO** 3 mg daily × 30 days, then 7 mg daily, may increase the dose to 14 mg daily after at least 30 days on 7 mg/day if additional glycemic control is needed
Obesity
Adult: SUBCUT 0.25 mg weekly × 4 wk, then 0.5 mg weekly × 4 wk, then 1 mg × 4 wk, 1.7 mg weekly × 4 wk, then 2.4 mg weekly onward
Available forms: Injection 2 mg/1.5 mL prefilled pen; tabs 3, 7, 14 mg

---

sertaconazole (Rx)

(ser-ta-KOE-na-zole)
Ertaczo
Func. class.: Antifungal, imidazole derivative

USES: Interdigital tinea pedis caused by Trichophyton rubrum, Trichophyton mentagrophytes, and Epidermophyton floccosum

CONTRAINDICATIONS
Hypersensitivity

DOSAGE AND ROUTES
Adult/child ≥12 yr
Topical: Apply to affected area(s) bid × 4 wk
Available forms: Topical cream 2%

---

sertraline (Rx)

(ser'tra-leen)

Zoloft

Func. class.: Antidepressant

Chem. class.: SSRI

Do not confuse:

sertraline/cetirizine

Zoloft/Zocor

ACTION: Inhibits serotonin reuptake in CNS; increases action of serotonin; does not affect dopamine, norepinephrine

USES: Major depressive disorder, obsessive-compulsive disorder (OCD), posttraumatic stress disorder (PTSD), panic disorder, social anxiety disorder, premenstrual dysphoric disorder (PMDD)

Unlabeled uses: Generalized anxiety disorder, premature ejaculation, pruritus (cholestatic liver disease), separation anxiety disorder

CONTRAINDICATIONS

Hypersensitivity to this product or SSRIs

Precautions: Pregnancy, breastfeeding, geriatric patients, renal/hepatic disease, epilepsy, recent MI, latex sensitivity (dropper of oral concentration)

Black Box Warning: Children, suicidal ideation

DOSAGE AND ROUTES

Major depression/OCD

• **Adult/geriatric patient/adolescent (unlabeled):** PO 25-50 mg/day; may increase to max of 200 mg/day; do not change dose at intervals of <1 wk; administer daily in AM or PM

• **Child 6-12 yr (unlabeled):** PO 25 mg/day, increase by 25-50 mg/wk, max 200 mg/day

PTSD/social anxiety disorder/panic disorder

• **Adult:** PO 25 mg/day, may increase by 50 mg/day after 7 days, range 50-200 mg

Premenstrual dysphoric disorder

• **Adult:** PO 50-150 mg nightly

Hepatic dose

• **Adult:** PO use lower dose or less frequent dosing intervals

Available forms: Tabs 25, 50, 100 mg; concentrate 20 mg/mL; capsules 25 ✦, 50 ✦, 100 mg ♣

Administer:

• Store at room temperature; do not freeze

• Increased fluids, bulk in diet for constipation, urinary retention

• With food, milk for GI symptoms

• Tablets crushed if patient is unable to swallow medication whole

• Sugarless gum, hard candy, frequent sips of water for dry mouth

• **Oral concentration:** dilute before use with 4 oz (½ cup) of water, orange juice, ginger ale, or lemon/lime soda; do not mix with other liquids

• Avoid use with other CNS depressants

• Dropper contains latex

SIDE EFFECTS

CNS: *Insomnia, agitation, dizziness, headache, fatigue,* confusion, gait abnormality (geriatric patients), neuroleptic malignant syndrome–like reaction, serotonin syndrome, suicidal ideation, anxiety, drowsiness

CV: Palpitations, chest pain

EENT: Vision abnormalities, yawning, tinnitus, intraocular pressure

ENDO: SIADH (geriatric patients); diabetes mellitus

GI: *Diarrhea, nausea, constipation, anorexia, dry mouth,* dyspepsia, *vomiting, flatulence,* weight gain/loss

GU: *Male sexual dysfunction,* menstrual disorders, urinary frequency

INTEG: Increased sweating, rash, hot flashes

MISC: Hyponatremia, neonatal abstinence syndrome

PHARMACOKINETICS

PO: Peak 4.5-8.4 hr; protein binding 98%; distribution to tissues, half-life 26 hr; extensively metabolized; metabolite excreted in urine, bile; weak inhibitor of CYP3A4, moderate inhibitor of CYP2D6

INTERACTIONS

• Altered lithium levels: lithium

• Disulfiram reaction: disulfiram and oral concentration due to alcohol content
• **Fatal reactions:** MAOIs, pimozide; avoid use within 2 wk

Increase: sertraline levels—cimetidine, warfarin, other highly protein-bound products

Increase: effects of antidepressants (tricyclics), diazepam, TOLBUTamide, warfarin, benzodiazepines, SUMAtriptan, phenytoin, cloZAPine

Increase: bleeding risk—anticoagulants, NSAIDs, thrombolytic, platelet inhibitors, salicylates

Increase: serotonin syndrome, neuroleptic malignant syndrome—SSRIs, SNRIs, serotonin-receptor agonists, tricyclics, cyclobenzaprine, sibutramine, traZODone, busPIRone, linezolid, traMADol; avoid concurrent use

Drug/Herb

Increase: SSRI, serotonin syndrome—St. John's wort, SAM-e, tryptophan; do not use together

Increase: CNS effect—kava, valerian

Drug/Lab Test

Increase: AST, ALT

False positive: urine screen for benzodiazepines

NURSING CONSIDERATIONS
Assess:

Black Box Warning: Depression/OCD/PTSD: mood, sensorium, affect, suicidal tendencies (child/young adult), increase in psychiatric symptoms, depression, panic attacks, OCD, PTSD, social anxiety disorder; symptoms usually occur in first few months of treatment

• **Premenstrual dysphoric disorder:** emotional lability, sad, hopelessness, insomnia, anxiety, food cravings, breast pain/tenderness
• **Serotonin syndrome** (hyperthermia, hypertension, rigidity, delirium, coma, myoclonus) or **neuroleptic malignant syndrome–like reaction** (muscle cramps, fever, unstable B/P, agitation, tremors, mental changes)
• **Bleeding (platelet serotonin depletion):** GI bleeding, ecchymoses, epistaxis, hematomas, petechiae, hemorrhage

• LFTs, thyroid function tests, growth rate, weight at baseline and periodically
• **Hypotension:** B/P (lying/standing), pulse q4hr; if systolic B/P drops 20 mm Hg, hold product, notify prescriber; VS q4hr in patients with CV disease
• Weight weekly; appetite may decrease with product
• Urinary retention, constipation, especially in geriatric patients
• Alcohol consumption; hold dose until morning
• **Beers:** avoid in older adults unless safer alternatives are unavailable; may cause ataxia, impaired psychomotor function
• **Pregnancy/breastfeeding:** use only if benefits outweigh fetal risk; serious complications may occur in neonates; cautious use in breastfeeding, excretion unknown

Evaluate:
• **Therapeutic response:** significant improvement in depression, OCD, PTSD, PMDD

Teach patient/family:
• That therapeutic effect may take ≥1 wk
• To use caution when driving, performing other activities requiring alertness because drowsiness, dizziness, blurred vision may occur
• Not to discontinue medication quickly after long-term use; may cause nausea, headache, malaise
• To avoid alcohol
• May be taken without regard to food
• That follow-up exams will be needed
• **Serotonin syndrome:** agitation, nausea, vomiting, diarrhea, twitching, sweating, shivering; report to prescriber immediately

Black Box Warning: Suicidal ideation: that suicidal thoughts/behaviors may occur in children/adolescents; to notify prescriber immediately if suicidal thoughts, panic attacks, severe anxiety occur

• To notify prescriber if pregnant or if planning to become pregnant, or if breastfeeding

---

Side effects: *italics* = common; red = life-threatening

S

sevelamer (Rx)

(se-vel'a-mer)

Renagel, Renvela

Func. class.: Phosphate binder

USES: Control of serum phosphorous in those with chronic kidney disease on hemodialysis

CONTRAINDICATIONS

Hypersensitivity to sevelamer or any component, bowel obstruction

DOSAGE AND ROUTES
Control of serum phosphorous
• **Adult: PO Those not taking a phosphate binder:** 800-1600 mg tid; if based on serum phosphorous levels: >5.5 mg/dL to <7.5 mg/dL: 800 mg tid; ≥7.5 mg/dL to <9 mg/dL: 1200-1600 mg tid; ≥9 mg/dL: 1600 mg tid
Maintenance dose adjustment based on serum phosphorous concentration:
>5.5 mg/dL: Increase by 400-800 mg per meal at 2-wk intervals; 3.5-5.5 mg/dL: Maintain current dose; <3.5 mg/dL: Decrease by 400-800 mg per meal
Dosage adjustment when switching between phosphate-binder products: 667 mg of calcium acetate is equivalent to 800 mg sevelamer
Conversion based on dose per meal: Calcium acetate 667 mg: Convert to 800 mg Renagel/Renvela; calcium acetate 1334 mg: Convert to 1600 mg as Renagel/Renvela (800-mg tablets × 2) or 1200 mg as Renagel (400-mg tablets × 3); calcium acetate 2001 mg: Convert to 2400 mg as Renagel/Renvela (800-mg tablets × 3) or 2000 mg as Renagel (400-mg tablets × 5)
Available forms: Tabs 400, 800 mg; oral suspension 0.8, 2.4 g packets

sildenafil (Rx)

(sil-den'a-fill)

LiQrev, Revatio, Viagra

Func. class.: Erectile agent, antihypertensive, pulmonary vasodilator
Chem. class.: Phosphodiesterase type-5 inhibitor

ACTION: Enhances the effect of nitric oxide (NO) by inhibiting phosphodiesterase type 5 (PDE5), which is necessary for degrading cGMP in the corpus cavernosum

USES: Treatment of erectile dysfunction; improvement in exercise ability, pulmonary hypertension
Unlabeled uses: Sexual dysfunction (women); altitude sickness, Raynaud's disease

CONTRAINDICATIONS

Hypersensitivity to this product or nitrates
Precautions: Pregnancy, anatomic penile deformities, sickle cell anemia, leukemia, multiple myeloma, retinitis pigmentosa, bleeding disorders, active peptic ulceration, CV/renal/hepatic disease, multiproduct antihypertensive regimens, geriatric patients

DOSAGE AND ROUTES
Erectile dysfunction (ED product only)
• **Adult male <65 yr: PO** 50 mg 1 hr before sexual activity; may be increased to 100 mg or decreased to 25 mg; max frequency 1×/day; use with alpha blockers: space 50-100-mg dose ≥4 hr of alpha blocker
• **Adult ≥65 yr (male): PO** 25 mg as needed about 1 hr before sexual activity
Renal/hepatic dose
• **Adult: PO** (Child-Pugh A, B) 25 mg, take 1 hr before sexual activity; max 1×/day; CCr <30 mL/min, 25 mg starting dose
Pulmonary hypertension (pulmonary hypertension product only)
• **Adult: PO** 20 mg tid; take 4-6 hr apart; **IV BOL** 10 mg tid
Pulmonary hypertension induced by altitude sickness (unlabeled)
• **Adult: PO** 50 mg 8 hr starting the day before accent and continuing for 5 days after reaching the target altitude or until descent is initiated

Available forms: ED: Tabs, 25, 50, 100 mg; pulomnary hypertension tabs 25 mg; sol for inj 10 mg/12.5 mL; powder for oral suspension 10 mg/mL

Administer:

• **Erectile dysfunction:** give approximately 1 hr before sexual activity; do not use more than 1×/day; give on empty stomach for better absorption

• **Pulmonary hypertension:** give 3×/day, 4-6 hr apart

IV Push Route

• Give undiluted, check that solution is not discolored or precipitate is present, give tid

SIDE EFFECTS

CNS: *Headache, flushing, dizziness,* transient global amnesia, seizures

CV: MI, sudden death, CV collapse, TIAs, ventricular dysrhythmias, CV hemorrhage

MISC: *Dyspepsia, nasal congestion, UTI, abnormal vision, diarrhea, rash,* nonarteritic ischemic optic neuropathy, hearing loss, priapism, sickle cell crisis

PHARMACOKINETICS

Rapidly absorbed; bioavailability 40%; metabolized by P45 CYP3A4, 2C9 in the liver (active metabolites); terminal half-life 4 hr; peak 15-30 min; reduced absorption with high-fat meal; excreted in feces, urine

INTERACTIONS

Do not use with nitrates, riociguat; fatal fall in B/P

Increase: sildenafil levels—cimetidine, erythromycin, ketoconazole, itraconazole, antiretroviral protease inhibitors, tacrolimus

Decrease: sildenafil levels—CYP450 inducers, rifampin, barbiturates, bosentan, carBAMazepine, dexamethasone, phenytoin, nevirapine, rifabutin, troglitazone; antacids

Decrease: B/P—α-blockers, alcohol, amLODIPine, angiotensin II receptor blockers

Drug/Food

Increase: product effect—grapefruit

Decrease: absorption—high-fat meal

NURSING CONSIDERATIONS

Assess:

• **For erectile dysfunction before use:** question about any failure to achieve erection or failure to maintain intercourse, anorgasmia

• **Phosphodiesterase type 5 inhibitors with lopinavir/ritonavir (Kaletra):** assess for hypotension, visual changes, prolonged erection, syncope; give only 25 mg q48hr and monitor for adverse reactions

• **Vision loss:** any severe loss of vision while taking this or any similar products; products should not be used

• Use of organic nitrates that should not be used with this product

• **MI, sudden death, CV collapse:** those with an MI within 6 mo, resting hypotension <90/50, resting hypertension >170/100, fluid depletion should use this product cautiously; may occur right after sexual activity to days afterward

• **Sickle cell crisis (vasoocclusive crisis):** when used for pulmonary hypertension; may require hospitalization

• **Pulmonary hypertension:** Cardiac status, hemodynamic parameters, exercise tolerance in pulmonary hypertension: B/P, pulse (Revatio)

Evaluate:

• **Therapeutic response:** decreasing pulmonary hypertension/improved exercise tolerance; ability to perform sexually (male)

Teach patient/family:

• That product does not protect against sexually transmitted diseases, including HIV

• That product absorption is reduced with a high-fat meal, to take on empty stomach for faster action; to take 30 min to 4 hr before sexual activity; peak is 2 hr

• That product should not be used with nitrates or soluble guanylate cyclase stimulators (riociguat) (PAH)

• That tabs may be split

• To notify prescriber immediately and to stop taking product if vision/hearing loss occurs or erection lasts >4 hr

S

Side effects: *italics* = common; red = life-threatening

- Do not use more than 100 mg in 24 hr
- To use only as directed
- That color vision may be altered
- **About cardiac risk:** usually in cardiac disease
- **Pregnancy/breastfeeding:** not indicated for women (ED Product), unknown in PAH, cautious use in breastfeeding

---

silodosin (Rx)
(si-lo′do-seen)

Rapaflo

Func. class.: Selective α_1-adrenergic blocker, BPH agent

Chem. class.: Sulfamoylphenethyl-amine derivative

ACTION: Binds preferentially to α_{1A}-adrenoceptor subtype located mainly in the prostate

USES: Symptoms of benign prostatic hyperplasia (BPH)

CONTRAINDICATIONS
Hypersensitivity, renal failure, hepatic disease
Precautions: Pregnancy, breastfeeding, children, females, geriatric patients, renal/hepatic disease, hypotension, ocular surgery, orthostatic hypotension, prostate cancer, syncope

DOSAGE AND ROUTES
BPH Adult: PO 8 mg daily with a meal
Renal dose
- **Adult: PO** CCr 30-49 mL/min, 4 mg/day; CCr <30 mL/min, not recommended
Available forms: Cap 4, 8 mg
Administer:
- Give with meal at same time each day
- Cap may be opened and sprinkled on applesauce, if unable to swallow, use water after applesauce
- Store at room temperature; protect from light and moisture

SIDE EFFECTS
CNS: *Dizziness, headache,* insomnia, syncope

CV: Orthostatic hypotension
EENT: Nasal congestion
GI: Diarrhea
GU: *Abnormal ejaculation,* urinary incontinence, priapism
INTEG: Rash, pruritus, allergic reactions

PHARMACOKINETICS
Decreased absorption with high-fat/high-calorie meal, half-life 13.3 hr of metabolite 24 hr, metabolized in liver extensively by CYP3A4, UGT2B7, excreted via urine, feces (55%) extensively protein bound (97%), onset rapid, peak up to 24 hr, duration up to 24 hr

INTERACTIONS
Increase: silodosin effect—CYP3A4 inhibitors (clarithromycin, itraconazole, ritonavir, antiretroviral protease inhibitors, aprepitant, chloramphenicol, conivaptan, dalfopristin, danazol, delavirdine, efavirenz, fosaprepitant, fluconazole, fluvoxaMINE, imatinib, isoniazid, miFEPRIStone, nefazodone, tamoxifen, telithromycin, troleandomycin, voriconazole, zileuton, zafirlukast); P-gb inhibitors
Drug/Food
Increase: silodosin effect—grapefruit juice
Drug Lab/Test
Increase: LFTs

NURSING CONSIDERATIONS
Assess:
- **Prostatic hyperplasia:** change in urinary patterns at baseline and throughout treatment; testing for prostate cancer before administration is recommended
- BUN, uric acid, urodynamic studies (urinary flow rates, residual volume), CCr; contraindicated in CCr <30 mL/min; I&O ratios, weight daily, edema, report weight gain or edema
- B/P (sitting, standing) during initial treatment; monitor for orthostatic hypotension; increased risk in elderly >65 yr

• **Pregnancy/breastfeeding:** not indicated for women

Evaluate:

• **Therapeutic response:** decreased symptoms of BPH

Teach patient/family

• Not to drive or operate machinery until effect is known; orthostatic hypotension occasionally occurs after first dose

• Not to use with grapefruit juice

• To take with same meal each day; contents of capsule may be sprinkled on room-temperature applesauce if consumed within 5 min; follow with 8 oz cool water

---

⚠ HIGH ALERT

siltuximab (Rx)
(sil-tux´-i-mab)

Sylvant

Func. class.: Antineoplastic: immune response modifier

USES: Multicentric Castleman disease (MCD) patients who are HIV-negative and human herpesvirus-8 (HHV-8)–negative

CONTRAINDICATIONS
Hypersensitivity

DOSAGE AND ROUTES

• **Adult:** **IV** 11 mg/kg over 1 hr q3wk until treatment failure

Available forms: Lyophilized powder for IV use: 100, 400 mg in single-dose vial

silver nitrate 1% ophthalmic
See Appendix B

silver nitrate 1% sulfacetamide sodium ophthalmic
See Appendix B

silver sulfADIAZINE topical
See Appendix B

simethicone (OTC, Rx)
(si-meth´i-kone)

Barriere ✿, Gas Relief ✿, Gas-Relief, Gas Relief Extra Strength, Gas Relief Infants, Gas Relief Ultra Strength, Gas Relief, Gas-X Childrens, Gas-X Extra Strength, Gas-X Infant Drops, Gas-X Ultra Strength, Infants Gas Relief, Mi-Acid Gas Relief, Ovol ✿, Phazyme

Func. class.: Antiflatulent

USES: Flatulence
Unlabeled uses: Dyspepsia

CONTRAINDICATIONS
Hypersensitivity, GI obstruction/perforation

DOSAGE AND ROUTES

• **Adult and child >12 yr:** **PO** 40-125 mg after meals and at bedtime prn, max 500 mg/day, 750 mg/day chewable

• **Child 2-12 yr:** **PO** 40-50 mg after meals and at bedtime prn, max 480 mg/day

• **Child <2 yr:** **PO** 20 mg qid prn, max 480 mg/day

simvastatin (Rx)
(sim-va-sta´tin)

FloLipid, Zocor

Func. class.: Antilipemic

Chem. class.: HMG-CoA reductase inhibitor

Do not confuse:
Zocor/Cozaar/Zoloft

ACTION: Inhibits HMG-CoA reductase enzyme, which reduces cholesterol synthesis

Side effects: *italics* = common; red = life-threatening

USES: As an adjunct for primary hypercholesterolemia (types IIa, IIb), isolated hypertriglyceridemia (Fredrickson type IV), and type III hyperlipoproteinemia, CAD, heterozygous familial hypercholesterolemia; MI/stroke prophylaxis

CONTRAINDICATIONS

Pregnancy, breastfeeding, hypersensitivity, active hepatic disease

Precautions: Past hepatic disease, alcoholism, severe acute infections, trauma, severe metabolic disorders, electrolyte imbalances, Chinese patients

DOSAGE AND ROUTES
Hyperlipidemia
Adult: PO 10-20 mg daily in the evening (range 5-40 mg)
Atherosclerosis (unlabeled)
• **Adult: PO** 20-40 mg/day in PM initially; usual range 5-40 mg/day in PM, max 40 mg/day for most patients, max 80 mg/day for patients taking 80 mg/day chronically without myopathy; dosage adjustments may be made in ≥4-wk intervals; those taking verapamil and amiodarone max 20 mg/day; max <80 mg for Chinese patients taking lipid-modifying niacin doses
Heterozygous familial hypercholesterolemia
• **Child/adolescent ≥10 yr including girls ≥1 yr postmenarche: PO** 10 mg in PM, range 10-40 mg/day
Renal dose
• **Adult: PO** 5 mg/day in the evening (severe renal disease)
Available forms: Tabs 5, 10, 20, 40, 80 mg
Administer:
• Discontinuing use before surgery is recommended in renal failure; restart afterward
• Avoid grapefruit juice
• Total daily dose in evening
• Store in cool environment in tight container protected from light

SIDE EFFECTS
CNS: Headache, cognitive impairment

GI: Nausea, constipation, diarrhea, dyspepsia, flatus, abdominal pain, liver dysfunction, pancreatitis, hyperglycemia
INTEG: Rash, pruritus
MS: Muscle cramps, myalgia, myositis, rhabdomyolysis, myopathy
RESP: Upper respiratory tract infection

PHARMACOKINETICS

Metabolized in liver (active metabolites); >98% protein bound; excreted primarily in bile, feces (60%), kidneys (15%); peak 1-2 hr; half-life 3 hr

INTERACTIONS
• Do not use with cycloSPORINE, gemfibrozil
Increase: effects of warfarin
Increase: rhabdomyolysis, myalgia; do not use concurrently—CYP3A4 inhibitors, niacin, erythromycin, clofibrate, clarithromycin, ketoconazole, itraconazole, protease inhibitors, macrolide antibiotics, danazol, delavirdine, nefazodone, verapamil, diltiaZEM, amiodarone, azole antifungals, telithromycin, voriconazole
Increase: simvastatin effect—ATP1B1 inhibitors
Increase: serum level of digoxin
Drug/Herb
Increase: effect—red yeast rice, kava, eucalyptus
Decrease: effect—St. John's wort
Drug/Food
Increase: simvastatin level—grapefruit juice (large amounts)
Drug/Lab Test
Increase: CK, LFTs, HbA1c

NURSING CONSIDERATIONS
Assess:
• **Diet history:** fat consumption; baseline and lipid profile: LDL, HDL, TG, cholesterol
• Hepatic studies at baseline, if clinically indicated; AST, ALT may increase
• **Rhabdomyolysis:** muscle tenderness, increased CPK levels (10 × ULN); therapy should be discontinued, more likely in those receiving >80 mg/day, first year of treatment, those ≥65 yr, females

---

sirolimus **1187**

• **Chinese patients:** avoid high doses (80 mg) if taking niacin >1 g/day due to increased risk of myopathies
• Renal studies in patients with compromised renal systems: BUN, I&O ratio, creatinine
• **Pregnancy/breastfeeding:** do not use in pregnancy, breastfeeding
Evaluate:
• **Therapeutic response:** decrease in LDL, total cholesterol, triglycerides; increase in HDL; slowing CAD
Teach patient/family:
• That blood work, follow-up exams will be necessary during treatment
• To report severe GI symptoms, headache
• That previously prescribed regimen will continue: low-cholesterol diet, exercise program, smoking cessation
• To take in evening, avoid using grapefruit juice
• To report muscle pain, weakness, abdominal pain, dark urine; yellowing of skin, eyes; memory loss
• This product may affect blood sugar levels in diabetes
• That compliance is needed for positive results, not to skip or double doses
• To notify prescriber if pregnancy is suspected or planned; not to breastfeed

---

siponimod (Rx)
Mayzent
Func. class.: MS agent

USES: MS

DOSAGE AND ROUTES
MS with CYP2C9 genotypes *1/*1, *1/*2, *2/*2
• **Adult: PO** Use the 5-day titration schedule: 0.25 mg on day 1, 0.25 mg on day 2, 0.5 mg on day 3, 0.75 mg on day 4, and 1.25 mg on day 5; begin maintenance dosage of 2 mg daily on day 6

Available forms: Tablet 0.25, 1, 2 mg; starter packs 0.25 mg (for 1-mg maintenance), 0.25 (for 2-mg maintenance)

⚠ HIGH ALERT

sirolimus (Rx)
(seer-oh-lie'mus)
Fyarro, Rapamune
Func. class.: Immunosuppressant
Chem. class.: Macrolide

ACTION: Produces immunosuppression by inhibiting T-lymphocyte activation and proliferation

USES: Organ transplants to prevent rejection; recommended use is with cycloSPORINE and corticosteroids

CONTRAINDICATIONS
Breastfeeding, hypersensitivity to this product, components of product
Precautions: Pregnancy, children <13 yr, severe cardiac/renal/hepatic disease; diabetes mellitus, hyperkalemia, hyperuricemia, hypertension, interstitial lung disease, hyperlipidemia, soya lecithin hypersensitivity

Black Box Warning: Lymphomas, infection, other malignancies, liver transplant, lung transplant; requires a specialized setting; requires an experienced clinician

DOSAGE AND ROUTES
Kidney transplant
• **Adult/adolescent ≥40 kg: PO** 2 mg/day with 6-mg loading dose; **IV infusion** 100 mg/m² over 30 min on days 1 and 8 of each 21-day cycle until disease progression or unacceptable toxicity
• **Child <13 yr weighing <40 kg (88 lb): PO** 1 mg/m²/day, 3 mg/m² loading dose
Hepatic dose
• **Adult/child ≥13 yr/<40 kg: PO** reduce by 33% for maintenance dose (mild to moderate hepatic impairment); reduce

---

Side effects: *italics* = common; red = life-threatening

by 50% for maintenance dose (severe hepatic impairment)

Lymphangioleimyotosis

Adult: PO 2 mg daily trough level (whole blood) after 10-20 days, titrate to 5-15 ng/mL, then monitor trough q3mo

Available forms: Oral sol 1 mg/mL; tabs 0.5 mg, 1 mg, 2 mg; lyophilized powder for injectable suspension 100 mg

Administer:

• Prophylaxis for *Pneumocystis jiroveci* pneumonia for 1 yr after transplantation; prophylaxis for CMV is recommended for 90 days after transplantation in those at increased risk for CMV

• All medications PO if possible; avoid IM inj; bleeding may occur

• For 3 days before transplant surgery; place in protective isolation; give at same time of day; give 4 hr after cycloSPORINE oral sol or caps; do not give with grapefruit juice

• Use amber oral syringe and withdraw amount needed; empty dose into plastic/glass container holding 60 mL of water/orange juice; stir vigorously and have patient drink at once; refill container with additional 120-mL water/orange juice; stir, have patient drink; if using a pouch, squeeze entire contents into container; follow above directions

• Store protected from light, refrigerate; stable for 30 days after opening (sol)

• Do not crush, chew; store tabs at room temperature

Black Box Warning: Only those experienced in immunosuppressant therapy and transplant should use this drug; must use in a specialized care setting with adequate medical equipment

SIDE EFFECTS

CNS: *Tremors, headache, insomnia, paresthesia,* chills, fever, progressive multifocal leukoencephalopathy (PML)

CV: Hypertension, *atrial fibrillation, HF, hypotension, palpitation, tachycardia,* peripheral edema, thrombosis

EENT: Blurred vision, photophobia

GI: Nausea, vomiting, diarrhea, constipation, hepatotoxicity, CDAD

GU: UTIs, albuminuria, hematuria, proteinuria, renal failure, nephrotic syndrome, increased creatinine, amenorrhea

HEMA: Anemia, leukopenia, thrombocytopenia

INTEG: *Rash, acne,* photosensitivity, exfoliative dermatitis

META: Hyperglycemia, increased creatinine, edema, hypercholesterolemia, *hyperlipemia,* hypophosphatemia, weight gain, hypo/hyperkalemia, hyperuricemia, hypomagnesemia, hypertriglyceridemia

MS: Arthralgia

RESP: Pleural effusion, atelectasis, *dyspnea,* pneumonitis, pulmonary embolism/fibrosis, pulmonary hypertension, interstitial lung disease

SYST: Lymphoma

PHARMACOKINETICS

Rapidly absorbed; peak 1 hr single dose, 2 hr multiple dosing; protein binding 92%; distribution to major organs, extensively metabolized by CYP3A4 excretion 91% feces, half-life 57-63 hr

INTERACTIONS

• **Increase:** Sirolimus metabolism strong CYP3A4 or P-gp inducers, avoid use

Increase: angioedema—ACE inhibitors, angiotensin II–receptor antagonists, cephalosporins, iodine-containing radiopaque contrast media, neuromuscular blockers, NSAIDs, penicillins, salicylates, thrombolytics

Increase: blood levels—antifungals, calcium channel blockers, cimetidine, danazol, erythromycin, cycloSPORINE, metoclopramide, bromocriptine, HIV-protease inhibitors

Decrease: Sirolimus metabolism causing toxicity, CYP3A4 inhibitors, avoid use

Decrease: blood levels—carBAMazepine, PHENobarbital, phenytoin, rifamycin, rifapentine

Decrease: effect of vaccines

Drug/Herb

• St. John's wort: may **decrease** the effect of sirolimus

Drug/Food

• Alters bioavailability; use consistently with/without food; do not use with grapefruit juice

Drug/Lab Test

Increase: LFTs, alk phos, lipids, triglycerides, total cholesterol, BUN, creatinine, LDH, phosphate

Decrease: platelets, sodium

Increase or decrease: magnesium, glucose, calcium

NURSING CONSIDERATIONS
Assess:

• High risk: those with Banff grade 3 acute rejection or vascular rejection before cycloSPORINE withdrawal, dialysis dependent, creatinine >4.5 mg/dL, African descent, retransplants, multiorgan transplant, high panel of reactive antibodies

• **Blood levels** in patients who may have altered metabolism, trough level ≥15 ng/mL is associated with increased adverse reactions; monitor trough concentrations in all patients

• **Renal status:** monitor fluid imbalance, edema, electrolytes, creatinine/BUN, CBC, serum potassium

• **Lipid profile:** cholesterol, triglycerides; lipid-lowering agent may be needed

Black Box Warning: Infection: immunosuppression may lead to susceptibility to infection, assess for infection

Black Box Warning: Neoplastic disease: lymphoma, skin cancer may occur; limit UV exposure; use protective clothing, sunscreen

Black Box Warning: Liver/lung transplant: not recommended; mortality and graft loss may occur

• **Pulmonary fibrosis, pulmonary effusion, pneumonitis:** dyspnea, cough, hypoxia; some fatal cases have occurred

• **Wound dehiscence and anastomotic disruption:** wound, vascular, airway, ureteral, biliary, inhibition of growth factors; do not combine with corticosteroids, not recommended in lung or liver transplant

• **Anaphylaxis, angioedema, exfoliative dermatitis:** more common when given with ACE inhibitors; do not use if a hypersensitivity reaction occurs

• **Bone marrow suppression:** HB, WBC, platelets during treatment each month; if leukocytes <3000/mm³ or platelets <100,000/mm³, product should be discontinued or reduced; decreased hemoglobin level

• **Hepatotoxicity:** alk phos, AST, ALT, amylase, bilirubin, dark urine, jaundice, itching, light-colored stools; product should be discontinued

• **Pregnancy/breastfeeding:** avoid use in pregnancy; obtain pregnancy test at baseline; use effective form of contraception, continue for 12 wk after discontinuing; notify prescriber if pregnancy occurs; unknown breastfeeding effects; weigh benefits, risks with prescriber

Evaluate:

• **Therapeutic response:** absence of graft rejection; immunosuppression with autoimmune disorders

Teach patient/family:

• To report fever, rash, severe diarrhea, chills, sore throat, fatigue; serious infections may occur; clay-colored stools, cramping (hepatotoxicity); fever, chills, sore throat (infection)

• To avoid crowds, persons with known infections to reduce risk for infection

• To use sunscreen, protective clothing to prevent burns, skin cancer

• Not to use with grapefruit juice

• To avoid live virus vaccines during treatment

• That lifelong use will be required to prevent rejection

• That continuing follow-up exams and blood work will be required

• To take with or without regard to food, at same time, consistently

• Take 4 hr after oral cycloSPORINE when used for renal transplant

• **Pregnancy/breastfeeding:** to use contraception before, during, for 12 wk after product discontinued; to avoid breastfeeding

⚠ HIGH ALERT

sitaGLIPtin (Rx)
(sit-a-glip′tin)

Januvia
Func. class.: Antidiabetic, oral
Chem. class.: Dipeptidyl-peptidase-4
inhibitor (DPP-4 inhibitor)

Do not confuse:
Januvia/Enjuvia/Jantoven/Janumet

ACTION: Slows the inactivation of
incretin hormones; improves glucose
homeostasis, improves glucose-dependent
insulin secretion, lowers glucagon secretions, and slows gastric emptying time

USES: Type 2 diabetes mellitus as
monotherapy or in combination with
other antidiabetic agents

CONTRAINDICATIONS

Angioedema, diabetic ketoacidosis (DKA)
Precautions: Pregnancy, geriatric
patients, GI obstruction, surgery, thyroid/
renal/hepatic disease, trauma, breastfeeding, pancreatitis, hypercortisolism,
hyperglycemia, hyperthyroidism, hypoglycemia, ileus, pituitary insufficiency,
surgery, type 1 diabetes mellitus, diabetic
ketoacidosis, adrenal insufficiency, burns

DOSAGE AND ROUTES

• **Adult: PO** 100 mg/day; lower dose
may be needed when used with a sulfo-
nylurea or insulin
Renal dose
• **Adult: PO** CCr 30-50 mL/min, 50 mg
daily; CCr <30 mL/min, 25 mg daily
Available forms: Tabs 25, 50, 100 mg
Administer:
• May be taken with/without food
• Do not split, crush, chew; swallow whole
• Conversion from other antidiabetic
agents: change may be made with grad-
ual dosage change
• Store in tight container at room tem-
perature

SIDE EFFECTS

CNS: *Headache*
ENDO: Hypoglycemia

GI: *Nausea, vomiting,* abdominal pain,
diarrhea, pancreatitis, constipation
GU: Acute renal failure, UTI
MISC: *Peripheral edema, upper respiratory infection*
SYST: Anaphylaxis, Stevens-Johnson syndrome, angioedema

PHARMACOKINETICS

Rapidly absorbed, excreted by the kidneys (unchanged 79%), half-life 12.4
hr, peak 1-4 hr, duration up to 24 hr

INTERACTIONS

Increase: levels of digoxin (minimal)
Increase: hypoglycemia—antidiabetics,
chloroquine, hydroxychloroquine,
androgens, beta-blockers, salicylates,
MAOIs
Increase: sitagliptin level—cimetidine,
disopyramide
Decrease: antidiabetic action thiazides,
ACE inhibitors, protease inhibitors,
estrogens, progestins, hormonal contra-
ceptives, sympathomimetics
Drug/Herb
Increase: antidiabetic effect—garlic,
green tea, horse chestnut
Drug/Lab Test
Increase: creatinine, LFTs

NURSING CONSIDERATIONS
Assess:
• **Hypoglycemic reactions:** sweating,
weakness, dizziness, anxiety, tremors, hunger; hyperglycemic reactions soon after
meals
• **Serious skin reactions:** swelling of
face, mouth, lips; dyspnea; wheezing
• **Pancreatitis:** severe abdominal pain,
nausea, vomiting; discontinue product,
monitor amylase, lipase
• **Renal studies:** BUN, creatinine during
treatment, especially in geriatric patients
or those with renal disease
• Glycosylated hemoglobin A1c; monitor
blood glucose (BG) as needed
Evaluate:
• **Therapeutic response:** decrease in
polyuria, polydipsia, polyphagia; clear
sensorium; absence of dizziness; stable
gait, blood glucose, A1c improvement

Teach patient/family:
• To perform regular self-monitoring of blood glucose using blood-glucose meter
• About the symptoms of hypo/hyperglycemia; what to do about each; to carry emergency ID
• To report severe joint pain immediately; may have a late onset
• That product must be continued on daily basis; about consequences of discontinuing product abruptly; to continue health regimen (diet, exercise)
• To avoid OTC medications, alcohol, digoxin, exenatide, insulins, nateglinide, repaglinide, and other products that lower blood glucose unless approved by prescriber
• That diabetes is a lifelong illness; that product is not a cure, only controls symptoms
• That all food included in diet plan must be eaten to prevent hypo/hyperglycemia
• To immediately notify prescriber of hypersensitivity reactions (rash, swelling of face, trouble breathing)
• To notify prescriber if pregnancy is planned, suspected

sitagliptin/metformin (Rx)

(sit-a-glip′tin/met-for′-min)

Janumet, Janumet XR

Func. class.: Antidiabetic

USES: Adjunct to diet and exercise to improve glycemic control in type 2 diabetes mellitus

CONTRAINDICATIONS

Hypersensitivity to sitagliptin, metformin, or any component, eGFR <30 mL/min/1.73 m^2); acute/chronic metabolic acidosis, diabetic ketoacidosis

Black Box Warning: Lactic acidosis

DOSAGE AND ROUTES
Diabetes mellitus, type 2, treatment
Total daily dose should be taken divided bid (immediate release) or daily (extended release)
• **Adult:** PO patients already on metformin: Sitagliptin 100 mg/day plus current daily dose of metformin. Patients currently on metformin 1.7 g/day (850 mg bid) may use sitagliptin 100 mg/metformin 2 g daily; **those not on metformin:** Sitagliptin 100 mg/metformin 1 g daily
Available forms: Tabs 50/500, 50/1000 mg; tabs ext rel 50/500, 50/1000, 100/1000 mg

sodium bicarbonate (Rx, OTC)

Baking soda, Alka-Seltzer ✦, Accusol ✦, Bibag ✦, Bicort ✦

Func. class.: Alkalinizer
Chem. class.: NaHCO$_3$

ACTION: Orally neutralizes gastric acid, which forms water, NaCl, CO$_2$; increases plasma bicarbonate, which buffers H$^+$ ion concentration; reverses acidosis IV

USES: Acidosis (metabolic), cardiac arrest, alkalinization (systemic/urinary), antacid, salicylate poisoning

CONTRAINDICATIONS
Metabolic/respiratory alkalosis, hypochloremia, hypocalcemia
Precautions: Pregnancy, children, HF, cirrhosis, toxemia, renal disease, hypertension, hypokalemia, breastfeeding, hypernatremia, Bartter's syndrome, Cushing syndrome, hyperaldosteronism

DOSAGE AND ROUTES
Conversions: 84 mg = 1 mmol (1 mEq) = 1 mmol (1 mEq) each of sodium and bicarbonate 10 ions
Acidosis, metabolic (not associated with cardiac arrest)
• **Adult/child:** IV INFUSION 2-5 mEq/kg over 4-8 hr depending on CO$_2$, pH, ABGs

S

Metabolic acidosis in chronic renal failure

Adults: PO 0.5-1 mEq/kg/day (42-84 mg/kg/day) in 2-3 divided doses or 650 or 1300 mg twice daily for a serum bicarbonate concentration of 19-21 mEq/L or 18 mEq/L or less, respectively. Titrate dose up to 1950 mg 3 times daily to target serum bicarbonate concentration (22 mEq/L or more)

Infants, children, and adolescents: PO 1-2 mEq/kg/day (84-168 mg/kg/day) in 2-3 divided doses. Titrate dose to target serum bicarbonate concentration

Cardiac arrest

• **Adult/child:** IV BOL 1 mEq/kg of 7.5% or 8.4% sol, then 0.5 mEq/kg q10min, then doses based on ABGs

• **Infant:** IV 1 mEq/kg over several min (use only the 0.5 mEq/mL [4.2%] sol for inj)

Alkalinization of urine

• **Adult:** PO 325 mg to 2 g qid or 48 mEq (4 g), then 12-24 mEq q4hr

• **Child:** PO 84-840 mg/kg/day (1-10 mEq/kg) in divided doses q4-6hr

Antacid

• **Adult:** PO 300 mg to 2 g chewed, taken with water daily-qid

Available forms: Tabs 300, 325, 600, 650 mg; inj 4.2%, 5%, 7.5%, 8.4%

Administer:

PO route

• Chew antacid tablets and drink 8 oz water

• Do not take antacid with milk because milk-alkali syndrome may result

Direct IV route

• Use for cardiac emergencies, not used often in cardiac arrest

• Use ampules or prefilled syringes only; give by rapid bolus dose; flush with NS before, after use

Continuous IV INFUSION route

• Diluted in an equal amount of compatible sol given 2-5 mEq/kg over 4-8 hr, max 50 mEq/hr; slower rate in children

• Extravasation with IV administration (tissue sloughing, ulceration, necrosis)

Y-site compatibilities: Acyclovir, amifostine, asparaginase, aztreonam, bivalirudin, bumetanide, ceFAZolin, cefepime, cefTAZidime, ceftizoxime, cefTRIAXone, chloramphenicol, cimetidine, cladribine, clindamycin, cyclophosphamide, cycloSPORINE, cytarabine, DAPTOmycin, DAUNOrubicin, dexamethasone sodium phosphate, dexmedetomidine, digoxin, DOCEtaxel, DOXOrubicin, enalaprilat, ertapenem, erythromycin, esmolol, etoposide, etoposide phosphate, famotidine, fentaNYL, filgrastim, fluconazole, fludarabine, furosemide, gallium nitrate, gemcitabine, gentamicin, granisetron, heparin, hydrocortisone sodium succinate, ifosfamide, indomethacin, insulin, ketorolac, labetalol, levoFLOXacin, lidocaine, linezolid, LORazepam, magnesium sulfate, melphalan, mesna, meperidine, methylPREDNISolone sodium succinate, metoclopramide, metoprolol, metroNIDAZOLE, milrinone, morphine, nafcillin, nitroglycerin, nitroprusside, PACLitaxel, palonosetron, pantoprazole, PEMEtrexed, penicillin G potassium, phenylephrine, phytonadione, piperacillin/tazobactam, potassium chloride, procainamide, propranolol, propofol, protamine, raNITIdine, remifentanil, tacrolimus, teniposide, thiotepa, ticarcillin/clavulanate, tirofiban, tobramycin, tolazoline, vasopressin, vit B complex with C, voriconazole

SIDE EFFECTS

CNS: Irritability, headache, confusion, stimulation, tremors, *twitching, hyperreflexia,* tetany, weakness, seizures of alkalosis

CV: Irregular pulse, cardiac arrest, water retention, edema, weight gain

GI: Flatulence, *belching, distention*

META: *Metabolic alkalosis*

MS: Muscular twitching, tetany, irritability

PHARMACOKINETICS

PO: Onset rapid, duration 10 min

IV: Onset 15 min, duration 1-2 hr, excreted in urine

INTERACTIONS

Increase: effects—amphetamines, mecamylamine, quiNINE, quiNIDine, pseudoephedrine, flecainide, anorexiants, sympathomimetics

Increase: sodium and decrease potassium—corticosteroids

Decrease: effects—lithium, chlorproPAMIDE, barbiturates, salicylates, benzodiazepines, ketoconazole, corticosteroids

Drug/Lab Test
Increase: sodium, lactate
Decrease: potassium

NURSING CONSIDERATIONS
Assess:
• Respiratory and pulse rate, rhythm, depth, lung sounds; notify prescriber of abnormalities
• **Fluid balance** (I&O, weight daily, edema); notify prescriber of fluid overload; assess for edema, crackles, shortness of breath
• Electrolytes, blood pH, PO_2, HCO_3^- during treatment; ABGs frequently during emergencies
• Weight daily with initial therapy
• **Alkalosis:** irritability, confusion, twitching, hyperreflexia stimulation, slow respirations, cyanosis, irregular pulse
• **Milk-alkali syndrome:** confusion, headache, nausea, vomiting, anorexia, urinary stones, hypercalcemia
• For GI perforation secondary to carbon dioxide in GI tract; may lead to perforation if ulcer is severe enough
• **Pregnancy/breastfeeding:** use as an antacid is considered unsafe; may breastfeed
Evaluate:
• **Therapeutic response:** ABGs, electrolytes, blood pH, HCO_3^- WNL
Teach patient/family:
• Not to take antacid with milk because milk-alkali syndrome may result; not to use antacid for >2 wk
• To notify prescriber if indigestion accompanied by chest pain; trouble breathing; diarrhea; dark, tarry stools; vomit that looks like coffee grounds; swelling of feet/ankles
• About sodium-restricted diet; to avoid use of baking soda for indigestion

---

sodium phenylbutyrate/ taurursodiol (Rx)

(SOE-dee-um FEN-il-BUE-ti-rate/ taur-UR-so-DYE-ol)

Relyvrio
Func. class.: Neuroprotective agent

USES: Amyotrophic lateral sclerosis (ALS)

DOSAGE AND ROUTES
Adults: PO 3 g sodium phenylbutyrate and 1 g taurursodiol (1 packet) once daily for the first 3 wk, then increase the dose to 3 g sodium phenylbutyrate and 1 g taurursodiol (1 packet) twice daily
Available forms: Powder for suspension 3 g/1 g

---

sodium polystyrene sulfonate (Rx)

(po-lee-stye′reen)

Kalexate ✦, Solystat ✦, Kionex, SPS
Func. class.: Potassium-removing resin, antidote
Chem. class.: Cation exchange resin

ACTION: Removes potassium by exchanging sodium for potassium in body, primarily in large intestine

USES: Hyperkalemia in conjunction with other measures

CONTRAINDICATIONS
Hypersensitivity to saccharin or parabens that may be in some products, GI obstruction, neonate (reduced gut motility)
Precautions: Pregnancy, geriatric patients, renal failure, HF, severe edema, severe hypertension, sodium restriction, constipation, GI bleeding, hypocalcemia

DOSAGE AND ROUTES
• **Adult: PO** 15 g daily-qid; **RECT** enema 30-50 g q1-2hr initially prn, then q6hr prn
• **Child (unlabeled): PO** 1 g/kg q6hr prn; **RECT** 1 g/kg q2-6hr prn
Available forms: Powder for susp 453.6 g, 454 g; oral susp 15 g/60 mL
Administer:
PO route
• **Powdered resin:** given as a suspension in water or syrup; the amount of fluid ranges from 20 to 100 mL, depending on the dosage, or 3-4 mL/g of resin; suspensions should be freshly prepared and not stored for >24 hr; the powder should not be mixed with foods or liquids that contain a large amount of potassium (bananas or orange juice)

Side effects: *italics* = common; red = life-threatening

Rectal route
- Precede retention enema with a cleansing enema
- Use the suspension retained in the colon for at least 30-60 min or for several hours, if possible
- After several hours have passed, administer a cleansing enema using a non–sodium-containing solution at body temperature; up to 2 quarts of fluid may be necessary; drain fluid through a Y-tube connection; observe the drainage if sorbitol was used

SIDE EFFECTS
GI: Constipation, anorexia, nausea, vomiting, diarrhea (sorbitol), fecal impaction, gastric irritation
META: Hypocalcemia, hypokalemia, hypomagnesemia, sodium retention

INTERACTIONS
Increase: hypokalemia—loop diuretics, cardiac glycosides
Increase: metabolic alkalosis—magnesium/calcium antacids
Increase: colonic necrosis—sorbitol; do not use concurrently
Decrease: effect of—lithium, thyroid hormones

NURSING CONSIDERATIONS
Assess:
- **Hyperkalemia:** serum potassium >5.5 mol/L; confusion, dyspnea, weakness, dysrhythmias; ECG for spiked T waves, depressed ST segments, prolonged QT and widening QRS complex
- **Hypokalemia:** serum potassium <3.5 mmol/L; muscle weakness, polyuria, cardiac hyperexcitability with poor contractility
- Bowel function daily; note consistency of stools, times/day
- **Hypotension:** confusion, irritability, muscular pain, weakness
- **Electrolytes:** serum potassium, calcium, magnesium, sodium; acid-base balance
- I&O ratio, weight daily; crackles, dyspnea, jugular venous distention, edema
- **Digoxin toxicity** (nausea, vomiting, blurred vision, anorexia, dysrhythmias) in those receiving digoxin

Evaluate:
- **Therapeutic response:** potassium level 3.5-5 mg/dL
Teach patient/family:
- About reason for medication and expected results
- To follow a low-potassium diet, provide sample diet
- To avoid laxatives, antacids, electrolyte-based products unless approved by prescriber

---

sodium zirconium cyclosilicate (Rx)
(sow'dee-um zir-koe'-nee-um sye'-kloe-sil'i-kate)
Lokelma
Func. class.: Antidote, potassium binder

USES: Treatment of hyperkalemia

CONTRAINDICATIONS
Hypersensitivity

DOSAGE AND ROUTES
Hyperkalemia
- **Adult: PO** 10 g tid for ≤48 hr; adjust dose by 5 g daily at 1-wk intervals as needed based on serum potassium; maintenance 10 g daily; max maintenance 15 g/day
Available forms: Powder for oral suspension 5-, 10-g packets

---

sofosbuvir (Rx)
(soe-fos'bue-vir)
Sovaldi
Func. class.: Antiviral, antihepatitis agent
Chem. class.: Nucleotide analog polymerase inhibitor

ACTION: Inhibits hepatitis C virus RNA polymerase by incorporating the polymerase into the viral RNA; also acts as a chain terminator

---

USES: Chronic hepatitis C (genotypes 1, 2, 3, 4) with compensated liver disease in combination

CONTRAINDICATIONS
Hypersensitivity, pregnancy in combination; male-mediated teratogenicity
Precautions: Breastfeeding, children, hepatic/renal disease

> Black Box Warning: Hepatitis B exacerbation

DOSAGE AND ROUTES
Chronic hepatitis C
Genotype 1, 4
• **Adult: PO** 400 mg daily with peginterferon alfa and ribavirin × 12 wk; may consider use for genotype 1 with only ribavirin × 24 wk
Chronic hepatitis C
Genotype 2
• **Adult: PO** 400 mg daily with ribavirin × 12 wk
Chronic hepatitis C
Genotype 3
• **Adult: PO** 400 mg daily with ribavirin or daclatasvir × 24 wk
Chronic hepatitis C with hepatocellular carcinoma in those waiting for liver transplant
• **Adult: PO** 400 mg daily with ribavirin × 48 wk or until transplant
Available forms: Tabs 400 mg
Administer:
• By mouth without regard to food
• Do not use as monotherapy
• Do not crush, break tabs

SIDE EFFECTS
CNS: Headache, chills, weakness, fatigue, fever, insomnia
GI: Diarrhea, hyperbilirubinemia, nausea
MISC: Rash, pruritus, neutropenia, anemia, myalgia

PHARMACOKINETICS
PO: Peak ½-2 hr, excreted by kidneys 80%, 61%-65% protein binding; half-life 0.4-27 hr

INTERACTIONS
Decrease: sofosbuvir-P-glycoprotein (P-gp) inducers (carBAMazepine, PHENobarbital, phenytoin, rifAMPin); OXcarbazepine, rifabutin, rifapentine, tipranavir; avoid concurrent use
Increase: bradycardia—amiodarone; avoid using together
Increase: sofosbuvir level—carvedilol, cobicistat
Drug/Herb
Decrease: sofosbuvir level—St. John's wort; do not use together

NURSING CONSIDERATIONS
Assess:
• Heart rate, B/P; severe bradycardia may occur with amiodarone used concurrently
• Serum HCV-RNA baseline and periodically
• Severe renal disease/GFR <30 mL/min/1.73 m^2: monitor BUN, creatinine
• Closer monitoring in geriatric patients; may develop renal, cardiac symptoms more rapidly
• **HBV reactivation:** test is required before beginning therapy; monitor throughout, monitor coinfected patients closely

> Black Box Warning: **Hepatitis B exacerbation:** monitor HBsAg, HBV DNA, hepatic enzymes, bilirubin

• **Pregnancy:** if planned or suspected; if pregnant, call the Antiretroviral Pregnancy Registry, 800-258-4263; obtain pregnancy test before starting treatment; women who have HIV-1 and HCV who are taking antiretrovirals also should enroll with the registry
Evaluate:
• **Therapeutic response:** decreased symptoms of chronic hepatitis C
Teach patient/family:
• That optimal duration of treatment is unknown; that product is not a cure; that transmission may still occur
• To avoid use with other medications unless approved by prescriber
• Not to stop abruptly unless directed; worsening of hepatitis may occur, not to use alone, keep in original container
• **Pregnancy/breastfeeding:** to notify prescriber if pregnancy is planned or

---

Side effects: *italics* = common; red = life-threatening

suspected; to use two forms of reliable contraception; to avoid breastfeeding

Black Box Warning: Hepatitis B exacerbation: to notify prescriber immediately of liver toxicity: yellow eyes or skin, fatigue, weakness, loss of appetite, nausea/vomiting, light-colored stools

---

sofosbuvir/velpatasvir (Rx)

(soe-fos′bue-vir/vel-pat′as-vir)

Epclusa

Func. class.: Antiviral, antihepatitis agent

ACTION: Sofosbuvir: A nucleotide prodrug that prevents hepatitis C viral (HCV) replication by inhibiting the activity of HCV NS5B RNA polymerase
Velpatasvir: Inhibits the HCV NS5A protein, which is required for viral replication

USES: Treatment of chronic hepatitis C infection, including genotypes 1, 2, 3, 4, 5, and 6, in those without cirrhosis and in patients with compensated cirrhosis (Child-Pugh A); treatment of chronic hepatitis C infection in patients with decompensated cirrhosis (Child-Pugh B or C)

CONTRAINDICATIONS
Hypersensitivity
Precautions: Breastfeeding, hepatitis C and HIV coinfection, male-mediated teratogenicity, pregnancy, renal failure/impairment

Black Box Warning: Hepatitis B exacerbation

DOSAGE AND ROUTES
Chronic hepatitis C infection without cirrhosis and with compensated cirrhosis (Child-Pugh A)
• **Adult: PO** 1 tablet (400 mg sofosbuvir; 100 mg velpatasvir) daily × 12 wk

Chronic hepatitis C infection in patients with decompensated cirrhosis (Child-Pugh B or C)
• **Adult/child/adolescent 3-17 yr and ≥30 kg: PO** 1 tablet (400 mg sofosbuvir; 100 mg velpatasvir) daily plus ribavirin × 12 wk. The dose of ribavirin is based on weight as follows: <75 kg give 500 mg bid; ≥75 kg give 600 mg bid
Available forms: Tabs 400 mg sofosbuvir-100 mg velpatasvir; granules 150 mg/37.5 mg, 200 mg/50 mg pellets

Administer:
• Take without regard to food
• If given with ribavirin, take ribavirin with food
• Pellets: may be poured in the mouth and swallowed without chewing, water may be taken after swallowing the pellets or may be taken with soft food

SIDE EFFECTS
CNS: *Fatigue, headache,* insomnia, depression, irritability, asthenia
GI: *Nausea, diarrhea*
INTEG: Rash
META: Hyperbilirubinemia
HEMA: Anemia

PHARMACOKINETICS
• **Sofosbuvir:** 61% to 65% protein binding, converted in the liver from the nucleotide prodrug to active nucleoside analog triphosphate; elimination via kidneys 80%, feces 14%, expired air 2.5%, terminal elimination half-life of 25 hr, peak 0.5-1 hr, high-fat meal increases bioavailability
• **Velpatasvir:** 99.5% protein binding, metabolized by CYP2B6, CYP2C8, and CYP3A4, excretion in bile 77% of the parent drug, 95% feces, 0.4% urine, terminal elimination half-life 15 hr, peak 3 hr, increased by high-fat meal

INTERACTIONS
Increase: velpatasvir level—CYP3A4 inhibitors (aldesleukin, aliskiren, amLO-DIPine, clarithromycin, aprepitant, fosaprepitant, atazanavir, bromocriptine, chloramphenicol, ciprofloxacin, cyclo-SPORINE, delavirdine, dasatinib, danazol, darunavir, diltiaZEM, dronedarone,

erythromycin, fluconazole, FLUoxetine, fluvoxaMINE, idelalisib, imatinib, indinavir, isavuconazonium, amprenavir, bocenavir, ketoconazole, itraconazole, dalfopristin/quinupristin, ritonavir, tipranavir, isoniazid, miconazole), P-gp inhibitors

Increase: bradycardia—amiodarone; avoid using together

Increase: myopathy, rhabdomyolysis—atorvastatin

Increase: sofosbuvir level—carvedilol, cobicistat

Increase: effect of both products—clarithromycin, azithromycin, boceprevir, canagliflozin, carvedilol, crizotinib

Decrease: velpatasvir level—CYP3A4 inducers (armodafinil, barbiturates, bexarotene, bosentan, carBAMazepine, dexamethasone, efavirenz, enzalutamide, eslicarbazepine, ethanol, etravirine, felbamate, flutamide, griseofulvin, lesinurad, modafinil, nafcillin, nevirapine, rifAMPin, rifapentine, rifabutin, phenytoin, PHENobarbital, pioglitazone, primidone); antacids, PPIs separate by 4 hr

Decrease: sofosbuvir level—P-glycoprotein (P-gp) inducers (carBAMazepine, PHENobarbital, phenytoin, rifAMPin); OXcarbazepine, rifabutin, rifapentine, tipranavir; avoid concurrent use

Decrease: levels of—ritonavir

Drug/Herb

Decrease: sofosbuvir level—St. John's wort; do not use together

NURSING CONSIDERATIONS
Assess

Black Box Warning: Hepatitis B exacerbation: monitor serum HCV-RNA baseline and periodically, monitor coinfected patients during and after treatment for signs of hepatitis B exacerbation (HBsAg, HBV DNA, hepatic enzymes, bilirubin), assess for signs of liver toxicity (yellow eyes or skin, fatigue, weakness, loss of appetite, nausea, vomiting, or light-colored stools); screen all potential recipients for current or prior HBV infection by testing HBsAg and anti-HBc concentrations. For

those whose screening reveals evidence of HBV infection, a baseline HBV DNA should be obtained before starting sofosbuvir/velpatasvir; monitor LFTs

• Heart rate, B/P; severe bradycardia may occur with amiodarone used concurrently

• Severe renal disease/GFR <30 mL/min/1.73 m^2; monitor BUN, creatinine

• Closer monitoring in geriatric patients; may develop renal, cardiac symptoms more rapidly

• **Anemia:** Monitor HB/Hct if anemia is suspected

• **Pregnancy/breastfeeding:** contraindicated in pregnant women and in the male partners of women who are pregnant; two reliable forms of effective contraception are needed during treatment and for 6 mo after use of these combination therapies. Pregnancy test immediately before initiation of therapy, monthly and for 6 mo post-therapy. To monitor maternal-fetal outcomes of pregnancies in female patients and female partners of male patients exposed to ribavirin during treatment and for 6 mo following cessation of treatment, report any cases to the Ribavirin Pregnancy Registry, 800-593-2214. For patients who are also infected with HIV and taking concomitant antiretrovirals, an Antiretroviral Pregnancy Registry is available at 800-258-4263; do not breastfeed

Evaluate:

• Decreased symptoms of chronic hepatitis C

Teach Patient/Family:

• That optimal duration of treatment is unknown; that product is not a cure, that transmission to others may still occur

• To avoid use with other products unless approved by prescriber

• Not to stop abruptly unless directed, worsening of hepatitis may occur; to keep in original container

• **Pregnancy/breastfeeding:** teach patients that they and their partners are required to use two reliable forms of effective contraception during treatment and for 6 mo after use; that pregnancy tests are needed immediately before, monthly during therapy, and for 6 mo post-therapy; not to breastfeed

Black Box Warning: Hepatitis exacerbation: report to provider immediately signs of liver toxicity (yellow eyes or skin, fatigue, weakness, loss of appetite, nausea, vomiting, or light-colored stools)

sofosbuvir/velpatasvir/voxilaprevir (Rx)

(soe-fos´-bue-vir/vel-pat´-as-vir/vox-i-la´pre-vir)

Vosevi

Func. class.: Antiviral, antihepatitis agent

USES: Treatment of chronic hepatitis C virus (HCV) infection without cirrhosis or with compensated cirrhosis (Child-Pugh class A) who have genotype 1, 2, 3, 4, 5, or 6 and have previously been treated with an HCV regimen containing an NS5A inhibitor or who have genotype 1a or 3 infection and have previously been treated with an HCV regimen containing sofosbuvir without an NS5A inhibitor

CONTRAINDICATIONS

Hypersensitivity, use with rifampin

Black Box Warning: Hepatitis B exacerbation

DOSAGE AND ROUTES

Chronic hepatitis C (without cirrhosis or with compensated cirrhosis) Child-Pugh class A

• **Adult: PO** Genotype 1, 2, 3, 4, 5, or 6 (previously treated with a combination therapy with a direct-acting antiviral): 1 tablet daily × 12 wk. For those with genotype 3 with prior NS5A inhibitor failure/cirrhosis, use ribavirin also; genotype 1a (previously treated with combination therapy containing

sofosbuvir without an NS5A inhibitor): 1 tablet daily × 12 wk

Available forms: Tabs 400/100/100 mg

solifenacin (Rx)

(sol-i-fen´a-sin)

VESIcare, Vesicare LS

Func. class.: Urinary antispasmodic, anticholinergic

Chem. class.: Antimuscarinic

Do not confuse:
Vesicare/Vesanoid

ACTION: Relaxes smooth muscles in urinary tract by inhibiting acetylcholine at postganglionic sites

USES: Overactive bladder (urinary frequency, urgency, incontinence), neurogenic detrusor overactivitiy (NDO) in pediatrics

CONTRAINDICATIONS

Hypersensitivity, uncontrolled closed-angle glaucoma, urinary retention, gastric retention

Precautions: Pregnancy, breastfeeding, children, geriatric patients, renal/hepatic disease, controlled closed-angle glaucoma, bladder outflow obstruction, GI obstruction, decreased GI motility, history of QT prolongation

DOSAGE AND ROUTES

• **Adult/Child ≥ 2yr, > 60 kg: PO** 5 mg/day, max 10 mg/day

• **Child: PO ≥2 yr 9 to 16 kg:** 2 mg (2 mL)/day, max 4 mg (4 mL)/day; **>15 kg to 30 kg:** 3 mg (3 mL/day), max 5 mg (5 mL)/day; **31-45 kg:** 3 mg (3 mL/day), max 6 mg (6 mL/day); **46-60 kg:** 4 mg (4 mL/day), max 8 mg (8 mL/day)

Renal/hepatic dose

• **Adult: PO** (Child-Pugh B) max 5 mg/day; CCr ≤30 mL/min, 5 mg/day

With CYP3A4 inhibitors: **Adult: PO** 5 mg/day (max)

Available forms: Tabs 5, 10 mg; oral solution 1 mg/mL

Administer:

PO route

• Without regard to meals

• Swallow product whole with water, liquid

SIDE EFFECTS
CNS: *Dizziness,* headache, confusion, depression, drowsiness
CV: Palpitations, sinus tachycardia, chest pain, QTc prolongation
EENT: *Vision abnormalities*
GI: *Nausea, anorexia,* abdominal pain, *constipation, dry mouth*
INTEG: Angioedema, exfoliative dermatitis

PHARMACOKINETICS
90% absorbed; 98% protein bound; extensively metabolized by CYP3A4; excreted in urine 69% (metabolites), feces 22%; half-life 45-68 hr (tablets), 26 hr (oral suspension); peak 4-8 hr (tablet), 2-6 hr (oral suspension), duration up to 24 hr

INTERACTIONS
Increase: QT prolongation—Class IA, III antidysrhythmias
Increase: CNS depression—sedatives, hypnotics, benzodiazepines, opioids
Increase: effects—CYP3A4 inhibitors (ketoconazole, clarithromycin, diclofenac, doxycycline, erythromycin, isoniazid, nefazodone, propofol, protease inhibitors, verapamil), max dose 5 mg
Decrease: effects—CYP3A4 inducers (carBAMazepine, nevirapine, PHENobarbital, phenytoin)
Drug/Herb
Decrease: effects—St. John's wort
Drug/Food
Increase: effect—grapefruit juice
Drug/Lab Test
Increase: LFTs

NURSING CONSIDERATIONS
Assess:
• **Urinary patterns:** distention, nocturia, frequency, urgency, incontinence
• **Allergic reactions:** rash
• **Cardiac patients:** monitor ECG for QTc prolongation, avoid products that cause QT prolongation
• **Angioedema** of the face, lips, tongue, larynx
• **Pregnancy/breastfeeding:** use only if benefits outweigh fetal risk; do not breastfeed, excretion unknown

Evaluate:
• **Therapeutic response:** decreasing dysuria, frequency, nocturia, incontinence
Teach patient/family:
• To avoid hazardous activities because dizziness may occur
• That constipation, blurred vision may occur; to notify prescriber if abdominal pain with constipation occurs
• To take without regard to food
• To swallow tab whole; do not split, crush, chew
• To call prescriber if severe abdominal pain or constipation lasts for ≥3 days
• That heat prostration may occur if used in hot environment, sweating is decreased
• About **anticholinergic effects:** blurred vision, constipation, urinary retention, hyperthermia

solriamfetol (Rx)
(sol'ri-am'fe-tol)
Sunosi
Func. class.: Narcolepsy agent
Chem. class.: Dopamine norepinephrine reuptake inhibitor
Controlled Substance Schedule IV

ACTION: Unknown, action may be due to its inhibitor of a dopamine and norepinephrine reuptake

USES: Excessive daytime sleepiness due to narcolepsy or obstructive sleep apnea

CONTRAINDICATIONS
Hypersensitivity, MAOIs
Precautions:
Alcoholism, bipolar disorder, cardiac disease, breastfeeding, diabetes mellitus, geriatrics, heart failure, hepatic disease, hypertension, MI, pregnancy, renal disease, schizophrenia, stroke, substance abuse, valvular heart disease, ventricular dysfunction

DOSAGE AND ROUTES
Narcolepsy
Adults: PO 75 mg daily on awakening; may increase to 150 mg after ≥3 days; max 150 mg/day
Obstructive sleep apnea
• **Adults: PO** 37.5 mg daily on awakening; double the dose at intervals of at least 3 days if needed; max 150 mg/day
Renal dose
Adult: PO 37.5 mg/day; may increase to 75 mg/day after ≥7 days
Available forms: Tablet 75, 150 mg
Administer:
• Without regard to food
• Take on awakening; avoid within 9 hr of bedtime

SIDE EFFECTS
CNS: *Insomnia, anxiety, headache,* dizziness
CV: Palpitations, chest discomfort
GI: *Anorexia, nausea, dry mouth, constipation,* abdominal pain
INTEG: Hyperhidrosis

PHARMACOKINETICS
Protein binding <20%, minimally metabolized; half-life 7.1 hr, increased in renal disease; excreted 95% unchanged, peak 1.2-3 hr

INTERACTIONS
Increased: hypertensive reaction—MAOIs; do not use within 14 days
Use caution when using dopaminergic agents or drugs that increase B/P or heart rate

NURSING CONSIDERATIONS
Assess:
• **Narcolepsy:** assess for trouble staying awake baseline and after 1 wk, 2 wk
• B/P and heart rate baseline and periodically; hypertension should be treated before starting this product
• **Psychiatric symptoms:** assess for symptoms baseline and periodically; those with renal disease may be at higher risk

• Abuse: assess for those with a recent history of drug abuse, especially alcohol, amphetamines, cocaine, methylphenidate; watch for drug-seeking behaviors
Evaluate:
• **Therapeutic response:** ability to stay awake
Teach patient/family:
• To discuss all Rx, OTC, herbs, and supplements taken and if taking an MAOI
• That if a dose is missed, skip missed dose and administer the next dose the following day in the morning on wakening
• To report to healthcare provider if inability to stay awake continues or if you develop anxiety, agitation, irritability, problems sleeping
• **Pregnancy/breastfeeding:** identify if pregnancy is planned or suspected, encourage to enroll in the pregnancy registry if she becomes pregnant; to enroll or obtain information from the registry, online at www.SunosiPregnancyRegistry.com or by calling 877-283-6220; present in breast milk

---

somapacitan-beco (Rx)
(soe′ma-pas′i-tan
Sogroya
Func. class.: Growth hormone

USES: Growth hormone deficiency

CONTRAINDICATIONS
Hypersensitivity, open heart/abdominal surgery, trauma; respiratory failure; malignancy; diabetic retinopathy

DOSAGE AND ROUTES
Growth hormone deficiency
• **Adult: SUBCUT** 1.5 mg weekly; may increase by 0.5-1.5 mg/wk q2-4wk based on response, max 8 mg/wk

---

⚠ HIGH ALERT

somatropin (Rx)

(soe-ma-troe′pin)

Genotropin, Genotropin MiniQuick, Humatrope, Norditropin FlexPro, Nutropin AQ, NuSpin 10, Nutropin AQ, NuSpin 20, Nutropin AQ, NuSpin 5, Omnitrope, Saizen, Saizenprep, Serostim, Zomacton, Zomacton

Func. class.: Pituitary hormone
Chem. class.: Growth hormone

Do not confuse:

somatropin/SUMAtriptan/somatrem

ACTION: Stimulates growth; somatropin is similar to natural growth hormone; both preparations were developed with the use of recombinant DNA

USES: Pituitary growth hormone deficiency (hypopituitary dwarfism), children with human growth hormone deficiency/growth failure, AIDS wasting syndrome, cachexia, adults with somatropin deficiency syndrome (SDS), short stature in Noonan syndrome, SHOX deficiency, Turner's syndrome, Prader-Willi syndrome

CONTRAINDICATIONS

Hypersensitivity to benzyl alcohol, creosol; closed epiphyses, intracranial lesions, acute respiratory failure, Prader-Willi syndrome with obesity, trauma
Precautions: Pregnancy, breastfeeding, newborn, geriatric patients, diabetes mellitus, hypothyroidism, prolonged treatment in adults, scoliosis, sleep apnea, chemotherapy, respiratory disease, glycerin hypersensitivity (with formulations that contain these products)

DOSAGE AND ROUTES
Genotropin

• **Child:** SUBCUT 0.16-0.24 mg/kg/wk divided into 6 or 7 daily inj; give in abdomen, thigh, buttocks

• **Adult:** SUBCUT 0.04-0.08 mg/kg/wk divided into 6-7 daily doses
Humatrope

• **Adult:** IM 0.006 international units/kg/day, max 0.0125 units/kg/day
• **Child:** SUBCUT/IM 0.18 mg/kg divided into equal doses either on 3 alternate days or 6×/wk, max weekly dose 0.3 mg/kg
Nutropin/Nutropin AQ (growth hormone deficiency)

• **Child:** SUBCUT 0.3 mg/kg/wk
Serostim

• **Adult:** SUBCUT at bedtime >55 kg, 6 mg; >45-55 kg, 5 mg; 35-45 kg, 4 mg
Norditropin

• **Child:** SUBCUT 0.024-0.034 mg/kg 6-7×/wk
GH deficiency

• **Adult:** SUBCUT (Saizen) 0.005 mg/kg/day; may increase after 4 wk to max 0.01 mg/kg/day

Available forms: Powder for inj (lyophilized) 1.5 mg (4 units/mL), 4 mg (12 units/vial), 5 mg (13 units/vial), 5 mg (15 units/vial) rDNA origin, 5.8 mg (15 units/mL), 6 mg (18 units/mL), 8 mg (24 units/vial), 10 mg (26 units/vial); inj 10 mg (30 units/vial), 5 mg/1.5 mL, 10 mg/1.5 mL, 15 mg/1.5 mL

Administer:
• Give IM or subcut; do not use IV
• Discontinue therapy if final height is achieved or epiphyseal fusion occurs
• Visually inspect parenteral products for particulate matter and discoloration

Reconstitution and storage
Genotropin
• Powder, available in a 5-mg cartridge (green tip) and a 12-mg cartridge (purple tip); the 5- and 12-mg cartridges may be used with the Genotropin Pen or the Genotropin Mixer; also in various doses ranging from 0.2 mg to 2 mg, in single use, auto-mix devices called Genotropin Miniquicks

• **Cartridges:** store cartridges refrigerated before reconstitution, do not freeze; protect from light; after the powder and diluent are mixed, gently tip the cartridge upside down a few times until

S

powder is dissolved; if solution is cloudy, do not use; following reconstitution, the 5-mg cartridge contains 5 mg/mL; the 12-mg cartridge contains 12 mg/mL; 5-mg and 12-mg cartridges contain overfill; the cartridges contain diluent with preservative (m-cresol) and may be stored refrigerated ≤28 days after reconstitution; do not use the 5-mg and 12-mg cartridges in patients with m-cresol hypersensitivity

• **Genotropin Miniquicks:** after dispensing but before reconstitution, store at ≤77° ≤3 mo; a reconstitution device is supplied; this product contains a diluent with no preservative, refrigerate after reconstitution and use within 24 hr; use reconstituted solution only once and discard remaining

Humatrope

• Before reconstitution, store refrigerated

• **Vials:** reconstitute each 5-mg vial with 1.5-5 mL of the diluent (contains m-cresol as a preservative) or bacteriostatic water for injection (contains benzyl alcohol as a preservative); swirl until contents are dissolved; do not shake; if the solution is cloudy, do not use; small, colorless particles may be present after refrigeration; vials reconstituted with the diluent or bacteriostatic water are stable for 14 days when refrigerated; for vials reconstituted with sterile water, use the vial only once and discard if not used immediately, refrigerate and use within 24 hr; avoid freezing

• **Cartridges:** reconstitute cartridges using *only* the supplied diluent syringe; once reconstituted, the cartridges are stable for up to 28 days when stored refrigerated; store the injection device without the needle attached; avoid freezing reconstituted solutions

Norditropin

• Do not use reconstituted solution if cloudy or contains particulate matter

• Before use, store refrigerated

• Reconstitution of the cartridges is not required; each cartridge size (5 mg, 10 mg, or 15 mg per 1.5-mL cartridge)

• After a cartridge has been inserted into the NordiPen injector or once a NordiFlex pen is in use, the pen should be stored refrigerated and used within 4 wk; alternatively, the 5-mg and 10-mg cartridges may be stored in the pen at room temperature, for ≤3 wk

Nutropin

• Before reconstitution, store refrigerated

• Reconstitute each 5-mg vial with 1-5 mL bacteriostatic water for injection (benzyl alcohol preserved) and each 10-mg vial with 1-10 mL of bacteriostatic water for injection (benzyl alcohol preserved); if using for newborns, reconstitute with sterile water for injection; swirl vial; do not shake; if the solution is cloudy after reconstitution or refrigeration, do not use; small, colorless particles may be present after refrigeration

• Solutions reconstituted with bacteriostatic water for injection are stable for 14 days refrigerated

• Solutions reconstituted with sterile water for injection should be used immediately and only once; discard any unused portions; avoid freezing reconstituted solutions

Nutropin AQ

• Does not require reconstitution; solution should be clear; small, colorless particles may be present after refrigeration; allow vial or pen cartridge to come to room temperature, and gently swirl; if solution is cloudy, do not use

• **Pen cartridge:** use only with Nutropin AQ Pen; the Nutropin AQ 10 pen allows use of a minimum 0.1-mg dose to a maximum 4-mg dose, in 0.1-mg increments; the Nutropin AQ 20 pen allows use of a minimum 0.2-mg dose to a maximum 8-mg dose, in 0.2-mg increments

• **Prefilled device:** a prefilled multidose, dial-a-dose device is available in 3 strengths; administer using disposable needles

• After initial use, products are stable for 28 days refrigerated; avoid freezing; protect from light

---

Omnitrope
- Before reconstitution, store vials refrigerated; store in the carton; Omnitrope is sensitive to light
- **Vials:** reconstitute with diluent provided; swirl do not shake; if the solution is cloudy after reconstitution, the contents must not be used; after reconstitution, the 1.5-mg vial may be refrigerated ≤24 hr; the 1.5-mg vial does not contain a preservative and should only be used once; discard remaining; the 5.8-mg vial diluent contains benzyl alcohol as a preservative; after reconstitution, the contents must be used within 3 wk; after the first injection, store the 5.8-mg vial in the carton, to protect from light, in the refrigerator; avoid freezing
- **Omnitrope Pen 5 cartridge:** each 5-mg cartridge must be inserted into the Omnitrope Pen 5 delivery system; the cartridge contains benzyl alcohol as a preservative; after the first use, store refrigerated ≤28 days; protect from light, avoid freezing
- **Omnitrope Pen 10 cartridge:** each 10-mg cartridge must be inserted into the Omnitrope Pen 10 delivery system; after the first use, store refrigerated ≤28 days; protect from light, avoid freezing

Saizen
- Before reconstitution, store at room temperature
- **Vials:** reconstitute each 5-mg vial/1-3 mL bacteriostatic water for injection; reconstitute each 8.8-mg vial/ 2-3 mL bacteriostatic water for injection (benzyl alcohol preserved); swirl until contents are dissolved completely; do not shake; the solution should be clear; if it is cloudy immediately after reconstitution or refrigeration, do not use; small colorless particles may be present after refrigeration; after reconstitution, store vials mixed with bacteriostatic water for injection refrigerated, use within 14 days; for vials mixed with sterile water for injection, use immediately, and any unused portion should be discarded; avoid freezing
- **Cartridges:** available in 4-mg and 8.8-mg Click.easy cartridges

Serostim
- Before reconstitution, store vials and diluent at room temperature (15° C-30° C; 59° F-86° F)
- **Vials:** reconstitute 5-mg or 6-mg vials/0.5-1 mL of supplied diluent (sterile water for injection); reconstitute the 4-mg vial with 0.5-1 mL of bacteriostatic water for injection (benzyl alcohol preserved), 8.8-mg vial with 1-2 mL of bacteriostatic water for injection (benzyl alcohol preserved); swirl; do not shake; the solution should be clear; if it is cloudy, do not use; small colorless particles may be present after refrigeration; if reconstituted with sterile water for injection, use within 24 hr; if reconstituted with bacteriostatic water for injection (benzyl alcohol preserved), the solution is stable for up to 14 days under refrigeration (2° C-8° C or 36° F-46° F); avoid freezing
- **Cartridges:** available in 8.8-mg Click. easy® cartridges after reconstitution, cartridges are stable refrigerated for ≤21 days; avoid freezing

Serostim LQ
- Before use, store refrigerated
- Available in 6-mg single-use cartridges that do not require reconstitution; administer using sterile disposable syringes and needles
- Bring to room temperature before use; discard single-use cartridge after use, discard cartridges after the expiration date; do not freeze; protect from light

Zomacton (formerly Tev-Tropin)
- Before reconstitution, store refrigerated
- Reconstitute each 5-mg vial with 1-5 mL bacteriostatic 0.9% sodium chloride (benzyl alcohol preserved) for injection; swirl; do not shake; the solution should be clear; if it is cloudy immediately after reconstitution, do not inject; small, colorless particles may be present after refrigeration; when administering to newborns, reconstitute with sterile normal saline for injection that is unpreserved
- Solution reconstituted with bacteriostatic 0.9% sodium chloride is stable

for 14 days when stored refrigerated; solution reconstituted with sterile normal saline should be used only once; discard remaining solution; avoid freezing

Valtropin
• Before dispensing, store vials and diluent refrigerated; after dispensing, may be stored at or below 77° F for up to 3 mo
• Reconstitute each 5-mg vial with the entire contents of the accompanying diluent, which contains metacresol as a preservative; swirl vial; do not shake; the solution should be clear, if it is cloudy or contains particulate matter, do not use; final concentration 3.33 mg/mL
• After reconstitution with the provided diluent, solutions may be stored refrigerated for up to 14 days; after reconstitution with sterile water for injection, use only one dose of Valtropin per vial and discard the unused portion

Zorbtive
• Unreconstituted vials of drug and diluent may be stored at room temperature until expiration date
• Reconstitute each vial of 4 mg, 5 mg, or 6 mg with 0.5-1 mL sterile water for injection, reconstitute each 8.8 mg with 1-2 mL bacteriostatic water for injection (0.9% benzyl alcohol preserved); in newborns or those with a benzyl alcohol hypersensitivity, sterile water for injection may be used; swirl; do not shake; the solution should be clear; if it is cloudy after reconstitution or refrigeration, do not use; small colorless particles may be present after refrigeration
• After reconstitution with sterile water for injection, use the solution immediately and discard any unused portion; when using bacteriostatic water for injection, reconstituted solutions are stable for up to 14 days refrigerated; avoid freezing
IM route
• Inject deeply into a large muscle; aspirate; rotate injection sites daily
SUBCUT route

• Volumes >1 mL of reconstituted solution are not recommended; do not inject intradermally
• Allow refrigerated solutions to come to room temperature before injection
• Subcutaneous injections may be given in the thigh, buttocks, or abdomen; rotate injection sites daily

SIDE EFFECTS
CNS: Headache, growth of intracranial tumor, fever, aggressive behavior
ENDO: Hyperglycemia, ketosis, hypothyroidism, thyroid hormone replacement may be needed
GI: Nausea, vomiting, pancreatitis
GU: *Hypercalciuria*
INTEG: Rash, urticaria, pain; inflammation at inj site, hematoma
MS: Tissue swelling, joint and muscle pain
SYST: Antibodies to growth hormone

PHARMACOKINETICS
Half-life 15-60 min, duration 7 days, metabolized in liver

INTERACTIONS
Increase: epiphyseal closure—androgens, thyroid hormones
Decrease: growth—glucocorticosteroids
Decrease: insulin, antidiabetic effect—dosage adjustment may be needed
Drug/Lab Test
Increase: glucose, urine glucose
Decrease: glucose, thyroid hormones

NURSING CONSIDERATIONS
Assess:
• Signs/symptoms of diabetes
• Growth hormone antibodies if patient fails to respond to therapy
• Thyroid function tests: T_3, T_4, TSH to identify hypothyroidism
• **Allergic reaction:** rash, itching, fever, nausea, wheezing
• **Hypercalciuria:** urinary stones; groin, flank pain; nausea, vomiting, urinary frequency, hematuria, chills
• Growth rate, bone age of child at intervals during treatment
• **Respiratory infection:** in those with Prader-Willi syndrome, may have sleep

apnea, upper airway obstruction; discontinue if obstruction occurs

• Rapid growth: assess for slipped capital femoral epiphysis; may also occur in endocrine disorders

• Monitor ophthalmologic status baseline and periodically; intracranial hypertension may occur

• **Beers:** avoid in older adults except as hormone replacement following pituitary gland removal

• **Pregnancy/breastfeeding:** effects unknown; cautious use in breastfeeding

Evaluate:

• **Therapeutic response:** growth in children

Teach patient/family:

• That treatment may continue for years; that regular assessments are required

• To maintain a growth record; to report knee/hip pain or limping

• That treatment is very expensive

• About subcut injection; to rotate injection site to avoid tissue atrophy; not to shake medication; to report peripheral edema, swelling to the provider

---

⚠ HIGH ALERT

sonidegib (Rx)
(soe´-ni-deg´-ib)

Odomzo

Func. class.: Antineoplastic

USES: Locally advanced basal cell carcinoma that has recurred after surgery or radiation therapy or in those who are not candidates for surgery or radiation therapy

CONTRAINDICATIONS

Hypersensitivity

Black Box Warning: Pregnancy, intrauterine fetal death, contraceptive requirement

DOSAGE AND ROUTES

• **Adult:** PO 200 mg daily until disease progression or unacceptable toxicity;

take on an empty stomach ≥1 hr before or 2 hr after a meal. Avoid use with strong CYP3A inhibitors or strong and moderate CYP3A inducers

Available forms: Capsules 200 mg

⚠ HIGH ALERT

sorafenib (Rx)
(sor-af´-e-nib)

NexAVAR

Func. class.: Antineoplastic, tyrosine kinase inhibitor

USES: Treatment of unresectable hepatocellular carcinoma, advanced renal cell carcinoma, progressive, differentiated thyroid carcinoma (refractory to radioactive iodine treatment)

CONTRAINDICATIONS

Hypersensitivity to sorafenib or any component

DOSAGE AND ROUTES

Adult

PO 400 mg bid; continue as long as beneficial

Available forms: Tabs 200 mg

⚠ HIGH ALERT

sotalol (Rx)
(sot´ah-lahl)

Betapace, Betapace AF, Sorine, Sotylize

Func. class.: Antidysrhythmic group III
Chem. class.: Nonselective β-blocker

Do not confuse:

sotalol/Sudafed

ACTION: Blockade of β_1- and β_2-receptors leads to antidysrhythmic effect, prolongs action potential in myocardial fibers without affecting conduction, prolongs QT interval, no effect on QRS duration

---

USES: Life-threatening ventricular dysrhythmias; Betapace AF: to maintain sinus rhythm with symptomatic atrial fibrillation/flutter

Unlabeled uses: Atrial fibrillation prophylaxis, cardiac surgery, PSVT, Wolff-Parkinson-White (WPW) syndrome

CONTRAINDICATIONS

Hypersensitivity to β-blockers, cardiogenic shock, heart block (2nd/3rd degree), sinus bradycardia, HF, bronchial asthma, CCr <40 mL/min, hypokalemia

> **Black Box Warning:** Congenital or acquired long QT syndrome

Precautions: Pregnancy, breastfeeding, major surgery, diabetes mellitus, renal/thyroid disease, COPD, well-compensated heart failure, CAD, nonallergic bronchospasm, electrolyte disturbances, bradycardia, peripheral vascular disease

> **Black Box Warning:** Cardiac dysrhythmias, torsades de pointes, ventricular dysrhythmias, ventricular fibrillation; requires a specialized care setting

DOSAGE AND ROUTES

Atrial fibrillation/atrial flutter

• **Adult: PO** Initially, 80 mg bid; may increase in increments of 80 mg/day q3days if QTc is <500 msec; most will have a satisfactory response with 120 mg twice daily; **IV** Initially, 75 mg bid; may increase by 75 mg/day q3days if the QTc is <500 msec; max 320 mg/day

Life-threatening tachycardia

• **Adult: PO** Initially, 80 mg bid; may increase by 80 mg/day q3days if the QTc is <500 msec to 160-320 mg/day. 480-640 mg/day may be used in refractory life-threatening arrhythmias; **IV** Initially, 75 mg bid; may increase by 75 mg/day q3days if the QTc is <500 msec to 150-300 mg/day. 550-600 mg/day may be used in refractory life-threatening arrhythmias

• **Adolescent/child 6-17 yr (unlabeled): PO** Initially, 30 mg/m^2/dose tid titrated up as needed at intervals of ≥36 hr (**max** 60 mg/m^2/dose tid)

Renal dose

• **Betapace/Betapace AF and Sorine (both for ventricular arrhythmias)**

• **Adult:** CCr ≥60 mL/min: no change; CCr 30-59 mL/min: extend dosage interval to q24hr. Dose may be titrated after at least 5 doses; CCr 10-29 mL/min: extend dosage interval to 36-48 hr according to clinical response. Dose may be titrated after at least 5 doses; CCr <10 mL/min: individualize

Betapace/Betapace AF (for atrial fibrillation/atrial flutter), Sotylize, and intravenous (IV) sotalol

• **Adult:** CCr ≥60 mL/min: no change; CCr 40-59 mL/min: extend dosage interval to q24hr. Dose may be titrated after at least 5 doses; CCr <40 mL/min: use is contraindicated

Available forms: Tabs 80, 120, 160, 240 mg; (Betapace AF) 80, 120, 160 mg; sol for inj 150 mg/10 mL (15 mg/mL); oral solution 5 mg/mL

Administer:

PO route

• Before, at bedtime; tab may be crushed or swallowed whole; give 1 hr before or 2 hr after meals

• Reduced dosage in renal dysfunction

• Betapace and Betapace AF are not interchangeable

• Do not give within 2 hr of antacids

• Store in dry area at room temperature; do not freeze

IV route

• Dilute to vol of either 120 mL or 300 mL with D$_5$W, LR

• **75-mg dose:** withdraw 6 mL sotalol inj (90 mg), add 114 mL diluent to make 120 mL (0.75 mg/mL); or withdraw 6 mL sotalol inj (90 mg), add 294 mL diluent to make 300 mL (0.3 mg/mL)

• **112.5-mg dose:** withdraw 9 mL sotalol inj (135 mL), add 111 mL diluent to make 120 mL (1.125 mg/mL); or withdraw 9 mL sotalol (135 mg), add 291 mL diluent to make 300 mL (0.45 mg/mL)

• **150-mg dose:** withdraw 12 mL of sotalol (180 mg), add 108 mL diluent to make 120 mL (1.5 mg/mL); or withdraw 12 mL sotalol (180 mg), add 288 mL diluent to make 300 mL (0.6 mg/mL)

• Use infusion pump and infuse 100 or 250 mL over 5 hr at a constant rate

SIDE EFFECTS

CNS: Dizziness, mental changes, drowsiness, fatigue, headache, depression, anxiety, paresthesia, insomnia, decreased concentration
CV: Prodysarrhythmia, prolonged QT, orthostatic hypotension, HF, ventricular dysrhythmias, AV block, palpitations, torsades de pointes; life-threatening ventricular dysrhythmias (Betapace AF)
EENT: Tinnitus, visual changes
GI: Nausea, vomiting, diarrhea, dry mouth, constipation, anorexia
GU: Impotence, dysuria
INTEG: Rash, alopecia, urticaria, pruritus, fever, diaphoresis
MS: Arthralgia, muscle cramps
RESP: Bronchospasm, wheezing

PHARMACOKINETICS

PO: Onset 1-2 hr, peak 2-4 hr, duration 8-12 hr; **IV:** onset 5-10 min, peak/duration unknown; half-life 12 hr, excreted unchanged in urine, crosses placenta, excreted in breast milk, protein binding 0%

INTERACTIONS

Black Box Warning: Increase: QT prolongation—class IA/III antidysrhythmics, some phenothiazines, β agonists, local anesthetics, tricyclics, haloperidol, chloroquine, droperidol, pentamidine; CYP3A4 inhibitors (amiodarone, clarithromycin, erythromycin, telithromycin, troleandomycin), arsenic trioxide; CYP3A4 substrates (methadone, pimozide, QUEtiapine, quiNIDine, risperiDONE, ziprasidone)

Increase: hypoglycemia effect—insulin
Increase: effects of lidocaine
Increase: hypotension—diuretics, other antihypertensives, nitroglycerin
Decrease: β-blocker effects—sympathomimetics
Decrease: bronchodilating effects of theophylline, β2-agonists
Decrease: hypoglycemic effects of sulfonylureas

Drug/Lab Test

False increase: urinary catecholamines
Interference: glucose, insulin tolerance tests
Drug/Herb
• Do not use with hawthorn

NURSING CONSIDERATIONS
Assess:
• I&O, weight daily; edema in feet, legs daily
• B/P, pulse q4hr; note rate, rhythm, quality
• Potassium, magnesium levels

Black Box Warning: Requires a specialized care setting: for a minimum of at least 3 days on maintenance dose with continuous ECG monitoring; calculate creatinine clearance before dosing

Black Box Warning: Cardiogenic shock, acute pulmonary edema: do not use, effect can further depress cardiac output

Black Box Warning: QT syndrome: apical/radial pulse before administration: notify prescriber of any significant changes; monitor ECG continuously (Betapace AF); use QT interval to determine patient eligibility; baseline QT must be ≤450 msec, if ≥500 msec, frequency or dosage must be decreased or drug discontinued

• Baselines of renal studies before therapy begins
• **Abrupt discontinuation:** do not discontinue abruptly, taper over 1-2 wk
• Dose should be adjusted slowly, with at least 3 days between changes; monitor ECG for QT interval
• Monitor electrolytes (hypokalemia, hypomagnesemia); may increase dysrhythmias
• **Pregnancy/breastfeeding:** use only if benefits outweigh fetal risk; do not breastfeed, excreted in breast milk
Evaluate:
• **Therapeutic response:** absence of life-threatening dysrhythmias
Teach patient/family:
• Not to discontinue product abruptly; to taper over 2 wk or may precipitate angina; to take exactly as prescribed
• Not to use antacids or OTC products containing α-adrenergic stimulants (na-

sal decongestants, OTC cold preparations) unless directed by prescriber

• To report bradycardia, dizziness, confusion, depression, fever

• To take pulse at home; advise patient when to notify prescriber

• To avoid alcohol, smoking, sodium intake

• To carry emergency ID to identify product being taken, allergies

• To avoid hazardous activities if dizziness present

• To report symptoms of HF, including difficulty breathing, especially on exertion or when lying down; night cough, swelling of extremities

• To wear support hose to minimize effects of orthostatic hypotension

• To monitor blood glucose if diabetic

• That hospitalization will be required for ≥3 days

---

spinosad (Rx)

(spin'oh-sad)

Natroba

Func. class.: Antiparasitic

USES: Topical treatment of head lice *(Pediculosis capitis)* infestation in adults and children ≥6 mo of age

CONTRAINDICATIONS

Hypersensitivity

DOSAGE AND ROUTES

Head lice

Adult/child: Topical: Apply needed amount to cover dry scalp and completely cover dry hair; if live lice are seen 7 days after first treatment, repeat

Available forms: Topical solution 0.9%

---

spesolimab (Rx)

(spes-o'li-mab)

Spevigo

Func. class.: Systemic antipsoriasis agent

Chem. class.: Monoclonal immunoglobulin antibody

ACTIONS: Humanized monoclonal immunoglobulin G1 (IgG1) antibody that inhibits interleukin-36 (IL-36) signaling by specifically binding to the IL-36 receptor (IL36R) and prevents downstream activation of proinflammatory and profibrotic pathways

USES: Generalized pustular psoriasis (GPP) flares

CONTRAINDICATIONS

Hypersensitivity, serious rash

Precautions: Pregnancy, breastfeeding, TB, infection, vaccination

DOSAGE AND ROUTES

Generalized pustular psoriasis (GPP) flares

Adults: IV INFUSION 900 mg over 90 min. A second 900-mg IV infusion may be given 1 wk after the initial dose if flare symptoms persist

Available forms: Solution for injection (IV) 450 mg/7.5 mL (60 mg/mL)

Administer:

IV infusion route

• Visually inspect for particulate matter and discoloration prior to use, the solution should be colorless to slightly brownish-yellow, clear to slightly opalescent. Do not use if the solution is cloudy, discolored, or contains large or colored particulates

• **Dilution:** Use aseptic technique; remove and discard 15 mL from a 100-mL container of sterile 0.9% sodium chloride injection; slowly add 15 mL of spesolimab solution (complete contents from two 450-mg/7.5-mL vials) into the 0.9% sodium chloride injection, gently mix; do not add or mix with other medications or diluents

• **Administer** diluted solution immediately, give as a continuous infusion over 90 min through an IV line containing a sterile, non-pyrogenic, low-protein-binding in-line filter (pore size of 0.2 microns)

• A preexisting IV line may be used for administration of the infusion if the line is flushed with sterile 0.9% sodium chloride injection prior to and at the end of the infusion. No other infusion should be administered in parallel via the same IV access

---

• If the infusion is slowed or temporarily stopped, the total infusion time (including stop time) must not exceed 180 min
• **Storage:** If not used immediately, the diluted solution may be stored 2 hr refrigerated at 36° F to 46° F (2° C to 8° C) for no more than 4 hr, protect from light

SIDE EFFECTS
GI: Diarrhea, nausea, vomiting, gastritis
INTEG: Pruritus, infusion-related reactions
MISC: Infection, Guillian-Barre syndrome, DRESS

PHARMACOKINETICS
Terminal half-life 25.5 days

INTERACTIONS
Do not give concurrently with live virus vaccines; immunizations should be brought up to date prior to treatment

NURSING CONSIDERATIONS
Assess:
• **Plaque psoriasis:** improvement in raised, red, inflamed lesions; dry skin with cracking and bleeding; itching, burning, or painful skin; silvery, scaly plaques; pitted nails or separation from the nail bed
• Infections (fever, flulike symptoms, dyspnea, change in urination, redness/swelling around any wounds), stop treatment if some serious infections occur, may be fatal; patients with active infections should not be started on this product
• Latent TB prior to therapy; obtain TB test, if positive, treat before starting this product
• Pregnancy/breastfeeding: identify if pregnancy is planned or suspected, effects in pregnancy or breastfeeding are unknown
Evaluate:
• **Therapeutic response:** improvement in symptoms of plaque psoriasis
Teach patient/family:
• Not to take any live virus vaccines during treatment
• To report signs of infection, allergic reaction, TB, immediately
• To advise all health care professionals of Rx, OTC, herbals, supplements taken

• Pregnancy/breastfeeding: to advise health care professional if pregnancy is planned or suspected or if breastfeeding
• To do regular skin assessments and report changes to provider

---

spironolactone (Rx)
(speer'on-oh-lak'tone)
Aldactone, CaroSpir
Func. class.: Potassium-sparing diuretic
Chem. class.: Aldosterone antagonist

Do not confuse:
Aldactone/Aldactazide

ACTION: Competes with aldosterone at receptor sites in distal tubule, thereby resulting in the excretion of sodium chloride and water and the retention of potassium and phosphate

USES: Edema of HF, hypertension, diuretic-induced hypokalemia, primary hyperaldosteronism (diagnosis, short-term treatment, long-term treatment), edema of nephrotic syndrome, cirrhosis of liver with ascites
Unlabeled uses: HF

CONTRAINDICATIONS
Hypersensitivity, anuria, severe renal disease, hyperkalemia
Precautions: Breastfeeding, dehydration, hepatic disease, renal impairment, electrolyte imbalances, metabolic acidosis, gynecomastia, pregnancy

Black Box Warning: Secondary malignancy

DOSAGE AND ROUTES
Edema/hypertension
• **Adult: PO** 25-100 mg/day in 1-2 divided doses
Heart failure (unlabeled)
• **Adult: PO** 12.5-25 mg/day; max 50 mg/day
Edema
• **Child: PO** 1-4 mg/kg/day as single dose or in divided doses

S

Hypertension
- **Child (unlabeled): PO** 1-4 mg/kg/day in divided doses

Hypokalemia
- **Adult: PO** 25-100 mg/day; if **PO**, potassium supplements must not be used

Primary hyperaldosteronism diagnosis
- **Adult: PO** 400 mg/day × 4 days or 4 wk depending on test, then 100-400 mg/day maintenance

Edema (nephrotic syndrome, HF, hepatic disease)
- **Adult: PO** 100 mg/day given as single dose or in divided doses, titrate to response, max 400 mg/day for hepatic disease, 200 mg/day for nephrotic syndrome
- **Child: PO** 1-4 mg/kg/day or 60 mg/m²/day given daily or in 2-4 divided doses

Renal dose
- **Adult: PO** CCr 10-50 mL/min, give dose q12-24hr; CCr <10 mL/min, avoid use

Available forms: Tabs 25, 50, 100 mg; oral suspension 25 mg/5 mL

Administer:
- In AM to avoid interference with sleep
- With food; if nausea occurs, absorption may be decreased slightly
- Effect may take 2 wk
- **Oral suspension:** Shake well, use calibrated measuring device

SIDE EFFECTS

CNS: *Headache,* confusion, drowsiness, lethargy, ataxia
ELECT: Hyperchloremic metabolic acidosis, hyperkalemia, hyponatremia
ENDO: Impotence, gynecomastia, irregular menses, amenorrhea, postmenopausal bleeding, hirsutism, deepening voice, breast pain
GI: *Diarrhea,* cramps, bleeding, gastritis, *vomiting,* anorexia, nausea, hepatocellular toxicity
HEMA: Agranulocytosis
INTEG: *Rash, pruritus,* urticaria

PHARMACOKINETICS

Onset 24-48 hr, peak 48-72 hr, metabolized in liver, excreted in urine, crosses placenta, protein binding >90%, terminal half-life 10-35 hr

INTERACTIONS

Increase: action of antihypertensives, digoxin, lithium
Increase: hyperchloremic acidosis in cirrhosis—cholestyramine
Increase: hyperkalemia—potassium-sparing diuretics, potassium products, ACE inhibitors, salt substitutes, angiotensin II receptor antagonists
Decrease: effect of anticoagulants, monitor INR/PT
Decrease: effect of spironolactone—ASA, NSAIDs

Drug/Food
Increase: hyperkalemia—potassium-rich foods, potassium salt substitutes

Drug/Herb
Increase: hypotension—hawthorn, horse chestnut
Decrease: antihypertensive effect—ephedra
Increase: severe photosensitivity—St. John's wort
Increase: BUN, potassium
Decrease: sodium, magnesium

Drug/Lab Test
Interference: 17-OHCS, 17-KS, radioimmunoassay, digoxin assay

NURSING CONSIDERATIONS

Assess:
- **Hypokalemia:** polyuria, polydipsia; dysrhythmias, including a U wave on ECG
- **Hyperkalemia:** weakness, fatigue, dyspnea, dysrhythmias, confusion, fatigue
- **Hyponatremia:** headache, weakness, lethargy, confusion, seizures, coma
- Electrolytes (sodium, chloride, potassium), BUN, serum creatinine, ABGs, CBC; potassium must be checked within 3 days, 1 wk, 1 mo × 3, then q3mo; recheck after starting products that alter potassium
- **HF assessment daily:** weight, I&O to determine fluid loss; effect of product may be decreased if used daily; ECG periodically with long-term therapy, breath sounds, edema, B/P
- Signs of metabolic acidosis: drowsiness, restlessness
- Confusion, especially in geriatric patients; take safety precautions if needed

• **Hydration:** skin turgor, thirst, dry mucous membranes

Black Box Warning: Secondary malignancy: assess periodically

• **Beers:** avoid in older adults with heart failure or CCr <30 mL/min
• **Pregnancy/breastfeeding:** use only if benefits outweigh fetal risk; fetal harm has occurred; do not breastfeed, excreted in breast milk
Evaluate:
• **Therapeutic response:** improvement in edema of feet, legs, sacral area daily if medication is being used in HF
Teach patient/family:
• To avoid foods with high potassium content: oranges, bananas, salt substitutes, dried apricots, dates; to avoid potassium salt substitutes
• That drowsiness, ataxia, mental confusion may occur; to observe caution when driving
• To notify prescriber of cramps, diarrhea, lethargy, thirst, headache, skin rash, menstrual abnormalities, deepening voice, breast enlargement
• To take in AM to prevent sleeplessness
• To avoid hazardous activities until reaction is known
• To notify prescriber if pregnancy is planned or suspected; not to breastfeed

TREATMENT OF OVERDOSE:
Lavage if taken orally; monitor electrolytes, administer IV fluids, monitor hydration, renal, CV status

spironolactone/hydrochlorothiazide (Rx)
(speer-on-oh-lak'tone/hye-droe-klor-oh-thye'-a-zide)
Aldactazide
Func. class.: Antihypertensive-diuretic

USES: Treatment of edema in CHF, nephrotic syndrome, cirrhosis of the liver with edema/ascites; treatment of mild-moderate hypertension

CONTRAINDICATIONS
Hypersensitivity to thiazides or sulfonamide-derived drugs; acute renal disease; anuria; renal decompensation; hypercalcemia; hyperkalemia; Addison disease; hepatic disease

DOSAGE AND ROUTES
Edema
• **Adult:** PO Hydrochlorothiazide 25-200 mg daily/spironolactone 25-200 mg daily or divided
Hypertension
• **Adult:** PO Hydrochlorothiazide 50-100 mg daily/spironolactone 50-100 mg daily
Available forms: Tabs 25 mg/25 mg, 50 mg/50 mg

stavudine (d4T) (Rx)
(sta'vyoo-deen)
Func. class.: Antiretroviral
Chem. class.: Nucleoside reverse transcriptase inhibitor (NRTI)

Do not confuse:
Zerit/ZyrTEC

ACTION: Prevents replication of HIV by the inhibition of the enzyme reverse transcriptase; causes DNA chain termination

USES: Treatment of HIV-1 in combination with other antiretrovirals

CONTRAINDICATIONS
Hypersensitivity to this product or zidovudine; didanosine, zalcitabine; severe peripheral neuropathy
Precautions: Breastfeeding, advanced HIV infection, bone marrow suppression, renal disease, peripheral neuropathy, osteoporosis, obesity

Black Box Warning: Pregnancy, hepatic disease, pancreatitis, lactic acidosis

DOSAGE AND ROUTES
• **Adult >60 kg:** PO 40 mg q12hr
• **Adult <60 kg:** PO 30 mg q12hr
• **Child <30 kg:** PO 1 mg/kg q12hr

Side effects: *italics* = common; red = life-threatening

- **Child ≥30 kg, ≤60 kg: PO** 30 mg q12hr
- **Child >60 kg: PO** 40 mg q12hr

Renal dose
- **Adult: PO** CCr 26-50 mL/min, reduce by 50%, give q12hr; CCr 10-25 mL/min, reduce by 50%, give q24hr

Available forms: Caps 15, 20, 30, 40 mg; powder for oral sol 1 mg/mL

Administer:
- With/without meals; absorption does not appear to be lowered when taken with food
- Use after hemodialysis
- Every 12 hr around the clock
- Shake suspension well before using

SIDE EFFECTS

CNS: *Peripheral neuropathy,* insomnia, anxiety, depression, dizziness, confusion, *headache,* chills/fever, malaise, neuropathy

CV: Chest pain, vasodilation, hypertension

EENT: Conjunctivitis, abnormal vision

GI: Hepatotoxicity, *diarrhea, nausea, vomiting,* anorexia, dyspepsia, constipation, stomatitis, pancreatitis

HEMA: Bone marrow suppression, leukopenia, macrocytosis

INTEG: *Rash,* sweating, pruritus, benign neoplasms

MISC: Lactic acidosis, asthenia, lipodystrophy

MS: Myalgia, arthralgia

RESP: Dyspnea, pneumonia, asthma

PHARMACOKINETICS

Excreted in urine, breast milk; peak 1 hr; half-life: elimination 1-1.6 hr

INTERACTIONS

Increase: myelosuppression—other myelosuppressants

Increase: peripheral neuropathy—lithium, dapsone, chloramphenicol didanosine, ethambutol, hydrALAZINE, phenytoin, vinCRIStine, zalcitabine

Increase: stavudine levels—probenecid

Decrease: stavudine effect—methadone, zidovudine

NURSING CONSIDERATIONS

Assess:

Black Box Warning: Lactic acidosis and severe hepatomegaly with steatosis: death may result; monitor LFTs

Black Box Warning: Pancreatitis: severe upper abdominal pain, radiating to back, nausea, vomiting usually when used in combination with didanosine

- Blood studies: WBC, differential, RBC, Hct, HB, platelets, serum amylase, lipase, blood glucose, plasma hepatitis C RNA, pregnancy test, serum cholesterol, serum lipids, hepatitis serology, baseline and periodically
- Renal tests: urinalysis, protein, blood, serum creatinine
- Lipoatrophy/lipodystrophy during treatment
- Bowel pattern before, during treatment
- Weakness, tremors, confusion, dizziness; product may have to be decreased, discontinued
- Viral load, CD4 counts, plasma HIV RNA at baseline and throughout treatment
- **Peripheral neuropathy:** tingling, pain in extremities; discontinue product, may not resolve after treatment is discontinued
- **Pregnancy/breastfeeding:** use only if benefits outweigh fetal risk; register patient in the Antiretroviral Pregnancy Registry, 800-258-4263; do not breastfeed

Evaluate:
- **Therapeutic response:** decreased symptoms of HIV

Teach patient/family:
- **About the signs of peripheral neuropathy:** burning, weakness, pain, prickling feeling in extremities
- That product should not be given with antineoplastics
- That product is not a cure for AIDS but will control symptoms
- To notify prescriber if sore throat, swollen lymph nodes, malaise, fever occur; that other products may be needed to prevent other infections
- That, even with use of product, patient may pass AIDS virus to others

• That follow-up visits are necessary; that serious toxicity may occur; that blood counts must be done q2wk
• That serious product interactions may occur if other medications are ingested; to discuss with prescriber before taking chloramphenicol, dapsone, CISplatin, didanosine, ethambutol, lithium, antifungals, antineoplastics
• To notify prescriber if pregnancy is planned or suspected; that fatal lactic acidosis may occur; to avoid breastfeeding
• That product may cause fainting or dizziness

---

stiripentol (Rx)

(stir-i-pen'tol)

Diacomit

Func. class.: Anticonvulsant—miscellaneous

ACTION: Several possible mechanisms of action, including effects on the gamma-aminobutyric acid (GABA) A receptor and novel inhibition of lactate dehydrogenase

USES: Seizures associated with Dravet syndrome in patients taking clobazam

CONTRAINDICATIONS

Hypersensitivity

Precautions: Abrupt discontinuation, breastfeeding, children, depression, driving or operating machinery, growth inhibition, hepatic disease, neutropenia, PKU, pregnancy, renal disease, suicidal ideation, thrombocytopenia

DOSAGE AND ROUTES

• **Adult/adolescent/child 12-17 yr: PO** 50 mg/kg/day in 2 or 3 divided doses; round to nearest possible dosage, which is usually within 50 to 150 mg of the recommended 50 mg/kg/day. Max 3000 mg/day

Available forms: Caps 250, 500 mg

Administer:
• Use seizure precautions

• Give during a meal, swallow whole with glass of water; do not break or open capsules
• Take missed doses as soon as possible; if it is almost time for the next dose, take only that dose, do not take double doses

SIDE EFFECTS

CNS: Suicidal ideation, depression, drowsiness, dizziness, ataxia, tremor, agitation, fatigue, insomnia, fever
GI: Anorexia, weight loss or gain, nausea, vomiting

HEMA: Neutropenia, thrombocytopenia
MISC: Infection, hypersalivation

PHARMACOKINETICS

Protein binding 99%, half-life 4.5-15 hr, peak 2-3 hr

INTERACTIONS

None known

NURSING CONSIDERATIONS
Assess:
• Monitor weight for increase or decrease; nausea, vomiting, anorexia; closely monitor growth rate, weight in pediatric patients
• **Depression, suicidal ideation:** assess for depression, suicidal thoughts and behaviors any time during treatment; monitor mental status (orientation, mood, behavior) baseline and often during treatment
• **Pregnancy/breastfeeding:** encourage pregnant patients to enroll in the North American Antiepileptic Drug (NAAED) Pregnancy Registry by calling 1-888-233-2334; no data on breastfeeding
• Monitor CBC baseline and periodically during treatment; significant neutropenia and thrombocytopenia may occur
Evaluate:
• **Therapeutic response:** lessening amount and duration of seizures with minimal sedation
Teach patient/family:
• To take only as prescribed, not to skip or double doses, to take at the same times of the day
• To notify all professional health care providers of products used, including OTC, Rx,

herbals, and supplements; not to change products unless approved by prescriber
• To notify health care providers before surgery of product use
• **Depression, suicidal thoughts/behaviors:** that suicidal thoughts and behaviors that may increase with use of this product
• **Pregnancy/breastfeeding:** to inform health care provider if pregnancy is planned or suspected or if breastfeeding
• To avoid driving or hazardous activities until reaction is known; dizziness, drowsiness may occur; resume driving only with prescriber clearance
• That exams and blood work will be needed throughout treatment
• To report excessive sedation, severe nausea/vomiting, depression, suicidal thoughts and behaviors

---

succimer (Rx)

(suks′-si-mer)

Chemet

Func. class.: Antidote

USES: Treatment of lead poisoning in children with serum lead levels >45 mcg/dL

CONTRAINDICATIONS
Hypersensitivity

DOSAGE AND ROUTES
Child/adolescent: PO 10 mg/kg/dose (or 350 mg/m²/dose) q8hr × 5 days, then 10 mg/kg/dose (or 350 mg/m²/dose) q12hr × 14 days; max 500 mg/dose; child <5 yr should be based on body weight
Available forms: Capsules 100 mg

⚠ HIGH ALERT

succinylcholine (Rx)

(suk-sin-ill-koe′leen)

Anectine, Quelicin

Func. class.: Neuromuscular blocker (depolarizing, ultra short)

ACTION: Inhibits transmission of nerve impulses by binding with cholinergic receptor sites, thus antagonizing action of acetylcholine; causes release of histamine

USES: Facilitation of endotracheal intubation, skeletal muscle relaxation during orthopedic manipulations

CONTRAINDICATIONS
Hypersensitivity, malignant hyperthermia, trauma
Precautions: Pregnancy, breastfeeding, geriatric or debilitated patients, cardiac disease, severe burns, fractures (fasciculations may increase damage), electrolyte imbalances, dehydration, neuromuscular/respiratory/cardiac/renal/hepatic disease, collagen diseases, glaucoma, eye surgery, hyperkalemia

Black Box Warning: Children <2 yr, myopathy, rhabdomyolysis

DOSAGE AND ROUTES
• **Adult: IV** 0.3-1.1 mg/kg, max 150 mg, maintenance 0.04-0.07 mg/kg q5-10min as needed; **CONT IV INFUSION** 0.5 to 10 mg/min; titrate to patient's twitch response. Usual dosage range: 2.5 to 4.3 mg/min
• **Child: IV** initially 1-2 mg/kg; **CONT IV INFUSION** not recommended
Available forms: Inj 20, 50, 100 mg/mL; powder for inj 100, 500 mg/vial, 1 g/vial
Administer:
• Give IV or IM; only experienced clinicians familiar with the use of neuromuscular blocking drugs should administer or supervise the use of this product
• Visually inspect parenteral products for particulate matter and discoloration before use
• Monitor heart rate and mechanical ventilator status during use
• Store in refrigerator, powder at room temperature; close tightly
IM route
• Recommended for infants and other patients in whom a suitable vein is not accessible
• Inject into a large muscle, preferably high into the deltoid muscle; aspirate before injection

Rapid IV injection route

• Owing to tachyphylaxis and prolonged apnea, this method is not recommended for prolonged procedures; rapid IV injection of succinylcholine can result in profound bradycardia or asystole in pediatric patients; as with adults, the risk increases with repeated doses; pretreatment with atropine may be needed

• No dilution of injection solution is necessary

• Inject rapidly IV over 10-30 sec

Continuous IV infusion route

• Not recommended for infants and children owing to risk of malignant hyperthermia

• This route is preferred for long surgical procedures

• Dilute succinylcholine to a concentration of 1-2 mg/mL with D$_5$W, D$_5$NS, NS, or 1/6 M sodium lactate injection; 1 g of the powder for injection or 20 mL of a 50-mg/mL solution may be added to 1 L or 500 mL of diluent to give solutions containing 1 or 2 mg/mL, respectively; alternatively, 500 mg of the powder for injection or 10 mL of a 50 mg/mL solution may be added to 500 mL or 250 mL of diluent to give solutions containing 1 or 2 mg/mL, respectively

• Infuse IV at a rate of 2.5 mg/min (range = 0.5-10 mg/min); adjust rate based on patient's response and requirements

Y-site compatibilities: Etomidate, heparin, potassium chloride, propofol, vit B/C

SIDE EFFECTS

CV: *Bradycardia, tachycardia; increased, decreased B/P;* sinus arrest, dysrhythmias, edema

EENT: Increased secretions, intraocular pressure

HEMA: Myoglobulinemia

INTEG: Rash, flushing, pruritus, urticaria

MS: *Weakness, muscle pain, fasciculations, prolonged relaxation, myalgia,* rhabdomyolysis

RESP: *Prolonged apnea,* bronchospasm, cyanosis, respiratory depression, wheezing, dyspnea

SYST: Anaphylaxis, angioedema

PHARMACOKINETICS

Hydrolyzed in blood, excreted in urine (active/inactive metabolites)

IM: Onset 2-3 min, duration 10-30 min

IV: Onset 1 min, peak 2-3 min, duration 6-10 min

INTERACTIONS

Increase: dysrhythmias: theophylline

Increase: neuromuscular blockade—aminoglycosides, β-blockers, cardiac glycosides, clindamycin, lincomycin, procainamide, quiNIDine, local anesthetics, polymyxin antibiotics, lithium, opioids, thiazides, enflurane, isoflurane, magnesium salts, oxytocin

Drug/Herb

• Blocks succinylcholine: melatonin

NURSING CONSIDERATIONS

Assess:

• Electrolyte imbalances (potassium, magnesium); may lead to increased action of product

• VS (B/P, pulse, respirations, airway) until fully recovered; rate, depth, pattern of respirations, strength of hand grip

• I&O ratio; check for urinary retention, frequency, hesitancy

• **Recovery:** decreased paralysis of face, diaphragm, leg, arm, rest of body

• **Allergic reactions:** rash, fever, respiratory distress, pruritus; product should be discontinued

Black Box Warning: Myopathy, rhabdomyolysis: in pediatric patients (rare)

• Assess temperature for malignant hyperthermia, previous reactions to anesthesia or paralytics

• Reassurance if communication is difficult during recovery from neuromuscular blockade; postoperative stiffness is normal, soon subsides

• **Pregnancy/breastfeeding:** use only if clearly needed; cautious use in breastfeeding, excretion unknown

S

Evaluate:
• **Therapeutic response:** paralysis of jaw, eyelid, head, neck, rest of body
Teach patient/family
• Reason for product, expected results

---

sucralfate (Rx)

(soo-kral′fate)

Carafate

Func. class.: Protectant, antiulcer
Chem. class.: Aluminum hydroxide, sulfated sucrose

ACTION: Forms a complex that adheres to ulcer site, adsorbs pepsin

USES: Duodenal ulcer, oral mucositis, stomatitis after radiation of head and neck
Unlabeled uses: Gastric/aphthous ulcers, gastroesophageal reflux, NSAID-induced ulcer prophylaxis, proctitis, stomatitis, stress gastritis prophylaxis, *C. difficile*

CONTRAINDICATIONS

Hypersensitivity
Precautions: Pregnancy, breastfeeding, children, renal failure; hypoglycemia (diabetics)

DOSAGE AND ROUTES
Duodenal ulcers
• **Adult: PO** 1 g qid 1 hr before meals, at bedtime
• **Child: PO** 40-80 mg/kg/day divided
Aphthous ulcer/stomatitis (unlabeled)
• **Adult: PO** 5-10 mL (500 mg-1 g) swished in mouth for several min; spit or swallow qid
Gastric ulcer/NSAID-induced ulcer prophylaxis/esophagitis/GERD (unlabeled)
• **Adult: PO** 1 g qid, 1 hr before meals and at bedtime
Available forms: Tabs 1 g; oral susp 1 g/10 mL
Administer:
PO route

• Do not crush or chew tabs; tabs may be broken or dissolved in water
• Do not take antacids 30 min before or after sucralfate
• On an empty stomach 1 hr before meals or other medications and at bedtime
• Store at room temperature
Side effects
GI: Dry mouth, constipation

PHARMACOKINETICS
PO: Duration up to 6 hr

INTERACTIONS
Decrease: action of tetracyclines, phenytoin, fat-soluble vitamins, digoxin, ketoconazole, theophylline
Decrease: absorption of fluoroquinolones
Decrease: absorption of sucralfate—antacids, cimetidine, raNITIdine

NURSING CONSIDERATIONS
Assess:
• **GI symptoms:** abdominal pain, blood in stools
• **Hypoglycemia:** may occur in patients with diabetes mellitus; monitor blood glucose carefully
Evaluate:
• **Therapeutic response:** absence of pain, GI complaints
Teach patient/family:
• To take on empty stomach
• To take full course of therapy; not to use for >8 wk; to avoid smoking
• To avoid antacids, milk, alkaline water within 1 hr of this product
• To increase fluids, bulk, exercise to lessen constipation

---

sugammadex (Rx)

(soo-gam′ma-dex)

Bridion

Func. class.: Antidote, selective relaxant binder

USES: Reversal of neuromuscular blockade induced by rocuronium/vecuronium in surgery

CONTRAINDICATIONS
Hypersensitivity

DOSAGE AND ROUTES
Routine reversal of rocuronium/vecuronium blockade
• **Adult: IV: Deep block:** 4 mg/kg as a single dose; **moderate block:** 2 mg/kg as a single dose
Immediate reversal of rocuronium-induced blockade
• **Adult: IV:** 16 mg/kg as a single dose given (3 min) after use of a single dose of rocuronium 1.2 mg/kg
Available forms: Injection 200 mg/2 mL, 500 mg/5 mL single-dose vials

---

sulfamethoxazole-trimethoprim (Rx)
(sul-fa-meth-ox′a-zole-trye-meth′oh-prim)
Bactrim, Bactrim DS, Septra, Septra DS, SMZ/TMP, Sulfatrim, Septra Pediatric ✦
Func. class.: Antiinfective
Chem. class.: Sulfonamide—miscellaneous

ACTION: Sulfamethoxazole (SMZ) interferes with the bacterial biosynthesis of proteins by competitive antagonism of PABA when adequate levels are maintained; trimethoprim (TMP) blocks the synthesis of tetrahydrofolic acid; the combination blocks 2 consecutive steps in the bacterial synthesis of essential nucleic acids and protein

USES: UTI, otitis media, acute and chronic prostatitis, shigellosis, chancroid, traveler's diarrhea, *Enterobacter* sp., *Escherichia coli, Haemophilus influenzae (beta-lactamase negative), Haemophilus influenzae (beta-lactamase*

positive), Klebsiella sp., *Morganella morganii, Pneumocystis carinii, Pneumocystis jiroveci, Proteus mirabilis, Proteus* sp., *Proteus vulgaris, Shigella flexneri, Shigella sonnei, Streptococcus pneumoniae;* **may also be effective for** *Acinetobacter baumannii, Actinomadura madurae, Actinomadura pelletieri, Bordetella pertussis, Burkholderia pseudomallei, Cyclospora cayetanensis, Haemophilus ducreyi, Isospora belli, Klebsiella granulomatis, Legionella micdadei, Legionella pneumophila, Listeria monocytogenes, Moraxella catarrhalis, Neisseria gonorrhoeae, Nocardia asteroides, Nocardia brasiliensis, Nocardia otitidiscaviarum, Pediculus capitis, Plasmodium falciparum, Providencia* sp., *Salmonella* sp., *Serratia* sp., *Shigella* sp., *Staphylococcus aureus (MRSA), Staphylococcus aureus (MSSA), Staphylococcus epidermidis, Stenotrophomonas maltophilia, Streptococcus pyogenes* (group A beta-hemolytic streptococci), *Streptomyces somaliensis, Toxoplasma gondii, Vibrio cholerae,* viridans streptococci, *Yersinia enterocolitica*

CONTRAINDICATIONS
Breastfeeding, infants <2 mo; hypersensitivity to trimethoprim or sulfonamides; pregnancy at term, megaloblastic anemia, CCr <15 mL/min
Precautions: Pregnancy, geriatric patients, infants, renal disease, G6PD deficiency, impaired hepatic/renal function, possible folate deficiency, severe allergy, bronchial asthma, UV exposure, porphyria, hyperkalemia, hypothyroidism

DOSAGE AND ROUTES
Based on TMP content
Most infections
• **Adult/child >2 mo:** PO/IV 6-12 mg TMP/kg/day divided q12hr
UTI
• **Adult: PO** 160 mg TMP q12hr × 10-14 days

• **Child:** PO 8 mg/kg TMP/day in 2 divided doses q12hr (treatment): 2 mg/kg/day (prophylaxis)

Otitis media

• **Child:** PO 8 mg/kg TMP/day in 2 divided doses q12hr × 10 days

Chronic bronchitis

• **Adult:** PO 160 mg TMP q12hr × 10-14 days

Serious infections/*Pneumocystis jiroveci* pneumonitis

• **Adult/child:** PO 15-20 mg/kg TMP daily in 4 divided doses q6hr × 14-21 days; **IV** 15-20 mg/kg/day (based on TMP) in 3-4 divided doses for ≤14 days

Renal dose

• **Adult:** PO CCr >30 mL/min, usual dose; CCr 15-30 mL/min, give 50% of usual dose; CCr <15 mL/min, not recommended

Available forms: Tabs 20 mg TMP/100 SMX ✿, 80 mg trimethoprim/400 mg sulfamethoxazole, 160 mg trimethoprim/800 mg sulfamethoxazole; susp 40 mg-200 mg/5 mL, 160 mg-800 mg/20 mL; IV 16 mg/80 mg/mL

Administer:

PO route

• Medication after C&S; repeat C&S after full course of medication

• With resuscitative equipment, EPINEPHrine available; severe allergic reactions may occur

• Without regard to meals

• With full glass of water to maintain adequate hydration; increase fluids to 2 L/day to decrease crystallization in kidneys

• Store in tight, light-resistant container at room temperature

Intermittent IV INFUSION route

• After diluting 5 mL of product/125 mL D₅W, run over 1-1½ hr, if using Septra ADD-Vantage vials dilute each 10-mL vial in ADD-Vantage diluent containers containing 250 mL of D₅W, infuse over 60-90 min, change site q48-72hr

Y-site compatibilities: Acyclovir, aldesleukin, allopurinol, amifostine, amphotericin B cholesteryl, atracurium, aztreonam, cefepime, cyclophosphamide, diltiaZEM, DOXOrubicin liposome, enalaprilat, esmolol, filgrastim, fludarabine, gallium, granisetron, HYDROmorphone, labetalol, LORazepam, magnesium sulfate, melphalan, meperidine, morphine, pancuronium, perphenazine, piperacillin/tazobactam, remifentanil, sargramostim, tacrolimus, teniposide, thiotepa, vecuronium, zidovudine

SIDE EFFECTS

CNS: Headache, insomnia, hallucinations, depression, vertigo, fatigue, anxiety, seizures, drug fever, chills, aseptic meningitis

CV: Allergic myocarditis

EENT: Tinnitus

GI: *Nausea, vomiting, abdominal pain,* stomatitis, hepatitis, glossitis, pancreatitis, diarrhea, enterocolitis, anorexia, CDAD

GU: Renal failure, toxic nephrosis; increased BUN, creatinine; crystalluria

HEMA: Leukopenia, neutropenia, thrombocytopenia, agranulocytosis, hemolytic anemia, hypoprothrombinemia, Henoch-Schönlein purpura, methemoglobinemia, eosinophilia

INTEG: Rash, dermatitis, urticaria, Stevens-Johnson syndrome, erythema, photosensitivity, pain, inflammation at inj site, toxic epidermal necrolysis, erythema multiforme

RESP: Cough, SOB

SYST: Anaphylaxis, SLE

PHARMACOKINETICS

PO: Rapidly absorbed; peak 1-4 hr; half-life 8-13 hr; excreted in urine (metabolites and unchanged), breast milk; crosses placenta; 68% bound to plasma proteins; TMP achieves high levels in prostatic tissue and fluid

INTERACTIONS

Increase: thrombocytopenia—thiazide diuretics

Increase: potassium levels—potassium-sparing diuretics, potassium supplements

Increase: hypoglycemic response—sulfonylurea agents

Increase: anticoagulant effects—oral anticoagulants
Increase: levels of dofetilide
Increase: crystalluria—methenamine
Increase: bone marrow depressant effects—methotrexate
Decrease: hepatic clearance of phenytoin, CYP2C9, CYP3A4 inducers
Decrease: response—cycloSPORINE
Drug/Lab Test
Increase: creatinine, bilirubin
Decrease: HB, platelets

NURSING CONSIDERATIONS
Assess:
• I&O ratio; note color, character, pH of urine if product administered for UTI
• Renal studies: BUN, creatinine, urinalysis with long-term therapy
• Type of infection; obtain C&S before starting therapy
• Blood dyscrasias, skin rash, fever, sore throat, bruising, bleeding, fatigue, joint pain
• **Allergic reaction:** rash, dermatitis, urticaria, pruritus, dyspnea, bronchospasm; product should be discontinued at 1st sign of rash; AIDS patients more susceptible, identify if patient has a sulfa allergy
Pregnancy/breastfeeding: use only if benefits outweigh fetal risk, may be harmful to fetus, do not breastfeed
Evaluate:
• **Therapeutic response:** absence of pain, fever; C&S negative
Teach patient/family:
• To take each oral dose with full glass of water to prevent crystalluria; to drink 8-10 glasses of water/day; to take product on an empty stomach 1 hr before meals, 2 hr after meals, not to treat diarrhea with OTC product, to notify health care professional if diarrhea lasts more than 2 days
• To complete full course of treatment to prevent superinfection
• To avoid sunlight; to use sunscreen to prevent burns
• To avoid OTC medications (aspirin, vit C) unless directed by prescriber
• To notify prescriber if skin rash, sore throat, fever, mouth sores, unusual bruising, bleeding occur; to notify prescriber

of CNS effects: anxiety, depression, hallucinations, seizures

sulfaSALAzine (Rx)
(sul-fa-sal′a-zeen)
Azulfidine, Azulfidine EN-tabs, Salazopyrin ♣, Salazopyrin EN-Tabs ♣
Func. class.: GI antiinflammatory, antirheumatic (DMARD)
Chem. class.: Sulfonamide

Do not confuse:
sulfaSALAzine/sulfiSOXAZOLE

ACTION: Prodrug to deliver sulfapyridine and 5-aminosalicylic acid to colon; antiinflammatory in connective tissue also

USES: Ulcerative colitis; RA; juvenile RA (Azulfidine EN-tabs)
Unlabeled uses: Crohn's disease
CONTRAINDICATIONS
Pregnancy at term, children <2 yr; hypersensitivity to sulfonamides or salicylates; intestinal, urinary obstruction; porphyria
Precautions: Pregnancy, breastfeeding, impaired renal/hepatic function, severe allergy, bronchial asthma, megaloblastic anemia
DOSAGE AND ROUTES
Ulcerative colitis
• **Adult: PO** 3-4 g/day in divided doses; maintenance 2 g/day in divided doses q6hr
• **Child ≥2 yr: PO** 40-60 mg/kg/day in 4-6 divided doses, then 30 mg/kg/day in 4 doses, max 2 g/day
Rheumatoid arthritis
• **Adult: PO** 0.5-1 g/day, then increase daily dose by 500 mg/wk to 2 g/day in 2-3 divided doses, max 3 gm/day
Juvenile rheumatoid arthritis
• **Child ≥6 yr: PO** 30-50 mg/kg/24 hr in 2 divided doses, max 4 gm/day
Renal dose
• Modify dose based on renal impairment, response
Crohn's disease (unlabeled)
• **Adult: PO** 1 g/15 kg, max 5 g/day

Available forms: Tabs 500 mg; oral susp 250 mg/5 mL; del rel tabs 500 mg

Administer:
• Do not break, crush, chew del rel tabs
• With full glass of water to maintain adequate hydration; increase fluids to 2 L/day to decrease crystallization in kidneys
• Total daily dose in evenly spaced doses and after meals to help minimize GI intolerance
• Store in tight, light-resistant container at room temperature

SIDE EFFECTS

CNS: Headache, neuropathy
GI: *Nausea, vomiting, abdominal pain,* stomatitis, hepatitis, glossitis, pancreatitis, diarrhea
GU: Orange-colored urine
HEMA: Leukopenia, neutropenia, thrombocytopenia, agranulocytosis, hemolytic anemia
INTEG: Rash, dermatitis, urticaria, Stevens-Johnson syndrome, erythema, photosensitivity
SYST: Anaphylaxis

PHARMACOKINETICS

PO: Partially absorbed; peak 1½-6 hr; duration 6-12 hr; half-life 6 hr; excreted in urine as sulfaSALAzine (15%), sulfapyridine (60%), 5-aminosalicylic acid, metabolites (20%-33%); excreted in breast milk; crosses placenta

INTERACTIONS

Increase: leukopenia risk—thiopurines (azaTHIOprine, mercaptopurine)
Increase: hypoglycemic response—oral hypoglycemics
Increase: anticoagulant effects—oral anticoagulants
Decrease: effect of cycloSPORINE, digoxin, folic acid
Decrease: renal excretion of methotrexate
Drug/Food
Decrease: iron/folic acid absorption
Drug/Lab Test
False positive: urinary glucose test

NURSING CONSIDERATIONS

Assess:
• **Ulcerative colitis, proctitis, other inflammatory bowel disease:** character, amount, consistency of stools; abdominal pain, cramping, blood, mucus
• **Rheumatoid arthritis:** assess mobility, joint swelling, pain, ability to complete activities of daily living
• Renal studies: BUN, creatinine, urinalysis (long-term therapy)
• **Blood dyscrasias:** skin rash, fever, sore throat, bruising, bleeding, fatigue, joint pain; monitor CBC before therapy and q3mo
• **Allergic reaction:** rash, dermatitis, urticaria, pruritus, dyspnea, bronchospasm; identify sulfa, salicylate allergy
• **Pregnancy/breastfeeding:** use only if clearly needed; cautious use in breastfeeding, excreted in breast milk

Evaluate:
• **Therapeutic response:** absence of fever, mucus in stools, pain in joints

Teach patient/family:
• To take each oral dose with full glass of water to prevent crystalluria
• That contact lenses, urine, skin may be yellow-orange
• To avoid sunlight or use sunscreen to prevent burns
• To notify prescriber of skin rash, sore throat, fever, mouth sores, unusual bruising, bleeding
• That decreased sperm production may occur; that it resolves after completion of medication
• To notify prescriber if enteric-coated tablets are seen in stool; discontinue if present

---

SUMAtriptan (Rx)

(soo-ma-trip′tan)

Imitrex, Imitrex STAT-Dose, Onzetra Xsail, Tosymra, Zembrace SymTouch

Func. class.: Antimigraine agent
Chem. class.: 5-HT$_{1B/D}$ receptor agonist, abortive agent, triptan

---

Do not confuse:
SUMAtriptan/somatropin

ACTION: Binds selectively to the vascular 5-HT$_1$B/D receptor subtype; exerts antimigraine effect; causes vasoconstriction in cranial arteries

USES: Acute treatment of migraine with/without aura and cluster headache

CONTRAINDICATIONS
Angina pectoris, history of MI, documented silent ischemia, Prinzmetal's angina, ischemic heart disease, IV use, concurrent ergotamine-containing preparations, uncontrolled hypertension, hypersensitivity, basilar or hemiplegic migraine
Precautions: Pregnancy, breastfeeding, children <18 yr, geriatric patients, postmenopausal women, men >40 yr, risk factors for CAD, hypercholesterolemia, obesity, diabetes, impaired renal/hepatic function, overuse

DOSAGE AND ROUTES
• **Adult: SUBCUT** ≤6 mg; may repeat in 1 hr; max 12 mg/24 hr; **PO** 25 mg with fluids, if no relief in 2 hr, give another dose, max 200 mg/day; **NASAL** single dose of 5, 10, or 20 mg in 1 nostril, may repeat in 2 hr, max 40 mg/24 hr; 1 puff each nostril q2hr; **nasal powder** 11 mg in each nostril may repeat after 2 hr
Hepatic dose
• **Adult: PO** 25 mg; if no response after 2 hr, give ≤50 mg
Available forms: Inj 4, 6 mg/0.5 mL; tabs 25, 50, 100 mg; nasal spray 5 mg/100 mcl-U; dose spray device 20 mg/100 mcl-U, prefilled syringes 6 mg/0.5-mL vials, 4 mg/0.5 mL, 3 mg/0.5 mL, 6 mg/0.5 mL autoinjector
Administer:
PO route
• Swallow tabs whole; do not break, crush, or chew
• Take tabs with fluids as soon as symptoms appear; may take a 2nd dose >4 hr; max 200 mg/24 hr

SUBCUT route
• SUBCUT only just below the skin; avoid IM or IV administration; use only for actual migraine attack
• Give 1st dose supervised by medical staff to patients with coronary artery disease or those at risk for CAD
Nasal route
• May give as 2 sprays of 5 mg in 1 nostril or 1 spray in each nostril (10 mg)
Nasal powder: fully press and release button, insert into nostril with tight seal, rotate mouthpiece to place in mouth, blow forcefully to deliver powder, discard nosepiece repeat

SIDE EFFECTS
CNS: *Tingling, hot sensation, burning, feeling of pressure, tightness, numbness, dizziness, sedation,* headache, anxiety, fatigue, cold sensation
CV: *Flushing,* MI, hypo/hypertension
EENT: Throat, mouth, nasal discomfort; vision changes
GI: Abdominal discomfort
INTEG: Inj-site reaction, sweating
MS: *Weakness, neck stiffness,* myalgia
RESP: Chest tightness, pressure

PHARMACOKINETICS
Onset of pain relief 10 min-2 hr, peak 2-4 hr, duration 24 hr; nasal onset 60 min, peak 2 hr; 10%-20% protein binding; metabolized in liver (metabolite); excreted in urine, feces; nasal spray half-life 2 hr

INTERACTIONS
Increase: vasospastic effects: ergot, ergot derivatives
Increase: serotonin syndrome—SSRIs, SNRIs, serotonin-receptor agonists, sibutramine
Increase: SUMAtriptan effect—MAOIs
Drug/Herb
• **Increase:** serotonin syndrome: SAM-e, St. John's wort

NURSING CONSIDERATIONS
Assess:
• **Migraine:** type of pain, aura; alleviating, aggravating factors; sensitivity to light, noise

S

- Increase: **serotonin syndrome:** delirium, coma, agitation, diaphoresis, hypertension, fever, tremors; may resemble neuroleptic malignant syndrome in patients taking SSRIs, SNRIs
- B/P; signs, symptoms of coronary vasospasms, ECG
- Tingling, hot sensation, burning, feeling of pressure, numbness, flushing, inj-site reaction
- Stress level, activity, recreation, coping mechanisms
- Neurologic status: LOC, blurring vision, nausea, vomiting, tingling in extremities preceding headache
- Ingestion of tyramine foods (pickled products, beer, wine, aged cheese), food additives, preservatives, colorings, artificial sweeteners, chocolate, caffeine, which may precipitate these types of headaches
- Renal function, urinary output
- Quiet, calm environment with decreased stimuli: noise, bright light, excessive talking
- **Pregnancy/breastfeeding:** use only if benefits outweigh fetal risk; avoid breastfeeding

Evaluate:
- **Therapeutic response:** decrease in frequency, severity of migraine

Teach patient/family:
- To report chest pain, tightness; sudden, severe abdominal pain; swelling of eyelids, face, lips; skin rash to prescriber immediately
- To notify prescriber if pregnancy is planned or suspected; to use contraception while taking product
- **Risk of medication overuse:** do not use for abortive headache treatments more than 10 days/mo (ergotamines, triptans, opioids, or combinations)
- **Nasal spray:** to use 1 spray in 1 nostril; may repeat if headache returns; not to repeat if pain continues after 1st dose
- To have a dark, quiet environment
- To avoid hazardous activities if dizziness, drowsiness occur
- To avoid alcohol; may increase headache
- To use SUBCUT inj technique, nasal route if prescribed

- That product does not reduce number of migraines; to be used for acute migraine; to use as symptoms occur
- **Nasal powder:** Use in each nostril using nosepiece and mouthpiece
- **SUBCUT:** provide pamphlet from manufacturer, review with patient

---

sumatriptan/naproxen (Rx)

(soo-ma-trip'tan/na-proks'-en)

Treximet

Func. class.: Antimigraine, NSAIDs

USES: Acute treatment of migraine with/without aura in adults/child ≥12 yr

CONTRAINDICATIONS

Hypersensitivity to sumatriptan, naproxen, or any component; asthma, urticaria, or allergic-type reactions after taking aspirin or other NSAIDs, angina pectoris, MI, Prinzmetal angina, CABG; Wolff-Parkinson-White syndrome stroke, hemiplegic/basilar migraine, PVD, uncontrolled hypertension; use within 24 hr of ergots or another 5-HT$_1$ agonist; use within 2 wk of a MAOI-A; third trimester of pregnancy; severe hepatic disease

DOSAGE AND ROUTES

- **Adult: PO** Sumatriptan 85 mg/naproxen 500 mg, may repeat after 2 hr, max Sumatriptan 170 mg/naproxen 1000 mg/24 hr

Available forms: Tabs 85 mg/500 mg

⚠ HIGH ALERT

SUNITinib (Rx)

(soo-nit'-in-ib)

Sutent

Func. class.: Antineoplastic—miscellaneous

Chem. class.: Multitargeted Protein-tyrosine kinase inhibitor

---

ACTION: Inhibits multiple receptor tyrosine kinases (RTKs); some are responsible for tumor growth

USES: Gastrointestinal stromal tumors (GIST) after disease progression or intolerance to imatinib; advanced renal carcinoma, pancreatic neuroendocrine tumors (pNET) in patients with unresectable locally advanced/metastatic disease

CONTRAINDICATIONS
Pregnancy, breastfeeding, hypersensitivity
Precautions: Children, geriatric patients, active infections, QT prolongation, torsades de pointes, stroke, heart failure

Black Box Warning: Hepatotoxicity

DOSAGE AND ROUTES
Gastrointestinal stromal tumors (GIST)/renal cell cancer
• **Adult: PO** 50 mg/day × 4 wk, then 2 wk off; may increase or decrease dose by 12.5 mg; if administered with CYP3A4 inducers, give 87.5 mg/day; if given with CYP3A4 inhibitors, give 37.5 mg/day
Pancreatic neuroendocrine (pNET)
• **Adult: PO** 37.5 mg daily continuously, increase or decrease by 12.5 mg based on tolerance, avoid potent CYP3A4 inhibitors/inducers; if used with CYP3A4 inhibitors, decrease SUNItinib dose to minimum of 25 mg/day; if used with CYP3A4 inducers, increase SUNItinib to max 62.5 mg/day
Available forms: Caps 12.5, 25, 37.5, 50 mg
Administer:
• With meal and large glass of water to decrease GI symptoms
• Store at 25° C (77° F)

SIDE EFFECTS
CNS: Headache, dizziness, insomnia, fatigue, reversible posterior leukoencephalopathy syndrome (RPLS)
CV: Hypertension, left ventricular dysfunction, QT prolongation, torsades de pointes, thrombotic microangiopathy, cardiac arrest, thromboembolism
ENDO: Hypo/hyperthyroidism
GI: *Nausea,* hepatotoxicity, vomiting, dyspepsia, *anorexia, abdominal pain,* altered taste, *constipation,* stomatitis, mucositis, pancreatitis, diarrhea, GI bleeding/perforation
GU: Nephrotic syndrome
HEMA: Neutropenia, thrombocytopenia, hemolytic anemia, leukopenia
INTEG: *Rash, yellow skin discoloration,* depigmentation of hair or skin, alopecia, necrotizing fasciitis, pyoderma gangrenosum
MS: Pain, arthralgia, myalgia, myopathy, rhabdomyolysis
RESP: Cough, dyspnea, pulmonary embolism
SYST: Bleeding, electrolyte abnormalities, hand-foot syndrome, serious infection, tumor lysis syndrome

PHARMACOKINETICS
Protein binding 95%; metabolized by CYP3A4; excreted in feces, small amount in urine; peak levels 6-12 hr; half-life 40-60 hr (SUNItinib); active metabolite 80-110 hr

INTERACTIONS
Increase: microangiopathic hemolytic anemia—bevacizumab; avoid concurrent use
Increase: QT prolongation—class IA/III antidysrhythmics, some phenothiazines, β agonists, local anesthetics, tricyclics, haloperidol, chloroquine, droperidol, pentamidine; CYP3A4 inhibitors (amiodarone, clarithromycin, erythromycin, telithromycin), arsenic trioxide; CYP3A4 substrates (methadone, pimozide, QUEtiapine, quiNIDine, risperiDONE, ziprasidone)
Increase: hepatotoxicity—acetaminophen
Increase: plasma concentrations of simvastatin, calcium channel blockers, warfarin; avoid use with warfarin, use low-molecular-weight anticoagulants instead
Decrease: SUNItinib concentrations—dexamethasone, phenytoin, carBAMazepine, rifAMPin, PHENobarbital
Drug/Herb
Decrease: SUNItinib concentration—St. John's wort
Drug/Food
Increase: plasma concentrations—grapefruit juice

S

Side effects: *italics* = common; red = life-threatening

NURSING CONSIDERATIONS
Assess:

• ANC and platelets; if ANC <1 × 10⁹/L and/or platelets <50 × 10⁹/L, stop until ANC >1.5 × 10⁹/L and platelets >75 × 10⁹/L; if ANC <0.5 × 10⁹/L and/or platelets <10 × 10⁹/L, reduce dosage by 200 mg; if cytopenia continues, reduce dosage by another 100 mg; if cytopenia continues for 4 wk, stop product until ANC ≥1 × 10⁹/L

• **CV status:** hypertension, QT prolongation can occur; monitor left ventricular ejection fraction (LVEF), MUGA at baseline, periodically; ECG

• **Renal toxicity:** if bilirubin >3 × IULN, withhold SUNItinib until bilirubin levels return to <1.5 × IULN; electrolytes

> **Black Box Warning: Hepatotoxicity:** monitor LFTs before treatment, monthly; if liver transaminases >5 × IULN, withhold SUNItinib until transaminase levels return to <2.5 × IULN

• **Nephrotic syndrome:** monitor urinalysis and proteinuria

• **Hand-foot syndrome:** redness, swelling, numbness, desquamation on palms and soles of the feet may occur days to months after use; if these occur, product should be discontinued

• **HF:** adrenal insufficiency in those experiencing trauma

• **QT prolongation:** those taking CYP3A4 inhibitors, those with sinus bradycardia, cardiac disease or electrolyte disturbances are at greater risk; monitor electrolytes, especially magnesium, potassium; monitor ECG

• **Osteonecrosis of the jaw:** dental disease or use of bisphosphonates may increase risk; invasive dental procedures should be avoided

• **Tumor lysis syndrome:** usually in renal cell carcinoma or GI stromal tumor; may be fatal, monitor for hyperkalemia, severe muscle weakness, hypocalcemia, hyperphosphatemia, myopathy, hyperuricemia; monitor serum electrolytes before each dose

• Bleeding: epistaxis; rectal, gingival, upper GI, genital, wound bleeding; tumor-related hemorrhage may occur rapidly

• Nutritious diet with iron, vitamin supplement, low fiber, few dairy products

• **Pregnancy/breastfeeding:** do not use in pregnancy, breastfeeding

Evaluate:

• **Therapeutic response:** decrease in size of tumor

Teach patient/family:

• **To report adverse reactions immediately:** SOB, bleeding

• About reason for treatment, expected result

• That many adverse reactions may occur: high B/P, bleeding, mouth swelling, taste change, skin discoloration, depigmentation of hair/skin

• To avoid persons with known upper respiratory infections; that immunosuppression is common

• To avoid grapefruit juice

• To report if pregnancy is planned or suspected or if breastfeeding

---

⚠ HIGH ALERT

suvorexant (Rx)
(soo'voe-rex'ant)

Belsomra

Func. class.: Psychotropic—sedative/hypnotic, anxiolytic

Chem. class.: Orexin receptor antagonist

Controlled Substance Schedule IV

ACTION: Suvorexant alters the signaling of neurotransmitters called orexins, which are responsible for regulating the sleep-wake cycle

USES: The treatment of insomnia characterized by difficulties with sleep onset and/or sleep maintenance

---

CONTRAINDICATIONS

Narcolepsy, hypersensitivity

Precautions: Preexisting respiratory disease, COPD, breastfeeding, pregnancy, labor, geriatrics, hepatic disease, sleep apnea, substance abuse, alcohol use, suicidal ideation, mental changes, depression

DOSAGE AND ROUTES

• **Adult: PO** 10 mg every night within 30 min of going to bed, and with ≥7 hr remaining before the planned time of awakening, may increase to maximum 20 mg every night

Available forms: Tabs 5, 10, 15, 20 mg

Administer:

• Give 30 min before bedtime
• Effect may be delayed if taken with food, take on empty stomach for faster effect

SIDE EFFECTS

CNS: Amnesia, suicidal ideation, anxiety, dizziness, drowsiness, hallucinations, headache, memory impairment, sleep paralysis

GI: Diarrhea

PHARMACOKINETICS

High protein binding, peak 2 hr, half-life 12 hr, excreted by feces (66%), urine (23%)

INTERACTIONS

Avoid use with CYP3A inhibitors

Increase: effects of both products—CNS depressants

Decrease: suvorexant effect—CYP3A inducers

Drug/Herb:

Increase: suvorexant effect—kava, valerian, melatonin

NURSING CONSIDERATIONS

Assess:

• **Sleeping patterns:** waking in the night, inability to fall asleep or stay asleep, amnesia
• **Beers:** avoid in older adults with delirium or at high risk for delirium
• **Pregnancy/breastfeeding:** use only if benefits outweigh fetal risk; cautious use in breastfeeding, excretion unknown

Evaluate:

• **Therapeutic response:** normalized sleeping patterns

Teach patient/family:

• To use on an empty stomach for faster effect
• To report immediately suicidal thoughts/behaviors or if depression worsens
• To avoid use with other products unless approved by prescriber
• To notify provider if pregnancy is planned or suspected, or if breastfeeding
• That complex sleep behaviors may occur (sleep driving, sleep eating)
• That daytime drowsiness or dizziness may occur; to avoid hazardous activities until response is known
• To avoid grapefruit juice

S

tacrolimus (Rx) (PO, IV) (NTI)

(tak-row'lim-us)

Advagraf ✦, Envarsus ER, Envarsus PA ✦, Astagraf XL, Prograf

tacrolimus (TOPICAL) (Rx)

Protopic

Func. class.: Immunosuppressant, calcineurin inhibitor

Chem. class.: Macrolide, calcineurin inhibitor

Do not confuse:

Prograf/PROzac/Proscar
tacrolimus/tamsulosin

ACTION: Produces immunosuppression by inhibiting T-lymphocytes

USES: Organ transplants to prevent rejection; **topical:** atopic dermatitis

CONTRAINDICATIONS

Children <2 yr (topical); hypersensitivity to this product or to some kinds of castor oil (IV); long-term use (topical)

Precautions: Pregnancy, breastfeeding, severe renal/hepatic disease; diabetes mellitus, hyperkalemia, hyperuricemia, hypertension, acute bronchospasm, African-American patients, heart failure, seizures, QT prolongation

Black Box Warning: Children <12, lymphomas, infection, neoplastic disease, neonates, infants, requires a specialized setting, requires an experienced clinician; liver transplant (ext rel)

DOSAGE AND ROUTES—NTI

Kidney transplant rejection prophylaxis

• **Adult:** IV 0.03-0.05 mg/kg/day as **CONT INFUSION,** begin within 24 hr of transplantation, delay until renal function has recovered; **PO** 0.2 mg/kg/day in 2 divided doses q12hr with azaTHIOprine

and corticosteroids, may give first dose within 24 hr of transplantation, delay until renal function has recovered; **EXT REL CAPS** 0.1 mg/kg daily preoperatively on empty stomach, 1st dose 12 hr before reperfusion and 0.2 mg/kg once daily postoperatively, 1st dose within 12 hr of reperfusion but ≥4 hr after preoperative dose in combination with mycophenolate and corticosteroids

Liver transplant rejection prophylaxis

• **Adult:** PO 0.1-0.15 mg/kg/day in 2 divided doses q12hr; give no sooner than 6 hr after transplantation; IV 0.03-0.05 mg/kg/day as **CONT INFUSION;** give no sooner than 6 hr after transplantation

Heart transplant rejection prophylaxis

• **Adult:** PO 0.075 mg/kg/day in 2 divided doses q12hr; give no sooner than 6 hr after transplantation; IV 0.01 mg/kg/day as **CONT INFUSION;** give no sooner than 6 hr after transplantation

Atopic dermatitis

• **Adult:** TOP use 0.03% or 0.1% ointment; apply bid × 7 days after clearing of signs

• **Child ≥2-15 yr:** TOP 0.03% ointment; apply bid × 7 days after clearing of signs

Graft-versus-host disease (orphan drug) (unlabeled)

• **Adult/adolescent:** IV 0.1 mg/kg/day in 2 divided doses given with other immunosuppressants or PO 0.3 mg/kg/day in 2 divided doses

• **Child:** CONT IV INFUSION 0.05 mg/kg/dose twice daily

Available forms: Inj 5 mg/mL; caps 0.5, 1, 5 mg; ext rel cap (Astragraf XL) 0.5, 1, 3, 5 mg; ointment 0.03%, 0.1%; ext rel cap (Envarsus XR) 0.75, 1.4 mg; granules for oral suspension 0.2, 1 mg unit dose packets

Administer

PO route

Conventional immediate-release capsules

• Give consistently with or without food

Extended-release capsules (Astagraf XL)
• Take in the AM, preferably on an empty stomach at least 1 hr before a meal or at least 2 hr after a meal
• Swallow whole; do not chew, divide, or crush capsules
• Do not administer with an alcoholic beverage
• If a dose is missed up to 14 hr from the scheduled time, take the dose; if a dose is missed at >14 hr from the scheduled time, skip the dose and take the next dose at the regularly scheduled time

Extended-release tablets (Envarsus XR)
• Take in the AM, preferably on an empty stomach at least 1 hr before a meal or at least 2 hr after a meal
• Swallow whole; do not chew, divide, or crush capsules
• Do not administer with an alcoholic beverage
• If a dose is missed up to 15 hr from the scheduled time, take the dose; if a dose is missed at >15 hr from the scheduled time, skip the dose and take the next dose at the regularly scheduled time

Topical route
• Apply thin layers to affected skin only; rub in gently
• Do not use occlusive dressings
• Use on small area of skin
• Topical ointment carries risk of developing cancer; use only when other options have failed

IV route
• Visually inspect for particulate matter and discoloration before use
• Because of the risk of hypersensitivity reactions, IV use should be reserved for those who cannot take tacrolimus orally. PO should replace IV therapy as soon as possible
• Observe patients for 30 min after beginning the infusion and frequently thereafter for possible hypersensitivity reactions
• Do not mix or infuse with solutions with a pH of 9 or more (acyclovir or ganciclovir)

Dilution
• The concentrate for injection must be diluted with NS or D₅W injection to a final concentration between 0.004 mg/mL and 0.02 mg/mL
• Prepare solutions in polyethylene or glass containers to allow storage for 24 hr; do not use polyvinyl chloride (PVC) containers, stability is decreased and the polyoxyl 60 hydrogenated castor oil in the formulation may leach phthalates from PVC containers

Continuous IV infusion
• Give through non-PVC tubing to minimize the potential for drug adsorption onto the tubing
• Infuse the required daily dose of the diluted IV solution over 24 hr

Y-site compatibilities: Alemtuzumab, alfentanil, amifostine, amikacin, aminophylline, amiodarone, amphotericin B colloidal, amphotericin B liposome, anidulafungin, argatroban, atracurium, aztreonam, benztropine, bivalirudin, bleomycin, bumetanide, buprenorphine, busulfan, butorphanol, calcium acetate/chloride/gluconate, CARBOplatin, carmustine, caspofungin, ceFAZolin, cefoperazone, cefotaxime, cefoTEtan, cefOXitin, cefTAZidime, ceftizoxime, cefTRIAXone, cefuroxime, chloramphenicol, chlorproMAZINE, cimetidine, ciprofloxacin, cisatracurium, CISplatin, clindamycin, cyclophosphamide, cycloSPORINE, cytarabine, DACTINomycin, DAPTOmycin, dexamethasone, dexmedetomidine, dexrazoxane, digoxin, diltiaZEM, diphenhydrAMINE, DOBUTamine, DOCEtaxel, dolasetron, DOPamine, doripenem, doxacurium, DOXOrubicin hydrochloride, doxycycline, droperidol, enalaprilat, ePHEDrine, EPINEPHrine, epiRUBicin, ertapenem, erythromycin, esmolol, etoposide, etoposide phosphate, famotidine, fenoldopam, fentaNYL, fluconazole, fludarabine, foscarnet, fosphenytoin, gemcitabine, gentamicin, glycopyrrolate, granisetron, haloperidol, heparin, hydrALAZINE, hydrocortisone, HYDROmorphone, IDArubicin, ifosfamide, imipenem/cilastatin, inamrinone, insulin, isoproterenol, ketorolac, labetalol, leucovorin, levoFLOXacin, levorphanol, lidocaine, linezolid, LORazepam, magnesium sulfate, mannitol, mechlorethamine, meperidine, meropenem, mesna, metaraminol, methotrexate, methyldopa, methylPREDNISolone, metoclopramide, metoprolol, metroNIDAZOLE, micafungin, midazolam, milrinone, mitoMYcin, mitoXANTRONE, mivacurium, morphine, multivitamins, nafcillin, nalbuphine, naloxone, nesiritide, niCARdipine, nitroglycerin, nitroprusside, norepinephrine, octreotide, ondansetron, oxacillin, oxaliplatin, oxytocin, PACLitaxel, palonosetron, pancuronium, PEMEtrexed, penicillin G, pentamidine, pentazocine, perphenazine, phentolamine, phenylephrine, piperacillin/tazobactam, potassium chloride/phosphates, procainamide, prochlorperazine, promethazine, propranolol, quinupristin/dalfopristin, raNITIdine, remifentanil, rocuronium, sodium acetate/bicarbonate/phosphates, streptozocin, succinylcholine, SUFentanil, teniposide, theophylline, thiotepa, ticarcillin/clavulanate, tigecycline, tirofiban, tobramycin, tolazoline, trimethobenzamide, vancomycin, vasopressin, vecuronium, verapamil, vinCRIStine, vinorelbine, voriconazole, zidovudine, zoledronic acid

SIDE EFFECTS

CNS: *Tremors, headache,* insomnia, paresthesia, chills, fever, seizures, BK virus-associated nephropathy, coma, posttransplant lymphoproliferative disorder (PTLD)
CV: Hypertension, myocardial hypertrophy, prolonged QTc, cardiomyopathy
EENT: Blurred vision, photophobia
GI: Nausea, vomiting, diarrhea, constipation, GI bleeding, GI perforation
GU: UTIs, albuminuria, hematuria, proteinuria, renal failure, hemolytic uremic syndrome
HEMA: Anemia, leukocytosis, thrombocytopenia, purpura
INTEG: Rash, flushing, itching, alopecia
META: Hyperglycemia, hyperuricemia, hypokalemia, hypomagnesemia, hyperkalemia
MS: Back pain, muscle spasms

RESP: Pleural effusion, atelectasis, dyspnea, interstitial lung disease, cough, asthma, bronchitis, pneumonia
SYST: Anaphylaxis, infection, malignancy, chills, fever

PHARMACOKINETICS
PO: Extensively metabolized, half-life 34.2 hr healthy, 11.7 hr liver transplant hr, 99% protein binding

INTERACTIONS
Increase: hyperkalemia -ACE inhibitors, Angiotensin II receptor blockers, potassium-sparing diuretics
Increase: QT prolongation—class IA/III antidysrhythmics, some phenothiazines, β agonists, local anesthetics, tricyclics, haloperidol, chloroquine, droperidol, pentamidine; CYP3A4 inhibitors (amiodarone, clarithromycin, erythromycin, telithromycin, troleandomycin), arsenic trioxide; CYP3A4 substrates (methadone, pimozide, QUEtiapine, quiNIDine, risperiDONE, ziprasidone); do not use together
Increased absorption, decrease tacrolimus dose by ⅔ with posaconazole, or voriconazole; monitor blood levels closely: CYP3A4 inhitors, strong (clarithromycin, ketoconazole, itraconazole, nefazodone, posaconazole, voriconazole):
Increase: toxicity—aminoglycosides, CISplatin, cycloSPORINE
Increase: blood levels—antifungals, calcium channel blockers, cimetidine, danazol, mycophenolate, mofetil
Decrease: blood levels—carBAMazepine, PHENobarbital, phenytoin, rifamycin
Decrease: effect of live virus vaccines
Drug/Herb
Decrease: immunosuppression—astragalus, echinacea, melatonin
Decreased tacrolimus levels: St. John's wort; avoid using together
Drug/Food
Increase: effect—grapefruit juice
Decreased absorption: food
Drug/Lab Test
Increase: glucose, BUN, creatinine
Increase or decrease: LFTs, potassium
Decrease: magnesium, HB, platelets

NURSING CONSIDERATIONS
Assess:

• **Blood studies:** HB, WBC, platelets during treatment monthly; if leukocytes <3000/mm³ or platelets <100,000/mm³, discontinue or reduce; decreased hemoglobin level may indicate bone marrow suppression

• **Hepatic studies:** alk phos, AST, ALT, amylase, bilirubin; for hepatotoxicity: dark urine, jaundice, itching, light-colored stools; product should be discontinued

• **Atopic dermatitis:** Check lesions baseline and during treatment

• Assess for castor oil allergy (HCO-60); do not use if present

• Serum creatinine/BUN, serum electrolytes, lipid profile, serum tacrolimus concentration

• **Anaphylaxis:** rash, pruritus, wheezing, laryngeal edema; stop infusion, initiate emergency procedures

• **QT prolongation:** ECG, ejection fraction; assess for chest pain, palpitations, dyspnea

• **PTLD:** Malaise, fever, weight loss, night sweats, decreased appetite can be fatal, allogenic hematopoietic stem cell transplant (HSCT) may be required

• **Blood level monitoring:** maintain tacrolimus whole blood (7-20 ng/mL) then 5-15 ng/mL for 1 yr in kidney transplant; 1-3 mo maintain whole blood at 8-20 ng/mL, then 6-18 ng/mL 3-18 mo after transplant (heart)

Black Box Warning: Liver transplant: ext rel product should not be used because of increased female mortality rate

Black Box Warning: Specialized care setting, experienced clinician: only use when equipped and staffed with adequate supportive services and by those experienced in immunosuppressive therapy and organ transplantation

Black Box Warning: Children, infants, neonates: not approved use of ointment in those <2 yr, ext rel in those <16 yr; not approved for pediatric kidney/heart transplant

• **Pregnancy/breastfeeding:** use only if benefits outweigh fetal risk; do not breastfeed, excretion unknown

Evaluate:

• **Therapeutic response:** absence of graft rejection; immunosuppression in patients with autoimmune disorders

Teach patient/family:
PO route

• To report fever, rash, severe diarrhea, chills, sore throat, fatigue; that serious infections may occur; to report clay-colored stools, cramping (hepatotoxicity), nephrotoxicity, signs of diabetes mellitus

• To avoid exposure to natural or artificial sunlight

• Not to breastfeed while taking product

• That repeated lab tests will be needed during treatment

• To avoid vaccines

• Not to use with alcohol, grapefruit, grapefruit juice

• **Organ rejection:** B/P, provide treatment for hypertension to help prevent rejection

Black Box Warning: To report symptoms of lymphoma, skin cancer; to avoid crowds, persons with known infections to reduce risk for infection; to avoid eating raw shellfish

Topical route

• To stop using topical product when atopic dermatitis is resolved; not to use >6 wk if symptoms do not improve; not to shower or swim after applying

• To report if pregnancy is planned or suspected

---

tadalafil (Rx)

(tah-dal'a-fil)

Adcirca, Cialis, Alyq

Func. class.: Impotence agent

Chem. class.: Phosphodiesterase type 5 inhibitor

ACTION: Inhibits phosphodiesterase type 5 (PDE5); enhances erectile function by increasing the amount of cGMP, which causes smooth muscle relaxation and increased

---

Side effects: *italics* = common; red = life-threatening

blood flow into the corpus cavernosum; improves erectile function for up to 36 hr

USES: Treatment of erectile dysfunction (Cialis), benign prostatic hyperplasia (BPH) with or without erectile dysfunction, pulmonary arterial hypertension (PAH) (Adcirca only)

CONTRAINDICATIONS
New-borns, children, women, hypersensitivity, patients taking organic nitrates either regularly and/or intermittently, patients taking any α-adrenergic antagonist other than 0.4 mg once-daily tamsulosin
Precautions: Pregnancy, anatomic penile deformities, sickle cell anemia, leukemia, multiple myeloma, CV/renal/hepatic disease, bleeding disorders, active peptic ulcer, prolonged erection

DOSAGE AND ROUTES
Erectile dysfunction
• **Adult: PO (Cialis)** 10 mg taken before sexual activity; dose may be reduced to 5 mg or increased to max 20 mg; usual max dosing frequency is 1×/day; once-daily dosing 2.5 mg once daily. May increase the dose to 5 mg/day if needed
BPH (Cialis)
• **Adult: PO** 5 mg daily at the same time every day
Pulmonary hypertension (Adcirca, Alyq)
• **Adult: PO** 40 mg (two 20-mg tablets) daily with or without food

Concomitant use with ketoconazole, itraconazole, ritonavir
• **Adult: PO** max 10 mg q72hr
Renal dose (Adcirca)
• **Adult: PO** CCr 51-80 mL/min: no adjustment for erectile dysfunction, 20 mg/day initially for pulmonary hypertension; CCr 31-50 mL/min, 5 mg/day, max 10 mg q48hr; CCr <30 mL/min, max 5 mg q72hr
Hepatic dose (Adcirca)
• **Adult: PO** (Child-Pugh A, B) max 10 mg/day or 20 mg/day (pulmonary hypertension) max 40 mg/day; (Child-Pugh C) not recommended
Available forms: Tabs (Cialis) 2.5, 5, 10, 20 mg; tabs (Adcirca Alyq) 20 mg

Administer:
• Product should not be used with nitrates in any form
• **Erectile dysfunction:** give before sexual activity; do not use more than 1×/day
• **Pulmonary hypertension:** give Adcirca, Alyq with/without meals

SIDE EFFECTS
CNS: *Headache, flushing, dizziness,* seizures, transient global amnesia
CV: Hypotension, QT prolongation
INTEG: Stevens-Johnson syndrome, exfoliative dermatitis, urticaria
MISC: Back pain/myalgia, *dyspepsia, nasal congestion, UTI,* blurred vision, changes in color vision, *diarrhea,* pruritus, priapism, nonarteritic ischemic optic neuropathy (NAION), hearing loss

PHARMACOKINETICS
Rapidly absorbed; metabolized by liver by CYP3A4; terminal half-life 17.5 hr; peak ½-6 hr; excreted primarily as metabolites in feces, urine; excreted 61% in feces, 36% in urine; 94% protein bound; rate and extent of absorption not influenced by food

INTERACTIONS
Do not use with nitrates because of unsafe drop in B/P, which could result in MI or stroke
Increase: tadalafil levels—itraconazole, ketoconazole, ritonavir (although not studied, may also include other HIV protease inhibitors)
Decrease: B/P—alcohol, α-blockers, amLODIPine, angiotensin II receptor blockers, enalapril
Decrease: effects of tadalafil—bosentan, antacids
Drug/Food
Increase: tadalafil effect—grapefruit

NURSING CONSIDERATIONS
Assess:
• **Cialis:** underlying cause of erectile dysfunction before treatment; use of organic nitrates that should not be used with this product; any severe loss of vision while taking this or any similar products

• **BPH:** urinary hesitancy, poor stream, dribbling baseline and periodically

- **Adcirca, Alyq:** hemodynamic parameters to exercise tolerance at baseline and periodically
- **Respiratory changes:** dyspnea, wheezing
- **CV status:** B/P, angina, palpitation, HR, edema, dizziness
- **Pregnancy/breastfeeding:** use only if clearly needed (Adcirca only); Cialis is not indicated for women; not used in breastfeeding
- **Beers:** use with caution in older adults; may exacerbate syncope; monitor frequently for syncope

Evaluate:
- **Therapeutic response:** ability to engage in sexual intercourse, improvement in exercise ability in pulmonary hypertension

Teach patient/family:
- To take 1 hr before sexual activity
- Not to drink large amounts of alcohol
- To discuss with provider all OTC, Rx, herbals, supplements taken
- That product does not protect against sexually transmitted diseases, including HIV
- That product has no effect in the absence of sexual stimulation; to seek medical help if erection lasts >4 hr
- To notify physician about all medicines, vitamins, herbs being taken, especially ritonavir, indinavir, ketoconazole, itraconazole, erythromycin, nitrates, α-blockers; that tadalafil is contraindicated for use with α-blockers except 0.4 mg/day tamsulosin
- To notify prescriber immediately and to stop taking product if vision, hearing loss occurs or if erection lasts >4 hr or if chest pain occurs

tafamidis (Rx)
(ta-fam′id-is)
Vyndamax, Vyndaqel
Func. class.: Metabolic agent

USES: Treatment of the cardiomyopathy of wild-type/hereditary transthyretin-mediated amyloidosis to reduce mortality and hospitalization

CONTRAINDICATIONS
Hypersensitivity

DOSAGE AND ROUTES
Amyloid cardiomyopathy
- **Adult:** PO **Vyndamax:** 61 mg daily; **Vyndaqel:** 80 mg daily

Available forms: Capsules 20 mg (tafamidis meglumine); capsules 61 mg (tafamidis)

tafenoquine (Rx)
(ta fen′oh-kwin)
Krintafel, Arakoda
Func. class.: Antimalarial
Chem. class.: 8-aminoquinoline

ACTION: Activity against the pre-erythrocytic liver stages of the parasite prevents the development of the erythrocytic forms, which are responsible for malarial relapse; may inhibit hematin polymerization, inducing apoptotic-like death of the parasite

USES: Prevention of relapse of *Plasmodium vivax* malaria in those receiving antimalarial therapy for acute *P. vivax* infection (Krintafel); for malaria prophylaxis (Arakoda)

CONTRAINDICATIONS
Hypersensitivity to this product or iodoquinol or primaquine, G6PD deficiency, psychosis

Precautions: Breastfeeding, contraception requirements, hepatic disease, methemoglobin reductase deficiency, pregnancy, pregnancy testing, psychiatric events, renal disease, reproductive risk

DOSAGE AND ROUTES
Prevention of relapse of *Plasmodium vivax* malaria (Krintafel)
- **Adult/adolescent ≥16 yr:** PO 300 mg as a single dose on the first or second day of the antimalarial therapy (chloroquine)

For malaria prophylaxis (Arakoda)
- **Adult:** PO 200 mg daily for 3 days before travel as loading dose, then 200 mg weekly starting 7 days after the last loading dose, continue during travel to area as maintenance, then 200 mg once at 7 days after the last maintenance dose in

the week after exit from area; may be given for ≤6 mo of continuous dosing

Administer:
• Give with food
• Swallow tablets whole. Do not break, crush, or chew
• If vomiting occurs within 1 hr after dosing, repeat the dose; do not attempt to redose more than once (prevention of relapse single-dose therapy)
• **Storage:** At room temperature in original container, protect from moisture

SIDE EFFECTS

CNS: Dizziness, headache, anxiety, abnormal dreams, insomnia, somnolence
EENT: Vortex keratopathy, photophobia
GI: Nausea, vomiting
HEMA: Decreased HB
INTEG: Angioedema, urticaria

PHARMACOKINETICS

Protein binding 99.5%, peak 12-15 hr, half-life 12-15 days (Krintafel). Affected cytochrome P450 isoenzymes and drug transporters: OCT2, MATE-1, MATE2-K

INTERACTIONS

• Avoid use with MATE (multidrug and toxin extrusion substrates) and OCT2 (organic cation transporter-2) (dofetilide, metformin); if these products must be given, monitor for toxicity

Drug/Lab:
Increase: methemoglobin, ALT, creatinine

NURSING CONSIDERATIONS

Assess
• **Malaria symptoms:** anemia, jaundice, diarrhea, sweating, vomiting, fast heart rate, low B/P; report symptoms to health care provider
• **Methemoglobinemia:** monitor for increased methemoglobin; report immediately shortness of breath, cyanosis, mental status changes; O_2 and methylene blue may be given
• **Psychiatric effects:** serious psychiatric adverse reactions have been observed in patients with a previous history of psychiatric conditions at doses higher than the approved dose; the effects may occur during or after treatment

• **Hypersensitivity reactions:** serious hypersensitivity reactions (angioedema) may occur; these reactions may occur during or after conclusion of therapy
• **Pregnancy/breastfeeding:** avoid use in pregnancy, a pregnancy test is required in all females of reproductive potential, adequate contraception is required during and for 3 mo after last dose; infant should be tested for G6PD deficiency before breastfeeding

Evaluate:
• **Therapeutic response:** prevention of relapse or prevention of malaria

Teach patient/family:
• **Pregnancy/breastfeeding:** not to use during pregnancy; adequate contraception should be used during and for 3 mo after last dose; infant should have a lab test performed before breastfeeding
• To swallow tablets whole, not to split or cut; to take with food
• To report immediately dark urine or lips as these may be symptoms of hemolytic anemia
• To use sunglasses in bright light to prevent photophobia

---

tafluprost (Rx)
(ta'floo-prost)
Zioptan
Func. class.: Ophthalmic, antiglaucoma

USES: Reduction of IOP in open-angle glaucoma/ocular hypertension

CONTRAINDICATIONS
Hypersensitivity

DOSAGE AND ROUTES
• **Adult:** Ophthalmic 1 drop in affected eye(s) daily in the PM
Available forms: Ophthalmic solution 0.0015%

⚠ HIGH ALERT

tagraxofusp-erzs
(tag-rax'oh-fusp)
Elzonris
Func. class.: Antineoplastic, miscellaneous

USES:
Treatment of blastic plasmacytoid dendritic cell neoplasm

CONTRAINDICATIONS
Hypersensitivity

Black Box Warning: Capillary leak syndrome

DOSAGE AND ROUTES
• **Adult/child ≥2 yr IV:** 12 mcg/kg daily on days 1-5 of a 21-day cycle; continue until disease progression or unacceptable toxicity
Available forms: Injection 1000 mcg/mL single-dose vial

⚠ HIGH ALERT

talazoparib (Rx)
(tal'a-zoe'pa-rib)
Talzenna
Func. class.: Antineoplastic
Chem. class.: Poly (ADP-ribose) polymerase (PARP) inhibitors

ACTION: An inhibitor of (ADP-ribose) (PARP) enzymes (PARP1 and PARP2) that are involved in DNA repair. Cytotoxicity involve inhibition of PARP enzymatic activity and increased formation of PARP-DNA, resulting in DNA damage, decreased cell proliferation, and apoptosis

USES: Deleterious/suspected deleterious germline BRCA-mutated (gBRCAm), HER2-negative locally advanced or metastatic breast cancer

CONTRAINDICATIONS
Hypersensitivity
Precautions: Anemia, bone marrow suppression, breastfeeding, contraception requirements, infertility, leukemia, leukopenia, male-mediated teratogenicity, myelodysplastic syndrome, neutropenia, new primary malignancy, pregnancy, pregnancy testing, reproductive risk, thrombocytopenia

DOSAGE AND ROUTES
• **Adult: PO** 1 mg daily until disease progression or unacceptable toxicity

Renal dose
• **Adult: PO** Moderate renal impairment (CrCL 30-59 mL/min): 0.75 mg daily; severe impairment (CCl 15-29 mL/min): 0.5 mg PO daily

Hematologic toxicity dose
• Do not start until patient has adequately recovered from hematologic toxicity caused by previous therapy
• Hemoglobin <8 g/dL: Hold, monitor blood counts weekly. When HB recovers to ≥9 g/dL, reduce daily dose by 0.25 mg and resume
• Neutrophil count <1000 cells/mm³: Hold, monitor blood counts weekly. When neutrophils recover to ≥1500 cells/mm³, reduce daily dose by 0.25 mg and resume
• Platelet count <50,000 cells/mm³: Hold, monitor blood counts weekly. When platelets recover to ≥75,000 cells/mm³, reduce daily dose by 0.25 mg and resume

Nonhematologic toxicity dose
• **Grade 3 or 4:** Hold; when toxicity resolves to grade ≤1, consider reducing dose by 0.25 mg and resuming
Available forms: Caps 0.25, 0.5, 0.75, 1 mg
Administer:
• Swallow capsules whole; do not open or dissolve
• May be taken with or without food
• If patient vomits or misses a dose, an additional dose should not be taken; take the next dose at regularly scheduled time
• **Storage:** At room temperature

SIDE EFFECTS
CNS: Fatigue, headache, dizziness
GI: Nausea, vomiting, diarrhea, anorexia, abdominal pain
HEMA: Anemia, neutropenia, thrombocytopenia
META: Hyperglycemia, hypocalcemia
MISC: New primary malignancy, leukemia, MDS/AML

Side effects: *italics* = common; red = life-threatening

PHARMACOKINETICS

74% protein binding, metabolized in liver, excretion in urine 68.7%, 19.8 % in feces

INTERACTIONS

• **Increase:** effect of talazoparib—P-gp inhibitors (amiodarone, carvedilol, clarithromycin, itraconazole, verapamil); monitor for potential increased adverse reactions

• **Increase:** effect of talazoparib—BCRP inhibitors; monitor for potential increased adverse reactions when coadministering

Drug/Lab:

• **Increase:** glucose, ALT, AST, alk phos
• **Decrease:** hemoglobin, platelets, neutrophils, lymphocytes, leukocytes, calcium

NURSING CONSIDERATIONS

Assess:

• Monitor CBC with differential baseline and monthly; serum creatinine; do not start until patient has recovered from hematologic toxicities from other chemotherapy

• **Pregnancy/breastfeeding:** obtain pregnancy test in females of reproductive potential before use; fetal harm may occur; effective contraception is needed during treatment and for ≥7 mo after the last dose; male patients with female partners of reproductive potential or pregnant partners should use effective contraception during treatment and for ≥4 mo following the last dose; fertility may be impaired in males

Evaluate:

• **Therapeutic response:** decreased growth, spread of breast cancer

Teach patient/family:

• **MDS/AML:** to report to health care provider if feeling tired or experiencing symptoms of weakness, fever, weight loss, frequent infections, bruising, bleeding easily, breathlessness, blood in urine or stool

• **Myelosuppression:** that product may cause anemia, leukopenia/neutropenia, and/or thrombocytopenia; that frequent lab testing will be required

• To take daily with or without food; that if a dose is missed, to take next normal dose at the usual time; to swallow each capsule whole; that capsules must not be opened or dissolved

• **Pregnancy/breastfeeding:** to notify health care provider if pregnant or planning to become pregnant; that females of reproductive potential must use effective contraception during treatment and for ≥7 mo after last dose; that females should not breastfeed during treatment or for ≥1 mo after receiving the last dose; that male patients with female partners of reproductive potential or who are pregnant should use effective contraception during treatment and for ≥4 mo after last dose

• To notify health care provider of nausea, vomiting to obtain options to lessen these side effects

• To notify health care provider of all Rx, OTC, herbals, or supplements taken; not to add or change medications unless approved by provider

---

⚠ HIGH ALERT

tamoxifen (Rx)

(ta-mox´i-fen)

Nolvadex-D ✤ Soltamox
Func. class.: Antineoplastic
Chem. class.: Antiestrogen hormone

ACTION: Inhibits cell division by binding to cytoplasmic estrogen receptors; resembles normal cell complex but inhibits DNA synthesis and estrogen response of target tissue

USES: Advanced breast carcinoma not responsive to other therapy in estrogen-receptor–positive patients (usually postmenopausal), prevention of breast cancer, after breast surgery/radiation for ductal carcinoma in situ
Unlabeled uses: Mastalgia, to reduce pain/size of gynecomastia, bipolar disorder, infertility, osteoporosis, ovarian cancer, precocious puberty

CONTRAINDICATIONS

Pregnancy, breastfeeding, hypersensitivity

Black Box Warning: Thromboembolic disease, endometrial cancer, stroke

Precautions: Women of childbearing age, leukopenia, thrombocytopenia, cataracts

Black Box Warning: Uterine cancer, new primary malignancy

DOSAGE AND ROUTES
Estrogen receptor-positive metastatic breast cancer (men/women)
• **Adult: PO** 20 mg/day for 5 yr; doses >20 mg/day, divide AM/PM
Early-stage estrogen receptor-positive breast cancer (adjuvant treatment)
• **Adult: PO** 20 mg/day × 5-10 yr
High risk for breast cancer
• **Adult: PO** 20 mg/day × 5 yr
Mastalgia/gynecomastia in men with prostate cancer (unlabeled)
• **Adult (male): PO** 20 mg/day for ≤1 yr
Available forms: Tabs 10, 20 mg; oral solution 10 mg/5 mL
Administer:
• Do not break, crush, or chew tabs
• Do not give antacid within 1-2 hr of dosing; give product after evening meal, before bedtime; give with food or fluids for GI symptoms
• Antiemetic 30-60 min before product to prevent vomiting
• Store in light-resistant container at room temperature
Oral solution: Use calibrated container, dose >20 mg/day should be divided morning and evening, may be used with food for gastric irritation

SIDE EFFECTS
CNS: *Hot flashes, headache, light-headedness,* depression, mood changes, stroke
CV: Chest pain, stroke, fluid retention, flushing
EENT: Blurred vision (high doses)
GI: *Nausea, vomiting,* altered taste
GU: Vaginal bleeding, uterine malignancies, *altered menses, amenorrhea*
HEMA: Thrombocytopenia, leukopenia, DVT
INTEG: *Rash,* alopecia

META: Hypercalcemia
RESP: Pulmonary embolism

PHARMACOKINETICS
PO: Peak 4-7 hr, half-life 7 days (1 wk terminal), metabolized in liver, excreted primarily in feces

INTERACTIONS
Increase: risk for death from breast cancer—PARoxetine
Increase: bleeding—anticoagulants
Increase: tamoxifen levels—bromocriptine
Increase: thromboembolic events—cytotoxics
Increase: toxicity—CYP3A4 inhibitors (aprepitant, antiretroviral protease inhibitors, clarithromycin, danazol, delavirdine, diltiaZEM, erythromycin, fluconazole, FLUoxetine, fluvoxaMINE, imatinib, ketoconazole, mibefradil, nefazodone, telithromycin, voriconazole)
Decrease: tamoxifen levels—aminoglutethimide, rifamycin
Decrease: letrozole levels—letrozole
Decrease: tamoxifen effect—CYP3A4 inducers (barbiturates, bosentan, carBAMazepine, efavirenz, phenytoins, nevirapine, rifabutin, rifampin)
Decrease: tamoxifen effects—CYP2D6 inhibitors (antidepressants)
Drug/Herb
• Avoid use with St. John's wort, dong quai, black cohosh
Drug/Lab Test
Increase: serum calcium, T_4, AST, ALT, cholesterol, triglycerides, BUN

NURSING CONSIDERATIONS
Assess:
• **Labs/diagnostics:** CBC, differential, platelet count baseline and weekly, withhold product if WBC is <3.5 × 10⁹/L or platelets <100 × 10⁹/L notify prescriber; breast exam, mammogram, pregnancy test, bone mineral density, LFTs, serum calcium, serum lipid profile, periodic eye exams (cataracts, retinopathy), pap smear

Black Box Warning: Bleeding q8hr: hematuria, guaiac, bruising, petechiae, mucosa, or orifices

---

Side effects: *italics* = common; red = life-threatening

• Effects of alopecia on body image; discuss feelings about body changes

Black Box Warning: Uterine malignancies, symptoms of stroke, pulmonary embolism that may occur in women with ductal carcinoma in situ (DCIS) and women at high risk for breast cancer; monitor gynecologic exams baseline and periodically

• **Severe allergic reactions:** rash, pruritus, urticaria, purpuric skin lesions, itching, flushing
• **Bone pain:** may give analgesics; pain usually transient
• **Pregnancy/breastfeeding:** do not use in pregnancy, breastfeeding
Evaluate:
• **Therapeutic response:** decreased tumor size, spread of malignancy
Teach patient/family:
• **About risk of stroke and PE:** to seek medical attention immediately in case of blurred vision, headache, weakness on one side of the body (stroke signs); or chest pain, fainting, sweating, difficulty breathing (PE)
• To report any complaints, side effects to prescriber; that use may be 5 yr
• To increase fluids to 2 L/day unless contraindicated
• To wear sunscreen, protective clothing, sunglasses
• That vaginal bleeding, pruritus, hot flashes are reversible after discontinuing treatment
• To immediately report decreased visual acuity, which may be irreversible; about need for routine eye exams; that care providers should be told about tamoxifen therapy
• To report vaginal bleeding immediately
• That **tumor flare**—increase in size of tumor, increase in bone pain—may occur and will subside rapidly; that analgesics may be taken for pain
• That hair may be lost during treatment; that a wig or hairpiece may make patient feel better; that new hair may be different in color, texture

• To use nonhormonal contraception during and for 2 mo after discontinuing treatment, that premenopausal women must use mechanical birth control because ovulation may be induced

---

tamsulosin (Rx)

(tam-sue-lo'sen)

Flomax, Flomax CR ✚

Func. class.: Selective α_1-peripheral adrenergic blocker, BPH agent
Chem. class.: Sulfamoylphenethylamine derivative

Do not confuse:
Flomax/fosamax
Tamsulosin/tacrolimus/tamoxifen

ACTION: Binds preferentially to α_{1A}-adrenoceptor subtype, which is located mainly in the prostate

USES: Symptoms of benign prostatic hyperplasia (BPH)
Unlabeled Uses: Ureteral stones as adjunctive treatment

CONTRAINDICATIONS
Hyper-sensitivity
Precautions: Pregnancy, breastfeeding, children, hepatic disease, CAD, severe renal disease, prostate cancer; cataract surgery (floppy iris syndrome)

DOSAGE AND ROUTES
BPH
• **Adult: PO** 0.4 mg/day increasing to 0.8 mg/day if required after 2-4 wk
Ureteral stones (unlabeled)
• **Adult: PO** 0.4 mg daily at bedtime up to 6 wk or expulsion of stones
Available forms: Caps 0.4 mg
Administer:
• Without regard to food
• Swallow caps whole; do not break, crush, or chew
• Give ½ hr after same meal each day
• If treatment is interrupted for several days, restart at lowest dose (0.4 mg/day)

• Store in tight container in cool environment

SIDE EFFECTS
CNS: *Dizziness, headache,* asthenia, insomnia
CV: Chest pain, orthostatic hypotension
EENT: Amblyopia, floppy iris syndrome
GI: Nausea, diarrhea, dysgeusia
GU: Decreased libido, abnormal ejaculation, priapism
INTEG: Rash, pruritus, urticaria
MS: Back pain
RESP: Rhinitis, pharyngitis, cough
SYST: Angioedema

PHARMACOKINETICS
Peak 4-5 hr, duration 9-15 hr, half-life 9-13 hr, metabolized in liver, excreted via urine, extensively protein bound (98%)

INTERACTIONS
Increase: B/P—prazosin, terazosin, doxazosin, α-blockers, vardenafil
Increase: toxicity—cimetidine

NURSING CONSIDERATIONS
Assess:
• **Prostatic hyperplasia:** change in urinary patterns at baseline and throughout treatment; I&O ratios, weight daily; edema; report weight gain or edema
• **Orthostatic hypotension:** monitor B/P, standing, sitting, significant fall in B/P may occur
• **Pregnancy/breastfeeding:** not to be used for women
Evaluate:
• **Therapeutic response:** decreased symptoms of benign prostatic hyperplasia
Teach patient/family:
• Not to drive or operate machinery for 4 hr after 1st dose or after dosage increase
• To continue to take even if feeling better
• To advise providers of all products, herbs taken
• To make position changes slowly because orthostatic hypotension may occur
• To take ½ hr after same meal each day
• To teach about priapism (rare)
• Not to crush, break, chew
• That decreased ejaculate or absence may occur; resolves after discontinuing product

---

▲ HIGH ALERT

tapentadol (Rx)
(ta-pen′ta-dol)
Nucynta, Nucynta ER
Func. class.: Analgesic, misc.
Chem. class.: μ-Opioid receptor agonist

Controlled Substance Schedule II

ACTION: Centrally acting synthetic analgesic; μ-opioid agonist activity is thought to result in analgesia; inhibits norepinephrine uptake

USES: Moderate to severe pain, diabetic peripheral neuropathy

CONTRAINDICATIONS
Hypersensitivity, asthma, ileus, respiratory depression

Black Box Warning: Respiratory depression

Precautions: Pregnancy, breastfeeding, children <18 yr, increased intracranial pressure, MI (acute), severe heart disease, respiratory depression, renal/hepatic disease, GI obstruction, ulcerative colitis, sleep apnea, seizure disorder

Black Box Warning: Accidental exposure, avoid ethanol, substance abuse, neonatal opioid withdrawal syndrome, potential for overdose, poisoning, coadministration with other CNS depressants

DOSAGE AND ROUTES
Acute pain
• **Adult: PO** 50-100 mg q4-6hr, may give 2nd dose ≥1 hr after 1st dose, max 700 mg on day 1, max 600 mg/day thereafter
Severe chronic pain
• **Adult: PO** ext rel 50 mg q12hr (opioid-naive), titrate to 50 mg/dose bid q3days, max 250 mg q12hr
Hepatic disease
• **Adult: PO** Immediate rel 50 mg q8hr, may titrate to response; ext rel 50 mg daily, max 100 mg/day
Available forms: Tabs 50, 75, 100 mg; tabs ext rel 50, 100, 150, 200, 250 mg; oral solution 20 mg/mL

T

Side effects: *italics* = common; red = life-threatening

Administer:

- With antiemetic if nausea, vomiting occur
- When pain is beginning to return; determine dosage interval by response
- Do not crush, chew, break ext rel product, or use with alcohol; swallow whole with sufficient liquid
- Preferred analgesic in those with altered cytochrome P450 or mild hepatic, mild to moderate renal disease
- Store in light-resistant area at room temperature

Black Box Warning: These products have high potential for overdose, poisoning; may be fatal because of respiratory depression

- **Oral solution:** measure using calibrated syringe

SIDE EFFECTS

CNS: *Drowsiness, dizziness, confusion, headache, euphoria,* hallucinations, restlessness, syncope, anxiety, flushing, psychological dependence, insomnia, lethargy, tremors, seizures
CV: Palpitations, bradycardia, hypo/hypertension, orthostatic hypotension, sinus tachycardia
GI: *Nausea, vomiting, anorexia, constipation, cramps,* gastritis, dyspepsia, biliary spasms
GU: Urinary retention/frequency
INTEG: *Rash,* urticaria, diaphoresis, pruritus
RESP: Respiratory depression, cough
SYST: Anaphylaxis, infection, serotonin syndrome

PHARMACOKINETICS

Bioavailability 32%, extensively metabolized by liver, excreted in urine 99%, terminal half-life 4 hr, protein binding 20%

INTERACTIONS

Black Box Warning: **Increase:** effects with other CNS depressants—alcohol, opioids, sedative/hypnotics, antipsychotics, skeletal muscle relaxants

Increase: toxicity—MAOIs
Increase: serotonin syndrome—SSRIs, SNRIs, serotonin-receptor agonists, tricyclics

Black Box Warning: Do not use with alcohol; fatal overdose may occur

Drug/Herb
Increase: sedative effect—kava, St. John's wort, valerian

NURSING CONSIDERATIONS
Assess:
- **Pain:** intensity, location, type, characteristics; need for pain medication by pain/sedation scoring; physical dependence
- I&O ratio; check for decreasing output; may indicate urinary retention
- CNS changes: dizziness, drowsiness, hallucinations, euphoria, LOC, pupil reaction
- **Serotonin syndrome:** increased heart rate, shivering, sweating, dilated pupils, tremors, high B/P, hyperthermia, headache, confusion; if these occur, stop product, administer serotonin antagonist if needed
- **Seizures:** history of seizures increased with SSRIs, SNRIs, tricyclic antidepressants
- Allergic reactions: rash, urticaria, anaphylaxis

Black Box Warning: **Addiction risk, previous substance abuse:** assess before using ext rel product; some may crush ext rel product and snort, inject product that is dissolved

Black Box Warning: **Accidental exposure:** identify if alcohol has been used before giving this product; may be fatal if used with tapentadol; keep from pets, children; avoid coadministration with other CNS depressants

Black Box Warning: **Respiratory dysfunction:** respiratory depression, character, rate, rhythm; notify prescriber if respirations are <10/min; B/P, pulse

Black Box Warning: **Neonatal opioid withdrawal syndrome:** may be fatal; monitor neonates for irritability, hyperactivity, abnormal sleep pattern, high-pitched crying, tremors, vomiting, diarrhea, failure to gain weight

• **Pregnancy/breastfeeding:** use only if benefits outweigh fetal risk, including neonatal opioid withdrawal syndrome; do not breastfeed, excretion unknown

Evaluate:

• **Therapeutic response:** decrease in pain

Teach patient/family:

• To report any symptoms of CNS changes, allergic reactions, seizures, serotonin syndrome

• That physical dependency may result from extended use

• That withdrawal symptoms may occur: nausea, vomiting, cramps, fever, faintness, anorexia

• To avoid CNS depressants, alcohol

• To avoid driving, operating machinery if drowsiness, dizziness occur

• To change positions slowly to decrease orthostatic hypotension

• Teach patient to take as directed, not to double doses, if breakthrough pain occurs, notify provider, do not discontinue abruptly, gradually taper

• **Seizures:** Teach patient that if seizure occurs, discontinue, notify provider

• Not to drive or perform other hazardous activities until response is known

• **Orthostatic hypertension:** To rise slowly to prevent orthostatic hypertension

• **Serotonin syndrome:** Teach patient symptoms of serotonin syndrome and when to contact provider

• To discuss with provider all OTC, Rx, herbals, supplements taken

Black Box Warning: Not to use with alcohol; may be fatal

• To notify prescriber if pregnancy is planned or suspected, or if breastfeeding

tapinarof
(ta-pin'ar-of)
Vtama
Func. class.: Antipsoriatic

USES: Plaque psoriasis

DOSAGE AND ROUTES
• **Adult: Topical** apply a thin layer to affected area qday
Available forms: Cream 1%

⚠ HIGH ALERT

tasimelteon
(tas'i-mel'tee-on)
Hetlioz, Hetlioz HQ
Func. class.: Hypnotic

USES: Non-24-hr sleep-wake disorder, nighttime sleep disturbances in Smith-Magenis syndrome

DOSAGE AND ROUTES
Non-24-hour sleep-wake disorder
• **Adult: PO** 20 mg each night before bed at same time
Nighttime sleep disturbance in Smith-Magenis syndrome
• **Adult/child ≥16 yr: PO** 20 mg each night 1 hr before bed
• **Child 3-15 yr, >28 kg: PO** Oral suspension 20 mg 1 hr before bed
• **Child 3-15 yr, <28 kg: PO** oral suspension 0.7 mg/kg 1 hr before bed
Available forms: Capsules 20 mg; oral suspension 4 mg/mL

tavaborole topical
See Appendix B

⚠ HIGH ALERT

tazemetostat (Rx)
(taz'e-met'oh-stat)
Tazverik
Func. class: Antineoplastic

USES: Epithelioid sarcoma, metastatic/locally advanced, follicular lymphoma, relapsed/refractory

CONTRAINDICATIONS
Hypersensitivity

Side effects: *italics* = common; red = life-threatening

DOSAGE AND ROUTES
• **Adult: PO** 800 mg bid until disease progression or unacceptable toxicity
Available forms: Tablet 200 mg

---

teclistamab (Rx)
(tek-LIS-tuh-mab)
Tecvayli
Func. class.: Antineoplastic
Chem. class.: Bispecific B-cell maturation antigen

ACTIONS: It is a T-cell antibody that binds to the receptor expressed on the surface of T cells to the B-cell antigen (BCMA) expressed on the surface of multiple myeloma cells

USES: Relapsed multiple myeloma; available only through restricted program (Tecvayli REMS)

CONTRAINDICATIONS
Hypersensitivity
Precautions: Anemia, contraception requirements, pregnancy, infection, neutropenia, requires a specialized care setting, requires an experienced clinician

> **Black Box Warning:** Cytokine release syndrome, neurotoxicity, restricted program only

DOSAGE AND ROUTES
• **Adult: SUBCUT** Step-up dosing day 1 0.06 mg/kg; day 4 0.3 mg/kg; day 7 first treatment 1.5 mg/kg; thereafter weekly 1.5 mg/kg
Available forms: Injection 30 mg/3 mL (10 mg/mL), 153 mg/1.7 mL (90 mg/mL) single-dose vial
Administer:
• Prior to each dose corticosteroid (PO/IV dexamethasone 16 mg); histamine-1 (H1) receptor antagonist (PO/IV diphenhydramine 50 mg or equivalent); antipyretics acetaminophen (650-1000 mg or equivalent)

• Remove from refrigerator and let warm at room temperature for 15 min
• Withdraw needed amount after swirling gently
• The appropriate injection volume is based on vial concentration, patient weight, and type of dose

SIDE EFFECTS
CNS: Fever, fatigue, headache, Gillian Barre syndrome, encephalopathy, seizures, peripheral neuropathy
CV: Hypotension/hypertension, edema
MS: MS pain, bone pain
GI: Nausea, increased LFTs, diarrhea, constipation, anorexia, vomiting, hepatic failure
HEMA: Lymphopenia, neutropenia, hypoalbuminemia, thrombocytopenia
INTEG: Injection site reaction
META: Hypophosphatemia, hyponatremia, hypocalcemia
SYST: Cytokine release syndrome, infection

PHARMACOKINETICS
Bioavailability 72%

INTERACTIONS
Decreased CYP enzyme activity, toxicity; monitor for toxicity and adjust the dose as needed for CYP substrates, especially during the first 2 wk

NURSING CONSIDERATIONS
Assess:
• For injection site pain, swelling, redness—usually occur after 2 injections (4-5 days); use cold compress to relieve pain/swelling
• Infections (fever, flulike symptoms, dyspnea, change in urination, redness/swelling around any wounds), stop treatment if some serious infections occur
• **Blood dyscrasias:** CBC, differential periodically
• Lab: LFTs, serum Ig concentrations will be drawn, and neurologic status will be reviewed periodically
Evaluate:
• **Therapeutic response:** Lessened spread of multiple myeloma

---

Teach patient/family:

• **Cytokine release syndrome:** discuss signs/symptoms (fever, hypoxia, chills, hypotension, sinus tachycardia, headache, elevated liver enzymes). Advise patients to immediately contact their health care provider if they experience any of these signs/symptoms

• Advise patients that hospitalization will be required × 48 hr after administration of all doses within the step-up dosing schedule

• **Hepatotoxicity:** advise patient to report dark urine, yellowing eyes, skin, fatigue, anorexia, right upper abdominal pain

• Not to take any live virus vaccines during treatment

• To report signs of infection, allergic reaction, immediately

• To advise all health care professionals of Rx, OTC, herbals, supplements taken

• **Pregnancy/breastfeeding:** To advise health care professional if pregnancy is planned or suspected or if breastfeeding, not to breastfeed or become pregnant during or for 5 mo after last dose, use effective contraception; that a pregnancy test may be done prior to starting treatment

• This product is available through a restricted program, Tecvayli REMS, that each patient is given a Tecvayli Patient Wallet Card that they should carry with them at all times and show to all of their health care providers. This card describes signs/symptoms of CRS and neurologic toxicity, which, and if experienced, the patient should seek medical attention immediately

tecovirimat (Rx)

(tek'oh-vir'i-mat)
Func. class.: Antiviral

USES: Treatment of human smallpox disease, variola virus
Unlabeled uses: Monkeypox virus

CONTRAINDICATIONS
Hypersensitivity

DOSAGE AND ROUTES
Smallpox

• **Adult 40 to <120 kg: PO:** 600 mg bid × 14 days; **IV** 200 mg q12hr × 14 days; **≥120 kg: PO** 600 mg (3 capsules) tid with meals for 14 days: **IV** 300 mg q12hr × 14 days

• **Child/adolescent: PO 13 to <25 kg:** 200 mg bid × 14 days; **25 to <40 kg:** 400 mg bid × 14 days; **≥40 kg:** 600 mg bid × 14 days
Available forms: Capsules 200 mg; solution for injection 200 mg/20 mL

tedizolid (Rx)

Sivextro
Func. class.: Antibiotic

USES: Skin and skin structure infections

DOSAGE AND ROUTES
Skin and skin structure infections:
• **Adult/child ≥12 yr: PO/IV** 200 mg daily × 6 days
Available forms: Tabs 200 mg; inj for IV 200 mg

teduglutide (Rx)

(te'due-gloo'tide)
Gattex, Revestive ✦
Func. class.: Functional GI disorder agent
Chem. class.: Recombinant glucagon-like peptide-2 analog

USES: Short bowel syndrome, dependent on parenteral support

DOSAGE AND ROUTES
• **Adult: SUBCUT** 0.05 mg/kg daily
Available forms: Injection (SUBCUT) 3.8 mg/0.38 mL (5 mg)

tegaserod (Rx)

(teg-a-seer'od)
Zelnorm
Func. class.: IBS agent

USES: IBS with constipation

CONTRAINDICATIONS
Hypersensitivity

Side effects: *italics* = common; red = life-threatening

DOSAGE AND ROUTES

• **Adult woman <65 yr: PO** 6 mg bid 30 min before meals, discontinue after 4-6 wk if poor response
Available forms: Tabs 6 mg

---

telavancin (Rx)

(tel-a-van′sin)

Vibativ

Func. class.: Antiinfective, miscellaneous
Chem. class.: Lipoglycopeptide

ACTION: Inhibits bacterial cell-wall synthesis, disrupts cell membrane integrity, blocks glycopeptides

USES: Complicated skin/skin structure infections caused by *Enterococcus faecalis, E. faecium, Staphylococcus aureus* (MRSA), *S. aureus* (MSSA), *S. epidermidis, S. haemolyticus, Streptococcus agalactiae* (group B), *S. dysgalactiae, S. pyogenes* (group A β-tremolytic), *S. anginosus, S. intermedius, S. constellatus;* hospital-acquired pneumonia caused by susceptible gram-positive bacteria
Unlabeled uses: Bacteremia

CONTRAINDICATIONS

Hyper-sensitivity
Precautions: Breastfeeding, children, geriatric patients, renal disease, antimicrobial resistance, diabetes mellitus, diarrhea, GI disease, heart failure, hypertension, pseudomembranous colitis, QT prolongation, vancomycin hypersensitivity

Black Box Warning: Pregnancy, renal disease

DOSAGE AND ROUTES
Complicated skin/skin-structure infections
• **Adult: IV INFUSION** 10 mg/kg over 60 min q24hr × 5-14 days

Hospital-acquired and ventilator-associated bacterial pneumonia
• **Adult: IV INFUSION** 10 mg/kg q24hr × 7-21 days
Renal dose
• **Adult: IV** CCr 30-50 mL/min 7.5 mg/kg q24hr; CCr 10-29 mL/min 10 mg/kg q48hr
Available forms: Lyophilized powder for inj 750 mg
Administer:
• Use only for susceptible organisms to prevent drug-resistant bacteria
• Antihistamine if red man syndrome occurs: decreased B/P; flushing of neck, face
• Avoid IM, subcut use
Intermittent IV INFUSION route
• After reconstitution with 15 mL D₅W sterile water for inj; 0.9% NaCl (15 mg/mL) **250-mg vial;** add 45 mL to **750-mg vial** (15 mg/mL) for dose of 150-800 mg; further dilute with 100-250 mL of compatible sol; for dose <150 mg or >800 mg, further dilute to concentration of 0.6-8 mg/mL with compatible sol; give over 60 min, avoid rapid IV; reconstituted or diluted sol is stable for 4 hr room temperature, 7 hr refrigerated; avoid rapid IV; may cause red man syndrome

Y-site compatibility: Amphotericin B lipid complex (Abelcet), ampicillin-sulbactam, azithromycin, calcium gluconate, caspofungin, cefepime, cefTAZidime, cefTRIAXone, ciprofloxacin, dexamethasone, diltiaZEM, DOBUTamine, DOPamine, doripenem, doxycycline, ertapenem, famotidine, fluconazole, gentamicin, hydrocortisone, labetalol, magnesium sulfate, mannitol, meropenem, metoclopramide, milrinone, norepinephrine, ondansetron, pantoprazole, phenylephrine, piperacillin-tazobactam, potassium chloride/phosphates, raNITIdine, sodium bicarbonate, sodium phosphates, tigecycline, tobramycin, vasopressin

SIDE EFFECTS
CNS: Anxiety, chills, flushing, headache, insomnia, dizziness
CV: QT prolongation, irregular heartbeat
EENT: Hearing loss
GI: Nausea, vomiting, CDAD, abdominal pain, constipation, diarrhea, metallic/soapy taste

---

GU: Nephrotoxicity, *increased BUN, creatinine,* renal failure, foamy urine

HEMA: Leukopenia, eosinophilia, anemia, thrombocytopenia

INTEG: Chills, fever, rash, thrombophlebitis at inj site; urticaria, pruritus, necrosis (red man syndrome)

SYST: Anaphylaxis, superinfection

PHARMACOKINETICS

Onset rapid, half-life 8-9 hr, excreted in urine (76%), protein binding 90%, hepatic metabolism

INTERACTIONS

Increase: otoxicity or nephrotoxicity—aminoglycosides, cephalosporins, colistin, polymyxin, bacitracin, CISplatin, amphotericin B, nondepolarizing muscle relaxants, cidofovir, tacrolimus, IV pentamidine, acyclovir, adefovir, cycloSPORINE, foscarnet, ganciclovir, pamidronate, streptozocin, zoledronic acid, NSAIDs, salicylates, ACE inhibitors, monitor closely

Increase: QT prolongation—class IA, III antidysrhythmics; some phenothiazines; chloroquine, clarithromycin, droperidol, dronedarone, erythromycin, haloperidol, methadone, pmozide, ziprasidone

May increase PTT: heparin, do not use together

Decrease: Vaccine effect—Vaccines (cholera, some typhoid)

Drug/Lab Test

False increase: INR, PT, PTT

NURSING CONSIDERATIONS

Assess:

• **Infection:** WBC, urine, stools, sputum, characteristics of wound throughout treatment, C&S

Black Box Warning: **Nephrotoxicity:** I&O ratio; report hematuria, oliguria; monitor BUN, CCr, avoid in those with CCr ≤50 mL/min; more common in those with diabetes, HF, hypertension, geriatric patients, renal disease

• **CDAD:** monitor for diarrhea, fever, blood in stools, abdominal pain; may happen several weeks after therapy ends, report to prescriber immediately

• **Anaphylaxis:** monitor for rash, itching, wheezing, laryngeal edema; discontinue

and notify prescriber immediately; emergency equipment and EPINEPHrine should be nearby

• **Auditory function during, after treatment;** hearing loss; ringing, roaring in ears; product should be discontinued

• **B/P during administration;** sudden drop may indicate red man syndrome; also flushing, pruritus, rash, use slow IV infusion to prevent

• **Respiratory status:** rate, character, wheezing, tightness in chest

• Adequate intake of fluids (2 L/day) to prevent nephrotoxicity

Black Box Warning: **Pregnancy:** obtain a pregnancy test before use; if a woman has taken this product during pregnancy, the national registry should be notified

Evaluate:

• **Therapeutic response:** negative culture

Teach patient/family:

• About all aspects of product therapy; that culture may be taken after completed course of medication

• To notify prescriber if infection continues

• That bitter taste, nausea, vomiting, headache may occur

• To report sore throat, fever, fatigue; could indicate superinfection; diarrhea (CDAD); hearing loss; rash, wheezing, tightness of chest, itching, tightening of throat (anaphylaxis)

Black Box Warning: To use contraception while taking this product; not to breastfeed; to notify prescriber if pregnancy is planned or suspected

telmisartan (Rx)

(tel-mih-sar'tan)

Micardis

Func. class.: Antihypertensive

Chem. class.: Angiotensin II receptor (Type AT$_1$) antagonist

ACTION: Blocks the vasoconstricting and aldosterone-secreting effects of angiotensin II; selectively blocks the binding of angiotensin II to the AT$_1$ receptor found in tissues

---

Side effects: *italics* = common; red = life-threatening

USES: Hypertension, alone or in combination; stroke, MI prophylaxis (>55 yr) in patients unable to take ACE inhibitors

CONTRAINDICATIONS
Hypersensitivity

Black Box Warning: Pregnancy

Precautions: breastfeeding, children, geriatric patients; hypersensitivity to ACE inhibitors; renal/hepatic disease, renal artery stenosis, dialysis, HF, hyperkalemia, hypotension, hypovolemia, African descent

DOSAGE AND ROUTES
Hypertension
• **Adult: PO** 40 mg/day; range 20-80 mg/day
Stroke, MI prophylaxis
• **Adult >55 yr: PO** 80 mg/day
Available forms: Tabs 20, 40, 80 mg
Administer:
• Without regard to meals
• Increased dose to African-American patients or consider alternative agent; B/P response may be reduced
• Do not remove from blister pack until ready to use

SIDE EFFECTS
CNS: *Dizziness, insomnia, anxiety, headache,* fatigue, syncope
CV: *Chest pain, edema, palpitations,* bradycardia, orthostatic hypotension
GI: Diarrhea, dyspepsia, *anorexia, vomiting*
META: Hyperkalemia
MS: Myalgia, pain
RESP: *Cough, upper respiratory infection,* sinusitis, pharyngitis
SYST: Angioedema

PHARMACOKINETICS
Onset of antihypertensive activity 3 hr, peak 0.5-1 hr, extensively metabolized, terminal half-life 24 hr, protein binding 99.5%, excreted in feces >97%, B/P response is less in Black patients

INTERACTIONS
Increase: digoxin peak/trough concentrations—digoxin

Increase: antihypertensive action—diuretics, other antihypertensives
Increase: hyperkalemia—potassium-sparing diuretics, potassium salt substitutes, ACE inhibitors
Decrease: antihypertensive effect—NSAIDs, salicylates
Drug/Lab Test
Increase: LFTs

NURSING CONSIDERATIONS
Assess:

Black Box Warning: Pregnancy/breast-feeding: if pregnancy test is positive, stop treatment; can cause death to fetus; do not breastfeed

• **Vitals:** B/P, pulse standing, lying; note rate, rhythm, quality; if severe hypotension occurs, place in supine position; usually occurs during first few weeks of treatment
• Baselines of renal, hepatic, electrolyte studies before therapy begins
• **Angioedema:** Monitor for facial swelling, swelling of eyes, dyspnea (rare)
• **Heart failure:** edema in feet, legs daily; jugular venous distention; dyspnea; crackles; weight increase >5 lb per week
Evaluate:
• **Therapeutic response:** decreased B/P
Teach patient/family:
• To comply with dosage schedule, even if feeling better; to take at same time of day; that therapeutic effect may take 2-4 wk
• To notify prescriber immediately of mouth sores, fever, swelling of hands or feet, swelling of face or lips, irregular heartbeat, chest pain, decreased urine output
• Not to stop abruptly; increased B/P will occur
• That excessive perspiration, dehydration, vomiting, diarrhea may lead to fall in blood pressure; to consult prescriber if these occur
• That product may cause dizziness, fainting, light-headedness; to avoid hazardous activities until response is known

---

Black Box Warning: To notify prescriber if pregnancy is planned or suspected; do not use in pregnancy, breastfeeding

• To notify prescriber of all prescriptions, OTC products, and supplements taken; to rise slowly from sitting to prevent drop in B/P
• **Overdose:** dizziness, bradycardia, or tachycardia

telmisartan/ hydrochlorothiazide (Rx)

(te-me-sar'tan/hye-droe-klor-oh-thye'-a-zide)

Micardis HCT

Func. class.: Antihypertensive, thiazide diuretic

USES: Treatment of hypertension

CONTRAINDICATIONS
Hypersensitivity

Black Box Warning: Pregnancy

DOSAGE AND ROUTES
Patients currently on telmisartan monotherapy
• **Adult: PO not currently controlled on telmisartan** 80 mg monotherapy: telmisartan 80 mg/hydrochlorothiazide 12.5 mg daily, may titrate up to telmisartan 160 mg/hydrochlorothiazide 25 mg daily after 2-4 wk
Patients currently on hydrochlorothiazide monotherapy
• **Adult: PO not currently controlled on hydrochlorothiazide** 25 mg daily monotherapy, hypokalemia while on hydrochlorothiazide 25 mg monotherapy: telmisartan 80 mg/hydrochlorothiazide 12.5 mg daily; may be titrated up to telmisartan 160 mg/hydrochlorothiazide 25 mg daily after 2-4 wk
Available forms: Tabs 40 mg/12.5 mg, 80 mg/12.5 mg, 80 mg/25 mg

telotristat (Rx)

(tel-oh'tri-stat)

Xermelo

Func. class.: Antidiarrheal

Chem. class.: Tryptophan hydroxylase inhibitor

Do not confuse:
Xermelo/Xarelto

ACTION: Reduces serotonin production; this decreases stools in carcinoid syndrome

USES: Carcinoid syndrome diarrhea; used with somatostatin analogue (SSA) when SSA alone does not control symptoms

CONTRAINDICATIONS
Hypersensitivity

Precautions: Abdominal pain, breastfeeding, constipation, GI perforation/obstruction, pregnancy

DOSAGE AND ROUTES
• **Adult: PO** 250 mg tid
Available forms: Tablet 250 mg
Administer:
• With food
• If dose is missed, give at regularly scheduled time, do not double
• Store at room temperature

SIDE EFFECTS
CNS: Headache, depression, fever
CV: Peripheral edema
GI: Nausea, constipation, flatulence, anorexia, abdominal pain

PHARMACOKINETICS
Peak 0.5-2 hr, half-life 0.6 hr, 99% plasma protein binding, excreted in urine (93.2%), affected by CYP3A4, P-glycoprotein (P-gp)

INTERACTIONS
Decrease: effect of—CYP3A4 substrates; monitor for ineffective results; dose of CYP3A4 may need to be increased
Decrease: effect of—octreotide; give short-acting octreotide 30-60 min after telotristat

T

Increase: telotristat effect—P-glycoprotein (P-gp) products
Drug/Lab
Increase: ALT, AST, alk phos

NURSING CONSIDERATIONS
Assess:
• **Stools:** volume, color, characteristics, frequency; bowel pattern before product; rebound constipation, abdominal pain; discontinue if abdominal pain or constipation is severe
• **Pregnancy/breastfeeding:** use only if benefits outweigh fetal risk, not studied in pregnancy; breastfeeding not recommended, effects unknown
Evaluate:
• **Therapeutic response:** decreased diarrhea without abdominal pain or severe constipation
Teach Patient/Family:
• To take with food
• That if dose is missed, do not double; take regular dose at next scheduled time
• **Pregnancy/breastfeeding:** to contact health care provider if pregnancy is suspected or planned, or if breastfeeding
• To discontinue and notify health care provider if abdominal pain or severe constipation occurs

---

⚠ HIGH ALERT

temazepam (Rx)
(te-maz´e-pam)

Restoril
Func. class.: Sedative/hypnotic
Chem. class.: Benzodiazepine, short to intermediate acting

Controlled Substance Schedule IV (USA), Schedule F (Canada)

Do not confuse:
Restoril/RisperDAL

ACTION: Produces CNS depression at limbic, thalamic, hypothalamic levels of the CNS; may be mediated by neurotransmitter γ-aminobutyric acid (GABA); results are sedation, hypnosis, skeletal muscle relaxation, anticonvulsant activity, anxiolytic action

USES: Insomnia, short-term treatment (generally 7-10 days)

CONTRAINDICATIONS
Pregnancy, breastfeeding, hypersensitivity to benzodiazepines
Precautions: Children <15 yr, geriatric patients, anemia, renal/hepatic disease, suicidal individuals, drug abuse, psychosis, acute closed-angle glaucoma, seizure disorders, angioedema, sleep-related behaviors (sleepwalking), intermittent porphyria, COPD, dementia, myasthenia gravis

Black Box Warning: Coadministration with other CNS depressants, abrupt discontinuation, substance abuse

DOSAGE AND ROUTES
Short-term treatment (7-10 days) of insomnia
• **Adult: PO** 7.5 to 30 mg at bedtime
• **Geriatric: PO** 7.5 mg at bedtime
Available forms: Caps 7.5, 15, 22.5, 30 mg
Administer:
• 15-30 min before bedtime for sleeplessness
• Without regard to food

Black Box Warning: Avoid use with CNS depressants; serious CNS depression may result

• Store in tight container in cool environment

SIDE EFFECTS
CNS: *Lethargy, drowsiness, daytime sedation,* dizziness, confusion, lightheadedness, headache, anxiety, irritability, complex sleep-related reactions (sleep driving, sleep eating), fatigue
CV: Chest pain, pulse changes, hypotension
EENT: Blurred vision
RESP: Apnea, respiratory depression, increased bronchial secretions

GI: Nausea, vomiting, diarrhea, heartburn, abdominal pain, constipation, anorexia
SYST: Severe allergic reactions

PHARMACOKINETICS

Onset 30 min, peak 1-2 hr, duration 6-8 hr, half-life 10-20 hr, metabolized by liver, excreted by kidneys, crosses placenta, excreted in breast milk, 98% protein binding

INTERACTIONS

Increase: effects of cimetidine, disulfiram, oral contraceptives

Black Box Warning: Increase: action of both products—alcohol, CNS depressants, opiates, benzodiazepines

Increase: effect of temazepam—probenecid
Decrease: effect of antacids, theophylline, rifAMPin
Drug/Herb
Increase: CNS depression—hops, kava, valerian, chamomile, skullcap
Drug/Food
Decrease: temazepam effect—caffeine
Drug/Lab Test
Increase: ALT, AST

NURSING CONSIDERATIONS
Assess:
• **Mental status:** mood, sensorium, affect, memory (long, short), orientation
• **Sleep patterns:** falling asleep, staying asleep, baseline, periodically
• **Dependency:** restrict amount given to patient, assess for physical/psychological dependency; high-level risk for abuse
• **Fall risk:** Assistance with ambulation after receiving dose
• **Beers:** avoid in older adults; increased sensitivity to benzodiazepines and decreased metabolism; may cause delirium
Evaluate:
• **Therapeutic response:** ability to sleep at night, decreased early morning awakening if taking product for insomnia
Teach patient/family:
• To avoid driving, other activities requiring alertness until stabilized; may cause dizziness, drowsiness

Black Box Warning: To avoid alcohol ingestion, other CNS depressants

• That effects may take 2 nights for benefits to be noticed
• To take as directed; not to increase dose unless approved by prescriber
• To limit to 7-10 days of continuous use
• About alternative measures to improve sleep: reading, exercise several hours before bedtime, warm bath, warm milk, TV, self-hypnosis, deep breathing
• Not to discontinue abruptly, withdraw gradually
• That complex sleep-related behaviors may occur: sleep driving/eating/walking
• That hangover, memory impairment are common in geriatric patients but less common than with barbiturates
• To notify prescriber if pregnancy is planned or suspected; to use contraception while taking this product; not to use in pregnancy; to use caution in breastfeeding, excretion unknown

TREATMENT OF OVERDOSE: monitor electrolytes, VS

⚠ HIGH ALERT

temozolomide (Rx)

(tem-oh-zole'oh-mide)
Temodar, Temodal ✦
Func. class.: Antineoplastic-alkylating agent
Chem. class.: Imidazotetrazine derivative

ACTION: Prodrug that undergoes conversion to MTIC; MTIC action prevents DNA transcription

USES: Anaplastic astrocytoma with relapse, glioblastoma multiforme, malignant glioma
Unlabeled uses: Metastatic malignant melanoma

CONTRAINDICATIONS

Preg-nancy, breastfeeding; hypersensitivity to this product, carbazine, or gelatin

---

Precautions: Geriatric patients, radiation therapy, renal/hepatic disease, bone marrow suppression, infection, myelosuppression

DOSAGE AND ROUTES
Glioblastoma multiforme
- **Adult: PO/IV** 75 mg/m²/day × 42-49 days with focal radiotherapy, then maintenance of 6 cycles; maintenance dose: 150 mg/m² on days 1-5 of a 28-day cycle

Refractory anaplastic astrocytoma
- **Adult: PO** 150 mg/day × 5 days, repeated q28days; **IV** 150 mg/m²/day over 90 min on days 1-5 q28days, may increase to 200 mg/m²/day on days 1-5 q28days if hematologic parameters permit

Available forms: Caps 5, 20, 100, 140, 180, 250 mg; powder for inj 100 mg/vial
Administer:
PO route
- Do not break, crush, chew, open caps
- Antiemetic 30-60 min before product to prevent vomiting
- Caps 1 at a time with 8 oz of water at same time of day
- Fluids IV or PO before chemotherapy to hydrate patient
- If caps accidentally damaged, do not allow contact with skin or inhale
- Use proper procedures for handling/disposing of chemotherapy products
- Give on empty stomach at bedtime to prevent nausea/vomiting
- Store in light-resistant container in a dry area

IV route
- Bring vial to room temperature; discard if cloudy
- Inject 41 mL sterile water for inj into vial (2.5 mg/mL)
- Gently swirl; do not shake

Intermittent IV INFUSION route
- Withdraw up to 40 mL from each vial to make total dose; transfer to empty 250-mL PVC infusion bag; flush before and after infusion
- Run over 90 min
- Use reconstituted sol within 14 hr, including infusion time
- Do not admix

SIDE EFFECTS
CNS: Seizures, *hemiparesis, dizziness, poor coordination, amnesia, insomnia, paresthesia, somnolence, paresis, ataxia, anxiety, dysphagia, depression, confusion*
GI: *Nausea, anorexia, vomiting,* abdominal pain, constipation
GU: Urinary incontinence, UTI, frequency
HEMA: Thrombocytopenia, leukopenia, anemia, myelosuppression, neutropenia
INTEG: *Rash, pruritus*
MISC: Headache, fatigue, asthenia, fever, edema, back pain, weight increase, diplopia
RESP: URI, pharyngitis, sinusitis, coughing
SYST: Anaphylaxis, secondary malignancy

PHARMACOKINETICS
Absorption complete, rapid; crosses blood-brain barrier; excreted in urine, feces; half-life 1.8 hr; peak 1 hr

INTERACTIONS
Increase: myelosuppression—radiation, other antineoplastics
Increase: bleeding risk—NSAIDs, anticoagulants, platelet inhibitors, thrombolytics
Decrease: antibody reaction—live virus vaccines, toxoids
Decrease: action of digoxin
Drug/Food
Decrease: drug absorption
Drug/Lab Test
Decrease: HB, platelets, WBC, neutrophils

NURSING CONSIDERATIONS
Assess:
- CBC on day 22 (21 days after 1st dose), CBC weekly until recovery if ANC <1.5 × 10⁹/L and platelets <100 × 10⁹/L; do not administer to patients who do not tolerate 100 mg/m²; myelosuppression usually occurs late during the treatment cycle
- Seizures throughout treatment; mental status
- Tumor response during treatment
- **Monitor temperature;** may indicate beginning infection
- **Hepatic studies** before, during therapy (bilirubin, AST, ALT, LDH), as needed or monthly

- **Bleeding:** hematuria, guaiac, bruising, petechiae, mucosa or orifices
- **Pregnancy/breastfeeding:** do not use in pregnancy, breastfeeding

Evaluate:
- **Therapeutic response:** decreased tumor size, spread of malignancy

Teach patient/family:
- To report signs of infection: fever, sore throat, flulike symptoms
- To report signs of anemia: fatigue, headache, faintness, SOB, irritability
- To report bleeding; to avoid use of razors, commercial mouthwash
- To notify prescriber if pregnancy is planned or suspected; not to breastfeed

⚠ HIGH ALERT

temsirolimus (Rx)
(tem-sir-oh'li-mus)
Torisel
Func. class.: Antineoplastic
Chem. class.: Kinase inhibitor, mTOR antagonist

USES: Renal cell carcinoma

CONTRAINDICATIONS
Pregnancy, breastfeeding; hypersensitivity to this product or to sirolimus; polysorbate 80
Precautions: Children <13 yr, females, severe pulmonary/renal/hepatic disease (bilirubin >1-1.5 × ULN or AST >ULN but bilirubin ≤ULN), diabetes mellitus, hyperkalemia, hyperuricemia, hypertension, bone marrow suppression, hypertriglyceridemia/hyperlipidemia, surgery, brain tumors

DOSAGE AND ROUTES
- **Adult: IV** 25 mg over 30-60 min weekly; treat until disease progression or severe toxicity occurs

Hepatic dose
- **Adult: IV** (mild impairment) bilirubin >1-1.5×ULN or AST >ULN but bilirubin ≤ULN: reduce to 15 mg/wk; moderate or severe impairment, do not use

Available forms: Solution (IV) 25 mg/mL

tenapanor (Rx)
(ten-a'pa-nor)
Ibsrela
Func. class.: IBS agent

USES: Irritable bowel syndrome with constipation in adults

CONTRAINDICATIONS
Hypersensitivity, GI obstruction

Black Box Warning: Children

DOSAGE AND ROUTES
- **Adult: PO** 50 mg bid immediately before breakfast or the first meal of the day and immediately before dinner

⚠ HIGH ALERT

tenecteplase (TNK-tPA) (Rx)
(ten-ek'ta-place)
TNKase
Func. class.: Thrombolytic/fibrinolytic
Chem. class.: Tissue plasminogen activator

Do not confuse:
TNKase/Activase

ACTION: Activates conversion of plasminogen to plasmin (fibrinolysin): plasmin breaks down clots (fibrin), fibrinogen, factors V, VII; occlusion of venous access lines

USES: Acute myocardial infarction, coronary artery thrombosis

CONTRAINDICATIONS
Hypersensitivity, arteriovenous malformation, aneurysm, active bleeding, intracranial/intraspinal surgery or trauma within 2 mo, CNS neoplasms, severe hypertension, severe renal/hepatic disease, history of CVA, increased ICP/stroke
Precautions: Pregnancy, breastfeeding, children, geriatric patients, arterial emboli from left side of heart, hypocoagulation, subacute bacterial endocarditis, rheumatic

Side effects: *italics* = common; red = life-threatening

valvular disease, cerebral embolism/thrombosis/hemorrhage, intraarterial diagnostic procedure or surgery (10 days), recent major surgery, dysrhythmias, hypertension

DOSAGE AND ROUTES
To reduce risk of death from an acute MI
Total dose, max 50 mg based on patient's weight
• **Adult <60 kg: IV BOL** 30 mg, give over 5 sec
• **Adult ≥60-<70 kg: IV BOL** 35 mg, give over 5 sec
• **Adult ≥70-<80 kg: IV BOL** 40 mg, give over 5 sec
• **Adult ≥80-<90 kg: IV BOL** 45 mg, give over 5 sec
• **Adult ≥90 kg: IV BOL** 50 mg, give over 5 sec, max 50 mg total dose
Available forms: Powder for inj, lyophilized 50 mg/vial
Administer:
IV bolus route
• Total dose is based on patient's weight, max 50 mg
• Refer to product insert for instruction on how to use product
• As soon as thrombi are identified; not useful for thrombi >1 wk old
• Cryoprecipitate or fresh frozen plasma if bleeding occurs
• Heparin after fibrinogen level >100 mg/dL; heparin infusion to increase PTT to 1.5-2× baseline for 3-7 days; IV heparin with loading dose is recommended
• Aseptically withdraw 10 mL of sterile water for inj from diluent vial; use red cannula syringe-filling device; inject all contents of syringe into product vial; direct into powder, swirl, withdraw correct dose; discard any unused sol; stand shield with dose vertically on flat surface and recap red cannula; remove entire shield assembly by twisting counterclockwise; give by IV BOL
• IV therapy: use upper-extremity vessel that is accessible to manual compression
• If product not used immediately, refrigerate; use within 8 hr; not compatible with dextrose; flush dextrose-containing lines with saline before and after administration

SIDE EFFECTS
CNS: Intercranial bleeding
CV: Dysrhythmias, hypotension, cardiogenic shock, cardiac arrest, heart failure, myocardial reinfarction, myocardial rupture, tamponade, pericarditis, pericardial effusion, thrombosis, CVA
RESP: Pulmonary edema/embolism
GI: GI bleed
GU: Hematuria
HEMA: Decreased Hct, bleeding
INTEG: Rash, urticaria, phlebitis at IV infusion site, itching, flushing
SYST: Retroperitoneal bleeding, surface bleeding, anaphylaxis

PHARMACOKINETICS
IV: Onset immediate, half-life 20-24 min, metabolized by liver

INTERACTIONS
Increase: bleeding—aspirin, indomethacin, phenylbutazone, anticoagulants, antithrombolytics, glycoprotein IIb/IIIa inhibitors, dipyridamole, clopidogrel, ticlopidine, NSAIDs, cefamandole, cefoperazone, cefoTEtan, SSRIs, SNRIs
Drug/Herb
Increase: risk of bleeding—feverfew, garlic, ginger, ginkgo, green tea, horse chestnut
Drug/Lab Test
Increase: INR, PT, PTT

NURSING CONSIDERATIONS
Assess:
• **Hypersensitivity:** fever, rash, itching, chills; mild reaction may be treated with antihistamines
• Cholesterol embolism, blue-toe syndrome, renal failure, MI, cerebral/spinal cord/bowel/retinal infarction, hypertension; can be fatal
• **Bleeding during 1st hr of treatment;** hematuria, hematemesis, bleeding from mucous membranes, epistaxis, ecchymosis; may require tranfusion (rare), continue to assess for bleeding for 24 hr

• **AVM, recent surgery, actual bleeding:** assess for contraindications before use

• **Blood studies:** Hct, platelets, PTT, PT, TT, aPTT before starting therapy; PT or aPTT must be <2× control before starting therapy; PTT or PT q3-4hr during treatment; also monitor CPK, ECG, fibrin degradation products (FDPs), fibrinogen, INR

• VS, B/P, pulse, respirations, neurologic signs, temperature at least q4hr; temperature >104° F (40° C) indicates internal bleeding; systolic pressure increase >25 mm Hg should be reported to prescriber

• **Neurologic changes** that may indicate intracranial bleeding; if suspected, a CT scan should be performed

• **Retroperitoneal bleeding:** back pain, leg weakness, diminished pulses

• Bed rest during entire course of treatment

• Avoidance of venous or arterial puncture, inj, rectal temperature, any invasive treatment, if possible; if arterial puncture is needed, use upper extremity, use pressure dressing for at least 30 min, monitor closely

• Treatment of fever with acetaminophen or aspirin

• Pressure for 30 sec to minor bleeding sites; inform prescriber if this does not attain hemostasis; apply pressure dressing

• **Pregnancy/breasfeeding:** use only if benefits outweigh fetal risk; cautious use in breastfeeding, excretion unknown

Evaluate:

• **Therapeutic response:** resolution of MI

Teach patient/family:

• About proper dental care to avoid bleeding

• To notify prescriber immediately of sudden, severe headache

• To notify prescriber of bleeding; hypersensitivity; fast, slow, or uneven heart rate; feeling of faintness; blood in urine, stools; nosebleeds

tenofovir alafenamide
Vemlidy
tenofovir disoproxil fumarate (Rx)
(ten-oh-foh′veer)
Viread
Func. class.: Antiretroviral
Chem. class.: Nucleoside reverse transcriptase inhibitor (NRTI)

ACTION: Inhibits replication of HIV virus by competing with the natural substrate and then incorporating into cellular DNA by viral reverse transcriptase, thereby terminating cellular DNA chain

USES: HIV-1 infection with at least 2 other antiretrovirals, hepatitis B

CONTRAINDICATIONS
Hypersensitivity, lactic acidosis
Precautions: Pregnancy, breastfeeding, children, geriatric patients, renal disease, CCr <60 mL/min, osteoporosis, immune reconstitution syndrome

Black Box Warning: Hepatitis B exacerbation

DOSAGE AND ROUTES
Chronic HIV infection (tenofovir alafenamide)
Adult: PO 25 mg/day
Human immunodeficiency virus (HIV) infection (tenofovir disoproxil fumarate)
• **Adult/adolescent/child weighing ≥35 kg: PO** Tablet: 300 mg once daily; Oral powder 300 mg/day (7.5 scoops) with 2-4 oz soft food
• **Adolescent/child weighing 28-34 kg: PO** Tablet: 250 mg/day
• **Child ≥2 yr and weighing 22-27 kg: PO** Tablet: 200 mg/day
• **Child ≥2 yr and weighing 17-21 kg: PO** Tablet: 150 mg/day
• **Child/adolescent ≥2 yr and weighing <35 kg: PO** Oral powder: 8 mg/kg/dose daily with 2-4 oz soft food. Round dose to nearest 20-mg increment

T

Hepatitis B infection

Adult/child/adolescent ≥35 kg: 300 mg/day × ≥12 mo

Renal dose

• **Adult: PO** CCr 30-49 mL/min, 300 mg q48hr; CCr 10-29 mL/min, 300 mg q72-96hr; CCr <10 mL/min, not recommended

Available forms: tenofovir disoproxil fumarate: Tabs 150, 200, 250, 300 mg; oral powder 40 mg/scoop; tenofovir alafenamide: tablets 25 mg

Administer

• Without regard to food

• Store at 25° C (77° F)

• **Missed dose:** take when remembered on same day, do not double doses

• **Oral powder:** use scoop provided, mix powder into 2-4 oz (¼-½ cup) of applesauce, yogurt, do not mix with liquid, product will not mix, product is bitter, use immediately after mixing, clean scoop

SIDE EFFECTS

CNS: *Headache, asthenia*

GI: *Nausea, vomiting, diarrhea,* anorexia, *flatulence, abdominal pain,* pancreatitis

GU: Renal failure, renal tubular acidosis/necrosis, Fanconi's syndrome

HEMA: Neutropenia, osteopenia

INTEG: *Rash,* angioedema

META: Lactic acidosis, hypokalemia, hypophosphatemia

MS: Arthralgia, myalgia, decreased bone mineral density, rhabdomyolysis

SYST: Lipodystrophy

PHARMACOKINETICS

Rapidly absorbed, distributed to extravascular space, excreted unchanged in urine 70%-80%, terminal half-life 17 hr, disoproxil fumarate alafenamide 0.5 hr, peak 1-2 hr (disoproxil fumarate), 0.5 hr (alafenamide)

INTERACTIONS

Increase: tenofovir level—cidofovir, acyclovir, valACYclovir, ganciclovir, valGANciclovir

Increase: level of didanosine when given with tenofovir

Increase: tenofovir level—any product that decreases renal function

NURSING CONSIDERATIONS

Assess:

• **HIV:** Viral load, CD4+ T-cell count, plasma HIV RNA, serum creatinine/BUN/phosphate

• Resistance testing at start of therapy and at treatment failure

> **Black Box Warning: Hepatitis exacerbations:** monitor hepatic studies: AST, ALT, bilirubin; amylase, lipase, triglycerides baseline and periodically during treatment, after treatment, assess for exacerbations for 6 mo after last dose

• **Bone, renal toxicity:** if bone abnormalities are suspected, obtain tests; serum phosphorus, creatinine

• **Lactic acidosis, severe hepatomegaly with steatosis, Fanconi's syndrome:** obtain baseline liver function tests; if elevated, discontinue treatment; discontinue even if liver function tests normal but lactic acidosis, hepatomegaly present; may be fatal

• **Pregnancy/breastfeeding:** use only if clearly needed; register patients in the Antiretroviral Pregnancy Registry, 800-258-4263; do not breastfeed

Evaluate:

• **Therapeutic response:** decrease in signs, symptoms of HIV; hepatitis B

Teach patient/family:

• To take without regard to food

• That GI complaints resolve after 3-4 wk of treatment

• Not to breastfeed while taking this product

• That product must be taken daily even if patient feels better

• That follow-up visits must be continued because serious toxicity may occur; that blood counts must be done q2wk

• That product will control symptoms but is not a cure for HIV; that patient is still infectious, may pass HIV virus on to others

• To discuss with provider all OTC, Rx, herbals, supplements taken

• **Hepatotoxicity:** To notify provider of yellow skin, eyes; dark urine, clay-colored stools, nausea, abdominal pain
• That other products may be necessary to prevent other infections
• If used for prophylaxis (PREP): does not prevent sexually transmitted infections; use appropriate barrier protection and safe sex practices
• That changes in body fat distribution; usually in the breasts, neck, and back, may occur
• To notify prescriber of symptoms of lactic acidosis (nausea, vomiting, weakness, abdominal pain)

teplizumab-mzwv (Rx)
Tzield
Func. class.: Antidiabetic

USES: To delay the onset of stage 3 type 1 diabetes (T1D) in adults and pediatric patients aged 8 yr and older with stage 2 T1D

DOSAGE AND ROUTES
See manufacturer's information
Available forms: Injection: 2 mg per 2 mL (1 mg/mL) single-dose vial

teprotumumab-trbw (Rx)
(tep′roe-toom′ue-mab)
Tepezza
Func. class.: Insulin-like growth factor-1 antagonist

USES: Treatment of thyroid eye disease

CONTRAINDICATIONS
Hypersensitivity

DOSAGE AND ROUTES
Thyroid eye disease
• **Adult: IV:** 10 mg/kg as a single dose, then 20 mg/kg q3wk × 7 more doses
Available forms: Powder for injection 500 mg

terazosin (Rx)
(ter-ay′zoe-sin)
Func. class.: Antihypertensive
Chem. class.: α-Adrenergic blocker

ACTION: Decreases total vascular resistance, which is responsible for a decrease in B/P; this occurs by the blockade of α₁-adrenoreceptors

USES: Hypertension, as a single agent or in combination with diuretics or β-blockers; BPH

CONTRAINDICATIONS
Hypersensitivity
Precautions: Pregnancy, breastfeeding, children, prostate cancer, syncope

DOSAGE AND ROUTES
Hypertension
• **Adult: PO** 1 mg at bedtime, may increase dose slowly to desired response; max 20 mg/day divided q12hr
Benign prostatic hyperplasia
• **Adult: PO** 1 mg at bedtime, gradually increase up to 5-10 mg; max 20 mg divided q12hr
Available forms: Caps 1, 2, 5, 10 mg
Administer:
• Give dose at bedtime; patient should not operate machinery because fainting may occur
• If treatment is interrupted for several days, restart with initial dose
• Without regard to food; feeding tube: place cap in 60 mL of warm tap water; stir until liquid spills from ruptured shell (5 min); stir until cap dissolves; draw solution into oral syringe; give through feeding tube; flush with water
• Store at room temperature

SIDE EFFECTS
CNS: *Dizziness, headache, drowsiness,* anxiety, depression, vertigo, weakness, fatigue, syncope

CV: *Palpitations, orthostatic hypotension,* tachycardia, *edema,* rebound hypertension

EENT: Blurred vision, epistaxis, tinnitus, dry mouth, red sclera, nasal congestion, sinusitis

GI: *Nausea,* vomiting, diarrhea, constipation, abdominal pain

GU: Urinary frequency, incontinence, impotence, priapism

RESP: Dyspnea, cough, pharyngitis, nasal congestion

PHARMACOKINETICS

Half-life 9-12 hr; protein binding 90%-94%; metabolized in liver; excreted in urine, feces; peak 2-3 hr, onset 15 min, duration 24 hr

INTERACTIONS

Increase: hypotensive effects—β-blockers, nitroglycerin, verapamil, other antihypertensives, alcohol, phosphodiesterase (PDE5) inhibitors (vardenafil, tadalafil, sildenafil)

Decrease: hypotensive effects—estrogens, NSAIDs, sympathomimetics, salicylates

Drug/Herb

Increase: antihypertensive effect—hawthorn

Decrease: antihypertensive effect—ephedra

Drug/Lab Test

Decrease: HB, WBC, platelets, albumin

NURSING CONSIDERATIONS

Assess:

• **BPH:** urinary patterns (hesitancy, frequency, change in stream, dribbling, dysuria, urgency)

• **Hypertension:** crackles, dyspnea, orthopnea q30min; orthostatic B/P, pulse, jugular venous distention q4hr; weight daily, I&O

• **First dose effect:** hypotension/syncope; orthostatic B/P

• **Labs:** BUN, uric acid if patient receiving long-term therapy

• **Beers:** avoid use in older adults as antihypertensive; high risk of orthostatic hypotension

• **Pregnancy/breastfeeding:** use only if benefits outweigh fetal risk; cautious use in breastfeeding, excretion unknown

Evaluate:

• **Therapeutic response:** decreased B/P, edema in feet, legs; decreased symptoms of BPH

Teach patient/family:

• That fainting occasionally occurs after 1st dose; not to drive or operate machinery for 4 hr after 1st dose or after an increase in dose; to take 1st dose at bedtime

• To rise slowly from sitting or lying position

• Not to discontinue abruptly; if doses have been missed for several days, notify prescriber; dose may need to be retitrated

• Not to drink alcohol

• **Hypertension:** to continue with regimen, including diet, exercise

---

terbinafine, oral (Rx)

(ter-bin′a-feen)

Func. class.: Antifungal

Chem. class.: Synthetic allylamine derivative

ACTION: Interferes with cell-membrane permeability of fungi such as *Trichophyton rubrum, Trichophyton mentagrophytes, Trichophyton tonsurans, Epidermophyton floccosum, Microsporum canis, Microsporum audouinii, Microsporum gypseum, Candida;* broad-spectrum antifungal

USES: (Oral) onychomycosis of toenail or fingernail due to dermatophytes, tinea capitis/corporis/cruris/pedis/versicolor

Unlabeled uses: Sporotrichosis, aspergillosis

CONTRAINDICATIONS

Hypersensitivity, chronic/active hepatic disease

Precautions: Pregnancy, breastfeeding, children, renal disease GFR ≤50 mL/min, immunosuppression, depression, HIV, insomnia, hemolytic-uremic syndrome, suicidal ideation, TTP

DOSAGE AND ROUTES

• **Adult: PO** 250 mg/day × 6 wk (fingernail); × 12 wk (toenail)

Available forms: Tabs 250 mg
Administer:
• **PO:** without regard to food
• Store at <25° C (77° F); protect from light

SIDE EFFECTS

CNS: Depression
EENT: Tinnitus, hearing impairment
GI: Diarrhea, dyspepsia, vertigo, abdominal pain, nausea, hepatitis
HEMA: Neutropenia
INTEG: Rash, pruritus, urticaria, Stevens-Johnson syndrome, photosensitivity
MISC: Headache, hepatic enzyme changes, taste, visual/olfactory disturbance

PHARMACOKINETICS

Peak 1-2 hr, >99% protein binding, half-life 36 hr

INTERACTIONS

Increase: levels of dextromethorphan
Increase: terbinafine clearance—rifAMPin
Increase: clearance of cycloSPORINE
Decrease: terbinafine clearance—cimetidine
Decrease: metabolism of—CYP2D6 (antidysrhythmics IC, III, amoxapine, atomoxetine, cloZAPine)
Drug/Herb
• Side effects: cola nut, guarana, yerba maté, tea (black, green), coffee
Drug/Lab Test
Increase: LFTs

NURSING CONSIDERATIONS

Assess:
• Hepatic studies (ALT, AST) before beginning treatment; do not use in presence of hepatic disease
• CBC in treatment >6 wk
• **Continuing infection:** increased size, number of lesions
• **Pregnancy/breastfeeding:** avoid during pregnancy and breastfeeding
Evaluate:
• **Therapeutic response:** decrease in size, number of lesions

Teach patient/family:
• That treatment may take 12 wk (toenail), 6 wk (fingernail)
• To notify prescriber of nausea, vomiting, fatigue, jaundice, dark urine, clay-colored stool, RUQ pain; may indicate hepatic dysfunction
• To take without regard to meals; granules may be sprinkled on soft food but not chewed; do not mix with fruit-based products

---

terbinafine topical
See Appendix B

---

terbutaline (Rx)
(ter-byoo´ta-leen)
Func. class.: Selective β₂-agonist; bronchodilator
Chem. class.: Catecholamine

ACTION: Relaxes bronchial smooth muscle by direct action on β₂-adrenergic receptors through the accumulation of cAMP at β-adrenergic receptor sites; bronchodilation, diuresis, CNS, cardiac stimulation occur; relaxes uterine smooth muscle

USES: Bronchospasm
Unlabeled uses: Premature labor, nonresponsive status asthmaticus in children (IV)

CONTRAINDICATIONS

Hypersensitivity to sympathomimetics, closed-angle glaucoma, tachydysrhythmias
Precautions: Pregnancy, breastfeeding, geriatric patients, cardiac disorders, hyperthyroidism, diabetes mellitus, prostatic hypertension, hypertension, seizure disorder

Black Box Warning: Premature labor

DOSAGE AND ROUTES
Asthma maintenance
• **Adult/adolescent ≥16 yr: PO** 2.5-5 mg q6h while awake, max 15 mg/day

---

• **Child/adolescent 12-15 yr: PO** 2.5 mg q6h while awake, max 7.5 mg/day
Bronchospasm
• **Adult/child ≥12 yr: SUBCUT** 0.25 mg q15-30min, max 0.5 mg in 4 hr
Renal dose
• **Adult: PO** CCr 10-50 mL/min, 50% of dose; CCr <10 mL/min, avoid use
Tocolytic (preterm labor) (unlabeled)
• **Adult: SUBCUT** 0.25 mg q20min to 6 hr, hold if pulse >120 bpm
Available forms: Tabs 2.5, 5 mg; inj 1 mg/mL
Administer:
• With food; may be crushed
• 2 hr before bedtime to avoid sleeplessness

IV route (unlabeled)
• Only used if subcut is ineffective
• IV after diluting each 5 mg/1 L D₅W for infusion
• IV, run 5 mcg/min; may increase 5 mcg q10min, titrate to response; after ½-1 hr, taper dose by 5 mcg; switch to PO as soon as possible
• Store at room temperature; do not use discolored sol

SIDE EFFECTS

CNS: Tremors, anxiety, insomnia, headache, dizziness, stimulation, restlessness
CV: Palpitations, tachycardia, hypertension, dysrhythmias, cardiac arrest, QT prolongation
GI: Nausea, vomiting
META: Hypokalemia, hyperglycemia
RESP: Paradoxical bronchospasm, dyspnea
MS: Muscle cramps
SYST: Angioedema, hypersensitivity

PHARMACOKINETICS

PO: Onset ½ hr, peak 1-2 hr, duration 4-8 hr, half-life 3.4 hr
SUBCUT: Onset 6-15 min, peak ½-1 hr, duration 1½-4 hr, half-life 5.7 hr

INTERACTIONS

Increase: hypertensive crisis—MAOIs
Increase: effects of both products—other sympathomimetics
Decrease: action—β-blockers; do not use together
Drug/Herb
Increase: effect—green tea (large amounts), guarana

NURSING CONSIDERATIONS

Assess:
• **Respiratory function:** vital capacity, forced expiratory volume (FEV), ABGs, B/P, pulse, respiratory pattern, lung sounds, sputum before and after treatment
• **CV status:** HR/rhythm, chest pain, palpitations
• **CNS:** tremors, anxiety, insomnia, dizziness
• Tolerance in patients receiving long-term therapy; dose may have to be changed; monitor for rebound bronchospasm
• **Paradoxical bronchospasm:** dyspnea, wheezing; keep emergency equipment nearby

Black Box Warning: Premature labor: maternal heart rate, B/P, contraction, fetal heart rate; can inhibit uterine contractions, labor; monitor for hypoglycemia; do not use injectable product for prevention or treatment over 72 hr in preterm labor; do not use oral product for preterm labor; avoid breastfeeding

Evaluate:
• **Therapeutic response:** absence of dyspnea, wheezing
Teach patient/family:
• Avoid cough/cold/allergy OTC medications because extra stimulation may occur
• About all aspects of product; to avoid smoking, smoke-filled rooms, persons with respiratory infections
• To maintain adequate hydration; to allow 15 min between inhalation of product and inhaled product containing steroid

• To take on time; if missed, not to make up after 1 hr; to wait until next dose

---

terconazole vaginal antifungal
See Appendix B

---

teriflunomide (Rx)
(ter´i-floo´noe-mide)
Aubagio
Func. class.: Multiple sclerosis agent
Chem. class.: Pyrimidine synthesis inhibitor

ACTION: Antiproliferative effects including peripheral T- and B-lymphocytes, might reduce inflammatory demyelination

USES: Reduction of the frequency of relapses or remitting MS

CONTRAINDICATIONS
Hypersensitivity to this product or leflunomide

Black Box Warning: Pregnancy

Precautions: Breastfeeding, alcoholism, diabetes mellitus, eosinophilic pneumonia, hepatitis, jaundice, male-mediated teratogenicity, pneumonitis, pulmonary disease/fibrosis, sarcoidosis, TB, vaccination, children, geriatrics

Black Box Warning: Hepatic disease, contraception requirements, male-mediated teratogenicity

DOSAGE AND ROUTES
• **Adult: PO** 7 or 14 mg/day, max 14 mg/day
Available forms: Tabs 7, 14 mg
Administer:
PO route
• May be taken without regard to food
• Use precautions in handling, use gloves

SIDE EFFECTS
CNS: Anxiety, headache

CV: Palpitations, hypertension, MI
EENT: Blurred vision, conjunctivitis, sinusitis
GI: Nausea, vomiting, diarrhea, cystitis, hepatotoxicity
HEMA: Leukopenia, lymphopenia, neutropenia
INTEG: Acne vulgaris, alopecia, pruritus
META: Weight loss
MISC: Infection, cystitis, Stevens-Johnson syndrome

PHARMACOKINETICS
Protein binding >99%, median half-life 18-19 days, peak 1-4 hr

INTERACTIONS
• Do not use with leflunomide, live virus vaccines
Increase: teriflunomide effect—cycloSPORINE, eltrombopag, gefitinib

Black Box Warning: Increase: hepatotoxicity—methotrexate, HMG-CoA reductase inhibitors

Increase: hematologic toxicity—zidovudine
Increase: effect of—oral contraceptives, repaglinide, pioglitazone, rosiglitazone, PACLitaxel, naproxen, topotecan, bosentan, furosemide
Decrease: effect of—warfarin, alosetron, DULoxetine, theophylline, tiZANidine, quiNINE, tamoxifen, bendamustine, rasagiline, rOPINIRole, selegiline, propafenone, mexiletine, lidocaine, anagrelide, cloZAPine, cinacalcet, caffeine; monitor closely
Decrease: effect of teriflunomide—cholestyramine

NURSING CONSIDERATIONS
Assess:
• **Labs:** ALT/AST, bilirubin, CBC within 6 mo of starting; measure ALT q6mo, CBC if infection is suspected, obtain TB test before beginning therapy
• **CNS symptoms:** anxiety, confusion, vertigo
• **GI status:** diarrhea, vomiting, abdominal pain

- **Cardiac status:** tachycardia, palpitations, vasodilation, chest pain; monitor B/P
- **Stevens-Johnson syndrome, toxic epidermal necrolysis:** Assess for fever, blisters, aches, fatigue, if these occur, stop product immediately
- **Hepatotoxicity:** Monitor LFTs after 6 mo or less of treatment, and monthly after start of treatment, do not use if ALT >2X ULN, discontinue if >3X ULN, monitor bilirubin
- **Blood dyscrasias:** Monitor CBC, platelets 6 mo before use and periodically, monitor for infection, monitor INR

Black Box Warning: **Pregnancy:** obtain pregnancy test in those of reproductive potential; this product should not be used during pregnancy or for 2 yr after last dose; those wishing to become pregnant must discontinue the product and undergo an accelerated elimination procedure with verification of teriflunomide plasma level <0.02 mg/L; do not use in breastfeeding

Evaluate:
- **Therapeutic response:** decreased symptoms of MS
Teach patient/family:
- That blurred vision can occur
- That hair may be lost, that a wig or hairpiece may be used
- Not to change dosing or stop taking without advice of prescriber
- To report skin changes, rashes immediately
- To avoid live virus vaccines; that updated vaccines should be done before use
- To report signs, symptoms of infection
- Teach patient to take as directed, provide "Medication Guide"
- Teach patient to notify provider of nausea, vomiting, loss of appetite, dark urine, yellow eyes or skin

Black Box Warning: To notify prescriber if pregnancy is planned or suspected; do not use in pregnancy or breastfeeding

teriparatide (Rx)
(tah-ree-par'ah-tide)
Forteo
Func. class.: Parathyroid hormone (rDNA)
Chem. class.: Teriparatide

ACTION: Contains human recombinant parathyroid hormone to stimulate new bone growth

USES: Postmenopausal women with osteoporosis, men with primary or hypogonadal osteoporosis who are at high risk for fracture, glucocorticoid-induced osteoporosis
Unlabeled uses: Hypoparathyroidism

CONTRAINDICATIONS
Hypersensitivity, increased baseline risk for osteosarcoma (Paget's disease, open epiphyses; previous bone radiation), bone metastases, history of skeletal malignancies, other metabolic bone diseases, preexisting hypercalcemia
Precautions: Pregnancy, breastfeeding, children, urolithiasis, hypotension, use >2 yr, cardiac disease

Black Box Warning: Secondary malignancy (osteogenic sarcoma)

DOSAGE AND ROUTES
- **Adult:** SUBCUT 20 mcg/day up to 2 yr
Available forms: Prefilled pen delivery device (delivers 20 mcg/day)
Administer:
SUBCUT route
- Solution should be clear/colorless
- Give by SUBCUT using disposable pen only; inject in thigh or abdomen; lightly pinch fold of skin; insert needle; release skin; inject at 90-degree angle over 5 sec; rotate inj sites
- Have patient sit or lie down; orthostatic hypotension may occur
- Protect from freezing, light; refrigerate pen
- Store refrigerated; do not freeze; may be used for 28 days after first inj

SIDE EFFECTS

CNS: Dizziness, headache, insomnia, depression, vertigo
CV: Hypertension, angina, syncope
GI: Nausea, diarrhea, dyspepsia, vomiting, constipation
INTEG: Rash, sweating
MISC: Pain, asthenia, hyperuricemia
MS: Arthralgia, leg cramps, back/leg pain, weakness, osteosarcoma (rare)
RESP: Rhinitis, cough, pharyngitis, pneumonia, dyspnea

PHARMACOKINETICS

SUBCUT: Extensively and rapidly absorbed, metabolized by liver, excreted by kidneys, terminal half-life 1 hr, onset rapid, peak ½ hr, duration 3 hr

INTERACTIONS

Increase: digoxin toxicity: digoxin
Drug/Lab Test
Increase: calcium, uric acid, urinary calcium
Decrease: phosphorous, magnesium

NURSING CONSIDERATIONS
Assess:

Black Box Warning: **Secondary malignancy:** osteosarcoma, dependent on length of treatment; those at higher risk for osteosarcoma should not use this product, monitor for bone pain, fracture risk

• **Labs:** Uric acid, magnesium, creatinine, BUN, urine pH, vit D, phosphate for normal serum levels; serum calcium may be transiently increased after dosing (max at 4-6 hr after dose)
• **Adverse reactions:** Bone pain, headache, fatigue, changes in LOC, leg cramps
• **Signs of persistent hypercalcemia:** nausea, vomiting, constipation, lethargy, muscle weakness
• **Nutritional status:** diet for sources of vit D (milk, some seafood), calcium (dairy products, dark green vegetables), phosphates (dairy products)

• **Pregnancy/breastfeeding:** use only if benefits outweigh fetal risk; not to be used in pregnant females; do not breastfeed
Evaluate:
• **Therapeutic response:** increased bone mineral density
Teach patient/family:
• About the symptoms of hypercalcemia
• About foods rich in calcium, vit D
• How to use delivery device, dispose of needles; not to share pen with others; to use at same time of day
• To sit or lie down if dizziness or fast heartbeat occurs after 1st few doses
• To report persistent bone pain, severe fatigue, weight loss, falls, swelling
• To rotate administration sites
• To store pen in refrigerator; pen may be used for 28 days

terlipressin (Rx)
(tur-luh-preh-sn)
Terlivaz
Func. class.: Pituitary hormone
Chem. class.: Vasopressin receptor agonist

ACTIONS: A vasopressin receptor agonist indicated to improve kidney function in adults with hepatorenal syndrome (HRS) with rapid reduction in kidney function

USES: Hepatorenal syndrome

CONTRAINDICATIONS
Acute myocardial ischemia, bowel ischemia, hypoxia, peripheral vascular ischemia

Black Box Warning: Acute-on-chronic liver failure, respiratory failure

Precautions: Volume overload, pregnancy, breastfeeding, liver failure, liver transplant

DOSAGE AND ROUTES
• **Adult:** IV Days 1-3 0.85 mg (1 vial) q6hr; day 4 assess serum creatinine vs.

T

baseline; if serum creatinine has decreased by ≥30%, continue 0.85 mg (1 vial) q6hr; if serum creatinine has decreased by <30%, give 1.7 mg (2 vials) q6hr; if no change in serum creatinine, discontinue; continue until 24 hr after 2 consecutive serum creatinine tests <1.5 mg/dL at least 2 hr apart, max 14 days

Available forms: Lyophilized powder for single dose IV 0.85 mg/vial

Administer:

• Reconstitute each vial with 5 mL of 0.9% NaCl injection for a 0.85 mg/5 mL solution

• Visually inspect for particulate matter and discoloration prior to administration

• Prior to initial dosing, assess patient for ACLF grade 3 and obtain patient baseline oxygenation level. Monitor patient oxygen saturation with pulse

• Intermittent IV push route

• Give by slow IV bolus over 2 min

• Administer through a peripheral or central line. A dedicated central line is not required

• Flush the line after use

• If not used immediately, store at 36° F to 46° F (2° C to 8° C) for up to 48 hr, do not freeze. The reconstituted solution does not need protection from light

PHARMACOKINETICS

Terminal half-life 0.9 hr, lysine 3 hr, max change in B/P and heart rate is 1.2-2 hr

INTERACTIONS

None known

NURSING CONSIDERATIONS

Assess:

• Oxygen saturation (SpO_2) prior to starting treatment; do not start in persons experiencing hypoxia (SpO_2 <90%) until improvement of oxygen saturation occurs

• Monitor for changes in respiratory status, including hypoxia, during therapy

using continuous pulse oximetry and regular clinical assessments

• Discontinue if SpO_2 decreases below 90% or if increased respiratory symptoms occur

• Pregnancy/breastfeeding: not to be used, as fetal harm may occur

Evaluate:

• Positive therapeutic outcome

Teach patient/family:

• Pregnancy/breastfeeding: to notify provider if pregnancy is planned or suspected or if breastfeeding. Not to be used in pregnancy and breastfeeding, effects are unknown

---

tesamorelin (Rx)

Egrifta

Func. class.: Pituitary hormone, growth hormone modifiers

ACTION: Binds to growth hormone (GH) releasing factor receptors on the pituitary somatotroph cells; binding stimulates the production, release of endogenous GH

USES: Treatment of excess abdominal fat in HIV-infected patients with lipodystrophy

CONTRAINDICATIONS

Hypersensitivity to this product or mannitol, neoplastic disease, pregnancy, disruption of the hypothalamic-pituitary axis (hypothalamic-pituitary-adrenal [HPA] suppression) due to hypophysectomy, hypopituitarism, pituitary tumor/surgery, radiation therapy of the head or head trauma, IV/IM administration

Precautions: Breastfeeding, CABG, diabetes, diabetic retinopathy, edema, geriatric patients, children, infants, adolescents

DOSAGE AND ROUTES

• **Adult:** SUBCUT 2 mg/day

Available forms: Powder for injection
1 mg
Administer:
Subcut route:
• Visually inspect parenteral products
for particulate matter and discoloration
before use
• To **reconstitute,** use 2, 1-mg vials,
inject 2.1 mL sterile water for inj into the
first 1-mg vial; use syringe with needle
attached; to avoid foaming, push plunger
in slowly and roll for 30 sec until mixed;
do not shake; withdraw 2.1 mL of the
reconstituted sol and add to second 1-mg
vial; roll, do not shake
• Use a 0.5-inch 27-G safety injection
needle; use immediately; **inject** subcut
into abdomen; avoid scar tissues, bruises,
navel; rotate sites; slowly push plunger
down until all sol has been injected
• Use a piece of sterile gauze to rub the
inj site clean; if bleeding, apply pressure
to site with gauze for 30 sec; if bleeding
continues, apply a bandage to site
• Properly dispose of used syringe, needles, vial, and sterile water for injection
bottle

SIDE EFFECTS
CNS: Depression, peripheral neuropathy
paresthesias, hypoesthesia, flushing,
night sweats, insomnia, headache
CV: Hypertension, edema, peripheral
edema, chest pain, palpitations
GI: *Nausea, vomiting,* upper abdominal
pain, dyspepsia, diarrhea, constipation
INTEG: *Pruritus,* urticaria, rash, flush-
ing, *injection site reactions*
MS: *Arthralgia, joint swelling, stiff-
ness, myalgias,* carpal tunnel syndrome
RESP: Upper respiratory tract infection
SYST: Secondary malignancy
META: Hypercalcemia, hyperuricemia

PHARMACOKINETICS
Half-life 26 min in healthy patients, 38 min
in those with HIV infection; peak 0.15 hr

INTERACTIONS
Decrease: effect of—simvastatin, ritonavir, cortisone, predniSONE

NURSING CONSIDERATIONS
Assess:
• **Lipodystrophy:** sunken cheeks, thinning arms and legs, fat accumulation in
the abdomen, jaws, and back of
neck; after treatment these should lessen
• Monitor for edema, joint pains, carpal
tunnel syndrome, therapy may need to be
discontinued
• Monitor glycosylated hemoglobin A1c
(HbA1c), serum IGF-1 concentrations,
ophthalmologic exam
• **Beers:** avoid in older adults except as
hormone replacement following pituitary
gland removal; may cause edema, arthralgia
• **Pregnancy/breastfeeding:** do not use
in pregnancy, breastfeeding

Evaluate:
• Decreasing lipodystrophy in HIV patients

Teach Patient/Family:
• That body fat distribution should
change
• That lab exams will be needed
• If dose is missed, skip and continue
with regular schedule
• About injection technique and preferred injection sites; to avoid bruised,
scarred, or broken skin
• About expectations; the product is
not indicated for weight-loss management
• **Hypersensitivity:** To report rash,
swelling of face, trouble breathing immediately
• **Fluid retention:** To report edema, joint
pain
• To notify prescriber if pregnancy is
planned or suspected, to avoid breastfeeding

testosterone cypionate
(Rx)
Depo-Testosterone
testosterone enanthate
(Rx)
Xyosted

T

testosterone topical (Rx)

Axiron, Vogelxo, AndroGel, Testim, Fortesta

testosterone nasal gel

Natesto

testosterone pellets (Rx)

Testopel

testosterone transdermal (Rx)

Androderm, AndroGel, Fortesta, Testim, Vogelxo

testosterone undecanoate

Aveed, Jatenzo

Func. class.: Androgenic anabolic steroid

Chem. class.: Halogenated testosterone derivative

Controlled Substance Schedule III

Do not confuse:
Testoderm/Testoderm TTS

ACTION: Increases weight by building body tissue; increases potassium, phosphorus, chloride, nitrogen levels, bone development

USES: Female breast cancer, hypogonadism, eunuchoidism, male climacteric, oligospermia, impotence, vulvar dystrophies, low testosterone levels, delayed male puberty (inj)

CONTRAINDICATIONS

Pregnancy, breastfeeding, severe cardiac/renal/hepatic disease, hypersensitivity, genital bleeding (rare), male breast/prostate cancer
Precautions: Diabetes mellitus, CV disease, MI, urinary tract disorders, prostate cancer, hypercalcemia

Black Box Warning: Children, accidental exposure, pulmonary oil microembolism, risk of serious hypersensitivity reactions or anaphylaxis

DOSAGE AND ROUTES
Replacement
• **Adult:** IM (enanthate or cypionate) 50-400 mg q2-4wk; **TOPICAL SOL (Axiron)** 60 mg (2 pump actuations); apply each AM
• **Adult (male)/child:** SUBCUT (pellets) 150-450 mg (2-6 pellets) inserted q3-6mo
• **Adult: TRANSDERMAL (Testoderm, Androderm)** 4-6 mg applied q24hr; **GEL (AndroGel)** 1% 5 mg applied q24hr, once daily; 1.62% 40.5 mg (2 pump actuations) every AM; topical sol **(Axiron)** 30 mg/actuation; **NASAL GEL** 1 pump actuation in each nostril tid
Breast cancer, palliative
• **Adult:** IM 200-400 mg q2-4wk (cypionate or enanthate)
Delayed male puberty
• **Adolescent males:** 50-200 mg q2-4wk for a limited period (cypionate or enathate)
Available forms: Enanthate: inj 200 mg/mL; **cypionate:** inj 100, 200 mg/mL; pellets 75 mg; **transdermal** 2, 4 mg/24 hr; **gel** 1%, 1.62%, 10 mg/actuation; **nasal gel** 5.5 mg/actuation
Administer:
• Titrated dose; use lowest effective dose
• IM inj deep into upper outer quadrant of gluteal muscle
• **Transdermal patches:** Testoderm to skin of scrotum; Androderm to skin of back, upper arms, thighs, abdomen; area must be dry shaved; may be reapplied after bathing, swimming
• **Gel:** products are not interchangeable; dosage and administration for

AndroGel 1% differs from that of AndroGel 1.62%; apply daily to clean, dry area on shoulders, upper arms, or abdomen; women, children should not touch treated skin

SIDE EFFECTS

CNS: Dizziness, headache, fatigue, tremors, paresthesias, flushing, sweating, anxiety, lability, insomnia, carpal tunnel syndrome
CV: Increased B/P
EENT: Conjunctival edema, nasal congestion
ENDO: Abnormal glucose tolerance test
GI: Nausea, vomiting, constipation, weight gain, cholestatic jaundice
GU: Hematuria, amenorrhea, vaginitis, decreased libido, decreased breast size, clitoral hypertrophy, testicular atrophy, gynecomastia, large prostate
HEMA: Polycythemia
INTEG: Rash, acneiform lesions, oily hair/skin, flushing, sweating, acne vulgaris, alopecia, hirsutism
MS: Cramps, spasms

PHARMACOKINETICS

PO: Metabolized in liver; excreted in urine, breast milk; crosses placenta

INTERACTIONS

• Edema: ACTH, adrenal steroids, buPROPion
Increase: effects of oxyphenbutazone
Increase: PT—anticoagulants
Decrease: glucose levels—may alter need for oral antidiabetics, insulin
Drug/Lab Test
Increase: serum cholesterol, blood glucose, urine glucose, Hct, Hgb, WBC
Decrease: serum calcium, serum potassium, T_4, T_3, thyroid ^{131}I uptake test, urine 17-OHCS, 17-KS, PBI

NURSING CONSIDERATIONS
Assess:
• **CV status:** B/P q4hr, HB/HCT; weight daily; notify prescriber if weekly weight gain >5 lb

• **Fluid volume:** I&O ratio; be alert for decreasing urinary output, increasing edema
• Growth rate, bone age in children; growth rate may be uneven (linear/bone growth) with extended use
• **Electrolytes:** potassium, sodium, chlorine, calcium; cholesterol
• **Hepatic studies:** ALT, AST, bilirubin
• Edema, hypertension, cardiac symptoms, jaundice

Black Box Warning: Anaphylaxis: usually with testosterone undecanoate (Aveed) oil for injection; may occur after any injection, observe for 30 min after each use; this product is contraindicated in those with castor oil, benzyl alcohol, benzoic acid hypersensitivity

Black Box Warning: Accidental exposure in children has occurred with topical product after contact with application site, with clothing; wash hands with soap, water

Black Box Warning: Pulmonary oil microembolism: occurs immediately after 1000 mg IM injected of testosterone undecanoate; symptoms include cough, dyspnea, chest pain, dizziness, throat tightening; some events resolve with supportive measures after a few minutes, some require emergency measures

• **Mental status:** affect, mood, behavioral changes, aggression
• **Signs of masculinization in female:** increased libido, deepening of voice, decreased breast tissue, enlarged clitoris, menstrual irregularities; **male:** gynecomastia, impotence, testicular atrophy

• **Hypercalcemia:** lethargy, polyuria, polydipsia, nausea, vomiting, constipation; product may have to be decreased

• **Hypoglycemia** in diabetic patients; oral antidiabetic action is increased

• Diet with increased calories, protein; decrease sodium if edema occurs

• **Beers:** avoid in older adults unless indicated for confirmed hypogonadism with clinical symptoms; potential for cardiac problems; do not use in prostate cancer

• **Pregnancy/breastfeeding:** do not use in pregnancy, breastfeeding

Evaluate:

• **Therapeutic response:** 4-6 wk in osteoporosis

Teach patient/family:

• That product must be combined with complete health plan: diet, rest, exercise

• To notify prescriber if therapeutic response decreases, if edema occurs

• About changes in sex characteristics: priapism, gynecomastia, increased libido

• That women should report menstrual irregularities, voice changes, acne, facial hair growth; if pregnancy is planned or suspected, or if breastfeeding

• That course of 1-3 mo is necessary for response with breast cancer

• About the proper application of patches and how to use gel, IM injection, intranasal gel; about SUBCUT implant complications

• **Nasal:** Teach patient to report nasal bleeding, irritation, pain

• **Topical:** Teach patient to avoid contact with area that has been treated, to wash area before contact

• **Transdermal:** Advise patient to notify provider of virilization in females

---

tetracaine ophthalmic
See Appendix B

---

tetracaine topical
See Appendix B

---

tetracycline (Rx)
(tet-ra-sye′kleen)
Func. class.: Broad-spectrum antiinfective
Chem. class.: Tetracycline

ACTION: Inhibits protein synthesis and phosphorylation in microorganisms; bacteriostatic

USES: Syphilis, *Chlamydia trachomatis,* gonorrhea, lymphogranuloma venereum; uncommon gram-positive, gram-negative organisms; rickettsial infections
Acinetobacter sp., *Actinomyces* sp., *Bacillus anthracis, Bacteroides* sp., *Balantidium coli, Bartonella bacilliformis, Borrelia recurrentis, Brucella* sp., *Campylobacter fetus, Chlamydia trachomatis, Chlamydophila psittaci, Clostridium* sp., *Entamoeba histolytica, Entamoeba* sp., *Escherichia coli, Francisella tularensis, Fusobacterium fusiforme, Haemophilus ducreyi, Haemophilus* influenzae (beta-lactamase negative), *Haemophilus influenzae* (beta-lactamase positive), *Klebsiella aerogenes, Klebsiella granulomatis, Klebsiella* sp., *Listeria monocytogenes, Mycoplasma pneumoniae, Neisseria gonorrhoeae, Rickettsia* sp., *Shigella* sp., *Streptococcus pneumoniae, Streptococcus pyogenes* (group A beta-hemolytic streptococci), *Treponema pallidum, Treponema pertenue, Vibrio cholerae, Yersinia pestis*

CONTRAINDICATIONS
Pregnancy, breastfeeding, children <8 yr, hypersensitivity to tetracyclines, severe renal/hepatic disease, myasthenia gravis

---

Precautions: Renal/hepatic disease, UV exposure, geriatrics

DOSAGE AND ROUTES
Susceptible infections
• **Adult: PO** 250-500 mg q6hr
• **Child >8 yr: PO** 25-50 mg/kg/day in divided doses q6hr, max 3 g/day
Chlamydia trachomatis
• **Adult: PO** 500 mg qid × 7 days
Syphilis
• **Adult and adolescent: PO** 500 mg qid × 2 wk; if syphilis duration >1 yr, must treat 28 days
Brucellosis
• **Adult: PO** 500 mg q6hr × 3 wk with **IM** 1 g streptomycin bid × 1st wk, then daily × 2nd wk
Urethral, endocervical, rectal infections *(C. trachomatis)*
• **Adult: PO** 500 mg qid × 7 days
Acne
• **Adult/adolescent: PO** 250 mg q6hr, then decrease slowly to 125-500 mg/day or every other day
Renal dose
• **Adult: PO** CCr 51-90 mL/min, give dose q8-12hr; CCr 10-50 mL/min, give dose q12-24hr; CCr <10 mL/min, give dose q24hr

Available forms: Caps 250, 500 mg
Administer:
• After C&S obtained, therapy may start before results are received
• 2 hr before or after iron products; 1 hr after antacid products
• Should be given on empty stomach (1 hr before or 2 hr after meals), avoid using at bedtime and take with a full glass of water to prevent irritation and ulceration
• Store in tight, light-resistant container at room temperature

SIDE EFFECTS
CNS: Fever, headache, paresthesia, ICP
CV: Pericarditis
EENT: Dysphagia, glossitis, decreased calcification, discoloration of deciduous teeth, oral candidiasis, oral ulcers

GI: *Nausea*, abdominal pain, *vomiting, diarrhea*, anorexia, enterocolitis, hepatotoxicity, flatulence, abdominal cramps, epigastric burning, stomatitis, hepatitis, CDAD
GU: *Increased BUN*, azotemia, acute renal failure
HEMA: Eosinophilia, neutropenia, thrombocytopenia, leukocytosis, hemolytic anemia
INTEG: *Rash, urticaria, photosensitivity, increased pigmentation*, exfoliative dermatitis, pruritus, angioedema, Stevens-Johnson syndrome
MISC: Increased intracranial pressure, candidiasis

PHARMACOKINETICS
PO: Peak 2-3 hr; duration 6 hr; half-life 6-12 hr; excreted in urine, breast milk; crosses placenta; 65% protein bound

INTERACTIONS
Fatal nephrotoxicity: methoxyflurane; do not use together
Do not take iron supplements, multivitamins, calcium supplements, antacids, laxatives within 2 hr of this product
Increase: Pseudotumor cerebri—ISOtretinoin; avoid concurrent use
Increase: effect of warfarin—digoxin
Decrease: hormonal contraceptive (possible but unlikely); use additional contraception
Decrease: effect of tetracycline—antacids, sodium bicarbonate, alkali products, iron, cimetidine
Decrease: effect of penicillins
Drug/Herb
• Photosensitivity: dong quai
Drug/Food
Decrease: tetracycline effect—dairy products
Drug/Lab Test
Increase: BUN, LFTs

NURSING CONSIDERATIONS
Assess:
• **CDAD:** diarrhea, abdominal pain, fever, fatigue, anorexia; possible anemia, elevated

T

WBC count, low serum albumin; stop product; usually either vancomycin or IV metroNIDAZOLE is given
• **Signs of anemia:** Hct, HB, fatigue
• **Fluid status:** I&O ratio
• **Blood studies:** PT, CBC, AST, ALT, BUN, creatinine if on prolonged therapy
• **Hypersensitivity:** rash, itching, pruritus, angioedema, Stevens-Johnson syndrome, exfoliative dermatitis; report immediately after stopping product
• **GI symptoms:** Nausea, vomiting, diarrhea; administer antiemetic, antacids as ordered
• **Superinfection:** fever, malaise, redness, pain, swelling, drainage, perineal itching, diarrhea, changes in cough or sputum if on prolonged therapy
• **Pregnancy/breastfeeding:** do not use in pregnancy, toxic to fetus; do not breastfeed, excreted in breast milk
Evaluate:
• **Therapeutic response:** absence of lesions, negative C&S, resolution of infection, prevention of malaria
Teach patient/family:
• To avoid sun exposure; that sunscreen does not seem to decrease photosensitivity
• That all prescribed medication must be taken to prevent superinfection
• To avoid milk products, antacids or to separate by 2 hr; to take with full glass of water; to take 1 hr before bedtime to prevent esophageal ulceration
• That tooth discoloration may occur, especially in children; not to use in child <8 yr, may cause bone formation abnormalities
• To notify prescriber immediately of diarrhea with pus, mucus, fever, abdominal pain
• To notify prescriber if pregnancy is planned or suspected
• Not to use outdated products; Fanconi's syndrome (nephrotoxicity) may occur

tetrahydrozoline nasal agent
See Appendix B

tetrahydrozoline ophthalmic
See Appendix B

thiamine (vit B₁) (PO-OTC; IV, IM-Rx)
Vitamin B₁
Func. class.: Vit B₁
Chem. class.: Water soluble

Do not confuse:
thiamine/Tenormin

ACTION: Needed for pyruvate metabolism, carbohydrate metabolism

USES: Vit B₁ deficiency or polyneuritis, cheilosis adjunct with thiamine beriberi, Wernicke-Korsakoff syndrome, pellagra, metabolic disorders, alcoholism

CONTRAINDICATIONS
Hypersensitivity
Precautions: Pregnancy

DOSAGE AND ROUTES
RDA
• **Adult: PO** (males) 1.2-1.5 mg; (females) 1.1 mg; (pregnancy) 1.4 mg; (breastfeeding) 1.4 mg
• **Child 9-13 yr: PO** 0.9 mg
• **Child 4-8 yr: PO** 0.6 mg
• **Child 1-3 yr: PO** 0.5 mg
• **Infant 7 mo-1 yr: PO** 0.3 mg
• **Neonate/infant ≤6 mo: PO** 0.2 mg
Beriberi
• **Adult: PO** 5-30 mg daily or in 3 divided doses × 1 mo; **IM/IV** 5-30 mg daily or in 3 divided doses, then convert to **PO**
• **Infant/child: PO** 10-50 mg daily × 2 wk, then 5-10 mg daily × 1 mo; **IV/IM** 10-25 mg/day × 2 wk, then 5-10 mg daily × 1 mo

Wernicke-Korsakoff syndrome
• **Adult:** IV 200 to 500 mg q8hr for at least 3 days
Available forms: Tabs 50, 100, 250, 500 mg; inj 100 mg/mL; enteric-coated tabs 20 mg
Administer:
IM route
• By IM inj; rotate sites if pain and inflammation occur; do not mix with alkaline sol; Z-track to minimize pain
Direct IV route
• Undiluted at 100 mg/mL over 5 min
Continuous IV INFUSION route
• Diluted in compatible IV sol

SIDE EFFECTS
CNS: Weakness, restlessness
CV: Collapse, pulmonary edema, hypotension
EENT: Tightness of throat
GI: Hemorrhage, *nausea, diarrhea*
INTEG: Angioneurotic edema, cyanosis, sweating, warmth
SYST: Anaphylaxis

PHARMACOKINETICS
PO/INJ: Unused amounts excreted in urine (unchanged)

NURSING CONSIDERATIONS
Assess:
• **Anaphylaxis (IV only):** swelling of face, eyes, lips, throat, wheezing
• **Alcoholism:** Give thiamine prior to glucose-containing IV fluids to chronic alcoholics
• **Thiamine deficiency:** anorexia, weakness/pain, depression, confusion, blurred vision, tachycardia
• Nutritional status: yeast, beef, liver, whole or enriched grains, legumes
• Application of cold to help decrease injection site pain
• **Pregnancy/breastfeeding:** considered compatible with pregnancy, breastfeeding
Evaluate:
• **Therapeutic response:** absence of nausea, vomiting, anorexia, insomnia, tachycardia, paresthesias, depression, muscle weakness

Teach patient/family:
• About the necessary foods to be included in diet: yeast, beef, liver, legumes, whole grains

thioridazine (Rx)
(thye-or-rid′a-zeen)
Func. class.: Antipsychotic (typical)
Chem. class.: Phenothiazine piperidine

USES: Psychotic disorders, schizophrenia, behavioral problems in children, anxiety, major depressive disorders, organic brain syndrome

CONTRAINDICATIONS
Children <2 yr, hypersensitivity, coma, CNS depression

Black Box Warning: QT prolongation, cardiac dysrhythmias, dementia-related psychosis, torsade de pointes

DOSAGE AND ROUTES
Schizophrenia
• **Adult:** PO 50-100 mg tid, max 800 mg/day; dose gradually increased to desired response, then reduced to minimum maintenance
Depression/behavioral problems/dementia
• **Geriatric:** PO 10-25 mg daily-tid, increase 4-7 days by 10-25 mg to desired dose, max 800 mg/day for short period
Available forms: Tablet 10, 25, 50, 100

thiotepa (Rx)
(thye-oh-tep′a)
Tepadina
Func. class.: Antineoplastic, alkylating agent

USES: To reduce the risk of graft rejection when used with busulfan and cyclophosphamide as a preparative regimen for allogeneic hematopoietic progenitor (stem) cell transplantation in children with class 3 beta-thalassemia

CONTRAINDICATIONS
Hypersensitivity, use with live/attenuated vaccines

DOSAGE AND ROUTES
• **Child: IV:** 5 mg/kg IV over 3 hours (via a central venous catheter) approximately 12 hours apart for 2 doses on day 6 prior to an allogeneic hematopoietic progenitor cell transplantation (HSCT) in combination with high-dose busulfan and cyclophosphamide

Available forms: Injection 15 mg

---

thyroid USP, porcine (desiccated) (Rx)
(thye′roid)
Armour Thyroid, Nature-Throid, NP Thyroid, Westhroid
Func. class.: Thyroid hormone
Chem. class.: Active thyroid hormone in natural state and ratio

---

USES: Hypothyroidism, cretinism (juvenile hypothyroidism), myxedema

CONTRAINDICATIONS
Adrenal insufficiency, MI, thyrotoxicosis, porcine protein hypersensitivity

Black Box Warning: Obesity treatment

DOSAGE AND ROUTES
Hypothyroidism
• **Adult:** PO 30 mg/day, increased by 15 mg/mo until desired response; maintenance dose 60-120 mg/day
• **Geriatric:** PO 7.5-15 mg/day, increase dose q6-8wk until desired response
Cretinism/juvenile hypothyroidism
• **Child:** PO 15 mg/day, then 30 mg/day after 2 wk, then 60 mg/day after another 2 wk; maintenance dose 60-180 mg/day
Myxedema
• **Adult:** PO 15 mg/day, double dose q2wk, maintenance 60-180 mg/day
Available forms: Tabs 15, 16.25, 30, 32.5, 60, 65, 90, 120, 130, 180, 195, 240, 300 mg

---

tiaGABine (Rx)
(tie-ah-ga′been)
Gabitril
Func. class.: Anticonvulsant

Do not confuse:
tiaGABine/tiZANidine

ACTION: Inhibits reuptake and metabolism of GABA, may increase seizure threshold; structurally similar to GABA; tiaGABine binding sites in neocortex, hippocampus

USES: Adjunct treatment of partial seizures in adults and children ≥12 yr

CONTRAINDICATIONS
Hypersensitivity
Precautions: Pregnancy, breastfeeding, children <12 yr, geriatric patients, renal/hepatic disease, suicidal thoughts/behaviors, status epilepticus, mania, bipolar disorder, abrupt discontinuation, depression

DOSAGE AND ROUTES
• **Adult (those receiving an enzyme-inducing antiepileptic product):** PO 4 mg/day in divided doses, may increase by 4-8 mg/wk until desired response, max 56 mg/day
• **Child 12-18 yr:** PO 4 mg/day, may increase by 4 mg at beginning of wk 2; may increase by 4-8 mg/wk until desired response; max 32 mg/day
Hepatic dose
• **Adult:** PO reduce dose or increase dosing interval
Available forms: Tabs 2, 4, 12, 16 mg
Administer:
• Store at room temperature, away from heat and light
• Use with food

SIDE EFFECTS
CNS: *Dizziness, anxiety,* somnolence, ataxia, confusion, *asthenia,* unsteady gait, depression, suicidal ideation, seizures, tremors, hostility, EEG changes, insomnia
CV: Vasodilation, tachycardia, hypertension

ENDO: Goiter, hypothyroidism
GI: Nausea, vomiting, diarrhea, increased appetite
INTEG: Pruritus, rash, Stevens-Johnson syndrome, alopecia, hyperhidrosis
MS: Myalgia
RESP: Pharyngitis, coughing

PHARMACOKINETICS
Absorption >95%; peak 45 min; protein binding 96%; metabolized in the liver via CYP3A4; half-life 7-9 hr without enzyme inducers, 2-5 hr with enzyme inducers

INTERACTIONS
• Lower doses may be needed when used with valproate
Increase: CNS depression—CNS depressants, alcohol
Decrease: tiaGABine effect—sevelamer
Decrease: effect—carBAMazepine, PHENobarbital, phenytoin, primidone
Drug/Food
Decrease: rate of absorption—high-fat meal

NURSING CONSIDERATIONS
Assess:
• Hepatic studies: ALT, AST, bilirubin at baseline and periodically
• **Seizures:** location, duration, presence of aura; assess for weakness
• Withdraw gradually to prevent seizures
• May cause status epilepticus and unexplained death
• **Mental status:** mood, sensorium, affect, behavioral changes, suicidal thoughts/behaviors; if mental status changes, notify prescriber, hypomania may be present before suicide attempt
• Assistance with ambulation during early part of treatment; dizziness occurs
• **Seizure precautions:** padded side rails; move objects that may harm patient
• **Pregnancy/breastfeeding:** use only if benefits outweigh fetal risks, may be fetal toxic; pregnant women should enroll in the North American Antiepileptic Drug Pregnancy Registry at 888-233-2334; avoid breastfeeding, likely to be excreted in breast milk

• **Beers:** avoid in older adults unless safer alternatives are unavailable; may cause ataxia, impaired psychomotor function
Evaluate:
• **Therapeutic response:** decreased seizure activity; document on patient's chart
Teach patient/family:
• To carry emergency ID stating patient's name, products taken, condition, prescriber's name and phone number
• To avoid driving, other activities that require alertness, until response is known
• Not to discontinue medication quickly after long-term use
• To take with food
• To notify prescriber if pregnancy is planned or suspected; to avoid breastfeeding
• To report suicidal thoughts, behaviors immediately

⚠ HIGH ALERT

ticagrelor (Rx)
Brilinta
Func. class.: Platelet inhibitor
Chem. class.: ADP receptor antagonist

ACTION: Reversibly binds to the platelet receptor, preventing platelet activation

USES: Arterial thromboembolism prophylaxis in acute coronary syndrome (ACS) (unstable angina, acute MI), including in patients undergoing percutaneous coronary intervention (PCI), stroke

CONTRAINDICATIONS
Hypersensitivity, severe hepatic disease

Black Box Warning: Bleeding, intracranial bleeding

Precautions: Pregnancy, breastfeeding, infants, neonates, children, GI bleeding, hepatic disease, abrupt discontinuation

Side effects: *italics* = common; red = life-threatening

Black Box Warning: Coronary artery bypass graft surgery (CABG), surgery, abrupt discontinuation, aspirin coadministration

DOSAGE AND ROUTES
Acute coronary syndrome
• **Adult: PO** loading dose 180 mg with aspirin (usually 325 mg PO); then give 90 mg bid with aspirin 75-100 mg/day, do not give maintenance doses of aspirin >100 mg/day
MI prophylaxis
• **Adult: PO** 60 mg bid with aspirin 75-100 mg daily
Available forms: Tab 60, 90 mg
Administer:
PO route
• May be taken without regard to food
• Discontinue 5-7 days before surgery
• May be crushed (90 mg tab) and mixed with purified water, 100 mL (PO) or 50 mL (NG); ensure entire dose is given by flushing mortar, syringe, NG tube with 2 additional 50 mL of water
• Store at room temperature, in original container in dry place

SIDE EFFECTS
CNS: *Headache,* dizziness, fatigue
CV: Hypertension, hypotension, chest pain, atrial fibrillation, bradyarrhythmias, syncope, ventricular pauses, HF
GI: Nausea, diarrhea
HEMA: Serious, fatal bleeding
MISC: Back pain, hyperuricemia, gynecomastia
RESP: Dyspnea, cough

PHARMACOKINETICS
Absolute bioavailability 36%, protein binding (>99%), metabolism by CYP3A4, weak P-glycoprotein substrates and inhibitors, elimination for product and metabolite are hepatic and biliary, 84% excreted in feces, 16% in urine, half-life is 7 hr for ticagrelor, 9 hr for metabolite, maximum inhibition of platelet aggregation (IPA) effect 2 hr, maintained ≥8 hr, peak 1.5 hr product, 2.5 hr metabolite

INTERACTIONS

Black Box Warning: Increase: bleeding risk—CYP3A4 inhibitors (ketoconazole, itraconazole, voriconazole, clarithromycin, telithromycin, nefazodone, ritonavir, lopinavir, ritonavir, saquinavir, nelfinavir, indinavir, atazanavir, delavirdine, isoniazid, dalfopristin, quinupristin, tipranavir); cycloSPORINE, anticoagulants, atazanavir, thrombolytics

Increase: effect of—simvastatin, lovastatin
Increase: bleeding risk—NSAIDs, anticoagulants, platelet inhibitors
Decrease: ticagrelor action—CYP3A4 inducers (rifAMPin, dexamethasone, phenytoin, carBAMazepine, PHENobarbital)
Increase or decrease: digoxin
Drug/Lab Test
Increase: serum creatinine

NURSING CONSIDERATIONS
Assess:
• **Thromboembolism:** Monitor CBC with differential with platelet count baseline and periodically during treatment

Black Box Warning: Bleeding: assess for bleeding that may occur when aspirin is combined with this product; some bleeding can be fatal, usually aspirin doses >100 mg/day; watch for frank bleeding, hypotension; avoid with active bleeding, history of intracranial hemorrhage

Black Box Warning: CABG: do not use in those undergoing CABG; discontinue ≥5 days before surgery

Black Box Warning: Aspirin coadministration: use with 75-100 mg of aspirin/day, avoid higher doses; ticagrelor efficacy is decreased with aspirin >100 mg/day

Black Box Warning: Abrupt discontinuation: do not discontinue abruptly; may increase risk for MI, stent thrombosis, death

• **Pregnancy/breastfeeding:** use only if benefits outweigh fetal risk, may be fetal toxic; do not breastfeed, excretion unknown

Evaluate:
• Prevention of thromboembolism

Teach patient/family:
• To take only as prescribed; not to skip or double doses; if a dose is missed, to take next dose at scheduled time

Black Box Warning: To notify prescriber of chills, fever, bruising, bleeding; not to use aspirin >100 mg/day

• Not to use any prescription, OTC products, herbs without approval of prescriber; products with aspirin, NSAIDs may cause bleeding; to be taken with aspirin; prescriber will order, do not alter dose
• To notify all health care providers of product use
• That product can be taken without regard to meals
• That it may take longer for bleeding to stop
• To notify prescriber if pregnancy is planned or suspected, not to breastfeed

ticlopidine (Rx)

Func. class.: Platelet aggregation inhibitors

USES: Prevention of thrombotic stroke, prevention of coronary artery stent thrombosis

DOSAGE AND ROUTES

Black Box Warning: Life-threatening adverse hematologic effects (neutropenia, agranulocytosis, thrombotic thrombocytopenic purpura, aplastic anemia)

Prevention of thrombotic stroke
• **Adult: PO** 250 mg bid

Prevention of coronary artery stent thrombosis
• **Adult: PO** 250 mg bid, beginning after stent implantation and for ≥30 days with aspirin

Available forms: Tabs 250 mg

tigecycline (Rx)

(tye-ge-sye′kleen)

Tygacil

Func. class.: Broad-spectrum antiinfective
Chem. class.: Glycylcyclines

ACTION: Inhibits protein synthesis and phosphorylation in microorganisms; bacteriostatic structurally similar to the tetracyclines

USES: Complicated skin/skin-structure infections (*Escherichia coli, Enterococcus faecalis* [vancomycin-susceptible only], *Staphylococcus aureus, Streptococcus agalactiae, S. anginosus* group, *S. pyogenes, Bacteroides fragilis*); complicated intraabdominal infections (*Citrobacter freundii, Enterobacter cloacae, E. coli, Klebsiella oxytoca, K. pneumoniae, E. faecalis* [vancomycin-susceptible only], *S. aureus* [methicillin-susceptible only], *S. anginosus* group, *B. fragilis, Bacteroides thetaiotaomicron, B. uniformis, B. vulgatus, Clostridium perfringens, Peptostreptococcus micros*); community-acquired pneumonia

CONTRAINDICATIONS

Pregnancy, breastfeeding, children <18 yr, hypersensitivity to tigecycline
Precautions: Renal/hepatic disease, hypersensitivity to tetracyclines, ventilator-associated/hospital-acquired pneumonias

Black Box Warning: Lab test interference due to maltose, mortality

DOSAGE AND ROUTES

• **Adult: IV infusion** 100 mg then 50 mg q12hr, **IV INFUSION** given over 30-60 min q12hr; × 5-14 days, depending on infection

Hepatic dose
• **Adult: IV** (Child-Pugh C) 100 mg, then 25 mg q12hr

T

Available forms: Powder for inj, lyophilized 50 mg

Administer:

• Tigecycline allergy test before using; obtain C&S, do not begin treatment before results or if susceptible organism is strongly suspected

Intermittent IV INFUSION route

• Reconstitute each vial with 5.3 mL of 0.9% NaCl or D₅ (10 mg/mL); swirl to dissolve; immediately withdraw 5 mL of reconstituted sol **dilute by adding** to 100-mL IV bag for infusion (1 mg/mL); may be yellow or orange; if not, sol should be discarded; do not give if particulate matter is present, use a dedicated IV line or Y-site, flush with NS before and after use, give over ½ hr

• Store in tight, light-resistant container at room temperature, diluted sol at room temperature for up to 24 hr, 6 hr in vial, and remaining time in IV bag, ≤48 hr refrigerated

Y-site compatibilities: Acyclovir, alfentanil, allopurinol, amifostine, amikacin, aminocaproic acid, aminophylline, amphotericin B liposome, ampicillin, ampicillin/sulbactam, argatroban, azithromycin, aztreonam, bivalirudin, bumetanide, buprenorphine, butorphanol, calcium chloride/gluconate, CARBOplatin, carmustine, caspofungin, ceFAZolin, cefepime, cefotaxime, cefoTEtan, cefOXitin, cefTAZidime, ceftizoxime, cefTRIAXone, cefuroxime, cimetidine, ciprofloxacin, cisatracurium, CISplatin, clindamycin, cyclophosphamide, cycloSPORINE, cytarabine, dacarbazine, DACTINomycin, DAPTOmycin, DAUNOrubicin hydrochloride, dexamethasone, dexmedetomidine, dexrazoxane, digoxin, diltiaZEM, diphenhydrAMINE, DOBUTamine, DOCEtaxel, dolasetron, DOPamine, doripenem, DOXOrubicin hydrochloride, DOXOrubicin liposome, droperidol, enalaprilat, EPINEPHrine, eptifibatide, ertapenem, erythromycin, esmolol, etoposide, etoposide phosphate, famotidine, fenoldopam, fentaNYL, fluconazole, fludarabine, fluorouracil, foscarnet, fosphenytoin, furosemide, ganciclovir, gemcitabine, gentamicin, glycopyrrolate, granisetron, haloperidol, heparin, hydrocortisone, HYDROmorphone, ifosfamide, imipenem/cilastatin, insulin, irinotecan, isoproterenol, ketorolac, labetalol, lansoprazole, lepirudin, leucovorin, levoFLOXacin, lidocaine, linezolid, LORazepam, magnesium sulfate, mannitol, mechlorethamine, melphalan, meperidine, meropenem, mesna, methohexital, methotrexate, methyldopa, metoclopramide, metoprolol, metroNIDAZOLE, midazolam, milrinone, mitoMYcin, mitoXANTRONE, morphine, moxifloxacin, mycophenolate, nafcillin, nalbuphine, naloxone, nesiritide, nitroglycerin, nitroprusside, norepinephrine, octreotide, ondansetron, oxaliplatin, oxytocin, PACLitaxel, palonosetron, pamidronate, pancuronium, pantoprazole, PEMEtrexed, pemtamidine, pentazocin, PENTobarbital, PHENobarbital, phenylephrine, piperacillin/tazobactam, potassium acetate/chloride/phosphate, procainamide, prochlorperazine, promethazine, propofol, propranolol, raNITIdine, remifentanil, rocuronium, sodium acetate/bicarbonate/phosphate, streptozocin, succinylcholine, SUFentanil, tacrolimus, teniposide, theophylline, thiopental, thiotepa, ticarcillin/clavulanate, tirofiban, tobramycin, topotecan, trimethoprim/sulfamethoxazole, vancomycin, vasopressin, vecuronium, vinBLAStine, vinCRIStine, vinorelbine, zidovudine, zoledronic acid

SIDE EFFECTS

CNS: Headache, dizziness, insomnia

CV: Hypo/hypertension, phlebitis

EENT: Tooth discoloration

GI: *Nausea, vomiting, diarrhea,* anorexia, constipation, dyspepsia, abdominal pain, hepatotoxicity, hepatic failure, CDAD

HEMA: Anemia, leukocytosis, thrombocytopenia

INTEG: *Rash,* pruritus, sweating, photosensitivity

META: Increased ALT, AST, BUN, lactic acid, alk phos, amylase; hyperglycemia, hypokalemia, hypoproteinemia, bilirubinemia

---

MISC: Back pain, fever, abnormal healing, abdominal pain, abscess, asthenia, infection, pain, peripheral edema, local reactions
RESP: Cough, dyspnea
SYST: Anaphylaxis, infection

PHARMACOKINETICS
Not extensively metabolized, 22% of unchanged product excreted in urine, terminal half-life 42 hr, primarily biliary excreted, protein binding 71%-89%

INTERACTIONS
Increase: effect of warfarin, monitor INR
Decrease: effect of oral contraceptives
Drug/Lab Test
Increase: amylase, LFTs, alk phos, BUN, creatinine, LDH, WBC, INR, PTT, PT
Decrease: potassium, calcium, sodium, HB/Hct, platelets

NURSING CONSIDERATIONS
Assess:

Black Box Warning: Increased mortality risk: use only with confirmation of strongly suspected bacterial infection; do not use as a prophylactic

• **CDAD:** diarrhea, abdominal pain, fever, fatigue, anorexia; possible anemia, elevated WBC level, low serum albumin; stop product; usually either vancomycin or IV metroNIDAZOLE is given
• **Signs of anemia:** Hct, HB, fatigue
• **Blood studies:** PT, CBC, AST, ALT, BUN creatinine
• **Hypersensitivity:** rash, itching, pruritus, angioedema, Stevens-Johnson syndrome, anaphylaxis
• **GI reactions:** Nausea, vomiting, diarrhea; administer antiemetic, antacids as ordered
• **Toxicity:** pseudotumor cerebri, photosensitivity, antianabolic actions (azotemia, BUN, hypophosphatemia, metabolic acidosis); tigecycline is structurally similar to tetracycline; pancreatitis, hyperamylasemia (may be fatal); if these occur,

discontinue, improvement usually occurs after product is discontinued
• **Overgrowth of infection:** fever, malaise, redness, pain, swelling, drainage, perineal itching, diarrhea, changes in cough or sputum
• **Pregnancy/breastfeeding:** do not use in pregnancy or breastfeeding; may cause fetal harm
Evaluate:
• **Therapeutic response:** decreased temperature, absence of lesions, negative C&S
Teach patient/family:
• To avoid sun exposure; sunscreen does not seem to decrease photosensitivity
• To avoid pregnancy while taking this product; fetal harm may occur; to avoid breastfeeding
• To report infection, increase in temperature; to report burning, pain at inj site
• To report diarrhea, fatigue, abdominal pain, severe nausea, vomiting

tildrakizumab-asmn (Rx)
(til-drakiz'ue-mab)
Ilumya
Func. class.: Antipsoriatic, interleukin-23 inhibitor

USES: Treatment of adults with moderate to severe plaque psoriasis

CONTRAINDICATIONS
Hypersensitivity

DOSAGE AND ROUTES
Plaque psoriasis
• **Adult: SUBCUT:** 100 mg at weeks 0, 4, and then q12wk
Available forms: Injection 100 mg/mL single-dose syringe

⚠ HIGH ALERT

timolol (Rx)
(tye'moe-lole)
Func. class.: Antihypertensive
Chem. class.: Nonselective β-blocker

ACTION: Competitively blocks stimulation of β-adrenergic receptor within vascular smooth muscle (decreases rate of SA node discharge, increases recovery time); slows conduction of AV node and decreases heart rate, which decreases O_2 consumption in myocardium; also decreases renin-aldosterone-angiotensin system; at high doses, inhibits $β_2$-receptors in bronchial system

USES: Mild to moderate hypertension, migraine prophylaxis, to decrease mortality after MI
Unlabeled uses: Tremors, angina pectoris

CONTRAINDICATIONS

Hypersensitivity to β-blockers, cardiogenic shock, heart block (2nd/3rd degree), sinus bradycardia, HF, cardiac failure, severe COPD, asthma
Precautions: Pregnancy, breastfeeding, major surgery, diabetes mellitus, COPD, well-compensated heart failure, nonallergic bronchospasm, peripheral vascular disease, thyroid/renal/hepatic disease

> Black Box Warning: Abrupt discontinuation

DOSAGE AND ROUTES
Hypertension
• **Adult:** PO 10 mg bid or 20 mg/day, may increase by 10 mg q7days, max 60 mg/day
• **Geriatric patients:** PO initiate dose cautiously
Myocardial infarction prophylaxis
• **Adult:** PO 10 mg bid beginning 1-4 wk after MI for ≥2 yr
Migraine headache prevention
• **Adult:** PO 10 mg bid or 20 mg/day; may increase to 30 mg/day, 20 mg in AM, 10 mg in PM; discontinue if not effective after 8 wk
Available forms: Tabs 5, 10, 20 mg
Administer:

• PO before or immediately after meals, at bedtime; tab may be crushed or swallowed whole
• Reduced dosage in renal dysfunction
• Store at room temperature; do not freeze

SIDE EFFECTS
CNS: *Insomnia, dizziness,* hallucinations, anxiety, fatigue, depression, headache
CV: Hypotension, bradycardia, HF, edema, chest pain, claudication, angina, AV block, ventricular dysrhythmias
EENT: *Visual changes;* sore throat; *double vision;* dry, burning eyes
GI: *Nausea,* vomiting, ischemic colitis, diarrhea, *abdominal pain,* mesenteric arterial thrombosis, flatulence, constipation
GU: Impotence, urinary frequency
HEMA: Agranulocytosis, thrombocytopenia, purpura
INTEG: Rash, alopecia, pruritus, fever
META: Hypoglycemia
MUSC: *Joint pain, muscle pain*
RESP: Bronchospasm, *dyspnea,* cough, crackles, nasal stuffiness

PHARMACOKINETICS
Peak 1-2 hr; half-life 4 hr; metabolized by liver; excreted in urine, breast milk; protein binding <10%

INTERACTIONS
Increase: hypotension, bradycardia—hydrALAZINE, methyldopa, prazosin, anticholinergics, alcohol, reserpine, nitrates
Increase: effects of β-blockers, calcium channel blockers
Decrease: antihypertensive effects—NSAIDs, sympathomimetics, thyroid, salicylates
Decrease: hypoglycemic effects—insulin, sulfonylureas
Decrease: bronchodilation—theophyllines
Drug/Lab Test
Increase: renal, hepatic studies, uric acid
Interference: glucose, insulin tolerance test

NURSING CONSIDERATIONS
Assess:

Black Box Warning: Abrupt discontinu-ation: may result in myocardial ischemia, MI, severe hypotension, ventricular dys-rhythmias in those with preexisting car-diovascular disease

• **Headaches:** location, severity, dura-tion, frequency at baseline and through-out treatment
• I&O; weight daily; edema in feet, legs daily
• B/P during initial treatment, periodi-cally thereafter, pulse q4hr; note rate, rhythm, quality
• Apical/radial pulse before administration; notify prescriber of any significant changes
• Baselines of renal, hepatic studies be-fore therapy begins
• Edema in feet, legs daily
• **Pregnancy/breastfeeding:** use only if benefits outweigh fetal risk, do not breastfeed, excreted in breast milk
Evaluate:
• **Therapeutic response:** decreased B/P after 1-2 wk
Teach patient/family:
• To take before or immediately after meals

Black Box Warning: Not to discontinue product abruptly; to taper over 2 wk; may precipitate angina

• Not to use OTC products containing α-adrenergic stimulants (nasal decon-gestants, cold preparations) unless di-rected by prescriber
• To report bradycardia, dizziness, con-fusion, depression, fever, sore throat, SOB to prescriber
• Product masks hypoglycemia; monitor blood sugar
• To take pulse at home; when to notify prescriber
• To avoid alcohol, smoking, sodium intake
• To comply with weight control, dietary adjustments, modified exercise program
• To carry emergency ID to identify product, allergies
• To avoid hazardous activities if dizzi-ness is present

• To report symptoms of HF: difficulty breathing, especially on exertion or when lying down; night cough; swelling of ex-tremities
• To take medication at bedtime; to wear support hose to minimize effect of ortho-static hypotension

TREATMENT OF OVERDOSE:
Lavage, IV atropine for bradycardia, IV theophylline for bronchospasm, digoxin, O_2, diuretic for cardiac failure, hemodialysis; administer vasopressor (norepinephrine)

timolol (ophthalmic) Rx
(tie-moe′lol)
Betimol, Istalol, Timop ✦, Timol ✦ Timoptic-XE, Timoptic
Func. class.: Antiglaucoma
Chem. class.: β-Blocker

ACTION: Can decrease aqueous humor and increase outflows

USES: Treatment of chronic open-angle glaucoma and ocular hypertension

CONTRAINDICATIONS
Hypersensitivity, AV block, heart failure, bradycardia, sick sinus syndrome, asthma
Precautions: Abrupt discontinuation, pregnancy, breastfeeding, children, COPD, depression, diabetes mellitus, myasthenia gravis, hyperthyroidism, pul-monary disease, angle-closure glaucoma

DOSAGE AND ROUTES
• **Adult:** instill 1 drop in each affected eye bid (0.25% solution) initially; if no response, 1 drop in each affected eye bid (0.5% solution) or 1 drop of gel in each affected eye daily
Available forms: Ophthalmic solu-tion 0.25, 0.5%; ophthalmic gel 0.25%, 0.5%
Administer:
• For ophthalmic use only

• Do not touch the tip of the dropper to the eye, fingertips, or other surface to prevent contamination
• Wash hands before and after use
• If >1 topical ophthalmic drug product is being used, the drugs should be administered at least 5 min apart
• Administer other topically applied ophthalmic medications at least 10 min before gel-forming solution
• To avoid contamination or the spread of infection, do not use dropper for more than one person
• Some products contain the preservative benzalkonium chloride, which can be absorbed by soft contact lenses; remove contact lenses before using solution; lenses may be reinserted 15 min after administration
• Decreased intraocular pressure can take several weeks, monitor IOP after a month

SIDE EFFECTS
CNS: *Insomnia,* headache, *dizziness,* anxiety, depression, headache, nightmares, *fatigue*
CV: Palpitations, heart failure, hypotension
EENT: Eye stinging/burning, tearing, photophobia, visual disturbances
GI: Nausea, dry mouth
RESP: Bronchospasm

PHARMACOKINETICS
Onset 30 min, peak 1-2 hr, duration 12-24 hr

INTERACTIONS
Increase: β-blocking effect—oral β-blockers
Increase: intraocular pressure reduction—topical miotics, dipivefrin, EPINEPHRine, carbonic anhydrase inhibitors; this may be beneficial
Increase: B/P, severe—when abruptly stopping cloNIDine
Increase: depression of AV nodal conduction, bradycardia, or hypotension—adenosine, cardiac glycosides, disopyramide, other antiarrhythmics, class 1C antiarrhythmic drugs (flecainide, propafenone, moricizine, encainide, quiNIDine, calcium-channel blockers, or drugs that significantly depress AV nodal conduction)
Increase: AV block nodal conduction, induce AV block—high doses of procainamide
Increase: antihypertensive effect—other antihypertensives

NURSING CONSIDERATIONS
Assess:
• **Systemic absorption:** when used in the eye, systemic absorption is common with the same adverse reactions and interactions
• Glaucoma: monitor intraocular pressure
• **Pregnancy/breastfeeding:** use only if benefits outweigh fetal risks; do not breastfeed, excreted in breast milk
Evaluate:
• Decreasing intraocular pressure
Teach patient/family:
• That product is for ophthalmic use only
• Not to touch the tip of the dropper to the eye, fingertips, or other surface to prevent contamination
• To wash hands before and after use
• To tilt the head back slightly and pull the lower eyelid down with the index finger to form a pouch; squeeze the prescribed number of drops into the pouch; close eyes to spread drops
• To apply finger pressure on the lacrimal sac for 1-2 min following use to prevent excessive systemic absorption
• To administer drugs at least 5 min apart if more than one topical ophthalmic drug product is being used
• To administer other topically applied ophthalmic medications at least 10 min before timolol gel-forming solution
• To not use dropper for more than one person to avoid contamination or the spread of infection
• That some products contain the preservative benzalkonium chloride, which may be absorbed by soft contact lenses; to remove contact lenses before administration of the solution; that lenses may be reinserted 15 min after administration

⚠ HIGH ALERT

tinidazole (Rx)

(tye-ni'da-zole)

Tindamax

Func. class.: Antiprotozoal
Chem. class.: Nitroimidazole derivative

ACTION: Interferes with DNA/RNA synthesis in protozoa

USES: Amebiasis, giardiasis, trichomoniasis
Unlabeled uses: Helicobacter pylori, prophylaxis against STDs following sexual assault, urethritis, nongonococcal

CONTRAINDICATIONS

Pregnancy, breastfeeding; hypersensitivity to this product or nitroimidazole derivative

Precautions: Children, geriatric patients, hepatic disease, CNS depression, blood dyscrasias, candidiasis, seizures, viral infection, alcoholism, pregnancy

Black Box Warning: Secondary malignancy

DOSAGE AND ROUTES
Intestinal amebiasis/amebic involvement of the liver
• **Adult: PO** 2 g daily × 3 days
• **Child ≥3 yr/adolescent: PO** 50 mg/kg/day × 3 days, max 2 g/day
Giardiasis
• **Adult: PO** 2 g as a single dose
• **Child ≥3 yr: PO** 50 mg/kg as a single dose, max 2 g
Trichomoniasis
• **Adult: PO** 2 g as a single dose
Bacterial vaginosis
• **Adult (nonpregnant woman): PO** 2 g/day × 2 days with food or 1 g/day × 5 days with food
Available forms: Tabs 250, 500 mg
Administer:
• Tabs can be crushed and mixed with artificial cherry syrup for children
• With food to increase plasma concentrations, minimize epigastric distress and other GI effects

SIDE EFFECTS
CNS: *Dizziness, headache,* seizures, *peripheral neuropathy,* malaise, fatigue
GI: *Nausea, vomiting,* anorexia, increased AST/ALT, constipation, abdominal pain, indigestion, altered taste
HEMA: Leukopenia, neutropenia
INTEG: Pruritus, urticaria, *rash,* oral candidiasis
SYST: Angioedema, cramping

PHARMACOKINETICS
Peak 1½ hr; metabolized extensively in liver; excreted unchanged (20%-25%) in urine, (12%) feces; half-life 12-14 hr; crosses blood-brain barrier

INTERACTIONS
• Do not use within 2 wk of disulfiram
Increase: tinidazole action—CYP3A4 inhibitors (cimetidine, ketoconazole): increased action of tinidazole
Increase: action of anticoagulants, cyclo-SPORINE, tacrolimus, fluorouracil, hydantoins, lithium
Decrease: tinidazole action—CYP3A4 inducers (PHENobarbital, rifampin, phenytoin); cholestyramine, oxytetracycline: decreased action of tinidazole
Drug/Herb
Increase or decrease: tinidazole level—St. John's wort
Drug/Lab Test
Increase: triglycerides, LDH, AST/ALT, glucose
Decrease: WBCs

NURSING CONSIDERATIONS
Assess:
• **Giardiasis:** obtain 3 stool samples several days apart beginning q3-4wk after treatment
• **Amebic liver abscess:** monitor CBC, ESR, amebic gel diffusion test, ultrasound; also total and differential leukocyte count

Black Box Warning: Secondary malignancy: avoid unnecessary use

• Signs of infection, anemia
• Bowel pattern before, during treatment
• **Pregnancy/breastfeeding:** contraindicated during first trimester; do not breastfeed

Evaluate:
• **Therapeutic response:** decrease in infection as evidenced by negative culture

Teach patient/family:
• To take with food to increase plasma concentrations, minimize epigastric distress and other GI effects; not to use alcoholic beverages during or for 3 days after treatment
• **Trichomoniasis:** that all partners should be notified and treated at the same time
• To avoid alcohol; may cause disulfiram reaction
• To avoid doing hazardous activities until reaction is known
• That product causes unpleasant taste
• Not to use OTC, Rx, or herbal products unless approved by prescriber

---

tioconazole vaginal antifungal
See Appendix B

---

tiotropium (Rx)
(ty-oh′tro-pee-um)
Spiriva HandiHaler, Spiriva Respimat
Func. class.: Anticholinergic, bronchodilator
Chem. class.: Synthetic quaternary ammonium compound

Do not confuse:
Spiriva/Apidra/Inspra

ACTION: Inhibits interaction of acetylcholine at receptor sites on the bronchial smooth muscle, thereby resulting in decreased cGMP and bronchodilation

USES: COPD; for the long-term treatment and once-daily maintenance of bronchospasm associated with COPD, including chronic bronchitis and emphysema

CONTRAINDICATIONS
Hypersensitivity to this product, atropine, or its derivatives
Precautions: Pregnancy, breastfeeding, children, geriatric patients, closed-angle glaucoma, prostatic hypertrophy, bladder neck obstruction, renal disease

DOSAGE AND ROUTES
• **Adult:** INH content of 1 cap/day (18 mcg) using HandiHaler inhalation device or 2 INH (spray) (2.5 mcg each) daily
Available forms: Powder for INH 18 mcg in blister packs containing 6 caps with inhaler; 30 caps with inhaler; spray inhaler (Respimat) 2.5 mcg/spray
Administer:
Inhalation route (caps)
• Not for acute bronchospasm or acute symptoms
• Caps are for INH only; do not swallow
• Check package insert for directions on how to use
• Rinse mouth after use
Inhalation route (spray)
• Insert cartridge into inhaler, prime inhaler, must reprime once if not used for >3 days, if not used for >21 days, prime until aerosol is visible, and 3 more times

SIDE EFFECTS
CNS: Depression, paresthesia
CV: Chest pain, increased heart rate, angina, atrial fibrillation, supraventricular tachycardia
EENT: Dry mouth, blurred vision, glaucoma
GI: Vomiting, abdominal pain, constipation, dyspepsia, paralytic ileus
GU: Urinary difficulty, urinary retention, UTI
INTEG: Rash, angioedema
MISC: Candidiasis, flulike syndrome, herpes zoster, infections, angina pectoris
MS: Arthritis, myalgic leg/skeletal pain

RESP: *Cough, sinusitis, upper respiratory tract infection,* epistaxis, pharyngitis

PHARMACOKINETICS
Half-life 5-6 days in animals, does not cross blood-brain barrier, very little metabolized in the liver, excreted in urine, 72% protein binding, peak 5 min

INTERACTIONS
• Other anticholinergics: avoid use with other anticholinergics
Drug/Lab Test
Increase: cholesterol, glucose

NURSING CONSIDERATIONS
Assess:
• **Respiratory status:** oral thrush, dyspnea, rate, breath sounds before and during treatment; pulmonary function tests at baseline and periodically; upper respiratory infections, cough, sinusitis
• **Tolerance over long-term therapy;** dose may have to be increased or changed
• Patient's ability to use HandiHaler
• **Pregnancy/breastfeeding:** use only if benefits outweigh fetal risk, cautious use in breastfeeding, unlikely to cause harm in the infant
Evaluate:
• **Therapeutic response:** ability to breathe easier
Teach patient/family:
• Signs of closed-angle glaucoma (eye pain, blurred vision, visual halos)
• That product is used for long-term maintenance, not for immediate relief of breathing problems; that effect takes 20 min, lasts 24 hr
• To avoid getting the powder in the eyes; may cause blurred vision and pupil dilation
• To breathe out completely; not to breathe into mouthpiece at any time
• To hold HandiHaler with mouthpiece upward; to press button in once, completely, and release; this allows for medication to be released
• To raise device to mouth and close lips tightly around mouthpiece
• With head upright, to breathe in slowly and deeply, but allow the cap to vibrate; to breathe until the lungs fill; to hold breath and remove mouthpiece; to resume normal breathing
• To rinse mouth after use; to use hard candy or regular oral hygiene to reduce dry mouth
• To report immediately blurred vision, eye pain, halos
• To keep caps in sealed blisters before use; to store at room temperature

tipranavir (Rx)
(ti-pran′a-veer)
Aptivus
Func. class.: Antiretroviral
Chem. class.: Protease inhibitor

ACTION: Inhibits human immunodeficiency virus (HIV) protease, thereby preventing the maturation of the virus

USES: HIV in combination with other antiretrovirals

CONTRAINDICATIONS
Hypersensitivity
Precautions: Pregnancy, breastfeeding, children, renal disease, history of renal stones, sulfa allergy, hemophilia, diabetes mellitus, pancreatitis, alcoholism, immune reconstitution syndrome, surgery, trauma, infection

Black Box Warning: Intracranial bleeding, hepatitis, hepatic disease (Child-Pugh B, C)

DOSAGE AND ROUTES
• **Adult: PO** 500 mg coadministered with ritonavir 200 mg bid with food
• **Adolescent and child ≥2 yr: PO** 14 mg/kg given with ritonavir 6 mg/kg bid or 375 mg/m² given with ritonavir 150 mg/m² bid, max 500 mg with ritonavir 200 mg bid
Available forms: Caps 250 mg; oral solution 100 mg/mL

Administer:

• Not to be used in those who are treatment-naive

• Swallow cap whole; do not break, crush, chew; store caps in refrigerator before use; after opening, store at room temperature; use within 60 days

• After meals

• In equal intervals around the clock to maintain blood levels

SIDE EFFECTS

CNS: *Headache, insomnia,* dizziness, somnolence, fatigue, *fever,* intracranial bleeding

GI: *Diarrhea, abdominal pain, nausea, vomiting,* anorexia, dry mouth, hepatitis B or C, pancreatitis, fatalities when given with ritonavir

GU: Nephrolithiasis

INTEG: *Rash,* urticaria, lipodystrophy, serious rash

MS: Pain

OTHER: Asthenia, insulin-resistant hyperglycemia, *hyperlipidemia,* ketoacidosis

PHARMACOKINETICS

Terminal half-life 6 hr, peak 3 hr, plasma protein binding 99.9%, steady state 7-10 days, metabolism CYP3A4, 80% fecal excretion

INTERACTIONS

Life-threatening dysrhythmias: amiodarone, astemizole, cisapride, ergots, flecainide, midazolam, pimozide, propafenone, quiNIDine, rifabutin, rifAMPin, terfenadine, triazolam

Increase: myopathy, rhabdomyolysis—HMG-CoA reductase inhibitors (lovastatin, simvastatin)

Increase: tipranavir levels—ketoconazole, delavirdine, itraconazole

Increase: levels of both products—clarithromycin, zidovudine

Increase: levels of tipranavir—oral contraception

Decrease: tipranavir levels—rifamycins, fluconazole, nevirapine, efavirenz

Drug/Herb

Decrease: tipranavir levels—St. John's wort; avoid concurrent use

Drug/Food

Decrease: tipranavir absorption—grapefruit juice; high-fat, high-protein foods

Drug/Lab Test

Increase: AST/ALT, cholesterol, blood glucose, amylase, lipase, triglycerides

NURSING CONSIDERATIONS

Assess:

• Signs of infection, anemia; presence of other sexually transmitted diseases

Black Box Warning: Hepatitis, pancreatitis: ALT, AST; total bilirubin, amylase; all may be elevated, discontinue in those with hepatic insufficiency or hepatitis or AST/ALT 10 × upper limit or AST/ALT 5-10 × ULN and total bilirubin 2.5 × ULN; assess for anorexia, nausea, jaundice, hepatomegaly, clay-colored stools

• **HIV:** Viral load, CD4, plasma HIV RNA, serum cholesterol profile, serum triglycerides during treatment

• Bowel pattern before, during treatment; if severe abdominal pain with bleeding occurs, product should be discontinued; monitor hydration

• **Serious rash:** if serious rash occurs, product should be discontinued

• **Immune reconstitution syndrome:** has been reported with combination antiretroviral therapy, patients may develop pain (MAC, CMV, PcP, TB) and autoimmune disease months after treatment

Black Box Warning: Intracranial bleeding: more common in those with trauma, surgery, or those taking antiplatelets or anticoagulants; assess for headache, nausea, vomiting, seizures, confusion, inability to speak, can be fatal

• Cushingoid symptoms: buffalo hump, facial/peripheral wasting, breast enlargement, central obesity

• **Pregnancy/breastfeeding:** use only if benefits outweigh fetal risk; enroll pregnant women in the Antiretroviral Pregnancy Registry, 800-258-4263; do not breastfeed

Evaluate:
• **Therapeutic response:** improving CD4 counts, viral load

Teach patient/family:
• To take as prescribed; if dose is missed, to take as soon as remembered up to 1 hr before next dose; not to double dose; that this product must be taken with other antivirals
• That product must be taken in equal intervals around the clock to maintain blood levels for duration of therapy
• That hyperglycemia may occur; to watch for increased thirst; weight loss; hunger; dry, itchy skin; to notify prescriber
• That product does not cure AIDS, only controls symptoms; not to donate blood
• That redistribution of body fat may occur
• Not to use with other products unless approved by prescriber, many drug interactions
• That product must be taken in combination with ritonavir
• To stop product and notify prescriber if anorexia, nausea, vomiting, yellowing of skin or eyes, clay-colored stools, fatigue, pain in upper abdomen

---

⚠ HIGH ALERT

tirofiban (Rx)

(tie-roh-fee′ban)

Aggrastat

Func. class.: Antiplatelet
Chem. class.: Glycoprotein IIb/IIIa inhibitor

Do not confuse:
Aggrastat/argatroban

ACTION: Antagonist of platelet glycoprotein (GP) IIb/IIIa receptor that prevents binding of fibrinogen and von Willebrand's factor, which inhibits platelet aggregation

USES: Acute coronary syndrome in combination with heparin

CONTRAINDICATIONS

Hypersensitivity, active internal bleeding, stroke, major surgery, severe trauma within 30 days, intracranial neoplasm, aneurysm, hemorrhage, acute pericarditis, platelets <100,000/mm³, history of thrombocytopenia, coagulopathy, systolic B/P >180 mm Hg or diastolic B/P >110 mm Hg

Precautions: Pregnancy, breastfeeding, children, geriatric patients, renal disease, bleeding tendencies, hypertension, platelets <150,000/mm³

DOSAGE AND ROUTES

• **Adult: IV** 25 mcg/kg within 5 min, then 0.15 mcg/kg/min for up to 18 hr after

Renal dose
• **Adult: IV** CCr <60 mL/min, 25 mcg/kg, then 0.075 mcg/kg/min

Available forms: Inj 50-mL vials; inj premixed bag 50 mcg/mL in 100, 250 mL

Administer:

Intermittent IV INFUSION route
• Discontinue no less than 2-4 hr before CABG
• Do not use if particulates are present
• Dilute inj: withdraw and discard 100 mL from 500-mL bag of sterile 0.9% NaCl or D₅W and replace this vol with 100 mL of tirofiban inj from 2 vials
• Tirofiban inj for sol is premixed in containers of 500 mL 0.9% NaCl (50 mg/mL), infuse over 30 min
• Minimize other arterial/venous punctures, IM inj, catheter use, intubation to reduce bleeding risk
• Discard unused solution after 24 hr from start of infusion

Y-site compatibilities: Acyclovir, alfentanil, allopurinol, amifostine, amikacin, aminocaproic acid, aminophylline, amiodarone, ampicillin, ampicillin/sulbactam, anidulafungin, argatroban, arsenic trioxide, atracurium, atropine, azithromycin, aztreonam, bivalirudin, bleomycin, bumetanide, buprenorphine, butorphanol, calcium chloride/gluconate, capreomycin, CARBOplatin, carmustine, caspofungin, ceFAZolin, cefepime, cefotaxime, cefoTEtan, cefOXitin, cefTAZidime, ceftizoxime, cefTRIAXone, cefuroxime, chloramphenicol, chlorproMAZINE, cimetidine, ciprofloxacin, cisatracurium, CISplatin, clindamycin, cyclophosphamide, cycloSPORINE, cytarabine, DACTINomycin, DAPTOmycin, dexamethasone, dexmedetomidine, dexrazoxane, digoxin, diltiaZEM, diphenhydrAMINE, DOBUTamine, DOCEtaxel, dolasetron, DOPamine, doxacurium, DOXOrubicin, DOXOrubicin liposome, doxycycline, droperidol, enalaprilat, ePHEDrine, EPINEPHrine, epiRUBicin, eptifibatide, ertapenem, erythromycin, esmolol, etoposide, etoposide phosphate, famotidine, fenoldopam, fentaNYL, fluconazole, fludarabine, fluorouracil, foscarnet, fosphenytoin, furosemide, ganciclovir, gemcitabine, gentamicin, glycopyrrolate, granisetron, haloperidol, heparin, hydrALAZINE, hydrocortisone, HYDROmorphone, IDArubicin, ifosfamide, imipenem/cilastatin, insulin, irinotecan, isoproterenol, ketorolac, labetalol, leucovorin, lidocaine, linezolid, LORazepam, magnesium sulfate, mannitol, mechlorethamine, melphalan, meperidine, meropenem, mesna, methylhexital, methotrexate, methyldopate, methylPREDNISolone, metoclopramide, metoprolol, metroNIDAZOLE, midazolam, milrinone, mitoXANTRONE, morphine, mycophenolate, nafcillin, nalbuphine, naloxone, nesiritide, niCARDipine, nitroglycerin, nitroprusside, norepinephrine, octreotide, ondansetron, oxaliplatin, oxytocin, PACLitaxel, palonosetron, pamidronate, pancuronium, pantoprazole, PEMEtrexed, PENTobarbital, PHENobarbital, phentolamine, phenylephrine, piperacillin/tazobactam, potassium acetate, potassium chloride/phosphates, procainamide, prochlorperazine, promethazine, propranolol, quinupristin/dalfopristin, raNITIdine, remifentanil, rocuronium, sodium acetate/bicarbonate, streptozocin, succinylcholine, SUFentanil, tacrolimus, teniposide, theophylline, thiopental, thiotepa, ticarcillin/clavulanate, tigecycline, tobramycin, topotecan, vancomycin, vasopressin, vecuronium, verapamil, vinBLAStine, vinCRIStine, vinorelbine, voriconazole, zidovudine, zoledronic acid

SIDE EFFECTS

CNS: Dizziness, headache
CV: Bradycardia, hypotension, edema
GI: Nausea, vomiting, GI hemorrhage
HEMA: Bleeding, thrombocytopenia
INTEG: *Rash*
MISC: Dissection, edema, pain in legs/pelvis, sweating
SYST: Anaphylaxis

PHARMOCOKINETICS

Half-life 2 hr; excretion via urine, feces; plasma clearance 20%-25% lower in geriatric patients with CAD; renal insufficiency decreases plasma clearance

INTERACTIONS

Increase: bleeding—aspirin, heparin, NSAIDs, abciximab, eptifibatide, clopidogrel, ticlopidine, dipyridamole, cefamandole, cefoTEtan, cefoperazone, valproic acid, heparins, thrombin inhibitors, SSRIs, SNRIs
Increase: tirofiban clearance—levothyroxine, omeprazole
Drug/Lab
Decrease: platelets, Hct, HB

NURSING CONSIDERATIONS
Assess:

• **Bleeding:** platelet counts, Hct, HB before treatment, within 6 hr of loading dose, and at least daily thereafter; watch for bleeding from puncture sites, catheters; or in stools, urine; discontinue if platelets (100 × 10 9/L); if platelets (<90 × 10 9/L) additional platelet counts should be performed to exclude pseudothrombocytopenia; if thrombocytopenia is confirmed, tirofiban and heparin should be discontinued

• Assess for contraindications to therapy: recent major surgery, active bleeding, peptic ulcer disease, trauma within 30 days

• **Pregnancy/breastfeeding:** do not use unless clearly needed; do not breastfeed, excretion unknown

Evaluate:
• **Therapeutic response:** treatment of acute coronary syndrome

Teach patient/family:
• That it is necessary to quit smoking to prevent excessive vasoconstriction

• About signs, symptoms of bleeding and low platelets; report bleeding (blood in stool/urine) to prescriber; use mechanical razors, soft-bristle toothbrush

• That there are many product and herbal interactions; do not use unless approved by prescriber

---

tirzepatide
(tir-zep′a-tide)
Mounjaro
Func. class.: Antidiabetics

USES: Adjunct to diet and exercise to improve glycemic control in diabetes type 2

DOSAGE AND ROUTES
• **Adult: SUBCUT** 2.5 mg qwk, after 4 wk, increase to 5 mg qwk, may increase q4wk by 2.5 mg if needed, max 15 mg/wk

---

⚠ HIGH ALERT

tisagenlecleucel (Rx)
(TIH-suh-jen-LEK-loo-sel)
Kymriah
Func. class.: Antineoplastic

USES: For the treatment of refractory B-cell precursor acute lymphoblastic leukemia

Black Box Warning: Cytokine release syndrome, infection, neurotoxicity

DOSAGE AND ROUTES
• **Adult ≤25 yr/adolescent/child/infant/neonate: IV (>50 kg):** Infuse a single dose of $0.1\text{-}2.5 \times 10^8$ CAR-positive viable

T cells (non–weight-based); **(≤50 kg):** Infuse a single dose of $0.2\text{-}5 \times 10^6$ CAR-positive viable T cells per kg of body weight. Give at 2-14 days after the completion of lymphocyte depletion with fludarabine and cyclophosphamide

Available forms: IV infusion single dose 10-50 mL with chimeric antigen receptor-positive viable T cell (infusion bag)

---

tisotumab vedotin-tftv (Rx)
(tye-sot′ue-mab ve-doe′tin)
Tivdak
Func. class.: Antineoplastic

USES:
Recurrent or metastatic cervical cancer

DOSAGE AND ROUTES
• **Adult: IV** 2 mg/kg (max 200 mg, weight of 100 kg or greater) give over 30 min q3wk until disease progression or unacceptable toxicity

Available forms: IV 40 mg single-dose vial

---

tiZANidine (Rx)
(ti-za′nih-deen)
Zanaflex
Func. class.: Skeletal muscle relaxant, α_2-adrenergic agonist
Chem. class.: Imidazoline

Do not confuse:
tiZANidine/tiaGABine

ACTION: Increases   presynaptic inhibition of motor neurons and reduces spasticity by α_2-adrenergic agonism

USES: Acute/intermittent management of increased muscle tone associated with spasticity, symptoms of MS
Unlabeled uses: Muscle spasm, MS pain

CONTRAINDICATIONS
Hypersensitivity
Precautions: Pregnancy, breastfeeding, children, geriatric patients, hypotension, renal/hepatic disease

---

Side effects: *italics* = common; red = life-threatening

DOSAGE AND ROUTES
• **Adult: PO** initial 2 mg every 6-8 hours, up to 3 doses in 24 hours; increase by 2-4 mg per dose at 1-4 day intervals, max 36 mg/day

Renal dose
• **Adult: PO** CCr <25 mL/min, start with lower dose

Available forms: Tabs 2, 4 mg; caps 2, 4, 6 mg

Administer
• Consistently either with/without food; food may affect absorption
• Titrate doses carefully
• Avoid use with other CNS depressants
• Caps, tabs are equivalent if used on empty stomach

SIDE EFFECTS
CNS: Somnolence, dizziness, speech disorder, dyskinesia, nervousness, hallucination, psychosis

CV: Hypotension, bradycardia, HF, CAD, MI

GI: Dry mouth, vomiting, increased ALT, abnormal LFTs, constipation

OTHER: Blurred vision, urinary frequency, pharyngitis, rhinitis, tremors, rash, muscle weakness, UTI

PHARMACOKINETICS
Completely absorbed, widely distributed, peak 1-2 hr, duration 3-6 hr, half-life 2.5 hr, protein binding 30%, metabolized by liver; excreted in urine, feces

INTERACTIONS
Increase: CNS depression—alcohol, other CNS depressants, opioids; do not use together unless absolutely needed

Increase: tiZANidine levels—other CYP1A2 inhibitors (acyclovir, amiodarone, famotidine, mexiletine, enoxacin, norfloxacin, propafenone, tacrine, verapamil, zileuton, oral contraceptives, ciprofloxacin), fluvoxaMINE; avoid concurrent use

Increase: hypotension—ACE inhibitors

Increase: effect of rasagiline

Increase: rebound hypertension risk—beta-blockers

Drug/Herb
Increase: CNS depression—kava, St. John's wort

Drug/Lab Test
Increase: alk phos, AST, ALT

NURSING CONSIDERATIONS
Assess:
• **Muscle spasticity** at baseline and throughout treatment
• **Hypotension:** gradual dosage increase should lessen hypotensive effects; have patient rise slowly from supine to upright; watch those patients receiving antihypertensives for increased effects
• **CNS:** Increased sedation, dizziness, hallucinations, psychosis; product may need to be discontinued
• Vision by ophthalmic exam; corneal opacities may occur
• **Hepatic studies:** baseline, at 1 mo after therapeutic dose is achieved and if clinically indicated during treatment and periodically thereafter
• **Pregnancy/breastfeeding:** use only if benefits outweigh fetal risk; no well-controlled studies; cautious use in breastfeeding, excretion unknown
• **Beers:** avoid in older men; may cause urinary retention

Evaluate:
• **Therapeutic response:** decreased muscle spasticity

Teach patient/family:
• To rise slowly from lying or sitting to upright position to prevent orthostatic hypotension
• To ask for assistance if dizziness, sedation occur; to avoid drinking alcohol; to avoid operating machinery, driving until effects known
• To discontinue gradually
• To avoid hazardous activities until reaction is known
• Not to use other products unless approved by prescriber; to avoid use with other CNS depressants, opioids; to get medical assistance if adverse reaction occurs
• To use gum, lozenges for dry mouth
• To report vision changes, hallucinations immediately to prescriber
• To always take consistently either with food or without food; effects may be altered by taking differently

tobramycin (Rx)

(toe-bra-mye′sin)

Bethkis, Kitabis Pak, Nebcin ✦
TOBI, TOBI Podhaler

Func. class.: Antiinfective
Chem. class.: Aminoglycoside

ACTION: Interferes with protein synthesis in bacterial cell by binding to ribosomal subunits, thereby causing inaccurate peptide sequences to form in protein chain causing bacterial death

USES: Severe systemic infections of CNS, respiratory, GI, urinary tract, bone, skin, soft tissues; cystic fibrosis (nebulizer) for *Acinetobacter calcoaceticus, Citrobacter* sp., *Enterobacter aerogenes, Enterobacter* sp., *Enterococcus* sp., *Escherichia coli, Haemophilus aegyptius, Haemophilus influenzae* (beta-lactamase negative), *Haemophilus influenzae* (beta-lactamase positive), *Klebsiella pneumoniae, Klebsiella* sp., *Moraxella lacunata, Morganella morganii, Neisseria* sp., *Proteus mirabilis, Proteus vulgaris, Providencia* sp., *Pseudomonas aeruginosa, Serratia* sp., *Staphylococcus aureus* (MSSA), *Staphylococcus epidermidis, Staphylococcus* sp., *Streptococcus pneumoniae, Streptococcus* sp.; may also be used for the following: *Acinetobacter* sp., *Aeromonas* sp., *Bacillus anthracis, Salmonella* sp., *Shigella* sp.

CONTRAINDICATIONS
Hypersensitivity to aminoglycosides

Black Box Warning: Pregnancy, severe renal disease

Precautions: Breastfeeding, geriatric patients, neonates, mild renal disease, myasthenia gravis, Parkinson's disease

Black Box Warning: Hearing deficits, neuromuscular disease

DOSAGE AND ROUTES
Serious infection
• **Adult:** **IM/IV** 3 mg/kg/day in divided doses q8hr; may give up to 6 mg/kg/day in divided doses q8-12hr; **once-daily dosing (pulse dosing)** (unlabeled) **IV** 5-7 mg/kg, dosing intervals determined using nomogram, based on random levels drawn 8-12 hr after 1st dose
• **Child ≥6 yr:** **NEB** 300 mg bid in repeating cycles of 28 days on/28 days off of product; give **INH** over 10-15 min using a handheld PARI LC PLUS reusable nebulizer with DeVilbiss Pulmo-Aide compressor
• **Neonate <1 wk:** **IM/IV** ≤4 mg/kg/day divided q12hr
Cystic fibrosis with *Pseudomonas aeruginosa*
• **Child:** **IM/IV** 6-7.5 mg/kg/day in 3-4 equal divided doses
Renal dose
Conventional dosing:
• Multiply the serum creatinine (mg/100 mL) by 6 to determine the dosing; to decrease the dose, divide the standard dose by the serum creatinine (mg/100 mL) to determine the lower recommended dose
Available forms: Inj 10, 40 mg/mL; powder for inj 1.2 g; neb sol 300 mg/5 mL; powder for inh 28 mg
Administer:
• After obtaining specimen for C&S; begin treatment before results
• Product in evenly spaced doses to maintain blood level; separate aminoglycosides and penicillins by ≥1 hr
• Use only on susceptible organisms to prevent development of product-resistant bacteria
IM route
• IM inj in large muscle mass; rotate inj sites, aspirate
Draw peak 1 hr after dose, trough right before next dose; absorption erratic
Inhalation route: (TOBI Podhaler)
• Use with Podhaler device; do not swallow caps; use device for 7 days, then discard
• Keep caps in blister pack until ready to use; administer other inhaled products or chest physiotherapy before

Intermittent IV INFUSION route

• Visually inspect sol; do not use if discolored or particulate is present
• **Vantage vials** are for IV only and only for exactly 60 or 80 mg
• Diluted in 50-100 mL 0.9% NaCl, D$_5$W (D$_{10}$W, Ringer's, LR); infuse over 20-60 min; volume for pediatric patients needs to be sufficient to allow for 20-60 min infusion

Y-site compatibilities: Acyclovir, aldesleukin, alfentanil, alprostadil, amifostine, aminophylline, amiodarone, amsacrine, anidulafungin, ascorbic acid, atracurium, atropine, aztreonam, bivalirudin, bretylium, bumetanide, buprenorphine, butorphanol, calcium chloride/gluconate, CARBOplatin, caspofungin, chloramphenicol, cimetidine, ciprofloxacin, cisatracurium, CISplatin, clindamycin, cyanocobalamin, cyclophosphamide, cycloSPORINE, cytarabine, DACTINomycin, DAPTOmycin, dexmedetomidine, digoxin, diltiaZEM, diphenhydrAMINE, DOBUTamine, DOCEtaxel, DOPamine, doripenem, doxacurium, DOXOrubicin hydrochloride, DOXOrubicin liposome, doxycycline, enalaprilat, ePHEDrine, EPINEPHrine, epiRUBicin, epoetin alfa, ertapenem, esmolol, etoposide, etoposide phosphate, famotidine, fenoldopam, fentaNYL, filgrastim, fluconazole, fludarabine, fluorouracil, foscarnet, furosemide, gemcitabine, gentamicin, glycopyrrolate, granisetron, HYDROmorphone, ifosfamide, imipenem/cilastatin, isoproterenol, ketorolac, labetalol, levoFLOXacin, lidocaine, linezolid, LORazepam, magnesium sulfate, mannitol, mechlorethamine, melphalan, meperidine, metaraminol, methicillin, methotrexate, methoxamine, methyldopate, methylPREDNISolone, metoclopramide, metoprolol, metroNIDAZOLE, miconazole, midazolam, milrinone, minocycline, mitoXANTRONE, morphine, moxalactam, multiple vitamins, nafcillin, nalbuphine, naloxone, niCARdipine, nitroglycerin, nitroprusside, norepinephrine, octreotide, ondansetron, oxaliplatin, oxytocin, PACLitaxel, palonosetron, pantoprazole, papaverine, penicillin G, pentazocine, perphenazine, PHENobarbital, phentolamine, phenylephrine, phytonadione, potassium chloride, procainamide, prochlorperazine, promethazine, propranolol, protamine, pyridoxime, quinupristin/dalfopristin, raNITIdine, remifentanil, riTUXimab, rocuronium, sodium acetate/bicarbonate, succinylcholine, SUFentanil, tacrolimus, teniposide, theophylline, thiamine, thiotepa, ticarcillin/clavulanate, tigecycline, tirofiban, tolazoline, trastuzumab, trimethaphan, urokinase, vancomycin, vasopressin, vecuronium, verapamil, vinCRIStine, vinorelbine, voriconazole, zidovudine

SIDE EFFECTS

CNS: Confusion, depression, numbness, tremors, seizures, muscle twitching, neurotoxicity, dizziness, vertigo
CV: Hypo/hypertension, palpitation
EENT: Ototoxicity, deafness, visual disturbances, tinnitus
GI: *Nausea, vomiting, anorexia;* increased ALT, AST, bilirubin, hepatomegaly, hepatic necrosis, splenomegaly
GU: Oliguria, hematuria, renal damage, azotemia, renal failure, nephrotoxicity
HEMA: Agranulocytosis, thrombocytopenia, leukopenia, eosinophilia, anemia
INTEG: *Rash*, burning, urticaria, dermatitis, alopecia

PHARMACOKINETICS

Plasma half-life 2-3 hr, prolonged in neonates; not metabolized; excreted unchanged in urine; crosses placental barrier; poor penetration into CSF
IM: Onset rapid, peak 1 hr, duration 8 hr
IV: Onset immediate, peak 30 min, duration 8 hr

INTERACTIONS

Black Box Warning: Increase: ototoxicity, neurotoxicity, nephrotoxicity—other aminoglycosides, amphotericin B, polymyxin, vancomycin, ethacrynic acid, furosemide, mannitol, methoxyflurane, CISplatin, cephalosporins, bacitracin, acyclovir, penicillins, cidofovir

Drug/Lab Test
Increase: eosinophils, BUN, creatinine, AST, ALT, LDH, alk phos, glucose

Decrease: potassium, calcium, sodium, magnesium, WBC, granulocytes, platelets

NURSING CONSIDERATIONS
Assess:
• Weight before treatment; dosage is usually based on ideal body weight but may be calculated on actual body weight
• **Fluid balance:** I&O ratio, urinalysis daily for proteinuria, cells, casts; report sudden change in urine output
• **VS** during infusion; watch for hypotension, change in pulse
• **IV** site for thrombophlebitis, including pain, redness, swelling; change site if needed; apply warm compresses to discontinued site

Black Box Warning: Serum aminoglycoside concentration; serum peak drawn at 30-60 min after IV infusion or 60 min after IM inj, trough drawn just before next dose, peak 4-10 mcg/mL, trough 0.5-2 mcg/mL, increased level may lead to serious toxicity

Black Box Warning: Renal impairment: CCr, BUN, serum creatinine; lower dosage should be given in renal impairment (CCr <80 mL/min); monitor electrolytes: potassium, sodium, chloride, magnesium monthly if patient receiving long-term therapy

Black Box Warning: Deafness by audiometric testing; ringing, roaring in ears; vertigo; assess hearing before, during, after treatment

• **Overgrowth of infection:** fever, malaise, redness, pain, swelling, perineal itching, diarrhea, stomatitis, change in cough, sputum
• **Vestibular dysfunction:** nausea, vomiting, dizziness, headache; product should be discontinued if severe
• Adequate fluids of 2-3 L/day unless contraindicated to prevent irritation of tubules

Black Box Warning: Pregnancy: identify if pregnancy is planned or suspected; do not use in pregnancy, breastfeeding

Evaluate:
• **Therapeutic response:** absence of fever, draining wounds, negative C&S after treatment
Teach patient/family:
• To promptly report headache, dizziness, symptoms of overgrowth of infection, renal impairment

Black Box Warning: To report loss of hearing; ringing, roaring in ears; feeling of fullness in head

Black Box Warning: To notify prescriber if pregnancy is planned or suspected; not to use in pregnancy, breastfeeding

• To avoid hazardous activities until response is known
Nebulizer
• To use other therapies first, then tobramycin, not to use if cloudy or contains particulates
Inhalation
• Teach patient how to use TobiPodhaler

TREATMENT OF OVERDOSE:
Hemodialysis; monitor serum levels of product

---

tobramycin ophthalmic
See Appendix B

T

---

tocilizumab (Rx)
(toe′si-liz′oo-mab)
Actemra, Actemra ACTPen
Func. class.: DMARDs (disease-modifying antirheumatoid drugs)/ tumor necrosis factor (TNF) modifier
Chem. class.: Interleukin-6 receptor antagonist

ACTION: Interleukin-6 (IL-6) receptor inhibiting monoclonal antibody, decreases inflammation in RA

Side effects: *italics* = common; red = life-threatening

USES: Rheumatoid arthritis, active systemic juvenile idiopathic arthritis

CONTRAINDICATIONS
Hypersensitivity

Precautions: Breastfeeding, pregnancy; risk for GI perforation, active hepatic disease, severe neutropenia/thrombocytopenia, demyelinating disorders

> **Black Box Warning:** Invasive fungal infection, active TB

DOSAGE AND ROUTES
For the treatment of coronavirus disease 2019 (COVID-19) due to severe acute respiratory syndrome
• **Adult/child 2-17 yr ≤30 kg:** IV 8 mg/kg (max: 800 mg/dose) via a single IV infusion. 1 additional dose may be given at least 8 hr after the initial infusion. Give with dexamethasone (with or without remdesivir) to treat hospitalized adults requiring supplemental oxygen

Moderate-severe rheumatoid arthritis
• **Adult:** IV 4 mg/kg over 1 hr q4wk, may increase to 8 mg/kg q4wk based on clinical response, max dose 800 mg/infusion; do not initiate if ANC <2000/mm³, platelets <100,000/mm³
• **Adult <100 kg:** SUBCUT 162 mg every other week (monotherapy or in combination); increase to 162 mg weekly based on response
• **Adult ≥100 kg:** SUBCUT 162 mg weekly (monotherapy or in combination)

Juvenile idiopathic arthritis
• **Child ≥2 yr/adolescent ≥30 kg:** IV 8 mg/kg over 1 hr q2wk
• **Child ≥2 yr/adolescent <30 kg:** IV 12 mg/kg every 2 wk

Active polyarticular juvenile idiopathic
• **Child 2-17 yr, ≥30 kg:** IV 8 mg/kg/dose every 4 wk; give over 1 hr
• **Child 2-17 yr, <30 kg:** IV 10 mg/kg/dose every 4 wk; give over 1 hr
• **Child 2-17 yr, ≥30 kg:** SUBCUT 162 mg/dose every 2 wk
• **Child 2-17 yr, <30 kg:** SUBCUT 162 mg/dose every 3 wk

Cytokine release syndrome (CRS)
• **Adult/adolescent/child ≥2 yr, ≥30 kg:** IV 8 mg/kg over 60 min for 1 dose, alone or in combination with corticosteroids. If no improvement, up to 3 additional doses may be given at least 8 hr apart; max 800 mg
• **Adult/adolescent/child ≥2 yr, <30 kg:** IV 12 mg/kg over 60 min for 1 dose, alone or in combination with corticosteroids. If no improvement up to 3 additional doses may be given ≥8 hr apart; max 800 mg

Giant cell arteritis (GCA)
• **Adult:** IV 6 mg/kg over 1 hr q4wk in combination with a tapering course of glucocorticoids, max 600 mg/infusion: **SUBCUT:** 162 mg once weekly, in combination with a tapering course of glucocorticoids; or 162 mg once every other week, in combination with a tapering course of glucocorticoids

Therapeutic drug monitoring
• Before initiation of treatment, check ANC, platelet count, and liver function tests (ALT/AST concentrations). In adults, not recommended for use in those with ANC <2,000/mm³, platelet count <100,000/mm³, or ALT or AST >1.5 × ULN

Hepatic dose
• **Adult patients with rheumatoid arthritis or giant cell arteritis with hepatic impairment**
Do not initiate treatment with tocilizumab if baseline AST/ALT is >1.5× ULN

Available forms: Sol for inj 20 mg/mL (80 mg/4 mL, 200 mg/10 mL, 400 mg/20 mL); prefilled syringes 162 mg/0.9 mL (SUBCUT)

Administer:
SUBCUT route
• Do not use discolored solution or those with particulates
• Remove syringe, allow to warm for 30 min at room temperature. Do not warm in any other way
• Use injection site such as the front of thigh, outer area of upper arm, or the abdomen except for the 2-inch area around the navel. Do not inject into

moles, scars; or areas where skin is tender, bruised, red, hard, or not intact. Rotate injection sites with each injection. Inject at >1 inch from the last area injected

Intermittent IV INFUSION route

• Visually inspect for particulate matter, discoloration before administration; should be colorless to pale yellow liquid
• From 100-mL infusion bag or bottle, withdraw vol of 0.9% sodium chloride inj equal to vol of tocilizumab sol required for patient's dose
• Slowly add tocilizumab from each vial into infusion bag or bottle; gently invert to avoid foaming; fully diluted sols are compatible with polypropylene, polyethylene, polyvinyl chloride infusion bags and polypropylene, polyethylene, glass infusion bottles
• Fully diluted sol for infusion may be stored refrigerated or at room temperature for ≤24 hr and should be protected from light; do not use unused product remaining in vials; no preservatives
• Allow to reach room temperature before infusion
• Give over 60 min with infusion set; do not administer as IV push or bolus
• Do not infuse concomitantly in same IV line with other drugs

SIDE EFFECTS

CNS: *Headache, dizziness*
CV: *Hypertension*
GI: Perforation, abdominal pain, gastritis, mouth ulcerations
HEMA: Neutropenia, thrombocytopenia
INTEG: Rash, infusion reactions
RESP: *Upper respiratory infections, nasopharyngitis, bronchitis*
SYST: Serious infections, anaphylaxis, infusion-related reactions, anti-tocilizumab antibody formation, secondary malignancy

INTERACTIONS

Decrease: product level—cycloSPORINE, theophylline, warfarin, monitor effects
Do not give with live virus vaccines, adverse reaction risk, decreased antibody response

Avoid use with TNF modifiers, DMARDs, immunosuppressives due to increased risk of infection
Increased hepatotoxicity risk: methotrexate

PHARMACOKINETICS

Half-life approx 6 days with single dose, approx 11 days with multiple (steady-state) doses

NURSING CONSIDERATIONS
Assess:

• **Rheumatoid arthritis:** ROM, pain, stiffness at baseline q1-2wk
• **Labs:** CBC with differential, LFTs, platelet count, serum lipid profile at baseline and periodically; LFTS 1-3 × ULN reduce dose, if 3-5 × ULN interrupt; platelets 50,000-100,000/mm^3 interrupt until platelets are >100,000/mm^3 then reduce at lower dose; monitor lipids after several weeks of therapy
• Before initiation of treatment, check ANC, platelet count, and liver function tests (ALT/AST concentrations). In adults, not recommended for use in those with ANC <2,000/mm^3, platelet count <100,000/mm^3, or ALT or AST >1.5 × ULN

Black Box Warning: **Infection:** Assess before treatment and periodically; obtain TB screening before beginning treatment; **invasive fungal infections:** discontinue if infection occurs during administration; may use antituberculosis therapy before tocilizumab in past history of latent or active TB when adequate course of treatment cannot be confirmed and those with a negative TB with risk factors for infections

• **Anaphylaxis/Stevens-Johnson syndrome:** Assess for rash, facial swelling, dyspnea, antihistamine, corticosteroids, emergency equipment should be available
• **Fungal infection:** Assess for flulike symptoms, dyspnea; antifungals may be needed; treatment may need to be discontinued until infection is resolved
• **Secondary malignancy:** assess for malignancy periodically
• **Pregnancy/breastfeeding:** use only if benefits outweigh fetal risk; pregnant patients

---

Side effects: *italics* = common; red = life-threatening

should enroll in the MotherToBaby Autoimmune Diseases in Pregnancy Registry; do not breastfeed, excretion unknown

Evaluate:

• **Therapeutic response:** ability to move more easily with less pain

Teach patient/family:

• That this treatment must continue unless safety or effectiveness is an issue
• About reason for use and expected results
• That labs will be needed including those for TB and hepatitis B before starting treatment
• To avoid live vaccines; to bring immunizations up-to-date before treatment
• Teach patient, caregiver how to administer SUBCUT injections, to identify allergic reactions after injection

Black Box Warning: To report signs, symptoms of infection, including TB and hepatitis B; to avoid others with infections

• To notify prescriber if pregnancy or suspected pregnancy; not to use if breastfeeding; to consider using a non-hormonal contraceptive because contraception may be decreased

---

tofacitinib (Rx)

(toe′fa-sye′ti-nib)

Xeljanz, Xeljanz XR

Func. class.: Antirheumatic agent (disease modifying), immunomodulator/biologic DMARD

Chem. class.: Janus kinase inhibitor

ACTION: Affects the signaling pathway of Janus kinase

USES: Rheumatoid arthritis (moderately to severely active) in those who have taken methotrexate with inadequate response or intolerance, juvenile arthritis, active psoriatic arthritis, ulcerative colitis, ankylosing spondylitis

CONTRAINDICATIONS

Hypersensitivity, use of live vaccines, severe liver disease, ANC <1000 cells/mm^3

Precautions: Pregnancy, breastfeeding, neonates, infants, children, geriatric patients, neoplastic disease, ulcerative colitis, neutropenia, peptic ulcer disease, active infections, risk of lymphomas/leukemias, TB, posttransplant lymphoproliferative disorder (PTLD), kidney disease, diabetes mellitus, HIV, hypercholesterolemia, herpes virus infection reactivation ♥⊕⋇, Asian patients

Black Box Warning: Infection, secondary malignancy

DOSAGE AND ROUTES
Psoriatic arthritis

• **Adult: PO** 5 mg bid with a DMARD if receiving potent CYP3A4 inhibitor, 5 mg/day if receiving moderate CYP3A4 inhibitor and 2C19 inhibitors; **EXT REL** 11 mg/day with a DMARD

Moderate to severe rheumatoid arthritis, ankylosing spondylitis

• **Adult: PO** 5 mg bid with or without methotrexate or a DMARD; **EXT REL** 11 mg/day

Juvenile arthritis

• **Child ≥2 yr and ≥10 kg/adolescents: PO** 10-19 kg: PO solution 3.2 mg bid; 20-39 kg: 4 mg bid; ≥40 kg (solution/tablet) 5 mg bid

Ulcerative colitis

• **Adult: PO** 10 mg bid × 8 wk or more, then 5 or 10 mg bid (immediate release)

Renal/hepatic dose

• **Mild impairment:** No change
• **Moderate to severe impairment:** If the current dose is 5 mg PO twice daily IR, reduce to 5 mg PO once daily. If the current dose is 11 mg PO once daily ER, reduce to 5 mg PO once daily IR

Available forms: Tabs 5 mg; ext rel tab 11, 22 mg; oral solution

Administer:

PO route

• Without regard to food
• Do not chew, crush, split XR tablet, swallow whole
• Do not take missed dose, resume normal schedule

SIDE EFFECTS

CNS: Headache, paresthesias, insomnia, fatigue

CV: Hypertension, increased PR interval

GI: Abdominal pain, nausea, liver damage, dyspepsia, vomiting, diarrhea, gastritis, GI perforation, steatosis

HEMA: Anemia, lymphocytosis, lymphopenia, neutropenia

INTEG: Rash, pruritus, angioedema

MISC: Increased cancer risk, risk of infection (TB, invasive fungal infections, other opportunistic infections), may be fatal, posttransplant lymphoproliferative disorder (PTLD), osteoarthritis

PHARMACOKINETICS

Bioavailability 70%, protein binding 40% (albumin), metabolism mediated by CYP3A4, half-life 3 hr, peak 0.5-1 hr

INTERACTIONS

Black Box Warning: Do not use with TNF modifiers, vaccines, potent immunosuppressants, other biologic DMARDS; serious infections may occur

Increase: tofacinib effect—CYP3A4 inhibitors (amprenavir, boceprevir, delavirdine, ketoconazole, indinavir, itraconazole, dalfopristin/quinupristin, ritonavir, tipranavir, fluconazole, isoniazid, miconazole)

Decrease: tofacinib effect—CYP3A4 inducers (rifAMPin, rifapentine, rifabutin, primidone, phenytoin, PHENobarbital, nevirapine, nafcillin, modafinil, griseofulvin, etravirine, efavirenz, barbiturates, bexarotene, bosentan, carBAMazepine, enzalutamide, dexamethasone)

Drug/Lab Test

Increase: LFTs, cholesterol, creatinine, lipids

Decrease: neutrophils, lymphocytes, HB

NURSING CONSIDERATIONS

Assess:

• **Labs:** Monitor lipid profile, Hct/HB, WBC, LFTs baseline and periodically

• **RA:** Pain; stiffness; ROM; swelling of joints before, during treatment

Black Box Warning: Active infection, including localized infection: Monitor for infection; fever; chills; flulike symptoms; red, oozing wounds; evaluate for latent or active TB before use; treat with antimycobacterials before use; may cause serious fatal infections (pulmonary or extrapulmonary TB; invasive fungal infections; and bacterial, viral, and opportunistic infections); during and after use, monitor for infection including TB in those who tested negative for latent TB before use; if a serious infection develops, interrupt therapy until the infection is controlled, reactivation of viral infections is higher in Asian patients

Black Box Warning: Secondary malignancy: lymphoma and other malignancies have been noted with product use

• **Epstein-Barr virus–associated posttransplant lymphoproliferative disorder (PTLD):** in kidney transplant patients when used with this product and immunosuppressives

• **Liver disease:** not recommended in severe liver disease, impairment; dose modification is needed with moderate liver impairment, monitor LFTs

• **GI perforation:** assess in those with diverticulitis, peptic ulcer disease, or ulcerative colitis

Black Box Warning: Immunosuppression: obtain neutrophil and lymphocyte counts before use; do not start the product in lymphocyte count <500 cells/mm³ or ANC <1000 cells/mm³; for ANC >1000 cells/mm³, monitor neutrophil counts after 4-8 wk and every 3 mo thereafter; lymphocyte count >500 cells/mm³, monitor lymphocyte counts every 3 mo

• **Anemia:** determine HB, do not start in HB <9 g/dL; in HB ≥9 g/dL, monitor HB after 4-8 wk and every 3 mo thereafter

• **Pregnancy/breastfeeding:** use during pregnancy only if the potential benefit justifies the potential risk to the fetus; if

---

Side effects: *italics* = common; red = life-threatening

pregnancy occurs, enrollment in the pregnancy registry is encouraged by calling 877-311-8972; discontinue product or breastfeeding; serious adverse reactions can occur in nursing infants

Evaluate:

• **Therapeutic response:** decreased inflammation, pain in joints, decreased joint destruction

Teach patient/family:

• Not to take any live virus vaccines during treatment; vaccines should be brought up-to-date before starting treatment

• To report signs of infection, allergic reaction

• **Pregnancy:** to report if pregnancy is planned or suspected; not to breastfeed

---

tolcapone (Rx)

(toll'cah'pone)

Tasmar

Func. class.: Antiparkinson agent
Chem. class.: COMT inhibitor

ACTION: Inhibits COMT; used as adjunct to levodopa/carbidopa therapy

USES: Parkinson's disease

CONTRAINDICATIONS

Hypersensitivity, rhabdomyolysis

Precautions: Pregnancy, breastfeeding, cardiac/renal disease, hypertension, asthma, history of rhabdomyolysis

  Black Box Warning: Hepatic disease

DOSAGE AND ROUTES

• **Adult: PO** 100 mg tid with levodopa/carbidopa therapy; max 600 mg/day, discontinue if no benefit after 3 wk

Available forms: Tabs 100 mg

Administer:

• Only to be used if levodopa/carbidopa does not provide satisfactory results

• Give without regard to food

SIDE EFFECTS

CNS: Dystonia, dyskinesia, dreaming, *fatigue, headache, confusion*, psychosis, hallucination, dizziness, sleep disorders

CV: *Orthostatic hypotension*, chest pain, hypotension

EENT: Cataract, eye inflammation

GI: *Nausea, vomiting, anorexia, abdominal distress*, diarrhea, constipation, fatal hepatic failure, increased LFTs

GU: UTI, urine discoloration, uterine tumor, micturition disorder, hematuria

HEMA: Hemolytic anemia, leukopenia, agranulocytosis

INTEG: Sweating, alopecia

MS: Rhabdomyolysis

PHARMACOKINETICS

Rapidly absorbed, peak 2 hr, protein binding 99%, extensively metabolized, half-life 2-3 hr, excreted in urine (60%)/feces (40%)

INTERACTIONS

Increase: CNS depression—CNS depressant

• May influence pharmacokinetics of α-methyldopa, DOBUTamine, apomorphine, isoproterenol

• Inhibition of normal catecholamine metabolism: MAOIs; MAO-B inhibitor may be used

NURSING CONSIDERATIONS

Assess:

  Black Box Warning: Hepatic disease: AST, ALT, alk phos, LDH, bilirubin, CBC; monitor ALT, AST q2wk × 1 yr, then q4wk × 6 mo, then q8wk thereafter; if LFTs elevated, product should not be used, if no improvement in 3 wk, discontinue; do not use in hepatic disease

• Involuntary movements of parkinsonism: akinesia, tremors, staggering gait, muscle rigidity, drooling

• B/P, respiration during initial treatment; hypo/hypertension should be reported

• Mental status: affect, mood, behavioral changes, avoid use in those with dystonia

Evaluate:

• **Therapeutic response:** decrease in akathisia, increased mood

Teach patient/family:

• To change positions slowly to prevent orthostatic hypotension

---

- That urine, sweat may change color
- That food taken within 1 hr before meals or 2 hr after meals decreases action of product by 20%; may be taken without regard to food
- To notify prescriber if pregnancy is planned or suspected
- That CNS changes may occur, hallucinations, involuntary movement
- To avoid hazardous activities until reaction is known; dizziness may occur
- To notify prescriber of poor impulse control, urges to gamble, spend money (rare)

Black Box Warning: To report signs of hepatic injury: clay-colored stools, jaundice, fatigue, appetite loss, lethargy, fatigue, itching, right upper abdominal pain

- To report diarrhea, nausea, vomiting, anorexia; that nausea may occur at beginning of treatment

tolnaftate topical
See Appendix B

tolterodine (Rx)
(toll-tehr´oh-deen)
Detrol, Detrol LA
Func. class.: Overactive bladder product
Chem. class.: Muscarinic receptor antagonist

ACTION: Relaxes smooth muscles in urinary tract by inhibiting acetylcholine at postganglionic sites

USES: Overactive bladder (urinary frequency, urgency), urinary incontinence

CONTRAINDICATIONS
Hypersensitivity, uncontrolled closed-angle glaucoma, urinary retention, gastric retention
Precautions: Pregnancy, breastfeeding, children, renal disease, controlled closed-angle glaucoma, bladder obstruction, QT prolongation, decreased GI motility

DOSAGE AND ROUTES
Overactive bladder
- **Adult and geriatric: PO** 2 mg bid; may decrease to 1 mg bid; **EXT REL** 4 mg/day, may decrease to 2 mg/day if needed, max 4 mg/day
Hepatic/renal dose
- **Adult: PO** 1 mg bid (50% dose) or **EXT REL** 2 mg/day; CCr ≤30 mL/min, reduce by 50%
CYP3A4 inhibitor dose
- **Adult: PO** 1 mg bid; **EXT REL** 2 mg/day
Available forms: Tabs 1, 2 mg; ext rel caps 2, 4 mg
Administer:
- Whole; take with liquids; do not crush, chew, or break ext rel product; without regard to meals

SIDE EFFECTS
CNS: Anxiety, paresthesia, fatigue, *dizziness, headache;* increasing dementia, memory impairment
CV: Chest pain, hypertension, QT prolongation
EENT: Vision abnormalities, xerophthalmia
GI: *Nausea, vomiting, anorexia,* abdominal pain, constipation, dry mouth, dyspepsia
GU: Dysuria, urinary retention, frequency, UTI
INTEG: Rash, pruritus
RESP: Bronchitis, cough, pharyngitis, upper respiratory tract infection
SYST: Angioedema, Stevens-Johnson syndrome

PHARMACOKINETICS
Rapidly absorbed; highly protein bound; extensively metabolized by CYP2D6; a portion of the population may be poor metabolizers; excreted in urine, feces half-life 2-3.7 hr

INTERACTIONS
- Do not use in those with known hypersensitivity to fesoterodine
- **Increase:** QT prolongation—class IA/III antidysrhythmics, some phenothiazines, β-agonists, local anesthetics, tricyclics, haloperidol, methadone, chloroquine, clarithromycin, droperidol, erythromycin, pentamidine

Side effects: *italics* = common; red = life-threatening

Increase: action of tolterodine—antiretroviral protease inhibitors, macrolide antiinfectives, azole antifungals

Increase: anticholinergic effect—antimuscarinics

Increase: urinary frequency—diuretics

Drug/Food

• Food increases bioavailability of tolterodine

Drug/Lab

Increase: LFTs, bilirubin

NURSING CONSIDERATIONS

Assess:

• **Urinary patterns:** distention, nocturia, frequency, urgency, incontinence, residual urine

• **Serious skin disorders:** angioedema, Stevens-Johnson syndrome; allergic reactions: rash; if this occurs, product should be discontinued; usually occurs in first few doses

• **QT prolongation:** ECG, ejection fraction; assess for chest pain, palpitations, dyspnea; may be compounded in those taking class IA/III dysrhythmics

Black Box Warning: Fatal hepatic injury: increased LFTs, bilirubin during first 18 mo of therapy in those with autosomal dominant polycystic kidney disease; assess for fatigue, anorexia, right upper abdominal pain, dark urine, jaundice; if these occur, discontinue product and do not restart if cause is liver injury

• **Beers:** avoid in older adults with delirium or at high risk for delirium; monitor for confusion, delirium frequently

Evaluate:

• Decreasing dysuria, frequency, nocturia, incontinence

Teach patient/family:

• To avoid hazardous activities; dizziness may occur

• Not to drink liquids before bedtime; to swallow ext rel product whole

• About the importance of bladder maintenance

• Not to breastfeed; to notify prescriber if pregnancy is planned or suspected

• To report signs of infection, skin effects, shortness of breath, urinary retention

---

tolvaptan (Rx)

(tole-vap′tan)

Jinarc, Jynarque, Samsca

Func. class.: Antihypertensive

Chem. class.: Vasopressin receptor antagonist, V2

ACTION: Arginine vasopressin (AVP) antagonist with affinity for V2 receptors; level of circulating AVP in circulating blood is critical for the regulation of water and the electrolyte balance, and it is usually elevated with euvolemic/hypervolemic hyponatremia

USES: Hypervolemic/euvolemic hyponatremia with heart failure, cirrhosis, SIADH

CONTRAINDICATIONS

Hypersensitivity, hypovolemia, anuria

Precautions: Pregnancy, breastfeeding, children, dehydration, geriatric patients, hyperkalemia, autosomal dominant PKD, malnutrition, alcoholism, hepatic disease

Black Box Warning: Osmotic demyelination syndrome; requires a specialized care setting

DOSAGE AND ROUTES

Hypovolemic/euvolemic hyponatremia

• **Adult: PO** 15 mg daily; after 24 hr, may increase to 30 mg daily; max 60 mg/day max 30 days

Polycystic kidney disease (ADPKD) (Jynarque) ⓓⓔⓡ

Adult: PO 60 mg/day, 45 mg q AM upon wakening and 15 mg daily 8 hr later, initially. Increase to 60 mg q AM upon wakening and 30 mg daily 8 hr later, then 90 mg q AM upon wakening and 30 mg daily 8 hr later at a minimum of weekly intervals, if tolerated. May downtitrate based on tolerability

Available forms: Tabs 15, 30, 45, 60, 90 mg

Administer:

• PO with/without food

• Avoid fluid restriction for first 24 hr

- Initiate in hospital setting
- Do not use with grapefruit, grapefruit juice

SIDE EFFECTS

CNS: Fever, dizziness
CV: Ventricular fibrillation, DIC, stroke, thrombosis
GI: *Nausea,* vomiting, *constipation,* colitis, hepatic injury
GU: Polyuria
HEMA: Bleeding
META: *Dehydration, hyperglycemia,* hyperkalemia, hypernatremia
MS: Rhabdomyolysis
RESP: Respiratory depression, pulmonary embolism

PHARMACOKINETICS

Peak 2-4 hr, protein binding 99%, metabolized by CYP3A4, terminal half-life 12 hr

INTERACTIONS

Increase: concentrations of tolvaptan—CYP3A4 inhibitors (efavirenz, fosamprenavir, quiNINE); P-gp inhibitors (cycloSPORINE, azithromycin, mefloquine, palperidone, propafenone, quiNIDine, testosterone)
Decrease: concentration of tolvaptan—CYP3A4 inducers (carBAMazepine, dexamethasone, etravirine, flutamide, griseofulvin, metyraPONE, modafinil, nafcillin, nevirapine, OXcarbazepine, phenytoin, rifAMPin, rifabutin, rifapentine, topiramate)
Drug/Herb
Decrease: tolvaptan effect—CYP3A4 inducer (St. John's wort)
Drug/Food
- Grapefruit/grapefruit juice; do not use together

NURSING CONSIDERATIONS

Assess:
- Renal, hepatic function

Black Box Warning: Osmotic demyelination syndrome: frequent sodium vol status; overly rapid correction of sodium concentration (>12 mEq/L per 24 hr); may occur in alcoholism, severe malnutrition, advanced liver disease, syndrome of inappropriate antidiuretic hormone; correct sodium levels slowly, may result in dysarthria, mutism, dysphagia, coma, seizure, death

- CV status: ventricular fibrillation, hypertension; monitor B/P, pulse
- Monitor electrolytes (sodium, potassium)

Black Box Warning: Specialized care setting: needed so that neurologic status and sodium can be monitored

- **Liver injury:** fatigue, abdominal pain, dark urine, clay-colored stools, jaundice
- **Pregnancy/breastfeeding:** use only if benefits outweigh fetal risk; do not breastfeed
Evaluate:
- **Therapeutic response:** correction of serum sodium levels
Teach patient/family:
- About administration procedure and expected results; that product will be used for ≤30 days
- To report difficulty swallowing, speaking, seizures, dizziness, drowsiness; embolism may be the cause
- To drink fluid in response to thirst
- Not to use grapefruit juice
- To notify prescriber before using other products
- To report right upper abdominal pain, nausea, vomiting, anorexia, dark urine, yellowing of skin, eyes (hepatic injury)
- That product will be started or restarted in the hospital when monitoring is possible
- To avoid pregnancy, breastfeeding while taking this product

---

topiramate (Rx)

(toh-pire′ah-mate)
Eprontia, Qudexy XR, Topamax, Topamax Sprinkle, Trokendi XR
Func. class.: Anticonvulsant—miscellaneous
Chem. class.: Monosaccharide derivative

Do not confuse:
Topamax/Toprol XL

ACTION: May prevent seizure spread as opposed to an elevation of seizure threshold, increases GABA activity

---

Side effects: *italics* = common; red = life-threatening

USES:
Partial seizures in adults and children 2-16 yr old; tonic-clonic seizures; seizures with Lennox-Gastaut syndrome; migraine prophylaxis

Unlabeled uses: Antipsychotic-induced weight gain, cluster headache, binge eating disorder, essential tremor

CONTRAINDICATIONS
Hypersensitivity, metabolic acidosis, pregnancy

Precautions: Breastfeeding, children, renal/hepatic disease, acute myopia, secondary closed-angle glaucoma, behavioral disorders, COPD, dialysis, encephalopathy, status asthmaticus, status epilepticus, surgery, paresthesias, maculopathy, nephrolithiasis

DOSAGE AND ROUTES
Adjunctive therapy for seizures

• **Adult/adolescent/child ≥10 yr:** PO 25-50 mg/day initially, titrate by 25-50 mg/wk, up to 200-400 mg/day in 2 divided doses

• **Adult/adolescent/child ≥10 yr:** PO (Qudexy XR, Trokendi XR) 50 mg daily; increase by 50 mg weekly during wk 2, 3, 4; increase by 100 mg weekly, wk 5, 6; final dose 400 mg daily

• **Child 2-9 yr:** PO wk 1: 25 mg in PM, then 25 mg bid if tolerated (wk 2), then increase by 25-50 mg/day each wk as tolerated over 5- to 7-wk titration period, maintenance given in 2 divided doses; <11 kg, minimum 150 mg/day, max 250 mg/day; 12-22 kg, minimum 200 mg/day, max 300 mg/day; 23-31 kg, minimum 200 mg/day, max 350 mg/day; 32-38 kg, minimum 250 mg/day, max 350 mg/day; >38 kg, minimum 250 mg/day, max 400 mg/day; Qudexy XR 25 mg daily at night, may increase to 50 mg wk 2, if tolerated, increase by 25-50 mg each wk over 5- to 7-wk titration period, max dose based on weight

• **Child ≤11 kg:** PO Qudexy XR minimum 150 mg daily, max 250 mg daily

• **Child 12-22 kg:** minimum 200 mg daily, max 300 mg daily

• **Child 23-31 kg:** minimum 200 mg daily, max 350 mg daily

• **Child 32-38 kg:** minimum 250 mg daily, max 350 mg daily

• **Child >38 kg:** minimum 250 mg daily, max 400 mg daily

Migraine prophylaxis

• **Adult:** PO 25 mg/day initially, increase by 25 mg/day/wk up to 100 mg/day in 2 divided doses

Renal dose

• **Adult:** PO CCr <70 mL/min, give ½ dose

Available forms: Tabs 25, 50, 100, 200 mg; ext rel caps 25, 50, 100, 200 mg; ext rel cap (sprinkles 24 hr) 25, 50, 100, 150, 200 mg; oral solution 25 mg/mL

Administer:

• Swallow tabs whole; do not break, crush, or chew tabs; very bitter

• May take without regard to meals

• Sprinkle cap can be given whole or opened and sprinkled on soft food; do not chew, drink water after sprinkle

• Store at room temperature away from heat, light

SIDE EFFECTS
CNS: *Dizziness, fatigue,* cognitive disorders, insomnia, *anxiety,* depression, paresthesia, *memory loss, tremors,* motor retardation, suicidal ideation, poor balance, ataxia

CV: Flushing, chest pain

EENT: Diplopia, *vision abnormality*

GI: Diarrhea, *anorexia, nausea, dyspepsia,* abdominal pain, constipation, dry mouth, pancreatitis

GU: Breast pain, dysmenorrhea, menstrual disorder

INTEG: Rash, alopecia

MISC: Weight loss, leukopenia, metabolic acidosis, increased body temperature; unexplained death (epilepsy)

RESP: Upper respiratory tract infection, pharyngitis, sinusitis

PHARMACOKINETICS
Well absorbed, peak 2 hr, terminal half-life 19-25 hr, excreted in urine (55%-97% unchanged), crosses placenta, excreted in breast milk, protein

binding (9%-17%), steady state 4 days

INTERACTIONS

Increase: renal stones—carbonic anhydrase inhibitors

Increase: effect of amitriptyline

Increase: CNS depression—alcohol, CNS depressants

Increase: topiramate levels—metFORMIN, hydroCHLOROthiazide, lamoTRIgine

Decrease: levels of hormonal contraceptives, estrogen, digoxin, valproic acid, lithium, risperiDONE

Decrease: topiramate levels—phenytoin, carBAMazepine, valproic acid, probenecid

NURSING CONSIDERATIONS

Assess:

• **Seizures:** location, type, duration, aura; **seizure precautions:** padded side rails; move objects that may harm patient

• **Bipolar disorder:** mood, behavior, activity

• **Renal studies:** urinalysis, BUN, urine creatinine, electrolytes q3mo; symptoms of renal colic

• **Hepatic studies:** ALT, AST, bilirubin if patient receiving long-term treatment

• CBC during long-term therapy (anemia); serum bicarbonate (metabolic acidosis)

• **Migraines:** pain location, duration; alleviating factors

• **Mental status:** mood, sensorium, affect, behavioral changes, **suicidal thoughts/behaviors;** if mental status changes, notify prescriber

• Body weight, perception of body image; eating disorders may occur or be exacerbated, especially in adolescents; evidence of cognitive disorder

• Assistance with ambulation during early part of treatment; dizziness occurs

• **Pregnancy/breastfeeding:** use only if benefits outweigh fetal risk, birth defects have occurred; pregnant patients should register with the Antiepileptic Drug Pregnancy Registry, 888-233-

2334; may decrease effectiveness of hormonal contraceptives; cautious use in breastfeeding, excretion unknown

• **Beers:** avoid in older adults unless safer alternative is unavailable; may cause ataxia, impaired psychomotor function

Evaluate:

• **Therapeutic response:** decreased seizure activity

Teach patient/family:

• To carry emergency ID stating patient's name, products taken, condition, prescriber's name, and phone number

• To avoid driving, other activities that require alertness, until response is known

• Not to discontinue medication quickly after long-term use; do not restart without close supervision if several doses are missed; to follow prescriber's directions closely

• To notify prescriber immediately of blurred vision, periorbital pain; that vision loss may occur

• To maintain adequate fluid intake

• About administration procedure and expected results

• To use nonhormonal contraceptive; that effect of oral contraceptives is decreased

• To drink plenty of fluids to prevent kidney stones

• May need to increase amount of food consumed; weight loss may occur

• To swallow ext rel product whole

• That minor hair loss may occur; to report to prescriber if severe

---

> ⚠ **HIGH ALERT**

topotecan (Rx)

(toh-poh-tee'kan)

Hycamtin

Func. class.: Antineoplastic, natural; topoisomerase inhibitor

Chem. class.: Camptothecin analog

ACTION: Antitumor product with topoisomerase-I–inhibitory activity; topoisomerase I relieves torsional strain in DNA by causing single-strand breaks; also causes double-strand DNA damage

USES: Metastatic ovarian cancer after failure of traditional chemotherapy; relapsed small-cell lung cancer; cervical cancer

CONTRAINDICATIONS
Pregnancy, breastfeeding, hypersensitivity, severe bone marrow depression

> **Black Box Warning:** Neutropenia, bone marrow suppression

Precautions: Children, renal disease, gelatin hypersensitivity, anemia, contraceptive requirements, dehydration, diarrhea, extravasation, herpes, infertility, neutropenia, pulmonary fibrosis, varicella

DOSAGE AND ROUTES
Metastatic carcinoma of the ovary
• **Adult: IV INFUSION** 1.5 mg/m^2, max 4 mg/dose, over 30 min daily × 5 days starting on day 1 of 21-day course × 4 courses
Persistent cervical cancer
• **Adult: IV INFUSION** 0.75 mg/m^2 on days 1, 2, 3 then 50 mg/m^2 cisplatin **IV** on day 1 then repeat q21days; adjust for toxicity
Relapsed small-cell lung cancer
• **Adult: PO** 2.3 mg/m^2/day × 5 days then repeat q21days
Renal dose
• **Adult: PO** CCr ≥50 mL/min: No change; CCr 30-49 mL/min: Reduce dose to 1.5 mg/m^2/day; dose may be increased by 0.4 mg/m^2/day after the first course if no severe hematologic or gastrointestinal toxicities occur; CCr <30 mL/min: Reduce dose to 0.6 mg/m^2/day; dose may be increased by 0.4 mg/m^2/day after the first course if no severe hematologic or gastrointestinal toxicities occur
• **Adult: IV** CCr 40-60 mL/min: No change; CCr 20-39 mL/min: Reduce dose to 0.75 mg/m^2; CCr <20 mL/min: unknown

Available forms
Lyophilized powder for inj 4 mg; injection solution 1 mg/mL, 4 mg/mL; caps 0.25, 1 mg
Administer:
• Store caps in refrigerator; IV INFUSION unopened at room temperature; protect both from light
PO route
• Do not break, crush, chew, or open caps; protect from light
• Take without regard to food
Intermittent IV INFUSION route
• Visually inspect for particulate matter and discoloration before use
• Reconstitute each 4-mg vial with 4 mL sterile water for injection; use immediately; no preservative
• Withdraw the appropriate volume of the reconstituted solution; dilute further; dilute in 0.9% NaCl or D$_5$W before administration
• The reconstituted solution is yellow or yellow-green
• Topotecan injection diluted for infusion is stable at room temperature with normal light for 24 hr
• Infuse over 30 min

SIDE EFFECTS
CNS: *Asthenia, headache,* myalgia, *pain,* weakness
GI: *Abdominal pain, constipation,* diarrhea, obstruction, *nausea,* stomatitis, *vomiting;* increased ALT, AST; anorexia
HEMA: Neutropenia, leukopenia, thrombocytopenia, anemia, sepsis
INTEG: *Total alopecia*
RESP: Dyspnea, cough, interstitial lung disease
MS: Arthralgia, myalgia

PHARMACOKINETICS
Rapidly and completely absorbed, excreted in urine and feces as metabolites, half-life 2.8 hr, 7%-35% bound to plasma proteins, PO peak 1-2 hr

INTERACTIONS
• **Avoid use with P-glycoprotein,** breast cancer resistance protein inhibitors (amiodarone, clarithromycin, diltiaZEM,

erythromycin, indinavir), quiNIDine, testosterone, verapamil, tamoxifen, itraconazole, mefloquine, RU-486, niCARdipine, vaccines, toxoids

Increase: myelosuppression when used with CISplatin

Increase: bleeding risk—NSAIDs, anticoagulants, thrombolytics, platelet inhibitors

Drug/Food

• Avoid use with grapefruit juice

NURSING CONSIDERATIONS
Assess:

• Hepatic studies: AST, ALT, alk phos, which may be elevated; creatinine, BUN

Black Box Warning: Bone marrow suppression: CBC, differential, platelet count weekly; withhold product if WBC is <3500/mm³ or platelet count is <100,000/mm³; notify prescriber of results; product should be discontinued

• **Pregnancy/breastfeeding:** do not use in pregnancy or breastfeeding, can cause fetal harm; use contraception during and for ≥1 mo after final dose (female), during and for 3 mo after final dose (males); may cause infertility in both males/females

• **Oral status:** Buccal cavity for dryness, sores or ulcerations, white patches, oral pain, bleeding, dysphagia

• **Interstitial lung disease (ILD):** fever, cough, dyspnea, hypoxia; may be fatal

• **Fluid balance:** Increased fluid intake to 2-3 L/day to prevent dehydration unless contraindicated

Evaluate:

• **Therapeutic response:** decreased tumor size, spread of malignancy

Teach patient/family:

• That total alopecia may occur; that hair grows back but is different in color and texture

• To avoid foods with citric acid, hot temperature, or rough texture if stomatitis is present; to drink adequate fluids

• To report stomatitis and any bleeding, white spots, ulcerations in mouth; to examine mouth daily; to report symptoms

Black Box Warning: To report signs of anemia: fatigue, headache, faintness, SOB, irritability

• Rinsing of mouth tid-qid with water, club soda; brushing of teeth bid-tid with soft brush or cotton-tipped applicator for stomatitis; to use unwaxed dental floss

• To use effective contraception during treatment and for 6 mo after; that males should use contraception during and for 3 mo after final dose; not to breastfeed

• To avoid OTC products without approval of prescriber

• To avoid driving or other activities requiring alertness

• To avoid vaccines, toxoids

• Not to crush, chew capsules

• Not to retake dose if vomiting occurs; to notify prescriber

toremifene (Rx)
(tor-em′ih-feen)
Fareston
Func. class.: Antineoplastic
Chem. class.: Antiestrogen hormone

USES: Advanced breast carcinoma not responsive to other therapy in estrogen receptor–positive patients (usually postmenopausal)

CONTRAINDICATIONS
Pregnancy, hypersensitivity, history of thromboembolism

Black Box Warning: QT prolongation

DOSAGE AND ROUTES
• **Adult: PO** 60 mg/day
Available forms: Tabs 60 mg

torsemide (Rx)
(tor′suh-mide)
Soaanz
Func. class.: Loop diuretic
Chem. class.: Sulfonamide derivative

ACTION: Acts on loop of Henle by inhibiting absorption of chloride, sodium, water

USES: Treatment of hypertension and edema with HF, ascites

CONTRAINDICATIONS

Infants, hypersensitivity to sulfonamides, anuria

Precautions: Pregnancy, breastfeeding, diabetes mellitus, dehydration, severe renal disease, electrolyte depletion, hypovolemia, syncope, ventricular dysrhythmias

DOSAGE AND ROUTES

HF diuresis
• **Adult: PO** 10-20 mg/day, may increase as needed, max 200 mg/day

Diuresis in chronic renal failure
• **Adult: PO** 20 mg/day, may increase to 200 mg/day

Hepatic cirrhosis
• **Adult: PO** 5-10 mg/day, may increase as needed, max 40 mg/day

Hypertension (except Soaanz)
• **Adult: PO** 5 mg/day, after 4-6 wk may increase to 10 mg/day

Available forms: Tabs 5, 10, 20, 100 mg

Administer:

PO route
• In AM to avoid interference with sleep if using product as diuretic
• With food or milk if nausea occurs; absorption may be decreased slightly

SIDE EFFECTS

CNS: *Headache, dizziness,* asthenia, insomnia, nervousness

CV: Orthostatic hypotension, chest pain, ECG changes, circulatory collapse, ventricular tachycardia, edema

EENT: *Loss of hearing,* ear pain, tinnitus, blurred vision

ELECT: *Hypokalemia, hypochloremic alkalosis, hyponatremia,* metabolic alkalosis

ENDO: *Hyperglycemia, hyperuricemia*

GI: *Nausea,* diarrhea, dyspepsia, cramps, constipation

GU: *Polyuria,* renal failure, glycosuria

INTEG: *Rash,* photosensitivity, pruritus

MS: Cramps, stiffness

RESP: Rhinitis, cough increase

PHARMACOKINETICS

PO: Rapidly absorbed; duration 6 hr; excreted in breast milk; crosses placenta; half-life 3.5 hr; protein binding 97%-99%, cleared through hepatic metabolism

INTERACTIONS

Increase: toxicity—lithium, nondepolarizing skeletal muscle relaxants, digoxin

Increase: action of antihypertensives, oral anticoagulants, nitrates; cautious use

Increase: ototoxicity—aminoglycosides, CISplatin, vancomycin; cautious use

Decrease: antihypertensive effect of torsemide—indomethacin, carBAMazepine, PHENobarbital, phenytoin, rifAMPin, NSAIDs

Decrease: hypoglycemic effect—antidiabetics; monitor blood glucose levels often

Drug/Herb
• Severe photosensitivity: St. John's wort

Drug/Lab Test
Increase: BUN, creatinine, uric acid, blood glucose, cholesterol

Decrease: potassium, magnesium, chloride sodium

NURSING CONSIDERATIONS

Assess:
• **Heart failure:** B/P lying, standing; postural hypotension may occur; weight, I&O daily to determine fluid loss; effect of product may be decreased if used daily
• **Fluid balance:** Increase fluid intake to 2-3 L/day to prevent dehydration unless contraindicated
• Hearing when giving high doses
• **Sulfa allergy:** determine before using product
• Electrolytes: potassium, sodium, chlorine; include blood glucose, CBC, blood pH, ABGs, uric acid; calcium, magnesium, potassium supplements may be required
• Blood glucose of diabetic patients, glycosuria
• **Renal failure:** monitor urinalysis, BUN, CCr
• **Hyperuricemia:** exacerbation of gout may occur
• **Metabolic alkalosis:** drowsiness, restlessness

• **Hypokalemia:** postural hypotension, malaise, fatigue, tachycardia, leg cramps, weakness

• Rashes, temperature elevation daily

• Confusion, especially in geriatric patients; take safety precautions if needed

• **Pregnancy/breastfeeding:** use only if clearly needed, no well-controlled studies; cautious use in breastfeeding

• **Beers:** use with caution in older adults; may exacerbate or cause SIADH or hyponatremia; monitor sodium levels frequently

Evaluate:

• **Therapeutic response:** improvement in edema of feet, legs, sacral area daily if medication is being used with HF

Teach patient/family:

• To rise slowly from lying, sitting position

• To recognize adverse reactions: muscle cramps, weakness, nausea, dizziness, tinnitus

• To take with food or milk for GI symptoms; to limit alcohol use

• To take early during the day to prevent nocturia

• To use sunscreen, protective clothing to prevent sunburn

• To notify prescriber if pregnancy is planned or suspected

• To report tinnitus immediately; may indicate toxicity

• Not to use any OTC medications, herbal products before approved by prescriber

TREATMENT OF OVERDOSE:

Lavage if taken orally; monitor electrolytes; administer dextrose in saline; monitor hydration, CV, renal status

---

⚠ HIGH ALERT

traMADol (Rx)

(tram′a-dole)

ConZip, Durela ✤, Qdolo, Ralivia ✤, Tridural ✤, Ultram, Zytram XL ✤

Func. class.: Analgesic—miscellaneous

Controlled Substance Schedule IV

Do not confuse:

traMADol/traZODone
Ultram/lithium

ACTION: Binds to μ-opioid receptors, inhibits reuptake of norepinephrine, serotonin

USES: Management of moderate to severe pain, chronic pain

Unlabeled uses: Restless legs syndrome (RLS), premature ejaculation

CONTRAINDICATIONS

Hypersensitivity, acute intoxication with any CNS depressant, alcohol, asthma, children, adenoidectomy, GI obstruction ileus, MAOIs

Black Box Warning: Respiratory depression

Precautions: Pregnancy, breastfeeding, geriatric patients, seizure disorder, renal/hepatic disease, head trauma, increased intracranial pressure, acute abdominal condition, drug abuse, depression, suicidal ideation, abrupt discontinuation, constipation

Black Box Warning: Coadministration with other CNS depressants, neonatal opioid withdrawal syndrome

DOSAGE AND ROUTES

Mild to moderate pain

• **Adult: PO** 25 mg daily, titrate by 25 mg ≥3 days to 100 mg/day (25 mg qid), then may increase by 50 mg ≥3 days to 200 mg (50 mg qid), then 50-100 mg q4-6hr, max 400 mg/day, use caution in geriatric patients

• **Geriatric >75 years: PO** <300 mg/day in divided doses

Moderate to severe chronic pain

• **Adult: PO-ER** (Ultram ER) 100 mg daily, titrate upward q5days in 100-mg increments, max 300 mg/day; (Ryzolt) 100 mg, titrate upward q2-3days in 100-mg increments, max 300 mg/day; products are not interchangeable

T

Side effects: *italics* = common; red = life-threatening

Renal dose
• **Adult: PO** CCr <30 mL/min, give regular dose q12hr, max 200 mg/day; do not use ext rel tab

Hepatic dose
• **Adult: PO** (Child-Pugh C) 50 mg q12hr; do not use ext rel tab

Restless legs syndrome (RLS) (unlabeled)
• **Adult: PO** 50-200 mg/day × 15-24 mo

Available forms: Tabs 50, 100 mg; ext rel tab 75 ♣, 100, 150 ♣, 200, 300, 400 ♣ mg; solution 5 mg/mL

Administer:
• Some ext rel products (Ultram ER) are not interchangeable
• Do not break, crush, or chew ext rel product
• With antiemetic for nausea, vomiting
• When pain is beginning to return; determine dosage interval by patient response
• With or without food; ER: always give with food, or always give on empty stomach
• Store in cool environment; protected from sunlight

SIDE EFFECTS

CNS: Dizziness, CNS stimulation, somnolence, headache, anxiety, confusion, euphoria, seizures, hallucinations, sedation, neuroleptic malignant syndrome–like reactions
CV: Vasodilation, orthostatic hypotension, tachycardia, hypertension, abnormal ECG
EENT: Visual disturbances
GI: Nausea, constipation, vomiting, dry mouth, diarrhea, abdominal pain, anorexia, flatulence, GI bleeding
GU: Urinary retention/frequency, menopausal symptoms, dysuria, menstrual disorder
INTEG: Pruritus, rash, urticaria, vesicles, flushing
SYST: Anaphylaxis, Stevens-Johnson syndrome, toxic epidermal necrolysis, serotonin syndrome

PHARMACOKINETICS

Rapidly and almost completely absorbed, steady state 2 days, peak 1.5 hr, duration 6 hr, half-life 7.9-8.8 hr (PO), 8-10 hr (ext rel), may cross blood-brain barrier, extensively metabolized, 30% excreted in urine as unchanged product, protein binding 20%

INTERACTIONS

• Inhibition of norepinephrine and serotonin reuptake: MAOIs; use together with caution

Black Box Warning: Increase: CNS depression—alcohol, sedatives, hypnotics, opiates

Increase: serotonin syndrome—SSRIs, SNRIs, serotonin-receptor agonists
Increase: traMADol levels—CYP3A4 inhibitors (aprepitant, antiretroviral protease inhibitors, clarithromycin, danazol, delavirdine, diltiaZEM, erythromycin, fluconazole, FLUoxetine, fluvoxaMINE, imatinib, ketoconazole, mibefradil, nefazodone, telithromycin, voriconazole)
Decrease: traMADol effects—CYP3A4 inducers (barbiturates, bosentan, carBAMazepine, efavirenz, phenytoins, nevirapine, rifabutin, rifAMPin)
Decrease: levels of traMADol—carBAMazepine

Drug/Herb
• Avoid use with St. John's wort
Increase: CNS depression—chamomile, hops, kava, skullcap, valerian

Drug/Lab Test
Increase: creatinine, hepatic enzymes
Decrease: HB

NURSING CONSIDERATIONS

Assess:
• **Pain:** location, type, character; give before pain becomes extreme

Black Box Warning: Respiratory depression: withhold if respirations <12/min; may be compounded by use of other CNS depressants

Black Box Warning: **Neonatal opioid withdrawal syndrome:** prolonged use of opioids in the mother may cause withdrawal in the neonate; can be fatal; assess for irritability, hyperactivity, abnormal sleep pattern, high-pitched cry, tremor, vomiting, diarrhea, failure to gain weight in the neonate

• **Fluid balance:** I&O ratio: check for decreasing output; may indicate urinary retention
• **Need for product;** dependency, toleration, need for upward titration
• **Bowel pattern;** for constipation; increase fluids, bulk in diet
• **CNS changes:** dizziness, drowsiness, hallucinations, euphoria, LOC, pupil reaction; avoid use with other CNS depressants
• **Hypersensitivity:** usually after beginning treatment
• Increased side effects in renal/hepatic disease
• **Serotonin syndrome, neuroleptic malignant syndrome:** increased heart rate, shivering, sweating, dilated pupils, tremors, high B/P, hyperthermia, headache, confusion; if these occur, stop product, administer serotonin antagonist if needed
• Safety: Assistance with ambulation; safety measures: side rails, nightlight, call bell within easy reach
• **Pregnancy/breastfeeding:** use only if benefits outweigh fetal risk, no well-controlled studies; do not use in labor/delivery; do not breastfeed
• **Beers:** avoid in older adults; may lower seizure threshold; monitor for seizures frequently in those with a seizure disorder
Evaluate:
• **Therapeutic response:** decrease in pain
Teach patient/family:
• Before taking, inform health care provider of any history of head injury; seizures; liver, kidney, thyroid problems; problems in urinating; pancreas or gallbladder problems; abuse of street or prescription drugs; alcohol addiction; or mental health problems

• Not to take other prescription medications, OTC products, vitamins, or herbal supplements without approval from health care provider
• To take exactly as prescribed by health care provider; not to take more than prescribed dose and not to take >8 tablets/day. If dose is missed, to take the next dose at usual time
• To notify health care provider if the prescribed does not control pain
• Not to stop product abruptly if taking regularly without talking to health care provider
• Not to drive or operate heavy machinery until effects of product are known; may cause dizziness or light-headedness
• Not to drink alcohol or use a prescription or OTC product that contains alcohol
• To notify health care provider of severe constipation, nausea, sleepiness, vomiting, tiredness, headache, dizziness, abdominal pain
• To get emergency medical help for difficulty in breathing, shortness of breath, fast heartbeat, chest pain; swelling of face, tongue, or throat; extreme drowsiness, light-headedness when changing positions, feeling faint, agitation, high body temperature, trouble walking, stiff muscles, or mental changes such as confusion
• To notify health care provider if pregnancy is planned or suspected. Prolonged use during pregnancy can cause withdrawal symptoms in neonate that could be life threatening if not recognized and treated. Do not breastfeed

⚠ HIGH ALERT

trametinib (Rx)
(tra-me′ti-nib)
MeKinist
Func. class.: Antineoplastic biologic response modifiers
Chem. class.: Signal transduction inhibitors (STIs), tyrosine kinase inhibitor

USES: Unresectable or metastatic BRAD V600E or BRAF V600K mutated malignant melanoma, non-small cell lung cancer, thyroid cancer

CONTRAINDICATIONS
Pregnancy, hypersensitivity

DOSAGE AND ROUTES
Unresectable or metastatic malignant melanoma
• **Adult: PO** 2 mg daily; may be used in combination with dacarbazine or PACLi-taxel in those with BRAF V600E
Unresectable or metastatic malignant melanoma
• **Adult: PO** 2 mg daily with dabrafenib 150 mg q12hr until disease progression, take both at same time
Available forms: Tabs 0.5, 2 mg

---

trandolapril (Rx)
(tran-doe'la-prill)
Func. class.: Antihypertensive
Chem. class.: Angiotension-converting enzyme inhibitor

USES: Hypertension, heart failure, left ventricular dysfunction post MI

CONTRAINDICATIONS
Breastfeeding, hypersensitivity, history of angioedema

Black Box Warning: Pregnancy

DOSAGE AND ROUTES
Hypertension
• **Adult: PO** 1 mg/day; 2 mg/day in African Americans; make dosage adjustment ≥1 wk; max 8 mg/day
Heart failure, left ventricular dysfunction post MI
• **Adult: PO** 1 mg/day, titrate upward to 4 mg/day if tolerated, continue for 2-4 yr
Renal/hepatic dose
• **Adult: PO** CCr <30 mL/min or hepatic disease, 0.5 mg/day
Available forms: Tabs 1, 2 ,4 mg

---

trandolapril/verapamil (Rx)
(tran-doe'la-pril/ver-ap'a-mil)
Tarka
Func. class.: Antihypertensive, calcium channel blocker

USES: Management of hypertension

CONTRAINDICATIONS
Hypersensitivity, severe left ventricular dysfunction; systolic pressure <90 mm Hg, cardiogenic shock, sick sinus syndrome, atrial flutter/atrial fibrillation, angioedema, use within 36 hr of switching to/from a neprilysin inhibitor, 2nd/3rd-degree AV block, use with aliskiren in those with diabetes, use with flibanserin

DOSAGE AND ROUTES
• **Adult: PO:** Trandolapril 1-4 mg/verapamil 180-240 mg daily
Available forms: Tabs, ext rel 1 mg/240 mg, 2 mg/180 mg, 2 mg/240 mg, 4 mg/240 mg

---

⚠ HIGH ALERT

trastuzumab (Rx)
(tras-tuz'uh-mab)
Herceptin
trastuzumab-anns
Kanjinti
trastuzumab-dkst
Ogivri
trastuzumab-dttb
Ontruzant
trastuzumab-pkrb
trastuzumab-gyyp
Trazimera
Func. class.: Antineoplastic—miscellaneous
Chem. class.: Humanized monoclonal antibody

ACTION: DNA-derived monoclonal antibody selectively binds to extracellular portion of human epidermal growth factor receptor 2; it inhibits the proliferation of cancer cells

USES: Breast cancer; metastatic with overexpression of 🔊 HER2, early breast cancer (adjuvant, neoadjuvant), gastric cancer; previously untreated HER2 over-expressing metastatic gastric or gastro-esophageal junction adenocarcinoma with CISplatin, 5-fluorouracil, or capecitabine

CONTRAINDICATIONS
Hypersensitivity to this product, Chinese hamster ovary cell protein
Precautions: Breastfeeding, children, geriatric patients, pulmonary disease, anemia, leukopenia

Black Box Warning: Respiratory distress syndrome, respiratory insufficiency, infusion-related reactions, cardiomyopathy, contraception requirement, pregnancy, pulmonary toxicity

DOSAGE AND ROUTES
HER2-positive, node-positive or node-negative (ER/PR negative) in combination (AC-TH)
• **Adult:** IV 4 mg/kg over 90 min on day 1, then 2 mg/kg over 30 min weekly for a total of 12 wk, with PACLitaxel (either 80 mg/m^2 IV wk or 175 mg/m^2 q3wk) beginning on day 1 for a total of 4 cycles (12 wk). On wk 13, begin trastuzumab 6 mg/kg over 30-90 min q3wk as monotherapy for a total of 52 wk of trastuzumab therapy; begin PACLitaxel plus trastuzumab after the completion of 4 cycles of AC chemotherapy (doxorubicin 60 mg/m^2 IV and cyclophosphamide 600 mg/m^2 IV q21days)
HER2-positive, node-positive or node-negative (ER/PR negative) in combination (AC-TH)
• **Adult:** IV 4 mg/kg over 90 min on day 1, then 2 mg/kg over 30 min weekly (total of 12 wk), with DOCEtaxel 100

mg/m^2 IV q21days beginning on day 1 for a total of 4 cycles (12 wk). On wk 13, begin trastuzumab 6 mg/kg IV over 30-90 min q3wk as monotherapy for a total of 52 wk of trastuzumab therapy. Begin DOCEtaxel plus trastuzumab after the completion of 4 cycles of AC chemotherapy (doxorubicin 60 mg/m^2 IV and cyclophosphamide 600 mg/m^2 IV q21days)
HER2-positive, node-positive or node-negative (ER/PR negative) in combination (TCH)
• **Adult:** IV 4 mg/kg over 90 min on day 1, then 2 mg/kg over 30 min weekly (total of 18 wk), with DOCEtaxel 75 mg/m^2 IV followed by CARBOplatin AUC 6 IV over 30-60 min beginning on day 1, q3wk, for a total of 6 cycles (18 wk). On wk 19, begin trastuzumab 6 mg/kg IV over 30-90 min q3wk as monotherapy (52 wk of trastuzumab)
HER2-positive, node-positive or node-negative (ER/PR negative) monotherapy
• **Adult:** IV 8 mg/kg over 90 min on day 1, followed by 6 mg/kg IV over 30-90 min q21days (total of 52 wk)
Available forms: Lyophilized powder 150, 440 mg
Administer:
• Check vial labels carefully, medication errors have occurred between Herceptin A and Kadcyla
• Acetaminophen as ordered to alleviate fever and headache
Intermittent IV INFUSION route
• Use cytotoxic handling procedures; avoid treatment >1 yr
• After **reconstituting** vial with 20 mL bacteriostatic water for inj, 1.1% benzyl alcohol preserved (supplied) to yield 21 mg/mL; mark date on vial 28 days from reconstitution date; if patient is allergic to benzyl alcohol, reconstitute with sterile water for inj; **Dilute:** withdraw amount of solution and add to 250 mL of 0.9% NaCl, use immediately; infuse over 90 min; subsequent 6 mg/kg dose may be given over 30-60 min
• Do not mix or dilute with other products or dextrose sol

Side effects: *italics* = common; red = life-threatening

SIDE EFFECTS

CNS: *Dizziness, numbness, paresthesias,* depression, *insomnia,* neuropathy, peripheral neuritis
CV: Tachycardia, heart failure
GI: Nausea, vomiting, *anorexia, diarrhea,* abdominal pain, hepatotoxicity, dysgeusia
HEMA: *Anemia,* leukopenia
INTEG: Rash, acne, herpes simplex
META: Edema, peripheral edema
MISC: *Flulike symptoms; fever, headache, chills*
MS: Arthralgia, *bone pain*
RESP: *Cough, dyspnea, pharyngitis, rhinitis,* sinusitis, pneumonia, pulmonary edema/fibrosis, acute respiratory distress syndrome (ARDS)
SYST: Anaphylaxis, angioedema

PHARMACOKINETICS

Half-life 1-32 days, 97% washout by 7 mo after end of treatment
Drug/Lab
Decrease: WBCs

INTERACTIONS

Increase: bleeding risk—warfarin
Increase: cardiomyopathy—anthracyclines, cyclophosphamide; avoid use
Decrease: immune response—vaccines, toxoids

NURSING CONSIDERATIONS

Assess:
• **Labs:** CBC, HER2 overexpression

Black Box Warning: HF, other cardiac symptoms: dyspnea, coughing; gallop; obtain full cardiac workup, ECG, baseline and q3mo during treatment and q6mo for ≥2 yr after adjuvant treatment (LVEF, MUGA, or ECHO); monitor for deterioration in those with decreased LVEF

• Symptoms of infection; may be masked by product
• **CNS reaction:** LOC, mental status, dizziness, confusion
• Hypersensitivity reactions, anaphylaxis

Black Box Warning: Infusion reactions that may be fatal: fever, chills, nausea, vomiting, pain, headache, dizziness, hypotension; discontinue product

• **Pulmonary toxicity:** dyspnea, interstitial pneumonitis, pulmonary hypertension, ARDS; can occur after infusion reaction, those with lung disease may have more severe toxicity
• **Benzyl alcohol hypersensitivity:** reconstitute with Sterile Water for Injection, USP; discard any unused portion
• **Hamster protein hypersensitivity** (Chinese hamster ovary cell hypersensitivity): increased risk of severe allergic reactions
• **Pregnancy/breastfeeding:** monitor for oligohydramnios. If oligohydramnios occurs, fetal testing should be done. Women should enroll in the MotHER Pregnancy Registry, 800-690-6720 or http://www.motherpregnancyregistry.com. Contraception should be used during and for ≥7 mo after last dose; pregnancy testing before use. Women who become pregnant while receiving or within 7 mo of the last dose should be apprised of potential hazard to the fetus. Unknown whether product is excreted into breast milk; advise women to discontinue breastfeeding during treatment and for 7 mo after last dose
Evaluate:
• **Therapeutic response:** decrease in size of tumors
Teach patient/family:
• To take acetaminophen for fever
• To avoid hazardous tasks because confusion, dizziness may occur
• To report signs of infection: sore throat, fever, diarrhea, vomiting
• That emotional lability is common; to notify prescriber if severe or incapacitating

Black Box Warning: Pregnancy/breastfeeding: to use contraception while taking this product and for 7 mo after last dose; breastfeed during and for 7 mo after treatment

Black Box Warning: To report pain at infusion site, usually with first dose

Black Box Warning: **Cardiomyopathy:** to report cough, swelling in extremities, shortness of breath; may occur during or after completion of treatment

⚠ HIGH ALERT

trastuzumab/ hyaluronidase (Rx)

(tras-tooz'ue-mab/hye-al-ur-on'i-dase)

Herceptin Hylecta
Func. class.: Antineoplastic, endoglycosidases

USES: Adjuvant treatment of HER2-overexpressing node positive/node negative (ER/PR negative or with one high-risk feature) in breast cancer, as part of a regimen with doxorubicin, cyclophosphamide, and either paclitaxel or docetaxel; as part of a regimen with docetaxel and carboplatin; as a single agent anthracycline-based therapy; HER2-overexpressing metastatic breast cancer (in combination with paclitaxel); single-agent treatment of HER2-overexpressing breast cancer

CONTRAINDICATIONS
Hypersensitivity

Black Box Warning: Pregnancy, CV toxicity, pulmonary toxicity

DOSAGE AND ROUTES
Breast cancer, adjuvant treatment, HER2+
• **Adult: SUBCUT:** Trastuzumab 600 mg/hyaluronidase 10,000 units once q3wk × 52 wk or until disease progression or unacceptable toxicity; give with doxorubicin, cyclophosphamide, and either paclitaxel or docetaxel; or in combination with docetaxel and carboplatin; or as a single agent following

multimodality anthracycline-based therapy
Breast cancer, metastatic, HER2+
• **Adult: SUBCUT:** Trastuzumab 600 mg/hyaluronidase 10,000 units once q3wk (with paclitaxel or as a single agent following one or more chemotherapy regimens for metastatic disease) until disease progression or unacceptable toxicity

Available forms: Injection 600 mg/10,000 units/5 mL in single-dose vial

travoprost ophthalmic
See Appendix B

traZODone (Rx)

(tray'zoe-done)
Func. class.: Antidepressant—miscellaneous
Chem. class.: Triazolopyridine

Do not confuse:
traZODone/traMADol

ACTION: Selectively inhibits serotonin uptake by brain; potentiates behavorial changes

USES: Major depressive disorder (unipolar)
Unlabeled uses: Aggressive or agitated behavior associated with dementia, insomnia

CONTRAINDICATIONS
Hypersensitivity to tricyclics
Precautions: Pregnancy, suicidal patients, severe depression, increased intraocular pressure, closed-angle glaucoma, urinary retention, cardiac/hepatic disease, hyperthyroidism, electroshock therapy, elective surgery, bleeding, abrupt discontinuation, bipolar disorder, breastfeeding, dehydration, hyponatremia, hypovolemia, recovery phase of MI, seizure disorders, prostatic hypertrophy, family history of long QT

Side effects: *italics* = common; red = life-threatening

Black Box Warning: Suicidal ideation in children/adolescents

DOSAGE AND ROUTES
Depression
• **Adult: PO** 150 mg/day in divided doses, may increase by 50 mg/day q3-4days, max 400 mg/day (outpatient), 600 mg/day (inpatient)
• **Geriatric: PO** 25-50 mg at bedtime, increase by 25-50 mg q3-7days to desired dose, usually 75-150 mg/day

Available forms: Tabs 50, 100, 150, 300 mg

Administer:
• Increased fluids, bulk in diet if constipation occurs, especially in geriatric patients
• With food, milk for GI symptoms
• Dosage at bedtime for oversedation during day; may take entire dose at bedtime; geriatric patients may not tolerate daily dosing
• Avoid use of CNS depressants
• Do not crush, break, chew ext rel product
• Store in tight, light-resistant container at room temperature

SIDE EFFECTS
CNS: *Dizziness, drowsiness,* confusion, headache, anxiety, tremors, stimulation, weakness, insomnia, nightmares, EPS (geriatric patients), increase in psychiatric symptoms, suicide in children/adolescents

CV: *Orthostatic hypotension, ECG changes, tachycardia,* hypertension, palpitations

EENT: *Blurred vision,* tinnitus, mydriasis

GI: *Diarrhea, dry mouth,* nausea, vomiting, paralytic ileus, increased appetite, cramps, epigastric distress, jaundice, hepatitis, stomatitis, constipation

GU: *Urinary retention,* acute renal failure, priapism

HEMA: Agranulocytosis, thrombocytopenia, eosinophilia, leukopenia

INTEG: Rash, urticaria, sweating, pruritus, photosensitivity

PHARMACOKINETICS
Peak 1 hr without food, 2 hr with food; metabolized by liver (CYP3A4); excreted by kidneys, in feces; half-life 4.4-7.5 hr

INTERACTIONS
Hyperpyretic crisis, seizures, hypertensive episode: MAOIs; do not use within 14 days of traZODone

Increase: toxicity, serotonin syndrome—FLUoxetine, nefazodone, other SSRIs, SNRIs, linezolid; methylene blue (IV)

Increase: effects of direct-acting sympathomimetics (EPINEPHrine), alcohol, barbiturates, benzodiazepines, CNS depressants, digoxin, phenytoin, carBAMazepine, traMADol

Increase: effects of traZODone—CYP3A4, 2D6 inhibitors (phenothiazines, protease inhibitors, azole antifungals)

Increase or decrease: effects of warfarin

Increase: QT prolongation—tricyclics

Decrease: effects of guanethidine, cloNIDine, indirect-acting sympathomimetics (ePHEDrine)

Drug/Herb
Increase: serotonin syndrome—SAM-e, St. John's wort

Increase: CNS depression—hops, kava, lavender, valerian

Drug/Lab Test
Increase: LFTs
Decrease: HB

NURSING CONSIDERATIONS
Assess:
• **CV status:** B/P lying, standing; pulse q4hr; if systolic B/P drops 20 mm Hg, hold product, notify prescriber; take vital signs q4hr in patients with CV disease
• **Blood studies:** CBC, leukocytes, differential
• **Hepatic studies:** AST, ALT, bilirubin
• Weight weekly; appetite may increase with product

• ECG for flattening of T wave, bundle branch block, AV block, dysrhythmias in cardiac patients
• **EPS,** primarily in geriatric patients: rigidity, dystonia, akathisia

Black Box Warning: Mental status changes: mood, sensorium, affect, suicidal tendencies, increase in psychiatric symptoms, depression, panic; observe for suicidal behaviors in children/adolescents, not approved for children; if worsening depression occurs, product may need to be tapered as rapidly as possible, without abrupt discontinuation

• Urinary retention, constipation; constipation most likely in children
• Alcohol consumption; hold dose until morning
• **Serotonin syndrome, neuroleptic malignant syndrome:** increased heart rate, shivering, sweating, dilated pupils, tremors, high B/P, hyperthermia, headache, confusion; if these occur, stop product, administer serotonin antagonist if needed
• **Pregnancy/breastfeeding:** use only if benefits outweigh fetal risk; no well-controlled studies; cautious use in breastfeeding, excreted in breast milk
Evaluate:
• **Therapeutic response:** decreased depression
Teach patient/family:
• That therapeutic effects may take 2-3 wk; to take ext rel product before bedtime; not to crush, chew ext rel product
• To use caution when driving, performing other activities requiring alertness because of drowsiness, dizziness, blurred vision
• To avoid alcohol ingestion
• Not to discontinue medication quickly after long-term use; may cause nausea, headache, malaise
• To report urinary retention, priapism >4 hr immediately
• To wear sunscreen or large hat because photosensitivity occurs

Black Box Warning: That suicidal thoughts/behaviors may occur (adolescents/children); to notify health care professional if there is an increase in depression, agitation

• To notify prescriber if pregnancy is planned or suspected; to avoid breastfeeding
• To rise slowly to prevent dizziness

TREATMENT OF OVERDOSE: ECG monitoring; administer anticonvulsant, atropine for bradycardia

> **⚠ HIGH ALERT**

tremelimumab (Rx)

(treh-meh-LIM-moo-mab)
Imjudo
Func. class.: Antineoplastic
Chem. class.: Monoclonal antibody

ACTIONS: Cytotoxic T-lymphocyte antigen blocking antibody

USES: Hepatocellular carcinoma in combination with durvalumab; non–small-cell lung cancer with durvalumab and platinum-based chemotherapy

CONTRAINDICATIONS

Hypersensitivity, pregnancy
Precautions: Immune-mediated pneumonitis, immune-mediated colitis, immune-mediated hepatitis, immune-mediated endocrinopathies, immune-mediated nephritis with renal dysfunction, immune-mediated pancreatitis, hypo/hyperthyroidism, active infections

DOSAGE AND ROUTES

• **Adults <30 kg: IV** 4 mg/kg on day 1. Observe the patient for signs of an infusion reaction for 60 min, then give durvalumab (20 mg/kg IV); continue durvalumab (4 mg/kg IV) as monotherapy q4wk until disease progression or unacceptable toxicity
• **Adults ≥30 kg: IV** 300 mg on day 1. Observe the patient for signs of an

infusion reaction for 60 min, then give durvalumab (1500 mg IV); continue durvalumab (1500 mg IV) as monotherapy q4wk until disease progression or unacceptable toxicity

Available forms: Solution for injection 25 mg/1.25 mL, 300 mg/15 mL

Administer:

IV route

• Inspect for particulate matter and discoloration. Discard if the solution is cloudy, discolored, or visible particles are observed

• Do not shake

• Give tremelimumab prior to durvalumab when given on the same day; use separate infusion bags and filters for durvalumab and tremelimumab

• Withdraw the required volume of drug and transfer into an IV bag of 0.9% sodium chloride injection or 5% dextrose injection

• The maximum diluent volume for patients weighing 30 kg or more (300-mg dose) is 150 mL

• The maximum diluent volume for patients weighing less than 30 kg (4 mg/kg dose) is 80 mL

• The final concentration should not exceed 10 mg/mL

• Mix by gentle inversion; do not shake

• Discard partially used or empty vials

• *Storage after dilution:* The storage time of diluted product from start of preparation until completion of the infusion max 24 hr under refrigeration (36° F to 46° F [2° C to 8° C]) or 24 hr at room temperature (up to 86° F [up to 30° C]). Do not freeze

• Give over 60 min using a sterile, low-protein-binding, 0.2- or 0.22-micron in-line filter

• Observe the patient for 60 min following completion of the infusion

• Do not coadminister with other drugs through the same intravenous line

SIDE EFFECTS

CNS: Fatigue
GI: Diarrhea, nausea, abdominal pain
MS: Pain
ENDO: Hypoparathyroidism
HEMA: Hemorrhage

INTEG: Infusion-related reactions, rash
SYST: Immune-mediated reactions

INTERACTIONS
None known

NURSING CONSIDERATIONS

Assess:

• For injection site pain, swelling, redness: use cold compress to relieve pain/swelling

• Infections (fever, flulike symptoms, dyspnea, change in urination, redness/swelling around any wounds), stop treatment if some serious infections, including sepsis, may occur, may be fatal; patients with active infections should not be started on this product

• Immune mediated reactions, may be fatal

• Pregnancy/breastfeeding: Not to use during pregnancy and for 3 mo after last dose and not to use during breastfeeding, confirm pregnancy status before using

Evaluate:

• **Therapeutic response:** decrease

Teach patient/family:

• To report signs of infection, allergic reaction, immediately

• To advise all health care professionals of Rx, OTC, herbals, supplements taken

• Pregnancy/breastfeeding: To advise health care professional if pregnancy is planned or suspected or if breastfeeding

---

treprostinil (Rx)
(treh-prah'stin-ill)
Orenitram, Remodulin, Tyvaso, Tyvaso Refill, Tyvaso Starter
Func. class.: Pulmonaryvasodilator
Chem. class.: Tricyclic benzidine prostacyclin analog

ACTION: Direct vasodilation of pulmonary, systemic arterial vascular beds; inhibition of platelet aggregation

USES: Pulmonary arterial hypertension (PAH) NYHA class II through IV

CONTRAINDICATIONS

Hypersensitivity to this product, other prostacyclin analogs

Precautions: Pregnancy, breastfeeding, children, geriatric patients, past renal/hepatic disease, thromboembolic disease, abrupt discontinuation, IV administration

DOSAGE AND ROUTES
Pulmonary arterial hypertension
• **Adult: SUBCUT CONT INFUSION/IV CONT INFUSION** 1.25 ng/kg/min. If not tolerated, reduce to 0.625 ng/kg/min. Increase dose by ≤1.25 ng/kg/min per wk × first 4 wk, then ≤2.5 ng/kg/min per wk; **ORAL INH:** 3 breaths (18 mcg) by Tyvaso Inhalation System qid 4 hr apart during waking hours; **PO:** 0.25 mg q12hr or 0.125 mg q8hr, increase by 0.25 or 0.5 mg bid or 0.125 mg tid q3-4days as tolerated

• **Adult taking gemfibrozil (or other strong CYP2C8 inhibitor): PO** 0.125 mg q12hr, increase by 0.125 mg bid q3-4days, as tolerated

For patients transitioning from IV or SUBCUT to PO
• **Adult: PO** For patients already receiving **IV** or **SUBCUT,** use the following equation: Total daily PO dose = 0.0072 × IV or SUBCUT dose (ng/kg/min) × Weight (kg). Reduce dose of IV or SUBCUT by up to 30 ng/kg/min per day while increasing dose of PO up to 6 mg/day (2 mg PO tid), if tolerated

Hepatic dose
• **Adult: SUBCUT INFUSION** 0.625 ng/kg ideal body weight/min; increase cautiously

Available forms: Inj 1, 2.5, 5, 10 mg/mL; neb sol 1.74 mg/2.9 mL; ext rel tab 0.125, 0.25, 2.5 mg

Administer:
• Sudden decreased doses, abrupt withdrawal may worsen pulmonary arterial hypertension symptoms

PO route
• Give with food

• Swallow tablets whole; use only intact tablets

Injectable route
• Visually inspect for particulate matter and discoloration before use
• Administer injection by continuous SUBCUT infusion. May be administered by continuous IV infusion in those who do not tolerate continuous SUBCUT (severe injection site pain or reaction)
• Have immediate access to a backup infusion pump and infusion sets. Avoid abrupt discontinuation. The infusion can be restarted after a few hours at the previous dose and rate; if the infusion is stopped for longer than a few hours, retitration may be needed
• The infusion pump used should be: small and lightweight; adjustable to approximately 0.002 mL/hr; have alarms for occlusion, end of infusion and low battery, programming error and motor malfunctions; accurate to +/−6% of the programmed rate; positive-pressure driven. The reservoir should be made of polyvinyl chloride, polypropylene, or glass
• **Opened vials:** A single vial should be used ≤30 days after the initial entry into the vial

CONTINUOUS IV route
• Given via a surgically placed central venous catheter via an ambulatory infusion pump. A peripheral IV cannula, placed into a large vein, may be used temporarily; use of a peripheral vein for more than a few hours may increase the risk of thrombophlebitis
• Infusion sets with an in-line 0.22- or 0.2-micron pore size filter should be used

IV infusion preparation
• May dilute with Remodulin sterile diluent for injection or similar approved high-pH glycine diluents (sterile diluent for Flolan or sterile diluent for epoprostenol sodium), sterile water for injection, or 0.9% NaCl for injection
• The concentration of diluted treprostinil should be calculated using the following formula: diluted concentration = [dose (ng/kg/min) × weight (kg) × 0.00006]/IV infusion rate (mL/hr)

T

• Typical ambulatory infusion pump reservoirs have volumes of 50 or 100 mL. The IV infusion rate is predetermined based on the volume of the reservoir with a desired infusion length of 48 hr (i.e., for a 50-mL reservoir, the infusion rate would be 1 mL/hr; for a 100-mL reservoir, the infusion rate would be 2 mL/hr)

• The reservoir should be filled with the calculated volume and a sufficient amount of diluent to achieve the total volume of the reservoir

• Once diluted with any diluent, may be given for 48 hr at 40° C

• **Storage:** If diluted with sterile water for injection or 0.9% NaCl, store up to 4 hr at room temperature or 24 hr if refrigerated. If diluted with an approved high-pH glycine diluent (sterile diluent for Remodulin, Flolan, or epoprostenol sodium), it may be stored for 14 days at room temperature at concentrations as low as 0.004 mg/mL

SUBCUT continuous infusion

• Give via a self-inserted SUBCUT catheter using an ambulatory infusion pump designed for subcutaneous drug delivery

SUBCUT infusion preparation

• Further dilution is NOT required before continuous SUBCUT use

• Do not mix or co-infuse with other medications

• The SUBCUT infusion rate can be calculated using the following formula: SUBCUT infusion rate = [dose (ng/kg/min) × weight (kg) × 0.00006]/treprostinil vial strength (mg/mL)

• During SUBCUT use, a single reservoir (syringe) of product can be given ≤72 hr at a max temperature of 37° C (98.6° F)

Oral inhalation administration

• Must be used only with the Tyvaso Inhalation System

• Avoid skin or eye contact with solution. Do not take PO

• Have access to a backup Optineb-ir device to avoid interruptions in therapy

• Do not mix with other medications in the Optineb-ir device

• One ampule contains a volume for all 4 treatment sessions in a single day

SIDE EFFECTS

CNS: Dizziness, headache, syncope

CV: Vasodilation, *hypotension, edema,* right ventricular heart failure

GI: Nausea, *diarrhea*

INTEG: *Rash,* pruritus

OTHER: Jaw pain, cough, throat irritation, UTI, leg cramps

SYST: Infusion site reactions, pain; increased risk for infection

PHARMACOKINETICS

Metabolized by liver; excreted in urine, feces; terminal half-life 2-4 hr; 90% protein binding

INTERACTIONS

• Excessive hypotension: diuretics, antihypertensives, vasodilators, MAOIs, β-blockers, calcium channel blockers

Increase: bleeding tendencies—anticoagulants, aspirin, NSAIDs, thrombin inhibitors, SSRIs

NURSING CONSIDERATIONS

Assess:

• Avoid abrupt discontinuation

• **CV status:** monitor B/P, baseline and periodically, HR and rhythm, S3, chest pain, edema, dyspnea, fatigue, ADLs, syncope

• **Hepatic studies:** AST, ALT, bilirubin, creatinine with long-term therapy

• **Blood studies:** CBC; CBC q2wk × 3 mo, Hct, HB, PT with long-term therapy, ABGs

• Bleeding time at baseline, throughout treatment; levels may be 2-5× normal limit

• **Beers:** use with caution in older adults; may exacerbate episodes of syncope; monitor frequently

• **Pregnancy/breastfeeding:** use only if clearly needed, no well-controlled studies; cautious use in breastfeeding, excretion unknown

Evaluate:

• **Therapeutic response:** decreased pulmonary arterial hypertension (PAH)

Teach patient/family:

• That blood work will be necessary during treatment; that treatment may last for years

- To report side effects such as diarrhea, skin rashes
- That therapy will be needed for prolonged periods of time, sometimes years
- To use aseptic technique for preparation, administration of treprostinil to prevent infection
- That there are many product, herbal interactions
- **Tablet:** to take with food; not to crush or chew tablets, not to skip doses
- **Subcut:** about injection technique; to rotate injection sites; to avoid irritated, scarred, or bruised skin
- **Inhalation:** to avoid contact of solution with skin or eyes; to wash hands after handling inhaler; to follow directions for use in package insert
- How to use inhaled solution; how to care for equipment
- About signs, symptoms of bleeding; blood in urine, stools

tretinoin (vit A acid, retinoic acid) (Rx)

(tret'i-noyn)

Altreno, Atralin, Avita, Refissa, Renova, Renova Pump, Retin-A, Retin-A Micro, Retin-A Micro Pump, StieVA-A ❖, Vesanoid ❖, Vitamin A Acid ❖

Func. class.: Vit A acid, acne product; antineoplastic (miscellaneous)
Chem. class.: Tretinoin derivative

ACTION: (Topical) Decreases cohesiveness of follicular epithelium, decreases microcomedone formation; (PO) induces maturation of acute promyelocytic leukemia, exact action is unknown

USES: (Topical) Acne vulgaris (grades 1-3); (PO) facial wrinkles, photoaging

CONTRAINDICATIONS
Hypersensitivity to retinoids or sensitivity to parabens

Black Box Warning: Pregnancy (PO)

Precautions: Pregnancy (topical), breastfeeding, eczema, sunburn, sun exposure

Black Box Warning: Rapid-evolving leukocytosis, respiratory compromise, acute promyelocytic leukemia differentiation syndrome, requires a specialized care setting, experienced clinician

DOSAGE AND ROUTES
- **Adult/child:** TOP cleanse area, apply 0.025%-0.1% cream or 0.05% liquid gel at bedtime, cover lightly
Available forms: Cream 0.01%, 0.02%, 0.025%, 0.05%, 0.1%; gel 0.01%, 0.025%, 0.04%, 0.05%, 0.1%; liquid 0.05%; caps 10 mg
Administer:
Topical route
- Once daily before bedtime; cover area lightly using gauze; use gloves to apply
- Store at room temperature
- Handwashing after application

SIDE EFFECTS
PO route
CNS: *Headache, fever, sweating,* fatigue
CV: Cardiac dysrhythmias, pericardial effusion
GI: *Nausea, vomiting,* hemorrhage, *abdominal pain, diarrhea, constipation, dyspepsia, distention, hepatitis*
Topical route
INTEG: Rash, stinging, warmth, redness, erythema, blistering, crusting, peeling, contact dermatitis, hypo/hyperpigmentation, dry skin, pruritus, scaly skin, retinoic acid syndrome (RAS)
META: Hypercholesterolemia, hypertriglyceridemia
RESP: Pneumonia, upper respiratory tract disease

PHARMACOKINETICS
PO: Terminal half-life 0.5-2 hr
TOPICAL: Poor systemic absorption

INTERACTIONS
- Use with caution: medicated, abrasive soaps; cleansers that have a drying effect;

products with high concentration of alcohol astringents (topical)

Increase: peeling—medication containing agents such as sulfur, benzoyl peroxide, resorcinol, salicylic acid (topical)

Increase: plasma concentrations of tretinoin—ketoconazole (PO)

Increase: ICP, risk of pseudotumor cerebri—tetracyclines; do not use together (PO)

Increase: photosensitivity—retinoids, quinolones, phenothiazines, sulfonamides, sulfonylureas, thiazide diuretics

Increase: thrombotic complications—aminocaproic acid, aprotinin, tranexamic acid

Drug/Lab Test

Increase: AST, ALT

NURSING CONSIDERATIONS
Assess:

Topical route

• Area of body involved, what helps or aggravates condition; cysts, dryness, itching; lesions may worsen at beginning of treatment

PO route

• Hepatic function, coagulation, hematologic parameters; also cholesterol, triglycerides

• **Pregnancy/breastfeeding:** do not use PO in pregnancy, breastfeeding

Evaluate:

• **Therapeutic response:** decrease in size, number of lesions

Teach patient/family:

Topical route

• To avoid application on normal skin; to avoid getting cream in eyes, nose, other mucous membranes; not to use product on areas with cuts, scrapes

• To use cream/gel by applying a thin layer to affected skin; to rub gently; to use liquid by applying with fingertip or cotton swab

• To avoid sunlight, sunlamps; to use protective clothing, sunscreen

• That treatment may cause warmth, stinging; that dryness, peeling will occur

• That cosmetics may be used over product; not to use shaving lotions

• That rash may occur during first 1-3 wk of therapy

• That product does not cure condition, only relieves symptoms

• That therapeutic results may be seen in 2-3 wk but may not be optimal until after 6 wk

PO route

Black Box Warning: To notify prescriber if pregnancy is planned or suspected

tretinoin topical
See Appendix B

triamcinolone (ophthalmic)
See Appendix B

triamcinolone (Rx)
(trye-am-sin'oh-lone)
Kenalog, Kenalog-80, P-Care K40, P-Care K80, Pod-Care 100K, Pro-C-Dure 5, Pro-C-Dure 6, Zilretta
Func. class.: Corticosteroid, synthetic
Chem. class.: Glucocorticoid, intermediate acting

ACTION: Decreases inflammation by suppression of migration of polymorphonuclear leukocytes, fibroblasts; reversal of increased capillary permeability and lysosomal stabilization

USES: Severe inflammation, immunosuppression, neoplasms, asthma (steroid dependent); collagen, respiratory, dermatologic/rheumatic disorders

CONTRAINDICATIONS
Hypersensitivity, neonatal prematurity; epidural/intrathecal administration (triamcinolone acetonide injections [Kenalog]), systemic fungal infections

Precautions: Pregnancy, breastfeeding, diabetes mellitus, glaucoma, osteoporosis, seizure disorders, ulcerative colitis, HF, myasthenia gravis, renal disease, esophagitis, peptic ulcer, acne, cataracts, coagulopathy, head trauma, children <2 yr, psychosis, idiopathic thrombocytopenia, acute glomerulonephritis, amebiasis, fungal infections, nonasthmatic bronchial disease, AIDS, TB, adrenal insufficiency, acute bronchospasm, acne rosacea, Cushing syndrome, acute MI, thromboembolism

DOSAGE AND ROUTES

• **Adult:** IM (acetonide) 40-80 mg q4wk; intraarticular (hexacetonide) 2-20 mg q3-4wk

• **Child:** IM acetonide 40 mg q4wk or 30-200 mcg/kg (1-6.25 mg/m^2) q1-7days (acetonide) 40-80 mg q4wk; intraarticular (hexacetonide) 2-20 mg q3-4wk

Available forms: Inj 3, 10, 40 mg/mL acetonide; inj 20, 5 mg/mL hexacetonide

Administer:

IM route

• After shaking susp (parenteral)
• Titrated dose; use lowest effective dose
• IM inj deep in large muscle mass; rotate sites; avoid deltoid; use 21-G needle
• Avoid SUBCUT administration, may damage tissue

SIDE EFFECTS

CNS: *Depression,* headache, mood changes

CV: *Hypertension,* circulatory collapse, embolism, tachycardia, edema

EENT: Fungal infections, increased intraocular pressure, blurred vision

GI: *Diarrhea, nausea, abdominal distention,* GI hemorrhage, *increased appetite,* pancreatitis

HEMA: Thrombocytopenia

INTEG: Acne, poor wound healing, ecchymosis, petechiae

MS: Fractures, osteoporosis, weakness

PHARMACOKINETICS

PO/IM: Peak 1-2 hr, half-life 2-5 hr

INTERACTIONS

Increase: side effects—alcohol, salicylates, indomethacin, amphotericin B, digoxin, cycloSPORINE, diuretics, quinolones

Increase: action of triamcinolone—salicylates, estrogens, indomethacin, oral contraceptives, ketoconazole, macrolide antiinfectives, carBAMazepine

Decrease: action of triamcinolone—cholestyramine, colestipol, barbiturates, rifAMPin, ePHEDrine, phenytoin, theophylline

Decrease: effects of anticoagulants, anticonvulsants, antidiabetics, ambenonium, neostigmine, isoniazid, toxoids, vaccines, anticholinesterases, salicylates, somatrem

Drug/Herb

• Hypokalemia: aloe, cascara, senna

Drug/Lab Test

Increase: cholesterol, sodium, blood glucose, uric acid, calcium, urine glucose

Decrease: calcium, potassium, T$_4$, T$_3$, thyroid ^{131}I uptake test, urine 17-OHCS, 17-KS, PBI

False negative: skin allergy tests

NURSING CONSIDERATIONS

Assess:

• Potassium, blood glucose, urine glucose while patient receiving long-term therapy; hypokalemia and hyperglycemia
• Weight daily; notify prescriber if weekly gain of >5 lb
• B/P, pulse; notify prescriber if chest pain occurs
• I&O ratio; be alert for decreasing urinary output, increasing edema
• Plasma cortisol levels during long-term therapy (normal level: 138-635 nmol/L SI units when drawn at 8 AM)
• **Infection:** increased temperature, WBC even after withdrawal of medication; product masks infection
• Potassium depletion: paresthesias, fatigue, nausea, vomiting, depression, polyuria, dysrhythmias, weakness
• Edema, hypertension, cardiac symptoms
• Mental status: affect, mood, behavioral changes, aggression
• Assistance with ambulation for patient with bone-tissue disease to prevent fractures
• **Beers:** avoid in older adults with delirium or at high risk for delirium; monitor for confusion, delirium
• **Pregnancy/breastfeeding:** use only if benefits outweigh fetal risk, cleft lip/palate

T

---

has occurred (1st trimester); cautious use in breastfeeding, excreted in breast milk

Evaluate:

• **Therapeutic response:** ease of respirations, decreased inflammation

Teach patient/family:

• That emergency ID as corticosteroid user should be carried; not to discontinue abruptly, taper dose

• To notify prescriber if therapeutic response decreases; that dosage adjustment may be needed

• To avoid OTC products: salicylates, alcohol in cough products, cold preparations unless directed by prescriber; to avoid live vaccines

• About cushingoid symptoms

• **About the symptoms of adrenal insufficiency:** nausea, anorexia, fatigue, dizziness, dyspnea, weakness, joint pain

---

triamcinolone nasal agent
See Appendix B

---

triamcinolone (topical)
(try-am-sin′oh-lone)
Kenalog, Sila III, Trianex, Triderm
Func. class.: Corticosteroid, topical

ACTION: Crosses cell membrane to attach to receptors to decrease inflammation, itching; inhibits multiple inflammatory cytokines

USES: Inflammation/itching in corticosteroid-responsive dermatoses on the skin or inflammation in the mouth

CONTRAINDICATIONS
Hypersensitivity, use on face or ear canal, infections
Precautions: Pregnancy, breastfeeding, children

DOSAGE AND ROUTES
• Apply to the affected areas bid-qid

Available forms: Aerosol 0.2 mg; paste (dental) 0.1%; lotion, cream, ointment 0.025%; ointment 0.05%; lotion, cream, ointment 0.1%; ointment, cream 0.5%

Administer:

Topical route

• May be used with occlusive dressings

• **Cream/ointment/lotion:** apply sparingly in a thin film and rub gently into the cleansed, slightly moist affected area; may use gloves to apply cream/ointment/lotion

• **Paste:** apply without rubbing, press into lesion until film develops

• **Spray:** spray a small amount of preparation onto the lesion

SIDE EFFECTS
ENDO: HPA axis suppression, Cushing's syndrome
INTEG: Burning, folliculitis, pruritus, dermatitis, hypopigmentation
META: Hyperglycemia; glycosuria

PHARMACOKINETICS
Absorption varies

INTERACTIONS
Increase: blood glucose

NURSING CONSIDERATIONS
Assess:
• Skin reactions: burning, pruritus, folliculitis, mouth lesions
Evaluate:
• Decreasing itching, inflammation on the skin, decreasing mouth lesions
Teach patient/family:
• How to use each product
• That long-term use may cause thinning skin, loss of fat tissue; avoid long-term use

---

triamcinolone (topical-oral) (Rx, OTC)
(trye-am-sin′oh-lone)
Kenalog in Orabase, Oralone Dental
Func. class.: Topical anesthetic
Chem. class.: Synthetic fluorinated adrenal corticosteroid

ACTION: Binds with steroid receptors, decreases inflammation

USES: Oral pain

CONTRAINDICATIONS
Hypersensitivity, application to large areas; presence of fungal, viral, or bacterial infections of mouth or throat
Precautions: Pregnancy, children <6 yr, sepsis, denuded skin, geriatric patients

DOSAGE AND ROUTES
• **Adult: TOP** Press ¼ inch into affected area until film appears, repeat bid-tid
Available forms: Paste 0.1%
Administer:
• After cleansing oral cavity after meals

SIDE EFFECTS
INTEG: Rash, irritation, sensitization

NURSING CONSIDERATIONS
Assess:
• Allergy: rash, irritation, reddening, swelling
• Infection: if affected area is infected, do not apply
Evaluate:
• **Therapeutic response:** absence of pain in affected area
Teach patient/family:
• To report rash, irritation, redness, swelling
• How to apply paste

---

triamterene (Rx)
(trye-am′ter-een)
Dyrenium
Func. class.: Antihypertensive, potassium-sparing diuretic

USES: Treatment of edema (CHF, cirrhosis of the liver, nephrotic syndrome, steroid-induced edema, idiopathic edema, edema due to secondary hyperaldosteronism)

CONTRAINDICATIONS
Hypersensitivity to triamterene or any component, anuria, severe renal/hepatic disease, hyperkalemia; use with other potassium-sparing products

Black Box Warning: Hyperkalemia

DOSAGE AND ROUTES
Edema
• **Adult: PO** 100 mg bid, titrate as needed; max 300 mg/day
Available forms: Capsules 50, 100 mg

---

triamterene/ hydrochlorothiazide (Rx)
(trye-am′ter-een/hye-droe-klor-oh-thye′a-zide)
Dyazide, Maxzide, Maxzide-25
Func. class.: Antihypertensive, potassium-sparing/thiazide diuretic

USES: Treatment of hypertension/edema (not initial treatment) when hypokalemia has developed on hydrochlorothiazide alone or when the development of hypokalemia must be avoided

CONTRAINDICATION
Hypersensitivity to hydrochlorothiazide, triamterene, sulfonamide-derived drugs, or any component, anuria; severe renal disease, use with potassium-sparing diuretics/potassium salt substitutes/potassium supplements, hyperkalemia

DOSAGE AND ROUTES
Hypertension/edema
• **Adult: PO** hydrochlorothiazide 25 mg/triamterene 37.5 mg: 1-2 tablets/capsules daily; hydrochlorothiazide 25 mg/triamterene 50 mg: 1-2 capsules daily; hydrochlorothiazide 50 mg/triamterene 75 mg: 1 tablet daily
Available forms: Capsules 37.5 mg/25 mg; tabs 37.5 mg/25 mg, 75 mg/50 mg

T

⚠ HIGH ALERT

triazolam (Rx)

(trye-ay′zoe-lam)

Halcion

Func. class.: Sedative-hypnotic, antianxiety

Chem. class.: Benzodiazepine, short acting

Controlled Substance Schedule IV (USA), Targeted (CDSA IV) (Canada)

Do not confuse:
Halcion/Haldol/halcinonide

ACTION: Produces CNS depression at limbic, thalamic, hypothalamic levels of CNS; may be mediated by neurotransmitter γ-aminobutyric acid (GABA); results in sedation, hypnosis, skeletal muscle relaxation, anticonvulsant activity, anxiolytic action

USES: Insomnia, sedative/hypnotic

CONTRAINDICATIONS

Pregnancy, breastfeeding, hypersensitivity to benzodiazepines

Precautions: Children <15 yr, geriatric patients, anemia, renal/hepatic disease, suicidal individuals, drug abuse, psychosis, acute closed-angle glaucoma, seizure disorders, angioedema, respiratory disease, depression, sleep-related behaviors (sleep walking), intermittent porphyria, myasthenia gravis, Parkinson's disease

Black Box Warning: Coadministration with other CNS depressants, respiratory depression, abrupt discontinuation, substance abuse

DOSAGE AND ROUTES

• **Adult: PO** 0.125-0.5 mg at bedtime, max 0.5 mg/day
• **Geriatric: PO** 0.0625-0.125 mg at bedtime, max 0.25 mg/day

Available forms: Tabs 0.125, 0.25 mg

Administer:

• After trying conservative measures for insomnia
• ½ hr before bedtime for sleeplessness
• On empty stomach for fast onset; may be taken with food if GI symptoms occur
• Avoid use with CNS depressants; serious CNS depression may result

SIDE EFFECTS

CNS: *Headache, lethargy, drowsiness, daytime sedation,* dizziness, confusion, light-headedness, anxiety, irritability, amnesia, poor coordination, complex sleep-related reactions: sleep driving, sleep eating

CV: Chest pain, pulse changes, ECG changes

GI: Nausea, vomiting, diarrhea, heartburn, abdominal pain, constipation

SYST: Severe allergic reactions

PHARMACOKINETICS

Onset 15-30 min, peak 1-2 hr, duration 6-8 hr, metabolized by liver, excreted by kidneys (inactive metabolites), crosses placenta, excreted in breast milk, half-life 1.5-5.5 hr

INTERACTIONS

• Smoking may decrease hypnotic effect

Increase: triazolam levels—CYP3A4 inhibitors (dilTIAZem, FLUoxetine, fluvoxaMINE, macrolides), protease inhibitors

Increase: effects of cimetidine, disulfiram, erythromycin, clarithromycin, probenecid, isoniazid, oral contraceptives; do not use concurrently

Black Box Warning: Increase: action of both products—alcohol, CNS depressants

Increase: triazolam levels—CYP2C19 inhibitors (fluconazole, ketoconazole, omeprazole, hormonal contraceptives, ticlopidine)

Decrease: triazolam levels—CYP3A4 inducers (carBAMazepine, phenobarbitol, phenytoin, rifamycins, valproate)

Decrease: effect of antacids, theophylline, rifAMPin

Drug/Herb

Increase: CNS depression—chamomile, hops, kava, lavender, valerian
Drug/Food
• Grapefruit may increase action; avoid concurrent use
Drug/Lab Test
Increase: ALT, AST, serum bilirubin
Decrease: RAI uptake
False increase: urinary 17-OHCS

NURSING CONSIDERATIONS
Assess:
• **Severe allergic reactions:** may occur during any use

Black Box Warning: Respiratory depression: may occur more frequently with coadministration of other CNS depressants; monitor respirations often

• **Mental status:** mood, sensorium, affect, memory (long, short term), insomnia, withdrawal symptoms, excessive sedation, impaired coordination
• Type of **sleep problem:** falling asleep, staying asleep
• **Safety:** Assistance with ambulation after receiving dose
• **Pregnancy/breastfeeding:** do not use in pregnancy; not recommended in breastfeeding
• **Beers:** avoid use in older adults; increased sensitivity to benzodiazepines and decreased metabolism; may cause or worsen delirium
Evaluate:
• **Therapeutic response:** ability to sleep at night, decreased amount of early morning awakening if taking product for insomnia
Teach patient/family:
• To use reliable contraception
• That dependence is possible after long-term use
• To avoid driving, other activities requiring alertness until product is stabilized

Black Box Warning: To avoid alcohol ingestion, sedatives, hypnotics

• That effects may take 2 nights for benefits to be noticed; that product is for short-term use only; to use for 7-10 continuous nights
• About alternative measures to improve sleep: reading, exercise several hours before bedtime, warm bath, warm milk, TV, self-hypnosis, deep breathing
• That complex sleep-related behaviors (sleep eating/driving) may occur
• That hangover is common in geriatric patients but less common than with barbiturates; that rebound insomnia may occur for 1-2 nights after discontinuing product; to discontinue by decreasing dose by 50% q2nights until 0.125 mg for 2 nights, then stop

TREATMENT OF OVERDOSE:
Lavage; monitor electrolytes, VS, flumazenil

triclabendazole (Rx)
(try-KLUH-bend-uh-zole)
Egaten
Func. class.: Anthelmintic

USES: Treatment of fascioliasis in children ≥6 yr

CONTRAINDICATIONS
Hypersensitivity to triclabendazole, other benzimidazoles, or any component

DOSAGE AND ROUTES
Fascioliasis
• **Child ≥6 yr: PO**
10 mg/kg q12hr × 2 doses
Available forms: Tabs 250 mg

trifarotene (Rx)
Aklief
Func. class.: Antiacne agent

USES: Acne vulgaris

DOSAGE AND ROUTES
• **Adult/child ≥9 yr: Topical** apply a layer to affected areas of face or torso daily in the evening

Available forms: Cream 0.005%

---

trifluridine ophthalmic
See Appendix B

> **⚠ HIGH ALERT**

trifluridine/tipiracil (Rx)
(trye-flure′i-deen/tye-pir′a-sil)
Lonsurf
Func. class.: Antineoplastic, antimetabolite

USES: Treatment of metastatic colorectal cancer in those previously treated with fluoropyrimidine/oxaliplatin/irinotecan, an anti-VEGF, and if RAS wild-type, an anti-EGFR; treatment of metastatic gastric/gastroesophageal junction adenocarcinoma in those previously treated with ≥ prior regimens of chemotherapy, with fluoropyrimidine/platinum/either a taxane/irinotecan, and HER2/neu-targeted therapy if needed

CONTRAINDICATIONS
Hypersensitivity

DOSAGE AND ROUTES
Metastatic colorectal cancer/metastatic gastric cancer
• **Adult: PO** 35 mg/m^2 (based on trifluridine component) bid on days 1-5 and 8-12 of a 28-day cycle, max per dose: trifluridine 80 mg; continue until disease progression or unacceptable toxicity
Available forms: Tabs 15 mg/16.4 mg; 20 mg/8.19 mg

---

trimethobenzamide (Rx)
(trye-meth-oh-ben′za-mide)
Tigan
Func. class.: Antiemetic, anticholinergic
Chem. class.: Ethanolamine derivative

USES: Nausea, vomiting

CONTRAINDICATIONS
Children (parenterally), hypersensitivity to opioids, shock

DOSAGE AND ROUTES
Nausea/vomiting
• **Adult: IM** 200 mg 3-4×/day; **PO** 300 mg 3-4×/day
Postoperative
• **Adult: IM** 200 mg followed by 2nd dose 1 hr later
Renal dose
• **Adult: IM** CCr 15-30 mL/min, give 50% of dose

Available forms: Capsules 300 mg; injection 100 mg/mL

---

trospium (Rx)
(trose′pee-um)
Trosec ✦
Func. class.: Anticholinergic, urinary antispasmodic
Chem. class.: Muscarinic receptor antagonist

ACTION: Relaxes smooth muscles in bladder by inhibiting acetylcholine effect on muscarinic receptors

USES: Overactive bladder (urinary frequency, urgency)

CONTRAINDICATIONS
Hypersensitivity, uncontrolled closed-angle glaucoma, urinary retention, gastric retention, myasthenia gravis
Precautions: Pregnancy, breastfeeding, children, geriatric patients, renal/hepatic disease, controlled closed-angle glaucoma, ulcerative colitis, intestinal atony, bladder outflow obstruction

DOSAGE AND ROUTES
• **Adult <75 yr: PO** 20 mg bid 1 hr before meals or on empty stomach; **EXT REL** 60 mg in AM

• **Geriatric ≥75 yr:** PO titrate down to 20 mg/day based on response and tolerance

Renal dose

• **Adult:** PO CCr <30 mL/min, 20 mg/day at bedtime, ext rel product not recommended

Available forms: Tabs 20 mg; caps ext rel 60 mg

Administer:

• 1 hr before meals or on empty stomach (reg rel); in AM (ext rel) ≥1 hr before meal

SIDE EFFECTS

CNS: Fatigue, dizziness, headache, confusion

CV: Tachycardia

EENT: Dry eyes, vision abnormalities

GI: Flatulence, abdominal pain, *constipation, dry mouth,* dyspepsia

GU: Urinary retention, UTI

INTEG: Dry skin, angioedema

MISC: Heat stroke, fever

PHARMACOKINETICS

Rapidly absorbed (10%); peak 5-6 hr; protein bound (50%-85%); extensively metabolized; excreted in urine, feces; excreted in urine by active tubular secretion; half-life 20 hr

INTERACTIONS

Increase: drowsiness—CNS depressants, alcohol

Increase or decrease: trospium effect—products excreted by active renal secretion (aMILoride, digoxin, morphine), metFORMIN, quiNIDine, procainamide, raNITIdine, tenofovir, triamterene, vancomycin

Drug/Food

Decrease: absorption—high-fat meal

NURSING CONSIDERATIONS

Assess:

• **Urinary patterns:** I&O ratio, CCr baseline and periodically, post-void residual distention, nocturia, frequency, urgency, incontinence, voiding patterns

• **Pregnancy/breastfeeding:** use only if benefits outweigh fetal risk; cautious use in breastfeeding, excreted in breast milk

• **Beers:** avoid in older adults with delirium or at high risk for delirium

Evaluate:

• **Therapeutic response:** correction of urinary status: absence of dysuria, frequency, nocturia, incontinence

Teach patient/family:

• To avoid hazardous activities because dizziness may occur

• That alcohol may increase drowsiness

• About anticholinergic effects that may occur

• That overheating may occur with strenuous exercise

• To avoid all other products unless approved by prescriber

• To use hard candy for dry mouth (most common side effect)

⚠ HIGH ALERT

tucatinib (Rx)

(too-ka′ti-nib)

Tukysa

Func. class.: Antineoplastic

USES: Breast cancer, human epidermal growth factor receptor 2 positive, advanced unresectable/metastatic

CONTRAINDICATIONS

Hypersensitivity, pregnancy, breastfeeding

DOSAGE AND ROUTES

• **Adult:** PO 300 mg bid with trastuzumab and capecitabine until disease progression or unacceptable toxicity

Available forms: Tablet 50, 150 mg

ubrogepant (Rx)

Ubrelvy

Func. class.: Calcitonin gene–related peptide (CGRP) receptor antagonist

USES: Acute migraine

CONTRAINDICATIONS
Hypersensitivity, strong CYP3A4 inhibitors

DOSAGE AND ROUTES
• **Adult: PO** 50 or 100 mg; if needed, may take second dose at least 2 hr after initial dose; max: 200 mg/24 hr; safety of treating more than 8 migraines in a 30-day period has not been established
Available forms: Tablet 50-100 mg

uliprista (Rx)

(ue-li-pris′tal)

Ella, Fibristal ♣

Func. class.: Contraceptive, progestin receptor modulator

USES:
Emergency contraception (ella): Prevention of pregnancy following unprotected intercourse or contraceptive failure
Uterine fibroids (Fibristal ♣): Treatment of moderate-severe signs/symptoms of uterine fibroids in those who are eligible for surgery; intermittent treatment of moderate-severe signs/symptoms of uterine fibroids

CONTRAINDICATIONS
Hypersensitivity, pregnancy

DOSAGE AND ROUTES
Emergency contraception (ella)
• **Adult women: PO:** 30 mg ASAP, but within 120 hr (5 days) of unprotected intercourse/contraceptive failure
Uterine fibroids (Fibristal ♣)
• **Adult women PO: (premenopausal):** 5 mg daily × 3, first course within the first 7 days of menstruation; start subsequent treatment courses, the 1st week of the 2nd

menstruation following completion of the prior course. The interval between courses is 2 menstrual cycles
Available forms: Tablet 30 mg

undecylenic acid topical
See Appendix B

unoprostone ophthalmic
See Appendix B

upadacitinib (Rx)

(Ue-pad′a-sye′ti-nib)

Rinvoq

Func. class.: Immunomodulating agent
Chem. class.: Janus associated kinase (JAK) inhibitor

ACTION: Oral JAK inhibitor; Janus kinase, a tyrosine kinase enzyme that transmits signals arising from cytokine or growth factor–receptor interactions on the cellular membrane to influence cellular processes of immune cell function and hematopoiesis

USES: Treatment of rheumatoid arthritis

CONTRAINDICATIONS
Hypersensitivity
Precautions: AIDS, anemia, breastfeeding, children, contraception requirements, corticosteroid use, diverticulitis, geriatrics, GI perforation, hepatic disease, hepatitis B exacerbation, herpes, HIV, neutropenia, pregnancy, pregnancy testing, vaccination

Black Box Warning: Infection, new primary malignancy, thrombosis, mortality, stroke

DOSAGE AND ROUTES
• **Adults: PO** 15 mg daily with or without methotrexate or other nonbiologic DMARDs

Available forms: Extended release tablet 15, 30, 45 mg
Administer:
• Give with or without food
• Swallow whole; do not split, crush, or chew

NURSING CONSIDERATIONS
Assess:
• **RA:** pain; stiffness; ROM; swelling of joints before, during treatment
• Infections (fever, flulike symptoms, dyspnea, change in urination, redness/swelling around any wounds)—stop treatment if present

Black Box Warning: Some serious infections including sepsis may occur, may be fatal; patients with active infections should not be started on this product

Black Box Warning: **Thrombosis (DVT, PE, arterial thrombosis):** Assess for symptoms and treat immediately, some have been fatal

May reactivate hepatitis B in chronic carriers; may be fatal

Black Box Warning: **Identify** latent TB before therapy; treat before starting this product

Blood dyscrasias: CBC, differential periodically

Black Box Warning: Assess for neoplastic disease (lymphomas/leukemia) monitor for these and skin cancer

• **Pregnancy/breastfeeding:** use only if clearly needed, no well-controlled studies; cautious use in breastfeeding, excreted in breast milk
Evaluate:
• **Therapeutic response:** decreased inflammation, pain in joints, decreased joint destruction

Teach patient/family:
• Not to take any live virus vaccines during treatment
• To report signs of infection, TB immediately

uridine (Rx)
(ure'i-deen)
Vistogard, Xuriden
Func. class.: Antidote

USES: Fluorouracil/capecitabine overdosage/toxicity; hereditary orotic aciduria

DOSAGE AND ROUTES
Fluorouracil/capecitabine overdosage or toxicity
• **Adult PO:** 10 g q6hr × 20 doses
• **Child PO:** 6.2 g/m^2 (max 10 g/dose) q6hr × 20 doses
Hereditary orotic aciduria
• **Adult PO:** 60 mg/kg daily; maintenance increase to 120 mg/kg daily
Available forms: Oral granules 2, 10 g packet

ustekinumab (Rx)
(us'te-kin'ue-mab)
Stelara
Func. class.: Immune response modifier, antipsoriatic agent
Chem. class.: Monoclonal antibody, interleukin-12 inhibitor

ACTION: Interleukin (IL)-12, IL-23 antagonist, binds to an interleukin protein, decreases inflammation

USES: Plaque psoriasis (adult/child), psoriatic arthritis

CONTRAINDICATIONS
Hypersensitivity, sepsis, active infections
Precautions: Pregnancy, breastfeeding, children ≤18 yr, geriatric patients, surgery, TB, diabetes mellitus, immunosuppression

DOSAGE AND ROUTES
Moderate to severe plaque psoriasis
• **Adult ≥100 kg with plaque psoriasis:** SUBCUT 90 mg, repeat in 4 wk, then 90 mg q12wk starting wk 16
• **Adult <100 kg SUBCUT** 45 mg, repeat in 4 wk, then 45 mg q12wk starting wk 16

U

- **Child 6-17 yr, >100 kg: SUBCUT** 90 mg, repeat in 4 wk, then q12wk
- **Child 6-17 yr, 60-100 kg: SUBCUT** 45 mg, repeat in 4 wk, then q12wk
- **Child 6-17 yr, <60 kg: SUBCUT** 0.75 mg/kg repeat in 4 wk, then q12wk

Crohn's disease/ulcerative colitis
- **Adult (weight-based dosing): IV** single induction dose **>85 kg,** 520 mg; **>55–85 kg,** 390 mg; **≤55 kg,** 260 mg; **maintenance:** 90 mg **SUBCUT** q8wk, starting 8 wk after induction dose

Available forms: Solutions for inj 45 mg/0.5 mL, 90 mg/mL, 130/25 mL

Administer:
- Do not shake the syringe or vial
- Visually inspect for particulate matter and discoloration before use; solution should be colorless to slightly yellow and may contain a few small translucent or white particles. Do not use if discolored, cloudy, or if foreign particulate matter is present

IV route
- **Preparation:** use an IV infusion only for the induction treatment of Crohn's disease
- Each vial is for single use only
- Calculate the dose and number of vials needed based on patient weight; each 26-mL vial contains 130 mg of product
- Withdraw and discard a volume of the 0.9% sodium chloride injection from a 250-mL infusion bag equal to the volume of needed product to be added
- Withdraw 26 mL of product from each vial needed and add it to 250-mL infusion bag. The final volume in the infusion bag should be 250 mL
- Gently mix; do not shake
- **Storage:** diluted solution must be used within 4 hr (no preservative). If administration is not immediate, store for up to 4 hr at room temperature up to 25° C (77° F). Do not freeze; discard unused portion

IV infusion route
- Give the diluted product over ≥1 hr
- Use only an infusion set with an in-line, sterile, nonpyrogenic, low protein-binding filter (pore size 0.2 micron)
- Do not infuse in the same line with other agents

SUBCUT route The first injection needs to be under the supervision of a qualified health care professional
- Inject in the front part of the middle thigh, the gluteal or abdominal region, and the outer area of the upper arm
- Do not give where skin is tender, bruised, red, or indurated
- Rotate injection sites. If a second injection is needed because two 45-mg vials or prefilled syringes are used for a 90-mg dose, repeat the injection process, and use a different injection site
- For the vial, use a 27-gauge, 0.5-inch needle to withdraw the dose
- The needle cover of the prefilled syringe contains latex. Persons allergic to natural rubber or latex should not handle the cover of the prefilled syringe

SIDE EFFECTS
CNS: Headache, leukoencephalopathy, depression, dizziness, fatigue
HEMA: Bleeding
INTEG: *Injection site reaction,* pruritus, skin irritation, erythema, exfoliative dermatitis, erythrodermic psoriasis
SYST: Serious infections, malignancies
MS: Myalgia, back pain
RESP: URI, oropharyngeal pain

PHARMACOKINETICS
Maximum serum concentration: 13.5 days after a single 45-mg subcut dose, 7 days after a single 90-mg subcut dose; half-life 14.9-45.6 days

INTERACTIONS
- Do not give concurrently with vaccines; immunizations should be brought up-to-date before treatment
- Avoid use with immunosuppressives

NURSING CONSIDERATIONS
Assess:
- Bring immunizations up-to-date before starting treatment; do not administer live vaccines during treatment and for 3 mo after treatment ends
- **Infection:** monitor for fever, sore throat, cough; do not use during active infections

---

• **Malignancy:** skin cancer may occur, especially in older patients who have used ultraviolet treatments with immunosuppressants

• **TB:** TB testing should be done before starting treatment

• For inj-site pain, swelling, rash

• **Pregnancy/breastfeeding:** pregnant patients should enroll in the Stelara pregnancy registry, 877-311-8972; use only if benefits outweigh fetal risk; cautious use in breastfeeding, excretion unknown

Evaluate:
• **Therapeutic response:** decreased plaque psoriasis

Teach patient/family:
• That product must be continued for prescribed time to be effective; to use as prescribed

• Not to receive live vaccinations during treatment

• To notify prescriber of possible infection (upper respiratory or other) or allergic reactions

• Injection techniques and disposal of equipment; not to reuse needles, syringes

• That follow-up will be needed

U

valACYclovir (Rx)
(val-a-sye′kloh-vir)
Valtrex
Func. class.: Antiviral
Chem. class.: Synthetic purine
nucleoside analog

Do not confuse:
valACYclovir/valGANciclovir/acyclovir
Valtrex/Valcyte

ACTION: Interferes with DNA synthesis
by conversion to acyclovir, thereby causing
decreased viral replication, time of lesional
healing

USES: Treatment or suppression of
herpes zoster (shingles), genital herpes,
herpes labialis (cold sores), varicella,
varicella zoster

CONTRAINDICATIONS
Hypersensitivity to this product or acyclovir, valGANciclovir
Precautions: Pregnancy, breastfeeding,
geriatric patients, hepatic/renal disease,
electrolyte imbalance, dehydration, penciclovir, famciclovir, ganciclovir, hypersensitivity, varicella

DOSAGE AND ROUTES
Herpes zoster (shingles)
• **Adult: PO** 1 g tid × 1 wk start within
48 hr of rash onset
Genital herpes (suppressive, initial)
• **Adult: PO** 1 g bid × 10 days initially
start at earliest sign or recurrence
Genital herpes (recurrent episodes)
• **Adult: PO** 500 mg bid × 3 days start at
earliest sign or recurrence
**Genital herpes (suppressive
therapy), long term**
• **Adult: PO** 1 g/day with **normal im-
mune function;** 500 mg/day for those with
≤9 recurrences/yr; 500 mg bid for **HIV-
infected patients with CD4 count ≥100**
Reduction of transmission
• **Adult: PO** 500 mg/day for source
partner up to 20 mo

Herpes labialis
• **Adult/child ≥12 yr: PO** 2 g bid × 1 day
at first sign of lesions
Varicella (chickenpox)
• **Adolescent and child ≥2 yr: PO** 20 mg/
kg/dose tid × 5 days, max 3 g/day
Renal dose
• **Adult: PO** CCr 30-49 mL/min, 1 g q12hr
(for regimens 1 g q8hr); 1 g q12hr × 1
day **(herpes labialis);** CCr 10-29 mL/min,
1 g q24hr **(genital herpes/herpes zoster);** 500 mg q24hr **(recurrent genital
herpes);** CCr <10 mL/min, 500 mg q24hr
(genital herpes/herpes zoster), 500 mg
q24hr **(recurrent genital herpes)**
Available forms: Tabs 500 mg, 1 g
Administer:
• As soon as possible (herpes labialis,
genital herpes); within 24 hr of rash
(varicella)
• Within 72 hr of outbreak (herpes
zoster), within 24 hr (chickenpox)
• Without regard to food
• Caps may be made into susp by pharmacy
• Store at room temperature; protect
from light, moisture

SIDE EFFECTS
CNS: Tremors, lethargy, *dizziness,
headache,* weakness, depression, hallu-
cinations, seizures, encephalopathy
GU: Crystalluria, renal failure
ENDO: *Dysmenorrhea*
GI: *Nausea,* vomiting, diarrhea, abdomi-
nal pain, constipation, *increased AST*
HEMA: Thrombocytopenic purpura,
hemolytic uremic syndrome
INTEG: *Rash*
MISC: Dehydration

PHARMACOKINETICS
Onset unknown, Peak 1.5-2.5 hr, duration up to 24 hr; half-life 2½-3½ hr;
converted to acyclovir in intestine, liver,
crosses placenta, enters breast milk;
excreted in urine primarily as acyclovir;
protein binding 13.5%-17.9%

INTERACTIONS
Increase: blood levels of valACYclovir—
cimetidine, probenecid; only significant
with renal disease

Drug/Lab Test
Increase: LFTs, creatinine
Decrease: WBC, platelets

NURSING CONSIDERATIONS
Assess:
• **Infection:** characteristics of lesions; therapy should be started at 1st sign or symptom of herpes; most effective within 72 hr of outbreak; C&S prior to product therapy; product may be taken as soon as culture is taken; repeat C&S after treatment; determine presence of other sexually transmitted diseases
• Thrombocytopenic purpura, hemolytic uremic syndrome; may be fatal
• **CNS/psychological status:** assess cognition, sleep patterns, mood affect; if seizures, encephalopathy occur, discontinue
• **Renal studies:** I&O, BUN/creatinine, GFR; hemolytic uremic syndrome (decreased output, fatigue, pallor) may occur in transplants (renal, bone marrow) or advanced HIV, hemodialysis may be used in renal failure
• Bowel pattern before, during treatment
• Skin eruptions: rash
• Allergies before treatment, reaction to each medication
• **Pregnancy/breastfeeding:** use only if benefits outweigh fetal risk; cautious use in breastfeeding, excreted in breast milk
Evaluate:
• **Therapeutic response:** absence of itching, painful lesions; crusting and healed lesions
Teach patient/family:
• To take as prescribed; if dose is missed, to take as soon as remembered up to 2 hr before next dose; not to double dose; to take without regard to meals
• That product may be taken orally before infection occurs; that product should be taken when itching or pain occurs, usually before eruptions
• To discuss all Rx, OTC, herbal supplements taken with health care professional
• That adequate hydration is needed to prevent crystalluria
• That partners need to be told that patient has herpes, they can become infected; that condoms must be worn to prevent reinfections
• That product does not cure infection, just controls symptoms; that product does not prevent infection of others

• To report CNS changes (tremors, weakness, lethargy, hallucinations, seizures) immediately
• **Pregnancy/breastfeeding:** Identify if pregnancy is planned or suspected or if breastfeeding

valbenazine (Rx)
(val-ben′-a-zeen)
Ingrezza
Func. class.: CNS agent; monoamine depletor

USES: For the treatment of tardive dyskinesia

DOSAGE AND ROUTES
Tardive dyskinesia
• **Adult: PO** Initially, 40 mg daily; after 1 wk, increase to 80 mg daily
Hepatic dose
• **Adult: Child-Pugh 7-15 or with CYP3A4 inhibitor (strong): PO** give 40 mg/day
Available forms:
Capsules 40, 60, 80 mg; capsule titration pack

valGANciclovir (Rx)
(val-gan-sy′kloh-veer)
Valcyte
Func. class.: Antiviral
Chem. class.: Synthetic nucleoside

Do not confuse:
valGANciclovir/valACYclovir
Valcyte/Valtrex

ACTION: Metabolized to ganciclovir; inhibits replication of human cytomegalovirus by selective inhibition of viral DNA synthesis

USES: Cytomegalovirus (CMV) retinitis in immunocompromised persons, including those with AIDS, after indirect ophthalmoscopy confirms diagnosis; prevention of CMV with transplantation; prevention of CMV in at-risk patient going through transplant (kidney, heart, pancreas)

CONTRAINDICATIONS
Breastfeeding, hypersensitivity to ganciclovir, valACYclovir; absolute neutrophil count <500/mm³; platelet count <25,000/mm³; hemodialysis; liver transplantation

Precautions: Children, geriatric patients, renal function impairment; hypersensitivity to acyclovir, penciclovir, famciclovir

Black Box Warning: Preexisting cytopenias, new primary malignancy, infertility, anemia, pregnancy

DOSAGE AND ROUTES
Treatment of CMV
• **Adult and adolescent: PO** 900 mg bid × 14-21 days with food; maintenance 900 mg/day with food

Transplant (CMV prophylaxis)
• **Adult/adolescent >16 yr: PO** 900 mg/day with food starting 10 days before transplantation until day 100 after transplantation (kidney/pancreas/heart); continue for 200 days (kidney)
• **Infant ≥4 mo/child/adolescent ≤16 yr: PO** give within 10 days of heart/kidney transplant; calculate dose as 7 × BSA × CCr, give as single daily dose

Renal dose
• **Adult: PO** CCr ≥60 mL/min, same as above; CCr 40-59 mL/min, 450 mg bid for 21 days, then 450 mg/day; CCr 25-39 mL/min, 450 mg/day, then 450 mg q2days; CCr 10-24 mL/min, 450 mg q2days, then 450 mg 2×/wk

Available forms: Tabs 450 mg, powder for oral sol 50 mg/mL

Administer:
• Do not get powder on skin, or handle broken tablets; potential carcinogen

PO tab
• With food for better absorption; avoid getting product on skin, wash hands if contact with skin; do not break, crush, or chew

Oral solution
• Oral with food
• Measure 9 mL purified water in graduated cylinder, shake bottle to loosen powder, add 1/2 liquid, shake well, add remaining water, shake; remove child-resistant cap and push bottle adapter into neck of bottle, close with cap, give using dispenser provided
• Store liquid in refrigerator; do not freeze; throw away any unused after 49 days

SIDE EFFECTS
CNS: *Fever,* chills, *confusion,* dizziness, *headache, insomnia,* psychosis, tremors, *paresthesia, weakness,* seizures
EENT: Retinal detachment with CMV retinitis
GI: *Nausea, vomiting, anorexia, diarrhea, abdominal pain*
GU: Hematuria, increased creatinine, BUN
HEMA: Thrombocytopenia, irreversible neutropenia, anemia, pancytopenia
INTEG: *Rash,* alopecia, *pruritus,* urticaria, pain at site, phlebitis, Stevens-Johnson syndrome
MISC: Local and systemic infections, sepsis

PHARMACOKINETICS
60% absorbed in GI tract, peak 1-3 hr, duration up to 24 hr. Metabolized to ganciclovir, which has a half-life of 3-4 1/2 hr; excreted by kidneys (unchanged); crosses blood-brain barrier, CSF

INTERACTIONS
Increase: Severe granulocytopenia: immunosuppressants, zidovudine, antineoplastics, radiation; do not use together
Increase: toxicity—dapsone, pentamidine, flucytosine, vinCRIStine, vinBLAStine, adriamycin, DOXOrubicin, amphotericin B, trimethoprim-sulfamethoxazole combinations or other nucleoside analogs, cycloSPORINE
Increase: effect of both drugs—mycophenolate
Increase: seizures—imipenem-cilastatin
Increase: effect of didanosine; monitor for adverse effects, toxicity
Decrease: renal clearance of valGANciclovir—probenecid

Drug/Food
Increase: absorption—high-fat meal

Drug/Lab Test
Increase: creatinine, BUN
Decrease: RBC/WBC, Hct/HB

NURSING CONSIDERATIONS
Assess:
• **CMV retinitis:** determine diagnosis by ophthalmoscopy before beginning treatment, culture may be used, negative results do not confirm that CMV retinitis is not present, use ophthalmoscopy q2wk during treatment

Black Box Warning: Leukopenia/ neutropenia/thrombocytopenia: WBCs, platelets q2days during 2×/day dosing, then q1wk, do not use if ANC <500 mm³, platelets <25,000/mm³, HB <8 g/ dL; leukopenia with daily WBC count in patients with prior leukopenia with other nucleoside analogs or for whom leukopenia counts are <1000 cells/mm³ at start of treatment

Black Box Warning: Malignancy: monitor for malignancy, avoid accidental exposure of broken, crushed tabs, powder; if these come in contact with skin, wash with soap and water

• Monitor serum creatinine or CCr, BUN ≥q2wk, I&O, and increase in fluid intake

Black Box Warning: Pregnancy/breastfeeding: Considered potentially teratogenic; adequate contraception should be used; do not breastfeed, obtain pregnancy test in those of childbearing potential prior to use

Evaluate:
• **Therapeutic response:** decreased symptoms of CMV
Teach patient/family:
• That product does not cure condition; that regular ophthalmologic q1mo and blood tests are necessary
• That major toxicities may necessitate discontinuing product
• To take with food, avoid high-fat meals

• **Blood dyscrasias:** bruising, bleeding, petechiae; seizures, dizziness; to avoid driving, hazardous activities
• To use sunscreen to prevent burns

Black Box Warning: Pregnancy/breastfeeding: To use contraception during treatment; that infertility may occur; that men should use barrier contraception for 90 days after treatment; not to breastfeed

valproate (Rx)
(val′proh-ate)
valproic acid (Rx)
(val′proh-ik)
divalproex sodium (Rx)
(dye-val′proh-ex)
Depakote, Depakote ER, Depakote Sprinkle, Epival ✦
Func. class.: Anticonvulsant, vascular headache suppressant
Chem. class.: Carboxylic acid derivative

ACTION: Increases levels of γ-aminobutyric acid (GABA) in the brain, which decreases seizure activity

USES: Simple (petit mal), complex (petit mal), absence, mixed seizures; manic episodes associated with bipolar disorder, prophylaxis of migraine, adjunct for schizophrenia, tardive dyskinesia, aggression in children with ADHD, organic brain syndrome, mania, migraines; tonic-clonic (grand mal), myoclonic seizures

CONTRAINDICATIONS
Hypersensitivity, urea cycle disorders, mitochondrial disease, hepatic disease
Precautions: Breastfeeding, geriatric patients, abrupt discontinuation, carnitine deficiency, coagulopathy, depression, diarrhea, encephalopathy, head trauma, organic brain syndrome, HIV, renal disease, suicidal ideation, surgery, thrombocytopenia

V

Black Box Warning: Children <2 yr, contraception requirements, hepatotoxicity, pancreatitis, pregnancy

DOSAGE AND ROUTES
Simple/absence seizures
• **Geriatrics: PO** Start at lower dose, titrate upward
• **Adult/adolescent/child ≥2 yr: PO/IV** Initially, 10-15 mg/kg/day; increase by 5-10 mg/kg/day weekly, max 60 mg/kg/day
Complex partial seizures
• **Adult/child ≥10 yr: PO/IV** 10-15 mg/kg/day, then increase by 5-10 mg/kg/day qwk, max 60 mg/kg/day

Acute mania
• **Adult: PO (delayed-release divalproex).** Initially, 750 mg/day in divided doses, then increase to the lowest effective dose, max 60 mg/kg/day; **PO (extended-release divalproex).** Initially, 25 mg/kg/day, to achieve the desired clinical effect, max 60 mg/kg/day

For migraine prophylaxis
• **Adult ≤65 yr: PO (delayed-release divalproex).** Initially, 250 mg bid, titrate as needed up to a max 500 mg bid; **PO (extended-release divalproex);** initially, 500 mg/day × 1 wk, then increasing to 1000 mg/day, max 1000 mg/day

Available forms: *Valproate:* inj 100 mg/mL; *valproic acid:* caps 250 mg; syrup 250 mg/5 mL; *divalproex:* del rel tabs 125, 250, 500 mg; ext rel tabs 250, 500 mg; sprinkle cap del rel 125 mg

Administer:
PO route
• Use safe handling procedures
• Do not confuse different forms
• Swallow tabs or caps whole; do not break, crush, or chew ext rel or del rel tabs
• Sprinkle cap contents on food or swallowed whole
• **Syrup:** Do not dilute with carbonated beverage; do not give syrup to patients with sodium restrictions, shake before use
• Give with food or milk to decrease GI symptoms
• Conversion from Depakote to Depakote ER, the ER product should be higher than immediate release

• Do not discontinue abruptly
• Give missed dose as soon as possible unless close to next dosing time
IV Infusion route
• Dilute dose with ≥50 mL D₅W, NS, LR (2 mg/mL)
• Run over 60 min (20 mg/min)
• Draw drug level, monitor, adjust dose as needed
• Use in those that cannot use PO

• **Y-site compatibilities:** cefepime, ceftazadime, cloxacillin, naloxone

SIDE EFFECTS
CNS: *Sedation, drowsiness,* dizziness, headache, depression, behavioral changes, tremors, aggression, weakness, coma, suicidal ideation, hypothermia
CV: Peripheral edema
EENT: Visual disturbances, taste perversion
GI: *Nausea, vomiting, constipation, diarrhea, dyspepsia,* anorexia, pancreatitis, stomatitis, weight gain, dry mouth, hepatotoxicity
HEMA: Thrombocytopenia, leukopenia
INTEG: *Rash,* alopecia, photosensitivity, dry skin, DRESS
META: Hyperammonemia, SIADH

PHARMACOKINETICS
Absorption complete (IV) well (PO); distribution widely, crosses blood-brain barrier. Metabolized by liver; excreted by kidneys, in breast milk; crosses placenta; half-life 6-16 hr; 90% protein binding; **PO:** Peak 4 hr (regular rel); 4-17 hr (ext rel)

INTERACTIONS
Increase: valproic acid toxicity level—erythromycin, felbamate, salicylates, NSAIDs, rifampin, carBAMazepine, cimetidine, monitor levels
Increase: CNS depression—alcohol, antidepressants, benzodiazepines, opioids, barbiturates, antihistamines, MAOIs, sedative/hypnotics, avoid concurrent use
Increase: action of, possible toxicity—phenytoin, carBAMazepine, ethosuximide, barbiturates, zidovudine, LORazepam, rufinamide, lamoTRIgine, assess for toxicity
Increase: bleeding—warfarin, monitor PT/INR
Decrease: valproate levels—carBAMazepine, cholestyramine, estrogen, hormonal contraceptives, carbapenem antibiotics

Drug/Lab Test
Increase: LFTs, bleeding time
Decrease: blood counts
False positive: ketones, urine
Interference: thyroid function tests
Increase: LFTs, bleeding time, ammonia
Decrease: sodium

NURSING CONSIDERATIONS
Assess:
• **Seizure disorder:** location, aura, activity, duration; seizure precautions should be in place
• **Mental status:** bipolar disorder: mood, activity, sleeping/eating, behavior; suicidal thoughts/behaviors
• **Migraines:** frequency, intensity, alleviating factors
• Blood studies: Hct, HB, RBC, serum folate, PT/PTT, serum ammonia, platelets, vit D if patient receiving long-term therapy, thrombocytopenia may occur at higher doses

Black Box Warning: Hepatotoxicity: AST, ALT, bilirubin, ammonia baseline and periodically during 6 mo or more, discontinue if hyperammonemia occurs; hepatic failure has occurred; monitor for fever, anorexia, vomiting, lethargy; jaundice of skin, eyes that may occur during treatment; those with organic brain disorders, mental retardation, children <2 yr are at greater risk, those with mitochondrial disease (contraindicated)

• **DRESS:** eosinophilia, changes in lab work, fever, rash, lymphadenopathy if present and condition confirmed, discontinue immediately, do not restart
• **Suicidal thoughts/behaviors:** usually occurs during beginning of therapy, limit amount of product that is given to the patient, assess for increasing suicidal thoughts, behaviors, anxiety, restlessness, hostility may proceed destructive behaviors
• **Hyperammonemic encephalopathy:** can be fatal in those with urea cycle disorders (UCD); lethargy, confusion, coma, CV, respiratory changes; discontinue
• **Trough/peak:** serum blood levels: therapeutic level 50-125 mcg/mL

Black Box Warning: Pancreatitis: may be fatal; report immediately nausea, vomiting, anorexia, abdominal pain; may occur anytime during treatment or for several months/years after discontinuing treatment, check risk factors before starting

• **Beers:** avoid in older adults unless safer alternative is unavailable; ataxia, impaired psychomotor function may occur

Black Box Warning: Pregnancy/breastfeeding: do not use in pregnancy (migraine prophylaxis), use only in pregnancy (epilepsy, manic episodes) if other alternatives are unavailable; major malformations may occur; enroll pregnant patients in the North American Antiepileptic Drug Pregnancy Registry, 888-233-2334; cautious use in breastfeeding, excreted in breast milk, male infertility may occur

Evaluate:
• **Therapeutic response:** decreased seizures
Teach patient/family:
• To avoid driving, other activities that require alertness
• To drink plenty of fluids
• To discuss all OTC, Rx, herbals, supplements taken with health care professional
• Not to discontinue medication quickly after long-term use, seizures may result; to take as directed; not to skip, double doses; not to chew capsules; to take with milk for GI upset
• That syrup may be mixed with fluids that are not carbonated; sprinkle cap can be opened and sprinkled on applesauce or soft food, and swallowed

Black Box Warning: To report visual disturbances, rash, diarrhea, abdominal pain, light-colored stools, jaundice, protracted vomiting, weakness to prescriber

• **DRESS:** to report fever, swelling of lymph glands, rash
• **Hepatotoxicity:** to report immediately, anorexia, nausea, vomiting, abdominal pain, fever

Side effects: *italics* = common; red = life-threatening

• That continuing follow-up exams and blood work will be needed
• To carry an emergency ID with condition, medications taken
• **Overdose symptoms:** Heart block, coma

Black Box Warning: Pancreatitis: to report immediately; may be fatal, abdominal pain, nausea, vomiting, anorexia

• To report immediately suicidal thoughts/behaviors, increased depression, changes in mood, anxiety, hostility

Black Box Warning: Pregnancy/breastfeeding: To use contraception while taking this product; to notify prescriber if pregnancy is planned or suspected

valsartan (Rx)

(val′sahr-tan)

Diovan

Func. class.: Antihypertensive
Chem. class.: Angiotensin II receptor antagonist (Type AT$_1$) (ARB)

Do not confuse:
Diovan/Zyban/Dioval

ACTION: Blocks the vasoconstrictor and aldosterone-secreting effects of angiotensin II; selectively blocks the binding of angiotensin II to the AT$_1$ receptor found in tissues

USES: Hypertension, alone or in combination in patients >6 yr, HF, post MI with left ventricular dysfunction/failure in stable patients

CONTRAINDICATIONS

Hypersensitivity, severe hepatic disease, bilateral renal artery stenosis

Black Box Warning: Pregnancy

Precautions: Breastfeeding, children, geriatric patients, hypersensitivity to ACE inhibitors; HF, hypertrophic cardiomyopathy, aortic/mitral valve stenosis, CAD, angioedema, renal/hepatic disease, hyperkalemia, hypovolemia, African descent

DOSAGE AND ROUTES
Hypertension

• **Adult: PO** 80 or 160 mg/day alone or with other antihypertensives, may increase to 320 mg/day
• **Geriatric: PO** adjust on clinical response; may start with lower dose
• **Child and adolescent 6-16 yr: PO** oral solution 0.65 mg/kg/dose (Max: 20 mg/dose) twice daily, initially. Adjust based on clinical response. Max: 1.35 mg/kg/dose (Max: 80 mg/dose) twice daily
• **Child 1-16 yr: PO** Tablet 1 mg/kg/dose, max 4 mg/kg/day

Heart failure, classes II to IV

• **Adult: PO** 20-40 mg bid, up to 160 mg bid

Post MI

• **Adult: PO** 20 mg bid as early as 12 hr post MI, may be titrated within 7 days to 40 mg bid, then titrate to maintenance of 160 mg bid

Available forms: Tabs 40, 80, 160, 320 mg; oral solution 4 mg/mL

Administer:

• Without regard to meals
• If dose is missed, give as soon as remembered; if close to next dose, skip

Oral Solution

Not equivalent to tablets, when solution is replaced by a tablet, dose may need to be increased

SIDE EFFECTS

CNS: *Dizziness, insomnia,* drowsiness, vertigo, headache, fatigue
CV: Angina pectoris, 2nd-degree AV block, cerebrovascular accident, hypotension, MI, *dysrhythmias*
EENT: Conjunctivitis
GI: *Diarrhea,* abdominal pain, nausea, hepatotoxicity
GU: Impotence, nephrotoxicity, renal failure
HEMA: *Anemia,* neutropenia
META: Hyperkalemia
MISC: Vasculitis, angioedema
MS: Cramps, myalgia, pain, stiffness
RESP: *Cough*

PHARMACOKINETICS

Onset up to 2 hr; peak 2-4 hr; duration 24 hr; extensively metabolized; protein binding 95%; half-life 6 hr; excreted in feces, urine, breast milk

INTERACTIONS

Do not use with aliskiren in diabetes or severe renal disease

Increase: effects of lithium, antidiabetics

Increase: hyperkalemia—potassium-sparing diuretics, potassium supplements, ACE inhibitors, cycloSPORINE

Increase: valsartan level—rifampin, ritonavir, gemfibrozil, telithromycin

Decrease: antihypertensive effects—NSAIDs, salicylates

Drug/Herb

Increase: antihypertensive effect—garlic, hawthorn

Decrease: antihypertensive effect—ephedra, ma huang

Drug/Food

Increase: hyperkalemia—salt substitutes with potasssium

Drug/Lab

Increase: potassium, creatinine

NURSING CONSIDERATIONS

Assess:

• **Vital signs:** B/P, pulse q4hr lying, sitting, standing; note rate, rhythm, quality periodically

• **Blood studies:** BUN, creatinine, LFTs, potassium, total/direct bilirubin before treatment

• **Angioedema:** facial swelling; SOB; edema in feet, legs daily

• **Dehydration:** Skin turgor, dryness of mucous membranes for hydration status; correct volume depletion before initiating therapy

Black Box Warning: Pregnancy/breastfeeding: Do not use in pregnancy, may cause fetal death; do not breastfeed

Evaluate:

• **Therapeutic response:** decreased B/P

Teach patient/family:

• To comply with dosage schedule, even if feeling better; that, if dose is missed, to take it as soon as possible unless it is within 1 hr of next dose

• To notify prescriber of fever, swelling of hands or feet, irregular heartbeat, chest pain, dizziness, persistent cough

• That excessive perspiration, dehydration, diarrhea may lead to fall in blood pressure; to consult prescriber if these occur; to maintain hydration

• That product may cause dizziness, fainting, light-headedness; to rise slowly to sitting or standing position to minimize orthostatic hypotension; to take B/P readings

• To avoid potassium supplements and foods, salt substitutes

Black Box Warning: Not to take product if pregnant or breastfeeding

• **Overdose symptoms:** bradycardia or tachycardia, circulatory collapse

---

valsartan/ hydrochlorothiazide (Rx)

(val-sar'tan/hye-droe-klor-oh-thye'a-zide)

Diovan HCT

Func. class.: Antihypertensive, thiazide diuretic

USES: Management of hypertension

Black Box Warning: Pregnancy

DOSAGE AND ROUTES

• **Adult: PO** Valsartan 160 mg/hydrochlorothiazide 12.5 mg daily; titrate as needed based after 1-2 wk, max valsartan 320 mg/hydrochlorothiazide 25 mg daily

Available forms: Valsartan 80 mg/hydrochlorothiazide 12.5 mg; valsartan 160 mg/hydrochlorothiazide 12.5 mg; valsartan 160 mg/hydrochlorothiazide 25 mg; valsartan 320 mg/hydrochlorothiazide 12.5 mg; valsartan 320 mg/hydrochlorothiazide 25 mg

---

vancomycin (Rx)

(van-koe-mye'sin)

Firvanq, Vancocin, Vancosol

Func. class.: Antiinfective—miscellaneous

Chem. class.: Tricyclic glycopeptide

ACTION: Inhibits bacterial cell-wall synthesis, damages bacterial plasma membrane and increases osmotic pressure

USES: *Actinomyces* sp., *Bacillus* sp., *Clostridium difficile, Clostridium* sp., *Enterococcus faecalis, Enterococcus faecium, Enterococcus* sp., *Lactobacillus*

V

Side effects: *italics* = common; red = life-threatening

sp., *Listeria monocytogenes, Staphylococcus aureus* (MRSA), *Staphylococcus aureus* (MSSA), *Staphylococcus epidermidis, Staphylococcus* sp., *Streptococcus agalactiae* (Group B), *Streptococcus bovis, Streptococcus pneumoniae, Streptococcus pyogenes* (group A beta-hemolytic streptococci), viridans streptococci; may be effective against *Corynebacterium jeikeium, Corynebacterium* sp., CDAD, staphylococcal enterocolitis, endocarditis prophylaxis for dental procedures, bacteremia, joint/bone infections, osteomyelitis, pneumonia, septicemia

Unlabeled uses: Anthrax, intraabdominal infections, diptheria, bone/joint infections, surgical infection prophylaxis

CONTRAINDICATIONS
Hypersensitivity to this product or corn
Precautions: Pregnancy, breastfeeding, neonates, geriatric patients, renal disease, hearing loss

DOSAGE AND ROUTES
Serious systemic infections
• **Adult: IV** 20 to 35 mg/kg/dose (Max: 3,000 mg/dose) loading dose, followed by 15 to 20 mg/kg/dose q 8 to 12 hr; adjust dose based on target PK/PD parameter. Consider loading dose in critically ill patients
• **Child: IV** 60 to 80 mg/kg/day divided q6hr (Usual Max: 3,000 mg/day); may require up to 3,600 mg/day); adjust dose based on target PK/PD parameter
• **Neonate: IV** 20 mg/kg initially, then 15 mg/kg q8-24hr
CDAD
• **Adult: PO** 125 mg qid × 10-14 days
• **Child: PO (unlabeled)** 40 mg/kg/day divided q6hr × 7-10 days, max 2 g/day
Staphylococcal endocarditis prophylaxis
• **Adult: IV** 25 to 30 mg/kg (actual body weight) loading dose for seriously-ill patients, then 15 to 20 mg/kg/dose (actual body weight) q 8 to 12 hr
• **Child: IV** 40 to 60 mg/kg/day divided q 6 to 12 hr
Staphylococcal enterocolitis
• **Adult: IV PO** 500-2000 mg/day in 3-4 divided doses × 7-10 days

• **Child PO:** 40 mg/kg/day in 3-4 divided doses × 7-10 days, max 2000 mg/day
Renal dose
• **Adult: IV** 15-20 mg/kg loading dose in seriously ill; individualize all other doses

Available forms: Cap 125, 250 mg; powder for inj 500 mg, 750 mg, 1 g; dextrose sol for inj 500 mg/100 mL, 750 mg/150 mL, 1 g/200 mL, powder for oral solution 25 mg/mL, 50 mg/mL
Administer:
• Obtain C&S before use, use only for susceptible organisms to prevent product-resistant bacteria
• Antihistamine if red man syndrome occurs: decreased B/P; flushing of neck, face; stop or slow infusion
• Dose based on serum concentration
IT route
• Dilute with preservative-free normal saline (1-5 mg/mL), give into ventricular cerebrospinal fluid
• **PO:** without regard to food, swallow whole (used only for *Clostridium difficile, staphylococcal enterocolitis*)
• Use calibrated measuring device for liquid
• IV form may be used NG after diluting in 30 mL water
• Store at room temperature for ≤2 wk after reconstitution
Intermittent IV INFUSION route
• After reconstitution with 10 mL sterile water for inj (500 mg/10 mL, 750 mg/15 mL, 1 g/20 mL); further dilution is needed for IV, 500 mg/100 mL, 750 mg/150 mL, 1 g/200 mL 0.9% NaCl, D₅W given as intermittent infusion over 1 hr; decrease rate of infusion if red man syndrome occurs
Continuous IV INFUSION route (unlabeled)
• May infuse 1-2 g in volume to give over 24 hr if intermittent IV route cannot be used
• A central line may be considered for long-term therapy, assess peripheral lines for phlebitis

Y-site compatibilities: Acetylcysteine, acyclovir, alatrofloxacin, aldesleukin, alemtuzumab, alfentanil, allopurinol, alprostadil, amifostine, amikacin, amino acids injection, aminocaproic acid, amiodarone, amoxicillin-clavulanate, amsacrine, anidulafungin, argatroban, ascorbic acid injection, atenolol, atracurium, atropine, azithromycin, benztropine, bleomycin, bretylium, bumetanide, buprenorphine, butorphanol, calcium chloride/gluconate, CARBOplatin, carmustine, caspofungin, cefpirome, chlorproMAZINE, cimetidine, ciprofloxacin, cisatracurium, CISplatin, clarithromycin, clindamycin, codeine, cyanocobalamin, cyclophosphamide, cycloSPORINE, cytarabine, DACTINomycin, DAUNOrubicin liposome, dexamethasone, dexmedetomidine, dexrazoxane, digoxin, diltiazem, diphenhydrAMINE, DOBUTamine, DOCEtaxel, dolasetron, DOPamine, doripenem, doxacurium, doxapram, DOXOrubicin, DOXOrubicin liposomal, doxycycline, enalaprilat, ePHEDrine, EPINEPHrine, epirubicin, eptifibatide, ertapenem, erythromycin, esmolol, etoposide, etoposide phosphate, famotidine, fenoldopam, fentaNYL, filgrastim, fluconazole, fludarabine, folic acid (as sodium salt), gallium, gemcitabine, gentamicin, glycopyrrolate, granisetron, HYDROmorphone, hydrOXYzine, ifosfamide, insulin (regular), irinotecan, isoproterenol, isosorbide, ketamine, labetalol, lactated Ringer's injection, lepirudin, levofloxacin, lidocaine, linezolid, LORazepam, magnesium sulfate, mannitol, mechlorethamine, melphalan, meperidine, meropenem, metaraminol, methyldopate, metoclopramide, metoprolol, metroNIDAZOLE, midazolam, milrinone, minocycline, mitoXANtrone, morphine, multiple vitamins injection, mycophenolate, nalbuphine, naloxone, nesiritide, netilmicin, niCARDipine, nitroglycerin, nitroprusside, norepinephrine, octreotide, ofloxacin, ondansetron, oxacillin, oxaliplatin, oxytocin, PACLitaxel (solvent/surfactant), palonosetron, pamidronate, pancuronium, papaverine, PEMEtrexed, penicillin G potassium/sodium, pentamidine, pentazocine, PENTobarbital, perphenazine, PHENobarbital, phentolamine, phenylephrine, phytonadione, piritramide, polymyxin B, potassium acetate/chloride, procainamide, prochlorperazine, promethazine, propranolol, protamine, pyridoxine, quiNIDine, ranitidine, remifentanil, rifampin, Ringer's injection, riTUXimab, sodium acetate/bicarbonate/citrate, succinylcholine, SUFentanil, tacrolimus, teniposide, thiamine, thiotepa, tigecycline, tirofiban, TNA (3-in-1), tobramycin, tolazoline, TPN (2-in-1), trastuzumab, urapidil, vasopressin, vecuronium, verapamil, vinBLAStine, vinCRIStine, vinorelbine, voriconazole, zidovudine, zoledronic acid

SIDE EFFECTS
CNS: Headache
CV: Hypotension, peripheral edema cardiac arrest, vascular collapse
EENT: *Ototoxicity,* permanent deafness, tinnitus, nystagmus
GI: Nausea, CDAD
GU: Nephrotoxicity
HEMA: Leukopenia, eosinophilia
INTEG: Chills, fever, rash, thrombophlebitis at inj site (red man syndrome), skin/subcutaneous tissue disorders
MS: Back pain
RESP: Wheezing, dyspnea
SYST: Anaphylaxis, superinfection

PHARMACOKINETICS
Widely distributed, crosses placenta, penetration in CSF (20%-30%)
PO: Absorption poor
IV: Onset rapid, peak 1 hr, half-life 4-8 hr, excreted in urine (active form)
Pediatric elimination half-lives: Newborns 6.7 hr, infant 1 mo-1 yr: 4.1 hr; child 2.5-11 yr: 5.6 hr

INTERACTIONS
Increase: ototoxicity/nephrotoxicity—aminoglycosides, cephalosporins, colistin, polymyxin, bactracin, cisplatin, amphotericin B, methotrexate, NSAIDs, cyclosporine, acyclovir, adefovir, foscarnet, ganciclovir, pamidroate, IV pentamine, streptozocin, tacrolimus, zoledronic acid; do not use with cholestyramine, colestipol, cidofovir
Increase: lactic acidosis—metformin
Increase: neuromuscular effects—nondepolarizing muscle relaxants

Drug/Lab Test
Increase: BUN/creatinine, eosinophils
Decrease: WBC

NURSING CONSIDERATIONS
Assess:

• **Infection:** WBC, urine, stools, sputum, characteristics of wound throughout treatment; obtain C&S before starting treatment, may start treatment before results are received

• **Nephrotoxicity:** I&O ratio; report hematuria, oliguria; nephrotoxicity may occur; BUN, creatinine

• Serum levels: peak 1 hr after 1-hr infusion 25-40 mg/L, trough before next dose 5-10 mg/L, especially in renal disease; no trough levels are needed for oral form

• **CDAD:** watery or bloody diarrhea, abdominal cramps, fever, pus, mucus, nausea, dehydration; discontinue immediately

• **Auditory function** during, after treatment; hearing loss; ringing, roaring in ears; product should be discontinued

• B/P during administration; sudden drop may indicate red man syndrome

• Skin eruptions

• **Red man syndrome:** flushing of neck, face, upper body, arms, back, may lead to anaphylaxis; slow IV infusion to >1 hr

• EPINEPHrine, suction, tracheostomy set, endotracheal intubation equipment on unit; anaphylaxis may occur

• Adequate intake of fluids (2 L/day) to prevent nephrotoxicity

Evaluate:

• **Therapeutic response:** absence of fever, sore throat; negative culture

Teach patient/family:

• About all aspects of product therapy; about the need to complete entire course of medication to ensure organism death (7-10 days); that culture may be taken after completed course of medication

• To report sore throat, fever, fatigue; could indicate superinfection

• That product must be taken in equal intervals around the clock to maintain blood levels

• That labs will need to be regularly monitored with IV infusion

• To notify prescriber if there is no change in 72-96 hr

• That antiinfectives must be taken before dental/medical invasive procedures in rheumatic heart disease

• **Pregnancy/breastfeeding:** identify if pregnancy is planned or suspected or if breastfeeding

⚠ HIGH ALERT

vandetanib (Rx)
(van-det′a-nib)
Caprelsa
Func. class.: Antineoplastic-tyrosine kinase inhibitor

USES: Treatment of metastatic/unresectable locally-advanced medullary thyroid cancer

Black Box Warning: QTc prolongation

DOSAGE AND ROUTES
• **Adult:** PO 300 mg daily, do not initiate treatment unless QTcF ≤450 msec
Renal dose
• **Adult:** PO *CCr ≥50 mL/min:* No change; *CCr 30-49 mL/min:* Reduce starting dose to 200 mg and monitor QT interval; *CCr <30 mL/min:* Do not use
Available forms: Tabs 100, 300 mg

vardenafil (Rx)
(var-den′a-fil)
Levitra, Staxyn
Func. class.: Erectile dysfunction agent
Chem. class.: Phosphodiesterase type 5 inhibitor

ACTION: Inhibits phosphodiesterase type 5 (PDE5), enhances erectile function by increasing the amount of cGMP, which in turn causes smooth muscle relaxation and increased blood flow into the corpus cavernosum

USES: Treatment of erectile dysfunction

CONTRAINDICATIONS

Hypersensitivity, coadministration of α-blockers or nitrates, renal failure, congenital or acquired QT prolongation, women, pregnancy, children

Precautions: Hepatic impairment, retinitis pigmentosa, anatomic penile deformities, sickle cell anemia, leukemia, multiple myeloma, bleeding disorders, active peptic ulceration, CV/renal disease

DOSAGE AND ROUTES
Levitra
• **Adult: PO** 10 mg taken 1 hr before sexual activity; dose may be reduced to 5 mg or increased to max 20 mg; max dosing frequency once daily; orally disintegrating tab 10 mg 60 min before sexual activity; do not use with potent CYP3A4 inhibitors
• **Geriatric >65 yr: PO** 5 mg initially, titrated as needed/tolerated, max: 1 dose/day and 20 mg/dose
Hepatic dose
• **Adult: PO** (Child-Pugh B) 5 mg, max 10 mg/day
Concomitant medications
• Ritonavir, max 2.5 mg q72hr; for indinavir, ketoconazole 400 mg/day and itraconazole 400 mg/day, max 2.5 mg/day; for ketoconazole 200 mg/day, itraconazole 200 mg/day and erythromycin max 5 mg/day
Staxyn
• **Adult: PO** 10 mg 1 hr before sexual activity, max 10 mg/24 hr
Available forms: Tabs 2.5, 5, 10, 20 mg; orally disintegrating tab 10 mg
Administer:
• Approximately 1 hr before sexual activity; do not use more than once daily; orally disintegrating tabs are not interchangeable with film-coated tabs
• Without regard to food; avoid taking with high-fat meal
• **Oral disintegrating tab:** place on tongue immediately after opening blister pack, allow to dissolve, do not use water

SIDE EFFECTS
CNS: *Headache, flushing, dizziness, insomnia*
EENT: Diminished vision, hearing loss
GU: Abnormal ejaculation, priapism

GI: Nausea
MISC: Flulike symptoms

PHARMACOKINETICS
Rapidly absorbed, bioavailability 15%, protein binding 95%, metabolized by liver by CYP3A4, distribution semen, terminal half-life 4-5 hr, onset 20 min, peak ½-1½ hr, duration <5 hr, reduced absorption with high-fat meal, primarily excreted in feces (91%-95%)

INTERACTIONS
• Do not use with nitrates because of unsafe decrease in B/P, which could result in MI or stroke
• **Serious dysrhythmias:** class IA/III antiarrhythmics, clarithromycin, droperidol, procainamide, quiNIDine, quinolones; do not use concurrently
Increase: hypotension—α-blockers, protease inhibitors, metoprolol, NIFEdipine, alcohol, amLODIPine, angiotensin II receptor blockers; do not use concurrently
Increase: vardenafil levels—erythromycin, azole antifungals (ketoconazole, itraconazole), cimetidine
Drug/Food
Decrease: absorption—high-fat meal
Increase: vardenafil level—grapefruit juice; avoid concurrent use
Drug/Lab Test
Increase: CK

NURSING CONSIDERATIONS
Assess:
• B/P, including orthostatic vasodilator properties
• Erectile dysfunction and cause before treatment
• Any severe loss of vision while taking this or similar products; products should not be used
• Use of organic nitrates, which should not be used with this product
• **Pregnancy/breastfeeding:** not used in women
Teach patient/family:
• That product does not protect against STDs, including HIV
• That product absorption is reduced with high-fat meal

Side effects: *italics* = common; red = life-threatening

• That product should not be used with nitrates in any form; to inform physician of all medications being taken

• That product has no effect in the absence of sexual stimulation; that patient should seek immediate medical attention if erections last >4 hr

• To notify prescriber immediately and stop taking product if vision loss occurs

• To take 1 hr before sexual activity and only once per day

• To notify prescriber of all OTC, prescription, and herbal products taken

---

varenicline (Rx)

(var-e-ni′kleen)

Champix ✦, Chantix, Tyrvaya

Func. class.: Smoking cessation agent
Chem. class.: Nicotine receptor agonist

ACTION: Partial agonist for nicotine receptors; partially activates receptors to help curb cravings; occupies receptors to prevent nicotine binding

USES: Adjunct to psychosocial interventions for tobacco cessation (smoking); dry eye disease (Tyrvaya)

CONTRAINDICATIONS

Hypersensitivity, eating disorders
Precautions: Pregnancy, breastfeeding, children <18 yr, geriatric patients, renal disease, recent MI, angioedema, bipolar disorder, depression, schizophrenia, suicidal ideation

DOSAGE AND ROUTES
Smoking cessation

• **Adult: PO** therapy should begin 1 wk before smoking stop date, take product plus tobacco for 7 days; titrate for 1 wk; days 1 through 3, 0.5 mg/day; days 4 through 7, 0.5 mg bid; day 8 through end of treatment, 1 mg bid; treatment is for 12 wk and may be repeated for another 12 wk

Dry eye disease

• **Adult: Nasal** 1 spray in each nostril q12h

Renal dose

• **Adult: PO** CCr ≤50 mL/min, titrate to max 0.5 mg bid

Available forms: Tabs 0.5, 1 mg; nasal spray 0.03 mg

Administer:

• Do not break, crush, or chew tabs

• Increased fluids, bulk in diet if constipation occurs

• After eating with a full glass of water

• Sugarless gum, hard candy, frequent sips of water for dry mouth

SIDE EFFECTS

CNS: Headache, agitation, dizziness, insomnia, abnormal dreams, fatigue, malaise, behavioral changes, depression, homicidal ideation, suicidal ideation, amnesia, hallucinations, hostility, mania, psychosis, tremors, seizures, stroke

CV: Dysrhythmias, MI

EENT: *Blurred vision*

GI: *Nausea, vomiting, dry mouth,* increased/decreased appetite, *constipation,* flatulence, GERD, diarrhea, gingivitis, dyspepsia, enterocolitis

GU: Erectile dysfunction, urinary frequency, menstrual irregularities

INTEG: Rash, pruritus, angioedema, Stevens-Johnson syndrome, flushing, dermatitis

MS: *Back pain,* myalgia, *arthralgia*

HEMA: Anemia

PHARMACOKINETICS

Elimination half-life 24 hr; metabolism minimal; 93% excreted unchanged in urine; steady state 4 days, onset 4 days, peak 3-4 hr

NURSING CONSIDERATIONS
Assess:

• **Smoking history:** motivation for smoking cessation, years used, amount each day; smoking cessation after 12 wk; if progress not made, product may be used for additional 12 wk

• Renal function in geriatric patients; cardiac status in cardiac disease

• **Neuropsychiatric symptoms:** mood, sensorium, affect; behavioral changes, agitation, depression, suicidal ideation; suicide has occurred; possible worsening

---

of depression, schizophrenia, bipolar disorder, risk is increased in adolescents

• **Angioedema, Stevens-Johnson syndrome:** rash during treatment; discontinue if rash, fever, fatigue, joint pain, lesions occur

• **CV reactions:** Stroke, MI more common in those with CV disease

• **Seizures:** May be increased in those with seizure disorders

• Risk of hypotension: take B/P baseline and periodically

• **Pregnancy/breastfeeding:** use only if benefits outweigh fetal risk, no well-controlled studies

Evaluate:

• **Therapeutic response:** smoking cessation

Teach patient/family:

• To set a date to quit smoking and to initiate treatment 1 wk before that date

• That treatment for smoking cessation lasts 12 wk and that another 12 wk may be required

• To use caution when driving, performing other activities requiring alertness; blurred vision may occur

• How to titrate product

• Not to use with nicotine patches unless directed by prescriber; may increase B/P

• That vivid dreams, insomnia may occur during beginning of treatment, but usually subside

• To notify prescriber of all OTC, prescription, or herbal products used

• To notify prescriber immediately of change in thought/behavior (suicidal ideation, hostility, depression); stop product

• Not to drive or operate machinery until effects are known

• To notify prescriber if pregnancy is planned or suspected or if breastfeeding

---

⚠ **HIGH ALERT**

vasopressin (Rx)

(vay-soe-press′in)

Vasostrict

Func. class.: Pituitary hormone

Chem. class.: Lysine vasopressin

Do not confuse:
vasopressin/desmopressin

ACTION: Promotes the reabsorption of water via action on the renal tubular epithelium; causes vasoconstriction

USES: Diabetes insipidus (nonnephrogenic/nonpsychogenic), hypotension, shock, septic shock, postcardiotomy cardiogenic shock

Unlabeled uses: Cardiac arrest, bleeding esophageal varices

CONTRAINDICATIONS

Hypersensitivity, chronic nephritis

Precautions: Pregnancy, breastfeeding, CAD, asthma, vascular/renal disease, migraines, seizures

DOSAGE AND ROUTES
Diabetes insipidus

• **Adult: IM/SUBCUT** 5-10 units bid-qid as needed; **CONT IV INFUSION** 0.0005 units/kg/hr (0.5 milliunit/kg/hr), double dose q30min as needed

• **Child: IM/SUBCUT** 2.5-10 units bid-qid as needed

Hypotension in septic shock

• **Adult:** IV 0.01 units/min, titrate by 0.005 units/min q10-15min until B/P target is achieved, to max 0.07 units/min after target B/P of 8 hr without use of catecholamines; taper 0.005 units/min q1hr to maintain B/P

GI hemorrhage (unlabeled)

• **Adult:** IV 0.2-0.4 units/min, titrate, max 0.8 units/min

Available forms: Sol for inj 20 units/mL

Administer

Continuous IV INFUSION route

• Dilute 2.5 or 5 mg/500 mL respectively of 0.9% NaCL or D₅W to 0.1 or 1 unit/mL in NS or D₅W. 1 unit/mL is suggested for those with fluid restrictions

• Discard unused solution after 18 hr at room temperature or 24 hr under refrigeration

IM route

• Inject deeply into a large muscle; aspirate prior to injection to avoid injection into a blood vessel

SUBCUT route:

• Inject SUBCUT, taking care not to inject intradermally

SIDE EFFECTS

CNS: Headache, lethargy, flushing, vertigo

CV: Chest pain, MI

GI: Nausea, heartburn, cramps, vomiting, flatus

MISC: urticaria

PHARMACOKINETICS

IM: Onset 1 hr; duration 3-8 hr; **IV** duration 60 min; half-life 15 min; metabolized in liver, kidneys; excreted in urine

INTERACTIONS

Increase: antidiuretic effect—tricyclics, SSRIs, carBAMazepine, chloropromide, fludrocortisone, clofibrate

Decrease: antidiuretic effect—lithium, demeclocycline, chlorpropamide, cyclophosphamide, enalapril, felbamate, haloperidol, pentamine

NURSING CONSIDERATIONS

Assess:

• Pulse, B/P, ECG periodically during treatment; if using for CPR, monitor continuously

• **Diabetes insipidus:** I&O ratio, weight daily; fluid/electrolyte balance, urine specific gravity; check for extreme thirst, poor skin turgor, dilute urine, large urine volume

• **Water intoxication:** lethargy, behavioral changes, disorientation, neuromuscular excitability

• Small doses may precipitate coronary adverse effects; keep emergency equipment nearby

• **Pregnancy/breastfeeding:** use only if benefits outweigh fetal risk; breastfeeding women should pump and discard milk for 1½ hr after receiving product

Evaluate:

• **Therapeutic response:** absence of severe thirst, decreased urine output, osmolality

Teach patient/family:

• To measure and record I&O

• To avoid herbals, supplements, all OTC medications unless approved by prescriber

• To report immediately hypersensitivity; wheezing; trouble breathing; rash; swelling of face, lips

• To report adverse reactions promptly

---

vedolizumab (Rx)

(ve'-doe-liz'ue-mab)

Entyvio

Func. class.: GI antiinflammatory

Chem class.: Integrin receptor antagonist

ACTION: A specific integrin receptor antagonist that inhibits the migration of specific memory T-lymphocytes across the endothelium into inflamed gastrointestinal parenchymal tissue, reduces chronic inflammation in ulcerative colitis and Crohn's disease

USES: For moderately to severely active ulcerative colitis/Crohn's disease

CONTRAINDICATIONS

Hypersensitivity

Precautions: Hepatic disease, infections, progressive multifocal leukoencephalopathy (PML), pregnancy, breastfeeding, live vaccines, TB, human antichimeric antibody (HACA)

DOSAGE AND ROUTES

• **Adult:** IV INFUSION 300 mg give over 30 min at wk 0, 2, and 6 as induction therapy, then 300 mg q8wk, continue if response occurs by wk 14

Available forms: Powder for injection 300-mg/20-mL vial

Administer:
• Full response by 6 wk; those who do not respond by week 14 are unlikely to respond
• Give as IV infusion only, do not use as an IV push or bolus
• Make sure all immunizations are up to date
• **Reconstitute** with 4.8 mL of sterile water for injection, using a syringe with a 21- to 25-gauge needle
• Insert the syringe needle into the vial and direct the stream of sterile water for injection to the glass wall of the vial, gently swirl, do not shake
• Allow the solution to stand up to 20 min at room temperature
• Once dissolved, product should be clear or opalescent, colorless to light brownish yellow, and free of visible particulates. Discard if discolored or if foreign particles are present
• Before withdrawing solution from vial, gently invert 3 times. Withdraw 5 mL (300 mg) using a 21- to 25-gauge needle. Discard remaining product
• **Dilute** by adding the 5 mL (300 mg) of reconstituted product to 250 mL of sterile 0.9% NaCl and gently mix bag. Do not mix with other medications. Give product if necessary, may be stored for up to 4 hr refrigerated, do not freeze. Infuse over 30 min; then, flush line with 30 mL of sterile 0.9% NaCl injection. Discard any unused solution

SIDE EFFECTS
CNS: *Headache,* fatigue, dizziness
GI: Nausea, vomiting
MISC: Rash, pruritus, infusion-related reactions
MS: *Arthralgia,* back pain
RESP: Cough, bronchospasm
SYST: Anaphylaxis, progressive multifocal leukoencephalopathy (PML), increased infection risk, pyrexia

PHARMACOKINETICS
Absorption complete, onset up to 6 wk, duration up to 8 wk, half-life 25 days

INTERACTIONS
Increase: infection risk—immunosuppressives, natalizumab, antineoplastics
Do not use with tumor necrosis factor (TNF) modifiers
Decrease: immune response—vaccines, toxoids

NURSING CONSIDERATIONS
Assess:
• **Ulcerative colitis/Crohn's disease:** monitor symptoms before and after treatment
• **Infection:** fever, fatigue, malaise; flu-like symptoms, UTI, URI signs/symptoms sore throat, cough, dyspnea, reaction at infusion site
• **Hypersensitivity:** swelling of lips, tongue, throat, face; rash; wheezing; hypertension; if serious reactions occur, discontinue product
• **Liver dysfunction:** elevated hepatic enzymes, jaundice, malaise, nausea, vomiting, abdominal pain, and anorexia are indication of severe liver injury, may be fatal or may require a liver transplant; if hepatic dysfunction is suspected, discontinue
• **Tuberculosis (TB) latent/active:** obtain TB skin test both before and during treatment; do not give in active infections
• **Progressive multifocal leukoencephalopathy (PML):** increased weakness on one side or clumsiness of limbs, visual disturbance, and changes in thinking, memory, and orientation leading to confusion and personality changes; severe disability or death can occur over weeks or months
Evaluate:
• **Therapeutic response:** lessening of ulcerative colitis and Crohn's disease
Teach patient/family:
• About the symptoms of infection and to report to health care provider immediately
• To report allergic reactions, PML; teach symptoms
• Not to use live virus vaccines while taking this product; to bring vaccinations up-to-date before starting this product

V

• The reason for product, expected result

• Risk of infection is increased, to notify health care professional of fever, chills, trouble breathing

• To discuss with health care professional all Rx, OTC, herbals, supplements taken

• To report planned or suspected pregnancy, or if breastfeeding; if pregnant, call 877-825-3327 to enroll in the Entyvia Pregnancy Registry

---

⚠ HIGH ALERT

vemurafenib (Rx)

Zelboraf

Func. class.: Antineoplastic
Chem. class.: Kinase inhibitor

ACTION: Inhibitor of mutated forms of BRAF serine threonine kinase, blocking cellular proliferation in melanoma cells; inhibits kinases including ⚕ CRAF, ARAF, wild-type BRAF, SRMA, ACK1, MAP4H5, and FGR

USES: Unresectable or metastatic malignant melanoma with ⚕ V600E mutation of the BRAF gene

CONTRAINDICATIONS

Hypersensitivity
Precautions: Pregnancy, breastfeeding, children, infants, neonates, hepatic disease, QT prolongation, secondary malignancy, torsades de pointes, hypokalemia, hypomagnesemia, sunlight exposure

DOSAGE AND ROUTES

• **Adult:** PO 960 mg (4 tabs) bid q12hr, continue until unacceptable toxicity or disease progression, if strong CYP3A4 inducers are used increase dose to 1200 mg (5 tablets)
Dose adjustments for toxicity from adverse reactions or QTc prolongation
• **Grade 1 or tolerable grade 2:** no dosage change; **intolerable grade 2 or grade 3**

(1st episode): interrupt treatment until toxicity resolves to grade ≤1, then reduce to 720 mg (3 tabs) bid; **grade 2 or grade 3 (2nd episode):** interrupt treatment until toxicity resolves to grade ≤1, then reduce to 480 mg (2 tabs) bid; **grade 2 or grade 3 (3rd episode):** discontinue treatment permanently; **grade 4 (1st episode):** discontinue permanently or interrupt until toxicity resolves to grade ≤1, then reduce to 480 mg (2 tabs) bid; **grade 4 (2nd episode):** discontinue permanently

Available forms: Tabs 240 mg
Administer:
• Continue until disease progresses or unacceptable toxicity occurs
• Missed doses can be taken up to 4 hr before the next dose is due; take about 12 hr apart, take without regard to meals
• Swallow whole with a full glass of water; do not crush or chew
• Store at room temperature in original container

SIDE EFFECTS

CNS: *Fatigue,* fever, headache, dizziness, peripheral neuropathy, *weakness*
CV: QT prolongation, atrial fibrillation, torsades de pointes
EENT: Uveitis, blurred vision, iritis, photophobia
GI: Nausea, diarrhea, dysgeusia, hepatotoxicity
INTEG: *Alopecia, pruritus,* hyperkeratosis, *maculopapular rash,* actinic keratosis, *xerosis/dry skin,* papular rash, palmar-plantar erythrodysesthesia (hand and foot syndrome), *photosensitivity*
MS: *Arthralgia, myalgias,* extremity pain, musculoskeletal pain, back pain, arthritis
GU: *Acute tubular necrosis, interstitial nephritis*
SYST: Secondary malignancy, anaphylaxis, Stevens-Johnson syndrome, toxic epidermal necrolysis, drug reaction with eosinophilia, anaphylaxis

PHARMACOKINETICS

>99% protein binding (albumin and alpha-1 acid glycoprotein), an inhibitor

---

of CYP1A2, 2A6, 2C9, 2C19, 2D6, 3A4/5 CYP1A2 inhibitor, a weak CYP2D6 inhibitor, and a CYP3A4 inducer; elimination 94% in feces, 1% in urine, half-life 57 hr, peak 3 hr, duration up to 12 hr

INTERACTIONS

Increase: vemurafenib effect—CYP3A4/CYP1A2 inhibitors (enoxacin, cimetidine, delavirdine, indinavir, isoniazid, itraconazole, dalfopristin, quinupristin, tipranavir)

Increase: QT prolongation, torsades de pointes—arsenic trioxide, certain phenothiazines (chlorproMAZINE, mesoridazine, thioridazine), grepafloxacin, pentamidine, probucol, sparfloxacin, troleandomycin, class IA antiarrhythmics (disopyramide, procainamide, quiNIDine), class III antiarrhythmics (amiodarone, dofetilide, ibutilide, sotalol), clarithromycin, ziprasidone, pimozide, haloperidol, halofantrine, quiNIDine, chloroquine, dronedarone, droperidol, erythromycin, methadone, posaconazole, propafenone, saquinavir, abarelix, amoxapine, apomorphine, asenapine, β-agonists, ofloxacin, eribulin, ezogabine, flecainide, gatifloxacin, gemifloxacin, halogenated anesthetics, iloperidone, levofloxacin, local anesthetics, magnesium sulfate, potassium sulfate, sodium, maprotiline, moxifloxacin, nilotinib, norfloxacin, ciprofloxacin, OLANZapine, paliperidone, some phenothiazines (fluPHENAZine, perphenazine, prochlorperazine, trifluoperazine), telavancin, tetrabenazine, tricyclic antidepressants, venlafaxine, vorinostat, citalopram, alfuzosin, cloZAPine, cyclobenzaprine, dolasetron, palonosetron, QUEtiapine, rilpivirine, SUNItinib, tacrolimus, vardenafil, indacaterol, dasatinib, fluconazole, lapatinib, lopinavir/ritonavir, mefloquine, octreotide, ondansetron, ranolazine, risperiDONE, telithromycin, vemurafenib

Decrease: vemurafenib effect—CYP3A4 inducers (rifampin, barbiturates, carBAMazepine, phenytoin, erythromycin, ketoconazole, fluvoxaMINE, alcohol, etravirine, ritonavir, bexarotene, rifabutin, OXcarbazepine, nevirapine, modafinil, metyraPONE)

Drug/Lab Test:
Increase: serum creatinine, LFTs, alkaline phosphatase, bilirubin

NURSING CONSIDERATIONS
Assess:

• **Hepatotoxicity:** liver function test (LFT) abnormalities, altered bilirubin levels may occur; monitor LFTs and bilirubin levels before treatment, then monthly; more frequent testing is needed in those with grade 2 or greater toxicities; laboratory alterations should be managed with dose reduction, treatment interruption, or discontinuation

• **Pancreatitis:** Nausea, vomiting, severe abdominal pain

• **QT prolongation:** avoid in patients with QT prolongation; monitor ECG and electrolytes in HF, bradycardia, electrolyte imbalance (hypokalemia, hypomagnesemia), or those taking concomitant medications known to prolong the QT interval; treatment interruption, dosage adjustment, treatment discontinuation may be needed in those who develop QT prolongation

• **Malignancy:** New melanoma

• Serum electrolytes, CCr, bilirubin, ECG

• **BRAF testing:** obtain testing before use; do not use in wild-type BRAF; confirm BRAF V600E mutation

• **Skin reactions:** assess for skin reaction

• **Pregnancy/breastfeeding:** identify whether pregnancy is planned or suspected; do not use in pregnancy; avoid breastfeeding

Evaluate:

• Decreased spread of malignancy

Teach patient/family:

• That missed doses can be taken up to 4 hr before the next dose is due to maintain the twice-daily regimen; that if vomiting occurs, do not retake dose, take next dose as scheduled

• Not to crush, chew tablets; use with water, take consistently with or without food

• To notify prescriber of new skin lesions

• To avoid sun exposure; to wear sunscreen, protective clothing

• **Hepatotoxicity:** To notify health care professional of yellow skin, eyes, dark

V

---

urine, clay-colored stool, nausea/vomiting, pain in right side of abdomen
• **Allergic reactions:** To report rash, trouble breathing; swelling of face, lips; blisters
• To discuss with health care professional all RX, OTC, herbals, supplements taken
• **Pregnancy:** to use reliable contraception; that both women and men of childbearing age should use adequate contraceptive methods during therapy and for at least 90 days after completing treatment

⚠ HIGH ALERT

venetoclax (Rx)
(veh-neh'toh-klax)

Venclexta
Func. class.: Antineoplastic, signal transduction inhibitor

USES: Treatment of CLL in patients with a 17p deletion who have received at least 1 prior therapy

CONTRAINDICATIONS
Hypersensitivity, pregnancy

DOSAGE AND ROUTES
• **Adult: PO** 20 mg/day × 7 days, increase dose weekly × 5 wk: wk 2, 50 mg/day; wk 3, 100 mg/day; wk 4, 200 mg/day; wk 5 and beyond, 400 mg/day. Continue therapy until disease progression
Available forms: Tablet 10, 50, 100 mg; starter pack

venlafaxine (Rx)
(ven-la-fax'een)

Effexor XR
Func. class.: Antidepressant—SNRI
Chem. class.: SNRI

ACTION: Potent inhibitor of neuronal serotonin and norepinephrine uptake, weak inhibitor of dopamine; no muscarinic, histaminergic, or α-adrenergic receptors in vitro

USES: Prevention/treatment of major depression; depression at the end of life; long-term treatment of general anxiety disorder, panic disorder, social anxiety disorder (Effexor XR only)
Unlabeled uses: Vasomotor symptoms in menopause, andropause, fibromyalgia

CONTRAINDICATIONS
Hypersensitivity, MAOIs
Precautions: Pregnancy, breastfeeding, geriatric patients, mania, hypertension, seizure disorder, recent MI, cardiac/renal/hepatic disease, eosinophilic pneumonia, desvenlafaxine hypersensitivity, bipolar disorder, interstitial lung disease, glaucoma

Black Box Warning: Children, suicidal ideation

DOSAGE AND ROUTES
Major Depression
• **Adult: PO** 75 mg/day in 2-3 divided doses; taken with food, may be increased to 150 mg/day; if needed, may be further increased to 225 mg/day; increments of 75 mg/day at intervals of ≥4 days; some hospitalized patients may require up to 375 mg/day in 3 divided doses; **EXT REL** 37.5-75 mg PO daily, max 225 mg/day; give XR daily
Anxiety disorders
• **Adult: PO** ER 75 mg/day or 37.5 mg/day × 4-7 days initially, max 225 mg/day
Social anxiety disorder (social phobia)
• **Adult: PO** ER 75 mg/day, may start at 37.5 mg/day × 4-7 days, then 75 mg/day
Panic disorder
• **Adult: PO** ER 37.5 mg/day × 7 days, titrate in increments of up to 75 mg/day at intervals of ≥7 days to max 225 mg/day if needed
Renal dose
• **Adult: PO** CCr 10-70 mL/min, reduce dose by 25%-50%; CCr <10 mL/min, reduce dose by 50%
Hepatic dose
• **Adult: PO** moderate impairment, 50% of dose

Hot flashes (unlabeled)
• **Adult (male, prostate cancer): PO** 12.5 mg bid × 4 wk; **females** 37.5-75 mg/day
Available forms: Tabs scored 25, 37.5, 50, 75, 100 mg; ext rel cap (Effexor XR) 37.5, 75, 150 mg, 225 mg
Administer:
• Once daily, AM or PM with food, milk for GI symptoms; do not crush, chew caps; caps can be opened and contents sprinkled on applesauce, given with full glass of water, use immediately
• Sugarless gum, hard candy, frequent sips of water for dry mouth
• Avoid use with CNS depressants
• Missed dose should not be made up by doubling, take next scheduled dose at usual time
• Give in small amounts because of suicide potential, especially at beginning of therapy
• Store in tight container at room temperature; do not freeze

SIDE EFFECTS

CNS: Emotional lability, *dizziness, weakness,* headache, hallucinations, insomnia, anxiety, suicidal ideation in children/adolescents, seizures, neuroleptic malignant syndrome–like reaction, *anxiety, abnormal dreams, paresthesia*
CV: Hypertension, chest pain, tachycardia, change in QTc interval, increased cholesterol, extrasystoles, syncope
EENT: *Abnormal vision,* taste, *ear pain*
GI: *Dysphagia, eructation, nausea,* anorexia, dry mouth, colitis, gastritis, gingivitis, *constipation,* stomatitis, stomach and mouth ulceration, *abdominal pain, vomiting, weight loss*
GU: *Anorgasmia,* abnormal ejaculation, urinary frequency, decreased libido, impotence, menstrual changes, *impaired urination*
INTEG: *Ecchymosis,* dry skin, photosensitivity, sweating, Stevens-Johnson syndrome; angioedema (ext rel)
META: *Peripheral edema, weight loss*

PHARMACOKINETICS

Well absorbed; extensively metabolized in liver by CYP2D6 to active metabolite, some are poor metabolizers ⊗⊗; 87% of product recovered in urine; 27% protein binding; half-life 5, 11 hr (active metabolite), respectively, onset up to 14 days, peak up to 4 wk

INTERACTIONS

Increase: Hyperthermia, rigidity, rapid fluctuations of vital signs, mental status changes, neuroleptic malignant syndrome: MAOIs
Increase: bleeding risk—salicylates, NSAIDs, platelet inhibitors, anticoagulants
Increase: venlafaxine effect—cimetidine
Increase: CNS depression—alcohol, opioids, antihistamines, sedative/hypnotics
Increase: levels of cloZAPine, desipramine, haloperidol, warfarin
Increase: serotonin syndrome—lithium, sibutramine, SUMAtriptan, traZODone, traMADol, SSRIs, serotonin receptor agonist, linezolid, methylene blue, tryptophan
Decrease: effect of indinavir
Decrease: venlafaxine effect—cyproheptadine

Drug/Herb
• **Increase: serotonin syndrome:** St. John's wort, tryptophan
Increase: CNS depression—chamomile, hops, kava, valerian

Drug/Lab Test
Increase: alk phos, bilirubin, AST, ALT, BUN, creatinine, serum cholesterol, CPK, LDH
False positive: amphetamines, phencyclidine

NURSING CONSIDERATIONS
Assess:

Black Box Warning: Mental status: mood, sensorium, affect, increase in psychiatric symptoms, depression, panic; assess for suicidal ideation in children/adolescents and in early treatment

• **Vital signs:** B/P lying, standing; pulse q4hr; if systolic B/P drops 20 mm Hg, hold product, notify prescriber; take VS q4hr in patients with CV disease
• **Bleeding:** GI, ecchymosis, epistaxis, hematomas, petechiae, hemorrhage

V

- **Blood studies:** CBC, differential, leukocytes, cardiac enzymes if patient is receiving long-term therapy
- **Hepatic studies:** AST, ALT, bilirubin
- Weight weekly; weight loss or gain; appetite may increase; peripheral edema may occur; monitor cholesterol
- **Withdrawal symptoms:** flulike symptoms, headache, nervousness, agitation, nausea, vomiting, muscle pain, weakness; not usual unless product is discontinued abruptly
- **Serotonin syndrome, neuroleptic malignant syndrome:** increased heart rate, shivering, sweating, dilated pupils, tremors, high B/P, hyperthermia, headache, confusion; if these occur, stop product, give serotonin antagonist if needed; usually worse if given with linezolid, methylene blue, tryptophan
- Assistance with ambulation during beginning therapy because drowsiness, dizziness occur
- **Beers:** use with caution in older adults; may exacerbate or cause syndrome of inappropriate antidiuretic hormone secretion (SIADH)
- **Pregnancy/breastfeeding:** use only if benefits outweigh fetal risk; use in late 3rd trimester has resulted in neonatal complications; do not breastfeed, excreted in breast milk

Evaluate:
- **Therapeutic response:** decreased depression, anxiety; increased well-being

Teach patient/family:
- To notify prescriber of rash, hives, allergic reactions, bleeding
- To use with caution when driving, performing other activities requiring alertness because of drowsiness, dizziness, blurred vision

Black Box Warning: That worsening of symptoms, suicidal thoughts/behaviors may occur in children or young adults; discuss with family members

- To avoid alcohol ingestion
- Not to discontinue medication abruptly after long-term use; may cause nausea, headache, malaise; taper over 14 days

- To wear sunscreen or large hat because photosensitivity occurs
- To avoid pregnancy or breastfeeding; birth defects have occurred when used in the 3rd trimester
- To monitor B/P for new hypertension or if patient has history of hypertension
- **Serotonin syndrome, neuroleptic malignant syndrome:** to report immediately shivering, sweating, tremors, fever, dilated pupils
- To take as prescribed, contents of capsule may be sprinkled on applesauce if unable to swallow whole

TREATMENT OF OVERDOSE: ECG monitoring; lavage; administer anticonvulsant; may require whole-bowel irrigation for ext rel product

⚠ HIGH ALERT

verapamil (Rx)
(ver-ap′a-mill)

Calan, Calan SR, Isoptin, Isoptin SR, Verelan, Verelan PM

Func. class.: Calcium channel blocker; antihypertensive; antianginal; antidysrhythmic (class IV)

Chem. class.: Diphenylalkylamine

ACTION: Inhibits calcium ion influx across cell membrane during cardiac depolarization; produces relaxation of coronary vascular smooth muscle; dilates coronary arteries; decreases SA/AV node conduction; dilates peripheral arteries

USES: Chronic stable, vasospastic, unstable angina; dysrhythmias, hypertension, supraventricular tachycardia, atrial flutter or fibrillation

Unlabeled uses: Acute MI, claudication, mania, atrial tachycardia, peripheral vascular disease

CONTRAINDICATIONS
Sick sinus syndrome, 2nd-/3rd-degree heart block, hypotension <90 mm Hg systolic, cardiogenic shock, severe HF,

Lown-Ganong-Levine syndrome, Wolff-Parkinson-White syndrome

Precautions: Pregnancy, breastfeeding, children, geriatric patients, HF, hypotension, hepatic injury, renal disease, concomitant β-blocker therapy

DOSAGE AND ROUTES
Hypertension
• **Adult: PO IR** 80 mg tid, may titrate upward, usual dose: 120 to 360 mg/day in 3 divided doses; **EXT REL** 120-240 mg/day as single dose, may increase to 240-480 mg/day
Angina
• **Adult: PO** 80-120 mg tid, increase weekly, max 480 mg/day
Atrial fibrillation/flutter (digitalized)
• **Adult: PO IR** 240-480 mg/day in 3-4 divided doses in digitalized patients
Atrial flutter/fibrillation; supraventricular dysrrthmias
• **Adult: IV BOL** 5-10 mg (0.075-0.15 mg/kg) over 2 min, may repeat 10 mg (0.15 mg/kg) 1/2 hr after 1st dose; maintenance infusion 0.005 mg/kg/min
• **Child 1-15 yr: IV BOL** 0.1-0.3 mg/kg over ≥2 min, repeat in 30 min, max 5 mg in single dose
• **Child 0-1 yr: IV BOL** 0.1-0.2 mg/kg over ≥2 min, may repeat after 30 min
To prevent paroxysmal supraventricular tachycardia
• **Adult: PO** IR 240-480 daily, divided in 3 or 4 doses, max 480 mg/day
Hepatic disease/geriatric patients/compromised ventricular function
• **Adult: PO** 40 mg tid initially, increase as tolerated
Available forms: Tabs 40, 80, 120 mg; ext rel tabs 120, 180, 240 mg; inj 2.5 mg/mL in ampules, syringes, vials; ext rel caps 100, 120, 180, 200, 240, 300, 360 mg
Administer:
PO route
• **IR:** Give without regard to food, give with meals or milk to prevent gastric upset
Ext rel route
• Do not crush or chew ext rel products; Verelan caps may be opened and contents sprinkled on food; do not dissolve chew cap contents

• Before meals, at bedtime; give ext rel product with food
Direct IV route
• Undiluted through Y-tube or 3-way stopcock of compatible sol; give over 2 min or 3 min for geriatric patients, with continuous ECG and B/P monitoring, discard unused solution
• Do not use IV with IV β-blockers; may cause AV nodal blockade

Y-site compatibilities: Alfentanil, amikacin, argatroban, ascorbic acid, atracurium, atropine, aztreonam, bivalirudin, bumetanide, buprenorphine, butorphanol, calcium chloride/gluconate, CARBOplatin, caspofungin, ceFAZolin, cefonicid, cefotaxime, cefoTEtan, cefOXitin, ceftizoxime, cefTRIAXone, cefuroxime, chlorproMAZINE, cimetidine, ciprofloxacin, clindamycin, cyanocobalamin, cyclophosphamide, cycloSPORINE, cytarabine, DACTINomycin, DAPTOmycin, dexamethasone, dexmedetomidine, digoxin, diltiazem, diphenhydrAMINE, DOBUTamine, DOCEtaxel, DOPamine, doxacurium, DOXOrubicin hydrochloride, doxycycline, enalaprilat, ePHEDrine, EPINEPHrine, epirubicin, epoetin alfa, eptifibatide, erythromycin, esmolol, etoposide, etoposide phosphate, famotidine, fenoldopam, fentaNYL, fluconazole, fludarabine, gemcitabine, gentamicin, glycopyrrolate, granisetron, heparin, hydrALAZINE, hydrocortisone, HYDROmorphone, ifosfamide, imipenem/cilastatin, inamrinone, insulin, isoproterenol, ketorolac, labetalol, levoFLOXacin, lidocaine, linezolid, LORazepam, magnesium sulfate, mannitol, mechlorethamine, meperidine, metaraminol, methotrexate, methoxamine, methyldopate, methylPREDNISolone, metoclopramide, metoprolol, metroNIDAZOLE, miconazole, midazolam, milrinone, mitoXANtrone, morphine, multivitamins, nalbuphine, naloxone, nesiritide, nitroglycerin, nitroprusside, norepinephrine, octreotide, ondansetron, oxaliplatin, oxytocin, PACLitaxel, palonosetron, papaverine, PEMEtrexed, penicillin G, pentamidine, pentazocine, phentolamine, phenylephrine, phytonadione, piperacillin/tazobactam, potassium chloride, procainamide, prochlorperazine, promethazine, propranolol, protamine, pyridoxime, quinupristin/dalfopristin, ranitidine, rocuronium, sodium acetate, succinylcholine, SUFentanil, tacrolimus, teniposide, theophylline, thiamine, ticarcillin/clavulanate, tirofiban, tobramycin, tolazoline, trimethaphan, urokinase, vancomycin, vasopressin, vecuronium, vinCRIStine, vinorelbine, voriconazole

SIDE EFFECTS

CNS: *Headache, drowsiness,* dizziness, anxiety, depression, weakness, insomnia, confusion, light-headedness, asthenia, fatigue

CV: *Edema,* HF, bradycardia, hypotension, palpitations, AV block, dysrhythmias

GI: *Nausea,* diarrhea, gastric upset, *constipation,* increased LFTs

GU: Impotence, gynecomastia, nocturia, polyuria

HEMA: Bruising, petechiae, bleeding

EENT: Blurred vision, tinnitus, equilibrium change, epistaxis

RESP: Cough

INTEG: Rash, bruising

MISC: Gingival hyperplasia

SYST: Stevens-Johnson syndrome

PHARMACOKINETICS

Metabolized by liver by CYP3A4, excreted in urine (70% as metabolites), protein binding 90%

PO: Onset variable; peak 3-4 hr; duration 17-24 hr; half-life 4 min, 3-12 hr

IV: Onset 3 min, peak 3-5 min, duration 10-20 min

INTERACTIONS

Increase: hypotension—prazosin, quiNIDine, fentaNYL, other antihypertensives, nitrates, monitor B/P

Increase: effects of verapamil—β-blockers, cimetidine, clarithromycin, erythromycin, monitor for CV effects

Increase: levels of digoxin, theophylline, cycloSPORINE, carBAMazepine, nondepolarizing muscle relaxants

Increase: HMG-CoA reductase inhibitors, (CYP3A4 substrates), avoid use or lower dose

Increase: cardiac effects—inhalation anesthetics, macrolide antibiotics monitor cardiac status

Decrease or increase: effects of lithium

Decrease: antihypertensive effects—NSAIDs, rifAMPin, strong CYP3A4 inducers

Drug/Food

Increase: hypotensive effects—grapefruit juice, avoid use

Drug/Herb

Increase: verapamil effect—ginseng, ginkgo

Increase: hypertension—ephedra (ma huang)

Decrease: verapamil effect—St. John's wort

Drug/Lab Test

Increase: AST, ALT, alk phos, BUN, creatinine, serum cholesterol

NURSING CONSIDERATIONS

Assess:

• **Cardiac status:** B/P, pulse, respiration, ECG intervals (PR, QRS, QT); notify prescriber if pulse <50 bpm, systolic B/P <90 mm Hg

• **HF:** I&O ratios, weight daily; crackles, weight gain, dyspnea, jugular venous distention

• Renal, hepatic studies during long-term treatment, serum potassium periodically

• **Stevens-Johnson syndrome:** rash with fever, fatigue, joint pain, lesions; discontinue immediately

• **Pregnancy/breastfeeding:** use only if benefit outweighs fetal risk; avoid breastfeeding

• **Beers:** avoid use in older adults; may cause fluid retention or exacerbate heart failure

Evaluate:

• **Therapeutic response:** decreased anginal pain, decreased B/P, dysrhythmias

Teach patient/family:

• To increase fluids, fiber to counteract constipation

• How to take pulse, B/P before taking product; to keep record or graph

• To avoid hazardous activities until stabilized on product, dizziness no longer a problem

• To limit caffeine consumption; to avoid alcohol products

• To avoid OTC or grapefruit products unless directed by prescriber

• To comply with all areas of medical regimen: diet, exercise, stress reduction, product therapy

- To change positions slowly to prevent syncope
- Not to discontinue abruptly; chest pain may occur
- To report chest pain, palpitations, irregular heartbeats, swelling of extremities, skin irritation, rash, tremors, weakness
- To notify prescriber if pregnancy is planned; to avoid breastfeeding

TREATMENT OF OVERDOSE:
Defibrillation, atropine for AV block, vasopressor for hypotension, IV calcium

---

vigabatrin (Rx)
(vye-ga′ba-trin)
Sabril, Vigadrone
Func. class.: Anticonvulsant
Chem. class.: GABA transaminase inhibitor

ACTION: May inhibit reuptake and metabolism of GABA; may increase seizure threshold; structurally similar to GABA

USES: Adjunct treatment of partial seizures in adults and children ≥12 yr, infantile spasm

CONTRAINDICATIONS
Hypersensitivity to this product
Precautions: Pregnancy, breastfeeding, children <2 yr, geriatric patients, renal/hepatic disease, suicidal thoughts/behaviors, abrupt discontinuation

Black Box Warning: Visual disturbance; requires an experienced clinician

DOSAGE AND ROUTES
Complex partial seizures
- **Adult/child ≥17 yr/>60 kg: PO** 500 mg bid, titrate in 500-mg increments at weekly intervals up to 1.5 g bid
- **Child 2 to 16 years, greater than 60 kg: PO** initial, 500 mg twice daily orally; may increase by 500 mg once weekly to MAX, 1500 mg twice daily
- **Child 2-16 yr, 26-60 kg: PO** 500 mg/day divided bid, increase weekly; max 2000/day divided bid

- **Child 2 to 16 years, >21 kg to 25 kg: PO** Initial, 500 mg/day orally given in 2 divided doses; may increase once weekly to MAX, 1500 mg/day given in 2 divided doses
- **Child 2-16 yr, ≥16-20 kg: PO** 450 mg/day divided bid, increase weekly to max 1300 mg/day divided bid
- **Child 2-16 yr, 10-15 kg: PO** 350 mg/day divided bid, increase weekly to max 1050 mg/day divided bid
Infantile spasm
- **Infant >1 mo/child ≤2 yr: PO** 50 mg/kg/day in 2 divided doses, titrate in increments of 25 to 50 mg/kg/day q3days, max 150 mg/kg/day
Renal dose
- **Adult: PO** CCr 50-80 mL/min, reduce dose by 25%; CCr 30-49 mL/min, reduce dose by 50%; CCr 10-29 mL/min, reduce dose by 75%

Available forms: Tabs 500 mg; powder for oral solution 500 mg
Administer:
- Use safe handling (hazardous)
- Give without regard to meals
PO route (tab)
- Use safe handling procedures
PO route (oral sol)
- Reconstitute immediately before using
- Empty contents of appropriate number of packets into clean cup
- For each packet, dissolve 10 mL water, concentration 50 mg/mL; do not use other liquids
- Stir until dissolved, sol should be clear
- Use calibrated oral syringe to measure correct dosage
- Discard any unused sol, or if particulates are present
- Store at room temperature

SIDE EFFECTS
CNS: Headache, memory impairment, *dizziness,* irritability, lethargy, malignant hyperthermia, insomnia, suicidal ideation
CV: Edema
EENT: Visual impairment
GI: Nausea, vomiting, diarrhea, increased appetite, abdominal pain, GI bleeding, hemorrhoids, weight gain, constipation

---

Side effects: *italics* = common; red = life-threatening

GU: Impotence, dysmenorrhea
HEMA: Anemia
INTEG: Pruritus, rash
RESP: Coughing, respiratory depression, pulmonary embolism

PHARMACOKINETICS
Absorption >95%, no protein binding, widely distributed, not metabolized, excretion in urine 80% parent drug, excretion slowed in renal disease, peak 2 hr, half-life 7.5 hr

INTERACTIONS
Increase: CNS depression—CNS depressants, cannabis, alcohol
Increase: Serious ophthalmic effects (glaucoma, retinopathy): azaTHIOprine, chloroquine, corticosteroids, deferoxamine, ethambutol, hydroxychloroquine, interferons, loxapine, mecasermin, rh-IGF-1, pentostatin, phenothiazine, phosphodiesterase inhibitors, tamoxifen, thiothixene, TCAs; avoid concurrent use

Drug/Lab Test
Decrease: ALT/AST

NURSING CONSIDERATIONS
Assess:

Black Box Warning: Visual impairment: Prescribers must be registered with the SHARE program due to risk of permanent vision loss; if no clinical response in 2-4 wk of pediatric patients or 3 mo in adults, discontinue; provide vision assessment before and after ≤4 wk at least q3mo, and 3-6 mo after last dose

• **Acute encephalopathy:** sedation, ataxia, confusion, disorientation, progressing to stupor; risk factors include high dose, rapid upward titration, renal impairment
• **Suicidal ideation:** changes in mood, increased depression, notify prescriber
• Renal studies: urinalysis, BUN, urine creatinine q3mo in those with renal disease
• Hepatic studies: ALT, AST, bilirubin
• Description of seizures: location, duration, presence of aura
• Mental status: mood, sensorium, affect, behavioral changes; if mental status changes, notify prescriber

• Assistance with ambulation during early part of treatment; dizziness occurs
• Seizure precautions: padded side rails; move objects that may harm patient
• **Pregnancy/breastfeeding:** use only if benefits outweigh fetal risk; pregnant patients should enroll in the North American Antiepileptic Drug Pregnancy Registry, 888-233-2334; do not breastfeed, excreted in breast milk

Evaluate:
• **Therapeutic response:** decreased seizure activity
• **Beers:** avoid in older adults unless safer alternatives are unavailable; may cause ataxia, impaired psychomotor function

Teach patient/family:
• To carry emergency ID stating patient's name, products taken, condition, prescriber's name and phone number
• To avoid driving, other activities that require alertness
• Not to discontinue medication quickly after long-term use
• To notify prescriber if pregnancy is planned or suspected
• To report suicidal thoughts/behaviors immediately
• To avoid alcohol; drowsiness, dizziness may occur

Black Box Warning: That drug may cause vision impairment; that regular exams will be needed; to notify prescriber at once if loss of vision occurs

• To notify prescriber if pregnancy is planned or suspected; not to breastfeed

---

vilazodone (Rx)
(vil-az′oh-done)
Viibryd
Func. class.: Antidepressant
Chem. class.: SSRI, benzofuran

ACTION: Novel antidepressant unrelated to other antidepressants, enhances serotonergic action by a dual mechanism

USES: Major depression

CONTRAINDICATIONS

Concomitant use of MAO inhibitors or within 14 days after discontinuing MAO inhibitor or within 14 days after discontinuing vilazodone

Precautions: Pregnancy, labor, infants, geriatric patients, abrupt discontinuation, bipolar disorder, bleeding, operating machinery, ECT, hepatic disease, hyponatremia, hypovolemia, substance abuse, history of seizures, serotonin syndrome, neuroleptic malignant syndrome; use with serotonin precursors or serotonergic drugs; suicidal ideation, worsening depression or behavior

Black Box Warning: Children, suicidal ideation

DOSAGE AND ROUTES
Major depressive disorder
• **Adult: PO** 10 mg × 7 days, then 20 mg × 7 days, then 40 mg/day; **if taking potent CYP3A4 inhibitor,** max 20 mg/day; **potent CYP3A4 inducer** increase dose up to double may be needed, max 80 mg/day

Available forms: Tabs 10, 20, 40 mg
Administer:
• With food to increase absorption
• Do not use within 2 wk of MAOIs
• Missed dose should be taken as soon as possible, unless it is almost time for next dose; do not double
• Store at room temperature, away from moisture, heat

SIDE EFFECTS
CNS: Restlessness, dizziness, drowsiness, fatigue, mania, insomnia, migraine, neuroleptic malignant syndrome–like reaction, paresthesias, seizures, suicidal ideation, tremors, night sweats, dream disorders
CV: Palpitations, ventricular extrasystole
EENT: Cataracts, blurred vision
GI: *Nausea*, vomiting, flatulence, *diarrhea, xerostomia*, altered taste, gastroenteritis, increased appetite
GU: Decreased libido, ejaculation disorder, increased frequency of urination, sexual dysfunction
HEMA: Bleeding, decreased platelets

INTEG: Sweating
MS: Arthralgia, fracture
SYST: Neonatal abstinence syndrome, withdrawal, serotonin syndrome

INTERACTIONS
Do not use within 2 wk of MAO inhibitors, linezolid, or methylene blue
Increase: serotonin syndrome—SSRIs, SNRIs, serotonin receptor agonists, selegiline, busPIRone, dextromethorphan, ergots, fenfluramine, dexfluramine, lithium, meperidine, fentaNYL, methylphenidate, dexmethylphenidate, metoclopramide, mirtazapine, nefazodone, pentazocine, phenothiazines, haloperidol, loxapine, thiothixene, molindone, amphetamines use cautiously
Increase: bleeding—anticoagulants, thrombolytics, platelet inhibitors, salicylates, NSAIDs, monitor for bleeding
Increase: vilazodone levels—CYP3A4 inhibitors (ketoconazole, erythromycin, efavirenz, dronedarone, clarithromycin, and others), dose decrease may be needed
Decrease: vilazodone effect—CYP3A4 inducers (carBAMazepine), dose increase may be needed
Drug/Food
• Avoid use with grapefruit juice
Drug/Herb
Increase: serotonin syndrome—St. John's wort
Drug/Lab Test
Decrease: sodium

PHARMACOKINETICS
Protein binding 96%-99%, metabolized by liver by CYP3A4 (major) and CYP2C19 and CYP2D (minor) and non-CYP pathways, peak 4-5 hr, half-life 25 hr

NURSING CONSIDERATIONS V
Assess:

Black Box Warning: Mental status: orientation, mood, behavior initially and periodically; initiate suicide precautions if indicated; history of seizures, mania

• **Bleeding risk:** assess for NSAIDs, ASA, anticoagulant use, check for bruising, black tarry stool, abdominal pain
• **Fracture risk:** assess diet for calcium, vitamin D; activity, bone density studies

Side effects: *italics* = common; red = life-threatening

• Renal/hepatic status: hyponatremia (confusion, weakness, headache); monitor serum sodium

• **Abrupt discontinuation:** do not discontinue abruptly, taper, monitor for symptoms of withdrawal; if intolerable, resume previous dose and decrease more slowly

• **Serotonin syndrome/NMS:** nausea, vomiting, sedation, sweating, facial flushing, high B/P; discontinue product, notify prescriber change in mental status, seizures, rigidity; discontinue product, notify prescriber immediately

• **Pregnancy/breastfeeding:** use only if benefits outweigh fetal risk; if used in 3rd trimester, fetal complications may occur; avoid breastfeeding, excreted in breast milk

Evaluate:

• **Therapeutic response:** remission of depressive symptoms, decreased anxiety

Teach patient/family:

• To take as directed, with food, not to double dose, follow-up will be needed

• To avoid abrupt discontinuation unless approved by prescriber

• Not to drive or operate machinery until effects are known

• Not to use other products unless approved by prescriber, do not use alcohol

• **To contact prescriber for** allergic reactions; personality changes (aggression, anxiety, anger, hostility); extreme sleepiness, confusion, nervous, restless, or clumsy; numbness, tingling, burning pain in hands, arms, legs, or feet; tremors; unusual behavior or thoughts about hurting oneself

Black Box Warning: Suicidal thoughts/ behaviors: discuss with family the possibility of suicidal thoughts/behaviors and that prescriber should be notified immediately if these occur

• To notify prescriber if pregnancy is planned or suspected; to avoid breastfeeding

---

⚠ HIGH ALERT

vinBLAStine (VLB) (Rx)
(vin-blast′een)
Func. class.: Antineoplastic
Chem. class.: Vinca alkaloid

Do not confuse:
vinBLAStine/vinCRIStine/vinorelbine

ACTION: Inhibits mitotic activity, arrests cell cycle at metaphase; inhibits RNA synthesis, blocks cellular use of glutamic acid needed for purine synthesis; vesicant

USES: Breast, testicular cancer, lymphomas, neuroblastoma; Hodgkin's/ non-Hodgkin's lymphoma; mycosis fungoides, histiocytosis, Kaposi's sarcoma, Langerhans cell histiocytosis
Unlabeled uses: Lung, bladder cancer; desmoid tumor

CONTRAINDICATIONS
Pregnancy, breastfeeding, infants, hypersensitivity, leukopenia, granulocytopenia, bone marrow suppression, infection
Precautions: Renal/hepatic disease, tumor lysis syndrome

Black Box Warning: Extravasation, intrathecal use

DOSAGE AND ROUTES
Doses vary greatly
Breast cancer
• **Adult:** IV 4.5 mg/m^2 on day 1 of every 21 days in combination with DOXOrubicin and thiotepa
Hodgkin's/lymphoma
• **Adult:** IV 6 mg/m^2 on days 1 and 15 of every 28 days with DOXOrubicin, bleomycin, dacarbazine (ABVD regimen)
• **Child:** IV 2.5-6 mg/m^2/day once q1-2wk × 3-6 wk, max weekly dose 12.5 mg/m^2
Non-Hodgkin's lymphoma
• **Adult/child:** IV 4 mg/m^2 or days 1 and 2 of a 28-day cycle with cisplatin and bleomycin

Letterer-Siwe disease
• **Child:** IV 6.5 mg/m^2
Testicular cancer (germ cell)
• **Adult:** IV 3.7 mg/m^2 on days 1-5 of each cycle in combination
• **Child:** IV 3 mg/m^2/day on days 1 through 5 with other antineoplastics
Bladder cancer (unlabeled)
• **Adult:** IV 3 mg/m^2 on day 2, q14days in combination with other antineoplastics
NSCLC (unlabeled)
• **Adult:** IV 4 mg/m^2 on days 1, 8, 15, 22, 29, then q2wk with cisplatin
Available forms: Inj, powder 10 mg for 10 mL IV; sol for inj 1 mg/mL
Administer:
• Use safe handling procedures

Black Box Warning: Extravasation: aspirate, give hyaluronidase 150 units/mL in 1 mL NaCl, through IV catheter or subcut in circular pattern around extravasated site, warm compress for vesicant activity treatment

Black Box Warning: Do not administer intrathecally; fatal

IV inj route
• Use a minibag if possible, or give through sideport or directly over 1 min

Y-site compatibilities: Acyclovir, alemtuzumab, alfentanil, allopurinol sodium, amifostine, amikacin, aminophylline, amiodarone, amphotericin B cholesteryl (Amphotec), amphotericin B lipid complex (Abelcet), ampicillin, ampicillin-sulbactam, anidulafungin, argatroban, arsenic trioxide, atenolol, atracurium, aztreonam, bivalirudin, bleomycin, bretylium, bumetanide, buprenorphine, busulfan, butorphanol, calcium chloride/gluconate, capreomycin, carboplatin, carmustine, caspofungin, cefazolin, cefoperazone, cefotaxime, cefotetan, cefOXitin, cefTAZidime, ceftazidime (ʟ-arginine), ceftizoxime, cefTRIAXone, cefuroxime, chloramphenicol sodium succinate, chlorproMAZINE, cimetidine, ciprofloxacin, cisatracurium, cisplatin, clindamycin, codeine, cyclophosphamide, cycloSPORINE, dacarbazine, DACTINomycin, DAPTOmycin, DAUNOrubicin, dexamethasone, dexmedetomidine, dexrazoxane, digoxin, diltiaZEM, diphenhydrAMINE, DOBUTamine, DOCEtaxel, dolasetron, DOPamine, DOXOrubicin, DOXOrubicin liposomal, doxycycline, droperidol, enalaprilat, ePHEDrine, EPINEPHrine, epiRUBicin, ertapenem, erythromycin, esmolol, etoposide, famotidine, fenoldopam, fentaNYL, filgrastim, fluconazole, fludarabine, fluorouracil, foscarnet, fosphenytoin, gallium, ganciclovir, garenoxacin, gatifloxacin, gemcitabine, gentamicin, glycopyrrolate, granisetron, haloperidol, heparin, hydrALAZINE, hydrocortisone, HYDROmorphone, hydrOXYzine, IDArubicin, ifosfamide, imipenem-cilastatin, inamrinone, insulin (regular), irinotecan, isoproterenol, ketorolac, labetalol, lepirudin, leucovorin, levoFLOXacin, levorphanol, lidocaine, linezolid, LORazepam, magnesium sulfate, mannitol, mechlorethamine, melphalan, meperidine, meropenem, mesna, metaraminol, methadone, methohexital, methotrexate, methyldopa, metoclopramide, metoprolol, metroNIDAZOLE, midazolam, milrinone, minocycline, mitoMYcin, mitoXANTRONE, morphine, moxifloxacin, nafcillin, nalbuphine, naloxone, nesiritide, nitroglycerin, nitroprusside, norepinephrine, octreotide, ofloxacin, ondansetron, oxaliplatin, PACLitaxel, palonosetron, pamidronate, pancuronium, PEMEtrexed, pentamidine, pentazocine, PENTobarbital, PHENobarbital, phentolamine, phenylephrine, piperacillin, piperacillin-tazobactam, polymyxin B, potassium acetate/chloride/phosphates, procainamide, prochlorperazine, promethazine, propranolol, quiNIDine, quinupristin-dalfopristin, raNITIdine, remifentanil, riTUXimab, sargramostim, sodium acetate/bicarbonate/phosphates, succinylcholine, SUFentanil, sulfamethoxazole-trimethoprim, tacrolimus, teniposide, theophylline, thiopental, thiotepa, ticarcillin, ticarcillin-clavulanate, tigecycline, tirofiban, tobramycin, tolazoline, topotecan, trastuzumab, trimethobenzamide, vancomycin, vasopressin, vecuronium, verapamil, vinCRIStine, vinorelbine, voriconazole, zidovudine, zoledronic acid

V

SIDE EFFECTS

CNS: Paresthesias, peripheral neuropathy, depression, headache, seizures, malaise
CV: Tachycardia, orthostatic hypo/hypertension
GI: *Nausea, vomiting,* ileus, *anorexia, stomatitis, constipation,* abdominal pain, GI/rectal bleeding, hepatotoxicity, pharyngitis
GU: Urinary retention, renal failure, hyperuricemia
HEMA: Thrombocytopenia, leukopenia, myelosuppression, agranulocytosis, granulocytosis, aplastic anemia, neutropenia, pancytopenia
INTEG: *Rash, alopecia,* photosensitivity, extravasation, tissue necrosis
META: SIADH
RESP: Fibrosis, pulmonary infiltrate, bronchospasm
SYST: Tumor lysis syndrome (TLS)

PHARMACOKINETICS

Half-life (triphasic) <5 min, 50-155 min, 23-85 hr; metabolized in liver; excreted in urine, feces; crosses blood-brain barrier

INTERACTIONS

Increase: synergism—bleomycin
• Do not use with radiation
Increase: bleeding risk—NSAIDs, anticoagulants, thrombolytics, antiplatelets
Increase: toxicity, bone marrow suppression—antineoplastics
Increase: action of methotrexate
Increase: adverse reactions—live virus vaccines
Increase: toxicity—CYP3A4 inhibitors (aprepitant, antiretroviral protease inhibitors, clarithromycin, danazol, delavirdine, diltiaZEM, erythromycin, fluconazole, FLUoxetine, fluvoxaMINE, imatinib, ketoconazole, mibefradil, nefazodone, telithromycin, voriconazole)
Decrease: vinBLAStine effect—CYP3A4 inducers (barbiturates, bosentan, carBAMazepine, efavirenz, phenytoins, nevirapine, rifabutin, rifAMPin)
Drug/Herb
• Avoid use with St. John's wort
Drug/Lab Test
Increase: uric acid, bilirubin

Decrease: HB, platelets, WBC

NURSING CONSIDERATIONS

Assess:
• B/P baseline and during use

• **Bone marrow toxicity:** CBC, differential, platelet count weekly; withhold product if WBC is <2000/mm³ or platelet count is <75,000/mm³; notify prescriber; RBC, Hct, HB may be decreased, nadir occurs on days 4-10 (leukopenia) and continues for another 1-2 wk
• **Infection:** check for sore mouth/throat, fever, rash, bruising, cough, flulike symptoms, diarrhea, nausea
• **Tumor lysis syndrome:** monitor for hyperkalemia, hyperphosphatemia, hyperuricemia; usually occurs with leukemia, lymphoma; alkalinization of the urine, allopurinol should be used to prevent urate nephropathy; monitor electrolytes and renal function (BUN, uric acid, urine CCR)
• **Hepatitis:** transient hepatitis may occur with continuous IV
• **Bleeding:** hematuria, guaiac, bruising, petechiae, mucosa, orifices
• **Bronchospasm:** can be life-threatening; usually occurs when giving mitoMYcin
• Effects of alopecia on body image; discuss feelings about body changes
• Sensitivity of feet/hands, which precedes neuropathy
• **Liver toxicity:** Jaundiced skin, sclera; dark urine, clay-colored stools, itchy skin, abdominal pain, fever, diarrhea
• Buccal cavity q8hr for dryness, sores, ulcerations, white patches, oral pain, bleeding, dysphagia
• Brushing of teeth bid-tid with soft brush or cotton-tipped applicator for stomatitis, use unwaxed dental floss

Black Box Warning: Extravasation: local irritation, pain, burning, discoloration at IV site (vesicant)

• **Severe allergic reaction:** rash, pruritus, urticaria, purpuric skin lesions, itching, flushing
• Increased fluid intake to 2-3 L/day to prevent urate deposits, calculi formation

---

• **Pregnancy/breastfeeding:** do not use in pregnancy; do not breastfeed

Evaluate:
• **Therapeutic response:** decreased tumor size, spread of malignancy

Teach patient/family:
• To report any bleeding, white spots, ulcerations in mouth to prescriber; to examine mouth daily
• To report any changes in breathing or coughing; to avoid exposure to persons with infection
• That hair may be lost during treatment; that a wig or hairpiece may make patient feel better; that new hair may be different in color, texture
• To report change in gait or numbness in extremities; may indicate neuropathy
• To avoid foods with citric acid, hot temperature, or rough texture
• To wear sunscreen, protective clothing, sunglasses
• To avoid receiving vaccinations
• **Infection:** to report sore throat, flulike symptoms; to avoid persons with known infections
• **Pregnancy:** not to breastfeed; that product may cause male infertility; to notify prescriber if pregnancy is planned or suspected

⚠ HIGH ALERT

vinCRISTine (VCR) (Rx)
(vin-kris′teen)
Func. class.: Antineoplastic—miscellaneous
Chem. class.: Vinca alkaloid

Do not confuse:
vinCRISTine/vinBLAStine/vinorelbine

ACTION: Inhibits mitotic activity, arrests cell cycle at metaphase; inhibits RNA synthesis, blocks cellular use of glutamic acid needed for purine synthesis; vesicant

USES: Lymphomas, neuroblastoma, Hodgkin's disease, acute lymphoblastic and other leukemias, rhabdomyosarcoma, Wilms' tumor, non-Hodgkin's lymphoma, malignant glioma, soft-tissue sarcoma; liposomal: Philadelphia chromosome—negative ALL in second or greater relapse or that has progressed after ≥2 antileukemia therapies

Unlabeled uses: trophoblastic tumors, multiple myeloma

CONTRAINDICATIONS
Pregnancy, breastfeeding, infants, hypersensitivity, radiation therapy

Black Box Warning: Intrathecal use

Precautions: Renal/hepatic disease, hypertension, neuromuscular disease

Black Box Warning: Extravasation

DOSAGE AND ROUTES
• **Adult:** IV 0.4-1.4 mg/m²/wk, max 2 mg
• **Child >10 kg:** IV 1-2 mg/m²/wk, max 2 mg

Available forms: Inj 1 mg/mL
Administer:
• **Cytotoxic:** Use safe handling procedures

Black Box Warning: Label syringes: IV use only, fatal if given intrathecally, vesicant

IV route
• Label syringe for "IV Use Only"
• Give by IV injection by those experienced with the product
• Give IV push through sidearm of free-flowing IV (D5 or NS), inject over at least 1 min, flush with NS
• May be mixed in 50 mL minibag D5 or NS, given over 15 min, use of minibag is recommended, central line is recommended
• Protect from light, use diluted solution within 6 hr (room temperature) or 24 hr (refrigerated)

Black Box Warning: Hyaluronidase 150 units/mL in 1 mL NaCl; apply warm compress for extravasation

Y-site compatibilities: Acyclovir, alemtuzumab, alfentanil, allopurinol, amifostine, amikacin, aminocaproic acid, aminophylline, amiodarone, amphotericin B cholesteryl, amphotericin B lipid complex, amphotericin B liposome, ampicillin, ampicillin-sulbactam, anidulafungin, argatroban, arsenic trioxide, asparaginase, atenolol, atracurium, azithromycin, aztreonam, bivalirudin, bleomycin, bumetanide, buprenorphine, butorphanol, calcium chloride/gluconate, capreomycin, CARBOplatin, carmustine, caspofungin, ceFAZolin, cefoperazone, cefoTEtan, cefOXitin, cefTAZidime, ceftizoxime, cefTRIAXone, cefuroxime, chlorproMAZINE, cimetidine, ciprofloxacin, cisatracurium, CISplatin, cladribine, clindamycin, codeine, cyclophosphamide, cycloSPORINE, cytarabine, D₅W-dextrose 5%, dacarbazine, DACTINomycin, DAPTOmycin, DAUNOrubicin, DAUNOrubicin citrate liposome, dexamethasone, dexmedetomidine, dexrazoxane, digoxin, diltiazem, diphenhydrAMINE, DOBUTamine, DOCEtaxel, dolasetron, DOPamine, doxacurium, doxapram, DOXOrubicin, DOXOrubicin liposomal, doxycycline, droperidol, enalaprilat, ePHEDrine, EPINEPHrine, epiRUBicin, ertapenem, erythromycin, esmolol, etoposide, famotidine, fenoldopam, fentaNYL, filgrastim, fluconazole, fludarabine, fluorouracil, foscarnet, fosphenytoin, gallium, ganciclovir, garenoxacin, gatifloxacin, gemcitabine, gentamicin, granisetron, haloperidol, heparin, hydrocortisone sodium phosphate/succinate, HYDROmorphone, hydrOXYzine, ifosfamide, imipenem-cilastatin, inamrinone, insulin (regular), isoproterenol, ketorolac, labetalol, lepirudin, leucovorin, levoFLOXacin, levorphanol, lidocaine, linezolid, LORazepam, magnesium sulfate, mannitol, mechlorethamine, melphalan, meperidine, meropenem, mesna, methadone, methohexital, methotrexate, methylPREDNISolone, metoclopramide, metoprolol, metroNIDAZOLE, midazolam, milrinone, minocycline, mitoMYcin, mitoXANtrone, mivacurium, morphine, moxifloxacin, nalbuphine, naloxone, nesiritide, niCARdipine, nitroglycerin, nitroprusside, norepinephrine, octreotide, ondansetron, oxaliplatin, PACLitaxel (solvent/surfactant), palonosetron, pamidronate, pancuronium, PEMEtrexed, pentamidine, pentazocine, PENTobarbital, PHENobarbital, phenylephrine, piperacillin, piperacillin–tazobactam, potassium acetate/chloride/phosphates, procainamide, prochlorperazine, promethazine, propranolol, quinupristin-dalfopristin, ranitidine, remifentanil, riTUXimab, rocuronium, sargramostim, sodium acetate/phosphates, succinylcholine, SUFentanil, sulfamethoxazole-trimethoprim, tacrolimus, teniposide, theophylline, thiopental, thiotepa, ticarcillin, ticarcillin-clavulanate, tigecycline, tirofiban, tobramycin, topotecan, trastuzumab, trimethobenzamide, vancomycin, vasopressin, vecuronium, verapamil, vinBLAStine, vinorelbine, voriconazole, zidovudine, zoledronic acid

SIDE EFFECTS

CNS: *Decreased reflexes, numbness, weakness, motor difficulties,* CNS depression, cranial nerve paralysis, seizures, peripheral neuropathy

CV: *Orthostatic hypotension*

EENT: *Diplopia*

GI: *Nausea, vomiting, anorexia, stomatitis, constipation,* paralytic ileus, *abdominal pain,* hepatotoxicity

GU: Renal tubular obstruction

HEMA: Thrombocytopenia, leukopenia, myelosuppression, anemia

INTEG: *Alopecia,* extravasation

SYST: Tumor lysis syndrome (TLS)

PHARMACOKINETICS

Half-life (triphasic) <5 min, 50-155 min, 23-85 hr; metabolized in liver; excreted in bile, feces; crosses placental, blood-brain barrier

INTERACTIONS

Decrease: immune response—vaccines, toxoids

Decrease: digoxin level—digoxin

Decrease: vinCRIStine effect—CYP3A4 inducers (barbiturates, bosentan, carBAMazepine, efavirenz, phenytoins, nevirapine, rifabutin, rifAMPin)

• Do not use with radiation

• **Acute pulmonary reactions:** mitoMYcin C

• **Increase:** toxicity—CYP3A4 inhibitors (aprepitant, antiretrovial protease inhibitors, clarithromycin, danazol, delavirdine, diltiaZEM, erythromycin, fluconazole, FLUoxetine, fluvoxaMINE, imatinib, ketoconazole, mibefradil, nefazodone, telithromycin, voriconazole)

Drug/Herb

• Avoid use with St. John's wort

Drug/Lab Test

Increase: uric acid

Decrease: HB, WBC, platelets, sodium

NURSING CONSIDERATIONS

Assess:

• CBC, differential, platelet count before each dose; withhold product if WBC is <4000/mm³ or platelet count is <75,000/mm³; notify prescriber; RBC, Hct, HB; may be decreased, nadir occurs on day 4-10 (leukopenia); continues for another 1-2 wk

• **Bronchospasm/dyspnea:** more common with mitoMYcin

• **GI autonomic neuropathy:** presents as severe constipation, cramps, ileus

• Hepatic studies before, during therapy (bilirubin, AST, ALT, LDH) as needed or monthly

• Sensitivity of feet/hands, which precedes neuropathy

• **Tumor lysis syndrome:** hyperkalemia, hyperphosphatemia, hyperuricemia, hypocalcemia; more common in leukemia, lymphoma; use alkalinization of urine with allopurinol, monitor electrolytes, renal function (BUN, urine, CCR, uric acid)

Black Box Warning: Extravasation: pain, swelling, poor blood return; if extravasation occurs, local inj of hyaluronidase and moderate heat to area may help disperse product

• **Bleeding:** hematuria, guaiac, bruising, petechiae, mucosa or orifices q8hr

• Effects of alopecia on body image; discuss feelings about body changes

• Buccal cavity q8hr for dryness, sores, ulcerations, white patches, oral pain, bleeding, dysphagia

• Symptoms indicating severe allergic reaction: rash, pruritus, urticaria, purpuric skin lesions, itching, flushing

• **Pregnancy/breastfeeding:** do not use in pregnancy, breastfeeding, contraception should be used during treatment

Evaluate:

• **Therapeutic response:** decreased tumor size, spread of malignancy

Teach patient/family:

• To brush teeth bid-tid with soft brush or cotton-tipped applicator for stomatitis; to use unwaxed dental floss

• To report change in gait or numbness in extremities; may indicate neuropathy

• To report any bleeding, white spots, or ulcerations in mouth to prescriber; to examine mouth daily

• To increase bulk, fluids, exercise to prevent constipation

• **Infection:** to report sore throat, fever, flulike symptoms; to avoid persons with known infection

• To avoid vaccinations

• That hair may be lost; that hair will grow back but with different texture, color

• **Pregnancy/breastfeeding:** to notify prescriber if pregnancy is planned or suspected; to use effective contraception during therapy; not to breastfeed

V

⚠ HIGH ALERT

vinorelbine (Rx)
(vi-nor'el-bine)
Navelbine
Func. class.: Antineoplastic—miscellaneous
Chem. class.: Semisynthetic vinca alkaloid

ACTION: Inhibits mitotic spindle activity, arrests cell cycle at metaphase; inhibits RNA synthesis, blocks cellular use of glutamic acid needed for purine synthesis; vesicant

USES: Unresectable advanced non–small-cell lung cancer (NSCLC) stage IV; may be used alone or in combination with CISplatin for stage III or IV NSCLC
Unlabeled uses: Hodgkin's disease, breast/ovarian/head/neck cancer, desmoid tumor

CONTRAINDICATIONS
Pregnancy, breastfeeding, infants, hypersensitivity, granulocyte count <1000 cells/mm^3 pretreatment

Black Box Warning: Severe neutropenia, intrathecal administration

Precautions: Children, geriatric patients, renal/hepatic/pulmonary/neurologic disease, anemia, bone marrow suppression, severe neutropenia, intrathecal administration, extravasation

Black Box Warning: Extravasation

DOSAGE AND ROUTES
• **Adult:** IV 30 mg/m^2/wk (monotherapy) or 25-30 mg/m^2 weekly with cisplatin 100 mg/m^2 q4wk

HER-2+ breast cancer (advanced) (unlabeled)
• **Adult:** IV 25 or 30 mg/m^2 q7days (monotherapy)
Available forms: Inj 10 mg/mL
Administer:

Black Box Warning: Do not give intrathecally, fatal; syringes with this product should be labeled "Warning, for IV use only, fatal if given intrathecally"

Intermittent IV INFUSION route
• Use minibag if possible
• Dilute to 0.5-2 mg/mL with 0.9% NaCl, 0.45% NaCl, D$_5$W, D$_5$/0.45% NaCl, LR, Ringer's sol, give over 6-10 min into side port of free-flowing IV line or central line, flush line with 75-125 mL of diluent or more

Black Box Warning: **Extravasation:** stop infusion, give hyaluronidase 150 units/mL in 1 mL NaCl through IV catheter or subcut in circular pattern around site, warm compress for extravasation for vesicant activity treatment

• If accidental exposure occurs to skin, mucosa, eye, immediately flush with large amounts of water/NS, wash skin with soap and water

Y-site compatibilities: Amikacin, aztreonam, bleomycin, bumetanide, buprenorphine, butorphanol, calcium gluconate, CARBOplatin, carmustine, cefotaxime, cefTAZidime, ceftizoxime, chlorproMAZINE, cimetidine, CISplatin, clindamycin, cyclophosphamide, cytarabine, dacarbazine, DACTINomycin, DAUNOrubicin, dexamethasone, diphenhydrAMINE, DOXOrubicin, DOXOrubicin liposome, doxycycline, droperidol, enalaprilat, etoposide, famotidine, filgrastim, floxuridine, fluconazole, fludarabine, gallium, gentamicin, granisetron, haloperidol, heparin, hydrocortisone, HYDROmorphone, hydrOXYzine, IDArubicin, ifosfamide, imipenem-cilastatin, LORazepam, mannitol, mechlorethamine, melphalan, meperidine, mesna, methotrexate, metoclopramide, metroNIDAZOLE, minocycline, mitoXANtrone, morphine, nalbuphine, netilmicin, ondansetron, plicamycin, streptozocin, teniposide, ticarcillin, ticarcillin-clavulanate, tobramycin, vancomycin, vinBLAStine, vinCRIStine, zidovudine

SIDE EFFECTS
CNS: Paresthesias, peripheral neuropathy, depression, headache, seizures, weakness, jaw pain, asthenia
CV: Chest pain
GI: *Nausea, vomiting,* ileus, *anorexia, stomatitis,* constipation, abdominal pain, *diarrhea,* hepatotoxicity, GI obstruction/perforation
HEMA: Neutropenia, anemia, thrombocytopenia, granulocytopenia
INTEG: *Rash, alopecia,* photosensitivity, inj site reaction, necrosis
META: SIADH
MS: Myalgia
RESP: SOB, dyspnea, pulmonary edema, acute bronchospasm, acute respiratory distress syndrome (ARDS)

PHARMACOKINETICS
Half-life 27-43 hr; peak 1-2 hr; highly bound to platelets, lymphocytes; metabolized in liver; excreted in feces; small amount unchanged in kidneys

INTERACTIONS
Increase: bleeding risk—NSAIDs, anticoagulants
Increase: toxicity—CYP3A4 inhibitors (aprepitant, antiretroviral protease inhibitors, clarithromycin, danazol, delavirdine, diltiaZEM, erythromycin, fluconazole, FLUoxetine, fluvoxaMINE, imatinib, ketoconazole, mibefradil, nefazodone, telithromycin, voriconazole)
Decrease: vinorelbine effect—CYP3A4 inducers (barbiturates, bosentan, carBAMazepine, efavirenz, phenytoins, nevirapine, rifabutin, rifampin)
Drug/Herb
• Avoid use with St. John's wort
Drug/Lab Test
Increase: LFTs, bilirubin
Decrease: HB, WBC, platelets

NURSING CONSIDERATIONS
Assess:
• B/P (baseline) during administration

Black Box Warning: Bone marrow suppression: CBC, differential, platelet count before each dose; withhold product if WBC is <4000/mm³ or platelet count is <75,000/mm³; notify prescriber of results; recovery will take 3 wk

• **Respiratory status: Bronchospasm:** more common with mitoMYcin; also dyspnea, wheezing; may be treated with oxygen, bronchodilators, corticosteroids, especially if there is underlying pulmonary disease
• **Neurologic status:** paresthesia, peripheral neuropathy, weakness; these may occur even after termination of treatment
• **Renal studies:** BUN; serum uric acid; urine CCr before, during therapy; I&O ratio; report fall in urine output to <30 mL/hr; decreased hyperuricemia
• **Infection,** cold, fever, sore throat; notify prescriber if these occur; effects of alopecia on body image
• **Bleeding:** hematuria, guaiac, bruising, petechiae, mucosa or orifices, no rectal temperatures; avoid IM inj; apply pressure to venipuncture sites
• **Hepatic function tests:** AST, ALT, bilirubin, LDH
• **Severe allergic reactions:** rash, pruritus, urticaria, itching, flushing, bronchospasm, hypotension; EPINEPHrine and crash cart should be nearby
• **Pregnancy:** determine pregnancy before starting treatment; do not use in pregnancy and for 6 mo after last dose; do not breastfeed
Evaluate:
• **Therapeutic response:** decreased tumor size, spread of malignancy
Teach patient/family:
• To report change in gait or numbness in extremities, continuing constipation; may indicate neurotoxicity

• To report pain, redness, inflammation at IV site

• To discuss all Rx, OTC, herbals, supplements taken

• To report change in respiratory status: Wheezing, cough, SOB, bronchospasm

• To brush teeth bid-tid with soft brush or cotton-tipped applicator for stomatitis; to use unwaxed dental floss

• To examine mouth daily for bleeding, white spots, ulcerations; to notify prescriber

• **Infection:** report sore throat, fever, flulike symptoms

• To avoid crowds, people with infections, vaccinations, OTC products

• That hair may be lost; that hair will grow back but with different texture, color

• **Pregnancy:** to notify prescriber if pregnancy is planned or suspected; to use effective contraception during treatment and for ≥6 mo after product is discontinued; male partners should use contraception during and for 3 mo after last dose; not to breastfeed

---

⚠ HIGH ALERT

vismodegib (Rx)

(vis′moe-deg′ib)

ERIVEDGE

Func. class.: Antineoplastic

Chem. class.: Hedgehog, pathway inhibitor

Do not confuse:
vismodegib/vemurafenib/vandatanib

ACTION: A hedgehog (Hh) signaling pathway inhibitor, slows growth of tumors

USES: Patients who have metastatic basal cell carcinoma, locally advanced

CONTRAINDICATIONS

Hypersensitivity, breastfeeding, females at risk of becoming pregnant; pregnancy, males who do not adhere to contraceptive measures, children/adolescents <18 yr

Black Box Warning: Intrauterine fetal death, male-mediated teratogenicity, pregnancy

Precautions: Children, blood donation renal/hepatic impairment, CV disease, history of pancreatitis, history of gallbladder disease, osteoporosis, respiratory disease

DOSAGE AND ROUTES

• **Adult: PO** 150 mg/day

Available forms: Cap 150 mg

Administer:

• Should be initiated and monitored only under the supervision of a health care provider qualified in the use of cancer therapies and with a full understanding of the risk of ERIVEDGE therapy and monitoring requirements

• Can cause embryo-fetal death or severe birth defects

• Not recommended for use in patients with severe renal or hepatic impairment; limited data are available for these patients

• Can cause irreversible premature fusion of the epiphyses in children

• Give without regard to food

• Swallow whole, do not open or crush caps

• If a dose is missed, do not take additional dose, take at usual time

• Store at 77°F (25°C)

SIDE EFFECTS

GI: *Nausea, vomiting, dysgeusia, constipation, anorexia, diarrhea*

GU: Amenorrhea, azotemia

INTEG: *Alopecia*

MISC: *Fatigue, decreased weight,* new primary malignancy, hypersensitivity reactions

MS: *Arthralgia,* muscle cramps

PHARMACOKINETICS

Protein binding >99%, elimination half-life 4 days

INTERACTIONS

None known

NURSING CONSIDERATIONS
Assess:

Black Box Warning: Pregnancy/breast-feeding: Obtain pregnancy test of all women within 7 days before therapy; contraception is needed during and for 24 mo after treatment; men receiving this product should use condoms with spermicide (even after vasectomy) during sexual intercourse with female partners and for 3 mo after the last dose; semen donation is contraindicated during treatment and for 3 mo after treatment; report exposure during pregnancy to the Genentech Adverse Event Line at 888-835-2555; do not breastfeed

GI toxicity: nausea, vomiting, anorexia, diarrhea, constipation

Evaluate:
• **Therapeutic response:** decreased spread of tumor

Teach patient/family:

Black Box Warning: Pregnancy/breastfeeding: Teach patients to notify providers immediately if pregnancy is suspected (or in a female partner for male patients); use effective contraception during and for 7 mo after treatment; men taking this product should use condoms with spermicide (even after vasectomy) and for 2 mo after the last dose; if product is used during pregnancy, should be apprised of the potential hazard to the fetus; encourage exposed women (either directly or through seminal fluid) to enroll in the ERIVEDGE pregnancy pharmacovigilance program; do not breastfeed

• About reason for treatment, expected results
• That if dose is missed, do not take, but resume scheduled doses; to swallow whole, not to crush or chew

• Not to donate blood during therapy or for ≥24 mo after conclusion of product
• **Amenorrhea:** it is unknown if reversible after completion of treatment

---

vitamin A (Rx, PO-OTC, Rx-IM)
Aquasol A
Func. class.: Vitamin, fat soluble
Chem. class.: Retinol

ACTION: Needed for normal bone, tooth development; visual dark adaptation; skin disease; mucosa tissue repair; assists with production of adrenal steroids, cholesterol, RNA

USES: Vit A deficiency

CONTRAINDICATIONS
Pregnancy (IM), hypersensitivity to vit A, malabsorption syndrome, hypervitaminosis A, IV administration

Precautions: Pregnancy (PO), breastfeeding, impaired renal function, children, hepatic disease, infants, alcoholism, hepatitis

DOSAGE AND ROUTES
• **Adult and child >8 yr: PO** 100,000-500,000 international units/day × 3 days then 50,000 international units/day × 2 wk; dose based on severity of deficiency; maintenance 10,000-20,000 international units for 2 mo
• **Child 1-8 yr: IM** 5000-15,000 international units/day × 10 days
• **Infant <1 yr: IM** 5000-15,000 international units/day × 10 days

Maintenance
• **Child 4-8 yr: IM** 15,000 international units/day × 2 mo
• **Child <4 yr: IM** 10,000 international units/day × 2 mo

Available forms: Caps 10,000, 25,000, 50,000 international units; drops 5000 international units; inj 50,000

international units/mL; tabs 10,000, 25,000, 50,000 international units

Administer:

PO route

• With food (PO) for better absorption
• Do not administer IV because of risk of anaphylactic shock; IM only
• Oral preparations not indicated for vit A deficiency in those with malabsorption syndrome
• Store in tight, light-resistant container

IM route

• Give deep in large muscle mass; do not use deltoid muscle for administration of >1 mL

SIDE EFFECTS

CNS: Headache, increased intracranial pressure, intracranial hypertension, lethargy, malaise
EENT: Gingivitis, papilledema, exophthalmos, inflammation of tongue and lips
GI: Nausea, vomiting, anorexia, abdominal pain, jaundice
INTEG: Drying of skin, pruritus, increased pigmentation, night sweats, alopecia
META: Hypomenorrhea, hypercalcemia
MS: Arthralgia, retarded growth, hard areas on bone

PHARMACOKINETICS

Stored in liver, kidneys, fat; excreted (metabolites) in urine, feces

INTERACTIONS

Increase: levels of vit A—corticosteroids, oral contraceptives
Decrease: absorption of vit A—mineral oil, cholestyramine, colestipol
Drug/Lab Test
False increase: bilirubin, serum cholesterol

NURSING CONSIDERATIONS

Assess:

• Nutritional status: yellow and dark green vegetables, yellow/orange fruits, vit A–fortified foods, liver, egg yolks
• **Vit A deficiency:** decreased growth; night blindness; dry, brittle nails; hair loss; urinary stones; increased infection; hyperkeratosis of skin; drying of cornea
• **Pregnancy/breastfeeding:** do not use IM in pregnancy, fetal complications may occur; breastfeeding is considered safe at recommended dietary levels

Evaluate:

• **Therapeutic response:** increased growth rate, weight; absence of dry skin and mucous membranes, night blindness

Teach patient/family:

• That if dose is missed, it should be omitted
• That ophthalmic exams may be required periodically throughout therapy
• Not to use mineral oil while taking this product
• To notify prescriber of nausea, vomiting, lip cracking, loss of hair, headache
• Not to take more than prescribed amount

TREATMENT OF OVERDOSE: Discontinue product

---

vitamin C (ascorbic acid) (otc, Rx)

(a-skor'bic)

Func. class.: Vit C—water-soluble vitamin

ACTION: Wound healing, collagen synthesis, antioxidant, carbohydrate metabolism

USES: Vit C deficiency, scurvy; delayed wound, bone healing; chronic disease; urine acidification; before gastrectomy; dietary supplement
Unlabeled uses: Common cold prevention

CONTRAINDICATIONS

Tartrazine, sulfite sensitivity; G6PD deficiency
Precautions: Pregnancy, gout, diabetes, renal calculi (large doses)

DOSAGE AND ROUTES
Dietary supplementation
- **Adult: PO** 50-500 mg/day
- **Child 14-18 yr: PO** 65 mg (female), 75 mg (male)
- **Child 9-13 yr: PO** 45 mg/day
- **Child 4-8 yr: PO** 25 mg/day
- **Child 1-3 yr: PO** 15 mg/day
- **Infant: PO** 40-50 mg/day

Scurvy
- **Adult: PO/SUBCUT/IM/IV** 100-250 mg/day × 2 wk, then 50 mg or more daily
- **Child: PO/SUBCUT/IM/IV** 100-300 mg/day × 2 wk, then 35 mg or more daily

Wound healing/chronic disease/fracture (may be given with zinc)
- **Adult: SUBCUT/IM/IV/PO** 200-500 mg/day for 1-2 mo
- **Child: SUBCUT/IM/IV/PO** 100-200 mg added doses for 1-2 mo

Urine acidification
- **Adult: PO** 4-12 g/day in divided doses
- **Child: PO** 500 mg q6-8hr

Available forms: Tabs 25, 50, 100, 250, 500, 1000, 1500 mg; effervescent tabs 1000 mg; chewable tabs 100, 250, 500 mg; timed-release tabs 500, 750, 1000, 1500 mg; timed-release caps 500 mg; crys 4 g/tsp; powder 4 g/tsp; liq 35 mg/0.6 mL; sol 100 mg/mL; syr 20 mg/mL, 500 mg/5 mL; inj SUBCUT, IM, IV 100, 250, 500 mg/mL

Administer:

PO route
- Do not crush or chew ext rel tabs or caps
- Caps may be opened and contents mixed with jelly

IV, direct route
- 100 mg undiluted by direct IV over at least 1 min; rapid infusion may cause fainting

Intermittent IV INFUSION route
- Diluted with D_5W, D_5NaCl, NS, LR, Ringer's, sodium lactate and given over 15 min

Syringe compatibilities: Metoclopramide, aminophylline, theophylline
Y-site compatibilities: Warfarin

SIDE EFFECTS
CNS: Headache, insomnia, dizziness, fatigue, flushing
GI: Nausea, vomiting, diarrhea, anorexia, heartburn, cramps
GU: Polyuria, urine acidification, oxalate/urate renal stones, dysuria
HEMA: Hemolytic anemia in patients with G6PD
INTEG: Inflammation at inj site

PHARMACOKINETICS
PO/INJ: Readily absorbed PO, metabolized in liver; unused amounts excreted in urine (unchanged), metabolites; crosses placenta, breast milk

INTERACTIONS
Drug/Lab Test
False negative: occult blood, urine bilirubin, leukocyte determination

NURSING CONSIDERATIONS
Assess:
- I&O ratio; urine pH (acidification)
- Ascorbic acid levels throughout treatment if continued deficiency is suspected
- Nutritional status: citrus fruits, vegetables
- Inj sites for inflammation
- Thrombophlebitis if receiving large dose
- **Pregnancy/breastfeeding:** use only recommended dietary allowances in pregnancy, breastfeeding

Evaluate:
- **Therapeutic response:** absence of anorexia, irritability, pallor, joint pain, hyperkeratosis, petechiae, poor wound healing

Teach patient/family:
- Necessary foods to include in diet, such as citrus fruits
- That smoking decreases vit C levels; not to exceed prescribed dose; that excesses will be excreted in urine, except when taking timed-release forms

V

vitamin E (otc)
Aquasol E
Func. class.: Vit E
Chem. class.: Fat soluble

ACTION: Needed for digestion and metabolism of polyunsaturated fats; decreases platelet aggregation, blood clot formation; promotes normal growth and development of muscle tissue, prostaglandin synthesis

USES: Vit E deficiency, impaired fat absorption, hemolytic anemia in premature neonates, prevention of retrolental fibroplasia, sickle cell anemia, supplement for malabsorption syndrome

CONTRAINDICATIONS

IV use in infants
Precautions: Pregnancy, anemia, breastfeeding, hypoprothrombinemia

DOSAGE AND ROUTES
Deficiency
• **Adult: PO** 60-75 units/day
• **Child: PO** 1 unit/kg/day (malabsorption)
Prevention of deficiency
• **Adult: PO** 30 units/day; **TOP** apply to affected areas
• **Infant: PO** 5 units/day
Available forms: Caps 100, 200, 400, 500, 600, 1000 units; tabs 100, 200, 400 units; drops 15 mg/0.3 mL; chew tabs 400 units; ointment; cream; lotion; oil
Administer:
PO route
• Administer with or after meals
• Chew chewable tabs well
• Sol may be dropped in mouth or mixed with food
• Store in tight, light-resistant container
Topical route
• To moisturize dry skin

SIDE EFFECTS
CNS: Headache, fatigue
CV: Increased risk for thrombophlebitis
EENT: Blurred vision
GI: Nausea, cramps, diarrhea
GU: Gonadal dysfunction
INTEG: Sterile abscess, contact dermatitis
META: Altered metabolism of hormones (thyroid, pituitary, adrenal), altered immunity

MS: Weakness

PHARMACOKINETICS
PO: Metabolized in liver, excreted in bile

INTERACTIONS
Increase: action of oral anticoagulants
Decrease: absorption—cholestyramine, colestipol, mineral oil, sucralfate

NURSING CONSIDERATIONS
Assess:
• Nutritional status: wheat germ; dark green, leafy vegetables; nuts; eggs; liver; vegetable oils; dairy products; cereals
• **Pregnancy/breastfeeding:** use only recommended dietary allowances in pregnancy, breastfeeding
Evaluate:
• **Therapeutic response:** absence of hemolytic anemia, adequate vit E levels, improvement in skin lesions, decreased edema
Teach patient/family:
• About the necessary foods for diet
• To omit dose if missed
• To avoid vitamin supplements unless directed by prescriber

⚠ HIGH ALERT

vorapaxar (Rx)
(vor′a-pax′ar)
Zontivity
Func. class.: Platelet aggregation inhibitor

ACTION: Antagonizes the protease-activated receptor-1 (PAR-1) expressed on platelets

USES: Secondary myocardial infarction prophylaxis or stroke prophylaxis or thrombosis prophylaxis for reduction of thrombotic cardiovascular events in patients with a history of myocardial infarction or with peripheral arterial disease

CONTRAINDICATIONS

Black Box Warning: Bleeding, intracranial bleeding, stroke

Precautions: Breastfeeding, coronary artery bypass graft surgery (CABG), geriatric patients, hepatic disease, labor, obstetric delivery, pregnancy, renal impairment, surgery

DOSAGE AND ROUTES
• **Adult: PO** 2.08 mg once daily with aspirin and/or clopidogrel
Available forms: Tab 2.08 mg
Administer:
• May be administered without regard to food
• May be given with clopidogrel in addition to ASA
• Give missed dose as soon as possible unless almost time for next scheduled dose, do not double

SIDE EFFECTS
HEMA: Bleeding
CNS: Depression, intracranial bleeding
EENT: Retinal changes, diplopia, epistaxis
INTEG: Rash
GI: GI bleed, melena
GU: Hematuria, rectal hemorrhage

PHARMACOKINETICS
Within 1 week of treatment reaches ≥80% inhibition of thrombin receptor, half-life is 8 days, protein binding 99%, primarily eliminated feces; peak 1 hr

INTERACTIONS
Increase: bleeding risk—anticoagulants, aspirin, NSAIDs, other platelet inhibitors, SSRIs, rifampin, SNRIs, thrombolytics, ethyl estradiol, calcium channel blockers
Decrease: vorapaxar effect—CYP3A inducers (carBAMazepine, phenytoin, rifAMPin)
Increase: vorapaxor effect—CYP3A4 inhibitors (clarithromycin, indinavir, itraconazole, ketoconazole, nefazodone, nelfinavir, posaconazole, ritonavir, saquinavir, teleprivar)

Drug/Herb
Decrease: vorapaxar level—St. John's wort; avoid concurrent use

NURSING CONSIDERATIONS
Assess:

Black Box Warning: For bleeding, intracranial bleeding/stroke during treatment; bleeding should be suspected in hypotension in those who have recently undergone surgery, coronary angiography, (PCI), CABG; avoid products that increase bleeding risk (salicylates, NSAIDs, SSRIs, SNRIs); avoid use in liver failure

• **Pregnancy/breastfeeding:** do not use in pregnancy; do not breastfeed, excretion unknown
Evaluate:
• **Therapeutic response:** absence of MI, stroke
Teach patient/family:
• To report any unusual bruising, bleeding to prescriber; that it may take longer to stop bleeding; that no true antidote exists and that there is an increased bleeding risk for 4 wk after last dose
• To take without regard to food
• To inform all providers that this product is being used; not to use OTC, prescription, or herbal products without approval of prescriber
• Not to breastfeed; to report if pregnancy is planned or suspected do not use in pregnancy
• To take as prescribed with aspirin or clopidogrel; not to use alone; not to discontinue without prescriber approval

---

voriconazole (Rx)
(vohr-i-kahn′a-zol)
Vfend, Vfend IV
Func. class.: Antifungal, systemic
Chem. class.: Triazole derivative

Do not confuse:
Vfend/Venofer

ACTION: Inhibits fungal ⍉ CYP450-mediation demethylation; needed for biosynthesis; causes leakage from cell membrane

USES: Invasive aspergillosis, serious fungal infections (*Candida* sp.,

---

Side effects: *italics* = common; red = life-threatening

Scedosporium apiospermum, Fusarium sp., *Monosporium apiospermum*)

CONTRAINDICATIONS
Pregnancy, breastfeeding, children, hypersensitivity, severe bone marrow depression, severe hepatic disease

Precautions: Renal disease (IV); ✖️☯️❀ patients of Asian/African descent; cardiomyopathy, cholestasis, chemotherapy, lactase deficiency, visual disturbances, renal failure, pancreatitis, QT prolongation, hypokalemia; ventricular dysrhythmias, torsades de pointes

DOSAGE AND ROUTES
Esophageal candidiasis
• **Adult/geriatric/child ≥12 yr and ≥40 kg: PO/IV** 200 mg q12hr; **<40 kg,** 100 mg q12hr

• **Child 2-12 yr; 12-14 yr <50 kg:** IV 4 mg/kg q12hr; minimum treatment 14 days, ≥7 days after resolution of symptoms

Candidemia of the skin, kidney, bladder wall, abdomen (nonneutropenic patients)
• **Adult/child ≥12 yr:** IV loading dose 6 mg/kg q12hr × 24 hr, then 3-4 mg/kg q12hr × ≥14 days and ≥7 days after resolution of symptoms; **PO** after loading dose **>40 kg** 200 mg q12hr × ≥14 days and ≥7 days after resolution of symptoms; **<40 kg** 100 mg q12hr × ≥14 days and ≥7 days after resolution of symptoms

Invasive aspergillosis
• **Adult/adolescent:** IV 6 mg/kg q12hr (loading dose), then 4 mg/kg q12hr, may reduce to 3 mg/kg q12hr if intolerable

• **Child 12-14 yr ≥50 kg; ≥15 yr:** IV: 6 mg/kg q12hr × 2, then 4 mg/kg q12hr. Continue IV ≥7 days, switch to PO when able

• Child 12-14 yr, < 50 kg and

• **Child 2-11:** IV 9 mg/kg/dose q12hr on day 1, followed by 8 mg/kg/dose q12hr

• **Child >12 yr, ≥40 kg: PO** loading dose 400 mg bid on day 1, then 200 mg bid × ≤6 mo

• **Child >12 yr, <40 kg: PO** loading dose 200 mg bid on day 1, then 100 mg bid × ≤6 mo

Renal dose
• **Adult: PO** CCr <50 mL/min, use orally only

Hepatic dose
• **Adult: PO/IV** (Child-Pugh Class A or B) standard loading dose, then 50% of maintenance dose; (Child-Pugh class C) avoid use

Available forms: Tabs 50, 200 mg; powder for inj, lyophilized 200 mg, powder for oral susp 45 g (40 mg/mL after reconstitution)

Administer:
PO route
• **Oral susp:** tap bottle; add 46 mL of water to bottle; shake well; remove cap; push bottle adapter into neck of bottle; replace cap; write expiration date (14 days); shake before each use; give using oral dispenser supplied, 1 hr before or after meals; tabs and susp may be interchanged

• Store at room temperature (powder, tabs)

Intermittent IV INFUSION route
• Product only after C&S confirms organism and product needed to treat condition; make sure product used only in life-threatening infections

• **Reconstitute** powder with 19 mL water for inj to 10 mg/mL; shake until dissolved

• **Further dilute** with NS, LR, D_5W by calculating dosing volume, infuse over 1-2 hr at concentration of ≤5 mg/mL; do not admix with other products

Y-site compatibilities: Acyclovir, alfentanil, allopurinol, amifostine, amikacin, aminocaproic acid, aminophylline, amiodarone, amphotericin B liposome, ampicillin, ampicillin/sulbactam, anidulafungin, azithromycin, aztreonam, bivalirudin, bleomycin, bumetanide, buprenorphine, butorphanol, calcium acetate/chloride/gluconate, CARBOplatin, carmustine, caspofungin, ceFAZolin, cefotaxime, cefoTEtan, cefOXitin, cefTAZidime, ceftizoxime, cefTRIAXone, chloramphenicol, chlorproMAZINE, cimetidine, ciprofloxacin, cisatracurium, CISplatin, clindamycin, cyclophosphamide, cytarabine, dacarbazine, DACTINomycin, DAPTOmycin, DAUNOrubicin, dexamethasone, dexmedetomidine, dexrazoxane, digoxin, diltiaZEM, diphenhydrAMINE,

DOBUTamine, DOCEtaxel, dolasetron, DOPamine, doripenem, doxacurium, doxycycline, droperidol, enalaprilat, ePHEDrine, EPINEPHrine, epirubicin, ertapenem, erythromycin, esmolol, etoposide, etoposide phosphate, famotidine, fenoldopam, fentaNYL, fluconazole, fludarabine, fluorouracil, foscarnet, fosphenytoin, furosemide, ganciclovir, gemcitabine, gentamicin, glycopyrrolate, granisetron, haloperidol, heparin, hydrALAZINE, hydrocortisone, ifosfamide, imipenem/cilastatin, inamrinone, insulin, irinotecan, isoproterenol, ketorolac, labetalol, leucovorin, levoFLOXacin, lidocaine, linezolid, LORazepam, magnesium sulfate, mannitol, mechlorethamine, melphalan, meperidine, meropenem, mesna, metaraminol, methohexital, methotrexate, methyldopate, methylPREDNISolone, metoclopramide, metoprolol, metroNIDAZOLE, midazolam, milrinone, mitoMYcin, morphine, nafcillin, nalbuphine, naloxone, niCARdipine, nitroglycerin, norepinephrine, octreotide, ondansetron, oxaliplatin, oxytocin, PACLitaxel, pamidronate, pancuronium, pentamidine, pentazocine, PENTobarbital, PHENobarbital, phentolamine, phenylephrine, piperacillin/tazobactam, potassium chloride/phosphates, procainamide, promethazine, propranolol, quinupristin/dalfopristin, remifentanil, rocuronium, sodium acetate/bicarbonate/phosphates, streptozocin, succinylcholine, SUFentanil, tacrolimus, teniposide, theophylline, thiotepa, ticarcillin/clavulanate, tirofiban, tobramycin, topotecan, trimethobenzamide, trimethoprim/sulfamethoxazole, vancomycin, vasopressin, vecuronium, verapamil, vinBLAStine, vinCRIStine, vinorelbine, zidovudine

SIDE EFFECTS

CNS: *Headache,* paresthesias, peripheral neuropathy, *hallucinations,* suicidal ideation, dizziness, fever, suicidal ideation, Guillian-Barre' syndrome

CV: Tachycardia, hypo/hypertension, vasodilation, peripheral edema
EENT: *Blurred vision,* eye hemorrhage, visual disturbances
GI: *Nausea, vomiting, anorexia, diarrhea,* cramps, hemorrhagic gastroenteritis, acute hepatic failure, hepatitis, intestinal perforation, pancreatitis
GU: *Hypokalemia,* azotemia, renal tubular necrosis, permanent renal impairment, anuria, oliguria
HEMA: Anemia, thrombocytopenia
INTEG: *Burning, irritation,* pain, necrosis at inj site with extravasation, dermatitis, *rash,* photosensitivity
MISC: cough, dyspnea, URI
SYST: Stevens-Johnson syndrome, toxic epidermal necrolysis, sepsis; melanoma, photosensitivity reactions

PHARMACOKINETICS

By CYP3A4, CYP2C9 enzymes; max serum concentration 1-2 hr after dosing; eliminated via hepatic metabolism; protein binding 58%; elimination half-life 6 hr (dose dependent)

INTERACTIONS

Increase: effects of benzodiazepines, calcium channel blockers, cycloSPORINE, ergots, HMG-CoA reductase inhibitors, pimozide, quiNIDine, prednisoLONE, sirolimus, sulfonylureas, tacrolimus, vinca alkaloids, warfarin, rifabutin, proton pump inhibitors, NNRTIs, protease inhibitors, phenytoin
Increase: nephrotoxicity—other nephrotoxic antibiotics (aminoglycosides, CISplatin, vancomycin, cycloSPORINE, polymyxin B)
Increase: hypokalemia—corticosteroids, digoxin, skeletal muscle relaxants, thiazides
Increase: QT prolongation—class IA/III antidysrhythmics, some phenothiazines, β agonists, local anesthetics, tricyclics, haloperidol, chloroquine, droperidol,

pentamidine; CYP3A4 inhibitors (amiodarone, clarithromycin, erythromycin, telithromycin, troleandomycin), arsenic trioxide; CYP3A4 substrates (methadone, pimozide, QUEtiapine, quiNIDine, risperiDONE, ziprasidone)

Drug/Herb

• Do not use with St. John's wort

Drug/Food

• Avoid use with high-fat meals, take 1 hr before or after meal

Drug/Lab Test

Increase: AST/ALT, alk phos, creatinine, bilirubin

Decrease: HB/Hct, platelets, WBC

NURSING CONSIDERATIONS

Assess:

• **Vitals:** VS q15-30min during first infusion; note changes in pulse, B/P

• **Renal:** I&O ratio; watch for decreasing urinary output, change in specific gravity; discontinue product to prevent permanent damage to renal tubules

• **Blood studies:** CBC, potassium, sodium, calcium, magnesium, q2wk; BUN, creatinine weekly

• Weight weekly; if weight increases >2 lb/wk, edema is present; renal damage should be considered

• **Renal toxicity:** increasing BUN, serum creatinine; if BUN is >40 mg/dL or if serum creatinine >3 mg/dL, product may be discontinued or dosage reduced

• **Hepatotoxicity:** increasing AST, ALT, alk phos, bilirubin, baseline and periodically

• **Allergic reaction:** dermatitis, rash; product should be discontinued, antihistamines (mild reaction) or EPINEPHrine (severe reaction) administered

• **Hypokalemia:** anorexia, drowsiness, weakness, decreased reflexes, dizziness, increased urinary output, increased thirst, paresthesias

• **Ototoxicity:** tinnitus (ringing, roaring in ears), vertigo, loss of hearing (rare); visual disturbance

• **QT prolongation:** ECG, ejection fraction; assess for chest pain, palpitations, dyspnea

• **Pregnancy/breastfeeding:** do not use in pregnancy, may cause fetal harm; do not breastfeed

Evaluate:

• **Therapeutic response:** decreased fever, malaise, rash, negative C&S for infecting organism

Teach patient/family:

• That long-term therapy may be needed to clear infection (2 wk-3 mo, depending on type of infection)

• To notify prescriber of bleeding, bruising, soft-tissue swelling, dark urine, persistent nausea or diarrhea, headache, rash, yellow skin/eyes

• Take 1 hr before or after meal (PO)

• Not to drive at night because of vision changes

• Avoid strong, direct sunlight

• Women of childbearing age should use effective contraceptive, do not breastfeed

---

vortioxetine (Rx)

(vor'tye-ox'e-teen)

Brintellix

Func. class.: Antidepressant

Chem. class.: Serotonin modulator

Do not confuse:

Brintellix/ Brilinta

ACTION: Reuptake inhibition at the serotonin transporter and agonist, or antagonist effects at serotonin receptors

USES: Major depressive disorder in adults

CONTRAINDICATIONS

Hypersensitivity, MAOI therapy

Precautions: Pregnancy, breastfeeding, seizure disorder, bipolar disorder,

---

hyponatremia, hypovolemia, abrupt discontinuation, anticoagulant therapy, bleeding, closed-angle glaucoma, geriatric patients, hepatic disease

Black Box Warning: Children, suicidal ideation

DOSAGE AND ROUTES
• **Adult: PO** 10 mg/day, may start with 5 mg/day initially, increase to 20 mg/day as tolerated, max 20 mg/day; poor metabolizers of CYP2D6 max 10 mg/day
Available forms: Tabs 5, 10, 20 mg
Administer: Without regard to food

SIDE EFFECTS
CNS: Flushing, mania, serotonin syndrome, vertigo, dizziness, suicidal attempts
GI: *Nausea, diarrhea,* dyspnea, constipation, vomiting, flatulence
GU: Impotence, *ejaculation/orgasm dysfunction*
INTEG: Pruritus
SYST: Serotonin syndrome, neonatal abstinence syndrome, angioedema, pulmonary hypertension of the newborn, SIADH

PHARMACOKINETICS
Protein binding 98%, excreted in urine (59%), feces (26%)

INTERACTIONS
Increase: effect of tricyclics; use cautiously
Increase: serotonin syndrome—serotonin receptor agonists, SSRIs, traMADol, lithium, MAOIs, traZODone, SNRIs (venlafaxine, DULoxetine)
Increase: bleeding risk—NSAIDs, salicylates, thrombolytics, anticoagulants, antiplatelets
Increase: CNS effects—barbiturates, sedative/hypnotics, other CNS depressants
Decrease: vortioxetine levels—carBAMazepine
Drug/Herb:
Increase: serotonin syndrome—St. John's wort

NURSING CONSIDERATIONS
Assess:

Black Box Warning: Mental status: mood, sensorium, affect, suicidal tendencies, increase in psychiatric symptoms, depression, panic

• **Serotonin syndrome:** increased heart rate, sweating, dilated pupils, tremors, twitching, hyperthermia, agitation
• Alcohol consumption; if alcohol is consumed, hold dose until AM
• **Sexual dysfunction:** impotence
• **Pregnancy/breastfeeding:** effects not known
Evaluate:
• **Therapeutic response:** decreased depression
Teach patient/family:
• That therapeutic effect may take several weeks
• That decrease in libido or impotence may occur
• To use caution when driving, performing other activities that require alertness because of drowsiness, dizziness, blurred vision; to report signs, symptoms of bleeding
• To avoid alcohol, other CNS depressants

Black Box Warning: That suicidal ideas, behaviors may occur in children or young adults

• About the effects of **serotonin syndrome:** nausea/vomiting, tremors; if symptoms occur, to discontinue immediately, notify prescriber
• To notify prescriber if pregnant, planning to become pregnant, or breastfeeding

---

vosoritide (Rx)
(voe-SOR-i-tide)
Voxzogo
Func. class.: Misc. agent affecting bone structure

USES:
Increase linear growth in pediatric patients with achondroplasia

DOSAGE AND ROUTES
• **Child:** SUBCUT based on body weight

Available forms: Lyophilized powder for injection 0.4 mg, 0.56 mg, 1.2 mg single-dose vial

USES: Hereditary transthyretin amyloidosis–associated polyneuropathy

DOSAGE AND ROUTES
• **Adults:** SUBCUT 25 mg q3mo, given by a health care professional

Available forms: Prefilled syringe solution for injection 25 mg/0.5 mL

---

vutrisiran (Rx)
(VUE-tri-SIR-an)
Amvuttra
Func. class.: Polyneuropathy agent

⚠ HIGH ALERT

warfarin (Rx)

(war´far-in)

Jantoven

Func. class.: Anticoagulant, vitamin K antagonist

Chem. class.: Coumarin derivative

Do not confuse:
Cardura/Avandia
Jantoven/Janumet/Januvia

ACTION: Interferes with blood clotting by indirect means; depresses hepatic synthesis of vit K–dependent coagulation factors (II, VII, IX, X)

USES: Antiphospholipid antibody syndrome, arterial thromboembolism prophylaxis, DVT, MI prophylaxis, after MI, stroke prophylaxis, thrombosis prophylaxis, pulmonary embolism

CONTRAINDICATIONS

Pregnancy, breastfeeding, hypersensitivity, hemophilia, leukemia with bleeding, peptic ulcer disease, thrombocytopenic purpura, hepatic disease (severe), malignant hypertension, subacute bacterial endocarditis, acute nephritis, blood dyscrasias, eclampsia, preeclampsia, hemorrhagic tendencies; surgery of CNS, eye; traumatic surgery with large open surface, bleeding tendencies of GI/GU/respiratory tract, stroke, aneurysms, pericardial effusion, spinal puncture, major regional/lumbar block anesthesia

Black Box Warning: Bleeding

Precautions: Geriatric patients, alcoholism, HF, debilitated patients, trauma, indwelling catheters, severe hypertension, active infections, protein C deficiency, polycythemia vera, vasculitis, severe diabetes, ☜ Asian patients (CYP2C9), protein C, S deficiency or VKORC1 AA genotype

DOSAGE AND ROUTES–NTI

• **Adult: PO** 2-5 mg/day × 2-4 days, then titrated to INR/PT

• **Adolescent/child/infant: PO** 0.2 mg/kg/day × 2 days titrated to INR, max 10 mg

Available forms: Tabs 1, 2, 2.5, 3, 4, 5, 6, 7.5, 10 mg

Administer:

PO route

• Obtain coagulation studies—INR, PT—before use; INR level should be 2.0-3.0

• At same time each day to maintain steady blood levels without regard to food; food decreases rate but not extent of absorption; do not change brands

• Tabs whole or crushed

• Avoiding all IM inj that may cause bleeding

• Store in tight container

SIDE EFFECTS

GI: Nausea, cramps, calciphylaxis

GU: Hematuria

HEMA: Hemorrhage, agranulocytosis, leukopenia, eosinophilia, anemia, ecchymosis, petechiae

INTEG: *Rash,* dermal necrosis

MISC: Fever

MS: Bone fractures

PHARMACOKINETICS

PO: Onset 12-24 hr, peak 1½-4 days, duration 3-5 days, effective half-life 20-60 hr; metabolized in liver; excreted in urine, feces (active/inactive metabolites); crosses placenta, 99% bound to plasma proteins

INTERACTIONS

Increase: warfarin action—allopurinol, amiodarone, azithromycin, chloral hydrate, chloramphenicol, cimetidine, clofibrate, cotrimoxazole, COX-2 selective inhibitors, dextrothyroxine, diflunisal,

W

disulfiram, erythromycin, ethacrynic acids, furosemide, glucagon, heparin, HMG-CoA reductase inhibitors, indomethacin, isoniazid, levoFLOXacin, mefenamic acid, metroNIDAZOLE, miFEPRIStone, NSAIDs, oxyphenbutazone, penicillins, phenylbutazone, quiNIDine, quinolone antiinfectives, RU-486, salicylates, sulfinpyrazone, sulfonamides, sulindac, SSRIs, steroids, thrombolytics, thyroid, tricyclics

Increase/decrease: effectiveness—assess for use of products that may increase or decrease effect

Increase: toxicity—oral sulfonylureas, phenytoin

Decrease: warfarin action—aprepitant, azaTHIOprine, barbiturates, bile acid sequestrants, bosentan, carBAMazepine, dicloxacillin, estrogens, ethchlorvynol, factor IX/VIIa, griseofulvin, nafcillin, oral contraceptives, phenytoin, rifAMPin, sucralfate, sulfaSALAzine, vit K, vit K foods

Drug/Herb

Increase: risk for bleeding—anise, chamomile, dong quai, evening primrose, feverfew, fish oil, garlic, ginger, ginkgo, ginseng, horse chestnut, licorice, melatonin, red yeast rice, saw palmetto

Decrease: anticoagulant effect—coenzyme Q10, St. John's wort

Drug/Lab Test

Increase: T_3 uptake, LFTs, INR, PT, PTT

NURSING CONSIDERATIONS
Assess:

Black Box Warning: **Blood studies** (Hct, PT, platelets, occult blood in stools) q3mo; INR: in hospital daily after 2nd or 3rd dose; when in therapeutic range (2-3) for 2 consecutive days, monitor 2-3× wk for 1-2 wk, then less frequently, depending on stability of INR results; *Outpatient:* monitor every few days until stable dose, then periodically thereafter, depending on stability of INR results, usually at least monthly

Black Box Warning: **Bleeding:** bleeding gums, petechiae, ecchymosis, black tarry stools, hematuria, occult bleeding (cerebral, intraabdominal; fatal hemorrhage can occur; do not use in uncontrolled bleeding

• Fever, skin rash, urticaria
• **Pregnancy/breastfeeding:** do not use in pregnancy; use effective contraception during and for 1 mo after final dose; cautious use in breastfeeding

Evaluate:

• **Therapeutic response:** decrease in deep venous thrombosis, absence of pulmonary embolism

Teach patient/family:

• To avoid OTC preparations that may cause serious product interactions unless directed by prescriber; to avoid alcohol, herbs, supplements
• To carry emergency ID identifying product taken
• About the importance of compliance with exams and doses

Black Box Warning: **Bleeding:** to report any signs of bleeding: gums, nosebleed, under skin, urine, stools; to use soft-bristle toothbrush to avoid bleeding gums; to use electric razor

• To avoid hazardous activities (e.g., football, hockey, skiing), dangerous work that can induce bleeding episodes
• To inform all health care providers of anticoagulant intake
• To take exactly as prescribed; dosage changes are common for desired effect; not to skip, double doses; take missed dose when remembered
• To eat a diet that is not varied; several foods contain vitamin K and can alter warfarin effect
• To report to prescriber fever, rash, trouble breathing
• That continuing follow-up exams and lab work will be needed

TREATMENT OF OVERDOSE:
Administer vit K

---

witch hazel (OTC)
(wich ha′zel)
A.E.R Witch Hazel, Medi Pads,
Preparation H Wipes
Func. class.: Astringents

USES: Anal/vaginal irritation

CONTRAINDICATIONS
None known

DOSAGE AND ROUTES
• **Adult/child ≥12 yr:** Topical, apply to affected area ≤6 times/day

zafirlukast (Rx)

(za-feer'loo-cast)

Accolate

Func. class.: Bronchodilator

Chem. class.: Leukotriene receptor antagonist

Do not confuse:

Accolate/Accupril/Accutane

ACTION: Antagonizes the contractile action of leukotrienes (LTD_4, LTE_4) in airway smooth muscle; inhibits bronchoconstriction caused by antigens

USES: Prophylaxis and chronic treatment of asthma in adults/children >5 yr

CONTRAINDICATIONS

Hypersensitivity, hepatic encephalopathy

Precautions: Pregnancy, breastfeeding, children, geriatric patients, hepatic disease, Churg-Strauss syndrome, acute bronchospasm

DOSAGE AND ROUTES

• **Adult/child ≥12 yr:** PO 20 mg bid
• **Child 5-11 yr:** PO 10 mg bid

Available forms: Tabs 10, 20 mg

Administer:

• 1 hr before or 2 hr after meals
• Protect from light

SIDE EFFECTS

CNS: Headache, dizziness, suicidal ideation, insomnia, fever

GI: Nausea, diarrhea, abdominal pain, vomiting, dyspepsia, hepatic failure, hepatitis

HEMA: Agranulocytosis

OTHER: Infections, pain, asthenia, myalgia, fever, increased ALT, urticaria, rash, angioedema

PHARMACOKINETICS

Rapidly absorbed, peak 3 hr, 99% protein binding (albumin), extensively metabolized, inhibits CYP2C9 and 3A4 enzyme systems, excreted in feces, clearance reduced in geriatric patients, hepatic impairment, half-life 10 hr

INTERACTIONS

Increase: plasma levels of zafirlukast—aspirin, acetaminophen

Increase: bleeding risk—warfarin, monitor INR closely

Decrease: plasma levels of zafirlukast—erythromycin, theophylline

Drug/Food

Decrease: bioavailability

Drug/Lab

Increase: ALT

NURSING CONSIDERATIONS

Assess:

• **Churg-Strauss syndrome** (rare): eosinophilia, vasculitic rash, worsening pulmonary symptoms, cardiac complications, neuropathy; may be caused by reducing oral corticosteroids

• **Respiratory status:** Respiratory rate, rhythm, depth; auscultate lung fields bilaterally; notify prescriber of abnormalities; not to be used for acute bronchospasm in acute asthma

• **Hepatic dysfunction:** right upper quadrant abdominal pain, nausea/vomiting, fatigue, lethargy, pruritus, jaundice, and flulike symptoms, discontinue; monitor LFTs; should be measured immediately and the patient managed if needed

• **Mental status:** depression, suicidal ideation, insomnia; product may need to be discontinued

• **Pregnancy/breastfeeding:** use only if clearly needed; do not breastfeed, excreted in breast milk

Evaluate:

• **Therapeutic response:** ability to breathe more easily

Teach patient/family:

• To check OTC medications, current prescription medications that may increase stimulation, do not stop other asthma medications unless instructed to do so

• To avoid hazardous activities because dizziness may occur

• That if GI upset occurs, to take product with 8 oz water; to take 1-2 hr after a meal; to avoid taking with food if possible because absorption may be decreased

• To notify prescriber of nausea, vomiting, diarrhea, abdominal pain, fatigue, jaundice, anorexia, flulike symptoms (hepatic dysfunction)
• Not to use for acute asthma episodes
• To take even if symptom free
• Not to take if breastfeeding

⚠ HIGH ALERT

zaleplon (Rx)
(zal'eh-plon)
Func. class.: Hypnotic, non-benzodiazepine
Chem. class.: Pyrazolopyrimidine

Controlled Substance Schedule IV

Do not confuse:
Zaleplon/Zelapron/Zemplar/Zolpidem

ACTION: Binds selectively to omega-1 receptor of the $GABA_A$, benzodiazepine receptor complex; results are sedation, hypnosis, skeletal muscle relaxation, anticonvulsant activity, anxiolytic action

USES: Insomnia (short-term treatment), up to 30 days

CONTRAINDICATIONS
Hypersensitivity, severe hepatic disease

Black Box Warning: Complex sleep-related behaviors

Precautions: Pregnancy, breastfeeding, children <15 yr, geriatric patients, respiratory/renal/hepatic disease, psychosis, angioedema, depression, CNS depression, suicidal ideation, sleep apnea; salicylate, tartrazine dye, hypersensitivity, opioid use, drug dependency

DOSAGE AND ROUTES
• **Adult:** PO 10 mg at bedtime; may increase to 20 mg if needed; 5 mg may be used in low-weight persons, use for only 7-10 days

• **Geriatric/hepatic dose:** PO 5 mg at bedtime; may increase if needed
Available forms: Caps 5, 10 mg
Administer:
• Immediately before bedtime for sleeplessness
• On empty stomach for fast onset
• Store in tight container in cool environment

SIDE EFFECTS

CNS: *Lethargy, drowsiness, daytime sedation,* dizziness, confusion, anxiety, amnesia, depersonalization, hallucinations, hyperesthesia, paresthesia, somnolence, tremors, vertigo, complex sleep-related reactions: sleep driving, sleep eating
CV: Chest pain, peripheral edema
EENT: Vision change, ear/eye pain, hyperacusis, parosmia
GI: Nausea, abdominal pain, constipation, anorexia, colitis, dyspepsia, dry mouth
MISC: Asthenia, fever, headache, myalgia, dysmenorrhea
MS: Myalgia, back pain, arthritis
RESP: Bronchitis
SYST: Severe allergic reactions

PHARMACOKINETICS
Rapid onset, metabolized by liver extensively, excreted by kidneys (inactive metabolites), half-life 1 hr, onset, peak 1 hr, duration 3-4 hr

INTERACTIONS
Increase: effect of zaleplon—cimetidine, use lower dose
Decrease: zaleplon bioavailability—CYP3A4 inducers (carBAMazepine, phenytoin, rifAMPin)
Increase: CNS depression—CNS depressants, monitor closely
Increase: respiratory depression, death—opioids, avoid concurrent use, or use lower dose of both
Drug/Food
• Prolonged absorption, sleep onset reduced: high-fat/heavy meal
Drug/Lab
Increase: lipids

Z

NURSING CONSIDERATIONS
Assess:

• **Mental status:** mood, sensorium, affect, memory (long, short term), excessive sedation, impaired coordination, aggression, confusion, hallucinations
• **Sleep disorder:** type of sleep problem: falling asleep, staying asleep

Black Box Warning: **Complex sleep-related behaviors:** Assess for previous complex sleep-related behaviors, and do not use with these patients, sleep eating, driving, walking, all while not fully awake

• **Respiratory status:** Any patient with compromised respiratory system is more prone to respiratory depression
• **Beers:** avoid in older adults with delirium or at high risk for delirium; potential for worsening or inducing delirium
Evaluate:
• **Therapeutic response:** ability to sleep at night, decreased amount of early morning awakening
Teach patient/family:
• To avoid driving or other activities requiring alertness until product is stabilized
• To avoid alcohol ingestion, advise prescriber of all other OTC/Rx/herbals taken

Black Box Warning: That product may cause memory problems, dependence (if used for longer periods of time), changes in behavior/thinking, complex sleep-related behaviors (sleep eating/driving)

• To report continuing insomnia even with product
• That product is for short-term use only and when patient can sleep ≥4 hr, dependence may occur if used for extended periods
• To take immediately before going to bed
• Not to ingest a high-fat/heavy meal before taking
• To be aware that allergic reactions may occur
• **Pregnancy/breastfeeding:** Identify if pregnancy is planned or suspected or if breastfeeding

---

zanamivir (Rx)
(zan′ah-mih-veer)
Relenza Diskhaler
Func. class.: Antiviral
Chem. class.: Neuraminidase inhibitor

USES: Treatment of influenza types A and B for patients who have been symptomatic for ≤2 days, seasonal influenza prophylaxis

DOSAGE AND ROUTES
Treatment of influenza A and B
• **Adult/child >7 yr: INH** 2 inhalations (two 5-mg blisters) q12hr × 5 days; on the 1st day, 2 doses should be taken with at least 2 hr between doses
Prophylaxis of influenza A and B
• **Adult/child >5 yr: INH** 10 mg (2 inhalations) daily × household prophylaxis: 10 days, community outbreak: 28 days
Available forms: Blisters of powder for inhalation: 5 mg for Diskhaler

---

zidovudine (Rx)
(zye-doe′-vue-deen)
Retrovir
Func. class.: Antiretroviral
Chem. class.: Nucleoside reverse transcriptase inhibitor (NRTI)

Do not confuse:
Retrovir/ritonavir

ACTION: Inhibits replication of HIV-1 virus by incorporating into cellular DNA by viral reverse transcriptase, thereby terminating the cellular DNA chain

USES: Used in combination with at least 2 other antiretrovirals for HIV-1 infection, prevention of perinatal HIV

CONTRAINDICATIONS
Hypersensitivity
Precautions: Pregnancy, breastfeeding, children, granulocyte count <1000/mm³ or HB <9.5 g/dL, severe renal disease, obesity

---

Black Box Warning: Hepatotoxicity, anemia, lactic acidosis, myopathy, neutropenia

DOSAGE AND ROUTES
HIV with other antiretroviral agents
• **Adult/adolescents: PO** 300 mg bid or 200 mg tid; **IV INFUSION** 1 mg/kg over 1 hr q4hr. Initiate oral therapy as soon as possible

• **Child 4 wk to <18 yr: PO** max adult dose; **≥30 kg:** 300 mg bid or 200 mg tid; **9-29 kg: PO** 9 mg/kg bid or 6 mg/kg tid; **4-8 kg: PO** 12 mg/kg bid or 8 mg/kg tid

Perinatal (HIV) prophylaxis
• **Adult >14 wk pregnant:** 100 mg 5 times/day until start of labor

• **Pregnant females (intrapartum): IV INFUSION** 2 mg/kg over 1 hr, followed by 1 mg/kg/hr **IV CONT INFUSION** until clamping of the umbilical cord

• **Neonate ≥35 wk gestational age: IV** 3 mg/kg q12hr beginning as soon as possible after birth, convert to PO as soon as possible

Renal dose
• **Adult: PO** CCr ≥15 mL/min: no change; CCr <15 mL/min, 100 mg q8hr or 300 mg/day

• **Pediatric patients: PO** GFR ≥10 mL/min/1.73 m^2: no change; GFR <10 mL/min/1.73 m^2: reduce dose by 50%

Available forms: Caps 100; tabs 300 mg; inj 10 mg/mL; syrup 50 mg/5 mL

Administer:
PO route
• By mouth; capsules should be swallowed whole, without regard to meals

• Trimethoprim-sulfamethoxazole, pyrimethamine, or acyclovir as ordered to prevent opportunistic infections; if these products are given, watch for neurotoxicity

• Missed doses: Should be taken as soon as remembered unless close to next dosing time

• Store in cool environment; protect from light

Syrup:
• Use calibrated measuring device

Intermittent IV INFUSION route
• Latex is in vial stopper
• After diluting in D$_5$W to ≤4 mg/mL; give over 1 hr (adult), 30 min (neonate)
• Discard any unused portions
• Protect unopened product from light; use diluted sol within 24 hr room temperature, 48 hr refrigerated, do not use discolored solutions
• Use only until PO can be taken
• Do not use by direct, bolus, or rapid IV

Y-site compatibilities: Acyclovir, alemtuzumab, allopurinol, amifostine, amikacin, amphotericin B, amphotericin B cholesteryl, anidulafungin, argatroban, aztreonam, cefepime, cefTAZidime, cefTRIAXone, cimetidine, cisatracurium, clindamycin, dexamethasone, DOBUTamine, DOPamine, DOXOrubicin liposome, erythromycin, filgrastim, fluconazole, fludarabine, gentamicin, granisetron, heparin, imipenem-cilastatin, LORazepam, melphalan, metoclopramide, morphine, nafcillin, ondansetron, oxacillin, PACLitaxel, pentamidine, phenylephrine, piperacillin, piperacillin-tazobactam, potassium chloride, raNITIdine, remifentanil, sargramostim, tacrolimus, teniposide, thiotepa, tobramycin, trimethoprim-sulfamethoxazole, trimetrexate, vancomycin, vinorelbine, zoledronic acid

SIDE EFFECTS
CNS: *Fever, headache, malaise,* diaphoresis, *dizziness, insomnia,* paresthesia, somnolence, chills, tremors, twitching, anxiety, confusion, depression, lability, vertigo, loss of mental acuity, seizures, malaise

EENT: Taste change, hearing loss, photophobia

GI: *Nausea, vomiting, diarrhea, anorexia,* cramps, *dyspepsia, constipation,* dysphagia, *flatulence,* rectal bleeding, mouth ulcer, abdominal pain, hepatomegaly

GU: Dysuria, polyuria, urinary frequency, hesitancy

HEMA: Granulocytopenia, anemia, severe bone marrow suppression

INTEG: *Rash,* acne, pruritus, urticaria

MS: Myalgia, arthralgia, muscle spasm

RESP: Dyspnea, cough, wheezing

SYST: Lactic acidosis, Stevens-Johnson syndrome

Z

PHARMACOKINETICS

PO: Rapidly absorbed from GI tract, peak ½-1½ hr; IV peak infusions end; metabolized in liver (inactive metabolites), excreted by kidneys, protein binding 38%, half-life½-3 hr

INTERACTIONS

Increase: bone marrow depression—antineoplastics, radiation, ganciclovir, valGANciclovir, trimethoprim-sulfamethoxazole

Increase: zidovudine level—methadone, atovaquone, fluconazole, probenecid, trimethoprim, valproic acid; may need to reduce zidovudine dose

Increase: toxicity-fluconazole, probenecid

Decrease: zidovudine levels—clarithromycin, interferons, NRTIs, DOXOrubicin, ribavirin, stavudine; avoid concurrent use

Drug/Lab Test

Decrease: platelets, granulocytes

Increase: LFTs, amylase, CPK

NURSING CONSIDERATIONS

Assess:

• **HIV:** monitor for symptoms of HIV, baseline and throughout treatment

Black Box Warning: Bone marrow suppression: monitor blood counts q2wk; watch for decreasing granulocytes, HB; if low, therapy may have to be discontinued and restarted after hematologic recovery; blood transfusions may be required; viral load, CD4 counts, LFTs, plasma HIV RNA, serum creatinine/BUN at baseline and throughout treatment

Black Box Warning: Lactic acidosis, severe hepatomegaly with steatosis (rare): Obtain baseline LFTs; if elevated, discontinue; discontinue even if liver function tests are normal but lactic acidosis, hepatomegaly are present; may be fatal; more common in females, may develop dyspnea, tachypnea

Black Box Warning: Myopathy may occur with long-term use, assess for myalgia, arthralgia during long-term use

• **Lipoatrophy:** May occur, another treatment may be needed to prevent it

• **Hypersensitivity:** Do not use if previous serious hypersensitivity to this product, Stevens-Johnson syndrome may occur

• **Immune reconstitution syndrome:** Assess for rash, fever, lymphadenopathy, abdominal pain due to opportunistic infections

• Monitor lipid profile, blood glucose, hepatitis B serology, plasma hepatitis C RNA, serum cholesterol, pregnancy test, urinalysis, serum lipase, amylase

• **Pregnancy/breastfeeding:** register pregnant patients at the Antiretroviral Pregnancy Registry, 800-258-4263; do not breastfeed, excreted in breast milk, max suppression of virus should be attained before pregnancy is considered; to be used near delivery even if HIV RNA status is unknown

Evaluate:

• **Therapeutic response:** decreased viral load, increased CD4 counts, decreased symptoms of HIV

Teach patient/family:

• That GI complaints and insomnia resolve after 3-4 wk of treatment

• **HIV:** That repeat testing in 4-6 wk is needed due to risk of false positive if used in newborn

• **Hypersensitivity:** To report rashes, some reactions may be fatal

• That product is not a cure for AIDS but will control symptoms; that compliance with treatment is required

• To notify prescriber of sore throat, swollen lymph nodes, malaise, fever, shortness of breath because other infections may occur; to avoid crowds or people with known infections

• That patient is still infective, may pass AIDS virus on to others

• That follow-up visits must be continued because serious toxicity may occur; that blood counts must be done q2wk; that blood transfusions may be needed for severe anemia

• That product must be taken bid or tid around the clock to prevent variations in blood levels

• To notify prescriber of rash, nausea, vomiting, weakness

• That serious product interactions may occur if OTC products are ingested; to check with prescriber before taking aspirin, acetaminophen, indomethacin
• That other products may be necessary to prevent other infections
• To take without regard to meals
• Not to take other antiretrovirals except those prescribed
• That product may cause fainting or dizziness; to avoid driving or other hazardous tasks until response is known
• That redistribution of body fat may occur
• Not to breastfeed during treatment, that use during pregnancy reduces transmission to neonate

---

zinc (Rx, OTC)
Galzin
Func. class.: Trace element; nutritional supplement

ACTION: Needed for adequate healing, bone and joint development (23% zinc)

USES: Prevention of zinc deficiency, adjunct to vit A therapy
Unlabeled uses: Wound healing
Precautions: Pregnancy, parenteral; breastfeeding, neonates, hypocupremia, neonatal prematurity, renal disease

DOSAGE AND ROUTES
Dietary supplement (elemental zinc)
• **Adult/adolescent/pregnant female:** PO 11-13 mg/day
• **Adult/lactating female:** PO 12-14 mg/day × 12 mo
• **Adult/adolescent male ≥14 yr:** PO 11 mg/day
• **Adult female ≥19 yr:** PO 8 mg/day
• **Adolescent female ≥14 yr:** PO 9 mg/day
• **Child 9-13 yr:** PO 8 mg/day
• **Child 4-8 yr:** PO 5 mg/day
• **Child 1-3 yr:** PO 3 mg/day
• **Infant 7-12 mo:** PO 3 mg/day
• **Infant birth to 6 mo:** PO 2 mg/day (adequate intake)

Nutritional supplement (IV)
• **Adult:** 2.5-4 mg/day; may increase by 2 mg/day if needed
• **Child 1-5 yr:** IV 50 mcg/kg/day
Wound healing
• **Adult:** PO 50 mg tid until healed (elemental zinc)
Available forms: Tabs 66, 110, 220 mg; inj 1 mg/mL, 5 mg/mL; caps 25, 50 mg
Administer:
• With meals to decrease gastric upset; avoid dairy products

SIDE EFFECTS
GI: Nausea, vomiting, cramps, heartburn, ulcer formation
OVERDOSE: Diarrhea, rash, dehydration, restlessness

INTERACTIONS
Decrease: absorption of fluoroquinolones—tetracyclines
Drug/Food
Decrease: absorption of PO zinc—dairy products, caffeine

NURSING CONSIDERATIONS
Assess:
• **Zinc deficiency:** poor wound healing, absence of taste, smell, slowing growth
• Alkaline phosphatase, HDL monthly in long-term therapy
• Zinc levels during treatment, CBC
• **Pregnancy/breastfeeding:** use only if benefits outweigh fetal risk (IV); considered safe in breastfeeding
Evaluate:
• **Therapeutic response:** absence of zinc deficiency
Teach patient/family:
• That element must be taken for 2-3 mo to be effective
• To immediately report nausea, diarrhea, rash, severe vomiting, restlessness, abdominal pain, tarry stools

---

ziprasidone (Rx)
(zi-praz'ih-dohn)
Geodon, Zeldox ✦
Func. class.: Antipsychotic/neuroleptic
Chem. class.: Benzisoxazole derivative

ACTION: Unknown; may be mediated through both dopamine type 2 (D_2) and serotonin type 2 (5-HT_2) antagonism

USES: Schizophrenia, acute agitation, acute psychosis, bipolar disorder, mania, psychotic depression

CONTRAINDICATIONS

Breastfeeding, hypersensitivity, acute MI, heart failure, QT prolongation, breastfeeding, drugs that increase QT interval

Precautions: Pregnancy, children, geriatric patients, cardiac/renal/hepatic disease, breast cancer, diabetes, seizure disorders, AV block, CNS depression, abrupt discontinuation, agranulocytosis, ambient temperature increase, suicidal ideation, torsades de pointes, strenuous exercise, diuretics, diarrhea

Black Box Warning: Increased mortality in geriatric patients with dementia-related psychosis

DOSAGE AND ROUTES
Schizophrenia

• **Adult: PO** 20 mg bid with food, adjust dosage every 2 days upward to max of 80 mg bid; **IM** 10-20 mg; may give 10 mg q2hr; doses of 20 mg may be given q4hr; max 40 mg/day (acute episodes)

Acute mania/mixed episodes bipolar disorder

• **Adult: PO** 20-40 mg bid with food; increase ≥q2days as needed **maintenance as adjunct to lithium/valproate** 40-80 mg bid

Rapid control of agitation in schizophrenia

• **Adult: IM** 10-20 mg as needed, max 40 mg/day

Available forms: Caps 20, 40, 60, 80 mg; inj 20 mg/mL (after reconstituting) single-dose vials

Administer:
PO route

• Take cap whole and with food, with plenty of fluid at same time of day

• Reduced dose in geriatric patients
• Anticholinergic agent to be used for EPS
• Store in tight, light-resistant container
IM route
• Add 1.2 mL sterile water for inj to vial; shake vigorously until dissolved; do not admix; give only IM; give deeply in large muscle; do not use if particulates are present, keep patient recumbent for 30 min after injection
• Do not give over 3 consecutive days, switch to PO as soon as possible
• Store injection at room temperature, protect from light, after reconstituting may be stored at room temperature × 24 hr, 7 days refrigerated

SIDE EFFECTS

CNS: *EPS, pseudoparkinsonism, akathisia, dystonia, tardive dyskinesia; drowsiness, insomnia, agitation, anxiety, headache,* seizures, neuroleptic malignant syndrome, dizziness, tremors, facial droop

CV: Orthostatic hypotension, tachycardia, prolonged QT/QTc, hypertension, sudden death, heart failure (geriatric patients), torsades de pointes

HEMA: Agranulocytosis

EENT: Blurred vision, diplopia

ENDO: Hypoglycemia

GI: *Nausea,* vomiting, *anorexia, constipation,* jaundice, weight gain, diarrhea, dry mouth, abdominal pain

GU: Priapism

INTEG: Rash, injection-site pain, sweating, DRESS, Steven's Johnson Syndrome photosensitivity

RESP: Infection, cough

PHARMACOKINETICS

IM: Peak 60 min

PO: Peak 6-8 hr, extensively metabolized by liver to major active metabolite, plasma protein binding 99%, half-life 7 hr

INTERACTIONS

Increase: respiratory depression-opioids, avoid concurrent use

Increase: ziprasidone level-CYP3A4 inhibitors (ketoconazole, itraconazole); dose may need to be reduced

Increase: QT prolongation—class IA/III antidysrhythmics, some phenothiazines, β-agonists, local anesthetics, tricyclics, haloperidol, methadone, chloroquine, clarithromycin, droperidol, erythromycin, pentamidine, moxifloxacin

Increase: sedation—other CNS depressants, alcohol

Increase: hypotension—antihypertensives, monitor B/P

Increase: serotonin syndrome, neuroleptic malignant syndrome—SSRIs, SNRIs

Decrease: ziprasidone effect—carbamazepine, may need ziprasidone dose increased

Drug/Lab
Increase: lipids, glucose
Decrease: WBCs

NURSING CONSIDERATIONS
Assess:
• Mental status before initial administration, AIMS assessment

Black Box Warning: Assess geriatric patient with dementia closely; heart failure, sudden death have occurred; this product is not approved for the treatment of dementia-related psychosis in the elderly

• **DRESS:** Assess for rash, fever, swollen lymph nodes, product should be discontinued
• **Steven's Johnson Syndrome:** rash with fever, aches, blisters, swelling of face, discontinue product immediately
• **Seizures:** Seizures in those with seizure disorders, provide seizure precautions, seizure threshold is lowered
• Assess for metabolic syndrome (hyperglycemia, hypertension, increased cholesterol/lipids, increased BMI/abdominal obesity)
• Watch for suicidal thoughts/behaviors
• Bilirubin, CBC, LFTs, fasting blood glucose, cholesterol profile; potassium, magnesium when taken with loop/thiazide diuretics monthly, not to be used with electrolyte abnormalities
• B/P standing and lying; also pulse, respirations; take these q4hr during ini-

tial treatment; establish baseline before starting treatment; report drops of 30 mm Hg; watch for ECG changes; QT prolongation may occur; discontinue product if QTc >500 msec
• Dizziness, faintness, palpitations, tachycardia on rising, may be serious dysrthmia
• **EPS,** including akathisia (inability to sit still, no pattern to movements), tardive dyskinesia (bizarre movements of the jaw, mouth, tongue, extremities), pseudoparkinsonism (rigidity, tremors, pill rolling, shuffling gait)
• **Neuroleptic malignant syndrome, serotonin syndrome:** hyperthermia, increased CPK, altered mental status, muscle rigidity
• Constipation, urinary retention daily; if these occur, increase bulk and water in diet or stool softener
• Fall risk assessment, supervised ambulation until patient is stabilized on medication; do not involve patient in strenuous exercise program because fainting is possible; patient should not stand still for a long time
• **Beers:** avoid use in older adults except for schizophrenia, bipolar disorder, or short term as an antiemetic during chemotherapy; increased risk of stroke and cognitive decline
• **Pregnancy/breastfeeding:** use only if benefits outweigh fetal risk, may cause EPS in the neonate, enroll pregnant women in the Atypical Antipsychotic Pregnancy Registry, 866-961-2388; avoid breastfeeding, excretion unknown

Evaluate:
• **Therapeutic response:** decrease in emotional excitement, hallucinations, delusions, paranoia; reorganization of patterns of thought, speech

Teach patient/family:
• That orthostatic hypotension may occur; to rise from sitting or lying position gradually
• To avoid hot tubs, hot showers, tub baths because hypotension may occur
• To avoid tanning beds, excessive sunlight, photosensitivity may occur

Side effects: *italics* = common; red = life-threatening

• To avoid abrupt withdrawal of product because EPS may result; that product should be withdrawn slowly
• To avoid OTC preparations (cough, hay fever, cold), herbals, supplements unless approved by prescriber because serious product interactions may occur; to avoid use with alcohol because increased drowsiness may occur
• To avoid hazardous activities if drowsy or dizzy
• To report impaired vision, tremors, muscle twitching, diarrhea
• That results may take up to 6 wk
• To notify prescriber if pregnancy is planned or suspected or if breastfeeding
• To report immediately mouth sores, rash, swollen face/mouth/eyes, swollen lymph nodes
• To take with food; not to break, crush, or chew capsules
• Not to use opioids with benzodiazepines, other CNS depressants; to seek emergency services for dizziness, severe sleepiness, change in breathing
• That continuing follow-up exams will be needed
• In hot weather, that heat stroke may occur; to take extra precautions to stay cool, take adequate liquids

TREATMENT OF OVERDOSE:
Provide airway; *do not induce vomiting*

⚠ HIGH ALERT

ziv-aflibercept (Rx)
(ziv-a-flih′ber-sept)

Zaltrap
Func. class.: Antineoplastic
Chem. class.: Signal transduction inhibitor (STI), fusion protein

USES: Metastatic colorectal cancer that is resistant or has progressed after an oxaliplatin-containing regimen in combination with 5-fluorouracil, leucovorin, irinotecan (FOLFIRI)

DOSAGE AND ROUTES
• **Adult:** IV 4 mg/kg over 1 hr on day 1 q2wk with the FOLFIRI regimen
• Do not use in severe hypertension until controlled, then use lower dose
Available forms: Solution for injection 100 mg/4 mL; 200 mg/8 mL single use

zoledronic acid (Rx)
(zoh′leh-drah′nick ass′id)

Aclasta ✦, Reclast, Zometa ✦
Func. class.: Bone-resorption inhibitor
Chem. class.: Bisphosphonate

USES: Moderate to severe hypercalcemia associated with malignancy; multiple myeloma; bone metastases from solid tumors (used with antineoplastics); active Paget's disease; osteoporosis, glucocorticoid-induced osteoporosis, osteoporosis prophylaxis in postmenopausal women

DOSAGE AND ROUTES
Hypercalcemia of malignancy
• **Adult:** IV INFUSION 4 mg, given as single infusion over ≥15 min; may re-treat with 4 mg if serum calcium does not return to normal within 1 wk
Multiple myeloma/metastatic bone lesions
• **Adult:** IV INFUSION 4 mg, give over 15 min q3-4wk
Osteoporosis
• **Adult:** IV INFUSION 5 mg over ≥15 min q12mo
Active Paget's disease
• **Adult:** IV INFUSION 5 mg over ≥15 min with 1500 mg elemental calcium in divided doses and 800 IU of vitamin D
Osteoporosis prophylaxis, postmenopausal women
• **Adult:** IV INFUSION 5 mg q2yr
Osteoporosis prophylaxis when taking systemic glucocorticoids
• **Adult:** IV 5 mg every year

Renal dose
• **Adult:** IV INFUSION CCr 50-60 mL/min, 3.5 mg; CCr 40-49 mL/min, 3.3 mg; CCr 30-39 mL/min, 3 mg; CCr <30 mL/min, do not use

Osteopenia prevention in androgen deprivation treatment (prostate cancer) (unlabeled)
• **Adult:** IV 4 mg q3mo × 1 yr or 4 mg q12mo
Available forms: Injection, ready-to-use IV solution 4 mg/100 mL, 5 mg/100 mL, injection IV 4 mg/ 5 mL

ZOLMitriptan (Rx)

(zole-mih-trip′tan)

Zomig

Func. class.: Migraine agent, abortive
Chem. class.: Serotonin 5-HT$_{1B}$/5HT$_{1D}$ receptor agonist (triptan)

ACTION: Binds selectively to the vascular 5-HT$_{1B}$/5HT$_{1D}$ receptor subtype, exerts antimigraine effect; causes vasoconstriction in cranial arteries

USES: Acute treatment of migraine with/without aura

CONTRAINDICATIONS

Angina pectoris, history of MI, documented silent ischemia, ischemic heart disease, uncontrolled hypertension, hypersensitivity, basilar or hemiplegic migraine, risk of CV events
Precautions: Pregnancy, breastfeeding, children, postmenopausal women, men >40 yr, geriatric patients, risk factors for CAD, hypercholesterolemia, obesity, diabetes, impaired renal/hepatic function

DOSAGE AND ROUTES

• **Adult:** PO start at 2.5 mg (tab may be broken), may repeat after 2 hr, max single dose 5 mg, max 10 mg/24 hr; NASAL 1 spray in 1 nostril at onset of migraine, repeat in 2 hr if no relief

Available forms: Tabs 2.5, 5 mg; nasal spray 2.5, 5 mg
Administer:
PO route (conventional tablet)
• Tablet may be split
• Take with fluids as soon as symptoms of migraine occur
• Not approved for more than 3-4 uses in a month
Nasal route
• Blow nose before use
• Remove top, insert in nostril, hold other nostril shut
• Do not prime
• Press on plunger while breathing gently through the nose
• Discard for single use only

SIDE EFFECTS

CNS: *Tingling, hot sensation, burning, feeling of pressure, tightness, numbness, dizziness, sedation*
CV: Palpitations, chest pain
GI: Abdominal discomfort, nausea, dry mouth, dyspepsia, dysphagia
MISC: Odd taste (spray)
MS: *Weakness, neck stiffness,* myalgia
RESP: Chest tightness, pressure

PHARMACOKINETICS

Peak 1 ½-3 hr (PO), 3 hr (nasal); 25% protein binding; half-life 3-3 ½ hr; metabolized in liver (metabolite); excreted in urine (60%-80%), feces (20%-40%)

INTERACTIONS

Increase: extended vasospastic effects: ergot, ergot derivatives, avoid using with ZOLMitriptan, space by 24 hr
Do not use within 2 wk of MAOIs
Increase: weakness, hyperreflexia, incoordination: SSRIs (FLUoxetine, fluvoxaMINE, PARoxetine, sertraline), SNRI, methylene blue, traMADol
Increase: half-life of ZOLMitriptan—cimetidine, oral contraceptives, monitor
Drug/Herb
Increase: serotonin syndrome: SAM-e, St. John's wort
Drug/Lab Test
Increase: ALP

Z

NURSING CONSIDERATIONS
Assess:

• **CNS/PANS:** Assess for tingling, hot sensation, burning, feeling of pressure, numbness, flushing
• **Neurologic status:** LOC, blurring vision, nausea, vomiting, tingling in extremities preceding headache
• **Diet and possible triggers:** Ingestion of tyramine foods (pickled products, beer, wine, aged cheese), food additives, preservatives, colorings, artifical sweeteners, chocolate, caffeine, which may precipitate these types of headaches, use over 10 day/mo may lead to exacerbation of headache
• **Serotonin syndrome** if also taking SSRI, SNRI (agitation, tachycardia, hypertension, diarrhea, sweating, spasms/rigidity)
• **Pregnancy/breastfeeding:** use only if benefits outweigh fetal risk; may cause harm, death to fetus; do not breastfeed, excreted in breast milk

Evaluate:
• **Therapeutic response:** decrease in frequency, severity of headache

Teach patient/family:
• To report any side effects to prescriber
• That product does not prevent or reduce number of migraines; not to use for other headaches
• To report chest pain, rash, swelling of face, slurred speech
• Discuss drug interactions with patient and effects of each
• Not to double doses; if second dose is needed, wait at least 2 hr
• **Pregnancy/breastfeeding:** Advise patient to report if pregnancy is planned or suspected or if breastfeeding

---

⚠ HIGH ALERT

zolpidem (Rx)
(zole'pih-dem)

Ambien, Ambien CR, Edluar, Sublinox ✦, Zolpimist, Intermezzo
Func. class.: Hypnotic
Chem. class.: Imidazopyridine

Controlled Substance Schedule IV

Do not confuse:
zolpidem/Zyloprim

ACTION: Produces CNS depression at limbic, thalamic, hypothalamic levels of CNS; may be mediated by neurotransmitter γ-aminobutyric acid (GABA), not a benzodiazepine; results are sedation, hypnosis, skeletal muscle relaxation, anticonvulsant activity, anxiolytic action

USES: Insomnia, short-term treatment

CONTRAINDICATIONS
Hypersensitivity to benzodiazepines
Precautions: Pregnancy, breastfeeding, children <18 yr, geriatric patients, anemia, hepatic disease, suicidal individuals, drug abuse, seizure disorders, angioedema, depression, respiratory disease, sleep apnea, myasthenia gravis, pulmonary disease, next-morning impairments; females (lower dose needed)

> **Black Box Warning:** Sleep-related behaviors (sleepwalking)

DOSAGE AND ROUTES
Sleep-maintenance insomnia, 7-8 hours planned sleep
• **Adult: PO** ER 6.25 mg (females) or 6.25-12.5 mg (males) immediately before bedtime with ≥7-8 hours of planned sleep before waking (max 12.5 mg); IR tablet, spray, ODT 5 mg (females) or 5-10 mg (males) immediately before bedtime with ≥7-8 hours of planned sleep before waking
Available forms: Tabs 5, 10 mg; ext rel tabs 6.25, 12.5 mg; ODT: 1.75, 3.5, 5, 10 mg; oral spray 5 mg/spray
Administer:
PO route
• Do not break, crush, or chew ext rel
• Take with full glass of water
• ½-1 hr before bedtime (PO); right before retiring (ext rel)
• On empty stomach for fast onset; may be taken with food if GI symptoms occur
• Store in tight container in cool environment

Spray route
• Prime before first use (5 sprays) or if pump is not used for ≥14 days (1 spray)
• Spray directly over tongue
• Do not use spray with or after a meal
ODT route
• Place product under tongue; allow to dissolve before swallowing; do not take with water

SIDE EFFECTS
CNS: Headache, lethargy, drowsiness, day-time sedation, dizziness, confusion, light-headedness, anxiety, irritability, amnesia, poor coordination, complex sleep-related reactions (sleep driving, sleep eating), depression, somnolence, suicidal ideation, abnormal thinking/behavioral changes
CV: Chest pain, palpitations
GI: Nausea, vomiting, diarrhea, heart-burn, abdominal pain, constipation
HEMA: Leukopenia, granulocytopenia (rare)
MISC: Myalgia
SYST: Severe allergic reactions, angio-edema, anaphylaxis

PHARMACOKINETICS
PO: Onset up to 1.5 hr, metabolized by liver, excreted by kidneys (inactive metabolites), crosses placenta, excreted in breast milk, half-life 2-3 hr

INTERACTIONS
Increase: action of both products—alcohol, CNS depressants, monitor carefully
Increase: zolpidem effect CYP3A4 inhibitors (ketoconazole, verapamil), dose may need to be reduced
Decrease: zolpidem effect CYP3A4 inducers (rifAMPin, phenytoin); dose may need to be increased
Drug/Herb
Increase: CNS depression—Chamomile, kava, valerian
St. John's wort: Decreased zolpidem effect, avoid use
Drug/Food
Food: Delayed action, absorption

NURSING CONSIDERATIONS
Assess:
• **Mental status:** mood, sensorium, af-fect, memory (long, short term), excessive sedation, impaired coordination, **suicidal thoughts/behaviors**
• Type of sleep problem: falling asleep, staying asleep
• **Pregnancy/breastfeeding:** use only if benefits outweigh fetal risk, may cause fetal harm; cautious use in breastfeeding

> **Black Box Warning:** Complex sleep disorders (rare): monitor for sleep eating/driving/walking, do not use if these occur with opioids

• **Beers:** avoid in older adults; CNS effects occur
Evaluate:
• **Therapeutic response:** ability to sleep at night, decreased amount of early morning awakening if taking product for insomnia
Teach patient/family:
• That dependence is possible after long-term use

> **Black Box Warning:** That complex sleep-related behaviors may occur (sleep driving/eating), to stop product if these occur

• To avoid driving or other activities re-quiring alertness until dosage is stabilized
• To avoid alcohol ingestion
• That effects may take 2 nights for benefits to be noticed; next-morning impairment may occur, to take immediately before bed
• Not to use during pregnancy, breast-feeding
• That hangover is common in geriatric patients but less common than with bar-biturates; that rebound insomnia may occur for 1-2 nights after discontinuing product; not to discontinue abruptly; to taper, avoid use
• **ODT:** Place tablet under tongue, allow to dissolve
• Not to crush, chew, break ext rel tabs
• **Spray:** To prime spray pump before us-ing (5 sprays before new use, 1 spray if not used ≥14 days), spray directly over tongue

TREATMENT OF OVERDOSE:
Monitor electrolytes, VS

zonisamide (Rx)

(zone-is′a-mide)

Zonegran, Zonisade

Func. class.: Anticonvulsant

Chem. class.: Sulfonamides

ACTION: May act through action at sodium and calcium channels, but exact action is unknown; serotonergic action

USES: Adjunctive therapy for partial seizures

CONTRAINDICATIONS

Hypersensitivity to this product or sulfonamides

Precautions: Pregnancy, breastfeeding, children <16 yr, geriatric patients, allergies, renal/hepatic disease; psychiatric condition, hepatic failure, pulmonary disease, suicidal ideation

DOSAGE AND ROUTES

• **Adult/child >16 yr:** 100 mg/day, may increase after 2 wk to 200 mg/day, may increase q2wk, max dose 600 mg/day

Available forms: Caps 25, 50, 100 mg; oral suspension 100 mg/5 mL

Administer:

• Without regard to food; swallow whole, do not crush or open

Oral suspension:

• Shake before using, use measuring device, discard 30 days after opening

SIDE EFFECTS

CNS: Dizziness, insomnia, paresthesias, depression, fatigue, headache, confusion, somnolence, agitation, irritability, speech disturbance, suicidal ideation, seizures, status epilepticus

EENT: Diplopia, verbal difficulty, speech abnormalities, taste perversion, amblyopia, pharyngitis, rhinitis, tinnitus, nystagmus

GI: Nausea, constipation, anorexia, weight loss, diarrhea, dyspepsia, dry mouth, abdominal pain

GU: Kidney stones

HEMA: Aplastic anemia, granulocytopenia (rare); ecchymosis

INTEG: Rash, pruritus

MISC: Flulike symptoms

SYST: Stevens-Johnson syndrome, metabolic acidosis

PHARMACOKINETICS

Peak 2-6 hr, half-life 63 hr, metabolized by liver, excreted by kidneys, protein binding 40%

INTERACTIONS

Increase: metabolic acidosis severity—other carbonic anhydrase inhibitors

Decrease: half-life of zonisamide—carBAMazepine, phenytoin, PHENobarbital

Increase: zonisamide clearance CYP3A4 inducers (phenytoin, valproate), monitor for continuing seizures

Increase: CNS depression—alcohol, other CNS depressants

Drug/Herb

Increase: effect of this product—St. John's wort

Drug/Food

• Do not use with grapefruit

Drug/Lab Test

Increase: BUN, creatinine

NURSING CONSIDERATIONS

Assess:

• **Seizures:** duration, type, intensity, precipitating factors

• Assess for hypersensitivity reactions

• **Renal function:** albumin concentration, BUN, urinalysis, creatinine, serum bicarbonate at baseline and periodically, renal failure may occur; increase fluid intake to prevent calculi

• **Mental status:** mood, sensorium, affect, memory (long-, short-term), **suicidal thoughts/behaviors,** assess often

• **Stevens-Johnson syndrome, aplastic anemia, fulminant hepatic necrosis (rare);** may cause death; monitor for rashes and hypersensitivity reactions, stop product immediately, notify prescriber

• Obtain bicarbonate level before treatment/periodically; metabolic acidosis may occur in children

• **Beers:** avoid in older adults unless safer alternative is unavailable; may cause ataxia, impaired psychomotor function

• **Pregnancy/breastfeeding:** use only if benefits outweigh fetal risk, may cause fetal harm; pregnant women should enroll in the North American Antiepileptic Drug Pregnancy Registry, 888-233-2334; do not breastfeed, excreted in breast milk, monitor for metabolic acidosis in mother and newborn, use contraception during and for at least 1 mo after last dose

Evaluate:

• **Therapeutic response:** decrease in severity of seizures

Teach patient/family:

• Not to discontinue product abruptly because seizures may occur

• To avoid hazardous activities until stabilized on product

• To use without regard to food, swallow capsule whole

• To carry emergency ID stating product use

• To notify prescriber of rash immediately; to notify prescriber of back pain, abdominal pain, blood in urine; to increase fluid intake to reduce risk of kidney stones

• To notify prescriber if pregnancy is planned, suspected, to use contraception during and for at least 1 mo after last dose

• To avoid grapefruit

• To notify prescriber of sore throat, fever, easy bruising

• To report suicidal thoughts, behaviors immediately, assess for mood changes, increase in depressive symptoms

Z

Appendix A

---

avacincaptad pegol (Rx)
A-va-sin-KAP-tad-PEG-ol

Izervay

Func. class.: Ophthalmic-complement inhibitor

USES: Geographic atrophy (GA) secondary to age-related macular degeneration (AMD)

CONTRAINDICATIONS
Ocular or periocular infections, active intraocular inflammation

DOSAGE AND ROUTES
Adult: Intravitreal injection 2 mg (0.1 mL of 20 mg/mL solution) to each affected eye once monthly (approximately 28 ± 7 days) for up to 12 mo

Available forms: Intravitreal solution: 20 mg/mL in a single-dose vial

---

bexagliflozin (Rx)
(bex'a-gli-floe'zin)

Brenzavvy

Func. class.: Oral antidiabetic

Chem. class.: Sodium-glucose cotransporter 2 (SGLT2) inhibitor

---

ACTION: Blocks glucose reabsorption by the kidney, increases glucose excretion, lowers blood glucose concentrations by inhibiting proximal renal tubular sodium glucose transporter 2 (SGLT2)

USES: Type 2 diabetes mellitus, with diet and exercise; may use in combination; to reduce CV events in type 2 diabetes mellitus with CV disease

CONTRAINDICATIONS
Dialysis, renal failure, hypersensitivity, breastfeeding, diabetic ketoacidosis, pregnancy 2nd/3rd trimester

Precautions: Pregnancy 1st trimester, children, renal/hepatic disease, hypothyroidism, hyperglycemia, hypotension, pituitary insufficiency, type 1 diabetes mellitus, malnutrition, fever, dehydration, adrenal insufficiency, geriatric patients, lower limb amputation

DOSAGE AND ROUTES
Type 2 diabetes mellitus

Adult: PO 20 mg once daily, taken in the morning

Renal dose

Adult: PO eGFR <30 mL/min/1.73 m^2 not recommended

Available forms: Tablets 20 mg

Administer:

PO route

• Once daily without regard to food
• Do not crush or chew the tablet
• Assess renal function prior to use
• Correct volume depletion before starting
• Not recommended if eGFR less than 30 mL/min/1.73 m^2
• Adjust dose in times of stress, surgery, trauma
• Store at room temperature

SIDE EFFECTS
CV: Hypotension, orthostatic hypotension

GI: Pancreatitis, nausea, vomiting dehydration

GU: Cystitis, candidiasis, urinary frequency, polydipsia, polyuria, renal impairment UTI, genital fungal infections

INTEG: Photosensitivity, rash, pruritus

META: Hypercholesterolemia, lipidemia, hypoglycemia, hyperkalemia, hypermagnesemia, hyperphosphatemia, hypersensitivity, ketoacidosis

MISC: Bone fractures

PHARMACOKINETICS
99% protein binding, metabolized by UGT1A9, UGT2B4, excreted 33% in urine, peak 1-2 hr, half-life 10.6-13 hr depending on dose

INTERACTIONS
Increase: hypoglycemia—sulfonylureas, insulin, MAOIs, salicylates, fibric acid

---

derivatives, bile acid sequestrants, ACE inhibitors, angiotensin II receptor antagonists, beta blockers, SSRIs; monitor for hypoglycemia, monitor blood glucose closely, dosage may need to be decreased
Increase: hyperkalemia—potassium-sparing diuretics, ACE inhibitors, ARBs, monitor potassium regularly
Increase or decrease: glycemic control—androgens, lithium, bortezomib, quinolones; monitor for glycemic control
Decrease: effect hyperglycemia—digestive enzymes, intestinal absorbents, thiazide diuretics, loop diuretics, corticosteroids, estrogen, progestins, hormonal contraceptives, sympathomimetics, isoniazid, phenothiazines; protease inhibitors, atypical antipsychotics, carbonic anhydrase inhibitors, cycloSPORINE, tacrolimus, baclofen, UGT inducers (PHENObarbital, phenytoin, rifAMPin, ritonavir); dose may need to be increased based on eGFR
Drug/Lab:
Increase: urine glucose, potassium, lipids, cholesterol, magnesium phosphate, uric acid, serum creatinine
Decrease: serum glucose, eGFR
Drug/Herb:
Decrease: bexagliflozin level—St. John's wort

NURSING CONSIDERATIONS
Assess:
• **Hypoglycemia** (weakness, hunger, dizziness, tremors, anxiety, tachycardia, sweating), hyperglycemia; even though product does not cause hypoglycemia, if patient is on sulfonylureas or insulin, hypoglycemia may be additive; if hypoglycemia occurs, treat with dextrose, or, if severe, with IV glucagon
• **Ketoacidosis:** Monitor for increased ketone levels; may occur with any glucose level, more common in those with severe illnesses
• **Necrotizing fasciitis (perineum):** Requires immediate surgery
• **Volume depletion:** Monitor for orthostatic hypotension, weakness, dizziness; may occur after beginning treatment; correct volume depletion before starting treatment
• For stress, surgery, or other trauma that may require a change in dose
• A1c q3mo; monitor serum glucose 1 hr PP throughout treatment; serum cholesterol, serum creatinine/BUN, serum electrolytes
• **Hyperkalemia (renal disease):** Monitor potassium closely
• **Bone fractures:** Monitor bone density, other conditions that may lead to bone fractures; fractures may occur within 3 mo of starting therapy
• **Renal impairment:** Monitor more frequently in those with renal disease; increased creatinine, eGFR may be decreased; BUN may occur
• **Lower limb amputation:** increased risk of amputation; monitor wound and feet closely for complications, provide foot care
• Monitor electrolytes, LDL, cholesterol and correct as needed
• **Fungal infections:** Usually in those with other infections
• **Pregnancy/breastfeeding:** Identify whether pregnancy is planned or suspected or if breastfeeding, use only if clearly needed, not to use in second/third trimester, do not breastfeed
Evaluate:
• Therapeutic response: Improved signs/symptoms of diabetes mellitus (decreased polyuria, polydipsia, polyphagia); clear sensorium, absence of dizziness, stable gait
Teach patient/family:
• The symptoms of hypo/hyperglycemia, what to do about each
• That medication must be taken as prescribed; explain consequences of discontinuing abruptly; that insulin may need to be used for stress, including trauma, fever, surgery; to take as soon as remembered if dose is missed unless close to next dose, then skip and take at next scheduled dose, do not double
• To avoid OTC medications and herbal supplements unless discussed with health care professional

- That diabetes is a lifelong illness; that the diet and exercise regimen must be followed; that this product is not a cure
- To carry emergency ID and glucose source
- That blood glucose monitoring is required to assess product effect
- **Renal injury:** Edema in extremities decreased, dark urine, seek care immediately
- **Necrotizing fasciitis:** Signs/symptoms of high temperature, genital swelling, pain, redness, seek care immediately
- **Hypersensitivity:** To notify prescriber immediately of itching, hives, rash, swelling of face/lips
- **Lower limb amputation risk:** Inspect feet; monitor for new ulcerations, wounds; educate about foot care, to report injury to limbs, sores
- **Ketoacidosis:** To notify prescriber immediately of nausea, vomiting, lack of appetite, sleepiness, difficulty breathing
- **Yeast infections (women/men):** That yeast infections can occur with this product (women, vaginal; men, penile); to report discharge, itching, swelling
- **UTI:** To report immediately burning, pain on urination, hematuria, back pain, decreased urine
- **Pregnancy/breastfeeding:** Not to breastfeed; to advise prescriber if pregnancy is planned or suspected

---

bimekizumab (Rx)
(bim'i-kiz'ue-mab)

Bimzelx

Func. class.: Immune response modifier

Chem. class.: Monoclonal antibody, interleukin-12 inhibitor

ACTION: Interleukin (IL)-17A (IL-17A), interleukin 17F (IL-17F), and interleukin 17-AF cytokine antagonist, binds to an IL protein, decreases inflammation

USES: Plaque psoriasis

CONTRAINDICATIONS
Hypersensitivity, active infections

Precautions: Pregnancy, breastfeeding, children ≤18 yr, geriatric patients, surgery, TB, diabetes mellitus, immunosuppression

DOSAGE AND ROUTES
Moderate-severe plaque psoriasis in persons who are candidates for systemic therapy or phototherapy:
Adults: SUBCUT 320 mg (two 160-mg injections) SUBCUT at wk 0, 4, 8, 12, and 16, then q8wk; for those ≥120 kg 320 mg q4wk after wk 16 may be used

Available forms: Solution for injection 160 mg/mL autoinjector or prefilled syringe

Administer:
- Administer by SUBCUT injection only
- Visually inspect parenteral products for particulate matter and discoloration prior to administration whenever solution and container permit. The solution should be free of visible particles, clear, and colorless to slightly yellow [69656]

SUBCUT administration
- Each 320-mg dose is given as 2 SUBCUT injections of 160 mg
- Administration sites for patient administration include upper arms, thighs, and any quadrant of the abdomen. Health care professionals may inject in the upper, outer arm
- Do not administer where the skin is tender, bruised, red, hard, thick, scaly, or affected by psoriasis
- Rotate sites of injection with each dose
- Wash hands before drug administration. Clean injection site with an alcohol wipe and let dry
- No preservatives; discard any unused product
- *Missed doses:* If a dose or administration time is missed, administer the missed dose as soon as possible, then resume dosing at the regularly scheduled time
- Remove from the refrigerator. To protect from light, do not remove the

---

prefilled syringes or autoinjectors from the carton. Allow 30-45 min to reach room temperature. DO NOT use any methods to speed the warming process, such as a microwave, hot water, or sunlight
• Inspect syringe or autoinjector for particulate matter and discoloration prior to use
• *Storage of unopened prefilled syringes and autoinjectors:* Protect from light and store refrigerated at 2-8° C (36-46° F) until time of use. Do not freeze and do not use the injection if it has been frozen. Do not shake
• If needed, a prefilled syringe or autoinjector may be stored at room temperature up to 25°C (77°F) for up to 30 days in the original carton to protect from light. Once the product has been stored at room temperature, do not return to the refrigerator; discard, if unused, within 30 days
• Record the date when first removed from the refrigerator in the spaces provided on the carton

SIDE EFFECTS
CNS: Headache, suicidal ideation
GI: Inflammatory bowel disease
INTEG: *Injection site reaction,* pruritus, skin irritation

PHARMACOKINETICS
Half-life 23 days

INTERACTIONS
• Monitor effect of CYP 3A4 substrates, adjust dose as needed
• Do not give concurrently with vaccines; immunizations should be brought up to date before treatment
• Avoid use with immunosuppressives

NURSING CONSIDERATIONS
Assess:
• Plaque psoriasis: Identify area of lesions and severity baseline and during treatment
• Labs: TB test, hepatitis B serology, LFTs, plasma hepatitis C RNA, plasma HIV RNA

• Bring immunizations up to date before starting treatment; do not administer live vaccines during treatment and for 3 mo after treatment ends
• **Infection:** Monitor for fever, sore throat, cough; do not use during active
• TB: TB testing should be done before starting treatment
• For injection site pain, swelling, rash
• **Pregnancy/breastfeeding:** Pregnant patients should enroll in the pregnancy registry, https://mothertobaby.org/pregnancy-studies/ or call 877-311-8972; use only if benefits outweigh fetal risk; avoid use in breastfeeding, excretion unknown
Evaluate:
• Therapeutic response: Decreased symptoms of plaque psoriasis
Teach patient/family:
• That product must be continued for prescribed time to be effective; to use as prescribed
• Not to receive live vaccinations during treatment
• To notify prescriber of possible infection (upper respiratory or other) or allergic reactions
• Injection techniques and disposal of equipment; not to reuse needles, syringes
• That follow-up will be needed

---

capivasertib (Rx)
(kap-EYE-va-SER-tib)
Truqap
Func. class.: Antineoplastic, kinase inhibitor
Chem. class.: EGFR/HER2/NEU inhibitor

ACTION: It is an irreversible inhibitor of the epidermal growth factor receptor (EGFR) and the human epidermal receptor type 2 (HER2) and HER4

USES: Hormone receptor (HR)-positive, HER2-negative, locally advanced or metastatic breast cancer with 1 or more PIK3CA/AKT1/PTEN alterations following progression on at least 1 endocrine-based regimen in the metastatic setting or recurrence on or within 12 mo of completing adjuvant therapy, in combination with fulvestrant

CONTRAINDICATIONS

Hypersensitivity

Precautions: Breastfeeding, contraception requirements, geriatric patients, hepatic disease, hepatotoxicity, infertility, pregnancy, pregnancy testing, reproductive risk

DOSAGE AND ROUTES

Adult: PO 400 mg bid daily on days 1-4 every 7 days, in combination with fulvestrant 500 mg IM on days 1, 15, 29, and every 28 days thereafter. Continue until disease progression or unacceptable toxicity. May add a luteinizing hormone–releasing hormone (LHRH) agonist for men and for pre- and perimenopausal women

Therapeutic drug monitoring

Dosage adjustments for treatment-related toxicities:

First dose reduction: 320 mg PO twice daily on days 1-4 every wk

Second dose reduction: 200 mg PO twice daily on days 1-4 every wk, permanently discontinue if this dose is not tolerated

Available forms: Tabs 160 mg, 200 mg

Administer:

• Swallow tablets whole; do not chew, crush, or split

• If a dose is missed within 4 hr, may take dose; if more than 4 hr do not replace the missed dose. Resume with the next scheduled daily dose

• If a patient vomits a dose, they should not take another dose. They may take the next dose at its usual scheduled time

SIDE EFFECTS

CNS: Fatigue

GI: Diarrhea, nausea, vomiting, stomatitis

INTEG: Rash, cutaneous reactions

PHARMACOKINETICS

Peak 1-2 hr, half-life 8.3 hr; fecal excretion 50%, urine 45%; metabolized by CYP3A4 and UGT2B7

INTERACTIONS

Increase: capivasertib effect—strong or moderate CYP3A4 inhibitors; avoid concomitant use, or reduce dose of capivasertib in moderate CYP3A4 inhibitors

Decrease: capivasertib effect—strong or moderate CYP3A4 inducers; avoid concomitant use

Drug/Lab

Increase: random glucose, fasting glucose, triglycerides, creatinine

Decrease: lymphocytes, HB, leukocytes, neutrophils

NURSING CONSIDERATIONS

Assess:

• **Hyperglycemia**: Monitor blood glucose levels baseline and throughout treatment; withhold, reduce dose, or permanently discontinue based on severity

• **Diarrhea:** Advise patients with diarrhea (common) to increase oral fluids, start antidiarrheal (loperamide) treatment, and consult with a health care provider if diarrhea occurs while taking; withhold, reduce dose, or permanently discontinue based on severity

• **Cutaneous adverse reactions:** Monitor for signs and symptoms of cutaneous adverse reactions; withhold, reduce dose, or permanently discontinue based on severity

• **Pregnancy/breastfeeding:** Avoid drug in females of reproductive potential; use contraception during treatment and for at least 1 mo after the last dose; can cause fetal harm or death; discontinue breastfeeding during treatment and for 1 mo after the final dose. Obtain a pregnancy test before starting treatment. Males with female partners of reproductive potential should avoid pregnancy and use effective contraception during treatment and ≥ mo after last dose

Evaluate:
• Therapeutic outcome: Decrease in breast cancer size and spread
Teach patient/family:
• **Diarrhea:** To report number of loose stools per day or change in stools to provider and may use antidiarrheals
• That follow-ups and lab work will be needed
• **Pregnancy/breastfeeding:** Not to use in pregnancy, breastfeeding; to use contraception during treatment and for at least 1 mo after last dose; do not breastfeed during and for 1 mo after last dose; men with a partner who may become pregnant should use contraception during treatment and for at least 4 mo after last dose

---

daprodustat (Rx)

(dap-ro-dus'-tat)

Jesduvroq
Func. class.: Antianemic agent

USES: Anemia due to chronic kidney disease in persons receiving dialysis for 4 mo or more

DOSAGES AND ROUTES

Black Box Warning: MI, stroke, thromboembolism, thrombosis

Adults with pretreatment hemoglobin concentration of less than 9 mg/dL: PO 4 mg once daily initially. Monitor Hb every 2 wk for the first mo and then every 4 wk, max: 24 mg/day
Adults with pretreatment hemoglobin concentration of 9-10 mg/dL: PO 2 mg once daily initially. Monitor Hb every 2 wk for the first mo and then every 4 wk, max: 24 mg/day
Adults with pretreatment hemoglobin concentration of more than 10 mg/dL: PO 1 mg once daily initially. Monitor Hb every 2 wk for the first mo and then every 4 wk, max: 24 mg/day
Available forms: Tablet 1 mg, 2 mg, 4 mg, 6 mg, 8 mg

---

efbemalenograstim (Rx)

Ryzneuta
Func. class.: Biologic modifier
C hem. class.: Granulocyte colony stimulating factor

ACTION: Stimulates proliferation and differentiation of neutrophils

USES: Chemotherapy-induced neutropenia prophylaxis, to decrease the incidence of febrile neutropenia, in patients with nonmyeloid malignancies receiving myelosuppressive anticancer drugs associated with a clinically significant incidence of febrile neutropenia

CONTRAINDICATIONS
Hypersensitivity
Precautions: Pregnancy, breastfeeding, children, myeloid malignancies, radiation therapy, sepsis, sickle cell disease, chemotherapy, respiratory disease

DOSAGE AND ROUTES
Chemotherapy-induced neutropenia prophylaxis, to decrease the incidence of febrile neutropenia, in patients with nonmyeloid malignancies receiving myelosuppressive anti-cancer drugs associated with a clinically significant incidence of febrile neutropenia
Adults: SUBCUT 20 mg once per chemotherapy cycle
Available forms: Injection: 20 mg/mL solution in a single-dose prefilled syringe
Administer:
• Given by SUBCUT injection
• Do not use within 14 days or 24 hr before or after cytotoxic chemotherapy
• Inject into the abdomen, the back or side of the upper arms, or the thighs; rotate injection sites
• Do not inject into scar tissue or areas that are reddened, inflamed, or swollen
• After injecting the entire dose, the needle safety device will be triggered and

---

the needle will be covered by the needle guard

• If a dose is missed, instruct the patient or caregiver to contact their health care provider

• Before injection, allow to reach room temperature for a maximum of 48 hr; any vial or syringe exposed to room temperature for more than 48 hr should be discarded

• Visually inspect for particulate matter and discoloration before use

• This product contains natural rubber latex, which may cause allergic reactions; the needle cap of the syringe contains natural rubber; persons with latex allergies should not administer this product

• Store in refrigerator; do not freeze, discard if frozen; protect from light, do not shake

SIDE EFFECTS

GI: *Nausea,* vomiting, anorexia, splenic rupture

HEMA: Thrombocytopenia, excessive leukocytosis

INTEG: Allergic reactions

RESP: Acute respiratory distress syndrome

PHARMACOKINETICS

SUBCUT: half-life 36.9 hr; metabolized via catabolic pathways into small peptides

INTERACTIONS

Increase: adverse reactions—do not use this product concomitantly with antineoplastics

NURSING CONSIDERATIONS

Assess:

• B/P, respirations, pulse before and during therapy

• Bone pain possible; give mild analgesics

• **Acute** respiratory distress syndrome (ARDS): Fever, dyspnea, lung infiltrates; discontinue in ARDS

• **Allergic reactions:** Rash, wheezing, facial edema, dyspnea, anaphylaxis; discontinue

• **Fatal splenic rupture:** Severe left upper abdominal, shoulder pain

• **Sickle cell crises** in those with sickle cell disorders: Discontinue if sickle cell crisis occurs

• **Glomerulonephritis:** Assess for pink/cola-colored, foamy urine, hypertension, edema, nausea, vomiting, muscle cramps; dose-reduction or interruption may be needed. Monitor for azotemia, hematuria (microscopic and macroscopic), proteinuria, and renal biopsy. Usually resolves after dose reduction or discontinuation of product

• **Thrombocytopenia:** Blood studies: CBC, platelet count before treatment and twice weekly; neutrophil counts drop by 50% if product is discontinued the next day

• **Capillary leak syndrome:** Monitor flulike symptoms, dizziness, and fatigue; intensive care may be required

• Myelodysplastic syndrome (MDS)/acute myeloid leukemia (AML) in breast/lung cancer: Assess for fatigue, dyspnea, pallor, easy or unusual bruising or bleeding, petechiae, low WBCs

• Pregnancy/breastfeeding: Unknown, use cautiously in pregnancy, and breastfeeding

Evaluate:

• Therapeutic response: Absence of neutropenia, infection

Teach patient/family:

• About dose, side effects, when to notify the health care provider

• Advise the patient to read the "Patient Information" sheet

• Advise patients of the following risks and potential risks: **Rupture or enlargement of the spleen**, to report immediately left upper quadrant abdominal pain or left shoulder pain; **ARDS** to report immediately dyspnea, with or without fever; **serious allergic reactions**, to report rash, facial edema, wheezing, dyspnea, hypotension, or tachycardia. Teach patient to seek immediate medical services; in those with **sickle cell disease**, sickle cell crisis and death have occurred, discuss potential risks and benefits; **glomerulo-nephritis**: report immediately swelling of the face or ankles, dark-colored urine or blood in the urine, or a decrease in urine amount. Capillary leak syndrome may occur. Symptoms include hypotension and edema. Advise patients to report signs and symptoms of capillary leak syndrome to their health care provider immediately [see Warnings and Precautions (5.9)].

• There may be an increased risk of myelodysplastic syndrome and/or acute myeloid leukemia in patients with breast and lung cancer who receive Ryzneuta in conjunction with chemotherapy and/or radiation therapy. Symptoms of MDS and AML may include tiredness, fever, and easy bruising or bleeding. Advise patients to report to their physician signs and symptoms of MDS/AML

---

eflornithine (Rx)
(ee-FLOOR-nih-theen)
Iwilfin
Func. class.: Antineoplastic
Chem. class.: Enzyme inhibitor of ODC

ACTION: An irreversible inhibitor of the enzyme ornithine decarboxylase (ODC), the first and rate-limiting enzyme in the biosynthesis of polyamines and a target of MYCN

USES: To reduce the risk of relapse in adult/pediatric patients with high-risk neuroblastoma (HRNB) who have demonstrated at least a partial response to prior multiagent, multimodality therapy including anti-GD2 immunotherapy

CONTRAINDICATIONS
Pregnancy, breastfeeding
Precautions: Myelosuppression, hepatotoxicity, hearing loss

DOSAGE AND ROUTES
Adult: PO Based on actual body weight. Given bid with or without food until disease progression, unacceptable toxicity, or max 2 yr
Available forms: Tablet 192 mg
Administer:
• Prior to use perform baseline audiogram, CBC, LFTs
• Recommended dosage is based on body surface area
• Tablet may be swallowed whole, chewed, or crushed and mixed with soft food or liquid

SIDE EFFECTS
EENT: Otitis media, sinusitis, conjunctivitis, allergic rhinitis, hearing loss
RESP: Pneumonia, URI, cough
INTEG: Skin infection
GU: UTI
GI: Diarrhea, vomiting
MISC: Fever

PHARMACOKINETICS
Peak 3.5 hr, half-life 3.5 hr, no protein binding

INTERACTIONS
None known
Lab/Drug
Increase: LFTs, glucose, potassium
Decrease: Potassium, glucose, sodium, neutrophils, WBC, platelets, HB

NURSING CONSIDERATIONS
Assess:
• **Myelosuppression:** Monitor CBC before and during treatment; withhold, reduce dose, or permanently discontinue based on severity. Assess for fatigue, dyspnea, dizziness
• **Hepatotoxicity:** Monitor LFTs before and during treatment; withhold, reduce dose, or permanently discontinue based on severity
• **Hearing loss:** Monitor hearing before and during treatment; withhold, reduce dose, or permanently discontinue based on severity
• **Pregnancy/breastfeeding**: Can cause fetal harm. Females of reproductive potential and males with partners of reproductive potential should use effective

contraception during and for 1 wk after last dose, do not breastfeed
Evaluate
• Therapeutic response: Decreasing tumor size
Teach patient/family
• **Myelosuppression:** Advise patient to report fatigue, shortness of breath, dizziness
• **Hepatotoxicity:** Advise patient to report yellowing of skin, eyes, dark urine, clay-colored stools
• **Hearing loss:** Advise patient to report hearing loss
• **Pregnancy/breastfeeding**: Can cause fetal harm. Advise females of reproductive potential and males with partners of reproductive potential to use effective contraception during and for 1 wk after last dose, do not breastfeed

---

elacestrant (Rx)
(EL-a-KES-trant)
Orserdu
Func. class.: Antineoplastic
Chem. class.: Estrogen-receptor antagonist

ACTION: Binds to estrogen receptor-alpha, inhibits 17β-estradiol–mediated cell proliferation

USES: Postmenopausal women or adult men, with ER-positive, HER2-negative, ESR1-mutated advanced or metastatic breast cancer with disease progression following at least one line of endocrine therapy

CONTRAINDICATIONS
Pregnancy, breastfeeding, children, hypersensitivity
Precautions: Hepatic disease, jaundice, thrombocytopenia, biliary tract disease

DOSAGE AND ROUTES
Adult: PO 345 mg tablet once daily, with food
Available forms: Tablet 86 mg, 345 mg

Administer:
PO route
• Antiemetic 30-60 min before product to prevent vomiting prn
• Store in refrigerator; protect from light

SIDE EFFECTS
CNS: *Headache,* depression, dizziness, insomnia, paresthesia, anxiety
GI: *Nausea, vomiting,* anorexia, constipation, diarrhea, abdominal pain, hepatitis, hepatic failure, hyperbilirubinemia
HEMA: Anemia
INTEG: *Rash,* sweating, *hot flashes,* inj site pain
MS: Bone pain, arthritis, back pain
RESP: Pharyngitis, dyspnea, cough
SYST: Angioedema

PHARMACOKINETICS
Half-life 40 days, metabolized by CYP3A4, excretion in feces 90%

INTERACTIONS
Drug/Lab Test
Increase: LFTs

NURSING CONSIDERATIONS
Assess:
• For anticoagulant use
• For side effects; report to prescriber
• **Pregnancy/breastfeeding:** Obtain a pregnancy test before dose, have patient use contraception during and for 1 wk after last dose, do not breastfeed during or for 1 wk after last dose; male patients with female partners of reproductive potential should use effective contraception during treatment and for 1 wk after the last dose; fertility may be impaired in females and males of reproductive potential
Evaluate:
• Therapeutic response: Decreased tumor size, spread of malignancy
Teach patient/family:
• To report any complaints, side effects to prescriber
• To report vaginal bleeding immediately

• That tumor flare (increase in size of tumor, increased bone pain) may occur, will subside rapidly; that analgesics may be taken for pain

• That premenopausal women must use mechanical birth control because ovulation may be induced; not to breastfeed

• To use contraception during and for 1 wk after last dose to prevent pregnancy, do not breastfeed during or for 1 wk after last dose; male patients with female partners of reproductive potential should use effective contraception during treatment and for 1 wk after the last dose; fertility may be impaired in females and males of reproductive potential

elranatamab (Rx)
(el'ra-nat'-a-mab)
ELREXFIO
Func. class.: Antineoplastic

USES: Relapsed or refractory multiple myeloma who have received at least 4 prior lines of therapy

Black Box Warning: Cytokine release syndrome, neurotoxicity

DOSAGE AND ROUTES
Adults: **SUBCUT Step-up dosing schedule:** dose 1, 12 mg on day 1; dose 2, 32 mg on day 4 (maintain a minimum of 2 days between step-up dose 1 and 2); first treatment dose, 76 mg on day 8 (maintain a minimum of 2 days between step-up dose 2 and the first treatment dose). At 1 wk after the first treatment dose, give 76 mg once weekly through wk 24. Maintain a minimum of 6 days between treatment doses. Starting on wk 25, give 76 mg every 2 wk until disease progression in patients who received at least 24 wk of treatment
Available forms: Solution for injection 44 mg/1.1 mL, 76 mg/1.9 mL

epcoritamab (Rx)
(ep-coh-rih'ta-mab)
Epkinly
Func. class.: Antineoplastics
Chem. class.: Monoclonal antibodies

ACTION: Bispecific T-cell engaging (BiTE) monoclonal antibody that binds to CD20 expressed on lymphoma cells and CD3 expressed on the surface of T-cells

USES: Relapsed or refractory diffuse large B-cell lymphoma (DLBCL) not otherwise specified (including DLBCL arising from indolent lymphoma) and high-grade B-cell lymphoma after 2 or more lines of systemic therapy

CONTRAINDICATIONS
Hypersensitivity, pregnancy, breastfeeding

Black Box Warning: Cytokine release syndrome, neurotoxicity

Precautions: Anemia, infection, neutropenia, driving/hazardous activities, thrombocytopenia, contraceptive requirements

DOSAGE AND ROUTES
Adult: **SUBCUT** Cycle 1: 0.16 mg on day 1 (step-up dose 1), 0.8 mg on day 8 (step-up dose 2), and 48 mg on days 15 and 22. Cycles 2 and 3: 48 mg on days 1, 8, 15, and 22 repeated every 28 days. Cycles 4-9: 48 mg on days 1 and 15 repeated every 28 days. Cycles 10 and beyond: 48 mg once every 28 days until disease progression
Available forms: Injection 4 mg/0.8 mL, 48 mg/0.8 mL
Administer:
SUBCUT route
• Prepare and administer by a health care professional with equipment capable of managing severe reactions

• Patients should be hospitalized for 24 hr after use of the first 48-mg dose scheduled on day 15 in cycle 1
• Premedicate with a corticosteroid, H1-antihistamine (diphenhydramine), and acetaminophen approximately 30-120 min prior to all doses in cycle 1

Preparation: 0.16-mg dose (2 dilutions required)

• Remove the 4 mg/0.8 mL vial from the refrigerator; allow the vial to come to room temperature for no more than 1 hr
• Gently swirl the vial; do not invert, shake

First dilution

• Transfer 0.8 mL from the 4-mg vial to an empty vial labeled Dilution A
• Add 4.2 mL of 0.9% NaCl injection into the Dilution A vial for a first diluted concentration of 0.8 mg/mL
• Gently swirl the Dilution A vial for 30-45 sec

Second dilution

• Transfer 2 mL of solution from the Dilution A vial into an empty vial labeled Dilution B; discard the remaining contents of the Dilution A vial
• Add 8 mL of 0.9% NaCl injection into the Dilution B vial for a second diluted concentration of 0.16 mg/mL
• Withdraw 1 mL from the Dilution B vial into a syringe labeled with the dose (0.16 mg) and time of day
• Discard the remaining contents of the Dilution B vial

0.8-mg dose (1 dilution required)

• Remove the 4 mg/0.8 mL vial from the refrigerator; allow the vial to come to room temperature for ≤1 hr
• Gently swirl the vial; do not invert, shake

Dilution

• Transfer 0.8 mL from the 4-mg vial to an empty vial labeled Dilution A
• Add 4.2 mL of 0.9% NaCl injection into the Dilution A vial for a first diluted concentration of 0.8 mg/mL
• Gently swirl the Dilution A vial for 30-45 sec

• Withdraw 1 mL from the Dilution A vial into a syringe labeled with the dose (0.8 mg) and time of day
• Discard the remaining contents of the Dilution A vial

48-mg dose (no dilution)

• Remove the 48 mg/0.8 mL vial from the refrigerator; allow the vial to come to room temperature for ≤1 hr
• Gently swirl the vial; do not invert, shake
• Withdraw 0.8 mL from the 48-mg vial into a syringe labeled with the dose (48 mg) and time of day
• Discard the remaining contents of the vial

Store:

• Use diluted solution immediately
• If not used immediately, store the solution in the refrigerator (2-8°C; 36-46°F) ≤24 hr or at room temperature (20-25°C; 68-77°F) ≤12 hr; protect from direct sunlight
• Max total storage time of 24 hr from the start of dose preparation to use

SUBCUT Injection:

• Inject dose into the subcutaneous tissue of the lower abdomen (preferred site) or the thigh
• Rotate the injection site from the left or right side (or vice versa) especially during the weekly administrations on cycles 1, 2, and 3
• Do not inject into tattoos, scars, or areas where the skin is red, bruised, tender, hard

PHARMACOKINETICS

Half-life 22 days, metabolized into small peptides via catabolic pathways

SIDE EFFECTS

CNS: *Headache, fever, fatigue,* immune effector cell–associated neurotoxicity syndrome (ICANS)

ENDO: Hypo/hyperkalemia, hypomagnesemia, hypophosphatemia

GI: *Nausea, vomiting, abdominal pain, diarrhea*

RESP: Pleural effusion
INTEG: Rash, injection site reaction
HEMA: Anemia, leukopenia, lymphopenia, thrombocytopenia
SYST: Tumor flare, tumor lysis syndrome, infection, sepsis, cytokine release syndrome

INTERACTIONS
Increase: CYP substrates—monitor for toxicity, adjust the dose as needed during the first month and during and after cytokine release syndrome
Drug/Lab Test
Increase: LFTs, renal function studies, potassium
Decrease: Hct, WBC, lymphocytes, platelets, neutrophils, magnesium, sodium, phosphate

NURSING CONSIDERATIONS
Assess:
• Labs: Pregnancy test, CBC with differential, neuro test
• **Hematologic toxicity:** Anemia, neutropenia, febrile neutropenia, thrombocytopenia may occur, monitor CBC baseline and during treatment; provide care as per institutional guidelines, interruption or discontinuation may be needed in severe myelosuppression, prophylactic use of granulocyte colony-stimulating factors may be required
• **Cytokine release syndrome:** Assess for pyrexia, hypotension, hypoxia, dyspnea, chills, tachycardia, headache, confusion, tremors, dizziness, ataxia; product should be discontinued
• **Tumor flare/tumor lysis syndrome**
• **Immune effector cell–associated neurotoxicity syndrome (ICANS):** Assess for confusion, lethargy, tremor, dysgraphia, aphasia, nonconvulsive status epilepticus; cognitive impairment or change in consciousness should be evaluated neurologically; these patients should not drive or operate dangerous machinery until resolution
• **Injection site reaction:** Monitor for redness, inflammation, swelling at site

• **Infection:** Monitor for sepsis, COVID-19, UTI, pneumonia, URI; do not use in active infections, provide PJP and herpes virus prophylaxis prior to starting treatment
• **Pregnancy/breastfeeding:** Assess whether pregnancy is planned or suspected or if breastfeeding; do not use in pregnancy, breastfeeding, obtain pregnancy test before starting treatment in pregnancy potential females
Evaluate:
• Therapeutic response: Decreased progression of B-cell lymphoma
Teach patient/family:
• Teach patient to report to health care professional flulike symptoms, fever, cough, cognitive changes, trouble breathing, chills, dizziness
• Advise patient not to drive or operate dangerous machinery if dizziness or changes in cognition occur
• **Pregnancy/breastfeeding:** To use highly effective contraceptive methods during and for 4 mo after treatment; to contact health care provider if pregnancy is suspected or confirmed; not to breastfeed during or for 4 mo after last dose

---

etrasimod (Rx)
(EH-trah-sih-mod)
Velsipity
Func. class.: Immunomodulator
Chem. class.: Oral sphingosine 1-phosphate receptor modulator

---

ACTION: Binds with high affinity to S1P receptors 1, 4, and 5, partially and reversibly blocks the capacity of lymphocytes to migrate from lymph nodes, reducing the number of lymphocytes in peripheral blood; the result is reduction of lymphocyte migration into the intestine

USES: Ulcerative colitis

CONTRAINDICATIONS
Hypersensitivity
Precautions: Pregnancy, breastfeeding, AIDS, angina, CV disease, RA, SLE

DOSAGE AND ROUTES
Moderate-severe active ulcerative colitis
Adult: PO 2 mg qday
Available forms: Tablets 2 mg
Administer:
• Swallow whole
• May be administered with or without food
• Administer live attenuated vaccines at least 1 mo prior to treatment
• Avoid vaccination with live vaccines during treatment and for 5 wk after last dose due to immunosuppression and increased risk of infection
• A diminished vaccine response may occur if vaccinations are administered during treatment

SIDE EFFECTS
CNS: Headache, migraine
CV: Hypertension
GI: Hepatotoxicity
INTEG: Skin cancer
MS: Arthralgia
SYST: Serious infections, anaphylaxis, sepsis

PHARMACOKINETICS
Half-life was 9.3 days

INTERACTIONS
• Do not give concurrently with vaccines; immunizations should be brought up-to-date before treatment
• Avoid use with immunosuppressives

NURSING CONSIDERATIONS
Assess:
• Ulcerative colitis: Diarrhea, mucus in stools, abdominal pain baseline and during treatment
• Test patients without a confirmed history of chickenpox or without documentation of a full course of vaccination against varicella-zoster virus (VZV) for antibodies to VZV prior to treatment
• Vaccinate antibody-negative patients prior to treatment, postpone treatment for 1 mo after vaccination to allow the full effect of vaccination to occur. Consider HPV vaccination prior to treatment
• Cancer screening, Papanicolaou (Pap) test in females is recommended
• **Infection:** Monitor for fever, sore throat, cough; do not use during active infections
• **Pregnancy/breastfeeding:** Women should use effective contraception during treatment and for 1 wk after last dose, pregnant patients should enroll in the pregnancy registry, calling 800-616-3791; do not use in pregnancy; avoid use in breastfeeding
Evaluate:
• Therapeutic response: Decreased symptoms of ulcerative colitis
Teach patient/family:
• That product must be continued for prescribed time to be effective; to use as prescribed
• To notify prescriber of possible infection (upper respiratory or other) or allergic reactions
• That follow-up will be needed

⚠ HIGH ALERT

exagamglogene (Rx)
(x-a-gam'gloh-jeen)
Casgevy
Func. class.: Gene modifier (sickle cell anemia)
Chem. class.: Stem cell gene replacement therapy

ACTION: A cellular gene therapy consisting of autologous CD34+ hematopoietic stem cells edited by CRISPR/Cas9 technology at the erythroid-specific enhancer region of the *BCL1A* gene. After exagamglogene autotemcel infusion, the edited CD34+ cells engraft in the bone marrow and differentiate to erythroid lineage cells with reduced BCL11A expression

---

Genetic warning

USES: Sickle cell disease with a history of vaso-occlusive events in adults and children ≥12 yr

CONTRAINDICATIONS
Pregnancy
Precautions: HIV, vaccination, breastfeeding

DOSAGE AND ROUTES
Adult/child ≥12 yr: IV infusion A minimum of 3×10^6 CD34+ cells/kg of body weight, single dose
Available forms: Suspension for infusion
Administer:
IV push route
• There is a risk of transmitting infectious diseases to health care professionals handling the product. Follow universal precautions and biosafety guidelines for handling and disposal of exagamglogene autotemcel
• Give between 48 hr and 7 days after the last dose of the myeloablative conditioning
• Give an antipyretic (acetaminophen) and an antihistamine (diphenhydramine) prior to use
• Visually inspect the vial(s) for any breaks or cracks before and after thawing. If a vial is compromised, do not infuse
• Coordinate the timing of thaw and infusion; confirm the infusion time in advance and adjust the start time for thaw so that the recipient and care team are ready
• Before thaw, confirm that exagamglogene autotemcel is printed on the vial label and that the recipient identity matches the unique personal ID information on the vial(s). Do not infuse if the information on the recipient-specific label on any of the vials does not match the intended recipient
• A dose may be contained in 1 or more cryopreserved recipient-specific vial(s); ensure that the correct number of vials are present. Use the accompanying Lot

Information Sheet to confirm the total number of vials to be administered, and confirm that each vial is within the expiration date prior to preparation for infusion
• Thaw each vial at 37° C (98° F) using a water bath. Thaw each vial holding the vial neck, gently agitating clockwise and counterclockwise. Thawing of each vial can take between 10 and 15 min; thawing is complete when ice crystals are no longer visible; ensure water bath temperature does not exceed 40° C (104° F) during thawing
• Do not leave unattended during thaw. Remove vial from water bath immediately once thawed. The thawed product should appear as a cellular suspension, which may contain proteinaceous particles or cellular aggregates. When the dose consists of multiple vials, thaw and administer 1 vial at a time. While thawing and administering a vial, remaining vials must remain in cryo-storage at −135° C or less (−211° F or less)
• Remove the flip-away tab of the vial cap; clean the septum with an alcohol swab; remove the cap on the vial adapter spike. With the thumb and forefinger of both hands, push the adapter into the vial septum, applying equal pressure until there is a single pop. Pull up on the adapter until you feel it lock. Attach the filter to the vial adapter
• Attach an empty 30-mL syringe to the filter and withdraw the entire vial volume. Remove the product-filled syringe from the filter and set aside
• Draw 5-10 mL of saline into the empty 10-mL syringe and attach the saline-filled syringe to the filter. Inject the saline into the vial and remove the empty syringe from the filter. Discard the empty syringe
• Attach the product-filled syringe to the filter and withdraw the contents of the vial into the syringe, then remove the syringe from the filter. Peel the product/

recipient identifier label from the Lot Information Sheet and affix to the product-filled syringe
• Do not wash, spin down, and/or re-suspend in new media prior to infusion
• Do not sample, alter, irradiate, or re-freeze
• Store: Infuse within 20 min of thaw
• Confirm the recipient's identity with the personal identifiers on the vial(s). Confirm the total number of vial(s) with the Lot Information Sheet
• If more than 1 vial is provided, thaw and administer each vial completely before proceeding to thaw the next vial
• Do not use an in-line blood filter or an infusion pump
• Give as an IV bolus/push within 20 min of product thaw. The total volume of product administered within 1 hr must not exceed 2.6 mL/kg
• Flush the primary line with 0.9% NaCl injection, using enough volume to flush the tubing and the length of the IV catheter, after administration of each vial
• Repeat steps for each vial

SIDE EFFECTS
HEMA: Thrombocytopenia, neutropenia, lymphopenia
GI: Stomatitis, nausea, constipation
INTEG: Infusion-related reactions
MISC: Sepsis, hyperbilirubemia

PHARMACOKINETICS
Not applicable

INTERACTIONS
• **Iron chelation:** avoid use for 6 mo after infusion due to risk of myelosuppression. If iron chelation is needed, consider administration of non-myelosuppressive iron chelators (deferoxamine) 3 mo after; phlebotomy can be used instead of iron chelation
• **G-CSF:** avoid administration of granulocyte colony–stimulating factors for 21 days after infusion
• **Vaccinations:** avoid vaccinations, as result is unknown

NURSING CONSIDERATIONS
Assess:
• Labs: CBC with differential, plasma HIV RNA, pregnancy test
• HIV: Do not use in those with HIV (HIV-1, HIV-2), hepatitis B virus (HBV), or hepatitis C virus (HCV). Screen for HIV-1, HIV-2, HBV, HCV, and any other infectious agents before collection of cells for manufacturing
• Pregnancy/breastfeeding: Women of childbearing potential should use adequate contraception during treatment, do not breastfeed, obtain a pregnancy test before use
Evaluate:
• Therapeutic response: Absence of sickle cell crisis
Teach patient/family:
• Advise the patient of the procedure for use, that follow-up exams and blood work will be needed
• Do not donate blood, tissues, cells
• Notify a health care professional of any side effects
• Pregnancy/breastfeeding: Identify if pregnancy is planned or suspected or if breastfeeding

---

fezolinetant (Rx)
(fez-oh-LIN-e-tant)
Veozah
Func. class.: Non-hormonal agent for menopause
Chem. class.: Neurokinin 3 (NK3) receptor antagonist

ACTION: Blocks neurokinin binding and modulates neuronal activity in the thermoregulatory center

USES: Moderate to severe vasomotor symptoms due to menopause

CONTRAINDICATIONS
Cirrhosis, severe renal impairment/end-stage renal disease, use with CYP1A2 inhibitors
Precautions: Hepatic disease

DOSAGE AND ROUTES
Adult female: PO 45 mg once daily
Available forms: Tablet 45 mg
Administer:
• Give with or without food

SIDE EFFECTS
GI: Abdominal pain, diarrhea, increases in LFTs
CNS: Insomnia, hot flush
MS: Back pain

PHARMACOKINETICS
Protein binding 51%, urine excretion 76.9%, metabolized by CYP1A2, minor metabolism by CYP2C9, CYP2C19, half-life 9.6 hr

INTERACTIONS
Increase: fezolinetant level—CYP1A2 inhibitor, do not use together

NURSING CONSIDERATIONS
Assess:
• Perform baseline bloodwork to evaluate for hepatic function and injury before beginning treatment; perform follow-up bloodwork at 3, 6, 9 mo after start of therapy and if hepatic symptoms occur; elevations in serum transaminase concentrations >3× ULN may occur; do not start if serum transaminase is equal to or exceeds 2× ULN
• Pregnancy/breastfeeding: No data available
Evaluate:
• Therapeutic response: Decreased hot flashes
Teach patient/family:
• Advise patient that continuing labs will be needed
• Pregnancy/breastfeeding: Identify if pregnancy is planned or suspected or if breastfeeding

---

fruquintinib
(froo-kwin'ti-nib)
Fruzaqla
Func. class.: Antineoplastic
Chem. class.: Tyrosine kinase inhibitor

ACTION: A small-molecule inhibitor of vascular endothelial growth factor receptor (VEGFR) that plays a role in angiogenesis, suppressing formation of new blood vessels, limiting the blood supply to tumors, and inhibiting their growth

USES: Metastatic colorectal cancer (mCRC) who have been previously treated with fluoropyrimidine, oxaliplatin, and irinotecan and those that have received anti-VEGF therapy and if RAS wild-type, an anti-EGFR treatment

CONTRAINDICATIONS
Hypersensitivity, severe hepatic disease, pregnancy, breastfeeding
Precautions: anticoagulat therapy, bleeding, cardiac disease

DOSAGE AND ROUTES
Adult: PO 5 mg qday, with or without food, for the first 21 days of each 28-day cycle
Available forms: Capsules 1 mg, 5 mg
Administer:
• Once a day without regard to food
• Swallow whole with water; do not crush, split

SIDE EFFECTS
CNS: Fatigue
CV: Hypertension
INTEG: Hand-foot reaction
GU: Proteinuria
GI: Diarrhea, perforation, fistulas, GI bleeding, reversible posterior leukoencephalopathy syndrome (RPLS)

PHARMACOKINETICS
Peak a few hours, metabolism—liver, by CYP3A4 enzyme, excreted—feces

INTERACTIONS
• Avoid use with CYP3A4 inducers/inhibitors
Increase: bleeding risk—anticoagulants, monitor INR
Drug/Lab
Increase: triglycerides, cholesterol, LFTs, bilirubin, alkaline phosphatase
Decrease: albumin, lymphocytes, platelets, aPTT, magnesium

Side effects: *italics* = common; red = life-threatening

NURSING CONSIDERATIONS
Assess:

• **Colorectal cancer (mCRC):** Monitor for diarrhea, alternating constipation and diarrhea, mucus colitis, abdominal pain, GI bleeding, perforation baseline and during treatment; permanently discontinue in patients who develop GI perforation or fistula

• **Hypertension: Monitor B/P** baseline and throughout therapy, control B/P prior to treatment, use antihypertensives and adjust dose, withhold, or permanently discontinue if severe

• **Hemorrhage:** Monitor for bleeding (hematuria, hematemesis, frank blood, blood in stools); withhold, reduce dose, or permanently discontinue if severe; monitor INR in patients receiving anticoagulants

• **Infections:** Monitor for infection (fever, flulike symptoms) and withhold during active infections; do not start in patients with active infections

• **Hepatotoxicity:** Monitor LFTs baseline and periodically; withhold, reduce the dose, or permanently discontinue if severe; assess for jaundice of skin, sclera, dark-colored urine, clay-colored stools, abdominal pain

• **Proteinuria:** Monitor 24-hr urine protein baseline and throughout treatment; discontinue for nephrotic syndrome

• **Palmar-plantar erythrodysesthesia**: Withhold based on severity

• **Posterior reversible encephalopathy syndrome (PRES):** Immediately discontinue if PRES is suspected and confirmed by MRI

• **Impaired wound healing:** Withhold for 2 wk before major surgery. Do not use for ≥2 wk following major surgery and until adequate wound healing.

• **Arterial thromboembolic events:** Monitor closely in those with a recent history of thromboembolic events; discontinue in those who develop arterial thromboembolism

• **Allergic reactions**: To FD&C Yellow No. 5 (tartrazine) and No. 6 (sunset yellow FCF): Contains FD&C Yellow No. 5 (tartrazine) and No. 6 (sunset yellow FCF) as color additives, which may cause allergic reactions (including bronchial asthma) in susceptible patients.

• **Pregnancy/breastfeeding:** Can cause fetal harm, determine pregnancy status before using. Advise females of childbearing potential and males with female partners of childbearing potential to use effective contraception during and for 2 wk after the last dose, do not breastfeed

Evaluate:

• Therapeutic response: Decreasing spread of mCRC

Teach patient/family:

• To contact health care provider for hepatotoxicity, symptoms of infection, changes in wound healing, allergic reactions, or bleeding

• Pregnancy/breastfeeding: To identify if pregnancy is planned or suspected or if breastfeeding; that females of childbearing potential and males with female partners of childbearing potential will need to use effective contraception during and for 2 wk after the last dose, not to breastfeed

---

ganaxolone (Rx)
(gan-AX-oh-lone)
Zytalmy
Func. class.: Anticonvulsant
Chem. class.: Neuroactive steroid gamma-aminobutyric acid (GABA) A receptor positive modulator

---

ACTION: Anticonvulsant effects are thought to result from positive allosteric modulation of the gamma-aminobutyric acid type A (GABA$_A$) receptor in the CNS

USES: Seizures associated with cyclin-dependent kinase-like 5 deficiency disorder (CDD)

CONTRAINDICATIONS
Hypersensitivity
Precautions: Hepatic disease, depression, pregnancy, breastfeeding, abrupt discontinuation, use with other CNS depressants

---

DOSAGE AND ROUTES
Adults: PO 150 mg tid × 7 days. Uptitrate per this schedule based on tolerability: 300 mg tid × 7 days, then 450 mg tid × 7 days. Increase to 600 mg tid and maintain dose. Max: 1800 mg/day

Children and adolescents 2-17 yr and >28 kg: PO 150 mg tid × 7 days. Uptitrate per this schedule based on tolerability: 300 mg tid × 7 days, then 450 mg tid × 7 days. Increase to 600 mg tid and maintain dose. Max: 1800 mg/day

Children and adolescents 2-17 yr and ≤28 kg: PO 6 mg/kg/dose tid × 7 days. Uptitrate per this schedule based on tolerability: 11 mg/kg/dose tid × 7 days, then 16 mg/kg/dose tid × 7 days. Increase to 21 mg/kg/dose tid and maintain dose. Max: 63 mg/kg/day

Available forms: Suspension 50 mg/mL
Administer:
• Administer with food
• Use an oral syringe to measure and administer the dose
• Shake for at least 1 min and then wait for 1 min before measuring and giving
• *Storage:* Discard any unused medication after 30 days after opening

SIDE EFFECTS
CNS: Seizures, fever, sedation, drowsiness, lethargy
GI: Hypersecretions
EEET: Seasonal allergy
MS: Gait disturbance
RESP: Bronchitis
MISC: Flulike symptoms

PHARMACOKINETICS
Protein binding 99%, half-life 34 hr, excretion 55% feces (2% as unchanged), 18% urine
Affected isoenzymes and drug transporters: CYP3A4/5, CYP2B6, CYP2C19, CYP2D6

INTERACTIONS
Increase: CNS depression—CNS depressants, alcohol
Decrease: ganaxolone effect—CYP3A4/5, CYP2B6, CYP2C19, and CYP2D6; CYP450 inducers, dosage increase may be needed

NURSING CONSIDERATIONS
Assess:
• **Seizures**: Identify type, character baseline and during treatment
• **CNS depressants**: Identify other CNS depressants taken, assess for increased sedation, lethargy
• **Hepatic disease**: Monitor for increased side effects, metabolism is decreased
Evaluate:
• Therapeutic response: Decreased amount and severity of seizures
Teach patient/family:
• Mental status: Advise family, caregivers, patient that suicidal thoughts, behaviors may increase beginning and during treatment
• Not to drive or engage in other hazardous activity until effect is known
• Not to discontinue abruptly, seizures may increase
• Pregnancy/breastfeeding: Identify if pregnancy is planned or suspected or if breastfeeding

---

gepirone (Rx)
(geh-PEE-rone)
Exxua
Func. class.: Antidepressant
Chem. class.: SSRI, benzofuran

ACTION: Novel antidepressant unrelated to other antidepressants, enhances serotonergic action by a dual mechanism

USES: Major depression

CONTRAINDICATIONS
Concomitant use of MAO inhibitors or within 14 days after discontinuing MAO inhibitor or within 14 days after discontinuing gepirone

Precautions: Pregnancy, geriatric patients, bipolar disorder, operating machinery, substance abuse, serotonin syndrome, use with serotonin precursors or serotonergic drugs; suicidal ideation, worsening depression or behavior

Black Box Warning: Children, suicidal ideation

DOSAGE AND ROUTES
Major depressive disorder
Adult: PO 18.2 mg qday with food, may increase to 36.3 mg/day on day 4. May further titrate to 54.5 mg/day after day 7 and to 72.6 mg/day after an additional week, if needed. Max: 72.6 mg/day.

Available forms: Tabs ER 18.2 mg

Administer:
- Swallow ER tablets whole. Do not split, crush, or chew
- Administer with food at approximately the same time each day
- Do not use within 2 wk of MAOIs
- Missed dose should be taken as soon as possible, unless it is almost time for next dose; do not double
- Store at room temperature, away from moisture, heat

SIDE EFFECTS
CNS: Dizziness, drowsiness, fatigue, mania, headache, insomnia, depression, suicidal ideation

CV: Persistent pulmonary hypertension

GI: *Nausea, diarrhea*

SYST: Neonatal abstinence syndrome, withdrawal, serotonin syndrome

INTERACTIONS
- Do not use within 2 wk of MAO inhibitors, linezolid, or methylene blue

Increase: serotonin syndrome—SSRIs, SNRIs, serotonin receptor agonists, selegiline, busPIRone, dextromethorphan, ergots, fenfluramine, dexfluramine, lithium, meperidine, fentaNYL, methylphenidate, dexmethylphenidate, metoclopramide, mirtazapine, nefazodone, pentazocine, phenothiazines, haloperidol, loxapine, thiothixene, molindone, amphetamines

Increase: gepirone levels—CYP3A4 inhibitors (ketoconazole, erythromycin, efavirenz, dronedarone, clarithromycin and others)

Decrease: gepirone effect—CYP3A4 inducers (carBAMazepine)

Drug/Food
Avoid use with grapefruit juice

Drug/Herb
Increase: serotonin syndrome—St. John's wort

PHARMACOKINETICS
Protein binding 72%, metabolized by liver by CYP3A4, excretion 60 % urine, half-life 5 hr

NURSING CONSIDERATIONS
Assess:

Black Box Warning: Mental status: Orientation, mood, behavior initially and periodically; initiate suicide precautions if indicated; history of seizures, mania

- Abrupt discontinuation: Do not discontinue abruptly, taper, monitor for symptoms of withdrawal; if intolerable, resume previous dose and decrease more slowly
- Serotonin syndrome/NMS: Nausea, vomiting, sedation, sweating, facial flushing, high B/P; discontinue product, notify prescriber change in mental status, seizures, rigidity; discontinue product, notify prescriber immediately
- Pregnancy/breastfeeding: Use only if benefits outweigh fetal risk; if pregnant, enroll in the National Pregnancy Registry for Antidepressants at 866-961-2388 or visiting online at https://womensmentalhealth. org/research/pregnancyregistry/ antidepressants/; fetal complications may occur; no data on breastfeeding

Evaluate:
- Therapeutic response: Remission of depressive symptoms

Teach patient/family:
- To take as directed, with food, not to double dose, follow-up will be needed
- Not to drive or operate machinery until effects are known

• Not to use other products unless approved by prescriber, do not use alcohol
• To contact prescriber for allergic reactions; personality changes (aggression, anxiety, anger, hostility); extreme sleepiness confusion, nervous, restless, or clumsy; numbness, tingling, burning pain in hands, arms, legs, or feet; tremors; unusual behavior or thoughts about hurting oneself

Black Box Warning: Suicidal thoughts/behaviors: Discuss with family the possibility of suicidal thoughts/behaviors and that prescriber should be notified immediately if these occur

• To notify prescriber if pregnancy is planned or suspected

glofitamab
(gloe-fit'-a-mab)
Columvi
Func. class.: Antineoplastic

USES: Diffuse large B-cell lymphoma, not otherwise specified, or large B-cell lymphoma arising from follicular lymphoma after 2 or more lines of systemic therapy

Black Box Warning: Cytokine release syndrome

DOSAGE AND ROUTES
Adult: IV infusion Cycle 1/day 1: Pretreat with obinutuzumab 1000 mg; cycle 1/day 8: 2.5 mg over 4 hr (step-up dose 1); cycle 1/day 15: 10 mg over 4 hr (step-up dose 2); cycle 2/day 1: 30 mg over 4 hr; cycles 3-12/day 1: 30 mg over 2 hr
Available forms: Injection concentrate: 2.5 mg/2.5 mL (1 mg/mL, 10 mg/10 mL [1 mg/mL]) in a single-dose vial for IV infusion after dilution

iptacopan
Fabhalta
Func. class.: Antineoplastic

USES: Adults with paroxysmal nocturnal hemoglobinuria (PNH)

Black Box Warning: Serious/life threatening infections

DOSAGE AND ROUTES
Adult: PO 200 mg bid
Available forms: Capsule 200 mg

lecanemab (Rx)
(lee-KAN-e-mab)
Leqembi
Func. class.: Alzheimer agent
Chem. class.: Amyloid beta–directed antibody

ACTION: A human immunoglobulin gamma 1 (IgG1) monoclonal antibody directed against amyloid beta, reduces amyloid beta plaques

USES: Alzheimer disease

CONTRAINDICATIONS
Serious hypersensitivity, anaphylaxis
Precautions: Pregnancy, breastfeeding, anticoagulant/thrombolytic therapy, hamster protein hypersensitivity, infusion-related reactions, stroke, aneurysm

Black Box Warning: Amyloid-related imaging abnormalities (ARIAs)

DOSAGE AND ROUTES
Adults: IV infusion 10 mg/kg every 2 wk
Available forms: Solution for infusion 200mg/2 mL, 500 mg/5 mL
Administer:
IV infusion route
• Visually inspect for particulate matter and discoloration prior to use, solution should be clear to opalescent and colorless to pale yellow; do not use if opaque particles, discoloration, or foreign particles are found

• *Missed dose:* Give as soon as possible

Preparation of IV infusion

• Each vial is for single-use only and is preservative-free, discard unused portions

• Calculate dose and total volume of solution required and the number of vials needed based on the patient's actual body weight (10 mg/kg). Each vial contains 100 mg/mL; more than 1 vial may be needed for a full dose. Select the correct number of vial(s) for the needed dose

• Withdraw the required volume from the vial(s) and add to an infusion bag of 250 mL of 0.9% NaCl only, gently invert to mix, do not shake

• *Store:* After dilution, immediate use is recommended. If not administered immediately, store the prepared infusion in the refrigerator at 2-8° C (36-46° F) for up to 4 hr or at room temperature up to 30° C (86° F) for up to 4 hr. Do not freeze

Administration

• Confirm amyloid beta pathology prior to treatment; MRI within 1 yr of beginning treatment then MRIs prior to the 5th, 7th, and 14th infusions to monitor for ARIA-E, ARIA-H

• Prior to infusion, allow the prepared IV infusion solution to warm to room temperature. Inspect before administration. Do not use if it is discolored, opaque, or foreign particles are seen. Do not shake

• Infuse IV over 1 hr through an IV line containing a terminal low-protein-binding 0.2-micron in-line filter, flush line

• Monitor for any signs or symptoms of an infusion-related reaction. Infusion rate may be reduced or infusion may be interrupted or discontinued and appropriate therapy administered as clinically indicated. Consider premedication with antihistamines, acetaminophen, nonsteroidal antiinflammatory drugs, or corticosteroids prior to future infusions

• Dosing interruptions for ARIA-E: Asymptomatic and mild ARIA-E on MRI:

continue; mild symptoms and mild ARIA-E on MRI: continue based on clinical judgment; moderate/severe symptoms (regardless of ARIA-E severity seen on MRI) or moderate or severe ARIA-E on MRI (regardless of symptoms): suspend until MRI demonstrates resolution and symptoms; use a follow-up MRI to assess for resolution 2-4 mo after initial MRI

• Dosing interruptions for patients with ARIA-H (based on clinical symptom severity and ARIA-H severity on MRI): Asymptomatic and mild ARIA-H on MRI: may continue; asymptomatic and moderate ARIA-H on MRI or symptomatic and mild or moderate ARIA-H on MRI: suspend until MRI demonstrates radiographic stabilization and symptoms resolve, follow-up MRI in 2-4 mo after initial episode; severe ARIA-H on MRI (regardless of symptoms): suspend until MRI demonstrates radiographic stabilization and symptoms

SIDE EFFECTS

CNS: Headache
HEMA: Microhemorrhage
RESP: Bronchospasm
SYST: ARIA, infusion-related reactions

INTERACTIONS

None known

PHARMACOKINETICS

Onset, peak, duration unknown

NURSING CONSIDERATIONS

Assess:

• ARIA: Assess for headache, confusion, dizziness, vision changes, nausea; notify prescriber

• Hypersensitivity: Assess for itching, rash, anaphylaxis

Evaluate:

• Therapeutic response: Decreasing symptoms of Alzheimer disease (confusion)

Teach patient/family:

• ARIA: Teach patient that ARIA may occur with temporary swelling in areas of the brain, small spots of bleeding on the brain; to report headache, confusion, dizziness, vision changes, nausea; that MRIs will be needed

• **Hypersensitivity:** Inform patient that serious hypersensitivity, including anaphylaxis, urticaria, may occur; to contact health care provider

---

⚠ HIGH ALERT

toripalimab
(to'se-li-zu'mab)

Loqtorzi
Func. class.: Antineoplastic

USES: Recurrent or metastatic nasopharyngeal carcinoma when used together with or following other therapies

DOSAGE AND ROUTES
Treatment of nasopharyngeal carcinoma:
Adults: IV 240 mg on day 1, every 3 wk until disease progression, unacceptable toxicity, or for up to 24 mo in patients without progression. Give with cisplatin (80 mg/m^2 IV on day 1) and gemcitabine (1000 mg/m^2 IV on days 1 and 8) every 3 wk for up to 6 cycles, give prior to chemotherapy when given on the same day
Available forms: Solution for injection 240 mg/6 mL

---

lotilaner (Rx)
(loti-lan-er)

Xdemvy
Func. class.: Ophthalmic, antiparasitic

USES: *Demodex* blepharitis

DOSAGE AND ROUTES
Adult: Ophthalmic Instill 1 drop in each eye twice daily (approximately 12 hr apart) for 6 wk
Available forms: Ophthalmic solution 0.25%

⚠ HIGH ALERT

lovotibeglogene autotemcel (Rx)
loh-voe-tee-BEG-loh-jeen aw-toh-TEM-sel)

Lyfgenia
Func. class.: Gene modifier (sickle cell anemia)
Chem. class.: Stem cell gene replacement therapy

ACTION: An autologous hematopoietic stem cell–based gene therapy that adds copies of a modified beta^A-globin gene (threonine [T] replaced with glutamine [Q] at position 87, T87Q or beta$^{A\text{-}T87Q}$-globin) into subjects' HSCs through transduction of autologous CD34+ cells with BB305 lentiviral vector (LVV), a cellular nonviral promoter that controls gene expression for RBCs and their precursors. BB305 LVV encodes beta$^{A\text{-}T87Q}$-globin

USES: Sickle cell disease and a history of vaso-occlusive events in adults and children ≥12 yr

CONTRAINDICATIONS
Pregnancy
Precautions: HIV, vaccination

Black Box Warning: New primary malignancy, α-thalassemia trait (−α3.7/−α3.7), delayed platelet engraftment, neutrophil engraftment failure, insertional oncogenesis, hypersensitivity, more than two α-globin gene deletions

DOSAGE AND ROUTES
Adult/child ≥12 yr: IV infusion A minimum of 3×10^6 CD34+ cells/kg of body weight in a 1-4 infusion bags, single dose
Available forms: Suspension for infusion

Administer:
- Allow a minimum of 48 hr after completion of myeloablative conditioning before infusion
- May carry the risk of transmitting infectious diseases to health care professionals handling the product. Follow universal precautions and biosafety guidelines for handling and disposal of the product

IV infusion route
- Visually inspect each infusion bag for any breaches of integrity before thawing and infusion
- Coordinate the timing of the thaw and infusion; confirm the infusion time in advance and adjust the start time for thaw so that the recipient and care team are ready
- Remove each metal cassette from liquid nitrogen storage and each infusion bag from the metal cassette. Confirm that lovotibeglogene autotemcel is printed on the infusion bag(s)
- Confirm that patient's identity matches the unique personal ID information located on the infusion bag(s). Do not infuse if the information on the recipient-specific label on the infusion bag does not match
- Ensure the correct number of infusion bags are present. Use the accompanying Lot Information Sheet to confirm that each infusion bag is within the expiration date
- Thaw the infusion bag(s) at 37°C (98.6°F) in a water bath or dry bath. Thawing of each infusion bag takes 2-4 min; do not leave unattended, and do not submerge the infusion ports in a water bath. If more than 1 infusion bag is provided, thaw and administer each infusion completely before proceeding to thaw the next infusion bag. Maintain any additional infusion bag(s), if applicable, at −140°C (−220°F) or less until time to thaw
- After thawing, mix the contents gently by massaging the infusion bag to disperse clumps of cellular material until all the contents are uniform; if visible clumps remain, continue to gently mix the contents
- Do not filter, wash, spin down, and/or resuspend new media before use; do not sample, alter, irradiate or refreeze
- *Store:* Do not store, infuse as soon as possible after thawing and complete the infusion within 4 hr
- Confirm the recipient's identity with the personal identifiers on the infusion bag. Confirm the total number of infusion bags with the Lot Information Sheet
- If more than 1 infusion bag is provided, thaw and administer each infusion completely before proceeding to thaw the next infusion bag
- Do not use an in-line blood filter or an infusion pump
- Give each bag by IV infusion over a period of less than 30 min
- Flush all remaining product in the infusion bag(s) and the tubing with at least 50 mL of 0.9% NaCl injection to ensure as many cells as possible are infused
- Repeat steps for each infusion bag

SIDE EFFECTS
CV: Hypotension, flushing, cardiac arrest
HEMA: Thrombocytopenia, neutropenia, febrile neutropenia, anemia, leukopenia, sickle cell anemia with crisis
GI: Stomatitis, nausea, decreased appetite
INTEG: Infusion-related reactions
META: Respiratory, thoracic, mediastinal disorders
MISC: Pyrexia, bacteremia, pharyngeal inflammation, hyperbilirubinemia, leukemia, new primary malignancy

PHARMACOKINETICS
Not applicable

INTERACTIONS
- **Hydroxyurea:** If used after apheresis, discontinue hydroxyurea ≤2 days prior to myeloablative conditioning

• **Iron chelation:** Avoid use for 6 mo after infusion due to risk of myelosuppression. If iron chelation is needed, consider administration of non-myelosuppressive iron chelators (deferoxamine) 3 mo after; phlebotomy can be used instead of iron chelation
• **G-CSF:** Avoid administration of granulocyte colony–stimulating factors for 21 days after infusion
• **Vaccinations:** Avoid vaccinations, as result is unknown
Lab/Drug
Increase: AST, ALT, GGT, bilirubin

NURSING CONSIDERATIONS
Assess:
• Labs: CBC with differential, plasma HIV RNA, pregnancy test
• **Hematologic malignancy:** Monitor patients for malignancy by CBCs at ≤6 months and through integration site analysis at months 6, 12, and as needed up to 15 yr
• **Delayed platelet engraftment:** Monitor often for thrombocytopenia and bleeding until platelet engraftment and platelet recovery occur
• Pregnancy/breastfeeding: Women of childbearing potential should use adequate contraception during treatment, do not breastfeed, obtain a pregnancy test before use
Evaluate:
• Therapeutic response: Absence of sickle cell crisis
Teach patient/family:
• Advise the patient of the procedure for use, that follow-up exams and blood work will be needed
• Do not donate blood, tissues, cells
• Notify a health care professional of abnormal bleeding, bruising, blood in urine/vomit/stools, coughing up blood, fatigue, fever, severe headache, abdominal/back pain; these could be evidence of a serious condition
• Pregnancy/breastfeeding: Identify if pregnancy is planned or suspected or if breastfeeding

maralixibat (Rx)
(mar-a-lix'i-bat)
Livmarli
Func. class.: GI agent, misc
Chem. class.: Ileal bile acid transporter (IBAT) inhibitor

ACTION: A reversible inhibitor of the IBAT, inhibition of the IBAT blocks the reabsorption of bile acids (primarily in the salt form) from the terminal ileum, interrupting enterohepatic circulation by shunting the bile acids away from the liver and toward fecal excretion

USES: Cholestatic pruritus associated with Alagille syndrome (ALGS) in those ≥1 yr

CONTRAINDICATIONS
Hypersensitivity
Precautions: Ascites, fat-soluble vitamin deficiencies, hepatic disease, pregnancy, breastfeeding, child <1 yr

DOSAGE AND ROUTES
Cholestatic pruritus in Alagille syndrome:
Adult/child ≥1 yr: PO Initially, 190 mcg/kg qday × 1 wk, then increase to 380 mcg/kg qday after a week, as tolerated, Max: 28.5 mg/day
Hepatic dose:
Interrupt treatment if new-onset hepatic function abnormalities occur. Once hepatic function returns to baseline or stabilizes at a new baseline, consider restarting maralixibat at 190 mcg/kg/day and increase to 380 mcg/kg/day as tolerated. Consider permanent discontinuation if abnormalities in liver tests recur or symptoms consistent with clinical hepatitis are observed. Permanently discontinue treatment if a patient experiences a hepatic decompensation event (variceal hemorrhage, ascites, hepatic encephalopathy)
Available forms: Oral solution 9.5 mg/mL
Administer:
• Give PO as a solution 30 min before the first meal of the day using provided

calibrated measuring device (0.5-mL, 1-mL, or 3-mL oral dispenser)

• If a dose is missed, take the missed dose as soon as possible within 12 hr of the time it is usually taken, and then resume normal dosing; if the dose is missed by >12 hr, skip the missed dose and take the next dose at regularly scheduled time

• Administer ≥4 hr before or after administration of bile acid sequestrants

• Store: After opening, store below 30° C (86° F). Discard remaining solution 100 days after opening

SIDE EFFECTS

GI: Diarrhea, abdominal pain, vomiting, liver-related effects, increased LFTs
INTEG: Rash
SYST: Fat-soluble vitamin deficiencies

PHARMACOKINETICS

91% protein bound; eliminated in the feces (73%, with 94% unchanged), half-life of 1.6 hr, serum bile acid may decrease by week 12, inhibits OATP2B1

INTERACTIONS

Decrease: maralixibat effect—bile acid sequestrants, separate by 4 hr
Decrease: HMG-CoA reductase inhibitors (statins), monitor statin effect and adjust dose, usually occurs in maralixibat doses >4.75 mg/day
Drug/Lab
Increase: AST, ALT, bilirubin, INR
Decrease: vitamins A, D, E, K

NURSING CONSIDERATIONS
Assessment:

• Pruritus: Monitor for decreasing pruritus in Alagille syndrome

• Monitor for the development of liver-related adverse reactions during therapy; monitor liver function (ALT, AST, total bilirubin, direct bilirubin, INR) baseline and during therapy

• Monitor for fat-soluble vitamin deficiency (vitamins A, D, E, and K [measured using INR levels]) during therapy; initiate vitamin supplementation if a deficiency is diagnosed

• Monitor for the development of adverse GI effects during treatment (diarrhea, abdominal pain, vomiting)

• Assess for systemic effects of propylene glycol, an inactive ingredient

• Pregnancy/breastfeeding: Use during pregnancy is not expected to result in measurable fetal exposure due to low systemic absorption after oral administration, may inhibit the absorption of fat-soluble vitamins; increased fat-soluble vitamin supplements may be needed

Evaluate:

• Therapeutic response: Decreasing pruritus after decreased serum bile acid

Teach patient/family:

• To notify health care provider of increasing abdominal pain, diarrhea, nausea, yellowing of eyes and skin, dark urine, clay-colored stools, increasing itching

• That continuing labs and follow-ups will be needed

• Pregnancy/breastfeeding: To notify health care provider if pregnancy is planned or suspected or if breastfeeding

---

> ## ⚠ HIGH ALERT
>
> ## maribavir (Rx)
> (ma-rye'ba-vir)
> Livtencity
> *Func. class.:* Antiviral
> *Chem. class.:* Kinase inhibitor

ACTION: A cytomegalovirus (CMV) pUL97 protein kinase inhibitor active against CMV

USES: CMV infection that is refractory to treatment (with or without genotype resistance) with ganciclovir, valganciclovir, cidofovir, or foscarnet in adult and pediatric transplant recipients ≥12 yr of age who weigh ≥35 kg

DOSAGE AND ROUTES
PCMV infection and disease in transplant recipients

Adult/adolescent ≥12 yeyrars of age weighing ≥35 kg: **PO** 400 mg (two 200-mg tablets) bid; if used with carbamazepine, increase to 800 mg bid; If used with PHENObarbital or phenytoin, increase dosage to 1200 mg bid
Available forms: Tablets 200 mg
Administer:
• Give PO without regard to meals
• IR: Taken whole, dispersed or crushed by mouth, or as dispersed tablets through a nasogastric (NG) or orogastric (OG) tube (French size 10 or larger). The suspension may be prepared ahead of time and stored at room temperature for up to 8 hr

SIDE EFFECTS
GI: Diarrhea, abdominal pain, vomiting, taste perversion
CNS: Fatigue
INTEG: Rash

PHARMACOKINETICS
Protein binding 98%, hepatic metabolism, metabolized by CYP3A4 with CYP1A2 as a minor metabolic pathway. The major circulating inactive metabolite is VP 44469 (N-dealkylated metabolite); 61% excreted as unchanged drug in the urine and 14% excreted as unchanged drug in the feces; half-life 4.32 hr; a substrate of CYP3A4, weak inhibitor of CYP3A4, P-glycoprotein (P-gp), and breast cancer resistance protein (BCRP)

INTERACTIONS
Increase: CYP3A4. P-gp, BCRP substrates, avoid using together
Increase: immunosuppressants, adjust dose as needed
Increase: digoxin levels, monitor for toxicity, digoxin dose may need reduction
Decrease: maribavir effect—CYP3A4 inducers, avoid using together
Drug/Herb
Decrease: maribavir effect—St. John's wort, avoid using together

NURSING CONSIDERATIONS
Assess:
• **CMV infection: Obtain an ophthalmology appointment baseline and periodically**; monitor CMV DNA

levels and check for resistance if the patient does not respond to treatment
• Identify medications taken and associated possible drug interactions prior to treatment
• Frequently monitor immunosuppressant drug levels throughout treatment, especially following initiation and after discontinuation
• Monitor for the development of liver-related adverse reactions during therapy
• Monitor liver function (ALT, AST, total bilirubin, direct bilirubin, INR) baseline and during therapy. Assess for yellowing eyes, sclera, clay-colored stools, dark urine, abdominal pain
• Monitor for the development of adverse GI effects during treatment
Patient family/teaching:
• Advise patient to take without regard to meals
• To discuss with health care provider all Rx, OTC, herbals, and supplements taken
• That continuing labs and exams will be needed
• Pregnancy/breastfeeding: Advise patient to report if pregnancy is planned or suspected or if breastfeeding

mavacamten (Rx)
(mav-a-kam-ten)
Camzyos
Func. class.: Cardiac agent
Chem. class: Cardiac myosin inhibitor

ACTION: A reversible inhibitor selective for cardiac myosin. Myosin inhibition reduces dynamic left ventricular outflow tract (LVOT) obstruction and improves cardiac filling pressures

USES: Adults with symptomatic New York Heart Association (NYHA) class II-III obstructive hypertrophic cardiomyopathy (HCM) to improve functional capacity and symptoms

CONTRAINDICATIONS
Hypersensitivity, use with moderate to strong CYP2C19 inhibitors, strong CYP3A4 inhibitors, moderate to strong CYP2C19 inducers, moderate to strong CYP3A4 inducers

Black Box Warning: HF

Precautions: Pregnancy, breastfeeding

DOSAGE AND ROUTES
Symptomatic NYHA class II-III obstructive hypertrophic cardiomyopathy:
Adults: PO 5 mg once daily initially. Adjust dose q4wk during initiation phase and q12wk during maintenance phase as needed

Available forms: Capsules 2.5, 5, 10, 15 mg
Administer:
• Swallow capsule whole. Do not break, open, or chew the capsules
• May administer without regard to food
• *Missed dose:* Administer a missed dose as soon as possible and the next scheduled dose at the usual time the following day. Exact timing of dosing during the day is not essential, but do not administer 2 doses on the same day

SIDE EFFECTS
CV: HF
CNS: Dizziness

PHARMACOKINETICS
Protein binding 98%, extensively metabolized, by CYP2C19 (74%), CYP3A4 (18%), and CYP2C9 (8%); 7% of the dose was recovered in the feces (1% unchanged) and 85% was recovered in the urine (3% unchanged). Variable half-life that depends on CYP2C19 metabolic status; affected cytochrome P450 isoenzymes and drug transporters: CYP2B6, CYP2C8, CYP2C9, CYP2C19, CYP3A4; a CYP2C19, CYP3A4 substrate and a CYP2B6, CYP2C8, CYP2C9, CYP2C19, CYP3A4 inducer, peak 1 hr

INTERACTIONS
Increase: mavacamten effect—increased risk of HF—CYP3A4 inhibitors, CYP2C19 inhibitors, avoid using together

Increase: mavacamten effect—digoxin, cimetidine, avoid using together
Decrease: mavacamten effect—CYP3A4 inducers, CYP2C19 inducers, avoid using together
Decrease: hormonal contraceptives, use additional nonhormonal contraception
Drug/Herb
Decrease: mavacamten effect—St. John's wort, avoid using together
Drug/Food
Increase: mavacamten effect—grapefruit juice, grapefruit, avoid using together

NURSING CONSIDERATIONS
Assess:
• **Cardiac parameters:** Left ventricular ejection fraction (LVEF) baseline and at 4 wk; if less than 55%, avoid use; if using a CYP3A4 inhibitor; echocardiogram (ECHO) baseline and at 4, 8, and 12 wk during initiation, then q12wk during maintenance
• **Dysrhythmias:** Assess for current and worsening dysrhythmias, dyspnea, chest pain
• **Drug interactions**: Review drug interactions before starting treatment. Coadministration of certain drugs may need to be avoided, or dosage adjustments may be necessary
• **Pregnancy/breastfeeding:** Identify pregnancy status before starting treatment, may cause fetal harm, use of nonhormonal contraceptives is needed during and for 4 mo after last dose; report pregnancy to Bristol Myers Squibb pregnancy outcome study (800-721-5072 or www.bms.com). No data on breastfeeding
Evaluate:
• Therapeutic response: Improvement in cardiac parameters in symptomatic NYHA class II-III obstructive hypertrophic cardiomyopathy
Teach patient/family:
• Use the *Patient Brochure* to discuss aspects of product use, have patient complete the *Patient Enrollment Form*
• **To report shortness of breath**, chest pain, fatigue, a racing sensation in

the heart (palpitations), swelling in the legs, rapid weight gain
• **Teach patient that continuing exams will be need to assess cardiac function**
• **Drug interactions:** Discuss all OTC, Rx, herbals, supplements taken; not to start or stop other products
• **Pregnancy/breastfeeding:** Identify if pregnancy is planned or suspected, discuss need for additional contraception, if hormonal contraceptives are used, must use contraception during and for 4 mo after last dose, avoid breastfeeding

---

mirikizumab (Rx)

(mir'i-kiz'ue-mab)

Omvoh

Func. class.: Immune response modifier
Chem. class.: Monoclonal antibody, interleukin-12 inhibitor

ACTION: Interleukin (IL)-12, IL-23 antagonist, binds to an interleukin protein, decreases inflammation

USES: Ulcerative colitis

CONTRAINDICATIONS
Hypersensitivity, sepsis, active infections
Precautions: Pregnancy, breastfeeding, children ≤18 yr, geriatric patients, surgery, TB, diabetes mellitus, immunosuppression

DOSAGE AND ROUTES
Moderate-severe active ulcerative colitis
Adult: IV INF (Induction) 300 mg over ≥30 min at wk 0, 4, and 8; (maintenance) after induction SUBCUT 200 mg (given as 2 consecutive injections of 100 mg each) at wk 12, then, 200 mg SUBCUT q4wk after that
Available forms: Solution for injection 300 mg/15 mL; prefilled pen solution for injection 100 mg/mL

Administer:
• Keep in original carton to protect from light
• Do not shake the syringe, vials, carton
• Visually inspect for particulate matter and discoloration before use; solution should be colorless to slightly yellow
• Do not use if discolored, cloudy, or foreign particulate matter is present
IV route
Preparation:
• Use IV infusion only for the induction treatment
• Each vial is for single use only
• Dilute prior to IV infusion administration. Using an 18-21G needle, withdraw 15 mL of mirikizumab solution from the vial and inject into an IV infusion bag (50-250 mL of 0.9% sodium chloride injection or 5% dextrose injection). Do not mix with other drugs. Do not dilute with solutions other than 0.9% sodium chloride or 5% dextrose injection
• Gently invert the infusion bag to mix, do not shake the prepared infusion bag
• *Store prepared infusion:* Start the infusion immediately after preparation. If not used immediately, store the diluted infusion solution in the refrigerator between 2° and 8° C (36° and 46° F). Use the diluted infusion solution within 48 total hr, of which no more than 5 hr are permitted at nonrefrigerated temperatures not to exceed 25° C (77° F), starting from the time of vial puncture. Protect from heat and light. Do not freeze
IV infusion administration (induction):
• Prime the line, give over ≥30 min
• Do not infuse through the same IV line with other drugs or solutions other than 0.9% sodium chloride or 5% dextrose injection
• At the end of the infusion, flush the line with 0.9% sodium chloride injection or 5% dextrose injection, give the flush at the same infusion rate as used for administration

---

Side effects: *italics* = common; red = life-threatening

Subcutaneous administration (maintenance):

• Each maintenance dose will require 2 prefilled pens. Each pen contains 100 mg/mL

• SUBCUT to be used with the guidance and supervision of a health care professional

• Patients may self-inject SUBCUT mirikizumab after training in SUBCUT injection technique. Provide proper training to patients and/or caregivers on the SUBCUT injection technique

• Refer to the manufacturer-provided "Instructions for Use" for detailed instructions on preparation and administration

• Before injection, remove the prefilled pen from the refrigerator and leave at room temperature for 30 min, do not shake the prefilled pens

• Sites for injection include the abdomen, thigh, and back of the upper arm. Instruct patients to inject in a different location every time

• Do not inject into areas where the skin is tender, bruised, indurated, or any lesions are present

• The prefilled syringe does not contain preservatives; discard any unused portion

• *Missed dose:* If a dose is missed, give as soon as possible, then resume dosing q4wk

• *Store:* The prefilled pen may be stored at room temperature up to 30° C (86° F) for up to 2 wk in the original carton to protect from light. Once a prefilled syringe has been stored at room temperature, do not return to the refrigerator

SIDE EFFECTS
CNS: Headache
GI: Hepatotoxicity
INTEG: *Injection site reaction,* pruritus, skin irritation
SYST: Serious infections, anaphylaxis, sepsis

PHARMACOKINETICS
Half-life was 9.3 days

INTERACTIONS
• Do not give concurrently with vaccines; immunizations should be brought up to date before treatment
• Avoid use with immunosuppressives

NURSING CONSIDERATIONS
Assess:
• Ulcerative colitis: Diarrhea, mucus in stools, abdominal pain baseline and during treatment
• Bring immunizations up to date before starting treatment; do not administer live vaccines during treatment and for 3 mo after treatment ends
• **Infection:** Monitor for fever, sore throat, cough; do not use during active infection
• TB: TB testing should be done before starting treatment
• For injection site pain, swelling, rash
• **Pregnancy/breastfeeding:** Pregnant patients should enroll in the pregnancy registry (877-302-2161); use only if benefits outweigh fetal risk; avoid use in breastfeeding, excretion unknown
Evaluate:
• Therapeutic response: Decreased symptoms of ulcerative colitis
Teach patient/family:
• That product must be continued for prescribed time to be effective; to use as prescribed
• Not to receive live vaccinations during treatment
• To notify prescriber of possible infection (upper respiratory or other) or allergic reactions
• Injection techniques and disposal of equipment; not to reuse needles, syringes
• That follow-up will be needed

---

mitapivat (Rx)
(MYE-ta-PIV-at)
Pyrukynd
Func. class.: Antianemic agent
Chem. class.: Pyruvate kinase activator

ACTION: Binds to the pyruvate kinase tetramer and increases pyruvate kinase (PK) activity. The red blood cell (RBC) form of pyruvate kinase (PK-R) is mutated in PK deficiency, which leads to reduced adenosine triphosphate (ATP), shortened RBC lifespan, and chronic hemolysis

USES: Hemolytic anemia in patients with pyruvate kinase (PK) deficiency

CONTRAINDICATIONS
None known
Precautions: Abrupt discontinuation, breastfeeding, hepatic disease, pregnancy

DOSAGE AND ROUTES
Adults: PO 5 mg bid, then increase dose to 20 mg bid and then 50 mg bid q4wk if hemoglobin (Hb) is below normal or patient has required a transfusion within the last 8 wk. Maintain current dose if Hb is within normal and patient has not required a transfusion within the last 8 wk
Available forms: Tablet 5, 20, 50 mg
Administer:
• May be administered with or without food. Swallow tablets whole; do not split, crush, chew, or dissolve the tablets
• *Missed dose:* If a dose is missed by 4 hr or less, administer as soon as possible. If a dose is missed by more than 4 hr, do not administer a replacement dose, and wait until the next scheduled dose. Then, return to the normal dosing schedule
• *Store:* Store between 68° and 77° F, store in carton until time of use

SIDE EFFECTS
CNS: Paresthesia
CV: Flushing, hot flashes, hypertension, atrial fibrillation, dysrhythmias
META: Hypertriglyceridemia
EENT: Dry mouth, oropharyngeal pain
GI: Constipation, gastroenteritis
MS: Back pain, arthralgia, flank pain

PHARMACOKINETICS
Protein binding 97.7%, metabolized by CYP3A4, excretion 49.6% in the urine (2.6% unchanged); 39.6% in the feces (less than 1% unchanged); half-life 3-5 hr, peak 30-60 min
Affected isoenzymes and drug transporters: CYP3A, CYP2B6, CYP2C9, CYP2C19, UGT1A1, and P-gp
Mitapivat is a CYP3A and P-gp substrate; CYP2B6, CYP2C8, CYP2C9, CYP2C19, and UGT1A1 inducer; and CYP3A and P-gp inhibitor

INTERACTIONS
Increase: mitapivat effect—increased risk with CYP3A4 inhibitors, avoid using together
Decrease: mitapivat effect—CYP3A4 inducers, avoid using together
Decrease: substrate level—CYP2B6 substrates, CYP2C substrates, CYP3A4 substrates
Drug/Lab
Increase: triglycerides, urates, Hb
Decrease: estradiol, estrone

NURSING CONSIDERATIONS
Assess:
• Monitor Hb/Hct baseline and periodically
• Identify drugs taken and drug interactions before use
Evaluate:
• Therapeutic response: Decreasing hemolytic anemia
Teach patient/family:
• Advise patient not to stop drug abruptly
• Discuss all OTC, Rx, herbals, supplements taken and not to add or remove product without discussing with prescriber
• **Pregnancy/breastfeeding:** Advise patient if using hormonal contraceptive that effect may be reduced, to use additional contraceptives

momelotinib (Rx)
(MOE-me-LOE-ti-nib)
Ojjaara
Func. class.: Kinase inhibitor

USES: Intermediate- or high-risk myelofibrosis (MF), including primary MF or secondary MF (postpolycythemia vera [PV] and postessential thrombocythemia [ET]), in adults with anemia

DOSAGE AND ROUTES
Adult: PO 200 mg once daily with or without food
Hepatic dose:
Adult, severe hepatic disease (Child-Pugh Class C): PO Reduce starting dose to 150 mg once daily
Available forms: Tablets 100 mg, 150 mg, 200 mg

---

motixafortide (Rx)
Aphexda
Func. class.: Hematopoietic stem cell mobilizer

USES: In combination with filgrastim (G-CSF) to mobilize hematopoietic stem cells to the peripheral blood for collection, autologous transplantation in multiple myeloma

DOSAGE AND ROUTES
Adult: SUBCUT Start treatment after filgrastim has been given daily for 4 days; then give 1.25 mg/kg actual body weight 10-14 hr prior to apheresis; a second dose can be given 10-14 hr prior to a third apheresis
Available forms: Lyophilized powder for injection: 62 mg in a single-dose vial (must reconstitute)

---

nedosiran (Rx)
(ned-oh-SIR-an)
Rivfloza
Func. class.: Metabolic disorder agent
Chem. class.: Primary hyperoxaluria type 1 (PH1) agent

ACTION: Reduces concentrations of hepatic LDH by degrading lactate dehydrogenase A (LDHA) mRNA in hepatocytes, leading to decreases in the production of oxalate by the liver

USES: Primary hyperoxaluria type 1

CONTRAINDICATIONS
Hypersensitivity
Precautions: Breastfeeding, pregnancy

DOSAGE AND ROUTES
Adult/child/adolescent 9-17 yr, ≥50 kg: SUBCUT 160 mg once monthly **Adult/adolescent 12-17 yr <50 kg: SUBCUT** 128 mg once monthly **Child 9-11 yr, <50 kg: SUBCUT** 3.3 mg/kg/dose (max: 128 mg/dose) once monthly
Available forms: 80 mg (0.5 mL) single-dose vial; 128 mg (0.8 mL) single-dose prefilled syringe; 160 mg (1 mL) single-dose prefilled syringe
Administer:
SUBCUT route
• Visually inspect for particulate matter and discoloration prior to use, product is colorless to yellow and particle free, preservative free
• *Store:* Store unused prefilled syringes or vials in the refrigerator at 2-8° C (36-46° F), prefilled syringes or vials can be stored at 15-30° C (59-86° F) ≤28 days (4 wk). Record the date of removal from the refrigerator on the carton and dispose of if not used within 28 days, avoid direct heat and light. Do not warm the prefilled syringe or vial using any heat sources, do not freeze
• *Missed dose:* If a dose is missed, give as soon as possible, if missed by >7 days, give as soon as possible and resume monthly dosing from most recent dose
• Remove prefilled syringe or vial(s) from refrigerator, wait 30 min before use
• **Prefilled syringe:** The prefilled syringe may be self-administered by persons 12 yr and older. A health care professional or caregiver may administer using a prefilled syringe for children 9-11 yr as well as for 2 yr and older
• **Vial:** The vial is intended for use under the guidance and supervision of a health care professional or caregiver

---

• **Administration:** Choose the injection site from the abdomen (at least 2 in. from the belly button) or the upper thigh. Do not inject into a vein or scarred or bruised skin

SIDE EFFECTS
INTEG: Rash, injection site reactions

PHARMACOKINETICS
Protein binding 85.6%, metabolized by endo- and exonucleases to shorter oligonucleotides, excretion unchanged urine (27% after 1 hr), half-life 15 hr, peak 6 hr

INTERACTIONS
None known

NURSING CONSIDERATIONS
Assess:
• Primary hyperoxaluria type 1: Monitor for urinary patterns, blood in urine, back pain, urgency, hesitancy before and during treatment
• Injection-site reactions: Monitor for redness, inflammation, pain
• Pregnancy/breastfeeding: Use cautiously, effects unknown
Evaluate:
• Therapeutic response: Decreasing pain from stones, blood in urine, back pain
Teach patient/family:
• Advise patient to read the Patient Information and Instructions for Use
• Instruct patients/caregivers on the dose to use, the timing of the dose, how and where to inject SUBCUT, what to do if a dose is missed, disposal of equipment
• Pregnancy/breastfeeding: Identify if pregnancy is planned or suspected or if breastfeeding

---

nirmatrelvir/ritonavir (Rx)
(nir-mat-rel-vir ri-toe′na-veer)
Paxlovid
Func. class.: Antiviral
Chem. class.: SARS-CoV-2 protease inhibitor

ACTION: Ritonavir is an HIV-1 protease inhibitor and a CYP3A inhibitor. Ritonavir does not have antiviral activity against SARS-CoV-2, but instead is used to boost nirmatrelvir; nirmatrelvir is an inhibitor of the SARS-CoV-2 main protease. By binding directly to the SARS-CoV-2 active site, nirmatrelvir prevents the virus from processing polyprotein precursors, thereby preventing viral replication

USES: Severe acute respiratory syndrome coronavirus 2 (SARS-CoV-2) infection resulting in mild to moderate coronavirus disease 2019 (COVID-19) in patients who are at high risk for progressing to severe COVID-19, including hospitalization or death

CONTRAINDICATIONS
Serious hypersensitivity, drugs metabolized by CYP3A4, CYP3A4 inducers
Precautions: Pregnancy, breastfeeding, hepatotoxicity, HIV-1 resistance development

DOSAGE AND ROUTES
Severe acute respiratory syndrome coronavirus 2 (SARS-CoV-2) infection resulting in mild to moderate coronavirus disease 2019 (COVID-19) in patients who are at high risk for progressing to severe COVID-19, including hospitalization or death:
Adults: PO 300 mg nirmatrelvir (two 150-mg tablets) and 100 mg ritonavir (one 100-mg tablet), with all 3 tablets taken together twice daily for 5 days
Available forms: Tablets 150 mg/100 mg, 300 mg/100 mg
Administer:
• Initiate treatment as soon as possible after the positive test for SARS-CoV-2 and within 5 days of symptom onset.
• Patients must complete the full 5-day treatment course and continue isolation in accordance with public health recommendations; treatment for longer than 5 consecutive days is not approved
• May administer tablets with or without food

• Swallow tablets whole with a sufficient amount of fluid.

• The prescribing information and the EUA recommend against crushing or chewing the tablets. However, the National Institutes of Health (NIH) COVID-19 treatment guidelines suggest the tablets can be split or crushed if necessary

SIDE EFFECTS

CNS: *Headache*

GI: Diarrhea, abdominal pain, nausea, vomiting, anorexia

INTEG: Rash

MISC: Anaphylaxis, Stevens-Johnson syndrome, toxic epidermal necrolysis

PHARMACOKINETICS

Half-life 3-5 hr (ritonavir)

INTERACTIONS

• Many drug interactions, check manufacturer's information

Increase: toxicity—amiodarone, astemizole, azole antifungals, benzodiazepines, buPROPion, CISapride, cloZAPine, desipramine, dihydroergotamine, encainide, ergotamine, flecainide, HMG-CoA reductase inhibitors, interleukins, meperidine, midazolam, pimozide, piroxicam, propafenone, propoxyphene, quiNIDine, ranolazine, saquinavir, terfenadine, triazolam, zolpidem; CYP2D6 inhibitors

Increase: QT prolongation—class IA/III antidysrhythmics, some phenothiazines, β-agonists, local anesthetics, tricyclics, haloperidol, chloroquine, droperidol, pentamidine, CYP3A4 inhibitors (amiodarone, clarithromycin, dasatinib, erythromycin, telithromycin, troleandomycin), arsenic trioxide, CYP3A4 substrates (methadone, pimozide, QUEtiapine, quiNIDine, risperiDONE, ziprasidone)

Increase: ritonavir levels—fluconazole

Increase: level of both products—clarithromycin, ddI

Increase: levels of—bosentan

Decrease: ritonavir levels—rifamycins, nevirapine, barbiturates, phenytoin

Decrease: levels of anticoagulants, atovaquone, divalproex, ethinyl estradiol, lamoTRIgine, phenytoin, sulfamethoxazole, theophylline, voriconazole, zidovudine

NURSING CONSIDERATIONS

Assess:

• SAR-CoV-2: Monitor LFTs and creatinine baseline and periodically during treatment

• Monitor for skin eruptions; rash

• **Serious skin disorders:** Stevens-Johnson syndrome, toxic epidermal necrolysis

• **Pregnancy/breastfeeding:** Use only if benefits outweigh fetal risk; do not breastfeed

Evaluate:

• Therapeutic response: Improvement in COVID symptoms, prevention of hospitalization

Teach patient/family:

• To take as prescribed; not to double dose

• To avoid OTC, prescription medications, herbs, supplements unless approved by prescriber, many drug interactions

---

nirogacestat

(NYE-roe-GAY-se-stat)

Ogsiveo

Func class.: Antineoplastic

USES: Adults with progressing desmoid tumors

DOSAGE AND ROUTES

Adult: PO 150 mg bid until disease progression or unacceptable toxicity

Available forms: Tablet 50 mg

---

nirsevimab-alip (Rx)

Beyfortus

Func. class.: Fusion inhibitor

USES: A respiratory syncytial virus (RSV) F protein–directed fusion inhibitor for the prevention of RSV lower

---

respiratory tract disease in neonates/infants born during or entering their 1st RSV season and children up to 24 mo who are vulnerable to severe RSV disease through their 2nd RSV season

DOSAGE AND ROUTES
Neonate/infant <5 kg: IM 50 mg;
>5 kg: 100 mg **Child ≤24 mo: IM** 200 mg (2 × 100 mg injections
Available forms: Injection 50 mg/0.5 mL in a single-dose prefilled syringe

---

perfluorohexyloctane (Rx)
Miebo
Func. class.: Ophthalmic

USES: Dry eye disease

DOSAGE AND ROUTES
Adult: Ophthalmic instill 1 drop 4 times daily into each eye
Available forms: Ophthalmic solution

---

pirtobrutinib (Rx)
(peer-toh-broo'-tin-ib)
Jaypirca
Func. class.: Antineoplastic
Chem. class: Tyrosine kinase inhibitor

ACTION: A small-molecule inhibitor of BTK, a signaling protein of the B-cell antigen receptor (BCR) and cytokine receptor pathways

USES: Adult patients with relapsed or refractory mantle cell lymphoma (MCL) after at least 2 lines of systemic therapy, including a BTK inhibitor

CONTRAINDICATIONS
Hypersensitivity
Precautions: Infections, hemorrhage, cytopenias, cardiac dysrhythmias, 2nd primary malignancies, pregnancy, breastfeeding

DOSAGE AND ROUTES
Adult: PO 200 mg orally once daily
Available forms: Tablets 50 mg, 100 mg
Administer:
• Once a day without regard to food
• Swallow whole with water, do not crush, split
• Manage toxicity by treatment interruption, dosage reduction, or discontinuation
• Reduce dose in severe renal impairment

SIDE EFFECTS
CNS: *Fatigue*
CV: Dysrhythmias
MS: *MS pain*
HEMA: *Decreased neutrophils, platelets, Hb, lymphocytes*
INTEG: *Bruising*
GI: *Diarrhea*
RESP: *Cough*
SYST: *COVID-19*

PHARMACOKINETICS
Half-life 19 hr, metabolism—liver by CYP3A4 enzyme and direct glucuronidation by UGT1A8 and UGT1A9, excreted—feces 37% and urine 57%, protein binding 96%

INTERACTIONS
• Avoid use with strong CYP3A4 inducers/inhibitors
Decrease: pirtobrutinib effect—moderate CYP3A inducers, increase the pirtobrutinib dose
Drug/Lab
Decrease: neutrophils, platelets, Hb, lymphocytes

NURSING CONSIDERATIONS
Assess:
• **Mantle cell lymphoma (MCL):** Assess for decreasing fatigue, stable blood counts, absence of nausea, vomiting, decrease in lymph nodes
• **Other malignancies:** Monitor patient for skin cancer and other cancers of the GU and breast, have patient use sunscreen and protective clothing when outside

• **Dysrhythmias:** Monitor for palpitations, dizziness, syncope, dyspnea that can indicate dysrhythmias; based on severity, dose may need reduction or withdrawal; those with hypertension or previous dysrhythmias are at higher risk

• **Cytopenias:** Neutropenia, thrombocytopenia, and anemia may occur; monitor CBC baseline and periodically

• **Hemorrhage:** Monitor those at risk for bleeding; withhold, reduce dose, or permanently discontinue if severe; may need to withhold product 3-7 days pre- and post-surgery; assess if antithrombotic agents are being used

• **Infections:** Monitor for infection (fever, flulike symptoms), some may be fatal (sepsis, pneumonia), opportunistic infections (*Pneumocystis jirovecii* pneumonia and fungal infection); withhold during active infections; do not start in patients with active infections; may use prophylaxis (vaccinations and antimicrobials) in patients who are at increased risk for infections

• **Pregnancy/breastfeeding:** Can cause fetal harm. Advise patients of potential risk to the fetus and to use effective contraception during and for 1 wk after last dose, do not breastfeed, verify pregnancy status before using

Evaluate:

• Therapeutic response: Blood counts improving

Patient/family teaching:

• To contact health care provider for symptoms of infection (chills, fever, weakness, flulike symptoms), palpitations, dizziness, fainting, chest discomfort, shortness of breath, bleeding, bruising, that product may need to be interrupted for surgery

• That continuing exams and blood work will be needed

• Advise patients to use sun protection and protective clothing and to monitor for other cancers

• To take once daily at the same time of the day with or without food, to swallow tablets whole with water, not to cut, crush, or chew

• **Pregnancy/breastfeeding:** To identify if pregnancy is planned or suspected or if breastfeeding; that females of child-bearing potential will need to use effective contraception during and for 1 wk after the last dose, not to breastfeed during and for 1 wk after last dose

---

> ⚠ **HIGH ALERT**
>
> ## quizartinib (Rx)
> (kwiz-ar'-tin-ib)
> Vanflyta
> *Func. class.*: Antineoplastic

USES: Used in combination with standard cytarabine and anthracycline induction and cytarabine consolidation and as maintenance monotherapy following consolidation chemotherapy for the treatment of adult patients with newly diagnosed acute myeloid leukemia (AML) that is FLT3 internal tandem duplication (ITD) positive as detected by an FDA-approved test

CONTRAINDICATIONS

Hypersensitivity, pregnancy, breastfeeding

Black Box Warning: Torsades de pointes, QT prolongation, cardiac arrest

DOSAGE AND ROUTES

Adult: PO Induction therapy: 35.4 mg orally once daily for 14 doses on days 8-21 (cycle 1) or days 6-19 (cycle 2) in combination with cytarabine and an anthracycline for up to 2 cycles. **Consolidation therapy:** 35.4 mg orally once daily for 14 doses on days 6-19 in combination with high-dose cytarabine for up to 4 cycles. **Maintenance therapy** following consolidation chemotherapy once the absolute neutrophil count is more than 500 cells/mm³ and the platelet count is more than 50,000 cells/mm³ as follows: quizartinib 26.5 mg orally once daily for 14 doses on days 1-14 on cycle 1, then increase the dosage to 53 mg

---

once daily starting on day 15 if the QTcF interval is 450 msec or less; continue at the 26.5 mg orally once-daily dosage if the QTcF interval was more than 500 msec during induction or consolidation. Continue maintenance therapy once daily until disease progression or for up to 36 cycles.

⚠ HIGH ALERT

repotrectinib (Rx)
(ree-poh-trek'-ti-nib)

Augtyro
Func. class.: Antineoplastic
Chem. class.: Tyrosine kinase inhibitor

ACTION: An inhibitor of proto-oncogene tyrosine protein kinase ROS1 (ROS1) and of the tropomyosin receptor tyrosine kinases (TRKs) TRKA, TRKB, and TRKC

CONTRAINDICATIONS
Hypersensitivity
Precautions: Fractures, pregnancy, breastfeeding, chronic lung disease, interstitial lung disease, myopathy, pneumonitis, hyperuricemia

DOSAGE AND ROUTES
Adult: PO 160 mg once daily for 14 days, then increase to 160 mg twice daily until disease progression or unacceptable toxicity
Available forms: Capsules 40 mg
Administer:
• Once a day without regard to food
• Swallow whole with water, do not crush, split
• *Missed dose:* If dose is missed or vomiting occurs, skip and give at next scheduled dose

SIDE EFFECTS
CNS: Dizziness, peripheral neuropathy, dysgeusia, cognitive changes, headache, fatigue,
CV: Edema

RESP: Dyspnea, cough
MS: Weakness, myalgia
EENT: Vision disorders
GI: Diarrhea, constipation, nausea, vomiting, weight change

PHARMACOKINETICS
Peak a few hours, metabolism-liver, by CYP3A4 enzyme, excreted-feces

INTERACTIONS
P-gp inhibitors: avoid concomitant use
Strong and moderate CYP3A inducers: avoid concomitant use
Decrease: some CYP3A substrates: avoid concomitant use with CYP3A substrates
Decrease: hormonal contraceptives, avoid concomitant use
Drug/Lab
Decrease: Hb, lymphocytes, leukocytes, neutrophils
Increase: aPTT, INR, creatine phosphokinase, GGT, AST, ALT, sodium, alkaline phosphatase, glucose, urate

NURSING CONSIDERATIONS
Assess:
• **ROS-1 positive non-small cell lung cancer**: Monitor for chest pain, cough, hoarseness, dyspnea, difficulty swallowing, baseline and during treatment
• **Hepatotoxicity**: Monitor LFTs baseline, every 2 wk during the 1st mo of treatment and periodically; withhold, reduce the dose, or permanently discontinue if severe; assess for jaundice of skin, sclera, dark-colored urine, clay-colored stools, abdominal pain
• **Myalgia (CPK elevation):** Monitor serum CPK levels during treatment in those with unexplained muscle pain, tenderness, or weakness; based on severity, withhold and resume at same or reduced dose upon improvement
• **Hyperuricemia**: Monitor serum uric acid levels baseline and periodically during treatment, may use urate-lowering medications as needed, withhold and resume at same or reduced dose, or permanently discontinue based on severity

---

• **Fractures:** Assess patient for skeletal pain, changes in mobility; may indicate fractures; assess fall risk

• **Central nervous system (CNS) effects:** Monitor for dizziness, ataxia, cognitive changes, consider withholding or permanently discontinuing based on severity

• **Interstitial lung disease (ILD)/pneumonitis:** Monitor for new or worsening pulmonary symptoms: dyspnea, dry cough, withhold in patients with suspected ILD/pneumonitis and permanently discontinue if ILD/pneumonitis is confirmed

• **Pregnancy/breastfeeding:** Can cause fetal harm. Advise patients of reproductive potential of the potential risk to the fetus and to use effective nonhormonal contraception during and for 2 mo after last dose, male patients with female partners of reproductive potential to use effective contraception during treatment and for 4 mo after the last dose. Do not breastfeed

Evaluate:

• Therapeutic response: Decreased symptoms of non-small cell lung cancer, prevention of spread

Teach patient/family:

• Advise patients not to drive or engage in other hazardous activities when experiencing CNS reactions

• Advise patient to notify health care provider of severe dyspnea, cough, clay-colored stools, dark urine, yellowing of skin or eyes, abdominal pain, muscle pain

• Hyperuricemia: Advise patients to inform their health care provider if they experience signs or symptoms associated with hyperuricemia

• Skeletal fractures: Inform patients that bone fractures have occurred in patients taking repotrectinib and advise patients to report symptoms to their health care provider [see Warnings and Precautions (5.6)]

• Embryo-fetal toxicity: Advise pregnant women and females of reproductive potential of the potential risk to a fetus. Advise females to inform their health care provider of a known or suspected pregnancy [see Warnings and Precautions (5.7), Use in Specific Populations (8.1, 8.3)]

• Advise females of reproductive potential to use effective nonhormonal contraception during treatment with repotrectinib and for 2 mo after the last dose, since repotrectinib can render some hormonal contraceptives ineffective [see Drug Interactions (7.2)]

• Advise male patients with female partners of reproductive potential to use effective contraception during treatment with repotrectinib and for 4 mo after the last dose [see Use in Specific Populations (8.1, 8.3)] Lactation: Advise females not to breastfeed during treatment with repotrectinib and for 10 days after the last dose [see Use in Specific Populations (8.2)]

• Drug interactions: Advise patients to inform their health care providers of all concomitant medications, including prescription medicines, over-the-counter drugs, vitamins, and herbal products [see Drug Interactions (7)]

• Advise patients to avoid grapefruit or grapefruit juice while taking repotrectinib [see Drug Interactions (7)]

• Advise patients that hormonal contraceptives can be ineffective while taking repotrectinib [see Drug Interactions (7)]

• Administration: Advise patients to swallow repotrectinib capsules whole with or without food [see Dosage and Administration (2.6), Pharmacokinetics (12.3)]

• Instruct patients if they miss a dose or vomit at any time after taking a dose of repotrectinib, not to "make it up," but take the next dose of repotrectinib at the next scheduled time [see Dosage and Administration (2.6)]. For more information, go to www.AUGTYRO.com or call 877-284-8976

⚠ HIGH ALERT

retifanlimab (Rx)
(RE-ti-FAN-li-mab)

Zynyz
Func. class.: Antineoplastic
Chem. class.: Monoclonal antibody

ACTION: A humanized IgG4 kappa monoclonal antibody that binds to the PD-1 receptor on T cells and blocks interaction with its ligands (PD-L1 and PD-L2), causing T-cell antitumor activity

USES: Metastatic or recurrent locally advanced Merkel cell carcinoma (MCC)

CONTRAINDICATIONS

Hypersensitivity, pregnancy, breastfeeding
Precautions: Anemia, infection, neutropenia, thrombocytopenia, contraceptive requirements, colitis, Crohn's disease, pneumonitis, transplant, nephritis

DOSAGE AND ROUTES
For the treatment of metastatic or recurrent locally advanced Merkel cell carcinoma (MCC):
Adult: IV infusion 500 mg every 4 wk until disease progression or ≤24 mo. Therapy may need to be temporarily withheld or permanently discontinued in immune-related reactions; permanently discontinue in life-threatening infusion-related reactions
Available forms: Solution for infusion 500 mg/20 mL
Administer:
IV infusion route
• Visually inspect for particulate matter and discoloration prior to use
• Product is a clear to slightly opalescent, colorless to pale yellow solution; discard if cloudy, discolored, or contains particulates
• For IV infusion only, do not give as an IV push or bolus
• Dilution is required prior to use

• May use premedication with an antipyretic and/or an antihistamine before use if the patient has a history of infusion-related reactions to therapeutic proteins
• **Withdraw** 20 mL from the vial and **dilute** in 0.9 % NaCl injection or D5 injection to a final concentration between 1.4 mg/mL and 10 mg/mL, discard unused portion
• Mix by gently inverting the bag; do not shake
• Use infusion bags made of polyvinylchloride (PVC) and di-2-ethylhexyl phthalate (DEHP), polyolefin copolymer, polyolefin with polyamide, or ethylene vinyl acetate
• *Storage following dilution:* Protect from light. Do not freeze or shake. Store at room temperature up to 25° C (77° F) ≤8 hr from the time of preparation to the end of infusion or refrigerated at 2-8° C (26-46° F) ≤24 hr from the time of preparation to the end of infusion. If refrigerated, allow to come to room temperature and give within 4 hr of removal from the refrigerator (including infusion time)
• **Administer** over 30 min
• Use a polyethylene or PVC with DEHP IV infusion set with a sterile, nonpyrogenic, low-protein-binding polyethersulfone, polyvinylidene fluoride, or cellulose acetate 0.2-micron to 5-micron in-line or add-on filter or 15-micron mesh in-line or add-on filter; do not use a polyurethane infusion set
• Do not co-administer other drugs through the same infusion line
• During use, monitor for infusion-related reactions

PHARMACOKINETICS
Half-life 19 days

SIDE EFFECTS
CNS: Fever, fatigue
GI: Nausea, vomiting
INTEG: Rash, injection-site reaction
MS: MS pain
HEMA: Anemia, leukopenia, lymphopenia, thrombocytopenia

INTERACTIONS
None known
Drug/Lab Test
Increase: LFTs, amylase, lipase, alkaline phosphatase
Decrease: Hct, lymphocytes, platelets, neutrophils, sodium, potassium

NURSING CONSIDERATIONS
Assess:
• Labs: Pregnancy test, CBC with differential
• Hematologic toxicity: Anemia, neutropenia, thrombocytopenia may occur, monitor CBC baseline and during treatment; provide care as per institutional guidelines, interruption or discontinuation may be needed in severe myelosuppression, prophylactic use of granulocyte colony-stimulating factors may be required
• Immune-mediated pneumonitis: May be fatal, systemic corticosteroids may be required or product withheld or discontinued
• Immune-mediated colitis: Cytomegalovirus infection/reactivation may occur in those with corticosteroid-refractory immune-mediated colitis, may require withholding or discontinuing
• Immune-mediated hepatitis, adrenal insufficiency, hypophysitis, thyroid disorders/type 1 diabetes: May requiring withholding or discontinuation
• May premedicate with an antipyretic and/or an antihistamine in patients who have had previous systemic reactions to infusions of therapeutic proteins
• Complications of allogeneic HSCT: Fatal and other serious complications can occur including hyperacute graft-versus-host disease (GVHD), acute GVHD, chronic GVHD, hepatic veno-occlusive disease, and steroid-requiring febrile syndrome; assess patients closely for transplant-related complications and intervene promptly
• **Injection-site reaction:** Monitor for redness, inflammation, swelling at site

• **Pregnancy/breastfeeding:** Assess whether pregnancy is planned or suspected or if breastfeeding; do not use in pregnancy, breastfeeding; obtain pregnancy test before starting treatment in females with pregnancy potential
Evaluate:
• Therapeutic response: Decreased progression of Merkel cell carcinoma
Teach patient/family:
• Advise patient to review the FDA-approved Medication Guide
• Advise patients to notify health care professional of worsening symptoms of cough, chest pain, shortness of breath, diarrhea, blood/mucus in stools, severe abdominal pain, dark urine, clay-colored stools, yellowing of skin, eyes, new rash, changes in urination
• Infusion-related reactions: Advise patients to contact their health care professional immediately for signs or symptoms of infusion-related reactions (redness, inflammation, pain at site)
• Advise patients to contact their health care professional immediately for symptoms after transplant
• **Pregnancy/breastfeeding:** To use highly effective contraceptive methods during and for 4 mo after treatment; to contact health care provider if pregnancy is suspected or confirmed; not to breastfeed during or for 4 mo after last dose

---

rezafungin (Rx)
(re-za-FUN-jin)
Rezzayo
Func. class.: Antifungal, systemic
Chem. class.: Echinocandin

ACTION: Inhibits an essential component in fungal cell walls; causes direct damage to fungal cell wall

USES: Candidemia and invasive candidiasis in persons who have limited or no alternative options

CONTRAINDICATIONS
Hypersensitivity
Precautions: Pregnancy, breastfeeding, children, severe hepatic disease, sunlight exposure

DOSAGE AND ROUTES
Candidemia and invasive candidiasis:
Adults: IV infusion loading dose 400 mg, then 200 mg once weekly
Available forms: Powder for infusion 200 mg, requires dilution
Administer:
Intermittent IV INFUSION route
• Visually inspect for particulate matter and discoloration prior to use; solution should be clear to pale yellow; do not use if cloudy or has precipitate
• **Reconstitute** each vial with 9.5 mL of sterile water for injection (20 mg/mL), swirl, do not shake, foaming will occur
• *Storage:* The reconstituted solution may be stored at 5-25° C (41-77° F) for 24 hr
• *Dilution:* Reconstituted solution must be diluted using 0.9% NaCl injection, 0.45% NaCl injection, or 5% dextrose injection
• Withdraw and discard the appropriate volume of diluent from a 250 mL infusion bag
• For the 400-mg loading dose: Remove 20 mL to obtain a total diluent volume of 230 mL
• For the 200-mg maintenance dose: Remove 10 mL to obtain a total diluent volume of 240 mL
• Transfer the indicated volume of the reconstituted solution into the infusion bag
• For the 400-mg loading dose: Add 20 mL of the reconstituted solution to an infusion bag containing 230 mL of diluent (1.6 mg/mL)
• For the 200-mg maintenance dose: Add 10 mL of the reconstituted solution to an infusion bag containing 240 mL of diluent (0.8 mg/mL)
• *Storage:* Diluted solution may be stored at 5-25° (41-77° F) for 48 hr, do not freeze

• **Administer** over 1 hr
• If infusion-related reactions occur, slow or pause, restart at a lower rate
• *Missed dose:* If a scheduled dose is missed, administer the missed dose as soon as possible. If the missed dose is administered within 3 days of the assigned day, the next weekly dose may be given on schedule. If the missed dose is administered more than 3 days after the assigned day, revise the dosing schedule to ensure at least 4 days before the next dose. If restarting after at least 2 wk of missed dosing, start the dosing again at the 400 mg loading dose

SIDE EFFECTS
CNS: *Headache,* fever, insomnia, peripheral neuropathy, tremor
GI: Abdominal pain, *nausea, anorexia, vomiting, diarrhea, increased AST/ALT, alkaline phosphatase,* GI bleeding
HEMA: Anemia, DIC
INTEG: *Rash,* urticaria, *injection site pain,* photosensitivity
META: Hypokalemia, hypophosphatemia, hypomagnesemia

PHARMACOKINETICS
Half-life130-180 hr; protein binding 87.5-93.6%

INTERACTIONS
None known
Drug/Lab:
Increase: LFTs
Decrease: magnesium, phosphate, potassium

NURSING CONSIDERATIONS
Assess:
• **Infection:** Clearing of cultures during treatment; obtain culture at baseline, throughout treatment; product may be started as soon as culture is taken (candidiasis
• Blood studies prior to, during treatment: bilirubin, AST, ALT, alkaline phosphatase, as needed; serum potassium, magnesium, phosphate
• **Hypersensitivity:** Rash, urticaria

• GI symptoms: Frequency of stools, cramping; if severe diarrhea occurs, electrolytes may need to be given
• **Pregnancy/breastfeeding:** No well-controlled studies; use in pregnancy only if benefits outweigh fetal risk; unknown if excreted in breast milk, use cautiously in breastfeeding
Evaluate:
• Therapeutic response: Decreased symptoms of *Candida* infections
Teach patient/family:
• To inform prescriber of hepatic disease
• To report GI bleeding, rash
• To use sunscreen, protective clothing to prevent photosensitivity
• **Pregnancy/breastfeeding:** To notify prescriber if pregnancy is suspected or planned; to use cautiously in breastfeeding

---

rozanolixizumab-noli (Rx)
(roz-an-oh-lix-IZ-ue-mab-noli)
Rystiggo
Func. class.: Myasthenia gravis agent

USES: Generalized myasthenia gravis with antiacetylcholine receptor or antimuscle-specific tyrosine kinase antibody positive

DOSAGE AND ROUTES
Adult: SUBCUT Infusion <50 kg: 420 mg 3 mL; 50 kg to <100 kg: 560 mg 4 mL; ≥100 kg: 840 mg 6 mL; give q 6 wk
Available forms: Injection: 280 mg/2 mL (140 mg/mL) in a single-dose vial

---

somatrogon-ghla (Rx)
(soe-MA-troe-gon-ghla)
Ngenla
Func. class.: Human growth hormone analog

USES: For pediatric patients aged 3 yr and older who have growth failure due to inadequate secretion of endogenous growth hormone

CONTRAINDICATIONS
Acute critical illness, hypersensitivity, closed epiphyses, active malignancy, active proliferative/severe nonproliferative diabetic retinopathy, Prader-Willi syndrome (severely obese or severe respiratory impairment)

DOSAGE AND ROUTES
Child ≥3 yr: SUBCUT 0.66 mg/kg qwk, on same day of the wk
Available forms: Injection 24 mg/1.2 mL (20 mg/mL) single-use prefilled pen (0.2-mg increments), 60 mg/1.2 mL (50 mg/mL) single-use prefilled pen that delivers a dose in 0.5-mg increments

---

sulbactam/durlobactam (Rx)
(sul-bak-tam dur-lo-bak-tam)
Xacduro
Func. class.: Antiinfective—miscellaneous
Chem. class.: β-lactam

ACTION: Sulbactam is a beta-lactam antibacterial and Ambler Class A serine beta-lactamase inhibitor of penicillin-binding proteins PB1 and PB3 in *Acinetobacter baumannii-calcoaceticus* (ABC); it inhibits the third and final stage of bacterial cell wall synthesis by preferentially binding to specific penicillin-binding proteins (PBPs) that are located inside the bacterial cell wall

USES: Nosocomial pneumonia (hospital-acquired pneumonia [HAP]), ventilator-associated pneumonia (VAP), due to *Acinetobacter baumannii*

CONTRAINDICATIONS
Hypersensitivity
Precautions: Pregnancy, breastfeeding, children, geriatric patients, renal disease; hypersensitivity to carbapenems, cephalosporins, penicillins, carbams,

cephalosporins, penicillins; CDAD, diabetes mellitus

DOSAGE AND ROUTES

Nosocomial pneumonia (hospital-acquired pneumonia [HAP]), ventilator-associated pneumonia (VAP), due to *Acinetobacter baumannii*

Adults: IV infusion 2 g (1 g sulbactam and 1 g durlobactam) over 3 hr every 6 hr for 7 days

Renal dose:

Adult: IV infusion **CCr 130 mL/min or more:** 2 g (1 g sulbactam and 1 g durlobactam) q4hr (augmented renal clearance); **CCr 45-129 mL/min:** 2 g (1 g sulbactam and 1 g durlobactam) q6hr (no dosage adjustments needed); **CCr 30-44 mL/min:** 2 g (1 g sulbactam and 1 g durlobactam) q8hr; **CCr 15-29 mL/min:** 2 g (1 g sulbactam and 1 g durlobactam) q12hr; **CCr <15 mL/min at initiation of therapy:** 2 g (1 g sulbactam and 1 g durlobactam) q12hr for the first 3 doses, then 2 g (1 g sulbactam and 1 g durlobactam) q24hr; **CCr declines to <15 mL/min while taking sulbactam; durlobactam:** 2 g (1 g sulbactam and 1 g durlobactam) q24hr

Available forms: Powder for injection 1 g/1 g

Administer:

• After C&S is taken, may start treatment before results are received

Intermittent IV infusion route

• Visually inspect for particulate matter and discoloration, solution should be clear to light yellow to orange, do not use if sulbactam or durlobactam appears cloudy or contains particulates

• Sulbactam; durlobactam is a co-packaged kit consisting of 1 single-dose sulbactam vial containing 1 g of sulbactam and 2 single-dose durlobactam vials each containing 0.5 g of durlobactam

• **Sulbactam: Reconstitute** each 1 g sulbactam vial/ 5 mL of sterile water for injection, gently shake

• Each reconstituted vial contains 1 g sulbactam/5 mL

• *Durlobactam:* **Reconstitute** each 0.5 g/2.5 mL of sterile water for injection, reconstitute both vials, gently shake

• Reconstituted sulbactam and durlobactam solutions are NOT for direct injection and MUST be diluted prior to IV infusion

• **Store:** Sulbactam and durlobactam reconstituted solutions must be further diluted within 1 hr of reconstitution

• **Dilution:** Prepare by withdrawing 5 mL reconstituted sulbactam and a total of 5 mL from both reconstituted durlobactam vials (2.5 mL each); add the withdrawn sulbactam and durlobactam volume to a 100-mL infusion bag of 0.9% NaCl for injection, USP; discard unused portion

• **Store:** Refrigerate the diluted solution at 2-8° C (36-46° F) solution prior to infusion, administer diluted solution within 24 hr of reconstitution, inclusive of infusion time, do not freeze

• Sulbactam; durlobactam should be brought to room temperature (20-25° C [68-77° F]) prior to use

• Do not admix

• Give over 3 hr

SIDE EFFECTS

CV: Increased dysrhythmias

GI: *Diarrhea,* CDAD, constipation

HEMA: Thrombocytopenia, anemia

GU: Renal failure

SYST: Anaphylaxis, superinfection

PHARMACOKINETICS

Sulbactam: Protein binding 38%, crosses placenta, minimal metabolism, a substrate for renal organic anion transporter (OAT)1, half-life 2.1 hr

Durlobactam: Protein binding 10 %, minimal metabolism, a substrate for renal organic anion transporter (OAT)1; excreted unchanged 78% in urine, half-life with normal renal function is 2.52 hr

INTERACTIONS

Increase: sulbactam level—OAT1 (fexinidazole, probenecid, sodium phenylbutyrate/taurursodiol), monitor for increased adverse reactions

NURSING CONSIDERATIONS

Assess:

• Renal disease: Monitor creatinine/BUN, lower dose may be needed

• **Infection:** Increased temperature, WBC, characteristics of wounds, sputum, urine or stool culture

• Sensitivity to penicillin, cephalosporins, carbapenems, may have sensitivity to this product

• **CDAD:** Bowel pattern daily; if severe diarrhea occurs, product should be discontinued; may indicate CDAD

• **Allergic reactions, anaphylaxis:** rash, urticaria, pruritus, wheezing, laryngeal edema; may occur a few days after therapy begins; have EPINEPHrine, antihistamine, emergency equipment available

• **Overgrowth of infection:** Perineal itching, fever, malaise, redness, pain, swelling, drainage, rash, diarrhea, change in cough, sputum

• **Pregnancy/breastfeeding:** Use only if benefit outweighs fetal risk; use caution in breastfeeding, excretion unknown

Evaluate:

• Therapeutic response: Negative C&S; absence of signs and symptoms of infection

Teach patient/family:

• To report severe diarrhea; may indicate CDAD

TREATMENT OF ANAPHYLAXIS:

EPINEPHrine, antihistamines; resuscitate if needed

---

talquetamab (Rx)

(tal-kwe'ta-mab)

Talvey

Func. class.: Antineoplastic

USES: Relapsed or refractory multiple myeloma who have received at least 4 prior therapies

Black Box Warning: Cytokine release syndrome, neurotoxicity

DOSAGE AND ROUTES

Multiple myeloma: Adults: SUBCUT
Step-up dose 1, 0.01 mg/kg on day 1; step-up dose 2, 0.06 mg/kg on day 4; and first treatment dose, 0.4 mg/kg on day 7. For step-up dose 2 and the first treatment dose, give between 2 and 4 days after the previous dose and up to 7 days after the previous dose to allow for resolution of adverse reactions. Begin the weekly dosing schedule starting 1 week after the first treatment dose as follows: 0.4 mg/kg once weekly until disease progression; maintain at least 6 days between weekly doses. Therapy interruption or discontinuation may be necessary in patients who develop toxicity. Administer dexamethasone 16 mg PO/IV, diphenhydramine 50 mg PO/IV, and acetaminophen 650-1000 mg PO/IV 1-3 hr prior to each dose in the step-up dosing schedule.

Adults: SUBCUT (every 2 wk schedule) Step-up dose 1, 0.01 mg/kg on day 1; step-up dose 2, 0.06 mg/kg on day 4; step-up dose 3, 0.4 mg/kg on day 7; and first treatment dose, 0.8 mg/kg on day 10. For step-up dose 2 and 3, may give between 2 and 4 days after the previous dose and up to 7 days after the previous dose to allow for resolution of adverse reactions; for the first treatment dose, may give between 2 and 7 days after step-up dose 3. Begin the biweekly dosing schedule starting 2 wk after the first treatment dose as follows: 0.8 mg/kg every 2 wk until disease progression; maintain at least 12 days between biweekly doses. Therapy interruption or discontinuation may be necessary in patients who develop toxicity. Administer premedication: dexamethasone 16 mg PO/ IV, diphenhydramine 50 mg PO/ IV or equivalent, and acetaminophen 650-1000 mg PO/IV or equivalent) at 1-3 hr prior to each dose

Available forms: Solution for injection 3 mg/1.5 mL, 40 mg/mL

⚕ Genetic warning

tapinarof (Rx)
(ta-pin'ar-of)

Vtama
Func. class.: Topical antipsoriasis
a gent
Chem. class.: Aryl hydrocarbon

ACTION: Regulates gene expression
in immune and epithelial cells

USES: Plaque psoriasis

CONTRAINDICATIONS
Hypersensitivity
Precautions: Child

DOSAGE AND ROUTES
Adult: TOPICAL Apply a thin layer of
cream to affected areas once daily
Available forms: Topical cream 1%
Administer:
• For topical use only, do not administer
via the oral, ophthalmic, or intravaginal
routes
• Apply as a thin layer to affected areas
• Wash hands after application, unless
the hands are included as an area to be
treated

SIDE EFFECTS
INTEG: Contact dermatitis, pruritus
CNS: Headache
MISC: Flulike symptoms

PHARMACOKINETICS
Unknown

INTERACTIONS
None known

NURSING CONSIDERATIONS
Assess:
• Psoriasis: Identify number and area
or lesions baseline and during treat-
ment
• Pregnancy/breastfeeding: Unknown
Evaluate:
• Therapeutic response: Decreasing
amount and severity of lesions
Teach patient/family:
• To wash hands after application

• Pregnancy/breastfeeding: To report if
pregnancy is planned or suspected or if
breastfeeding

tofersen (Rx)
(TOE-fur-sen)

Qalsody
Func. class.: ALS agent

USES: Amyotrophic lateral sclerosis
(ALS) in adults who have a mutation in
the superoxide dismutase 1 (*SOD1*) gene

DOSAGE AND ROUTES
Adult: Intrathecally 100 mg every 14
days for 3 doses, followed by 100 mg
intrathecally every 28 days
Available forms: Solution for injection
(intrathecally) 100 mg/15 mL

⚠ HIGH ALERT

toripalimab (Rx)
(tor-ee-pa-li-mab)

Loqtorzi
Func. class.: Antineoplastic

USES: Recurrent or metastatic locally
advanced nasopharyngeal carcinoma

DOSAGE AND ROUTES
Adult: IV 240 mg q2wk until disease
progression or unacceptable toxicity or
up to 24 mo; recurrent: 3mg/kg q3wk
until disease progression or unacceptable toxicity
Available forms: Injection 240 mg/6
mL (40 mg/mL)

vamorolone
(va-MOR-oh-lone)

Agamree
Func. class.: Corticosteroid

USES: To treat Duchenne muscular
dystrophy

DOSAGE AND ROUTES

Adult/child >2 yr: PO 6 mg/kg qday, max 300 mg/day

Available forms: Oral solution 40 mg/mL

---

velmanase (Rx)

(vel-ma'-nase)

Lamzede

Func. class.: Metabolic disorder agent

USES: Non–central nervous system manifestations of alpha-mannosidosis in adult and pediatric patients

DOSAGE AND ROUTES

Black Box Warning: Serious allergic reactions

Adult female: IV infusion 1 mg/kg (actual body weight) once every week

Available forms: Injection, single-dose vial for reconstitution 10 mg

---

zavegepant (Rx)

Zavzpret

Func. class.: Antimigraine agent

Chem. class.: Calcitonin gene-related peptide (CGRP) receptor antagonist, antibody

---

ACTION: Calcitonin gene-related peptide (CGRP) receptor antagonist

USES: For the acute treatment of migraine with or without aura in adults, not used for preventive treatment of migraine

CONTRAINDICATIONS

Hypersensitivity

Precautions: Breastfeeding, pregnancy

DOSAGE AND ROUTES

Adult: Nasal 10 mg as a single spray in 1 nostril as needed, max 10 mg (1 spray)/24 hr

Available forms: Nasal solution 10 mg/0.1 mL

Administer:

• Only in 1 nostril

ADVERSE EFFECTS

MISC: Taste disorders, nausea, nasal discomfort, vomiting, anorexia

PHARMACOKINETICS

Peak 30 min, half-life 6.55 hr

INTERACTIONS

• Avoid use with drugs inhibit the OATP1B3 or NTCP transporters

• Avoid use of intranasal decongestants

NURSING CONSIDERATIONS

Assess:

• **Migraines:** Time of day, aggravating and ameliorating effects, auras or halos, sensitivity to light, noise, diet

• **Pregnancy/breastfeeding:** Data are lacking

Evaluate:

• Therapeutic response: Decrease in severity of migraines

Teach patient/family:

• To read the FDA-approved patient labeling (Patient Information and Instructions for Use)

• Hypersensitivity: Inform patients about the signs and symptoms of hypersensitivity (rash, itching, trouble breathing), to contact their health care provider immediately if signs or symptoms of hypersensitivity reactions occur

• To discuss all Rx, OTC, herbals, and supplements taken or plan to take, to use intranasal decongestants ≥1 hr after use

---

zilucoplan (Rx)

(zil-ue-KOE-plan)

Zilbrysq

USES: Generalized myasthenia gravis in those who are anti-acetylcholine receptor antibody positive

DOSAGE AND ROUTES

Adult ≥77 kg: SUBCUT 32.4 mg once daily

Adult 56-76 kg: SUBCUT 23 mg once daily
Adult <56 kg: SUBCUT 16.6 mg once daily

---

zuranolone (Rx) rems
(zoo-RAN-oh-lone)
Zurzuvae
Func. class.: Antidepressant
Chem. class.: GABA modulator

ACTION: Not fully known but thought to be related to its positive modulation of γ-aminobutyric acid A (GABA-A) receptors; GABA is a major inhibitory neurotransmitter in the brain

USES: Postpartum depression

CONTRAINDICATIONS
Hypersensitivity
Precautions: Abrupt discontinuation, driving or hazardous activities, breastfeeding, coadministration with other CNS depressants, alcohol use, hypoxia, pregnancy, renal failure, suicidal ideation

Black Box Warning: CNS depression, driving or hazardous activities

DOSAGE AND ROUTES
Postpartum depression
Adult female: PO 50 mg once daily in the evening, with a fatty meal or food, for 14 days. If a patient experiences CNS depression during the 14-day course, may reduce the dose to 40 mg PO once daily in the evening
Available forms: Capsule 20 mg, 25 mg, 30 mg
Administer:
• Give capsules once daily in the evening with fat-containing food (such as a fatty meal containing 400-1,000 calories, 25-50% fat).
• *Missed dose:* If a dose is missed, the dose should be skipped and take at the regular time the following evening, then continue taking once daily in the evening

until the remainder of the 14-day treatment course is completed

SIDE EFFECTS
CNS: Sedation, drowsiness, dizziness, memory impairment, somnolence, fatigue, suicidal ideation
GI: Diarrhea,
EENT: Nasopharyngitis
GU: UTI

PHARMACOKINETICS
Steady state 3-5 days, peak 5-6 hr, protein binding >99%, extensively metabolized by CYP3A4 enzyme, half-life 19.7-24.6 hr; excreted as 45% urine as metabolites, 41% feces as metabolites

INTERACTIONS
Increase: CNS depression—CNS depressants, avoid using together or reduce dose
Increase: adverse reactions—strong CYP3A4 inhibitors, reduce the zuranolone dosage to 30 mg once daily in the evening for 14 days
Decrease: zuranolone effect—CYP3A4 inducers, avoid concomitant use

NURSING CONSIDERATIONS
Assess:
• Postpartum depression: Assess baseline and frequently for change in mood

Black Box Warning: Assess for excessive sedation, patient should avoid driving, other hazardous tasks

• **Suicidal ideation:** Assess for suicidal thoughts and behavior; more common in young adults
Evaluate:
• Therapeutic response: Decrease in postpartum depression, improved mood
Teach patient/family:
• Reason for product and expected result
• To discuss all Rx, OTC, herbals, and supplements with health care provider
• To report pain, inflammation at injection site
• Excessive sedation, have caregiver or family member check frequently

---

• Not to drive or engage in hazardous tasks for at least 12 hr after taking a dose and also for the duration of the 14-day treatment course

• Not to use alcohol or other CNS depressants

• **Pregnancy/breastfeeding:** To identify if pregnancy is planned or suspected or if breastfeeding; to use effective contraception during and for 1 wk after last dose, use cautiously in breastfeeding; if pregnant, register with the National Pregnancy Registry for Antidepressants at 844-405-6185 or visit https://womensmentalhealth.org/clinical-and-research-programs/pregnancyregistry/antidepressants/

Appendix B

Ophthalmic, Nasal, Topical, and Otic Products

OPHTHALMIC PRODUCTS

ANESTHETICS

chloroprocaine (Rx)
(klor'-o-proe-kane)
Iheezo

lidocaine (Rx)
(lye'doe-kane)
Akten

proparacaine (Rx)
(proe-par'a-kane)
Alcaine, Ocu-Caine, Ophthetic, Parcaine

tetracaine (Rx)
(tet'ra-kane)

ANTIHISTAMINES

alcaftadine
(al-caf'tah-deen)
Lastacaft

azelastine (Rx)
(ay-zell'ah-steen)
Optivar

epinastine (Rx)
(ep-een-as'teen)
Elistat

ketotifen (OTC)
(kee-toh-tif'en)
Alaway, Zaditor

levocabastine (Rx)
(lee-voh-cab'ah-steen)
Livostin

olopatadine (OTC, Rx)
(oh-loh-pat'ah-deen)
Pataday, Patanol

ANTIINFECTIVES

azithromycin (Rx)
(ay-zi-thro-my'sin)
AzaSite

besifloxacin (Rx)
(be'si-flox'a-sin)
Besivance

ciprofloxacin (Rx)
(sip-ro-floks'a-sin)
Ciloxan

erythromycin (Rx)
(er-ith-roe-mye'sin)

ganciclovir (Rx)
(gan-sye'kloe-vir)
Zirgan

gatifloxacin (Rx)
(gat-ih-floks'ah-sin)
Zymaxid

gentamicin (Rx)
(jen-ta-mye'sin)
Gentak

levofloxacin (Rx)
(lee-voh-flock'sah-sin)

moxifloxacin (Rx)
(mox-i-flox'a-sin)
Moxeza, Vigamox

Side effects: *italics* = common; red = life-threatening

natamycin (Rx)
(nat-a-mye'sin)

Natacyn

ofloxacin (Rx)
(oh-floks'a-sin)

Ocuflox

silver nitrate 1% (Rx)

sulfacetamide sodium (Rx)
(sul-fa-seet'a-mide)

Bleph-10

tobramycin (Rx)
(toe-bra-mye'sin)

Tobrex

trifluridine (Rx)
(trye-floor'i-deen)

Viroptic

β-ADRENERGIC BLOCKERS

betaxolol (Rx)
(beh-tax'oh-lole)

Betoptic-S

carteolol (Rx)
(kar-tee'oh-lole)

levobetaxolol (Rx)
(lee-voh-beh-tax'oh-lohl)

Betaxon

levobunolol (Rx)
(lee-voe-byoo'no-lole)

Betagen

metipranolol (Rx)
(met-ee-pran'oh-lole)

timolol (Rx)
(tym'moe-lole)

Betimol, Timoptic, Timoptic Ocudose, Timoptic-XE

CARBONIC ANHYDRASE INHIBITORS

brinzolamide (Rx)
(brin-zoh'la-mide)

Azopt

dorzolamide (Rx)
(dor-zol'a-mide)

Trusopt

CHOLINERGICS (direct-acting)

acetylcholine (Rx)
(ah-see-til-koe'leen)

Miochol-E

carbachol (Rx)
(kar'ba-kole)

Isopto Carbachol, Miostat

pilocarpine (Rx)
(pye-loe-kar'peen)

Isopto Carpine, Vuity

CHOLINESTERASE INHIBITORS

physostigmine (Rx)
(fi-zoe-stig'meen)

CORTICOSTEROIDS

dexamethasone (Rx)
(dex-a-meth'a-sone)

Dextenza, Maxidex, Ozurdex

fluorometholone (Rx)
(flure-oh-meth'oh-lone)

Flarex, FML, FML Forte, FML S.O.P.

loteprednol (Rx)
(loe-tee-pred-nole)

Alrex, EYsuVIS, Inveltys, Lotemax, Lotemax SM

prednisoLONE (Rx)
(pred-niss'oh-lone)

Pred-Forte, Pred Mild

MYDRIATICS
atropine (Rx)
(a'troe-peen)
cyclopentolate (Rx)
(sye-kloe-pen'toe-late)
Cyclogyl
homatropine (Rx)
(home-a'troe-peen)
phenylephrine (OTC)
(fen-ill-ef'rin)

NONSTEROIDAL ANTI-INFLAMMATORIES
bromfenac (Rx)
(brome'fen-ak)
BromSite, Prolensa
diclofenac (Rx)
(dye-kloe'fen-ak)
flurbiprofen (Rx)
(flure-bi'pro-fen)
Ocufen
ketorolac (Rx)
(kee-toe'role-ak)
Acular, Acular LS, Acuvail
nepafenac (Rx)
(ne-pa-fen'ak)
Ilevro, Nevanac

PROSTAGLANDIN RECEPTOR AGONIST
omidenepag (Rx)
Omlonti

SYMPATHOMIMETICS
apraclonidine (Rx)
(a-pra-klon'i-deen)
Iopidine
brimonidine (Rx)
(brem-on'i-dine)
Alphagan P, Lumify
latanoprostene bunod (Rx)
(la-tan-oh-pros'teen bu'nod)
Vyzulta

OPHTHALMIC DECONGESTANTS/VASOCONSTRICTORS
Iodoxamide
(loe-dox'ah-mide)
Alomide
naphazoline (OTC)
(naf-az'oh-leen)
AK-Con, All Clear Eye Drops, All Clear AR Maximum Strength Ophthalmic Solution, Clear Eyes Redness Relief, GoodSense Redness Relief Plus
tetrahydrozoline (OTC)
(tet-ra-hye-dro'zoe-leen)
Eye Drops, Visine Red Eye

MISCELLANEOUS OPHTHALMICS
bimatoprost (Rx)
(bih-mat'o-prost)
Durysta, Latisse, Lumigan
cyclosporine
(sye'kloe-spor-een)
Cequa, Restasis, Verkazia
latanoprost (Rx)
(la-tan'oh-prost)
Xalatan, Xelpros
travoprost (Rx)
(tra'voe-prost)
Travatan Z
unoprostone (Rx)
(yoo-noe-pros'tone)
Rescula

β-ADRENERGIC BLOCKERS

ACTION: Reduces production of aqueous humor by unknown mechanism

USES: Ocular hypertension, chronic open-angle glaucoma

Side effects: *italics* = common; red = life-threatening

ANESTHETICS

ACTION: Decreases ion permeability by stabilizing neuronal membrane

USES: Cataract extraction, tonometry, gonioscopy, removal of foreign objects, corneal suture removal, glaucoma surgery (ophthalmic); pruritus, sunburn, toothache, sore throat, cold sores, oral pain, rectal pain and irritation, control of gagging (topical)

ANTIINFECTIVES

ACTION: Inhibits folic acid synthesis by preventing PABA use, which is necessary for bacterial growth

USES: Conjunctivitis, superficial eye infections, corneal ulcers, prophylaxis against infection after removal of foreign matter from the eye

ANTIINFLAMMATORIES

ACTION: Decreases inflammation, resulting in decreased pain, photophobia, hyperemia, cellular infiltration

USES: Inflammation of eye, eyelids, conjunctiva, cornea; uveitis, iridocyclitis, allergic conditions, burns, foreign bodies, postoperatively in cataract

CARBONIC ANHYDRASE INHIBITOR

ACTION: Converted to epINEPHrine, which decreases aqueous production and increases outflow

USES: Open-angle glaucoma, ocular hypertension

DIRECT-ACTING MIOTIC

ACTION: Acts directly on cholinergic receptor sites; induces miosis, spasm of accommodation, fall in intraocular pressure, caused by stimulation of ciliary, pupillary sphincter muscles, which leads to pulling away of iris from filtration angle, resulting in increased outflow of aqueous humor

USES: Primary glaucoma, early stages of wide-angle glaucoma (less useful in advanced stages), chronic open-angle glaucoma, acute closed-angle glaucoma before emergency surgery; also neutralizes mydriatics used during eye exam; may be used alternately with mydriatics to break adhesions between iris and lens

CONTRAINDICATIONS: Hypersensitivity

Precautions: Pregnancy, breastfeeding, children, aphakia, hypersensitivity to carbonic anhydrase inhibitors, sulfonamides, thiazide diuretics, ocular inhibitors, renal/hepatic insufficiency

Administer
• Storage at room temperature away from light

ADVERSE EFFECTS
CNS: Headache
CV: Hypertension, tachycardia, dysrhythmias
EENT: Burning, stinging
GI: Bitter taste

NURSING CONSIDERATIONS
Assess
• Monitor ophthalmic exams and intraocular pressure readings
• Monitor blood counts; renal/hepatic function tests and serum electrolytes during long-term treatment

Teach patient/family
• Teach how to instill drops
• Advise patient that product may cause burning, itching, blurring, dryness of eye area

Evaluate

Positive therapeutic outcome
• Absence of increased intraocular pressure

NASAL AGENTS

NASAL ANESTHESIAS
Cocaine (Rx)

Numbrino

NASAL ANTIHISTAMINES
olopatadine (Rx)
(oh-low-pat'uh-deen)

Patanase

NASAL DECONGESTANTS
azelastine (Rx)
(ay-zell'ah-steen)

Astelin, Astepro, Astepro Allergy

EPINEPHrine (Rx)
(ep-i-neff'rin)

Adrenalin Nasal Solution

oxymetazoline (OTC)
(ox-i-met-az'oh-leen)

12-Hour Decongestant, Afrin No Drip Severe Congestion, Afrin Nasal Spray, Afrin No Drip Extra Moisture, Afrin No Drip Original, Afrin No Drip Sinus, Afrin Sinus, Dristan 12-Hour, Dristan Spray, Mucinex Children's Stuffy Nose, Mucinex Sinus-Max Clear & Cool, Mucinex Sinus-Max Sinus/Allergy, Nasal Decongestant Spray, Nasal Spray 12 Hour, Vicks QlearQuil, Vicks Sinex 12-Hour Decongestant, Vicks Sinex Moisturizing, Vicks Sinex Severe Decongestant

phenylephrine (OTC)
(fen-ill-eff'rin)

4-Way Fast Acting, Neo-Synephrine Mild, Neo-Synephrine Cold/Allergy Ext, Neo-Synephrine Reg

tetrahydrozoline (OTC)
(tet-ra-hye-dro'zoe-leen)

NASAL STEROIDS
beclomethasone (Rx)
(be-kloe-meth'a-sone)

Beconase AQ Nasal, Qnasl, Qnasl Childrens

budesonide (Rx)
(byoo-des'oh-nide)

Rhinocort Allergy

flunisolide (Rx)
(floo-niss'oh-lide)

fluticasone (OTC)
(floo-tic'a-son)

Flonase Sensimist, Flonase Sensimist Children's

triamcinolone (OTC)
(trye-am-sin'oh-lone)

GoodSense Nasal Allergy Spray, Nasacort Allergy 24HR Children's, Nasacort Allergy 24HR, Nasal Allergy 24 Hour

NONSTEROIDAL ANTIINFLAMMATORY
ketorolac (Rx)
(kee'toe-role-ak)

Sprix

ACTION: Produces vasoconstriction (rapid, long acting) of arterioles, thereby decreasing fluid exudation, mucosal engorgement by stimulation of α-adrenergic receptors in vascular smooth muscle

Therapeutic outcome: Absence of nasal congestion

USES: Nasal congestion

CONTRAINDICATIONS: Hypersensitivity to sympathomimetic amines

Precautions: Pregnancy, children <6 yr, geriatric patients, diabetes, CV disease, hypertension, hyperthyroidism, increased ICP, prostatic hypertrophy, glaucoma

---

Administer

• Have patient tilt head back, squeeze bulb to create a vacuum, and draw correct amount of sol into dropper; insert 2 gtt of sol into nostril; repeat in other nostril
• Store in light-resistant container; do not expose to high temperature or let sol come into contact with aluminum
• Give for <4 consecutive days
• Provide environmental humidification to decrease nasal congestion, dryness

ADVERSE EFFECTS

CNS: Anxiety, restlessness, tremors, weakness, insomnia, dizziness, fever, headache
EENT: Irritation, burning, sneezing, stinging, dryness, rebound congestion
GI: Nausea, vomiting, anorexia
INTEG: Contact dermatitis

NURSING CONSIDERATIONS
Assess

• Assess for redness, swelling, pain in nasal passages before, during treatment
• Assess for systemic absorption; hypertension, tachycardia; notify prescriber; systemic absorption occurs at high doses or after prolonged use

Teach patient/family

• Advise patient that stinging may occur for several applications; drying of mucosa may be decreased by environmental humidification
• Caution patient to notify prescriber if irregular pulse, insomnia, dizziness, or tremors occur
• Teach patient proper administration to avoid systemic absorption
• Advise patient to rinse dropper with very hot water to prevent contamination

Evaluate
Positive therapeutic outcome

• Decreased nasal congestion

TOPICAL GLUCOCORTICOIDS

alclometasone (Rx)
(al-kloe-met'a-sone)
Aclovate

amcinonide
(am-sin'oh-nide)

betamethasone (Rx)
(bay-ta-meth'a-sone)
Beta Derm, Betanate, Del-Beta, Diprolene, Luxiq, Sernivo

betamethasone (augmented) (Rx)
(bay-ta-meth'a-sone)
Diprolene AF

clobetasol (Rx)
(kloe-bay'ta-sol)
Clobetavix, Clobex, Clodan, Impoyz, Olux, Olux-E, Tasoprol, Temovate, Tovet

desonide (Rx)
(dess'oh-nide)
Desonate, DesRx, LoKam, Tridesilon, Verdeso Foam

desoximetasone (Rx)
(dess-ox-i-met'a-sone)
Topicort

diflorasone (Rx)
(dye-flor'a-sone)
Apexicon E, Psorcon

fluocinolone (Rx)
(floo-oh-sin'oh-lone)
Derma-Smoothe/FS, Synalar

flurandrenolide (Rx)
(flure-an-dren'oh-lide)
Cordran, Nolix

fluticasone (Rx)
(floo-tik'a-sone)
Beser, Cutivate

halcinonide (Rx)
(hal-sin'oh-nide)
Halog

hydrocortisone (Rx)
(hye-droe-kor'ti-sone)
Ala-Cort, Ala-Scalp, Anti-Itch Maximum Strength, Anucort-HC, Anusol HC, Aquanil HC,

Maximum Strength, Cortifoam, Instacort 5, Locoid, MiCort-HC, NuCort, Pandel, Preparation H, Procto-Med HC, Procto-Pak, Proctocort, Proctozone-HC, Recort Plus, Sarnol-HC, Scalacort DK, Scalpicin Maximum Strength, Sarna HC , Uremol HC

triamcinolone (Rx)

(trye-am-sin'oh-lone)

Aristocort C, Aristocort R, Kenalog, Oralone, Sila III, Trianex, Triaderm, Triderm

ACTION: Antipruritic, antiinflammatory

Therapeutic outcome: Decreased itching, inflammation

USES: Psoriasis, eczema, contact dermatitis, pruritus; usually reserved for severe dermatoses that have not responded to less potent formulation

CONTRAINDICATIONS: Hypersensitivity, viral infections, fungal infections

Precautions: Pregnancy

DOSAGE AND ROUTES
Adult and child: Apply to affected area

Administer
• Apply only to affected areas; do not get in eyes
• Apply and leave site uncovered or lightly covered; occlusive dressing is not recommended—systemic absorption may occur
• Use only on dermatoses; do not use on weeping, denuded, or infected area
• Cleanse area before application of product
• Continue treatment for a few days after area has cleared
• Store at room temperature

ADVERSE EFFECTS
INTEG: *Acne, atrophy, epidermal thinning, purpura, striae*

NURSING CONSIDERATIONS
Assess
• Monitor temp; if fever develops, product should be discontinued
• Monitor for systemic absorption, increased temp, inflammation, irritation

Teach patient/family
• Teach patient to avoid sunlight on affected area; burns may occur
• Teach patient to limit treatment to 14 days

Evaluate
Positive therapeutic outcome
• Absence of severe itching, patches on skin, flaking

TOPICAL ANTIFUNGALS

clotrimazole (OTC)
(kloe-trye'ma-zole)
Alevazol, Antifungal Clotrimazole, Cruex, Lotrimin AF

econazole (OTC)
(ee-kon'a-zole)
Ecoza, Zolpak

efinaconazole (Rx)
(ef-in-a-kon'a-zole)
Jublia

ketoconazole (Rx, OTC)
(kee-toe-kon'a-zole)
Extina

luliconazole (Rx)
(loo-li-kon'a-zole)
Luzu

miconazole (OTC)
(mye-kon'a-zole)

Aloe Vesta Antifungal, Aloe Vesta Clear Antifungal, Antifungal, Azolen Tincture, Carrington Antifungal, Cavilon, Cruex Prescription Strength, DermaFunga, Desenex Jock Itch, Desene, Fungoid Tincture, Lotrimin AF Deodorant

---

Powder, Lotrimin AF Jock Itch
Powder, Lotrimin AF Powder,
Lotrimin AF, Micaderm, Micatin,
Podactin Remedy Antifungal,
Soothe & Cool INZO Antifungal,
Triple Paste AF, Zeasorb

naftifine (Rx)
(naff'ti-feen)

Naftin

nystatin (Rx)
(nye-stat'in)

Nyamyc, Nystop

oxiconazole (Rx)
(ox-i-kon'a-zole)

Oxistat

sulconazole (Rx)
(sul-kon'a-zole)

Exelderm

tavaborole (Rx)
(ta'va-bor'ole)

Kerydin

terbinafine (OTC)
(ter-bin'a-feen)

LamISIL AT Jock Itch, LamISIL AT

tolnaftate (OTC)
(tole-naf'tate)

Absorbine Junior, Anti-Fungal,
Antifungal, Athletes Foot Spray,
Dr Gs Clear Nail, Fungi-Guard,
Fungoid-D, Jock Itch Spray,
Mycocide Clinical NS, Podactin,
Proclearz, Tinactin Deodorant,
Tinactin, Tinaspore

undecylenic acid (OTC)
(un-deh-sih-len'ik)

ACTION: Interferes with fungal cell
membrane permeability

Therapeutic outcome: Absence
of itching and white patches of the skin

USES: Tinea cruris, tinea pedis, diaper
rash, minor skin irritations; amphotericin B is used for *Candida* infections

CONTRAINDICATIONS: Hypersensitivity

Precautions: Pregnancy, breastfeeding, children

DOSAGE AND ROUTES
Massage into affected area, surrounding
area daily or bid, continue for 7-14 days,
max 4 wk

Administer
• Apply to affected area, surrounding
area; do not cover with occlusive dressings
• Store below 30° C (86° F)

ADVERSE EFFECTS
INTEG: Burning, stinging, dryness,
itching, local irritation

NURSING CONSIDERATIONS
Assess
• Assess skin for fungal infections: peeling, dryness, itching before, throughout
treatment
• Assess for continuing infection;
increased size, number of lesions

Teach patient/family
• Instruct to apply with glove to prevent
further infection; not to cover with occlusive dressings
• Teach patient that long-term therapy
may be needed to clear infection (2 wk-6
mo depending on organism); compliance is needed even after feeling better
• Teach patient proper hygiene: handwashing technique, nail care, use of concomitant top agents if prescribed
• Caution patient to avoid use of OTC
creams, ointments, lotions unless directed by prescriber
• Instruct patient to use medical asepsis
(hand washing) before, after each application; to change socks and shoes once a
day during treatment of tinea pedis
• Advise patient to report to health care
prescriber if infection persists or recurs;
if blisters, burning, oozing, swelling occur

• Caution patient to avoid alcohol because nausea, vomiting, hypertension may occur

• Caution patient to use sunscreen or avoid direct sunlight to prevent photosensitivity

• Advise patient to notify prescriber of sore throat, fever, skin rash, which may indicate overgrowth of organisms

Evaluate

Positive therapeutic outcome

• Decrease in size, number of lesions

TOPICAL ANTIINFECTIVES

azelaic acid (Rx)
(a-zuh-lay'ic)
Finacea
bacitracin (OTC)
(bass-i-tray'sin)
clindamycin (Rx)
(klin-da-my'sin)
Cleocin, Cleocin-T, Clindacin ETZ, Evoclin
erythromycin (Rx)
(er-ith-roe-mye'sin)
Ery, Erygel, Emcin, Emgel
gentamicin (Rx)
(jen-ta-mye'sin)
mafenide (Rx)
(ma'fe-nide)
Sulfamylon
metronidazole (Rx)
(met-roh-nye'da-zole)
MetroGel, MetroCream, MetroLotion, Nydamax, Rosaden
mupirocin (Rx)
(myoo-peer'oh-sin)
Centany, Centany AT
retapamulin (Rx)
(re-tap'a-mue'lin)

Altabax
salicylic acid (OTC, Rx)
(sal'i-sil'ik)
Bensal HP, Betasa, Clear Away 1-Step Wart Remover, Corn Remover One Step, Gordofilm, Ionil, Keralyt, Keralyt Scalp, Keralyt, Mediplast, Neutrogena Oil-Free Acne Wash, P & S, Psoriasin, Sal-Plant, SalAc, Salex, Salicylic Acid Wart Remover, Salimez, Salimez Forte, Salva, UltraSal-ER, Virasal, Xalix
silver sulfADIAZINE (Rx)
(sul-fa-dye'a-zeen)
Silvadene, SSD
tretinoin (Rx)
(treh'tih-noyn)
Altreno, Atralin, Avita, Refissa, Retin-A, Renova, Tretin-X

ACTION: Interferes with bacterial protein synthesis

Therapeutic outcome: Resolution of infection

USES: Skin infections, minor burns, wounds, skin grafts, primary pyodermas, otitis externa

CONTRAINDICATIONS: Hypersensitivity, large areas, burns, ulcerations

Precautions: Pregnancy, breastfeeding, impaired renal function, perforated eardrum

Administer

• Apply enough medication to cover lesions completely

• Apply after cleansing with soap, water before each application; dry well

• Apply to less than 20% of body surface area when patient has impaired renal function

• Store at room temperature in dry place

Side effects: *italics* = common; red = life-threatening

ADVERSE EFFECTS

INTEG: Rash, urticaria, scaling, redness

NURSING CONSIDERATIONS
Assess

• Assess for allergic reaction: burning, stinging, swelling, redness

• Assess for signs of nephrotoxicity or ototoxicity

Evaluate

Positive therapeutic outcome

• Decrease in size, number of lesions

TOPICAL ANTIVIRALS

acyclovir (Rx)
(ay-sye′kloe-ver)
Sitavig, Zovirax Topical

penciclovir (Rx)
(pen-sye′kloe-ver)
Denavir

ACTION: Interferes with viral DNA replication

Therapeutic outcome: Resolution of infection

USES: Simple mucocutaneous herpes simplex, in immunocompromised clients with initial herpes genitalis

CONTRAINDICATIONS: Hypersensitivity

Precautions: Pregnancy, breastfeeding

Administer

• Apply with finger cot or rubber glove to prevent further infection

• Apply enough medication to cover lesions completely

• Apply after cleansing with soap, water before each application; dry well

• Store at room temperature in dry place

ADVERSE EFFECTS

INTEG: Rash, urticaria, stinging, burning, pruritus, vulvitis

NURSING CONSIDERATIONS
Assess

• Assess for allergic reaction: burning, stinging, swelling, redness, rash, vulvitis, pruritus

• Assess for signs of nephrotoxicity or ototoxicity

Teach patient/family

• Teach patient not to use in eyes or when there is no evidence of infection

• Advise patient to apply with glove to prevent further infection

• Advise patient to avoid use of OTC creams, ointments, lotions unless directed by prescriber

• Advise patient to use medical asepsis (hand washing) before, after each application and to avoid contact with eyes

• Advise patient to adhere strictly to prescribed regimen to maximize successful treatment outcome

• Advise patient to begin taking product when symptoms arise

Evaluate

Positive therapeutic outcome

• Decrease in size, number of lesions

TOPICAL ANESTHETICS

benzocaine (OTC)
(ben′zoe-kane)
Americaine Anesthetic, Anbesol Maximum Strength, Hurracaine, Mycinettes

dibucaine (OTC)
(dye′byoo-kane)
Nupercainal

lidocaine (Rx, OTC)
(lye′doe-kane)
Astero, Glydo, Lidomar, LidoRx, Zilactin-L

pramoxine (OTC)
(pra-mox′een)
Preparation H, Proctofoam, Vagisil Medicated

---

tetracaine (OTC, Rx)
(tet′ra-cane)
Pontocaine, Supracaine, Viractin

ACTION: Inhibits conduction of nerve impulses from sensory nerves

Therapeutic outcome: Decreasing inflammation, itching, pain

USES: Oral irritation, sore throat, toothache, cold sore, canker sore, sunburn, minor cuts, insect bites, pain, itching

CONTRAINDICATIONS: Hypersensitivity, infants <1 yr, application to large areas

Precautions: Pregnancy, children <6 yr, sepsis, denuded skin

DOSAGE AND ROUTES
Adult and child: TOP apply qid as needed; RECT insert tid and after each BM

Administer
• Store in tight, light-resistant container; do not freeze, puncture, or incinerate aerosol container

ADVERSE EFFECTS
INTEG: Rash, irritation, sensitization

NURSING CONSIDERATIONS
Assess
• Assess pain: location, duration, characteristics before, after administration
• Assess for infection: redness, drainage, inflammation; this product should not be used until infection is treated

Teach Patient/Family
• Teach patient to avoid contact with eyes
• Teach patient not to use for prolonged periods: use for <1 wk; if condition remains, prescriber should be contacted

Evaluate
Positive therapeutic outcome
• Decreased redness, swelling, pain

TOPICAL MISCELLANEOUS

birch triterpenes (OTC)
Filsuvez

docosanol (OTC)
(doh-koh′sah-nohl)
Abreva

pimecrolimus (Rx)
(pim-eh-kroh-ly′mus)
Elidel

oxymetazoline (Rx)
(ox-ee′meh-taz-oh-lin)
Rhofade

ACTION: Docosanol unknown; pimecrolimus may bind with macrophilin and inhibit calcium-dependent phosphatase

Therapeutic outcome: Decreased redness, swelling, pain

USES: Docosanol applied to fever blisters to promote more rapid healing; pimecrolimus used to treat mild to moderate atopic dermatitis in nonimmunocompromised patients ≥2 yr who are unresponsive to other treatment

CONTRAINDICATIONS: Hypersensitivity

Precautions: Pregnancy, breastfeeding, dermal infections

DOSAGE AND ROUTES
Docosanol
Adult: TOP rub into blisters 5×/day until healing occurs

Pimecrolimus
Adult and child ≥2 yr: TOP apply thin layer 2×/day and rub in; use as long as needed

Administer
• Apply to skin, rub in gently

ADVERSE EFFECTS
Docosanol
NONE known

Pimecrolimus
INTEG: Burning

NURSING CONSIDERATIONS
Assess

• Assess skin condition (color, pain, inflammation) before, after administration
• Assess for signs and symptoms of skin infections (redness, draining lesions); if present, avoid use of product (pimecrolimus)

Teach patient/family

• Advise patient to avoid contact between medication and eyes
• Instruct patient to discontinue use of product when condition clears

Evaluate

Positive therapeutic outcome
• Decreased inflammation, redness

VAGINAL ANTIINFECTIVES

ANTIBACTERIALS
clindamycin (Rx)
(klin-da-my′sin)
Xaciato

ANTIFUNGALS
butoconazole (OTC)
(byoo-toh-kone′ah-zole)
Gynazol-1

clotrimazole (OTC)
(kloe-trye′ma-zole)
Gyne-Lotrimin

miconazole (OTC)
(mye-kon′a-zole)
Monistat 3, Monistat 7,
Monistat-1 Day or Night,
Vagistat-3

terconazole (OTC)
(ter-kone′ah-zole)

tioconazole (OTC)
(tye-oh-kone′ah-zole)
Vagistat-1

ACTION: Interferes with fungal DNA replication; binds sterols in fungal cell membranes, which increases permeability, leaking of nutrients

Therapeutic outcome: Fungistatic/fungicidal against susceptible organisms: *Candida* only

USES: Vaginal, vulval, vulvovaginal candidiasis (moniliasis)

CONTRAINDICATIONS: Hypersensitivity

Precautions: Pregnancy, breastfeeding, children <2 yr

Administer
Topical route
• Administer one full applicator every night high into the vagina
• Store at room temperature in dry place

ADVERSE EFFECTS
GU: Vulvovaginal burning, itching, pelvic cramps
INTEG: Rash, urticaria, stinging, burning
MISC: *Headache,* body pain

NURSING CONSIDERATIONS
Assess

• Assess for allergic reaction: burning, stinging, itching, discharge, soreness

Teach patient/family

• Instruct patient in asepsis (hand washing) before, after each application
• Teach patient to apply with applicator only; to avoid use of any other vaginal product unless directed by prescriber; sanitary napkin may prevent soiling of undergarments
• Instruct patient to abstain from sexual intercourse until treatment is completed; reinfection and irritation may occur
• Advise patient to notify prescriber if symptoms persist

Evaluate

Positive therapeutic outcome
• Decrease in itching or white discharge (vaginal)

OTIC ANTIINFECTIVES

---

ciprofloxacin (Rx)
(sip′roe-flox′a-sin)
Cetraxal, Otiprio
Ofloxacin (Rx)

ACTION: Inhibits protein synthesis in susceptible microorganisms

USES: Ear infection (external), short-term use

CONTRAINDICATIONS: Hypersensitivity, perforated eardrum

Precautions: Pregnancy

Administer
• After removing impacted cerumen by irrigation
• After cleaning stopper with alcohol
• After restraining child if necessary
• After warming sol to body temp

ADVERSE EFFECTS
EENT: Itching, irritation in ear
INTEG: Rash, urticaria

NURSING CONSIDERATIONS
Assess
• Assess for redness, swelling, fever, pain in ear, which indicates superinfection

Teach patient/family
• Teach patient correct method of instillation using aseptic technique, including not touching dropper to ear
• Inform patient that dizziness may occur after instillation

Evaluate

Positive therapeutic outcome
• Decreased ear pain

Appendix C   Vaccines and Toxoids

GENERIC NAME	TRADE NAME	USES	DOSAGE AND ROUTES	CONTRAINDICATIONS
anthrax vaccine	BioThrax	Pre-/postexposure prophylaxis	**Preexposure** Adult: SUBCUT 0.5 mL at 0, 2, 4 wk, then 0.5 mL at 6, 12, 18 mo **Postexposure** Adult: SUBCUT 0.5 mL 0, 2, 4 wk, with antibiotics	Hypersensitivity
BCG vaccine	TICE BCG	TB exposure	Adult and child ≥1 mo: 0.2–0.3 mL Child <1 mo: Reduce dose by 50% using 2 mL of sterile water after reconstituting	Hypersensitivity, hypogammaglobulinemia, positive TB test, burns
COVID-19 vaccine	Moderna COVID-19 vaccine	COVID-19 (EUA)	Adult: IM 0.5 mL × 2, 1 mo apart, booster 0.25 mL ≥6 mo after last dose	Severe hypersensitivity
COVID-19 vaccine	Booster 6 mon-5 yrs (Dark pink cap) Booster (Dark blue cap) Comirnaty (Pfizer) Tozinameran	COVID-19	Adult/child 12-18 yr: IM 30 mcg × 2 given 21 days apart Child 5-11 yr: IM 10 mcg × 2 given 21 days apart 6 mon-≤4yr (maroon cap/border) 5 yr-≤11yr (Gray cap/border)	Severe hypersensitivity
dengue tatravalent vaccine, live	Dengvaxia	Prevention of dengue disease	Child 9-16 yr SUBCUT 0.5 mL × 3 doses, 6 mo apart at mo 1, 6, 12	Hypersensitivity
diphtheria and tetanus toxoids, adsorbed	Tenivac	Induces antitoxins to provide immunity to diphtheria and tetanus	Adult and child ≥7 yr: IM (adult strength) 0.5 mL q4-8wk × 2 doses, then 3rd dose 6-12 mo after 2nd dose, booster IM 0.5 mL q10yr Child 1-6 yr: IM (pediatric strength) 0.5 mL q4wk × 2 doses, booster 6-12 mo after 2nd dose Infant 6 wk-1 yr: IM (pediatric strength) 0.5 mL q4wk × 3 doses, booster 6-12 mo after 3rd dose	Hypersensitivity to mercury, thimerosal; immunocompromised patients; radiation; corticosteroids; acute illness

diphtheria and tetanus toxoids and whole-cell pertussis vaccine (DPT, DTP)	DTwP, Tri-Immunol	Prevention of diphtheria, tetanus, pertussis	Doses vary Check product information	Hypersensitivity, active infection, poliomyelitis outbreak, immunosuppression, febrile illness
diphtheria and tetanus toxoids and acellular pertussis vaccine	Adacel, Boostrix, Daptacel, Infanrix	Prevention of diphtheria, tetanus, pertussis	Doses vary Check product information	Hypersensitivity, active infection, poliomyelitis outbreak, immunosuppression, febrile illness
diphtheria, tetanus, pertussis, haemophilus, polio IPV	Pentacel	Immunity to diphtheria, tetanus, pertussis, haemophilus, polio IPV	Infant >6 wk and child ≤5 yr: IM 0.5 mL at 2, 4, 6, and 15-18 mo	Hypersensitivity, polio outbreak, acute infection, immunosuppression
diphtheria, tetanus, pertussis, polio vaccine IPV	Kinrix, Quadracel	Immunity to diphtheria, tetanus, pertussis, polio vaccine IPV	Child: IM 0.5 mL.	Hypersensitivity, polio outbreak, acute infection, immunosuppression
ebola zaire vaccine, live	Ervebo		1 mL (single-dose vial) once	Hypersensitivity
encephalitis, tick-borne vaccine	TicoVac	Prevention of tick-borne encephalitis	Child: 1-15 yr: IM 0.25 mL × 3 doses Adult/adolescent >16 yr: 0.50 mL × 3 doses	
Influenza A (H1N1)	Influenza A (swine flu) virus vaccine	Immunity to H1N1	Adult <50 yr, adolescent, child ≥2 yr: Intranasal 1 dose (roughly 0.1 mL) into each nostril; child 2-9 repeat dose ≥4 wk later Adult, adolescent, child ≥3 yr: IM 0.5 mL as a single dose; child 3-9 yr repeat dose ≥4 wk later (Novartis) (CSL); child 4-9 yr repeat dose ≥4 wk later (Sanofi); infants ≥6 mo, child <36 mo: IM 0.25 mL, repeat in 4 wk (Sanofi) Adult: IM 0.5 mL as a single dose (GSK)	
haemophilus b conjugate vaccine, diphtheria CRM₁₉₇ protein conjugate (HbOC)	HibTITER	Polysaccharide immunization of children 2-6 yr against H. influenzae b, conjugate	**HibTITER (IM only)** Child: IM 0.5 mL Child 2-6 mo: 0.5 mL q2mo × 3 inj	Hypersensitivity, febrile illness, active infection

Continued

Appendix C Vaccines and Toxoids—cont'd

GENERIC NAME	TRADE NAME	USES	DOSAGE AND ROUTES	CONTRAINDICATIONS
haemophilus b conjugate vaccine, meningococcal protein conjugate (PRP-OMP)	PedvaxHIB	Immunization of child 2, 4, 6 mo	Child 7-11 mo: Previously unvaccinated 0.5 mL (2mo inj) Child 12-14 mo: Previously unvaccinated 0.5 mL × 1 inj **PedvaxHIB (IM only)** Child 2-14 mo: 0.5 mL × 2 inj at 2, 4 mo of age (6 mo dose not needed) then booster at 12-18 mo against invasive disease Child ≥15 mo: Previously unvaccinated 0.5 mL inj	
hepatitis A vaccine, inactivated	Havrix, VAQTA	Active immunization against hepatitis A virus	Adult: IM 1440 EL units (Havrix) or 50 units (VAQTA) as a single dose; booster dose the same given at 6, 12 mo Child 2-18 yr: IM 720 EL units (Havrix) or 25 units (VAQTA) as a single dose, booster dose is the same given at 6, 12 mo	Hypersensitivity
hepatitis B vaccine, recombinant	Engerix-B, Prefterbrion, Recombivax HB	Immunization against subtypes of hepatitis B virus	Varies widely	Hypersensitivity to this vaccine or yeast
human papillomavirus recombinant vaccine, quadrivalent	Gardasil 9	Prevention of HPV types 6, 11, 16, 18, cervical cancer, genital warts, precancerous dysplastic lesions, anal cancer/anal intraepithelial neoplasia	Adult up to 26 yr and child >9 yr to 26 yr: IM give as 3 separate doses; 1st dose as elected; 2nd dose 2 mo after 1st dose; 3rd dose 6 mo after 1st dose	Child <9 yr, pregnancy, breastfeeding, geriatric patients, active disease, hypersensitivity
influenza virus vaccine	Afluria, FluMist, Fluvirin, Fluzone	Prevention of seasonal influenza	Adult and child >12 yr: IM 0.5 mL in 1 dose Adult 18-64 yr: ID 0.1 mL as a single dose Child 3-12 yr: IM 0.5 mL, repeat in 1 mo (split) unless 1978-1985 vaccine was given; also given nasal Child 6 mo to 3 yr: IM 0.25 mL, repeat in 1 mo (split) unless 1978-1985 vaccine was given; also given nasal child ≤2 yr	Hypersensitivity, active infection, chicken egg allergy, Guillain-Barré syndrome, active neurologic disorders
Japanese encephalitis virus vaccine, inactivated	Ixiaro	Active immunity against Japanese encephalitis (JE)	Adult and child >3 yr: IM 0.5 mL (deltoid), then 0.5 mL 28 days later. Give the second dose ≥1 wk before potential exposure Child ≥2 mo to <3 yr: IM 0.25 mL (anterolateral aspect of the thigh or deltoid for children 1-2 yr with adequate muscle mass), then 0.25 mL 28 days later	Hypersensitivity to murine, thimerosal; allergic reactions to previous dose

measles, mumps, and rubella vaccine, live	M-M-R-II	Prevention of measles, mumps, rubella	Adult: SUBCUT 1 vial; 2 vials separated by 1 mo, in person born after 1957 Child >15 mo and adult: SUBCUT 0.5 mL	Hypersensitivity, blood dyscrasias, anemia, active infection, immunosuppression; egg, chicken allergy; pregnancy, febrile illness, neomycin allergy, neoplasms
measles, mumps, rubella, varicella	ProQuad	Immunity to measles, mumps, rubella, varicella	Child: SUBCUT 0.5 mL	Hypersensitivity to eggs, neomycin, cancer, radiation, corticosteroids, blood dyscrasias, active untreated TB
meningococcal groups A, C, Y, W conjugate vaccine	MenQuadfi	Meningitis	Adult: IM 0.5 mL	Hypersensitivity to this product or any tetanus toxoid
meningococcal polysaccharide vaccine	Menomune-A/C	Prophylaxis to meningococcal meningitis	Adult and child >2 yr: SUBCUT 0.5 mL.	Hypersensitivity to thimerosal, pregnancy, acute illness
pneumococcal 7-valent conjugate vaccine	Prevnar	Immunity against *Streptococcus pneumoniae*	Child: IM 0.5 mL × 3 doses (7-11 mo); × 2 doses (12-23 mo); × 1 dose >2-9 yr	Hypersensitivity to diphtheria toxoid or this product
pneumococcal 15-valent conjugate vaccine	Vaxneuvance	Pneumococcal immunization	Adult: IM 0.5 mL	
pneumococcal 20-valent conjugate vaccine	Prevnar 20	Pneumococcal immunization	Adult: IM 0.5 mL	
pneumococcal vaccine, polyvalent	Pneumovax 23	Pneumococcal immunization	Adult and child >2 yr: IM/SUBCUT 0.5 mL.	Hypersensitivity, Hodgkin's disease, ARDS
poliovirus vaccine (IPV)	IPOL	Prevention of polio	Adult and child >2 yr: PO 0.5 mL, given q8wk × 2 doses, then 0.5 mL ½-1 yr after dose 2 Infant: PO 0.5 mL at 2, 4, 18 mo; booster at 4-6 yr; may also be given: IPV at 2, 4 mo, then TOPV at 12-18 mo, booster at 4-6 yr	Hypersensitivity, active infection, allergy to neomycin/streptomycin, immunosuppression, vomiting, diarrhea
rabies vaccine, human diploid cell (HDCV)	Imovax, RabAvert	Active immunity to rabies	Preexposure Adult and child: IM 1 mL day 0, 7, 21, or 28 (total 4 doses) Postexposure Adult and child: IM 1 mL on day 0, 3, 7, 14, 28 (total 5 doses)	No contraindications

Continued

Appendix C   Vaccines and Toxoids—cont'd

GENERIC NAME	TRADE NAME	USES	DOSAGE AND ROUTES	CONTRAINDICATIONS
rotavirus	RotaTeq, Rotarix	Prevents rotavirus	Infant: PO 3 doses given between 6 and 32 wk of age; 1st dose between 6-12 wk of age; 2nd and 3rd doses q4-10wk	Hypersensitivity to this product or latex, immunocompromised, blood products given within 6 wk, lymphatic disorders
smallpox and monkeypox vaccine, live, nonreplicating	Jynneos	Prevention of smallpox and monkeypox disease	Adult: SUBCUT 0.5 mL × 2 doses, 4 wk apart	Hypersensitivity
tetanus toxoid, adsorbed	No trade name	Tetanus toxoid: Used for prophylactic treatment of wounds	Adult and child: IM 0.5 mL q4-6wk × 2 doses, then 0.5 mL 1 yr after dose 2 (adsorbed); SUBCUT/IM 0.5 mL q4-8wk × 3 doses, then 0.5 mL ½-1 yr after dose 3, booster dose 0.5 mL q10yr	Hypersensitivity; active infection, poliomyelitis outbreak, immunosuppression
typhoid vaccine, parenteral typhoid vaccine, oral	Typhim Vi Vivotif Berna Vaccine	Active immunity to typhoid fever	Adult: PO 1 cap 1 hr before meals × 4 doses, booster q5yr Adult and child >10 yr: SUBCUT 0.5 mL, repeat in 4 wk, booster q3yr Child 6 mo-10 yr: SUBCUT 0.25 mL, repeat in 4 wk, booster q3yr	Parenteral: Systemic or allergic reaction, acute respiratory or other acute infection, intensive physical exercise in high temperatures Oral: Hypersensitivity; acute febrile illness, suppressive or antibiotic products
typhoid Vi polysaccharide vaccine	Typhim Vi	Active immunity to typhoid fever	Adult and child ≥2 yr: IM 0.5 mL as a single dose, reimmunize q2yr 0.5 mL IM, if needed	Hypersensitivity, chronic typhoid carriers
varicella-zoster virus vaccine	Varivax, Zostavax	Prevention of varicella zoster (chickenpox)	Adult and child ≥13 yr: SUBCUT 0.5 mL, 2nd dose SUBCUT 0.5 mL 4-8 wk later	Hypersensitivity to neomycin; blood dyscrasias, immunosuppression, active untreated TB, acute illness, pregnancy, diseases of lymphatic system
yellow fever vaccine	YF-Vax	Active immunity to yellow fever	Adult and child ≥9 mo: SUBCUT 0.5 mL deeply; booster q10yr Child 6-9 mo: same as above if exposed	Hypersensitivity to egg or chicken embryo protein, pregnancy, child <6 mo, immunodeficiency
zoster vaccine recombinant, adjuvanted	Shingrix	Prevention of herpes zoster (shingles)	Adult: IM 2 doses (0.5 mL each) at 0 and 2 to 6 months	History of severe allergic reaction (e.g., anaphylaxis) to any component of the vaccine or after a previous dose

Appendix D

GENERIC	TRADE	USE
eplontersen	Wainua	To treat transthyretin-mediated amyloidosis
immune globulin IV	Alyglo	To treat primary immunodeficiency syndrome
Travoprost implant	iDose TR	To treat glaucoma

Index

Note: Page numbers followed by "f" indicate figures and "t" indicate tables.

Entries can be identified as follows: DISEASES/DISORDERS, *DRUG CATEGORIES*, generic names,
Trade Names.

Entries can be identified as follows: DISEASES/DISORDERS, *DRUG CATEGORIES*, generic names, Trade Names.

Entries can be identified as follows: DISEASES/DISORDERS, *DRUG CATEGORIES*, generic names,
Trade Names.

Entries can be identified as follows: DISEASES/DISORDERS, *DRUG CATEGORIES*, generic names,
Trade Names.

Entries can be identified as follows: DISEASES/DISORDERS, *DRUG CATEGORIES*, generic names,
Trade Names.

INDEX

Entries can be identified as follows: DISEASES/DISORDERS, *DRUG CATEGORIES*, generic names, Trade Names.

Entries can be identified as follows: DISEASES/DISORDERS, *DRUG CATEGORIES*, generic names,
Trade Names.

INDEX

Entries can be identified as follows: DISEASES/DISORDERS, *DRUG CATEGORIES*, generic names, Trade Names.

Entries can be identified as follows: DISEASES/DISORDERS, *DRUG CATEGORIES*, generic names, Trade Names.

INDEX

Entries can be identified as follows: DISEASES/DISORDERS, *DRUG CATEGORIES*, generic names,
Trade Names.

INDEX

Entries can be identified as follows: DISEASES/DISORDERS, *DRUG CATEGORIES*, generic names,
Trade Names.

Entries can be identified as follows: DISEASES/DISORDERS, *DRUG CATEGORIES*, generic names,
Trade Names.

INDEX

Entries can be identified as follows: DISEASES/DISORDERS, *DRUG CATEGORIES*, generic names, Trade Names.

Entries can be identified as follows: DISEASES/DISORDERS, *DRUG CATEGORIES*, generic names,
Trade Names.

Entries can be identified as follows: DISEASES/DISORDERS, *DRUG CATEGORIES*, generic names,
Trade Names.

Entries can be identified as follows: DISEASES/DISORDERS, *DRUG CATEGORIES*, generic names,
Trade Names.

INDEX

INDEX

Entries can be identified as follows: DISEASES/DISORDERS, *DRUG CATEGORIES*, generic names, Trade Names.

Entries can be identified as follows: DISEASES/DISORDERS, *DRUG CATEGORIES*, generic names, Trade Names.

INDEX

Entries can be identified as follows: DISEASES/DISORDERS, *DRUG CATEGORIES*, generic names, Trade Names.

Entries can be identified as follows: DISEASES/DISORDERS, *DRUG CATEGORIES*, generic names, Trade Names.

INDEX

Entries can be identified as follows: DISEASES/DISORDERS, *DRUG CATEGORIES*, generic names, Trade Names.

Entries can be identified as follows: DISEASES/DISORDERS, *DRUG CATEGORIES*, generic names,
Trade Names.

INDEX

Entries can be identified as follows: DISEASES/DISORDERS, *DRUG CATEGORIES*, generic names,
Trade Names.

Entries can be identified as follows: DISEASES/DISORDERS, *DRUG CATEGORIES*, generic names,
Trade Names.

INDEX

Entries can be identified as follows: DISEASES/DISORDERS, *DRUG CATEGORIES*, generic names, Trade Names.

Entries can be identified as follows: DISEASES/DISORDERS, *DRUG CATEGORIES*, generic names,
Trade Names.

Entries can be identified as follows: DISEASES/DISORDERS, *DRUG CATEGORIES*, generic names, Trade Names.

INDEX

Entries can be identified as follows: DISEASES/DISORDERS, *DRUG CATEGORIES*, generic names,
Trade Names.

Entries can be identified as follows: DISEASES/DISORDERS, *DRUG CATEGORIES*, generic names, Trade Names.

Entries can be identified as follows: DISEASES/DISORDERS, *DRUG CATEGORIES*, generic names, Trade Names.

Entries can be identified as follows: DISEASES/DISORDERS, *DRUG CATEGORIES*, generic names, Trade Names.

Entries can be identified as follows: DISEASES/DISORDERS, *DRUG CATEGORIES*, generic names,
Trade Names.

Entries can be identified as follows: DISEASES/DISORDERS, *DRUG CATEGORIES*, generic names,
Trade Names.

INDEX

Entries can be identified as follows: DISEASES/DISORDERS, *DRUG CATEGORIES*, generic names, Trade Names.

Entries can be identified as follows: DISEASES/DISORDERS, *DRUG CATEGORIES*, generic names,
Trade Names.

Entries can be identified as follows: DISEASES/DISORDERS, *DRUG CATEGORIES*, generic names, Trade Names.

Entries can be identified as follows: DISEASES/DISORDERS, *DRUG CATEGORIES*, generic names, Trade Names.

INDEX

Entries can be identified as follows: DISEASES/DISORDERS, *DRUG CATEGORIES*, generic names,
Trade Names.

1498 Index

Entries can be identified as follows: DISEASES/DISORDERS, *DRUG CATEGORIES*, generic names, Trade Names.

INDEX

Entries can be identified as follows: DISEASES/DISORDERS, *DRUG CATEGORIES*, generic names,
Trade Names.

Entries can be identified as follows: DISEASES/DISORDERS, *DRUG CATEGORIES*, generic names,
Trade Names.

Entries can be identified as follows: DISEASES/DISORDERS, *DRUG CATEGORIES*, generic names, Trade Names.

Entries can be identified as follows: DISEASES/DISORDERS, *DRUG CATEGORIES*, generic names, Trade Names.

INDEX

Entries can be identified as follows: DISEASES/DISORDERS, *DRUG CATEGORIES*, generic names,
Trade Names.

Entries can be identified as follows: DISEASES/DISORDERS, *DRUG CATEGORIES*, generic names, Trade Names.

INDEX

Entries can be identified as follows: DISEASES/DISORDERS, *DRUG CATEGORIES*, generic names, Trade Names.

Entries can be identified as follows: DISEASES/DISORDERS, *DRUG CATEGORIES*, generic names, Trade Names.

INDEX

Entries can be identified as follows: DISEASES/DISORDERS, *DRUG CATEGORIES*, generic names,
Trade Names.

Entries can be identified as follows: DISEASES/DISORDERS, *DRUG CATEGORIES*, generic names, Trade Names.

INDEX

Entries can be identified as follows: DISEASES/DISORDERS, *DRUG CATEGORIES*, generic names, Trade Names.

Entries can be identified as follows: DISEASES/DISORDERS, *DRUG CATEGORIES*, generic names, Trade Names.

vandetanib, 1336
Vanflyta, 1422
VAP. *See* VENTILATOR-
	ASSOCIATED PNEUMO-
	NIA (VAP)
Vaprisol, 302
VAQTA, 1450
vardenafil, 1336
varenicline, 1338
VARIANT ANGINA
	NIFEdipine, 928
VARICEAL BLEEDING
	octreotide, 950
VARICELLA INFECTION
	acyclovir, 17
	famciclovir, 534
	immune globulin IM (IMIG/
		IGIM), 679
	valACYclovir, 1326
VARICELLA ZOSTER
	peginterferon alfa-2a, 1009
	valACYclovir, 1326
varicella-zoster virus vaccine,
	1452
VARIOLA
	peginterferon alfa-2a, 1009
	tecovirimat, 1240
Varivax, 1452
Varubi, 1155
Vascepa, 666, 965
VASCULAR DEMENTIA
	rivastigmine, 1151
VASCULAR HEADACHE
	ergotamine/caffeine, 486
VASCULITIS
	azaTHIOprine, 123
Vaseretic, 461
VASOMOTOR SYMPTOMS
	estradiol, 510
	estrogens, conjugated, 513
vasopressin, 1339
Vasostrict, 1339
Vasotec, 460
Vaxneuvance, 1451
Vectibix, 999
Vectical, 203
vedolizumab, 1340
Veklury. 1118
Velcade, 167
velmanase, 1432
Velphoro, 705
Velsipity, 1399
Veltassa, 1006
Vemlidy, 1251
vemurafenib, 1342
Venclexta, 1344

venetoclax, 1344
venlafaxine, 1344
Venofer, 548, 705
VENOUS THROMBOEMBOLISM
	(VTE)
	aspirin, 99
	dalteparin, 329
	fondaparinux, 588
VENOUS THROMBOSIS
	protein C concentrate, 1086
Ventavis, 672
VENTILATOR-ASSOCIATED
	PNEUMONIA (VAP)
	sulbactam/durlobactam,
		1428
Ventolin Diskus, 30
Ventolin HFA, 30
Ventolin Nebules, 30
VENTRICULAR DYSRHYTH-
	MIA. *See also*
	SUPRAVENTRICULAR
	DYSRHYTHMIA
	amiodarone, 59
	flecainide, 558
	lidocaine (parenteral), 769
	procainamide, 1066
	sotalol, 1205
VENTRICULAR TACHYCARDIA
	amiodarone, 59
	lidocaine (parenteral), 769
	propafenone, 1076
	quiNIDine gluconate, 1097
VENTRICULITIS
	cefotaxime, 246
Veozah, 1402
VePesid, 521
verapamil, 1346
Verdeso Foam, 1440
Verelan, 1346
Verelan PM, 1346
Veripred, 1057
Verkazia, 1437
Vermox, 813
Versacloz, 295
VERTIGO
	meclizine, 814
Verzenio, 4
Vesanoid, 1313
VESIcare, 1198
Vesicare LS, 1198
VESICULAR STOMATITIS
	peginterferon alfa-2a, 1009
Vfend, 1365
Vfend IV, 1365
Viagra, 1182
Vibativ, 1242

Viberzi, 448
Vibramycin, 423
Vicks Formula, 44, 373
Vicks QlearQuil, 1439
Vicks Sinex 12-Hour Decon-
	gestant, 1439
Vicks Sinex Moisturizing, 1439
Vicks Sinex Severe Decongest-
	ant, 1439
Victoza, 777
Vidaza, 121
Videx EC, 380
Viekira Pak, 964
Viekira XR, 964
Vienva, 303
vigabatrin, 1349
Vigadrone, 1349
Vigamox, 897, 1435
Viibryd, 1350
Vijoice, 42
vilazodone, 1350
Vimovo, 914
Vimpat, 730
vinBLAStine (VLB), 1352
vinCRIStine, 1355
vinorelbine, 1358
Viokase, 997
VIPoma
	octreotide, 950
Viracept, 918
Viractin, 1445
Viramune, 922
Viramune XR, 922
Virasal, 1443
Virazole, 1126
Viread, 1251
VIRIDANS STREPTOCOCCI
	cefditoren, 246
	linezolid, 775
	meropenem, 829
Viroptic, 1436
VISCERAL LEISHMANIASIS
	amphotericin B liposomal
		(LAmB), 73
	miltefosine, 873
Visine Red Eye, 1437
vismodegib, 1360
Vistaril, 655
Vistogard, 1323
vit A acid, 1313
vit B₁, 1266
vit B₂, 1129
vit B₆, 1090
vit B₉, 586
vitamin A, 1361

INDEX

Entries can be identified as follows: DISEASES/DISORDERS, *DRUG CATEGORIES*, generic names,
Trade Names.

INDEX

Entries can be identified as follows: DISEASES/DISORDERS, *DRUG CATEGORIES*, generic names,
Trade Names.

Formulas

Surface area rule:

$$\text{Child dose} = \frac{\text{Surface area (m}^2)}{1.73 \text{ m}^2} \times \text{Adult dose}$$

Calculating strength of a solution:

$$\begin{array}{cc} \textit{Solution Strength}: & \textit{Desired Solution}: \\ \dfrac{x}{100} & = \dfrac{\text{Amount of drug desired}}{\text{Amount of finished solution}} \end{array}$$

Calculating flow rate for IV:

$$\text{Rate of flow} = \frac{\text{Amount of fluid} \times \text{Administration set calibration}}{\text{Running time}}$$

$$\frac{x}{1} = \frac{\text{(mL) (gtt/min)}}{\text{min}}$$

Calculation of medication dosages:

Formula method:

$$\frac{\text{Amount ordered}}{\text{Amount on hand}} \times \text{Vehicle} = \text{Number of tablets, capsules, or amount of liquid}$$

Vehicle is the drug form or amount of liquid containing the dosage. Amounts used in calculation by formula must be in same system.

Ratio–proportion method:

1 tablet:tablet in mg on hand::*x* tablet order in mg
            Know or have::Want to know or order

Multiply means and extremes, divide both sides by known amount to get *x*. Amounts used in equation must be in same system.

Dimensional analysis method:

$$\text{Order in mg} \times \frac{\text{1 tablet or capsule}}{\text{What 1 tablet or capsule is in mg}} = \text{Tablets or capsules to be given}$$

If amounts are in different systems:

$$\text{Order in mg} \times \frac{\text{1 tablet or capsule}}{\text{What 1 tablet or capsule is in g}} \times \frac{1}{1000 \text{ mg}} = \text{Tablets or capsules to be given}$$

Temperature conversion:

$F = C \times \frac{9}{5} + 32$

$C = \frac{5}{9} (F - 32)$

Nomogram for calculation of body surface area

Place a straight edge from the patient's height in the left column to the patient's weight in the right column. The point of intersection on the body surface area column indicates the body surface area (BSA). (Reproduced in Behrman RE, Kliegman RM, Jenson HB: *Nelson textbook of pediatrics,* ed 18, Philadelphia, 2011, WB Saunders; Nomogram modified from data of E. Boyd by CD West.)

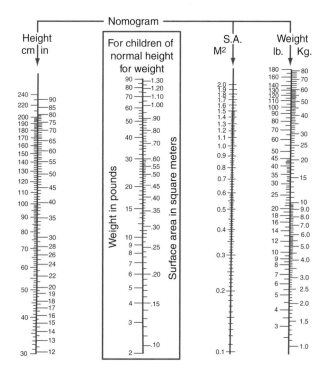

Alternative (Mosteller's formula):

$$\text{Surface area (m}^2) = \sqrt{\dfrac{\text{Height (cm)} \times \text{Weight (kg)}}{3600}}$$

Antitoxins and antivenins

GENERIC NAME	TRADE NAME	USES	DOSAGE AND ROUTES	CONTRAINDICATIONS
Black widow spider antivenin (*Lactrodectus mactans*)	No trade name	Black widow spider bite	Adult and child: IM 2.5 ml, 2nd dose may be given if severe; give in anterolateral thigh, obtain test for sensitivity before inj	Hypersensitivity to this product or horse serum
Crotalidae antivenom, polyvalent	No trade name	Rattlesnake bite	Adult and child: IV 20-150 ml depending on seriousness of bite, may give additional doses based on response	Hypersensitivity
Diphtheria antitoxin, equine	No trade name	Diphtheria	Adult and child: IM/slow IV 20,000-120,000 units, may give additional doses after 24 hr	Hypersensitivity
Micrurus fulvius antivenin	No trade name	East/Texas coral snake bite	Adult and child: IV 30-50 ml, give through running IV line of normal saline, give 1st 1-2 ml over 4-5 min, watch for allergic reaction	Hypersensitivity
Scorpion antivenin (centruroides sculpturatus equine)	Anascorp	Scorpion stings	Adult and child: IV 3 vial/50 ml NS given over 10 min, may give other doses 1 vial/50 ml NS over 10 min q30-60min	N/A

Abbreviations

ABG	arterial blood gas		**GVHD**	graft-versus-host disease
ADA	American Diabetes Association		**H$_2$**	histamine$_2$
ADH	antidiuretic hormone		**hCG**	human chorionic gonadotropin
ALT	alanine aminotransferase		**Hct**	hematocrit
ANA	antinuclear antibody		**HDCV**	human diploid cell rabies vaccine
APLA	antiphospholipid antibody syndrome		**Hgb**	hemoglobin
APTT	activated partial thromboplastin time		**H & H**	hematocrit and hemoglobin
ASA	acetylsalicylic acid, aspirin		**5-HIAA**	5-hydroxyindoleacetic acid
AST	aspartate aminotransferase (SGOT)		**HIV**	human immunodeficiency virus (AIDS)
AV	atrioventricular		**HR**	heart rate
bid	twice a day		**IBD**	inflammatory bowel disease
BPH	benign prostatic hypertrophy		**IC**	intracardiac
BPM	beats per minute		**ICP**	intracranial pressure
BUN	blood urea nitrogen		**ID**	intradermal
CAD	coronary artery disease		**IgG**	immunoglobulin G
CBC	complete blood cell count		**IM**	intramuscular
CCr	creatinine clearance		**INF**	infusion
CHF	congestive heart failure		**INH**	inhalation
CNS	central nervous system		**inj**	injection
CONT	continuous		**I&O**	intake and output
COPD	chronic obstructive pulmonary disease		**INT**	intermittent
CPAP	continuous positive airway pressure		**IPPB**	intermittent positive-pressure breathing
CPK	creatine phosphokinase		**IT**	intrathecal
CPS	carbamoyl phosphate synthetase		**ITP**	idiopathic thrombocytopenic purpura
C&S	culture and sensitivity		**IUD**	intrauterine device
CSF	cerebrospinal fluid		**IV**	intravenous
CTCL	cutaneous T-cell lymphoma		**IVP**	intravenous pyelogram
CV	cardiovascular		**K**	potassium
CVA	cerebrovascular accident		**LDH**	lactic dehydrogenase
CVP	central venous pressure		**LE**	lupus erythematosus
D&C	dilatation and curettage		**LFT**	liver function test
DIC	diffuse intravascular coagulation		**LH**	luteinizing hormone
DIR INF	direct infusion		**LOC**	level of consciousness
D$_5$W	5% glucose in distilled water		**LR**	lactated Ringer's solution
DVT	deep vein thrombosis		**LT**	leukotriene
ECG	electrocardiogram (EKG)		**m**	minim
EDTA	ethylenediamine tetraacetic acid		**m^2**	square meter
EEG	electroencephalogram		**MAC**	monitored anesthesia care
EPS	extrapyramidal symptom		**MAOI**	monoamine oxidase inhibitor
ESR	erythrocyte sedimentation rate		**mcg**	microgram
EXT REL	extended release		**mEq**	milliequivalent
FBS	fasting blood sugar		**mg**	milligram
FHT	fetal heart tones		**MI**	myocardial infarction
FSH	follicle-stimulating hormone		**ml**	milliliter
GABA	γ-aminobutyric acid		**mm**	millimeter
GPC	giant papillary conjunctivitis		**mo**	month
gr	grain		**Na**	sodium
GT	glucose tolerance test		**ng**	nanogram
GU	genitourinary		**NGU**	non-gonococcal urethritis